The LIPPINCOTT manual of MEDICAL-SURGICAL NURSING

Second Edition

Adapted for use in the United Kingdom and the Republic of Ireland by:

William Blows

Barbara Dunn

Leonard Evans

Bernadette Frawley

Cynthia Gilling

Rosemarie Hawkins

Morgan Hicks

Elizabeth Keighley

Brian Lake

Geraldine Matthison

Carol March

Neal Mellon

Anna Serra

Allison Speedie

Lynette Stone

David Thompson

Rosemary Webster

The LIPPINCOTT manual of MEDICAL-SURGICAL NURSING

– Second Edition –

Lillian Sholtis Brunner
RN, MSN, ScD, LittD, FAAN

Vice-Chairman (Education and Research):
Board of Trustees; Consultant in Nursing,
Presbyterian–University of Pennsylvania Medical
Center, Philadelphia, Pennsylvania

Member, Board of Overseers,
School of Nursing, University of Pennsylvania,
Philadelphia, Pennsylvania

Formerly Assistant Professor of Nursing,
Yale University School of Nursing,
New Haven, Connecticut

Doris Smith Suddarth
RN, BSNE, MSN

Formerly Consultant in Health Occupations,
Job Corps Health Office, U.S. Department of Labor

Formerly Coordinator of the Curriculum,
The Alexandria Hospital School of Nursing,
Alexandria, Virginia

Harper & Row, Publishers
London

Philadelphia
New York
St. Louis
Sydney

San Francisco
London
Singapore
Tokyo

Reprint 1990
Copyright © 1989 Harper & Row Ltd, London

Adapted from The Lippincott Manual of Nursing Practice,
Fourth Edition Copyright © 1986 J B Lippincott Company

Harper & Row Ltd
Middlesex House
34–42 Cleveland Street
London W1P 5FB

British Library Cataloguing in Publication Data

Brunner, Lillian Sholtis
 The Lippincott manual of medical surgical
 nursing 2nd ed.
 1. Medicine. Nursing. Manuals
 I. Title   II. Suddath, Doris Smith
 610.73

 ISBN 0-06-318435-4

Typeset by Rowland Phototypesetting Ltd
Bury St Edmunds, Suffolk
Printed in Malta by Interprint Limited

NOTE:
The publishers wish to state that, whilst every effort has been made
to ensure the accuracy and correctness of the information contained
herein, the authors of the original work from which this adaptation
is taken cannot be held responsible for any changes made to the
original text in the course of the adaptation.

Contents

Adaptors for the UK edition

William Blows RMN, RGN, RNT, OStJ, Tutor, Dartford School of Nursing

Barbara Dunn RGN, SCM, RCNT, RNT, Formerly Tutor, Guildford Nurse Education Centre

Leonard Evans MEd, BA, RGN, ONC, RCNT, RNT, Director of Nurse Education, West Thames School of Nursing

Bernadette Frawley RGN, RCNT, Clinical Teacher, AMI Harley Street Clinic

Cynthia Gilling MA, BEd(Hons), RGN, SCM, RNT, Director of Nurse Education, The Royal Free Hospital School of Nursing

Rosemarie Hawkins RGN, Formerly Senior Nurse, Department of Occupational Medicine, Brompton Hospital

Morgan Hicks RGN, OND, RCNT, Cert Ed, RNT, Senior Tutor, National Heart and Chest Hospitals

Elizabeth Keighley BEd(Hons), RGN, RSCN, Dip(Lond), RCNT, DipNEd, Assistant Director of Nurse Education–Continuing Education, City and Hackney Health Authority, St Bartholomews Hospital

Brian Lake BEd(Hons), RGN, RN, RNT, BTACert, Director of Education and Training, The Royal Marsden Hospital and Institute of Cancer Research

Geraldine Matthison RGN, Formerly Clinical Nurse Specialist, Bethnal Green Hospital

Carol March RGN, SCM, RCNT, Nurse Teacher, Pembury Hospital

Neal Mellon RGN, Manager, Critical Care Services, Papworth Hospital

Anna Serra RGN, RNT, Formerly Senior Tutor, The Royal National Throat, Nose and Ear Hospital

Allison Speedie RGN, ONC, Ward Sister, Oncology Unit, St Luke's Hospital

Lynette Stone BA, RGN, RM(NSW), Senior Nurse, Dermatology, St John's Hospital for Diseases of the Skin and St Thomas' Hospital

David Thompson BSc, PhD, RGN, RMN, ONC, Lecturer, Department of Nursing, University of Liverpool

Rosemary Webster BSc, RGN, Sister, Coronary Care Unit, Leicester General Hospital

Contributors for the US edition

Brenda G. Bare RN, MSN, Acting Director, The Alexandria Hospital School of Nursing, Alexandria, Virginia

Elizabeth W. Bayley RN, MS, Director: Burn, Emergency and Trauma Nursing, Widener University School of Nursing, Chester, Pennsylvania

Susan M. Foster RN, MS, Educational Coordinator, Critical Care, The Alexandria Hospital, Alexandria, Virginia

Marilyn Hravnak RN, MSN, CCRN, CRTT, Clinical Instructor, Surgical Intensive Care Unit, Presbyterian–University Hospital of Pittsburgh, Pittsburgh, Pennsylvania

Donna D. Ignatavicius RN, MS, Instructor, University of Maryland School of Nursing, Baltimore, Maryland

Leslie H. Kirilloff RN, PhD, Associate Professor, Pulmonary Nursing Specialty, University of Pittsburgh, Pittsburgh, Pennsylvania

Dorothy B. Liddel RN, MSN, Curriculum Coordinator, The Alexandria Hospital School of Nursing, Alexandria, Virginia

Rita Nemchik RN, MS, Director, Center for Continuing Education, University of Pennsylvania School of Nursing, Philadelphia, Pennsylvania

Janet N. Pavel RN, Supervisory Nurse, Clinical Center Blood Bank, National Institutes of Health, Bethesda, Maryland

Suzanne C. O'Connell Smeltzer RN, EdD, Assistant Professor, Adult Health and Illness Section, University of Pennsylvania School of Nursing, Philadelphia, Pennsylvania; and Robert Wood Johnson Clinical Nursing Scholar, University of Rochester School of Nursing, Rochester, New York

Loretta Spittle RN, MS, CCRN, Clinical Specialist, Cardiovascular Nursing, The Alexandria Hospital, Alexandria, Virginia

Preface

The pressures to maintain a high standard of nursing care, in this time of constraint on resources of manpower shortages and with the demand for value for money, is the dilemma every practising nurse faces today. The rapid change in the use of techniques and treatments that are now less invasive and more accurate, has led to a high turn-over of patients for those working in hospitals and has increased the demands on community services.

This second edition of The Lippincott Manual of Medical–Surgical Nursing aims to assist nurses to maintain that high standard of care. It is a useful, easy reference book and covers most situations likely to be encountered in a general hospital.

It has incorporated an individualized approach to care and offers a guide to assessing patients' needs and identifying possible problems. This is introduced in Chapter 1 and continued throughout the text. In describing clinical procedures, care has been taken to adhere to principles and nursing research when giving the rationale for action. More emphasis has been given to aspects of health education and advice on discharge, including useful addresses of support groups. For more specialized nursing care, readers are given suggestions for further reading from the many texts and articles now available.

The contents of each chapter have been completely revised by the adaptors and consideration given to the useful comments and suggestions forwarded by reviewers and readers. The three previous volumes have been brought together into one volume for this new edition and many new sections have been added. Care has been taken to adapt text and content to nursing practice in the United Kingdom.

We hope this manual will be useful to students and qualified nursing staff in enhancing their nursing practice and maintaining clinical competence.

Cynthia Gilling

1

Total Patient Care – A Holistic Approach

THE AIM OF NURSING

The aim of nursing is to assist a patient in overcoming problems which have caused a disturbance in normal physical or psychological functioning.

To reach this aim, it is necessary for the nurse to acknowledge the individuality of the patient, to identify the cause and extent of the problem, and to provide nursing interventions which will alleviate or solve the problem. This must be done logically and methodically.

One framework in which this can be accomplished is by the use of the nursing process, alternatively referred to as 'a systematic approach to planning nursing care'.

This framework should be regarded as a circle, with four main stages.

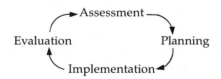

These stages may be subdivided further.

1. *Assessment.*
   a. Recognition of the unique identity of the individual patient.
   b. Assessment of the individual needs.
   c. Appraisal of physical, psychological and social problems.

   These steps involve an interview between the nurse and the patient, or a relative, in order to obtain relevant information, which must be documented. This information is gathered together in the form of a nursing history (data collection).
2. *Planning nursing intervention* – taking into account the medical care which is prescribed.
3. *Implementing nursing care.*
4. *Evaluating the care* which has been given and the outcome. This leads back to reassessment.

The time scale for this cycle of events will be dictated by any significant change in the physical, psychological or social status of the patient; thus it may occur from hour to hour, or weekly.

OBTAINING A NURSING HISTORY

GENERAL PRINCIPLES

1. The first step in caring for a patient and gaining his active co-operation, is to gather a complete and accurate nursing history.
2. Time spent in establishing a good nurse–patient relationship, as early as possible, will enable the patient to feel more relaxed, and be able to talk about the particular problems which are causing him concern.
3. Skill in interviewing will affect both the accuracy

of the information which is obtained, and also the quality of the nurse–patient relationship. This point cannot be overemphasized.

4. The purpose of the interview is to encourage an exchange of information between patient and nurse. In order to do this, some basic conditions are necessary. These include:
   a. The provision of privacy for the interview, in as quiet a place as possible, with a comfortable situation for both patient and nurse.
   b. Beginning the interview with a courteous greeting and an introduction. Explain who you are and why you are there.
   c. A pleasant tone of voice, with unhurried words, and the attitude of a sensitive listener, so that the patient will feel free to express his thoughts and feelings.
   d. The patient must feel that his words are being understood.
   e. A sympathetic attitude. At times, the patient may hint at underlying problems, but may be unable to put them into words. The nurse should help the patient to overcome this difficulty by altering her method of approach and reassuring the patient about the necessity for this particular information.
   f. Guidance of the interview, so that the necessary information is obtained, but without inhibiting the patient from expressing anxieties not covered by the questions.
   g. In some circumstances, the patient may be unable to give any information himself, and this should be sought from a relative or carer. This is obviously the case if the patient is unconscious. If there is some physical or psychological difficulty in communication, the nurse should endeavour to allow the patient to participate or show agreement with the information which is being given about them.
   h. The timing of this interview will be variable, according to the condition of the patient and the availability of a relative. For instance, if the patient is admitted as an emergency, unaccompanied by a relative, and in a breathless and exhausted state, very minimal information will be sought immediately, and a full nursing history may have to be deferred for 24 hours.

TYPES OF INFORMATION NEEDED
Personal details, e.g., name, address, age, date of birth, general practitioner. The patient will usually be able to answer these questions fluently, and will gain confidence in doing so.

PERSONAL AND SOCIAL HISTORY
The purpose of this is:
1. To identify the patient's lifestyle, as this may have some bearing on the present condition, and also the present and future ability of the patient to cope with the condition.
2. To have a basis for developing a plan of care which will be suitable for this particular patient, for instance, involving personal, family or financial resources.
3. To gain knowledge about living patterns, e.g. sleep, meals, exercise, so that a plan of care can be devised which will not disrupt these patterns as far as possible.
4. To help the patient develop a workable plan of care at home, based on knowledge of the home conditions.
5. To discover if the patient's occupation is directly or indirectly related to the present problems.
6. To determine if the religious convictions of the patient may necessitate any modification of the normal nursing procedures or therapy, e.g. dietary requirements, refusal of blood transfusions.

FAMILY HISTORY
The purpose of this is:
1. To picture the patient's family health. This may reveal a hereditary or a familial tendency to a disease.
2. To supplement the social history of the patient. When enquiring about brothers and sisters, for example, information will usually be forthcoming about the closeness or estrangement of members of the family. This is often a useful point when considering resources that are available for future care.

MEDICAL HISTORY
The purpose of this is:
1. To gain a subjective view from the patient about his interpretation of his specific problems, and also his expectations of the possible diagnosis and outcome.
2. To gain an objective view by observation of the patient, and by examination and tests which are carried out by the doctor.

Principles of obtaining a medical history
Obtaining a medical history does not mean that the nurse will undertake a full physical examination of the patient.
1. It does mean that the nurse will find out from the patient the particular problems that have occurred, which necessitated medical advice and admission to hospital.

2. When talking to the patient, the nurse will use her ears, not only for listening to the actual words spoken by the patient, but also for the tone of voice and, for instance, signs of breathlessness.

3. The nurse will use her eyes for observing signs of physical or psychological discomfort, for example, painful movements or unwillingness to make eye contact, also, any signs of abnormalities of the skin or underlying tissues.

4. The nurse will use her sense of smell, not only to detect problems of maintaining cleanliness, but also problems of incontinence, discharges or ketotic breath.

5. Before obtaining a medical history, the nurse will have already gained information about the personal and social background of the patient. When asking about bodily dysfunctions, it is important to put the questions using appropriate language for the individual patient.

6. It is vital that the nurse never 'talks down' to the patient or appears to underestimate his intelligence. It is also necessary for her to use words which are clearly understood.

7. The interview must be conducted in a relaxed, unhurried manner, and the nurse must not appear to the patient to be merely interested in filling in a complicated form. However, in order that a comprehensive and accurate history is obtained, the information must be recorded in a methodical manner. A relatively unstructured form may be used. For example:

PROBLEM CHART		NAME	
Respiration	Mobility	Nutrition and digestion	Communication [physical and psychological problems]
Circulatory	Sleeping and rest	Elimination	Establishing and maintaining relationships

RECORDING THE INFORMATION

GENERAL GUIDELINES

1. Keep in mind the purpose of recording the information and the audience for whom it is intended. This serves to guide the form and content of the record.

2. Remember that the patient's record is a legal document. Facts must be identified and stated precisely and accurately. Bias and misinterpretation must be avoided.

3. Avoid duplication of material. This makes careful reading of the record very time consuming, and so scanning over the facts is likely, with the possibility of errors occurring.

4. The facts must be recorded clearly and in a logical sequence.

5. Avoid using abbreviations unless they are in common usage, and well known to any readers using the record.

6. Record the information as soon as it is obtained, to minimize the chance of errors or omissions.

IDENTIFYING PROBLEMS

After recording the information which has been obtained (a) subjectively from the patients themselves and (b) objectively from the observations made by the nurse, the next step is to identify the particular problems which are preventing the patient from achieving his maximum efficiency, and develop a plan of nursing care to help the patient to overcome these problems.

These problems can be identified by using a recognized model of nursing care. There are many models which have been formulated, and these should be regarded as tools to aid the nurse in her assessment of the total needs of her patient. Just as one tool is more useful for a particular job, so one model may be found to be more appropriate for a particular patient; for instance, whether the patient is highly dependent in an intensive care unit or of low dependency in a long-stay ward. A model of nursing should be a useful aid, not a constricting device, and it is to be hoped that nurses will feel free to adapt a model, if necessary, to help them identify the needs of their patients.

Examples of three widely used models of nursing are given here. Virginia Henderson (1960) has listed the components of basic nursing care, which highlight the points with which the patient may need help:

1. With respiration.
2. With eating and drinking.
3. With elimination.
4. With maintaining a desirable posture in walking, sitting and lying; and helping him move from one position to another.
5. With resting and sleeping.
6. With selecting clothing, dressing and undressing.
7. With maintaining body temperature within normal limits.
8. With keeping the body clean and well groomed and protecting the skin.
9. Avoiding dangers in the environment; and protecting others from any potential danger from the patient, such as infection or violence.
10. To communicate with others – to express his needs and feelings.
11. To practise his religion or conform to his concept of right and wrong.
12. With work, or with productive occupation.
13. With recreational activities.
14. With learning.

Roper, Logan and Tierney (1985) have used the concept of activities of living. These are: maintaining a safe environment; communicating; breathing; eating and drinking; eliminating; personal cleansing and dressing; controlling body temperature; mobilizing; working and playing; expressing sexuality; sleeping; dying.

It is obvious from this list and that of Henderson that these factors cannot be considered in isolation from one another, but are interdependent. Also, Roper et al. described groups of factors which influence activities of living. These are: physical; psychological; sociocultural; environmental; politico-economic.

Factors such as these help the nurse to broaden her view of the patient and to take into account the patient's place in the local community and society as a whole.

Roy (Riehl and Roy, 1980) formulated the adaptation model. Among the assumptions contained in this are: 'the person is in constant interaction with a changing environment; health and illness are an inevitable dimension of the person's life; the person must respond positively to environmental changes.'

It is the failure of the person to adapt to these external or internal environmental changes that will necessitate medical and nursing intervention.

Roy also stated that the person is conceptualized as having four modes of adaptation or response, and that these can be classified as: the physiological mode; the self-concept mode; the interdependence mode; the role–function mode.

In order to identify problems when working to these models, the nurse will need to have acquired experience of people of differing age groups, social, cultural and intellectual backgrounds, and understand their reactions to the change of environment when they are admitted to hospital or are unable to be normally mobile at home. The nurse will need good interpersonal skills in order to establish a trusting relationship. She will also need cognitive skills to understand normal bodily functions and the changes which bring about disordered functioning.

Planning and implementation

Having identified the problems, it is then necessary to plan the appropriate nursing care. This should be done, whenever possible, with the full consent and co-operation of the patient and relatives.

The aim at this stage is to:

1. Pick out from the nursing history those problems which can be solved or alleviated by nursing intervention.
2. Determine the order of priority in which these problems require attention.
3. Set goals for the expected outcomes of the nursing intervention.
4. Decide the method and frequency of the specific nursing intervention that is required.
5. Determine at what intervals the previous points should be evaluated and the patient situation reassessed.
6. Write a care plan, so that all members of the care team can see clearly the aims of care for the particular patient, and can judge the progress which has been made.

The implementation of nursing care is given in detail throughout the book, either under 'Rehabilitation Concepts', or in the chapters on specific conditions.

Evaluation and reassessment
The purpose of this is:
1. To make one's own assessment and discuss with other members of the care team the adequacy of the observations that were made.
2. To measure the effectiveness of the nursing care. This may be an objective measurement, e.g. by recording the improved nutritional status of a patient by a weekly weight gain. It may be a subjective measurement involving a consensus of opinions of colleagues about an improvement in the psychological state of the patient occurring as the physical state also improves.
3. To identify whether:
   a. A goal has been reached and the problem has been solved.
   b. Further time should be allowed for continuation of present nursing care.
   c. The existing care is inappropriate or ineffective and should be modified or radically altered.
   d. New problems have arisen which may necessitate alteration of priorities.

Total patient care using the nursing process and a model of care is an on-going method of adapting to the individual needs of each patient. In different clinical areas, the method of recording the history and the pattern of nursing care may vary, but the personalized approach to the care of the patient remains.

PATIENT EDUCATION AND THE NURSING PROCESS

PATIENT EDUCATION

Patient education is an essential component of nursing care and is directed toward promotion, maintenance and restoration of health, and towards adaptation to the residual effects of illness.

OBJECTIVE
To teach people to live life to its healthiest – that is, to strive toward achieving one's maximum health potential.

PRINCIPLES OF TEACHING AND LEARNING
1. The teaching–learning process requires the active involvement of both the teacher and the learner.
2. The desired outcome of the teaching–learning process is a change in the learner's behaviour.
3. The teacher serves as a facilitator of learning.
4. Learning is facilitated by progressing from the simple to the complex and from the known to the unknown.
5. Learning is facilitated when the learner is aware of his progress towards the learning goals.

VARIABLES THAT AFFECT LEARNING
READINESS
Physical readiness
1. Physical distress that absorbs the patient's attention prevents effective learning.
2. Readiness to learn can be promoted by alleviating or at least minimizing as much as possible the patient's physical distress.

Emotional readiness
1. Motivation to learn depends upon:
   a. Acceptance of the illness or acceptance of the fact that illness is a threat.
   b. Recognition of the need to learn.
   c. A therapeutic regimen compatible with the patient's lifestyle or altered lifestyle.
2. Motivation to learn can be promoted by:
   a. Creating a warm, accepting, positive atmosphere.
   b. Encouraging the patient to participate in the establishment of acceptable, realistic, attainable learning goals.
   c. Providing feedback about progress, that is, positive reinforcement when the patient is successful, constructive criticism when he is unsuccessful.

Experimental readiness
1. The patient's previous experiences, especially learning experiences, affect the learning process.
   a. Success in past learning experiences usually serves to motivate future learning.
   b. Failure in past learning experiences often causes the learner to be hesitant to make new attempts to learn; this learner must be helped to gain confidence in his ability to learn.
2. Learning is dependent upon attainment of those behaviours that are prerequisites to the specific learning task, for example, knowledge of the basics of normal nutrition is a prerequisite to understanding a special diet.

THE LEARNING ATMOSPHERE
1. The physical environment should be conducive to learning: quiet, uninterrupted, and comfortable. Consider the following variables:
   a. Temperature;
   b. Lighting;
   c. Noise level;
   d. Traffic in the ward e.g. trolleys;
   e. Seating facilities and arrangement.
2. The time of the teaching–learning session should be scheduled to meet the patient's needs.
   a. Encourage the patient and his family to participate in the scheduling of the teaching–learning session.
   b. Select a time when the patient is most alert, most comfortable and least fatigued.
   c. Select a time when the patient is not anticipating immediate diagnostic or therapeutic procedures.
   d. Select a time when family members who are to be included in the teaching plan are available.

TEACHING STRATEGIES
Learning is facilitated by selecting teaching techniques and methods that are most appropriate to meet the individual patient's needs.

One-to-one teaching
This is most useful for:
1. Teaching patients who are only just starting to come to terms with a change of body image.
2. Where the teaching involves such personal matters as catheter care or changing stoma bags.
3. Teaching patients who are very reserved, elderly or embarrassed about a particular disability.
4. Teaching those with learning difficulties who require repeated reinforcement of learning and who may feel intimidated in a group situation.

Lecture
1. Is most useful in teaching groups of patients who share the same learning needs.
2. Should always be accompanied by discussion, which allows the individual patient to:
   a. Express his feelings and concerns.
   b. Ask questions.
   c. Clarify information.

Group discussion
1. Is most useful for patients who relate well in groups.
2. Allows patients to experience security through being a member of a group of patients with similar problems or learning needs.

3. Provides patients with the opportunity to gain support, assistance, and encouragement from group members.

Demonstration and practice
1. Is most useful when skills are to be learned.
2. Ample opportunity must be provided for practice sessions.
3. Equipment should be the same as that which the patient will use after leaving the hospital.

Teaching aids
1. Are useful to supplement the resources of the nurse in helping the patient to learn.
2. Include books, pamphlets, pictures, films, slides, tapes and models.
3. Must be reviewed before presentation to ensure that they are appropriate for meeting the patient's individual learning needs.

Reinforcement and follow-up
1. Allow ample time for the patient to learn and to have his learning reinforced.
2. Follow-up sessions promote the patient's confidence in his ability to retain his newly learned behaviours.
3. Evaluate the patient's progress, which is imperative, and plan additional teaching sessions, as necessary.
4. Follow-up sessions after discharge may be needed to assist the patient in transferring what he has learned in the hospital to his home setting.

THE NURSING PROCESS IN PATIENT TEACHING

The teaching–learning process is an integral part of the nursing process. With a focus on learning and with regard for the principles, variables, techniques and strategies of teaching and learning, the steps of the nursing process – assessing, planning, implementing, and evaluating – are used for the purpose of meeting the teaching and learning needs of the patient and his family.

Assessment
1. Assess the patient's learning needs and his physical, emotional and experiential readiness for health education.
   a. What are his health beliefs and behaviours?
   b. What psychosocial adaptations is he making?
   c. Is he ready to learn?
      (i) Is he able to learn these behaviours?

(ii) What are his expectations?

(iii) What additional information is needed about him?

2. Assess the patient's need for education and preparation related to the self-care activities for which he will be responsible after discharge.

3. Use appropriate assessment guides to facilitate data collection. Adapt such guides to the individual responses, problems and needs of the patient.

4. Formulate nursing care plans that relate to the patient's learning needs.

   a. Organize, analyse, synthesize and summarize the collected data.

   b. Identify the patient's learning need(s), its particular characteristic(s) and aetiology(ies).

   c. State nursing problems concisely and precisely.

Planning

1. Assign priority to the nursing problems.

2. Specify the short-term, intermediate and long-term learning goals established by both the nurse and patient.

3. Identify teaching actions appropriate for goal attainment.

4. Establish expected outcome criteria.

5. Identify critical time periods for the attainment of outcomes.

6. Develop a written teaching plan.

   a. Include problems (in order of priority), goals, teaching strategies, outcome criteria, and critical time periods.

   b. Write entries precisely, concisely and systematically.

   c. Include a topical outline of the information to be presented.

   d. Select appropriate teaching techniques and methods.

   e. Keep the plan current and flexible to meet the patient's changing learning needs.

7. Involve the patient, his family and/or significant others, nursing team members and other health team members in all aspects of planning.

Implementation

1. Put the teaching plan into action.

2. Know the material to be presented.

3. Provide an atmosphere conducive to learning.

4. Use language the patient can understand.

5. Use appropriate teaching techniques and methods.

6. Use the same equipment that the patient will use after discharge.

7. Encourage the patient and his family to participate actively in learning.

8. Co-ordinate the activities of the patient, his family and/or significant others, nursing team members and other health team members.

9. Emphasize the importance of learning to care for self after discharge.

10. Record the patient's responses to the teaching actions.

Evaluation

1. Collect objective data:

   a. Observe the patient.

   b. Ask questions to determine if the patient understands.

   c. Use rating scales, checklists, anecdotal notes and written tests when appropriate.

2. Compare the patient's behavioural outcomes with the outcome criteria. Determine the extent to which the goals were achieved.

3. Include the patient, his family and/or significant others, nursing team members and other health team members in the evaluation.

4. Identify alterations that need to be made in the teaching plan.

5. Make referrals to appropriate resource persons or agencies for reinforcement of learning after discharge.

6. Continue all steps of the teaching–learning process: assessing, planning, implementing and evaluating.

FURTHER READING

BOOKS

Henderson, V. (1960) *Basic Principles of Nursing Care*, International Council for Nurses, Geneva.

Hunt, J.M. and Marks-Maran, D. (1980) *Nursing Care Plans*, HM&M Nursing Publications, John Wiley, Chichester.

Kershaw, B. and Salvage, J. (1986) *Models for Nursing*, HM&M Nursing Publications, John Wiley, Chichester.

Kratz, C. (ed.) (1979) *The Nursing Process*, Baillière Tindall, London.

Lewis, L.W. and Timby, B.K. (1987) *Fundamental Skills and Concepts in Patient Care* (4th edn), J.B. Lippincott, Philadelphia.

Little, D.E. and Carnevalli, D.L. (1976) *Nursing Care Planning*, J.B. Lippincott, Philadelphia.

Matheney, R.V. (ed.) (1978) *Fundamentals of Patient Centred Nursing*, C.V. Mosby, St Louis.

Mayers, M.G. (1978) *A Systematic Approach to the Nursing Care Plan*, Prentice Hall, New Jersey.

McFarlane, J. and Castledine, G. (1982) *A Guide to the Practice of Nursing Using the Nursing Process*, C.V. Mosby, London.

Orem, D.E. (1985) *Nursing Concepts of Practice* (3rd edn), McGraw-Hill, New York.

Riehl, J.P. and Roy, C. (1980) *Conceptual Models for Nursing Practice*, Prentice Hall, New Jersey.

Roper, N., Logan, W. and Tierney, A.J. (1985) *The Elements of Nursing* (2nd edn), Churchill Livingstone, Edinburgh.

Thompson, B. and Bridge, W. (1981) *Teaching Patient Care*, HM&M Nursing Publications, John Wiley, Chichester.

Wright, S.G. (1986) *Building and Using a Model of Nursing*, Edward Arnold, London.

Yura, H. and Walsh, M.B. (1978) *The Nursing Process*, Appleton-Century-Crofts, New York.

ARTICLES

Communication

MacLeod Clark, J. (1985) Communication – why it can go wrong, *Nursing*, June, Vol. 2, No. 38, pp. 1119–20.

Maguire, P. (1985) Consequences of poor communication between nurses and patients, *Nursing*, June, Vol. 2, No. 38, pp. 1115–18.

Mallows, D. (1985) Communication – A patient's view, *Nursing*, June, Vol. 2, No. 38, pp. 1112–14.

Tomlinson, A. and Williams, A. (1985) Communication skills in nursing. A practical account, *Nursing*, June, Vol. 2, No. 38, pp. 1121–23.

Patient education

Bracey, J. and Blythe, J. (1985) Promoting positive health, *Nursing Mirror*, 7 August, Vol. 161, No. 6, p. 17.

Coroman, S. (1984) Prevention is better than cure, *Nursing Mirror*, 26 September, Vol. 159, No. 11, p. 35.

Kratz, C. (1985) Matters for concern – Health education is our business, *Community Outlook*, 10 April, p. 6.

Webb, P. (1985) Getting it right – Patient teaching, *Nursing*, June, Vol. 2, No. 38, pp. 1132–34.

Nursing process and individualized patient care

Aggleton, P. and Chalmers, H. (1984) Models and theories. Defining the terms, *Nursing Times*, 5 September, Vol. 80, No. 36, pp. 24–8.

— (1984) Models and theories 2. The Roy adaptation model, *Nursing Times*, 3 October, Vol. 80, No. 40, pp. 45–8.

— (1984) Models and theories 3. The Riehl interaction model, *Nursing Times*, 7 November, Vol. 80, No. 45, pp. 58–61.

— (1984) Models and theories 4. Roger's unitary field model, *Nursing Times*, 12 December, Vol. 80, No. 50, pp. 35–9.

— (1985) Models and theories 5. Orem's self-care model, *Nursing Times*, January, Vol. 81, No. 1, pp. 36–9.

— (1985) Models and theories 6. Roper's activities of living model, *Nursing Times*, 13 February, Vol. 81, No. 7, pp. 59–61.

— (1985) Models and theories 7. Henderson's model of nursing, *Nursing Times*, 6 March, Vol. 81, No. 10, pp. 33–5.

— (1985) Models and theories 8. Critical examination, *Nursing Times*, 3 April, Vol. 81, No. 14, pp. 38–9.

Castledine, G. (1982) The patient's progress, *Nursing Mirror*, 20 October, Vol. 155, No. 16, p. 14.

Clark, J. (1985) The nursing process – Delivering the goods, *Community Outlook*, 9 January, pp. 23–8.

Crow, J. (1977) The nursing process 2. How and why to take a nursing history, *Nursing Times*, 30 June, Vol. 73, pp. 950–7.

— (1977) The nursing process 3. A nursing history questionnaire for patients, *Nursing Times*, 30 June, Vol. 73, pp. 978–94.

Crow, S. (1985) Putting the process into practice, *Nursing Times*, 6 March, Vol. 81, No. 10 (suppl.), p. 11.

Ellis, B. (1985) The nursing process. Making it work, *Community Outlook*, 9 January, pp. 19–22.

Fitton, J. (1985) The nursing process. For the record, *Community Outlook*, 12 June, pp. 19–22.

Martin, L. and Glasper, A. (1986) Core plans: Nursing models and the nursing process in action, *Nursing Practice*, Vol. 4, pp. 268–73.

Miller, A.F. (1984) Nursing process and patient care, *Nursing Times*, Occasional Paper, 27 June, Vol. 80, No. 13, pp. 56–80.

Roe, S. and Farrell, P. (1986) Shaping the nursing process, *Nursing Practice*, Vol. 1, pp. 274–8.

2
Rehabilitation Concepts

REHABILITATION

Rehabilitation is the process whereby anyone who has suffered a physical or psychological illness or accident regains complete normal functioning, or accepts the limits imposed by the illness. By adapting and strengthening his powers, and with aid from various professional and voluntary agencies, he is able to achieve the highest level of physical, mental, social and vocational activity of which he is capable.

Rehabilitation is necessary for a person who has suffered a myocardial infarction or other medical condition, just as much as someone who has had an amputation of his leg.

REHABILITATION TEAM

Rehabilitation is a creative process which calls for a team of health care professionals working together and contributing their specialized services towards a common goal, for the benefit of the individual patient.

The multidisciplinary team, under the guidance of the doctor or surgeon, should: assess the needs and strengths of the patient; plan the necessary action; ensure that resources, both human and material, are available for implementing the plan; at appropriate intervals, evaluate the progress that has been made and reassess the situation. All this should be done with the co-operation of the patient and, where possible, his family.

1. The patient should be encouraged to set his own realistic goals, after explanation, teaching and discussion have occurred.
2. The nursing staff are responsible for developing a plan of care, directed towards the achievement of these goals. Ideally, there should be a 'primary nurse', who will co-ordinate the nursing team and facilitate the other health care professionals.
3. The physiotherapist will work with the patient in regaining mobility, by strengthening muscle action, and by preventing deformities and other complications that can occur due to immobility (see p. 16).
4. The occupational therapist will assess the ability of the patient to undertake the activities of daily living and will provide new or specially adapted equipment to enable the patient to be as independent as possible, both in the home or at work. She will provide opportunities for the patient to practise skills while in hospital and, if necessary, will visit the patient at home, to evaluate progress.
5. The social worker will assess the background of the patient. It may be necessary to give information about: the social security benefits that are available for people suffering from long-term illnesses; those who are unable to continue with their previous occupation and may need retraining; those who need special diets or structural alterations to their homes, for example, that could cause financial difficulty; perhaps the need to move into accommodation where varying amounts of care are provided. Also, the family may be in financial difficulties if the patient is unable to make his normal contribution to the family income.
6. Specialist psychological support should be available. In some cases this may mean the intervention of a psychiatrist. However, it is desirable that a trained counsellor should be accessible to the patient with a particular problem, both before and after treatment is carried out, in hospital and at home. Examples of this would be a mastectomy counsellor, stoma therapist, prosthetic adviser, sexual counsellor, etc.

REHABILITATION NURSING FUNCTIONS

1. Identify the problems which are preventing the patient from achieving his maximum efficiency, and develop a plan of nursing care to help the patient to overcome these problems. Methods of identifying problems have been discussed in Chapter 1.
2. Provide direct nursing care 'that will maintain optimum physical and mental health for the patient and meet his medical treatment needs.
3. Supply nursing care that prevents the complications that may occur because of lack of mobility, and eliminate the possibility of cross-infection.
4. Establish a sustained, supporting nurse–patient relationship.
5. Participate in the retraining of the patient in self-care activities.
6. Provide health care and teaching that will meet the needs of the individual patient and also the family.
7. Record and report nursing observations of the patient's condition, progress and personal needs, as well as the action taken to meet these needs.
8. Assist with patient discharge plans and ensure continuity of home care or follow-up care with the community services or outpatient department.
9. Evaluate the nursing care in terms of the overall goals.

CAUSES OF DISABILITY

1. *Primary disability* – the result of a pathological process (congenital, trauma, inflammatory, etc.).
2. *Secondary disability* – the result of either inactivity or contraindicated and injurious activity.
3. *Disuse syndrome* – disabilities due to inactivity.
   For causes and prevention of disability see Table 2.1.

Table 2.1   Causes and prevention of disability

Condition	Cause	Prevention
1. *Muscle atrophy* (diminution in muscle strength and size)	Lack of exercise	Exercise
2. *Joint contracture* (limited range of movement)	Lack of joint movement	Passive movements, splinting, positioning
3. *Metabolic disturbances* Osteoporosis	Lack of weight-bearing ability Postmenopausal problems	Active movements Tilt table
Urinary tract stones	Immobilization Dehydration/concentrated urine Urinary tract infection	Mobilization High fluid intake High fluid intake Prompt treatment of infections. Avoid catheterization

4. *Circulatory disturbances*
   Orthostatic hypotension
   Venous thrombosis
	Recumbent position
	Slowing of venous return
	Varicose veins
	Poor positioning in operating theatre
	Lack of motion in lower extremities
		Tilt table and stand-up exercises
		Foot and leg exercises
		Elastic stockings
		Appropriate padding on theatre table
		Early mobilization

Hypostatic pneumonia	Poor position. Prolonged rest in one position	Frequent change of position. Breathing exercises. Early mobilization.
Pressure sores	Pressure. Immobility	Frequent change of position. Appropriate padding on theatre table. Assessment of patients at risk. See p. 30

5. *Sphincter disturbances*
   Urinary incontinence
   Urinary retention
	Lack of opportunity
	Lack of opportunity
	Fear and embarrassment
		Regular toilet routine
		Regular toilet routine
		Provision of privacy and comfort. See p. 15

Constipation	Lack of suitable diet Lack of exercise Lack of opportunity	Adequate fluids and roughage Early mobilization Regular toilet routine
6. *Psychological disturbance*	Separation from accustomed environment. Institutional routine Inactivity Sleeplessness Depression	Nursing care is planned to take into account patient's normal living routine Early mobilization Suitable environment. See p. 40 Correct psychological preparation before hospitalization and explanation of treatment and future care

PSYCHOLOGICAL REACTIONS OF A PATIENT TO PROLONGED ILLNESS OR DISABILITY

Prolonged illness or disability has a tremendous impact on a patient's image of himself. There may be an actual change of body shape or function, e.g. amputation or colostomy. There will be a change of psychological and social status – from being a person able to manage the normal physical functions, to a person who is wholly or partially dependent upon someone else. A patient with illness or disability has normal needs which have to be met by different methods.

NURSING OBJECTIVES
1. Be aware of the factors influencing the patient's behaviour.
2. Help the patient to feel worthwhile.

NURSING INSIGHT
The way in which the patient relates to others will be affected by the way in which he perceives changes in his body image.

Assessment
STAGES OF PSYCHOLOGICAL REACTION
Period of confusion, disorganization and denial
1. The patient may be in a state of conflict, having to cope with problems of forced dependence, loss of self-esteem and with feelings that personal and family integrity are threatened.
2. The patient may use the mechanism of denial by refusing to accept new limitations:
   a. May have false hopes for a speedy and complete recovery;
   b. May regress and become self-centred and childlike;
   c. May attempt to remain 'normal' and nondisabled. Denial is the mechanism used particularly by those who have placed great value on strength, attractive appearance and social status.

Period of depression and grief
This is a period of reaction.
1. Appears to grieve for his lost functions or altered body image.

2. Depression is also due to inactivity and sensory deprivation, because of restricted environmental stimulation.
3. Limited mobility and sensory stimulation may produce behavioural disruption.

Period of adaptation and adjustment
1. Redirection of energies towards coping with physical functioning.
2. The patient reviews his body image and modifies the former picture of himself. He has a reorientation to himself.
3. The patient accepts a degree of dependency.
4. He accepts the limitations imposed by the condition.
5. He begins to make realistic goals for the future.

PATIENT PROBLEMS
1. Depression and grief related to losses.
2. Ineffective individual coping related to effects of disability.

Planning and implementation
NURSING INTERVENTIONS
1. Provide an atmosphere of acceptance.
   a. Develop a trusting relationship.
   b. Use open-ended questions to elicit and clarify information.
   c. Allow open expression of feelings; assist the patient to identify sources of hostility/anger.
   d. Avoid displaying value judgments regarding the patient's feelings.
   e. Give emotional support to help the patient work through shock, anger and grief.
   f. Clarify and validate reality.
2. Determine the patient's remaining resources for maintaining an effective lifestyle.
   a. Find out about previous interests, values and goals.
   b. Assist the patient in identifying positive coping patterns used in the past that can be used in the present.
   c. Work with the patient, emphasizing his assets, while, at the same time, listening, encouraging and sharing his problems and triumphs.
   d. Help the patient to think of substitutions and of attaining goals of 'being' (new joys, attitudes, perspectives, opportunities for fulfilment).
   e. Help the patient to think about and resume previously rewarding activities.

f. Encourage the patient to assume increasing responsibility for his rehabilitation programme.

g. Reassure the patient that the support of other caring professionals/family/friends is available.

Evaluation

EXPECTED OUTCOMES

The patient has been able to:

1. Work through the grieving process.
   a. Use thought-stopping techniques when grief seems intolerable.
   b. Express anger and frustration.
   c. Reveal less emotional lability (i.e. less frequent periods of crying).
2. Demonstrate beginning ability to cope with situation:
   a. Verbalize feelings about disability.
   b. Verbalize alternate methods of dealing with problems.
   c. Begin to structure a daily programme.
   d. Accept suggestions from rehabilitation personnel.
   e. Discuss the future in more optimistic terms.

HELPING THE PATIENT WITH RESPIRATION

NURSING OBJECTIVES

1. Enable the patient to breathe sufficiently well to allow adequate oxygenation of the tissues.
2. Provide necessary aid for normal respiration, or artificial ventilation if needed (see Chapter 4, Care of the Patient with a Respiratory Disorder).
3. Assist the patient to perform for himself the activities of living as far as possible, without getting breathless and exhausted.

Assessment

1. Impairment of the ability of the patient to maintain clear air passages, or an adequate ventilation of the lungs. Observations will be made of the colour of the skin (peripheral or central cyanosis), respiratory rate and depth, respiratory distress on exertion or at rest.
2. Impairment of exercise tolerance, e.g. restricted breathing when walking up stairs or on the flat.

3. Difficulty in clearing the airways of sputum, aided or unaided.
4. Assessment of the likely time span of the problem. Does this require:
   a. Short-term assistance, with no residual disability?
   b. Long-term assistance with the probability of further acute episodes or chronic degeneration?

Planning

1. Provide immediate assistance to relieve dyspnoea.
2. Arrange for medical and physiotherapy help.
3. Provide for the relief of secondary problems, e.g. inability to maintain nutrition, hygiene and mobility because of exhaustion, dehydration, confusion.

Implementation

1. Provide adequate support for the patient to maintain an upright position, by the use of special pillows, backrests or comfortable high-backed chairs.
2. Arrange for appropriate physiotherapy, and plan for other nursing activities to fit in with this, e.g. meal times may have to be adjusted so that they do not come immediately before physiotherapy, as this may cause vomiting, and not immediately afterwards, as the patient may be too tired to eat. (If analgesia is required to enable the patient to breathe more freely and without pain, it should be given 20 to 30 minutes before treatment.)
3. Give help, or perform tasks for the patient which he would normally do for himself, but which are now too difficult and cause dyspnoea. e.g. help with washing and dressing.
4. In consultation with the patient, arrange for meals which are nourishing, and do not require too much mastication.
5. Any anxiety or overexcitement will increase the respiration rate, thus requiring more muscular effort and therefore an increased oxygen demand. This may lead to a feeling of panic by the patient, who may find it difficult to speak and make his fears known to the nurse. She must anticipate the need for explanation and reassurance, and give practical help to restore quiet, rhythmic respirations.
6. Encourage a good fluid intake. This is essential because:
   a. A patient with respiratory difficulties may breathe constantly through his mouth, resulting in a dry, coated tongue and mouth.

b. It is an aid to the prevention of constipation, which results in straining to defaecate, causing anxiety and dyspnoea.

7. Arrange for a home visit to be made, before the patient is discharged from hospital, so that aids can be provided: e.g. easy access to cooking facilities and utensils, so that unnecessary bending or stretching is avoided; good heating facilities, and the provision of financial support for this if necessary; easily accessible indoor toilet facilities; oxygen equipment if medically prescribed. Detailed treatment for specific respiratory disorders is found in Chapter 4.

Evaluation
EXPECTED OUTCOME
1. The patient is able to maintain adequate oxygenation.
2. The patient is aware of the reason for his problems.
3. The patient is able to adjust his lifestyle if necessary.
4. The patient is able to perform the appropriate breathing exercises, and to use the prescribed drugs and any equipment that can contribute to his recovery and prevent a recurrence or deterioration of his condition.

HELPING THE PATIENT WITH EATING AND DRINKING

NURSING OBJECTIVES
1. Enable the patient to ingest the correct amount and type of nourishment.
2. Maintain the dignity of the patient.

Assessment
1. Impairment of the manual dexterity of the patient, e.g. short-term problems such as fractures of arms, or operations on the hands, where normal use of hands and arms will be regained later. Long-term problems such as rheumatoid arthritis affecting the hands, Parkinson's disease or paralysis mean that the patient will require a careful and frequent assessment of progress, and provision of special aids and help from the occupational therapist as well as the nursing staff.

2. Sensory deprivation, e.g. blindness. A blind patient who is admitted to hospital for some medical or surgical condition will find his normal routine and method of coping drastically affected. Lack of taste or smell will diminish the patient's appetite and desire for food.
3. Lack of motivation to eat or drink, e.g. severe depression, anorexia nervosa, fear and anxiety.
4. Physical discomfort, e.g. having to remain in a supine position, pain or discomfort which has not been controlled, discomfort due to mouth infections, diseases, operations or badly fitting dentures, breathlessness or exhaustion.
5. Cultural or religious beliefs.
6. Disruption of normal eating pattern.

Planning
To provide: necessary feeding aids; comfortable positioning with pillows or supports; congenial environment; suitable and acceptable diet; psychological support and encouragement.

Implementation
1. Allow the patient to state his preferences and give as wide a choice of food as possible. Guidance may be needed to ensure that a well balanced diet is chosen.
2. Ensure that the catering department send the correct food, well presented, at the correct time. Encourage relatives to bring any specialities which the patient enjoys, if these are appropriate.
3. Ensure that the environment is as pleasant as possible. Ideally, there should be a separate dining area, where patients can sit at the table. A patient who is unable to get up should be made as comfortable as possible, e.g. a bed-pan or commode offered, handwashing facilities, and mouth care if needed. The room should be well aired and cleared of used equipment and utensils. The patient should be helped into a suitable position, with a convenient table at hand. This should be done well in advance of the arrival of the meal, so that the food does not get cold and unappetizing.
4. A drink must always be easily available in a suitable container.
5. An unhurried atmosphere is essential.
6. Cutlery with large handles may be beneficial for a patient with a special difficulty, e.g. Parkinson's disease, rheumatoid arthritis, cerebrovascular accident or multiple sclerosis. Table napkins should be provided for all patients, but some may need further protection of their clothing. This must not diminish the dignity of the patient. Some may be reluctant to have their meals at the

main table because they are liable to spill food and cause embarrassment to themselves and to others. If they wish, a more secluded area of the room may be provided.

7. If the patient is unable to feed himself at all, the nurse should ensure his comfort before bringing the meal, and should allow the patient to make his choice from the menu. The nurse should sit down by the bed or chair if possible, in order to promote an unhurried atmosphere. The patient should be consulted about the addition of salt or pepper to the food, then ample time should be allowed for each mouthful of food to be chewed and swallowed. A rest between mouthfuls may be necessary if the patient is breathless or easily exhausted. Drinks should be offered. A mouthwash should be given at the end of the meal.

Evaluation
EXPECTED OUTCOMES
The patient is able to:
1. Achieve and maintain a partial or complete independence in feeding himself.
2. Consume a well-balanced diet, in adequate quantity, suitable for his individual needs.
3. Enjoy meal times.
4. Achieve an improvement in nutritional status.

HELPING THE PATIENT WITH ELIMINATION

PROBLEMS WITH MICTURITION

NURSING OBJECTIVES
1. Enable the patient to empty his bladder at suitable intervals.
2. Prevent urinary tract infection, and preserve renal function.
3. Help the patient to maintain his dignity and be socially acceptable.

Assessment
1. Urinary infection.
2. Diminished or lack of nerve control of the bladder, e.g. due to cerebrovascular accident, multiple sclerosis, paraplegia.

3. Bladder problems, e.g. enlarged prostate gland, uterine prolapse, cystocele.
4. Inability to reach the toilet easily because of mobility problems.
5. Lethargy and depression.

Planning
1. Encourage the patient to have a positive attitude to the problem, and to co-operate in working out a plan.
2. Acquire any aids which may help.
3. Maintain the dignity of the patient.

Implementation
1. Make a plan of definite times for the patient to empty his bladder, and ensure that he is able to get to the toilet at these times.
2. Whenever possible, the patient should be encouraged to go out to the toilet to ensure privacy. If this is not possible, a commode may be provided, and the bed well screened from other patients.
3. Give sufficient oral fluids at regular intervals. If the patient has difficulty passing urine, wait for 30 minutes, then ask the patient to attempt to pass urine; he may apply pressure on the lower abdomen if necessary. The interval should be two-hourly to begin with, and this may be increased to three-hourly during the day time. The patient may be woken during the night if this is thought to be desirable.
4. The patient should be encouraged to dress in his own clothes. If necessary, incontinence appliances or garments may be provided, as a form of reassurance, until the patient has confidence in his ability to control micturition.
5. It is essential that the patient is able to get to the toilet easily, without delay, and that any garments can be removed without difficulty. It may be necessary to change the fastening on some garments to a device such as Velcro for a patient with rheumatoid athritis in the hands.
6. Frequent urine testing is necessary, because of the possibility of infection.
7. Encourage the patient to make decisions concerning his future care. Try to involve him in a social group. Boredom and apathy must be avoided at all costs. Stimulate an interest in the environment and current events.

Evaluation
EXPECTED OUTCOMES
1. The patient empties his bladder at the first sensation of pressure and remains dry.
2. There is no residual urine.

3. No urinary infection.
4. Good fluid intake.
5. Maintenance of social contacts.

PROBLEMS WITH DEFAECATION

NURSING OBJECTIVES
1. Develop regular bowel habits in the patient, if possible by natural methods.
2. Prevent faecal incontinence, impaction or irregularity.

Assessment
1. Infrequent and irregular defaecation.
2. Frequent soiling.
3. Painful defaecation.
4. Assessment should be made of the patient's dietary habits, fluid intake and use of aperients.

Planning
1. Keep a record of the time of defaecation.
2. Encourage the patient to have a positive attitude to the problem.
3. Involve the dietitian and physiotherapist in the plan of care.

Implementation
1. Establish a definite time for encouragement to defaecate.
   a. Note must be taken of the patient's normal bowel habits, as wide variations can occur in individuals.
   b. Attempts should be made within 15 minutes of a meal, usually breakfast, as this maximizes the stimulation of peristalsis, and the gastrocolic reflex.
2. Promote good dietary habits.
   a. Adequate fluid intake.
   b. Addition of fibre to the diet. An acceptable form is the use of bran cereals at breakfast.
   c. Provision of raw and cooked vegetables, and plenty of fruit. It is essential to check the patient's teeth or dentures, and to ensure that he is happy to eat this type of food.
3. In a case of soiling, a rectal examination should be done, to eliminate the possibility of faecal impaction causing spurious diarrhoea.
4. Encourage as much mobility and muscular exercise as the patient can manage.
5. The use of suppositories may be necessary at first, to stimulate the anorectal reflex.

6. Make sure that the patient can attain a comfortable position, either on a commode or in the toilet. The provision of a footstool may help the patient to make the best use of his muscles, as this position most nearly approximates the physiological position for defaecation.
7. The temporary use of aperients may be necessary, but these should not be used routinely.
8. The provision of privacy, an odour-free atmosphere, absolute cleanliness and facilities for personal hygiene are essential.

Evaluation
EXPECTED OUTCOMES
1. The patient achieves regular bowel functioning, with minimal use of aperients.
2. There is no faecal soiling or incontinence.

HELPING THE PATIENT WITH MOBILITY

NURSING OBJECTIVES
1. Prevent contractures.
2. Strengthen muscles and promote independence.
3. Prevent pressure sores by relieving pressure and stimulating the circulation.
4. Promote lung expansion and drainage of respiratory secretions.

Assessment
1. Muscle weakness or paralysis due to disuse or disease.
2. Nerve damage or disease.
3. Amputation.
4. Fear or depression.

Planning
1. Gain the co-operation and confidence of the patient in planning his achievable goals, in conjunction with the physiotherapy team.
2. Plan his day so that he will not get fatigued.
3. Give encouragement and praise for reaching a goal.

Implementation
1. Achieve good posture in bed.

POSITIONING

PRINCIPLES OF BODY ALIGNMENT

Dorsal or supine position
1. The head is in line with the spine, both laterally and anteroposteriorly.
2. The trunk is positioned so that flexion of the hips is minimized.
3. The arms are slightly flexed with the hands resting on the bed.
4. The legs are extended.
5. The heels may be suspended in a space between the mattress and footboard.
6. The toes are pointing upwards.

Side-lying or lateral position
1. The head is in line with the spine.
2. The uppermost hip joint is slightly forward and supported by a pillow in a position of slight abduction.
3. A pillow supports the arm, which is flexed at both the elbow and shoulder joints.

Prone position
1. The head is turned laterally and is in alignment with the rest of the body.
2. The arms are abducted and externally rotated at the shoulder joint; the elbows are flexed.
3. A small flat support may sometimes be needed to be placed under the pelvis, extending from the level of the umbilicus to the upper third of the thigh.
4. The lower extremities remain in a neutral position.
5. The toes are suspended over the edge of the mattress.

THERAPEUTIC EXERCISES

Exercise involves the function of muscles, nerves, bones and joints as well as the cardiovascular and respiratory systems. The return of function depends on the strength of the musculature that controls the joint.

NURSING OBJECTIVES
1. Develop and retrain deficient muscles.
2. Restore as much normal movement as possible.
3. Maintain and build muscle strength.
4. Maintain joint function.
5. Prevent deformity.
6. Retrain for muscular co-ordination.
7. Stimulate circulation.
8. Build up tolerance and endurance.

TYPES OF EXERCISE
1. Passive.
2. Active assisted.
3. Active.
4. Resisted.
5. Isometric or static.

Passive
An exercise carried out by the therapist or the nurse without assistance from the patient.
1. Purposes:
   a. To retain as much joint range of movement as possible.
   b. To maintain circulation.
2. Action:
   a. Stabilize the proximal joint and support the distal part.
   b. Move the joint smoothly, slowly and gently through its full range of movement.
   c. Avoid producing excessive pain.

Active assisted
An exercise carried out by the patient with assistance from the therapist or the nurse.
1. Purpose: to encourage normal muscle action.
2. Action:
   a. Support the distal part and encourage the patient to take the joint actively through its range of movement.
   b. Give only the amount of assistance necessary to accomplish the action.
   c. Short periods of activity should be followed by adequate rest periods.

Active
An exercise accomplished by the patient without assistance.
1. Purpose: to maintain and increase muscle strength.
2. Action:
   a. When possible, active exercise should be done against gravity.
   b. The joint is moved through its full range of movement without assistance from nurse or therapist.
   c. The patient should not substitute another joint movement for the one intended.

Resisted
An active exercise carried out by the patient working against resistance produced by either manual or mechanical means.
1. Purpose: to provide resistance in order to increase muscle power.

2. Action:
   a. The patient moves the joint through its full range of movement while the therapist provides slight resistance at first and then progressively increases resistance.
   b. Sandbags and weights can be used and are supplied at the distal part of the involved joint.
   c. The movements should be done smoothly.

Isometric or static
Alternately contracting and relaxing a muscle while keeping the part in a fixed position. This exercise is performed by the patient.
1. Purpose: to maintain strength when a joint is immobilized or when it should not be put through a range of movement.
2. Action:
   a. The patient contracts or tightens the muscle as much as possible without moving the joint.
   b. He holds for several seconds, then 'lets go' and relaxes.

RANGE OF MOVEMENT EXERCISES

Range of movement is the movement of a joint through its full range in all appropriate planes. It may be passive, active or resisted.

NURSING OBJECTIVES
1. Maintain function and prevent deterioration.
2. Maintain or increase the maximal movement of a joint.

UNDERLYING PRINCIPLES
1. Range of movement testing is done by the doctor or physiotherapist to determine the movement that exists at the joint areas. Testing sets realistic and positive goals.
2. The patient's range of movement is affected by his physical condition, the disease process and his genetic make-up.
3. Each joint in the body has a normal range of movement.
4. Joints may lose their normal range of movement, stiffen, and produce a permanent disability.
5. Range of movement exercises are individually planned since there is a wide variety in the degree of movement which patients of different body builds and from different age groups are capable.
6. Range of movement exercises should be carried out whenever there is physical inactivity, provided the patient's clinical condition allows such activity.

TECHNIQUES OF RANGE OF MOVEMENT
1. Place the patient in a supine position with his arms to the side and the knees extended.
2. Hold the extremity either side of the joint, e.g. elbow, wrist or knee, and move the joint slowly, smoothly and gently through its range. This is repeated about three times.
3. Avoid moving a joint beyond its free range of movement; avoid forcing movement. The movement should be stopped at the point of pain.
4. When spasticity is present, move the joint slowly to the point of resistance.
5. Refer to Figure 2.1 for joint movement, and Figure 2.2 for a pictorial review of range of movement exercises.

DEFINITIONS
Abduction – movement away from the midline of the body.
Adduction – movement towards the midline of the body.
Flexion – bending of a joint so that the angle of the joint diminishes.
Extension – the return movement from flexion; the joint angle is increased.
Inversion – movement that turns the sole of the foot inwards.
Eversion – movement that turns the sole of the foot outwards.
Dorsiflexion – flexing or bending the ankle towards the leg.
Plantar flexion – flexing or bending the ankle in the direction of the sole.
Pronation – rotating the forearm so that the palm of the hand is downwards.
Supination – rotating the forearm so that the palm of the hand is upwards.
Rotation – turning or movement of a part around its axis.
Internal rotation – turning inwards towards the centre.
External rotation – turning outwards, away from the centre.

PREVENTING EXTERNAL ROTATION OF HIP

Patients on prolonged bed rest may develop external rotation deformity of the hip. The hip (being a ball-and-socket joint) has a tendency to rotate outward when the patient lies on his back.

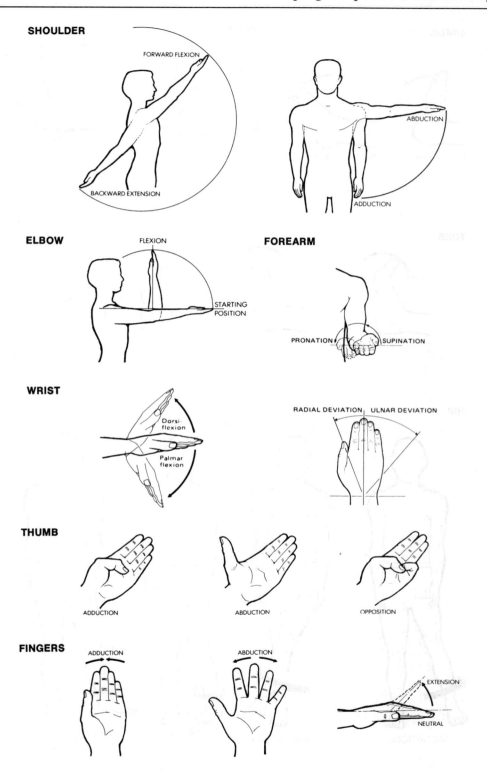

Figure 2.1. Range of joint movement

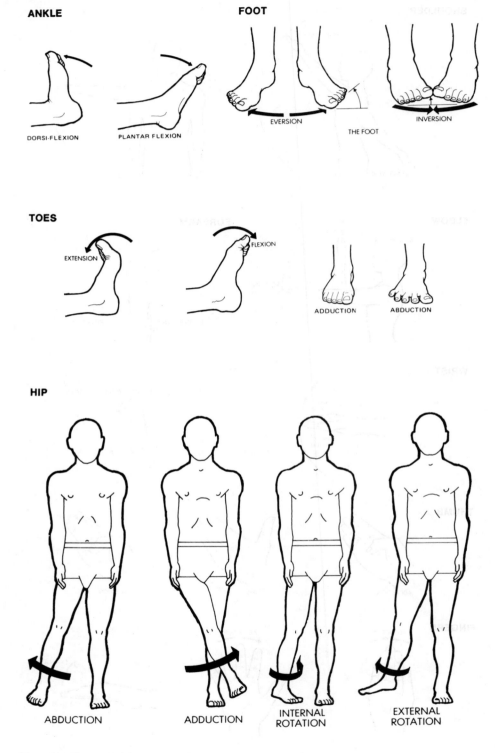

ANKLE

DORSI-FLEXION   PLANTAR FLEXION

FOOT

EVERSION   THE FOOT   INVERSION

TOES

EXTENSION   FLEXION

ADDUCTION   ABDUCTION

HIP

ABDUCTION   ADDUCTION   INTERNAL ROTATION   EXTERNAL ROTATION

Figure 2.1. Range of joint movement (cont.)

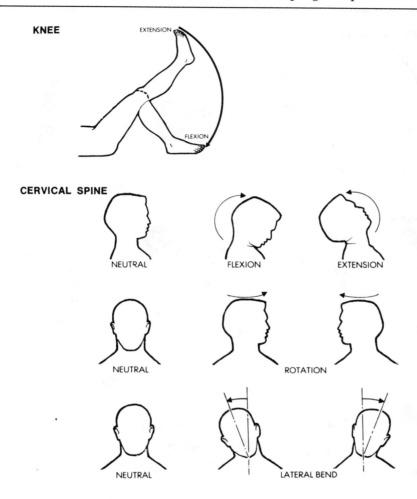

Figure 2.1. Range of joint movement (cont.)

SHOULDER: Flexion

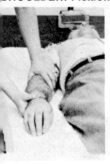 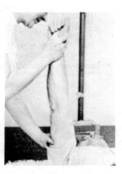 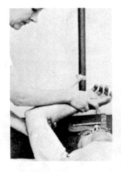 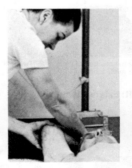 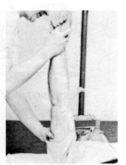

1. Start by placing one hand above the patient's elbow. Hold the patient's hand with your other hand.

2. Lift his arm up from the side of his body.

3. Move the arm slowly and gently toward his head as far as possible without causing pain.

4. If the headboard prevents full forward flexion, bend the arm at the elbow.

5. Lift arm again before returning to side or neutral position. Repeat the exercise.

Figure 2.2. Range of movement exercises (from Nursing '72, April, 1972)

SHOULDER: Abduction and Adduction

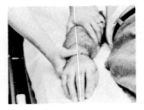
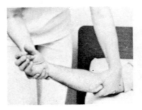
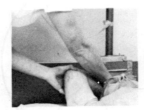
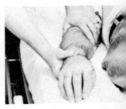

1. Place one hand above the patient's elbow. Hold his hand with your other hand.

2. Keeping his arm straight, move it sideways away from his body.

3. Bend and move the arm slowly around toward the patient's head. Move his arm back as far as possible without pain.

4. Return the arm to the side neutral position. Repeat the exercise.

SHOULDER: Internal and External Rotation

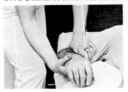
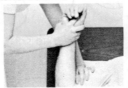
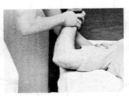
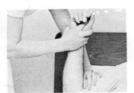

1. Place the patient's arm pointed away from his body, elbow bent. Hold his upper arm against the mattress.

2. Lift his lower arm and hand.

3. Move his lower arm and hand slowly and gently back toward his head as far as possible without causing pain.

4. Return his arm to the starting position. Repeat exercise.

SHOULDER: Cross Adduction

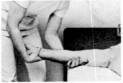
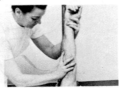
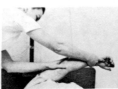
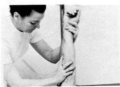

1. Place one hand on the patient's arm above his elbow. Hold his hand with your other hand.

2. Lift his arm.

3. With arm at shoulder height move arm across the body as far as possible toward the other shoulder.

4. Return the arm to the starting position. Repeat the exercise.

FOREARM: Supination and Pronation

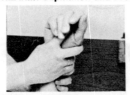
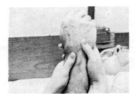
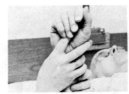

1. Starting position: Note the position of the patient's hand and the nurse's hands.

2. Twist the palm of the patient's hand toward his face.

3. Then, twist the palm of his hand back toward his feet. Repeat.

WRIST AND FINGER: Extension and Flexion

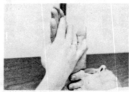
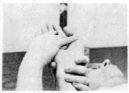
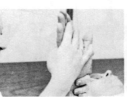
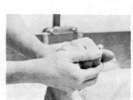

1. Hold the patient's wrist with one hand and his hand with your other hand.

2. Bend his hand backward while keeping his fingers straight.

3. Straighten the hand.

4. Bend his hand forward, closing his fingers to make a fist. Open his hand and repeat the exercise.

Figure 2.2. Range of movement exercises (cont.)

THUMB: Flexion and Extension

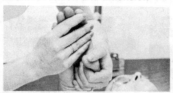
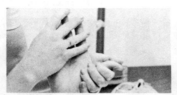
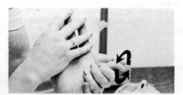

1. Hold the patient's fingers straight within one of your hands. Bend the patient's thumb into the palm of his hand with your other hand.

2. Pull his thumb back so that it points away from his palm. Repeat the exercise.

3. Move his thumb around in a circle. (circumduction)

KNEE AND HIP: Flexion and Extension

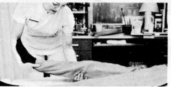
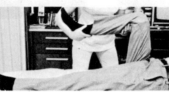
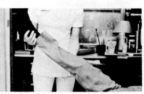

1. Place one of your hands under the patient's knee. Place your other hand on the heel of his foot.

2. Lift his leg and bend it at the knee. Move his leg slowly back toward his head as far as it will go without hurting him.

3. Then straighten his knee by lifting the foot upward. Lower his leg to the starting position and repeat the exercise.

HIP: Internal and External Rotation

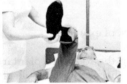
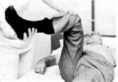
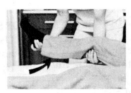
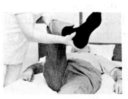

1. Place one hand under the patient's knee and your other hand on the heel of his foot. Lift his leg and bend it to a right angle at the knee.

2. Hold his knee in place and pull his foot toward you.

3. Move his foot back to the starting position.

4. Then push his foot away from you. Move his foot back to the starting position and repeat the exercise.

HIP: Abduction and Adduction

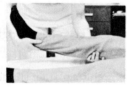

1. Place one hand under the patient's knee. Place your other hand under his heel. Hold the leg straight and then lift it up about 5cm from the mattress.

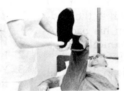
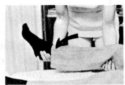

2. Pull the leg out toward you (abduction).

3. Push the leg back to the starting position (adduction). Repeat the exercise.

ANKLE: Dorsiflexion and Plantar Flexion

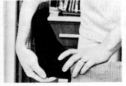
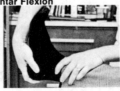
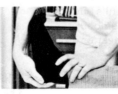
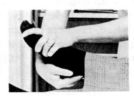

1. Hold the patient's heel with your hand, letting the sole of his foot rest against your arm.

2. Press your arm against the bottom of the foot, moving it back toward the leg (dorsiflexion). At the same time, pull on the heel.

3. Move your arm back to the starting position.

4. Move your hand up to the top of the foot, below the toes. Push down on the foot to point the toes and at the same time, push up against the heel (plantar flexion).

Figure 2.2. Range of movement exercises (cont.)

FOOT: Eversion and Inversion

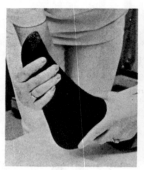
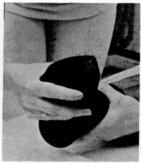

1. Start by turning the whole foot so that the sole is facing outward (eversion).

2. Then turn the foot so that the sole is facing inward (inversion).

TOE: Extension and Flexion

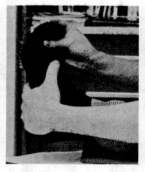
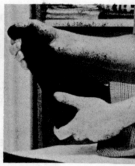

1. Start by pulling up on the toes.

2. Then push down on the toes.

Figure 2.2. Range of movement exercises (cont.)

NURSING INTERVENTIONS

1. To prevent this deformity, use a trochanter roll extending from the crest of the ilium to the mid-thigh when the patient is lying on his back. A trochanter roll serves as a mechanical wedge under the projection of the greater trochanter.
2. Use a footboard when the patient is in the dorsal position.
3. To make and position a trochanter roll:
   a. Take both ends of a large towel and bring them to the centre. The towel is now folded in half with the edges at the centre.
   b. Turn the towel over so that the ends are facing downward.
   c. Turn the patient on his side with his upper leg flexed.
   d. Place one side of the towel in the midline of the buttock. The towel should extend from the crest of the ilium to the mid-thigh.
   e. Then place the patient in a dorsal position with his leg extended.
   f. Grasp the remaining side of the towel and roll inward in an underneath fashion until the entire roll is well under the patient's buttocks. The roll should be kept taut and smooth.
   g. For the larger patient, a drawsheet or a bath blanket may be used.

PREVENTING FOOTDROP

Footdrop (plantar flexion) is a deformity caused by contraction of both the gastrocnemius and the soleus muscles; it may be produced by loss of flexibility of the Achilles tendon.

CAUSES
1. Prolonged bed rest and lack of exercise.
2. Incorrect positioning in bed.
3. Weight of bedding forcing the toes into plantar flexion (ankle bends in the direction of the sole of the foot).

CLINICAL PROBLEM
If footdrop continues without correction, the patient will walk on his toes without the heel of his foot touching the ground.

NURSING INTERVENTIONS
1. Use a footboard or pillows to keep feet at right angles to the legs when the patient is lying on his back.
   a. Position the feet with the entire plantar surface firmly against the footboard.
   b. Maintain the legs in a neutral position. Use a trochanter roll.
2. Encourage the patient to flex and extend (curl and stretch) his feet and toes frequently.
3. Have the patient rotate ankles clockwise and anti-clockwise several times each hour.

PREPARATION FOR TRANSFER OF PATIENT

NURSING OBJECTIVE
Develop the ability to raise and move the body in different positions.

EXERCISES TO STRENGTHEN ARM AND SHOULDER MUSCLES
1. Ask the patient to sit upright in bed.
2. Place a book under each hand.
3. Ask the patient to push down on the book, thus raising his body weight.

TECHNIQUE FOR MOVING A HELPLESS PATIENT TO THE EDGE OF THE BED
1. Move the patient's head and shoulders towards the edge of the bed.
2. Move his feet and legs to the edge of the bed. (The patient is now in a crescent position giving good range of movement to the lateral trunk muscles.)
3. Place both your arms well under the patient's hips. (Before the next manoeuvre, tighten or set the muscles of your back and abdomen.)
4. Straighten your back while moving the patient towards you.

NONWEIGHT-BEARING TRANSFERS
These transfers are carried out by double lower-extremity amputees, or paraplegics who are not wearing braces (Figure 2.3).

CRUTCH WALKING

Crutches are artificial supports that assist patients who need aid in walking because of disease, injury or a birth defect.

PREPARATION FOR CRUTCH WALKING
Nursing objectives
1. Develop power in the shoulder girdle and upper extremities that bear the patient's weight when crutch walking.
2. Obtain the correct type and size of crutches for the individual.

Strengthen the muscles needed for ambulation
1. For quadriceps contraction:
   a. With the patient's leg flat on the bed, ask the patient to dorsiflex the foot and raise the heel off the bed.
   The next points will vary according to the capabilities of each patient. These are average times.
   b. Maintain the muscle contracture for a count of five.
   c. Relax for a count of five.
   d. Repeat this exercise 10 to 15 times hourly.
2. For gluteal contraction:
   a. Contract or pinch the buttocks together for a count of five.
   b. Relax for a count of five.
   c. Repeat 10 to 15 times hourly.

Strengthen the muscles of the upper extremities
1. Ask the patient to flex and extend arms slowly while holding traction weights. Gradually increase the poundage of the weights.
2. Do push-ups while lying in the prone position.
3. Squeeze rubber ball – this increases grasping strength.

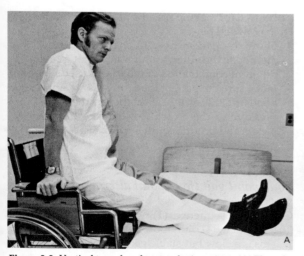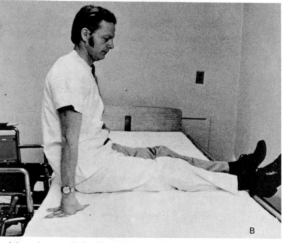

Figure 2.3. Vertical transfer of a paraplegic patient. (A) Place the wheelchair facing the bed as close to the bed as possible. Lock brakes. Instruct the patient to push up on his hands and arms and slide his body forward onto the bed. (B) This is a nonweight-bearing transfer in which the patient learns to transfer on the same level. Later this type of nonweight-bearing transfer can be done to a higher and lower level by the push-up method

4. Raise head and shoulders from the bed, stretch hands as far forward as possible.
5. Sit up on bed or chair:
    a. Raise body from chair by pushing hands against the chair seat.
    b. Raise body out of seat and hold position. Relax.

Measure for axillary crutches

1. When the patient is lying down (this gives an approximate measurement):
    a. Ask the patient to wear the shoes normally used for walking.
    b. Measure from the anterior fold of the axilla to the sole of the foot, then add 5cm.
    c. Alternatively, subtract 40cm from the patient's height.
2. When the patient is standing erect:
    a. Stand the patient against the wall with feet slightly apart and away from the wall.
    b. Mark 5cm out from the side to the tip of the toe.
    c. Measure 15cm straight ahead from the first mark. Mark this point.
    d. Measure from 5cm below axilla to the second mark. This measurement is the crutch length.

Crutch stance

1. Ask the patient to wear well-fitting shoes with firm soles.
2. The crutches should be fitted with large rubber suction tips.
3. Ask the patient to stand by a chair with his weight on the unaffected leg to achieve balance.
4. Position the patient against a wall with his head in a neutral position.
5. Place crutches 5cm in front of the patient and 10cm to the side (Figure 2.4).
    a. The hand piece should be adjusted to allow a 30° elbow flexion.
    b. There should be a four-finger width insertion between the axillary fold and the arm piece.
    c. A foam rubber pad on the underarm piece should relieve pressure on the upper arm and thoracic cage.

TEACHING THE CRUTCH GAIT

1. The selection of the crutch gait depends on the type and severity of the disability and the patient's physical condition, arm and trunk strength and/or body balance.
2. Teach the patient at least two gaits – a faster gait to

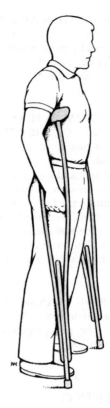

Figure 2.4. Crutch stance

be used for making speed and a slower one for use in crowded places.
3. Show the patient how to change gait from one method to the other, as this relieves fatigue since a different combination of muscles is used.
4. Make sure the patient is bearing his weight on his hands. If the weight is borne on the axilla, the pressure of the crutch can damage the brachial plexus and produce crutch paralysis.

CRUTCH GAITS

Four-point gait (four-point alternate crutch gait)

Crutch–foot sequence: (1) right crutch, (2) left foot, (3) left crutch, (4) right foot.

1. This is a slow but stable gait; the patient's weight is constantly being shifted.
2. Four-point gait can be used only by patients who can move each leg separately and bear a considerable amount of weight on each of them.

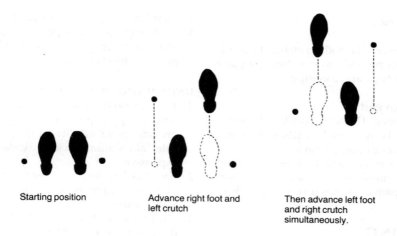

Starting position

Advance right foot and
left crutch

Then advance left foot
and right crutch
simultaneously.

Figure 2.5. Two-point gait

Two-point gait (two-point alternate crutch gait)

Crutch–foot sequence (Figure 2.5): (1) right crutch and left foot, (2) left crutch and right foot simultaneously.

1. This is a faster gait but requires more balance since there are only two points of contact with the floor.

Three-point gait

Crutch–foot sequence: (1) both crutches and the weaker lower extremity simultaneously, (2) then the stronger lower extremity.

1. This is a fairly rapid gait but requires more strength and balance.
2. The patient's arms must be strong enough to support his entire body weight.

Tripod crutch gait
Tripod alternative crutch gait

Crutch–foot sequence: (1) right crutch, (2) left crutch, (3) swing body and legs forward.

Tripod simultaneous crutch gait

Crutch–foot sequence (Figure 2.6): (1) both crutches, (2) swing body and legs forward.

1. The patient constantly maintains a tripod position.
2. At the start, both crutches are held fairly widespread out in front while both feet are held together at the back.
3. These gaits are slow and laboured.

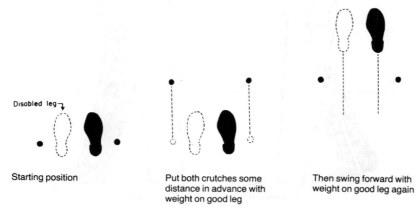

Disabled leg

Starting position

Put both crutches some
distance in advance with
weight on good leg

Then swing forward with
weight on good leg again

Figure 2.6. Tripod simultaneous crutch gait

Swinging crutch gaits
Swinging-to gait
Crutch–foot sequence: (1) both crutches forward, (2) then lift and swing body *to* crutches, (3) place crutches in front of body and continue.

Swinging-through gait
Crutch–foot sequence: (1) both crutches forward, (2) lift and swing body *beyond* crutches, (3) place crutches in front of body and continue.

1. In the swinging crutch gaits, both legs are lifted off the ground simultaneously and swung forward while the patient pushes up on the crutches.

CANE WALKING

PURPOSES
A cane is used for balance and support.
1. To assist the patient to walk with greater balance and support and less fatigue.
2. To compensate for deficiencies of function normally performed by the neuromuscular skeletal system.

3. To relieve pressure on weight-bearing joints.
4. To provide forces to push or pull the body forward or to restrain the forward motion of the patient while walking.

UNDERLYING PRINCIPLES
1. A firm wooden stick fitted with a 3.75cm rubber suction tip to provide traction while walking, provides good stability for the patient. An adjustable, aluminium stick is available, but is very expensive.
2. The stick handle should be level with the greater trochanter when the patient is wearing his normal walking shoes.
3. The patient's elbow should be flexed 25–30° when the stick is the correct length.

TECHNIQUE FOR WALKING WITH A STICK
Teach the patient as follows:
1. Hold the stick in the hand opposite to the affected extremity, i.e. the stick should be held on the good side.
2. Move the cane at the same time that the affected leg is moved (Figure 2.7).

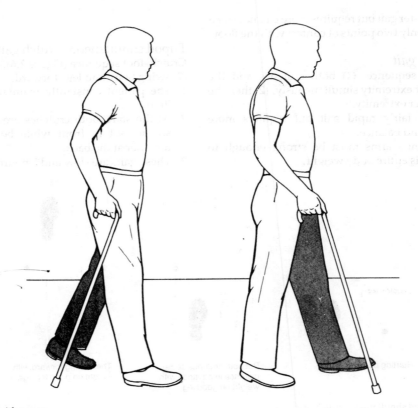

Figure 2.7. Walking with a cane

3. Keep the stick fairly close to the body to prevent leaning.
4. When climbing stairs:
   a. Step up with unaffected leg, with both stick and affected leg on lower step.
   b. Then place stick and affected leg on higher step.
   c. Reverse this procedure for descending steps. The unaffected, or stronger, leg goes up first and comes down last.

Evaluation
EXPECTED OUTCOMES
1. The patient has regained the maximum amount of mobility with help and encouragement from the care team, and is motivated to continue to make efforts to improve further.
2. The patient has achieved a degree of independence and can make social contacts.
3. He can maintain a good posture.

HELPING THE PATIENT TO KEEP HIS BODY CLEAN AND WELL GROOMED AND TO PROTECT THE SKIN

NURSING OBJECTIVES
1. Assist the patient in maintaining a high standard of personal hygiene.
2. Protect the integrity of the skin in patients at risk.
3. Encourage the patient to take an interest in care of the hair, face and nails.

Assessment
1. Physical inability to maintain own hygiene due to:
   a. Restricted movement of hands and arms.
   b. Restricted body movement because of paralysis or weakness or traction.
   c. Breathlessness on exertion.
2. Psychological problems, such as severe depression, mental impairment.
3. Physical problems compounded by inadequate toilet and washing facilities.

Planning
1. Provide facilities for the patient to wash himself as much as possible and to give help when needed.

2. Provide special aids for those with disability with hand or arm movements.
3. Arrange home assessment visits if necessary, before the patient goes home, to ensure adequate toilet and bathing facilities.

Implementation
1. Provide facilities for cleanliness of the skin. This may necessitate:
   a. A complete bed bath for a helpless, or very ill patient.
   b. Provision of a bowl of water and the necessary toilet requisites, placing the patient in a well-supported position, and encouraging him to wash and dry his face and hands, and perhaps arms and chest as well, if this can be done without causing undue fatigue or strain.
   c. Assisting the patient with a bath or shower, using mechanical lifts or bath appliances as necessary.
   d. Supervising the patient attending to his own personal hygiene and only providing assistance when needed.
2. Providing aids for those with a disability of hands or arms, or those with limited movement.
3. Remember that the nurse is also a teacher, and some patients with a low standard of personal hygiene need tactful guidance and encouragement. *However*, apparent lack of cleanliness may be due to physical or psychological incapacity, and may be a cause of distress to the patient.
4. The hair must be thoroughly brushed and combed. Women should be encouraged to take an interest in the styling of their hair and a hairdresser should make frequent visits. It is important for the nurse to ascertain if any patient is unwilling to ask for a visit from the hairdresser because of financial difficulties, and to tactfully arrange for this through hospital funds. If the patient's own hairdresser wishes to come, this should be encouraged.
5. The nurse should be able to shampoo the patient's hair either in bed or in the bathroom as frequently as needed.
6. All men should be encouraged to shave themselves. If this is not possible, a barber or the nurse should perform this.
7. Mouth cleanliness is essential. This can usually be accomplished by the patients themselves using a normal shaped toothbrush and paste, but a large handle may be needed for those who have difficulty in holding thin articles.
8. Although the aim of rehabilitation is to achieve as much independence as possible, many patients

may find cutting and care of finger and toe nails is beyond their capability, and a chiropodist should visit.

9. Advice and practical help must be available for a patient who needs special cosmetics, e.g. for covering scar tissue, or for provision of wigs or prostheses.

Evaluation
EXPECTED OUTCOMES
1. The patient is motivated and helped to maintain his own hygiene, with help if necessary.
2. The patient takes pride in his appearance.

PREVENTION AND TREATMENT OF PRESSURE SORES (DECUBITUS ULCERS)

Pressure sores are localized areas of necrosis occurring in the skin and subcutaneous tissues as a result of pressure.

ALTERED PHYSIOLOGY
Pressure; tissue anoxia and ischaemia; necrosis of tissue cells; sloughing and ulceration; infection; sepsis; involvement of underlying tissues; rapidly irreversible condition.

Two types of lesions can occur: (a) superficial lesions which are visible immediately; (b) lesions which occur in deeper tissues due to prolonged pressure, which may not be visible for 24 to 48 hours after the pressure occurs, e.g. bad positioning on an operating table, with only a thin layer of padding.

CAUSES
Pressure
Pressure exerted on skin and subcutaneous tissues by bony prominences and by the object on which the body rests (mattress, stretcher, plaster bed, etc.) interferes with the blood supply of the tissues and if it is prolonged will cause tissue death.

Contributing factors
1. Immobilization and lack of normal movement, particularly if associated with neurological, circulatory and orthopaedic conditions.
2. Sensory and motor deficits.
   a. Sensory loss produces lack of awareness of pain and pressure.
   b. Motor paralysis with associated muscular atrophy causes lack of movement and reduction in padding between overlying skin and underlying bone.

3. Poor nutrition – negative nitrogen, phosphorus, sulphur and calcium balance will produce wasting of tissue, osteoporosis and loss of weight.
   a. Anaemia.
   b. Hypoproteinaemia.
   c. Vitamin deficiencies, particularly that of ascorbic acid.
4. Oedema which interferes with supply of nutrients to the cells.
5. Friction, moisture and heat irritate the skin, making it less resistant to injury.
6. Infection lowers the resistance of skin to breakdown; destroys tissue.
7. Shearing force – caused by gravitational forces that pull the patient's body down towards the foot of the bed, and by resisting forces creating friction on the skin surface.
   a. Pulling tissues so that surface tissues and blood vessels are stretched and injured.
   b. It happens when a patient: is pulled up in the bed instead of being lifted clear of the sheets; is allowed to slump down in a chair or bed; moves in bed by digging heels and elbows into the mattress.
8. Advancing age and debility may cause changes in skin due to reduced production of sebum.
9. Equipment – traction, plaster casts, badly designed chairs or beds.
10. Concurrent illnesses, particularly diabetes mellitus.

SITES
1. Weight-bearing bony prominences which are covered only by skin and small amounts of subcutaneous fat. Most (75 per cent) pressure sores occur at such sites (Figure 2.8).
2. Other bony promontories – knees, malleoli, heels and elbows.

SIGNS AND SYMPTOMS
1. Redness.
2. Dusky, cyanotic blue-grey area indicating capillary occlusion and subcutaneous weakening.
3. Blistering.
4. Break in the skin progressing to tissue necrosis.

Planning and implementation
NURSING INTERVENTIONS
Identify patients at particular risk
This can be undertaken conveniently using the Doreen Norton Risk Scoring System (Table 2.2). Any patient who scores 12 or less needs very specialized care. The frequency with which the score should be assessed varies with individual patients, but all

MAJOR PRESSURE SITES

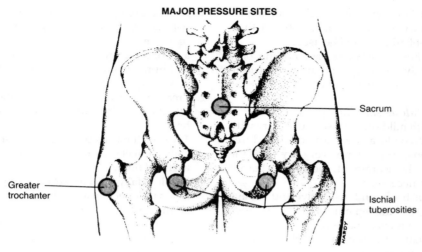

Sacrum

Greater trochanter

Ischial tuberosities

Figure 2.8. Pressure areas

Table 2.2   Pressure sore risk assessment scoring system (Doreen Norton)

A Physical condition		B Mental condition		C Activity		D Mobility		E Incontinent	
Good	4	Alert	4	Ambulant	4	Full	4	Not	4
Fair	3	Apathetic	3	Walk/help	3	Slightly limited	3	Occasionally	3
Poor	2	Confused	2	Chairbound	2	Very limited	2	Usually/urine	2
Very bad	1	Stuporous	1	Bedfast	1	Immobile	1	Doubly	1

Norton, D. 1975. Research on the Problem of Pressure Sores. *Nursing Mirror*, 13 Feb, 1975. Vol. 140, No. 7, pp. 65–67.

nurses should be alert to the fact that a significant change in the condition of the patient means a reassessment of the score.

Relieve pressure
1. By encouraging the patient to keep active.
2. Turn the patient regularly, at one-, two- or four-hourly intervals to allow the blood to flow back into the tissues which are affected by pressure. If possible, position the patient on all four sides in sequence, laterally, dorsal and prone.
3. Use pillows or pads to relieve pressure around particular areas, e.g. heels. Sheepskins, natural or synthetic, can be placed under the patient's buttocks, and sheepskin bootees can be used to prevent friction on heels.
4. Use devices to support specific areas of the body; the supporting medium should mould to the patient to ensure uniformly distributed pressure and should allow evaporation of perspiration.

a. Gel-type flotation pad – reduces pressure, since the gel-like material (similar in consistency to human adipose tissue) 'gives' with the patient's weight.
b. Fleeces (synthetic; wool) – softness and resilience of padding provides resistance to shearing force and results in even distribution of pressure; provides freedom from wrinkles and friction, and dissipation and absorption of moisture.
c. Fluid-supported mattresses (waterbeds) and fluid-supported seats – eliminate pressure points; as the body sinks into the fluid, additional surface area becomes available for weight-bearing, thereby further decreasing body weight per unit area.
5. Use a bedcradle to lift the weight of the bedclothes off the limbs so that there is no impediment to free movement.
6. Avoid placing the patient on a poorly ventilated

mattress that is covered with plastic or impermeable material. If this is unavoidable, a thick cotton under-blanket should be used.
7. Drawsheets should not be used as a routine, only when absolutely necessary. This applies to cotton drawsheets as well as plastic sheets.

Maintain meticulous skin hygiene
1. Wash skin with mild soap, rinse and *blot* dry with a soft towel. Keep local areas dry, clean and free from excretions. If the skin is very dry, or if the patient is doubly incontinent, the use of a barrier cream may be necessary.
2. If the patient is bedbound, use active and passive exercises to aid movement, and to improve muscular, skin and vascular tone.
3. Mobilize the patient as soon as possible. If actual ambulation is not possible, a change of position from a bed to a chair will help.
4. Use alternating pressure mattresses or chairs, which help to improve the circulation as well as relieving pressure.
5. Inspect the skin frequently for signs of pressure. A patient with paraplegia must be taught to inspect his skin, using a mirror.
6. Keep the patient's weight off reddened areas until it has completely cleared.
7. Relieve pressure over the ischial area for patients sitting in wheelchairs for any length of time. Teach paraplegic patients to do push-ups every hour for intermittent relief of pressure over ischial tuberosities.
8. Inspect any areas where friction may occur from the edge of plaster casts, splints and bandages.

Improve nutritional state of the patient
1. Sufficient protein and vitamin C intake are essential.
2. A check on the general health of the patient, to exclude anaemia, diabetes and cardiovascular disorders.

TREATING PRESSURE SORES
Goals
1. Relieve all pressure from the area.
2. Continue with preventive measures of a more vigorous nature.
3. Encourage restoration of circulation and cellular function.
4. Prevent necrosis of deeper structures.

Principles
Treatment is related to the extent and depth of the wound and any associated infection.

1. Relieve pressure from the area; a pressure sore will not heal when subjected to continuous pressure.
   a. Continue preventive measures.
   b. Improve general health of the patient to provide optimal healing.
2. Treat the underlying disorder – underlying conditions must be managed to allow the ulcer to heal.
3. Take bacterial cultures (and sensitivity studies) early if infection is present; pressure sores contain bacterial flora.
4. Employ daily mechanical cleansing of the ulcer – clears up infection and stimulates regeneration of epithelium.
   a. Deep ulcers may need to be irrigated with prescribed sterile solution or cleansed in a whirlpool.
   b. Debride ulcer – devitalized tissue promotes infection, delays granulation, and impedes healing.
      (i) Use sharp dissection (scalpel blade) to remove eschar covering the ulcer.
      (ii) Cross-hatching of the eschar with the scalpel blade may facilitate penetration of enzymatic debriding agent (collagenase therapy).
      (iii) Debridement of deep necrotic ulcers is performed in the operating room.
5. Control infection – may be a precipitating cause and may inhibit healing of ulcer; chronic infection contributes to anaemia, hypoalbuminaemia, and malnutrition.
   a. Assess for systemic infection – fever, cellulitis, lymphangitis.
   b. Give systemic antibiotic therapy based on identification of pathogens and antibiotic sensitivity determinations.
   c. Place the patient on drainage and secretion precautions if the decubitus ulcer is infected, minor or limited, and on contact isolation if the ulcer is draining.
6. Utilize physical types of treatment.
   a. Expose ulcer to air and sunlight.
   b. Employ light stroking around lesion – promotes venous return and reduces oedema.
   c. Use ultraviolet irradiation:
      (i) Clean discharges from surface of ulcer.
      (ii) Cover normal skin surrounding ulcer during irradiation.
   d. Whirlpool treatments – increase circulation and have debriding action.
   e. Use oxygen under pressure applied directly on ulcer (hyperbaric oxygen therapy) – directs

more oxygen to tissues; hastens metabolic processes and reduces healing time.

7. Utilize topical applications as directed. There is a wide variety of opinion concerning these agents.
   a. Skin barriers – Karaya powder, Stomahesive, etc.
   b. Antiseptic plastic sprays.
   c. Aerosol spray containing a corticosteroid and an antibiotic.
   d. Absorbable gelatin sponges (Gelfoam) – placed at base of ulcer to improve healing and decrease plasma loss from pressure sores.
   e. Enzymatic debriding agents (collagenase therapy) – digests necrotic tissue and purulent exudate and is applied using the following procedure:
      (i) Remove eschar covering ulcer or cross-hatch eschar with scalpel blade to allow enzyme to come in contact with the material to be digested.
      (ii) Remove loose debris with forceps.
      (iii) Irrigate with prescribed sterile solution.
      (iv) Assess wound for inflammation, pus, odour.
      (v) Apply enzymatic debriding ointment in thin, even layer over surface of ulcer.
      (vi) Cover with dry sterile dressing secured with hypoallergenic tape or gauze bandage.
   f. Transparent, elastic, self-adhesive film (Op-Site) – purported to seal in body's normal defences (leucocytes, plasma, fibrin).
   g. Dextranomer (Debrisan) – useful when depth of ulcer exceeds 2mm or for a moist sloughing wound.
      (i) Cleanse ulcer thoroughly with prescribed solution for each treatment and damp-dry.
      (ii) Apply dextranomer directly onto lesion – contains dry porous beads with hydrophilic (water-absorbing) properties; also absorbs debris, allowing granulation tissue to develop.
      (iii) Cover with a dry porous dressing and secure with a gauze bandage.
   h. Absorption (co-polymer starch) dressing.
8. Ensure good nutrition – to reverse catabolism, correct anaemia and oedema, and increase tissue oxygenation and perfusion.
   a. High-protein feedings may be employed to correct protein deficiency; loss of serum from a draining ulcer depletes the body stores of protein, specifically albumin.
   b. Iron and ascorbic acid (vitamin C) given as

directed – vitamin C is necessary for collagen formation. Wound healing is dependent on collagen.)
   c. Zinc supplements – to accelerate healing.
9. Prepare the patient for surgical intervention if ulcer does not respond to conservative measures.
   a. Prepare the patient for lying prone before surgery is performed.
   b. Assist with diagnostic work-up in addition to pre-surgical management for spasticity and contractures.
   c. Surgical procedures:
      (i) Incision and drainage – if ulcer is not draining properly, is suppurating or is not undermined.
      (ii) Grafting procedures – different types of grafts are used according to size of ulcer.
      (iii) Closure of defect – removal of ulcer, surrounding scar, underlying bursa, affected bone.
   d. Postoperative nursing intervention:
      (i) Relieve pressure by proper positioning and elimination of shearing forces for four to six weeks.
      (ii) Allow controlled pressure on site (after six weeks) for 10 to 15 minutes, two to three times a day under close nursing surveillance; watch for redness or abrasion.

Evaluation
EXPECTED OUTCOMES
1. The skin will achieve and maintain a healthy colour, with no signs of redness, bruising or pallor.
2. No lesions will appear. Any which are present will show a progressive diminution in depth and area.
3. The patient is able to participate in his own care by changing position regularly, if he is able.
4. Regular reassessment of the general condition of the patient will be recorded.

HELPING THE PATIENT WITH SELECTING CLOTHING, DRESSING AND UNDRESSING

NURSING OBJECTIVES
1. Help the patient to obtain clothes which:
   a. Express his own personal preference;

b. Are easy for that individual to put on or take off;
c. Are in keeping with the environment;
d. Are fresh and clean.
2. Teach the patient and relatives the best way of putting on garments and removing them, and the use of any special aids which can help.

Assessment

1. Psychological problems, e.g. depression, when the patient may have lost interest in his own appearance.
2. Physical weakness and loss of willpower following a severe illness.
3. Difficulty in buying clothes, e.g. lack of mobility, blindness, financial problems.
4. Difficulty in finding clothes to fit, due to some physical problem.

Planning

1. Obtain financial assistance for those in need.
2. Encourage the patient to choose his own clothes.
3. Encourage the patient to enjoy social contacts.

Implementation

1. Arrange shopping expeditions to appropriate stores whenever possible. As more stores have late night shopping, relatives or clubs may be able to assist with this.
2. If the patient is unable to get to the shops, a range of catalogues should be available. It may be possible for a retailer to visit a hospital and bring a selection of clothes. The patient may have relied on relatives or friends giving him clothes for Christmas or birthday presents, and these may not have been exactly what he likes. Choice should be given whenever possible.
3. The patient may be unable to, or have great difficulty in, obtaining clothing which is suitable for a particular disability, e.g. garments with front or extra large openings.
4. Financial difficulties may have prevented the patient from buying new clothes.
5. Always encourage the patient to choose the clothes which he wishes to wear that day. If the patient has his own clothes, provision must be made for these to be kept in a suitable cupboard, and hung up if possible. If hospital clothes are worn, there should be a sufficient variety of size, colour and style so that individuality is retained.
6. Ensure that laundering facilities are available for personal clothes if the relatives are unable to take these home for washing.

7. Obtain advice from the occupational therapy department for special problems.
8. Encourage the patient to be as independent as possible. Although dressing may take a considerable time, it will give the patient a feeling of achievement.
9. No patient must be left without suitable underwear, even though there may be a problem with incontinence. This is degrading and unnecessary.

Evaluation
EXPECTED OUTCOMES
1. The patient takes pride in his appearance.
2. There is an adequate supply of clean, well ironed clothes, specially chosen by the patient.
3. The patient takes an interest in selecting new clothes.
4. Relatives and friends co-operate in encouraging the patient to make his own choice.

HELPING THE PATIENT TO EXPRESS SEXUALITY

Sexuality is part of a person's self-concept and involves feelings of self-worth, acceptance, sharing, affection and intimacy, as well as feelings of masculinity or femininity. It includes physical, psychological, emotional and social elements and is reflected in everything a person says and does.

The handicapped person is also a sexual human being.

Assessment
SEXUAL HISTORY
This includes present sexual activity, level of satisfaction and concerns.

PATIENT PROBLEMS
Potential for sexual dysfunction related to disability, problems in self-esteem, effects of treatment and inability to have sexual intercourse.

Planning and implementation
NURSING INTERVENTIONS
1. Be comfortable with your own sexuality; avoid imposing your values on the patient.
2. Establish an atmosphere that is conducive to acceptance and open communication.
3. Let the patient know that sexual rehabilitation is part of the total rehabilitation programme.

4. Inform the patient that there is a breadth and depth of sexual expression possible and that he is a person of value.
5. Recognize that feelings of warmth, approval and friendship, as well as sharing and touching, are important.
6. Be aware that patients with longstanding disabilities may need training in communication and assertiveness skills.
7. Inform the patient of the availability of the following services:
   a. Social skills training;
   b. Sex education/counselling services (individual, couples, and family);
   c. Genetic/contraceptive counselling;
   d. Sex therapy;
   e. Reading materials; audiovisual materials;
   f. Group discussion.
8. See the further reading section at the end of this chapter, p. 41.

Evaluation
EXPECTED OUTCOMES
Patient feels more positive about self:
1. Demonstrates improvement in hygiene and grooming.
2. Discusses alternate methods of sexual pleasure.
3. Expresses satisfaction over changes in social relationships.
4. Plans to join a support group.

HELPING THE PATIENT TO AVOID DANGERS IN THE ENVIRONMENT

NURSING OBJECTIVES
1. Encourage the patient to be involved in self-care without causing himself any injury.
2. Alert the patient to dangers inherent in a disabled person, e.g. through lack of mobility.
3. Provide a safe environment without restricting the patient's initiative.

Assessment
The patient may have problems with:
1. Sensory deprivation:
   a. Touch and pain;
   b. Sight;
   c. Hearing;
   d. Consciousness;
   e. Balance;
   f. Intellectual functioning.
2. Loss of normal body defences, e.g. immunosuppression.
3. Loss of strength:
   a. Lack of willpower due to illness;
   b. Lack of physical strength (very young or elderly).
4. Badly designed or maintained furniture, equipment or utensils.

Planning
1. Provide a hazard-free environment, by providing suitable supports, protections or guards for vulnerable patients in hospital or at home. Ensure regular servicing of electrical equipment, and plan for regular safety inspections.
2. Provide appropriate and repeated teaching/demonstrations for slow learners.
3. Strengthen the physical and psychological abilities of the patient in order to compensate for those which are lacking.

Implementation
1. Ensure freedom from potential hazards:
   a. At floor level, e.g. trailing flexes, slip mats, spilt water or food;
   b. Unguarded fires, wheelchairs or beds without fixed castors or brakes;
   c. Overhanging shelves, dazzling lights, inconvenient steps.
2. Clothing must not restrict free movement.
3. Shoes must be well fitting. It is important to avoid the wearing of slippers, as they do not afford a firm footing.
4. No trailing belts or ties, as these can cause falls.
5. Safety in the bathroom. There should be aids for the patient to get in and out of the bath, and a non-slip mat in the bottom of the bath.
6. Safety in the kitchen. There should be easy access to shelves and cupboards. The cooking hob must be at a suitable level. If gas is used a self-igniting device should be provided. There must be a suitable storage cupboard for food, as well as a refrigerator. This is essential, because people who have a disability may not be able to get to the shops very easily, and may have to buy food to last for several days at a time. This must be stored in a cool airy place, free from contamination.
7. A patient with sight problems will need special devices in the kitchen. Details of these will be found in Chapter 15, Care of the Patient with an Eye Disorder.

8. Drugs must be clearly labelled, with the name and the time at which they should be taken. Various methods may be employed to clarify this, e.g. colour coding or the use of bubble packs, so that the times can actually be written on them. Avoid unnecessary medication; destroy unfinished drugs or those which are out of date.

9. The young, elderly or people with impaired intelligence may need protection from unscrupulous members of society, or they may be abused by their own family. The nurse should be aware that problems could occur, and should be alert to any signs of abnormal tension, or any physical or mental deterioration that seems unusual. For elderly people or disabled people living on their own, a safety chain should be fitted to the front door.

10. For details of the care of the unconscious patient, see Chapter 16, Care of the Patient with a Neurological Disorder.

Evaluation
EXPECTED OUTCOMES
The patient is able to:
1. Be aware of particular potential hazards, and take appropriate steps to avoid them.
2. Use the aids which are available, and know how these should be maintained.
3. Be confident in his ability to be as independent as possible.
4. Know how to call for assistance if it is required.

HELPING THE PATIENT TO COMMUNICATE WITH OTHERS

NURSING OBJECTIVES
1. Form a channel of communication between the patient and the nurse, preferably by verbal or, if necessary, nonverbal means.
2. Encourage the patient to communicate willingly with staff, other patients and relatives.
3. Combat apathy and provide a stimulating environment.
4. Monitor the amount of nurse–patient interaction.

Assessment
1. Physical problems, such as impairment of speech due to:

a. Neurological disorders such as cerebrovascular accident, cerebral palsy, motor neurone disease;
b. Local problems, such as a fractured jaw that has been wired, operations or treatment of the tongue, laryngectomy, tracheostomy.
2. Deafness.
3. Blindness.
4. Language problems.
5. Psychological problems, such as severe depression, mistrust, or problems stemming from mental subnormality.

Planning
1. Plan to spend time with the patient to establish a good relationship.
2. Provide appropriate aids to communication.
3. Involve others, e.g. speech therapist, interpreter, local groups for the deaf, stroke clubs, laryngectomy counsellors, etc.
4. Ensure that all staff and relatives understand the methods of communication being used.

Implementation
1. One nurse should act as a 'primary nurse' for the patient, to form a trusting relationship; to introduce other members of the care team and ensure that they understand the means of communication. This will avoid considerable frustration, embarrassment and loss of dignity of both the patient and staff.
2. An unsuspected or unacknowledged degree of deafness may be present. An appointment with the audiometry department should be made as a hearing aid may be necessary. It is important that the hearing aid is in good repair, that new batteries are available and that both the patient and relatives understand its use. The nurse should stand in front of the patient, and speak slowly and clearly, not necessarily louder than normal. Patience and encouragement are essential. For profoundly deaf people, communication by sign language may be used.
3. A patient with aphasia due to a cerebrovascular accident suffers considerable frustration because of the lack of ability to form the words that he wishes to. Specialist care from the speech therapist is essential. Picture or word cards may help the patient to make his immediate needs known.
4. Note must be taken of anyone who withdraws from communicating with others. This may be a sign of deterioration of his mental or physical state and may need medical intervention.
5. Even though a patient may be unable or unwilling

to communicate with others, it is necessary for people to talk to him as a sensible human being, even though no relation may be present, e.g. as in an unconscious patient. On discharge from hospital, care must be taken that the patient will have social contacts. If he is housebound, CB radio contacts or amateur radio society groups for the disabled may give links. With the latter groups, communication can be by morse code, and can be helpful for those with speech difficulties.

6. All nurses working in the ward situation must be aware of the time which is actually spent communicating with each patient. In some cases this may be less than one hour a day giving personal attention to a patient.
7. Encourage the patient to be with other people, e.g. clubs, outings and church attendance, but allow him to express preferences.
8. A pad and pencil or a 'magic slate' should be available for patients who have had a laryngectomy or tracheostomy in the immediate postoperative period.
9. It is essential for the patient to have a means of calling for aid or attracting the attention of the staff. This must be considered before the patient is sent home, as well as during the time he is in hospital.

Evaluation
EXPECTED OUTCOMES
The patient is able to:
1. Communicate with others and make his needs known, by verbal or nonverbal means.
2. Participate in social contacts.
3. Live as independently and with as much self-fulfilment as possible.

HELPING THE PATIENT TO PRACTISE HIS RELIGION OR TO CONFORM TO HIS CONCEPTS OF RIGHT AND WRONG

NURSING OBJECTIVES
1. Understand the aspects of a patient's religion which may need special consideration.
2. Encourage the patient to practise his religion as he wishes.

Assessment
1. The patient who belongs to an ethnic minority group.
2. The patient who belongs to a religious group, which requires a particular way of behaviour.
3. A patient who has a conscientious objection to certain types of treatment, procedures or operations.

Planning
1. Ensure that information is available for all staff about religious customs and requirements.
2. Ensure that the patient is able to establish contact and receive visits from his clergyman/priest/minister/religious leader when he wishes.
3. Involve the patient in decision-making at all levels.

Implementation
1. Acknowledge the uniqueness of the individual and respect his freedom to adhere to his religious beliefs.
2. Any ethical issues which arise should be treated with sympathy, but also with a knowledge of the issues involved, and the possible effects on the patient in the future.
3. Arrange for the hospital chaplain or appropriate religious adviser to visit if the patient wishes. Provide a quiet place, free from interruption for them, with privacy.
4. Make arrangements for the patient to receive the sacraments which are part of his religious life, without making him feel that he is causing trouble or disrupting the ward routine.
5. The nurse must not deliberately set out to impose her own beliefs on a patient or his family.
6. Wherever possible, the patient should be involved as a part of his own religious group or community; visits to his own church should be arranged if possible and visits from other church members should be encouraged.
7. Special diets should be available. Explanation should be given about medical restrictions.

Evaluation
EXPECTED OUTCOMES
1. The patient feels confident that no treatment or procedures will be carried out without his knowledge and consent.
2. His religious principles regarding diet and observances are respected.
3. He has access to his religious advisers when he wishes.

HELPING THE PATIENT WITH WORK OR PRODUCTIVE OCCUPATION

NURSING OBJECTIVES

1. Enable the patient to achieve a feeling of independence by accomplishing some form of employment.
2. Help the patient to fulfil the more basic physiological and psychological needs in order to reach higher levels of self-fulfilment. These have been described by Maslow (Figure 2.9).

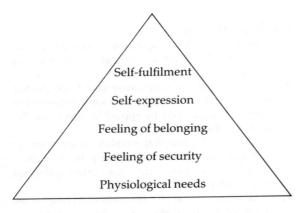

Figure 2.9. Maslow's hierarchy of needs

Assessment

1. Problems with movement of arms and hands.
2. Problems with mobility.
3. Problems with mental impairment and/or lack of concentration.

Planning

1. Obtain the most appropriate aids or appliances for the patient.
2. Teach him how to use these to his best advantage, and how to maintain them.
3. Help the patient to strengthen the abilities that he has.

Implementation

1. Discuss with the patient the type of work which he has previously done, and his wishes and hopes for the future. Encourage him to make full use of special abilities.
2. Co-operate with the occupational therapy and physiotherapy departments in helping the patient to make a realistic plan of goals, and to acquire the most suitable aids for him, e.g. special prostheses will be needed for upper or lower limb amputees. For a patient who is severely disabled, such as with tetraplegia, an electronic machine may be provided which will enable him to operate various machinery and use a typewriter, known as patient operated selector mechanism (POSSUM). Even if he is completely immobile, this would enable the patient to make use of his brain and even run a business.
3. Some form of mobility may be needed. (See 'Helping the patient with mobility', page 16). Each individual must be assessed carefully to see which form of transport is most suitable, e.g. hand-controlled chairs, battery-operated chairs or a car adapted for a particular disability. A Disability Mobility Allowance may be available. Also, there may be concessions on hire purchase for a car, with motor insurance and some public transport. Useful addresses include: The Disablement Income Group, Atlee House, Toynbee Hall, 28 Commercial Street, London, EC1; Disabled Drivers Association, Ashwellthorpe Hall, Ashwellthorpe, Norwich NR16 1EX; The Royal Association for Disability and Rehabilitation, 23/25 Mortimer Street, London W1N 8AB; The Disability Alliance, 5, Netherhall Gardens, London NW3 5RN.
4. One of the most important people who may help is the disablement rehabilitation officer (DRO), who can provide information about retraining schemes and sheltered workshops. However, many people are able to use their own initiative and find productive employment themselves.

Evaluation

EXPECTED OUTCOMES

1. The patient is able to achieve a sense of independence and self-fulfilment by undertaking a productive occupation.
2. The patient understands the immediate and potential use of equipment which is available to help him.

HELPING THE PATIENT WITH RECREATIONAL ACTIVITIES

NURSING OBJECTIVES

1. Encourage the patient to participate in some activity which will provide enjoyment, without necessarily yielding an end product.
2. Provide the necessary equipment or environment for this activity.

Assessment

1. Physical disability, blindness, deafness, lack of mobility.
2. Lack of facilities, lack of social contacts.
3. Psychological problems, depression, apathy.

Planning

1. Arrange for up-to-date information about recreational and sports facilities in the locality, as well as any clubs within the hospital itself.
2. Arrange with the occupational therapist to obtain special equipment or furniture which could help the patient.
3. Encourage social contacts.

Implementation

1. Identify the type of recreational activity which will give most enjoyment to the patient. The nurse may wish to persuade the patient to undertake some activity which she thinks will be beneficial, but this may be quite against the inclinations of the patient. For instance, Bingo sessions may be considered an ideal recreational activity by some people, and fill others with horror.
2. If physical recreation is needed, there are several possibilities. Many sports centres have a special time set aside for handicapped people so that help can be given with transporting them to the centre and helping with the special sport. This may include swimming or the use of the gymnasium for various ball games. There are 450 branches of Riding for the Disabled, and special archery groups. There is the possibility of competitive sport.
3. Libraries are available (either public ones or Red Cross libraries) which may provide mobile facilities.

4. Further study may be a form of recreation. The Open University provides many courses and excellent tutorial contacts for those people who cannot attend the normal tutorial sessions, and may require special help, e.g. with writing down the assignments.
5. Social clubs of all kinds are available. It is often possible for the patient to join a club which provides a specialist interest, e.g. music societies, archaeological societies, chess clubs. Most of these are only too willing to provide help with transport to club meetings.
6. If the patient is housebound, a visiting occupational therapist may help to provide materials for recreational activities. Amateur radio may enable a disabled person to literally keep in contact with the rest of the world.

Evaluation

EXPECTED OUTCOMES

1. The patient is able to enjoy mental and physical activities which will not only prevent boredom, but give satisfaction and relieve stress. Gooch (1984) states:

> The anxiety of how to fill the time when one is denied the normal work or leisure activities can be very real. Boredom and frustration result in greater problems. . . . A day room with books, games and television can provide diversion for a short stay, but more needs to be done for the long-stay patients.

HELPING THE PATIENT TO LEARN

NURSING OBJECTIVES

1. Enable the patient to learn the best way of coping with his problem.
2. Enable the patient to be aware of the medical background of his problem, as far as possible, and to encourage him to ask questions about available treatments or future plans.
3. Teach the patient any necessary modifications of his former lifestyle which may be needed. This topic is covered in Chapter 1, 'Patient Education and the Nursing Process' (page 5).

HELPING THE PATIENT TO REST AND SLEEP

NURSING OBJECTIVES

1. Identify and overcome particular problems which are preventing rest and sleep.
2. Enable the patient to establish a routine which will allow time for mental and physical relaxation as well as actual sleeping time.
3. Substitute physiological methods and habits for drug use.
4. Promote a positive attitude to relaxation.

Assessment

1. Fear of a strange environment and apprehension regarding the future.
2. Noisy surroundings and too many lights.
3. Uncomfortable bed (too hard or soft), heavy or tight bedclothes.
4. Inability to attain usual posture for sleeping.
5. Pain.
6. Insufficient exercise or stimulation during the day, or frequent 'naps'.
7. Frequency of micturition or fear of incontinence.

Planning

1. Plan a suitable environment for the patient.
2. Arrange for a programme during the day which will allow time for rest, but also some stimulating activity.
3. Plan for the administration of any diuretic drugs early in the day, whenever possible.
4. Review the use of night sedation.

Implementation

1. Establish a good nurse–patient relationship. This will encourage the patient to express his anxieties and fears, and enable the nurse to give full explanations of procedures and plans of care, both immediate and in the future. Encourage the patient to make suggestions for his future rehabilitation.
2. Provide an environment which will prove interesting for the patient. Do not assume that the best means of achieving this is for the patient to watch the television all day. Mental and physical activity should be encouraged. The occupational therapist may be able to help by providing equipment.
3. Pain must be relieved by the appropriate means

for the individual patient. Fear and anxiety increase pain, and should be eliminated. Analgesic drugs should be available for patients who will obviously need them, e.g. postoperatively. Patients with a terminal illness must have a realistic regimen provided, which is constantly being reassessed, so that pain is prevented rather than being allowed to cause distress. Specialist advice in conjunction with the pain clinic must be available (see Chapter 18, Care of the Patient with Cancer).
4. Arrange for individualized patient care, so that treatments, procedures and observations can be carried out at one time, as far as possible, allowing for an uninterrupted rest time, for instance, after lunch.
5. During rest and sleeping times, ensure quietness, dimmed lights, adequate warmth and ventilation. Obtain the co-operation of all the staff.
6. Check that discomfort is not caused by full bladder or bowels, and that an anxious patient is able to call for help or independently get to the toilet easily.
7. Give encouragement to the patient about the progress made during the day to induce a relaxed frame of mind.
8. For anxious, very ill patients or children, the presence of a nurse or relative sitting near them will provide a feeling of confidence and companionship which is conducive to relaxation.
9. Discuss with the patient their previous sleeping habits, and try to provide a plan of care which coincides as far as possible with this.

Evaluation

EXPECTED OUTCOMES

The patient will be able to:
1. Relax, physically and mentally.
2. Attain a comfortable position in bed.
3. Have uninterrupted sleep for a satisfying length of time.
4. Decrease the amount of sedative drugs needed.

HELPING THE PATIENT TO MAINTAIN BODY TEMPERATURE WITHIN NORMAL LIMITS

NURSING OBJECTIVES

1. Provide an environment with a stable temperature and satisfactory humidity.

2. Provide specialized nursing intervention for those patients in whom the physiological control of body temperature has been affected, causing either hypo- or hyperthermia.

Assessment

1. Decreased homeostatic mechanisms due to ageing process or pathological conditions.
2. Inability to maintain a suitable environment, e.g. lack of heating due to breakdown of appliances, poor financial means, difficulty of control of appliance.
3. Unsuitable clothes, possibly due to lack of money.
4. Inability to have hot meals due to lack of interest in food, difficulty in handling cooking utensils, badly designed or positioned equipment.

Planning

1. Arrange for medical aid in the diagnosis and treatment of pathological conditions.
2. Plan for home assessment visits as appropriate.
3. Provide liaison with other hospital, community and social services staff.

Implementation

1. Ensure a constant temperature within the whole area in which the patient will be moving around. This includes bathrooms and sleeping area as well as the day room. It is important to consider the provision of adequate heating in the home well before the time of transfer of the patient to his home. This is particularly important in very vulnerable patients, e.g. very young or old, or those with limited mobility. The constant temperature should be maintained throughout the whole 24-hour span.
2. Regularly record temperature levels of those patients who are at risk of developing a pyrexia, e.g. those with a metabolic disturbance, such as hypo- or hyperthyroidism, or cerebral lesions.
3. Close observation is needed for a patient suffering from a rigor: light but warm coverings during the shivering stage; the provision of a fan during the hot stage; and tepid sponging of the skin to allow reduction of temperature by evaporation.
4. Provide clothing of suitable material. Cotton is the most comfortable material for those with a raised temperature. Several layers of light, non-constricting wool material are most suitable for those who need warmth.
5. Increased fluid intake is essential for a patient with pyrexia.
6. Hot drinks and food with a sufficient energy

content are necessary for those with a temperature below normal. Remember, a sudden rise in temperature or a drop to a subnormal level may indicate a deterioration in the condition of the patient and should be reported to the doctor.

Evaluation
EXPECTED OUTCOMES

1. The patient regains a temperature within normal limits.
2. The patient has received any practical or financial help which is needed, and is confident in his ability to maintain a suitable environment, as independently as possible.

FURTHER READING

BOOKS

Adams, A. *et al.* (1980) *Assessing Vital Functions Accurately*, Nursing Skillbooks, Intermed Communications, Pennsylvania.

Altschul, A. (1972) *Patient–Nurse Interaction*, Churchill Livingstone, Edinburgh.

Brechin, A., Liddiard, P. and Swain, J. (1980) *Handicap in a Social World*, Open University, Milton Keynes.

Campbell, A.V. (1975) *Moral Dilemmas in Nursing*, Churchill Livingstone, Edinburgh.

Darnborough, A. and Kinrade, J. (1986) *Directory of Aids for Disabled and Elderly People*, Woodhead-Faulkner, Cambridge.

Dartington, T., Miller, E. and Gwynne, G. (1981) *A Life Together. The Distribution of Attitudes around the Disabled*, Tavistock Publications, London.

Downie, P.A. and Kennedy, P. (1981) *Lifting, Handling and Helping Patients*, Faber, London.

Downie, R.S. and Telfer, E. (1980) *Caring and Curing*, Methuen, London.

Glover, J. (1985) *Human Sexuality in Nursing Care*, Croom Helm, Beckenham.

Gooch, J. (1984) *The Other Side of Surgery*, Macmillan Press, London.

Greenwood, J. (1984) *Coping with Sexual Relationships*, McDonald, Edinburgh.

Matheney, R.V. (1972) *Fundamentals of Patient-Centred Nursing*, C.V. Mosby, St Louis.

Meredith Davies, B. (1982) *The Disabled Child and Adult*, Baillière Tindall, London.

Roper, N., Logan, W.W. and Tierney, A.J. (1985) *The*

Elements of Nursing (2nd edn), Churchill Livingstone, Edinburgh.

Shopland, A. *et al.* (1979) *Refer to Occupational Therapy*, Churchill Livingstone, Edinburgh.

Tarling, C. (1980) *Hoists and Their Uses*, Heinemann Medical, London.

ARTICLES

General

Devlin, R. (1985) Disability – Coping in the kitchen, *Community Outlook*, March, pp. 11–14.

Gould, D. (1985) Measuring recovery, *Nursing Mirror*, 27 March, Vol. 160, No. 13, pp. 17–18.

Huddleston, J. (1986) First the mind and then the body, *Geriatric Nursing*, July–Aug, Vol. 6, No. 4, pp. 14–15.

Price, B. (1986) Giving the patient control; a model of rehabilitation, *Nursing Times*, 14 May, Vol. 82, No. 20, pp. 28–31.

Rankin Box, D.F. (1986) Comfort, *Nursing*, Series 3, No. 8, pp. 340–2.

Feeding

Lask, S. (1986) The nurses' role in nutrition education, *Nursing*, Vol. 3, No. 7, pp. 296–300.

Wilson, M. (1986) Eating and drinking, *Nursing*, Vol. 3, No. 7, pp. 265–7.

Yates, E.J. and Whitehead, G. (1986) Aids to feeding, *Nursing*, Vol. 3, No. 7, pp. 244–8.

Pressure area care

Anthony, D. and Bannes, E. (1985) Measure pressure sores accurately, *Nursing Times*, 5 September, Vol. 80, No. 36, pp. 33–5.

DHSS (1979) The prevention of pressure sores, Proceedings of the conference at the Nursing Practice Research Unit.

Johnson, A. (1984) Towards rapid healing, *Nursing Times*, 24 November, Vol. 80, No. 48, pp. 39–43.

Jones, J. (1986) An investigation into the diagnostic skills of nurses in an acute medical unit, relating to the identification of risk of pressure sore development in patients, *Nursing Practice*, Vol. 1, pp. 257–67.

Mitchell, A. (1985) Pressure sores. Healing through teamwork, *Nursing Times*, 29 May, Vol. 81, No. 22, pp. 53–7.

Pritchard, V. (1986) Calculating the risk, *Nursing Times Supplement*, 19 February, pp. 59–61.

Torrance, C. (1981) Pressure sores: Pathogenesis, prophylaxis and treatment, *Nursing Times Supplement*, 8 April, pp. 13–16.

— (1984) Pressure sore fact sheet, *Community Outlook*, 12 December, pp. 442–3.

Versluysen, M. (1986) Pressure sores, prevention and treatment, *Nursing*, June, Vol. 3, No. 6, pp. 216–18.

Viner, C. (1986) Floating on a bed of beads, *Nursing Times Supplement*, 19 February, pp. 62–6.

Incontinence

Blannin, J. (1986) Incontinence and the individual, *Nursing*, Series 3, October, pp. 1–2.

Jones, V. (1986) The continence advisor, a key role in the team, *Nursing*, Series 3, October, pp. 8–9.

Sleep

Canavan, T. (1986) The functions of sleep, *Nursing*, Vol. 3, No. 9, pp. 333–4.

Carter, D. (1985) Sleepless nights – In need of a good night's sleep. Hospital patients, *Nursing Times*, 13 November, Vol. 18, No. 46, pp. 24–6.

Hanning, C.D. (1986) Sleep and breathing: 'To sleep perchance to breathe', *Intensive Care Nursing*, Vol. 2, No. 1, pp. 8–15.

Jahanshahi, M. (1986) Insomnia, *Nursing*, Vol. 3, No. 9, pp. 328–32.

3

Care of the Surgical Patient

CONCEPT OF THE PATIENT UNDERGOING SURGERY

For the patient undergoing surgery, the total experience (perioperative nursing care) can be divided into three phases:

1. Preoperative phase – from the time the decision is made for surgical intervention to the transferen of the patient to the operating room.
2. Intraoperative phase – from the time the patient received in the operating room until he is admited to the recovery room.
3. Postoperative phase – from the time of admissio to the recovery room to the follow-up clinic an evaluation.

Examples of nursing intervention during thes phases are presented in Table 3.1.

Table 3.1   Examples of nursing interventions

Preoperative phase	Intraoperative phase	Postoperative phase

Preoperative assessment
Home/clinic
1. Initiates initial preoperative assessment
2. Plans teaching methods appropriate to patient's needs
3. Involves family in interview if possible
 	
Surgical unit
1. Completes preoperative assessment
2. Co-ordinates patient teaching with other nursing staff
3. Explains phases in operative period and expectations
4. Develops a plan of care
 	
Anaesthetic room
1. Assesses patient's level of consciousness
2. Reviews chart
3. Identifies patient
4. Verifies surgical site
 	
Planning
1. Determines a plan of care
 	
Psychological support
1. Tells patient what is happening
2. Determines psychological status
3. Gives prior warning of noxious stimuli
4. Stands near/touches patient during procedures/induction
5. Communicates patient's emotional status to other appropriate members of the health care team
	Maintenance of safety
	1. Assures that the sponge, needle and instrument counts are correct
	2. Positions the patient
	  a. Functional alignment
	  b. Exposure of surgical site
	  c. Maintenance of position throughout procedure
	3. Provides physical support
	
	Physiological monitoring
	1. Calculates effects on patient of excessive fluid loss
	2. Distinguishes normal from abnormal cardiopulmonary data
	3. Reports changes in patient's pulse, respirations, temperature, and blood pressure
	
	Psychological monitoring (prior to induction and if patient conscious)
	1. Provides emotional support to patient
	2. Continues to assess patient's emotional status
	3. Communicates patient's emotional status to other appropriate members of the health care team
	
	Nursing management
	1. Provides physical safety for the patient
	2. Maintains aseptic, controlled environment
	3. Effectively manages human resources
		Communication of intraoperative information
		1. Gives patient's name
		2. States type of surgery performed
		3. Provides contributing intraoperative factors, i.e. drain, catheters
		4. States physical limitations
		5. States impairments resulting from surgery
		6. Reports patient's preoperative level of consciousness
		7. Communicates necessary equipment needs
		
		Postoperative evaluation
		Recovery area
		1. Determines patient's immediate response to surgical intervention
		
		Surgical unit
		1. Evaluates effectiveness of nursing care in the operating room
		2. Determines patient's level of satisfaction with care given during operative period
		3. Evaluates products used on patient in the operating room
		4. Determines patient's psychological status
		5. Assists with discharge planning
		
		Home/clinic
		1. Seeks patient's perception of surgery in terms of the effects of anaesthetic agents. Impact on body image, distortion, immobilization
		2. Determines family's perceptions of surgery

(Source: Operating room nursing: perioperative role. AORN J (1978) May; Vol. 27; reprinted with permission.)

NURSING PROCESS OVERVIEW IN THE PREOPERATIVE PERIOD

Preoperative assessment

NURSING HISTORY, PHYSICAL EXAMINATION AND DIAGNOSTIC DETERMINATIONS

1. Engage the patient in conversation to determine his reaction to and concerns about hospitalization and the forthcoming operation.
2. Take a nursing history (see Chapter 1).
3. Assess nutritional status.
4. Prepare the patient for various diagnostic tests by explaining why and how they are done and how the patient may contribute to the success of the test. Record reactions to tests, as well as the outcome of such tests. (Diagnostic studies are specific for each patient and are presented in detail in each condition discussed in following chapters.)
5. Ascertain risk factors and develop individualized preventive strategies (see p. 49).
6. Determine the patient's level of understanding of his condition; develop a plan for preoperative patient education (see right-hand column).

PATIENT PROBLEMS

1. Knowledge deficit: inadequate or insufficient information about the operation.
2. Fear, worry and depression related to the diagnosis, to the outcome of surgery and to risk factors and postoperative pain.
3. Disturbance in self-concept (body image and role performance) related to surgery and postoperative care.
4. Possible risk factors related to lifestyle and health status.

Planning and implementation

NURSING INTERVENTIONS

1. Assist the patient in understanding the physical and psychosocial aspects of the surgery he is about to undergo.
2. Acquaint the patient and his family with the environment, protocols and expectations as surgery is anticipated.
3. Teach the patient certain procedures that will help in reducing postoperative complications and in increasing comfort and enhancing recovery.
4. Prepare the patient physically and psychologically for the anaesthetic and operative procedure.

5. Collaborate with other members of the health team in co-ordinating all preoperative preparations.

Evaluation

EXPECTED OUTCOMES

1. Approaches planned surgery with a positive attitude.
2. Demonstrates and explains the major postoperative activities he will be required to perform.
3. Reduces potential risks to acceptable levels.
4. Co-operates during immediate presurgical preparation and tells why he is receiving presurgical medication.

PREOPERATIVE PATIENT EDUCATION

Preoperative patient education is the giving of information to the patient who is scheduled to have an operation; such instruction may be offered through conversation, discussion, the use of audiovisual aids, and demonstrations. It is designed to help the patient understand what he is about to experience so that he can participate intelligently and recover more effectively from surgery and anaesthesia.

Note: Parts of this programme may be initiated before hospitalization.

PATIENT EDUCATION

This may include the family or significant others.

Obtain information and plan care

1. Determine what the patient already knows and what he wishes to know. This can be accomplished by reading the patient's chart, by interviewing the patient and by communicating with his surgeon, family and other members of the health team.
2. Plan this presentation or series of presentations for this individual patient or a group of patients.
3. Encourage active participation of patients in their care and recovery.
4. Demonstrate essential techniques; provide opportunity for patient practice and return demonstration.
5. Provide time for and encourage patient to ask questions and express his concerns; make every effort to answer all queries truthfully and in basic agreement with the overall therapeutic plan.

Constantly assess needs of patient as teaching progresses

1. Begin at the patient's level of understanding and proceed from there.
2. Correct misinformation – provide opportunity for him to express himself.
3. Provide general information and be alert for patient needs as intercommunication takes place. Assess his ability to absorb, his curiosity or lack of it:
   a. Explain details of preoperative preparation.
   b. Offer general information on his specific surgery. (Surgeon is the resource person.)
   c. Tell when surgery is scheduled (if known) and how long it will take; explain that afterwards he will go to the recovery room.
   d. Let him know that his family will be kept informed and that they will be told where to wait and when they can see him; note visiting hours.
   e. Explain to him how a procedure or test may *feel* during or after.
   f. Describe the recovery room; what personnel and equipment the patient may expect to see and hear (specially trained personnel, monitoring equipment, tubing for various functions and a moderate amount of activity by nurses and surgeons).
   g. Explain the importance of his participation in his postoperative recovery. Tell him you will demonstrate to him some of the activities he will be doing postoperatively.
   h. Utilize other resource persons: surgeons, therapists, chaplain, interpreters and so on.
   i. Document in outline form what has been taught, as well as the patient's reaction and level of understanding.

NURSING ALERT
Touch is a useful action in preoperative teaching of patients that appears to reduce anxiety significantly.

Use audiovisual aids if available

1. Videotapes with sound or film strips with narration are effective in giving basic information to a single patient or group of patients.
2. Booklets, brochures and models, if available, are helpful.
3. Demonstrate any equipment that will be specific for the particular patient. For example: drainage equipment; side rails; ostomy bag; monitoring equipment.

NURSING ALERT
The extent of preoperative patient teaching is determined on an individual basis; determinants are the patient's previous knowledge, his desire to learn and willingness to use this new knowledge, his psychoemotional and physical condition, the amount of time available and the quality of teaching. Effectiveness is greater when time is provided for patient participation and discussion.

PREOPERATIVE PRACTICE OF POSTOPERATIVE ACTIVITIES

Activities that the patient will practice and do postoperatively include the following.

Diaphragmatic breathing

This is a mode of breathing in which the dome of the diaphragm is flattened during inspiration, resulting in enlargement of the upper abdomen as air rushes into the chest. During expiration, abdominal muscles and the diaphragm relax (also see p. 115).

For the patient:

1. Assume bed position similar to that most likely to be used postoperatively (upright).
2. Place both hands over lower rib cage; make a loose fist and rest the flat surface of the fingernails against the chest (to feel chest movement).
3. Exhale gently and fully; ribs will sink downward and inward toward midline.
4. Inhale deeply through mouth and nose; permit abdomen to rise as lungs fill with air.
5. Hold this breath for a count of 5.
6. Exhale and let *all* air out through mouth and nose.
7. Repeat 15 times with a brief rest following each group of five.
8. Practice this twice each day preoperatively.

Spirometry

Preoperatively, the patient may be asked to use a spirometer to measure his deep breaths (inspired air) while exerting his maximum effort.

The preoperative measurement becomes the goal to be achieved as soon as possible after the operation.

1. Postoperatively, the patient is encouraged to use the spirometer frequently depending on condition.
2. Deep inhalations expand alveoli, which, in turn, prevents atelectasis and other pulmonary complications.
3. There is less pain with inspiratory concentration than with expiratory concentration, such as with coughing.

Coughing
Coughing promotes the removal of chest secretions.
1. Interlace the fingers and place the hands over the proposed incision site; this will act as a splint during coughing and not harm the incision.
2. Lean forward slightly while sitting in bed.
3. Breathe, using the diaphragm as described under diaphragmatic breathing.
4. Inhale fully with the mouth slightly open.
5. Let out three or four sharp 'hacks'.
6. Then, with mouth open, take in a deep breath and quickly give one or two strong coughs.
7. Secretions should be readily cleared from the chest to prevent respiratory complications (pneumonia, obstruction, etc.).

Turning
Changing positions from the patient's back to side-lying (and vice versa) stimulates circulation, encourages deeper breathing and relieves pressure areas.
1. Assist the patient to move onto his side if he is unable to do this himself.
2. Place the uppermost leg in a more flexed position than that of the lower leg and place a pillow comfortably between the legs.
3. Ensure that the patient is turned from one side to his back and onto the other side every two hours.

Foot and leg exercises
Moving the legs improves circulation and muscle tone.
1. Ask the patient to lie on his back; instruct him to bend the knee and raise the foot – hold it for a few seconds, extend the leg, and lower it to the bed.
2. Repeat the above for about five times with one leg and then with the other. Repeat the procedure five times every three to five hours.
3. Then ask the patient to lie on his side; exercise the legs by pretending to pedal a bicycle.
4. Suggest the following foot exercise: trace a complete circle with the big toe.

INFORMED CONSENT

A consent form is signed by the patient, granting permission to have the operation performed as described by the surgeon. This is a medico-legal requirement and the patient's signature must be witnessed by the appropriate doctor.

PURPOSES
1. Ensure that the patient understands the nature of the treatment, including potential complications.
2. Indicate that the patient's decision was made without pressure.
3. Protect the patient against unauthorized procedures.
4. Protect the surgeon and hospital against legal action by a patient who claims that an unauthorized procedure was performed.

Before signing a consent form, the patient should:
1. Be told in clear and simple terms by the surgeon what is to be done (drawings or audiovisual aids may help).
2. Be aware of the risks, possible complications, disfigurement and removal of parts.
3. Have a general idea of what to expect in the early and late postoperative periods.
4. Have a general idea of the time involved from surgery to recovery.
5. Have an opportunity to ask any questions.
6. Sign a separate form for each operation.

CONSENT AND THE ADOLESCENT PATIENT
In Great Britain 16 years is taken as the age of consent.

CIRCUMSTANCES REQUIRING CONSENT
1. Any surgical procedure where scalpel, scissors, suture or electrocoagulation may be used.
2. Entrance into a body cavity – paracentesis, bronchoscopy, cystoscopy.
3. General anaesthesia, local infiltration and regional block (e.g. for reduction of a fracture).

OBTAINING CONSENT
1. *Written* permission is best and is legally acceptable.
2. The patient's signature is obtained with his complete understanding of what is to occur; it is obtained before he receives sedation and is secured without pressure or duress.
3. The form is witnessed by the appropriate doctor. It is the doctor's ultimate responsibility.
4. If no parent or guardian is available, the duty administrator may be authorized to give the consent.
5. For female sterilization, the consent of the husband is preferable but not essential.
6. For a minor (or a patient who is unconscious or irresponsible), permission is required from a responsible member of the family – parent or legal guardian.
7. For a married minor, permission from the husband or wife is acceptable.

8. If the patient is unable to write, an 'X' to indicate his sign is acceptable if there are two signed witnesses to his mark.

TYPES OF SURGERY AND SURGICAL INCISIONS

Types of surgery
1. Optional: surgery is scheduled completely at the preference of the patient (e.g. cosmetic surgery).
2. Elective: the approximate time for surgery is at the convenience of the patient; failure to have surgery is not catastrophic (e.g. superficial cyst).
3. Required: the condition requires surgery within a few weeks (e.g. eye cataract).
4. Urgent: surgical problem requires attention within 24 to 48 hours (e.g. cancer).
5. Emergency: requires immediate surgical attention without delay (e.g. intestinal obstruction).
6. Day surgery (see next section).

Regions and incisions of the abdomen
These are shown in Figure 3.1.

DAY SURGERY (AMBULATORY)

Day surgery, in-and-out surgery and outpatient surgery are not new ideas but are becoming more prevalent. The nurse is in a key role to assess patient status, plan operative care, monitor, instruct and evaluate the patient.

ADVANTAGES
1. Reduces the time spent in hospital for the patient and this also reduces the cost to the hospital.
2. Reduced psychological stress to the patient.
3. Less evidence of hospital-acquired infection.
4. Less time lost from work by patient; minimal disruption of patient's activities and family life.

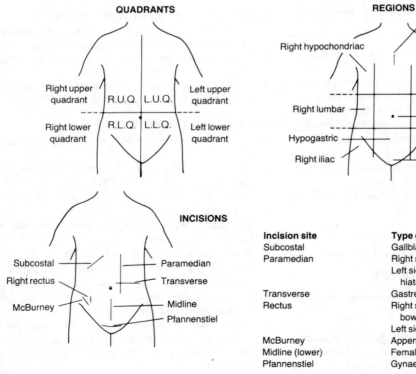

Incision site	Type of surgery
Subcostal	Gallbladder and biliary tract surgery
Paramedian	Right side – biliary tract, gallbladder
	Left side – splenectomy, gastrectomy, hiatal hernia repair
Transverse	Gastrectomy
Rectus	Right side – appendicectomy, small bowel resection
	Left side – sigmoid colon resection
McBurney	Appendicectomy
Midline (lower)	Female reproductive tract
Pfannenstiel	Gynaecological surgery

Figure 3.1. Regions and incisions of the abdomen

DISADVANTAGES

1. Less time to assess and evaluate patient.
2. Less time to establish rapport between patient and health personnel.
3. No opportunity to assess for late postoperative complications (this is in the hands of the patient and lay individuals).

PATIENT SELECTION

Criteria for selection include:

1. Surgery of short duration (15 to 90 minutes).
2. Noninfected conditions.
3. Type of operation in which postoperative complications are predictably low.
4. Age is usually not a factor, although too risky in a premature infant.
5. Patient should be willing and have a positive outlook (someone frightened or unwilling to have the surgery is a poor risk).
6. Types of frequently performed procedures include:
    a. Dilatation and curettage;
    b. Tubal ligation;
    c. Myringotomy;
    d. Excision of skin lesions;
    e. Oral surgery (tonsillectomy and adenoidectomy);
    f. Dental surgery;
    g. Cystoscopy;
    h. Diagnostic laparoscopy;
    i. Vasectomy.

NURSING MANAGEMENT

Initial assessment

1. Develop a nursing history for the day surgical patient.
2. Ensure consent form has been signed and witnessed by the appropriate doctor.
3. Explain what laboratory studies are needed and why.
4. Determine patient's physical and psychological status during initial assessment: Calm or agitated? Overweight? Disabilities or limitations? Clean or dirty? Allergies? Medications being taken? Condition of teeth (dentures, caps, crowns)? Blood pressure problems? Major illnesses? Other surgeries? Seizures? Severe headaches?
5. Begin patient education. Instructions to patient:
    a. Notify surgical unit immediately if you get a cold, have a fever or have any illness before date of surgery.
    b. Arrive at specified time.
    c. No food or fluid since midnight before the day of surgery.

d. No make-up or nail polish.
e. Comfortable, loose clothing; low-heeled shoes.
f. No valuables or jewellery.
g. Brush teeth in morning, rinse, but do not swallow liquid.
h. Have a responsible adult accompany you and drive you home – have person stay with you for 24 hours after surgery.

Preoperative preparation

1. Take baseline records of temperature, pulse, respiration and blood pressure.
2. Ask patient to provide a urine specimen and perform routine analysis.
3. Administer preanaesthetic medication; check vital signs.
4. Escort the patient to surgery after he has emptied his bladder.

Postoperative care

1. Check vital signs frequently until stable.
2. Administer oxygen if necessary; check temperature.
3. Change patient's position as he progresses in activity – head of bed elevated, ambulating with no dizziness or nausea.
4. Ascertain, using the following criteria, that the patient has recovered adequately to be discharged:
    a. Vital signs stable.
    b. Stands without dizziness and nausea; begins to walk.
    c. Comfortable and free of excessive pain.
    d. Able to void urine.
    e. Oriented as to time, place, person.
    f. Understands postoperative instructions and takes instruction sheet home.

SURGICAL RISK FACTORS AND PREVENTIVE STRATEGIES

Obesity

1. Danger:
    a. Increases difficulty involved in technical aspects of performing surgery (e.g. sutures are difficult to tie because of fatty secretions); incidence of burst abdomen is greater.

b. Increases likelihood of infection because of lessened resistance.

c. Postoperatively, more difficult to turn and ventilate the patient when he is lying on his side. This leads to hypoventilation, pneumonia and other pulmonary problems.

d. Increases demands on the heart, leading to cardiovascular embarrassment.

e. Increases possibility of renal, biliary, hepatic and endocrine disorders.

2. Therapeutic approach: encourage weight reduction if time permits.

Fluid, electrolyte, and nutritional status

1. Danger: dehydration and malnutrition have adverse effects in terms of a general anaesthetic, the shock of surgery, and postoperative recovery – can disturb fluid and electrolyte balance and lead to shock.

2. Therapeutic approach:
   a. Administer fluids (parenteral) as prescribed.
   b. Keep a detailed input and output record.
   c. Provide high-calorie diet to alleviate malnutrition; supplement with protein and vitamin C – helps repair tissue and serves as a deterrent to infection.
   d. Recommend repair of dental caries and proper mouth hygiene to prevent respiratory tract infection.
   e. Assist with administration (and surveillance) of blood transfusion or protein hydrolysates if there is a protein deficiency.
   f. Assist with hyperalimentation.
   g. Monitor for evidence of electrolyte imbalance (Na^+, K^+, Ca^{++}, etc).

Ageing

1. Danger:
   a. Recognize that reactions to injury are not as obvious and are slower in appearing.
   b. Be aware that the cumulative effect of medications is greater in the older person than it is in younger people.
   c. Note that medications such as morphine and barbiturates in the usual dosages may cause confusion and disorientation; morphine may cause respiratory depression.

2. Therapeutic approach:
   a. Consider using lesser doses for desired effect.
   b. Anticipate problems from long-standing chronic disorders such as anaemia, obesity, diabetes, hypoproteinaemia.
   c. Adjust nutritional intake to conform to higher protein and vitamin needs.
   d. When possible, cater to set patterns in older

patients (sleeping and eating patterns, use of alcohol and laxatives).

Presence of disease

1. Cardiovascular:
   a. Increased diligence is required when surgical problem is complicated by a cardiovascular problem.
   b. Avoid overloading the body with fluids (oral, parenteral, blood) because of possible congestive failure and pulmonary oedema.
   c. Prevent prolonged immobilization, which results in stasis of circulating fluids.
   d. Encourage change of position but avoid sudden exertion.
   e. Note evidence of hypoxia and initiate therapy.

2. Diabetes:
   a. Be aware that hypoglycaemia due to inadequate carbohydrate intake or insulin overdosage is life-threatening in uncontrolled diabetes.
   b. Recognize the signs and symptoms of ketoacidosis and glycosuria (p. 562), which can threaten an otherwise smooth surgical experience.
   c. Reassure the diabetic patient that when his disease is controlled, the surgical risk may be no greater than it is for the nondiabetic person.

3. Alcoholism:
   a. Anticipate the additional problem of malnutrition in the presurgical alcoholic patient.
   b. Recognize that the acutely intoxicated person is susceptible to injury and may receive serious injuries without being aware of them.
   c. Be prepared to perform gastric washout on the intoxicated patient if surgery cannot be postponed; this may lessen the chance of vomiting and aspiration during anaesthesia induction.
   d. Note that risk due to surgery is greater for the individual who is a chronic alcoholic.
   e. Anticipate the acute withdrawal syndrome (delirium tremens).

4. Pulmonary and upper respiratory disease:
   a. Surgery may be contraindicated in the patient who has an upper respiratory infection because such an infection may be the forerunner of more serious illness, such as pneumonia.
   b. Patients with chronic pulmonary problems such as emphysema, bronchiectasis, etc. should be treated for several days preoperatively with bronchodilators, aerosol medications and conscientious mouth care, along with a reduction in weight and smoking, and methods to control secretions.

5. Concurrent or prior drug therapy:
   a. Hazards exist when certain medications are given concomitantly with others; therefore, an awareness of prior drug therapy is essential. (Example: interaction of some drugs with anaesthetics can lead to arterial hypotension and circulatory collapse.)
   b. The anaesthetist should be informed if the patient is taking any of the following drugs:
      (i) Certain antibiotics* – may, when combined with a curariform muscle relaxant, interrupt nerve transmission, causing respiratory paralysis and apnoea.
      (ii) Antidepressants, particularly monoamine oxidase inhibitors (MAOIs), increase hypotensive effects of anaesthesia.
      (iii) Phenothiazines increase hypotensive action of anaesthetics.
      (iv) Diuretics, particularly thiazides, cause electrolyte imbalance and respiratory depression during anaesthesia.
   This should be indicated in the nursing notes.

PREOPERATIVE PROPHYLAXIS TO PREVENT POSTOPERATIVE VENOUS THROMBOSIS

It is suggested that low-dose heparin be administered to all *haemostatically competent* patients over the age of 40 who are to undergo major elective abdominal or thoracic surgical procedures, as this will effect an 80 per cent reduction in postoperative pulmonary emboli.

PREOPERATIVE SCREENING
1. Administer no aspirin or other platelet anti-aggregating drugs for five days before an operation.
2. Note laboratory results for haematocrit, prothrombin time, partial thromplastin time and platelet count; these should be within normal ranges before operation.

*Neomycin, streptomycin, polymyxin A and B, colistin, viomycin, and kanamycin.

DOSE AND DURATION OF PROPHYLAXIS
1. Administer 5,000 international units (IUs) of heparin (subcutaneously) 2 hours before operation.
2. Repeat above dosage every 12 hours until discharge from hospital.

LIMITATIONS AND CONTRAINDICATIONS
1. Of limited value in:
   a. Repair of femoral fracture.
   b. Hip and knee joint reconstruction.
   c. Open prostatectomy.
2. Not recommended for operations:
   a. On the eye.
   b. On the brain.
   c. With spinal anaesthesia.
3. *The regimen is ineffective in patients with an active thrombotic process.*
4. This regimen is followed only at the discretion of the surgeon.

MONITORING HEPARIN THERAPY
1. Since low-dose heparin does not significantly prolong coagulation time, no laboratory test (whole blood clotting time, partial thromboplastin time, antithrombin III assay) is necessary during therapy.
2. With this regimen, there may be a *slight increase in minor wound haematoma*. Report this immediately.
3. Employ adjunctive measures – early ambulation, leg exercises and elastic stockings.
4. Avoid positioning of legs that could compromise venous return.

SKIN PREPARATION OF SPECIFIC OPERATIVE AREAS

PHYSIOLOGICAL EMPHASIS
1. Human skin normally harbours transient and resident bacterial flora, some of which are pathogenic.
2. Skin cannot be sterilized without destroying skin cells.
3. Friction enhances the action of detergent antiseptics.
4. No existing antiseptic produces instant skin disinfection.
5. Numerous studies indicate that shaving the skin may produce nicks and breaks in the skin, which, in turn, breaks down the skin barrier to infection. Many surgeons will indicate how they wish the skin to be prepared.

GUIDELINES: PREPARING THE PATIENT'S SKIN FOR SURGERY BY DEPILATION CREAM, e.g. SURGEX CREAM*

GOAL
To cleanse the skin and reduce the number of organisms on the skin to eliminate as far as possible the transference of such organisms into the incision site.

There are a number of creams on the market and the appropriate instructions should be followed. Guidelines given here are for Surgex Cream.

FOR SPECIFIC AREAS
This is shown in Figure 3.2.

EQUIPMENT
1 tube (100g) Surgex Cream with wooden spatula
1 foil basin
1 disposable glove
1 pair of blunt-ended scissors, if required (for long hair)
2 paper towels
1 polythene sheet
2 disposable flannels

PROCEDURE
Preparatory phase
1. Explain to the patient the purpose of the activity.
2. Instruct the patient to assume the most comfortable and satisfactory position for the required skin preparation.
3. Cover patient with a sheet and expose area to be depilated.
4. Place polythene sheet under area to be prepared.

NURSING ALERT
Patients with known allergies, red or fair hair and/or sensitive skin, should be 'patch' tested, using a small amount of cream applied to a limb for five minutes. If the patient complains of burning, irritation or blistering, wash cream off immediately. Avoid applying cream to open wounds, mucous membranes and eyes. Such areas must be occluded using dry gauze squares before application of the cream.

Performance phase

Nursing action	Rationale
1. If hair is long, clip hair using scissors.	Cream acts more quickly on short hair and is easier to apply.
2. Squeeze approximate amount of cream into foil basin (if whole tube is to be used, squeeze cream onto gloved hand).	One tube will depilate a whole limb.

---

* Surgex Cream is manufactured by Cooper Cosmetics, S.A. Switzerland.

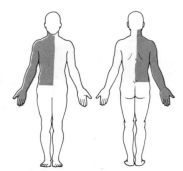

Shoulder prep. Prepare area from fingertips to hair line, midline chest to midline spine on operative side and to iliac crest, including axilla.

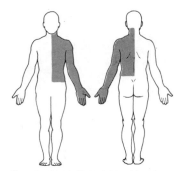

Upper arm prep. Prepare area from fingertips to neckline (hairline), on operative side from midline chest to midline spine on operative side from axilla to iliac crest. Trim and clean fingernails. Use brush on hand and nails.

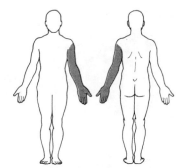

Hand prep. Prepare area from fingertips to shoulder. Trim and clean fingernails. Use brush on hand and nails.

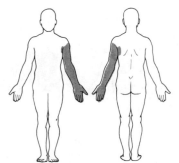

Forearm and elbow prep. Prepare area from fingernails to shoulder including axilla. Trim and clean fingernails. Use brush on hand and nails.

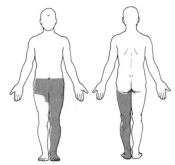

Saphenous vein ligation prep. Prepare area from umbilicus to toes of affected leg, or both legs. Include pubis and perineal area. Prepare entire leg posteriorly.

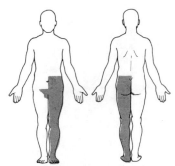

Thigh prep. Prepare area from toes to 7.5cm above the umbilicus, midline front and back. Complete pubic preparation. Clean and trim toenails. Use brush on foot and nails.

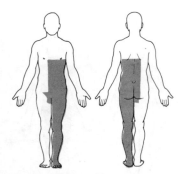

Hip prep. Prepare area from toes to nipple line and at least 7.5cm beyond midline back and front. Complete pubic preparation. Clean and trim toe nails. Use brush on foot and nails. Hip fractures – all preparations are made in the operating room.

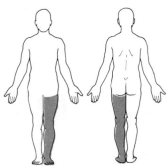

Knee and lower leg prep. Prepare entire leg, toes to groin. Clean and trim toenails. Use brush on foot and nails.

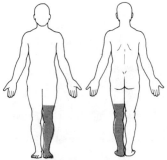

Ankle and foot prep. Prepare entire leg, toes to 7.5cm above the knee. Clean and trim toenails. Use brush on foot and nails.

Figure 3.2. Preparing the patient's skin for surgery (from Committee on Control of Surgical Infections of the Committee on Pre- and Postoperative Care (1977) *American College of Surgeons: Manual on Control of Infection in Surgical Patients*, J. B. Lippincott, Philadelphia)

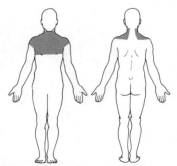

Thyroid prep. Prepare area from chin line to nipples including axillary region. Extend to back of neck and upper shoulder as sketched.

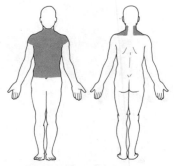

Parathyroid prep. Prepare area (as for sternal splitting) from chin line to umbilicus, shoulder to shoulder in the front. Extend to back of neck and upper shoulder in back as shown. Prepare laterally for chest tubes if so prescribed.

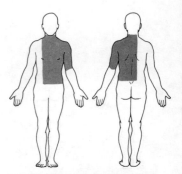

Thoractomy prep. Prepare area from chin line to iliac crest, from nipple on unaffected side to at least 5cm beyond the midline in back. Include axilla and entire arm to elbow.

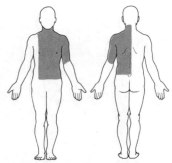

Mastectomy prep. Prepare area from upper neck to iliac crest, from nipple line on unaffected side to midline of back (affected side). Prepare axilla and entire arm to elbow on affected side.

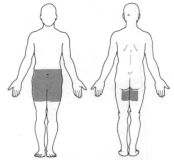

Lower abdominal prep (as for hernia, femoral vein ligation, femoral embolectomy). Prepare area from 5cm above the umbilicus to mid-thigh, including the pubic area. Femoral ligation – prepare area to midline of thigh posteriorly. Hernia and embolectomy – prepare skin to costal margin and down to knees as prescribed.

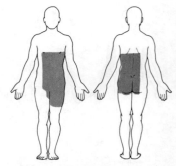

Flank prep (as for renal procedures, adrenalectomy, sympathectomy). Prepare area from nipple line to pubis and 7.5cm beyond the midline in back. Prepare pubic area. Prepare upper thigh on the affected side.

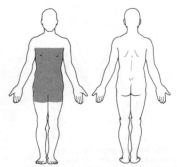

Abdominal prep. Prepare area from 7.5cm above the nipple line to upper thighs, including pubis.

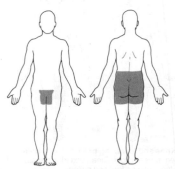

Perineal prep (as for haemorrhoidectomy, fistula-in-ano). Prepare pubis, perineum and perianal areas: Prepare area from the waist in back to at least 7.5cm below the groin.

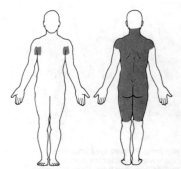

Spine prep. Prepare area of entire back, including shoulders and neck, to hair line and down to knees and to both sides, including axillae.

Figure 3.2. (cont.)

3. If whole leg is to be depilated, support heel on pillows.

Prevents back of leg touching sheet and cream being removed.

4. Leave for 10 to 20 minutes depending on area and amount of hair to be depilated.

Do not leave cream on until it is hard in an attempt to get a better depilation.

5. a. If patient confined to bed use wooden spatula to scrape off cream and hair onto towel. Wash depilated area.
   b. If patient ambulant, give patient disposable flannels and ask to shower using Hibiscrub to wash away cream and hair.

6. Check prepared area. Never shave off any remaining hair and cream. Patients who are particularly hairy may require two applications.

To ensure all hair is removed.

7. Patients may be depilated up to 48 hours prior to surgery using Surgex.

Follow-up phase
1. Remove all equipment and dispose of expendable materials according to local policy.
2. Remind the patient of the necessity for keeping the prepared area clean for surgery.

GUIDELINES: PREPARING THE PATIENT'S SKIN FOR SURGERY BY SHAVING

GOAL
To cleanse the skin and reduce the number of organisms on the skin to eliminate as far as possible the transference of such organisms into the incision site.

FOR SPECIFIC AREAS
See Figure 3.2. For head surgery, obtain specific instructions from the surgeon concerning the extent of shaving.

EQUIPMENT
Disposable tray
Gallipot
5 per cent soft soap solution
1 packet of cotton wool balls or gauze squares (10 × 10cm)
Disposable razor
Kleenex wipes
Bag for rubbish
1 pair of blunt-ended scissors, if required (for long hair)
Cotton-tipped applicators (cotton buds)
Absorbent pad (to protect bedding)

PROCEDURE

Preparatory phase

1. Explain to patient the purpose of the activity.
2. Instruct patient to assume the most comfortable and satisfactory position for the required skin preparation.
3. Cover patient with sheet and expose area to be shaved.
4. Place absorbent pad under area to be shaved.
5. The patient should be shaved as near to the time of operation as possible, at least within 12 hours of surgery. Note: communal electric razors should *not* be used.

Performance phase

Nursing action	**Rationale**
1. Cut long hairs with scissors, if necessary.	Much easier and quicker than with a razor.
2. Pour 5 per cent soft soap solution into gallipot and, using cotton wool balls and soap solution, lather the operation site. Begin at the incision site and, in a circular pattern, work outward from the centre.	Oils, soil and organisms are removed from skin surfaces. Working away from incision site prevents the clean area from becoming re-contaminated.
3. Provide extra attention to areas where there are folds of skin (e.g. axillae, pubic area, umbilicus). Use cotton tipped applicators, where necessary.	Greater numbers of organisms are harboured in folds of skin; removal requires extra effort.
4. Use a disposable or sterilized razor and a sharp new blade.	Avoids risk of infectious hepatitis from contaminated razor.
5. Draw loose skin taut. Shave with the direction of hair growth – not the opposite direction to hair growth. Use tissue to clean razor.	This leaves a blunt rather than a sharp hair stub, which could penetrate the wall of hair follicle and inject itself into the skin (risking postoperative pseudofolliculitis).
6. If the operative area includes calloused areas or the nails, use a soft bristled brush.	Facilitates cleansing.
7. Avoid nicking the skin; report any skin abrasions.	An opening in the skin increases the hazard of infection.
8. Gently dry the patient.	Prevents chapping.

NURSING ALERT

Pseudofolliculitis barbae is a papulopustular inflammation of hair follicles in areas that have been shaved so closely that the sharp-pointed tip may inject itself into the side of the hair follicle, carrying bacteria into the skin. It simulates folliculitis barbae, which develops in bearded areas. Note above items 5 and 6 to prevent this condition.

Follow-up phase

1. Remove all equipment and dispose of expendable materials according to local policy.

2. Remind the patient of the necessity for keeping the prepared area clean for surgery; ensure his comfort.

SHOWER/BATHING
1. Unless contraindicated, a shower or bath should be taken as near as possible to the time of the operation (i.e. after depilation or shaving).
2. When having a shower, patients may be asked by the surgeon to use Hibiscrub (4 per cent chlorhexidine). Again, special attention should be paid to axillae, umbilicus and perineal area.
3. When bathing, a 14ml sachet of Steribath (0.4 per cent iodine) may be added to the water. Check with the surgeon.
4. Patients who have been hospitalized for a long time undergoing neck, head and/or facial surgery should wash their hair using Hibiscrub, followed by a normal shampoo.

IMMEDIATE PRESURGICAL PREPARATION OF THE PATIENT

PHYSICAL AND PSYCHOLOGICAL ATTENTION TO THE PATIENT
1. Provide patient with a short gown to be worn to the operating room.
2. Remove hairpins; plait long hair; cover hair with a cap.
3. Remove dentures or plates and place in appropriate labelled container (unless anaesthetist requests that they be left in to reduce respiratory tract obstruction); inspect mouth for foreign material such as chewing gum.
4. Remove jewellery, identify properly and place in the hospital safe; if wedding ring cannot be removed, cover with non-allergic tape.
5. Remove contact lenses; ask the patient to place them in properly marked receptacle (left and right), identify properly and deposit in the hospital safe. Record presence of prosthesis if not removed, e.g. artificial eye.
6. Have the patient void urine before receiving preoperative medication and immediately before leaving for the operating room; measure amount and note time of voiding; document.
7. Continue to support the patient emotionally and correct any misconceptions he may have.
8. Permit the patient to relax as the medication becomes effective prior to his being called to the operating room; warn patient of effects, e.g. dry mouth; instruct the patient to call for assistance if necessary. Raise side rails if necessary.

PREANAESTHETIC MEDICATION
Prescribed to meet individual needs.

GOALS
1. Facilitate the administration of any anaesthetic.
2. Minimize respiratory tract secretions and changes in heart rate.
3. Relax the patient and reduce anxiety.

NURSING ALERT
Administer preanaesthetic medication precisely at the time it is prescribed. If given too early, the maximum potency will have passed before it is needed; if given too late, the action will not have begun before anaesthesia is started.

'On call' medications
1. Have medication ready and administer as soon as call is received.
2. Proceed with remaining preparation activities.
3. Indicate on the chart or preoperative checklist the time when medication was administered.

TRANSPORTING PATIENT TO THE OPERATING ROOM
1. Adhere to the principle of maintaining the comfort and safety of the patient.
2. Accompany circulating nurse to the patient's bedside for introduction and proper identification.

3. Assist in transferring the patient from bed to stretcher (unless the bed goes to the operating room).
4. Complete chart and preoperative check list; include laboratory reports and X-rays as required in the operating room.
5. Recognize importance of co-ordinating team effort to ensure arrival of the patient in the operating room at the proper time.

THE PATIENT'S FAMILY

1. Direct the patient's family to the proper waiting room where magazines, television and coffee may be available if required.
2. Acquaint the family with the fact that a long interval of waiting does not mean the patient is in the operating room all the while; anaesthesia preparation and induction take time, and after surgery the patient is taken to the recovery room.
3. Tell the family what to expect postoperatively when they see the patient – tubes, monitoring equipment and blood transfusions, suctioning and oxygen equipment.

THE NURSING PROCESS IN THE IMMEDIATE POSTOPERATIVE PERIOD

Assessment

IMMEDIATE NURSING ASSESSMENT

Upon receiving a patient in the recovery room from the anaesthetist and circulating nurse, the following determinations are made:

1. Appraise the air-exchange status of the patient and note his skin colour.
2. Verify the patient's identity, the operative procedure and the surgeon who performed the procedure.
3. Request a briefing on problems encountered in the operating room and those that may arise in the recovery period.
4. Determine vital signs and establish with the anaesthetist an agreement as to their meaning.
5. Examine the operative site and check dressings for drainage.
6. Perform safety checks to verify that padded side rails are in place and restraints properly applied for infusions, transfusions, etc.

PATIENT PROBLEMS

1. Possible ineffective airway clearance related to effects of general anaesthesia.
2. Possible fluid volume deficit related to blood loss, food and fluid deprivation, potential vomiting.
3. Alteration in sensory perception related to effects of medications and anaesthesia.
4. Alteration in comfort (pain) related to surgical incision and tissue trauma.
5. Impairment of skin integrity related to operative incision.
6. Alteration in nutrition related to reduced intake preoperatively and during day of surgery.
7. Potential for injury due to sensory deprivation as a result of preanaesthetic medications and anaesthesia.

Planning and implementation
NURSING INTERVENTIONS
Ensure the maintenance of a patent airway and adequate respiratory function

1. Place the patient in the lateral position with neck extended (if not contraindicated) – this permits the best possible expansion of the lungs.
2. Allow metal, rubber or plastic airway to remain in place until the patient begins to waken and is trying to eject the airway.
   a. The airway keeps the passage open and prevents the tongue from falling backward and obstructing the air passages.
   b. Leaving the airway in after the pharyngeal reflex has returned may cause the patient to choke and vomit.
   Note: Many seriously ill patients return from the operating room with a tracheal tube in place; this may be left in place for hours or days and requires special management.
3. When the patient is partially awake and the airway is removed, he may show signs of choking, nausea or vomiting; place him in the lateral position with the upper arm supported on a pillow.
   a. This will promote chest expansion.
   b. Turn the patient every hour or two to facilitate breathing and ventilation.
4. Aspirate excessive secretions when they are heard in the nasopharynx and oropharynx.
   a. Using a Y-connecting tube with catheter, turn suction machine on, wearing disposable gloves insert catheter into pharynx 15–20cm, then close Y-tube outlet with finger to activate suction; withdraw slowly while rotating catheter.
   b. If secretions are lower in the tracheobronchial tree, intratracheal suctioning may be necess-

ary. (See procedure for tracheal suctioning, p. 107.)

5. Encourage patient to take deep breaths to aerate lungs fully and prevent hypostatic pneumonia.
6. Administer humidified oxygen if required.
   a. Heat and moisture are normally lost during exhalation.
   b. Dehydrated patients may require oxygen and humidity because of higher incidence of irritated respiratory passages in these patients.
   c. Secretions can be kept soft to facilitate removal.
7. Employ mechanical ventilation to maintain adequate pulmonary ventilation if required (see p. 160).

Assess status of circulatory system

1. Take vital signs (blood pressure, pulse and respiration) frequently, as clinical condition indicates, until the patient is well stabilized. Then check every four hours thereafter.
   a. Know the patient's preoperative blood pressure in order to make significant comparisons.
   b. Report immediately a falling systolic pressure.
   c. Variations in blood pressure and cardiac dysrhythmias are reportable.
   d. Respirations over 30 should be reported.
   e. Evaluate pulse pressure to determine status of perfusion.
2. Recognize the variety of factors that may alter circulating blood volume.
   a. Reactions to anaesthesia and medications.
   b. Blood loss and organ manipulation during surgery.
   c. Moving the patient from one position on the operating table to another on the stretcher.
3. Monitor temperature hourly to be alert for hyperthermia and to detect hypothermia. A temperature over 37.7°C or under 36.1°C is reportable.
4. Be aware of early symptoms of shock or haemorrhage.
   a. Cool extremities, decreased urine output and narrowing of pulse pressure may be indicative of decreased cardiac output.
   b. Rapid, thready pulse and a falling blood pressure may indicate haemorrhage, leading to a decrease in blood volume.
   c. Initiate oxygen therapy to increase oxygen availability from the circulating blood.
   d. Place the patient in shock position with feet elevated (unless contraindicated).
   e. See page 63 for more detailed consideration of shock.

Promote comfort and maintain safety

1. Provide a therapeutic environment with proper temperature and humidity; remove unnecessary blanket, which might cause loss of body fluid through excessive perspiration; when cold, provide warm blankets.
2. Place side rails in protecting position until the patient is fully awake.
3. Protect the extremity into which intravenous fluids are running so that the needle will not become accidentally dislodged.
4. Turn the patient frequently and maintain good body alignment.
5. Avoid nerve damage and muscle strain by properly supporting and padding pressure areas.
6. Assess pain by observing behavioural and physiological manifestations.
7. Administer analgesics (low blood pressure may be a result of pain).

Continue constant surveillance of the patient until he is completely out of the anaesthestic

NURSING ALERT

This phase of nursing care is geared to recognizing the significance of signs and anticipating and preventing postoperative difficulties.

Carefully monitor the patient coming out of general anaesthesia until:

1. *Vital signs are stable for at least 30 minutes and are within his normal range.*
2. *He is breathing easily.*
3. *Reflexes have returned to normal.*
4. *He is out of anaesthesia, responsive and oriented to time and place.*

For the patient who had regional anaesthesia, observe carefully until:

1. *Sensation has been recovered.*
2. *Reflexes have returned.*
3. *Vital signs have stabilized for at least 30 minutes.*

1. Be aware of the fact that the patient cannot complain of injury such as the pricking of an open safety pin or a clamp that is exerting pressure.
2. Examine dressings for unexpected drainage or bleeding.
3. Check dressings for constriction.
4. Observe drainage tubes and catheters for proper connection and patency.
5. Note proper functioning of monitoring and suctioning devices, oxygen therapy equipment, etc.
6. Observe the patient for bladder distension.
7. Monitor infusion rate, amount and type of fluid.

8. Inspect skin and tissue surrounding intravenous needles to detect early infiltration.
9. Evaluate periodically the patient's status of orientation – how he responds to being addressed by his name or performs simple movements upon receiving a command.
   Note: Alterations in cerebral function may suggest impaired oxygen delivery to tissues.
10. Determine return of motor control following spinal anaesthesia – indicated by how the patient responds to a pinprick or a request to move a body part.

Recognize stress factors that may affect the patient in the recovery room and attempt to minimize them

1. Know that the ability to hear returns more quickly than other senses as the patient emerges from anaesthesia.
2. Avoid saying anything in the patient's presence that may disturb him; he may appear to be sleeping but still consciously hears what is being said.
3. Explain procedures and activities at the patient's level of understanding.
4. Minimize the patient's exposure to emergency treatment of nearby patients by drawing curtains and lowering voice and noise levels.
5. Treat the patient as a person who needs as much attention as the equipment and monitoring devices.
6. Respect his feeling of sensory deprivation and simultaneous bombardment of sensory stimuli; make any necessary adjustments to minimize this problem.
7. Make every effort to demonstrate concern for and understanding of this patient – anticipate his needs and feelings.
8. Tell the patient repeatedly that the surgery is over and that he is in the recovery room.

Transfer the patient from the recovery room to the ward

1. Relay appropriate information to the ward nurse regarding the patient's condition; point out significant needs (e.g. drainage, fluid therapy, incision and dressing requirements, intake needs, urinary output).
2. Assure the patient of his value as a person and reinforce his positive thoughts of recovering.

Evaluation
EXPECTED OUTCOMES
(Criteria for leaving recovery unit.)
1. Breathes easily.

2. Reaches stable vital signs and achieves adequate circulatory perfusion.
3. Responds well to commands when asked to cough, breathe deeply or move extremities.
4. Approaches a satisfactory level of awareness and consciousness.
5. Complains minimally of pain that is being controlled with increasingly less potent medications.
6. Maintains acceptable levels of urinary output (at least 30ml/h).
7. Appears to have vomiting well under control, if not absent.

POSTOPERATIVE DISCOMFORTS

Many patients experience some discomforts postoperatively. These are usually related to the general anaesthetic and/or the surgical procedure. The most common discomforts are nausea, vomiting, restlessness, sleeplessness, thirst, constipation and pain.

NAUSEA AND VOMITING

INCIDENCE
1. Occurs in many postoperative patients.
2. Results from an accumulation of fluid or food in the stomach before peristalsis returns.
3. May occur as a result of abdominal distension, which follows manipulation of abdominal organs.
4. Induced during anaesthesia from inadequate ventilation.
5. Likely to occur if the patient believes preoperatively that he will vomit (psychological induction).
6. May be a side effect of narcotics.

PREVENTIVE MEASURES
1. The surgeon will usually request that a nasogastric tube is inserted for operations on the gastrointestinal tract to prevent abdominal distension, which triggers vomiting (see Chapter 7).
2. Determine whether patient is sensitive to morphine and pethidine (Demerol), since they may induce vomiting in some patients.
3. Be alert for any significant comment such as, 'I just know I will vomit under anaesthesia'. Report such a comment to the anaesthetist, who may

prescribe an antiemetic drug and also talk to the patient before the operation.

NURSING INTERVENTIONS

1. Encourage patient to breathe deeply to facilitate elimination of anaesthetic.
2. Support the wound during retching and vomiting; turn head to side to avoid aspiration.
3. Discard vomit and refresh patient – mouthwash for mouth, clean linens for bed, etc.
4. Suspect idiosyncratic response to a drug if vomiting is worse when a medication is given (but diminishes thereafter).
5. Administer antiemetic medication such as prochlorperazine (Stemetil).
6. Offer hot tea with lemon or small sips of a carbonated beverage such as soda water, if tolerated.
7. Report excessive or prolonged vomiting so that the cause may be investigated.
8. Detect presence of abdominal distension, hiccoughs, suggesting gastric retention.
9. Suspect the possibility of paralytic ileus.

RESTLESSNESS AND SLEEPLESSNESS

See Table 3.2

THIRST

CAUSES

1. Inhibition of secretions by preoperative medication with atropine.
2. Fluid lost via perspiration, blood loss and dehydration due to preoperative fluid restriction.

NURSING INTERVENTIONS

1. Administer fluids by vein or by mouth if tolerated.
2. Offer sips of hot tea with lemon juice to dissolve mucus.
3. Apply a moistened gauze square over lips occasionally to humidify inspired air.
4. Allow the patient to rinse mouth with mouthwash; lemon juice and glycerin swabbing of the mouth is also refreshing.
5. Obtain hard sweets or chewing gum to help in stimulating saliva flow and in keeping the mouth moist.

CONSTIPATION

CAUSES

1. Trauma and irritation to the bowel during surgery.
2. Local inflammation, peritonitis or abscess.
3. Long-standing bowel problem: this may lead to faecal impaction.

Table 3.2 Combating restlessness and sleeplessness

Promoting factors	Relief measures
1. Discomfort such as back pain, headache and thirst	1. Massage the back gently. Administer acetylsalicylic acid as prescribed
2. Tight dressings or drainage-soaked dressings	2. Change dressings and check for tightness
3. Urinary retention	3. Use nursing measures to initiate micturition (see p. 15)
4. Abdominal distension	4. Ambulation; insert rectal tube to relieve flatus – stimulates peristalsis and propels gas to rectum
5. Noise and environmental stimuli	5. Keep noise level at a minimum. Limit visitors to those who may promote rest in the patient. For rest periods, provide privacy, darkness, and quiet. Schedule treatments with this in mind
6. Worry and anxiety	6. Attempt to find cause of concern. Provide time to talk with the patient and permit him to vent his feelings. Seek advice of spiritual counsellor or psychologist if necessary Offer sedatives or hypnotics as required/prescribed

PREVENTIVE MEASURES

1. Early ambulation to aid in promoting peristalsis.
2. Adequate fluid intake to keep stool soft and promote hydration.
3. Proper diet to promote peristalsis and maintain adequate fluid balance.
4. Query patient as to his usual remedy for constipation; try this.

TREATMENT OF FAECAL IMPACTION

(See also p. 499).
1. Insert a gloved finger and break up the impaction manually.
2. Administer an oil enema (180–200ml) to help soften the mass and facilitate evacuation.

PAIN

Pain is a subjective symptom in which the patient exhibits a feeling of distress caused by stimulation of certain nerve endings; usually it indicates that tissue damage is beginning to take place or has taken place as a result of surgery.

INCIDENCE

1. Pain is one of the earliest symptoms that the patient expresses upon return to consciousness.
2. Maximal postoperative pain occurs between 12 and 36 hours after surgery and usually disappears by 48 hours.
3. Soluble anaesthetic agents are slow to leave the body and therefore control pain for a longer time than agents that are insoluble; the latter produce rapid recovery, but the patient is more restless and complains more of pain.
4. Older persons seem to have a higher tolerance for pain than younger or middle-aged persons.
5. There is no documented proof that one sex tolerates pain better than the other.

CLINICAL FEATURES

1. Autonomic:
   a. Outpouring of adrenaline.
   b. Elevation of blood pressure.
   c. Increase in heart and pulse rate.
   d. Rapid and irregular respiration.
   e. Increase in perspiration.
2. Skeletal muscle:
   a. Increase in muscle tension or activity.
3. Psychological:
   a. Increase in irritability.
   b. Increase in apprehension.
   c. Increase in anxiety.

   d. Attention focused on pain.
   e. Complaints of pain.

Patient's reaction depends upon:
1. Previous experience.
2. Anxiety or tension.
3. State of health.
4. His ability to concentrate away from the problem or be distracted.
5. Meaning that pain has for him.

NURSING INTERVENTIONS

1. Employ comfort measures in caring for the patient.
   a. Provide therapeutic environment – proper temperature and humidity, ventilation, visitors.
   b. Increase the patient's bodily comfort by adding a blanket if he is cold, and vice versa.
   c. Massage the patient's back in soothing strokes – move him easily and gently.
   d. Offer diversional activities, soft radio music or favourite quiet television programme.
   e. Provide for fluid needs by giving a cool drink, offering a bedpan.
   f. Investigate possible causes of pain such as bandage or adhesive that is too tight, full bladder, cast that is too snug or elevated temperature suggestive of inflammation or infection.
2. Initiate measures to reduce the likelihood of pain.
   a. Encourage the patient to turn frequently.
   b. Massage pressure areas; support vulnerable areas – strategic placement of pillow, anchoring a footboard, placing a pillow between legs in the Sims's lateral position.
   c. Determine the patient's need to micturate and need for relief from intestinal distension.
   d. Loosen constricting dressings.
   e. Keep bedding clean, dry and free from crumbs.
   f. Maintain the patient in correct physiological position.
   g. Encourage the patient to verbalize – to ease pain reaction, raise threshold.
   h. Give analgesic drugs as prophylaxis to prevent pain.
3. Relieve localized pain.
   a. Carefully support the painful area and elevate painful extremities.
   b. Apply medications or antipruritics as prescribed.
   c. Encourage and assist the patient to follow prescribed exercise programme.
4. Recognize the power of suggestion; mention that

relief of pain will take place when a 'reasonable' method is selected and used.

a. Combine chosen method of pain relief with verbal assurance that it will help.

b. Explain why the method chosen will help in relieving pain – positive assurance has been recognized as enhancing the effect of the 'reasonable' action.

c. Indicate to the patient that you understand that he has pain, that you have time to listen and to help him, and that you care.

5. Be selective in administering pain-relieving agents; recognize individual differences.

a. First determine the patient's respiratory rate and level of activity (arousal); use this information in making subsequent assessments.

b. Administer tranquillizers to relieve anxiety.

c. Use narcotic analgesics when postoperative pain justifies such medication.

d. Patients who have had abdominal or chest surgery are more likely to need narcotics. The exchange of respiratory gases can be reduced by pain that causes reflex chest–muscle contraction.

e. Potent drugs such as morphine may produce depression of the patient's respiratory centre thereby reducing rate and depth of breathing; also, such drugs tend to constrict bronchiolar smooth muscles and increase tracheal bronchial secretions – leading to atelectasis and pneumonia.

f. Give narcotic agonist–antagonist (capable of reversing effects of narcotics, but in absence of narcotic, they produce a narcotic-like action) when prescribed.

g. Provide soporifics for sleep induction.

h. Administer muscle-relaxant and antispasmodic medications for uncontrolled muscle tension.

i. Utilize specific medications for specific conditions such as relief of nausea, relief of undesirable coughing, relief of headache.

j. Administer naloxone hydrochloride (Narcan) to relieve significant respiratory depression when brought about by a narcotic or narcotic agonist–antagonist.

NURSING ALERT
'Potentiators' (hydroxyzine, promethazine) appear to sedate the patient, but it has not been proven that they are effective in potentiating the effects of an analgesic.

6. Recognize desired effects and untoward reactions of all medications given.

a. Observe patient for desired effect of medication.

b. Note respiratory rate; compare it with rate noted before medication was given. Assess the difference. A narcotic is more likely to cause respiratory depression.

c. Be alert to toxic manifestations and hypersensitivity reactions.

   (i) Unpleasant psychic reactions (anxiety, hallucinations) may occur in some patients after taking a narcotic agonist–antagonist.

d. Be knowledgeable about drug interactions.

e. Note signs of respiratory embarrassment, adverse vital signs, rashes.

POSTOPERATIVE COMPLICATIONS

SHOCK

Shock is a response of the body to a decrease in the circulating volume of blood; tissue perfusion is impaired culminating, eventually, in cellular hypoxia.

CLASSIFICATION

1. *Oligaemic* (haematogenic) – shock resulting from loss of plasma or whole blood; this may be external or internal. When 10 per cent of the blood volume is lost, *hypovolaemic* shock occurs.

2. *Bacteraemic* (septic or toxic shock) – characterized by a change in the capillary endothelium, permitting loss of blood and plasma through capillary walls into surrounding tissues; no actual fluid volume is lost from the body.

3. *Cardiogenic* – observed when there is interference with heart pumping action, as might occur in myocardial infarction, cardiac tamponade, which results in inadequate vascular circulation.

4. *Neurogenic* (vasogenic) – marked vasodilation and reflex inhibition, which results in a sluggish circulating system, depriving vital centres of proper blood supply.

5. *Psychic* – results from extreme pain or deep fear.

ALTERED PHYSIOLOGY AND CLINICAL FEATURES

1. Loss of effective circulating blood volume – initiates metabolic and physiological reactions resulting in poor tissue perfusion (Table 3.3).

Table 3.3   Correlation of magnitude to volume deficit and clinical presentation

Approximate deficit	Decrease in blood volume	Shock	
		Degree	Signs
ml 0–500	per cent 0–10	None	None
500–1,200	10–25	Mild (compensated)	Slight tachycardia Mild hypotension Mild peripheral vasoconstriction
1,200–1,800	25–35	Moderate	Thready pulse, 100–120 beats/min Blood pressure, 90–100mmHg systolic Marked vasoconstriction Diaphoresis Anxiety, restlessness Decreased urinary output
1,800–2,500	35–50	Severe	Thready pulse, 120 beats/min Blood pressure, 60mmHg systolic Marked vasoconstriction Marked diaphoresis No urinary output

Source: Wilkins, E.W. Jr (ed.) (1983) *MGH Textbook of Emergency Medicine* (2nd edn), Williams & Wilkins, Baltimore, p. 40.

2. Hyperventilation, caused by stress, leads to respiratory alkalosis; this is the earliest acid–gas change of shock.
3. Pituitary hormones are released:
   a. ACTH (adrenocorticotropic) – stimulates the adrenal cortex to secrete glucocorticoids.
   b. ADH (antidiuretic) – stimulates kidney tubules to absorb more fluid.
   c. ASH (aldosterone-stimulating) – stimulates potassium excretion by kidney, stimulates sodium chloride retention and water retention.
4. Adrenaline and noradrenaline promote capillary vasoconstriction – increases flow through vital organs but diminishes flow through peripheral tissues. Later, peripheral vasoconstriction produces *pale, cold, clammy skin.*
5. Acidosis causes lung to compensate – increased rate and volume.
6. Heart rate accelerates; diastole lessens. With lessened coronary perfusion during diastole, cardiac output falls, resulting in *reduced systolic pressure, lowered pulse pressure,* and generalized vasoconstriction.
7. Weak, thready pulse and subnormal temperature.
8. Lip cyanosis, surrounding pallor; decreased salivary secretions.
9. At first patient appears *nervous* and *apprehensive*; later, *apathy develops* and *sensations are dulled. Muscle weakness* and *fatigue* become apparent.

EFFECTS OF SHOCK
1. *Anoxia* (hypoxia) – lack of oxygen in the body.
2. *Anoxaemia* – decreased amount of oxygen in the blood.
3. *Hyperpyrexia* – an excessive fever, about 42.2–42.8°C, which occurs shortly before death.
4. *Oliguria* – decreased kidney secretion and urinary output.
5. *Anuria* – absence of urinary secretion.
6. *Thrombosis* with subsequent emboli due to blood stasis.

NURSING INTERVENTIONS
Prevention of shock
1. Prepare adequately the mental as well as the physical condition of the patient.
2. Anticipate any complications that may arise during and after surgery.

3. Have blood available if there is any indication that it may be needed.
4. Measure accurately any blood loss.
5. Keep operative trauma to a minimum; minimize postoperative disturbance of the patient.
6. Anticipate progression of symptoms upon earliest manifestation.
7. Monitor vital signs frequently until they are stable.
8. Assess vital sign deviations; evaluate blood pressure in relation to other parameters.
9. Institute therapy immediately following an injury, etc., that is likely to lead to shock.
10. Recognize that blood pressure limits vary with individuals; in some patients 90/60mmHg may be normal, whereas in others it may indicate severe shock.
11. Prevent infection; this will prevent septic shock.

Definitive management

1. KEEP THE AIRWAY PATENT
   a. Use an airway or the doctor will insert an endotracheal tube.
   b. Remove oral and tracheal secretions.
   c. Institute resuscitative measures if necessary.
2. Arrest haemorrhage (not present in septic shock). Ascertain where haemorrhage is occurring; if external, utilize pressure control.
3. Place patient in most physiologically desirable position for shock (Figure 3.3).
   a. Elevate the head on a pillow.
   b. Keep the trunk horizontal.
   c. Elevate lower extremities about 20 to 30 degrees, keeping knees straight.

NURSING ALERT

Do not use Trendelenburg head-low position because (1) after initial increase of blood to the head, a reflex compensatory action takes place causing vasoconstriction and thereby decreasing blood supply to the brain; and (2) viscera tend to fall against the diaphragm, causing increased resistance to breathing and inadequate ventilation.

4. Call medical officer who will ensure an adequate venous return by:
   a. Inserting intravenous catheter for infusion in upper extremities; two may be required.
   b. Placing a central venous pressure catheter in or near right atrium (see Chapter 5 Guidelines p. 221).
      (i) Notice direction and degree of change from initial reading.
      (ii) Utilize route established by the central venous pressure catheter for emergency fluid volume and electrolyte replacement.
   c. Start plasma expanders, if needed, until whole blood is available.
5. The medical officer may obtain blood for determinations of pH, Po_2, Pco_2 and haematocrit.
   a. pH – may indicate acidosis resulting from anaerobic metabolism.

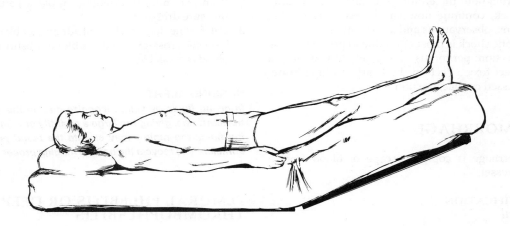

Figure 3.3. Proper positioning of the patient who shows signs of shock. Elevate the lower extremities about 20 degrees, keeping the knees straight, trunk horizontal and head slightly elevated

b. Pco_2 – assesses function of pulmonary alveolar membrane.

c. Po_2 – determines level of oxygen tension.

d. Haematocrit – reveals losses due to obstruction or peritonitis.

6. The doctor may request that a urinary catheter is inserted to monitor hourly urine output. The objective is to maintain a 1ml/kg/h urinary volume output to ensure adequate kidney perfusion.

7. Antibiotics may be prescribed or broad-spectrum chemotherapeutic agents may be used, in order to offset infection, which can occur due to stagnant hypoxia in wounds and in peripheral tissues.

8. Support the defence mechanisms of the patient.
   a. Comfort and reassure the patient if he is conscious.
   b. Resort to sedation and analgesia with discriminating judgment.
   c. Keep the patient warm, but do not apply too much external covering, since it will produce unnecessary vasodilation resulting in more fluid loss.

9. Recognize signs of impending cardiac failure – increasing central venous pressure, distended neck veins, pulmonary crackles, etc. The doctor will initiate prophylactic digitalization.

10. If the patient does not respond to fluid loading and cardiac drugs, expect steroids to be prescribed.

11. If response to conventional methods fails, it may be necessary to resort to mechanical assistance, such as use of intra-aortic balloon pump to increase diastolic aortic pressure.

12. Throughout the entire panorama of impending shock, continue flow sheet, recording of vital signs, observations and interventions.

13. Septic shock is most often due to gram-negative infection: peritonitis, meningitis; it may have a direct toxic effect on the heart resulting in depressed cardiac function.

HAEMORRHAGE

Haemorrhage is copious escape of blood from a blood vessel.

CLASSIFICATION
General

1. *Primary* – occurs at the time of operation.
2. *Intermediary* – occurs within the first few hours after surgery. Blood pressure returns to normal and causes loosening of poorly tied vessels and flushing out of weak clots from untied vessels.
3. *Secondary* – occurs some time after surgery, and is due to infection which exudes the clot in the end of a major vessel.

According to blood vessels

1. *Capillary* – slow general oozing from capillaries.
2. *Venous* – bleeding that is dark in colour and bubbles out.
3. *Arterial* – bleeding that spurts and is bright red in colour.

According to location

1. *Evident or external* – visible bleeding on the surface.
2. *Concealed or internal* – bleeding that cannot be seen.

CLINICAL FEATURES

1. Apprehension, restlessness, thirst; cold, moist, pale skin.
2. Pulse increases, respirations become rapid and deep ('air hunger'), temperature drops.
3. With progression of haemorrhage:
   a. Decrease in cardiac output.
   b. Rapidly decreasing arterial and venous blood pressure as well as haemoglobin.
   c. Pallor around the mouth, spots appear before the eyes, ringing in the ears.
   d. Patient grows weaker until death occurs.

NURSING INTERVENTIONS

1. Treat the patient as described for shock (p. 63).
2. Inspect the wound as a possible site of bleeding. If an extremity is bleeding, apply a gauze-pad pressure dressing.
3. Call for the doctor who will administer blood that has been cross-matched or a blood substitute until blood is available.

NURSING ALERT

In giving fluids by vein, recognize that, in the case of haemorrhage, giving too large a quantity or administering fluids too rapidly may elevate the blood pressure sufficiently to recycle the haemorrhaging process.

FEMORAL PHLEBITIS OR DEEP THROMBOPHLEBITIS

Phlebitis often occurs after operations on the lower abdomen or during the course of septic conditions such as ruptured ulcer or peritonitis. (See Chapter 5.)

CAUSES
1. Injury – damage to vein resulting from:
   a. Tight straps or leg holders during surgery.
   b. Compression of a blanket roll under the knees.
2. Fluid loss or dehydration leading to concentration of blood.
3. Lowered metabolism and circulatory depression after surgery leading to slowing of blood flow.
4. Combinations of the above.
5. Venous stasis due to immobility.

CLINICAL FEATURES
1. Left leg appears to be affected more frequently than right.
2. Pain or cramp in the calf, progressing to painful swelling of entire leg.
3. Slight fever, chills, perspiration.
4. Marked tenderness over anteromedial surface of thigh.
5. Limb feels warm to touch.
6. Intravascular clotting without marked inflammation may develop, leading to phlebothrombosis.

NURSING ALERT
A complaint of slight soreness of the calf is never ignored. The danger inherent in femoral thrombosis is that a clot may be dislodged and produce an embolus.

NURSING INTERVENTIONS
Prophylaxis
1. Hydrate the patient adequately postoperatively to prevent blood concentration.
2. Encourage leg exercises and ambulate the patient as soon as permitted by the surgeon. (Exercises are taught preoperatively – see p. 47.)
3. Avoid any restricting devices such as tight straps that can constrict and impair circulation.
4. Prevent the use of bed rolls, knee garters, even 'dangling' over the side of the bed, because there is danger of constricting the vessels under the knee.

Active intervention
1. The doctor will initiate anticoagulant therapy either intravenously, intramuscularly, or subcutaneously (see p. 51).
2. Prevent swelling and stagnation of venous blood by wrapping the legs from the toes to the groin with elastic bandage or elastic stockings.
3. Control pain in the extremities by bandaging.

PULMONARY COMPLICATIONS

PREVENTIVE MEASURES
1. Report any evidence of upper respiratory infection to the surgeon.
2. Postoperatively, initiate measures to prevent chilling.
3. Aspirate secretions that might cause respiratory embarrassment.
4. Recognize the predisposing causes of pulmonary complications:
   a. Infections – mouth, nose, throat.
   b. Aspiration of vomitus.
   c. History of heavy smoking, chronic respiratory disease.
   d. Obesity.

COMPLICATIONS
1. *Atelectasis* – collapse of pulmonary alveoli caused by a mucous plug closing a bronchus.
2. *Bronchitis* – inflammation of bronchi, causing a cough with considerable mucous secretion.
3. *Bronchopneumonia* – a chest complication with elevated temperature, pulse, and respiratory rate plus a productive cough.
4. *Lobar pneumonia* – onset of a chill followed by a high temperature, pulse and respiration elevation, flushed cheeks, respiratory embarrassment.
5. *Hypostatic pulmonary congestion* – more common in the debilitated or elderly patient, whose weakened heart and vascular system permit stagnation of secretions at base of lungs.
6. *Pleurisy* – knife-like pain in the chest on the affected side, particularly on intake of a deep breath, and elevated temperature, pulse and respirations.

NURSING INTERVENTIONS
1. Appraise the patient's progress very carefully on a daily basis for the first postoperative week to detect early signs and symptoms of respiratory difficulties:
   a. Slight temperature, pulse and respiration elevations.
   b. Apprehension and restlessness.
   c. Complaints of chest pain, signs of dyspnoea or cough.
2. Promote full aeration of the lungs:
   a. Turn the patient frequently.
   b. Encourage the patient to take 10 deep breaths hourly.
   c. Utilize a spirometer or any device that encourages the patient to ventilate. Inspiratory

exercises are more effective than expiratory.
  d. Assist the patient in coughing in an effort to bring up mucous secretions.
  e. Assist the patient to ambulate as early as the doctor will allow.
3. Initiate specific measures for particular pulmonary problems:
  a. Provide cool mist or steam (electric vaporizer) for the patient who exhibits signs of bronchitis.
  b. Encourage the patient to take fluids and expectorants if he appears to be developing pneumonia.
  c. Administer antibiotics to patients with pulmonary infections.
  d. Prevent abdominal distension – causes pulmonary and circulatory embarrassment.
  e. Provide analgesics for discomfort.
  f. Note that the patient who has pleurisy with effusion may need chest aspiration; have equipment ready and be prepared to assist.
  g. Be prepared to administer oxygen to assist in aeration of the lungs for oxygenation of blood.
  h. Obtain sputum specimen for bacteriology.

PULMONARY EMBOLISM

An embolus is a foreign body in the bloodstream – usually a blood clot that has become dislodged from the original site. When such a clot is carried to the heart, it is forced into the pulmonary artery or one of its branches. (See also p. 189.)

CLINICAL FEATURES
1. Sharp, stabbing pains in the chest.
2. Anxiousness and cyanosis.
3. Pupillary dilation, profuse perspiration.
4. Rapid and irregular pulse becoming imperceptible – leads rapidly to death.
5. Dyspnoea.

IMMEDIATE TREATMENT
1. Administer oxygen and inhalations with the patient in an upright sitting position.
2. Reassure and quieten the patient.
3. Administer morphine to control panic and pain as prescribed, if not contraindicated.

URINARY DIFFICULTIES

RETENTION OF URINE
1. Incidence – occurs most frequently after oper-

ations on the rectum, anus, vagina or lower abdomen; caused by spasm of bladder sphincter.
2. Nursing measures:
  a. Assist male patients to sit or even stand up (if permissible), or female patients to use the commode since many patients are unable to micturate while lying in bed.
  b. Provide the patient with privacy.
  c. Use the psychological aid of running the tap water – frequently the sound or sight of running water relaxes the spasm of the bladder sphincter.
  d. Catheterize only when all other measures are unsuccessful:
    (i) May lead to possible bladder infection.
    (ii) Subsequent catheterizations are often required.

NURSING ALERT
Recognize that when a patient micturates small amounts (30 to 60 ml every 15 to 30 minutes) this may be a sign of overdistended bladder ('retention' with overflow).

URINARY INCONTINENCE
1. Cause – loss of tone of the bladder sphincter.
2. Incidence – occurs as a complication in the aged after surgery or shocking injury.
3. Recovery – disappears as patient gains strength and muscle tone.
4. Management:
  a. Offer a bedpan hourly.
  b. Provide extra padding under patient; use special disposable pants.
  c. Initiate a consistent plan for special care of the skin to avoid skin breakdown.

INTESTINAL OBSTRUCTION

CAUSES
1. May occur following surgery on lower abdomen and pelvis, especially when there is drainage.
2. A loop of intestines may kink because of inflammatory adhesions.
3. A loop of intestine may become involved in the drainage tract.

CLINICAL FEATURES
1. Most commonly occurs between the third and fifth postoperative day.
2. Sharp, colicky abdominal pains with pain-free intervals.
3. Pain is localized and should be noted, since it may

become more generalized later; location may pinpoint source of difficulty.

4. Peristaltic activity can be assessed by listening to the abdomen with a stethoscope.
5. Pain-free intervals grow shorter as time advances.
6. With completion of obstruction, intestinal contents back up into stomach and cause vomiting (faecaloid).
7. Abdominal distension and perhaps hiccoughs occur, but no bowel movements, if obstruction is complete; if obstruction is partial or incomplete, diarrhoea may occur.
8. Following a simple enema, returns are clear, indicating very small amount of intestinal contents has reached large intestines.
9. If obstruction is not relieved, vomiting continues, distension becomes more pronounced, pulse increases, shock develops and death occurs.

MANAGEMENT

1. Relieve abdominal distension by passing a naso-gastric suction tube.
2. Administer body-deficient electrolytes per intravenous infusion as prescribed.
3. Consider preparing the patient for surgical intervention if obstruction continues unresolved (see p. 490).

HICCOUGHS

Hiccoughs are intermittent spasms of the diaphragm causing a sound ('hic') that results from the vibration of closed vocal cords as air rushes suddenly into the lungs.

CAUSES

Irritation of phrenic nerve between spinal cord and terminal ramifications on undersurface of. diaphragm.

1. Direct – distended stomach, peritonitis, abdominal distension, chest pleurisy, tumours pressing on nerves or surgery performed near the diaphragm.
2. Indirect – toxaemia, uraemia.
3. Reflex – exposure to cold, drinking very hot or very cold liquids, intestinal obstruction.

MANAGEMENT

1. Remove the cause if possible:
   a. Gastric lavage for gastric distension.
   b. Treatment for pleurisy.
   c. Removal of drainage tubes causing irritation.

2. When removal of cause is not possible, favourite simple remedies may be tried:
   a. Holding breath while taking a large swallow of water.
   b. Applying finger pressure on the eyeballs through closed lids for several minutes.
   c. Inhaling carbon dioxide (breathing in and out of a paper bag).
3. Medications may be prescribed (chlorpromazine, perphenazine). The degree of success with these drugs varies widely, usually used for intractable hiccoughs.
4. Introduce a catheter (16 CH/FG) into the patient's pharynx about 7–10cm; rotate gently and jiggle back and forth; this action interrupts impulses from vagus nerve, and hiccoughs stop.
5. For intractable hiccoughs, an extreme procedure is surgical crush of the phrenic nerve.

WOUND INFECTION

Infection in a wound occurs when there is growth of bacteria; infection may be limited to a single area or may affect a patient systemically.

EXAMPLES OF CAUSATIVE ORGANISMS

1. *Staphylococcus aureus*.
2. *Escherichia coli*.
3. *Proteus vulgaris*.
4. *Pseudomonas aeruginosa*.
5. Anaerobic bacteria (e.g. *Bacteroides fragilis*). Anaerobes have become more prominent in wound infections, particularly following bowel surgery; a characteristic odour can be detected. Often this infection is detected only if anaerobic cultures are performed.

CLINICAL FEATURES

1. Redness, excessive swelling, tenderness.
2. Red streaks in the skin near the wound.
3. Pus or other discharge from the wound.
4. Tender lymph nodes in axillary region or groin closest to wound.
5. Foul smell from wound.
6. Generalized body chills or fever.
7. Elevated temperature and pulse.

NURSING ALERT

A useful rule of thumb is that an elevated temperature occurring within 24 hours suggests a pulmonary infection: within 48 hours suggests a urinary tract infection; after 72 hours suggests a wound infection.

FACTORS AFFECTING THE EXTENT OF AN INFECTION

1. The kind, virulence and quantity of contaminating micro-organisms.
2. Presence of foreign bodies or devitalized tissue.
3. Location and nature of the wound.
4. Amount of dead space or presence of haematoma.
5. Immune response of the patient.
6. Presence of ischaemia leading to wound compression.
7. Condition of the patient, such as whether he is elderly, alcoholic, diabetic, malnourished.

PREVENTIVE MEDICAL AND NURSING INTERVENTIONS

1. Insist on housekeeping cleanliness in the surgical environment.
2. Instruct the patient in how to keep a wound clean; not to interfere with the dressing or wound; include aseptic technique in the handling of dressings if required.

Preoperative

1. Encourage the patient to achieve an optimal nutritional level. If hypoproteinaemic with weight loss, provide oral or parenteral alimentation.
2. Reduce preoperative hospitalization to barest minimum to avoid acquiring 'hospital infection'.
3. When the risk of developing an infection is high (or when infection would have grave consequences), antibiotic therapy is initiated preoperatively.
4. Most clinically effective antibiotics given as prophylaxis are the cephalosporins (spectrum includes gram-positive and gram-negative).
5. Antibiotic bowel preparation for colon surgery may benefit from a combination of oral and possibly preoperative systemic antibiotics.

Operative

1. Follow strict asepsis when the wound is made and thereafter until it is completely healed.
2. When a wound has exudate, fibrin, desiccated fat or nonviable skin, it should not be approximated by primary closure but should be delayed for secondary closure.

Postoperative care of an infected wound

1. Surgeon removes one or more stitches, separates wound edges and examines for infection using a probe.
2. A culture is taken and sent to the bacteriology laboratory.

3. Wound irrigation may be done; have sterile syringe and saline available.
4. A drain (rubber or gauze) may be inserted.
5. Antibiotics are prescribed.
6. Hot, wet dressings may be suggested.

WOUND COMPLICATIONS

HAEMORRHAGE AND HAEMATOMA

Features

1. Inspect dressings frequently during the first 24 hours postoperatively:
   a. Note evidence of bright red blood on dressings.
   b. Look for bulging, which may indicate bleeding and clot formation (haematoma) under the skin.
   c. Examine bedding directly underneath incision site for evidence of trickling ooze.
   d. Check drainage bottle for undue amount of red drainage.
2. Check vital signs for evidence of bleeding – elevated pulse, apprehension, air hunger (see p. 66).

Management

1. Notify doctor.
2. If bleeding continues, it may be necessary for the patient to return to surgery to have bleeding vessel ligated, to remove large haematoma, to resuture wound.

RUPTURE (DEHISCENCE, DISRUPTION, EVISCERATION, ABDOMINAL CATASTROPHE)

Causes

1. The wounds of elderly patients do not heal as readily as those of younger patients.
2. Pulmonary and cardiovascular diseases contribute to wound breakdown, since they impede delivery of nutritional essentials to the wound (circulatory and pulmonary difficulties).
3. Abdominal distension, obesity, infection, poor nutritional status and systemic diseases (e.g. diabetes).

Prophylaxis

1. Apply abdominal binder for heavy or elderly patients or those with weak or pendulous abdominal walls.
2. Encourage proper nutrition with emphasis on adequate amounts of protein and vitamin C.

Clinical features

1. Patient complains that something suddenly 'gave way' in his wound.
2. In an intestinal wound, the edges of the wound may part and the intestines may gradually push out – observe for drainage of peritoneal fluid on dressings (clear or serosanguineous fluid).

Management

1. Stay with the patient and have someone notify the surgeon immediately.
2. If intestines are exposed, cover with sterile, moist saline dressings.
3. Keep the patient on absolute bed rest.
4. Instruct the patient to bend his knees – relieves tension on abdomen.
5. Assure the patient that his wound will be properly cared for; keep him quiet and relaxed.
6. Prepare the patient for surgery and repair of the wound.

POSTOPERATIVE PSYCHOLOGICAL DISTURBANCES

Delirium is a mental aberration that occurs only occasionally in some postoperative patients.

CLASSIFICATION

Toxic

1. Incidence – occurs in combination with symptoms of general toxaemia (e.g. peritonitis, sepsis).
2. Symptoms – acutely ill, restless patient with elevated temperature and pulse, flushed face, bright and roving eyes – indicates mental confusion.
3. Management:
   a. Administer fluids to aid in elimination of toxins.
      Note: Not all delirious patients can tolerate fluids. It is also inappropriate to administer fluids if it may lead to cerebral fluid retention and delirium; treatment in this instance is fluid restriction.
   b. Control infection by giving the proper antibiotics.

Traumatic

1. Incidence – develops following sudden trauma, particularly in the highly nervous person.
2. Symptoms – manifests itself by wild excitement, hallucinations, delusions or melancholic depression.

3. Management:
   a. Administer tranquillizing medications; chloral hydrate, paraldehyde.
   b. This state of delirium begins and ends abruptly.

Delirium tremens

1. Incidence – patients who have used alcohol excessively are poor surgical risks and take anaesthetic agents poorly.
2. Symptoms – postoperatively, after continued abstinence from alcohol, patient shows signs of delirium tremens:
   a. Restless, nervous, easily irritated.
   b. Sleeps poorly, disturbed by unreal dreams, momentarily appears to be in a strange place and does not know nursing or medical staff.
   c. Later, loses control of mental functions; his mind is filled with haunting hallucinations that torment him constantly.
   d. Additional symptoms include sleeplessness, excessive perspiration and marked tremor of the extremities. Patient eventually becomes stuporous.
3. Medical and nursing management:
   a. Administer sedatives to keep the patient quiet and comfortable; stimulation may be required by older patients with alcoholism.
   b. Give glucose intravenously and concentrated vitamins by mouth to control nutritional deficiencies.
   c. Recommend that the patient remain in bed; it may be necessary to restrain him so that injuries are minimized. (Bear in mind that restraining should be a last resort, since this often makes such a patient quite rebellious.)
   d. Encourage ambulation as soon as the surgical condition permits.
   e. See also pp. 1094–1095.

THE PATIENT RECEIVING INFUSION THERAPY

GOALS

1. Maintain or replace body stores of water, electrolytes, vitamins, proteins, calories and nitrogen in the patient who cannot maintain an adequate intake by mouth.
2. Restore acid–base balance.

3. Replenish blood volume.
4. Provide avenues for the administration of medications.

PHYSIOLOGICAL ASSIMILATION OF INFUSION SOLUTIONS

Principles

1. Blood cells (erythrocytes, etc) are surrounded by a semipermeable membrane.
2. Osmotic pressure is the pressure demonstrated when a solvent moves through the semipermeable membrane from weaker to stronger concentrations.
3. Osmotic characteristics of different solutions are often determined by the way they affect red blood cells.

Types of fluid

1. Isotonic – a solution that has the same osmotic pressure externally as that found across the semipermeable membrane within the cell:
   a. Normal saline 0.9 per cent.
   b. Dextrose 5 per cent in water.
   c. Ringer's lactate.
   d. Balanced isotonic.
2. Hypotonic – a solution that has less osmotic pressure than that of blood serum; this causes the cells to expand or swell, for example, sodium chloride 0.45 per cent.
3. Hypertonic – a solution that has higher osmotic pressure than that of blood serum; this causes the cells to shrink:
   a. Dextrose 5 per cent in saline.
   b. Dextrose 10 per cent in saline.
   c. Dextrose 10 per cent in water.
   d. Dextrose 5 per cent in half-strength saline.
   e. Dextrose 20 per cent in water.

Composition of fluids

1. Saline solution – fluids and electrolytes (Na^+, Cl^-).
2. Dextrose – fluid and calories.
3. Ringer's – fluid, electrolytes (Na^+, K^+, Cl^-, Ca^{++}, lactate).
4. Balanced isotonic – fluid, electrolytes, some calories (Na^+, K^+, Mg^{++}, Cl^-, HCO_3^-, gluconate).
5. Whole blood and blood components (see Chapter 6).
6. Plasma expanders – albumin, dextran, haemaccel. These improve circulating blood volume.
7. Parenteral hyperalimentation nutrients.
8. Administration of a particular medication or combination and medications.

NURSING PROCESS OVERVIEW

Assessment

DIAGNOSIS AND NEED FOR FLUID THERAPY

It is important to know the major and minor medical problems of the patient as indicated in the doctor's diagnostic evaluation and the nurse's assessment of the patient.

1. Can the patient's illness affect his fluid balance?
2. What medication or treatment is he receiving that can affect fluid components? How?
3. What is the relation of his fluid intake to fluid output?
4. Does he have dietary restrictions?
5. Is he taking adequate fluids by mouth?
6. What is the doctor's plan of treatment?

EVIDENCE OF FLUID IMBALANCE IN THE PATIENT

1. Determine body temperature – febrile conditions suggest loss of body fluids through perspiration.
2. Is he thirsty? Possible dehydration.
3. Observe for dry, warm skin, cracked lips – signs of dehydration.
4. Check skin for elasticity – lightly pull up a pinch-fold of skin, release it. Does it rapidly resume its normal position? In an elderly patient, check for tongue furrows – this may be more significant than skin turgor.
5. Note colour and amount of urine – concentrated, scanty urine indicates lack of fluids.
6. Compare present weight with admission weight – it may indicate fluid change.
7. Absence of moisture in axillae or groin may indicate dehydration.

INSPECTION OF PRESCRIBED FLUID AND EQUIPMENT TO BE USED FOR THE INFUSION

1. Observe fluid for discolouration, foreign particles, cloudiness, film – if present, do not use.
2. Fluid in a bag:
   a. Gently squeeze and observe for leakage.
3. Fluid in a glass bottle:
   a. Hold flask up to light.
   b. Slowly rotate flask in upright position and then on its side; carefully inspect for a flash of light that could indicate a crack.
4. Check IV tubing for discolouration or defects; if noted, secure new equipment.

5. Follow instructions for assembling equipment, using aseptic technique when inserting drip chamber spike into flask; flush equipment with 20–30 ml of fluid from receptacle before using.
6. Return defective equipment with a note describing defect to the proper department.

PATIENT PROBLEMS
1. Fluid volume deficit related to possible dehydration, shock, haemorrhage, decreased venous filling, use of diuretics, etc.
2. Knowledge deficit; unfamiliarity with intravenous or infusion procedures.
3. Fear related to expected discomfort of procedure.
4. Potential for injury related to intravenous (IV) infiltration.

NURSING ALERT
In the UK a nurse (student or qualified) is not trained or covered by insurance to perform a venepuncture in order to administer intravenous fluids. This procedure is carried out by the doctor. However, some hospital authorities may allow doctors to delegate this procedure to a qualified nurse, who has received specific instruction, but it still remains the doctor's responsibility. This includes venepuncture for taking blood samples and the administration of intravenous drugs direct into a cannula. Nurses should check local hospital policy.

Planning and implementation
NURSING INTERVENTIONS
1. Acquaint the patient with the requirements for intravenous infusion and his need for it.
2. Adjust rate of flow of fluids appropriate to needs of patient as prescribed.
3. See 'Stabilizing extremity' below.

STABILIZING EXTREMITY WITH A PADDED ARMBOARD
1. This is done if the patient is restless, disoriented, elderly or a child and if motion could result in infiltration into tissues or phlebitis.
2. Various kinds of armboards are available; an armboard should be padded.

NURSING ALERT
If hand and arm are to be immobilized, place in normal functional position. Contractures may occur if hand is immobilized in flat position.
For hand:
Dorsiflexion of wrist about 20–25 degrees.
Flexion of metacarpophalangeal joint about 45–50 degrees.

Palm slightly cupped with finger flexion increasing from index to little finger.
Thumb should be extended in relaxed position and not flexed under fingers.

3. Prevent compression of nerves or blood vessels; check pulse and ask patient if pressure is too great.

ADJUSTING RATE OF FLOW OF FLUID IN INFUSION THERAPY
The doctor prescribes the flow rate. However, the nurse is responsible for regulating and maintaining the proper rate.

Patient determining factors
1. Surface area of the patient: the larger the person, the more fluid he requires and the faster he uses it.
2. Patient condition: if patient has cardiovascular or renal problems, the rate should be carefully monitored.
3. Age of patient: administer intermittent medication more slowly to the very young or elderly.
4. Tolerance to solutions: example – test protein sensitivity by administering protein hydrolysates slowly.
5. Fluid composition for this particular patient: when drugs are administered via infusion, the effect desired often depends on speed of administration.
6. Patient movement and activity.

Factors affecting rate of flow
1. Pressure gradient – the difference between two levels in a fluid system.
2. Friction – the interaction between fluid molecules and surfaces of inner wall of tubing.
3. Diameter and length of tubing; gauge of cannula.
4. Height of column of fluid.
5. Size of opening through which fluid leaves receptacle.
6. Characteristics of fluid:
   a. Viscosity;
   b. Temperature – refrigerated fluids may cause diminished flow and vessel spasm; bring fluid to room temperature.
7. Vein trauma, clots, plugging of vents, venous spasm, vasoconstriction, etc.
8. Flow-control-clamp difficulties:
   a. Some clamps may slip and loosen, resulting in a very rapid, or 'runaway', infusion.
   b. Plastic tubing may distort, causing 'creep' or

'cold flow' – the inside diameter of tubing will continue to change long after clamp is tightened or relaxed.
  c. Marked stretching of tubing may cause distortions of tubing and render clamp ineffective (may occur when patient turns over and pulls on a short tubing).
9. Kinking of the tubing.
10. If there is any question regarding rate of fluid administration, check with the doctor.

Calculation of flow rate

1. Drops per millilitre vary with commercial parenteral sets. (Check directions on set or calculate by timing for one minute.) (Also, see Table 3.4 on calibrating IV fluids, below.)
2. Utilize the following formula:

$$\text{Drops/min.} = \frac{\text{Total volume infused} \times \text{drops/ml}}{\text{Total time for infusion in minutes}}$$

Example:
Infuse 1,000ml of 5 per cent D/S in two hours (set indicates 10 drops in 1ml)

$$\frac{1,000 \times 10}{120 \text{ min.}} = 80 \text{ drops/min.}$$

Note: Convenient calculators are available from manufacturers of parenteral solutions.

ELECTRONIC FLOW RATE REGULATORS

TYPES

1. Controller – an electronic device that is mechanically different from the pump; it regulates by electronically monitoring drop rate or regulating fluid passage by a magnetically activated metal ball valve. The advantages are:
   a. More accurate than nonelectronic regulators.
   b. Has alarms to alert for problems.
   c. Takes care of a wide range of fluid and medication needs of patients.
2. Infusion pump – an electronic device that exerts pressure (1) on tubing or (2) on fluid.

Table 3.4 Calibrating intravenous fluids

Prescription	Regular (15 drops/ml)		Microdrip (60 drops/ml)		Macrodrip (10 drops/ml)	
	Drops/min	Drops/¼ min	Drops/min	Drops/¼ min	Drops/min	Drops/¼ min
40ml/h	10	2¼	40	10	7	2
50ml/h	12	3	50	12½	8	2
60ml/h	15	4	60	15	10	2½
80ml/h	20	5	80	20	13	3
100ml/h	25	6	100	25	16	4
125ml/h	30	7½	125	30	20	5
150ml/h	38	9½	150	38	25	6

24-hour fluids	
ml/24 hr	ml/hr
1,000	40
1,500	60
2,000	80
2,500	100
3,000	125
3,500	145

Source: Norcross, M. B. (1975), *American Journal of Nursing*, November, Vol. 75, p. 2003.

By pumping against pressure gradients, a constant, accurate and preselected fluid rate and volume can be maintained. Types are:

a. Peristaltic – moves fluid by exerting externally applied forces on tubing:
   (i) Linear;
   (ii) Rotary.
b. Piston–cylinder – exerts pressure on fluid in a cylinder by pumping action of a piston.
c. Syringe – a motor-driven device in which plunger is depressed at a constant preset rate to eject medication.
d. Volumetric – a device that uses the piston–cylinder principle. Chief advantage is that most models will not pump air (a safeguard against air emboli).

ADVANTAGES

1. Ability to infuse large volumes of fluid with accuracy.
2. Usually an alarm warns of problems.
3. Can be used for intra-arterial infusions.

DISADVANTAGES

1. Cost considerations; it has been demonstrated that not only are these devices cost-effective, but complications (such as infiltration, postinfusion phlebitis and the necessity for infusion restarts) are reduced significantly.
2. Some require special tubing.

INDICATIONS FOR USE OF CONTROLLED INFUSIONS

1. Intra-arterial infusions.
2. Critical care fluid and medication management.
3. Forcing fluids – total parenteral nutrition, enteral alimentation.
4. Closed wound irrigation.
5. Antacid titration via nasogastric tube.
6. Continuous heparin administration.
7. Minute doses of medications for systemic use.
8. Chemotherapy and oxytocic drugs.
9. Regional arterial perfusion.
10. Antidysrhythmic drugs; pressor agents.
11. Bronchoactive and hypoglycaemic agents.

COMPLICATIONS OF INTRAVENOUS THERAPY

INFECTION

A local reaction due to contamination; this may spread systemically.

1. Causes (Figure 3.4):
   a. Fluid contamination; this may be due to faulty preparation, crack in flask, puncture in plastic container, fluid additives. No container should hang longer than 24 hours; some solutions expire in less time.
   b. Peripheral IV catheters are changed in 48–72 hours; when catheter is in place for a longer period, there is greater chance of infection. IV administration sets should also be changed frequently according to hospital policy.
   c. Failure to 'prep' skin rigorously – to remove dead skin, dirt, mucus, etc. before inserting cannula.
   d. Ineffective handwashing technique can result in cross-contamination.

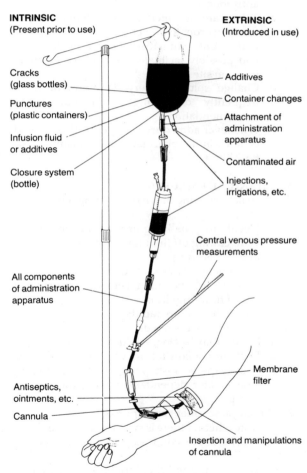

INTRINSIC (Present prior to use)

Cracks (glass bottles)

Punctures (plastic containers)

Infusion fluid or additives

Closure system (bottle)

All components of administration apparatus

Antiseptics, ointments, etc.

Cannula

EXTRINSIC (Introduced in use)

Additives

Container changes

Attachment of administration apparatus

Contaminated air

Injections, irrigations, etc.

Central venous pressure measurements

Membrane filter

Insertion and manipulations of cannula

Figure 3.4. Potential mechanisms for contamination of intravenous infusion systems (Source: Maki, D. G. (1976) Preventing infection in intravenous therapy, *Hospital Practice*, April)

e. Use of contaminated bar soap, liquid soap, and hand lotion may result in infection.
f. May be transmitted within the patient from another infected part of his body to the catheter site.
g. The practice of manipulating the system for administration of medication, tubing changes, dressing changes, etc. may provide the opportunity for introducing contaminants.
2. Preventive nursing:
   a. Practice rigid aseptic technique when changing bags/containers, when inserting a cannula; the doctor should consider the procedure a minor operation.
   b. The doctor should thoroughly cleanse the infusion site; follow this with an iodine-base antiseptic.
   c. Take care to anchor the catheter/cannula firmly in order to prevent excessive movement that might traumatize the cannulated vein and possibly facilitate entry of organisms at infusion site.
   d. Change solution every 24 hours or more frequently depending on manufacturer's recommendations.
   e. Whenever admixtures are made, they should be done in the pharmacy under a laminar–air flow hood.

MECHANICAL FAILURES

Solution flow slowing down or stopping, etc.
1. Causes:
   a. Needle may be lying against the side of the vein, cutting off fluid flow. (Patient may have moved his arm.)
   b. The tubing may be kinked.
   c. Level of intravenous receptacle may change rate of flow (gravity):
      (i) Higher – more rapid;
      (ii) Lower – less rapid.
   d. Needle may be clogged due to clotting.
   e. Regulator of flow rate may be faulty; the clamp with a tapered V-shaped groove seems to provide greater dependability than the regular clamp.
2. Nursing assessment and approach:
   a. Note whether there is swelling at needle site; if oedema is present, it suggests infiltration (see p. 77).
   b. Remove tape and check for kinking of tubing.
   c. Pull back cannula because it may be lying against wall of vein.
   d. Move the patient's arm to a new position.
   e. Elevate or lower needle to prevent occlusion of

bevel of needle; if necessary to maintain a slightly different position, use a gauze pad or cotton ball as a prop and maintain position by placing a few adhesive straps.
   f. Try pulling the needle or catheter back a short distance, since it may be occluded at a bifurcation.
   g. Check for infiltration; apply tourniquet to stop venous flow; if catheter is in vein, IV flow will also stop.
   h. Never irrigate (override undue resistance) a cannula or needle with syringe since it may force a clot into the circulation.
   i. If none of the preceding steps produces the desired flow, call the doctor.

NURSING ALERT

Sterile distilled water is never added to an intravenous infusion because it is hypotonic.

BACTERAEMIA

A generalized reaction due to contaminated equipment or solutions (less apparent with disposable equipment).
1. Symptoms (occur about 30 minutes to one hour after start of infusion):
   a. Abrupt temperature elevation, chills.
   b. Face flushing, sudden pulse rate change.
   c. Complaints of backache, headache.
   d. Nausea and vomiting.
   e. Hypotension – vascular collapse.
   f. Cyanosis – vascular collapse.
2. Preventive nursing:
   a. Solutions never hang more than 24 hours or even less as recommended by manufacturer's directives.
   b. Use of 0.22 micron filter decreases risk of IV-related complications.
   c. Cannula site is to be changed every 48–72 hours.
   d. Change IV administration set every 24–48 hours.
3. Nursing treatment:
   a. Notify doctor.
   b. Discontinue infusion and IV cannula as directed.
   c. Check vital signs; reassure patient.
   d. Save all equipment for further laboratory study.
   e. Record name, lot number and information, i.e. manufacturer of solution and any medications that have been added.

NERVE DAMAGE

May result from bandaging the arm too tightly to the splint.

1. Symptoms: numbness of fingers or hands.
2. Preventive nursing: place padding around arm where bandage is to be applied.
3. Nursing treatment:
   a. Massage arm and move shoulder through its range of motion.
   b. Instruct the patient to open and close hand several times each hour.
   c. Physiotherapy may be required.

INFILTRATION

Dislodging of needle will cause fluid to infiltrate tissues.

1. Symptoms at site:
   a. Oedema, blanching of skin – also check under-surface of arm for puffiness.
   b. Discomfort, depending on nature of solution.
   c. Fluid flows more slowly or stops.
   d. Note temperature of skin; since solution is much cooler than patient, infiltration site will feel cool to touch.
   e. With a vasoconstrictor, such as noradrenaline infiltration can cause serious injury leading to necrosis and sloughing of tissues.
2. Preventive nursing:
   a. Fasten needle securely.
   b. Check IV site for complications hourly.
   c. Check IV flow rate at least hourly.
   d. Avoid looping of tubing below bed level.
3. Nursing treatment:
   a. Stop infusion.
   b. Notify doctor, intravenous therapist, etc.
   c. Place a sterile 7.5 × 7.5cm gauze pad over needle and vein; withdraw needle and apply firm pressure over venepuncture site for several minutes.
   d. Apply warm compresses to increase fluid absorption if not contraindicated.
   e. Infusion may be restarted by a doctor elsewhere.

CIRCULATORY OVERLOAD

Patient receives an excessive amount of solution (happens more frequently in elderly patients or in infants).

1. Symptoms:
   a. Headache, flushed skin, rapid pulse.
   b. Venous distension (engorged neck veins).
   c. Increased blood pressure.
   d. Increased venous pressure.
   e. Coughing, shortness of breath, increased respirations.
   f. Syncope, shock.
   g. Pulmonary oedema leading to dyspnoea and cyanosis.
2. Preventive nursing:
   a. Know whether patient has existing heart condition – more prone to develop acute pulmonary oedema.
   b. Monitor solution flow.
   c. Place patient in semi-sitting position during infusion.
   d. Be especially attentive to the elderly or the infant.
   e. Monitor fluid balance.
3. Nursing treatment:
   a. Slow infusion to a 'keep-open' rate (available for emergency medication); notify doctor.
   b. Raise patient to sitting position – will ease the breathing problem.

DRUG OVERLOAD

Patient receives an excessive amount of fluid containing drugs.

1. Toxic concentrations of drug are collected in main organs: brain and heart.
2. Symptoms:
   a. Dizziness, fainting leading to shock.
   b. Specific symptoms related to the offending drug.
3. Preventive nursing interventions – monitor flow rate carefully.
4. Nursing treatment – related to the nature of the medication.

SUPERFICIAL THROMBOPHLEBITIS

1. Causes:
   a. Overuse of a vein, which may cause vasospasm; this may lead to an inflammatory process.
   b. Irritating infusion solution (strong acids or alkalis, hypertonic glucose solutions and certain drugs such as cytotoxic agents, methacillin, barbiturates).
   c. Clot formation in an inflamed vein.
   d. Anatomical location – veins of the lower extremities (relatively sluggish blood flow) are more vulnerable than cephalic vessels.
   e. Length of time the cannula is in place – the longer the cannulation, the greater the possibility of infection.
   f. Polyvinyl chloride catheters appear to be associated with infection more often than steel needles.

g. Catheter diameter: large-bore catheters are more often associated with phlebitis than small-bore.
2. Symptoms:
   a. Tenderness at first, then pain along course of the vein.
   b. Oedema and redness at injection site.
   c. Arm feels warmer than other arm.
3. Preventive nursing:
   a. Advise doctor to change intravenous site so that the same vein is used no longer than 72 hours (preferably no longer than 48 hours).
   b. Use large veins for irritating fluids because of higher rate of blood flow, which rapidly dilutes irritant.
   c. Stabilize venepuncture at area of flexion.
   d. Use the appropriate filter for infusions that may be irritating.
4. Nursing treatment:
   a. Apply cold compresses immediately to relieve pain and inflammation.
   b. Later follow with moist warm compresses to stimulate circulation and promote absorption.

AIR EMBOLISM
Air manages to get into the circulatory system.

NURSING ALERT
Recognize the high possibility of air embolism when a doctor pumps in blood (e.g. 500ml in 10 minutes), since this builds high pressure in blood receptacle.

1. Symptoms:
   a. Hypotension, cyanosis, tachycardia.
   b. Increased venous pressure, loss of consciousness.
2. Preventive nursing:
   a. Replace initial bag before it is completely empty with a fresh, full bag; check attachment to be certain it is tight.
   b. In 'Y' type sets, tightly clamp the nearly empty bag to prevent air from being sucked into the tubing.
   c. Allow fluid to flow through tubing and needle or catheter to force air out – before starting infusion.
   d. Use an appropriate filter.
3. Nursing treatment:
   Unless prompt action is taken, the patient may die within minutes.
   a. *Immediately* turn patient on left side in Trendelenburg position – air will rise to feet or right atrium. The trapped air will be slowly absorbed.

Evaluation
EXPECTED OUTCOMES
1. Receives adequate intravenous therapy as prescribed.
2. Shows no untoward side effects of intravenous therapy.
3. Communicates an understanding of the reason for intravenous therapy.
4. Experiences a comfortable and safe intravenous infusion with no signs of infiltration or pain.

CARE OF THE WOUND

A wound is an injury to the tissues of the body causing disruption of the normal tissue pattern; such an injury is caused by physical means.

CLASSIFICATION
According to the manner in which it is made:
1. Incised – made by a clean cut with a sharp instrument; e.g. a surgeon's incision with a scalpel.
2. Contused – made by a blunt force, which does not break through the skin but causes considerable soft tissue damage (e.g. a rock, when thrown, bruises a person).
3. Lacerated – made by an object that tears tissues, producing jagged irregular edges (e.g. blunt knife, jagged wire, glass).
4. Puncture – made by a pointed instrument, such as an ice pick, bullet, knife stab, nail.

SURGICAL CLASSIFICATION
1. Clean – an aseptically made wound, as in surgery, in which all bleeding vessels have been ligated (tied).
2. Contaminated – exposed to excessive amounts of bacteria (e.g. unprepared colon surgery, dirty laceration). These wounds are not grossly infected but have been exposed to bacteria (contaminated) and have higher risk of infection.
3. Infected – a wound that may not be closed may contain devitalized or infected material.
4. Debridement – the process whereby devitalized or necrotic tissue is cut out and flushed clean with saline solution.

PHYSIOLOGY OF WOUND HEALING
This is shown in Figure 3.5.

First intention healing (primary union)
Healing that takes place aseptically with a minimum of tissue damage and tissue reaction; this is the ideal

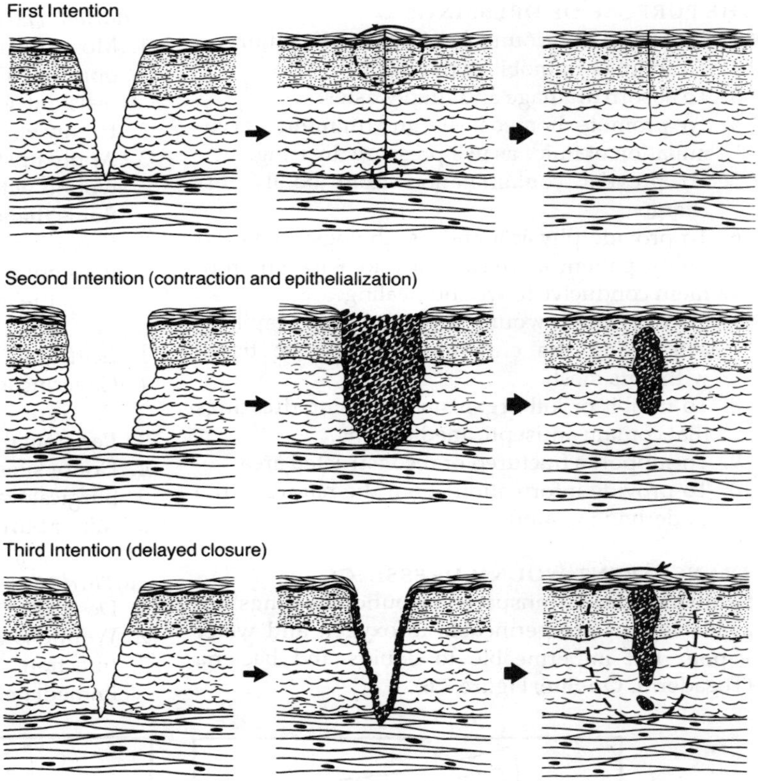

First Intention

Second Intention (contraction and epithelialization)

Third Intention (delayed closure)

Figure 3.5. Classification of wound healing. *First intention:* A clean incision is made with primary closure; there is minimal scarring. *Second intention* (contraction and epithelialization): The wound is left open to granulate in with resultant large scab and abnormal dermal–epidermal junction. *Third intention* (delayed closure): The wound is left open and closed secondarily when there is no evidence of infection. (Hardy, V. D. (1983) *Hardy's Textbook of Surgery*, J. B. Lippincott, Philadelphia, p. 109)

sought by the surgical staff; surgically closed (sutures or surgical tapes).   ·

Second intention healing (granulation)

Wounds that are left open to heal spontaneously; not surgically closed. They need not be infected.

1. If infected, pus forms; drainage is accomplished by incision and perhaps insertion of drains.
2. Necrotic material disintegrates and sloughs off.
3. Cavity fills with a red, soft, sensitive tissue, which bleeds easily.
4. Buds, called granulation tissue, enlarge to fill area formerly destroyed and thus form a scar.

Third intention healing (secondary suture)

1. Occurs when a wound breaks down and is re-sutured or when a wound has been kept open and fills with granulation tissue and then is closed with sutures (two faces of granulation tissue are brought together in apposition).
2. Scar tissue formation is deeper, wider and more pronounced.

WOUND HEALING WITHOUT DRESSINGS

Preferred by some surgeons; may be desirable for a simple, clean wound.

Advantages

1. Permits better observation and early detection of problems.
2. Promotes cleanliness and facilitates bathing.
3. Eliminates conditions necessary for growth of organisms:
   a. Warmth;
   b. Moisture;
   c. Darkness.
4. Avoids adhesive tape reaction.
5. Facilitates patient activity.
6. Is economical.

Disadvantages

1. Psychologically, a patient may object to an exposed wound.
2. Wound is more vulnerable to injury.
3. Bedding and clothing may catch on stitches.

THE PURPOSE OF DRESSINGS
1. To protect the wound from mechanical injury.
2. To splint or immobilize the wound.
3. To absorb drainage and fluid wastes.
4. To promote homeostasis and minimize accumulation of fluid, as in a pressure dressing.
5. To prevent contamination from bodily discharges.
6. To provide physical and psychological comfort for the patient as well as a physiological environment conducive to wound healing.
7. To debride a wound by combining capillary action and the entwining of necrotic tissue within its mesh.
8. To inhibit or kill organisms by using dressings that contain antiseptic medications.
9. To support a fractured or reconstructed area.
10. To provide information about the nature of the underlying wound.

TRANSPARENT WOUND DRESSINGS
Synthetic, clear, transparent wound dressings are available that are permeable to oxygen and water vapour but impermeable to liquids and bacteria (Tegaderm, Op-Site; Figure 3.6).

Characteristics
1. Most are made of polyurethane film with the opposite side coated with hypoallergenic water-resistant adhesive.
2. Highly elastic and conforms to body contours.
3. Apply unstretched and unwrinkled to dry, clean wound with sufficient margin to avoid leakage of fluids that may accumulate under the dressing.
4. If excessive fluid does not accumulate or infection does not occur, dressing may be left in place until re-epithelialization is complete.

Indications
1. Covering arterial and venous catheter sites.
2. Pressure sores.
3. Peristomal and peri-fistulas.
4. Donor sites for skin grafts.
5. Surgical wounds.
6. Minor burn areas.

Advantages
1. Decreased pain noted.
2. Wound is visible.
3. Infection can be noted early and treated immediately.

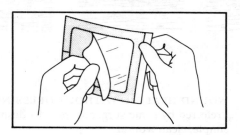

1. Clean and thoroughly dry application area; remove and discard centre cut-out window.

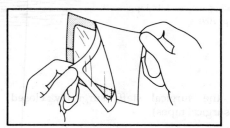

2. Peel paper liner from paper-framed dressing, exposing adhesive surface.

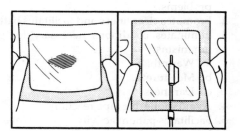

3. Position over wound or intravenous site. Smooth dressing from centre toward edges.

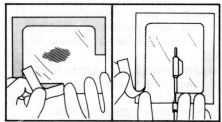

4. Remove paper frame. Smooth dressing edges. Over intravenous, seal dressing securely around intravenous tubing or hub.

Figure 3.6. These diagrams show how Tegaderm Transparent Dressing is applied. *Part 3:* indicates the placement of Tegaderm Transparent IV Dressing. *Part 4:* below the dressing the adaptor and intravenous tubing are stabilized with Transpore Surgical Tape to provide a neat, secure visible peripheral intravenous site (Source: courtesy of 3M Medical Products Division)

4. Greater freedom of movement.
5. Patient bathing is facilitated.

NURSING PROCESS OVERVIEW

Assessment
FACTORS THAT AFFECT WOUND HEALING
1. What type of surgery did patient have?
2. Where is the wound? How extensive?
   a. Was haemostasis in the operating room effective?
   b. What is nature of vascularity (e.g. adequate blood supply)?
   c. Evidence of oedema? Inflammation?
3. How is the wound held together? Butterfly tapes, wire sutures, tension sutures, clips?
4. Are there drains in place? What kind? How many? Portable suction?
5. What kinds of dressings are being used?
   a. Are they saturated with exudate?
   b. Is drainage consistent with nature of surgery?
6. How does the patient appear? Signs or complaints of wound pain or discomfort? Fever?
7. How old is the patient?
   a. What is his nutritional status?
   b. Has his intake of protein and vitamin C been adequate? (These are needed for wound healing.)
8. Was he given packed cells to maintain adequate levels of red blood cells?
9. What conditions does patient have, and what medications is he taking that could affect wound healing?
   a. Check his medications – steroids, etc.
   b. Note all listed diagnoses – diabetes mellitus, etc.
10. How long has patient been in the hospital preoperatively? (Longer preoperative hospitalization increases risk of nosocomial infections.)
11. Does he understand principles of asepsis and importance of not touching sterile parts of dressing and the incision line?

PATIENT PROBLEMS
1. Alteration in comfort (pain) related to incision site, drains, nature of surgery, dressing changes, etc.
2. Knowledge deficit: lack of understanding of principles of asepsis and potential for contaminating wound.
3. Potential for infection related to incision.
4. Fear related to possibility of rupturing skin stitches.
5. Potential for injury related to unhealed wound and altered mobility.

Planning and implementation
NURSING INTERVENTIONS
1. Ensure patient comfort by changing dressings when required.
2. Minimize strain put on wound by tape or bandage, in order to promote proper healing.
3. Maintain asepsis during dressing change and wound cleansing.
4. Discard soiled dressings in proper receptacle for incineration.
5. Monitor incision site for signs of irritation, inflammation.
6. Support the patient's need for mobility by providing adequate support of incision site.
7. Document condition of incision site (drainage, if present, colour, smoothness, etc.) when dressings are changed.

Evaluation
EXPECTED OUTCOMES
1. Relates that incision site is comfortable, looks clean, improves each day.
2. Enumerates restrictions on certain physical activities to prevent wound dehiscence.
3. Tells why it is important to wash hands when changing dressings.
4. Demonstrates how to change his own dressings.
5. Indicates the need for proper disposition of soiled dressings to avoid contamination or spread of infection, if wound is still draining.
6. Lists conditions that need to be reported: dehiscence, bleeding when wound appeared to have approximated; oozing or drainage after wound appeared to be dry; heat, redness, pain, swelling.

PROCEDURAL CONSIDERATIONS IN WOUND CARE

INTRODUCTION
Before undertaking the care of any wound the following should be adhered to:

1. The principles of asepsis.
2. An awareness of cross-infection and how pathogenic micro-organisms may be introduced into the wound by the nurse/dresser.
3. Appropriate and thorough handwashing before, during and after the procedure.
4. An awareness of the ward environment and its potential to cause infection. (A room specifically allocated for dressings is preferable.)
5. Hospital policy regarding the disposal of soiled dressings and instruments.
6. Seek advice from infection control adviser as appropriate.
7. An awareness of the present increase in hospital-caused infections (including methicillin-resistant *Staphylococcus aureus*), resulting in prolonged admission for the patient and the need for expensive antibiotic therapy.

GUIDELINES: CHANGE OF SURGICAL DRESSINGS

SURGICAL DRESSING TECHNIQUE
The procedure of changing dressings, examining and cleansing the wound, utilizing principles of asepsis.

1. This is usually performed by a nurse alone, unless the wound is complicated.
2. The condition of the wound is noted in order to understand the nature of the patient's surgical recovery.
3. The healing process is facilitated by keeping the wound clean.
4. The date for the removal of stitches or clips depends on the location of wound, the operation and the surgeon's instructions (usually five or six days).

EQUIPMENT
Dressing pack contains scissors, forceps, gallipots, gauze and cotton wool swabs (some of these items may be packed individually).
Antiseptic solution/sterile saline, if required.
For a wound with a drainage tube, add sterile safety pin if shortening is required. Equipment for irrigating the wound may be required; also equipment for taking a swab, if indicated.
Sterile disposable gloves may be used.

Unsterile equipment
Bag for discarding dressing and disposable items.
Adhesive tape of the appropriate size.
Pads to protect the patient's bed, if necessary.

PROCEDURE
Preparatory phase
1. Inform the patient that his dressing is to be changed. Explain procedure to him. Have him lie in bed in comfort.
2. Avoid changing dressings at meal times and when ward cleaning is in progress.
3. Ensure his privacy by drawing the curtains or closing the door; expose the dressing site.
4. If the dressings have a foul odour, they should be changed in a separate treatment area that is adequately ventilated.
5. Prevent undue exposure of the patient; respect his modesty and prevent him from being chilled.
6. Wash your hands thoroughly; this should be done before and after each patient.

Remove adhesive tape

Nursing action	**Rationale**
1. Remove tape along longitudinal axis, slowly and gently.	Removing tape in the same plane is less injurious and less painful.
2. Peel back edges by holding skin taut and pushing away from tape.	It is less traumatic to push skin away from tape than to pull tape from skin.
3. Remove tape near a wound by pulling toward the wound.	Pulling away from a wound may tear some of the delicate, newly formed tissues.
4. Use a suitable solvent, such as baby oil, if the tape does not pull away easily.	Oil is safe, works as well as true solvents and, in addition, lubricates and soothes the sensitive skin beneath.

Remove old dressing

Method A (using disposable gloves)

Nursing action	**Rationale**
1. Don sterile disposable gloves, remove top dressings carefully, and discard into plastic bag.	Dressings are not to be handled by ungloved hands because of the possibility of transmitting pathogenic organisms.
2. Gradually loosen last dressing and observe skin and wound site.	If dressings adhere, moisten them with sterile saline and slowly withdraw dressing.
3. Remove and discard disposable gloves into plastic bag.	This will go to the incinerator later.

Method B (using a sterile plastic bag)

Nursing action	**Rationale**
1. After washing hands, open package containing sterile plastic bag.	Bag should extend several centimetres above wrist.
2. Put right hand into sterile bag, being careful not to touch outside of bag (this bag acts as a sterile glove).	Bag acts as a glove to protect hand from the dressings.
3. Pick up all soiled dressings as above and hold them in right hand; use left hand to grasp top edge of bag and pull it down over the hand and dressings.	This encloses soiled dressings in a plastic container; this bag can be used to receive soiled cotton balls or dressings used to clean wound.

Cleansing a simple wound

Nursing action	**Rationale**
1. Use aseptic technique.	To prevent contamination of a clean wound or to prevent further contamination of a dirty wound. Also to prevent transmission of pathogenic organisms to clean area.
2. Open sterile pack containing scissors, forceps, swabs, etc. Make sure the contents are not handled.	
3. Open any accessory packs as required, including pack of sterile fluid, if used, and empty into sterile container.	
4. Using forceps (or gloved hand) cleanse wound using a fresh swab each time and in one direction. Dry with fresh dry swab.	Applying a one-way direction prevents recontamination of the wound. Leaving the wound moist aids suitable media for pathogenic organism.
5. With sterile forceps apply gauze and dressing suitable for the wound.	
6. Secure dressing with tape, if necessary.	

FOLLOW-UP CARE

Nursing action	**Rationale**
1. Make patient comfortable.	
2. Discard disposable items and soiled dressings into the bag provided then place into designated receptacle for burning. Clean equipment which is to be re-used.	To prevent transmission of pathogenic organisms.
3. Record nature of procedure and condition of wound, as well as patient reaction.	

GUIDELINES: DRESSING A DRAINING WOUND

REINFORCEMENT OF DRESSINGS

Draining wounds may require frequent changes of dressings. Outer layers may be removed and fresh dressings applied without disturbing wound site.
1. Saturated dressings cause discomfort to the patient.
2. Dressing edges may become dry, hard and scratchy.
3. Odour may be unpleasant.

AUXILIARY AIDS TO FACILITATE DRESSING CHANGES
Montgomery straps

Strips of adhesive tape, the edges of which have been folded back for a short distance with a small hole cut in the folded portion and threaded with gauze strips or cotton tape. Two opposing strips are brought together and the tapes tied (Figure 3.7).

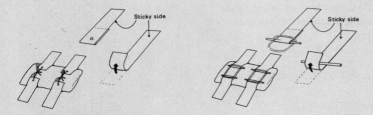

Figure 3.7. Montgomery straps; two styles are shown

REMOVAL OF ADHERENT DRESSINGS

1. To prevent the discomfort of removing dry, sticking dressings, moisten the dressing with sterile saline or hydrogen peroxide.
2. Provide a disposable bowl or towel to catch excessive fluid.

ANCHORING AND GRADUAL WITHDRAWAL OF DRAINAGE TUBES

1. When the dressing is changed, the drainage tube is often pulled out of the wound a few centimetres and the excess tube is cut off.
2. The shortening of the drainage tube will depend on the amount of drainage and is done on the advice of the surgeon.
3. Hollow, hard rubber or polythene tubes are used occasionally to drain a cavity. The tube is usually anchored with a suture.
4. When shortening the drainage tube for the first time, the suture holding the tube in place is removed. The tube is then gently drawn out of the wound a few centimetres, using forceps, the sterile safety pin is inserted into the drainage tube and closed. The safety pin prevents the drainage tube from slipping back into the wound. The excess tubing is then cut off and a clean dressing applied.

SKIN CARE

1. Drainage is often irritating to surrounding skin tissues, particularly if it contains gastrointestinal secretions.
2. Apply protective ointment if prescribed (caution – ointments may cause maceration and may prevent drainage).
3. Recognize value of portable wound suction in maintaining cleanliness of surrounding tissues (see p. 86).
4. Attach drainage tubing to suction bottle. Check tubing frequently for kinking or looping which would restrict flow of drainage.

GUIDELINES: USING PORTABLE WOUND SUCTION
(Redivac, Portovac)

Portable wound suction is a suction system that gently removes excess fluid and debris from a wound by means of a perforated catheter connected to a portable suction apparatus.

PURPOSE
To speed healing of the wound by removing fluids that could retard tissue granulation and by exerting negative pressure, which permits two layers of tissue to adhere and thus eliminates dead space.

ADVANTAGES
1. Tubing rarely becomes occluded because it is siliconized and has multiple perforations.
2. Pressure exerted is gentle and even; suction is quiet.
3. Equipment is lightweight, permitting patient to move easily.
4. It is easy to measure amount of wound drainage.

EQUIPMENT REQUIRED FOR INSERTION
1. A long (0.25–0.5cm) malleable stainless steel introducing needle with a cutting edge on one end and a fine screw thread at the other.
2. A long 0.25cm calibre, siliconized, noncollapsible, polyethylene catheter with many small perforations in the centre.
3. A noncollapsible, siliconized, polyethylene connecting tube. The wound catheter fits snugly into the lumen of this tube.
4. A vacuum source (evacuator) consisting of an unbreakable plastic container with rigid ends and collapsible sides (may be a size to collect 200, 400, or 800ml of fluid). Box has one cuffed hole into which the connecting tube fits snugly and an airhole supplied with a plug. This box may be of accordion-like collapsible plastic, or it may have steel coil springs on the inside to hold the ends of the box apart.
5. A plastic Y-connector, which fits between wound catheters and connecting tube and allows two wound tubes to be connected to one evacuator if desired.

METHOD OF INSERTING DRAINAGE TUBE(S)
1. In the operating room, the surgeon places the perforated drainage tubing in the desired wound area.
2. A stab wound is made with the needle, and excess tubing is drawn through the wound (stab wound is preferred because a more tightly sealed porthole is created; if the wound opening is used, drainage may seep through the incision line).
3. Needle is cut off, and tubing is attached via adapter to evacuator tubing (Figure 3.8).

METHOD OF INITIATING SUCTION

Nursing action	Rationale
1. Connect tubes to evacuator.	
2. Squeeze ends of box together.	This will expel air.

Figure 3.8. (A) Two perforated catheters are draining the incisional area, following a radical neck dissection. By means of a Y-tube, drainage is drawn into a portable wound-suction receptacle. When full, open top plug of receptacle and empty. (B) To re-establish negative pressure, compress receptacle as indicated and replace plug; suction drainage will resume

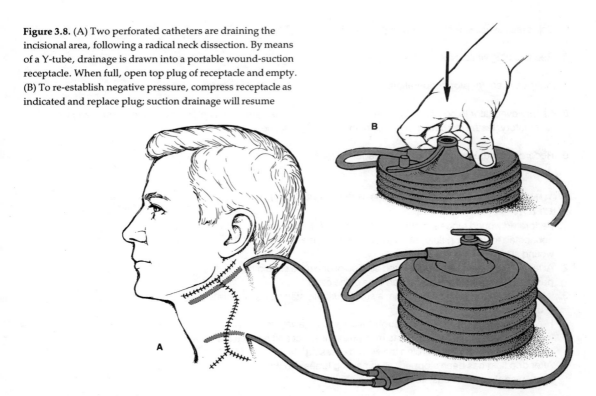

Nursing action	Rationale
3. Plug air hole.	To create a negative pressure.
4. As spring expands, a negative pressure of approximately 45mmHg is produced.	Any fluid and blood in tissues is sucked into evacuator. Negative pressure is not great enough to suck the soft tissues into the holes of the catheters.
5. When evacuator is full (200, 400, or 800ml – depending on size of evacuator), it is time to empty. A good rule is to empty every eight hours, or more frequently if necessary.	Negative pressure has been fully dissipated.

EMPTYING EVACUATOR

Nursing action	**Rationale**
1. Carefully remove plug, maintaining its sterility.	
2. Empty contents of evacuator into calibrated container.	Measure drainage.
3. Place evacuator on flat surface.	To permit adequate compression.
4. Cleanse opening, as well as plug, with an alcohol swab.	To maintain cleanliness of outlet.

5. Compress evacuator completely (Figure 3.8B).	To remove air.
6. Replace plug while evacuator is compressed.	To re-establish negative pressure (suction).
7. Check system for proper operation.	Look for fluid entering receptacle.
8. Secure evacuator to bedding; if patient is ambulatory, fasten evacuator to his clothing.	This permits patient to move without disturbing closed suction.
9. Record character and amount of drainage.	

WOUND IRRIGATION COMBINED WITH PORTABLE WOUND SUCTION

1. Perforated wound tubes are placed side by side in wound. One is connected to irrigating fluid (or antibiotic solution), the other to portable wound suction.
2. At least 30 per cent of the perforated section of one tube should be positioned parallel to the perforated area of the other.
3. If tubes are to remain for some time, a suture (usually stainless steel wire) is used.
4. Having the drainage tube exit through a stab wound (away from main incision line) makes it convenient to manipulate, inspect and remove the drainage tube without disturbing the wound dressing.
5. After drip fluid has been stopped, all remaining tubes should have suction applied for at least 48 hours.

TUBE REMOVAL
At conclusion of use, discard tubing and evacuator by placing in a paper bag and depositing in container for incineration.

GUIDELINES: SUTURE REMOVAL

The timing of stitch removal (of nonabsorbable stitches) depends on the location of the stitch on the body usually: head and neck, three to five days; chest and abdomen, five to seven days; lower extremities, seven to ten days, and the instruction of the surgeon.

EQUIPMENT
Stitch removal tray containing:
    Swabs
    Smooth forceps
    Scissors or stitch cutter
    Dressing

PROCEDURE

Nursing action	**Rationale**
1. Cleanse the stitch area carefully and thoroughly, if required, using forceps and swabs wrung out in antiseptic solution. Repeat using a fresh dry swab. (Some surgeons prefer dry wounds and prefer sutures not to be swabbed with lotion as it is said this allows organisms to enter.)	Stitches provide pathways for micro-organisms to invade tissues; therefore, skin surface must be rendered as clean as possible.
2. Hydrogen peroxide may be used if there are dried blood encrustations.	In the process of liberating oxygen, peroxide will loosen dried serum.
3. Grasp the knot of the suture with a pair of smooth forceps and gently pull upwards.	This will pull stitch away from skin.
4. Cut the shortened end of the stitch as close to the skin as possible.	This will allow the stitch to be pulled free of wound so that only that part of the stitch which is under the skin touches subcutaneous tissues.

NURSING ALERT
Note that no segment of the stitch that is on the surface of the skin should be drawn below the skin surface. To permit this would introduce skin-surface contaminants subcutaneously with risk of infection.

5. For continuous suture removal, cut the suture at each skin orifice on one side and remove the suture through the opposite side.	The objective here again is to avoid subcutaneous contamination.
6. If there is any oozing, apply a small dressing.	Any orifice is a potential site for infection.
7. Avoid injury to the tender and newly healed wound.	

CLIP REMOVAL
This is a similar procedure to suture removal.

EQUIPMENT
As above plus appropriate clip removers.

PROCEDURE
Michael clips
The curved blade of the clip removers is gently inserted below the middle of the clip. The pressure exerted on bringing the blades of the clip remover together will cause the clip to be released. Ease points of the clip out of skin.

FURTHER READING

BOOKS

Bickerton, J. (1985) *Surgical Nursing*, Heinemann, London.

David, J.A. (1986) *Wound Management – A Comprehensive Guide to Dressing and Healing*, Dunitz, London.

Faulder, C. (1985) *Whose Body Is It? The Trouble of Informed Consent*, Virago Press, London.

Hosking, J. and Welchew, E. (1985) *Postoperative Pain – Understanding Its Nature and How to Treat It*, Faber and Faber, London.

Middleton, D. (1985) *Nursing I (Part 4): Care of the Surgical Patient*, Blackwell Scientific, London.

Westaby, S. (1985) *Wound Care*, Heinemann, London.

ARTICLES

Intravenous therapy

Bowell, E. and Armstrong, J. (1980) Management of intravenous therapy, *Nursing*, Vol. 13, pp. 579–83.

Cheung, P. (1986) Learning your tables (use of dosage-rate charts for calculating intravenous infusion dosage rates), *Nursing Times*, Vol. 82, No. 42, 15 October, pp. 40–1.

Krakowska, G. (1986) Practice versus procedure (a study to examine current practice and attitudes in setting up intravenous infusions), *Nursing Times*, Vol. 82, No. 49, pp. 64–66, 69.

Nelson, R. and Miller, H. (1986) Keeping air out of IV lines, *Nursing*, Vol. 86, 16 March, pp. 57–9.

Pre- and postoperative care

Alcock, P. (1986) Preoperative information and visits promote recovery of patients, *National Association of Theatre Nurses News*, 23 July, pp. 17–18.

Closs, S.J., MacDonald, I.A. and Hawthorn, P.J. (1986) Factors affecting perioperative body temperature, *Journal of Advanced Nursing*, Vol. 11, No. 6, pp. 739–44.

Davies, B.D. (1981) Communications in nursing – preoperative information given in relation to patient outcome, *Nursing Times*, Vol. 77, No. 14, pp. 599–601.

Editorial (1983) Preoperative depilation, *Lancet*, June, 11 1(8337), p. 1311.

Farmer, G. (1985) The role of the anaesthetic nurse, *NATN News*, 22 November, pp. 10–12.

Jones, J. (1986) Hearing and memory in anaesthetised patients, *British Medical Journal*, 17 May, Vol. 292, pp. 1291–2.

Leeson, C. (1985) Pain and the postoperative patient, *Nursing Add On*, Vol. 2, No. 43, November, pp. 1289–90.

Melia, K. (1986) Informed consent. Dangerous territory, *Nursing Times*, Vol. 82, No. 21, p. 27.

Pyne, R. (1986) Informed consent – tell me honestly, *Nursing Times*, Vol. 82, No. 21, pp. 25–6.

Saxey, S. (1986) The nurse's response to postoperative pain, *Nursing Add On*, Vol. 3, 10 October, pp. 377–81.

Wells, R. (1986) Informed consent. The great conspiracy, *Nursing Times*, Vol. 82, No. 21, pp. 22–5.

Wound healing

Dowding, C.M. (1986) Nutrition in wound healing, *Nursing Add On*, 3 May, Vol. 786, pp. 174–6.

Fraser, I. (1982) Removing starch powder from gloves, *British Medical Journal*, 19 June, Vol. 284, No. 6332, p. 1835.

Ingleston, L. (1986) Wound care. Make haste slowly, *Nursing Times*, Vol. 82, No. 37, pp. 28–30.

Jaber, F. (1986) Charting wound healing, *Nursing Times*, Vol. 82, No. 37, pp. 24–7.

Johnson, A. (1986) Wound care – cleansing infected wounds, *Nursing Times*, Vol. 82, No. 37, pp. 30–4.

Leaper, D. (1986) Antiseptics and their effects on healing tissue, *Nursing Times*, Vol. 82, 28 May, pp. 45–7.

Moir-Bussy, B.R. (1986) The surgical wound, *Nursing Add On*, 3 March, pp. 92–4.

O'Brien, D.K. (1986) Postoperative wound infections, *Nursing Add On*, 3 May, pp. 180–2.

Stewart, A. (1986) The choice of dressing for wound healing, *Professional Nurse*, Vol. 1, March, pp. 155–6.

4

Care of the Patient with a Respiratory Disorder

CONCEPTS UNDERLYING RESPIRATORY FUNCTION, DISEASE AND THERAPY

FUNCTIONS OF THE RESPIRATORY SYSTEM
1. Uptake of oxygen.
2. Elimination of carbon dioxide, thereby helping to maintain the pH of the blood.

ANATOMICAL COMPONENTS OF THE RESPIRATORY SYSTEM
1. Air passages through which air passes from the external environment to the alveolar–capillary membrane, and returns.
2. Alveolar–capillary membrane – through which diffusion of carbon dioxide and oxygen occurs between the gases in the alveolar air and in the blood.
3. Respiratory muscles, which enlarge the capacity of the thoracic cavity, thereby drawing air down the air passages to the lungs. These muscles are normally the diaphragm and intercostal muscles. The accessory muscles which may be used for forceful inspiration are the sternocleidomastoid and the anterior serratus muscles.
4. Pleura, to transmit the movement of the respiratory muscles to the lung tissue, thus varying the negative pressure within the thoracic cavity.
5. Intact nerve pathway to the muscles, i.e., intercostal nerves to the intercostal muscles and phrenic nerve to the diaphragm.
6. Respiratory centre in the medulla.

BASIC TERMINOLOGY
1. *Ventilation* – movement of air in and out of the lungs by means of inspiration and expiration.
2. *Tidal volume* – amount of air moved in and out of the lungs and air passages with each breath under normal conditions. In an adult this is normally about 400ml.
3. *Vital capacity* – the maximum volume of air that can be expelled from the lungs by forceful effort following a maximum inspiration.
4. *Perfusion* – filling of the pulmonary capillaries with venous blood which has returned to the heart from the systemic circulation, and is pumped from the right ventricle via the pulmonary artery to the lungs. Normally about 2 per cent of this blood bypasses the alveoli and does not participate in gaseous exchange. This bypass is called shunting.

CONTROL OF RESPIRATION
The rate and depth of respiration is controlled by the respiratory centre in the medulla oblongata. The rhythmicity of respiration is controlled by the pneumotaxic centre in the pons (Figure 4.1).

ABBREVIATIONS
P_{ACO_2} – partial pressure of alveolar carbon dioxide.
P_{aCO_2} – partial pressure of arterial carbon dioxide.
P_{AO_2} – partial pressure of alveolar oxygen.
P_{aO_2} – partial pressure of arterial oxygen.

PHYSIOLOGY OF GAS EXCHANGE – CONCEPT OF PARTIAL PRESSURE
Gases are exchanged through a thin membrane by diffusion, i.e. the gas of high pressure passes through the membrane to the lower pressure, in order to equalize the pressure on either side of the membrane.

There are two areas in the body where this gaseous exchange occurs:
1. The exchange of gases between the alveoli and the capillary network which closely surrounds them. This exchange is known as external respiration.
2. The exchange of gases between the capillaries and

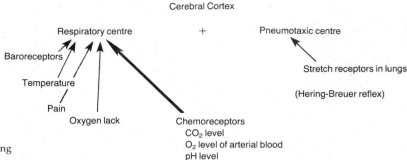

Figure 4.1. Afferent impulses affecting the control of respiration

the tissue cells in every part of the body. This is known as internal respiration.

In atmospheric air, which is a mixture of gases, and which at sea level exerts a total pressure equal to 760mmHg (101.3kPa), each of the gases exerts a pressure or tension in proportion to its percentage of the whole. (As well as the gases, there is a variable amount of water vapour. Due to the specialized structure of the lining of the air passages, air is saturated with water vapour by the time it has reached the lungs.)

The pressure, or tension, exerted by the individual gases in a mixture is known as the partial pressure.

The composition of air is approximately: nitrogen, 79 per cent; oxygen, 21 per cent; carbon dioxide, 0.04 per cent.

To estimate the partial pressure of these gases, it is necessary to calculate their proportion of the total air pressure. For example, nitrogen, 79 per cent of 760 = 600.

Therefore the partial pressure of nitrogen P_{N_2} is 600mmHg. In order to convert this to SI units, divide by 7.5, which gives 80kPa.

The partial pressure of oxygen is 21 per cent of 760 = 159.6. Therefore, P_{O_2} 159.6mmHg = 21.3kPa.

EXTERNAL RESPIRATION (EXCHANGE OF GASES BETWEEN THE LUNGS AND THE BLOOD)

The composition of alveolar air is:

Nitrogen, 80 per cent:	573mmHg = 76.7kPa
Oxygen, 14 per cent:	100mmHg = 13.0kPa
Carbon dioxide, 5.5–6 per cent:	40mmHg = 5.3kPa
Water vapour:	47mmHg = 6.3kPa

The blood arriving at the capillary network surrounding the alveoli has the following composition:

$$P_{O_2} = 40\text{mmHg} = 5.3\text{kPa}$$

$$P_{CO_2} = 46\text{mmHg} = 6.1\text{kPa}$$

Therefore, it is obvious that by diffusion, oxygen will pass from the alveoli into the capillaries, and carbon dioxide will pass from its higher pressure in the capillaries to the lower pressure in the alveoli. Due to this exchange, the blood leaving the lungs contains P_{O_2} 100mmHg = 13kPa, P_{CO_2} 40mmHg = 5.3kPa, that is, in equilibrium with the alveolar air.

INTERNAL RESPIRATION (EXCHANGE OF GASES BETWEEN THE BLOOD AND THE CELLS)

The blood in the capillaries arriving at the tissues has a higher pressure of oxygen than the tissue fluid, and a lower pressure of carbon dioxide, so that oxygen diffuses out of the capillaries and carbon dioxide passes back into them (Figure 4.2).

PULMONARY VENTILATION

The amount of air which is taken in with each breath under resting conditions is about 400ml. This is known as the tidal volume. In order to establish the pulmonary ventilation, the tidal volume is multiplied by the number of breaths per minute. The usual range of pulmonary ventilation is from about 400ml × 15 breaths = 600ml, to 400ml × 20 breaths = 800ml, i.e. 6–8 litre/min. This can be increased considerably during vigorous exercise to 50 litre/min. Not all the air which is taken in with a breath reaches the alveoli. Out of 400ml which is taken in, about 150ml remains in the air passages, where no gaseous exchange occurs. This area is known as the dead space.

It is sometimes necessary to know the alveolar ventilation, which is calculated by respiratory rate × (tidal volume − dead space):

$$\text{Alveolar volume} = 15 \times (400 - 150) = 3{,}750\text{ml/min}$$

CARRIAGE OF OXYGEN

Oxygen is carried by the haemoglobin contained in the red blood cells: 1g of haemoglobin has the ability to combine with 1.34ml of oxygen. Thus, a person

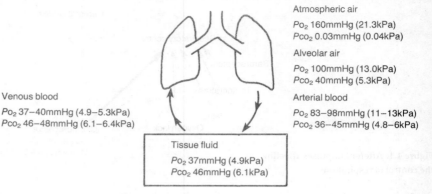

Atmospheric air

Po_2 160mmHg (21.3kPa)
Pco_2 0.03mmHg (0.04kPa)

Alveolar air

Po_2 100mmHg (13.0kPa)
Pco_2 40mmHg (5.3kPa)

Arterial blood

Po_2 83–98mmHg (11–13kPa)
Pco_2 36–45mmHg (4.8–6kPa)

Venous blood

Po_2 37–40mmHg (4.9–5.3kPa)
Pco_2 46–48mmHg (6.1–6.4kPa)

Tissue fluid

Po_2 37mmHg (4.9kPa)
Pco_2 46mmHg (6.1kPa)

Figure 4.2. Internal respiration

with 15g haemoglobin/100ml blood would, theoretically, be able to carry $1.34 \times 15 = 20$ml oxygen/100ml blood. This is known as the oxygen capacity.

At a tension of 100mmHg (13.0kPa), the oxygen capacity is very close to this amount, i.e. 95–97 per cent of the oxygen capacity, where there is 19ml oxygen/100ml blood.

When internal respiration takes place under resting conditions, about 5ml oxygen per 100ml blood are given up. During exercise, more oxygen is given up, increasing to 15ml oxygen/100ml blood. This can be shown on a graph and is known as the oxygen dissociation curve (Figure 4.3).

During vigorous exercise, there is an increase in temperature and hydrogen ion production; this decrease in the pH of the blood has the effect of moving the curve to the right, i.e. proportionately more oxygen is extracted.

Hypoxia. This is a situation in which there is lack of oxygen in the body.
Hypoxaemia. This is an oxygen deficiency in the blood.

$$\text{Normal } Pao_2 = 83\text{--}98\text{mmHg (11--13kPa)}$$

Causes of hypoxaemia

1. Most common cause in diseases which affect the alveolar membrane so that diffusion of gases is impaired, although perfusion of the lungs is normal. This can occur, for example, in pneumonia and emphysema.
2. A low partial pressure of oxygen in the inspired air, e.g. at high altitudes.
3. Some of the blood bypasses the pulmonary circulation, as in ventricular septal defects.
4. Decrease in the amount of haemoglobin available

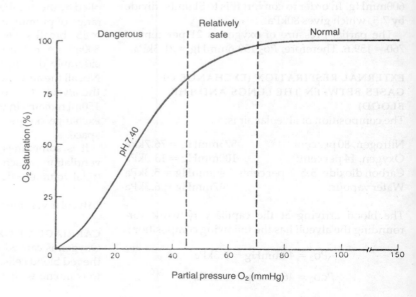

Figure 4.3. Oxygen–haemoglobin dissociation curve

for the carriage of oxygen, e.g. in anaemia, and also in carbon monoxide poisoning (carbon monoxide has a very great affinity for haemoglobin, so that only a small amount of inspired carbon monoxide may decrease by half the available haemoglobin for the carriage of oxygen).

Hypoxia will occur for these reasons, plus a sluggish circulation which occurs in cardiac failure or shock. In this case, the amount of oxygen passing into the blood and the amount of haemoglobin are both normal, but the circulation is inadequate to supply the needs of the tissues.

HYPERCAPNIA

This is retention of carbon dioxide in the blood, i.e. the $Paco_2$ is above 45mmHg (60kPa) at rest.

Causes of hypercapnia

1. Diseases which affect the alveolar membrane, such as pneumonia.
2. Interference with the respiratory centre, e.g. by drugs.
3. Mechanical difficulties, or interference with the nerves or the neuromuscular junction.

ACID–BASE BALANCE

The pH of the blood has to be maintained within narrow limits of 7.35 to 7.45, and a balance has to be made between the amount of acid produced as a result of metabolic processes, and the amount excreted by (a) the lungs in the form of carbon dioxide + water (carbonic acid), and (b) actively excreted by the kidney tubules.

In order for carbonic acid to be carried in the blood, it is buffered by bicarbonate, and in order for this to happen, the normal bicarbonate/carbonic acid ratio is 20:1. However, if respiration is inadequate, and carbon dioxide cannot be excreted, hypercapnia will result, causing a drop in the pH of the blood. This is known as *respiratory acidosis*. Conversely, if hyperventilation occurs, and too much carbon dioxide is 'washed out' of the blood, the pH will rise (*respiratory alkalosis*).

Metabolic acidosis occurs when the production of acid is increased, e.g. in diabetes mellitus, or when kidney function is impaired, e.g. in chronic renal disease and renal failure.

Metabolic alkalosis occurs when acid is lost from the body, e.g. from prolonged vomiting, or nasogastric suction, or when there is increased ingestion of alkali, which may occur by self-medication of patients with indigestion by taking antacid drugs containing sodium bicarbonate.

The respiratory system is able to compensate for a change in the pH level by altering the rate and depth of respirations.

MAJOR FEATURES OF BRONCHOPULMONARY DISEASE

COUGH AND SPUTUM PRODUCTION
Causes
1. Coughing is a protective mechanism that serves to clear the airways.
2. Cough-producing stimuli may be inflammatory, mechanical, chemical or thermal.
3. Clinical problems producing cough are infection, inflammation, neoplasms, cardiovascular disorders, trauma, physical agents and allergic disorders.
4. Violent coughing may cause bronchial obstruction and syncope, and cause further irritation of the bronchi.
5. Thick, mucopurulent sputum, which is difficult to remove, is more apt to cause violent coughing.

Nursing assessment
1. Evaluate the character of the patient's cough:
   a. Throat-clearing cough – postnasal drip.
   b. Dry and hacking – may be due to nervousness, viral infections, bronchogenic carcinoma, early congestive heart failure.
   c. Loud and harsh – irritation in upper airway.
   d. Wheezing – associated with bronchospasm.
   e. Severe or changing in character or with position – may be bronchogenic cancer (cough, chest pain, haemoptysis).
   f. Loose – indicates problems in peripheral bronchi and lung parenchyma.
   g. Painful – may indicate pleural involvement, chest wall disease.
   h. Chronic, productive – sign of bronchopulmonary disease.
2. Note relationship of cough to time, to patient's position and to environmental exposure:
   a. Recent onset of cough (hours or days) suggests infection.
   b. Cough most noticeable upon awakening – suppurative lung disease; bronchitis.
   c. Coughing paroxysms at night – may indicate bronchial asthma or left-sided heart failure.
   d. Cough that worsens when patient is supine –

may be due to postnasal drip from sinusitis, bronchiectasis.

e. Cough associated with food intake – may be the result of aspiration into tracheobronchial tree.

f. Cough of recent onset or gradually progressive over a period of weeks or months suggests tuberculosis or bronchogenic carcinoma.

3. Determine the patient's:

a. Smoking history: Current? Past?

b. Environmental or occupational exposure to dusts, fumes or gases?

c. Allergies, asthma, sinusitis, upper respiratory infection?

4. Observe character, quantity, and colour of expectorated material and ability of patient to clear his secretions. Ask if there has been a change in the character or frequency of coughing.

a. Clear or mucoid – stems from viral infection, chronic bronchitis, postnasal drip.

b. Thick yellow or green sputum – due to primary or secondary bacterial infections.

c. Rusty – may indicate bacterial pneumonia (if patient not receiving antibiotics).

d. Malodorous – due to lung abscess, infection from fusospirochaetal or anaerobic organisms.

e. Frothy pink sputum – indicates acute pulmonary oedema.

f. Note amount of sputum produced daily. A sudden decrease in the quantity of sputum may indicate inspissation (drying and thickening) in tracheobronchial tree and may lead to respiratory insufficiency and failure.

g. Layering of sputum in sputum cup occurs in lung abscess or bronchiectasis.

Nursing interventions

1. Give cough suppressants, expectorants and mucolytic agents, as prescribed.

2. Make sure the patient is adequately hydrated to liquefy sputum.

3. Assist the patient to cough productively by controlled coughing, postural drainage and chest percussion.

4. Discourage smoking – interferes with lung defence mechanisms: interferes with ciliary action, increases bronchial secretions, causes inflammation and hyperplasia of mucous glands, reduces production of surfactant, impairs function of alveolar macrophages (scavenger cells).

5. Encourage oral hygiene – odour and taste of sputum depresses appetite.

DYSPNOEA

Breathlessness or difficult breathing. May be acute, chronic, progressive, recurrent or paroxysmal.

Causes

1. In lung disease, shortness of breath is due to change in lung rigidity or increased airway resistance.

2. Lung disease places strain on the right ventricle – may cause right ventricular failure.

Clinical implications

1. In general, the acute lung diseases produce a more severe grade of dyspnoea than do the chronic diseases.

2. Sudden dyspnoea in a healthy person may indicate pneumothorax (air in pleural cavity).

3. Sudden dyspnoea in ill or postoperative patient may indicate pulmonary embolus; pneumothorax.

4. Orthopnoea – characteristic of cardiogenic pulmonary congestion.

5. Expiratory wheeze – arises from obstructive disease in peripheral airways (asthma, chronic bronchitis, emphysema).

6. Noisy respirations – related to localized obstruction of major branches, tumour, foreign body or narrowing of smaller airways.

7. Inspiratory stridor – indicates partial obstruction at laryngeal or tracheal level.

8. Paroxysmal wheezing unrelated to exertion – may arise from bronchial (allergic) asthma or bronchitis.

Nursing assessment

Ascertain circumstances that cause dyspnoea:

1. Relation to exertion, position or environmental exposure.

2. Quantify exertion and specify type producing dyspnoea (housework, mowing lawn, walking a set distance).

3. Mode of onset? Sudden? Gradual?

4. Quantify change in dyspnoea. (What could patient do a year ago, a month ago, that he cannot do now?)

5. Can the patient take a deep breath?

6. At what time of day/night is it obvious?

7. Is there associated cough?

8. Is there expiratory wheeze?

9. Is dyspnoea associated with other symptoms?

Nursing interventions

The treatment depends on alleviating the cause:

1. Place the patient on rest with his head elevated.

2. Administer oxygen as prescribed.

HAEMOPTYSIS
Coughing up or expectoration of blood or blood-stained sputum from the respiratory tract.

Causes
1. Chronic bronchitis; bronchiectasis.
2. Bronchial carcinoma.
3. Bronchial or parenchymal infections.
4. Cardiovascular conditions (mitral stenosis).

Nursing assessment
1. Question the patient about ingestion of aspirin or aspirin-containing medication within the past 24 hours.
2. Ascertain whether blood is coming from nose or throat, gastrointestinal tract or lungs.
   a. Nose (*epistaxis*) – usually there is a discharge of blood from nose:
      (i) During severe epistaxis, the patient may swallow or aspirate blood.
      (ii) Look for dried blood in nose or nasopharynx.
   b. Gastrointestinal trace (*haematemesis*):
      (i) Usually preceded by nausea and accompanied by retching and vomiting.
      (ii) Blood appears dark red in colour; may contain food particles.
      (iii) Blood is acid in reaction (pH less than 7.0).
   c. Lungs (*haemoptysis*)
      (i) Blood is *coughed* up; patient may have tickling in throat, salty taste, burning or bubbling sensation in chest.
      (ii) Usually bright red and frothy; blood-tinged sputum may persist for days.
      (iii) Blood is alkaline in reaction (pH greater than 7.0).

Nursing interventions
1. Place the patient on bed rest and give mild sedation as prescribed.
   a. Place on affected side (if known) – to avoid flooding the unaffected lung.
   b. Maintain a calm, reassuring approach – fright in a patient promotes hyperventilation.
2. Recognize the patient's fear and apprehension due to this threatening symptom and give him understanding and support.
3. Record quantity, colour and character (mixed with mucus, pure blood).
4. Save all coughed up blood for inspection by the doctor.

CHEST PAIN
Causes
1. Parietal pleura has rich supply of sensory nerves coming from intercostal nerves to the diaphragm. These nerve endings may be stimulated by inflammation and stretching of membranes and by respiratory movements – produces a characteristic sharp, knife-like pain.
2. Pleuropulmonary pain – bacterial pneumonia, infarction, spontaneous pneumothorax.

Clinical features and nursing assessment
1. Pleural pain is a common manifestation of inflammatory and malignant disease, but also accompanies pneumothorax and pulmonary embolism.
2. Pleural pain (usually well localized, sharp and stabbing) occurs at end of inspiration.
3. Assess quality, intensity and radiation of pain.
4. Note factors that precipitate pain.
5. Evaluate whether position of the patient changes character of pain.
6. Determine the effect of inspiration and expiration on the patient's pain.

Nursing interventions
1. Should be directed towards relieving underlying causes.
2. Give prescribed analgesic, taking care not to depress respiratory centre or productive cough.
3. Assist with regional anaesthetic block – procaine is injected along the intercostal nerves that supply the painful area in cases where pain is intractable.

HOARSENESS
Causes
1. Acute: when associated with febrile episode, suggests viral laryngotracheobronchitis.
2. Persistent: may indicate intrinsic neoplasm of vocal cord, bronchogenic cancer, mediastinal lesion.

SYMPTOMS OF BRONCHOPULMONARY DISEASE
1. Anorexia.
2. Fever.
3. Weight loss.
4. Fatigue, malaise, weakness. } related to duration and severity of disease
5. Sweats.
6. Chills.

SIGNS OF BRONCHOPULMONARY DISEASE
1. Cyanosis.
2. Clubbing of fingers.
3. Wasting.

RESPIRATORY FAILURE AND INSUFFICIENCY
Terminology
1. *Respiratory insufficiency* – altered function of the respiratory system which produces clinical symptoms (usually includes dyspnoea).
2. *Chronic respiratory failure:*
   a. Hypoxia (decreased Pao_2) or hypercapnia (increased $Paco_2$).
   b. Due to disorder of any component of the respiratory system.
   c. Occurs usually over a period of months to years – allows for activation of compensatory mechanisms.
3. *Acute respiratory failure:*
   a. Hypoxia (Pao_2 less than 6.6–8.0kPa; 50–60mmHg) or hypercapnia ($Paco_2$ greater than 6.6kPa; 50mmHg).
   b. Occurs rapidly, usually in minutes to hours or days.
4. *Ventilatory failure:*
   a. Respiratory failure due to decreased alveolar ventilation.
   b. Characterized by elevated $Paco_2$.
   c. Relationship to *minute volume* (amount of air inhaled and exhaled in one minute).
      (i) Alveolar ventilation + *dead space ventilation* = minute volume. (Dead space is amount of air moving in and out of conducting airways and other areas of lung which are ventilated but not perfused with blood.)
      (ii) Ventilatory failure may be present even if minute volume is normal or even high. The lung disorder causes an increase in dead space ventilation.
      (iii) In ventilatory failure due to disorders of the respiratory control centre or disorders of the thoracic cage and muscles, the minute volume and alveolar ventilation are reduced.
5. *Oxygenation failure:*
   a. Consists purely of a decreased Pao_2.
   b. Found primarily in localized or diffuse infiltrative or vascular pulmonary disorders.
6. *Obstructive disorder:*
   a. Ventilatory insufficiency or failure due to impaired airflow in conducting airways.
   b. Results from airway narrowing (bronchitis, asthma) or loss of lung elasticity required to expel air (emphysema).
7. *Restrictive disorder* – ventilatory insufficiency or failure due to impaired movement of the thoracic cage or musculature or to increased lung stiffness.

Causes of respiratory failure
1. Disorders of the respiratory control centre:
   a. Drug intoxication (general anaesthetics, narcotics, barbiturates, hypnotics, excessive oxygen administration to patients with chronic obstructive lung disease).
   b. Vascular disorders (brainstem infarction and haemorrhage, decreased perfusion due to shock).
   c. Trauma (head injury, increased intracranial pressure).
   d. Infection (meningitis, encephalitis).
   e. Others ('primary alveolar hypoventilation', myxoedema coma, status epilepticus).
2. Disorders of impulse transmission:
   a. Drug intoxication (curariform drugs, anticholinesterases).
   b. Degenerative disorders (amyotrophic lateral sclerosis, multiple sclerosis).
   c. Infection (poliomyelitis, Guillain-Barré syndrome, tetanus, rabies).
   d. Trauma (transection of the spinal cord).
   e. Others (myasthenia gravis).
3. Disorders of the thoracic wall and musculature:
   a. Skeletal (scoliosis, flail chest, multiple rib fractures, thoracotomy).
   b. Muscular (polymyositis, muscular dystrophies).
   c. Pleural (effusion, haemothorax, empyema, fibrothorax, pneumothorax).
4. Disorders of conducting airways:
   a. Upper airways (foreign body, epiglottitis, laryngitis, smoke and noxious gas inhalation, acute laryngeal oedema, tumour).
   b. Peripheral airways (chronic bronchitis, emphysema, asthma).
5. Disorders involving the alveolar–capillary membrane.
   a. Infection (lobar, aspiration or interstitial pneumonia).
   b. Vascular (thromboemboli, fat emboli, polyarteritis, Wegener's granulomatosis, pulmonary oedema).
   c. Neoplasm (lymphogenous spread of carcinoma).
   d. Others (interstitial fibrosis, uraemic pneumonitis, shock lung, noncardiac pulmonary oedema).

CLINICAL FEATURES OF RESPIRATORY FAILURE

Nursing history	Interpretation
Cough, dyspnoea, wheezing, sputum production and colour	*Any* recent *change* should point to an abnormality of the lung and raise suspicion of respiratory insufficiency or failure.
Drug usage	May point to depression of the respiratory control centre and raise the likelihood of ventilatory failure.
Oxygen administration	Oxygen administration, particularly in patients with chronic bronchitis or emphysema who are dependent on hypoxaemia as a stimulus to breathing and who have grown insensitive to carbon dioxide as a stimulus to breathing, may bring about ventilatory failure.
Weakness or paralysis	Weakness or paralysis in any other part of the body indicates the possibility of weakness or paralysis of the thoracic muscles and actual or impending ventilatory failure.
State of responsiveness	Coma occurs early in disorders of the respiratory control centre but may be a late manifestation of other causes of respiratory failure; *any otherwise unexplained change in the level of consciousness should raise the possibility of respiratory failure.*
Respiratory rate	Reduced in disorders of the respiratory control centre; rapid respiratory rate occurs early in disorders of the thoracic cage and musculature and of the lung proper.
Pattern of respiration	Abnormalities of rhythm (Cheyne-Stokes respiration, Biot's respiration) are found in disorders of the respiratory control centre.
Depth of respiration	Shallow in disorders of the respiratory control centre, disorders of impulse transmission and weakness of the thoracic musculature; *may be deceptively normal* in disorders of the lung.
Use of accessory muscles of breathing (scalene, sternomastoid and pectoralis) and intercostal retraction	Laboured breathing usually seen in disorders of the lung parenchyma, skeletal deformities.
Pulse	Usually rapid in acute respiratory failure, but may be deceptively normal in disorders of the respiratory control centre (drug intoxication) and disorders of impulse transmission (Guillain-Barré syndrome).

| Cyanosis | Useful only when present; absence of cyanosis, however, does not exclude respiratory failure. |
| Chest auscultation | Abnormalities may indicate lung disease; *breath sounds may be decreased in intensity or deceptively 'normal' in severe airway obstruction.* |

NURSING ALERT

1. *Any of the abnormalities outlined above should point to the possibility of actual or impending respiratory failure.*
2. *Arterial blood gases should be obtained by the doctor whenever the nursing history or patient assessment suggests respiratory insufficiency or failure.*
3. *Even if arterial blood gas studies are normal, respiratory insufficiency may still be present and may progress to respiratory failure.*
4. *Bedside measurement of the vital capacity at frequent intervals is helpful in following the progress of patients with disorders of the respiratory control centre, or impulse transmission, or of the thoracic musculature.*

VENTILATORY FAILURE WITH NORMAL LUNGS

AETIOLOGY

1. Insufficient respiratory centre activity (drug intoxication – drug overdose, general anaesthesia; vascular disorders – cerebral vascular insufficiency, cerebral tumour; trauma – head injury, increased intracranial pressure).
2. Insufficient chest wall function (neuromuscular disease – Guillain-Barré, myasthenia gravis, poliomyelitis, demyelinating disease, muscular dystrophy; trauma to the chest wall resulting in multiple fractures; spinal cord trauma; kyphoscoliosis)

Assessment

CLINICAL FEATURES

1. Hypoxaemia and hypercapnia.
2. Decreased vital capacity, decreased inspiratory force.
3. Decreased respiratory rate (insufficient respiratory centre activity) *or* increased respiratory rate (insufficient chest wall function).

PATIENT PROBLEMS

1. Impaired gas exchange related to inadequate respiratory centre activity or chest wall movement.
2. Potential alteration in airway clearance related to inability to cough and breathe deeply.
3. Impaired physical mobility related to underlying disorder.

Planning and implementation

NURSING INTERVENTIONS

1. Give specific treatment for cause of respiratory failure (i.e. narcotic antagonist for narcotic or narcotic analogue intoxication, pyridostigmine for myasthenia gravis, as prescribed).
2. Initiate measures to prevent atelectasis and promote chest expansion.
3. Monitor adequacy of alveolar ventilation by frequent measurement of respiratory rate, vital capacity and inspiratory force.
4. If respiratory rate is >35/minute, vital capacity <15/ml/kg body weight, or inspiratory force is less than $-25 cmH_2O$, the patient may require intubation and mechanical ventilation.
5. Assist patient with maintaining activities of living, e.g. hygiene needs.

Evaluation

EXPECTED OUTCOMES

1. Patient demonstrates reversal of symptomatology related to underlying disorder: achieves normal respiratory rate, vital capacity and inspiratory force.
2. Achieves normal Pao_2 and $Paco_2$.
3. Prevents development of atelectasis and secretion retention: coughs and breathes deeply at frequent intervals.
4. Regains optimal physical mobility.

VENTILATORY FAILURE WITH INTRINSIC LUNG DISEASE

AETIOLOGY

1. Chronic obstructive airways disease (chronic bronchitis, emphysema).
2. Severe asthma.

Assessment

CLINICAL FEATURES

1. Hypoxaemia and hypercapnia that is increased in relation to patient's normal values.
2. Use of accessory muscles (scalene, sternomastoid and pectoralis) and intercostal retraction – reflects difficulty moving air through passages in bronchospasm or obstructed by secretions.
3. Crackles (râles) or wheezing – indicates fluid in alveoli and airways, bronchospasm.
4. Altered level of consciousness – indicates decreased cerebral perfusion.

PATIENT PROBLEMS

1. Ineffective airway clearance related to increased or tenacious secretions.
2. Impaired gas exchange related to lung parenchyma damage and/or airway obstruction.
3. Alteration in fluid volume (excess) related to right ventricular failure.
4. Weakness and impaired mobility related to disorder.

Planning and implementation

NURSING INTERVENTIONS

1. Administer oxygen at 24 to 38 per cent by Venturi mask, or 1 to 2 litres per minute by nasal cannula, as prescribed.
2. Begin intravenous fluids to reduce sputum viscosity, as prescribed.
3. Initiate measures to increase alveolar ventilation – bronchodilators to reduce bronchospasm, corticosteroids to reduce airway inflammation, as directed. Chest physical therapy to remove mucus, slow respiratory rate with pursed-lip breathing.
4. Give specific treatment for cause of the exacerbation (i.e. antibiotics for respiratory infection, as prescribed).
5. Prepare for intubation and mechanical ventilation only if patient is apnoeic on admission – usually from sedative drugs or excessive oxygen concentration (>28 per cent); patient becomes increasingly lethargic, cannot cough or expectorate secretions, or cannot co-operate with therapy; or pH falls below 7.25 and the $Paco_2$ continues to increase despite use of the above therapy.
6. Assist patient as necessary with activities of living, e.g. hygiene needs.

Evaluation

EXPECTED OUTCOMES

1. Patient demonstrates ability to clear airway of secretions (decrease in volume and tenacity of respiratory secretions).
2. Achieves blood gas values that are within the patient's normal limits.
3. Demonstrates normal fluid balance.
4. Patient regains optimal physical mobility.

DIAGNOSTIC PROCEDURES FOR RESPIRATORY CONDITIONS

AUSCULTATION OF THE CHEST

A stethoscope is an instrument for conveying sounds from the chest wall to the ears of the listener.

PURPOSE

To recognize and localize abnormalities in lungs or pleura and heart and pericardium by sound.

EQUIPMENT

Stethoscope – may have bell chest piece, diaphragm chest piece, or both.

Bell – transmits relatively low-pitched sounds best.

Diaphragm – transmits relatively high pitched sounds best (Figure 4.4).

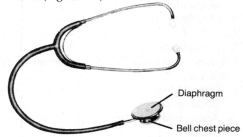

Figure 4.4. Stethoscope with diaphragm and bell chest piece (courtesy: Bard Parker)

UNDERLYING PRINCIPLES

1. The doctor will need as quiet an environment as possible. All surplus clothing should be removed, so that nothing is touching the end or the tubing of the stethoscope.
2. If possible, have the patient sitting upright, and leaning slightly forward. A very ill patient may have to be gently turned from side to side.
3. Ask the patient to breathe with his mouth open while the doctor is listening to his chest.

EXPLANATION OF DIFFERENT BREATH SOUNDS

1. The sound of normal breathing that is detected on the chest wall is generated by the rate at which air flows through the higher passages of the bronchial tree.
2. Since inspiration is shorter than expiration, air flows at a higher rate of speed during inspiration. The inspiratory sound is louder than the expiratory sound.
3. The character of normal breath sounds varies over different lung areas even in normal individuals.
4. A localized decrease in or absence of breath sounds may be noted in abnormal conditions.

Abnormal breath sounds

In diseases involving the bronchial tree and alveoli in such a way that fluid or mucus obstructs air flow, certain sounds, termed *adventitious sounds* (sounds not normally occurring), may be heard:

1. *Râles* – crackling or bubbling (discontinuous) noises; may also be called *crackles*. Râles sound like the crackling of tissue paper or the rubbing together of hairs at the end of the stethoscope. Râles may be fine, medium or coarse. Significance: pneumonia, pulmonary fibrosis or congestive heart failure.
2. *Rhonchi* – musical (continuous) sounds or vibrations, usually of longer duration; may also be called *wheezes*. Significance: airways obstruction.
   a. Generated from larger bronchi; heard in both inspiration and expiration.
   b. May vary in pitch, quality, and intensity.
3. *Pleural rub*, or *pleural friction rub* – leathery, grating, rough sound heard in both inspiration and expiration; induced by inflammation of pleural surfaces.
   a. Heard 'close' to the ear; sounds louder when stethoscope is pressed against the chest.
   b. Associated with breathing and unaffected by cough.

PALPATION
Purpose
1. To identify areas of tenderness, masses or inflammation.
2. To assess mobility of ribs and spine.
3. To assess fremitus (palpable vibrations transmitted through the bronchopulmonary system on speaking).

PERCUSSION
Purpose
To identify areas of dullness in the thorax, and to compare resonance on inspiration and expiration.

DIAGNOSTIC STUDIES

If the patient has to undergo any of the following investigations, the nurse should explain the procedure to the patient in terms he will understand, and the nurse should answer any questions that the patient may have. For further information regarding the nurses' responsibilities before and after these investigations, observe individual hospital policies and procedures.

RADIOGRAPHY
Chest X-ray
1. Normal pulmonary tissue is radiolucent. Thus densities produced by tumours, foreign bodies and so on can be detected.
2. Shows position of normal structures, displacement and presence of abnormal shadows.
3. Chest X-rays may reveal extensive pathology in the lungs in the absence of symptoms.

Tomography
1. Provides films of sections of lungs at different levels within the thorax.
2. Useful in demonstrating presence of small, solid lesions, calcification or cavitation within a lesion.

Computed tomography
Computed tomography is an imaging method in which the lungs are scanned in successive layers by a narrow beam X-ray. A computer printout is obtained of the absorption values of the tissues in the plane that is being scanned.

It may be used to define pulmonary nodules, small tumours adjacent to pleural surfaces (which may be invisible on routine X-ray) and to demonstrate mediastinal abnormalities and hilar adenopathy.

Fluoroscopy
Enables radiologist to view heart, lungs and diaphragm in the dynamic (moving) state.

Barium swallow
Outlines the oesophagus, revealing displacement of oesophagus and encroachment on its lumen, since cardiac, pulmonary and mediastinal abnormalities can be seen as deviations of the oesophagus.

Bronchography
A radiopaque medium is instilled directly into the trachea and bronchi, and the entire bronchial tree or selected areas may be visualized. This is a diagnostic test for any disease that alters the calibre or patency of the bronchial tree or that causes its displacement.

1. Patient is assessed for allergic reaction to anaesthetic agent or contrast media before the test is started.
2. Topical anaesthesia is sprayed in the mouth, on the tongue and posterior pharynx.
3. Local anaesthetic is injected into the larynx and tracheal tree.
   a. Extreme caution is indicated in patients with respiratory insufficiency, since these patients may experience temporary problems with ventilation and diffusion.
   b. Oxygen, antispasmodic agents and cortisone should be available.
4. Nursing responsibilities after bronchogram:
   a. Withhold fluids and food until patient demonstrates a cough reflex.
   b. Encourage patient to cough and clear his bronchial tree; postural drainage may be required.
   c. A slight elevation of temperature is common following a bronchogram.
5. Physiotherapy is essential before and after this procedure.

Angiographic studies of pulmonary vessels (radio-opacification of pulmonary blood vessels)

1. Contrast media is injected into following blood vessels:
   a. Antecubital veins of one or both arms.
   b. Superior vena cava, right atrium, right ventricle or main pulmonary artery.
   c. Right or left pulmonary artery or one of its branches.
2. Films are taken in rapid sequence after injection.
   a. Useful in diagnosis of pulmonary vascular abnormalities (arterial aneurysm, thromboemboli, congenital disorders) and to detect abnormal vasculature arising from tumours.
3. Aortography – opacification studies of either thoracic aorta or abdominal aorta; taken when aneurysm of thoracic aorta is suspected.

RADIOISOTOPE DIAGNOSTIC PROCEDURES
Perfusion lung scan
Following injection of a radioactive isotope, scans are made with a scintillation camera.
1. Measures blood perfusion through the lungs; evaluates lung function on a regional basis.
2. Useful in perfusion (vascular) abnormalities.

Ventilation scan
1. Inhalation of radioactive gas (xenon), which diffuses throughout the lungs.

2. Useful in detecting ventilation abnormalities (emphysema).

ENDOSCOPIC PROCEDURES
Bronchoscopy
The direct inspection and observation of the larynx, trachea and bronchi through a bronchoscope that is designed for passage through the trachea. It has both diagnostic and therapeutic purposes.
1. Uses:
   a. Inspection of pathological changes in the bronchial tree.
   b. Removal of secretions (sputum) and tissue for cytological and bacteriological study.
   c. Removal of a foreign body.
   d. Improvement of drainage.
   e. Treatment by application of chemotherapeutic agent.
2. Local (topical) or general anaesthesia is used.

Nursing responsibilities:
1. Ensure that the patient understands the procedure, and that the consent form is signed.
2. Administer medication to reduce secretions and prevent vasovagal syncope and relieve anxiety. Give encouragement and nursing support.
3. Restrict fluid and food for six hours before procedure – to reduce risk of aspiration when reflexes are blocked.
4. Remove dentures, contact lenses and other prostheses.
5. After the procedure, wait until patient demonstrates that he can cough before giving him cracked ice or fluids. A return to his usual diet is resumed in a few hours.
6. Following bronchoscopy:
   a. Ensure correct position before and after return of cough reflex.
   b. Assist productive coughing.
7. Following bronchoscopy, watch patient for:
   a. Cyanosis.
   b. Hypotension.
   c. Tachycardia and dysrhythmia.
   d. Haemoptysis.
   e. Dyspnoea.
   f. Bronchospasm.
   g. Blocked airways.

Flexible fibreoptic bronchoscopy
Passage of thin, flexible and bronchofibrescope that can be directed into segmental bronchi; by its smaller size, flexibility and excellent optical system, it allows increased visualization of peripheral airways.

1. May be done with patient resting in sitting or supine position.
2. Causes very little discomfort; better patient acceptance even under local anaesthetic only.
3. Allows for bronchial brush biopsy (see below).
4. Clinical applications for flexible fibreoptic bronchoscopy are similar to those for rigid bronchoscopy (see below); allows diagnostic visualization of enlarged area for observation and biopsy; therapeutic removal of secretions, evaluation of haemoptysis.
5. Possible complications: reaction to anaesthetic agent, penumothorax, bleeding.

Bronchial brush biopsy
Bronchofibrescope is introduced into the target bronchus under fluoroscopic monitoring. It is used to evaluate lung lesions and to identify pathogenic organisms.
1. Small brush attached to end of flexible wire is inserted through the fibrescope.
2. Tumour area is brushed back and forth to desquamate some of the mucosal cells.
   a. Smears and culture are made.
   b. Catheter is irrigated with saline for additional cultures and cytology material.

Nursing responsibilities:
1. See that consent form has been signed.
2. Patient may have a mild sore throat and transient haemoptysis after procedure.
3. Possible complications: anaesthetic reactions, laryngospasm, pneumothorax (rare), haemoptysis.

EXAMINATION OF SPUTUM
Purpose
1. Sputum is obtained for evaluation of gross appearance, for microscopic examination, for Gram staining and culture to identify the predominant organisms and for cytological examination.
   a. Direct smear – shows presence of pathogenic bacteria.
   b. Sputum culture – to make diagnosis, to determine drug sensitivity and to serve as a guide for drug treatment (choice of antibiotic).
   c. Sputum cytology (exfoliative cytology) – used to identify tumour cells.
2. Patients receiving antibiotics, steroids and immunosuppressive agents for prolonged periods may have periodic sputum examinations since these agents may give rise to opportunistic pulmonary infections.

Methods of obtaining sputum
(Ensure patient is supported in correct position.)
1. By deep breathing and coughing:
   a. Instruct patient to take several deep breaths, exhale and then clear his throat.
   b. Repeat three or four times.
   c. Ask patient to cough vigorously and expectorate into sterile container.
   d. See that specimen is transported to laboratory immediately; allowing it to stand in a warm room will result in overgrowth of contaminating organisms, and make culture more difficult and may alter cellular morphology.
   e. Give oral hygiene frequently, especially if patient has foul sputum.
2. By ultrasonic or heated hypertonic saline nebulization:
   a. Patient inhales through mouth slowly and deeply for 10 to 15 minutes.
   b. Increases the moisture content of air going to lower tract; particles will condense on tracheobronchial tree and aid in expectoration.
3. Tracheal aspiration.
4. Bronchoscopic removal.
5. Bronchial brushing guided by fluoroscopy.
6. Gastric aspiration:
   a. Nasogastric tube is inserted into the stomach to siphon out swallowed pulmonary secretions.
   b. This test is useful for culture of tubercle bacilli.

EXAMINATION OF PLEURAL FLUID AND PLEURAL BIOPSY
Pleural fluid
A thin layer of fluid remains in the pleural space; abnormal amounts of pleural fluid (effusion) have varied aetiologies and the pleural fluid is studied along with other tests to determine underlying cause.
1. Pleural fluid is obtained by aspiration or by tube thoracotomy.
2. Pleural fluid is examined for protein content, specific gravity and presence or absence of formed elements. (Sediment may demonstrate malignant cells.)
   a. Pleural fluid is usually light straw colour.
   b. Purulent fluid – suggests empyema.
   c. Blood-tinged fluid – pulmonary infarction; neoplastic disease.
   d. Milky fluid (chylothorax) – invasion of thoracic duct by tumour or inflammatory process; traumatic rupture of thoracic duct.
3. Observe and record total amount of fluid with-

drawn, nature of fluid and its colour and viscosity.

4. Prepare sample of fluid for laboratory evaluation if ordered.

5. Routine studies include Gram-stain culture and sensitivity; acid-fast stain and culture for acid-fast bacilli; cell count and differential; cytology; specific gravity; total protein; lactic dehydrogenase.

Pleural biopsy

Accomplished via needle biopsy of pleura or via pleuroscopy (visual exploration of pleural space through a bronchofibrescope inserted into pleural space).

BIOPSY PROCEDURES OF THE LUNG
Objective
Obtain histological material from lung.

Transbronchoscopic biopsy

Flexible forceps inserted through bronchoscope and specimen of lung tissue obtained.

Percutaneous needle biopsy

1. Skin site cleansed and anaesthetized.
2. Small skin incision is made and a needle is advanced under fluoroscopic control to the desired site.
3. With the needle in the periphery of the lesion, the stylet is removed, the syringe attached and suction applied.
4. Specimen is smeared and fixed on a slide.

Open lung biopsy

1. Used in making a diagnosis when other biopsy methods fail.
2. Usually done by a small anterior thoracotomy; does not usually involve a rib resection.
3. Subsequent pneumothorax controlled by chest tube connected to a water-seal drainage system.

LYMPH NODE BIOPSY (SCALENE OR CERVICOMEDIASTINAL NODES)
Objective
To detect lymph node spread of pulmonary disease. It is used as a diagnostic and prognostic measure.

1. Scalene lymph nodes are enmeshed in deep cervical pad of fat; these nodes drain lungs and mediastinum and may show histological changes from intrathoracic disease.

2. Mediastinoscopy – surgery of superior mediastinum for exploration and biopsy of mediastinal nodes.
   a. Done to detect mediastinal involvement of pulmonary malignancy and to obtain tissue for diagnosis of other conditions (e.g. sarcoidosis).
   b. Biopsy usually done through a suprasternal incision.

PULMONARY FUNCTION STUDIES
These are shown in Table 4.1.
1. Static lung volumes – low lung volumes indicate restrictive abnormalities (fibrosis, sarcoidosis, scoliosis). High residual volume (air remaining after maximal exhalation) indicates air trapping (emphysema).
2. Dynamic lung volumes (ventilatory studies) – reduction generally indicates airway obstruction (emphysema, bronchitis, asthma).
3. Diffusing capacity – reduction indicates loss of lung surface effective in transfer of gas (sarcoidosis, fibrosis, emphysema).

ESSENTIALS OF ARTERIAL BLOOD GAS EVALUATION
Purpose
1. Are a measurement of the amount of oxygen and carbon dioxide present in arterial blood, as well as the pH of the blood.
2. Provide a means of assessing the adequacy of ventilation, i.e. the lungs supplying O_2 to the body and removing CO_2.
3. Helps assess the acid–base status in the body – whether acidosis or alkalosis is present and to what degree.

Clinical uses of arterial blood gas studies
Arterial blood gas studies are helpful in diagnosis and treatment in the presence of the following:
1. Unexpected tachypnoea, dyspnoea (especially in patients with cardiopulmonary disease).
2. Unexpected restlessness and anxiety in bed patients.
3. Drowsiness and confusion in patients receiving oxygen therapy.
4. Before thoracic and other major surgery.
5. Before and during prolonged oxygen therapy and during ventilator support of patients.
6. Critically ill cardiopulmonary patients; tissue oxygenation and acid–base balance eventually affected.

Table 4.1 Ventilatory function tests*

Description	Terms used	Symbol	Remarks
The largest volume measured on complete expiration after the deepest inspiration without forced or rapid effort	Vital capacity	VC	This may be normal or even high in patients with chronic obstructive airways disease and is *of little value by itself*
The vital capacity performed with expiration as forceful and rapid as possible	Forced vital capacity	FVC	This volume is often significantly reduced in chronic obstructive airways disease due to air-trapping, and is an important standard measurement
Volume of gas exhaled over a given time interval during the performance of forced vital capacity	Forced expiratory volume (qualified by subscript indicating the time interval in seconds)	FEV_T ($FEV_{1.0}$)	If below predicted normal values, this is a valuable clue to the severity of the expiratory airway obstruction
FEV_T expressed as a percentage of the forced vital capacity: $\dfrac{FEV_{T \times 100}}{FVC}$	Percentage expired (in T seconds)	$FEV_{T\%}$	This time–volume relationship is another way of expressing the presence of airway obstruction
The average rate of flow for a specified portion of the forced expiratory volume, usually between 200 and 1,200ml	Forced expiratory flow	$FEF_{200-1200}$	Formally called maximum expiratory flow rate (MEFR). A slowed rate is an early manifestation of chronic obstructive airways disease
Average rate of flow during the middle half of the forced expiratory volume	Forced mid-expiratory flow	$FEF_{25-75\%}$	Formerly called maximum mid-expiratory flow rate. This is slowed early in the course of ventilatory impairment
Volume of air which a subject can breathe with voluntary maximal effort for a given time	Maximal voluntary ventilation	MVV	Formerly called maximum breathing capacity. Another valuable test, usually correlating well with the patient's complaint of dyspnoea

* Source: American Lung Association: *Chronic Obstructive Airways Disease*, 1972.

GUIDELINES: TRACHEAL ASPIRATION

PURPOSE
To obtain a sputum specimen; to relieve obstruction.

EQUIPMENT
Tracheal aspirate specimen collection set.

PROCEDURE

Nursing action	Rationale
Note: Tracheal aspiration requires education and clinical practice under expert supervision.	

1. Use sterile equipment:
  a. Sterile catheter No. 16 F, connecting tubing to tracheal aspirate specimen collection set.
  b. Sterile gloves
  c. Explain procedure to patient.
	To prevent introduction of organisms into the respiratory system. A clear explanation will enable the patient to co-operate where possible.

2. Oxygenate patient before and after each passage of the catheter.	
3. Using one hand, pass the catheter (suction turned off) through the patient's nose; place the other hand on the patient's forehead. Alternatively, a catheter can be passed via an oral airway, through the patient's mouth.	To stabilize the patient's head and to reassure the patient.
4. When the catheter reaches the larynx, coughing may be stimulated. Gently advance the catheter into the trachea.	At this point, coughing is unproductive.
5. Pull catheter slightly forward; this will initiate vigorous coughing. Provide tissues for patient's expectorations.	Irritation of trachea triggers coughing reflex.
6. Apply suction and remove catheter gently.	
7. Send specimen to laboratory.	
8. Comfort patient.	

GUIDELINES: ASSISTING THE PATIENT UNDERGOING CHEST ASPIRATION

Chest aspiration (thoracentesis) is the aspiration of fluid or air from the pleural space. It may be a diagnostic or a therapeutic procedure.

PURPOSES
1. Remove fluid and air from the pleural cavity.
2. Obtain diagnostic aspiration of pleural fluid.
3. Obtain pleural biopsy.

EQUIPMENT
Syringes: 5, 20, 25, 50ml syringes
Needles: Nos. 22, 26, 16 (7.5cm long)
Three-way tap and rubber tubing
Local anaesthetic
Biopsy needle
Antiseptic lotion for skin cleansing
Sterile pack containing: gauze swabs, gallipots, dissecting forceps, wool
   swabs, sterile towels, sterile jug
Three sterile specimen containers
Sterile gloves
Spencer Wells artery forceps

PROCEDURE
Preparatory phase

Nursing action	Rationale
1. Ascertain in advance if chest X-rays have been ordered and completed. These should be available at the bedside.	Posteroanterior and lateral chest X-rays are used to localize fluid and air in the pleural cavity and to aid in determining the puncture site.
2. See if consent form has been explained and signed.	
3. Determine if the patient is allergic to the local anaesthetic agent to be used. Give sedation if prescribed.	
4. Inform the patient about the procedure and indicate how he can be helpful. Explain: a. The nature of the procedure. b. The importance of remaining immobile. c. Pressure sensations to be experienced, but he should indicate if he is in pain. d. That no discomfort is anticipated after the procedure.	The patient should be encouraged to ask questions before the procedure. If he wishes to speak or cough during the procedure, he should warn the doctor, before doing so, by raising the hand on the opposite side to the aspiration.

5. Make the patient comfortable with adequate supports (Figure 4.5). If possible place him upright and in one of the following positions:
   a. Sitting on the edge of the bed with feet supported and head on a padded over-the-bed table.
   b. Straddling a chair with his arms and head resting on the back of the chair.
      If he is unable to assume a sitting position have him lie on the unaffected side.

The upright position facilitates the removal of fluid that usually localizes at the base of the chest. A comfortable position helps the patient to relax.

6. Support and reassure the patient during the procedure.
   a. Prepare the patient for sensations of cold from skin cleanser and for pressure and sting from infiltration of local anaesthetic agent.
   b. Encourage the patient to refrain from coughing. A cough linctus may be needed.

Sudden and unexpected movement by the patient can cause trauma to the visceral pleura with possible penetration of the lung.

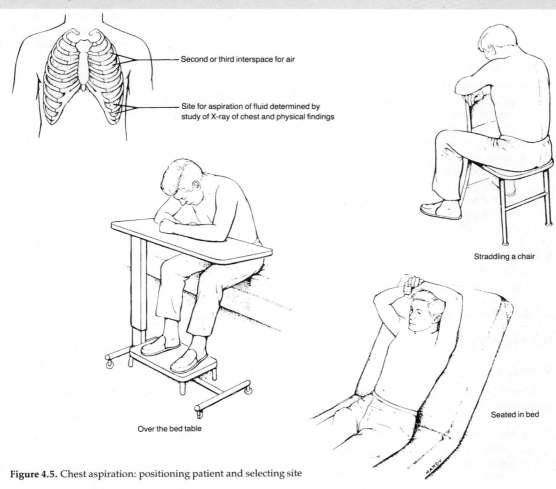

Second or third interspace for air

Site for aspiration of fluid determined by study of X-ray of chest and physical findings

Straddling a chair

Over the bed table

Seated in bed

Figure 4.5. Chest aspiration: positioning patient and selecting site

Performance phase

Nursing action

1. Expose the entire chest. The site for aspiration is determined from chest X-rays and by percussion. If fluid is in the pleural cavity, the thoracocentesis site is determined by study of the chest X-ray and physical findings, with attention to the site of maximal dullness on percussion.

2. The procedure is done under aseptic conditions. After the skin is cleansed, the doctor slowly injects a local anaesthetic with a small-calibre needle into the skin, then into the deeper tissues.

3. The doctor advances the aspiration needle with the syringe attached. When the pleural space is reached, suction may be applied with the syringe.
   a. A 20 or 50ml syringe with a three-way adapter (stopcock) is attached to the needle. (One end of the adapter is attached to the needle and the other to the tubing leading to a receptacle that receives the fluid being aspirated.)
   b. If a considerable quantity of fluid is to be removed, the needle is held in place on the chest wall with a small pair of artery forceps.

4. After the needle is withdrawn, pressure is applied over the puncture site and a small sterile dressing is fixed in place.

5. Observe patient for faintness or shock.

Rationale

If air is in the pleural cavity, the aspiration site is usually in the second or third intercostal space in the mid-clavicular line. Air rises in the thorax because the density of air is much less than the density of liquid.

An intradermal wheal is raised slowly; rapid intradermal injection causes pain. The parietal pleura is very sensitive and should be well infiltrated with anaesthetic before the aspiration needle is passed through it.
When a large quantity of fluid is withdrawn, a three-way adapter serves to keep air from entering the pleural cavity.
The artery forceps steady the needle on the chest wall. Sudden pleuritic pain or shoulder pain may indicate that the visceral or diaphragmatic pleura are being irritated by the needle point.

Follow-up phase

Nursing action

1. A chest X-ray is usually obtained following chest aspiration.

2. Record the total amount of fluid withdrawn and the nature of the fluid and carefully label the specimen jars. A specimen container with formalin may be needed if a pleural biopsy is being performed.

Rationale

Chest X-ray verifies that there is no pneumothorax.

The fluid may be clear, serous, bloody, purulent, etc.

3. Observe the patient frequently for increasing respirations, faintness, vertigo, tightness in the chest, uncontrollable cough, blood-tinged, frothy mucus and rapid pulse.

Pneumothorax, tension pneumothorax, subcutaneous emphysema or pyogenic infection may result from an aspiration. Pulmonary oedema or cardiac distress can be produced by a sudden shift in mediastinal contents when large amounts of fluid are aspirated.

CHEST PHYSIOTHERAPY

NURSING ALERT
The following exercises are normally carried out by a physiotherapist. However, nurses working in a specialized unit should fully understand the principles of these exercises, and be able to carry out basic physiotherapy in the absence of an expert.

POSTURAL DRAINAGE EXERCISE
Postural drainage is the use of specific positions so that the force of gravity can assist in the removal of bronchial secretions from the affected bronchioles into the bronchi and trachea (Figure 4.6).

UNDERLYING PRINCIPLES
1. The patient is positioned so that the diseased area(s) are in a vertical position, and gravity is used to assist drainage of the specific segment(s).
2. The positions assumed are determined by the location, severity and duration of mucus obstruction.
3. The exercises are usually performed two to four times daily, before meals and at bedtime.

NURSING MANAGEMENT
1. Make the patient comfortable before the procedure starts and as comfortable as possible while he assumes each position.
   a. Bronchodilator medications may be inhaled before postural drainage to reduce bronchospasm, decrease thickness of mucus and sputum, and combat oedema of the bronchial walls.
   b. Use a back rest to prop up patient to desired height if his bed is not adjustable; have a sputum pot ready.
2. Use a stethoscope to determine the areas of needed drainage.
3. Upper lobes are generally drained by upright positions; lower and middle lobes are drained by head-down positions.
4. Place patient in left prone and left oblique positions (simultaneously) – this will give additional drainage to middle lobe and lateral segments of the right lower lobe; assuming the right prone and right oblique position (simultaneously) will give additional drainage to middle lobe and lateral segments of the left lower lobe.
5. Encourage the patient to cough after he has spent the allotted time in each position.
6. Encourage diaphragmatic breathing throughout postural drainage exercises; this helps widen airways so that secretions can be drained.
7. Chest wall percussion (by another person) may be desirable to loosen and propel sputum in the direction of gravity drainage.
8. Evaluate patient's colour and pulse the first few times he performs these exercises.
9. Help the patient to brush his teeth and use mouthwash after postural drainage.
10. Encourage patient to rest in bed following the procedure.

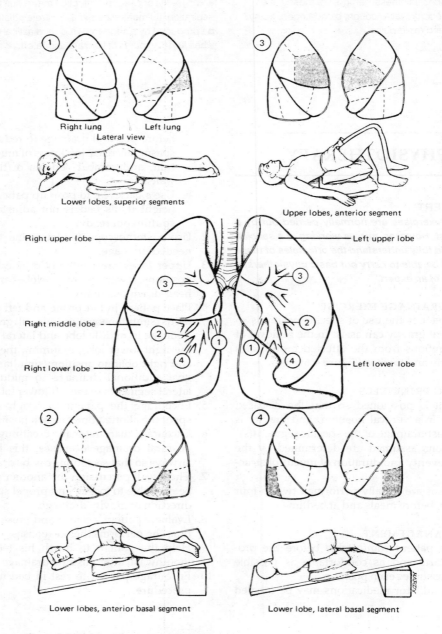

Figure 4.6. Positions for postural drainage

GUIDELINES: PERCUSSION (CLAPPING) AND VIBRATION

Percussion and vibration are manual techniques designed to loosen secretions and promote drainage of mucus and secretions from the lungs while the patient is in the position of postural drainage indicated for his specific lung problem. The procedure requires trained personnel.

1. Percussion – Movement done by striking the chest wall in a rhythmical fashion with cupped hands over the chest segment to be drained. The wrists are alternatively flexed and extended so that the chest is cupped or clapped in a painless manner.
2. Vibration – Technique of applying manual compression and tremor to the chest wall during the exhalation phase of respiration.

OBJECTIVES

1. Dislodge mucus adhering to the bronchioles and bronchi.
2. Help mobilize secretions.

CLINICAL INDICATIONS

Lung conditions that cause increased production of secretions:

1. Bronchiectasis.
2. Empyema.
3. Cystic fibrosis.
4. Chronic bronchitis.
5. Post-thoracic surgery (with analgesics).

CONTRAINDICATIONS

1. Lung abscess or tumours.
2. Pneumothorax.
3. Disease of the chest wall.
4. Lung haemorrhage.
5. Painful chest conditions.
6. Tuberculosis.

PROCEDURE
Performance phase

Nursing action	Rationale
1. Tell the patient to use diaphragmatic breathing.	Diaphragmatic breathing helps the patient to relax and helps to widen airways.
2. Position the patient in prescribed postural drainage position(s). The spine should be straight to promote rib cage expansion.	The patient is positioned according to which area of the lung is to be drained.
3. Percuss (or clap) with cupped hands over the chest wall for one or two minutes from: a. The lower ribs to shoulders in the back. b. The lower ribs to top of chest in front.	This action helps to dislodge mucous plugs and mobilize secretions toward the main bronchi and trachea. The air trapped between the operator's hand and chest wall will produce a characteristic hollow sound.

4. Avoid clapping over the spine, liver, kidneys or spleen.

Percussion over these areas may cause injuries to the spine and internal organs.

5. Instruct the patient to inhale slowly and deeply. Vibrate the chest wall as the patient exhales slowly through pursed lips.

This sets up a vibration that carries through the chest wall and helps free the mucus.
This manoeuvre is performed in the direction in which the ribs move upon expiration.
Contracting the abdominal muscles while coughing increases cough effectiveness. Coughing aids in the movement and expulsion of secretions.

   a. Place one hand on top of the other over affected area or place one hand on each side of the rib cage.
   b. Tense the muscles of the hands and arms causing the arms to vibrate in a rapid motion.
   c. Relieve pressure on the thorax as the patient inhales.
   d. Encourage the patient to cough, using his abdominal muscles, after three or four vibrations.

6. Allow the patient to rest for several minutes.

7. Listen with a stethoscope to changes in breath sounds.

The appearance of moist sounds (râles, rhonchi) indicates movement of air around mucus in the bronchi.

8. Repeat the percussion and vibration cycle according to the patient's tolerance and his clinical response; usually 15 to 20 minutes.

NURSING ALERT
Postural drainage and percussion may result in hypoxia and should only be used if secretions are believed to be present.

GUIDELINES: TEACHING THE PATIENT BREATHING EXERCISES

Breathing exercises are exercises and breathing practices that are utilized to correct respiratory deficits and to increase efficiency in breathing.

PURPOSES
1. Relax muscles and relieve anxiety.
2. Eliminate useless unco-ordinated patterns of respiratory muscle activity.
3. Slow the respiratory rate.
4. Decrease the work of breathing.
5. Expand lower lobe and prevent hypostatic pneumonia and facilitate venous return.

GENERAL INSTRUCTIONS
1. Clear the nasal passages before beginning breathing exercises.
2. Always inhale through the nose – permits filtration, humidification and warming of air.

3. Breathe slowly in a rhythmical and relaxed manner – permits more complete exhalation and emptying of lungs; helps overcome anxiety associated with dyspnoea and decreases oxygen requirement.
4. Avoid sudden exertion.
5. Practise breathing exercises in several positions, since air distribution and pulmonary circulation vary according to position of the chest.

DIAPHRAGMATIC BREATHING
Purpose
To increase the use of the diaphragm during breathing.

Teaching procedure	Rationale
Instruct the patient as follows:	
1. Place one hand on stomach just below the ribs and the other hand on the middle of the chest.	This helps the patient to become aware of the diaphragm and its function in breathing.
2. Breathe in slowly and deeply through the nose, letting the abdomen protrude as far as it will (Figure 4.7). The abdomen enlarges during inspiration and decreases in size during expiration.	Slow inhalation provides ventilation and hyperinflation of the lungs.
3. Breathe out through pursed lips while contracting (tightening) the abdominal muscles.	Contracting the abdominal muscles assists the diaphragm in rising to empty the lung.
4. The chest should move as little as possible; attention should be directed to the abdomen, not the chest.	Contraction of the abdominal muscles should take place during expiration.

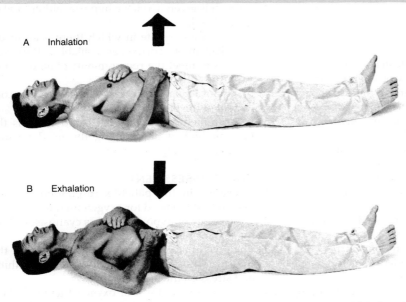

A   Inhalation

B   Exhalation

Figure 4.7. Breathing exercises for inhalation and exhalation (Source: *Living with Asthma, Chronic Bronchitis and Emphysema*, Riker Laboratories, Northridge, California)

5. Repeat for approximately one minute (followed by a rest period of two minutes). Work up to 10 minutes, four times daily.

6. Learn to do diaphragmatic breathing while lying, then sitting and ultimately standing and walking.

Diaphragmatic breathing should become automatic with sufficient practice and concentration. If the patient becomes short of breath have him stop the exercises until his breathing pattern comes under control.

Other exercises

Lateral costal breathing
1. Place hands on sides on lower ribs.
2. Inhale deeply and slowly while sides expand, moving hands outward.
3. Exhale slowly and feel the hands and ribs move in.
4. Rest.

Posterior basal breathing
1. Sit in a chair. Place hands behind back; hold flat against lower ribs.
2. Inhale deeply and slowly while rib cage expands backward; the hands will move outward.
3. Keep hands in place. Blow out slowly; hands will move in.

OXYGEN THERAPY

GENERAL CONSIDERATIONS
1. Oxygen is an odourless, tasteless, colourless transparent gas that is slightly heavier than air.
2. Oxygen supports combustion, so there is always danger of fire when oxygen is being used:
   a. Avoid using oil or grease around oxygen connections.
   b. Eliminate antiseptic tinctures, alcohol and ether in immediate oxygen environment.
   c. Do not permit any electrical devices (radios, heating pads, electric razors) in or near an oxygen tent.
   d. Keep the oxygen cylinder (if used) secured in an upright position away from heat.
   e. Post 'NO SMOKING' signs on the patient's door and in view of the patient's visitors.
   f. Have fire extinguisher available.
3. Oxygen is dispensed from a cylinder or piped-in system and requires:
   a. Reduction gauge – reduces pressure to that of the atmosphere.
   b. Flow meter (flow gauge, flow control) – regulates control of oxygen in litres per minute.
4. Oxygen is given to relieve hypoxia, either local or generalized.
   a. Hypoxia – a state in which there is an insufficient amount of oxygen available in the tissue cells to meet the requirements of an organ or tissue at that moment.
   b. Hypoxaemia – a decrease in the oxygen content of the blood.
5. Measurement of the arterial blood gases is the best method of determining the need for and adequacy of oxygen therapy.

CLINICAL ASSESSMENT
1. A change in the patient's respiration is often evidence of the need for oxygen therapy.
2. Other signs of hypoxia, such as cyanosis, may or may not be present.
3. The goal in administering oxygen is to treat the hypoxia while decreasing the work of breathing and stress on the myocardium.
4. The appropriate form of oxygen therapy is best ascertained after obtaining arterial blood gases, which will indicate the patient's oxygenation status and acid–base balance.

5. Oxygen must be given with extreme caution to some patients. In certain conditions (chronic obstructive airways disease) the administration of a high oxygen concentration will remove the respiratory drive that has been created largely by the patient's low oxygen tension:
   a. Ventilation is reduced.
   b. Acute acidosis and carbon dioxide narcosis may follow.

Note: Oxygen toxicity should always be of concern in the patient receiving inspired concentrations over 60 per cent for over 24 hours.

OXYGEN DELIVERY SYSTEMS

1. Oxygen may be administered by nasal cannula, oropharyngeal catheter (nasal catheter), various types of face masks and tent. It may also be applied directly to endotracheal or tracheal tube via a 'T' piece.

2. The method selected depends on the concentration of oxygen required.

MONITORING OXYGEN THERAPY

NURSING ALERT

1. *Arterial blood gas evaluations are the best means of gauging the effectiveness of oxygen therapy and guiding appropriate changes. Of particular importance is the effect of oxygen therapy on the patient who has chronic obstructive lung disease and who may retain carbon dioxide if given too much oxygen. Frequent blood gas evaluations may be necessary in this type of patient to make sure that his respiratory drive is not suppressed. Also continue clinical observations, as above.*

2. *Various types of oxygen analysers are available which allows the nurse to measure the concentration of oxygen delivered to the patient. Oxygen analysers are especially useful in measuring the amount of oxygen delivered by the various types of masks.*

GUIDELINES: ASSISTING THE PATIENT RECEIVING OXYGEN BY NASAL CANNULA

This is shown in Figure 4.8.

PURPOSE

To administer a low-to-medium concentration of oxygen, when precise accuracy is not essential.

EQUIPMENT

Oxygen source
Plastic nasal cannula with connecting tubing (disposable)
Humidifier filled with sterile distilled water to indicated level
Flowmeter
'NO SMOKING' signs

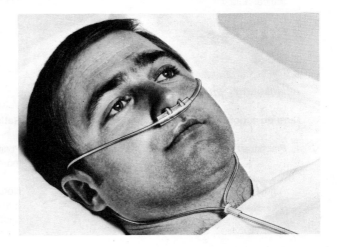

Figure 4.8. Administering oxygen by nasal cannula (courtesy: Hudson Oxygen Therapy Sales Company)

Assessment

Nursing action

1. Assess the patient's respiratory rate and level of consciousness.

2. Determine current arterial blood gases if available.

Rationale

Nasal cannula oxygen administration is often used for patients prone to CO_2 retention. Oxygen may depress the hypoxic drive of these patients (evidenced by a decreased respiratory rate, altered mental status, and further $Paco_2$ elevation).

Note: If $Paco_2$ is decreased or normal, the patient is not experiencing CO_2 retention and can use oxygen without fear of the above consequences.

Planning and implementation
Preparatory phase

Nursing action

1. Post 'NO SMOKING' signs on the patient's door and in view of patient and visitors.

2. Show the nasal cannula to the patient and explain the procedure.

3. Make sure that the humidifier is filled to the appropriate mark.

4. Attach the connecting tube from the nasal cannula to the humidifier outlet.

5. Set the flow rate at prescribed litres/minute. Feel to determine if oxygen is flowing through the tips of the cannula.

Rationale

If the humidifier bottle is not sufficiently full, less moisture will be delivered.

Approximate oxygen concentrators delivered by nasal cannula are:

   1 litre = 24 per cent
   2 litres = 28 per cent
   3 litres = 32 per cent
   4 litres = 36 per cent
   5 litres = 40 per cent

Performance phase

Nursing action

1. Place the tips of the cannula in the patient's nose.

2. Adjust flow to prescribed rate.

Rationale

Position the cannula so that the tips do not extend more than 2.5cm into the nares.

Note: Because a nasal cannula is a low-flow system (patient's tidal volume supplies part of the inspired gas), oxygen concentration will vary, depending on the patient's respiratory rate and tidal volume.

NURSING ALERT

Patients who require low, constant concentrations of oxygen and whose breathing pattern varies greatly may need to use a Venturi mask, particularly if they are carbon dioxide retainers.

Follow-up phase

Nursing action

1. Change cannula, humidifiers, tubing and other equipment exposed to moisture frequently.

2. Assess patient's condition, arterial blood gases and the functioning of equipment at regular intervals.

Rationale

Contaminated equipment may cause infection in debilitated patients.

Depression of hypoxaemic drive is most likely to occur within the first hours of oxygen use.

Evaluation/outcome

Nursing action

1. Record flow rate used, patient response.

2. Determine patient comfort with oxygen use.

Rationale

Note the patient's tolerance of treatment. Notify the doctor if intolerance is noted.

Flow rates in excess of four litres/minute may lead to air swallowing and cause irritation to the nasal and pharyngeal mucosa. If higher concentrations are required, consider an alternate form of therapy.

GUIDELINES: ASSISTING THE PATIENT RECEIVING OXYGEN BY VENTURI MASK

A Venturi mask is a face mask designed to administer precisely controlled low oxygen concentrations (24, 28, 32, 35 and 40 per cent). It is used primarily to increase the comfort and breathing efficiency of the patient with chronic lung disease, but may safely be used by other patients if they need it and if their oxygen need is met (Figure 4.9).

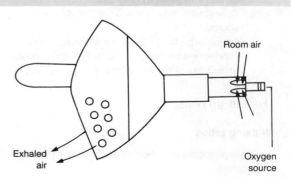

Room air

Exhaled air

Oxygen source

Figure 4.9. Venturi mask (courtesy: *Manual of Clinical Nursing Procedures*, The Royal Marsden Hospital, Harper & Row)

Assessment

Nursing action

1. Assess patient's respiratory rate and level of consciousness.

2. Determine current arterial blood gases if available.

Rationale

Venturi masks are used for patients prone to CO_2 retention. Oxygen may depress the hypoxic drive of these patients (evidenced by a decreased respiratory rate, altered mental status and further $Paco_2$ elevation).

Planning and implementation
Preparatory phase

Nursing action

1. Post 'NO SMOKING' signs on the door of the patient's room and in view of patient and visitors.

2. Show the Venturi mask to the patient and explain the procedure.

3. Connect the mask by lightweight tubing to the oxygen source.

4. Turn on the oxygen flowmeter and adjust to the prescribed rate (usually indicated on the mask). Check to see that oxygen is flowing out the vent holes in the mask.

Rationale

To ensure the correct air/oxygen mix, oxygen must be set at the prescribed flow rate. Prescribed flow rates differ for different oxygen concentrations. Usually this information is printed on the mask or interchangeable colour-coded adapter.

Performance phase

Nursing action

1. Place Venturi mask over the patient's nose and mouth and under the chin. Adjust elastic strap.

2. Check to make sure holes for air entry are not obstructed by the patient's bedding.

3. If high humidity is used:
   a. Connect the nebulizer to a compressed air source.
   b. Attach large-bore tubing to the nebulizer and connect the tubing to the fitting for high humidity at the base of the Venturi mask.

Rationale

Proper mask function depends on mixing of sufficient amount of air and oxygen.

When a Venturi mask is used with high humidity, both an oxygen source and compressed air source are required. The compressed air source provides air for the air/oxygen mix. Excessive oxygen would be inspired if both tubings were connected to an oxygen source.

Follow-up phase

Nursing action

1. Change the mask, nebulizer and tubing at frequent intervals.

Rationale

Nebulizers, tubing and masks may become contaminated and cause infections.

2. Assess the patient's condition and arterial blood gases, and the functioning of the equipment at regular intervals.

Depression of hypoxic drive is most likely to occur within the first hours of oxygen use.

3. Offer the patient frequent mouth care.

Oxygen has a 'drying' effect.

Evaluation/outcome

Nursing action

Rationale

1. Record inspired oxygen concentration, patient response.

Note the patient's tolerance of treatment. Notify the doctor if intolerance occurs.

2. Determine patient comfort with oxygen use.

Venturi masks are best tolerated for relatively short periods of time because of their size and appearance. They also must be removed for eating and drinking. With improvement in patient condition, a nasal cannula may often be substituted.

GUIDELINES: ADMINISTERING OXYGEN BY AEROSOL MASK

PURPOSE
To provide oxygen in concentrations of 35 per cent or greater with high humidity by administering aerosol mist either heated or unheated, or when high humidity compressed air therapy is desired (Figure 4.10).

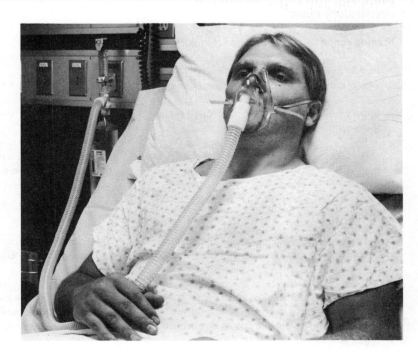

Figure 4.10. Administering oxygen by simple face mask with aerosol (courtesy: Photography Department Montefiore Hospital, Pittsburgh, Pennsylvania)

EQUIPMENT
Oxygen source
Nebulizer bottle with sterile distilled water
Plastic aerosol mask
Large-bore tubing (if high humidity is being used) or small-bore tubing
Flowmeter
'NO SMOKING' signs

Assessment

Nursing action	**Rationale**
1. Assess the patient's respiratory rate, level of consciousness and arterial blood gases, if available.	Because the aerosol face mask is a low-flow system (patient's tidal volume may supply part of inspired gas), oxygen concentration will vary depending on the patient's respiratory rate and rhythm. Oxygen delivery may be inadequate for tachypnoeic patients (flow does not meet peak inspiratory demand) or excessive for patients with slow respirations.
2. Assess viscosity and volume of sputum produced.	Aerosol is given to assist in mobilizing retained secretions.

Planning and implementation
Preparatory phase

Nursing action	**Rationale**
1. Post 'NO SMOKING' signs on patient's door and in view of the patient and visitors.	
2. Show the aerosol mask to the patient and explain the procedure.	
3. Make sure the nebulizer is filled to the appropriate mark.	If the nebulizer bottle is not sufficiently full, less moisture will be delivered.
4. Attach the large-bore tubing from the mask to the nebulizer outlet.	
5. Set desired oxygen concentration on nebulizer bottle and plug in the heating element, if used.	The inspired oxygen concentration is determined by the nebulizer setting. Usual percentages are 35 to 40 per cent.
6. If the patient is tachypnoeic and a concentration of 50 per cent oxygen or greater is desired, two nebulizers and flowmeters should be attached together.	The aerosol mask is a low-flow system. Attaching two nebulizers together doubles nebulizer flow but does *not* change the inspired oxygen concentration.

Performance phase

Nursing action

1. Adjust the flow rate until the desired mist is produced (usually 10 to 12 litres/minute).

2. Apply the mask to the patient's face and adjust the straps so that the mask fits securely and there are no leaks.

Rationale

This ensures that the patient is receiving flow sufficient to meet inspiratory demand and maintains a constant, accurate concentration of oxygen.

Follow-up phase

Nursing action

1. Change mask, tubing, nebulizer and other equipment exposed to moisture at frequent intervals.

2. Assess the patient's condition and the functioning of equipment at regular intervals.

3. If the patient's condition changes, assess arterial blood gases.

4. Drain the tubing frequently. If a heating element is used, the tubing will have to be drained more often.

5. If a heating device is used, the temperature must be checked often.

6. Offer the patient frequent mouth care.

Rationale

Contaminated equipment may cause infection in debilitated patients.

Assess the patient for change in mental status, diaphoresis, changes in blood pressure and increasing heart and respiratory rates.

Inadequate flow rates may cause symptoms of hypoxaemia and hypoxia.

The tubing must be kept free of condensate. Condensate allowed to accumulate in the delivery tube will block flow and alter oxygen concentration.

Excessive temperatures can cause airway burns; patients with elevated temperatures should be humidified with an unheated device.

Condensate may collect around patient's face. Oxygen also has drying effect on the mouth.

Evaluation/outcome

Nursing action

1. Record inspired oxygen concentration and patient response.

2. Record changes in volume and tenacity of sputum produced.

Rationale

Note the patient's tolerance of treatment. Notify the doctor if intolerance occurs.

Indicates effectiveness of therapy.

GUIDELINES: ASSISTING THE PATIENT RECEIVING OXYGEN VIA ENDOTRACHEAL AND TRACHEOSTOMY TUBES

A T-tube is a device which connects directly to the patient's endotracheal or tracheostomy tube; it delivers oxygen and humidity from a nebulizer source (Figure 4.11).

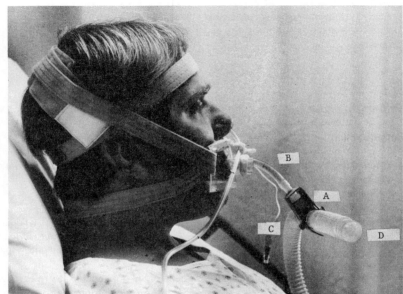

Figure 4.11. Administering oxygen via an endotracheal tube with a T-piece. A T-piece (A) is attached to the endotracheal tube (B) and a large-bore tubing (C) serves as a source for oxygen and humidity with (D) as reservoir tubing

PURPOSE
To administer oxygen in conjunction with humidity to the patient whose upper airway (and its humidification) has been bypassed either by a tracheostomy or by an endotracheal tube.

EQUIPMENT
Oxygen or compressed air source
Flowmeter
Nebulizer and sterile distilled water (heating element may be used as
    described in aerosol masks)
Large bore tubing
T-piece
'NO SMOKING' signs

Planning and implementation
1. Post 'NO SMOKING' signs on the patient's door and in view of patient and visitors.
2. Show the T-tube to the patient and explain the procedure.
3. Make sure the nebulizer is filled to the appropriate mark.
4. Attach the large bore tubing from the T-tube to the nebulizer outlet.
5. Set desired oxygen concentration.

Performance phase

Nursing action

Rationale

1. Adjust the flow rate until desired mist is produced and meets the patient's inspiratory demand.

2. The tubing should be positioned so that it is not pulling on the tracheostomy tube and so that it allows a comfortable range of movement for the patient.

If the tracheostomy or endotracheal tube is pulled, damage can be caused to the trachea.

Follow-up phase

Nursing action

Rationale

1. Change mask, tubing, nebulizer and other equipment exposed to moisture daily.

Contaminated equipment may cause virulent infections in debilitated patients.

2. Assess patient's condition and the functioning of equipment at regular intervals.

Assess the patient for mental aberration, disturbed consciousness, abnormal colour, perspiration, changes in blood pressure and increasing heart and respiratory rates.

3. Drain the tubing frequently. If a heating element is used, the tubing will have to be monitored and drained more often.

The tubing must be kept free of condensate. Condensate allowed to accumulate in the delivery tube will block flow and alter oxygen concentration.

4. If a heating device is used, the temperature must be checked often.

Excessive temperatures can cause airway burns; patients with elevated temperatures will be better humidified with an unheated device.

5. If the patient appears tachypnoeic, increase flow rate and monitor the oxygen concentration with an oxygen analyser.

Inadequate flow rates may cause inaccurate oxygen concentrations in patients who are tachypnoeic.

Evaluation/outcome

Nursing action

Rationale

1. Record inspired oxygen concentration and note patient's response.

Observe the patient's tolerance to the treatment. Notify the doctor if intolerance occurs.

GUIDELINES: ASSISTING THE PATIENT RECEIVING OXYGEN BY TRACHEOSTOMY COLLAR

A tracheostomy collar (Figure 4.12) is a device that fits over the tracheostomy and delivers humidity and oxygen.

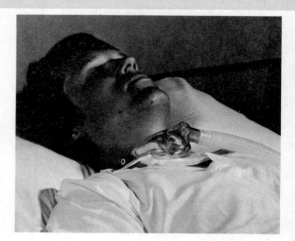

Figure 4.12. Administering oxygen by tracheostomy collar

PURPOSE
To administer humidity (either with or without oxygen) to the tracheostomized patient. If the patient does not require either precise or high concentrations of oxygen he is usually more comfortable with a tracheostomy collar than with a T-tube.

EQUIPMENT
Oxygen or compressed air source
Flowmeter
Nebulizer and sterile distilled water
Large bore tubing
Tracheostomy collar
'NO SMOKING' signs

Planning and implementation
Performance phase

Nursing action	Rationale
1. Adjust the flow rate until the desired mist is produced and meets the patient's inspiratory demand.	The aerosol mist in the tracheostomy collar should not be completely withdrawn on the patient's inspiration.

Follow-up phase

Nursing action	Rationale
1. Change mask tubing, nebulizers and other equipment exposed to moisture daily.	Contaminated equipment may cause virulent infections in delibitated patients.

GUIDELINES: ASSISTING THE PATIENT USING OXYGEN WITH CPAP

Continuous positive airway pressure (CPAP) is used in the spontaneously breathing patient in conjunction with oxygen. It maintains the alveoli in an 'open' state to allow adequate oxygenation of the patient (Figure 4.13).

CPAP provides expiratory and inspiratory positive airway pressure in a manner similar to positive end-expiratory pressure (PEEP) during mechanical ventilation but without endotracheal intubation. The mask has (1) an inflatable cushion and head strap designed to tightly seal the mask against the face, (2) a PEEP valve incorporated into the exhalation port to maintain positive pressure on exhalation, and (3) uses high inspiratory flow rates to maintain positive pressure on inspiration.

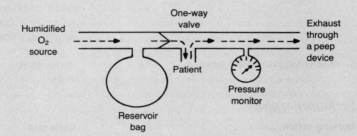

Figure 4.13. A CPAP circuit

EQUIPMENT
Oxygen blender
Flowmeter
CPAP mask
Valve for prescribed PEEP (2.5, 5, 7.5, 10, or 12.5cm H_2O)
Nebulizer with sterile distilled water
Large-bore tubing
Nasogastric tube
Sealing pad to accommodate nasogastric tube

Assessment

Nursing action	Rationale
1. Assess the patient's level of consciousness and gag reflex.	CPAP by face mask may lead to aspiration in patient not sufficiently alert to swallow oral secretions.
2. Determine current arterial blood gases.	Provides a baseline for evaluating response.

NURSING ALERT
1. *CPAP is used when patients have not responded to attempts to increase Pao_2 with other types of masks.*
2. *The patient will require frequent assessment to detect changes in respiratory status, cardiovascular status and level of consciousness.*
3. *If the patient's level of consciousness decreases or arterial blood gases deteriorate, intubation may be necessary.*

Planning and implementation
Preparatory phase

Nursing action	Rationale
1. Post 'NO SMOKING' signs on the patient's door and in view of the patient and visitors.	
2. Show the mask to the patient and explain the procedure.	
3. Make sure nebulizer is filled to the appropriate mark.	
4. Insert nasogastric tube.	With CPAP, the patient may swallow air, causing gastric distension, emesis and/or distension or gastric suture line. Prophylactic nasogastric suction diminishes this risk.
5. Attach nasogastric tube adapter.	Use of adapter may decrease air leak around the mask.

Performance phase

Nursing action	Rationale
1. Set prescribed concentration of oxygen blender and adjust flow rate so that it is sufficient to meet the patient's inspiratory demand.	O_2 blenders are devices that mix air and O_2 using a proportioning valve. Concentrations of 21 to 100 per cent may be delivered at flows of 2 to 100 litres per minute, depending on the model. Because the patient will be receiving all of his minute volume from this 'closed system', it is essential that the flow rate be adequate to meet changes in the patient's breathing pattern.
2. Place the mask on the patient's face, adjust the head strap and inflate the mask cushion to ensure a tight seal.	To maintain CPAP, an airtight seal is required. Head straps and the inflatable cushion help to ensure that difficult areas, such as the nose and chin, are sealed with greater comfort to the patient.
3. Stay with the patient to observe his reaction.	If the CPAP level is too high for a particular individual (CPAP is usually not used in levels above 10cm), the patient's work of breathing may actually be increased rather than diminished.

Follow-up phase

Nursing action	Rationale
1. Assess patient's mental status, respiratory status, cardiovascular status and fluid balance frequently.	Provides objective documentation of patient response. CPAP may increase work of breathing, resulting in patient tiring and inability to maintain ventilation without intubation. CPAP may also decrease venous return (PEEP effect), resulting in decreased cardiac output.

2. Assess patency of nasogastric tube at frequent intervals.

May become obstructed, causing gastric distension.

3. Organize care to remove the mask as infrequently as possible.

If mask is removed (for coughing, suctioning), CPAP is not maintained and inspired oxygen concentrations drop.

4. Assess patient comfort and functioning of the equipment frequently.

Tight fit of the mask may predispose to skin breakdown. System may develop leaks, resulting in air escaping between the patient's face and mask.

Evaluation/outcome

Nursing action

Rationale

1. Record patient response. With improvement, oxygen therapy without positive airway pressure can be substituted. With deterioration, intubation and mechanical ventilation may be required.

Face mask CPAP is usually continued only for short periods (72 hours) because of patient tiring and the necessity to remove mask for suctioning and coughing. Note the patient's tolerance of treatment. Notify doctor if intolerance occurs.

2. Determine patient comfort with oxygen use.

Moisture accumulation and tight fit of the mask predispose to skin breakdown.

GUIDELINES: ASSISTING THE PATIENT RECEIVING OXYGEN BY TENT

An oxygen tent is a device that circulates filtered and cooled air within the environment of a plastic canopy (tent). It is used infrequently and generally only with children.

PURPOSE
To provide a low-to-moderate concentration of oxygen in a temperature-controlled environment.

EQUIPMENT
Oxygen source
Oxygen tent
Special tent call bell

Wrench
'NO SMOKING' signs (2)
Drawsheet

Planning and implementation
Preparatory phase
1. Place 'NO SMOKING' signs on patient's door and on equipment in view of patient and visitors.
2. Explain the benefits of oxygen therapy. To allay anxiety offer this explanation before bringing the equipment into the room.
3. Support the patient in upright position, using back rest and pillows.

4. Connect regulator to oxygen tank or wall outlet.
   a. Plug cord into wall.
   b. Turn on motor.
   c. Adjust temperature control to 18.5 to 22.2°C.
   d. Turn on oxygen tank and flush with high litre rate until desired concentration is reached.

Performance phase

Nursing action	Rationale

1. Extend the rod. Drape canopy over patient and over a half to two-thirds of bed.
   a. Tuck top and side edges of canopy under mattress.
   b. Use a folded drawsheet across patient's legs to improve the seal.
   c. Tuck drawsheet under mattress.
	A tight seal must be made between the canopy and bed to prevent oxygen leaks.

2. Turn flowmeter to 12 to 15 litre/min.	
3. Give the patient the special call bell.	Sparks from an electrical call bell are exceedingly dangerous since oxygen supports combustion.
4. Plan nursing care so that the patient and tent are disturbed as little as possible.	Oxygen is lost by displacement of incoming gas when the canopy is opened and by diffusion of gas molecules through minute leaks around the console.

a. When bathing patient, slide the canopy towards the patient's neck.
   b. Flood the tent with oxygen after readjusting the canopy.
   c. Wrap the patient's head and shoulders if the circulating air causes an uncomfortable draught.
   d. Take the patient's temperature via rectum.
	The oxygen environment is disrupted when the canopy is opened. The patient thereby receives only room air.

5. Use an oxygen analyser to determine oxygen concentration within the tent every four hours.	An oxygen analyser monitors oxygen concentration and permits the nurse or therapist to evaluate the operating efficiency of the tent.

Follow-up phase

Nursing action	Rationale

1. **Note:** Assess the patient every 30 to 45 minutes to determine his condition and to check the following:
   a. Temperature of the tent.
   b. Litre flow.
   c. Amount of oxygen in the tank.
   d. If oxygen vent is unobstructed.
	Assess the patient for drowsiness, mental aberration, disturbed consciousness, abnormal colour, perspiration, changes in blood pressure and increasing heart and respiratory rates.

GUIDELINES: ADMINISTERING OXYGEN BY AMBU-BAG OR BAG–AIRWAY SYSTEMS

An Ambu-bag is used when a patient is not intubated. This situation usually occurs only during a cardiopulmonary arrest (Figure 4.14).

Bag–airway systems are used on an intubated patient and commonly are used to hyperinflate ventilator patients during suctioning and when being transported (Figure 4.15).

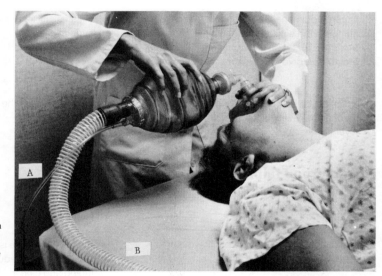

Figure 4.14. Administering oxygen by bag mask. The bag is connected to an oxygen source (A) and supplied with a reservoir tubing (B) (courtesy: Photography Department, Montefiore Hospital, Pittsburgh, Pennsylvania)

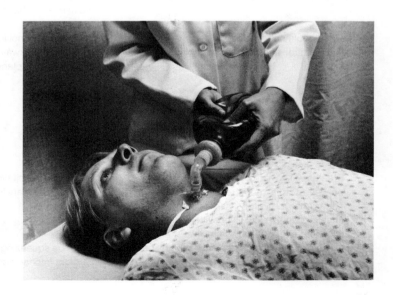

Figure 4.15. Using a resuscitation bag connected to an artificial airway (courtesy: Photography Department, Montefiore Hospital, Pittsburgh, Pennsylvania)

EQUIPMENT
Oxygen source
Resuscitation bag and mask
O_2 connecting tubing
Flowmeter

Assessment

Nursing action

1. In cardiopulmonary arrest, shout for help and place ear to patient's nose and mouth to determine presence/absence of respirations. If respirations are absent, give four breaths, then palpate carotid pulse.

2. If using tracheal suction on a patient who is mechanically ventilated, assess the heart rate, level of consciousness and respiratory status.

Rationale

Initiates call for assistance. Gives initial ventilatory support.

Provides a baseline to estimate patient's tolerance of procedure.

Planning and implementation
Preparatory phase

Nursing action

1. Attach connecting tubing from flowmeter to resuscitation bag.

2. Turn flowmeter to a high flow rate.

3. In a cardiopulmonary arrest situation, every effort should be made to establish a patent airway.

Rationale

A humidifier bottle is not used, since the high flow rates of oxygen required would force water into the tubing and clog it.

A high flow rate or 'flush' position is necessary to meet the minute ventilation of the patient.

If the patient is not intubated, attach mask to the bag, insert an oral airway and, while tilting back the patient's head, place the mask over the patient's face.

Performance phase

Nursing action

1. If cardiac massage is being given:
   a. Breaths will have to be quickly interposed between cardiac compressions. If the patient needs only respiratory assistance, watch for chest expansion and listen with the stethoscope to ensure adequate ventilation.
   b. A rate of approximately 14 to 18 breaths per minute is used unless the patient is being given external cardiac compressions.

Rationale

Squeeze resuscitation bag with sufficient force and at the rate necessary to maintain adequate minute ventilation.

Continue squeezing bag at appropriate intervals until cardiopulmonary resuscitation is no longer required.

2. If hyperinflation is being used with suctioning, ventilate the patient before and after each suctioning pass (*including* after the last suction pass).

Hyperinflation prior to suctioning helps prevent hypoxaemia. Hyperinflation after suctioning replaces O_2 removed during the procedure and helps to prevent atelectasis. The larger tidal volumes may also assist in mobilizing secretions and promote surfactant secretion.

Evaluation/outcome

Nursing action

1. In cardiopulmonary arrest, verify return of spontaneous pulse and respirations. Initiate further support as needed.

2. In tracheal suctioning, return patient to previous support. Note patient tolerance of procedure.

Rationale

Establishes patient's need for definitive therapy (drugs, defibrillation, intensive care).

Note heart rate, rate and ease of respirations, arterial blood pressure (if monitored), level of consciousness. Notify doctor if intolerance occurs.

OTHER RESPIRATORY THERAPEUTIC METHODS

GUIDELINES: ASSISTING THE PATIENT UNDERGOING INTERMITTENT POSITIVE PRESSURE BREATHING (IPPB)

The intermittent positive pressure breathing unit is a piece of equipment that supplies air or oxygen under positive pressure (above atmospheric) during inspiration (Figure 4.16).

PURPOSES
1. Administer aerosolized medication.
2. Mobilize secretions and aid expectoration.
3. Improve alveolar ventilation and prevent atelectasis.
4. Assist respiration via positive pressure on inspiration.

CONTRAINDICATIONS
1. Uncompensated pneumothorax.
2. Mediastinal and subcutaneous emphysema.
3. Untreated active tuberculosis.
4. Use with caution in patients with gastrointestinal surgery, haemoptysis, bullous disease.

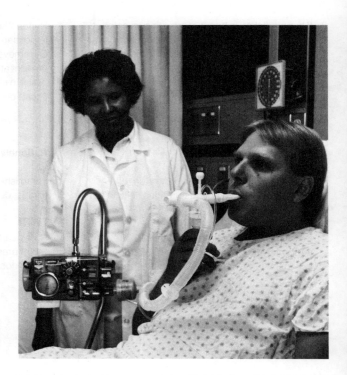

Figure 4.16. Assisting the patient undergoing intermittent positive pressure breathing (IPPB) (courtesy: Photography Department, Montefiore Hospital, Pittsburgh, Pennsylvania)

EQUIPMENT
Intermittent positive pressure breathing (IPPB) circuitry according to the type of machine used
Prescribed medication
'NO SMOKING' signs if oxygen is used as the drive gas

Assessment

Nursing action

1. Monitor the patient's heart rate, especially if the medication prescribed is a bronchodilator.

Rationale

Bronchodilators may produce tachycardia, palpitations, dizziness, nausea and excessive perspiration.

Planning and implementation
Preparatory phase

Nursing action

1. Post 'NO SMOKING' signs. Explain the procedure to the patient.

2. Place the patient in a comfortable sitting or semi-Fowler's position.

Rationale

Proper explanation of the procedure helps to ensure the patient's cooperation.

The diaphragmatic excursion is greater in this position, and the upright position helps prevent air-swallowing.

3. Turn on the pressure source (oxygen, compressed air).

4. Place the prescribed medication in the nebulizer/or sterile distilled water.

An IPPB treatment should not be given with dry gas.

5. Adjust all controls on tentative settings (usually 15). Select the inspiratory flowrate according to the machine being used (and doctor's request).

Positive pressure is measured in centimetres of water pressure; the pressure delivery is usually in the range of 10 to 20cmH$_2$O. Each unit should be tested to see whether the predetermined setting is accomplished before treating the patient.

6. Check the nebulizer for mist.

Adequate fog and particle size is essential to effective distribution of medication.

Performance phase

Nursing action

Rationale

1. Instruct the patient to bite down gently on the mouthpiece and to seal the mouthpiece with his lips.

The mouthpiece (or mask) must constitute a closed circuit if the unit is to cycle. (If the patient exhales through his nose while using the mouthpiece the unit will not reach the desired pressure.)

2. Tell the patient to breathe slowly and normally and let the machine do the work.

A slight inspiratory effort will activate the positive pressure phase, and the lungs will be inflated with a rapid rate of flow until the predetermined pressure is reached and pressure expiration takes place.

3. Observe expansion of the patient's chest and measure exhaled tidal volume to ensure adequate ventilation.
   a. Patient should breathe at own rate.

   b. Instruct him to hold his breath for three to four seconds at the end of each inspiration.

Measurement of tidal volumes is particularly useful in the patient who has a high arterial Pco$_2$ and needs high tidal volumes to lower it.
The machine will exert a regulated pressure on inhalation, helping him to breathe more deeply.
This ensures settling of aerosol particles on bronchiolar mucosa.

4. Remind the patient to exhale completely and slowly in a relaxed manner. The patient controls exhalation.

This type of breathing encourages good diaphragmatic motion and reduces residual air volume.

5. After several breaths, tell the patient to push all the air out, count 1, 2, 3, and stop inhaling (on the machine) for a few seconds to assess extent of improvement.

The treatment should take 10 to 20 minutes depending on the clinical problem.

6. Encourage the patient to continue this type of breathing until all the medication is given.

The medication should be completely nebulized to ensure effectiveness of treatment.

Evaluation/outcome

Nursing action	Rationale
1. Record medication used, patient's respiratory rate and effort and description of secretions expectorated (also pressure limit and flow rate).	Note the patient's tolerance of the treatment. Notify the doctor if intolerance occurs.
2. Disassemble and clean the exhalation unit and nebulizer after each use. Keep this equipment in the patient's room. This equipment is changed every 24 hours.	Each patient has his own breathing circuit (exhalation valve, nebulizer, tubing, mouthpiece and mask). By proper cleaning, sterilization and storage of equipment infection can be prevented from entering already diseased lungs.

GUIDELINES: ASSISTING THE PATIENT UNDERGOING NEBULIZER THERAPY WITHOUT POSITIVE PRESSURE

A nebulizer is a device that produces a stable aerosol of fluid particles; it is powered by either oxygen or compressed air.

CONTRAINDICATIONS
Inability of patient to co-operate in taking deep breaths; adverse reactions encountered with medication.

HAZARDS
Swelling of dried, retained secretions; precipitation of bronchospasm.

EQUIPMENT
Air compressor or oxygen/air flowmeter
Oxygen nipple adapter
Nebulizer manifold
Medication or saline solution

Assessment

Nursing action	Rationale
1. Monitor the heart rate before and after the treatment for patients using bronchodilator drugs.	Bronchodilators may produce tachycardia, precordial distress, palpitation, dizziness, nausea and excessive perspiration.

Planning and implementation
Preparatory phase

Nursing action	Rationale
1. Explain the procedure of the patient. *This therapy depends on patient effort.*	Proper explanation of the procedure helps to ensure the patient's co-operation.

2. Place the patient in a comfortable sitting or a semi-Fowler's position. Check peak-flow reading.

The diaphragmatic excursion and lung compliance is greater in this position. This ensures maximal distribution and deposition of aerosolized particles to basilar areas of the lungs.

3. Connect the nebulizer (containing medication or saline) and connecting tubing to the oxygen flowmeter and set flow at 4 to 5 litres/minute, or to the air compressor.

A fine mist from the device should be visible.

Performance phase

Nursing action

Rationale

1. Instruct the patient to exhale.

2. Tell the patient to take in a deep breath from the mouthpiece, hold his breath briefly, then exhale.

This encourages optimal dispersion of the medication.

3. Nose clips are sometimes used if the patient has difficulty breathing only through his mouth.

4. Observe expansion of the patient's chest to ascertain that he is taking deep breaths.

This will ensure that medication is deposited below the level of the oropharynx.

5. Instruct the patient to breathe slowly and deeply until all the medication is nebulized.

Medication usually will be nebulized within 10 to 15 minutes at a gas flow of 4 to 5 litres/minute.

6. Upon completion of the treatment, encourage the patient to cough after several deep breaths.

The deep lung inflation will allow forceful coughing and facilitate the expectoration of secretions.

Follow-up phase

Nursing action

Rationale

1. Disassemble and clean nebulizer after each use. Keep this equipment in the patient's room. The equipment is changed every 24 hours.

Each patient has his own breathing circuit (nebulizer, tubing and mouthpiece). Through proper cleaning, sterilization and storage of equipment, organisms can be prevented from entering the lungs.

Evaluation/outcome

Nursing action

Rationale

1. Record medication used, patient's respiratory rate and effort, pre- and post-treatment heart rate, and description of secretions.

Note the patient's tolerance of the treatment. Notify doctor of any intolerance.

2. Re-check peak-flow reading and compare with pre-nebulizer reading.

Establishes any improvement in peak-flow following administration of nebulizer.

GUIDELINES: ASSISTING THE PATIENT USING AN ULTRASONIC NEBULIZER

Ultrasonic nebulizers employ fluid contained in a chamber, which is rapidly vibrated, causing the fluid to break into small particles. A flow of gas then carries these particles to the patient to be inhaled. This treatment will be administered to the patient at atmospheric pressures, or may be incorporated into an intermittent positive pressure breathing (IPPB) treatment or mechanical ventilation.

EQUIPMENT
Ultrasonic nebulizer and nebulizer cup
Circuitry set-up (according to manufacturer's instructions)
Disposable aerosol mask

Assessment

Nursing action	Rationale
1. Auscultate the chest and monitor vital signs.	The patient's baseline is established.

Planning and implementation
Preparatory phase

Nursing action	Rationale
1. Explain the procedure to the patient.	
2. Fill the coupling compartment (water reservoir) of the machine with tap water.	
3. Place the nebulizer chamber in the coupling compartment and fill with the prescribed fluid.	Normal saline is usually used.
4. Assemble circuitry according to manufacturer's instruction.	
5. Plug in the machine and adjust the setting until the desired amount of mist is obtained.	
6. Check peak-flow reading.	

Performance phase

Nursing action	Rationale
1. Place the mask on the patient's face. Instruct the patient to breathe in slowly through his mouth and to exhale the same way.	This allows maximal particle deposition.
2. Have the patient continue to breathe in this manner for the prescribed length of the treatment.	The procedure usually lasts approximately 15 minutes.

3. Observe the patient for any adverse reaction to the treatment:
   a. Wheezing (bronchospasm)
   b. Excessive fluid deposition, causing suffocation

The patient may develop wheezing because of the irritating effects of the fluid on the airways, or may not be able to expectorate the delivered fluid and secretions. The fluid may also cause dried retained secretions to swell, resulting in airway narrowing or closure. He may need assistance in draining his secretions by suctioning or postural drainage.

4. Encourage the patient to periodically cough and expectorate any secretions loosened during the treatment.

Follow-up phase

Nursing action

1. Keep this equipment in the patient's room. The equipment should be changed every 24 hours.

Rationale

Ultrasonic nebulizers have a high contamination rate. It is desirable that each patient have his own device in his room.

Outcome/evaluation

Nursing action

1. Record the medication used, the patient's respiratory rate and effort and description of secretions expectorated.

2. Re-check peak-flow reading and compare with pre-nebulizer reading.

Rationale

Note any adverse reactions. Notify doctor of any patient intolerance of the treatment.

Establishes any improvement in peak flow following administration of nebulizer.

ARTIFICIAL AIRWAY MANAGEMENT

An artificial airway is a tube that is inserted at the mouth or nose (endotracheal tube) or level of the second or third tracheal ring (tracheostomy) to permit mechanical ventilation and/or facilitate secretion removal. The distal end of the tube is located in the trachea below the vocal cords.

INDICATIONS

1. Acute respiratory failure, central nervous system depression, neuromuscular disease, pulmonary diseases, chest wall injury.
2. Upper airway obstruction (tumour, inflammation, foreign body, laryngeal spasm).

3. Anticipated upper airway obstruction from oedema or soft tissue swelling due to head and neck trauma, some postoperative head and neck procedures involving the airway, facial or airway burns, decreased level of consciousness.
4. Aspiration pneumonia.
5. Fractured cervical vertebrae with spinal cord injury requiring ventilatory assistance.

ROUTE OF INSERTION
Endotracheal

May be inserted through the nose or the mouth. A cuff is always located at the distal end of the tube.

1. Orotracheal – insertion of an oral tube is technically easier, since it is done under direct visualization. Disadvantages are increased oral secretions, decreased patient comfort, difficulty with stabilization and inability of patient to use lip movement as a communication means.

2. Nasotracheal – may be more comfortable to the patient and is easier to stabilize. Disadvantages are that blind insertion is required; possible development of pressure necrosis of the nasal airway, sinusitis and otitis media.

Tube types:
1. Vary according to length and inner diameter in millimetres. Usual sizes for adults are 6, 7, 8 and 9mm.
2. Vary according to cuff. Most are high volume, low pressure, with self-sealing inflation valves, or the cuff may be of foam rubber.

Tracheostomy

Inserted into the trachea via an incision created at the level of the second or third cartilage ring; totally bypasses the upper airway. These tubes may or may not be cuffed. Patients with tracheostomies requiring mechanical ventilation are given cuffed tracheostomy tubes. Patients who are awake and alert, are able to protect the airway and do not require mechanical ventilation may be given a cuffless tracheostomy tube. This same group of patients may be given cuffed tracheostomy tubes, with the cuff inflated only during feeding.

Tube types (see Figure 4.20, p. 154).
1. Vary according to composition and cuff type: synthetic Teflon, nylon, polyvinyl chloride, polyethylene or silastic. May or may not have inner cannula. Usually are cuffed:
   a. Tubes with high-volume, low-pressure cuffs, self-sealing inflation valves. With or without inner cannula;
   b. Pressure-limiting cuffs;
   c. Polyurethane foam-filled cuffs;
   d. Speaking tracheostomy tube;
   e. Fenestrated;
   f. Silver (rarely used).
2. May vary according to length and inner diameter in millimetres. Usual sizes for an adult are 6, 7, 8 and 9mm.

NURSING MANAGEMENT
1. Ensure adequate ventilation and oxygenation through the use of mechanical ventilation, continuous positive airway pressure (CPAP) device or Gilstin T-piece adapter.
2. Provide adequate humidity, since the natural humidifying pathway of the oropharynx is bypassed. Clear airway of secretions as needed with suctioning.
3. Use aseptic technique when entering the artificial airway. The artificial airway bypasses the upper airway, and the lower airways are sterile below the level of the vocal cords.
4. Frequently assess the patient's need for ventilatory assistance.
5. Elevate the patient to a semi-Fowler's or sitting position, when possible, since these positions result in improved lung compliance. The patient's position, however, should be changed at least every two hours to ensure ventilation of all lung segments and prevention of secretion stagnation. Position changes are also necessary to avoid skin breakdown.
6. Nutrition:
   a. Only the inflated cuff of the endotracheal/ tracheostomy tube prevents the aspiration of oropharyngeal contents into the lungs. *The patient must not receive oral feeding.* Nutrition must take the form of enteral tube feedings, or parenteral hyperalimentation.
   b. Tracheostomy – if the tracheostomy tube is cuffed, the nurse should determine whether the patient is able to eat with the cuff inflated or deflated.
   Note: Patients on mechanical ventilation or CPAP must have the cuff inflated at all times. The inflated cuff prevents aspiration of food contents into the lungs, but bulging of the tracheal wall caused by the inflated cuff may push against the oesophagus and make swallowing more difficult. Patients who are not on mechanical ventilation and are awake, alert and able to protect the airway are candidates for eating with the cuff deflated.
      (i) To assess ability to protect the airway: (a) sit the patient upright; (b) feed the patient coloured gelatine; (c) if colour from gelatine can be suctioned from the tracheostomy tube, aspiration is occurring and the cuff must be inflated during feeding and for one hour afterward.
7. Be aware of the complications and damage that inflated cuffs may have on the tracheal mucosa. Endotracheal tube cuffs should be inflated continuously and deflated only during intubation, extubation and tube reposition. The internal cuff pressure should be checked every two hours. Tracheostomy tube cuffs also should be inflated continuously in patients on mechanical ventilation or CPAP. Tracheostomized patients who are breathing spontaneously may have the cuffs inflated continuously (in the patient having suppressed levels of consciousness with an inability to protect airway), deflated continuously or in-

flated only for feeding if the patient is at risk for aspiration.

3. External tube site care:

a. Endotracheal tubes – patients with endotracheal tubes have mouth care every shift, or as frequently as needed. Oral secretions tend to stagnate, and risk of oral infection is increased. An oral endotracheal tube may also stimulate an increase in the production of oral secretions. The tube must be secured at all times and the ventilator, CPAP or T-piece tubing supported so that traction is not applied to the tube. .

b. Tracheostomy tube – the stoma should be cleaned once a shift, or more frequently if needed, and the tracheostomy ties changed once a day. The ventilator, CPAP or T-piece tubing must be supported so that traction is not applied to the tracheostomy tube.

9. Have available at all times at the patient's bedside a resuscitation bag, oxygen source and mask to ventilate the patient in the event of accidental tube removal. Anticipate your course of action in such an event.

a. Endotracheal tube – know location and assembly of reintubation equipment. Know method of contact of personnel capable of reintubation.

b. Tracheostomy – have extra tracheostomy tube at bedside. Be aware of reinsertion technique, or know method of contacting personnel capable of reinserting the tube.

Note: Remember that with tracheostomized patients, as long as the airway is patent (from upper to lower), it is possible to bag/mask ventilate with the resuscitation bag if the stoma is covered. Only patients with complete airway obstruction, an open stoma or laryngectomy need have mouth to stoma ventilation performed.

PSYCHOLOGICAL CARE OF THE PATIENT

1. Recognize that the patient is usually apprehensive, particularly about choking, inability to communicate verbally, being unable to remove secretions, difficulty in breathing or mechanical failure.

2. Explain the function of the equipment carefully.

3. Inform the patient and his family that he will not be able to speak while the tube is in place (the exception being a tracheostomy tube with a deflated cuff, a fenestrated tube or a speaking tracheostomy tube). Develop with the patient the best method of communication (e.g. sign language, lip movement, letter boards, paper and pencil, magic slate or coded messages). Patients with tracheostomy tubes or nasal endotracheal tubes may effectively use orally operated electrolarynx devices. Devise a means for the patient to get the nurse's attention when someone is not immediately available at the bedside, such as call bell, hand-operated bell, rattle, etc.

4. Anticipate some of the patient's questions by discussing 'Is it permanent?' 'Will it hurt to breathe?' 'Will someone be with me?'

COMPLICATIONS

1. Mechanical:
   a. Cuff leaks;
   b. Cuff herniation;
   c. Tube obstruction (biting, kinking, mucus plug, blood clot);
   d. Tube displacement;
   e. Inadvertent extubation;
   f. Right main stem intubation (endotracheal tube).

2. Laryngeal and tracheal:
   a. Sore throat;
   b. Hoarse voice;
   c. Glottic oedema;
   d. Ulceration of tracheal mucosa;
   e. Vocal cord ulceration, granuloma or polyps;
   f. Vocal cord paralysis;
   g. Laryngotracheal web – formation of a web of fibrin and cellular debris initiated by necrotic tissue at the glottic or subglottic level. Most often seen four to five days after tracheal extubation;
   h. Postextubation tracheal stenosis;
   i. Tracheal dilatation;
   j. Formation of tracheal–oesophageal fistula;
   k. Formation of tracheal–arterial fistula;
   l. Inominate artery erosion;
   m. See additional complications under specific procedures dealing with artificial airways.

GUIDELINES: ENDOTRACHEAL INTUBATION

This is shown in Figure 4.17.

NURSING ALERT
This procedure is normally only undertaken by the doctor. However, trained nurses in specialized units who have received the appropriate training can intubate patients, provided it is in accordance with hospital policy and with the consent of the medical staff.

EQUIPMENT

Laryngoscope with curved or straight blade and working light source (check batteries and bulb periodically)

Endotracheal tube with low-pressure cuff and adapter to connect tube to ventilator or resuscitation bag

Stylet to guide the endotracheal tube

Oral airway (assorted sizes) or bite block to keep patient from biting into and occluding the endotracheal tube

Adhesive tape or tapes

Sterile anaesthetic lubricant jelly (water-soluble)

Syringe

Suction source

Suction catheter and tonsil suction

Resuscitation bag and mask connected to oxygen source

Anaesthetic spray

Sterile towel

Assessment

Nursing action	Rationale
1. Monitor the patient's heart rate, level of consciousness and respiratory status.	Provides a baseline to estimate patient's tolerance of procedure.

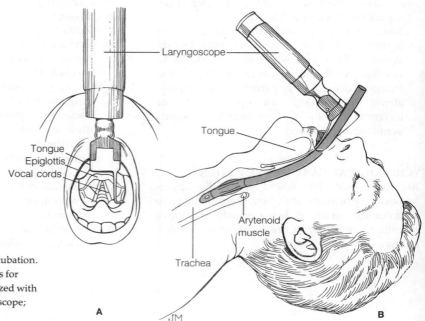

Figure 4.17. Endotracheal intubation. (A) Primary glottic landmarks for tracheal intubation as visualized with proper placement of laryngoscope; (B) Positioning the endotube

Planning and implementation

Nursing action	Rationale
1. Remove the patient's dental bridgework and plates.	May interfere with insertion. Will not be able to remove easily from patient once intubated.
2. Remove headboard of bed (optional).	
3. Prepare equipment a. Ensure function of resuscitation bag with mask, and suction.	Patient may require ventilatory assistance during procedure. Suction should be functional, since gagging and emesis may occur during procedure.

b. Assemble the laryngoscope – make sure the light bulb is tightly attached and functional.
  c. Select an endotracheal tube of the appropriate size (6 to 9mm for average adult).
  d. Place the endotracheal tube on a sterile towel.
	Although the tube will pass through the contaminated mouth or nose, the airway below the vocal cords is sterile, and efforts must be made to prevent contamination of the distal end of the tube and cuff. The proximal end of the tube may be handled, since it will reside in the upper airway.

e. Inflate the cuff to make sure it assumes a symmetrical shape and holds volume without leakage. Then deflate maximally.	Malfunction of the cuff must be ascertained before tube placement occurs.
f. Lubricate the distal end of the tube liberally with the sterile, anaesthetic, water-soluble jelly.	Aids in insertion.
g. Insert the stylet into the tube (if oral intubation is planned; nasal intubation does not employ use of the stylet).	Stiffens the soft tube, allowing it to be more easily directed into the trachea.
4. Aspirate stomach contents if nasogastric tube is in place.	
5. If time allows, inform the patient of impending inability to talk and discuss alternate means of communication.	
6. If the patient is confused, it may be necessary to apply soft wrist restraints.	Restraint of the confused patient may be necessary to promote patient safety and maintain sterile technique.
7. The doctor will then insert the endotracheal tube via laryngoscope and inflate the cuff with the appropriate amount of air.	
8. Insert oral airway or bite block if necessary.	This keeps patient from biting down on the tube and obstructing the airway.
9. Ascertain expansion of both sides of the chest by observation and auscultation of breath sounds.	Observation and auscultation help in determining that tube remains in position and has not slipped into the right main stem bronchus.

10. Mark proximal end of tube with marking pen or tape at the point where the tube reaches the corner of the patient's mouth.

This will allow for detection of any later change in tube position.

11. Secure tube to the patient's face with adhesive tape.

The tube must be fixed securely to ensure that it will not be dislodged. Dislodgement of a tube with an inflated cuff may result in damage to the vocal cords.

12. Obtain chest X-ray to verify tube position.

Follow-up phase

Nursing action

Rationale

1. Make adjustment in tube placement on the basis of the chest X-ray results.

The tube may be advanced or removed several centimetres for proper placement on the basis of the chest X-ray results.

Evaluation/outcome

Nursing action

Rationale

1. Record tube type and size and patient tolerance of the procedure. Auscultate breath sounds every one to two hours or if signs and symptoms of respiratory distress occur. Assess arterial blood gases after intubation if requested by the doctor.

Arterial blood gases may be prescribed to ensure adequacy of ventilation and respiration. Tube displacement outward may result in extubation (cuff above vocal cords).

GUIDELINES: EXTUBATION

Extubation consists of removal of the oral or nasal endotracheal tube.
Note: Extubation may be performed only if personnel qualified to reintubate are available. The occurrence of laryngospasm or tracheal oedema postextubation may require immediate tube replacement.

EQUIPMENT

Tonsil suction (surgical suction instrument)
10ml syringe
Resuscitation bag and mask with oxygen flow
Aerosol face mask connected to aerosol tubing and nebulizer with oxygen
 source
Sterile towel
Suction catheter and Yankaeur sucker

Assessment

Nursing action

Rationale

1. Monitor heart rate, lung expansion and breath sounds pre-extubation.

2. Assess the patient for other signs of recovered muscle power.
   a. Instruct the patient to tightly squeeze the index and middle fingers of your hand. Resistance to removal of your fingers from the patient's grasp must be demonstrated.
   b. Ask the patient to lift his head from the pillow and hold for two to three seconds.

Adequate muscle strength is necessary to ensure maintenance of a patent airway.

Planning and implementation
Preparatory phase

Nursing action

Rationale

1. Obtain directions for extubation and postextubation oxygen therapy from the doctor.

Do not attempt extubation until postextubation oxygen therapy is available and functioning at the bedside.

2. Explain the procedure to the patient:
   a. He will have the artificial airway removed.
   b. He will be suctioned prior to extubation.
   c. He will be asked to take deep breaths on command.
   d. He will be asked to cough after extubation.

Increases patient co-operation.

3. Prepare necessary equipment for extubation. Have ready for use: tonsil suction, 10ml syringe, bag/mask unit and oxygen via face mask.

4. Place patient in sitting or semi-Fowler's position (unless contraindicated).

Increases lung compliance and decreases work of breathing. Facilitates coughing.

Performance phase

Nursing action

Rationale

1. Suction endotracheal tube.

2. Suction oropharyngeal airway above the endotracheal cuff as thoroughly as possible.

Secretions left above the cuff may be aspirated when the cuff is deflated.

3. Loosen tape or endotracheal tube securing device.

4. Extubate the patient:
   a. Ask the patient to take as deep a breath as possible (if the patient is not following commands, give a deep breath with the resuscitation bag).
   b. At peak inspiration, deflate the cuff completely and pull the tube out in the direction of the curve (out and downward).

At peak inspiration, the trachea and vocal cords will dilate, allowing atraumatic tube removal.

5. Once the tube is fully removed, ask the patient to cough or exhale forcefully to remove secretions. Then suction the back of the patient's airway with the tonsil suction.

Frequently, old blood is seen in the secretions of newly extubated patients. Monitor for the appearance of bright red blood due to trauma occurring during extubation.

6. Evaluate immediately for any signs of airway obstruction, stridor or difficult breathing. If the patient develops any of the above problems, attempt to ventilate the patient with the resuscitation bag and mask and prepare for reintubation.

Immediate complications:
Laryngospasm may develop causing obstruction of the airway.
Oedema may develop at the cuff site. Signs of narrowing airway lumen are high-pitched crowing sounds, decreased air movement, and respiratory distress.

7. Administer oxygen as directed.

Follow-up phase

Nursing action

Rationale

1. Observe patient closely postextubation for any signs and symptoms of airway obstruction or respiratory insufficiency.

Tracheal or laryngeal oedema may develop postextubation (a possibility for up to 24 hours). Signs and symptoms include high-pitched, crowing upper airway sounds and respiratory distress.

2. Observe character of voice.

Hoarseness is a common postextubation complaint. Observe for worsening hoarseness or vocal cord paralysis.

Evaluation/outcome

Nursing action

Rationale

1. Note patient tolerance of procedure, upper and lower airway sounds postextubation, description of secretions.

Establishes a baseline to assess improvement/development of complications.

GUIDELINES: ASSISTING WITH TRACHEOSTOMY INSERTION

A tracheostomy is an external opening made into the trachea (Figure 4.18).

EQUIPMENT
Tracheostomy tube (sizes 6 to 9mm for most adults)
Sterile instruments: scalpel and blade, forceps, suture
    material, scissors, tracheal dilator
Sterile gown and drapes, gloves
Cap and mask
Antiseptic solution
Gauze sponges
Shave kit

Sedation
Local anaesthetic and syringe
Resuscitation bag and mask with oxygen source
Suction source and catheters
Syringe for cuff inflation
Respiratory support available for post-tracheostomy
    (mechanical ventilation, tracheal oxygen mask,
    continuous positive airway pressure CPAP, T-piece)

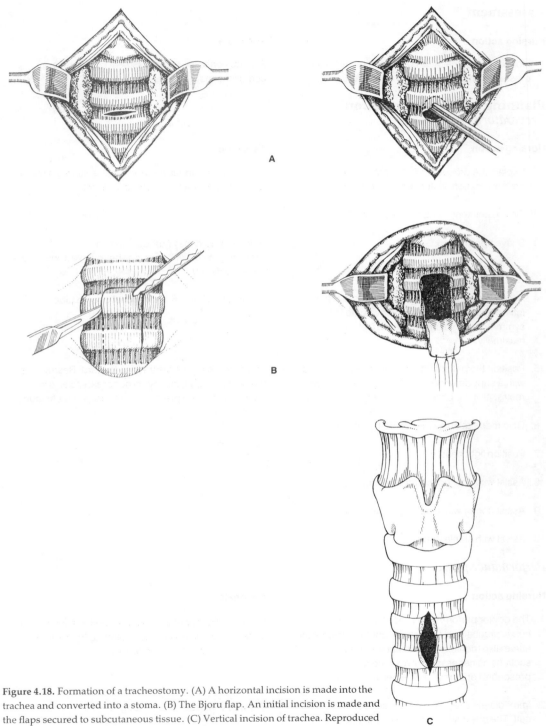

Figure 4.18. Formation of a tracheostomy. (A) A horizontal incision is made into the trachea and converted into a stoma. (B) The Bjoru flap. An initial incision is made and the flaps secured to subcutaneous tissue. (C) Vertical incision of trachea. Reproduced with permission of Portex Ltd.

Assessment

Nursing action

1. Monitor vital signs (heart rate, respiration, blood pressure, temperature) before insertion.

Rationale

Provides baseline for assessment of progress or complications.

Planning and implementation
Preparatory phase

Nursing action

1. Explain the procedure to the patient. Discuss a communication system with the patient.

2. Obtain consent for operative procedure.

3. Shave neck region.

4. Assemble equipment. Using aseptic technique, inflate tracheostomy cuff and evaluate for symmetry and volume leakage. Deflate maximally.

5. Position the patient (supine with head extended, with a support under shoulders). Apply soft wrist restraints if the patient is confused.

6. Give medication as requested by doctor.

7. Position light source.

8. Assist with antiseptic preparation.

9. Assist doctor with gowning and gloving.

10. Assist with sterile draping.

Rationale

Apprehension about inability to talk is usually a major concern of the tracheostomized patient.

Hair and beard may harbour harmful micro-organisms. If beard is to be removed, inform the patient or family.

Ensures that the cuff is functional prior to tube insertion.

This position brings the trachea forward. Restraint of the confused patient may be necessary to ensure patient safety and preservation of aseptic technique.

Performance phase

Nursing action

1. The doctor performs the procedure with the nurse circulating. He or she or another designated nurse also monitors the patient's vital signs, suctions as necessary, gives medication as prescribed or administers emergency care.

2. Immediately after the tube is inserted, inflate the cuff. The chest should be auscultated for the presence of bilateral breath sounds.

Rationale

Bradycardia may result from vagal stimulation due to tracheal manipulation or hypoxaemia. Hypoxaemia may also cause cardiac irritability.

Ensures ventilation of both lungs.

Follow-up phase

Nursing action

Rationale

1. Apply respiratory assistive devices (mechanical ventilation, tracheostomy oxygen mask, CPAP, T-piece adapter).

2. Check the tracheostomy tube cuff pressure.

   Excessive cuff pressure may cause tracheal damage.

3. 'Tie sutures' or 'stay sutures' of oo silk may have been placed through either side of the tracheal cartilage at the incision and brought out through the wound. Each is to be taped to the skin at a 45-degree angle laterally to the sternum (Figure 4.19).

   Should the tracheostomy tube become dislodged, the stay sutures may be grasped and used to spread the tracheal cartilage apart, facilitating placement of the new tube.

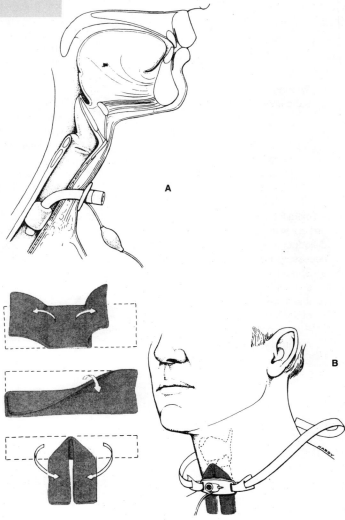

Figure 4.19. (A) How tracheostomy tube fits within tracheal wall; (B) appropriate dressing for a tracheostomy

Evaluation/outcome

Nursing action	Rationale
1. Assess vital signs and ventilatory status; note tube size used, doctor performing procedure, type, dose and route of medications given.	Provides baseline.
2. Obtain chest X-ray.	Documents proper tube placement.
3. Assess and chart condition of stoma: a. Bleeding;	Some bleeding around the stoma site is not uncommon for the first few hours. Monitor and inform the doctor of any increase in bleeding. Clean site aseptically when necessary (see 'Care of the Patient with Tracheostomy', p. 151). Do not change tracheostomy ties for first 24 hours, since accidental dislodgement of the tube could result when the ties are loose, and tube reinsertion through the as yet unformed stoma may be difficult or impossible to accomplish.
b. Swelling; c. Subcutaneous air.	When positive pressure respiratory assistive devices are used (mechanical ventilation, CPAP) before the wound is healed, air may be forced into the subcutaneous fat layer. This can be seen as enlargement of the neck and facial tissues and felt as crepitus or 'crackling' when the skin is depressed. The doctor should be informed.
4. An extra tube, obturator and tracheal dilator should be kept at the bedside. In the event of tube dislodgement, reinsertion of a new tube may be necessary. For emergency tube insertion: a. Spread the wound with a tracheal dilator or stay sutures; b. Insert replacement tube (containing the obturator) at an angle; c. Point cannula downward and insert the tube maximally; remove the obturator.	The tracheal dilator will open the airway and allow ventilation in the spontaneously breathing patient. Avoid inserting the tube horizontally, as the tube may be forced against the back wall of the trachea.

GUIDELINES: CARE OF THE PATIENT WITH TRACHEOSTOMY

Tracheostomy care keeps the area clean and dry, preventing skin irritation and infection. Secretions collected above the tracheostomy tube cuff ooze out of the surgical incision. The resultant wetness promotes irritation of the skin, and the wetness, coupled with the transmission of bacteria via the secretions, sets up a medium for infection to occur.

EQUIPMENT

Assemble the following equipment or obtain a prepackaged tracheostomy care kit:

Sterile towel
Sterile gauze sponges (12)
Sterile cotton swabs
Sterile gloves
Hydrogen peroxide
Sterile water
Antiseptic solution and ointment (optional)
Tracheostomy tie tapes

Assessment

Nursing action	Rationale
1. Assess condition of stoma prior to tracheostomy care (redness, swelling, character of secretions, presence of purulence or bleeding).	The presence of skin breakdown or infection must be monitored. Culture of the site may be warranted by appearance of these signs.

Planning and implementation
Preparatory phase

Nursing action	Rationale
1. Suction the trachea and pharynx thoroughly prior to tracheostomy care.	Removal of secretions prior to tracheostomy care keeps the area clean longer.
2. Explain procedure to the patient.	
3. Wash hands thoroughly.	
4. Assemble equipment:	
a. Place sterile towel on patient's chest under tracheostomy site.	Provides sterile field.
b. Open four gauze sponges and pour hydrogen peroxide on them.	For removing mucus and crust, which promotes bacterial growth.
c. Open two gauze sponges and pour antiseptic solution on them.	May be applied to fresh stoma or infected stoma – not necessary for clean, healed stoma.
d. Open two gauze sponges, keep dry.	
e. Open two gauze sponges and pour sterile water on them.	

f. Place tracheostomy tube tapes on field.

g. Put on sterile gloves.

Sterile gloves prevent contamination of the wound by nurse's hands and also protect the nurse's hands from infection.

Performance phase

Nursing action

Rationale

1. Clean the external end of the tracheostomy tube with 2 gauze sponges with hydrogen peroxide; discard sponges.

2. Clean the stoma area with two peroxide-soaked gauze sponges. Make only a single sweep with each gauze sponge before discarding.

Hydrogen peroxide may help loosen dry crusted secretions.

3. Loosen and remove any crust with sterile cotton swabs.

4. Repeat second step using the sterile water-soaked gauze sponges.

Ensures that all hydrogen peroxide is removed.

5. Repeat two using dry sponges.

Ensures dryness of the area – wetness promotes infection and irritation.

6. (Optional) An infected wound may be cleaned with gauze saturated with an antiseptic solution, then dried. A thin layer of antibiotic ointment may be applied to the stoma with a cotton swab.

May help clear infection of the wound.

7. Change the tracheostomy tie tapes:
    a. Cut soiled tape while holding tube securely with other hand.

Stabilization of the tube helps prevent accidental dislodgement and keeps irritation and coughing due to tube manipulation at a minimum. Two people may participate in the procedure at this point.

    b. Remove old tapes carefully.
    c. Grasp slit end of clean tape and pull it through opening on side of the tracheostomy tube.
    d. Pull other end of tape securely through the slit end of the tape.
    e. Repeat on the other side.
    f. Tie the tapes at the side of the neck in a square knot. Alternate knot from side to side each time tapes are changed.

To prevent irritation and rotate pressure site.

    g. Tape should be tight enough to keep tube securely in the stoma but loose enough to permit two fingers to fit between the tapes and the neck.

Excessive tightness of tapes will compress jugular veins and decrease blood circulation to the skin under the tape, as well as being uncomfortable for the patient.

8. Some surgeons elect to place a gauze pad between the stoma site and the tracheostomy tube to absorb secretions and prevent irritation of the stoma. Others feel that this is unnecessary. Many surgeons feel that gauze should not be used around the stoma. In their opinion, the dressing keeps the area moist and dark, promoting stomal infection. They believe the stoma should be left open to the air and the surrounding area kept dry. A dressing is used only if secretions are draining onto subclavian or neck intravenous sites or chest incisions.

Follow-up phase

Nursing action

1. Cleaning of the fresh stoma should be performed every eight hours, or more frequently if indicated by accumulation of secretions. Ties should be changed every 24 hours, or more frequently if soiled or wet.

Rationale

The area must be kept clean and dry to prevent infection or irritation of tissues.

Evaluation/outcome

Nursing action

1. Document procedure performance, observations of stoma (irritation, redness, oedema, subcutaneous air), and character of secretions (colour, purulence).

Rationale

Provides a baseline. Notify doctor of changes in stoma appearance or secretions.

GUIDELINES: STERILE TRACHEOBRONCHIAL SUCTION VIA TRACHEOSTOMY OR ENDOTRACHEAL TUBE (SPONTANEOUS OR MECHANICAL VENTILATION)

INDICATIONS

1. When secretions can be seen or sounds resulting from secretions are heard with or without the use of a stethoscope.
2. Following postural drainage or chest physiotherapy.
3. Following respiratory treatments aimed at liquefying secretions (i.e. ultrasonic nebulization).
4. Following a sudden rise or the 'popping off' of the peak airway pressure in mechanically ventilated patients that is not due to kinking of the artificial airway or ventilator tube, patient biting the tube, the patient coughing or struggling against the ventilator or pneumothorax.

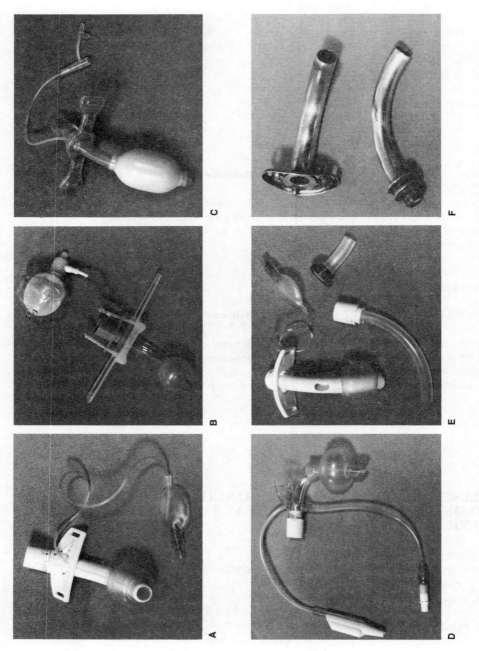

Figure 4.20. Types of tracheostomy tubes. A, Low pressure cuff (Shiley); B, Pressure limiting cuff (Lanz); C, Polyurethane foam filled cuff (Fome-Cuff); D, Speaking tube (Pitt); E, Fenestrated tube (Shiley); F, Silver tube. (Courtesy of Photography Department, Montefiore Hospital, Pittsburgh, Pennsylvania)

EQUIPMENT

Assemble the following equipment or obtain a prepackaged suctioning kit:

Sterile suction catheters – No. 14 or 16 (adult), No. 8 or 10 (child). The outer diameter of the suction catheter should be no greater than two-thirds of the inner diameter of the artificial airway

Two sterile gloves

Sterile towel

Suction source set at −80 to −120mmHg

Sterile water

Resuscitation bag connected to 100 per cent oxygen source (if patient is on PEEP or CPAP, add positive end-expiratory pressure (PEEP) valve to exhalation valve on resuscitation bag in an amount equal to that on the ventilator or CPAP device)

Normal saline solution (in syringe or single-dose packet)

Sterile cup for water

Alcohol swabs

Sterile, water-soluble lubricant jelly

Assessment

Nursing action	Rationale
1. Monitor heart rate, colour, ease of respiration. If the patient is monitored, continuously monitor heart rate and arterial blood pressure. If arterial blood gases are done routinely, know baseline values. (It is important to establish a baseline, since suctioning should be discontinued and oxygen applied or manual ventilation reinstituted if, during the suction procedure, the heart rate decreases by 20 beats per minute or increases by 40 beats per minute, blood pressure drops or cardiac dysrhythmia is noted.)	Suctioning may cause: a. Hypoxaemia, initially resulting in tachycardia and increased blood pressure, progressing to cardiac ectopy, bradycardia, hypotension and cyanosis. b. Vagal stimulation, which may result in bradycardia.

Planning and implementation
Preparatory phase

Nursing action	Rationale
1. Explain to the patient the importance of performing the suction procedure in an aseptic manner.	Thorough explanation lessens patient's anxiety and promotes co-operation.
2. Assemble equipment. Check function of suction and manual resuscitation bag connected to 100 per cent O_2 source.	Make sure that all equipment is functional before sterile technique is instituted to prevent interruption once the procedure is begun. Use of 100 per cent O_2 will help to prevent hypoxaemia.
3. Wash hands thoroughly.	

Performance phase

Nursing action	Rationale
1. Open sterile towel – place in a bib-like fashion on patient's chest. Open alcohol wipes and place on corner of towel. Place small amount of sterile water-soluble jelly on towel.	

2. Open sterile gloves – place on towel.

3. Open suction catheter package.

4. If the patient is on mechanical ventilation, test to make sure that disconnection of ventilator attachment may be made with one hand.

5. Don sterile gloves. Designate one hand as contaminated for disconnecting, bagging and working the suctioning control. Usually the dominant hand is kept sterile and will be used to thread the suction catheter.

The hand designated as sterile must remain uncontaminated so that organisms are not introduced into the lungs. The contaminated hand must also be gloved to prevent sputum from contacting the nurse's hand, possibly resulting in an infection for the nurse.

6. Use the sterile hand to remove carefully the suction catheter from the package, curling the catheter around the gloved fingers.

7. Connect suction source to the suction fitting of the catheter with the contaminated hand.

8. Using the contaminated hand, disconnect the patient from the ventilator, CPAP device or other oxygen source. (Place the ventilator connector on the sterile towel and flip a corner of the towel over the connection to prevent fluid from spraying into the area.)

Prevents contamination of the connection.

9. Ventilate and oxygenate the patient with the resuscitator bag, compressing firmly and as completely as possible approximately five to six times (try to approximate the patient's tidal volume). This procedure is called 'bagging' the patient. In the spontaneously breathing patient, co-ordinate manual ventilations with the patient's own inspiratory effort.

Ventilation prior to suctioning helps prevent hypoxaemia. When possible, two nurses work as a team to suction. Attempting to ventilate against the patient's own respiratory efforts may result in high airway pressures, predisposing the patient to barotrauma (lung injury due to pressure).

10. Lubricate the tip of the suction catheter. Gently insert suction catheter as far as possible into the artificial airway without applying suction. Most patients will cough when the catheter touches the trachea.

Suctioning on insertion would unnecessarily decrease oxygen in the airway.

11. Apply suction and quickly rotate the catheter while it is being withdrawn.

Failure to rotate catheter may result in damage to tracheal mucosa. Release suction if a pulling sensation is felt.

12. Limit suction time to 10 to 15 seconds. Discontinue if heart rate decreases by 20 beats per minute or increases by 40 beats per minute, or if cardiac ectopy is observed.

Suctioning removes oxygen as well as secretions and may also cause vagal stimulation.

13. Bag patient between suction passes with approximately four to five manual ventilations.

The oxygen removed by suctioning must be replenished before suctioning is attempted again.

14. At this point, sterile nonbacteriostatic saline may be instilled into the trachea via the artificial airway if secretions are tenacious.

Some surgeons feel that secretion removal may be facilitated with saline instillation. Others feel that saline does not mix with mucus and that suctioning of the saline just instilled is the only effect produced by performing this step.

   a. Remove needle from syringe and inject 3 to 5ml nonbacteriostatic saline into the artificial airway during spontaneous inspiration. Alternately, a saline 'bullet' or small prepackaged container of saline may be used.

   a. Removal of the needle will prevent accidental loss of the needle into the airway. Instillation of the saline during inspiration will prevent the saline from being blown back out of the tube.

   b. Bag vigorously and then suction.

   b. Bagging stimulates cough and distributes saline to loosen secretions.

15. Rinse suction tubing between suction passes by inserting tip in cup of sterile water and applying suction.

16. Continue making suction passes, bagging the patient between passes, until the airways are clear of accumulated secretions. No more than four suction passes should be made per suctioning episode.

Repeated suctioning of a patient in a short time interval predisposes to hypoxaemia, as well as being tiring and traumatic to the patient.

17. Return the patient to the ventilator or apply CPAP or other oxygen-delivery device.

18. Suction oral secretions from the oropharynx above the artificial airway cuff.

Follow-up phase

Nursing action

Rationale

1. Clean connection of resuscitation bag with alcohol; wipe before storing.

2. Assess need for further suctioning at least every two hours, or more frequently if secretions are copious.

Evaluation/outcome

Nursing action

Rationale

1. Note any change in vital signs or patient's intolerance to the procedure. Record amount and consistency of secretions (Figure 4.21).

Evaluate the effectiveness of procedure.

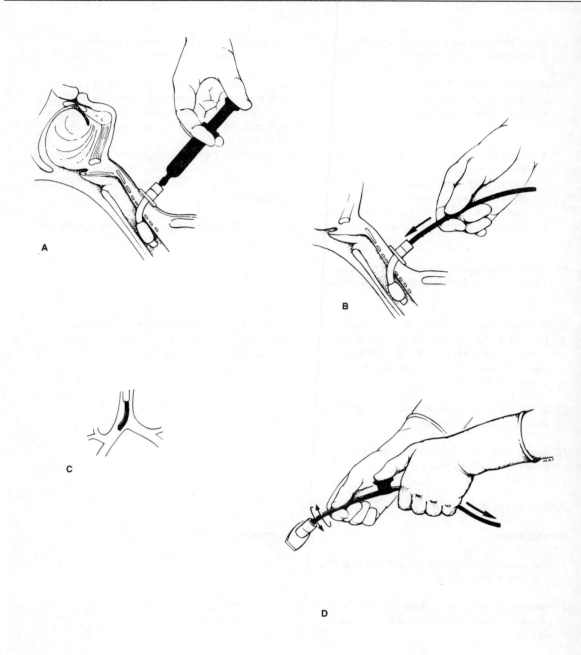

Figure 4.21. Care of the tracheostomy patient. (A) After the tracheostomy cuff is deflated (note that the cuff does not touch the sides of the trachea) 3–5ml of sterile saline can be instilled into the tube to loosen secretions. (B) After donning sterile gloves, the nurse introduces a sterile catheter without applying suction. (C) To remove secretions from the bronchus, insert tube 20–30cm. (D) Suction is applied by sealing the button outlet with the thumb. Gradually withdraw the catheter with a rotating motion

GUIDELINES: ARTIFICIAL AIRWAY CUFF INFLATION/DEFLATION

The cuffs of endotracheal and tracheostomy tubes must be inflated continuously when the patient is on mechanical ventilation or CPAP. The cuff is then deflated only for tube removal or repositioning. The cuffs of spontaneously breathing tracheostomized patients may require inflation at all times if the patient has a sufficiently depressed level of consciousness, or neuromuscular deficiency that does not permit the patient to protect his airway. The cuffs of spontaneously breathing tracheostomized patients not on mechanical ventilation or CPAP may be deflated:

1. At times when the patient can adequately protect the airway.
2. Between meals, if the patient is at aspiration risk only during feeding. The cuff may be inflated prior to feeding and for one hour after feeding.

COMPLICATIONS OF EXCESSIVE CUFF PRESSURE

Tracheal swelling
Tracheal ulceration
Tracheal fistula

Tracheal necrosis
Tracheal malacia

EQUIPMENT
Suction catheter
Tonsil suction
Suction source
10ml syringe
Manual resuscitation bag connected to 100 per cent oxygen at 10–15 litres/minute.

PROCEDURE
May require a doctor's request: usually the cuff is initially inflated by the doctor.

DEFLATING A CUFF

Nursing action	Rationale
1. Explain procedure to the patient. Suction pharynx (oral and nasal).	Removes secretions which could be aspirated during the process of deflation.
2. Deflate cuff slowly.	On endotracheal tube, a small test balloon at end of tubing remains inflated as long as cuff is inflated.
3. Suction through the tracheostomy or endotracheal tube.	Removes secretions which may have been present above inflated cuff and around exterior of tube and may now have seeped downwards. The coughing reflex may be stimulated during deflation, which helps to mobilize secretions.
4. Provide adequate ventilation while cuff is deflated.	
a. If the patient does not require assisted ventilation: provide humidified warm air.	a. Continue observation of patient: pulse, colour, etc. If any signs of distress, place patient back on mechanical ventilator.

b. If the patient requires assisted ventilation; provide a manually inflating breathing bag or respirator if patient has been on a mechanical ventilator.

b. If patient is apnoeic, cuff should not be deflated for more than 30 or 45 seconds.

INFLATING A CUFF (SLOWLY)

Nursing action

Rationale

1. Stipulations:
   a. To be done when patient requires mechanical ventilation or is being fed.
      (i) Semi-Fowler's position is most comfortable if permissible, and is required for half an hour after feeding.
      (ii) On right side.
   b. Inflate cuff during inspiration (positive pressure phase).

   a. To prevent aspiration of food into lungs.

      (i) Gravity assists in moving food into the stomach.

      (ii) To prevent regurgitation of feeding.

2. Method A:
   a. Inject air into cuff until complete seal is achieved or to selected pressure, following doctor's orders. By listening with a stethoscope placed just below the chin one may determine that no leak exists.
   b. Clamp tube leading to cuff.

   a. The pressure-cycled ventilator will turn off; air will not escape around tube or from nose or mouth. In the conscious patient, a leak-free system is present when he is aphonic.

3. Method B (minimal leak inflation):
   a. Inject air until full seal is acquired; withdraw 0.5ml of air and clamp tube.
   b. Note and record amount of air required to inflate cuff.

   a. A partial leak is purposely created so that ventilator can be set to compensate for it.
   b. If at subsequent times more air is required to inflate cuff, tracheal dilatation or other serious problem (erosion of a large blood vessel or tracheo-oesophageal diverticulum or fistula) may be the cause.

MECHANICAL VENTILATION

A mechanical ventilator is a positive pressure breathing device which can maintain respiration automatically for prolonged periods of time. It is indicated when the patient is unable to maintain safe levels of arterial carbon dioxide or oxygen by spontaneous breathing.

TYPES OF VENTILATOR

1. *Pressure-cycled* – the ventilator delivers a predetermined pressure, then turns off.
   a. Gas flows result from this pressure and increases lung volume.
   b. Volume delivered is dependent on lung compliance and varies from breath to breath.
   c. Blockage at any point between machine and lungs will not stop the on-off cycling of the ventilator – but the patient will receive *no volume*.

d. Volume-based alarms should always be used with this ventilator.

2. *Volume-cycled* – the ventilator delivers a predetermined volume of air to the patient regardless of any changing lung condition. If machine is unable to deliver such volume, the operator is alerted by an audible and visible alarm.

MODES OF OPERATION
Controlled ventilation
1. Cycles automatically at rate that is selected by operator.
2. A fixed level of ventilation is provided. Will not cycle or have gas available or circuitry to respond to patient's own inspiratory efforts (may result in increase in work of breathing for patients attempting to breathe spontaneously).
3. Possibly indicated for patients whose respiratory drive is absent.

Assist ventilation
1. Inspiratory cycle of ventilator activated by detection of decrease in airway pressure caused by the patient's voluntary inspiratory activity.
2. Once inspiration initiated, ventilator will deliver gas flow until desired volume, pressure or time limit is reached.
3. No minimum level of minute ventilation is provided. Indicated for the patient who is making regular inspiratory efforts but who cannot achieve an adequate tidal volume.

Assist/control
1. Inspiratory cycle of ventilator activated by detection of the patient's voluntary inspiratory effort.
2. Ventilator additionally cycles at a rate predetermined by the operator. Should the patient stop breathing, or breathe so weakly that the ventilator cannot function as an assister, this mandatory baseline rate will prevent apnoea. A minimum level of minute ventilation is provided.
3. Indicated for patients who are breathing spontaneously but who have the potential to lose their respiratory drive or muscular control of ventilation. In this mode, the patient's work of breathing is greatly reduced.

Intermittent mandatory ventilation
1. Allows patient to breathe spontaneously through ventilator circuitry.
2. Periodically, at preselected rate and volume, cycles to give a 'mandated' ventilator breath. A minimum level of ventilation is provided.
3. Gas provided for spontaneous breathing usually flows continuously through the ventilator circuitry.
4. Indications – patients requiring ventilator assistance in whom it may be desirable to do some of the work of breathing.

Synchronized intermittent mandatory ventilation
1. Allows patient to breathe spontaneously through the ventilator circuitry.
2. Periodically, at a preselected time, a mandatory breath is delivered. The patient may initiate the mandatory breath with his own inspiratory effort, and the ventilator breath will be synchronized with the patient's efforts, or will be 'assisted'. If the patient does not provide inspiratory effort, the breath will still be delivered, or be 'controlled'.
3. Gas provided for spontaneous breathing is usually delivered through a demand regulator which is activated by the patient.
4. Indicated for patients who needs ventilator assistance, but in whom it may be desirable to perform some of the work of breathing.

SPECIAL POSITIVE PRESSURE VENTILATION TECHNIQUES
Positive end-expiratory pressure (PEEP)
1. Manoeuvre by which pressure during mechanical ventilation is maintained above atmospheric at end of exhalation, resulting in an increased functional residual capacity. Airway pressure is therefore positive throughout the entire ventilatory cycle.
2. Purpose – the increase in functional residual capacity (or the amount of air left in the lungs at the end of expiration) is greater than atmospheric pressure:
   a. Increasing the surface area for gas exchange.
   b. Preventing collapse of alveolar units and development of atelectasis.
3. Benefits:
   a. Positive intra-airway pressure may be helpful in reducing the transudation of fluid from the pulmonary capillaries in situations where capillary pressure is increased (i.e. left heart failure).
   b. Increased lung compliance resulting in decreased work of breathing.
4. Hazards:
   a. Since the mean airway pressure is increased by PEEP, venous return is impeded. This may result in a decrease in cardiac output (especially noted in hypovolaemic patients).
   b. The increased airway pressure may possibly

result in alveolar rupture. The likelihood is greater in patients with noncompliant lungs. This trauma may result in pneumothorax, tension pneumothorax or development of subcutaneous emphysema.

c. The decreased venous return may cause anti-diuretic hormone formation to be stimulated, resulting in decreased urine output.

5. Precautions:
   a. Monitor frequently for signs and symptoms of pneumothorax (decreased lung movement, hyperresonant percussion note, diminished breath sounds).
   b. Monitor for signs of decreased venous return:
      (i) Decreased arterial blood pressure;
      (ii) Decreased cardiac output;
      (iii) Decreased urine output; formation of peripheral oedema.
   c. Abrupt discontinuance of PEEP is not recom-mended. The patient should not be without PEEP for longer than 15 seconds. The manual resuscitation bag used for ventilation during suction procedure or patient transport should be equipped with a PEEP device. Some clin-icians feel that loss of PEEP for short periods of time is not detrimental in the lower ranges (less than 10cmH₂O). An exception might be patients with increased intracranial pressure.
   d. Intrapulmonary blood vessel pressure may in-crease because of compression of the vessels by increased intra-airway pressure. This may cause a rise in the central venous pressure and pulmonary wedge pressure, a point to be noted when interpreting the significance of these pressures.

Continuous positive airway pressure (CPAP)

1. Also provides for positive airway pressure during all parts of a respiratory cycle but refers to spontaneous ventilation rather than mechanical ventilation.
2. May be delivered through ventilator circuitry when ventilator rate is at '0', or may be delivered through a separate CPAP circuitry that does not require the ventilator.
3. Indicated for patients who are capable of main-taining an adequate tidal volume, but have pathology preventing maintenance of adequate levels of tissue oxygenation.
4. CPAP has the same benefits, hazards and pre-cautions noted with PEEP. Mean airway press-ures may be lower because of lack of mechanical ventilation breaths. This results in less risk of trauma and impedance of venous return.

UNDERLYING PRINCIPLES

1. Variables that control ventilation and oxygen-ation:
   a. Ventilator rate – adjusted by rate knob. On some ventilators, it is set by adjusting the inspiratory and expiratory times.
   b. Tidal volume – set by tidal volume knob. Measured as inhaled volume.
   c. Fraction inspired oxygen concentration (F_1O_2) – set on ventilator or with an oxygen blender. Measured with an oxygen analyser.
   d. Ventilator dead space – circuitry common to inhalation and exhalation.
   e. PEEP – set within the ventilator or with the use of external PEEP devices. Measured at the proximal airway.
2. CO_2 elimination – controlled by tidal volume, rate and dead space.
3. Oxygen tension – controlled by oxygen concen-tration and PEEP (also by rate and tidal volume).
4. The duration of inspiration should not exceed exhalation. Rate, tidal volume, gas flow in litres per minute, and inspiratory pause all control in-spiratory time. Inverse inspiration–exhalation ratio results in 'stacking' of breaths or build-up of pressure within the airway. Trauma and decreased cardiac output can result.
5. The inspired gas must be warmed and humidified to prevent thickening of secretions and decrease in body temperature. Sterile distilled water is warmed and humidified via a heated humidifier or nebulizer.

CLINICAL INDICATIONS

1. Mechanical failure of ventilation:
   a. Neuromuscular disease;
   b. Central nervous system disease;
   c. Central nervous system depression (drug intoxication, respiratory depressants, cardiac arrest);
   d. Musculoskeletal disease;
   e. Inefficiency of thorax cage in generating press-ure gradients necessary for ventilation (chest injury, thoracic malformation).
2. Disorders of pulmonary gas exchange:
   a. Acute respiratory failure;
   b. Chronic respiratory failure;
   c. Left ventricular failure;
   d. Pulmonary diseases resulting in diffusion abnormality;
   e. Pulmonary diseases resulting in ventilation/ perfusion mismatch.

COMPLICATIONS

1. Airway obstruction (thickened secretions, mechanical problem with artificial airway or ventilator circuitry).
2. Tracheal damage.
3. Pulmonary infection.
4. Trauma (pneumothorax or tension pneumothorax).
5. Cardiac embarrassment.
6. Atelectasis.
7. Gastrointestinal malfunction (dilation, bleeding).
8. Renal malfunction.
9. Central nervous system malfunction.

GUIDELINES: MANAGING THE PATIENT REQUIRING MECHANICAL VENTILATION

EQUIPMENT
Artificial airway
Mechanical ventilator
Ventilator circuitry
Humidifier
See manufacturer's directions for specific machine

Assessment

Nursing action	Rationale
1. Obtain baseline samples for blood gas determinations (pH, Pao_2, $Paco_2$, HCO_3) and chest X-ray.	Baseline measurements serve as a guide in determining progress of therapy.

Planning and implementation
Preparatory phase

Nursing action	Rationale
1. Give a brief explanation to the patient.	Emphasize that mechanical ventilation is a temporary measure. The patient should be prepared psychologically for weaning the day the ventilator is first used.
2. Establish the airway by means of a cuffed endotracheal tube.	Endotracheal intubation provides access to the lower part of the airway for removal of secretions. The cuffed tube prevents leakage of air into mouth during ventilation and permits control of pressure and lung inflation.
a. Inflate the cuff to the pressure prescribed by the doctor to achieve a proper seal. Inflation pressure should not normally exceed 20 mmHg as measured by a cuff pressure manometer.	a. Pressure greater than 20mmHg can compromise circulation in the trachea. Insufficient cuff pressure may allow gas leakage and a diminished volume of air may be delivered to the patient.
b. Secure the tube in place with surgical adhesive. Insert an oral airway as a bite block to prevent the patient from occluding an orotracheal tube.	b. Securing the tube prevents dislodgement into the right or left mainstem bronchus.

3. Prepare ventilator according to manufacturer's directions:
   a. Turn on machine.
   b. Adjust volume control; establish tidal and minute volumes as determined by the doctor.
   c. Set the oxygen concentration.

   d. Adjust respiratory rate of ventilator to 12 to 14 respirations/minute.

   e. Adjust flow state (velocity of gas flow during inspiration) to 30 to 40 litres/minute.

   f. Couple the patient's endotracheal tube to the ventilator.

Maintenance of ventilation depends on correct machine settings.

b. Arterial blood pH, carbon dioxide and oxygen tensions serve as guides in adjusting the ventilator.
c. This is generally based on the arterial oxygen levels obtained as a baseline.
d. This setting approximates normal respiration. The patient who has respiratory stimulus will cycle machine by himself; set the control to a rate slightly lower than the patient's actual rate. These machine settings are subject to change according to patient's condition and response and the make of the machine being used.
e. The slower the flow rate the lower will be the pressure required to deliver the patient's gas volume. This results in a lower intrathoracic pressure and less impedance of venous return and cardiac output.
f. Be sure connections are secure. Watch for accidental disconnection between the patient's airway and the ventilator; observe for separation of ventilator tubings from nebulizer, electrical wall-plug slippage, etc.

4. Carry out arterial blood gas determinations approximately 20 minutes after patient is on ventilator. Arterial blood sampling is carried out repeatedly during the acute period.

The only effective way to attain and maintain normal oxygen and carbon dioxide tensions is to measure these tensions frequently in arterial blood and adjust the settings of the ventilator accordingly. Arterial blood gases are monitored to assess the effectiveness of therapy. There are no reliable clinical signs of CO_2 retention or alkalosis.

5. The patient is never left unattended or unobserved.

Positioning

Nursing action

1. Turn patient from side to side hourly.

2. Lateral turns of 120 degrees are desirable; from right semiprone to left semiprone.

3. Sit the patient upright at regular intervals.

4. Position the patient in postural drainage positions as requested.

5. Carry out passive range of motion exercises of all extremities.

Rationale

Prevents skin breakdown.

Upright posture increases ventilation of lower lobes.

Adequate postural drainage decreases the need for deep tracheobronchial catheter aspiration by preventing retention of secretions in the periphery of the lungs.

Deep breaths

Nursing action

1. Augment the patient's spontaneous tidal volume by periodically giving him six to eight deep breaths with a hand resuscitator bag or use sigh mechanism available on some ventilators. Provide patient with adequate oxygenation during this manoeuvre.

Rationale

Periodic sighing with greater than normal tidal volumes helps to prevent alveolar collapse. Provision of deep breaths by mechanical hyperinflation also helps to promote coughing and reveals the presence of retained secretions.

Aspiration of secretions

Nursing action

1. Aspirate secretions from the trachea using sterile technique.

2. Oxygenate patient for one to two minutes before each suctioning episode and before second passage of the catheter.

3. Note the amount, colour and consistency of tracheal secretions obtained.

4. Inform the doctor if there is appreciable change.

Rationale

Ventilation and nebulization liquefy secretions, causing them to rise into the upper airways.

Do not prolong aspiration more than 15 seconds because cardiac arrest may ensue in patients with borderline oxygenation.

Chest auscultation

Nursing action

1. Listen with a stethoscope to the chest from bottom to top on both sides (hourly).

2. Determine whether breath sounds are present or absent, normal or abnormal, and whether a change has occurred.

3. Observe the patient's diaphragmatic excursions and changes in the use of accessory muscles of respiration.

Rationale

Auscultation of the chest is a means of assessing airway patency and ventilatory distribution. It also confirms the proper placement of the endotracheal or tracheostomy tube.

Humidification

Nursing action

1. Check the water level in the humidification reservoir to ensure that the patient is never ventilated with dry gas. Empty the water that condenses in the delivery tubing. Humidifier or nebulizer and tubing must be changed every 24 hours.

Rationale

Water condensing in the delivery tubing may cause obstruction and sudden flooding of the trachea. Warm, moist tubing is a perfect breeding area for bacteria.

Airway pressure

Nursing action

1. Check the airway pressure gauge at frequent intervals in patients on volume-limited ventilators.

Rationale

Since these ventilators deliver a fixed volume, a sudden drop in pressure indicates a leak in the system. A sudden rise in pressure indicates obstruction of the delivery of gas to the patient. Could indicate (a) blockage by secretions; (b) tube slippage into a mainstem bronchus; (c) pneumothorax; or (d) pulmonary oedema.

Tidal volumes

Nursing action

1. Measure the tidal volume with a respirometer for patients on pressure-limited ventilators.

Rationale

An abrupt fall in tidal volume indicates increase in airway resistance (e.g. bronchospasm or other obstruction), an increase in tissue resistance (pulmonary oedema) or a leak in the patient circuit of the ventilator.

Cuff inflation

Nursing action

1. Clean the pharynx and larynx of accumulated secretions by either suction or postural drainage.

2. Release air slowly from the cuff, using a syringe, while maintaining positive pressure via the ventilator or a self-inflating manual resuscitator.

3. Reinflate the cuff with just enough air to prevent gross leakage when positive pressure is again applied to airway.

Rationale

If the tube becomes blocked the patient will not be able to breathe.

The cuff is deflated periodically to prevent necrosis of the tracheal mucosa. However, with soft cuffs or atmospheric seal cuffs, deflation of cuffs is not usually necessary.

Excessive cuff inflation may cause pressure necrosis over a period of time.

Tracheostomy

Nursing action

1. Tracheostomy care should be given as needed, using sterile technique.

Rationale

To continue ventilation while the inner cannula is removed, a substitute sterile inner cannula or adapter should be inserted into the outer cannula and connected to the ventilator.

Bacteriological specimens

Nursing action

1. Aspirate tracheal secretions into a sterile container and send to laboratory for culture and sensitivity tests.

Rationale

This technique allows the earliest detection of infection or change in infecting organisms in the tracheobronchial tree.

a. This is done immediately after endotracheal intubation.
b. Gram-staining of secretion is done, as required.

Circulatory measurements

Nursing action

1. Monitor pulse rate and arterial blood pressure; intra-arterial pressure monitoring may be carried out.

Rationale

To accomplish intra-arterial pressure monitoring a catheter is introduced into an artery, usually the radial or femoral, and the pressure at the catheter tip is transmitted to a pressure transducer that converts the pressure wave into an electrical signal that is displayed for continuous visual observation on an oscilloscope.

2. Measure the central venous pressure as directed.

This measurement provides a guide for the administration of blood and other intravenous fluids and is also a criterion for determining the presence of right ventricular failure.

Sedation and muscle relaxants

Nursing action

1. Administer sedatives and muscle relaxants as directed.

Rationale

Sedatives and muscle relaxants eliminate spontaneous breathing efforts between ventilator cycles and reduce oxygen consumption. Morphine and curare (or similar drugs) produce vasodilatation. Measure arterial blood pressure before their administration to detect hypotension.

2. Explain procedures to patient and provide reassurance.

The patient may be awake although not capable of any motor response while these drugs are being given.

Fluid balance

Nursing action

1. Record intake and output precisely and obtain an accurate daily weight.

Rationale

Positive fluid balance resulting in increase in body weight and interstitial pulmonary oedema is a frequent problem in patients requiring mechanical ventilation. Prevention requires early recognition of fluid accumulation. Average adult who is dependent on parenteral nutrition can be expected to lose 0.25kg/per day; therefore, *constant body weight indicates positive fluid balance*.

Nutrition

Nursing action

1. Start nasogastric feeding.

Rationale

Patients on mechanical ventilation have their artificial airway cuff inflated at all times.

Abdominal complications

Nursing action	**Rationale**
1. Test all stools and gastric drainage for occult blood.	About a quarter of patients requiring mechanical ventilation develop gastrointestinal bleeding; many of these patients require blood transfusions.
2. Measure abdominal girth daily.	Abdominal distension occurs frequently with respiratory failure and further hinders respiration by elevation of the diaphragm. Measurement of abdominal girth provides objective assessment of the degree of distension.

Communication
1. Provide writing paper and pad. A patient on mechanical ventilation with tracheostomy tube is unable to talk.
2. Establish some form of nonverbal communication if patient is too sick to write. Give patient the call light.
3. Reassure patient and family that normal speech will return upon removal of tracheal tube.
4. Ensure that the patient has adequate rest and sleep.
5. Keep the patient in touch with reality; explain that mechanical ventilation is only temporary.

Recording
Maintain a flow sheet to record ventilation patterns, arterial blood studies, venous chemical determinations, haematocrit, status of fluid balance, weight and assessment of patient's condition.

GUIDELINES: WEANING THE PATIENT FROM THE MECHANICAL VENTILATOR

Weaning is the process by which the patient is gradually allowed to assume the responsibility for regulating and performing his own ventilation. Before weaning is instituted, the patient should have acceptable arterial blood gases while on the ventilator, have no evidence of acute pulmonary complication or dead space ventilation, have an intrapulmonary shunt less than 30 per cent and be haemodynamically stable while on the ventilator.

EQUIPMENT
Varies according to technique used
T-piece (see p. 124)
Intermittent Mandatory Ventilation (IMV) or Synchronized Intermittent
   Mandatory Ventilation (SIMV) equipment (set up in addition to ventilator or
   incorporated in ventilator and circuitry)

Assessment

Nursing action

1. For weaning to be successful, the patient must be physiologically capable of maintaining spontaneous respirations. Assessments must ensure that:
   a. The underlying disease process is significantly reversed, as evidenced by pulmonary examination, arterial blood gas, chest X-ray.
   b. The patient can mechanically perform ventilation and should: have vital capacity greater than 10–15ml/kg; have tidal volume greater than 5ml/kg; have spontaneous respiratory rate of less than 25 breaths per min.; be without significant tachycardia; not be hypotensive; have optimal haemaglobin for his condition.

2. Assess for other factors that may cause respiratory insufficiency:
   a. Acid–base abnormality.
   b. Caloric depletion.
   c. Electrolyte abnormality.
   d. Exercise intolerance.
   e. Fever.
   f. Abnormal fluid balance.
   g. Hyperglycaemia.
   h. Infection.
   i. Pain.
   j. Protein loss.
   k. Sleep deprivation.
   l. Decreased level of consciousness.

Rationale

Provides baseline; ensures that patient is capable of having adequate neuromuscular control to provide adequate ventilation.

Weaning is difficult when these conditions are present.

Planning and implementation
Preparatory phase

Nursing action

1. Ensure psychological preparation. Explain procedure. Explain that weaning is not always successful on the initial attempt.

2. Prepare appropriate equipment:
   a. T-tube.
   b. IMV or SIMV circuitry (frequently incorporated in ventilator circuitry)

3. Position the patient in sitting or semi-Fowler's position.

Rationale

Explaining procedure to patient will decrease patient anxiety and promote co-operation. The patient should not be discouraged if weaning is unsuccessful on the first attempt.

Increases lung compliance, decreases work of breathing.

4. Pick optimal time of day.

The patient should be rested.

5. Perform bronchial hygiene necessary to ensure that the patient is in best condition (postural drainage, chest physical therapy and suctioning) prior to weaning attempt.

The patient should be in best pulmonary condition for weaning to be successful.

Performance phase
T-piece
This system provides oxygen enrichment and humidity to a patient with an endotracheal or tracheostomy tube while allowing completely spontaneous respirations (for set-up and function, see oxygen therapy section, p. 116).

Nursing action

Rationale

1. Discontinue mechanical ventilation and apply T-piece adapter.

Stay with the patient during weaning time to decrease patient anxiety and monitor for tolerance of procedure.

2. Monitor the patient for factors indicating need for reinstitution of mechanical ventilation:
   a. Blood pressure increase or decrease greater than 20mmHg systolic or 10mmHg diastolic.
   b. Heart rate increase of 20 beats/minute or rate greater than 110.
   c. Respiratory rate increase greater than 10 breaths per minute or rate greater than 30.
   d. Tidal volume less than 250–300ml (in adults).
   e. Appearance of new cardiac ectopy, or increase in baseline ectopy.
   f. Pao_2 less than 60, $Paco_2$ greater than 55, or pH less than 7.35 (may accept lower Pao_2 and pH, and higher $Paco_2$ in patients with chronic obstructive airways disease).

Indicates intolerance of weaning procedure.

3. Institute other techniques helpful in encouraging weaning:
   a. Mental stimulation.
   b. Biofeedback.
   c. Participation in care.

Provides motivation and positive feedback.

IVM or SIMV weaning

Nursing action

Rationale

1. Set ventilator to IMV or SIMV mode.

2. Set rate interval.

This determines the time interval between machine-delivered breaths, during which the patient will breathe on his own.

3. If the patient is on continuous flow IMV circuitry, observe reservoir bag to be sure that it remains mostly inflated during all phases of ventilation.

The gas flow rate into the bag must be adequate to prevent the bag from collapsing during inspiration. Flow rates of 6 to 10 litres per minute are usually adequate.

4. If gas for the patient's spontaneous breath is delivered via a demand valve regulator, ensure that machine sensitivity is at maximum setting.

Aids in decreasing work of breathing necessary to open demand valve.

5. Evaluate for tolerance of procedure. Monitor for factors indicating need for increase or decrease of mandatory respiratory rate. In rapid weaning, changes may be made approximately every 20 to 30 minutes.

Indicates intolerance of weaning procedure.

6. If intolerance is not indicated, decrease mandatory rate as patient tolerates.

May be done as frequently as every 20 to 30 minutes with arterial blood gas monitoring, documentation of successful weaning.

7. Institute other techniques helpful in encouraging weaning.

Provides motivation and positive feedback.

Evaluation/outcome

Nursing action

Rationale

1. Record at each weaning interval: heart rate, blood pressure, respiratory rate, F_1O_2, and arterial blood gas.

Provides record of procedure and assessment of progress.

RESPIRATORY CLINICAL CONDITIONS

THE PNEUMONIAS

Pneumonia is an inflammatory process, involving the terminal airways and alveoli of the lung, because of an infection (bacteria, viruses, *Mycoplasma*, fungi).

PREDISPOSING FACTORS AND FEATURES

1. Pneumonia may be community-acquired (due to a limited number of organisms, namely *Streptococcus pneumoniae*) or hospital-acquired, due primarily to aerobic Gram-negative bacilli and staphylococci.
2. Pathogens producing pneumonia may be carried in the nasopharynx of a healthy person.
3. Pathogens may invade tissues when the host's natural resistance is lowered by severe underlying illness.
4. Colds and upper respiratory tract infections lead to more serious illnesses by allowing bacterial invasion of lower respiratory tract.
5. Immunocompromised patients (those receiving corticosteroids; those with cancer; those being treated with chemotherapy or radiotherapy; those undergoing organ transplantation) have an increased chance of developing overwhelming infection.
6. A wide variety of pulmonary infections may develop in patients receiving immunosuppressive drugs (aerobic and anaerobic Gram-negative bacilli, *Staphylococcus*, *Nocardia*, fungi, *Candida*, viruses, *Pneumocystis carinii*, reactivation of tuberculosis and others).
7. Any condition interfering with normal drainage

of the lung will predispose the person to pneumonia (e.g., cancer of the lung).

8. Postoperative patients may develop broncho-pneumonia, since anaesthesia impairs respiratory defences and decreases diaphragmatic movement.

9. Depression of the central nervous system (from drugs [including alcohol], head injury) predispose the patient to pneumonia.

10. People over 50 have a higher fatality rate even with appropriate antibiotic therapy.

NURSING ALERT

Recurring pneumonia often indicates underlying disease (cancer of the lung, multiple myeloma).

HEALTH MAINTENANCE AND PREVENTIVE MEASURES

1. Natural resistance should be maintained (adequate nutrition, rest, exercise).
2. Avoid contract with people who have upper respiratory infections.
3. Obliteration of cough reflex and aspiration of secretions should be avoided.
4. Adequate bronchial hygiene should be employed.
5. Immobilized patients should be turned every two hours and encouraged to breathe deeply, sigh and cough.
6. Use every measure to reduce bacterial colonization and superinfection of the hospitalized patient.
7. Highly susceptible people (elderly and chronically ill) should be immunized against influenza.
8. Pneumococcal vaccine should be given to those at greatest risk – persons over 50 with chronic systemic diseases, chronic obstructive airways disease, sickle cell anaemia, absence of spleen, immunosuppression patients who have had a pneumonectomy.

Assessment
CLINICAL FEATURES
See Tables 4.2 and 4.3.

DIAGNOSTIC EVALUATION

1. Chest auscultation and percussion – listen for dullness to percussion, bronchial breath sounds, crackles.
2. Lateral and posteroanterior chest X-rays – to localize the process and determine presence or absence of fluid.
3. Gram stain, culture and sensitivity studies of sputum.
4. Blood culture – to recover causative organism; bloodstream invasion (bacteraemia) occurs frequently with bacterial pneumonia.
5. Thoracocentesis – if pleural effusion is present.
6. Other serological tests for *Legionella pneumophila*, psittacosis, etc.
7. Counterimmunoelectrophoresis and immunofluorescence microscopy – for immunological detection of microbial antigens or their products.

PATIENT PROBLEMS

1. Ineffective breathing patterns and cough related to infection of lung.
2. Potential for complications (pain, alteration in tissue perfusion, impaired gas exchange, fluid volume deficit) related to respiratory toxicity and pneumonic disease process.
3. Knowledge deficit of therapeutic and preventive programme.

Planning and implementation
NURSING INTERVENTIONS
For a patient with bacterial pneumonia

Assessment

1. Take a careful history to help establish aetiology:
   a. What was the mode of onset?
   b. Number, frequency and duration of chills.

Table 4.2   Commonly encountered nonbacterial pneumonias

Type (nonbacterial)	Organism responsible	Manifestations	Clinical features	Treatment	Complications
Mycoplasmal pneumonia	*Mycoplasma pneumoniae*	Gradual onset, severe headache, irritating hacking cough productive of scanty, mucoid sputum Anorexia; malaise Low grade fever	Occurs most commonly in children and young adults Cold agglutinin antibody titre elevated	Tetracycline	Rare: pleural effusion meningoence- phalitis myelitis Guillain-Barré syndrome
Viral pneumonia	Influenza viruses Parainfluenza viruses Respiratory syncytial viruses Adenovirus Varicella, rubella, rubeola, herpes simplex, cytomegalo- virus, Epstein–Barr virus	Cough Constitutional symptoms may be pronounced (severe headache, anorexia, fever and myalgia)	In majority of patients influenza begins as an acute coryza; others have bronchitis, pleurisy, etc, while still others develop gastrointestinal symptoms Risk of developing influenza related to crowding and close contact of groups of individuals	Treat symptomatically Does not respond to treatment with presently available antibiotics Prophylactic vaccination recommended for high risk persons (over 65; chronic cardiac or pulmonary disease, diabetes and other metabolic disorders)	May develop a superimposed bacterial infection Bronchopneumonia Pericarditis; endocarditis
Pneumocystis carinii pneumonia	*Pneumocystis carinii*	Insidious onset Increasing dyspnoea and nonproductive cough Tachypnoea; progresses rapidly to intercostal retraction, nasal flaring and cyanosis Lowering of arterial oxygen tension Chest X-ray will reveal diffuse, bilateral interstitial pneumonia	Usually seen in host whose resistance is compromised Organism invades lungs of patients who have suppressed immune system (from cancer, leukaemia) or following immunosuppres- sive therapy for cancer, organ transplant or collagen disease Frequently associated with concurrent infection by viruses (cytomegalo- virus), bacteria and fungi Diagnosis made by lung biopsy	Pentamide isethionate	Patients are critically ill Death may be due to asphyxia
Legionnaire's disease	*Legionella pneumophila*	Cough Toxaemia Gastrointestinal symptoms Hyponatraemia		Erythromycin	

Table 4.3   Commonly encountered bacterial pneumonias

Type (bacterial)	Organism responsible	Manifestations
Streptococcal pneumonia	*Streptococcus pneumoniae*	May be history of previous respiratory infection Sudden onset, with shaking and chills Rapidly rising fever Cough, with expectoration of rusty or green (purulent) sputum Pleuritic pain aggravated by cough Chest dull to percussion; râles, bronchial breath sounds
Staphylococcal pneumonia	*Staphylococcus aureus*	Often prior history of viral infection Insidious development of cough, with expectoration of yellow, bloodstreaked mucus Onset may be sudden if patient is outside hospital Fever Pleuritic chest pain Pulse varies; may be slow in proportion to temperature
Klebsiella pneumonia	*Klebsiella pneumoniae* (Friedländer's bacillus – encapsulated Gram-negative aerobic bacillus)	Onset sudden with high fever, chills, pleuritic pain, haemoptysis Dyspnoea, cyanosis Pink, gelatinous or loose, thin sputum expectorated Profound prostration and toxicity
Pseudomonas pneumonia	*Pseudomonas aeruginosa*	Apprehension, confusion, cyanosis, bradycardia, reversal of diurnal temperature curve

Clinical features	Treatment	Complications
Herpes simplex lesions often present Usually involves one or more lobes	Penicillin G Alternate drug therapy in penicillin-allergic patient (erythromycin, clindamycin, cephalothin)	Shock Pleural effusion Superinfections Pericarditis
Frequently seen in hospital setting Staphyloccocal pneumonia is a necrotizing infection Treatment must be vigorous and prolonged due to disease's tendency to destroy the lungs Organism may develop rapid lung resistance Prolonged convalescence usual	Methicillin, nafcillin, clindamycin, lincomycin	Effusion/pneumothorax Lung abscess Empyema Meningitis
Tends to attack chronically ill, debilitated, alcoholic and elderly people or those with chronic obstructive pulmonary disease Tissue necrosis occurs rapidly in lungs May be rapidly fulminating, progressing to fatal outcome	Gentamicin, cephalothin, cefazolin, kanamycin	Multiple lung abscesses with cyst formation Persistent cough with expectoration remains for prolonged period Empyema Pericarditis
High mortality rate Susceptible persons: those with pre-existing lung disease, cancer (particularly leukaemia); those with homograft transplants, burns; debilitated persons; patients receiving prolonged courses of antibiotics	Gentamicin, carbenicillin	Multiple lung abscess formation High fatality rate
Positive pressure breathing equipment may be contaminated with these organisms		

   c. Description of chest pain.

   d. Patient taking any recent antibiotic treatment?

   e. Any family illness?

   f. Alcohol, tobacco, drug abuse?

2. Identify the aetiological agent causing the pneumonia and determine the drug sensitivity:

   a. Obtain freshly expectorated sputum for direct smear (Gram stain) and culture.

     (i) Be sure the patient *coughs* up sputum, not saliva.

     (ii) Instruct the patient to expectorate into sterile container for culture. The expectorate may become contaminated with colonizing upper respiratory flora.

   b. Use of physiotherapy, as directed; tenacious sputum may be liquefied by inhaling nebulized aerosol of water or saline solution by mask.

   c. Aspirate trachea with catheter if patient is too ill to expectorate sputum.

3. Give prescribed antibiotic agent – the therapy of pneumonia depends on laboratory identification of the agent causing the infection and on the drainage of purulent secretions.

Clearing the bronchi of collected secretions

This is important as retained secretions interfere with gas exchange and may cause slow recovery.

1. Encourage high level of fluid intake within limits of patient's cardiac reserve – adequate hydration thins mucus and serves as an effective expectorant; replaces fluid losses due to fever, diaphoresis, dehydration and dyspnoea.

2. Humidify air to loosen secretions and improve ventilation.

3. Encourage the patient to cough; avoid suppressing the cough reflex, especially in patients who sound 'bubbly'.

4. Employ chest wall percussion and postural drainage to mobilize secretions.

5. Utilize tracheal aspiration in patients with poor cough response.

6. Assist in bronchoscopic removal of thickened mucous plugs if patient is too weak to cough effectively.

7. Auscultate the chest for crackles.

8. Control cough when coughing is nonproductive and paroxysms cause serious hypoxaemia; give moderate doses of codeine as prescribed.

9. Avoid hypoxaemia, especially in patients with existing heart disease.

Careful and continuous observation of the patient until clinical condition improves

1. Remember that fatal complications may develop during the early period of antibiotic treatment.

2. Monitor temperature, pulse, respiration, and blood pressure at regular intervals to assess the patient's response to therapy.

3. The doctor will listen to the lungs and heart for heart murmurs or friction rub as this may indicate acute bacterial endocarditis, pericarditis or myocarditis.

4. Assess for resistant fever or return of fever from:

   a. Drug allergy – usually skin eruptions appear seven to ten days after the beginning of treatment.

   b. Drug resistance or slow response to therapy.

   c. Inadequate or inappropriate antibiotic therapy.

   d. Inadequate lung drainage.

   e. Superinfection (infection with a second organism resistant to antibiotics used).

   f. Failure of pneumonia to resolve; raises suspicion of underlying carcinoma of bronchus.

   g. Pneumonia caused by unusual bacteria, fungi, tuberculosis or *Pneumocystis carinii*.

5. Obtain chest X-rays to follow subsidence of pneumonic process.

Supportive methods of treatment

1. Blood gas analysis to determine oxygen need and patient response to the concentration of oxygen selected. An arterial oxygen tension (Pao_2) below 55mmHg indicates hypoxaemia.

2. Administer oxygen at concentration to maintain Pao_2 at acceptable level – hypoxaemia may be encountered because of abnormal ventilation/perfusion ratios in affected lung segments.

3. Avoid high concentrations of oxygen in patients with chronic obstructive airways disease (chronic bronchitis, emphysema) – *the use of high oxygen concentrations may worsen alveolar ventilation by removing the patient's only remaining ventilatory drive.*

4. Observe the patient for cyanosis, dyspnoea, hypoxaemia, and confusion.

5. Patients with pneumonia and coexisting chronic ventilatory insufficiency may require mechanical ventilation.

6. Relieve the pleuritic pain:

   a. Avoid suppressing a productive cough.

   b. Avoid narcotics in patient with history of chronic obstructive airways disease.

   c. Administer moderate doses of analgesics to relieve pleuritic pain.

d. Treat dry cough and laryngospasm with aerosolized water produced by an ultrasonic nebulizer.

e. Evaluate the patient's response, before administering sedatives or tranquillizers, to assess for signs and symptoms suggestive of meningitis.

NURSING ALERT

Restlessness, confusion, aggressiveness may be due to cerebral hypoxia. In such instances, sedatives are inappropriate.

7. Maintain adequate hydration, since fluid loss is high from fever, dehydration, dyspnoea and diaphoresis.
8. Encourage modified bed rest during febrile period.
9. Treat abdominal distension or ileus, which may be due to swallowing of air during intervals of severe dyspnoea.
   a. Pass nasogastric tube for acute gastric distension.
10. Assist patient as necessary with activities of living.

Prevention of complications

1. Patients should respond to treatment within 24 to 48 hours. However, be on the alert for complications such as the following:
   a. Pleural effusion.
   b. Sustained hypotension and shock, especially in Gram-negative bacterial disease, particularly in the elderly.
   c. Delayed recovery.
   d. Superinfection: pericarditis, bacteraemia, meningitis.
   e. Atelectasis – from obstruction of bronchus by accumulated secretions; may occur at any stage of acute pneumonia.
   f. Delirium – *this is considered a medical emergency*.
   g. Congestive heart failure, cardiac dysrhythmias, pericarditis, myocarditis.
   h. Peripheral thrombophlebitis, with or without pulmonary emboli.
   i. Acute respiratory insufficiency.
2. Employ special nursing surveillance for patients with the following conditions:
   a. Alcoholism or chronic obstructive airways disease; these people, as well as elderly patients, may have little or no fever.
   b. Chronic bronchitis; it is difficult to detect subtle changes in condition, since the patient may have seriously compromised pulmonary function.
   c. Epilepsy: pneumonia may result from aspiration following a seizure.
   d. Delirium, which may be caused by hypoxia, meningitis, delirium tremens of alcoholism.
      (i) Prepare for lumbar puncture; meningitis may be lethal.
      (ii) Ensure adequate hydration and give mild sedation, as prescribed.
      (iii) Give oxygen.
      (iv) Delirium must be controlled to prevent exhaustion and cardiac failure.
3. Assess these patients for *unusual behaviour*, alterations in mental status, stupor and congestive heart failure.

DISCHARGE PLANNING AND PATIENT EDUCATION

1. Fatigue, weakness and depression may be prolonged after pneumonia.
2. Encourage chair rest after fever subsides; gradually increase activities to bring energy level back to pre-illness stage.
3. Encourage breathing exercises to clear lungs and promote full expansion and function after the fever subsides.
4. Explain that a chest X-ray is taken four to six weeks after discharge; should show cleared lungs.
5. It is wise to stop smoking. Cigarette smoking destroys tracheobronchial cilial action, which is the first line of defence of lungs; also irritates mucosa of bronchi and inhibits function of alveolar scavenger cells (macrophages).
6. Advise the patient to keep up natural resistance with good nutrition, adequate rest – one episode of pneumonia may make the individual susceptible to recurring respiratory infections.
7. Instruct the patient to avoid fatigue, sudden extremes in temperature, and excessive alcohol intake, which lower resistance to pneumonia.
8. Encourage the patient to obtain influenza vaccine at prescribed times. Influenza increases susceptibility to secondary bacterial pneumonia.
9. Encourage the patient to seek medical advice about receiving pneumococcal vaccine against *Streptococcus pneumoniae*, which is effective against the majority of bacteraemic pneumococcal diseases.

Evaluation
EXPECTED OUTCOMES
1. Patient demonstrates improved respiratory

function – normal blood gases, respiratory rates, breathing patterns.
2. Is free of complications – diminished cough and sputum production, improved chest X-rays, decline in fever.
3. Adheres to therapeutic and preventive programme. Takes prescribed antibiotic drug and does breathing exercises; stops smoking and understands preventive measures.

ASPIRATION PNEUMONIA

Aspiration is the inhalation of oropharyngeal secretions and/or stomach contents into the lungs. It may produce an acute form of pneumonia.

AETIOLOGY
Patients at risk and factors associated with risk:
1. Loss of protective airway reflexes – swallowing, laryngeal, cough.
   a. Altered state of consciousness (general anaesthesia, head injury, stroke, coma, convulsions);
   b. Alcohol; drug overdose;
   c. During resuscitation procedures;
   d. Seriously ill, debilitated patients;
   e. Abnormalities of normal pharyngeal and gag reflexes.
2. Nasogastric tube feedings.
3. Obstetrical patients – from general anaesthesia, lithotomy position, delayed emptying of stomach from enlarged uterus, labour contractions.
4. Oesophageal disease – hiatus hernia.
5. Delayed emptying time of stomach – intestinal obstruction, abdominal distension.
6. Prolonged endotracheal intubation/tracheostomy – can depress glottic and laryngeal reflexes from disuse.

PREVENTION
1. Be on guard constantly and monitor patients at risk as described above.
2. Elevate head of bed for debilitated patients, for those receiving tube feedings, and for those with motility diseases of the oesophagus.
3. Place patients with impaired reflexes in a lateral position.
4. Be sure that nasogastric tube is patent.
5. Give tube feedings slowly, with patient sitting up in bed.
   a. Check position of tube in stomach before feeding.

b. Check seal of cuff of tracheostomy or endotracheal tube before feeding.
6. Keep the patients in a fasting state before anaesthesia (at least eight hours).
7. Place the unconscious patient on his side and elevate the foot of the bed 15–23cm unless medically contraindicated.

Assessment
CLINICAL FEATURES
1. Depends on volume and character of aspirated contents:
   a. Food particles – mechanical blockage of airways and secondary infection;
   b. Pathogenic bacteria – from oropharyngeal secretions containing bacteria;
   c. Gastric juice – destructive to alveoli and capillaries; results in outpouring of protein-rich fluids into the interstitial and intra-alveolar spaces – impairs exchange of oxygen and carbon dioxide, producing hypoxaemia, respiratory insufficiency and failure;
   d. Faecal contamination – endotoxins may be absorbed or thick proteinaceous material found in the intestinal contents may obstruct airway, leading to atelectasis and secondary bacterial infection.
2. Tachycardia tachypnoea.
3. Dyspnoea and cough.
4. Cyanosis.
5. Crackles, rhonchi, wheezing.
6. Pink, frothy sputum (may simulate acute pulmonary oedema).
7. Fever.

NURSING ALERT
The morbidity and mortality rate of aspiration pneumonia remains high even with optimum treatment. Prevention is the key to the problem.

PATIENT PROBLEMS
1. Ineffective airway clearance and alteration in breathing pattern (dyspnoea) related to aspiration of secretions or stomach contents into lungs.
2. Impaired gas exchange.
3. Potential fluid volume deficit.
4. Potential for complications (infection, respiratory or metabolic acidosis).

Planning and implementation
NURSING INTERVENTIONS
Improvement of respiratory function
(The therapy depends on the material aspirated.)
1. Clear the obstructed airway:

a. If foreign body becomes lodged in the patient's throat, remove object with forceps.

b. Place the patient in tilted head-down position on right side (right side more frequently affected if patient has aspirated solid particles).

c. Suction tracheal/endotracheal tube – to remove any particulate matter.

d. Prepare for laryngoscopy/bronchoscopy if the patient is asphyxiated by solid material.

2. Correct hypoxia by immediate ventilation:

a. Give oxygen.

b. Place patient on assisted ventilation – if adequate Po_2 cannot be maintained with other means of administering oxygen.

3. Correct hypotension (usually the result of hypovolaemia and hypoxia) by fluid volume replacement.

Prevention or resolution of complications

1. Monitor for fever, purulent sputum and X-ray evidence of pulmonary infiltrate.

2. Give supportive therapy as prescribed.

a. Antibiotics – if there is evidence of superimposed bacterial infection; pulmonary infection usually occurs one to two weeks after initial insult.

b. Correct acidosis – respiratory acidosis and metabolic acidosis indicate a severe reaction due to aspiration of gastric contents.

c. Monitor arterial blood gases.

3. Watch for development of later complications; lung abscess, empyema.

Evaluation
EXPECTED OUTCOMES

1. Patient demonstrates improved respiratory function: normal blood gases, respiratory rate, breathing pattern.

2. Shows no signs of complications: no fever or acidosis, no coughing or dyspnoea, no evidence of pneumonitis on chest X-ray.

PLEURISY

Pleurisy is a clinical term to describe *pleuritis* (inflammation of the pleura). Fibrinous pleurisy is deposition of a fibrinous exudate on the pleural surface.

CAUSES

May occur in the course of many pulmonary diseases:

1. Pneumonia (bacterial, viral);

2. Tuberculosis;

3. Pulmonary infarction, embolism;

4. Pulmonary abscess;

5. Upper respiratory tract infection;

6. Pulmonary neoplasm.

CLINICAL FEATURES

1. Chest pain – becomes severe, sharp and knife-like upon inspiration (pleuritic pain).

a. Pain may become minimal or absent when breath is held.

b. Pain may be localized or radiate to shoulder or abdomen.

2. Intercostal tenderness.

3. Pleural friction rub – grating or leathery sounds heard in both phases of respiration; heard low in the axilla or over the lung base posteriorly; may be heard only for a day or so.

4. Evidence of infection; fever, malaise, increased white cell count.

DIAGNOSTIC EVALUATION

Explain to the patient what is involved in the following investigations:

1. Chest X-ray;

2. Sputum examination;

3. Examination of pleural fluid obtained by thoracocentesis for smear and culture;

4. Pleural biopsy (selected patients).

TREATMENT AND NURSING MANAGEMENT

1. Implement treatment for the underlying primary disease (pneumonia, infarction, etc). Inflammation usually improves when the primary disease subsides.

2. Relieve the pain:

a. Give prescribed analgesics;

b. Splint the rib cage when the patient coughs;

c. Apply heat or cold – to provide symptomatic relief;

d. Instruct the patient to lie on affected side occasionally – to splint chest wall;

e. Assist with procaine intercostal block.

3. Watch for signs of development of pleural effusion (collection of fluid in pleural space): shortness of breath, pain, local decreased expansion of chest wall.

4. Assist the patient as necessary with the activities of living, e.g. hygiene needs.

PLEURAL EFFUSION

Pleural effusion refers to a collection of fluid in the

pleural space. It is rarely a primary disease, but is usually secondary to other diseases.

AETIOLOGY
Complication of:
1. Disseminated cancer (particularly lung and breast); lymphoma;
2. Infection: tuberculosis, bacterial pneumonia, pulmonary infection;
3. Congestive heart failure;
4. Cirrhosis;
5. Kidney disease;
6. Others: sarcoidosis, systemic lupus erythematosus, peritoneal dialysis, etc.

CLINICAL FEATURES
(Usually caused by underlying disease.)
1. Increasing dyspnoea.
2. Dullness or flatness to percussion (over areas of fluid) with minimal or absent breath sounds.

DIAGNOSTIC EVALUATION
Explain to the patient what is involved in the following investigations:
1. Chest X-ray;
2. Thoracocentesis – biochemical, bacteriological and cytological studies of pleural fluid;
3. Physical examination;
4. Pleuroscopy (visual exploration of pleural space through a thoracoscope inserted into the pleural space); pleural biopsy.

TREATMENT
1. The treatment depends on the cause.
2. The following methods of treatment have been advocated for malignant effusions:
   a. Thoracocentesis (aspiration) of fluid removal and relief of dyspnoea. In malignant diseases, thoracocentesis may provide only transient benefits since effusion may re-accumulate within a few days.
   b. Tube drainage (chest catheter) connected to underwater seal drainage system or suction; instillation of sclerosing agent (tetracycline; cytotoxic agent) into pleural space to obliterate pleural space by formation of adhesions between the visceral and parietal pleura (pleurodesis).
      (i) Chest tube inserted into pleural space to drain the fluid and re-expand the lung.
      (ii) Drug is introduced through tube into pleural space; tube is clamped; patient is helped to assume the following positions for one to five minutes each to ensure uniform distribution of the drug and maximize drug contact with pleural surfaces: prone, left side down, supine, right side down, knee to chest (if able).
      (iii) Tube is unclamped as prescribed.
      (iv) Chest drainage continued for 24 hours or longer.
      (v) Resulting pleural irritation, inflammation and fibrosis causes fusion of the visceral and parietal surfaces when they are brought together by the negative pressure caused by chest suction.
   c. Radiation of the chest wall.
   d. Surgical procedures to control malignant effusions – parietal pleurectomy; pleural abrasion.

LUNG ABSCESS

A lung abscess is a localized, pus-containing, necrotic lesion in the lung characterized by cavity formation.

AETIOLOGY
1. Aspiration of vomitus or infected material from upper respiratory tract.
2. Aspiration of foreign body into lung.
3. Bronchial obstruction (usually a tumour causes obstruction to the bronchus, causing distal stasis and infection of secretions, or there is necrosis within the tumour mass).
4. Necrotizing pneumonias.
5. Tuberculosis.
6. Pulmonary embolism.

CLINICAL FEATURES
1. The right lung is involved more frequently than the left – owing to dependent position of the right bronchus, the less acute angle which the right main bronchus forms within the trachea and its larger size.
2. In the initial stages, the cavity in the lung may or may not communicate with the bronchus.
3. Eventually the cavity becomes surrounded or encapsulated by a wall of fibrous tissue, except at one or two points where the necrotic process extends until it reaches the lumen of some bronchus or pleural space and establishes a communication with the respiratory tract, the pleural cavity (bronchopleural fistula), or both.

Assessment
CLINICAL SIGNS
1. Cough.

2. Fever and malaise – from segmental pneumonitis and atelectasis.
3. Headache, anaemia, weight loss.
4. Pleuritic chest pain – from extension of suppurative pneumonitis to pleural surface.
5. Production of mucopurulent sputum – often foul-smelling; blood streaking common; may become profuse after abscess ruptures into bronchial tree.

DIAGNOSTIC EVALUATION
1. History of patient.
2. X-ray of chest – for diagnosis and location of lesion.
3. Direct bronchoscopic visualization – to exclude possibility of tumour or foreign body; bronchial washings and brush biopsy may be done for cytology.
4. Bronchogram – may be necessary to differentiate between lung abscess and bronchiectasis.
5. Leucocytosis in acute stage.
6. Sputum culture and sensitivity – to determine causative organism(s) and antibiotic sensitivity.
7. Dullness and bronchial breath sounds – may be heard over diseased segment.

PATIENT PROBLEMS
1. Alteration in respiratory function (cough, dyspnoea, sputum production) related to presence of suppurative lung disease.
2. Alteration in comfort (chest pain and headache) related to underlying condition.
3. Potential nonadherence to therapeutic regimen related to extended course of treatment.
4. Potential for infection and nutritional imbalance.

Planning and implementation
NURSING INTERVENTIONS
1. Carry out drainage procedures:
   a. Postural drainage (hastens resolution) – positions to be assumed depend on the segmental localization of the abscess.
   b. Percussion, coughing and breathing exercises.
   c. Prepare patient for therapeutic bronchoscopy – to drain abscess.
2. Give prescribed antibiotics based on culture and sensitivity studies of organisms – mixed infections are common and may require multiple antibiotics.
3. Measure and record the volume of sputum – to follow the course of healing.
4. Utilize supportive measures during the acute phase of illness:
   a. Support respiratory and cardiac function.

   b. Give a high-protein, high-calorie diet – chronic infections are associated with catabolic state, which requires calories and protein to facilitate healing.
   c. Care for the patient having blood component therapy – anaemia may be advanced in the patient with infection.
5. Prepare the patient for serial X-rays – to judge effectiveness of therapy.
6. Prepare for surgical intervention if indicated – done only if the patient fails to respond to adequate medical treatment.
   a. Excision – usually lobectomy (occasionally segmental resection); usually performed when there is a thick-walled abscess with purulent drainage.
   b. Thoracotomy tube drainage – usually done for patients who cannot tolerate major thoracotomy (elderly, patients with alcoholism and those with low pulmonary functional reserve).

PATIENT EDUCATION
1. Teach the patient that an extended course of antibiotic therapy (four to eight weeks) is usually necessary, depending on demonstration of improved/clear chest film.
2. Encourage the patient to have patience.
3. Encourage the patient to assume responsibility for attaining and maintaining an optimal state of health through a planned programme of good nutrition, rest and exercise.

Evaluation
EXPECTED OUTCOMES
1. Patient achieves improved respiratory function: temperature in normal range, less purulent sputum coughed up, improved X-ray.
2. Adheres to therapeutic regimen by taking antibiotics and reporting for follow-up care.

BRONCHIECTASIS

Bronchiectasis is a chronic dilation of the bronchi and bronchioles due to inflammation and destruction of their walls.

CAUSES
1. Pulmonary infections and obstruction of bronchi.
2. Aspiration of foreign bodies, vomitus or material from upper respiratory tract.
3. Extrinsic pressure from tumours, dilated blood vessels, enlarged lymph nodes.

ALTERED PHYSIOLOGY

Impairment of bronchial clearance → increased bronchial secretions → stasis → infection → weakening and further destruction of bronchial walls → increased dilation → atelectasis → inflammatory scarring → fibrosis of involved areas → respiratory insufficiency → ventilation and perfusion imbalance → hypoxaemia.

HEALTH MAINTENANCE AND PREVENTION

1. Treat all respiratory infections promptly.
2. Teach the family to seek medical treatment and ongoing surveillance if child has recurrent respiratory infections; more than half of cases start in childhood.
3. All unconscious patients should be turned (prone position to lateral) – to drain all bronchial segments.
4. Encourage individual immunization programme to prevent pertussis and measles (which can lead to bronchiectasis).

Assessment

CLINICAL FEATURES

The patient experiences symptoms when he has superimposed infection.

1. Persistent and/or productive cough with mucopurulent sputum.
2. Intermittent haemoptysis.
3. Recurrent fever and bouts of localized pulmonary infection/pneumonia.
4. Crackles (râles) and rhonchi over involved areas.
5. Dyspnoea (depending on amount of lung tissue involved).
6. Wheezing.
7. Clubbing of fingers (long-standing disease).

DIAGNOSTIC EVALUATION

1. Bronchogram (to map the entire bronchial tree to determine narrowing, dilation or obstruction of the bronchi).
2. Bronchoscopy – to rule out obstructive lesion.
3. Sputum examination.

PATIENT PROBLEMS

1. Ineffective airway clearance and breathing patterns related to copious sputum production and irreversible dilation of the bronchial tree.
2. Potential for infection.
3. Potential for nonadherence to therapeutic regimen related to prolonged course of disease.
4. Weight loss, weakness, dyspnoea and cyanosis related to advanced disease.

Planning and implementation

NURSING INTERVENTIONS

1. Empty the bronchi of their accumulated secretions:
   a. Use postural drainage suitable to segment(s) involved to drain the bronchiectatic areas by gravity, thus reducing degree of infection and amount of secretions.
      (i) Postural drainage should be done for 20 minutes twice daily, or more frequently as clinical condition indicates.
      (ii) Affected chest area may be percussed or 'cupped' to assist in raising secretions.
   b. Encourage copious fluid intake to reduce viscosity of sputum and make expectoration easier.
   c. Utilize vaporizer to provide humidification and to keep secretions liquid.
   d. Eliminate smoking and dusts, which are bronchial irritants that increase secretions.
   e. Give expectorants and bronchodilator drugs, as prescribed.
   f. Prepare patient for bronchoscopy when necessary to drain sputum and/or remove foreign body.
2. Implement treatment for the patient during periods of acute infection.
   a. Employ antibiotic therapy, as prescribed, guided by sensitivity studies on organisms cultured from sputum.
   b. Patients with repeated infections may be given short courses of antibiotics prophylactically during the winter months.
3. Prepare patient for surgical intervention when conservative treatment is inadequate.
   a. Segmental resection to spare as much healthy, functioning lung parenchyma as possible.
   b. Evaluate for postoperative complications:
      (i) Pneumonia;
      (ii) Empyema.

PATIENT EDUCATION

1. Instruct the patient to avoid noxious fumes, dusts and other pulmonary irritants (cigarette smoking).
2. Teach the patient to monitor sputum. Report to local GP if change in quantity (increase/decrease) or character occurs.
3. Instruct the patient and family about importance of pulmonary drainage:
   a. Teach drainage exercises and chest physical therapy techniques;
   b. Encourage postural drainage before rising in

the morning, since sputum accumulates during night;

c. Engage in physical activity throughout day to help move mucus.

4. Encourage regular dental care.

5. Emphasize the importance of influenza immunization.

6. For other patient education aspects, see 'Care of the Patient With Emphysema' (p. 186).

Evaluation

EXPECTED OUTCOMES

1. Patient demonstrates ability to clear airway of secretions.

2. Breathes with increased ease.

3. Adheres to therapeutic programme: takes prescribed medications, carries out pulmonary drainage exercises, has regular check-up.

CHRONIC OBSTRUCTIVE AIRWAYS DISEASE (COAD)

Chronic obstructive airways disease (COAD) is a term that refers to a group of conditions associated with chronic obstruction of airflow in the lungs. It includes:

1. Bronchitis.
2. Emphysema.
3. Asthma.

ALTERED PHYSIOLOGY

1. Basically, the person with COAD may have:

   a. Excessive secretion of mucus and chronic infection within the airways not due to specific causes (bronchitis);

   b. An increase in size of air spaces distal to the terminal bronchioles, with loss of alveolar walls and elastic recoil of the lungs (emphysema);

   c. Narrowing of the bronchial airways that changes in severity (asthma, since the triggering device in asthma is allergic in origin);

   d. There may be an overlap of these conditions.

2. As a result of these conditions, there is a subsequent derangement of airway dynamics (e.g. obstruction to airflow).

CAUSES OF COAD

1. Cigarette smoking.
2. Air pollution.
3. Occupational exposure.
4. Allergy.
5. Autoimmunity.

6. Infection.
7. Genetic predisposition.
8. Ageing.

CHRONIC BRONCHITIS

Chronic bronchitis is a chronic infection of the lower respiratory tract characterized by excessive mucus secretion, cough and dyspnoea associated with recurring infections of the lower respiratory tract. There is often reduced ability to ventilate the lungs.

A World Health Organization (WHO) definition of chronic bronchitis is 'cough and sputum on most days of over three months over two consecutive years, in the absence of other major lung disease'.

ALTERED PHYSIOLOGY

Infection, irritation, hypersensitivity → local hyperaemia → hypertrophy of mucous glands → increase in size and number of mucus-producing elements in bronchi (mucous glands and goblet cells) → inflammation and changes in bronchial and bronchiolar walls.

HEALTH MAINTENANCE AND PREVENTION

1. Avoid respiratory irritants, particularly tobacco smoke; chronic bronchitis is most often a smoker's disease.

2. People who are prone to respiratory infections should be immunized against influenza and *Streptococcus pneumoniae*.

3. Acute respiratory infections should be treated.

CLINICAL FEATURES

1. A wide range of viral, bacterial and mycoplasmal infections can produce acute exacerbations of bronchitis.

2. Exacerbations of chronic bronchitis are most apt to occur during winter months – patients have bronchospasm due to inhalation of cold air.

3. Secretions must be expelled; otherwise they produce chronic bronchial obstruction, air trapping, hypoxaemia, carbon dioxide retention and localized infection.

4. Chronic bronchitis often progresses to emphysema.

5. Hypoxaemia may lead to right ventricular failure (cor pulmonale).

6. Usually insidious, developing over a period of years.

   a. Persistent bouts of cough and sputum production.

b. Recurrent acute respiratory infections followed by persistent cough.

c. Production of thick, gelatinous sputum (greater amounts produced during superimposed infections).

d. Wheezing and dyspnoea as disease progresses.

DIAGNOSTIC EVALUATION
1. Chest X-ray – to exclude other diseases of the chest.
2. Pulmonary function and arterial blood gas studies.

MANAGEMENT
Goals
1. Maintain patency of peripheral bronchial tree.
2. Facilitate removal of bronchial exudates.
3. Prevent disability.
4. See below (emphysema) for management, health education and evaluation.

PULMONARY EMPHYSEMA

Pulmonary emphysema is a complex lung disease characterized by destruction of the alveoli, enlargement of distal airspaces and a breakdown of alveolar walls. There is a slowly progressive deterioration of lung function for many years before the development of illness.

CAUSES
(See 'Causes of COAD', p. 183.)

Assessment
CLINICAL FEATURES
1. Dyspnoea; slow in onset and steadily progressive.
2. Cough – may be minimal, except with respiratory infection.
3. Fatigue, sleep difficulties, irritability, anorexia, weight loss – due to hypoxia, increased respiratory muscular effort and respiratory acidosis.

DIAGNOSTIC EVALUATION
1. Clinical assessment of patient.
2. History of cough, exertional dyspnoea, wheezing, smoking, exposure to dusts, fumes, gases.
3. Pulmonary function tests.
4. Chest X-ray – abnormal only in advanced disease.
5. Arterial blood gas analysis (with exercise if possible) to detect hypoxaemia.

6. Alpha$_1$-antitrypsin assay – useful in identifying person at risk.
7. Explain the above investigations to the patient and why they are necessary.

COMPLICATIONS
1. Respiratory acidosis.
2. Cor pulmonale.
3. Congestive heart failure.
4. Spontaneous pneumothorax.
5. Overwhelming respiratory infections.
6. Cardiac dysrhythmias.
7. Profound depression.
8. Malnutrition.

PATIENT PROBLEMS
1. Hypoxaemia related to severe chronic obstructive pulmonary disease.
2. Faulty breathing patterns related to effects of disease.
3. Activity intolerance related to impaired pulmonary function and fatigue.
4. Potential for infection related to compromised pulmonary function.
5. Alteration in nutrition (less than body requirements) related to shortness of breath at meal times, loss of muscle mass, tenacious sputum, potassium depletion.
6. Coping difficulties and emotional lability related to shortness of breath and fatigue.
7. Sleep pattern disturbance related to hypoxia.

Planning and implementation
NURSING INTERVENTIONS
Removal of bronchial secretions to improve pulmonary ventilation and gas exchange
1. *Eliminate all pulmonary irritants, particularly cigarette smoking.*
   a. Cessation of smoking usually results in decreased pulmonary irritation, sputum production and cough.
   b. Avoid outside physical activities when air pollutants are high.
   c. Keep bedroom as dust-free as possible.
   d. Consider the use of air filters to remove particles and pollutants from air in areas where this is a problem.
   e. Use a room humidifier during winter months – allows dust particles to settle and makes air less irritating.
2. Control bronchospasm to decrease the work of breathing – many patients with chronic obstructive pulmonary disease have some degree of bronchospasm.

a. Bronchospasm is detected by auscultation with a stethoscope.

b. Administer prescribed bronchodilators, which dilate airways by relieving bronchial mucosal oedema and smooth muscle contraction.

(i) Drugs may be administered orally, sub-cutaneously, intravenously or rectally; or via nebulization (by pressurized aerosols, hand-held nebulizers, pump-driven nebulizers, metered-dose devices, ultrasonic unit).

(ii) Assess patient for unwanted side-effects – tremulousness, tachycardia, cardiac dysrhythmias, central nervous system stimulation, hypertension.

(iii) Follow inhalation of bronchodilator drug with inhalation of moisture – to thin secretions.

(iv) Avoid excessive use of bronchodilators.

(v) Auscultate the chest after administration of aerosol bronchodilators to assess improvement of air entry and reduction of adventitious breath sounds.

(vi) Assess if patient has reduction in dyspnoea.

3. Keep secretions liquid.
a. Encourage high level of fluid intake (8 to 10 glasses; 2 to 2½ litres daily) within level of cardiac reserve.
b. Give inhalations of nebulized water to humidify bronchial tree and liquefy sputum.

4. Use postural drainage positions to aid in clearance of secretions, since mucopurulent secretions are responsible for airway obstruction.
a. Positions that drain lower and middle lobes appear to be most helpful in patients with COAD.
b. Other patients achieve effective cough and sputum clearance while seated and leaning forward.
c. Employ percussion of thorax to assist in propulsion of sputum through the bronchi, when necessary.

5. Use controlled coughing.
a. Inhale slowly and deeply.
b. Exhale through pursed lips – empties lungs of residual volume.
c. Cough in short bursts of 'huffing' rather than vigorously forcing cough which causes airways to collapse.
d. Inhale slowly.

6. Prepare patient for bronchosopic removal of secretions if he is unable to cough and raise his sputum.

7. Prepare patient for endotracheal intubation or tracheostomy if indicated, to permit more effective suctioning of secretions and to provide ventilatory assistance.

NURSING ALERT

Patients with acute respiratory failure along with acute ventilatory failure and rapid CO_2 retention will require mechanical ventilation.

Control of infection

1. Recognize early manifestations of respiratory infection – increased dyspnoea, fatigue; change in colour, amount and character of sputum; nervousness; irritability; low-grade fever.

2. Obtain sputum for smear and culture.

3. Give prescribed antibiotics (ampicillin; erythromycin; tetracycline) at first sign of respiratory infection to control secondary bacterial infection in the bronchial tree, thus clearing the airways.

4. Periodic sputum cultures for possible superinfection should be done for patients on long-term antibiotic therapy.

5. Advise patient to avoid exposure to persons with respiratory tract infections.

6. Give corticosteroids as prescribed; these drugs have an anti-inflammatory effect, and thus help to relieve airway obstruction.
a. Short course of corticosteroids may be beneficial to persons who have acute attacks of bronchial obstruction, severe wheezing, or marked eosinophilia in sputum or blood.
b. Antacids may be prescribed to prevent development of an ulcer.

NURSING ALERT

Watch for increased susceptibility to infections, for gastrointestinal discomfort, and for bleeding tendencies.

Nutritional considerations

1. Dyspnoea, with accompanying air swallowing, cough, and sputum production, combined with intake of medications, contributes to loss of appetite and weight loss. Nutritional depletion may influence rate of decline in lung function.

2. Encourage six small meals daily if patient is dyspnoeic – even a small increase in abdominal contents may press on diaphragm and cause dyspnoea.

3. Offer high-protein diet with between-meal snacks to improve caloric intake and counteract weight loss.

4. Avoid foods producing abdominal discomfort.

5. Give supplemental oxygen while patient is eating to relieve dyspnoea (when directed).

Relief of severe hypoxaemia and related symptoms

1. Give low-flow oxygen to selected patients with severe, chronic, obstructive airways disease – to correct hypoxaemia in a controlled manner and thereby minimize CO_2 retention.
   a. In patients with COAD, poor exchange of gases may result in chronically elevated CO_2 (which is then a less effective stimulus to respiration). Giving a high concentration of oxygen may remove the hypoxic drive – leading to increased hypoventilation, respiratory decompensation and the development of a worsening respiratory acidosis.
   b. Low-flow oxygen dosage is individualized and is given after analysis of arterial blood gases.
   c. Graded exercises with low-flow oxygen may be given to increase exercise capacity.
2. Avoid narcotics, sedatives, and tranquillizers. Watch for excessive somnolence, restlessness, aggressiveness, anxiety, or confusion which is frequently caused by acute respiratory insufficiency.

Techniques of breathing retraining to strengthen diaphragm and muscles of expiration and to decrease the work of breathing

1. Relaxation exercises – to reduce stress, tension and anxiety.
2. Teach lower costal, diaphragmatic and abdominal breathing, using a slow and relaxed breathing pattern to reduce respiratory rate and decrease energy cost of breathing.
3. Use pursed-lip breathing at intervals and during periods of dyspnoea to control rate and depth of respiration and improve respiratory muscle coordination.

Reconditioning of patient and increase in physical activity

1. Employ graded exercise and physical conditioning programmes (enhances delivery of oxygen to tissues; allows functioning at a higher level of activity with greater comfort) – walking, stationary bicycle. Portable oxygen system for low-flow oxygen may be used for ambulation in selected patients – useful for patients with hypoxaemia with marked disability.
2. Encourage patient to carry out regular exercise training programme to increase physical endurance and promote sense of well-being and independence.
3. Train patient in energy-saving methods.

Psychosocial support

1. Understand that the constant shortness of breath and fatigue makes the patient irritable, apprehensive, anxious and depressed, with feelings of helplessness/hopelessness.
2. Assess the patient for reactive behaviours (anger, depression, acceptance).
3. Demonstrate a positive and interested approach to the patient:
   a. Be a good listener and show that you care.
   b. Be sensitive to his fears, anxiety and depression; helps give emotional relief and insight.
4. Strengthen the patient's self-image.
5. Allow the patient to express his feelings and retain (within a controlled degree) the mechanisms of denial and repression.
6. Be aware that sexual dysfunction is common in patients with COAD.
7. Support spouse/family members.

PATIENT EDUCATION

1. Give the patient a clear explanation of his disease, what to expect, how to treat and live with it. Reinforce by frequent explanations, reading material, demonstrations, and question and answer sessions.
2. Review with the patient the objectives of treatment and nursing management.
3. Work with the patient to set goals (i.e. stair climbing, return to work, etc).

Instruct the patient as follows:

1. Avoid exposure to respiratory irritants – cigarette smoke, pollens, fumes, aerosols, dust, cold.
   a. Stop smoking and avoid smoke-filled rooms.
   b. Avoid sweeping, dusting and exposure to paint, aerosols, bleaches, and other respiratory irritants.
   c. Keep kitchen ventilated.
   d. Stay out of extremely hot/cold weather to avoid aggravating bronchial obstruction and sputum production.
      (i) Keep a warming mask or scarf over nose and mouth to warm inspired air in cold weather.
      (ii) Stay indoors with air conditioning when pollution level is high.
      (iii) Try to avoid abrupt environmental changes.

(iv) Shower in warm (not too hot or too cold) water.

e. Humidify indoor air in winter; maintain 30 to 50 per cent humidity for optimal mucociliary function.

2. Prevent and treat respiratory infections.

a. Avoid exposure to persons with respiratory infections; a respiratory infection makes symptoms worse and can produce further irreversible damage.

b. Avoid crowds and areas with poor ventilation.

c. Take influenza immunization (if not allergic) to decrease likelihood of developing infection.

d. Recognize and report evidence of respiratory infection *promptly* to the local GP – chest pain, changes in character of sputum (amount, colour, or consistency), increasing difficulty in raising sputum, increasing cough/wheezing, increasing shortness of breath.

e. Take prescribed antibiotic at first sign of infection.

(i) Have a home supply available.

(ii) Have periodic sputum cultures when receiving long-term antibiotic therapy.

3. Reduce bronchial secretions.

a. Maintain an adequate fluid intake (8 to 10 glasses daily); mark down the amount of liquid consumed daily.

b. Take bronchodilators only as directed.

c. Follow postural drainage exercises as prescribed.

(i) Stay in each position five to fifteen minutes.

(ii) Utilize controlled cough after each position.

d. Take medications prescribed for cough and expectoration.

e. Avoid drugs that suppress cough and dry secretions (certain cough medicines, antihistamines).

4. Increase pulmonary ventilation.

a. Use respiratory therapy consistently and faithfully.

(i) Learn how to assemble and disassemble equipment.

(ii) Do the procedure immediately upon arising in the morning, before retiring, and as prescribed. Use the *exact* amount of medication prescribed.

(iii) Inhale and exhale as evenly as possible during the treatment.

(iv) Try to cough *productively* (with *controlled coughing*) after the treatment.

(a) Breathe slowly and deeply, using diaphragmatic breathing.

(b) Hold breath several seconds.

(c) Cough – two short, forceful coughs with the mouth open; the first cough loosens mucus, and the second cough moves it.

(d) Pause and inhale by sniffing quietly. (Inhaling vigorously may initiate unproductive coughing, which is energy consuming.)

(e) Rest.

(v) Practice oral hygiene after each treatment.

(vi) Clean respiratory therapy equipment daily to prevent contamination and secondary infection and ensure equipment functioning.

(a) Allow equipment to dry thoroughly before reassembling.

(b) Do not reuse medications/solution/water left standing in a humidifier/nebulizer.

5. Do breathing exercises to strengthen muscles of expiration, to strengthen and co-ordinate muscles of breathing, and to lessen fatigue and to help empty lungs more completely.

a. Learn the importance of slow and relaxed breathing (controlled breathing).

b. Practice diaphragmatic breathing and pursed-lip breathing.

c. Consciously use pursed-lip breathing during episodes of dyspnoea and stress.

d. Maintain muscle tone of the body by regular exercise.

6. Maintain general health at highest attainable level.

a. Follow good habits of nutrition – patients with COAD may have loss of muscle mass with poor nutritional status, poor appetite, potassium depletion, sodium retention and dehydration.

b. Follow high-protein diet with adequate mineral, vitamin and fluid intake.

c. Avoid excessive hot or cold fluids/foods that may provoke an irritating cough.

d. Avoid hard-to-chew foods (causes tiring) and gas-forming foods, which cause distension and restrict diaphragmatic movement.

e. Eat five to six small meals daily – to ease shortness of breath during and after meals.

f. Have rest periods before and after meals if eating produces shortness of breath.

g. Do not eat when upset/angry.

h. Avoid potassium depletion – patients with

COAD tend to have low potassium levels; also patient may be taking diuretics.
  (i) Watch for weakness, numbness, tingling of fingers, leg cramps.
  (ii) Foods high in potassium include bananas, dried fruits, dates, figs, orange juice, grape juice, milk, peaches, potatoes.
  i. Restrict sodium as directed.
  j. Use community resources (meals on wheels) if energy level is low.
7. Avoid activities that produce excessive shortness of breath.
  a. Live with the limitations that emphysema imposes.
  b. Learn to relax and work at a slower pace.
  c. Obtain vocational counselling to secure a sedentary job if presently in a demanding manual job.
  d. Avoid overfatigue, which is a factor in producing respiratory distress.
  e. Adjust activities according to individual fatigue patterns.
  f. Use pursed-lip breathing in a slow and relaxed manner during periods of breathlessness and physical exertion.
  g. Try to cope with emotional stress as positively as possible – such stress triggers attacks of dyspnoea.
  h. Study individual lifestyle and avoid energy-wasting activities.
  i. Exercise to improve physical condition.
8. Understand the importance of preserving existing function.
  a. Become familiar with the nature of emphysema and reasons for a therapeutic programme.
  b. Accept the fact that therapy and medical supervision must be continued for a lifetime.

Evaluation
EXPECTED OUTCOMES
1. Patient increases activity level: takes broncho-dilators/medications as prescribed, demonstrates improved exercise tolerance (walks longer distances; climbs more stairs), identifies time when energy levels are high/low.
2. Avoids and seeks treatment for infection.
3. Improves nutritional status; times meals to coincide with periods of improved breathing; rests before and after meals.
4. Demonstrates some relief of hypoxaemia with low-flow oxygen and graded exercises as prescribed.

5. Works to breathe more effectively; performs breathing exercises at scheduled periods.
6. Demonstrates improved emotional outlook; expresses feelings; seeks support group.
7. Adheres to therapeutic programme for controlling respiratory environment, preventing infection, reducing bronchial secretions, increasing pulmonary ventilation, practising breathing exercises, maintaining health, avoiding tiring activities and continuing with follow-up care.

PULMONARY HEART DISEASE (COR PULMONALE)

Pulmonary heart disease (cor pulmonale) is an alteration in the structure or function of the right ventricle resulting from disease affecting lung structure or function or its vasculature (except when this alteration results from disease of the left side of the heart or from congenital heart disease).

AETIOLOGY
1. Chronic obstructive airways disease – chronic bronchitis, emphysema most common.
2. Conditions that restrict ventilatory function – kyphoscoliosis.
3. Pulmonary vascular disease – pulmonary emboli.

PATHOPHYSIOLOGY
Chronic obstructive airways disease → hypoxia → hypercapnia → acidosis → circulatory complications → pulmonary hypertension → right heart enlargement → right heart failure.

Assessment
CLINICAL FEATURES
1. Peripheral oedema.
2. Respiratory insufficiency; progressive dyspnoea (orthopnoea, paroxysmal nocturnal dyspnoea), chronic cough.
3. Right heart enlargement demonstrated by:
  a. Physical examination;
  b. ECG changes;
  c. Chest X-ray – shows change in heart size.
4. Manifestations of carbon dioxide narcosis – headache, confusion, somnolence, coma.
5. Central cyanosis.

DIAGNOSTIC EVALUATION
1. Arterial blood gas analysis.
2. Pulmonary function tests.

PATIENT PROBLEMS
. Ineffective breathing pattern (dyspnoea) related to right ventricular hypertrophy and pulmonary hypertension.
. Impaired gas exchange.
. Potential fluid volume excess.
. Activity intolerance.

Planning and implementation
NURSING INTERVENTIONS
. Improve ventilation and correct hypoxaemia with its consequent pulmonary hypertension.
   a. Use oxygen with mechanical ventilatory aids as directed or continuous low-flow oxygen to reduce pulmonary artery pressure and pulmonary vascular resistance.
   b. Monitor arterial blood gases as a guide in assessing adequacy of alveolar ventilation.
   c. Avoid central nervous system depressants (narcotics, barbiturates, hypnotics) – have depressant action on respiratory centres.
   d. See management of respiratory failure (p. 98).
. Combat respiratory infection, which commonly precipitates pulmonary heart disease – respiratory infection causes carbon dioxide retention and hypoxaemia, resulting in constriction of pulmonary arterioles and subsequent pulmonary hypertension.
. Implement measures to treat heart failure when it exists.
   a. Reverse the patient's hypoxaemia and hypercapnia. (See above treatment first in order to improve cardiac action.)
   b. Limit physical activity.
   c. Restrict sodium intake.
   d. Give diuretics as prescribed to lower pulmonary artery pressure by reducing total blood volume.
   e. Watch electrolyte levels, especially potassium, as hypokalaemia increases risk of dysrhythmias.
   f. Give digitalis as prescribed if right ventricular failure is present. Digitalis is given with caution, since digitalis toxicity is a serious problem in management of respiratory failure because of hypoxaemia, acidosis and electrolyte abnormalities.
   g. Employ ECG monitoring when necessary – high incidence of dysrhythmias in these patients.
   h. Administer vasodilators and beta-adrenergic drugs as directed.

PATIENT EDUCATION
1. Emphasize the importance of stopping cigarette smoking; cigarette smoking is a major cause of pulmonary heart disease.
   a. Query the patient about his smoking habits.
   b. Inform the patient of risks of smoking and benefits to be gained when smoking is stopped.
2. Teach the patient to recognize and treat infections immediately.
3. Inform the patient of interrelationship between infection, air pollution and cardiopulmonary disease.
4. Explain to the patient/family that restlessness, depression and poor sleeping, as well as irritable and angry behaviour, may be characteristic; patient should improve with rise in O_2 and fall in CO_2 levels in arterial blood gas values.
5. Explain that if the patient has chronic lung disease it may be necessary to have continuous low-flow oxygen therapy at home.

Evaluation
EXPECTED OUTCOMES
1. Patient demonstrates improved respiratory function: decreased hypoxaemia, improved breathing patterns, normal blood gas values, etc.
2. Demonstrates increased activity tolerance and less fatigue
3. Follows diet protocol for reducing salt intake.

PULMONARY EMBOLISM

Pulmonary embolism refers to the obstruction of one or more pulmonary arteries by a thrombus (or thrombi) originating somewhere in the venous system or in the right side of the heart, which becomes dislodged and is carried to the lungs.

Pulmonary infarction refers to necrosis of lung tissue that can result from interference with blood supply.

PREDISPOSING FACTORS
1. Stasis of venous circulation, especially in blood vessels with injury to the endothelial lining – leads to intravascular clotting. Immobilization, sitting, prolonged standing contribute to venous stasis of lower extremities.
2. Injury to the vessel wall.
3. Hypercoagulability of the blood.
4. Septic foci related to drug abuse.
5. Most emboli originate in the deep veins of the lower extremities or pelvis, where they become detached and are carried to the lungs.

HEALTH MAINTENANCE AND PREVENTION

1. Assess each patient with a high risk factor for pulmonary embolism.
2. Be aware of high-risk patients – immobilization, trauma to pelvis (especially surgical) and lower extremities (especially hip fracture), obesity, history of thromboembolic disease, varicose veins, pregnancy, congestive heart failure, myocardial infarction, malignant disease, postoperative patients, elderly.
3. Prevent stasis of blood in extremities due to dependent position of legs, prolonged sitting, immobility, constricting clothing.
   a. Encourage early mobilization and weight bearing.
   b. Elevate legs 15 to 20 degrees at intervals – to minimize stasis and increase venous return.
   c. Apply fitted elastic stockings – to increase blood flow to deep leg veins.
   d. Instruct the patient to wiggle toes, move feet, raise and lower legs frequently – to increase venous return.
   e. Do not allow the patient's legs and feet to dangle in a dependent position; have the patient place his feet on a chair when sitting on the edge of the bed (if bed is in a high position). Instruct the patient to avoid crossing the legs.
   f. External pneumatic compression of calves – boots alternately inflate and deflate to pump blood from calf veins; used postoperatively.
4. Avoid haemoconcentration and immobilization of patients confined to bed.
5. Encourage higher levels of fluid intake during periods of immobility.
6. Avoid leaving catheters in veins (parenteral therapy, measurement of central venous pressure) for prolonged periods.
7. Examine the patient's legs carefully, since thrombi frequently originate in deep veins of legs, particularly those of the calf. Assess for swelling of leg, duskiness, pain upon pressure over calf muscle, pain upon dorsiflexion of the foot (positive Homan's sign).
8. Use agents for preventing venous thrombi and pulmonary embolism in high-risk patients; the approach depends on the patient's status.
   a. Oral anticoagulants, as prescribed (warfarin sodium) – antithrombotic agent useful in hip surgery.
   b. Low dose heparin as prescribed for patients over 40 undergoing major surgery.
   c. Antiplatelet agents, as prescribed (aspirin; dipyridamole).

Assessment

CLINICAL FEATURES

Underlying considerations:
1. The size and location of the embolus determines the physiological effect. Symptoms therefore vary from none to cardiovascular collapse.
2. The physiological effects develop from pulmonary artery obstruction and heightened resistance to blood flow through partially obstructed vessels.
3. Small emboli tend to be multiple and recurrent.
4. Chest pain with apprehension and a sense of impending doom; occurs when most of the pulmonary artery is obstructed.
5. Dyspnoea, pleuritic pain, cough; tachypnoea.
6. Subtle deterioration in patient's condition with no explainable cause.
7. Pallor, cyanosis, tachydysrhythmias, clinical shock.
8. Engorgement of neck veins.
9. Pleural friction rub.

NURSING ALERT

Be suspicious if there is a subtle deterioration in the patient's condition and unexplained cardiovascular and pulmonary findings.

DIAGNOSTIC EVALUATION

1. Physical findings: clinical signs and symptoms are elusive.
2. Arterial blood gases – systemic arterial hypoxaemia is usually found, due to perfusion abnormality of the lung.
3. Radioisotope lung scans – perfusion scan investigates regional blood flow to determine presence of perfusion defects; ventilation scan may be done in patient with large perfusion defects.
4. Pulmonary angiogram (most definitive) – emboli seen as 'filling defects'.
5. Contrast phlebography or impedance phlebography – for detecting deep vein thrombosis of the legs.

PATIENT PROBLEMS

1. Ineffective breathing pattern (dyspnoea) related to acute increase in alveolar dead space and possible changes in lung mechanics from embolism.
2. Alterations in tissue perfusion related to decreased blood circulation.
3. Potential for recurrence.
4. Potential for bleeding related to thrombolytic/anticoagulant therapy.
5. Anxiety related to inability to breathe.

Planning and implementation
NURSING INTERVENTIONS
Restoration of pulmonary function

1. Provide respiratory assistance to eliminate hypoxaemia.
   a. Oxygen via face mask or nasal catheter.
   b. Monitor vital signs, ECG and arterial blood gases.
2. Give intravenous fluids as prescribed to preserve right ventricular filling pressure and increase blood pressure.
3. Treat patient for heart failure when present.
4. Give analgesics and sedatives as directed for pain control and apprehension.

Preventing recurrence and extension of thromboembolism

1. Administer heparin (intravenously) as directed – stops further thrombus formation and extends the clotting time of the blood; it is an anticoagulant and antithrombotic.
   a. IV loading dose usually followed by continuous pump or drip infusion or given intermittently every four to six hours.
   b. Dosage adjusted to maintain the activated partial thromboplastin time at 1.5 and 2.5 times the pretreatment value (if the value was normal).
   c. Assess patient for untoward bleeding; major bleeding may occur from gastrointestinal tract, brain, lungs, nose, and genitourinary tract.
   d. Have protamine available to neutralize heparin during episodes of acute bleeding.
2. Give warfarin sodium as anticoagulant, as prescribed (prevents formation and extension of stasis thrombi in the venous system); may be given simultaneously at the beginning or after five to six days of heparin therapy.
   a. Dosage is controlled by monitoring serial tests of prothrombin time; desired prothrombin time is 2 to 2.5 times the normal value.
   b. Have vitamin K available to counteract effects of prothrombin depressant drugs (warfarin sodium) – bleeding is the most important side effect.
   c. Anticoagulants may be contraindicated in certain situations: recent brain, spinal cord, joint or urinary surgery; certain bleeding tendencies; fracture of pelvis or extremity; recent bleeding from peptic ulceration.
   d. Be aware that many drugs interact with anticoagulants.
3. Give thrombolytic agents (streptokinase; urokinase) as directed – lyse thrombi in deep venous system and emboli in pulmonary circulation, causing more rapid resolution of the thrombi/emboli and restoring pulmonary circulation to normal; improve circulatory and haemodynamic status.
   a. Effective in acute pulmonary embolism and thrombosis in popliteal and proximal deep veins.
   b. Administered intravenously in a loading dose followed by constant infusion.
   c. Limit invasive procedures (central venous pressure line, arterial puncture, intramuscular injections) during infusion to minimize bleeding.
      (i) Essential arterial blood gas studies should be taken on upper extremities; apply digital compression at puncture site for 30 minutes.
      (ii) Apply pressure dressing to previously involved sites.
      (iii) Maintain patient on strict bed rest during thrombolytic therapy.
      (iv) Take vital signs every four hours during infusion.
      (v) Discontinue infusion in the event of uncontrolled bleeding.
   d. Thrombolytic therapy usually followed with heparin and warfarin treatment to prevent additional thrombus formation.
4. Prepare patient for surgical intervention when anticoagulation is contraindicated or has failed, or when the patient has a major embolization.
   a. Inferior venacaval interruption – reduces channel size to prevent passage of emboli and at the same time permits some blood to flow. One of the following may be done:
      (i) Plication with suture or clips.
      (ii) Intraluminal obstruction achieved with umbrella filters, balloon catheters, trapping catheters. All methods of venacaval interruption may produce venous insufficiency of lower extremities with subsequent stasis and leg swelling.
   b. Embolectomy by:
      (i) Transvenous pulmonary embolectomy – transvenous suction catheter introduced into affected pulmonary artery to aspirate emboli.
      (ii) Surgical removal of embolus from pulmonary artery; performed with cardiopulmonary bypass in patient with massive embolism with shock.

PATIENT EDUCATION

1. See preventive measures, p. 190.
2. Patient may have to continue taking anticoagulant therapy for six weeks to six months following his initial episode.
3. Female patients who have experienced thromboembolism should be advised against taking oral contraceptives.
4. Instruct the patient to watch for signs of over-anticoagulation: bleeding gums, nosebleeds, bruising, haematuria, blood in stools, etc.
5. Patient should avoid taking any medications unless approved by the doctor, since many drugs interact with anticoagulants.
6. The patient should notify the dentist that he is on an anticoagulant.
7. Avoid inactivity for prolonged periods or sitting with legs crossed.
8. Wear a Medic-Alert bracelet identifying patient as anticoagulant user.
9. Lose weight if applicable; obesity is an important risk factor for women.

Evaluation
EXPECTED OUTCOMES

1. Patient shows improved respiratory function: absence of dyspnoea, tachypnoea or pleural friction rub; normal breath sounds upon auscultation.
2. Demonstrates need to avoid bleeding: applies pressure to puncture site after laboratory tests; verbalizes the need for regular laboratory monitoring during treatment; participates in self-monitoring for bleeding (bruising, blood in urine/stools, etc); wears identification bracelet.
3. Prevents recurrence: takes prescribed anticoagulant to protect against further thromboembolism; avoids sitting for prolonged periods; avoids alcohol and over-the-counter drugs; wears gradient support stockings.

CANCER OF THE LUNG (BRONCHOGENIC CANCER)

Bronchogenic cancer refers to a malignant tumour of the lung arising within the wall or epithelial lining of the bronchus. The lung is also a common site of metastasis from cancer elsewhere in the body via venous circulation or lymphatic spread. Primary cancer of the pleura is uncommon, except in asbestos workers.

CLASSIFICATION (ACCORDING TO CELL TYPE)

1. Squamous cell – most common.
2. Undifferentiated (includes variety of anaplastic or poorly differentiated cells):
   a. Small cell undifferentiated carcinoma (oat cell);
   b. Large cell undifferentiated carcinoma.
3. Adenocarcinoma.
4. Bronchiolar or alveolar carcinoma.

PREDISPOSING FACTORS

1. Cigarette smoking – amount, frequency and duration of smoking have positive relationship to cancer of the lung.
2. Industrial exposure to asbestos, arsenic, chromium, nickel, iron, radioactive substances, isopropyl oil, coal tar fumes, petroleum oil mists.

PREVENTIVE MEASURES

1. Maintain close watch of patients who are smokers – disease is insidious and exists before producing symptoms.
2. Encourage patients to abstain from cigarette smoking.
3. Recognize the presence of the tumour before symptoms appear:
   a. Continuous surveillance of smokers, especially those over 40;
   b. Chest X-rays at prescribed intervals.

NURSING ALERT

Suspect cancer of the lung in patients who belong to a susceptible age group and who have repeated unresolved respiratory infections.

Assessment
CLINICAL FEATURES

Usually occur late and are related to size and location of tumour, extent of spread and involvement of other structures.

1. Cough – especially a new type or changing cough.
2. Haemoptysis.
3. Thoracic discomfort; chest pain.
4. Wheezing.
5. Repeated infection of upper respiratory tract.
6. General symptoms; weight loss, fatigue, anorexia.
7. Usual sites of metastases: regional nodes, liver, adrenals, brain, bones, kidneys.
8. Signs of superior venacaval obstruction.
9. Change of voice.

DIAGNOSTIC EVALUATION

1. X-ray of chest – including fluoroscopy and

tomography; lung cancers may be partly or completely hidden by other structures.
2. Cytological examination of sputum/chest fluids for malignant cells.
3. Bronchoscopic evaluation. Fluorescence bronchofibreoscopy – intravenous injection of a haematoporphyrin derivative given 72 hours before bronchoscopy; this is accumulated and retained in malignant tissue and emits a red fluorescence upon excitation by violet light during bronchofibreoscopy.
4. Lymph node biopsy; mediastinoscopy – to establish lymphatic spread; to plan treatment.
5. Lung, brain and bone scans, if indicated.
6. Computed tomography – sensitive in detecting small pulmonary nodules and metastatic lesions.
7. Pulmonary function tests combined with split-function perfusion scan to determine if patient will have adequate pulmonary reserve to withstand surgical procedure.

MANAGEMENT
1. The treatment depends on the cell type, the stage of disease and the physiological status of the patient.
2. Treatment includes surgery (pneumonectomy, lobectomy, sleeve resection [removal of portion of a main bronchus with re-establishment of tracheobronchial continuity]), radiotherapy, chemotherapy and immunotherapy (see below), used separately or in combination.

Immunotherapy
1. Patients with lung cancer tend to be immunosuppressed; severe immunodeficiency may exist before operation.
2. Immunotherapy may be tried to reverse this immunosuppression; in theory this may lead to tumour rejection.
3. Objective of immunotherapy: to restore or augment the normal mechanisms of host defence against the tumour cells or suppression of tumour cell proliferation.
4. Immunotherapeutic approaches:
   a. BCG (bacille Calmette Guérin), an immune stimulating agent, is injected into pleural space (either into clamped pleural drainage system, via thoracocentesis), or via needle injection into peripheral lung tumour through a fibreoptic bronchoscope. Theoretical rationale: immunostimulating agent is brought into contact with tumour antigens; also allows stimulation of regional lymph nodes draining tumour.

b. Levamisole – theoretically restores depressed immune responses to normal.
c. Transfer factors – material extracted from sensitized lymphocytes of lymphocyte donors; injected into patient to stimulate cell-mediated immunity.

PATIENT PROBLEMS
1. Cough and dyspnoea related to lung tumour, possible obstructive injection, superior venacaval obstruction, invasion of adjacent structures.
2. Malnutrition related to hypermetabolic state, taste aversion, anorexia from radiotherapy/chemotherapy.
3. Potential for complications.
4. Anxiety and depression related to uncertain outcome and possible recurrence of disease.

Planning and implementation
NURSING INTERVENTIONS
Relief of respiratory symptoms
1. Prepare patient physically, emotionally and intellectually for prescribed therapeutic programme.
2. Elevate head of bed to promote gravity drainage and prevent fluid collection in upper body (from superior vena cava syndrome).
3. Teach breathing retraining exercises to increase diaphragmatic excursion with resultant reduction in work of breathing.
4. Give appropriate treatment for productive cough (expectorant; antibiotic agent) to prevent inspissated secretions and subsequent dyspnoea.
5. Support patient undergoing removal of pleural fluid (by thoracocentesis or tube thoracostomy) and instillation of sclerosing agent to obliterate pleural space and prevent fluid recurrence.

Improvement of nutritional status
1. Emphasize that nutrition is an important part of the treatment of lung cancer:
   a. Eat small amounts of high-calorie and high-protein foods frequently, rather than three daily meals.
   b. Eat major meal in the morning if rapidly becoming satiated and feeling full are problems.
   c. Be sure protein intake is adequate.
      (i) Substitute milk, eggs, chicken, fowl, fish and oral nutritional supplements if aversion to meat is present.
      (ii) Take prescribed vitamin supplement to avoid deficiency states.
2. Give enteral or total parenteral nutrition for a malnourished patient who is unable or unwilling to eat.

Prevention of complications

Monitor for complications:

1. Superior vena cava syndrome – interference in the return of blood through superior vena cava to the right atrium; manifested by facial and upper extremity oedema, dyspnoea/orthopnoea and cough, dilated venous collateral channels.
2. Hypercalcaemia, manifested by polyuria, nocturia, gastrointestinal symptoms, mental obtusion, profound weakness.
3. Pleural effusion.
4. Infectious complications, especially upper respiratory infections.

Other nursing interventions

1. See 'Patient education', below, for emotional support of patient.
2. Encourage sufficient hydration to thin secretions and to return calcium levels to normal if hypercalcaemia is present.
3. Encourage patient to use muscles (range of motion and other exercises) to avoid complications of inactivity and disuse.
4. Use all known safeguards, including meticulous handwashing techniques, to reduce incidence of infections since the patient with lung cancer tends to be immunosuppressed.

PATIENT EDUCATION

Quality of life

1. Focus on carrying on as normal a life as possible; an improved quality of life can be maintained.

Concerns about pain

1. Realize that not every ache and pain is due to the results of lung cancer; some patients do not even experience pain.
2. Use aspirin or prescription medication as necessary. Do not be concerned about 'addiction'.
3. Radiotherapy may be used for pain control if tumour has spread to bone.
4. Report any new or persistent pain; it may be due to some other cause, such as arthritis.

Emotional reactions

1. Shock, disbelief, denial, anger and depression are all normal reactions to the diagnosis of lung cancer.
2. Try to get the patient to express any concerns; share these concerns with health professionals.
3. Encourage the patient to communicate feelings to significant persons in his life.
4. Expect some feelings of anxiety and depression to recur during illness.

5. Encourage the patient to keep busy and remain in the mainstream. Continue with usual activities (work, recreation, sexual) as much as possible.
6. Secure services of a trained counsellor if emotional stresses become overwhelming.
7. Talk to social service worker about financial assistance as money problems are a major concern to many.
8. Be aware that the various voluntary organizations offer services and support to people with cancer.

Evaluation

EXPECTED OUTCOMES

1. Patient achieves relief of cough and dyspnoea.
2. Maintains nutritional balance; absence of excessive weight loss.
3. Absence of preventable complications.
4. Copes with emotional distress; communicates feelings about lung cancer.

OCCUPATIONAL LUNG DISEASES

Diseases of the lungs can occur in a variety of occupations as a result of exposure to organic or inorganic (mineral) dusts and noxious gases.

ALTERED PHYSIOLOGY

1. Effects of inhaling noxious particles, gases or fumes depends on composition of inhaled substance, its antigenic (precipitating an immune response) or irritating properties, the dose inhaled, the length of time inhaled and the host's response.
2. Exposure to inorganic dusts stimulates pulmonary interstitial fibroblasts, resulting in pulmonary interstitial fibrosis.
3. Noxious fumes may cause acute injury to alveolar wall with increasing capillary permeability and pulmonary oedema.
4. Occupational lung diseases usually develop slowly (20 to 30 years) and are asymptomatic in the early stages.

PREVENTION AND HEALTH MAINTENANCE

Objective

Reduce exposure of workers to industrial products that may be hazardous to breathing.

1. Preserve, in every way possible, the general

health of the worker/miner exposed to occupational dusts.
2. Enclose toxic substances, and reduce their concentration in the air:
   a. Engineering controls to reduce exposure;
   b. Monitoring of air samples.
3. Ventilate properly to reduce dust content of work atmosphere.
4. Have workers use protective devices (face masks, respirators, hoods, etc).
5. Monitor workers who are exposed to high concentrations of industrial dusts.
6. Encourage workers to stop smoking.

PNEUMOCONIOSES

The pneumoconioses refer to a non-neoplastic alteration of the lung resulting from exposure to inorganic dust (e.g. 'dusty lung') and the tissue reaction to its presence. The most common pneumoconioses are silicosis, asbestosis and coal worker's pneumoconiosis.

SILICOSIS
Silicosis is a chronic pulmonary fibrosis caused by inhalation of silica dust.

Aetiology and altered physiology
1. Exposure to silica dust is encountered in almost any form of mining because the earth's crust is composed of silica and silicates (gold, coal, tin, copper mining); also stone cutting, quarrying, manufacture of abrasives, ceramics, pottery and foundry work.
2. When silica particles (which have fibrogenic properties) are inhaled, nodular lesions are produced throughout the lungs. These nodules undergo fibrosis, enlarge and fuse.
3. Dense masses form in the upper portion of the lungs; restrictive and obstructive lung disease results.

Clinical features
1. Chronic productive cough.
2. Dyspnoea upon effort.
3. Susceptibility to lower respiratory tract infections.

Management
1. There is no specific treatment; the patient is treated symptomatically.
2. Give prophylactic isoniazid, as prescribed, to patients with positive skin tests; silicosis is associated with tuberculosis.

3. Prevention: see 'Prevention and health maintenance', p. 194.

ASBESTOSIS
Asbestosis is a diffuse pulmonary fibrosis caused by inhalation of asbestos dust and particles.

Altered physiology
1. Asbestos fibres are inhaled and enter alveoli, which in time are eventually obliterated by fibrous tissue that surrounds the asbestos particles.
2. Fibrous pleural thickening and pleural plaque formation produce restrictive lung disease, decrease in lung volume, diminished gas transfer and hypoxaemia with subsequent development of cor pulmonale.

Aetiology
1. Found in workers involved in manufacture, cutting and demolition of asbestos-containing materials; there are over 4,000 known uses of asbestos fibre (asbestos mining and manufacturing, construction, roofing, demolition work, brake linings, floor tiles, paints, plastics, shipyards, insulation).

NURSING ALERT
Asbestosis is strongly associated with bronchogenic cancer, also with mesotheliomas of the pleura and peritoneum and probably with neoplasms in other sites.

Clinical features
These may develop 20 to 40 years after exposure.
1. Dyspnoea on exertion: severe, progressive, irreversible.
2. Cough.
3. Crackles heard at lung bases.
4. Clubbing of fingers and toes; cor pulmonale.

Treatment
1. No treatment will affect the progressive fibrosis. Most of the asbestos fibres already in the lungs will remain there.
2. Persuade people who have been exposed to asbestos fibres to stop smoking. The risk of developing lung cancer for an asbestos worker who smokes is considered to be 50 to 100 times greater than that for a nonexposed nonsmoker.
3. Keep worker under cancer surveillance; watch for changing cough, haemoptysis, weight loss, melaena, etc.
4. Continuous low-flow oxygen may be prescribed

for patients with severe gas transport abnormalities.

5. Prevention: see 'Prevention and health maintenance', p. 194.

COAL WORKER'S PNEUMOCONIOSIS

Coal worker's pneumoconiosis ('black lung') is a variety of respiratory disease found in coal workers in which there is an accumulation of coal dust in the lungs, causing a tissue reaction in its presence.

Altered physiology

1. Dusts (coal, kaolin, mica, silica) are inhaled and deposited in the alveoli and respiratory bronchioles.
2. There is an increase of macrophages that engulf the particles and transport them to terminal bronchioles.
3. When normal clearance mechanisms no longer can handle the excessive dust load, the respiratory bronchioles and alveoli become clogged with coal dust, dying macrophages and fibroblasts, which lead to the formation of the coal macule, the primary lesion of coal worker's pneumoconiosis.
4. As macules enlarge, there is dilation of the weakening bronchiole with subsequent development of focal or centrilobular emphysema.

Clinical features

1. Progressive dyspnoea.
2. Cough and sputum production; expectoration of varying amounts of black fluid.

Management

1. There is no specific treatment; the treatment is symptomatic (e.g. bronchodilator drugs, antibiotics for infection).
2. See also treatment of emphysema, p. 184.
3. Prevention: see p. 194.

CHEST TRAUMA

Chest trauma is an injury to the chest caused by any form of violence.

1. Chest injuries are potentially life-threatening because of (1) immediate disturbances of cardiorespiratory physiology and haemorrhage, and (2) later developments of infection, damaged lung and thoracic cage.
2. Patients with chest trauma may have injuries to multiple organ systems.
3. The patient should be examined for intra-abdominal injuries, which must be treated aggressively.

ALTERED PHYSIOLOGY

1. In penetrating injuries, some air escapes into the pleural space. (Negative intrapleural pressure is replaced by atmospheric pressure.)
2. The loss of normal negative pressure within the pleural cavity causes collapse of the lung.

Assessment

CLINICAL FEATURES

1. Dyspnoea.
2. Asymmetrical chest movement.
3. Pain with breathing.
4. Cyanosis.

EMERGENCY MANAGEMENT

Objective

Restore normal cardiorespiratory function as quickly as possible. This is accomplished by performing effective resuscitation while simultaneously assessing the patient, restoring chest wall integrity and re-expanding the lung. The order of priority is determined by the clinical status of the patient.

NURSING INTERVENTIONS

Relief of acute respiratory distress

1. Evaluate the status of the respiratory and circulatory systems:
   a. Examiner's ear is placed close to patient's mouth and nose, allowing him to listen at the airway, watch uncovered chest movements and monitor pulse – this provides a rough estimate of the adequacy of ventilation.
   b. Assess for signs of obstruction, sternal retraction, stridor, wheezing and cyanosis.
   c. Check neck for position of trachea, subcutaneous emphysema and distended neck veins.
2. Establish and maintain an open airway and ventilation:
   a. Aspirate secretions, vomitus and blood from nose and throat via:
      (i) Tracheal aspiration, if patient is unable to clear the tracheobronchial tree by coughing.
      (ii) Utilize endotracheal tube if patient is

bleeding from nasopharynx or if trachea is injured (short-term use).

(iii) Employ bronchoscopic aspiration if necessary.

(iv) Prepare for tracheostomy if necessary:
  (a) Tracheostomy helps to obtain clear, dry tracheobronchial tree, helps the patient breathe with less effort, decreases amount of dead air space in the respiratory tree, and helps reduce paradoxical motion.
  (b) The use of a cuffed tracheostomy tube permits a closed system for air exchange when connected to a ventilator.

b. Stabilize the chest wall.

c. Free the pleural cavity of blood and air.

d. Sucking chest wounds should be closed with an emergency dressing. The presence of lung injury and chest tube drainage must also be considered.

3. Control haemorrhage.

4. Treat for shock (may be due to blood loss, impairment of cardiorespiratory function):
a. Use one or more intravenous infusion lines; obtain blood for baseline studies.
b. Restore blood volume to adequate levels – plasma expanders, electrolyte solutions.
c. Give infusion rapidly.
d. Monitor serial central venous pressure readings to prevent hypovolaemia and circulatory overload.

5. Apply electrodes for ECG monitoring – dysrhythmias are a frequent cause of death in chest trauma victims.

6. Assist with treatment of specific type of injury (see following discussion).

7. Ongoing nursing surveillance includes:
a. Monitoring of arterial blood pressure, central venous pressure and respirations.
b. Arterial blood gas measurements obtained by the doctor to determine need for mechanical ventilation.
c. Urinary output (hourly) – to evaluate tissue perfusion.
d. Thoracic drainage – to provide information about rate of blood loss, whether or not bleeding has stopped, whether surgical intervention is necessary.
e. ECG monitoring – for early detection and treatment of cardiac dysrhythmias.

8. Complications of chest injuries: aspiration, atelectasis, pneumonia, mediastinal/subcutaneous emphysema, respiratory failure.

HAEMOTHORAX

Blood in the pleural space as a result of penetrating or blunt chest trauma.

1. Blood in the pleural cavity produces a compression of the lungs and can result in hidden blood loss, causing signs and symptoms of shock.

2. Patient may be asymptomatic; or he may be dyspnoeic, apprehensive or in shock.

3. Management:
a. Blood and air are aspirated via needle thoracocentesis by the doctor, *or*
b. An intercostal catheter (thoracotomy tube) is inserted and drainage instituted to accomplish more complete and continuous removal of blood and air – effects re-expansion of lung and permits monitoring of blood loss. The chest catheter is sutured in position and connected to a water-seal drainage bottle.
c. Record the volume of fluid drained into the collection bottle hourly for the first several hours to alert for a sudden increase in drainage.
d. Prepare the patient for immediate blood replacement and thoracotomy if bleeding continues.

PNEUMOTHORAX

Air in the pleural space occurring spontaneously from injury or disease. In patients with chest trauma, it is usually the result of a laceration to the lung parenchyma, tracheobronchial tree or oesophagus.

The patient's clinical status depends on the rate of air leakage and size of wound.

1. Assessment:
a. Hyperresonance; diminished breath sounds.
b. Reduced mobility of affected half of thorax.

2. Spontaneous pneumothorax:
a. May occur in healthy individuals; is usually due to rupture of an overdilated air sac in the lung.
b. Treatment is generally nonoperative if pneumothorax is not too extensive; needle aspiration or chest tube drainage may be necessary to achieve re-expansion of collapsed lung.
c. Surgical intervention (thoracotomy) is advised for patients with recurrent spontaneous pneumothorax.

3. Tension pneumothorax – build-up of pressure in the pleural space, resulting in compromise of ventilation; produces a collapse of the lung and decreased ventilation of other lung because of

compression, and decreased venous return to the heart.

   a. Clinical picture is one of air hunger, agitation, hypotension and cyanosis; there is an *acute threat to life*.

   b. Management:

     (i) Insert chest tube drain immediately to allow air to escape (chest tube then connected to underwater-seal suction).

     (ii) Use thoracocentesis for emergency decompression of pleural space until tube thoracostomy can be accomplished.

OPEN PNEUMOTHORAX

Also called sucking wound of chest, this implies an opening in the chest wall large enough to allow air to pass freely in and out of thoracic cavity with each attempted respiration; the rush of air through the hole in the chest wall produces a 'sucking sound'. This represents an acute threat to life.

1. When there is a large open hole in the chest wall, the patient will have a 'steal' in ventilation of other lung.
2. A portion of the tidal volume will move back and forth through the hole in the chest wall rather than the trachea as it normally does.
3. Management:

   a. Close the chest wound immediately to restore adequate ventilation and respiration.

   b. Instruct the patient to inhale and exhale forcefully against a closed glottis (Valsalva manoeuvre) as the pressure dressing (petroleum gauze secured with elastic adhesive) is laid in place. (This manoeuvre helps to expand collapsed lung.)

   c. Prepare for chest tube insertion and drainage to permit evacuation of fluid/air and produce re-expansion of the lung. Surgical intervention may be necessary.

   d. If condition permits, place patient in semi-sitting position to permit greater ventilatory efficiency.

FRACTURE OF RIBS AND STERNUM

This is the most common chest injury.

NURSING ALERT
Rib fractures should be regarded as potentially serious because they may result in underlying lung contusion.

Older individuals with pre-existing pulmonary disease may develop atelectasis and pneumonia following a rib fracture. If rib fragments are driven inward, there may be lacerations of the pleura, a pneumothorax, haemothorax, or haemopneumothorax.

1. Manifestations:

   a. Localized tenderness or crepitus (crackling) over fracture site.

   b. Chest pain referred to the fracture site.

   c. Painful, shallow respirations (due to splinting of involved chest).

2. Management:

   a. Give analgesics (usually non-narcotic) to assist in effective coughing and deep breathing.

   b. Encourage deep-breathing with strong inspiration; give local support to injured area with nurse's hands.

   c. Assist with intercostal nerve block – to relieve pain so that coughing and deep breathing may be accomplished.

   d. For multiple rib fractures, epidural anaesthesia may be used.

FLAIL CHEST

This is loss of stability of chest wall, with subsequent respiratory impairment, and this is usually the result of multiple rib fractures or combined fractures of the sternum and ribs.

1. Pathophysiology:

   a. When this occurs, one portion of the chest has lost its bony connection to the rest of the rib cage.

   b. During respiration, the detached part of the chest will be pulled in on inspiration and blown out on expiration (paradoxical movement).

   c. Normal mechanics of breathing are impaired to a degree that seriously jeopardizes ventilation.

   d. Generally associated with some degree of lung contusion (see below).

2. Clinical manifestations:

   a. Pain, dyspnoea, cyanosis.

   b. Paradoxical (reverse of normal) movements of involved chest wall.

3. Management:

   a. Stabilize the flail portion of the chest with the hands; apply a pressure dressing and turn the patient on his injured side, or place a 4.5kg sandbag at site of flail.

   b. If respiratory failure is present, prepare for immediate endotracheal intubation and ventilation therapy with controlled ventilation or positive-end expiratory pressure – treats underlying pulmonary contusion and serves to stabilize the thoracic cage for healing of fractures, improves alveolar ventilation and restores thoracic cage stability and intrathoracic volume by decreasing work of breathing, *or*

c. Thoracic epidural analgesia may be used for some patients to relieve pain and improve ventilation.

d. See also treatment for lung contusion, which follows.

PULMONARY (LUNG) CONTUSION

Damage to the lung parenchyma that results in leakage of blood and fluid into the interstitial space of the lung.

1. Clinical manifestations:
   a. Tachypnoea, tachycardia.
   b. Crackles (râles) on auscultation.
   c. Pleuritic chest pain.
   d. Copious secretions.
   e. Cough – constant, loose, rattling.
2. Management (for moderate lung contusion):
   a. Employ endotracheal intubation and ventilatory support; place the patient on ventilator with low concentration of oxygen and positive-end expiratory pressure (PEEP) – to maintain the pressure and keep lungs inflated.
   b. Administer diuretics as prescribed – to reduce oedema.

c. Correct metabolic acidosis with intravenous sodium bicarbonate as prescribed.

d. Utilize pulmonary artery pressure monitoring.

CARDIAC TAMPONADE

This is compression of the heart as a result of accumulation of fluid within the pericardial space.

1. Clinical manifestations:
   a. Falling blood pressure.
   b. Rising venous pressure/distended neck veins/ elevated venous pressure.
   c. Distant heart sounds.
   d. Pulsus paradoxus (systolic blood pressure drops and fluctuates with respiration).
   e. Dyspnoea, cyanosis, shock.

NURSING ALERT
A rapidly developing effusion interferes with ventricular filling and causes impairment of circulation. Thus, there is a reduced cardiac output and poor venous return to the heart. Cardiac collapse can result. In the patient with hypovolaemia due to associated injuries, the venous pressure may not rise, thus masking the signs of cardiac tamponade.

2. Management (for penetrating injuries):
   a. Emergency thoracotomy to control bleeding and to repair cardiac injury.
   b. Pericardial aspiration (pericardiocentesis), aspiration or drainage of the pericardium; to transiently improve haemodynamic function enabling transfer to operating theatre.
      (i) Repeated aspirations may be necessary.

UNDERWATER-SEAL CHEST DRAINAGE

GUIDELINES: ASSISTING WITH CHEST DRAIN INSERTION

A tube thoracostomy is the insertion of one or more flexible tubes into the pleural space to evacuate air, blood or fluid collections.

EQUIPMENT
Tube thoracostomy tray:
   Syringes
   Needles/trocar
   Basins/skin germicide
   Sponges
   Scalpel/sterile drape/gloves
   Two large clamps

Suture material
Local anaesthetic
Chest tube (appropriate size); connector
Chest drainage system – connecting tubes and
   tubing, collection bottles or commercial system,
   vacuum pump (if required)

SITES FOR CHEST TUBE PLACEMENT
For pneumothorax – interspace along midclavicular or anterior axillary line.
For pleural effusion or haemothorax – sixth to seventh lateral interspace in
   the midaxillary line.

PROCEDURE
Preparatory phase

Nursing action	Rationale
1. Assess patient for pneumothorax, haemothorax, presence of respiratory distress.	
2. Obtain a chest X-ray. Other means of localization of pleural fluid include ultrasound and/or fluoroscopic localization.	To evaluate extent of lung collapse or amount of bleeding in pleural space.
3. Assemble drainage system.	
4. Reassure the patient and explain the steps of the procedure. Tell the patient to expect a needle prick and a sensation of slight pressure during infiltration anaesthesia.	The patient can cope by remaining immobile and doing relaxed breathing during tube insertion.
5. Position the patient according to the doctor's preference:	
a. Have the patient sit up, bend forward, and hug a pillow, *or*	This posture moves the scapulae forward and out of the way.
b. Place the patient prone with pillow under his chest, *or*	The prone position helps immobilize the patient.
c. Have the patient lie on his unaffected side with his upper arm hanging over the side of the table.	This pulls the scapula out of the way.

Performance phase
Trocar technique for chest tube insertion
A trocar catheter is used for the insertion of a large-bore tube for removal of a
modest to large amount of air leak or for the evacuation of a serious effusion.

Doctor's action	Rationale
1. A small incision is made over the prepared, anaesthetized site. Blunt dissection (with a haemostat) through the muscle planes in the interspace to the parietal pleura is performed.	To admit the diameter of the chest tube.
2. The trocar is directed into the pleural space, the cannula removed and a chest tube inserted into the pleural space and connected to a drainage system.	There is a trocar catheter available equipped with an indwelling pointed rod for ease of insertion.

Haemostat technique using a large-bore chest tube
A large bore chest tube is used to drain blood or thick effusions from the pleural space.

Doctor's action	**Rationale**
1. After skin preparation and anaesthetic infiltration, an incision is made through the skin and subcutaneous tissue.	The skin incision is usually made one interspace below proposed site of penetration of the intercostal muscles and pleura.
2. A curved haemostat is inserted into the pleural cavity and the tissue is spread with the clamp.	To make a tissue tract for the chest tube.
3. The tract is explored with an examining finger.	Digital examination helps confirm the presence of the tract and penetration of the pleural cavity.
4. The tube is held by the haemostat and directed through the opening up over the rib and into the pleural cavity.	
5. The clamp is withdrawn and the chest tube is connected to a chest drainage system.	The chest tube has multiple openings at the proximal end for drainage of air/blood.
6. The tube is sutured in place and covered with a sterile dressing.	

Follow-up care

Nursing action	**Rationale**
1. Observe the drainage system for blood/air. Observe that there is free fluctuation in the tube upon respiration (see water-seal drainage p. 204).	If a haemothorax is draining through a thoracostomy tube into a bottle containing sterile normal saline, the blood is available for autotransfusion.
2. Secure a follow-up chest X-ray.	To confirm correct chest tube placement and re-expansion of the lung.
3. Look for bleeding, infection, leakage of air and fluid around the tube.	

CHEST DRAINAGE

PATHOPHYSIOLOGY

1. The normal breathing mechanism operates on the principle of negative pressure (the pressure in the chest cavity is lower than the pressure of the outside air, causing air to move into the lungs during inspiration).
2. Whenever the chest is opened, from any cause, there is loss of negative pressure, which can result in collapse of the lung. The collection of air, fluid or other substances in the chest can compromise cardiopulmonary function and even cause collapse of the lung, because these substances take up space.
3. Pathological substances that collect in the pleural space include: fibrin, or clotted blood, liquids (serous fluids, blood, pus, chyle) and gases (air from the lung, tracheobronchial tree or oesophagus).
4. Surgical incision of the chest wall almost always causes some degree of pneumothorax. Air and

fluid collect in the intrapleural space, restricting lung expansion and reducing air exchange.

5. It is necessary to keep the pleural space evacuated postoperatively and to maintain negative pressure within this potential space. Therefore, during or immediately after thoracic surgery, chest tubes are positioned strategically in the pleural space, sutured to the skin, and connected to some type of drainage apparatus to remove the residual air and drainage fluid from the pleural or mediastinal space. This assists in the re-expansion of remaining lung tissue.

PRINCIPLES OF CHEST DRAINAGE

1. A chest drainage system must be capable of removing whatever collects in the pleural space so that a normal pleural space and normal cardiopulmonary function may be restored and maintained.
2. There are many types of commercial chest drainage systems in use, most of which use the water-seal principle. The chest catheter is attached to a bottle, using a one-way valve principle. Water acts as a seal and permits air and fluid to drain from the chest, but air cannot re-enter the submerged tip of the tube.
3. Chest drainage can be categorized into three types of mechanical systems, as follows (Figure 4.22).

The single-bottle water-seal system

1. The end of the drainage tube from the patient's chest is covered by a layer of water, which permits drainage of air and fluid from the pleural space, but does not allow air to move back into the chest. Functionally, drainage depends on gravity, on the mechanics of respiration and, if desired, on suction by the addition of *controlled* vacuum.
2. The tube from the patient extends approximately 2.5cm below the level of the water in the container. There is a vent for the escape of any air that is drained from the lung. The water level fluctuates as the patient breathes; it goes up when the patient inhales and down when the patient exhales.
3. At the end of the drainage tube, bubbling may or may not be visible. Bubbling can mean either persistent leakage of air from the lung or other tissues or a leak in the system.

The two-bottle system

1. The two-bottle system consists of the same water-seal chamber, plus a fluid-collection bottle.
2. Drainage is similar to that of a single unit, except

that when pleural fluid drains, the underwater-seal system is not affected by the volume of drainage.

3. Effective drainage depends on gravity or on the amount of suction added to the system. When vacuum (suction) is added to the system from a vacuum source, such as wall suction, the connection is made at the vent stem of the underwater-seal bottle.
4. The amount of suction applied to the system is regulated by the wall gauge.

The three-bottle system

1. The three-bottle system is similar in all respects to the two-bottle system, except for the addition of a third bottle to control the amount of suction applied.
2. The amount of suction is determined by the depth to which the tip of the venting glass tube is submerged in the water.
3. In the three-bottle system (as in the other two systems), drainage depends on gravity or the amount of suction applied. The amount of suction in the three-bottle system is controlled by the manometer bottle. The mechanical suction motor or wall suction creates and maintains a negative pressure throughout the entire closed drainage system.
4. The manometer bottle regulates the amount of vacuum in the system. This bottle contains three tubes: (1) a short tube above the water level comes from the water-seal bottle; (2) another short tube leads to the vacuum or suction motor, or to wall suction; (3) the third tube is a long tube that extends below the water level in the bottle and opens to the atmosphere outside the bottle. This tube regulates the amount of vacuum in the system, depending on the depth to which the tube is submerged – the usual depth is 20cm.
5. When the vacuum in the system becomes greater than the depth to which the tube is submerged, outside air is sucked into the system. This results in constant bubbling in the manometer bottle, which indicates that the system is functioning properly.

Note: When the motor or the wall vacuum is turned off, the drainage system should be open to the atmosphere so that intrapleural air can escape from the system. This can be done by detaching the tubing from the suction port to provide a vent.

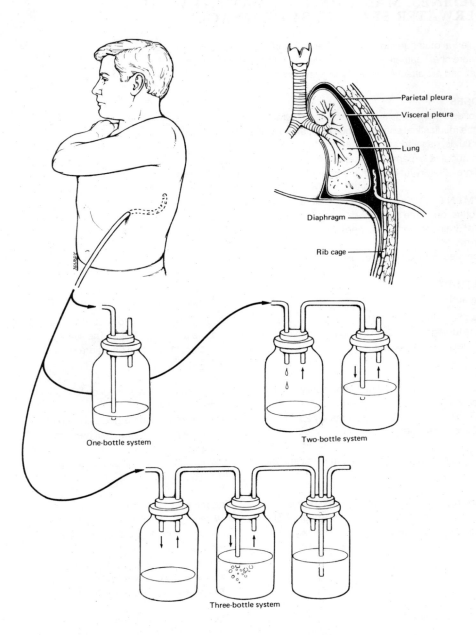

Figure 4.22. One-bottle, two-bottle and three-bottle chest drainage systems

GUIDELINES: MANAGING THE PATIENT WITH UNDERWATER-SEAL CHEST DRAINAGE*

An intrapleural drainage tube is used after most intrathoracic procedures. One or more chest catheters are held in the pleural space by suture to the chest wall and are attached to a drainage system.

PURPOSES

1. Remove solids, liquids and gas from the pleural space or thoracic cavity and the mediastinal space (serous fluid, blood, pus and occasionally other fluids; gas and air from the lung, tracheobronchial tree).
2. Bring about re-expansion of the lung and restore normal cardiorespiratory function after surgery, trauma or medical conditions.

EQUIPMENT

Closed chest drainage system
Holder for drainage system (if needed)
Vacuum motor
Sterile connector for emergency use

PROCEDURE

Nursing action

Rationale

1. Attach the drainage tube from the pleural space to the tubing that leads to a long tube with end submerged in sterile water.

    Water-seal drainage provides for the escape of air and fluid into a drainage bottle. The water acts as a seal and keeps the air from being drawn back into the pleural space.

2. Check the tube connections periodically. Tape if necessary:
    a. The tube should be approximately 2.5cm below the water level.

    b. The short tube is left open to the atmosphere.

    Tube connections are checked to ensure tight fit and patency of the tubes:
    a. If the tube is submerged too deep below the water level, a higher intrapleural pressure is required to expel air.
    b. Venting the short glass tube lets air escape from the bottle.

3. Mark the original fluid level with tape on the outside of the drainage bottle. Mark hourly/daily increments (date and time) at the drainage level.

    This marking will show the amount of fluid loss and how fast fluid is collecting in the drainage bottle. It serves as a basis for blood replacement, if the fluid is blood. Grossly bloody drainage will appear in the bottle in the immediate postoperative period and, if excessive, may necessitate reoperation. Drainage usually declines progressively after the first 24 hours.

4. Make sure that the tubing does not loop or interfere with the movements of the patient.

    Fluid collecting in the dependent segment of the tubing will decrease the negative pressure applied to the catheter. Kinking, looping or pressure on the drainage tubing can produce back pressure, thus possibly forcing drainage back into the pleural space, or impedes drainage from the pleural space.

* There are numerous commercial disposable chest drainage devices available for collecting pleural fluid that use the water-seal principle.

5. Encourage the patient to assume a position of comfort. Encourage good body alignment. When the patient is in a lateral position, place a rolled towel under the tubing to protect it from the weight of the patient's body. Encourage the patient to change his position frequently.

The patient's position should be changed frequently to promote drainage and his body kept in good alignment to prevent postural deformity and contractures. Proper positioning helps breathing and promotes better air exchange. Pain medication may be indicated to enhance comfort and deep-breathing.

6. Put the arm and shoulder of the affected side through range-of-motion exercises several times daily. Some pain medication may be necessary.

Exercise helps to avoid ankylosis of the shoulder and assist in lessening postoperative pain and discomfort.

7. 'Milk' the tubing in the direction of the drainage bottle hourly. (Some polyvinyl tubes are too rigid to be 'milked'.)

'Milking' the tubing prevents it from becoming plugged with clots and fibrin. Constant attention to maintaining the patency of the tube will facilitate prompt expansion of the lung and minimize complications.

8. Make sure there is fluctuation of the fluid level in the long glass tube.

Fluctuation of the water level in the tube shows that there is effective communication between the pleural space and the drainage bottle, provides a valuable indication of the patency of the drainage system and is a gauge of intrapleural pressure.

9. Fluctuations of fluid in the tubing will stop when:
   a. The lung has re-expanded;
   b. The tubing is obstructed by blood clots or fibrin;
   c. A dependent loop develops (see point 4 opposite);
   d. Suction motor or wall suction is not operating properly.

10. Watch for leaks of air in the drainage system as indicated by contant bubbling in the water-seal bottle:
    a. Report excessive bubbling in the water-seal chamber immediately.
    b. 'Milking' of chest tubes in patients with air leaks should be done only if requested by surgeon.

Leaking and trapping of air in the pleural space can result in tension pneumothorax.

11. Observe and report immediately signs of rapid, shallow breathing, cyanosis, pressure in the chest, subcutaneous emphysema or symptoms of haemorrhage.

Many clinical conditions may cause these signs and symptoms, including tension pneumothorax, mediastinal shift, haemorrhage, severe incisional pain, pulmonary embolus and cardiac tamponade. Surgical intervention may be necessary.

12. Encourage the patient to breathe deeply and cough at frequent intervals. If there are signs of incisional pain, adequate pain medication is indicated.

Deep breathing and coughing help to raise the intrapleural pressure, which allows emptying of any accumulation in the pleural space and removes secretions from the tracheobronchial tree so that the lung expands and atelectasis is prevented.

13. Stabilize the drainage-bottle on the floor or in a special holder. *Caution visitors and personnel against handling equipment or displacing the drainage bottle.*

If any part of the apparatus is damaged, the closed system of drainage will be destroyed and the patient will be endangered by atmospheric pressure in the pleural space and resultant collapse of the lung. The drainage system must be kept airtight to re-establish negative intrapleural pressure.

14. If the patient has to be transported to another area, place the drainage bottle below the chest level (as close to the floor as possible) if he is lying on a stretcher. If the tube becomes disconnected, cut off the contaminated tips of the chest tube and tubing, insert a sterile connector in the chest tube and tubing and reattach to the drainage system.

The drainage apparatus must be kept at a level lower than the patient's chest to prevent backflow of fluid into the pleural space.

15. When assisting the surgeon in removing the tube:
   a. Instruct the patient to perform the Valsalva manoeuvre (forcible exhalation against a closed glottis, holding one's breath).
   b. The chest tube is clamped and quickly removed.
   c. Simultaneously, a small bandage is applied and made airtight with petrolatum gauze covered by 10 × 10cm gauze and thoroughly covered and sealed with tape.

The chest tube is removed as directed when the lung is re-expanded (usually 24 hours to several days). During removal of the tube, the chief priorities are prevention of entrance of air into the pleural space as the tube is withdrawn and prevention of infection.

THORACIC SURGERY

NURSING ALERT
Meticulous attention must be given to the preoperative and postoperative care of patients undergoing thoracic surgery. These operations are wide in scope and represent a major stress on the cardiorespiratory system; patients requiring thoracotomy often have pre-existing pulmonary disease with a limited cardiopulmonary reserve.

PREOPERATIVE CARE

Goals
1. Determine if the patient can survive planned procedure.
2. Ensure optimal condition of the patient for surgery.

Determine preoperative status of the patient and his physical state
1. Assist the patient undergoing diagnostic studies
   a. History and physical examination.
   b. Chest X-rays.
   c. Pulmonary function studies to ascertain patient will have adequately functioning lung tissue postoperatively; incidence of postoperative pulmonary complications is closely correlated with preoperative pulmonary disease.
   d. Special diagnostic studies as required; lung scanning may show if gas exchange will be affected by procedure.
   e. Baseline studies to ascertain any unsuspected abnormalities and to serve as a baseline reference during the postoperative period:

(i) ECG – to disclose presence of athero-sclerotic heart disease or conduction defect;

(ii) Prothrombin time, partial thromboplastin time, platelet count – to confirm integrity of coagulation system;

(iii) Blood urea nitrogen (BUN), serum creatinine – to obtain a 'rough' measure-ment of renal function;

(iv) Blood sugar or glucose tolerance – to detect unrecognized diabetes;

(v) Blood electrolytes, serum protein studies and blood volume determinations, as indicated;

(vi) Arterial blood gas studies to determine presence of hypoxaemia/hypercapnia.

2. Nursing assessment of the patient:

a. What signs and symptoms are present (cough, expectoration, wheeze, haemoptysis, chest pain)?

b. What is his smoking history (amount and duration)? How much is he presently smoking?

c. What is the patient's cardiopulmonary toler-ance while bathing, eating, walking, etc?

d. What is the 'physiological age' of the patient (general appearance, mental alertness, be-haviour, degree of nutrition)?

e. What other medical conditions exist?

f. What is his breathing pattern?

g. How much exertion is required to produce dyspnoea?

h. What are his personal preferences and dislikes?

Improve alveolar ventilation and overall respiratory function

1. Encourage the patient to stop smoking, since this increases bronchial irritation.

2. Teach an effective coughing technique:

a. Sit the patient upright with knees flexed and body bending slightly forward.

b. Splint the proposed incision site with your hands; show the patient how to splint the painful area with firm hand pressure or sup-port it with a pillow or folded towel while coughing.

c. Instruct the patient to take three short breaths, followed by a deep inspiration, inhaling slowly and evenly through the nose.

d. Instruct him to contract (pull in) his abdominal muscles and cough twice forcefully with his mouth open and tongue out.

e. Have the patient lie on his side with his hips and knees flexed if he is unable to sit.

f. 'Huffing technique' for the patient with dimin-ished expiratory flow rate or for the patient who refuses to cough:

(i) Take a deep diaphragmatic breath and exhale forcefully against your hand; exhale in a quick distinct pant, or 'huff'.

(ii) Practise doing small 'huffs' and progress to one strong 'huff' while exhaling.

3. Employ all measures to minimize pulmonary secretions:

a. Measure sputum daily in patients with large volume of secretions to determine if volume of secretion is decreasing.

b. Encourage patient to cough effectively (see above).

c. Humidify the air to loosen secretions.

d. Administer bronchodilators for broncho-spasm.

e. Give antibiotics for infection.

f. Encourage deep breathing with the use of incentive spirometer or blow bottles.

g. Teach diaphragmatic breathing pre-operatively.

h. Set up a schedule of breathing exercises that encourage the use of abdominal muscles.

i. Carry out postural drainage in patients having increased mucus production.

Evaluate cardiovascular and pulmonary status so that complications may be anticipated and prevented

1. Study the results of diagnostic tests to learn of existing deviations from normal.

2. Observe the patient and his reactions to various activities of daily living.

3. Give cardiac drugs as prescribed to patients with congestive heart failure.

4. Correct anaemia, dehydration and hypoprotein-aemia – intravenous infusions, tube feedings, blood transfusions as directed.

5. Give prophylactic anticoagulant (low-dose hepar-in) as prescribed to reduce postoperative inci-dence of deep vein thrombosis and pulmonary embolism.

Prepare patient for surgery by offering reassurance, explanations and skilful preoperative nursing care

1. Orientate the patient to events in the post-operative period:

a. Coughing with chest support and breathing routine.

b. Presence of chest tube and drainage bottles.

c. Oxygen therapy; ventilator therapy.

d. Measures used to control discomfort.

e. Leg exercises and range of motion exercises for affected shoulder.

f. Coping measures (breathing, turning, analgesics) for postoperative discomfort.

2. Encourage expression of psychological and safety needs.

3. See that consent form has been explained and signed.

POSTOPERATIVE CARE

Assessment
PATIENT PROBLEMS

1. Ineffective breathing pattern related to altered physiology secondary to opening the pleural cavity and ineffective airway clearance.

2. Pain related to chest incision and presence of chest tubes.

3. Impaired mobility of affected shoulder and arm related to location of incision and presence of chest tubes.

4. Potential for complications.

Planning and implementation
NURSING INTERVENTIONS
Maintenance of effective respiration and gas exchange

1. Maintain an open airway and assure adequate respiratory function:

a. Look and listen at the patient's open mouth as he breathes for evidence of obstruction, and listen to his chest (auscultation) with a stethoscope.

b. Monitor for adequacy of pulmonary function:

(i) Measure Pao_2, $Paco_2$ and tidal volume.

(ii) Use indwelling arterial line to facilitate drawing arterial blood samples and provide a continuous measurement of systemic arterial pressures.

c. Most patients have endotracheal tubes in place with ventilatory support until adequate respiratory function and stable cardiovascular status is attained. Ventilatory weaning is started as early as possible.

d. Aspirate all secretions with suctioning until the patient is able to raise secretions effectively – endotracheal secretions are present in excessive amounts in post-thoracotomy patients because of trauma to the tracheobronchial tree

during operation, diminished lung ventilation and diminished cough reflex.

(i) Excessive secretions will produce airway obstruction; air in the alveoli distal to the obstruction will become absorbed, and the lung will collapse.

NURSING ALERT

Look for changes in colour and consistency of aspirated sputum. Colourless, fluid sputum is not unusual; opacification or colouring of sputum may mean dehydration or infection.

2. Maintain continuing nursing surveillance of the patient's haemodynamic status:

a. Take blood pressure, pulse and respiration every 15 minutes or more frequently as indicated; extend the time intervals according to the patient's clinical status.

b. Evaluate *character* of respirations and patient's colour – depth of respiration is an important criterion in evaluating whether lungs are being adequately expanded.

c. Auscultate and percuss chest frequently to determine adequacy of ventilation – detects early respiratory embarrassment.

d. Monitor heart rate and rhythm via auscultation and ECG, since arrhythmias are more frequently seen after thoracic surgery.

(i) Dysrhythmias can occur anytime and contribute significantly to postoperative mortality rate.

(ii) *Rate of occurrence of dysrhythmias increases with patients over 50 and with those undergoing pneumonectomy or oesophageal surgery.*

(iii) Begin anti-dysrhythmic measures immediately if indicated.

e. Monitor the central venous pressure for prompt recognition of hypovolaemia and for evidence of excessive fluid administration.

f. Monitor cardiac output and pulmonary artery wedge or left atrial mean pressures.

g. Elevate the head of the bed 30 to 40 degrees when patient is orientated and his blood pressure stabilized.

3. Maintain surveillance and careful management of the chest drainage system, which is used to eliminate any residual air or fluid following thoracotomy:*

---

* A patient with a pneumonectomy usually does not have water-seal chest drainage, since it is desirable that the pleural space fill with an effusion, which eventually obliterates this space. Some surgeons do use a 'modified' water-seal system.

a. Chest tube(s) inserted at time of surgery to prevent fluid and air from accumulating in pleural or mediastinal space and to assist in re-expansion of remaining lung tissue.

b. Check amount and character of drainage immediately postoperatively and at necessary intervals thereafter – drainage should progressively decrease after first 12 hours.

c. The drainage is usually bloody immediately after surgery but becomes serous in 24 hours or so.

d. Persistence of bloody drainage indicates bleeding. Prepare for blood replacement and possible reoperation to achieve haemostasis.

e. See summary of the nurse's role in the management of water-seal drainage (p. 204).

. Give humidified, warmed oxygen in immediate postoperative period to ensure maximum oxygenation – respirations are still depressed, and residual secretions in the peripheral respiratory passages may partially block gas exchange. Warming and humidification of inspired gases promotes ciliary action and prevents loss of body heat. Monitoring by means of arterial blood gas analysis is the most accurate method of detecting existing or impending hypoxaemia.

a. Assess for respiratory distress and a feeling of tightness in the chest.

b. Watch for restlessness – often the first sign of hypoxia.

?ain relief

. Provide regular pain relief – pain limits chest excursions, thereby decreasing ventilation.

a. Severity of pain varies with type of incision and with the patient's reaction to and ability to cope with pain. Usually a posterior-lateral incision is the most painful.

b. Give narcotics (usually in frequent small doses) for pain relief, to permit patient to breathe more deeply and cough more effectively; place on oral analgesic as soon as possible.

c. Avoid depressing respiratory and vascular systems with too much narcotic; patient should not be so somnolent that he does not cough.

. Position the patient in bed correctly.

a. Position patient upright (15 to 30 degrees) if cardiovascular system is stable to facilitate optimal ventilation; allows diaphragm to descend and lung volume to increase; this also helps residual air to rise in upper portion of pleural space where it can be removed by the chest tube.

b. Patients with limited respiratory reserve may not be able to turn on unoperated side as this may limit ventilation of the operated side.

c. Vary the position from horizontal to semi-erect; remaining in one position tends to promote the retention of secretions in the dependent portion of the lungs.

3. Encourage and promote an effective cough routine; a persistent and ineffective cough exhausts the patient, and retained secretions lead to atelectasis and pneumonia.

a. Sit the patient on side of bed with feet supported on a chair if his condition permits.

b. Support the chest firmly over the operated side and against opposite chest to lessen incisional pain or support the thorax with one hand pressing on the midsternum and the other arm around the back if there is a median sternotomy incision.

c. Instruct the patient to take a deep breath (to increase cough pressure), to pull in his abdominal muscles and to cough vigorously.

d. Assist the patient to cough at least every one to two hours during the first 24 hours and when necessary thereafter (Figure 4.23).

Mobility of the affected shoulder

1. Restore normal range of motion and function of shoulder and trunk.
2. Encourage breathing exercises to mobilize thorax.
3. Encourage skeletal exercises to promote abduction and mobilization of the shoulder.
4. Ambulate as soon as pulmonary and circulatory systems are compensated.
5. Encourage progressive activities according to diminution of fatigue.

Prevention of complications

1. Anticipate and forestall complications.

a. Hypoxia; watch for restlessness, tachycardia, tachypnoea and elevated blood pressure.

b. Postoperative bleeding; watch for restlessness, anxiety, pallor, tachycardia and hypotension.

c. Low cardiac output syndrome.

d. Pneumonitis; atelectasis.

e. Cardiac dysrhythmias, myocardial infarction, pulmonary oedema.

f. Gastric distension.

g. Renal failure.

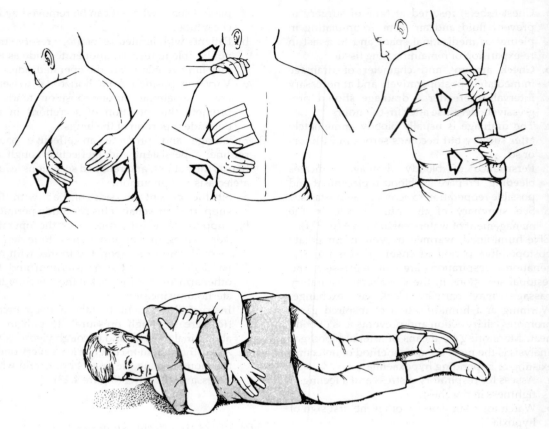

Figure 4.23. Promotion of an effective cough

Other nursing interventions

1. Administer blood and parenteral fluids as directed, at a slower rate after thoracic surgery – pulmonary oedema due to transfusion/infusion overload is an ever-present threat; following pneumonectomy, the pulmonary vascular system has been greatly reduced.
2. Continue to monitor blood gas and serum electrolyte values.
3. Monitor hourly urine output from indwelling catheter, since urine volume reflects cardiac output and organ perfusion.

PATIENT EDUCATION

1. There will be some intercostal pain for a period of time, which can be relieved by local heat and oral analgesia.
2. Weakness and fatigue are common during the first three weeks following a thoracotomy.
3. Range-of-motion exercises for the arm and shoulder on the affected side should be carried out several times daily to avoid ankylosis of the shoulder ('frozen shoulder').
4. Carry out deep-breathing exercises for the first few weeks at home.
5. Consciously practise good body alignment, preferably in front of a full-length mirror.
6. The chest muscles may be weaker than normal for three to six months following surgery. Avoid lifting more than 9kg until complete healing has taken place.
7. Alternate walking and other activities with frequent short rest periods. Walk at a moderate pace and gradually extend walking time and distance.
8. Stop any activity immediately that causes undue fatigue, increased shortness of breath or chest pain.
9. Because all or part of one lung has been re

moved, stay away from respiratory irritants (smoke, fumes, high level of air pollution).

   a. Avoid anything that may cause spasms of coughing.

   b. Sit in nonsmoking areas in public places.

10. Have an annual influenza injection (pneumonectomy patients).

11. Report for follow-up care by the surgeon or clinic as necessary.

Evaluation

EXPECTED OUTCOMES

1. Maintains effective respiration: normal respiratory rate and blood gas measurements, absence of wheezes and crackles; able to cough up secretions.
2. Achieves pain relief by requesting pain medication and splinting incision with hands when coughing.
3. Attains/maintains mobility of affected shoulder: extends arm at hourly intervals; checks posture; consciously tries to use affected arm; ambulates increasing distances.
4. Avoids preventable complications: absence of bleeding, hypoxia.

FURTHER READING

BOOKS

Campbell, D. and Spence, A.A. (1983) *A Nurse's Guide to Anaesthetics, Resuscitation and Intensive Care*, Churchill Livingstone, Edinburgh.

Crofton, J. and Douglas, A. (1981) *Respiratory Diseases*, Blackwell Scientific Publications, Oxford.

Flower, C. (1981) *Radiology of the Respiratory System*, Update Publications, MTP Press, Lancaster.

Geddes, D.M. (1981) *Airway Obstruction*, Update Publications, MTP Press, Lancaster.

Harper, R.W. (1981) *A Guide to Respiratory Care. Physiology and Clinical Application*, J.B. Lippincott, Philadelphia.

Hudak, C.M., Gallo, B.M. and Lohr, T. (1986) *Critical Care Nursing. A Holistic Approach*. J.B. Lippincott, Philadelphia.

Martz, K.V., Joiner, J.W. and Shepherd, R.M. (1984) *Management of the Patient Ventilator System. A Team Approach*, CV Mosby, St Louis.

Mathers, R.G. (1983) *The Respiratory System*, Churchill Livingstone, Edinburgh.

Nursing Now Series (1984), *Respiratory Emergencies*, Springhouse, Pennsylvania.

Tortora, G.J. and Anagnostakos, N.P. (1986) *Principles of Anatomy and Physiology*, Harper and Row, New York.

The Royal Marsden Hospital (1988) *Manual of Clinical Nursing Procedures 2nd edn*, Harper and Row, London.

Webber, B.A. and Gaskell, D.V. (1980) *The Brompton Hospital Guide to Chest Physiotherapy*, Blackwell Scientific Publications, Oxford.

ARTICLES

Artificial airway management

Fuchs, P.L. (1983) Providing endotracheal tube care, *Nursing*, Vol. 13, September, pp. 6–7.

— (1983) Providing tracheostomy care, *Nursing*, Vol. 13, July, pp. 19–23.

Chest physiotherapy

Thompson, M.C. (1984) Physiotherapy – essentials of chest care, *Nursing*, Vol. 2, No. 27, July, pp. 796–800.

Clinical conditions

Bain, R. (1984) Management of chest trauma, *Nursing*, Vol. 2, No. 27, July, pp. 788–91.

Coleman, D.A. (1986) Pneumonia: where nursing care really counts, *R.N.*, Vol. 49, February, pp. 22–9.

Duffy, B. (1985) Chronic breathing difficulties, *Nursing Mirror*, 25 September, Vol. 161, No. 13, pp. 40–2.

James, B. (1984) Adult respiratory distress syndrome, *Nursing*, Vol. 2, No. 27, July, pp. 792–5.

Meloche, A.T. (1986) Pulmonary embolism, *The Canadian Nurse*, Vol. 82, August, pp. 23–6.

Mortimer, B. and Froud, A. (1984) Respiratory infections, *Nursing*, Vol. 2, No. 28, August, pp. 831–5.

Peddie, M. (1985) Left-sided empyema, *Nursing Times*, Vol. 81, 27 March, pp. 31–4.

General

Boylan, A. and Brown, P. (1985) Student observations: respiration, *Nursing Times*, Vol. 81, 13 March, pp. 35–8.

Durie, M. (1984) Respiratory problems and nursing intervention, *Nursing*, Vol. 2, No. 28, August, pp. 826–8.

Lake Taylor, D. (1985) Assessing breath sounds, *Nursing*, Vol. 15, No. 3, March, pp. 60–2.

Shrake, K. (1979) The ABCs of ABGs, or how to interpret a blood gas value, *Nursing*, Vol. 9, No. 9, September, pp. 26–33.

Twohig, R.G. (1984) Respiratory function tests, *Nursing*, Vol. 2, No. 27, July, pp. 807–810.

Mechanical ventilation

Fuchs Carroll, P. (1986) Caring for ventilator patients, *Nursing*, Vol. 16, No. 2, February, pp. 34–40.

Sykes, K. (1986) Advances in ventilatory support in acute lung disease, *Care of the Critically Ill*, Vol. 2, No. 2, March, pp. 50–2.

Worthington de Toledo, L. (1980) Caring for the patient – instead of the ventilator, *R.N.*, Vol. 43, December, pp. 21–3.

Oxygen therapy

D'Agostino, J.S. (1983) Set your mind at ease on oxygen toxicity, *Nursing*, Vol. 13, July, pp. 55–6.

Domigan-Wentz, J. (1985) The CPAP mask: a comfortable approach to ARDS, *American Journal of Nursing*, Vol. 85, July, pp. 813–5.

Cox, D. and Gillbe, C. (1981) Fixed performance oxygen masks, *Anaesthesia*, Vol. 36, pp. 958–64.

McMillan, E. (1984) Oxygen therapy, *Nursing*, Vol. 2, No. 28, August, pp. 822–5.

Other respiratory therapeutic methods

Fuchs, P.L. (1983) Using humidifiers and nebulizers, *Nursing*, Vol. 13, June, pp. 6–11.

Mumford, S.P. (1986) Using jet nebulizers, *The Professional Nurse*, Vol. 1, January, pp. 95–7.

Thoracic surgery

Fuchs, P. (1983) Before and after surgery stay right on respiratory care, *Nursing*, Vol. 13, May, pp. 47–50.

Glenn, S. (1986) Aiding recovery from a lobectomy, *Nursing Times*, Vol. 82, 18 June, pp. 50–3.

Mims, B.C. (1984) Helping your patient breathe easier after chest surgery, *R.N.*, Vol. 47, December, pp. 25–9.

Underwater-seal drainage

Dalrymple, D. (1984) Setting up for thoracic drainage, *Nursing*, Vol. 14, June, pp. 12–14.

Erickson, R. (1981) Chest tubes: they're really not that complicated, *Nursing*, Vol. 11, No. 5, May, pp. 34–43.

Mumford, S.P. (1986) Draining the pleural cavity, *The Professional Nurse*, Vol. 1, June, pp. 240–2.

Nicoll, J. (1983) Management of underwater chest drainage, *Nursing Times*, Vol. 79, 23 February, pp. 58–9.

5

Care of the Patient with a Cardiovascular Disorder

Heart Disorders

MANIFESTATIONS OF HEART DISEASE

The patient's symptoms of heart disease depend on the nature of cardiac pathology and the resultant physiological disturbances in circulation.

DYSPNOEA
Dyspnoea is undue breathlessness, an awareness of discomfort associated with breathing.

General features
1. Cardiac dyspnoea – failure of left ventricle characterized by increased left atrial, pulmonary venous and capillary pressures; as left atrial pressure rises, the lungs become congested, resulting in dyspnoea.
2. Dypsnoea due to heart disease is usually characterized by rapid and shallow respirations.
3. The threshold (tolerance) for dyspnoea varies with the individual.

Types of dyspnoea
1. *Exertional dyspnoea* – breathlessness upon moderate exertion which is relieved by rest; seen in heart failure, chronic pulmonary disease.
2. *Orthopnoea* – shortness of breath when lying down which is relieved by promptly sitting upright.
   a. Usually due to stasis of blood in lungs, indicating left ventricular failure, mitral disease.
   b. May be from cardiac incompetence or pulmonary incompetence.
3. *Paroxysmal nocturnal dyspnoea* – sudden dyspnoea at night while lying down, due to left ventricular failure, pulmonary oedema, mitral stenosis.
4. *Cheyne-Stokes respiration* – periodic breathing characterized by gradual increase in depth of respiration followed by a decrease in respiration resulting in apnoea; periods of hyperpnoea alternating with periods of apnoea.
   a. Cheyne-Stokes respiration is usually considered a serious sign.
   b. Associated with left ventricular failure (severe), cerebral vascular disease.

Nursing assessment
1. What precipitates or relieves the dyspnoea?
2. What position does the patient assume?
3. What is the skin colour? Pallor? Cyanosis?
4. What is the nature of respiration, e.g., depth, frequency?
5. Is there any sputum? Is it frothy?

CHEST PAIN
Cardiac causes of chest pain
1. Tight crushing chest pain which may radiate to arms, neck and jaw – ischaemia caused by an increase in demand for coronary blood flow and oxygen delivery, which exceeds available blood supply; due to coronary artery disease (angina pectoris, myocardial infarction); or reduced supply due to coronary artery spasm.
2. Excruciating pain radiating to back and flanks – from acute dissecting aneurysm of the aorta.
3. Sharp precordial pain (over heart area) radiating to left shoulder and upper back, aggravated by respirations – indicates acute pericarditis.

Nursing assessment
1. Where is pain located? Does it radiate? To neck? Face? Back? Abdominal area?
2. What is the character of the pain – dull, sharp, boring, crushing?
3. Are there associated symptoms and signs? Sweating? Light-headedness? Nausea? Shortness of breath?
4. What are the time and mode of onset?

5. How long does the episode last?
6. What factors precipitate pain (breathing, coughing, swallowing, rapid walking, emotional stress, exposure to cold)?
7. What factors alleviate pain (rest, change in position, glyceryl trinitrate (GTN))?

PALPITATION

Palpitation is a rapid, forceful or irregular heartbeat felt by the patient.

General features
1. The patient complains of pounding, jumping, stopping sensations in his chest.
2. May be associated with heart disease – enlargement of heart, disturbances of rhythm.
3. Other causes – anxiety, fever, anaemia, thyroid disturbances, and reactions to certain drugs.

Nursing assessment
1. Take blood pressure to check for haemodynamic changes.
2. Note concomitant symptoms – dizziness, chest pain, dyspnoea.
3. Compare apical and a peripheral pulse.
4. Notify doctor and take ECG during episodes of palpitation – for later interpretation.

OEDEMA

Oedema is an abnormal accumulation of serous fluid in the connective tissues and/or cutaneous tissues.

General features
1. Cardiac causes of oedema – heart failure.
2. Other causes of oedema – sodium retention, liver disease, renal disease, hypoproteinaemia, venous or lymphatic obstruction.

Types
1. Ascites – excessive fluid in peritoneal cavity.
2. Pleural effusion – excessive fluid in the pleural cavity.
3. Anasarca – gross generalized oedema.

Nursing implications
1. In heart conditions the location of oedema is influenced by gravity. Fluid collects in the lower parts of the body (dependent oedema).
   a. Assess for oedema of ankles and feet in the ambulant patient.
   b. Assess for oedema of sacral area and posterior thighs in patients confined to bed.
2. Avoid undue pressure on oedematous areas. Oedematous patients are prone to develop pressure sores.

3. Oedema causes stretching of the tissue spaces and is detectable by applying finger pressure to the skin.
   a. Oedema is present if the finger leaves a small depression.
   b. With gross oedema it may not be possible to displace the fluid and the skin will appear taut and shiny and feel hard.
4. Excessive weight gain is likely and daily weights can be correlated to the volume of fluid retention.

HAEMOPTYSIS

Haemoptysis is the coughing up of blood.
1. Small quantities of dark clotted blood – may indicate mitral stenosis, but more commonly associated with pulmonary embolism and pulmonary infarction.
2. Frank haemoptysis – due to lung pathology.
3. Pink, frothy sputum – indicates acute pulmonary oedema.
4. Blood-streaked sputum – indicates acute pulmonary congestion.

FATIGUE
1. Fatigue associated with heart disease is produced by low cardiac output.
2. Undue fatigue related to effort – indicates advanced heart disease, heart failure, mitral stenosis.

SYNCOPE AND FAINTING
1. May be caused by anoxaemia or reduced cardiac output with resulting inadequate circulation.
2. Also seen in dysrhythmias, atrioventricular block, carotid–sinus sensitivity.

CYANOSIS
Cyanosis is a bluish discolouration of the skin and mucous membranes.

Types of cyanosis
1. Central cyanosis – low oxygen saturation of arterial blood.
2. Peripheral cyanosis – reduction of oxyhaemoglobin in capillaries from slow circulation – results from reduced cardiac output due to mitral stenosis, pulmonary stenosis, heart failure.

Cardiac causes of cyanosis
1. Congenital heart disease – due to mixing of arterial stream with venous blood.
2. Heart failure and pulmonary oedema – due to circulatory hypoxia resulting from circulatory failure.

Nursing implications

1. Look at lobes of ears, fingernail beds, cutaneous surfaces of the lips, mucous membranes.
2. Give oxygen when indicated.

ABDOMINAL PAIN OR DISCOMFORT

1. Epigastric (upper abdominal) pain – due to myocardial infarction, distension of liver capsule from heart failure.
2. Severe abdominal pain – may be due to dissecting abdominal aorta, rupture of aortic aneurysm.
3. Intermittent abdominal pain (related to food intake) – indicates circulatory insufficiency of mesenteric arteries or noncardiac pain.

OTHER FEATURES OF HEART DISEASE

1. Distension of neck veins – may be produced by pressure on liver (hepatojugular reflux), heart failure, pericardial compression due to effusion or constrictive pericarditis.
2. Clubbing of fingers – due to cyanotic congenital heart disease, bacterial endocarditis, certain forms of lung pathology; may also be familial.
3. Jaundice – heart failure associated with severe liver congestion.

DIAGNOSIS IN HEART DISEASE

PHYSICAL ASSESSMENT
Arterial pulse

1. Examine the pulses bilaterally; peripheral pulses should be equal.
   a. Note amplitude (fullness), which depends on pulse pressure (difference between systolic and diastolic pressures); this gives an estimate of stroke volume.
      (i) Small volume pulse may be from low stroke volume and peripheral vasoconstriction (myocardial infarction, shock, constrictive pericarditis, vasoconstrictive drugs).
      (ii) Large volume pulse produced by large stroke volume (aortic regurgitation, pregnancy, thyrotoxicosis, bradycardia, patent ductus arteriosus).
   b. Palpate carotid artery – reveals character of pulse in the proximal aorta and provides in-

dication of any abnormality causing disease of left ventricle.

Blood pressure

1. Take on both arms; subsequently blood pressure is taken on right arm.
2. Measure blood pressure with patient supine and standing.
3. Document site of blood pressure measurement and position of patient. (See also pages 356–357 for further discussion of technique.)

Respiration

Note rate, depth and respiratory pattern.

Jugular venous pulse

1. Venous pulsation can be more easily seen than felt.
2. Identification of venous pulse permits assessment of height of venous pressure.

Heart auscultation

1. Heart auscultation requires knowledge, experience and a 'listening ear' tuned to hear each event of the cardiac cycle.
2. Heart auscultation should be systematic.
3. Listen for rate and regularity of rhythm.
   a. Determine if an irregularity is related to respiratory movements.
   b. Evaluate the sequence in which an irregularity occurs.
4. During auscultation, the examiner assesses the venous pulse, feels the pulsation of the right carotid artery and the radial artery, feels precordial movement and listens to the heart (Figure 5.1).

CARDIAC INVESTIGATIONS
Electrocardiography

Electrocardiogram (ECG) – a visual representation of the electrical activity of the heart as reflected by changes in electrical potential at the skin surface.

1. ECG is obtained by placing leads on various body parts (Figure 5.2) and recording the electrical impulse as a tracing on a strip of paper or on the screen of an oscilloscope.
2. Clinical usefulness – evaluation of conditions that interfere with normal electrophysiological function – disturbances of rhythm, disorders of cardiac muscle, enlargement of chambers of heart, electrolyte disturbances.

   See p. 300 for a more detailed account of electrocardiography.

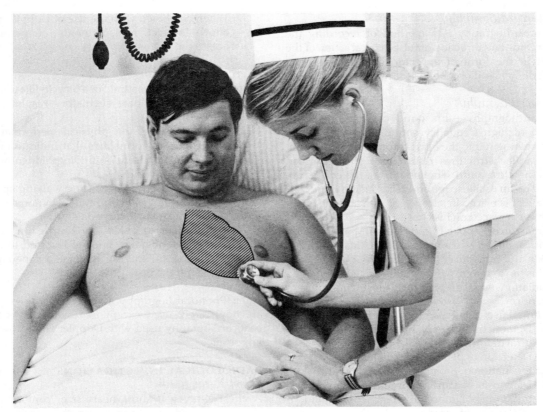

Figure 5.1. Heart auscultation

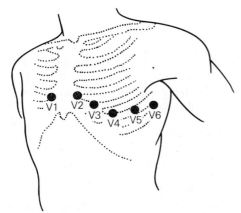

V1 Fourth intercostal space at right sternal border.
V2 Fourth intercostal space at left sternal border.
V3 Equidistant between V2 and V4.
V4 Fifth intercostal space in left mid-clavicular line.
All subsequent leads are taken in the same horizontal plane as V4.
V5 Anterior axillary line.
V6 Mid-axillary line.

Figure 5.2. Locations of unipolar precordial leads

Ambulatory electrocardiographic monitoring
The patient wears miniaturized tape-recording device using a single or double lead system attached to belt or worn on a shoulder device.

1. Various systems are available which record continuously patient's ECG for up to 24 hours while he is going about his daily activities.
2. Patient keeps a diary – records his activities and any symptoms that are noted; useful when symptoms are provoked by specific activities (jogging, stress); used for assessing patients who suffer from transient dizziness, syncope or near syncope; detecting dysrhythmias; assessing response to therapy; and evaluating patients after myocardial infarction.

Phonocardiography
A graphic recording of the occurrence, timing and duration of sounds in the cardiac cycle. (An electrocardiogram may be recorded simultaneously.)

1. Identifies and differentiates various sounds.
2. Affords permanent record for future comparison.
3. Takes approximately 20 minutes.

Vectorcardiography

Vectorcardiography is a method of recording the magnitude and direction of the electrical action of the heart in the form of a vector loop display on a cathode-ray oscilloscope.

Echocardiography

Echocardiography (ultrasound cardiography) is a record of high frequency sound vibrations which have been sent into the heart through the chest wall. The cardiac structures return the echoes derived from the ultrasound. The motions of the echoes are traced on an oscilloscope and recorded on film.
1. Patient is placed in supine position and the transducer is placed on his chest.
2. Transducer applied (left sternal border) with ultrasonic gel to maintain airless contact between skin and transducer (Figure 5.3).
3. This is a noninvasive, painless technique; no radiation exposure; takes 30 to 60 minutes to perform.
4. Clinical usefulness:
   a. Demonstration of valvular and other structural deformities.
   b. Detection of pericardial effusion.
   c. Evaluation of prosthetic valve function.
   d. Diagnosis of cardiac tumours; asymmetrical thickening of interventricular septum.
   e. Diagnosis of cardiomegaly (heart enlargement).

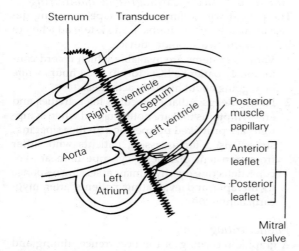

Figure 5.3. Echocardiography. With the transducer as shown, the echocardiogram will record echoes from the chest wall, right ventricular wall, ventricular septum, anterior and posterior leaflets of the mitral valve, and posterior left ventricular wall

f. When combined with the use of Doppler will allow indirect measurements of gradient across the valves.

Exercise stress testing

Exercise testing on a treadmill or a bicycle-like device is carried out to evaluate circulatory response to stress.
1. Evaluates capacity for physical performance; evaluates ECG abnormalities that indicate myocardial ischaemia; useful in finding hidden heart conditions.
2. Patient is exercised by increasing walking speed and the incline of the treadmill or by increasing the load against which he pedals.
3. Instruct patient to avoid smoking, eating and drinking for four hours prior to test and to rest and avoid stimulants or extreme temperature changes after the test.

Note: Phonocardiography and vectorcardiography are now rarely used except in research, whereas echocardiography used with Doppler is of growing importance.

RADIOLOGICAL INVESTIGATIONS
Chest X-ray

A chest X-ray will show heart size, contour and position; reveals cardiac and pericardial calcifications and demonstrates early interstitial pulmonary oedema.

Fluoroscopy

Fluoroscopy assesses unusual cardiac contours, cardiac and vascular pulsations on a luminescent X-ray screen. Also useful in verifying position of intravenous pacemaking electrodes and for guidance of catheter in cardiac catheterization.

Cinefluorography

Cinefluorography involves a fluoroscopic image photographed on motion picture film.

Angiocardiography

Angiocardiography is the injection of contrast medium into the vascular system (to outline the heart and blood vessels) accompanied by serial X-rays or photographed using high-speed motion picture films; provides information regarding structural abnormalities (occlusions, defects or fistulas or abnormal heart valve function).
1. Selective angiocardiography – contrast medium is injected through a catheter directly into one of the heart chambers, coronary arteries or greater ves-

sels, and the angiocardiogram is recorded by means of a rapid film changer or motion picture camera.

2. Aortography – a form of angiography that outlines the lumen of the aorta and major arteries arising from it.

   In thoracic aortography, contrast medium is introduced and the aortic arch and its great vessels are studied by means of rapid serial X-rays. The intravenous, translumbar or retrograde approach may be used.

Coronary arteriography

A radio-opaque catheter is introduced into the right brachial artery via open arteriotomy (or femoral artery via percutaneous puncture), passed into the ascending aorta and manipulated into appropriate coronary artery under fluoroscopic control.

1. Used as a diagnostic tool before coronary artery surgery or myocardial revascularization and after surgery to evaluate graft patency.
2. Used to study suspected congenital anomalies of the coronary arteries.
3. Nursing implications:
   a. Keep the patient in a fasting state prior to the examination.
   b. Limit patient's activities for approximately 12 hours after procedure.
   c. Record blood pressure, pulse, respirations every 15 minutes (or more often as patient's condition indicates) until all are stable.
   d. Check for bleeding at puncture or cutdown site.
   e. Patient may complain of mild headache and of discomfort at puncture site.

Cardiac catheterization

Catheter(s) is (are) introduced into the heart and blood vessels to (1) measure oxygen concentration, saturation, tension and pressure in the various heart chambers; (2) detect shunts; (3) provide blood samples for analysis; and (4) determine cardiac output and pulmonary blood flow. Angiography is usually combined with heart catheterization for coronary artery visualization.

1. Right-heart catheterization – a radio-opaque catheter is passed from an antecubital or femoral vein into the right atrium, right ventricle and pulmonary vasculature under direct visualization with a fluoroscope.
   a. Right atrium and right ventricle pressures measured; blood samples taken for haematocrit and oxygen saturation.
   b. Catheter introduced into pulmonary artery and as far as possible beyond that point; capillary samples and capillary (wedge) pressures are then recorded.

2. Left-heart catheterization – may be accomplished using four sites: (1) percutaneous needle puncture of the left atrium, (2) percutaneous needle puncture of left ventricle, (3) transseptal puncture or (4) retrograde catheterization of left ventricle.
   a. Permits flow and pressure measurements (haemodynamic data) of the left heart.
   b. Useful in evaluating status of mitral and aortic valves and coronary arteries.

3. Complications of heart catheterization.
   a. Dysrhythmias (ventricular fibrillation), syncope, vasospasm.
   b. Pericardial tamponade, myocardial infarction, pulmonary oedema.
   c. Thrombophlebitis of vein used for catheterization.
   d. Allergic reaction to contrast medium.
   e. Perforation of great vessels of heart; systemic emboli.
   f. Loss of pulse distal to arteriotomy and possible ischaemia of lower arm and hand.

4. Nursing implications.

   Preceding heart catheterization:
   a. Know which approach is to be used in order to anticipate possible complications.
   b. Patient to fast six hours before procedure – to prevent vomiting and aspiration.
   c. Ascertain history of previous allergies.
   d. Explain to the patient that he will be lying on an examining table for a prolonged period and that he may experience certain sensations:
      (i) Occasional thudding sensations in the chest – from ectopic beats, particularly when the catheter tip is manipulated in ventricles.
      (ii) Strong desire to cough – may occur during dye injection into right heart during angiography.
      (iii) Transient feeling of heat, particularly in head – from injection of contrast medium.
   e. Ask patient to remove dentures.
   f. Be sure that patient has received premedication as prescribed.

   Following heart catheterization:
   a. During the procedure the patient is attached to a cardiac monitor. Appropriate resuscitative equipment should be readily available.
   b. Record the blood pressure and apical pulse every 15 minutes (or more frequently), until stable after the procedure – to detect dysrhythmias.

c. Check peripheral pulses in affected extremity (dorsalis pedis, posterior tibial pulse in the lower extremity and radial pulse in upper extremity); evaluate extremity temperature and colour and complaints of pain, numbness or tingling sensation – to determine signs of arterial insufficiency.

d. Patient rests in bed until following morning.

e. Watch puncture (cutdown) sites for haematoma formation. Question patient about increase in pain/tenderness at site.

f. Assess for complaints of chest pain and report occurrence immediately.

Indicator dilution curves

Injection of dye into one of the heart chambers and the evaluation of its appearance in a peripheral artery.

1. Gives information concerning presence or absence of intracardiac shunts.
2. Is a means of calculating cardiac output.

Myocardial imaging (radionuclide imaging)

With the use of radionuclides and scintillation cameras, radionuclide angiograms can be utilized to assess left ventricular performance.

1. 'Hot spot' or positive imaging:
   a. Technetium-99m is a radionuclide most commonly utilized. Necrosed or ischaemic myocardium takes up the phosphate and produces a 'hot spot' indicative of a positive scan.
   b. Scans become positive within 12 to 36 hours and are usually negative after seven days.
   c. Utilized when diagnosis of myocardial infarction (MI) is unclear. Not used in routine work-up for diagnostic evaluation of MI.
2. 'Cold spot' imaging:
   a. Thallium-201 most common isotope utilized. Thallium-201 concentrates in myocardial cells relative to blood flow. Areas of low concentration are termed 'cold spots'.
   b. Differentiation between old and new infarctions cannot be determined with this method and no distinction can be made between areas of infarction and ischaemia.
   c. A normal thallium scan is likely to rule out the diagnosis of myocardial infarction. Usually not employed in routine diagnostic evaluation of MI.
3. Radionuclide ventriculogram:
   a. A non-invasive method for accurate assessment of ventricular haemodynamics and regional wall motion.
   b. Provides measurements of right and left ventricular ejection fraction, distinguishes regional from global ventricular wall motion and allows for subjective analysis of cardiac anatomy to detect intracardiac shunts and valvular or congenital abnormalities.
   c. A radiopharmaceutical (usually technetium-99m) is injected rapidly through a central venous catheter, Swan–Ganz catheter or antecubital vein.
   d. Indices of ventricular performance are measured from the initial transit of the radiotracer through the heart.

TESTS OF CIRCULATION TIME

Circulation time measures the velocity of blood flow and helps diagnose both right-heart and left-heart failure. Two methods are used:

1. Arm-to-tongue – rapid injection (intravenously) of dehydrocholic acid in a peripheral vein. Interval between time when the injection is given and time when the patient complains of a bitter taste is measured with a stopwatch.
2. Arm-to-lung – intravenous injection of either ether or paraldehyde. The end point is reached when the odour of the drug is detected on the patient's breath or when the patient begins to cough.
   a. Normal arm-to-tongue time – 8 to 16 seconds.
   b. Normal arm-to-lung time – 4 to 8 seconds.

BLOOD STUDIES

1. Antistreptolysin titre – measurement of blood antibodies against streptococcus; shows whether a patient has had a recent infection.
2. Erythrocyte sedimentation rate (ESR) – speed of sedimentation of red cells of blood expressed in millimetres per hour. The rate is elevated when an inflammatory process is present; also used as a test for rheumatic fever. May be reduced in heart failure.
3. C-reactive protein (CRP) – a blood test that is a sensitive (but nonspecific) indicator of inflammation of infectious or noninfectious origin.
4. Blood culture – test to detect presence of bacteria in circulating blood. Clinical usefulness in cardiology – indicates infective endocarditis.
5. Blood electrolytes (potassium, sodium, calcium) to identify patients with heart failure or renal disease (especially if treated with digitalis or diuretics).
6. Serum enzyme tests – heart muscle is rich in enzymes which may cause different biochemical reactions.
   a. Serum activity of enzymes increases sig-

nificantly following myocardial infarction because enzymes are released by injured or dead myocardial cells.

b. The following enzyme studies are frequently used (normal values differ according to type of test used):
   (i) Serum lactic dehydrogenase (LDI I).
   (ii) Serum glutamic oxaloacetic transaminase (SGOT).
   (iii) Serum glutamic pyruvic transaminase (SGPT).
   (iv) Creatine phosphokinase (CPK) (measures presence of heart muscle damage more specifically since it is found only in myocardium, skeletal muscle and brain tissue).
   (v) Hydroxybutyric dehydrogenase (HBD).

Note: Serum enzymes are measured in different combinations as some show up quicker than others.

c. However, these enzymes may be widely distributed in tissues and elevated in conditions not associated with myocardial infarction (i.e., damage to skeletal muscles, liver, brain, kidneys and other organs).

d. Isoenzymes – forms of protein species that promote the same biochemical action as enzymes but differ chemically, physically and/or immunologically.
   (i) Isoenzymes can be identified by laboratory methods to reveal the specific tissue that is damaged; creatine kinase can be separated into three isoenzymes, known as MM, MB and BB.
   (ii) An elevation of serum CK-MB activity signifies that an adverse effect on myocardial cells has taken place; thus, it is the most specific and sensitive enzymatic criterion of myocardial injury now available. CK-MB greater than 5 IU is significant.

HAEMODYNAMIC MONITORING

Haemodynamic monitoring is the assessment of the patient's circulatory status; it includes measurements of heart rate, intra-arterial pressure, pulmonary artery and pulmonary capillary wedge pressures, central venous pressure, cardiac output and blood volume. Continued on p. 229.

GUIDELINES: CENTRAL VENOUS PRESSURE

Central venous pressure (CVP) is the pressure within the right atrium or in the great veins within the thorax.
Central venous pressure monitoring serves as a guide for assessment of right-sided cardiac function.
Central venous pressure monitoring serves as a guide for assessment of left-sided cardiac function only in the absence of cardiorespiratory disease.

OBJECTIVES
1. Serve as a guide for fluid replacement in seriously ill patients.
2. Estimate blood volume deficits.
3. Determine pressures in the right atrium and central veins.
4. Evaluate for circulatory failure (in context with total clinical picture of patient).

VEIN SITES FOR CATHETER PLACEMENT
The most commonly used sites are:
1. Subclavian.
2. Internal or external jugular.
3. Median basilic.

EQUIPMENT

Venous pressure tray
Cutdown tray
Infusion solution and infusion set

3- or 4-way stopcock (a pressure transducer may be used)
IV pole attached to bed; arm board; adhesive tape
ECG monitor
Spirit level (for establishing zero point)

PROCEDURE

See Figure 5.4.

Preparatory phase

Nursing action

Rationale

1. Assemble equipment according to manufacturer's directions.
2. Explain that the procedure is similar to an intravenous infusion and that the patient may move in bed as desired after the passage of the CVP catheter.

3. Place the patient in a position of comfort. This is the baseline position used for subsequent readings.

Serial CVP readings should be made with the patient in the same position.

4. Attach manometer to the intravenous pole The zero point of the manometer should be on a level with the patient's right atrium.

The right atrium is at the midaxillary line, which is about one-third of the distance from the anterior to the posterior chest wall (see Figure 5.4). The midaxillary line is an external reference point for the zero level of the manometer (which coincides with the level of the right atrium).

5. The CVP catheter is connected to a three-way stopcock which communicates with an open intravenous infusion (saline or heparin) and with a manometer (the measuring device).
6. Start the intravenous flow and fill the manometer 10cm above anticipated reading (or until the level of 20cmH$_2$O is reached). Turn the stopcock and fill the tubing with fluid.

7. The CVP site is surgically cleansed. CVP catheter (line) is introduced percutaneously or by direct venous cutdown and threaded through an antecubital, subclavian or internal or external jugular vein into the superior vena cava just before it enters the right atrium.

The correct catheter placement can be confirmed by fluoroscopy or chest X-ray or by observing the fluctuations in the manometer with respirations (respiratory swing).

8. When the catheter enters the thorax an inspiratory fall and expiratory rise in venous pressure are observed.

The fluid level fluctuates with respiration. It rises sharply with coughing, straining.

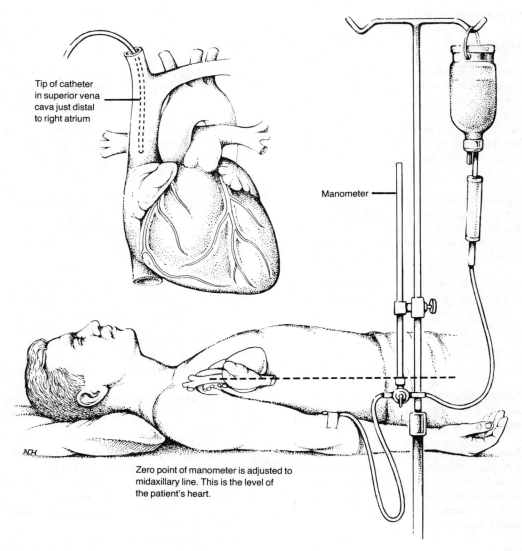

Tip of catheter
in superior vena
cava just distal
to right atrium

Manometer

Zero point of manometer is adjusted to
midaxillary line. This is the level of
the patient's heart.

Figure 5.4. Central venous pressure

9. The patient may be monitored by ECG during catheter insertion.	When the tip of the catheter contacts the wall of the right atrium (or right ventricle) it may produce aberrant impulses and disturb cardiac rhythm.
10. The catheter may be sutured and taped in place. A sterile dressing is applied. Label dressing with time and date of catheter insertion.	
11. The infusion is adjusted to flow into the patient's vein by a slow continuous drip.	The infusion may cause a significant increase in venous pressure if permitted to flow too rapidly.

To measure the CVP

Nursing action

1. Place patient in the identified position (as mentioned under Preparatory Phase) and confirm the zero point.

2. Turn the stopcock to open the connection between the patient and the manometer. Close the flow from the intravenous solution (Figure 5.5).

3. Observe the fall in the height of the column of fluid in manometer. Record the level at which the solution stabilizes. This is the central venous pressure. Record CVP and the position of the patient.

4. The CVP may range from 5–12cmH$_2$O. (Absolute numerical values have not been agreed upon.)

5. Turn the stopcock again to allow intravenous solution to flow from solution bottle into patient's veins.

6. Assess the patient's clinical condition. Frequent changes in measurements (interpreted within the context of the clinical situation) will serve as a guide to detect whether the heart can handle its fluid load and whether hypovolaemia or hypervolaemia are present.

7. Observe the patient for complications.
   a. From catheter trauma:
      (i) Pneumo/haemo/hydrothorax.
      (ii) Haematoma.
      (iii) Cardiac tamponade.
   b. Secondary to presence of catheter:
      (i) Thrombophlebitis.
      (ii) Sepsis.
      (iii) Embolus or clot at catheter tip.
      (iv) Dysrhythmia.

Rationale

The zero point or baseline for the manometer should be on a level with the patient's right atrium.

When the stopcock is turned to connect the manometer to the intravenous catheter, fluid in the manometer column falls until it balances the central venous pressure in the superior vena cava.

The CVP reading is reflected by the height of a column of fluid in the manometer when there is open communication between the catheter and the manometer.

The change in CVP is a more useful indication of adequacy of venous blood volume and alterations of cardiovascular function. CVP is a dynamic measurement. The normal values may change from patient to patient. The management of the patient is not based on one reading but on repeated serial readings in correlation with patient's clinical state.

When readings are not being made, flow is from a very slow microdrip to the catheter, bypassing the manometer.

CVP is interpreted by considering the patient's entire clinical picture; hourly urine output, heart rate, blood pressure, cardiac output measurements.
a. A CVP near zero indicates that the patient is hypovolaemic (verified if rapid intravenous infusion causes patient to improve).
b. A CVP above 15–20cmH$_2$O may indicate hypervolaemia, poor cardiac contractility, cardiac tamponade or haemo/pneumothorax.

Inspect entry site twice daily, or as directed by the doctor, for signs of local inflammation/phlebitis. Inform the doctor immediately if there are any signs of infection.

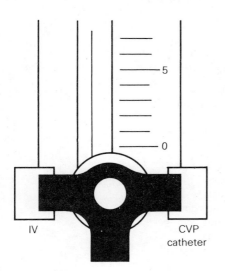

A. Position for IV fluid administration

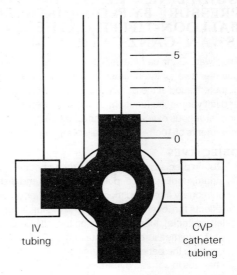

B. Position for filling CVP manometer

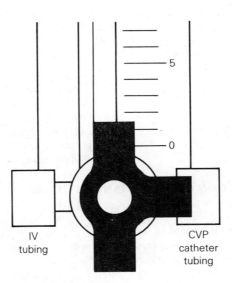

C. Position for CVP measurement

Figure 5.5. Valve positions for intravenous fluid administration and central venous pressure measurement

GUIDELINES: MEASURING PULMONARY ARTERY PRESSURE BY FLOW-DIRECTED BALLOON-TIPPED CATHETER (SWAN–GANZ CATHETER)*

The Swan–Ganz catheter is a flow-directed, balloon-tipped, four-lumen catheter (two- or three-lumen also available), allowing for ease of right heart catheterization at the bedside and permitting continuous monitoring of right and left ventricular function, pulmonary artery pressures, cardiac output and arterial venous oxygen difference. The catheter is 110cm long, marked at increments of 10cm, and is available in diameters of No. 5 and 7 French.

OBJECTIVES

1. Obtain precise haemodynamic data concerning pressures in the right atrium, right ventricle, pulmonary artery and distal branches of the pulmonary artery (pulmonary capillary wedge pressure). The latter reflects the level of the pressure in the left atrium (or filling pressure in the left ventricle), thus pressures on the left side of the heart are inferred from pressure measurements obtained on the right side of the circulation.
2. Evaluate the patient and permit rational selection of therapy when critical changes in cardiac dynamics occur.
3. Evaluate the patient's response to implemented therapy.
4. Obtain measurement of cardiac output through thermodilution.
5. Obtain mixed venous blood samplings from pulmonary artery.

UNDERLYING CONSIDERATIONS

1. Left atrial pressure is closely related to left ventricular end-diastolic pressure (LVEDP) (filling pressure of the left ventricle) and is therefore an indicator of left ventricular function.
2. Pulmonary artery pressures are important in evaluating patients with cardiogenic shock, severe left ventricular failure with pulmonary oedema, mitral regurgitation and/or ventricular-septal rupture, etc.

EQUIPMENT

Swan–Ganz catheter set
ECG; monitor and display unit
Defibrillator
Pressure transducer; transducer holder
Cutdown tray

2.5ml syringe
Sterile saline solution
Heparin
Lignocaine drip (for standby)
Local anaesthetic
Skin antiseptic

PROCEDURE FOR INSERTION OF SWAN–GANZ CATHETER (PERFORMED BY DOCTOR)
Preparation

1. Explain procedure to patient as condition allows.
2. Shave and prepare the skin over the insertion site. Cover with sterile towels.
3. Test the catheter under sterile water for balloon leakage.
4. A transducer/monitor for the determination of pressures will be prepared by the doctor.
5. An intravenous infusion will also be required.

---

* Although the term 'Swan–Ganz' is widely used to describe any balloon flow-directed catheter, they should more properly be called pulmonary artery flotation catheters. Swan–Ganz is a registered trademark of Edwards Laboratories, a division of the American Hospital Supply Corporation.

Insertion

1. The Swan–Ganz catheter is inserted through an antecubital vein or through an internal jugular vein by either percutaneous puncture or intravenous cutdown. (Other veins, e.g. brachial, subclavian, femoral, may be used.)
2. The catheter is advanced to the superior vena cava. Oscillations of the pressure waveforms will indicate when the tip of the catheter is within the thoracic cavity (Figure 5.6). (Catheter placement may be determined by fluoroscopy, by evaluation of the pressure waves and also by the markings on the catheter.)
3. When the catheter is in the superior vena cava it is inflated with air and advanced gently. The amount of air to be used is indicated on the catheter.
4. The inflated balloon at the tip of the catheter will be guided by the flowing stream of blood through the right atrium and tricuspid valve into the right ventricle. From this position it finds its way into the main pulmonary artery.

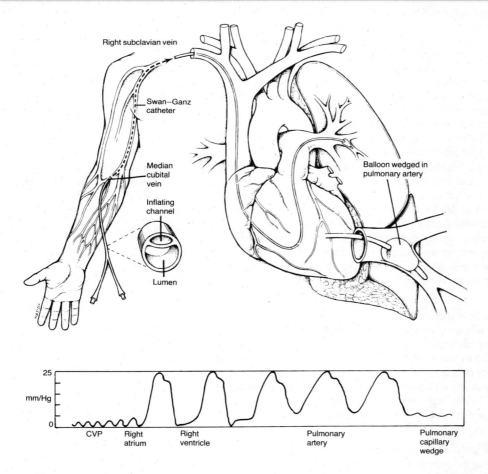

Figure 5.6. Insertion of Swan–Ganz catheter. The position of the catheter is reflected by the pressure tracings. Capillary wedge pressure is obtained by inflating the balloon

(Watch ECG monitor for signs of ventricular irritability as catheter enters the right ventricle. The balloon will flow from the right atrium to the pulmonary artery in approximately 10 to 20 seconds).

5. The flowing blood will continue to direct the catheter more distally into the pulmonary tree. When the catheter reaches a pulmonary vessel that is approximately the same size or slightly smaller in diameter than the inflated balloon, it cannot be advanced any further. This is the wedge position.

6. The pressure is recorded with the balloon wedged in the pulmonary vascular bed.
   a. Normal wedge pressure is less than 12mmHg.
   b. In patients with myocardial infarction the optimal wedge pressures are 15–18mmHg. In these patients pressures below 15mmHg may indicate intravascular hypovolaemia, whereas pressures over 18 indicate left ventricular failure (congestive heart failure) in the absence of mitral stenosis.

7. The balloon is deflated, causing the catheter to retract spontaneously into a larger pulmonary artery. This gives the pulmonary artery pressure reading.
   a. The upper limit of normal pressure in the pulmonary artery is approximately 30/12mmHg.
   b. The normal mean pulmonary artery pressure (average pressure in pulmonary artery throughout the entire cardiac cycle) is approximately 10–15mmHg. Increased pulmonary artery pressure readings indicate:
      (i) Pulmonary hypertension from many causes.
      (ii) Chronic obstructive airways disease.
      (iii) Acute respiratory insufficiency.
      (iv) Long-standing congenital heart disease with large shunts.
      (v) Left ventricular failure.
      (vi) Mitral stenosis.
      The causes for decreased pulmonary artery pressure are relatively the same as those for a low wedge pressure.

8. The catheter is sutured in place. Antibiotic ointment may be placed around the site and covered with a sterile dressing.

9. The catheter is kept patent by a low-flow (3ml/hr) continuous irrigation of heparinized saline.

To obtain a wedge pressure reading

1. Note amount of air to be injected into balloon.
2. Inflate the balloon slowly until the contour of the pulmonary arterial pressure changes to that of pulmonary wedge pressure. As soon as a wedge pattern is observed, no more air is introduced. Do not introduce more air into balloon than specified. Pulmonary capillary wedge pressure is only measured intermittently. Do not allow the catheter to remain in the wedge position for more than one or two minutes.

For removal of the catheter

1. Be sure the balloon is not inflated.
2. The catheter is removed slowly; pressure dressing is applied over the site. The site should be checked periodically for bleeding.

3. The catheter tip should be sent for culture and sensitivity once it is removed.

Complications
1. Pulmonary infarction.
2. Dysrhythmias.
3. Thromboembolus.
4. Balloon rupture or knotting of catheter.

CARDIAC OUTPUT

Cardiac output is the amount (volume) of blood ejected by one ventricle in one minute.

CLINICAL ASSESSMENT OF CARDIAC OUTPUT
A low cardiac output may be detected by:
1. Cyanosis or duskiness of buccal mucosa, nailbeds and ear lobes.
2. Cool, moist skin.
3. Low urine output.
4. Falling blood pressure.

UNDERLYING CONCEPTS
1. Cardiac output depends on cardiac function, tone of the blood vessels and blood volume.
2. Cardiac output is expressed in litres per minute and is equal to the stroke volume × heart rate (SV × HR).
   a. SV = amount of blood ejected from ventricle per beat.
   b. HR = number of cardiac contractions/minute.
   c. Normal cardiac output = 5 to 6 litres/minute.
3. Cardiac output is usually expressed as the cardiac index (CI).
   a. CI = indicator for peripheral perfusion of organs.
   b. CI = CO divided by body surface area; the body surface area is determined by standard charts.
   c. Normal CI = 2.7–4.3 litres/min/m^2 indicates normal peripheral perfusion.
4. Cardiac output is measured by a variety of techniques. In the clinical setting, it is usually measured by the thermodilution techniques used in conjunction with a flow-directed balloon catheter (Swan–Ganz catheter).

METHOD
1. The Swan–Ganz catheter is positioned in its final position in a branch of the pulmonary artery; it has a thermistor (external heat-sensing device) situated 4cm from the tip of the catheter, which measures the temperature of the blood that flows by it.
2. Sterile dextrose or saline solution at 0°C is injected through one lumen of the catheter. The solution mixes with the blood in the right side of the heart and flows to the pulmonary artery where blood temperature is detected by the thermistor.
3. A small computer converts the temperature changes into a direct reading of cardiac output.

SPECIAL MEDICAL AND NURSING MEASURES

GUIDELINES: ASSISTING THE PATIENT UNDERGOING PERICARDIAL ASPIRATION (PERICARDIOCENTESIS)

Pericardial aspiration is the puncturing of the pericardial sac in order to aspirate fluid and thereby relieve cardiac tamponade.

Cardiac tamponade is compression of the heart by blood, effusion or a foreign body in the pericardial sac which restricts normal heart action.

CLINICAL FEATURES OF CARDIAC TAMPONADE

1. Rising venous pressure (a CVP of 20cmH$_2$O or more).
2. Falling arterial blood pressure.
3. Small, quiet heart; muffled heart sounds (detected by fluoroscopy and chest auscultation).
4. Narrowing pulse pressure (difference between systolic and diastolic pressures).
5. Paradoxical pulse (lessening of pulse amplitude during inspiration).
6. Distention of neck veins and rise in neck veins with inspiration (Kussmaul's sign).
7. Apprehension; dyspnoea.
8. Tachypnoea; pallor or cyanosis.
9. Characteristic posture – sitting upright and leaning forward.
10. Clinical shock.

OBJECTIVES

1. Remove fluid from the pericardial sac caused by:
   a. Pericarditis.
   b. Effusion from malignant neoplasm or lymphoma.
   c. Trauma to heart or chest.
   d. Acute rheumatic fever.
   e. Uraemia.
2. Obtain fluid for diagnosis.
3. Instil certain therapeutic drugs.

EQUIPMENT

Pericardial aspiration tray
Aspiration catheter
Skin antiseptic, e.g. chlorhexidine 0.5 per cent in spirit
Lignocaine 1 or 2 per cent
Sterile gloves

ECG machine for monitoring purposes
Sterile earth wire – to be connected between pericardial needle and V lead of ECG machine (use alligator clip type connectors)
Apparatus for resuscitation including thoracotomy and pacemaker equipment

SITES FOR PERICARDIAL ASPIRATION

1. Subxiphoid – needle inserted in the angle between left costal margin and xiphoid.
2. Near cardiac apex, 2cm inside left border of cardiac dullness.
3. To the left of the fifth or sixth interspace at the sternal margin.
4. Right side of fourth intercostal space just inside border of dullness.

PROCEDURE

See Figure 5.7.

Preparation

1. Explain the procedure to the patient and give premedication as prescribed, e.g. diazepam.
2. Assist the doctor with the setting up of an intravenous infusion (can be used as a route for intravenous drugs in event of an emergency).
3. Place the patient in a comfortable position with the head of the bed or

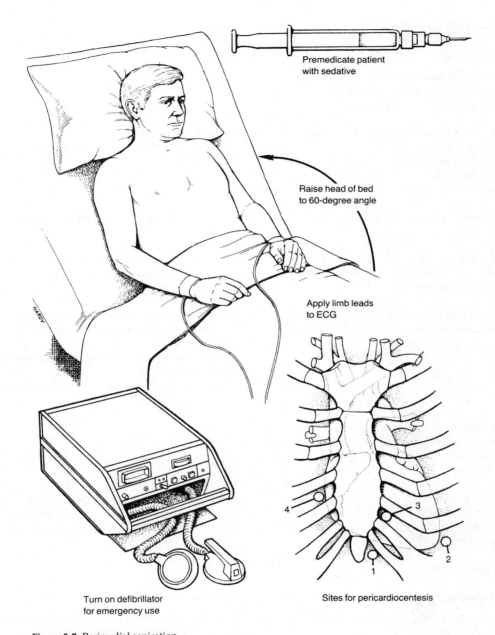

Premedicate patient
with sedative

Raise head of bed
to 60-degree angle

Apply limb leads
to ECG

Turn on defibrillator
for emergency use

Sites for pericardiocentesis

Figure 5.7. Pericardial aspiration

treatment table raised to a 60° angle. (This position makes it easier to
insert needle into pericardial sac.)
4. Apply the limb leads of the ECG machine to the patient.
5. Prepare emergency equipment as per protocol, e.g. turn on defibrillator,
have pacemaker available.
6. Open the pericardial aspirator tray, using aseptic technique.

Performance phase

Doctor's action	Rationale
1. The site is prepared with skin antiseptic, the area covered with sterile towels. Lignocaine is infiltrated into the area.	
2. The pericardial aspiration needle is attached to a 50ml syringe by a three-way stopcock. The V lead (precordial lead wire) of the ECG machine is attached to the hub of the aspirating needle by a sterile wire and alligator clips or clamp.	There is a danger of laceration of myocardium/coronary artery and of cardiac dysrhythmias.
3. The needle is advanced slowly until fluid is obtained.	Fluid is generally aspirated at a depth of 2.5–4cm.
4. When the pericardial sac has been entered, a haemostat is clamped to the needle at the chest wall just where it penetrates the skin.	This prevents movement of the needle and further penetration while fluid is being removed.
5. The patient's ECG monitor, blood pressure and venous pressure must be observed constantly.	a. The ST segment rises if the point of the needle contacts the ventricle; there may be ventricular ectopic beats. b. The PR segment is elevated when the needle touches the atrium. c. Large, erratic QRS complexes indicate penetration of the myocardium.
6. If a large amount of fluid is present, a polythene catheter may be inserted through a needle and left in the pericardial sac and attached to a drainage bottle.	
7. Watch for presence of bloody fluid. If blood accumulates rapidly, an immediate thoracotomy and cardiorrhaphy (suturing of heart muscle) may be indicated.	Bloody pericardial fluid may be due to trauma. Bloody pericardial effusion fluid does not clot, whereas blood obtained from inadvertent puncture of one of the heart chambers *does* clot.

Follow-up phase

Nursing action	Rationale
1. Place patient in intensive care unit or cardiac care unit, as available.	Following pericardial aspiration careful monitoring of blood pressure and venous pressure will be necessary to indicate possible recurrence of tamponade. A repeated aspiration is then necessary.
2. Watch for rising venous pressure and falling arterial pressure.	In the presence of these signs the patient is probably experiencing cardiac tamponade.
3. Call the doctor immediately if observations vary only minimally.	

4. Be prepared for further treatment at all times.

5. Observe for complications:
   a. Inadvertent puncture of heart chamber.
   b. Dysrhythmias.
   c. Puncture of lung, stomach or liver.
   d. Laceration of coronary artery or myocardium.

GUIDELINES: CARDIOPULMONARY RESUSCITATION FOR CARDIAC ARREST*

Cardiac arrest is a sudden and unexpected cessation of the heartbeat and effective circulation.

CAUSES
1. Cardiac:
   a. Ventricular fibrillation.
   b. Ventricular asystole.
   c. Electromechanical dissociation.
2. Asphyxia (drowning, carbon monoxide poisoning, drug overdose, smoke from fires).
3. Anaphylactic reaction (to insects, medications, food).
4. Accidents (electrocution, drowning, inhalation of toxic gases).
5. Complication of surgery.
6. Acute airway obstruction.

SIGNS AND SYMPTOMS
1. Immediate collapse followed by loss of consciousness.
2. Absence of palpable carotid or femoral pulse.
3. Absence of audible heart sounds.
4. Apnoea.
5. Convulsions (may or may not be present).
6. Dilation of pupils of eyes (unreliable sign).
7. Ashen grey colour.

OBJECTIVES
1. Establish *promptly* effective circulation and ventilation.
2. Prevent irreversible cerebral anoxic damage.

EQUIPMENT
Arrest board (if on unsupported mattress)
Oral airway
O_2 supply
Bag and mask device, e.g., rebreathing circuit
Intubation equipment

Suction equipment
Defibrillator
Emergency cardiac drugs
Intravenous equipment

---

* Adapted from Jowett, N. I. and Thompson, D. R. (1988) Basic life support – the forgotten skills? *Intensive Care Nursing*, No. 4, pp. 9–17; and Jowett, N. I. and Thompson, D. R. (1988) Advanced cardiac life support: current perspectives. *Intensive Care Nursing*, No. 4, pp. 71–81.

UNDERLYING PRINCIPLES

1. Basic cardiopulmonary resuscitation (CPR) consists of the following ABC sequence: Airway, Breathing and Circulation.
2. Cardiopulmonary resuscitation consists of maintaining an open airway, providing artificial ventilation by means of rescue breathing and providing artificial circulation by external cardiac compression.

PROCEDURE FOR CARDIOPULMONARY RESUSCITATION

Nursing action

1. Note the time as soon as the cardiac arrest is determined. Summon help immediately. Place the patient in a horizontal position on a firm surface.

2. In a witnessed cardiac arrest, a precordial thump may be administered: deliver a single sharp blow over the midportion of the sternum using the fleshy portion of the fist; strike from a distance of 20.3–30.5cm above the chest (Figure 5.8).

3. If patient is not breathing, open the airway and quickly ventilate the lungs four times. (See Artificial Ventilation, which follows.)

4. Palpate for carotid pulse for 5 to 10 seconds.

5. Start external cardiac compression immediately if carotid pulse is absent or questionable.

Rationale

NURSING ALERT
Lack of effective circulation to the central nervous system for more than 3 to 5 minutes may result in irreversible damage.

The precordial thump is useful when the pulse cannot be detected following a witnessed cardiac arrest or when dealing with a patient who is being monitored or is being paced for a known AV block. The precordial thump should be administered within the first minute after cardiac arrest.

Carotid artery is always immediately accessible whereas femoral artery is not. Brachial/radial palpation of lesser value.

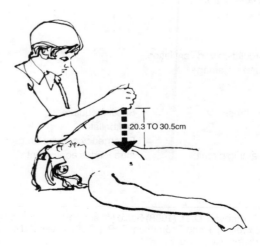

Figure 5.8. Precordial thump

PROCEDURE FOR ARTIFICIAL VENTILATION

Nursing action	Rationale
Carry out artificial ventilation and external cardiac compression *simultaneously*.	
1. Clear airway of material, e.g. saliva, vomit.	
2. Tilt the head back and pull the jaw forward.	This manoeuvre lifts the tongue off the back wall of the pharynx and opens the airway.
3. Insert oropharyngeal airway if available.	
4. Ventilate the patient. Inflate the patient's lungs by a forceful expiration of a full breath through a mouth-to-mouth airtight seal. Or ventilate the patient by bag and mask technique.	Forceful ventilation helps overcome airway obstruction by increasing the pressure gradient of air movement and dilating the upper airway. With each attempted inflation the patient's chest should rise to a visible degree. Absence of chest expansion indicates airway obstruction.
5. Keep the jaw pulled forward during ventilation to relieve obstruction.	
6. Provide 12 breaths per minute.	

PROCEDURE FOR EXTERNAL CARDIAC COMPRESSION (MUST BE ACCOMPANIED BY ARTIFICIAL VENTILATION)

Nursing action	Rationale
1. Place the heel of one hand on the lower half of the sternum 3.8cm from the tip of the xiphoid and towards the patient's head.	Proper placement of the hands reduces possible complications of fractured ribs or injury to adjacent abdominal organs.
2. Place the other hand on top of the first one. The fingers should not touch the chest wall (Figure 5.9).	
3. Using your weight while keeping the elbows straight, quickly and forcefully depress the lower sternum 3–5cm towards the spine and then suddenly release the sternal pressure.	Each compression forces the blood from the heart into the arterial system. Relaxation immediately follows compression and is of equal duration.
a. Do not allow the hands to lose contact with the sternum.	
b. The body weight should be carried by the arm muscles.	
4. Use 80–100 compression per minute for two people performing CPR.* Compressions should be smooth, regular and uninterrupted.	If done correctly this rate can maintain adequate blood flow and pressure and allows cardiac refill.

* This procedure is done best by two people. If only one is available, he must perform both artificial ventilation and external cardiac compression, using a 15:2 ratio consisting of two quick lung inflations after each 15 chest compressions. The single rescuer must perform each series of chest compressions at a faster rate of 80–100 compressions per minute because of interruptions for lung inflation.

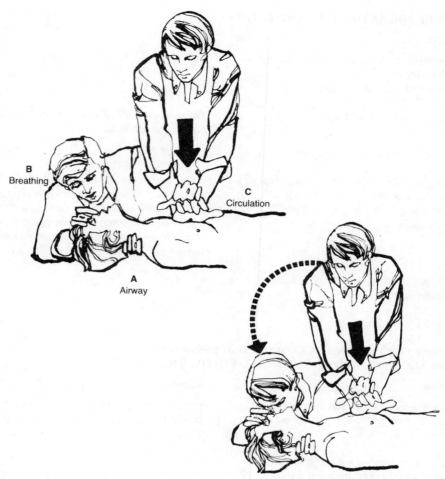

Figure 5.9. Two-rescuer cardiopulmonary resuscitation: five chest compressions – rate of 60/minute, no pause for ventilation; one lung inflation – after each five compressions, interposed between compressions. One-rescuer cardiopulmonary resuscitation: 15 chest compressions – rate of 80–100/minute

5. The second person delivers one deep breath for each five cardiac compressions, without interruption of the compression cycle.

If only one person is available, he must give two lung inflations before each 15 chest compressions.

6. Palpate for carotid or femoral pulse periodically and note size of pupils as an indication of response.

The presence of a palpable carotid pulse and constriction of pupils are evidence of effective circulation and oxygenated blood. If pupils remain widely dilated and do not react to light and if the patient is deeply unconscious with absence of spontaneous respirations, serious brain damage is imminent or has occurred.

7. While resuscitation proceeds, simultaneous efforts are made to start an intravenous infusion.

Have suction ready and attach ECG electrodes to the patient.

8. If ventricular fibrillation occurs, conversion to a normal sinus rhythm must be effected by electric countershock delivered by a defibrillator.

9. The decision to terminate resuscitation is made medically and takes into consideration the cerebral and cardiac state of the patient. Cardiac compression should continue until the patient can maintain blood pressure, etc., or the situation becomes hopeless.

10. Drug therapy — see Table 5.1 for major drugs commonly used in cardiopulmonary resuscitation.

GUIDELINES: DIRECT CURRENT DEFIBRILLATION PROCEDURE FOR VENTRICULAR FIBRILLATION/VENTRICULAR TACHYCARDIA

Defibrillation (countershock) is the use of electrical discharge to patient's chest wall to terminate ventricular fibrillation or ventricular tachycardia.

A defibrillator is an instrument that delivers an electric shock to the heart to convert ventricular fibrillation to normal sinus rhythm. (Defibrillators are also used electively to convert other abnormal cardiac rhythms.)

OBJECTIVE
Terminate ventricular fibrillation or ventricular tachycardia.

EQUIPMENT
DC defibrillator with paddles
Conduction jelly (electrode gel) or special pads which have been
    impregnated with gel
Resuscitative equipment

Note: The technique of defibrillation is performed by the medical staff. Nurses working in special units, e.g. CCU or ITU, are trained to use a defibrillator and are allowed to do so.

PROCEDURE

Nursing action	Rationale
1. Expose the patient's anterior chest.	This procedure should be carried out immediately after ventricular fibrillation is detected to minimize cerebral and circulatory deterioration.
2. Start cardiopulmonary resuscitation immediately.	Cardiopulmonary resuscitation is essential before and after defibrillation to assure blood supply to the cerebral and coronary arteries.

Table 5.1   Major drugs commonly used in cardiopulmonary resuscitation

Drugs and dosages	Major effects	Indications
Adrenaline: 0.5–1.0ml of 1:1000 solution (0.5–1.0mg) administered intravenously or intracardially; repeat every 5 minutes if needed	Positive inotropic, positive chronotropic and pressor effects; makes fine fibrillation coarse and thereby facilitates defibrillation	1. Ventricular asystole 2. Ventricular fibrillation (fine)
Isoprenaline: 2mg in 500ml dextrose 5 per cent at 2–4μg/min (i.e. 0.5–1.0ml/min)	Positive inotropic and positive chronotropic effects; causes vasodilation rather than vasoconstriction	1. Ventricular asystole 2. Speeds up a slow AV block
Calcium chloride: 5–10ml (0.5–1.0g) of 10 per cent solution administered slowly, intravenously, over a period of 5 minutes or Calcium gluconate: 10–20ml of 10 per cent solution (1–2g), administered slowly, intravenously	Positive inotropic and chronotropic effects; use with caution in patients receiving digoxin	1. Electromechanical dissociation 2. Ventricular asystole 3. Ventricular fibrillation (fine)
Atropine: 0.5mg administered every 5 minutes, to a total of 2mg, intravenously	Decreases vagal tone	Slow cardiac rate with supraventricular rhythm, if accompanied by hypotension or ventricular escape beats
Sodium bicarbonate: 1mEq/kg of body weight within 2 minutes of cardiac arrest; repeat every 10 minutes in the absence of functional circulation	Combats acidosis produced by inadequate tissue perfusion; too much bicarbonate can lead to plasma alkalosis and hyperosmolality with cerebral acidosis	Absent functional circulation
Lignocaine: 1–2mg per kg body weight in bolus doses administered intravenously; 4g in 1,000ml (4:1 drip) at continuous intravenous drip at 2–4mg/minute for maintenance	Raises fibrillation threshold and increases the electrical stimulation threshold of the ventricle during diastole	1. Ventricular fibrillation resistant to direct current defibrillation or successful defibrillation reverting repeatedly to fibrillation 2. Control of multifocal ventricular ectopic beats and episodes of ventricular tachycardia
Procainamide HCl: 50–100mg/minute administered intravenously, reaching a maximum of 1g in 15 minutes	Raises fibrillation threshold; slows conduction, and decreases excitability of the ventricles	Same as for lignocaine

Adapted from Vijay, N.K. and Schoonmaker, F.W. (1975). Major drugs commonly used in cardiopulmonary resuscitation, *American Family Physician*.

3. A second person should turn on the defibrillator to the prescribed setting.

The shock is measured in Watt seconds or joules – from 50 to 400.

4. Apply electrode paste/pads liberally to the paddle electrodes.

The electrode paste/pads helps to provide better contact and prevents skin burns. Do not allow any paste on the skin between electrodes. If the paste areas touch, the current may short circuit, severely burning the patient, and may not penetrate the heart.

5. Apply one electrode just to the right of the upper sternum below the clavicle and the other electrode just to the left of the cardiac apex or left nipple (Figure 5.10).

If anteroposterior paddles are used, the anterior paddle is held with pressure on the middle sternum while the patient lies on the posterior paddle under the left infrascapular region. With this method the defibrillation more directly traverses the heart.

6. Grasp the paddles only by the insulated handles.

7. GIVE THE COMMAND TO STAND CLEAR OF THE PATIENT AND THE BED.

If a person touches the bed, he may act as a ground for the current and receive a shock.

8. Push the discharge buttons in both paddles simultaneously.

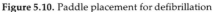

Figure 5.10. Paddle placement for defibrillation

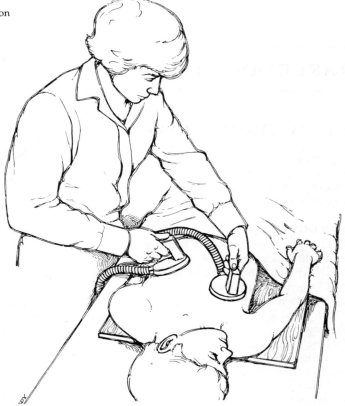

9. Remove the paddles from the patient *immediately* after the shock is administered.

10. Resume cardiopulmonary resuscitation efforts until stable rhythm, spontaneous respirations, pulse and blood pressure return.

After discharge of the defibrillation, cardiopulmonary resuscitation efforts should be resumed, total delay should be no more than five seconds in order to oxygenate the patient and restore circulation.

11. Look at the ECG monitor to determine the specific therapy for the resultant electrical mechanism. Further high-energy countershocks may be necessary.

Follow-up phase

Nursing action

Rationale

1. After the patient is defibrillated and rhythm is restored, lignocaine may be given for recurrent episodes, and sodium bicarbonate *may* be administered to treat metabolic acidosis.

Any resultant dysrhythmia may require appropriate drug intervention. Metabolic acidosis is due to accumulation of acidic products in blood because of cessation of respiration.

2. Continue with intensive monitoring/care.

HEART DISORDERS

CARDIAC DYSRHYTHMIAS

Dysrhythmia is a clinical disorder to the heart beat; it may include a disturbance of rate, rhythm (sequence) or both. Dysrhythmias are derangements of heart function and not of heart structure.

AETIOLOGY
1. Dysrhythmias due to organic heart disease:
   a. Inflammatory heart disease.
   b. Degenerative heart disease (atherosclerosis).
   c. Congenital heart disease.
   d. Hypertensive heart disease.
2. Dysrhythmias due to disturbances of other organ systems:
   a. Disease of central nervous system – from sympathetic and vagal stimulation.
   b. Pulmonary disease.
   c. Endocrine disorders (hyperthyroidism and hypothyroidism, hypoglycaemia, diabetic ketoacidosis).
   d. Gastrointestinal disorders (fluid and electrolyte imbalance).
   e. Renal disorders (renal failure).
3. Dysrhythmias from other causes:
   a. Drugs (digitalis intoxication, quinidine, procainamide).
   b. Infection.
   c. Disturbances of electrolyte balance.
   d. Anaemia.
   e. Following cardiac surgery.
   f. Hypoxia.

CLASSIFICATION OF DYSRHYTHMIAS BASED ON DISTURBED PHYSIOLOGY
1. Disturbance of impulse formation – heartbeat activated for one or more beats by a pacemaker other than the sinus node.
2. Disturbances of conduction – due to delayed transmission of impulse, the failure of some impulses to be conducted or to a block at the affected site.
3. Combined disorders – combination of abnormally rapid impulse formation and decreased ability to conduct the impulses.

CLINICAL FEATURES

Depends on ventricular rate, condition of heart and patient's psychological reaction.

1. Symptoms and signs of rapid dysrhythmias:
   a. Palpitation.
   b. Dizziness and fainting.
   c. Throbbing in head and neck.
   d. Shortness of breath.
   e. Precordial discomfort and pain.
   f. Anxiety.
2. Symptoms and signs of slow heart action (brady-dysrhythmia/bradycardia)
   a. Shortness of breath.
   b. Fatigue on exertion.
   c. Dizziness and fainting – may indicate syncopal attacks, leading to convulsive seizures.

CLINICAL EFFECTS

1. Some dysrhythmias are relatively harmless while others are forerunners of cardiac arrest.
2. Cardiac dysrhythmias can reduce cardiac output, lower the blood pressure and decrease blood perfusion of the brain, heart, kidneys, gastro-intestinal tract, muscles and skin.
3. Cardiac dysrhythmias often produce attacks of transient cerebral ischaemia or complete stroke.
4. Dysrhythmias can precipitate heart failure or angina pectoris in certain patients.
5. Bradydysrhythmias/bradycardia (rate below 60) predispose to electrical instability of the heart.
6. A marked degree of disability may accompany a dysrhythmia.

NURSING ASSESSMENT

1. How does the patient describe his symptoms?
2. What is the duration and frequency of the dysrhythmia? Any previous occurrence?
3. Evaluate the patient's general appearance: pallor, cyanosis, sweating – may indicate peripheral arteriolar constriction.
4. Observe carotid pulsation: Rapid and vigorous? Irregular with varying amplitude?
5. Listen to the heartbeat with a stethoscope.
   a. Listen for rate, presence of irregularity, increase in intensity of first heart sound.
      (i) 30 beats or lower – complete AV block, partial AV block or sinus bradycardia.
      (ii) 40–60 beats/min – varying degrees of AV block, sinus bradycardia.
      (iii) 60–110 beats/min – sinus arrhythmia, ectopic beats, AV heart block, atrial fibrillation, atrial flutter, atrial tachycardia with block.
      (iv) 140–180 beats/min – atrial tachycardia, atrial flutter, junctional or ventricular tachycardia.

   Note: see section 2 for basics of electrophysiology to explain electrophysiological terms.

   b. If possible have an ECG taken during an episode of dysrhythmia.
   c. Take the blood pressure and pulse – distal pulses give clue to heart's ability to perfuse the periphery.
6. Take respiratory rate: note depth and effort.
7. Evaluate for:
   a. Mental confusion with dysrhythmia – indicates cerebral ischaemia.
   b. Presence of signs and symptoms of congestive heart failure – may indicate dysrhythmia causing serious effect.
   c. Chest pains with dysrhythmia – due to myocardial ischaemia.
   d. Weakness.
8. Use portable cardiac monitoring for persons with suspected dysrhythmias (patients with dizzy spells, palpitations, chest pain) and to evaluate antidysrhythmic therapy.
   a. One lead sensor is taped to patient's chest and connected to portable recording equipment. Recorder is started.
   b. Patient goes about his daily routine while keeping a diary of times and activities during which he feels his symptoms.
   c. After eight to 24 hours the tape is put through a scanner for oscilloscope reading (computer scanning now available).
9. See p. 240 and p. 307 for a complete discussion of the most common dysrhythmias and their treatment.
10. See section for clinical effect on blood pressure (p. 354).

NURSING MANAGEMENT

1. Offer calm explanations and convey optimism – patients with dysrhythmias are likely to be anxious, and anxiety tends to aggravate symptoms; fear and anxiety can outweigh all other factors.
2. The treatment of dysrhythmias includes pharmacological, electrical (pacing; cardioversion) and surgical (excision of the 'foci', etc) therapy. See p. 240 and p. 307 for a complete discussion of the most common dysrhythmias, their ECG interpretations and treatment.

PATIENT EDUCATION
Involve family in the teaching as follows:
1. Take prescribed medication on schedule.
2. Stop smoking.
3. Modification of the diet may be indicated; in general, avoid caffeine (coffee, cola, cocoa, chocolate, tea) and pain medications that contain caffeine or stimulants.

CARDIAC PACING

A cardiac pacemaker is an electronic device that delivers direct stimulation to the heart, causing electrical depolarization and cardiac contraction. The pacemaker initiates and maintains the heart rate when the natural pacemakers of the heart are unable to do so.

Cardiac pacing is accomplished through stimulation of either the atrium, the ventricle or both.

Cardiac pacing can be internal or external.
1. Internal – electrical stimulation of endocardium or epicardium.
2. External – external electrical stimulation through electrodes applied to chest wall or the oesophageal wall (transoesophageal pacing). Requires large amount of electrical current to cause significant muscle contraction. Rarely used because of complications of pain and skin burns.

UNDERLYING PRINCIPLES
Pacemakers consist of two component parts:
1. *Pulse generator*, which contains the circuitry and batteries that generate the electrical signal; the battery cells are usually lithium cell units with a projected life of eight to 12 years, or less frequently, mercury–zinc batteries with a projected life of two to five years and isotopic (nuclear) batteries with a projected life of 20 years.

    For temporary pacing, the pulse generator is outside the body (Figure 5.11). For permanent pacing it is implanted within the body (Figure 5.12).
2. *Pacemaker electrodes*, which transmit the pacemaker impulses to the heart. The stimuli from the pacemaker travel through a flexible catheter electrode (lead or wire) that is threaded through a vein into the right ventricle (endocardial approach), or introduced by direct penetration of the chest wall (requires thoracotomy or upper abdominal surgical approach – epicardial approach).
    a. Pacemaker electrode may be unipolar or bipolar: *unipolar* catheter has one electrode in

contact with heart; *bipolar* has two electrodes i contact with heart. Bipolar may be converte to unipolar. Unipolar catheters sense intrinsi cardiac signals better and produce a large pacer spike on an ECG recording.

CLINICAL INDICATIONS
1. Symptomatic bradydysrhythmias (slow hear rates):
    a. Sinoatrial bradydysrhythmias.
    b. Sinoatrial arrest.
    c. Sick sinus syndrome.
2. Heart block:
    a. Mobitz I – second-degree AV block (Wenc kebach phenomenon); rate variable, usually 6 to 100 beats per minute;
    b. Mobitz II – second-degree AV block; rat usually 30 to 55 per minute;
    c. Complete heart block.
3. Prophylaxis:
    a. Following acute myocardial infarction dys rhythmia and conduction defects;
    b. Before or following cardiac surgery;
    c. During coronary arteriography;
    d. Before permanent pacing.
4. Tachydysrhythmias (fast heart rates) to brea rapid rhythm disturbances:
    a. Supraventricular;
    b. Ventricular.

PACING MODES
1. Demand (synchronous, noncompetitive) atria ventricular.

    Most commonly used; has the advantage o working only when the heart rate goes below certain level. Therefore, it does not compete wit the heart's basic rhythm. If the patient's heart rat falls below a predetermined level (programmec into pulse generator), an electrical stimulus i delivered to the heart.
2. Fixed rate (asynchronous, competitive) atria ventricular.

    This unit delivers an electrical stimulus at present constant rate that is independent o the patient's own rhythm. However, it car compete with the patient's own rhythm. Usec infrequently, usually in patients with complete and unvarying heart block. Does not allow atria contribution to cardiac output.
3. Synchronous atrial/ventricular.

    A demand form of pacing, which is able tc increase heart rate to accompany the physio logical demands of the body. An atrial electrode senses the patient's atrial depolarization, wait

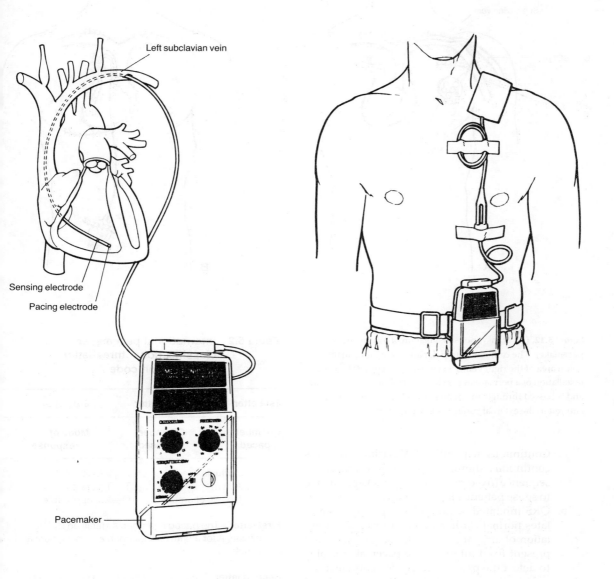

Left subclavian vein

Sensing electrode

Pacing electrode

Pacemaker

Figure 5.11. Temporary pacemaker: the transvenous catheter electrode is attached to a battery-powered external pacemaker. The catheter is wedged in the apex of the right ventricle

for a preset interval and triggers firing of ventricular pacer. If rapid atrial rhythm occurs, the ventricular pacemaker stimulates the ventricle at a fixed rate independent of atrial activity.

4. Bifocal atrioventricular sequential.

Mode of choice for pacing patients with borderline cardiac function and selected dysrhythmias. Offers stimulation of both atria and ventricles.

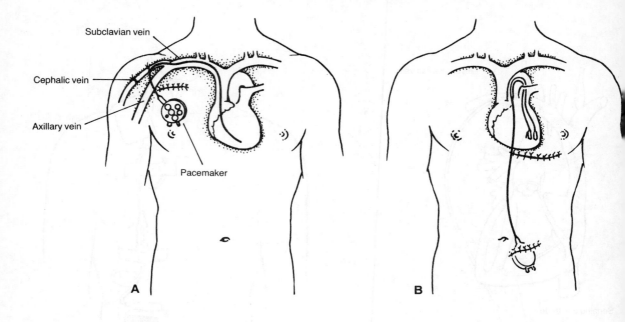

Figure 5.12. (A) Transvenous installation of a permanent pacemaker. The catheter is unipolar and is threaded to the apical area of the right ventricle via a major vein. (B) Epicardial installation of a permanent pacemaker. The catheter is bipolar and is passed through an opening in the chest wall and is sutured to the external surface of the left ventricle

a. Continuous sequential A-V pacing – delivers continuous stimuli to atria and ventricles in sequence (fixed rate). The pacemaker is unable to sense patient's intrinsic rhythm.

b. QRS inhibited sequence A-V pacing – simulates normal cardiac function through stimulation of atria and ventricles sequentially at a present fixed interval. The pacemaker is able to detect the patient's intrinsic ventricular depolarization and will shut off both atrial and ventricular pacing stimuli. (**Note:** QRS is the terminology used to describe the electrical changes in the cardiac cycle.)

5. New developments.

   Programmable pacemaker allows non-invasive adjustment (programming) of implanted pacemaker.

See Table 5.2 for the International Pacemaker Classification – three-letter identification code.

Table 5.2   International pacemaker classification – three-letter identification code

1st Letter	2nd Letter	3rd Letter
Chamber paced	**Chamber sensed**	**Mode of response**
V – Ventricle A – Atrium D – Double chamber		I – Inhibited T – Triggered O – Not applicable

First letter – The paced chamber is identified by V for ventricle, A for atrium or D for double – both atrium and ventricle

Second letter – The sensed chamber of either is again V for ventricle, A for atrium

Third letter – The mode of response, if any, is either:
I for inhibited, a pacemaker whose output is blocked by a sensed signal, or
T for triggered, a unit whose output is discharged by a sensed signal.
O indicates a specific comment is not applicable.

(Parsonnet, V., Furman, S. and Smyth, N.P.D. (1974) Implantable cardiac pacemakers status report and resource guidelines, *Circulation*, Vol. 50, No. 4, p. A21. Used by permission of the American Heart Association.)

APPROACHES TO PACEMAKER IMPLANTATION

1. *Temporary transvenous pacing* – insertion of catheter electrode threaded through a vein into the apex of the right ventricle under the guidance of an image intensifier; the distal electrode is connected to a negative terminal of a battery-powered external pacemaker (see Figure 5.11).
   a. The catheter electrode is secured in the vein with suture.
   b. Antibiotic ointment is applied around the incision and catheter.
   c. Catheter electrode position confirmed by X-ray.
   d. Patient placed in cardiac care unit for monitoring.
      (i) Temporary pacing may be done for hours, days or weeks; it is continued until patient improves or a permanent pacemaker is implanted.
      (ii) Improves cardiac output and coronary, cerebral and renal blood flow.
      (iii) Controls ventricular tachycardia and fibrillation.
      (iv) Allows complete control of heart rate during surgery.
      (v) Permits observation of effects of pacing on heart function so that optimum pacing rate for the patient can be selected before permanent pacemaker is implanted.

2. *Permanent pacemakers:*
   a. *Transvenous* – electrodes (unipolar or bipolar) are threaded through cephalic or external jugular vein and into the right ventricle. The peripheral end of the electrode is connected to the pulse generator which is implanted underneath the skin below the right or left pectoral region or below the clavicle (Fig. 5.12A).
      Advantages:
      (i) Performed under local anaesthesia.
      (ii) Thoracotomy unnecessary.
   b. *Epicardial* – electrodes are applied directly to the myocardium and the pulse generator is usually placed underneath the skin of the subcostal area (Fig. 5.12B).
      Advantages:
      (i) Offers electrode stability.
      (ii) Greater selection of pacing modes.
      (iii) Method of choice for children to allow for vertical growth.

Assessment
PATIENT PROBLEMS

1. Potential for injury related to pacemaker malfunction and from the presence of the pacemaker within the body.
2. Potential for infection related to foreign body implantation.
3. Anxiety related to pacemaker insertion and hospitalization.
4. Fear of death related to pacemaker failure.
5. Body image disturbances (potential) related to pacemaker implant.
6. Powerlessness related to perceived dependence on pacemaker.

Planning and implementation
NURSING INTERVENTIONS
Maintaining optimal cardiac rhythm

1. Observe for complications of pacemaker malfunction – failure in one or more components of the pacing system; battery exhaustion; wire (electrode) fractures; failure to capture and/or sense properly.
   a. Monitor ECG following implantation (high risk if electrode is displaced soon after insertion).
   b. Take pulse regularly for one full minute to assess rate and rhythm.
   c. Assess for dizziness, light-headedness, chest pain, shortness of breath (may indicate pacemaker malfunction).
2. Record the following information after insertion of pacemaker:
   a. Note the data about the model, date of insertion, location of pulse generator, stimulation threshold and pacemaker rate on the patient's record. Report and record changes in these parameters.
   b. Place a card at the head of the bed indicating that the patient has a pacemaker.
3. Assist the patient in and out of bed when ambulatory – a fall can dislodge an electrode. (There is a high incidence of associated disease in elderly patients; the mean age of these patients is 70 years – have associated arteriosclerotic heart disease and heart failure, hypertension and diabetes.)
4. Observe for complications related to presence of pacemaker in body: dysrhythmias – ventricular ectopic activity – from irritation of the ventricular wall by the electrode. Pacemakers can create baffling dysrhythmias. Complications from electrode malposition or perforation; high ventricular threshold may cause abrupt loss of pacing.
   a. Maintain intravenous infusion to have an accessible vein in the event of dysrhythmia.
   b. Make sure all equipment is grounded with three-pronged plugs inserted into a proper

outlet – improperly grounded equipment can generate currents capable of producing ventricular fibrillation.

Note: A clinical engineer, electrician or other qualified person should make certain that the patient is in an electrically safe environment.

c. Avoid using electrocautery, electrocoagulating equipment and electric razors – external interference may suppress output of temporary pacemaker. Check to see that no metal parts are exposed and electrode insulation is intact – to prevent accidental ventricular fibrillation from stray electrical currents.
d. Monitor blood pressure and haemodynamic status.
e. Question the patient about symptoms experienced.
f. Observe for hiccoughs – may be caused by chest/diaphragmatic stimulation.
g. Implement passive range of motion to side of pacemaker implant to avoid pain and stiffness of muscles and joints.

Avoidance of infection
1. Observe wound for infection – local infection (sepsis or haematoma formation) – occurs at the site of venous cutdown or subcutaneous pacemaker placement.
   a. Inspect the incision site under the pressure dressings for bleeding and haematoma – haematoma appears to be a contributing factor to wound infection.
   b. Observe the vein through which the pacing catheter has been placed for evidence of phlebitis.
2. Utilize sterile technique for dressing changes.
3. Take temperature regularly (note elevations – 38.5°C).
4. Observe for signs/symptoms of bacteraemia (see Endocarditis, Clinical Features, pp. 271–272).

Reduction in anxiety
1. Assess anxiety level of patient preoperatively and postoperatively: *mild* – increased alertness; *moderate* – decreased ability to communicate; *severe* – drastic decrease in ability to communicate; and *panic* – inability to communicate, distortion of reality. Learning cannot take place in severe or panic level of anxiety.
2. Offer careful explanations regarding anticipated procedures and treatments and answer the patient's questions with concise explanations.

Repeat as necessary. Information is geared to level of patient. (Patients have difficulty processing input – give thought to timing and amount of information.)
a. Preoperatively – reinforce explanation of procedure to the patient and family. Explain that the patient will be awake (for transvenous pacing), will lie on a hard table 20 to 30 minutes, but discomfort will be minimal.
b. Postoperatively – explain to the patient the nature and purpose of monitoring equipment (ECG). Monitoring will be continuous for several days, but the patient will be able to walk around in room and use bedside commode while being monitored.
   Explain to the patient that analgesics will be administered for pain at implantation site.
3. Explore with patient (preoperatively and postoperatively) those factors that evoke feelings of anxiety. Converse with the patient frequently and convey willingness to listen.
4. Encourage the patient to utilize coping mechanisms to overcome anxieties – talking, crying, walking.
5. Offer measures to ensure patient comfort – prescribed analgesics, backrubs.
6. Discuss with the patient the plan of care, allowing the patient to make decisions where appropriate.
7. Encourage family members to offer support and understanding to the patient through a willingness to listen to the patient's concerns.

Perceptions as to cause of fears
1. Encourage patient expression regarding pacemaker implantation – 'What do you think about receiving and living with a pacemaker?'
2. Listen and encourage the patient's attempt to discuss fears.
3. Assess for unwarranted fears expressed by the patient (commonly, pacemaker failure) and provide explanations to alleviate fear. Explain to the patient life expectancy of batteries and the measures taken to check for failure (see Patient Education).
4. Talk to family members about their fears and offer explanations to help allay the fears (avoids the transmission of unwarranted fears to the patient).

Maintaining a positive body image
1. Assess for verbal and nonverbal cues (inability to look at insertion site) indicative of nonacceptance of pacemaker.
2. Encourage the patient to express concerns regarding self-image and pacer implant.

3. Reassure the patient that sexual activity and modes of dressing will not be altered by pacemaker implantation.
4. Offer the patient the opportunity to talk to others who have had a pacemaker implantation.
5. Encourage spouse of patient or significant other to discuss concerns of self-image with the patient.

Resumption of previous roles and activities prior to pacemaker implantation with minimal limitations

1. Explore with the patient his feelings toward limitations secondary to illness.
   a. Discuss with the patient current lifestyle prior to need for pacemaker.
   b. Discuss with the patient areas of independence and dependence in his life.
   c. Discuss with the patient the importance of learning how to live with a pacemaker.
   d. Encourage family members to offer support and express to the patient their willingness to help.
2. Encourage the patient's readiness to learn.
   a. Assess the patient's readiness to learn about his pacemaker.
   b. Offer literature to the patient to review as desired (e.g. British Heart Foundation booklets).
3. Encourage the patient to accept responsibility for care.
   a. Review plan of care with the patient.
   b. Encourage the patient to make decisions regarding a daily schedule of self-care activities.
   c. Engage the patient in goal-setting – establish with the patient priorities of care, time frames to accomplish goals up until discharge.
4. See Patient Education, below.

PATIENT EDUCATION
General principles
1. Patient teaching should be individualized, provide for active participation by patient and, if possible, include at least one significant other of patient.
2. To evaluate the patient's retention of material, the patient should be asked to repeat in his own words the concepts discussed and return a demonstration of the skills presented.

Anatomy and physiology of the heart
Use diagrams to identify heart structure, conduction system and area where pacemaker is inserted.

Introduction to pacemaker
1. Give the patient the manufacturer's instructions (for his particular pacemaker) and help him to become familiar with his pacemaker.
2. If available, give the patient a pacemaker to hold and identify unique features of patient's pacemaker.
3. Reassure the patient so that he will develop confidence in his pacemaker and new lifestyle.
   a. Physical activity does not usually have to be curtailed because of an implanted pacemaker.
   b. Sexual activity may be resumed when desired.
   c. Caution the patient not to manipulate pulse generator by twisting or retracting electrode catheter ('twiddler's syndrome').

Pacemaker failure
1. Teach the patient to check his own pulse rate daily for one full minute at rest to be certain that preset rate remains constant.
2. Teach the patient to evaluate daily pulse rate by comparing it with a normal pulse range.
   a. To identify normal pulse range, tell the patient to record pulse rate every day for one month after returning to normal living pattern.
   b. Tell the patient to use the one-month record of pulse to evaluate his daily pulse rates.
3. Teach the patient to:
   a. Report *immediately* any sudden slowing of pulse greater than four to five beats per minute, or any increase in pulse rate.
   b. Report signs and symptoms of dizziness, fainting, palpitation, prolonged hiccoughs and chest pain to doctor immediately – indicative of pacemaker failure.
   c. Take pulse while these feelings are being experienced.
4. Encourage the patient to wear identification bracelet and carry pacemaker identification card that lists his pacemaker type, rate, doctor's name and the hospital where the pacemaker was inserted.

Electromagnetic interference
1. Advise the patient that improvements in pacemaker design have reduced problems of electromagnetic interference (EMI). Give general instructions to the patient unless specific instructions are included with pacemaker.
   a. Sources of electromagnetic interference that still affect a number of pulse generators include high-energy radar, television and radio transmitters, industrial arc welders, certain

electrocautery machines used in hospitals, airport screening devices (metal triggers alarm), anti-theft devices found in jewellery and department stores, microwave oven.

b. Teach the patient that if dizziness occurs, he should move 1.5 to 3.0m away from source (0.9m from microwave) and check pulse. Pulse should return to normal. Patient should explain to appropriate individual that he has a pacemaker.

c. Advise the patient to sit in the back of airplanes away from the kitchens (microwaves present).

d. Advise the patient to inform his dentist that he has a pacemaker.

Care of pacemaker site

1. Advise patient to wear loose-fitting clothing around the area of pacemaker implantation until healing has taken place.
2. Watch for signs and symptoms of infection around generator and leads – fever, heat, pain, skin breakdown at implant site.
3. Advise patient to keep incision clean and dry. Avoid showers until healing has taken place (bath may be taken).

Follow-up

1. See that the patient has a copy of his ECG tracing (according to hospital policy) – for future comparisons. Encourage patient to have regular pacemaker check-up (preferably at a pacemaker clinic) for monitoring function and integrity of his pacemaker.
2. Transtelephonic evaluation of implanted cardiac pacemakers for battery and electrode failure is available.
3. Review medications with the patient prior to discharge.
4. Inform the patient that the pulse generator will have to be removed surgically for a variety of reasons (battery failure) and replaced; improved power sources and circuitry make reoperation less frequent.
   a. Relatively simple procedure performed under local anaesthesia.
   b. Incision made; old generator disconnected from electrode catheter.
   c. New generator connected and placed in existing subcutaneous pocket; incision closed.
   d. Prophylactic antibiotics usually administered.
   e. Patient discharged from hospital one to three days postoperatively.

Evaluation

EXPECTED OUTCOMES

1. Maintains an optimal cardiac output; does not demonstrate signs and symptoms of pacemaker malfunction.
2. Remains free of infection – exhibits no signs/symptoms of septicaemia or phlebitis; temperature normal; incision free of redness.
3. Achieves a reduction in anxiety – identifies sources of anxiety and communicates ability to cope with anxiety.
4. Recognizes factors causing fears – identifies fears related to pacemaker implant, utilizes family members for support, communicates ability to cope with fears.
5. Resumes previous roles and activities (prior to pacemaker insertion) – demonstrates independence with daily self-care activities, asks for assistance when appropriate.
6. Maintains a positive body image – expresses feelings of well-being.

ARTERIOSCLEROSIS AND ATHEROSCLEROSIS

Arteriosclerosis is an arterial disease manifested by a loss of elasticity and a hardening of the vessel wall.

Atherosclerosis is the most common type of arteriosclerosis, manifested by the formation of atheroma (patchy lipoidal degeneration of the intima).

The volume of blood that can flow through the artery is reduced. Atherosclerosis usually develops in high-flow, high-pressure arteries such as those in the heart, brain, kidneys and aorta, especially at bifurcation points (where vessels divide into two branches).

Atherosclerosis causes 90 per cent of all ischaemic heart disease (IHD). IHD is a collective term for disturbances of blood flow within the coronary arteries giving rise to altered perfusion of the heart muscle (myocardium) and disruption of the normal electrical cycle controlling heart rhythm.

IHD develops in three stages:

1. Childhood – fatty streaks appear in the arterial wall.
2. Fibrous plaques develop, reflecting a low-grade inflammatory reaction and a healing response.
3. Complications develop – necrosis, calcification and vascularization with or without haemorrhage into the plaque. These changes predispose to thrombosis.

IHD presents in a number of forms, the main groups of which are:
1. Angina pectoris.
2. Myocardial infarction (MI).
3. Sudden death.

SIGNIFICANCE
1. Arteriosclerosis is the chief cause of death in the UK.
2. One of the major clinical features of atherosclerosis is ischaemic heart disease (IHD).
3. Studies indicate that atherosclerotic heart disease is partially preventable if attention is paid to 'risk' factors.

AETIOLOGY
There is much debate and controversy about the causation of atheroma, ischaemic heart disease and related disorders. However, there is some general agreement that the cause is multifactorial – genetic factors interacting with biological, environmental, social and occupational factors and lifestyle. Although the term 'risk' factor is commonly used, in itself the term is controversial as the assumption is made that such factors may be modified or preventable. However, the majority of risk factors are genetic and nonmodifiable.

COMMON RISK FACTORS
1. Age.
2. Sex – death rate greater in males than in females.
3. Impaired glucose tolerance (diabetes mellitus).
4. Hypertension.
5. A relatively large amount of cholesterol in the low-density lipoprotein fraction (serum).
6. Obesity.
7. Cigarette smoking.
8. Physical inactivity – since substantial collateral circulation is not established.
9. Emotional tension.
10. High salt intake.
11. Soft water.

ALTERED PHYSIOLOGY
1. Arteriosclerosis → narrowing of arterial vessels → malnutrition of tissue cells → ischaemic necrosis → fibrosis → sclerosis.
2. Sclerosis → degeneration of major organs because of lack of blood supply (nutrition): brain, myocardium, kidney.
3. Fatty streaks develop in the subintimal region.
4. Fibrous plaques of cholesterol, fatty acids and often calcium form an intima of arterial vessels (atherosclerosis).

5. Dislodging of plaque may occur, or a thrombus may be formed near the plaque; subsequent embolus may cause arterial occlusion and infarction in distant body sites.
6. After menopause, women are no longer protected by oestrogen.

GENERAL PATIENT ASSESSMENT
1. Arteriosclerosis is a generalized vascular disease; however, it varies from patient to patient in that it may affect one area more than another.
2. Often, it limits itself to a segment of the vascular tree.
3. Five areas that are the most dangerous and cause disturbing symptoms are:
   a. Brain – cerebroarteriosclerosis.
   b. Heart – ischaemic artery disease.
   c. Gastrointestinal tract.
   d. Kidneys.
   e. Extremities.
4. Prognosis depends on extent of pathology and area of involvement.

TREATMENT
1. Since arteriosclerosis and atherosclerosis affect many different parts of the body, treatment is described where the major condition occurs. For example, angina pectoris and myocardial infarction are brought about by atherosclerosis of coronary arteries; treatment is discussed under the disease entity.
2. Operative reconstruction of involved vessels.

PATIENT EDUCATION
Attention is directed to reducing risk factors by avoiding tension, reducing excess weight, giving up cigarette smoking, controlling diabetes and adjusting diet to reduce cholesterol intake (Table 5.3).

ANGINA PECTORIS

Angina pectoris is a clinical symptom characterized by paroxysms of pain or oppression in the anterior chest produced as a result of insufficient coronary blood flow and/or coronary myocardial hypoxia.

ALTERED PHYSIOLOGY
Atherosclerosis of major vessels → critical obstruction with diminution of coronary blood flow → decreased myocardial oxygen delivery in response to myocardial oxygen demand → anginal pain. Disparity between myocardial oxygen supply and demand.

Table 5.3   Fat- and cholesterol-controlled diet. (A variety of foods may be selected from each of the basic four food groups. Emphasize those foods listed in the 'suggested' column.)

Meat, poultry, fish, dried beans and peas, eggs

Suggested	Avoid or use infrequently
For 100mg cholesterol diet, limit flesh foods to 85g daily. For 200mg cholesterol diet, limit flesh foods to 170–226g daily Most often: chicken, turkey, veal, fish, shellfish (except shrimp) A few times a week: very lean beef, lamb, pork, ham if all visible meat fat is discarded *Dried peas, beans, lentils – prepared with allowed ingredients *Peanut butter (count as a fat choice) *Egg whites as desired *Egg substitute	Duck, goose, shrimp Fatty meats (e.g. spare ribs, frankfurters, sausage, bacon and lunch meats, hamburger, canned corn beef) Egg yolks, whole eggs

Vegetables and fruit – at least four servings daily, including sources of vitamins C and A

Suggested	Avoid or use infrequently
All types of fruits and vegetables may be used (unless prepared with restricted ingredients): fresh, frozen, canned, dried	Vegetables in butter, cream or cheese sauce Vegetables fried in saturated fat

Bread and cereals (wholegrain, enriched or fortified) – at least four servings daily

Suggested	Avoid or use infrequently
*Breads: whole wheat, rye, oatmeal, white enriched, French, Italian, raisin, English muffins, hard rolls *Cereal (hot or cold), rice, barley *Pasta: spaghetti, macaroni Biscuits, muffins and so forth, made at home using allowed ingredients, in moderation (a source of fat)	Commercial biscuits, muffins, doughnuts, butter rolls, sweet rolls Crackers Commercial mixes containing dried eggs, whole milk and/or fat

Milk products – adults should use 500ml or the equivalent daily

Suggested	Avoid or use infrequently
Skim milk dairy products: fortified skim (nonfat) milk or milk powder, buttermilk, evaporated skim milk, chocolate-flavoured skim milk, yogurt made with skim milk Cheeses made from skim milk: cottage cheese Cheese substitutes made with corn oil, in moderation	Whole milk and whole milk products: chocolate milk, canned evaporated whole milk, ice cream, cream of any type, whole milk yogurt Most nondairy cream substitutes Cheeses made from cream or whole milk

Fats and oils (polyunsaturated) – limit total amount used, including that used in cooking, so that fat content of diet does not exceed prescribed amount (e.g. 20 or 30 per cent of calories)

Suggested	Avoid or use infrequently
*Polyunsaturated vegetable oils: corn oil, sesame seed oil, soya bean oil, sunflower seed oil, walnut oil	Solid fats and shortenings: butter, hard margarine and vegetable shortening with a low P/S ratio (i.e. 3:2 or lower),

*Margarines and liquid oil shortenings made with an allowed oil and having a high P/S ratio (i.e. about 2:1 or above)	lard, salt pork, meat fat, coconut oil, palm oil
Salad dressings made with allowed ingredients, mayonnaise (omitted on 100mg cholesterol diet)	(Peanut oil and olive oil are not saturated or polyunsaturated. They may be used occasionally for flavour)
Soups and sauces: clear fat-free broth, fat-free vegetable soup	Creamy and cheese salad dressings Cream soup

Desserts, beverages, snacks, condiments

Acceptable if calories allow	*Avoid or use infrequently*
*Cocoa powder, fruit whip, gelatin, puddings made with nonfat milk, water ice	Chocolate, whole milk puddings, ice cream (ice milk is sometimes allowed)
*Jelly, jam, marmalade, honey, most types of nuts	Chocolate, caramels, butterscotch
Homemade baked desserts using allowed ingredients	Coconut, cashews
*Carbonated beverages, fruit drinks, wine, beer, whisky	Commercial cakes, pies, biscuits and mixes
	Potato chips and other commercial fried snacks

Negligible calorie content

*Tea, herb tea, coffee, decaffeinated coffee
Herbs, spices, vinegar, mustard, small amounts of ketchup, horseradish, meat sauce, soy sauce

* Free of cholesterol
(Suitor, C.W. and Hunter, M.F. (1984) *Nutrition: Principles and Application in Health Promotion* (2nd ed.) J.B. Lippincott, Philadelphia, pp. 608–9).

AETIOLOGY
1. Usually due to atherosclerotic heart disease – is almost invariably associated with a significant obstruction of a major coronary artery.
2. May be from various other conditions such as severe aortic stenosis or insufficiency, aortitis, hyperthyroidism, anaemia, tachycardia.
3. Coronary artery spasm.

CLINICAL FEATURES
Pain – probably caused by metabolic changes produced by ischaemia.
1. *Location* – behind middle or upper third of sternum (retrosternal) felt deep in chest. Patient may make a fist over site of pain.
2. *Radiation* – usually radiates to neck, jaw, shoulders and upper extremities (on left side more often than on right).
   a. Frequently may be localized.
   b. Patient often experiences tightness, choking or a strangling sensation.
3. *Character* – constrictive, oppressive, strangling, vice-like, insistent.
   a. May be mild to severe.
   b. May produce numbness or weakness in arms, wrist, hands.

c. Accompanied by severe apprehension and feeling of impending death.
4. *Duration* – attack usually lasts less than three minutes.
   Attacks occurring when patient is at rest – persist five to 15 minutes.

NURSING ALERT
Suspect an impending myocardial infarction if anginal pain lasts more than 20 to 30 minutes.

5. *Factors precipitating pain:*
   a. Exertion.
   b. Exposure to cold.
   c. Eating a heavy meal.
   d. Emotion and excitement. In this case, the pain may be delayed for 24 hours or so.

TREATMENT
The objective of treatment is to reduce the workload of the heart, thereby decreasing myocardial oxygen demands, to relieve pain and to prevent myocardial infarction.

Drug therapy combined with lifestyle modification and/or surgical intervention (coronary artery bypass graft surgery) are employed for the treatment of symptoms.

DRUG THERAPY
Nitrates
Mainstay of treatment – tablets and spray.
1. Objective – to reduce myocardial oxygen consumption.
2. Effects – decreases ischaemia and relieves anginal pain.
3. Mechanism of action (not clearly established):
   a. Glyceryl trinitrate (GTN) has an effect on peripheral circulation – by increasing the capacity of the venous bed, it causes venous pooling of blood throughout the body.
   b. As a result, less blood is returned to the heart, and there is a reduction in ventricular volume, stroke volume and cardiac output.
   c. Nitrates also relax the systemic arteriolar bed and thus may cause a fall in blood pressure.
   d. Nitrates also increase coronary blood flow and oxygen supply by dilation of coronary collaterals.
4. GTN should be taken *before* pain develops. The patient regulates the drug usage, taking the smallest dose that relieves pain.
5. GTN is usually given sublingually (under tongue) or in buccal pouch while the patient is seated (see Patient Education, pp. 254–255).
   a. Pain relief usually begins within three minutes.
   b. Caution the patient not to take more than two to three sublingual GTN tablets over a 15-minute period.
6. Side-effects – headaches, transient dizziness, weakness, syncope (may be caused by cerebral ischaemia from postural hypotension); some side-effects may subside with continued therapy.

GTN ointment
Appears to protect against anginal pain and promote its relief. Useful for patients experiencing nocturnal angina or whose angina occurs frequently.
1. Ointment is measured with a calibrated strip of paper that comes with the product and is smoothed onto the skin in a thin uniform layer; can be applied on any convenient skin surface, since it is topically absorbed.
2. May be covered with plastic film – protects clothing and enhances absorption.
3. Appears to have beneficial effects persisting up to four to six hours.

Transdermal GTN
Impregnated on an adhesive circular bandage and applied topically to skin to provide 24-hour constant drug absorption through the skin into the systemic circulation.

1. The circular discs are applied daily to skin that is free of hair and in an area not subject to excessive movement. The site of application should be changed slightly each time to avoid undue skin irritation.

Beta-adrenergic blocking drugs
To decrease myocardial oxygen need.
1. Propranolol – reduces oxygen consumption by blocking sympathetic impulses to the heart. This produces a reduction in heart rate, systemic blood pressure and myocardial contractility, which is associated with a decrease in myocardial oxygen consumption. This allows the patient to work or exercise while requiring less myocardial oxygen delivery.
2. Given daily in divided doses at equally spaced intervals; dosage titrated to the patient's symptoms.
3. Side-effects – fatigue, hypotension, severe bradycardia, mental depression, bronchospasm in susceptible individual; may precipitate congestive heart failure.
4. Take blood pressure and heart rate with the patient in upright position two hours after administration to assess for postural hypotension.
5. Do not give if pulse rate drops below 50 beats per minute.
6. Propranolol also used in conjunction with sublingual isosorbide mononitrate for anti-anginal and anti-ischaemia prophylaxis.
7. Exercise ECG testing may be used to determine when optimal therapy has been achieved.

Calcium channel blockers (calcium antagonists)
1. Objective – to reduce myocardial oxygen demand and decrease net myocardial oxygen consumption.
2. Effect – alter the electrochemical function of myocardial cells by blocking the influx of calcium. This causes a reduction in the mechanical activity of the cells, since the myocardial cells are unable to respond vigorously to the electrical stimulation of the pacemaker cells.
3. Mechanism of action:
   a. *Coronary arterial dilatation* – calcium channel blockers decrease smooth muscle tone in the coronary arteries, causing a decrease in coronary vascular resistance and a resultant increase in coronary blood flow. Coronary collateral circulation is also increased.
   b. *Negative inotropic effect* – calcium channel blockers (verapamil and diltiazem only) exert a dose-dependent negative inotropic effect, re-

sulting in a decrease in myocardial contractility and a lowering of myocardial oxygen consumption. A low dose produces a negative inotropic effect. High doses produce substantial peripheral dilatation, resulting in a reflex positive inotropic effect. The net myocardial oxygen consumption, however, remains decreased.

c. *Peripheral arterial dilatation* – calcium channel blockers cause widespread vasodilatation with a resultant decrease in systemic vascular resistance.

d. *Automaticity* – calcium channel blockers (verapamil and diltiazem only) reduce the rate of sinus node discharge and inhibit conduction through the AV node.

4. Calcium channel blockers are used alone, in combination with either nitrates or beta-adrenergic blocking agents, or in combination with nitrates and beta-adrenergic blocking agents. Calcium channel blockers used after therapy with nitrates or beta-adrenergic blocking agents have been ineffective or only partially effective in relieving angina. Calcium channel blockers are usually added when angina occurs at rest or there is evidence of coronary spasm.

a. *Verapamil* – side-effects include dizziness, headache, constipation, hypotension, AV conduction disturbances; may increase serum concentration of digoxin.

NURSING ALERT
Caution should be observed when combining verapamil with beta-adrenergic blocking agents, since the potency of the drugs is enhanced.

b. *Nifedipine* – side-effects include dizziness, headache, constipation, nausea, fatigue and hypotension; may increase serum digoxin levels.

c. *Diltiazem* – side-effects include dizziness, headaches, fatigue, nausea, constipation and rash; may produce AV conduction disturbances (to a lesser degree than verapamil).

Assessment
Assess and record all facets of the patient's activities that precede or precipitate attacks of anginal pain

1. When do attacks tend to occur? Following a meal? After engaging in certain activities? After physical activities in general? After visits of family/others?
2. Where is the pain located?
3. How does the patient describe the pain?

4. Was the onset of pain sudden? Gradual?
5. How long did it last – seconds? minutes? hours?
6. Was the pain steady and unwavering in quality?
7. Is the discomfort accompanied by other symptoms? Sweating? Light-headedness? Nausea? Palpitations? Shortness of breath?
8. How many minutes after taking GTN did the pain last?
9. What was the mode of abatement?

Try to take an ECG during episodes of pain
ECG may show transient ST segment shifts or T wave changes that revert to normal when pain is relieved. (See section 2 in this chapter for essentials of basic electrophysiology.)

PATIENT PROBLEMS
1. Chest pain related to myocardial ischaemia.
2. Anxiety related to fear of impending death and uncertainty of aetiology and prognosis.
3. Activity intolerance related to loss of balance between myocardial oxygen supply and demand.

Planning and implementation
NURSING INTERVENTIONS
Relief of pain and avoidance of complications
1. Administer medication as prescribed. (For details see Drug Therapy, pp. 252–253.)
2. Assess effect of drug therapy, especially upon initiation of therapy or an increase in dosage.
   a. Take frequent vital signs to evaluate the haemodynamic effects of the drugs.
   b. Notify doctor if diastolic pressure falls below 60mmHg.
   c. Monitor ECG for conduction disturbances in patients receiving diltiazem or verapamil.
   d. Observe for side-effects of medications and be alert to possible hazard of drug interactions.
   e. Review manufacturer's instructions before administering agents, noting mechanism of action, dosage and side-effects (agents are still being studied and dosage, side-effects may change).
3. Assess for development of unstable angina (progressive increase in frequency, intensity and duration of anginal attacks); these patients are at high risk for myocardial infarction and sudden death; may be admitted to coronary care unit.
   a. Assessment of acute anginal attack:
      (i) How long did it take for the GTN to relieve discomfort?
      (ii) Was the relief partial or complete?
      (iii) Take blood pressure every three minutes (one to two minutes after drug adminis-

tration) to evaluate adequacy of drug effect (should be a moderate decline in systolic pressure).

(iv) Assess for dizziness and faintness after drug administration; check blood pressure and heart rate with the patient in upright position.

b. If anginal pain undergoes a change in pattern, intensifying, lasting longer or becoming more easily provoked, suspect an acute myocardial infarction.

4. Watch for development of heart failure and dysrhythmias.

5. Correct other problems in order to decrease oxygen demands of myocardium – hypertension, hyperthyroidism, aortic stenosis, anaemia.

6. Prepare for surgical intervention (angioplasty, coronary artery bypass surgery) to bring a new blood supply to ischaemic myocardium when symptoms cannot be controlled (see pp. 293–300).

Decrease in anxiety

1. Explain to the patient and family reasons for hospitalization, diagnostic tests and therapies administered.

2. Encourage the patient to express fears and concerns regarding illness through frequent conversations – conveys to the patient a willingness to listen.

3. Answer the patient's questions with concise explanations.

4. Continually assess the patient's and family's level of anxiety and utilization of appropriate coping mechanisms.

5. Explain to the patient the importance of anxiety reduction to assist in control of angina. (Anxiety and fear put an increased stress on the heart, requiring the heart to use more oxygen. The result may be an imbalance of myocardial oxygen supply and demand, causing pain.)

6. Administer drugs to relieve patient anxiety. *Sedatives and tranquillizers* – may be used to prevent attacks precipitated by aggravation, excitement or tension.

7. Support the patient having coronary arteriography to determine if surgical intervention is advisable.

Modification of activity level

Activity considerations:

1. Help the patient to participate in self-assessment to determine the provoking factors/events that precipitate the onset of angina – including physical activity, emotional pressures, worries, family, financial problems.

2. Reduce activity to below the point at which anginal pain occurs.

3. GTN should be used prophylactically to avoid pain known to occur with certain activities (stair climbing, sexual intercourse, exposure to cold).

4. See Patient Education, below.

PATIENT EDUCATION

Instruct the patient as follows:

1. Chest discomfort or pain may be provoked by any activity that puts too much load on the heart and increases heart rate and blood pressure.

2. Use moderation in all activities to prevent an episode of anginal pain.
   a. Participate in a normal daily programme of activities that do not produce chest discomfort, shortness of breath and undue fatigue.
   b. Avoid activities known to cause anginal pain – sudden exertion, walking against the wind, extremes of temperature, high altitude, emotionally stressful situations; may accelerate heart rate, raise blood pressure and increase cardiac work.
   c. Refrain from engaging in physical activity for two hours after meals. Rest after each meal if possible.
   d. Do not undertake activities requiring heavy effort (carrying heavy objects).
   e. Try to avoid cold weather if possible; dress warmly and walk more slowly. Wear scarf over nose and mouth when in cold air.
   f. Reduce weight, if necessary, to reduce cardiac load.
   g. Avoid overeating.
      (i) Avoid excessive caffeine intake (coffee, cola drinks) that can increase the heart rate and produce angina.
      (ii) Do not use 'diet pills', nasal decongestants or any over-the-counter medications that can increase the heart rate or stimulate high blood pressure.
      (iii) Avoid the use of alcohol or drink alcohol only in moderation (alcohol can increase hypotensive side-effects of drugs).

3. Use prescribed GTN effectively.
   a. Carry GTN at all times.
      (i) GTN is volatile and is inactivated by heat, moisture, air, light and time.
      (ii) Keep GTN in original dark glass container, tightly closed – to prevent absorption of drug by other pills or pillbox.

(iii) Do not carry GTN in a plastic or metal pillbox or mixed with other pills.

(iv) Renew supply every two or three months.

(v) GTN should cause a slight burning or stinging sensation under the tongue when it is potent.

b. Place GTN under tongue at first sign of chest discomfort.

(i) Stop all effort/activity; sit, and take GTN tablet – relief should be obtained in a few minutes.

(ii) Do not swallow saliva until tablet is dissolved.

(iii) Bite the tablet between front teeth and slip under tongue to dissolve if quick action is desired.

(iv) Repeat dosage in a few minutes for total of three tablets if relief is not obtained.

(v) Keep a record of number of tablets taken – to evaluate any change in anginal pattern.

(vi) Take GTN prophylactically to avoid pain known to occur with certain activities.

4. If taking a beta-blocker, do not interrupt therapy without first consulting the doctor – abrupt withdrawal can produce exacerbation of angina, myocardial infarction.

5. Seek medical help if pain persists more than 20 minutes or becomes more intense or widespread. (Do not drive yourself.)

6. If dizziness or faintness occurs, lower head between legs and breathe deeply to enhance recovery from symptoms.

7. Mild headaches are common. If severe headaches occur (lasting longer than 15 minutes) consult doctor. Dosage may have to be reduced.

8. Provide information to the patient regarding vocational rehabilitation if a less stressful job is needed.

9. Inform the patient of available cardiac rehabilitation programmes.

10. Inform the patient of available methods of learning stress management: biofeedback, transcendental meditation, etc.

11. Involve partner and family members in educating patient.

Evaluation

EXPECTED OUTCOMES

1. Maintains balance between myocardial oxygen supply and demand; absence of chest pain, takes appropriate measures to relieve pain, calls nurse, takes GTN and stops activity.

2. Experiences no complications; normal sinus rhythm, chest pain duration less than five minutes, chest pain relieved with GTN.

3. Achieves a decrease in anxiety; expresses lessening anxiety, expresses ability to cope.

4. Adheres to modified activity level; avoids activities that precipitate angina attacks.

GUIDELINES: PERCUTANEOUS TRANSLUMINAL CORONARY ANGIOPLASTY (PTCA)

Percutaneous transluminal coronary angioplasty (PTCA) is a technique utilized for the treatment of ischaemic heart disease (IHD) unresponsive to medical therapy. A balloon-tipped catheter is introduced through a guidewire into a coronary vessel with a proximal, accessible, noncalcified atheromatous lesion. The balloon of the catheter is then inflated, causing disruption of the intima and changes in the atheroma. The result is an increase in the diameter of the lumen of the coronary vessel (as judged by angiographic criteria) and improvement of blood flow below the lesion. Balloon inflation/deflation may be repeated until satisfactory results are achieved (Figure 5.13).

CONTRAINDICATIONS

1. Patients with left main coronary artery disease are generally not good candidates for this procedure.

2. Patients with multi-vessel disease (role of procedure remains unclear).

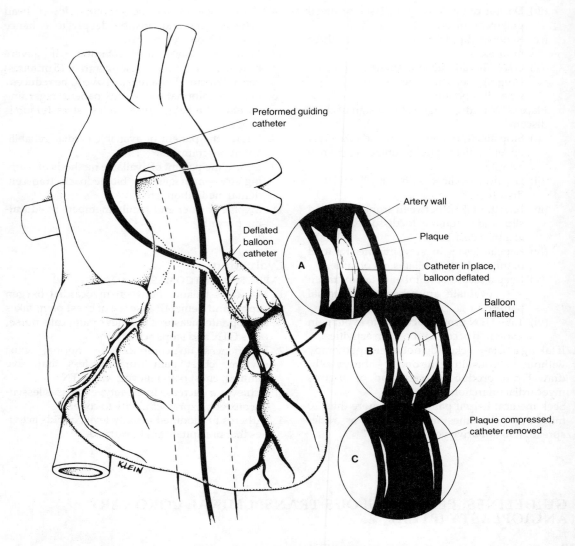

Figure 5.13. Percutaneous transluminal coronary angioplasty. (A) The balloon-tipped catheter is passed into the affected coronary artery. (B) The balloon is then rapidly inflated and deflated with controlled pressure. (C) The balloon disrupts the intima and causes changes in the atheroma, resulting in an increase in the diameter of the lumen of the vessel and improvement of blood flow. (Redrawn after Purcell, J.A. and Giffen, P.A. (1981) Percutaneous transluminal coronary angioplasty, *American Journal of Nursing*, Vol. 81, No. 9, pp. 1620–6)

COMPLICATIONS
Coronary occlusion occurs in approximately 5 per cent of patients. Necessitates immediate coronary artery bypass graft surgery to avert myocardial infarction. A cardiac surgical team must be on standby during all PTCA procedures.

PROCEDURE
Preparatory phase

Nursing action	Rationale
1. Assess the patient's level of understanding of PTCA procedure.	Cardiologist will initially explain procedure to the patient. Teaching is geared to the patient's comprehension level to minimize stress.
2. Reinforce all information about the procedure and accompanying events. Instruct the patient as follows:	Preparation for procedure minimizes anxiety and enhances recovery.
a. Procedure will be performed in cardiac catheterization laboratory and will take approximately two hours (see Heart Catheterization, pp. 219–220).	Procedure similar to coronary arteriography. All tactile and auditory stimuli should be explained to the patient.
b. Discuss diagnostic tests to be done prior to procedure – angiography etc.	Chest X-ray, ECG, blood tests: coagulation, complete blood count, electrolytes; urinalysis, myocardial imaging.
c. The location of coronary vessels and a description of the patient's lesion.	Ensures understanding.
d. Local anaesthesia will be given at catheter insertion site.	Promotes patient comfort.
e. The patient will be alert throughout procedure and will be asked to cough.	Coughing enhances catheter placement.
f. A temporary pacemaker will be inserted.	Used for emergency pacing if necessary.
g. Medication (heparin, GTN) will be given.	Heparin prevents clot formation. GTN reduces incidence of coronary spasm.
h. Stress importance of reporting chest pain to nurse or doctor before, during, or after procedure.	Indicates myocardial ischaemia, which could precipitate complications.
i. Food and fluid will be restricted the night and morning before procedure.	Reduces incidence of stomach upset during procedure.
j. Bed rest will be maintained for six to 12 hours after procedure, with head of bed elevated no more than 30 degrees, and immobilization of affected extremity.	Activity may cause bleeding and prolong healing of vessel lining.
k. Patient may eat after procedure.	Intravenous access will remain in place for six hours.
l. Vital signs will be observed frequently.	Necessary for detection of complications.
m. Discharge will be the following day.	
3. Prepare the patient for complications of procedure. (Before procedure, patient must be a suitable candidate for heart surgery and have consented to heart surgery as alternative treatment.)	Coronary artery occlusion, coronary artery rupture or acute coronary artery spasm may necessitate cardiopulmonary bypass graft surgery.
a. Provide preoperative teaching to the patient and family regarding heart surgery (see pp. 294–295).	
4. Record the patient's vital signs before going to catheterization laboratory.	Provides baseline data for comparison after procedure.
a. Assess peripheral pulses and colour and temperature of extremities.	

Post-procedure phase

Nursing action	Rationale
1. Check vital signs every 15 minutes for one hour, then every half-hour for two hours, and finally every hour for four hours.	Allows for frequent assessment of possible complications – bleeding, bradycardia, hypotension.
2. Check peripheral pulse of affected extremity and insertion site after each vital sign check.	Because intraprocedure heparinization is not reversed, there is increased chance of bleeding after procedure.
a. Look for presence of haematoma and mark haematoma to note change in size.	Notify doctor if haematoma continues to enlarge or if bleeding is not controlled after pressure is applied at
b. Check bed linen for blood under patient.	site with fingers.
c. Mark peripheral pulse of affected extremity with water-soluble ink.	Facilitates pulse checks.
d. Observe colour and temperature of affected extremity.	Notify doctor if extremities become cool and pale, and pulses become significantly diminished or absent.
3. Record intake and output and monitor serum electrolytes.	Contrast medium used during procedure causes diuresis and potassium depletion.

Follow-up phase

Nursing action	Rationale
1. Instruct the patient as follows:	
a. Modification of cardiac risk factors as means of controlling progression of coronary artery disease.	PTCA is palliative treatment for ischaemic heart disease, not a cure. Refer patient to outpatient cardiac rehabilitation programme.
b. Name of medications, action, dosage and side-effects.	Common medications prevent clot formation (e.g. aspirin); increase blood flow to heart (isosorbide); or slow heart rate/decrease chest pain (propranolol).
c. Dates and importance of follow-up tests – exercise ECG, thallium-201 perfusion imaging.	Stenosis can recur within six months. Second angioplasty usually successful for more than one year.
d. Symptoms for which patient should seek medical attention – side-effects of medications, chest pain or weight increases greater than 2.2kg.	Chest pain unrelieved with GTN and persisting longer than 15 minutes after rest is significant.

MYOCARDIAL INFARCTION

Myocardial infarction (MI) refers to the process by which myocardial tissue is destroyed in regions of the heart that are deprived of their blood supply because of an interruption of coronary blood flow.

INCIDENCE OF CARDIOVASCULAR DISEASE IN THE UK

In the past three decades the incidence of cardiovascular disease in the UK has risen at a steady rate and now accounts for 250,000 deaths per annum. Approximately 180,000 (70 per cent) of these deaths are attributable to the effects of ischaemic heart disease, and of this number, 50 per cent are sudden deaths (MI). Almost half the number of deaths occur in people who have had no recognizable features of ischaemic heart disease.

CAUSES

1. Atherosclerotic heart disease – usually with superimposed thrombosis – coronary artery

disease with proximal obstruction to coronary flow in one or more major vessels.

. Coronary artery embolism.

. Decreased coronary blood flow with shock/haemorrhage.

. Coronary artery spasm.

Assessment

CLINICAL FEATURES

. Chest pain – steady, constrictive pain (central portion of chest and epigastrium) not relieved by rest or nitrates; pain may radiate widely; may produce dysrhythmias, hypotension, shock, cardiac failure.

. Profuse perspiration; moist, clammy skin with pallor.

. Drop in blood pressure.

. Dyspnoea, weakness and fainting.

. Nausea and vomiting.

. Anxiety and restlessness.

. Tachycardia or bradycardia.

NURSING ALERT

Many patients do not have symptoms; these are the 'silent infarcts'. Nevertheless there is still resultant damage to the myocardium.

. Atypical symptoms – extreme fatigue, epigastric or abdominal distress, shortness of breath.

DIAGNOSTIC EVALUATION

. Clinical history and findings from physical examination.

. ECG changes (within two to 12 hours, but may take as long as 72 to 96 hours). See pages 306–307 for ECG interpretation of MI.

. Elevation of serum isoenzymes (see CPK-MB test).

. Radionuclide imaging – see page 220; allows recognition of areas of decreased perfusion as 'cold spots', which are seen in areas of ischaemia and infarction.

AREAS OF TRAUMA

Knowledge of the coronary blood supply will help in understanding the areas traumatized by infarction and to predict specific patient problems which may occur (Figure 5.14; Table 5.4).

TREATMENT

The objective of treatment is to promote adequate circulatory function with healing of the myocardium, to limit size of infarct and to prevent death.

PATIENT PROBLEMS

1. Alteration in cardiac output related to mechanical factors (preload, afterload, contractility).
2. Pain related to myocardial ischaemia.
3. Anxiety related to fear of death, complex environment and uncertainty of aetiology and prognosis.
4. Activity intolerance related to imbalance between myocardial oxygen supply and demand.
5. Altered pattern of elimination; constipation related to restricted activity level.
6. Potential for depression related to threats to self-esteem and disturbances in sleep–rest patterns.

Planning and implementation

NURSING INTERVENTIONS

Maintaining haemodynamic stability

1. Admit to coronary care unit for constant monitoring.
   a. Lift patient from stretcher to bed; place in position of comfort.
   b. Insert an intravenous cannula to keep vein open for administration of intravenous medications in event of a dysrhythmia.
2. Attach ECG monitoring electrodes to monitor the heart rhythm and to confirm clinical impression of MI. Explain to patient that:
   a. He is able to move about the bed when attached to cardiac monitor.
   b. Cardiac monitor only monitors heart rhythm, and does not affect it.
   c. Movement may cause bizarre patterns (artefacts) on the screen.
   d. It is common for electrodes to become loose – they will be replaced.
3. Continually assess peripheral perfusion (blood supply to organs and tissues).
   a. Measure and record vital signs every one or two hours to determine presence of impending cardiogenic shock and other complications.
      (i) Note on record, method of taking blood pressure (palpation/auscultation).
      (ii) Evaluate both apical and radial pulse rates. Note strength of femoral pulse.
   b. Count respirations – tachypnoea may indicate heart failure, pulmonary embolism.
   c. Monitor body temperature – gives some indication of tissue perfusion.
   d. Assess skin temperature and colour.
   e. Assess neck veins for distension – elevation of venous pressure may indicate failure of heart to pump effectively.
   f. Assess for changes in mental status (apathy,

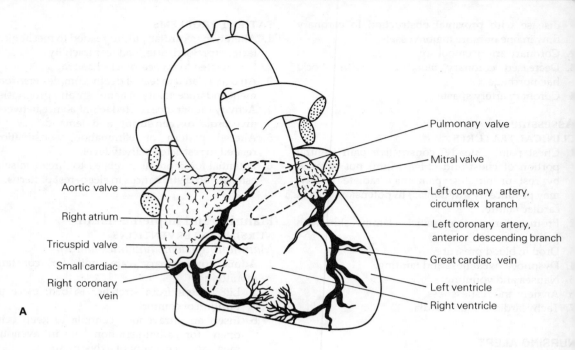

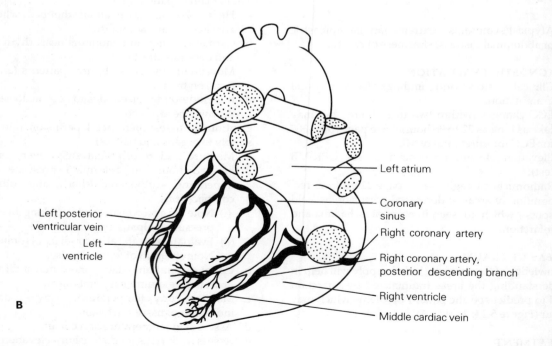

Figure 5.14. Coronary blood vessels. (A) Anterior view. (B) Posterior view

Table 5.4   Major coronary arteries and structures perfused

Coronary artery	Chambers	Structures
Right	Right atrium	Sinus node (60 per cent of population)
		AV* node, AV bundle (90 per cent of population)
	Right ventricle	Inferior wall, posterior wall
	Left ventricle	Posterior left papillary muscle
	Interventricular septum, posterior portion	Left bundle branch, posterior fascicle
Left anterior descending	Left ventricle	Anterior wall
		Apex
		Anterior left papillary muscle
	Interventricular septum, anterior portion	AV bundle
		Right bundle branch
		Left bundle branch, anterior and septal fascicles
Left circumflex	Left atrium	
	Left ventricle	Lateral wall
		Posterior wall
	Interventricular septum, posterior portion	Left bundle branch, posterior fascicle
	Right atrium	Sinus node (40 per cent of population)
		AV node, AV bundle (10 per cent of population)

AV = atrioventricular.

confusion, restlessness) – from inadequate cerebral perfusion.

g. Evaluate urine output (30ml/hour) – decrease in urine volume reflects a decrease in renal blood flow.

. Prepare for thrombolysis if indicated.

. Be alert for indications of complications.

  a. *Cardiogenic shock:*
   (i) Falling arterial blood pressure.
   (ii) Reduced urinary volume (30ml/hour or less).
   (iii) Cool, moist skin; may be peripheral cyanosis – due to systemic vasoconstriction caused by reduction in cardiac output.
   (iv) Restlessness, apathy, lessening of responsiveness – from systemic vasoconstriction.
   (v) See p. 266 for management of cardiogenic shock. A patient with cardiogenic shock should, ideally, be transferred to coronary care unit with haemodynamic monitoring capabilities.

  b. *Heart failure* – myocardial infarction reduces ability of left ventricle to eject blood, diminishes cardiac output, produces an elevation of left ventricular end pressure with ensuing pulmonary vascular complications.
   (i) Assess for tachycardia and gallop rhythm, dyspnoea, orthopnoea, oedema, hepatomegaly.
   (ii) Watch for development of pulmonary oedema (see pp. 291–293) – represents extreme left ventricular failure. Assess for extreme dyspnoea, frothy, blood-stained mucus, tachycardia, distended neck veins and diffuse crackles.
   (iii) See pp. 283–291 for treatment of heart failure and acute pulmonary oedema.

  c. *Other complications:*
   (i) Papillary muscle rupture, ventricular septal rupture, ventricular aneurysm.
   (ii) Postmyocardial infarction syndrome (Dressler's syndrome) – a recurrent febrile illness with pericarditis, pleuritis and pneumonitis.
   (iii) Cerebral and peripheral emboli; pulmonary emboli.

  d. *Prepare for surgical intervention if indicated* – insertion of intra-aortic counterpulsation device, coronary artery bypass, repair of ventricular septal defect, mitral valve replacement. (See nursing management of patient undergoing heart surgery, pp. 294–300.)

6. Monitor dietary intake.
  a. Diet is prescribed according to status of circulatory condition.
  b. Avoid large meals, which increase demand for splanchnic blood flow and increase cardiac workload.

Avoidance of life-threatening dysrhythmias

1. *Dysrhythmias* – occur frequently in first few days after infarction. The reduction in myocardial oxygenation produces myocardial ischaemia. Ischaemic muscle is electrically unstable and produces dysrhythmias. Risk of ventricular fibrillation and death is greatest in first few hours following MI.
   a. Assess, prevent and treat conditions that may initiate a dysrhythmia – heart failure, pulmonary embolus, inadequate pulmonary ventilation, electrolyte disturbances, underoxygenation of blood.
   b. Draw arterial blood for blood gas analysis.
   c. Watch for ventricular fibrillation, ventricular tachycardia, AV block, asystole.
   d. See pp. 307–327 for management of dysrhythmias.
2. Be vigilant for occurrence of any type of ventricular ectopic beats – may presage ventricular tachycardia and ventricular fibrillation. (See pp. 317–320 for discussion of dysrhythmias.)
   a. Correct dysrhythmia immediately – may unfavourably alter the balance between oxygen supply and demand at the periphery of the infarct.
   b. Lignocaine may be given prophylactically – to protect patient against ventricular fibrillation.
   c. Other antidysrhythmic drugs include procainamide, quinidine, propranolol, atropine, etc – selected by classification.
   d. Prepare patient for prophylactic pacing (pp. 242–248), if indicated.
3. Administer oxygen by nasal cannula (p. 117) and encourage patient to take deep breaths – may decrease incidence of dysrhythmias by allowing the myocardium to be less ischaemic and thus less irritable; may reduce size of infarct.

Establishing balance between myocardial oxygen supply and demand

1. Offer psychological support and reassurance to patient to decrease anxiety.
2. Give analgesic, morphine or diamorphine – decreases sympathetic activity and reduces myocardial oxygen consumption with subsequent decreases in heart rate, blood pressure and muscle tension.
3. Give in small intravenous doses until relief is obtained (if vital signs are within safe parameters).
4. Evaluate analgesic effect with patient.

NURSING ALERT

Assess for persistent or recurring pain, which suggests an extension or threatened extension of infarct; urgent and aggressive intervention is required. Notify doctors immediately.

5. Monitor blood pressure, pulse and respiratory rate before administering narcotics – narcotics depress arterial pressure and may contribute to development of shock and dysrhythmias.
6. Assess for complications of narcotic administration, such as respiratory impairment (especially in patients with chronic obstructive airways disease) and hypotension.
7. Avoid intramuscular injections of analgesic agents, since they may cause falsely elevated serum CK values, resulting in an incorrect diagnosis of myocardial infarction.

Decreasing anxiety

1. Assess levels of anxiety and coping mechanisms of patient and his family.
2. Relieve the patient's pain and anxiety – anxiety and fear increase the heart rate (which puts heart under more stress), raise the blood pressure, and cause the adrenal glands to release adrenaline which may produce dysrhythmias.
3. Discuss with patient coronary care unit environment and what can be anticipated in the coming days, to allay anxiety and help him mobilize his resources for coping.
4. Explain all procedures to the patient and invite questions.
5. If severe anxiety is present, try to maintain consistency of care, with one or two nurses assisting patient regularly. Calm environment.
6. Before discharge from coronary care unit, prepare the patient for non-intensive care environment through discussions with family and patient focusing on the decreased need to monitor patient continually.
7. Administer antianxiety agents – anxiety is associated with increased sympathetic drive.

Adjustment in activity level

1. Promote rest with increased mobilization.
   a. Place the patient at rest – to lower heart rate and blood pressure and oxygen demands on heart and to maintain cardiac work at its lowest level. The following is an example of an activity schedule:
      (i) Day 1 – bed rest with commode; requires less cardiovascular work than bedpan.
      (ii) Day 2 – out of bed to chair, as tolerated.
      (iii) Day 3 – ambulation as tolerated.

2. Assist with implementation of self-care activities on a gradual basis.
   a. Assist with hygiene needs as necessary.
   b. After discharge from coronary care unit, a warm shower may be taken with assistance.
3. Instruct patient to avoid any sudden effort.
4. Offer patient diversional activities, such as light reading and listening to the radio.
5. Maintain optimum independence.

Establishing normal elimination pattern
1. Offer diet with bulk and fibre.
2. Allow use of bedside commode rather than bedpan.
3. Administer stool softeners as required.

Developing adaptive coping abilities
1. Use of nursing history to give knowledge of previous experience.
2. Assess the patient's stage of grieving.
3. Give intelligent reassurance and assist the patient in establishing a positive attitude towards his illness.
   a. Most people use the mechanism of denial during initial stages of MI.
   b. Depression is commonly encountered on about the third day in the coronary care unit, although it may not surface until the patient returns home.
      (i) Depression following MI is normal; the patient is grieving over his losses – health, confidence, independence.
      (ii) The patient may feel pressure from having to alter his lifestyle (i.e., eating, drinking, smoking).
4. Assess for maladaptive coping patterns – inappropriate denial, withdrawal, changes in usual communicative patterns, destructive behaviour. Ask the patient what he is thinking about and feeling; try to draw out specific concerns.
5. Involve family in support and education.
   a. The family, especially the partner is likely to feel more anxious than the patient.
   b. They may experience feelings of loss, guilt, anger, denial.
   c. They are likely to benefit from being given information, made to feel involved, being given hope, feeling their needs are recognized.
   d. Visitors may be a source of support for the patient, but visiting times can also be exhausting and stressful – need to consider the needs of the patient and other patients in close proximity.

6. Allow the patient to have control over plan of care as much as possible; include the patient in decision-making when appropriate. Give realistic expectations.
7. Compliment the patient on activities he is able to do; avoid false reassurance.
8. Discuss with the patient usual sleep patterns – onset of sleep, usual waking time, number of hours of rest needed daily.
9. Manipulate environment to provide and maintain the patient's normal sleep patterns.

PATIENT EDUCATION
Objectives
Restore patient to his optimal physical, emotional, social and work level.

Aid in restoring confidence and self-esteem.

Prevent progression of underlying disease (atherosclerosis).

Ensure family members are adequately prepared.

Health education needs to be geared to the individual patient and his family. During the initial 24 to 48 hours, the patient may not be able to retain much information. Information needs to be reinforced later in the hospital stay. Advice sheets and booklets are a useful source of reference.

1. Inform the patient about what has happened to his heart and explain that myocardial healing starts early but is not complete for six to eight weeks.
2. A myocardial infarction may require some modification of lifestyle. Patient should be able to drive after four to six weeks although HGV and PSV drivers lose their licences.
3. Exercise tolerance testing will be done after myocardial healing to determine optimal level of activity and to plan rehabilitation programme.
4. A programme of exercise training will be prescribed at this time to improve cardiovascular functional capacity.
5. Physical limitations are usually only temporary. The following guidelines usually apply until the patient is re-evaluated after complete myocardial healing:
   a. Expect to feel weak and tired for a period of time; depression is not uncommon.
   b. Walk daily, gradually increasing the distance and time.
   c. Avoid doing anything that tenses the muscles (isometric exercises, weight lifting, straining, lifting heavy objects, pushing/pulling heavy loads) – may place strain on coronary reserve.

d. Rest after meals and before doing any exercise.
e. Space activities throughout the day to alternate rest and work.
   (i) Stop as soon as fatigued. Have an afternoon nap.
   (ii) Avoid tenseness and rushing.
f. Avoid working with arms above shoulder level.
g. Shorten work hours when first returning to work.
   (i) Most patients return to work after six to eight weeks.
   (ii) Heavy manual workers may need to change their job.
   (iii) Retirement may be realistic alternative for some.
   (iv) Need to consider financial aspects – wife may need to go out to work, for example.
   (v) Patient may feel inadequate if no longer being the breadwinner.
6. Advise the patient to eat three to four meals daily (each containing about the same amount of food).
   a. Avoid large meals.
   b. Avoid hurrying while eating.
   c. Limit caffeine intake (coffee and cola) and cigarette smoking.
   d. Maintain prescribed diet (modifications in calories, fats and sodium).
7. Extremes in temperature and walking against the wind should be avoided.
   a. Stop immediately for shortness of breath.
   b. Sit down and take GTN for chest pain.
8. Sexual relations may be resumed when the patient feels able.
   a. If patient can walk briskly or climb two flights of stairs, he can usually resume sexual activity with familiar partner; resumption of sexual activity parallels resumption of usual activities.
   b. Sexual activity should be avoided after eating a heavy meal, after drinking alcohol or when tired.
   c. Myocardial infarction during sexual intercourse is extremely rare.
   d. The spouse may have more anxieties than the patient.
9. Instruct the patient to notify the doctor if the following symptoms appear:
   a. Chest pressure or pain not relieved in 15 minutes by GTN or rest.
   b. Shortness of breath.
   c. Unusual fatigue.
   d. Swelling of feet and ankles.
   e. Fainting, dizziness.
   f. Very slow or rapid heart beat.
10. Explain drug regimen.

Evaluation
EXPECTED OUTCOMES
1. Maintains haemodynamic stability; exhibits no signs/symptoms of heart failure – diaphoresis, hypotension, change in mental status, cool, clammy skin.
2. Experiences no life-threatening dysrhythmias; heart rate 60 to 100 beats per minute; rhythm – normal sinus rhythm.
3. Maintains balance between myocardial oxygen supply and demand; experiences no chest pain, calls nurse if experiences pain.
4. Experiences a decrease in anxiety; exhibits calm speech pattern, relaxed facial expression, expresses feelings about death.
5. Adheres to limited activity prescription; engages in appropriate levels of activity.
6. Maintains normal elimination pattern; soft, formed stool per normal pattern for patient.
7. Copes adaptively to illness; communicates self-confidence in future lifestyle; requests information regarding illness, environment and routines; participates in self-care activities.

GUIDELINES: THROMBOLYTIC THERAPY

Thrombolytic therapy is a recent development which has revolutionized the treatment of acute myocardial infarction patients. The aim is to induce dissolution of the thrombus and provide subsequent reperfusion to the ischaemic zone. It involves intracoronary, or more commonly, intravenous administration of a thrombolytic agent. Success rate is 70 to 80 per cent for reperfusion.

The currently available thrombolytic agents are:
1. Streptokinase (most common).

2. Urokinase.
3. Recombinant tissue-type plasminogen activator (rTPA).
4. Anisoylated plasminogen – streptokinase activator complex (APSAC).
5. Prourokinase.

CONTRAINDICATIONS
1. Active bleeding.
2. Surgery, trauma, CVA or neurosurgical procedure performed within six months.
3. Gastrointestinal bleeding, or biopsy predisposing to bleeding within the last 14 days.
4. Traumatic or prolonged cardiopulmonary resuscitation within 14 days.
5. Allergy to selected thrombolytic agent.

Other relative contraindications include severe systemic arterial hypertension, severe hepatic or renal disease, pregnancy or menorrhagia.

COMPLICATIONS
1. Bleeding episodes – frequently from puncture sites, haematuria, less common is bleeding from gums and recent cuts and abrasions.
2. Reperfusion dysrhythmias.
3. Allergic reactions including fever, rash, anaphylaxis.

PROCEDURE
Patient selection

Nursing action	Rationale

1. Be alert for possible candidates for treatment. Identified by:
  a. Recent onset of chest pain of at least 30 minutes duration and not longer than six hours.
  b. Electrocardiographic changes reflecting acute myocardial injury.
  c. No contraindications.
	Necrosis of ischaemic myocardium is virtually complete within six hours of coronary occlusion.

2. Explain procedure to patient including probable need for angiography later.	The procedure is relatively new and potentially stressful.
3. Observe for complications – hydrocortisone may be given before administration.	Anaphylaxis is a possible complication.

Post-procedure

Nursing action	Rationale
1. Antiplatelet therapy (e.g. aspirin) and calcium antagonists (e.g. nifedipine) may be prescribed.	Strategies are aimed at limiting the circumstances that caused the thrombus formation.
2. Full anticoagulation and percutaneous transluminal coronary angioplasty (PTCA) may be performed within 10 days.	May help ensure that the affected area remains patent.
3. Be aware of possible complications, and explain expected outcome.	Patient is likely to want to know the outcome of the procedure.

CARDIOGENIC SHOCK

Cardiogenic shock (power failure), the end stage of left ventricular dysfunction, occurs when the left ventricle is extensively damaged by myocardial infarction. The heart muscle loses its contractile power, and there is marked reduction in cardiac output with decreased perfusion (lack of blood and oxygen) to vital organs (heart, brain and kidneys). The degree of pump dysfunction is related to the extent of damage to the heart muscle.

Cardiogenic shock now accounts for the majority of hospital deaths from myocardial infarction and has a high mortality rate.

Assessment

CLINICAL FEATURES
1. Low systolic pressure (90mmHg or 30mmHg less than previous levels).
2. Oliguria – urine output less than 30ml/hour – from impaired renal circulation.
3. Cold, clammy skin, weak pulse, cyanosis – from circulatory insufficiency.
4. Mental lethargy, confusion – from poor cerebral perfusion.

DIAGNOSTIC EVALUATION
1. Physical examination – signs/symptoms of decrease in cerebral, renal and peripheral perfusion, pulmonary congestion and hypotension.
2. Medical history – reduction in cardiac output unrelated to hypovolaemia, significant dysrhythmias, depressive drug therapy, arterial hypoxia or acute pain.
3. Diagnosis of MI – ECG, medical history, physical examination.

TREATMENT
1. The management of cardiogenic shock is directed at decreasing pulmonary congestion, improving cardiac output and decreasing systemic congestion, while preserving the borderline areas of the myocardium and limiting infarct size.
2. Measures to decrease pulmonary congestion focus on reduction of venous return or reduction of circulating blood volume. Cardiac output is improved through therapy that decreases cardiac workload and stimulates cardiac contractility while maintaining balance of myocardial oxygen supply and demand. Systemic congestion is treated by decreasing circulating blood volume.

PATIENT PROBLEMS
1. Impaired cardiac output related to massive ischaemic damage to the left ventricle.
2. Impaired gas exchange related to pulmonary congestion.
3. Alteration in mental status related to impaired cerebral blood flow.
4. Impaired tissue perfusion related to decreased peripheral blood flow.

Planning and implementation
NURSING INTERVENTIONS
Improvement in cardiac output
1. Start haemodynamic monitoring at the *first* indication of deterioration of the patient's condition – haemodynamic monitoring is necessary for continuing patient evaluation and serves as a guideline for therapy. Measure left ventricular pressure – oxygen demands of ischaemic myocardium are determined by left ventricular pressure and heart rate, myocardial contractility size, shape and wall thickness of left ventricle.
   a. Measurement of left ventricular end-diastolic pressure is estimated by the pulmonary arterial wedge pressure as measured by the Swan–Ganz catheter.
      (i) Values are elevated in patients with left ventricular failure, mitral valve disease, pulmonary hypertension.
      (ii) See pages 226–229 for technique.
   b. Pulmonary capillary wedge pressure (PCWP) provides an accurate estimate of left ventricular filling pressure only in the absence of mitral valve disease.
      (i) Used also as a guide for infusion therapy, pulmonary congestion is indicated by PCWP greater than 18mmHg; the increase signifies that the left side of the heart is in failure.
      (ii) See pages 226–229 for technique.
   c. Evaluate cardiac output – pulmonary artery catheters are also used to evaluate cardiac output by thermodilution technique.
2. Measure intra-arterial pressure by direct arterial cannulization – more accurate measurement of blood pressure.
3. Administer continuous oxygen at percentage needed to combat hypoxaemia.
4. Correct hypovolaemia.
   a. Administer IV fluids until left ventricular pressure increases to 18–20mmHg (the value associated with highest cardiac output).
   b. Watch for development of pulmonary oedema, which may occur abruptly.

5. Give appropriate drug therapy if the patient is still in shock – to lessen ischaemia and limit size of infarct and decrease the work of the heart.
   a. *Vasodilator therapy* – vasodilator drugs dilate capacitance vessels (veins and venules) and/or resistance vessels (arterioles), reducing impedance to left ventricular outflow and venous return to the heart; decreases myocardial oxygen consumption; improves perfusion to organs. Vasodilators in current use include sodium nitroprusside, phentolamine and GTN.
   b. *Inotropic agents* – used to increase cardiac output by direct effect on myocardium. Include digitalis, dopamine and dobutamine.
   c. *Diuretics* – may reduce tissue oedema at site of infarct and improve myocardial perfusion and oxygenation.
6. Measure urine volume via indwelling catheter every half to one hour – urine flow reflects renal blood flow and the status of central circulation.
7. Relieve psychological stress and anxiety – explain all procedures to the patient, allow family members to visit, administer sedation if necessary (anxiety may cause an increase in myocardial oxygen demand).
8. Be alert for significant dysrhythmias.
9. Utilize counterpulsation to decrease ventricular work of the patient with severe shock. (See description of method which follows.)
10. Prepare the patient for surgical intervention to correct defects that are interfering with pump function and to reperfuse the heart (see Patient Undergoing Heart Surgery, pp. 293–300).

Decrease in pulmonary congestion

1. Assess for signs/symptoms of acute pulmonary congestion. Note and record respiratory rate of patient, evidence of dyspnoea, cough, haemoptysis, orthopnoea.
2. Monitor arterial blood gases to assess for hypoxia and metabolic acidosis.
3. Place the patient in semi-upright or upright position (decreases venous return).
4. Administer drug therapy as directed.
   a. Morphine – aids in decreasing venous return.
   b. Aminophylline – reduces bronchospasm caused by severe congestion; also can act as peripheral vasodilator.
   c. Vasodilators – dilate venous and arterial beds to varying degrees, causing a decrease in venous return and systemic vascular resistance (nitroprusside, GTN).
   d. Diuretics – decrease circulating blood volume

and may have an effect on decreasing venous return.
5. Be alert for complications of drug therapy (aminophylline may cause nausea, vomiting, tachydysrhythmias).
6. Monitor the patient closely during administration of mechanical ventilation (positive end-expiratory pressure [PEEP] may be implemented to aid in decreasing venous return and to improve arterial oxygenation) and plasmapheresis (decreases blood volume by removing blood from circulation).

Improvement in level of consciousness

1. Assess for mental status changes every two hours utilizing a systematic approach (i.e. Glasgow Coma Scale).
2. Report changes to doctor immediately.

Adequate tissue perfusion

1. Assess for tissue symptoms indicative of heart failure progressing to shock (see Clinical Features, point 3).
2. Report symptoms to doctor immediately.

Evaluation
EXPECTED OUTCOMES

1. Demonstrates improved cardiac output – CO greater than 2.5 litre/min, CI (cardiac index) greater than 2.2 litre/min/m^2, PCWP less than 18mmHg, urine output greater than 30ml/hour.
2. Exhibits a decrease in pulmonary congestion – spontaneous respirations in range of 14 to 18, breath sounds clear on auscultation, blood gas values (arterial) within normal limits for patient.
3. Demonstrates improved level of consciousness – alert (follows commands), absence of confusion, pupils equal and reactive to light.
4. Exhibits adequate tissue perfusion – skin warm and dry, nailbeds and lips with normal colouring.

COUNTERPULSATION (MECHANICAL CARDIAC ASSISTANCE)

Counterpulsation (diastolic augmentation) is a method of assisting the failing heart and circulation by mechanical support that may be accomplished by (1) intra-aortic balloon pump or (2) external counterpulsation pressure. Counterpulsation with an intra-aortic balloon pump (IABP) during the acute phase of myocardial infarction eases the workload of a damaged heart and if started before irreversible change takes place, may limite infarct size by increasing coronary blood flow.

INTRA-AORTIC BALLOON PUMP

A balloon catheter is introduced via the femoral artery or via a percutaneous route into the descending thoracic aorta; it is inflated and deflated in sequence with the cardiac cycle and acts as an auxiliary pump assisting forward blood flow (Figure 5.15). This provides an augmentation of diastole, which results in an increase in coronary blood flow and cardiac output, and it reduces left ventricular end pressure (by causing a more complete emptying of the left ventricle). This decreases the resistance in the arterial tree against which the heart must pump and reduces myocardial oxygen requirements.

1. Using synchronization with the patient's ECG, the balloon is inflated at the onset of diastole ('diastolic augmentation'); this results in increased diastolic pressure, which increases coronary blood flow and myocardial nutrition.
2. The balloon is deflated at the onset of cardiac

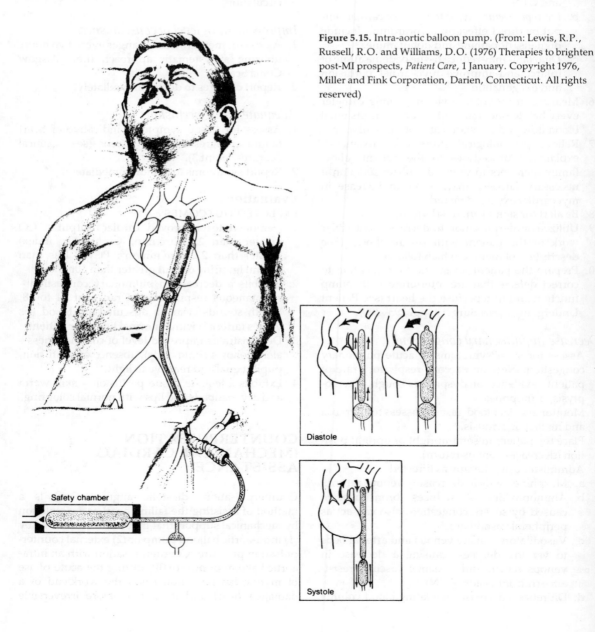

Figure 5.15. Intra-aortic balloon pump. (From: Lewis, R.P., Russell, R.O. and Williams, D.O. (1976) Therapies to brighten post-MI prospects, *Patient Care*, 1 January. Copyright 1976, Miller and Fink Corporation, Darien, Connecticut. All rights reserved)

Safety chamber

Diastole

Systole

systole to lower the aortic blood pressure so that the work of the left ventricle is reduced (reduction in left ventricular impedance and afterload).

3. A bedside console provides gas for balloon inflation and controls the inflation/deflation cycle to accommodate variations in the patient's heart rate. It is timed by the ECG and triggered by the arterial pulse wave.

4. Once stabilized the patient is weaned off IABP by reducing the ratio of inflations to diastoles or by reducing balloon volumes.

5. Clinical uses:
   a. Treatment of cardiogenic shock following myocardial infarction.
   b. Low cardiac output states – following open heart surgery; life-threatening dysrhythmias.
   c. High cardiac output states – sepsis, haemorrhage.

d. Myocardial ischaemia unresponsive to medical therapy and external counterpulsation pressure.

EXTERNAL COUNTERPULSATION PRESSURE (ECP)

A non-invasive method of assisting the circulation, it is designed to boost the heart temporarily during a period of pump failure (Figure 5.16). It helps maintain adequate perfusion of vital organs and tissues until the heart is able to resume its function.

1. The counterpulsation device is positioned around the lower extremities from thighs to ankles; the

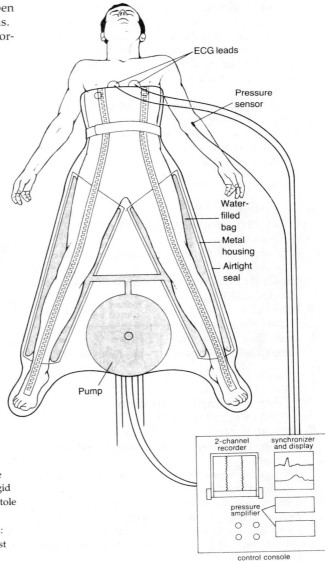

Figure 5.16. External counterpulsation pressure; a pressure sensor is threaded into a radial artery. Bags contained in rigid cylinders that encase both legs are filled with water on diastole and emptied on systole with a pump – placed between the patient's ankles – which is triggered by ECG signals. (From: Putting the counterpressure on, *Emergency Medicine*, August 1975)

legs are encased in two rigid troughs, and the system is closed to make an airtight seal.
2. A pump is positioned between the patient's ankles.
3. Water is pumped through the system during diastole in response to an electronic signal triggered by the ECG; squeezing the legs during diastole forces a column of arterial blood back to the heart, which provides diastolic augmentation and improves coronary arterial filling pressure.
4. The pressure is released (application of negative pressure) during cardiac systole, which lowers the systolic pressure (and thus the peak left ventricular pressure).
5. In cardiogenic shock, ECP increases the coronary blood flow by raising diastolic pressure, which may improve cardiac function; compression of the legs also increases venous return to the heart and thus increases cardiac output. Left ventricular work is thus reduced.
6. Clinical uses:
   a. Chest pain associated with MI unrelieved by medical therapy.
   b. Mild to moderate heart failure.
7. See Myocardial Infarction, pp. 258–265 and Cardiogenic Shock, pp. 266–270.

Assessment
PATIENT PROBLEMS (PATIENT RECEIVING IABP THERAPY)
1. Fear related to invasive therapy, environment and death.
2. Impaired cardiac output related to refractory left ventricular failure.
3. Potential for injury related to thrombus formation, thrombocytopenia and infection.
4. Immobility related to IABP therapy.
5. Sleep pattern disturbance related to environment.

Planning and implementation
NURSING INTERVENTIONS
Reduction of fear
1. Explain procedure to the patient and invite questions.
2. Allow the patient to express fears regarding illness and therapy.
3. Offer reassurance and comfort measures.
4. Explain therapy to family and encourage them to visit and discuss fears with the patient.
5. Obtain consent form from patient or authorized family member before procedure.

Establishing haemodynamic stability
1. Assist doctor and patient during insertion of IABP catheter.
2. Monitor haemodynamic parameters with Swan–Ganz catheter and intra-arterial line (see Haemodynamic Monitoring, pp. 226–229).
   a. Record central venous pressure (CP), pulmonary capillary wedge pressure (PCWP), pulmonary arterial pressure (PAP), cardiac output (CO), heart rate (HR) and blood pressure (BP).
   b. Record date, time, and the patient's tolerance of procedure.
3. Start IABP immediately after insertion according to doctor's request.
   a. Note timing of inflation and deflation of balloon every hour and adjust as necessary.
   b. Record vital signs every 15 to 30 minutes for four to nine hours and then hourly.
   c. Record gas utilized for pumping (CO_2 or helium).
   d. Review manufacturer's manual for IABP equipment in use.
4. Monitor and record urine output from indwelling catheter every hour.
5. Record daily intake and output.
6. Treat dysrhythmias as directed by doctor.
7. Report any chest pain experienced by patient.
8. Record effectiveness of therapy.
9. See Cardiogenic Shock, pp. 266–270.

Avoiding complications
1. Check peripheral pulses with Doppler every hour (especially left brachial, radial and popliteal arteries).
2. Assess colour and temperature of extremities every hour. Notify doctor if extremities are dusky or cold.
3. Monitor rectal temperature every two to four hours and report temperature greater than 38.5°C.
4. Obtain blood, sputum and urine cultures per doctor request.
5. Utilize sterile technique for all dressing changes.
6. Assess for redness, swelling, warmth and intravenous sites.
7. Incorporate good handwashing techniques during care.
8. Administer prescribed anticoagulation therapy.
9. Evaluate prothrombin times daily.

Normal skin integrity and joint motion
1. Implement passive range of motion exercises with exception of extremity with IABP catheter.

2. Turn patient from side to side as a unit every two hours (patients are usually debilitated and prone to pressure sores).
3. Keep head of bed elevated 15 to 30 degrees or flat (catheter may migrate upward and obstruct left subclavian artery).

Minimum sleep deprivation
1. Manipulate environment to allow patient uninterrupted rest periods.
2. Monitor for signs/symptoms of ICU psychosis (hallucinations, disorientation).
3. Orient the patient to time and place as appropriate.
4. Keep the patient informed of progress of therapy.

Evaluation
EXPECTED OUTCOMES
1. Maintains hemodynamic stability: CI (cardiac index) greater than 2.4 litre/min/m^2, urine output greater than 30ml/hour, no chest pain.
2. Recognizes factors causing fear – expresses ability to cope with fears.
3. Free of preventable complications – peripheral pulses present, skin warm and colour normal, temperature within normal limits.
4. Maintains normal skin integrity and joint motion – absence of skin breakdown, able to perform active range of movements of extremities.
5. Experiences minimum sleep deprivation – sleeps five hours daily without interruption.

ENDOCARDIAL DISEASE

Endocarditis is an exudative and proliferative inflammatory alteration of the endocardium.

Infective endocarditis (bacterial endocarditis) is an infection of the valves and inner lining of the heart caused by direct invasion of bacteria or other organisms; leads to deformity of the valve leaflets.

AETIOLOGY
1. Bacteria:
   a. *Streptococcus viridans* – bacteraemia occurs after dental work or upper respiratory infection.
   b. *Staphylococcus aureus* – bacteraemia occurs after cardiac surgery or parenteral drug abuse.
   c. *Enterococci* (penicillin-resistant group D streptococci) – bacteraemia usually occurs in elderly (over 60) with genitourinary tract infection.
2. Fungi (*Candida albicans, Aspergillus*).
3. Rickettsiae.

ALTERED PHYSIOLOGY
1. Characterized by bacteria lodging on endocardium of valves (usually mitral and aortic). The bacteria multiply – fibrin and platelet thrombi are deposited, forming vegetations. The vegetations on the affected endocardial surface may embolize to various organs and tissues.
2. Formation of emboli may occur in spleen, kidney, central nervous system and lungs. Observe patient for petechiae of skin and mucous membranes.

CHARACTERISTICS
1. Infective endocarditis develops on a heart valve already injured by other disease or congenital defects.
2. May follow cardiac surgery, especially when prosthetic heart valves are used. (Foreign bodies, such as prosthetic valves, predispose to infection.)
3. High incidence among heroin addicts in whom the disease affects, for the most part, normal valves.
4. Hospitalized patients with indwelling catheters, those on prolonged intravenous therapy or prolonged antibiotic therapy, and those on immunosuppressive drugs or steroids may develop fungal endocarditis.
5. Rapid valvular destruction may lead to death.

Assessment
CLINICAL FEATURES
General
1. Fever, chills, sweats (fever may be absent in elderly or in patients with uraemia).
2. Anorexia, weight loss.
3. Cough; back and joint pain.
4. Splenomegaly.

Skin and nails
1. Splinter haemorrhages in nail beds.
2. Petechiae – conjunctiva, mucous membranes.
3. Roth's spots (haemorrhages with pale centres in the fundi of eyes).
4. Osler's nodes (painful red nodes on pads of fingers and toes).
5. Janeway's lesions (purplish macules on palms or soles).

Heart
Murmur – appearance of a new murmur or change in an old one.

Central nervous system

Headaches, transient cerebral ischaemia, focal neurological lesions, cerebrovascular accidents, encephalopathy, meningitis.

Embolic phenomena

Lung (recurrent pneumonia); kidney (haematuria); spleen; heart (myocardial infarction); brain (stroke); or peripheral vessels.

DIAGNOSTIC EVALUATION

1. Blood culture – serial blood cultures are drawn to document the presence of continuous bacteraemia and to determine aetiological agent.
2. Sensitivity studies – to determine the antibiotic for treatment.
3. Elevated erythrocyte sedimentation rate; anaemia; mild leucocytosis.
4. ECG.
5. Echocardiography – to follow ventricular dimensions, progressive cardiomegaly.

PATIENT PROBLEMS

1. Reduction in cardiac output related to structural factors (incompetent valves).
2. Impaired tissue perfusion related to embolic lesions/vasculitis.
3. Inadequate nutritional intake related to anorexia.
4. Anxiety related to acute illness and hospitalization.
5. Potential for injury related to complications of disease and therapy.

Planning and implementation

TREATMENT

Objectives

To eradicate the invading organisms by adequate doses of appropriate agent to kill every organism in every vegetation.

To prevent development of endocarditis in susceptible people.

1. Determine the causative organism by obtaining serial blood cultures.
2. Treat with bactericidal or other appropriate drugs based on proven sensitivity to causative agent.
   a. Bactericidal serum levels of selected antibiotic are monitored by titrating it against the causative organism; if the serum does not have adequate bactericidal activity more antibiotic or a different antibiotic is given.
   b. Blood cultures are taken periodically – to monitor adequacy of therapy.
   c. Intravenous route usually used for long-term administration of parenteral antibiotics.
      (i) Apply antibiotic ointment at needle entry site and cover with sterile dressing.
      (ii) Note the date of needle or cannula insertion on nursing care plan.
   d. Adequate dosages are necessary to kill every organism in every vegetation.
   e. Combinations of drugs may be used if adequate serum levels are not achieved with one drug.
   f. Treatment with amphotericin and surgery usually required for patient with fungal endocarditis.
3. Take temperature at regular intervals – course of fever is evaluated as one determinant of effectiveness of treatment.
4. Place patient in cardiac monitoring unit if patient is in heart failure or to detect cardiac dysrhythmias (secondary to involvement of heart conduction system of myocarditis).
5. Prepare for surgical intervention for:
   a. Heart failure secondary to perforation of aortic valve or to ruptured chordae tendinae or papillary muscle.
      (i) Onset of congestive heart failure carries a grave prognosis and is a major indication for surgery.
      (ii) Aortic valve predominantly involved.
   b. Excision of infected valves – for patients refractory to antibiotic therapy (particularly if resistant organisms involve either mitral or aortic valves).
   c. Excision of tricuspid valves – encountered with drug abusers.
   d. Removal of prosthetic valve or patch for patient with prosthetic valve endocarditis. (Be alert for new or changing murmurs.)
   e. Formation of emboli.
   f. Drainage of abscess/empyema – for patient with localized abscess or empyema.
   g. Repair of peripheral or cerebral mycotic aneurysm.

NURSING INTERVENTIONS

Attaining haemodynamic stability

1. Monitor blood pressure and pulse.
2. Assess jugular venous distention.
3. Record intake and output.
4. Record daily weight.
5. Place the patient on cardiac monitor if dysrhythmia is present.

Adequate tissue perfusion

1. Assess the patient for altered mentation, haemoptysis, haematuria, aphasia, loss of muscle strength, complaints of pain.
2. Observe for splinter haemorrhages of nailbeds, Osler's nodes, and Janeway's lesions.
3. Notify doctor of observed changes in the patient's status.

Improvement in nutritional status

1. Assess the patient's daily caloric intake.
2. Discuss food preferences with the patient.
3. Consult with a dietitian regarding nutritional needs of patient and food preferences.
4. Encourage small meals and snacks throughout the day.
5. Record daily caloric intake and weight.
6. Educate family members about the patient's caloric needs.
7. Encourage family members to assist the patient with meals and bring in the patient's favourite foods.

Reduction in anxiety

1. Encourage the patient to express fears regarding illness and hospitalization.
2. Educate the patient about disease process and therapy needed.
3. Explain all procedures to patient before initiation.
4. Offer the patient literature, if available, about his disease.
5. Encourage diversional activities for the patient such as television, reading and interaction with other patients.
6. Contact social worker to assist the patient with financial planning and home discharge arrangements if applicable.
7. Educate family members about the patient's disease and therapy.
8. Encourage family members to interact with the patient as frequently as possible.

Prevention of complications of disease

1. Observe basic principles of asepsis, good handwashing techniques and continuity of patient care by primary nurse.
2. Employ meticulous intravenous care for long-term antibiotic therapy.
   a. Note the date of needle or cannula insertion on nursing care plan.
3. Develop chart for rotation of sites for intramuscular administration of antibiotic therapy.
4. Take the patient's temperature at least twice a day and mark a graph.

5. Observe for side-effects of long-term antibiotic therapy – ototoxicity, renal failure.
6. Monitor laboratory values – hematocrit, creatinine, white blood cells.
7. Observe for signs and symptoms of embolic phenomena (see Clinical Features, p. 271), heart failure, mycotic aneurysms and neurological, haematological, and renal complications.
8. Prepare for surgical intervention for:
   a. Acute destructive valvular lesion – excision of infected valves or removal of prosthetic valve.
   b. Haemodynamic impairment.
   c. Recurrent emboli.
   d. Infection that cannot be eliminated with antibiotic therapy.
   e. Drainage of abscess/empyema – for patient with localized abscess or empyema.
   f. Repair of peripheral or cerebral mycotic aneurysm.

PATIENT EDUCATION

1. Develop in depth formal programme to educate individuals at risk regarding disease process, pathological manifestations, therapy and preventions.
   a. Discuss anatomy of heart and changes that occur during endocarditis, using diagrams of the heart.
   b. Give the patient written literature on early signs and symptoms of disease; review these with the patient.
   c. Discuss with individual the mode of entry of infection.
   d. Antibiotic prophylaxis is recommended for people at risk who are undergoing procedures most likely to cause bacteraemia (dental procedures causing gingival bleeding, surgery on or instrumentation of gastrointestinal tract, certain genitourinary procedures, etc).
   e. Identify individual steps necessary to prevent infection.
      (i) Good oral hygiene, regular tooth brushing and flossing.
      (ii) Notification to health-care staff of any history of congenital heart disease or valvular disease.
      (iii) Discuss importance of carrying emergency identification with information of medical history at all times.
      (iv) Take temperature if infection is suspected and notify doctor of elevation.
      (v) Teach individual to inspect soles of feet for Janeway's lesions indicative of possible relapse.

(vi) Educate people at risk to look for and treat symptoms of illness indicating bacteraemia – injuries, sore throats, furuncles, etc.

f. Discuss antibiotic prophylaxis – what it means and what individual must do to ensure his safety.

g. Encourage susceptible individuals to receive pneumococcal vaccine and influenza vaccines.
   (i) Teach that vaccines reduce the risk of severe infections that could precipitate heart failure.

h. Teach women in childbearing years the risks of utilizing IUDs for birth control (source of infection) and that antibiotic therapy is not necessary for individuals having normal deliveries.

2. Educate individuals who have had endocarditis regarding possible relapse.

a. Discuss importance of keeping follow-up appointments after hospital discharge (infection can recur in one to two months).

b. Review the tests that will be performed after hospital discharge – blood cultures, physical examination.

Evaluation
EXPECTED OUTCOMES
1. Maintains haemodynamic stability – exhibits no symptoms of heart failure.
2. Maintains satisfactory tissue perfusion – lack of signs/symptoms of embolic phenomena.
3. Demonstrates decrease in anxiety.
4. Achieves improved nutritional status – increases daily caloric intake compatible with height/weight/age.
5. Remains free of complications – normal temperature, negative blood cultures, normal white blood cell count, and creatinine, no hearing impairments.

RHEUMATIC HEART DISEASE

Rheumatic heart disease is the condition of progressive endocardial damage which occurs as a consequence of acute rheumatic fever. There is valvular deformity with associated compensatory changes in the size of the heart chambers and the thickness of their walls.

ROLE OF STREPTOCOCCAL INFECTION
Rheumatic fever is a self-limiting condition resulting from infection by group A haemolytic streptococci. Onset is usually one to three weeks post acute streptococcal respiratory infection. Period of latency and persistence of circulating antibodies to streptococci long after acute infection has subsided suggests an autoimmune or hyperimmune reaction.

Symptoms of haemolytic streptococcal infection
1. Sudden onset of sore throat; throat reddened with exudate.
2. Swollen, tender lymph nodes at angle of jaw.
3. Headache and fever 38.9–40°C.
4. Abdominal pain (children).

Note: Some cases of streptococcal throat infection are relatively asymptomatic.

Diagnostic evaluation
1. Throat culture – to determine presence of streptococcal organisms.
2. Increased sedimentation rate; white blood cell count and differential and C-reactive protein – increase during acute phase of infection.
3. Elevated antistreptolysin titre.

Treatment of streptococcal infection
1. Benzathine penicillin (single dose intramuscularly) or oral penicillin for 10 full days – to eradicate streptococci.
2. Erythromycin for patients sensitive to penicillin.

CLINICAL FEATURES OF RHEUMATIC FEVER
1. Polyarthritis; warm and swollen joints.
2. Carditis.
3. Chorea (irregular, jerky, involuntary, unpredictable muscular movements).
4. Erythema marginatum (wavy, thin red-line skin rash on trunk and extremities).
5. Subcutaneous nodules.
6. Fever.
7. Prolonged PR interval demonstrated by ECG.
8. Friction rub; mitral systolic murmur; aortic diastolic murmur.

LABORATORY TESTS
1. Increased erythrocyte sedimentation rate; white blood cell and differential and C-reactive protein – increase during acute phase of infection.
2. Positive antistreptolysin O (ASO) titre.

TREATMENT
The objectives of treatment are targeted toward eradicating the involved microorganism through antibiotic therapy, maintaining optimal cardiac function through rest, controlling fever and pain with salicylates, and preventing recurrent episodes of rheumatic fever in susceptible individuals.

NURSING MANAGEMENT

1. Limit physical activity during the acute phase – patient should rest in bed as long as there is fever or signs of active carditis.
2. Administer penicillin therapy – to eradicate haemolytic streptococcus; erythromycin may be used if the patient is allergic to penicillin.
3. Give salicylates to suppress rheumatic activity by controlling toxic features, to reduce fever, and to relieve joint pain.
4. Assess for effectiveness of drug therapy.
   a. Take and record temperature every 3–4 hours.
   b. Evaluate the patient's comfort level.
5. Monitor the patient's dietary intake (symptoms of disease inhibit the patient's ability to take in nutrients).
   a. Record the patient's daily caloric intake.
   b. Supplement diet with high-carbohydrate liquids if indicated.
6. Assess for signs/symptoms of acute rheumatic carditis.
   a. Be alert to the patient's complaints of chest pain, palpitations, and/or precordial 'tightness'.
   b. Monitor for tachycardia (usually persistent when the patient sleeps) or bradycardia.
   c. Be alert to development of second degree heart block or Wenckebach syndrome (acute rheumatic carditis causes PR interval prolongation).
7. Be aware of the possible complication of chronic rheumatic endocarditis. Chronic rheumatic endocarditis is a complication of rheumatic fever, which frequently produces progressive disability and a shortened life span. Every structural component of the heart is likely to be the site of an inflammatory reaction.
   a. Although the patient is symptom-free for a time, the damage to the valves (rigidity and deformity, thickening and fusion of the commissures, or shortening and fusion of chordae tendinae) will produce heart sounds that are characteristic of valvular stenosis, regurgitation, or both.
   b. The myocardium will compensate for these valvular defects for a while, but in time it fails to compensate, and the patient develops symptoms of congestive heart failure.
   c. See pp. 279–281 for treatment of valvular heart disease and pp. 285–291 for treatment of congestive heart failure.

PATIENT EDUCATION

1. Teach the patient the importance and ways of preventing a recurrence of rheumatic heart disease.
   a. Counsel the patient to maintain good nutrition.
      (i) Provide teaching on basic food groups.
      (ii) Assist with planning several daily meal plans.
      (iii) Discuss proper preparation of food (clean utensils and kitchen area) and proper storage of food.
      (iv) Discuss with the patient his financial situation and home facilities relative to nutritional health maintenance. If appropriate, contact social services for the patient.
   b. Counsel the patient on hygienic practices.
      (i) Discuss proper handwashing, disposal of tissues, laundering of handkerchiefs (decrease chance of exposure to microbes).
      (ii) Discuss importance of using patient's own tootbrush, soap and wash cloths when living in group situations.
   c. Counsel the patient on importance of receiving adequate rest.
   d. Counsel the patient to seek treatment immediately should sore throat occur.
2. Instruct the patient to utilize prophylactic penicillin therapy before undergoing surgery of genitourinary tract, lower intestinal tract, and respiratory tract.
3. See Patient Education, Endocarditis, pp. 273–274.

MYOCARDITIS

Myocarditis is an inflammatory process involving the myocardium.

AETIOLOGY
Follows infection:
1. Bacterial – beta-haemolytic streptococcus.
2. Viral – Coxsackie group, influenza, viral pneumonia, mumps, infectious mononucleosis.
3. Mycotic – blastomycosis, moniliasis.
4. Parasitic – trichinosis.
5. Protozoal – trypanosomiasis (Chagas' disease), malaria.
6. Spirochaetal – syphilis.

Assessment
CLINICAL FEATURES
Symptoms
1. Depend on type of infection, degree of myocardial damage, capacity of myocardium to recover and host resistance.
2. Fatigue and dyspnoea.
3. Palpitations.
4. Occasional precordial discomfort.

Clinical findings
1. Cardiac enlargement.
2. Cardiac murmur – abnormal heart sound; sounds like fluid passing an obstruction.
3. Pericardial friction rub.
4. Gallop rhythm – a tripling or quadrupling of heart sounds (resembling the galloping of a horse) heard upon auscultation.
5. Pulsus alternans – a pulse in which there is regular alternation of weak and strong beats.
6. Fever with tachycardia.
7. Evidence of development of heart failure.

Diagnostic evaluation
1. History of recent infection
2. Transient ECG changes – ST segment flattened, T wave inversion, conduction defects, supraventricular and ventricular ectopic beats.
3. Elevated white blood cells count and sedimentation rate.
4. Chest X-ray – may show heart enlargement and lung congestion.
5. Elevated antibody titres (antistreptolysin O [ASO titre] as in rheumatic fever).
6. Stool and throat cultures isolating bacteria or a virus.

PATIENT PROBLEMS
1. Potential complications of disease – heart failure and dysrhythmias.
2. Activity intolerance related to myocardial tissue damage.
3. Potential for ineffective coping (individual) related to life-threatening illness and hospitalization.

Planning and implementation
TREATMENT
Treatment objectives are targeted toward management of complications.
1. Diuretic and digoxin therapy for heart failure and atrial fibrillation.
2. Antidysrhythmic therapy (usually quinidine or procainamide).
3. Strict bed rest to promote healing of damaged myocardium.
4. Antibiotic therapy if causative bacteria is isolated.

NURSING INTERVENTIONS
Maintaining haemodynamic stability
1. Evaluate for clinical evidence that disease is subsiding – monitor pulse, auscultate for abnormal heart sounds (murmur or change in existing murmur), check temperature, auscultate lung fields, monitor respirations.
2. Record daily intake and output.
3. Record weight daily.
4. Check for peripheral oedema.
5. Elevate head of bed, if necessary, to enhance respiration.
6. Treat the symptoms of heart failure (see p. 284).
   a. Give digitalis – augments myocardial contractility and slows heart rate.
   b. Administer diuretics – to control pulmonary or systemic congestion.

NURSING ALERT
Patients with myocarditis may be sensitive to digitalis – assess for toxic symptoms (see pp. 316–317).

7. Evaluate the patient's pulse and apical rate for signs of tachycardia and gallop rhythm – indications that heart failure is recurring.
8. Evaluate for evidences of dysrhythmias – *patients with myocarditis are prone to develop dysrhythmias*.
   a. Place patient in unit with continuous cardiac monitoring if evidence of a dysrhythmia develops.
   b. See pp. 307–330 for management of dysrhythmias.
   c. Have equipment for resuscitation, cardiac defibrillation and cardiac pacing available in event of life-threatening dysrhythmia.

Strict bed rest
1. Place patient on bed rest to reduce heart rate, stroke volume, blood pressure and heart contractility; also helps to decrease residual damage and complications of myocarditis, and promotes healing.
   Prolonged bed rest may be required – until there is reduction in heart size and improvement of function.
2. Provide diversional activities for patient.
3. Allow the patient to use bedside commode rather than bedpan (reduces cardiovascular workload).

Effective coping with illness
1. Explore with the patient his fears, anxieties and concerns regarding illness and hospitalization.

2. Answer questions with a straightforward approach.
3. Discuss with the patient activities that can be continued after discharge.
   a. Discuss need to modify activities in immediate future.
   b. Explore with the patient lifestyle modifications and discuss adequacy of self-concept.
4. Emphasize the patient's strengths rather than limitations.
5. Encourage family members to support the patient and learn about his illness.
6. Discuss with family members their fears and anxieties relative to the patient's illness so that they will be able to communicate positively with the patient.

PATIENT EDUCATION
Instruct the patient as follows:
1. There is usually some residual heart enlargement; physical activity may be increased *slowly*, begin with chair rest for increasing periods of time; follow with walking in the room and then outdoors.
2. Report any symptom involving rapidly beating heart.
3. Avoid competitive sports, alcohol and other myocardial toxins.
4. Pregnancy is not advisable for women with cardiomyopathies (diseases that affect structure and function of myocardium).
5. Prevention – prevent infectious diseases by means of appropriate immunizations.

Evaluation
EXPECTED OUTCOMES
1. Maintains haemodynamic stability – respirations within range of 14 to 20, lung sounds clear on auscultation, normal sinus rhythm.
2. Adheres to strict bed rest.
3. Copes adaptively to illness – expresses ability to adapt to change in lifestyle imposed by illness, participates in self-care activities and health education programme, avoids maladaptive coping mechanisms such as strong denial, inappropriate grief, anger, depression.

PERICARDITIS

Pericarditis is an inflammation of the pericardium, the membranous sac enveloping the heart. It is a manifestation of a more generalized disease.

Pericardial effusion is an outpouring of fluid into the pericardial cavity.

Constrictive pericarditis is a condition in which a chronic inflammatory thickening of the pericardium compresses the heart so that it is unable to fill normally during diastole.

AETIOLOGY
1. Nonspecific:
   Usually occurs secondarily or as a complication of some other disease – uraemia, metastatic tumours, etc.
2. Infection:
   a. Bacteria – staphylococcus, meningococcus, streptococcus, pneumococcus, gonococcus, *Mycobacterium tuberculosis* (commonly follows rheumatic fever and pneumonia).
   b. Virus.
   c. Fungus.
3. Disorders of connective tissues and allergies – lupus erythematosus, periarteritis nodosa.
4. Myocardial infarction; early, 24 to 72 hours; or late, one week to two years (Dressler's syndrome).
5. Neoplastic processes; following irradiation of mediastinal tumours.
6. Chest trauma, particularly after heart surgery.
7. Drugs (procainamide; phenytoin).

Assessment
CLINICAL FEATURES
1. Pain in anterior chest, aggravated by thoracic motion – may vary from mild to sharp and severe; located in precordial area (may be felt beneath clavicle, neck, scapular region) – may be relieved by leaning forward.
2. Pericardial friction rub – scratchy, grating or creaking sound.
3. Dyspnoea – from compression of heart and surrounding thoracic structures.
4. Fever, sweating, chills – due to inflammation of pericardium.
5. Dysrhythmias.

DIAGNOSTIC EVALUATION
1. Echocardiogram – most sensitive method for detecting pericardial effusion.
2. Chest X-ray – may show heart enlargement.
3. ECG – to evaluate for myocardial infarction.
4. White blood cell and differential.
5. Antinuclear antibody serological tests and lupus erythematosus cell preparation – to rule out lupus erythematosus.
6. Purified protein derivative test – for tuberculosis; ASO titres – for rheumatic fever.

7. Pericardial aspiration for examination of peri-cardial fluid for aetiological diagnosis.
8. Serum urea and creatinine to evaluate uraemia.

NURSING ALERT

Normal pericardial sac contains less than 25–30ml of fluid; pericardial fluid may accumulate slowly without noticeable symptoms. However, a rapidly developing effusion can produce serious haemodynamic altera-tions.

TREATMENT

The objectives of treatment are targeted toward determining the aetiology, when known, and being alert to the possible complication of cardiac tamponade.

PATIENT PROBLEMS

1. Chest pain related to pericardial inflammation.
2. Potential for complications – cardiac tamponade and constrictive pericarditis.

Planning and implementation

NURSING INTERVENTIONS

Reducing discomfort

1. Evaluate the patient's complaint of chest pain.
   a. Ask the patient if pain is aggravated by breathing, turning in bed, twisting body, coughing, yawning or swallowing.
   b. Elevate head of bed; position pillow on over-the-bed table so that the patient can lean on it.
      (i) Assess if above intervention relieves the patient's chest pain (associated pleuritic pain of pericarditis is usually relieved by sitting up and/or leaning forward).
      (ii) Be alert to the patient's medical diagnoses when assessing pain. Postmyocardial in-farction patients may experience a dull, crushing pain radiating to neck, arm, and shoulders, mimicking an extension of in-farction (Dressler's syndrome).
2. Give prescribed drug regimen for pain and symptomatic relief.
   a. Nonsteroidal anti-inflammatory drugs (NSAIDs, aspirin, indomethacin) – suppress inflammatory symptoms of acute pericarditis.
   b. Corticosteroids – for more severe symptoms.
3. Give specific therapy when the cause is known.
   a. Bacterial pericarditis – penicillin or other anti-microbial agents.
   b. Rheumatic fever – procaine penicillin, pred-nisone.
   c. Tuberculosis – antituberculosis chemotherapy

(see p. 984). (There is a high incidence of con-striction in tuberculosis pericarditis.)
   d. Fungal pericarditis – amphotericin B.
   e. Disseminated lupus erythematosus – adrenal steroids.
   f. Uraemic pericarditis – dialysis, indomethacin, biochemical control of uraemia.
   g. Neoplastic pericarditis – intrapericardial in-stillation of chemotherapy: radiotherapy.
   h. Postmyocardial infarction syndrome – bed rest, aspirin, prednisone.
      (i) Relieve anxiety of the patient and family by explaining the difference between pain of pericarditis and pain of recurrent myocardial infarction (patients may fear extension of myocardial tissue damage).
      (ii) Explain to the patient and family that peri-carditis does not indicate further heart damage.
   i. Postpericardiotomy syndrome (after open heart surgery) – treat symptomatically.
4. Encourage the patient to remain on bed rest when chest pain, fever and friction rub occur.

Avoiding complications

1. Be alert to the possibility of cardiac tamponade (see Pericardiocentesis, pp. 229–233).
   a. Assess for falling arterial pressures and rising venous pressure.
   b. Note presence of paradoxical pulse.
   c. Prepare the patient for immediate pericardio-centesis (see Pericardiocentesis, pp. 229–233).
2. Be cognizant of other complications of pericarditis – heart failure, dysrhythmias, haemopericardium (complication in postmyocardial infarction pa-tients on anticoagulation therapy).
3. Be alert for signs/symptoms of pericarditis when administering procainamide or phenytoin (agents may induce a lupus-like syndrome with peri-carditis).
4. Prepare the patient for surgical intervention (direct pericardial decompression) – for patient with cardiac embarrassment associated with con-strictive pericarditis.

PATIENT EDUCATION

1. Teach patient the aetiology of pericarditis.
2. Instruct patient about signs/symptoms of peri-carditis and the need for long-term medication therapy to help relieve symptoms.
3. Review all medications with the patient – pur-pose, side-effects, dosage and special pre-cautions.
4. Evaluate the patient's understanding by asking

the patient to define understanding by asking the patient to define pericarditis, the medications necessary for therapy, and the side-effects and correct dosage of medications.

Evaluation
EXPECTED OUTCOMES
. Experiences minimal discomfort – no chest pain.
. Experiences no complications – respirations 14 to 18 times per minute, no dyspnoea, no apprehension or acute anxiety.

ACQUIRED VALVULAR DISEASE OF THE HEART

CAUSES
. Rheumatic fever.
. Congenital aortic stenosis.
. Traumatic lesions of aortic valve.
. Syphilis.

ALTERED PHYSIOLOGY
. Inflammatory process→thickening and retraction of valve cusps→fusion and shortening of chordae tendinae→inadequate closure of valve.
. Mitral valve most commonly involved, followed by aortic, tricuspid and pulmonary valves.
. Patients with valvular disease usually develop heart failure in time.

TYPES OF VALVULAR DISEASE
. Aortic stenosis.
. Aortic incompetence.
. Mitral stenosis.
. Mitral incompetence.
. Tricuspid stenosis.
. Tricuspid incompetence.

Assessment
DIAGNOSTIC EVALUATION
. Chest X-ray – to determine size and shape of heart.
. ECG – to detect atrial and ventricular hypertrophy, myocardial infarction; to diagnose disturbances of rhythm.
. Fluoroscopy – to detect intracardiac calcification.
. Echocardiography – can visualize abnormal valves (mitral, aortic) and chamber enlargement.
. Cardiac catheterization.
   a. To observe and record intracardiac pressure and oxygen saturation of blood in each heart chamber.

   b. To receive information regarding presence of shunts.
   c. To calculate cardiac output.
6. Angiography – used as part of diagnostic cardiac catheterization and to confirm diagnosis.

PATIENT PROBLEMS
1. Decreased cardiac output related to mechanical factors (preload, afterload, contractility).
2. Activity intolerance related to reduced oxygen available for energy.
3. Potential for ineffective coping related to acute and chronic illness.

Planning and implementation
NURSING INTERVENTIONS
Maintaining adequate cardiac output
1. Assess the patient for possible complications that would compromise cardiac function. Implement treatment protocols for these complications (heart failure, infective endocarditis, rheumatic heart disease).
2. Prepare the patient for surgical intervention, if indicated (see Management of Patient for Heart Surgery, pp. 293–300).

Improvement in coping ability
1. Instruct the patient regarding specific valvular dysfunction, possible aetiology, and therapies implemented to relieve symptoms.
   a. Include family members in discussions with the patient.
   b. Stress the importance of adapting lifestyle to cope with illness.
   c. Discuss with the patient surgical intervention as the treatment method, if applicable (see Heart Surgery, pp. 293–300).
2. Assess the patient's use of appropriate coping mechanisms to deal with illness.
   Spend some time daily with the patient, allowing him to express concerns and ask questions.
3. Refer the patient to appropriate counselling services, if indicated (vocational, social work, cardiac rehabilitation).

PATIENT EDUCATION
See Patient Education, Heart Failure, pp. 288–291; Infective Endocarditis, pp. 273–274; and Rheumatic heart disease, p. 275.

Evaluation
EXPECTED OUTCOMES
1. Maintains adequate cardiac output – blood pressure and heart rate within normal limits for

patient, respirations unlaboured on exertion at 14 to 18 per minute, no cough or sputum production, no chest pain, fatigue minimal (rests between activities of daily living, says that fatigue has not worsened).
2. Copes adaptively to illness.

AORTIC STENOSIS

Aortic stenosis is a narrowing of the orifice between the left ventricle and the aorta. The obstruction to the aortic outflow places a pressure load on the left ventricle that results in hypertrophy and failure. It is often caused by rheumatic fever or arteriosclerosis, or it may be congenital.

CLINICAL FEATURES
1. Exertional dyspnoea and fatigue.
2. Dizziness and fainting – from reduced blood supply to brain.
3. Angina pectoris.
4. Low blood pressure and low pulse pressure – from diminished blood flow.
5. Dysrhythmias.
6. Symptoms of heart failure.

DIAGNOSTIC EVALUATION
1. Chest X-ray – usually shows left ventricular enlargement.
2. Cardiac catheterization
3. Angiocardiography
4. Echocardiography

will reveal the pressures in the left ventricle and aorta.

TREATMENT
1. Surgical replacement of aortic valve – prosthetic device or aortic valve homograft. See pp. 294–300 for care of patient undergoing heart surgery.
2. Treat angina and heart failure as dictated by patient's condition.

AORTIC INCOMPETENCE

Aortic incompetence (regurgitation) is caused by inflammatory lesions that deform the flaps so that they fail to completely seal the aortic orifice during diastole and thus permit a backflow of blood from the aorta into the left ventricle.

It may be caused by rheumatic endocarditis, bacterial endocarditis or congenital malformation, or from diseases which cause dilatation or tearing of the ascending aorta (syphilitic disease, rheumatoid spondylitis, dissecting aneurysm).

CLINICAL FEATURES
1. Dyspnoea: exertional dyspnoea, paroxysmal nocturnal dyspnoea.
2. Chest pain.
3. Palpitations; patient is aware of overactivity of heart.
4. Diastolic murmur.
5. Symptoms of heart failure.

DIAGNOSTIC EVALUATION
1. ECG – shows pattern of left ventricular hypertrophy.
2. Chest X-ray – reveals varying degrees of cardiomegaly from left ventricular enlargement.
3. Echocardiography – estimates size and thickness of left ventricle.
4. Cardiac catheterization and angiography.

TREATMENT
Surgical intervention – replacement of damaged aortic valve. See pp. 294–300 for nursing management of patient undergoing heart surgery.

MITRAL STENOSIS

Mitral stenosis is the progressive thickening and contracture of valve cusps with narrowing of the orifice and progressive obstruction to blood flow. It is a late manifestation of rheumatic damage to the endocardium.

CLINICAL FEATURES
1. Dyspnoea; excessive fatigue.
2. Pulmonary congestion, haemoptysis, cough, orthopnoea.
3. Characteristic murmurs – increased first heart sound, opening snap and low pitched rumbling diastolic murmur heard at the apex.
4. Dysrhythmias – palpitations during exercise; atrial fibrillation.
5. Angina pectoris.
6. Systemic embolism.
7. Hoarseness (due to compression of left recurrent largyngeal nerve).

DIAGNOSTIC EVALUATION
1. ECG – shows evidence of left atrial enlargement, right ventricular hypertrophy.
2. Echocardiography – can demonstrate valve

thickening, calcification and abnormal, slowed diastolic valve excursion.
. Cardiac catheterization and angiocardiography.

TREATMENT
. Medical treatment.
   a. Prevent rheumatic recurrences with antibiotic therapy.
   b. Treat the developing heart failure – digitalis, sodium restriction, limitation of activity (see pp. 285–290).
   c. Control atrial fibrillation.
2. Surgical intervention may be accomplished by:
   a. Closed mitral valvotomy – introduction of dilator or fingers through left ventricular apex into valve to split its commissures.
   b. Open mitral valvotomy – direct incision of the commissures.
   c. Mitral valve replacement.
   d. See pp. 294–300 for the management of the patient undergoing heart surgery.

MITRAL INCOMPETENCE

Mitral incompetence (regurgitation) is the result of incompetence and distortion of the mitral valve so that the free margins can no longer come into apposition during systole. The chordae tendinae may become shortened, preventing complete closure of the leaflets. This may be caused by mitral value prolapse, chronic rheumatic heart disease, post-infarction or infective endocarditis.

CLINICAL FEATURES
1. Shortness of breath on exertion, fatigue, cough.
2. Dysrhythmias.
3. Systolic murmur – heard in left axilla.
4. Cardiac enlargement.

DIAGNOSTIC EVALUATION
1. Chest X-ray – shows enlarged left atrium.
2. ECG – may reveal evidence of both left ventricular and left atrial enlargement.
3. Angiocardiography and cardiac catheterization – confirm diagnosis.

TREATMENT
Surgical intervention – replacement with prosthetic device, either ball valve or disc type. This procedure is done when there is extensive calcification and destruction of the chordae tendinae.

TRICUSPID STENOSIS

Tricuspid stenosis is restriction of the tricuspid valve orifice due to commissural fusion and fibrosis usually following rheumatic fever. It is commonly associated with diseases of the mitral valve.

CLINICAL FEATURES
1. Dyspnoea, nocturnal dyspnoea, orthopnoea.
2. Haemoptysis.
3. Visible pulsations of neck veins.
4. Murmurs – similar to those of rheumatic mitral disease; blowing diastolic murmur along left sternal border.
5. Symptoms of right-sided heart failure (late).

DIAGNOSTIC EVALUATION
1. ECG – may reveal atrial fibrillation.
2. Cardiac catheterization and angiocardiography – to confirm diagnosis.

TREATMENT
1. Patient may have mitral and aortic disease which must be corrected.
2. Surgical treatment of accompanying tricuspid valve disease may be carried out at the time of operation after correction of mitral valve disease.

TRICUSPID INCOMPETENCE

Tricuspid incompetence allows the regurgitation of blood from the right ventricle into the right atrium during ventricular systole.

CLINICAL FEATURES
1. Right-sided heart failure – from overload of right ventricle.
2. Oedema – with congestion of liver and hepatic malfunction, ascites, hydrothorax.
3. Elevated venous pressure.
4. Atrial fibrillation.
5. Pansystolic murmur in tricuspid area.

TREATMENT
1. Surgical treatment of mitral valve disease or combined mitral and aortic valve disease – may reverse pulmonary hypertension and produce disappearance of tricuspid regurgitation.
2. Replacement of tricuspid valve may be indicated.

NORMAL AND ABNORMAL HEART SOUNDS

NORMAL HEART SOUNDS

1. The 'lub-dub' of the heart is heard clearly through the stethoscope and are usually described as S_1 and S_2.
   a. S_1, the first sound, is the closing of both the atrioventricular valves, and the mitral and tricuspid just before ventricular systole, i.e. S_1 is the 'lub' of the 'lub-dub'.
   b. S_2, the second sound, is the closing of both semilunar valves, the aortic and the pulmonary, just before diastole, i.e. S_2 is the 'dub' of 'lub-dub'.

2. The sounds of S_1 and S_2 differ in loudness at each valve location.
   a. Begin listening at the apex of the heart by listening to the mitral and tricuspid valves for S_1.
   b. Then move to the base over the aortic and pulmonary valves for S_2.

3. Note location, timing, quality, intensity and pitch of any murmur.
   a. Murmurs are graded I to VI, grade I being the faintest.
   b. **Note:**
      (i) The rate and rhythm of the heart.
      (ii) The quality of the first heart sound – normal, accentuated, diminished.

Table 5.5 Abnormal heart sounds*

Sound	Abnormality	Mechanism	Examples
S_1	Louder than normal	1. Valve wide open	Short PR interval, ectopic beats, tachycardia, mitral or tricuspid stenosis
		2. Prolonged ventricular filling	Left to right shunts
	Softer than normal	1. Valve partly closed	First degree AV block
		2. Valve prematurely closed	Severe hypertension
		3. Normal tensing impossible due to leak	Mitral or tricuspid incompetence.
		4. Damping of sound	Thick chest, pericardial effusion
S_2	Persistent or paradoxical split	1. Asynchronous ventricular activation	
		a. Block of bundle branch	RBBB (persistent split), LBBB (paradoxical split)
		b. Ectopy	Left ventricular (persistent), right ventricular (paradoxical)
		2. Prolonged ejection on one side of heart	
		a. Systolic overload	Pulmonary stenosis or hypertension (persistent), aortic stenosis or systemic hypertension (paradoxical)
		b. Diastolic overload	Pulmonary incompetence (persistent), atrial septal defect (persistent), ventricular septal defect (persistent), aortic incompetence (paradoxical), patent ductus arteriosus (paradoxical)
		c. Other	Right ventricular failure (persistent), left ventricular failure (paradoxical), myocardial infarction (paradoxical), angina (paradoxical)
		3. Two outlets for ventricular ejection	Mitral incompetence (persistent), ventricular septal defect (persistent), tricuspid incompetence (paradoxical)

Single sound	1. One component decreased	Severe aortic or pulmonary stenosis
	2. Aortic valve anterior	Tetralogy of Fallot
	3. Murmur obscuring A$_2$	Atrial septal defect, patent ductus arteriosus, pulmonary stenosis
Presence	1. Diastolic overloading of ventricles	Valvular incompetence, atrial septal defect (RV), left to right shunts (LV), high output states†
	2. Decreased ventricular compliance and/or increased ventricular diastolic pressure	Ventricular failure, ischaemic heart disease, constrictive pericarditis, cardiomyopathies
Presence	1. Systolic overloading of ventricles	Aortic or pulmonary stenosis, hypertension (systemic or pulmonary)
	2. Systolic overloading of right atrium	Tricuspid stenosis
	3. Decreased ventricular compliance and/or increased ventricular diastolic pressure	Mitral incompetence, ventricular failure, ischaemic heart disease, cardiomyopathies
	4. Systemic diseases	Severe anaemia, severe infections
	5. First degree AV block	

Adapted from Marriott, H. (1967) *Differential Diagnosis of Heart Disease*, Oldmar, Tampa Tracings, Florida.
RV = right ventricular overloading; LV = left ventricular overloading.

(iii) Compare the second sound at the aortic valve (A$_2$) with the second sound at the pulmonary valve (P$_2$) – A$_2$ is normally louder than P$_2$ in normal young adults, but in older people they are equal.

ABNORMAL HEART SOUNDS

See Table 5.5.

A third heart sound, S$_3$, may be heard early in diastole.

a. S$_3$ is a ventricle flow sound that usually occurs in a dilated ventricle.
b. It is caused by rapid return of blood from the vena cava.
c. Is best heard when the patient is lying on his left side.
d. With slow heart rate S$_3$ sounds like the 'Y' in Kentucky.
   With fast heart rate S$_1$, S$_2$ and S$_3$ sound like a galloping horse, hence the term 'gallop rhythm'.
e. S$_3$ is normal in young adult or adolescent. In any other case it probably means left ventricular failure.

A fourth heart sound, S$_4$, may be heard late in diastole.

a. S$_4$ is an atrial flow sound.

b. It is best heard under the same conditions as S$_3$.
3. a. S$_3$ occurs just after S$_2$; S$_4$ occurs just before S$_1$.
   b. A combination of S$_3$ and S$_4$ (a summation gallop) is a loud single sound that occurs in mid-diastole.
   c. **Note:**
      (i) Listen to one sound at a time.
      (ii) Use bell and diaphragm of the stethoscope when examining the heart.
      (iii) Auscultation is not fully established as part of the nurses' role in the UK except in some specialist units.

HEART FAILURE

Heart failure is the inability of the heart to pump the amount of oxygenated blood necessary to effect venous return and to meet the metabolic requirements of the body.

Bilateral heart failure is the occurrence of circulatory congestion due to decreased myocardial contractility; as a result, cardiac output is inadequate to maintain the blood flow to body organs and tissues. This ultimately causes sodium and water retention and elevation of left atrial pressure, which results in pulmonary vascular congestion.

CAUSES
1. Secondary to heart disease: coronary athero-sclerosis, hypertension, valvular heart disease, congenital heart disease, diffuse myocardial disease, dysrhythmias.
2. Pulmonary embolism; chronic lung disease.
3. Haemorrhage and anaemia.
4. Anaesthesia and surgery.
5. Transfusions or infusions.
6. Thyrotoxicosis.
7. Pregnancy.
8. Infections.
9. Physical and emotional stress.
10. Excessive sodium intake.

Assessment
CLINICAL FEATURES
Initially there may be either left or right ventricular failure, but in time the other ventricle fails because of the additional workload. The patient usually has a combination of symptoms; any system may be involved.

Left-sided heart failure
1. Congestion occurs mainly in the lungs from dam-ming back of blood into pulmonary veins and capillaries.
   a. Shortness of breath, dyspnoea on exertion, paroxysmal nocturnal dyspnoea (due to re-absorption of dependent oedema that has de-veloped during day), orthopnoea, pulmonary oedema.
   b. Cough – may be dry, unproductive; often occurs at night.
2. Fatigue – from insomnia, nocturia, dyspnoea, cough, low cardiac output.
3. Insomnia.
4. Tachycardia – S_3 ventricular gallop.
5. Restlessness.

Right-sided heart failure
Signs and symptoms of elevated pressures and congestion in systemic veins and capillaries:
1. Oedema of ankles; unexplained weight gain.
   Pitting oedema – is obvious only after retention of at least 4.5kg of fluid.
2. Liver congestion – may produce upper abdominal pain.
3. Distended neck veins.
4. Abnormal fluid in body cavities (pleural space, abdominal cavity).

5. Anorexia and nausea.
6. Nocturia – diuresis occurs at night with rest an improved cardiac output.
7. Weakness.
8. Oliguria.
9. Confusion.

COMPLICATIONS
1. Intractable or refractory heart failure – patie becomes progressively refractory to therapy (n yielding to treatment).
2. Cardiac dysrhythmias.
3. Myocardial failure.
4. Digitalis toxicity – from decreased functio potassium depletion, etc.
5. Pulmonary infarction; pneumonia.

DIAGNOSTIC EVALUATION
1. Cardiovascular findings.
   a. Cardiomegaly (hypertrophy of heart) – d tected by physical examination and che X-ray.
   b. Ventricular gallop – evident on auscultatio ECG.
   c. Rapid heart rate.
   d. Development of pulsus alternans.
   e. Distended neck veins.
   f. Hepatomegaly (enlargement of the liver).
2. ECG.
3. Chest X-ray – to evaluate heart size; show lur fields (for pleural effusion) and vascular conge tion.
4. Arterial blood gas studies.
5. Liver function studies – may be altered due hepatic congestion.

PATIENT PROBLEMS
1. Decreased cardiac output related to mechanic factors (contractility, preload, afterload).
2. Impaired gas exchange related to inadequa ventilation/perfusion ratio.
3. Body fluid excess related to continued sodiu and water retention.
4. Activity intolerance related to inability of heart deliver adequate oxygen supply to muscle.
5. Disturbance in sleep pattern related to anxie and restlessness.

Planning and implementation
TREATMENT
The objectives of treatment are targeted toward r ducing the work of the heart through promotion rest, increasing the force and efficiency of myocardi contraction through administration of pharma

biological agents, and eliminating excessive accumulation of body water by use of diuretics and sodium
restriction.

NURSING INTERVENTIONS
Maintaining adequate cardiac output

Place patient at physical and emotional rest to
reduce work of heart.

a. Provide rest in semi-recumbent position or in
armchair in air-conditioned environment – reduces work of heart, increases heart reserve,
reduces blood pressure, decreases work of
respiratory muscles and oxygen utilization,
improves efficiency of heart contraction; recumbency promotes diuresis by improving
renal perfusion.

b. Provide bedside commode – to reduce work of
getting to bathroom and for defaecation.

c. Provide for psychological rest – emotional
stress produces vasoconstriction, elevates
arterial pressure, and speeds the heart.

  (i) Promote physical comfort.

  (ii) Avoid situations that tend to promote
  anxiety/agitation.

  (iii) Offer careful explanations and answers to
  the patient's questions.

d. Assess the patient's response to rest; are his
symptoms alleviated?

Evaluate frequently for progression of left ventricular failure.

a. Take frequent blood pressure readings.

  (i) Observe for lowering of systolic pressure.

  (ii) Note narrowing of pulse pressure.

b. Assess peripheral arterial pulses frequently.

  (i) Note alternations in strong and weak
  pulsations (pulsus alternans).

  (ii) Document findings of assessment.

  (iii) Monitor for premature ventricular beats.

c. Observe for signs/symptoms of reduced
peripheral tissue perfusion – cool temperature
of skin, facial pallor, poor capillary refill of
nailbeds.

Administer drugs as described below.

Digitalis therapy

Administer digitalis (a cardiac glycoside) as prescribed – to increase the force of myocardial contraction and produce a stronger systolic contraction of
the heart and to slow the heart rate. This results in
increased cardiac output; decreased heart size,
venous pressure and blood volume; diuresis and
relief of oedema. Digitalis is also used to slow the
ventricular rate in the setting of supraventricular
dysrhythmias.

1. A loading (digitalizing) dose may be given in
order to induce the full therapeutic effect of the
drug when rapid digitalization is necessary.

2. Otherwise, the patient is started without a loading dose. The patient is then given a daily dose
just adequate to replace the drug that is destroyed
or excreted – to maintain digitalis effect without
toxicity.

3. *Digitalis preparations* (choice of drug depends on
speed of onset and duration of action required
and on individual patient response):

a. Oral –
Digoxin
Digitoxin
Lanatoside C

b. Parenteral –
Digoxin
Ouabain
Digitoxin

4. Be alert to factors that may cause increased sensitivity to digitalis:

a. Myocardial infarction, particularly ischaemia.

b. Potassium depletion.

c. Kidney or hepatic disease.

d. Diuretic therapy.

e. Diarrhoea.

f. Loss of appetite.

g. Advancing age.

h. Hypoxia and hypercapnia in pulmonary
disease.

i. Acidosis; alkalosis.

5. Monitor serum concentration of digitalis. Digitalis
assay may be measured by laboratory for
therapeutic guidance and to assess for toxicity.

6. Monitor serum potassium levels and ECGs, especially in patients receiving digitalis and diuretics. *There is a predisposition to dysrhythmias if the
state of potassium balance is not evaluated and corrected.*

7. Assess clinical response of patient with respect to
relief of symptoms (lessening dyspnoea and
orthopnoea, decrease in crackles, relief of
peripheral oedema).

8. Watch for toxic effects – *dysrhythmias* (most important toxic effect), *anorexia,* nausea, vomiting,
diarrhoea, bradycardia, headache, malaise,
behavioural changes, increasing failure.

NURSING ALERT
*The incidence of digitalis toxicity is high because of the
narrow margin between therapeutic and toxic doses.
Toxic effects do not always appear in a predictable
manner. Digitalis toxicity has a high mortality rate.*

9. Take pulse and apical heart rate before administering each dose of digitalis.
   Withhold digitalis and notify doctor if following is noted:
   a. Slowing of rate.
   b. Change in rhythm – bradycardia, ventricular ectopic beat, bigeminy (two pulse beats following in rapid succession), atrial fibrillation.*
   c. Dangerous cardiac dysrhythmias require immediate treatment (see pp. 317–327).

Vasodilator therapy and inotropic agents (for heart failure unresponsive to usual therapy)

1. Rationale: vasodilators are used to increase cardiac output by dilating the peripheral vascular vessels and reducing impedance (resistance) to left ventricular outflow.
   a. By relaxing capacitance vessels (veins and venules), vasodilators reduce ventricular filling pressures (preload) and volumes.
   b. By relaxing resistance vessels (arterioles), vasodilators can reduce impedance to left ventricular ejection and improve stroke volume.
2. Vasodilators used in congestive heart failure:
   a. Nitrates (GTN, isosorbide dinitrate) – predominantly dilates systemic veins.
   b. Nitroprusside – dilator effect on both arterial and venous beds.
   c. Hydralazine – predominantly affects arterioles; reduces arteriolar tone.
   d. Prazosin – balanced effects on both arterial and venous circulation.
3. Invasive haemodynamic monitoring is often used to guide drug administration (see pp. 221–229).

NURSING ALERT
Watch for sudden unexpected hypotension, which can cause myocardial ischaemia and decrease perfusion to vital organs.

---

* Regularization of the rate in a patient with chronic atrial fibrillation should be a warning that digitalis intoxication may be present.

4. Inotropic agents:
   a. Dobutamine – directly increases myocardial contractility.
   b. Digitalis.
5. Combinations of above drugs used.

Achieving an improved ventilation/perfusion ratio

1. Raise head of bed 20–30cm – reduces venous return to heart and lungs; alleviates pulmonary congestion.
   a. Support lower arms with pillows – to eliminate pull of their weight on shoulder muscles.
   b. Sit orthopnoeic patient on side of bed with feet supported by a chair, head and arms resting on an over-the-bed table, and lumbosacral area supported with pillows.
2. Observe for increased rate of respirations (could be indicative of falling arterial pH).
3. Observe for Cheyne-Stokes respirations (may occur in elderly because of a decrease in cerebral perfusion stimulating a neurogenic response).
4. Position the patient every two hours (or encourage the patient to change position frequently) – to help prevent atelectasis and pneumonia.
5. Encourage deep breathing exercises every one to two hours – to avoid atelectasis.
6. Offer small, frequent feedings – to avoid excessive gastric filling and abdominal distention with subsequent elevation of diaphragm that causes decrease in lung capacity.

Decreasing excessive body fluid

Administer prescribed diuretic (agent that increases the rate of urine flow).

1. Type and dosage of diuretic administered depends on degree of heart failure and state of renal function (Table 5.6).
2. Give diuretic early in the morning – night-time diuresis disturbs sleep.
3. Keep input and output record – the patient may lose large volume of fluid after a single dose of diuretic.

Table 5.6   Frequently used diuretics

Definition
1. Diuretics are agents which increase rate of urine flow

Action
1. Dependent on functionally active kidneys; most diuretics decrease the reabsorption of electrolytes (principally sodium) by the kidneys and promote water loss as a secondary action
2. In the treatment of hypertension the natriuretic (sodium excretion) effect is probably the action of importance
3. In oedema states the salt and water effects are both important

Dosage determination
(1) Patient's daily weight; (2) clinical signs and symptoms; (3) physical examination; (4) state of renal function

Diuretic	Action	Nursing implications
Thiazides (benzothiazine derivatives)		
Chlorothiazide Hydrochlorothiazide Hydroflumethiazide Bendrofluazide	Increases renal excretion of sodium (natriuresis), potassium, chloride, bicarbonate (alkaline urine) with accompanying 'osmotic' water loss Most widely used for prolonged administration	Watch for side-effects from electrolyte imbalance; hypokalaemia (weakness and fatigue), hyperuricaemia, hyperglycaemia, nausea and vomiting diarrhoea, abdominal cramps, dizziness, paraesthesias Give supplementary potassium
Potassium-sparing diuretics		
Spironolactone	Inhibits action of aldosterone in distal tubule and reduces reabsorption of sodium and chloride Gives gradual diuretic effect Used in treatment of cirrhosis and oedema when other diuretics are toxic or ineffective	Usually used in combination with thiazide diuretic Watch for side-effects – skin rash, gynaecomastia
Triamterene	Appears to interfere with exchange of sodium for potassium and H^+ in the distal tubule	Usually used as an adjunct to thiazide therapy May cause elevation in blood urea levels Watch for nausea, vomiting, diarrhoea, weakness, headache and skin rash
Potent diuretics		
Frusemide Ethacrynic acid	Usually reserved for patients who do not respond to classical thiazide diuretics Blocks the reabsorption of sodium and water in proximal renal tubule and interferes with reabsorption of sodium in ascending limb of loop of Henle and in the most proximal portion of the distal tubule Associated with sodium, potassium, chloride and hydrogen on loss (acid urine) Frusemide has an almost immediate action when given intravenously Ethracynic acid; maximum activity is reached in 2 hours and diuresis persists 6–8 hours	Potent and rapid-acting Especially useful in acute pulmonary oedema *May produce profound diuresis* with elevation of blood urea Watch for nausea, vomiting, diarrhoea, skin rash, pruritis, blurring of vision, postural hypotension, vertigo, hearing loss Frusemide is chemically related to sulphonamides; consider cross allergies Administer early in the day to avoid nocturia and consequent loss of sleep
Osmotic diuretics		
Urea Mannitol (most commonly used)	Substances given in hypertonic solution by vein, excreted by the kidneys; because of limitation of kidney to reabsorb or concentrate them, water loss is obligatory Substances given by vein in hypertonic solutions that slowly cross the blood–brain barrier; thus the osmotic gradient across the blood–brain barrier results in an outward translocation of water from the brain tissue	May be used to treat oedema of the brain, especially in acute head injury with rapid swelling of the brain

4. Weigh the patient daily – to determine if oedema is being controlled; weight loss should not exceed 0.45–0.9kg per day.
5. Assess for weakness, malaise, muscle cramps – diuretic therapy may produce hypovolaemia and electrolyte depletion, namely *hypokalaemia*. Hypokalaemia may cause weakening of cardiac contractions and may precipitate digitalis toxicity in the form of dysrhythmias.
6. Give oral potassium as prescribed.
7. Be aware that problems associated with diuretic administration include disorders of potassium balance, hyperuricaemia, volume depletion and hyponatraemia, magnesium depletion, hyperglycaemia and diabetes mellitus.
8. Watch for signs of bladder distension in the elderly male with prostatic hyperplasia.
9. Assess for symptoms of electrolyte depletion – lassitude, apathy, mental confusion, anorexia, decreasing urinary output.
10. Limit intravenous fluid administration through use of heparin lock (allows for periodic drug administration without increasing excessive fluid intake).
11. Assess for pitting oedema of lower extremities and sacral area.
    Use aids such as sheepskin to prevent pressure sores (poor blood flow and oedema increase susceptibility).
12. Observe for the complications of bed rest – pressure sores (especially in oedematous patients), phlebothrombosis, pulmonary embolism.
13. Be alert to complaints of right upper quadrant abdominal pain, poor appetite, nausea and abdominal distension (may indicate hepatic and visceral engorgement).
14. Monitor the patient's diet. Diet may be limited in sodium – to prevent, control, or eliminate oedema; may also be limited in calories.
    a. Patients on diuretics may not be on sodium-restricted diet.
    b. Caution patients to avoid added salt in food and foods with high sodium content.

Establishing a balance between oxygen supply and demand

1. Increase the patient's activities gradually. Alter or modify the patient's activities – to keep within the limits of his cardiac reserve.
   a. Assist the patient with self-care activities early in the day (fatigue sets in as day progresses).
   b. Be alert to complaints of chest pain or skeletal pain during or after activities.

2. Observe the pulse, symptoms and behavioural response to increased activity.
   a. Monitor the patient's heart rate during self care activities.
   b. Allow heart rate to decrease to pre-activity level before initiating a new activity.
      (i) Note time lapse between cessation of activity and decrease in heart rate (decreased stroke volume causes immediate rise in heart rate).
      (ii) Document time lapse and revise patient care plan as appropriate (progressive increase in time lapse may be indicative of increased left ventricular failure).
   c. Ask the patient about degree of fatigue experienced during and after activities.

Achieving adequate rest

1. Relieve night-time anxiety and provide for rest and sleep – patients with heart failure have a tendency to be restless at night because of cerebral hypoxia with superimposed nitrogen retention.
   a. Give oxygen during acute stage – to diminish work of breathing and increase the comfort of the patient.
   b. Give appropriate sedation – to relieve insomnia and restlessness.
      (i) Give small doses of diamorphine as prescribed for extreme dyspnoea.
      (ii) Give mild sedation as needed for sleep. Use sedation carefully to prevent respiratory depression; detoxification of drugs is delayed because of hepatic congestion and immobility of patient.
   c. Keep a night light on in the room; the presence of a family member provides reassurance to some persons.
   d. Avoid restraints – resistance to restraints increases cardiac load.

PATIENT EDUCATION

1. Explain the disease process to the patient; the term 'failure' may have terrifying implications.
   a. Explain the pumping action of the heart – 'to move blood through the body to provide nutrients and aid in the removal of waste material'.
   b. Explain the difference between 'heart attack' and heart failure.
2. Teach the signs and symptoms of recurrence.
   a. Ask patient to recall how he felt when he first became ill.
   b. Watch for:
      (i) Gain in weight – report weight gain of

more than 0.9–1.4kg in a few days. Weigh at same time daily to detect any tendency toward fluid retention.

  (ii) Swelling of ankles, feet or abdomen.

  (iii) Persistent cough.

  (iv) Tiredness; loss of appetite.

  (v) Frequent urination at night.

Review medication regiment.

a. Label all medications.

b. Give written instructions concerning digitalis and diuretic therapy.

c. Inform patient not to substitute another brand of digitalis for the one he is taking.

  (i) Make sure the patient has a check-off system that will show that he has taken his medications.

  (ii) Teach the patient to take and record his pulse rate.

  (iii) Inform the patient of the signs and symptoms of digitalis toxicity and potassium depletion.

d. Tell the patient to weigh himself daily and log his weight if he is on diuretic therapy.

Review activity programme.

Instruct the patient as follows:

a. Increase walking and other activities gradu-ally, provided they do not cause fatigue and dyspnoea.

b. In general, continue at whatever activity level can be maintained without the appearance of symptoms.

c. Avoid excesses in eating and drinking.

d. Undertake a weight reduction programme until optimal weight is reached.

e. Avoid extremes in heat and cold – which increase the work of the heart; air conditioning may be essential in a hot, humid environment.

f. Keep *regular* appointment with doctor or clinic.

5. Restrict sodium as directed (Table 5.7).

a. Give patient a booklet containing sodium content of common foods.

b. Give patient a written diet plan with list of permitted and restricted foods.

c. Advise patient to look at all labels to ascertain sodium content (antacids, laxatives, cough remedies, etc).

  (i) Teach the patient to rinse the mouth well after using tooth cleansers and mouthwashes – some of these contain large amounts of sodium.

  (ii) Teach the patient that sodium is present in

Table 5.7 Sodium-restricted diet* (500 mg; 1,800 calories)†

Category	Allowed	To be avoided
Dairy products		
Milk	2 glasses	Salt or monosodium glutamate
Cheese	¼ cup unsalted cottage cheese	Ice cream
	130 gm low sodium dietetic cheese	Sherbet
Fat	Unsalted butter or margarine	Malted milk
	Unsalted cooking fat or oil	Milk shakes
	Unsalted French dressing	Chocolate milk
	Unsalted mayonnaise	Condensed milk
	Unsalted nuts	Butter or margarine
	Heavy or light cream	Commercial salad dressing
Eggs	1 egg daily	Bacon or bacon fat
		Olives
		Salted nuts
		Party spreads and dips
Meat, fish, fowl	Fresh, frozen or dietetic canned meat or poultry; beef, lamb, pork, veal, fresh tongue, liver, chicken, duck, turkey, rabbit	Brains or kidneys
		Canned, salted or smoked meat (bacon, salami, corned or chopped beef, frankfurters, ham, meats koshered by salting, luncheon meats, salt pork, sausage, smoked tongue)
	Fresh or dietetic canned (not frozen) fish	Frozen fish fillets; canned, salted or smoked fish; canned tuna or salmon
		Shellfish – clams, crabs, lobsters, oysters, scallops, prawns, shrimps, etc

Table 5.7   Continued

Category	Allowed	To be avoided
Vegetables	Fresh, frozen or canned dietary vegetables (except those listed)	Canned vegetables or vegetable juices unless they are low sodium dietetic Frozen vegetables if processed with sa[lt] Artichokes, carrots, celery, spinach, white turnips
Fruits	Any fruit or fruit juice (if sugar has not been added)	Fruits canned or frozen in sugar (because of the extra calories)
Breads, cereals, cereal products	Low sodium bread, rolls, crackers Dry cereals (puffed rice, puffed wheat, shredded wheat) Unsalted melba toast Macaroni or noodles Spaghetti, rice, barley Unsalted popcorn Flour	Regular breads, crackers Commercial mixes Cooked cereals containing a sodium compound Dry cereals other than those listed or those having more than 6mg of sodium in 100g of cereal Self-raising flour Potato crisps
Miscellaneous	Coffee, tea, coffee substitutes, lemons. limes, plain unflavoured gelatine, vinegar, cream of tartar, potassium bicarbonate, sodium-free baking powder, yeast	Instant cocoa mixes; other beverage mixes, including fruit-flavoured powders; malted milk; soft drinks (both regular and low calorie); sodium cyclamate and sodium saccharin; commercial sweets; commercial gelatin desserts; regular baking powder; baking soda (sodium bicarbonate); rennet tablets; molasses; pudding mixes

* From Sodium-restricted diet, 500mg, American Heart Association.

† For a 250mg sodium diet, use low sodium milk (either low sodium whole milk or low sodium powdered milk) instead of ordinary milk.

For 1,000mg sodium diet, follow 500mg sodium diet, plus one of the following for the additional 500mg of sodium:

¼ teaspoon salt
¾ teaspoon monosodium glutamate
1 cup tomato juice

Average serving of cooked cereal, rice, spaghetti, noodles, etc., seasoned with salt
1 average frankfurter
42g ham

cough remedies, laxatives, pain relievers, oestrogens, etc.

d. Ascertain the amount of sodium in the local drinking water through inquiry to local water authority.

6. Advise the patient to accept the fact that restricting sodium and taking digitalis will be permanent part of his lifestyle.

7. Teach the patient the importance of adhering to

the low-sodium diet.

a. Sodium is present in many types of natura[l] foods and in varying amounts in processe[d] foods.

b. Make the diet as palatable as possible.
   (i) Use flavourings, spices, herbs and lemo[n] juice.
   (ii) Avoid salt substitutes in the presence o[f] renal disease.

Evaluation
EXPECTED OUTCOMES
1. Maintains adequate cardiac output – normal blood pressure and heart rate (no hypotension, tachycardia or cool clammy skin).
2. Exhibits improved ventilation/perfusion ratio – respiratory rate 16 to 20, arterial blood gases within normal limits, no signs of crackles or wheezes in lung fields.
3. Demonstrates a decrease in body fluid – weight decrease of 2.2kg daily, no pitting oedema of lower extremities and sacral area.
4. Maintains balance between oxygen supply and demand – heart rate within normal limits, rests between activities – checks heart rate after activities, if elevated more than 10 beats above pre-activity heart rate, waits until heart rate decreases before next activity.

ACUTE PULMONARY OEDEMA

Acute pulmonary oedema refers to the presence of excess fluid in the lung, either in the interstitial spaces or in the alveoli. It usually follows acute left ventricular failure.

NURSING ALERT
Acute pulmonary oedema is a true medical emergency since it is a life-threatening condition.

CAUSES
1. Heart disease: acute left ventricular failure, myocardial infarction, aortic stenosis, severe mitral valve disease, hypertension, heart failure.
2. Circulatory overload – transfusions and infusions.
3. Drug hypersensitivity; allergy; poisoning.
4. Lung injuries – smoke inhalation, shock lung, pulmonary embolism or infarct.
5. Central nervous system injuries – stroke, head trauma.
6. Infection and fever.

Assessment
CLINICAL FEATURES
1. Coughing and restlessness during sleep (premonitory symptoms).
2. Extreme dyspnoea and orthopnoea – patient usually uses accessory muscles of respiration with retraction of intercostal spaces and supraclavicular areas.
3. Cough with varying amounts of white- or pink-tinged frothy sputum.
4. Extreme anxiety and panic.
5. Noisy breathing – inspiratory and expiratory wheezing and bubbling sounds.
6. Cyanosis with profuse perspiration.
7. Distended neck veins.
8. Tachycardia.
9. Cardiac asthma.

DIAGNOSTIC EVALUATION
1. Medical history, physical examination.
2. Chest X-ray.
3. Echocardiogram (suspected valvular disease).
4. Measurement of pulmonary artery wedge pressure by Swan–Ganz catheter (differentiates aetiology of pulmonary oedema – cardiogenic or altered alveolar-capillary membrane).
5. Blood cultures (suspected infection).
6. Cardiac enzymes (suspected myocardial infarction).

PATIENT PROBLEMS
1. Impaired gas exchange related to inadequate ventilation/perfusion ratio.
2. Altered breathing patterns (dyspnoea, orthopnoea, wheezing) related to excess fluid in the lungs.
3. Anxiety related to sensation of suffocation.

Planning and implementation
TREATMENT
The objective of treatment is to improve ventilation and oxygenation and to reduce pulmonary congestion. Strategy for management is initiation of nonspecific measures* (i.e. oxygen therapy, diamorphine sulphate administration, patient in upright position), identification of precipitating factors (i.e. myocardial infarction, infection), and correction of factors contributing to underlying condition.

NURSING INTERVENTIONS
Improved oxygenation
1. Give oxygen in high concentration – to relieve hypoxia and dyspnoea.
   a. Oxygen may be given with high enough pressure to provide blood oxygenation and to overcome the pressure barrier of the oedema fluid.
   b. This is accomplished by giving oxygen by intermittent or continuous pressure.
2. *Take steps to reduce venous return to the heart.*
   Place patient in upright position; head and

---

* Many of the nonspecific measures are implemented simultaneously.

shoulders up, feet and legs hanging down – to favour pooling of blood in dependent portions of body by gravitational forces; to decrease venous return.

3. Give diamorphine in small titrated intermittent doses (intravenously) until dyspnoea lessens – to allay acute anxiety and decrease respiratory effort, allowing better oxygen exchange; this also decreases peripheral resistance so that blood can be redistributed from the pulmonary circulation to the periphery.
   a. Diamorphine is *not* given if pulmonary oedema is caused by cerebrovascular accident or occurs in the presence of chronic pulmonary disease or cardiogenic shock.
   b. Watch for excessive respiratory depression.
   c. Monitor blood pressure, since diamorphine may intensify hypotension.
   d. Have diamorphine antagonist available – naloxone hydrochloride (Narcan).

4. Give injections of diuretic intravenously (ethacrynic acid; frusemide) – to reduce blood volume and pulmonary congestion by producing prompt diuresis.
   a. Insert an indwelling catheter – large urinary volume will accumulate rapidly.
   b. *Watch for falling blood pressure, increasing heart rate and decreasing urinary output – indications that the total circulation is not tolerating diuresis and that hypovolaemia may develop.*
   c. Check electrolyte levels, since potassium loss may be significant.
   d. Watch for signs of urinary obstruction in men with prostatic hyperplasia.

5. Administer vasodilator if patient fails to respond to therapy – to reduce impedance (resistance) to left ventricular ejection of blood; allows more complete ventricular emptying and increases venous capacity so that left ventricular filling pressure is reduced. Patient monitored by measuring pulmonary artery pressure and cardiac output.
   Nitroprusside or sublingual GTN usually prescribed by doctor (see Failure, p. 286).

6. Assist doctor with phlebotomy if indicated for treatment.
   a. *Phlebotomy* is the rapid withdrawal of approximately 500 ml of blood from peripheral vein.
   b. Phlebotomy aids in decreasing venous return and produces a corresponding decline in right ventricular output.
   c. Phlebotomy is usually done to reduce intravascular pressure when attack is precipitated

by overadministration of blood or infusion fluids.

7. Administer dobutamine as prescribed by doctor.
8. Aminophylline may be given when indicated to relieve bronchospasm.
   a. Monitor blood levels of drug.
   b. Assess the patient for side effects of drug – ventricular dysrhythmias, hypotension, headache.
9. Administer cardiac glycosides (digitalis) (usually prescribed in treating pulmonary oedema secondary to myocardial infarction).
10. Assist with cardioversion if indicated (pulmonary oedema precipitates tachycardias).
11. Give appropriate drugs for severe, sustained hypertension.
12. Continually evaluate the patient's response to therapy.

Decrease in anxiety

1. Stay with the patient and display a confident attitude – the presence of another person is therapeutic, since the acute anxiety of the patient may tend to intensify the severity of his condition. (Arterial vasoconstriction diminishes as anxiety is relieved.)
2. Explain to the patient in a calm manner all therapies administered and the reason for their use.
   a. Give brief explanations related to goal of therapies (i.e. 'Diamorphine will help you relax and ease your work of breathing').
   b. Explain to the patient the importance of wearing oxygen mask. Assure the patient that mask will not increase sensation of suffocation.
3. Inform the patient and family of progress toward resolution of pulmonary oedema.
4. Allow time for the patient and family to ventilate concerns and fears.

PATIENT EDUCATION
During convalescence, instruct the patient as follows in order to prevent recurrences of pulmonary oedema:

1. Ask: What symptoms did you have before the attack? (He should be aware of these.)
2. If coughing develops (a wet cough), sit with legs dangling over side of bed.
3. See Patient Education, Heart Failure, pp. 288–291.

Evaluation
EXPECTED OUTCOMES
1. Attains improved oxygenation – unlaboured respirations at 14 to 18 times per minute, lungs clear

on auscultation, blood gases within normal limits for patient, no cough or sputum.
2. Achieves decrease in anxiety – appears calm; rests comfortably.

HEART SURGERY

NURSING PROCESS OVERVIEW

Assessment

PATIENT HISTORY

1. Review the patient's record to learn past history and present condition, paying close attention to pulmonary, renal, hepatic, haematological and metabolic systems.
   a. Cardiac history; *history of cardiac dysrhythmias*.
   b. Pulmonary health – patients with COAD (chronic obstructive airways disease) may require prolonged postoperative respiratory support.
   c. Depression – can produce a serious postoperative depressive state and can affect postoperative morbidity and mortality.
   d. Ask about previous/present alcohol intake; smoking history.
2. Assess laboratory studies.
   a. Complete blood count; serum electrolytes; lipid profile; a nose, throat, sputum and urine cultures.
   b. Antibody screen.
   c. Preoperative coagulation survey (platelet count, prothrombin time, partial thromboplastin time) – extracorporeal circulation will affect certain coagulation factors.
   d. Renal and hepatic function tests.
3. Assess the patient's reactions to medications – these patients are usually on multiple drugs.
   a. Digitalis:
      (i) Patient may be receiving large doses to improve myocardial contractility.
      (ii) Drug may be stopped several days before surgery – to avoid digitoxic dysrhythmias from cardiopulmonary bypass.
   b. Diuretics:
      (i) Assess the patient for potassium depletion and volume depletion (weakness, postural hypotension) – diuretics may produce potassium loss, and severe diuresis may cause a decrease in blood volume.
      (ii) Give potassium supplement if the patient is on prolonged diuretic therapy – to replenish body stores.
      (iii) Diuretics may be omitted several days preoperatively to avoid electrolyte imbalance and consequent dysrhythmias postoperatively. Salt and water restriction may be advised.
   c. Beta-adrenergic blockers (propranolol) – continue as directed.
   d. Psychotropic drugs (diazepam; chlordiazepoxide) – postoperative withdrawal may cause extreme agitation.
   e. Antihypertensives (reserpine) – omitted as far in advance of procedure as possible to allow noradrenaline repletion.
   f. Alcohol – sudden withdrawal may produce delirium.
   g. Anticoagulant drugs – discontinued several days before operation to allow coagulation mechanism to return to normal.
   h. Determine if the patient has taken corticosteroids within the year prior to surgery – patients on steroids are given supplemental doses to cover stress of surgery.
   i. Prophylactic antibiotics may be given preoperatively.
   j. Determine whether the patient has any drug sensitivities.
4. Be aware of the preoperative conditions that predispose to postoperative respiratory complications:
   a. Pulmonary hypertension.
   b. Pulmonary congestion or oedema.
   c. Pre-existing lung disease.
   d. Pulmonary sepsis.
   e. Elderly or debilitated patient.
5. Encourage the patient to stop smoking – smoking increases incidence of postoperative respiratory complications.
6. Surgical preparation:
   a. Shave anterior and lateral surfaces of trunk and neck; shave entire body down to ankles (for coronary bypass).
   b. Shower/bathe with antiseptic soap.

PATIENT PROBLEMS

1. Anxiety related to fear of unknown, fear of death and fear of pain.
2. Potential for impaired gas exchange related to inadequate ventilation/perfusion ratio.
3. Potential for decreased cardiac output related to manipulation of heart during surgery.

4. Potential for fluid and electrolyte disturbances related to heart–lung machine.
5. Potential for sensory overload related to excessive environmental stimuli.
6. Potential for complications – dysrhythmias, cardiac tamponade, myocardial infarction, hypovolaemia and embolization.
7. Pain related to sternotomy and leg incisions.

Planning and implementation
PREOPERATIVE NURSING INTERVENTIONS
Decrease in anxiety
1. Evaluate the patient's emotional state and try to reduce his anxieties – patients undergoing heart surgery are more anxious and fearful than other surgical patients. (Moderate anxiety assists patient to cope with stresses of surgery. Low anxiety level may indicate that the patient is using denial. High anxiety may impair the patient's ability to learn and listen.)
    a. Offer support to patients with low or high anxiety states. Give support by being present, by listening, and by showing interest – patient is called upon to deal with a stressful and life-threatening crisis.
    b. Encourage the patient to express what he feels and thinks – ventilation of feelings and fantasies relieves sense of isolation and facilitates a growing and supportive relationship.
        (i) Try to elicit special concerns.
        (ii) Patients with unusual degree of anxiety and history of mental illness may require psychiatric consultation.
        (iii) Patients with low levels of anxiety may have stormy postoperative course – have not prepared themselves for stress of surgery.
        (iv) Patients with characteristics of type A personality (competitive striving for achievement, sense of time urgency, aggressiveness and hostility) may be extremely anxious because of sudden role reversal; attempt to meet needs with explanations of objectives of surgery and probable postoperative experience.
    c. Help the patient and family to mobilize defences and cope with fears.
    d. Clarify the information given the patient previously by the cardiovascular surgeon.
        (i) Ask the patient to state why surgery is necessary.
        (ii) Give the patient pamphlet on heart surgery to reinforce discussions with

health care team and to review with family members.
    e. Anticipate and answer the patient's questions.
        (i) Ask the patient what he wants to know.
        (ii) Establish a relationship of trust.
    f. Support the patient undergoing diagnostic studies to determine type and severity of specific lesions; tests also provide a baseline for postoperative evaluation.
        (i) Cardiac catheterization and angiography.
        (ii) Pulmonary function studies.
        (iii) ECG, echocardiogram, phonocardiogram.
        (iv) Exercise stress testing.
        (v) Chest X-ray.
    g. Expect some patients to have psychological and psychiatric problems from prolonged illness.

Preoperative teaching
1. Prepare the patient for events in the postoperative period.
    a. Take the patient and family on tour of intensive care unit – lessens anxiety about being there.
        (i) Introduce the patient to staff personnel who will be caring for him.
        (ii) Give family a schedule of visiting hours and times for phone contact.
    b. Teach chest physical therapy procedures – to optimize pulmonary function.
        (i) Encourage the patient to practise with incentive spirometer.
        (ii) Show and practise diaphragmatic breathing techniques.
        (iii) Encourage the patient to practise effective coughing, leg exercises.
    c. Prepare patient for presence of monitors, chest tubes, intravenous lines, blood transfusion, endotracheal tube, nasogastric tube, pacing wires, arterial line, indwelling catheter.
        (i) Explain to the patient that two chest tubes will be inserted below incision into chest cavity for drainage and maintenance of negative pressure.
        (ii) Explain to the patient that endotracheal tube will prevent speaking, but that he will be able to communicate through writing until tube is removed (usually within 24 hours).
        (iii) Explain to the patient that his diet will consist of liquids until 24 hours after surgery.
        (iv) Explain to the patient that monitoring equipment and intravenous lines will re-

strict movement, and nursing staff will position the patient comfortably every two hours and as necessary.

d. Discuss with the patient the need to monitor vital signs frequently and the likelihood of frequent disturbances of the patient's rest.

e. Discuss pain management with the patient.

   (i) Explain to the patient that median sternotomies require one-third as much analgesia for relief of the patient's pain than do abdominal incisions.

   (ii) Assure the patient that analgesics will be administered as necessary to control pain.

2. Tell the patient that both hands may be loosely restrained for a number of hours after surgery to eliminate possibility of pulling out tubes and intravenous lines inadvertently.

3. Discuss with the patient surgical preparation for the day of scheduled surgery and the night prior to it.

   a. Shave anterior and lateral surfaces of trunk and neck. (Shave entire body down to ankles for coronary bypass.)

   b. Explain to the patient that sedatives will be given before he goes to the operating room.

4. Encourage the patient to stop smoking – smoking increases chance of postoperative respiratory complications.

5. Document preoperative teaching done and the patient's behaviour and level of understanding before and after teaching. Record specifically what the patient was taught.

POSTOPERATIVE NURSING INTERVENTIONS

1. Orient the patient to surroundings as soon as he awakens from surgical procedure. Tell the patient that operation is over, where he is, the time of day and your name.

2. Allow family members to visit the patient as soon as his condition stabilizes. Encourage family members to talk to and touch the patient (family members may be overwhelmed by critical care environment).

3. As the patient becomes more alert, remind him of the purpose of all the equipment in his environment. Continually orient the patient to time and place (let the patient know if it is day or night).

Adequate oxygenation

1. Secure all connections for lines and tubes (arterial, Swan–Ganz, CVP, chest tubes, urinary catheter to collecting bottle, endotracheal tube to ventilator, ECG to monitoring system, pacing wires, etc).

2. Provide for tissue oxygenation and assess respiratory status. Ensure adequate oxygenation in early postoperative period; respiratory insufficiency is common following open heart surgery.

a. Use assisted or controlled ventilation (see p. 116) – respiratory support is used during first 24 hours to provide airway in the event of cardiac arrest, to decrease work of heart, to maintain effective ventilation.

   (i) Adequacy of ventilation is assessed by the patient's clinical status and by direct measurement of tidal volume and arterial blood gases.

   (ii) Check endotracheal tube placement.

   (iii) Arterial blood gas analysis (see p. 105) is usually performed during first hour postoperatively and whenever necessary thereafter.

   (iv) Sedate patient adequately – to help him tolerate endotracheal tube and cope with ventilatory sensations.

   (v) Use chest physiotherapy for patients with lung congestion to prevent retention of secretions and atelectasis.

       (a) Promote coughing, deep breathing and turning – to keep airway patent, prevent atelectasis, and facilitate lung expansion.

   (vi) Suction tracheobronchial secretions carefully (see p. 153) – prolonged aspiration leads to hypoxia and possible cardiac arrest.

   (vii) Restrict fluids for first few days – danger of pulmonary congestion from excessive fluid intake.

   (viii) Chest X-ray taken immediately after surgery and daily thereafter – to evaluate state of lung expansion and to detect atelectasis; to demonstrate heart size and contour, confirm placement of central line, endotracheal tube, and chest drains.

   (ix) See p. 168 for weaning process and endotracheal tube removal.

Adequate cardiac output

1. Use haemodynamic monitoring* during immediate postoperative period, especially for cardiovascular and respiratory status and fluid and

---

* Monitoring equipment is valuable only when it is understood and used correctly. The clinical assessment of the patient by the nurse is indispensable to patient care.

electrolyte balance – to prevent complications or to recognize them as early as possible.

2. Monitor cardiovascular status to determine effectiveness of cardiac output with haemodynamic monitoring. Serial readings of blood pressure and arterial pressure, heart rate, central venous pressure and left atrial or pulmonary artery pressure from monitor modules are observed, correlated with the patient's condition and recorded.

   a. Assess arterial pressure every 15 minutes until stable and as directed thereafter – blood pressure is one of the most important physiological parameters to follow.

      (i) Take direct measurement (arterial line, transducer) – most accurate blood pressure.

      (ii) Extreme vasoconstriction following extracorporeal circulation makes auscultatory blood pressure unobtainable.

   b. Check peripheral pulses (pedal, tibial, radial) as a further check on heart action.

      (i) Palpate the carotid, brachial, popliteal and femoral pulses; absence of these pulses may be due to recent catheterization of the extremity.

   c. Measure left atrial pressure or pulmonary artery wedge pressure – to determine the left ventricular end-diastolic volume and to assess cardiac output (see pp. 226–229).

      (i) Rising pressures may indicate heart failure or pulmonary oedema.

   d. Take central venous pressure readings hourly (see pp. 221–225) – indicate blood volume, vascular tone and pumping effectiveness of the heart.

      (i) High central venous pressure reading may result from hypervolaemia, heart failure, cardiac tamponade. Ventilator may elevate central venous pressure.

      (ii) If blood pressure drop is due to low blood volume, central venous pressure will show corresponding drop.

      (iii) *Changes* in values are more important than isolated readings.

3. Check urine output every half to one hour (from indwelling catheter) – urine output is an index of cardiac output and renal perfusion. Continue with ongoing patient assessment.

   a. Observe buccal mucosa, nail beds, lips, ear lobes and extremities for duskiness/cyanosis – signs of low cardiac output.

   b. Feel the skin; cool, moist skin reveals lowered cardiac output. Note temperature and colour of extremities.

   c. Note fullness and tone of superficial veins of feet; evaluate pedal and femoral pulses.

   d. Assess for venous distention of neck veins or veins of dorsal surface of hands (raised above level of heart) – may signal a changing demand or diminishing capacity of heart.

   e. Evaluate temperature.

4. Assess neurological status – the brain is dependent on a continuous supply of oxygenated blood and must rely on adequate and continuous perfusion by the heart.

   a. Hypoperfusion or microemboli (air debris) may produce CNS damage after heart surgery.

   b. Observe for symptoms of hypoxia – restlessness, headache, confusion, dyspnoea, hypotension and cyanosis.

   c. Assess the patient's neurological status hourly in terms of:

      (i) Level of responsiveness.

      (ii) Response to verbal commands and painful stimuli.

      (iii) Pupillary size and reaction to light.

      (iv) Movement of extremities; handgrasp ability.

   d. Treat postoperative convulsive seizures. Give medications according to therapeutic directives – coronary vasodilators, antibiotics, analgesics, anticoagulants (patients with prosthetic valves).

Fluid and electrolyte balance

1. Maintain fluid and electrolyte balance – adequate circulating blood volume is necessary for optimal cellular activity; metabolic acidosis and electrolyte imbalance can occur after use of pump oxygenator.

   a. Fluids may be limited to avoid overloading.

   b. Keep intake and output flow sheet – as a method of determining positive or negative fluid balance and the patient's fluid requirements.

      (i) Intravenous fluids (including flush solutions through arterial and venous lines) considered intake.

      (ii) Assess hydration status of patient – evaluation of pulmonary wedge, left atrial pressure and central venous pressure readings; weight, electrolyte levels, hematocrit readings, distention of neck veins, tissue oedema, liver size, breath sounds.

      (iii) Record urine output every half to one hour.

(iv) Measure postoperative chest drainage – should not exceed 200ml/hour for first four to six hours.

    (a) Watch for sudden cessation of chest drainage – from kinked or blocked chest tube.

    (b) See page 204 for management of patient with water-seal drainage.

2. Be alert to changes in serum electrolytes – a specific concentration of electrolytes is necessary in both extracellular and intracellular body fluids in order to sustain life.

  a. *Hypokalaemia* (low potassium level):

    (i) May be caused by inadequate intake, diuretics, vomiting, excessive nasogastric drainage, stress from surgery.

    (ii) Effects of low potassium level – dysrhythmias, digitalis toxicity, metabolic alkalosis, weakened myocardium, cardiac arrest.

    (iii) Watch for specific ECG changes.

    (iv) Give intravenous potassium replacement as directed.

  b. *Hyperkalaemia* (high potassium level):

    (i) May be caused by increased intake, red cell breakdown from the pump, acidosis, renal insufficiency, tissue necrosis and adrenal cortical insufficiency.

    (ii) Effects of high potassium level – mental confusion, restlessness, nausea, weakness and paraesthesia of extremities.

    (iii) Be prepared to administer an ion-exchange resin, sodium polystyrene sulphonate, which binds the potassium, or give intravenous sodium bicarbonate or intravenous insulin and glucose to drive the potassium back into the cells from the extracellular fluid.

  c. *Hyponatraemia* (low sodium):

    (i) May be due to reduction of total body sodium or to an increased water intake causing a dilution of body sodium.

    (ii) Assess for weakness, fatigue, confusion, convulsions and coma.

  d. *Hypocalcaemia* (low calcium level):

    (i) May be due to alkalosis (which reduces the amount of Ca^{++} in the extracellular fluid) and multiple blood transfusions.

    (ii) Signs and symptoms of reduced calcium levels – numbness and tingling in the fingertips, toes, ear and nose, carpopedal spasm, muscle cramps and tetany.

    (iii) Give replacement therapy as directed.

  e. *Hypercalcaemia* (high calcium level):

    (i) May cause dysrhythmias imitating those caused by digitalis toxicity.

    (ii) Assess for signs of digitalis toxicity.

    (iii) Institute treatment as directed – this condition may lead to asystole and death.

Decrease in discomfort

1. Examine sternotomy incision and leg dressings.

2. Relieve the patient's pain – cardiac surgical patients experience pain caused by sternotomy incision and irritation of pleura by chest tubes.

  a. Record nature, type, location, and duration of pain – pain and anxiety increase pulse rate, oxygen consumption and cardiac work.

  b. Differentiate between incisional pain and anginal pain.

  c. Watch for restlessness and apprehension – may be from hypoxia or a low-output state; analgesics or sedatives do not correct this problem.

  d. Administer medication as often as prescribed – to reduce amount of pain and to aid the patient in performing deep breathing and coughing exercises more effectively.

    (i) Reassure the patient that staff understands that treatment is painful and that it is acceptable to be angry.

    (ii) Encourage the patient to talk about his experience.

Mental and psychological orientation

Postcardiotomy delirium – may appear after a brief lucid period.

1. Symptoms:

  a. Psychotic disturbances are more frequent after heart operations with extracorporeal circulation than after general surgery.

  b. Signs and symptoms include delirium (impairment of orientation, memory, intellectual function, judgement), transient perceptual distortions, visual and auditory hallucinations, disorientation and paranoid delusions.

  c. Symptoms may be related to sleep deprivation, increased sensory input, disorientation to night and day, prolonged inability to speak because of endotracheal intubation, age, preoperative cardiac status, etc.

2. Keep the patient oriented to time and place; notify the patient of procedures and expectations of his co-operation. Give repeated explanations of what is happening.

3. Encourage family to come in at regular times – helps the patient regain sense of reality.

4. Plan care to allow rest periods, day–night pattern, and uninterrupted sleep.

5. Encourage mobility as soon as possible. Keep environment as free as possible of excessive auditory and sensory input. Prevent bodily injury.
6. Reassure the patient and his family that psychiatric disorders following cardiac surgery are usually transient.
7. Remove the patient from intensive care unit as soon as possible. Allow patient to express events of his psychotic episode – helps him deal with and assimilate experience.

Avoidance of complications

1. *Cardiac dysrhythmias:*
   a. Watch ECG monitor – cardiac dysrhythmias frequently occur after heart surgery.
      (i) Ventricular ectopic beats occur most frequently following aortic valve replacement and coronary bypass surgery. May be treated with pacing, lignocaine, potassium.
      (ii) Dysrhythmias also apt to occur with ischaemia, hypoxia, alterations in serum potassium, oedema, bleeding, acid–base or electrolyte disturbances, digitalis toxicity, myocardial failure.
      (iii) Observe other parameters in correlation with monitor information – a low serum potassium level makes the heart susceptible to ventricular dysrhythmias.
      (iv) See pp. 307–327 for discussion of cardiac dysrhythmias.
2. *Cardiac tamponade* – results from bleeding into the pericardial sac or accumulation of fluids in the sac, which compresses the heart and prevents adequate filling of the ventricles.
   a. Assess for signs of tamponade – arterial hypotension, rising central venous pressure, rising left atrial pressure, muffled heart sounds, weak, thready pulse, neck vein distention, falling urinary output.
   b. Check for diminished amount of drainage in the chest-collection bottle; may indicate that fluid is accumulating elsewhere.
   c. Prepare for pericardiocentesis (see pp. 229–233).
3. *Myocardial infarction:*
   a. Check cardiac enzymes daily – elevations may indicate myocardial infarction.
   b. Symptoms may be masked by the usual postoperative discomfort.
      (i) Watch for decreased cardiac output in the presence of normal circulating volume and filling pressure.
      (ii) Obtain serial ECGs and isoenzymes to determine extent of myocardial injury.
      (iii) Assess pain to differentiate myocardial pain from incisional pain.
   c. Treatment is individualized. Postoperative activity level may be reduced to allow heart adequate time for healing.
4. *Cardiac failure* (low-output syndrome) – causes deficient blood perfusion to different organs.
   a. Observe for falling mean arterial pressure, rising filling pressures (central venous pressure, PCW, or LAP), and increasing tachycardia; the patient may exhibit signs of restlessness and agitation, cold and blue extremities, venous distention, laboured respirations, tissue oedema and ascites.
5. *Persistent bleeding* – from cardiac incision, tissue fragility, trauma to tissues, clotting defects; blood clotting disturbances usually transitory following cardiopulmonary bypass; however, a significant platelet deficiency may be present.
   a. Watch for steady and continuous drainage of blood; watch central venous pressure and left atrial pressures.
   b. Treatment – protamine sulphate, vitamin K, or blood components.
   c. Prepare for potential return to surgery for bleeding persisting (over 300ml per hour) for four to six hours.
6. *Hypovolaemia* (decreased circulating blood volume):
   a. Low central venous pressure is an indication of hypovolaemia.
   b. Assess for arterial hypotension, low central venous pressure, increasing pulse rate, and low left atrial and pulmonary artery wedge pressures.
   c. Prepare to administer blood, intravenous solutions.
7. *Renal failure* – urine output depends on cardiac output, blood volume, state of hydration and condition of kidneys.
   a. Renal injury may be caused by deficient perfusion, haemolysis, low cardiac output prior to and following open heart surgery; use of vasopressor agents to increase blood pressure.
   b. Measure urine volume; less than 20ml/hour can indicate decreased renal function.
   c. Carry out specific gravity tests to determine kidneys' ability to concentrate urine in renal tubules.
   d. Watch urea, creatinine and electrolyte levels.
   e. Give rapid-acting diuretics and/or inotropic

drugs (dopamine, dobutamine) to increase cardiac output and renal blood flow.

f.   Prepare the patient for peritoneal dialysis or haemodialysis if indicated. (Renal insufficiency may produce serious cardiac dysrhythmias.)

8. *Hypotension* – may be caused by inadequate cardiac contractility and reduction in blood volume or by mechanical ventilation (when the patient 'fights' the ventilator, or PEEP is used), all of which can produce a reduction in cardiac output.

a.   Monitor vital signs, left atrial pressure, central venous pressure and arterial pressure.

b.   Note chest tube drainage – hypotension may be caused by excessive bleeding.

c.   Give blood as directed to maintain left atrial pressure at a level which will provide an adequate circulating volume for good tissue perfusion.

9. *Embolization* – may result from injury to the intima of the blood vessels, dislodgement of a clot from a damaged valve, venous stasis aggravated by certain dysrhythmias, loosening of mural thrombi and coagulation problems.

a.   Common embolic sites are lungs, coronary arteries, mesentery, extremities, kidneys, spleen, and brain.

b.   Symptoms of embolization (vary according to site) – midabdominal or midback pain; pain, cessation of pulses, blanching, numbness, coldness of extremity; chest pain and respiratory distress with pulmonary embolus or myocardial infarction; and one-sided weakness, pupil changes, as in stroke.

c.   Initiate preventive measures – antiembolic stockings; omit pressure on popliteal space (leg crossing, raising knee gatch); start passive and active exercises.

10. *Postpericardiotomy syndrome* – a group of symptoms occurring following cardiac and pericardial trauma and myocardial infarction.

a.   Cause is not certain – may be from anticardiac antibodies, viral aetiology, etc.

b.   Features – fever, malaise, arthralgias, dyspnoea, pericardial effusion, pleural effusion, friction rub.

c.   Treatment is symptomatic (bed rest, aspirin), since condition is self-limiting but recurrence is not uncommon.

11. *Postperfusion syndrome:*

a.   Signs and symptoms – fever, splenomegaly, lymphocytosis.

b.   Draw blood for culture – postperfusion syndrome can mimic bacterial endocarditis or hepatitis.

c.   Treatment is symptomatic, since syndrome is self-limiting.

d.   Reassure patient that this is only a temporary setback in his convalescence.

12. *Febrile complications* – probably from body's reaction to tissue trauma or accumulation of blood and serum in pleural and pericardial spaces.

a.   Control higher degrees of fever by use of hypothermia mattress.

b.   Evaluate for atelectasis, pleural effusion or pneumonia if fever persists.

c.   Evaluate for urinary tract infection/wound infection.

d.   Bear in mind the possibility of infective endocarditis if fever persists (see pp. 271–274).

13. *Hepatitis.*

PATIENT EDUCATION, DISCHARGE PLANNING AND REHABILITATION FOLLOWING CARDIAC SURGERY

Objective

Assume a normal life as promptly as possible.

1. Begin discussing long-range plans with patient during convalescence in order to help him make modifications in his lifestyle.

2. Give written guidelines:

a.   *Activities:*

   (i)   Increase activities gradually within limits. Avoid strenuous activities until after exercise stress testing.

   (ii) Take short rest periods.

   (iii) Avoid lifting more than 9kg.

   (iv) Participate in activities that do not cause pain or discomfort.

   (v)   Increase walking time and distance each day.

   (vi) Stairs (one to two times daily) the first week; increase as tolerated.

   (vii) Avoid large crowds at first.

   (viii) Driving – avoid driving until after first postoperative check-up. At this time ask doctor when you may drive.

   (ix) Sexual relations – resumption of sexual relations parallels ability to participate in other activities. Usually may resume sexual activities two weeks after surgery. Avoid if tired or after heavy meal. Consult doctor if chest discomfort, difficult breathing or palpitations occur and last longer than 15 minutes after intercourse.

   (x)   Return to work – after first postoperative check-up, as advised by doctor.

(xi) Expect some chest discomfort.

b. *Diet:*

    (i) Some patients are placed on minimum salt restriction (e.g. no salt added at table); cholesterol may be limited.

    (ii) Weigh daily and report weight gain of more than 2.2kg per week.

c. *Medications:*

    (i) Label all medications; give purposes and side-effects.

    (ii) Patients with prosthetic valves may continue warfarin regimen indefinitely.

3. Patients with prosthetic valves:

  a. Pregnancy usually discouraged in women with prosthetic valves.

  b. Caution patient about need for antibiotic coverage following dental and surgical procedures.

  c. Patients on anticoagulants should watch for bleeding and should avoid use of aspirin (and many other drugs) – interferes with action of warfarin.

4. Advise the patient to carry an identification card stating cardiac condition and medications being taken.

5. The patient may be placed on rehabilitation and exercise programme after exercise stress testing.

6. Inform the patient whom to contact (and how) in case of an emergency.

7. See also Patient Education after Myocardial Infarction, pp. 263–264 and Patient Education, Infective Endocarditis, pp. 273–274.

Evaluation
EXPECTED OUTCOMES

1. Experiences a decrease in anxiety – expresses a lessening of anxiety, listens to and learns preoperative content taught (states reasons for operation, events to occur prior to and after surgery, need for follow-up rehabilitation after surgery).

2. Maintains adequate oxygenation – arterial blood gases within normal limits for patient, extubated 24 hours after surgery, spontaneous, unlaboured respirations 14 to 18 per minute.

3. Demonstrates adequate cardiac output – blood pressure and heart rate within normal limits for patient, skin warm and dry, urine output greater than 50ml per hour.

4. Achieves fluid and electrolyte balance – serum electrolytes normal, lungs clear on auscultation, absence of oedema.

5. Adapts to intensive care environment – no hallucinations, oriented to time and place consistently when asked, sleeps five hours without interruption.

6. Remains free of complications – absence of life-threatening dysrhythmias, heart sounds normal, cardiac enzymes normal, temperature within normal limits for patient, absence of bleeding.

7. Experiences minimal discomfort; absence of incisional pain.

Essentials of Basic Electrocardiography

THE ECG AND HEART PHYSIOLOGY

These are shown in Figure 5.17.

HEART PHYSIOLOGY

1. Heart tissue is highly specialized muscle mass, which possesses the special properties of automaticity, rhythmicity, conductivity and excitability.

2. These properties makes it possible for the heart to initiate a rhythmic wave of impulse with the subsequent conduction of that impulse resulting in a single heart contraction.

3. The site of normal impulse origin is referred to as the *sinus node* and is located in the right atrium. The sinus node is the natural pacemaker of the heart because it possesses the fastest intrinsic rate above all other heart muscle. The sinus node paces between 60 and 100 times per minute. The atrioventricular (AV) node has an intrinsic rate of between 40 and 60 times per minute; the ventricles' intrinsic rate is 20 to 40 times per minute.

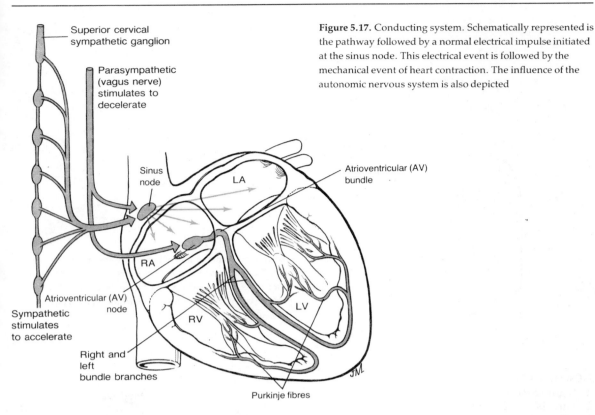

Figure 5.17. Conducting system. Schematically represented is the pathway followed by a normal electrical impulse initiated at the sinus node. This electrical event is followed by the mechanical event of heart contraction. The influence of the autonomic nervous system is also depicted

4. Once excited by the sinus node, the wave of impulse spreads over the thin walls of the atria to the atrioventricular node. The impulse is physiologically delayed at the AV node to allow for ventricular filling.
5. The AV node, as the name implies, lies at the junction of the atria and ventricles.
6. The wave of impulse then traverses the AV bundle and the left and right bundle branches of the ventricles and finally terminates in the Purkinje fibres of the ventricles. This electrical activity leads to a single heart contraction and is referred to as *depolarization of the ventricles* (see Figure 5.19).
7. The conduction system of the heart is under the control of the autonomic nervous system.
   a. Sympathetic – speeds the heart rate and strengthens contractions.
   b. Parasympathetic – slows the heart rate (vagal nerve).
8. The relaxation phase, which follows contraction, is referred to as *repolarization*.

THE ELECTROCARDIOGRAPH
1. Machine capable of transcribing to graph paper the electrical activity of the heart.

2. Electrical activity is generated by the cells of the heart as ions are exchanged across cell membranes.
3. Electrodes that are capable of conducting electrical activity from the heart to the ECG machine are placed at strategic positions on the extremities and chest precordium.
4. The electrical energy sensed is then converted to a graphic display by the ECG machine. This display is referred to as the *electrocardiogram* (ECG) (Figure 5.20).

CLINICAL USE OF ECG
An electrocardiogram can be helpful in diagnosing and following the progress of many disorders such as:
1. Myocardial infarction and ischaemic heart disease.
2. Cardiac dysrhythmias.
3. Cardiac enlargement.
4. Electrolyte abnormalities (especially potassium and calcium).
5. Pericarditis (inflammation of the pericardial sac which surrounds the heart).
6. Pericardial effusion (fluid in the pericardial sac which can restrict the heart's pumping ability).

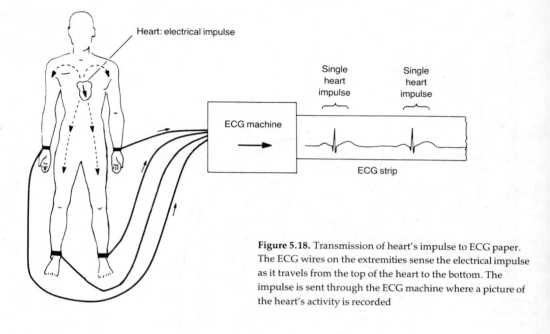

Heart: electrical impulse

Single heart impulse

Single heart impulse

ECG machine

ECG strip

Figure 5.18. Transmission of heart's impulse to ECG paper. The ECG wires on the extremities sense the electrical impulse as it travels from the top of the heart to the bottom. The impulse is sent through the ECG machine where a picture of the heart's activity is recorded

NORMAL ECG

1. Figure 5.21 represents a normal ECG.
2. Each heart beat manifests as three major deflections:
   a. P wave.
   b. QRS complex.
   c. T wave.
3. The QRS complex is composed of three parts:
   a. Q wave – the first downward deflection. A Q wave of significant deflection (pathological) is not normally present in the healthy ECG and usually indicates an old myocardial infarction.
   b. R wave – the first upward deflection.
   c. S wave – the first downward deflection after the R wave.

4. Beats come at regular intervals and the deflections in correct sequence (normal sinus rhythm), indicating that the impulse is originating properly from the sinus node.

ECG WAVES RELATED TO HEART ANATOMY

This is shown in Figure 5.20.

1. *P wave* – begins in the sinus node and can be thought of as representing the cardiac electrical impulse travelling through the *atria*, i.e. atrial depolarization.
2. *QRS complex* – represents the impulse going through the *ventricles*, i.e. ventricular depolarization. It begins in the AV node which lies above the ventricular chambers.
3. *T wave* – represents ventricular repolarization.

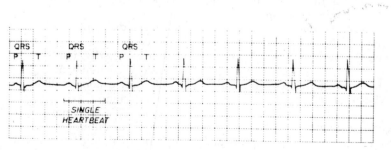

QRS   QRS   QRS
P   T   P   T   P   T

SINGLE HEARTBEAT

Figure 5.19. A normal ECG. A single heart beat is represented

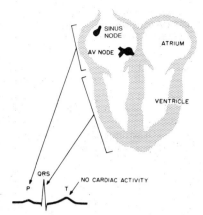

Figure 5.20. ECG waves related to heart anatomy. The electrical impulse is shown travelling through the chambers of the heart and thus inscribing the normal ECG of one heart beat. The P wave represents atrial activity and the QRS complex is derived from ventricular stimulation

ECG PAPER

This is shown in Figure 5.21.

1. Vertical lines – measure the *magnitude* of the electrical impulse.
2. Horizontal inscriptions – represent the *time* it takes for an impulse to travel over cardiac tissue.

3. In vertical and horizontal axes, each small block is 1mm and one darker large block is 5mm.
4. In horizontal axis, one small block represents 0.04 and one darker large block represents 0.20 seconds when paper speed is set at 25mm/second.

DETERMINATION OF CARDIAC RATE ON ECG PAPER

1. Cardiac rate can be obtained by dividing the number of heavily lined large blocks that lie between every two QRS complexes into 300.
2. The number 300 is used because 300 large blocks represent one minute on the ECG paper. Examples:
   a. If there are three large blocks between every two QRS complexes, the rate would be 100 beats/minute (300 divided by 3 = 100) (Figure 5.22).
   b. If there are two and one-half blocks between every two QRS complexes, the rate would be 120 beats/minute.

ECG LEADS

1. Standard ECG machines have a dial which turns to 1 to 12 leads (I, II, III, AVR, AVL, AVF, V1, V2, V3, V4, V5, V6).

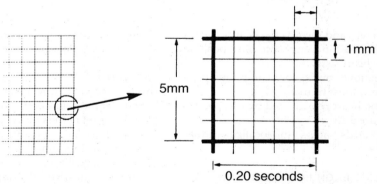

Figure 5.21. Meaning of blocks on ECG paper. It is necessary to remember one small block is 1mm tall and 1mm wide

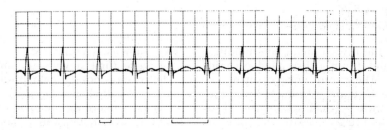

Figure 5.22. Determination of rate. There are three large blocks between every two QRS complexes. By dividing 300 by 3 the rate is 100 beats/minute

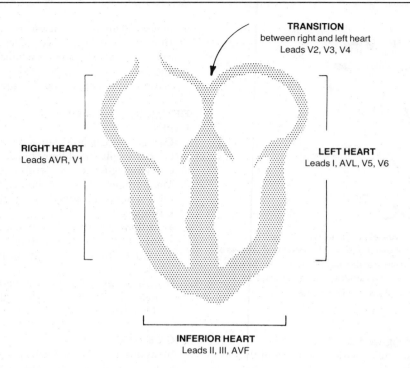

TRANSITION
between right and left heart
Leads V2, V3, V4

RIGHT HEART
Leads AVR, V1

LEFT HEART
Leads I, AVL, V5, V6

INFERIOR HEART
Leads II, III, AVF

Figure 5.23. ECG leads related to heart anatomy

2. Each lead receives and records the heart's electrical impulse from a different anatomical position relative to the heart's surface.
3. Letter designations can be confusing; thus position of each lead must be memorized.
4. The area of the heart represented by each lead is shown in Figure 5.23.
5. Location of leads helps to localize cardiac pathology.

SIGNIFICANCE OF EACH ECG WAVE AND INTERVAL

P wave
This is shown in Figure 5.24a.
1. The P wave represents the atrial contraction (depolarization).
2. Enlargement of the P wave deflection indicates enlargement of the atrium such as might occur in mitral stenosis. (The atrium enlarges in mitral stenosis because the mitral opening between the atrium and ventricle is small, causing blood to dam back, which in turn forces the atrial wall to hypertrophy.)
3. The P wave is considered enlarged if it is over

3mm tall (three small blocks) or 0.12 seconds wide (three small blocks).

PR interval
This is shown in Figure 5.24b.
1. Starts at the beginning of the P wave and extends to the onset of the Q wave.
2. At normal rates, the PR interval ranges between 0.12 and 0.20 seconds.
3. A prolonged PR interval may be a precursor to a variety of heart blocks (types of conduction defects); causes include myocardial disease or ischaemia, digitalis toxicity or electrolyte disturbances.

QRS complex
This is shown in Figure 5.24c.
1. Q wave (first downward stroke a significant deflection is not normally present in the healthy heart. A pathological Q wave is usually indicative of an old myocardial infarction.
2. The R wave (first upward deflection).
   a. Increases in amplitude when the ventricle hypertrophies, as in most types of heart

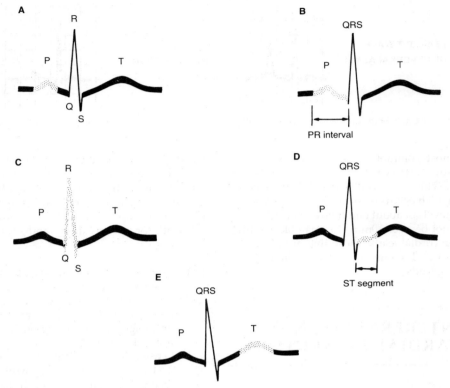

Figure 5.24. Parts of a heart beat. (A) The P wave. (B) The PR interval (extends from the beginning of the P wave to the onset of the Q wave). (C) The QRS complex. Even when the complex does not have a discrete Q or S wave it is still referred to as the QRS complex to denote a ventricular impulse and to provide simplicity and uniformity. (D) The ST segment begins at the termination of the S wave and ends at the beginning of the T wave. (E) The T wave

disease. (Overwork of a specific part of the heart causes hypertrophy.)
  b. May become small when the heart is compressed by fluid, as in a pericardial effusion.

ST segment
This is shown in Figure 5.24d.
1. Begins at the end of the S wave (the first downward deflection after the R wave) and terminates at the beginning of the T wave.
2. Is elevated above the baseline on the ECG strip in states of acute injury, e.g. in an acute myocardial infarction or in pericarditis.
3. Is depressed in ischaemic states (when the heart muscle is getting a decreased supply of oxygen) or when a patient is taking digitalis.
4. Becomes long in hypocalcaemia. (Hypocalcaemia occurs most commonly in chronic renal disease because the scarred kidneys cannot excrete phosphate. Since phosphate and calcium maintain a reciprocal balance in the body fluid, the elevated

phosphate causes a depression in the calcium level.)
5. Becomes shorter in hypercalcaemia, which is most commonly seen in metastatic carcinoma because the tumour erodes the bones and spills calcium into the serum.

T wave
This is shown in Figure 5.24e.
1. Represents no cardiac activity, but reflects the electrical recovery of the ventricular contraction (repolarization). (An electrical impulse is the flow of electrons; the T wave is inscribed when these electrons migrate back to their resting position after traversing the heart muscle to make it contract.)
2. Is flat when the heart is not receiving enough oxygen (ischaemic heart disease).
3. May be inverted in a myocardial infarction.
4. May be made tall by an elevated serum potassium.

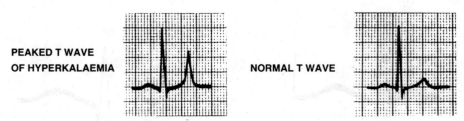

PEAKED T WAVE
OF HYPERKALAEMIA

NORMAL T WAVE

Figure 5.25. The ECGs show the difference between the tall peaked T wave of hyperkalaemia and the normal rounded T wave

The most common cause of elevated serum potassium levels is renal disease; the most frequent ECG finding is a tall, peaked, narrow-based T wave which begins to form when the potassium reaches levels of about 6mEq/litre (Figure 5.25).

5. Should not be over 10mm (10 small blocks) high in the precordial leads (those that are placed on the chest) and should not be over 5mm in the remaining leads.

ECG INTERPRETATION OF MYOCARDIAL INFARCTION

ECG INTERPRETATION
This is shown in Figure 5.26.

Note: The ECGs of some patients suffering myocardial infarctions may show *no specific changes* on the initial tracing. Therefore, if a person has symptoms compatible with a heart attack and has a normal ECG, he should nevertheless be admitted to the hospital for observation and further electrocardiograms.

1. Elevation of ST segment is usually a first finding.
2. T wave inversion follows.
   Then a large pathological Q wave appears.
   a. As infarct heals, Q wave may remain as the only sign of an old coronary occlusion. (In AVR a large Q wave is normal.)
   b. Q wave can be considered abnormal if it is over 0.04 seconds wide (one small block is 0.04 seconds) or if it is greater in depth than one-third the height of the QRS complex (Figure 5.27).

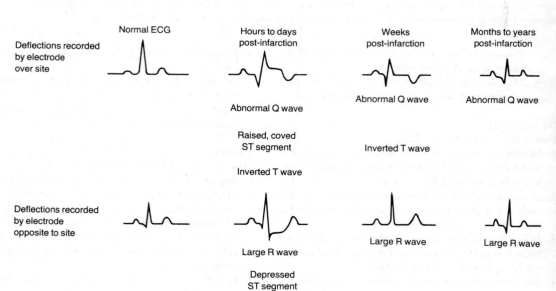

Figure 5.26. Evolutionary changes in myocardial infarction

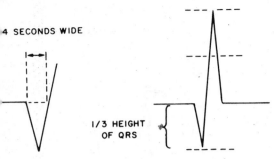

4 SECONDS WIDE

1/3 HEIGHT
OF QRS

Figure 5.27. Abnormal Q wave. A Q wave is considered abnormal when it is over 0.04 seconds (one small block on the ECG paper) or over one-third the height of the QRS complex. This usually indicates an old myocardial infarction

ECG INTERPRETATION OF CARDIAC DYSRHYTHMIAS

Dysrhythmias (irregular rhythms) are a symptom of an underlying process and should be regarded as a symptom, not a diagnosis.

Note: All heart muscle tissue is capable of exciting impulses when the normal pacemaker is compromised. This fact serves as the basis for dysrhythmia formation.

Dysrhythmias are generally evaluated continuously by placing at-risk patients on a bedside monitor.

The rhythm strips obtained from the monitor should not be used for diagnostic purposes.

If a question should arise regarding a rhythm that requires diagnostic data, a standard 12-lead ECG is always done.

NURSING ALERT

Cardiac output, which is defined as the volume of blood ejected from the ventricle per minute, is a function of heart rate times the stroke volume. Dysrhythmias, which are alterations in rate or rhythm of heart contraction, can seriously alter cardiac output. This concept must be considered each time a patient experiences a dysrhythmia.

FORMAT FOR ASSESSMENT AND INTERPRETATION OF DYSRHYTHMIAS

When reviewing a dysrhythmia, one should develop a systematic approach to assist in accurate interpretation. There is a variety of approaches that may be taken. One format that is particularly helpful is as follows:

1. Determine the rate. Is it fast, slow, or normal?
2. Determine the rhythm. Is it regular, irregular, regularly irregular, or irregularly irregular?
3. Find the P waves. Is one present for each QRS complex? Are they absent? Are they replaced by other wave forms? What is the configuration like? Are they identical, well-formed, or do they change shape?
4. Measure the PR interval. The normal interval should be between 0.12 and 0.20 seconds.
5. Measure the QRS complex. The normal QRS complex should be between 0.06 and 0.10 seconds. Are they identical in configuration? Do they fall early? Does the configuration vary?
6. Look at the T wave. Is it positively or negatively deflected? Is it peaked?
7. Measure the QT interval. The normal QT interval should be less than half the R to R interval.

By following a format, one can, through deductive reasoning, arrive at a correct interpretation by associating each part of the format with anatomical and physiological function of the heart.

Dysrhythmias may be classified as disturbances in either impulse formation or in conduction (heart blocks). The following dysrhythmias are considered disturbances of impulse formation. Heart blocks are reviewed later (see pp. 320–325).

Note: The lower the ectopic focus resides in the heart, the more lethal the dysrhythmia becomes.

SINUS TACHYCARDIA

Sinus tachycardia can be defined as a cardiac rate of over 100 beats/minute. All the complexes are normal, but their rate is excessive.

AETIOLOGY

The sinus node is under the influence of the autonomic nervous system. The sympathetic fibres, which act to speed up excitation of the sinus node, are stimulated by underlying causes.

UNDERLYING CAUSES

1. Exercise.
2. Anxiety.
3. Fever.
4. Shock.
5. Drugs.
6. Altered metabolic states, such as hyperthyroidism.
7. Electrolyte disturbances.

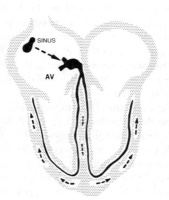

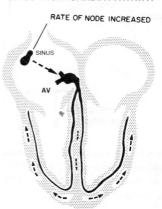

Figure 5.28. The pathway of sinus tachycardia is the same as that of a normal sinus rhythm, but the number of impulses per minute is greater in sinus tachycardia

MECHANISM OF SINUS TACHYCARDIA
This is shown in Figure 5.28. The pathway of sinus tachycardia is the same as that of a normal sinus rhythm, but the number of impulses per minute is greater in sinus tachycardia.

ECG OF SINUS TACHYCARDIA
This is shown in Figure 5.29. The P wave, the QRS complex and the T wave are all normal. The only abnormality is a rate of over 100 beats/minute.

TREATMENT
Since sinus tachycardia is usually a compensatory rhythm, treatment is directed at the primary causes, which usually are not cardiac.

SINUS BRADYCARDIA

Sinus bradycardia is defined as a heart rate below 60/minute. All the complexes are normal.

AETIOLOGY
The parasympathetic fibres (vagal tone) are stimu lated and cause the sinus node to slow.

UNDERLYING CAUSES
1. Can be expected in the well-trained athlete.
2. Drugs.
3. Altered metabolic states, such as hypo thyroidism.
4. The process of ageing, which causes increasin fibrotic tissue and scarring of the sinus node.
5. Certain cardiac diseases, such as acute myocardia infarction.

COMPLICATIONS
Slow rate and low cardiac output can cause:
1. Fainting (Stokes–Adams syndrome), or
2. Heart failure. (Heart cannot pump all the flui presented to it, resulting in stasis or 'congestion of the blood in the lungs and other body tissues.

MECHANISM OF SINUS BRADYCARDIA
See Figure 5.30.

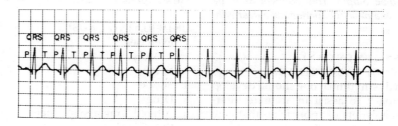

Figure 5.29. ECG of sinus tachycardia

NORMAL PATHWAY

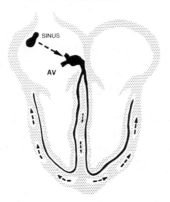

SINUS BRADYCARDIA PATHWAY

RATE OF NODE DECREASED

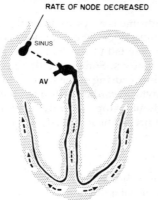

Figure 5.30. Mechanism of sinus bradycardia

ECG OF SINUS BRADYCARDIA

See Figure 5.31. The only abnormality is a rate below
[60] beats/minute.

TREATMENT

Rarely has to be treated.

If heart failure or fainting occurs, treatment
should be initiated immediately to increase the
heart rate.

a. Give 0.3–1.2mg of atropine intravenously (inhibits the vagal or 'slowing' nerve and therefore allows the heart go faster).

b. If patient becomes resistant to atropine, the
rate can be increased by adding 1mg of isoprenaline hydrochloride to 250ml of 5 per
cent glucose in water and initially running the
solution at about 10 drops/minute. (Stimulates
the sympathetic or 'fast' nerve of the heart.)
(Atropine can be prepared more quickly and is
less toxic to the heart than isoprenaline hydrochloride.)

c. The heart rate can be increased or decreased by
adjusting the rate of fluid administered.

d. An electrical pacemaker may be necessary in
unresponsive cases or when the fluid load
becomes excessive.

SINUS ARRHYTHMIA

Sinus arrhythmia is normally found in children and
young adults and is characterized by a heart rhythm
that is normal in every way except for irregularity.

AETIOLOGY

1. On inspiration the heart rate increases and on
expiration the heart rate decreases.

2. Inspiration tends to inhibit the vagus nerve (slows
the heart) and causes an acceleration of the
cardiac rate.

MECHANISM OF SINUS ARRHYTHMIA

See Figure 5.32. The pathway of sinus arrhythmia is
the same as that of the normal sinus rhythm, the only
difference being the regularity of the impulses.

ECG OF SINUS ARRHYTHMIA

See Figure 5.33. All the complexes are normal, only
the rate is irregular – varying with respiration. The
rate increases with inspiration and decreases with
expiration.

TREATMENT

Since sinus arrhythmia is usually normal, no treatment is necessary.

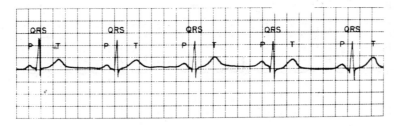

Figure 5.31. ECG of sinus bradycardia

SICK SINUS SYNDROME

Sick sinus syndrome is a dysrhythmia that is caused by a diseased sinus node. The sinus node conducts at a slow rate or may fail to conduct at all, producing sinus block or pauses. Sometimes there is a related tachycardia, thus causing some to refer to this syndrome as 'bradytachycardia syndrome'. If the related tachycardia should stop abruptly, and the sinus node does not fire, all heart activity will cease (asystole).

AETIOLOGY
1. Arteriosclerotic heart disease.
2. Acute myocardial infarction.

MECHANISM OF SICK SINUS SYNDROME
1. When the sinus node fails to fire for whatever reason, the end result is a lack of impulse conducted to the atria or ventricles. Thus, there is a long pause before another impulse is discharged.
2. Whether or not the patient is affected depends on the length of the pause.

3. Ischaemia is a common cause of sick sinus syndrome.

ANALYSIS OF SICK SINUS SYNDROME
1. Rate – may be slow or within normal limits. Rhythm will be regular except when a pause occurs; when the rhythm resumes, it will be regular.
2. P wave – present before each QRS complex; normal configuration and identical, the P wave will suddenly not appear when expected. No QRS complex will follow.
3. P–R interval – within normal limits.
4. QRS complex – follow each QRS except when there is no P wave. The QRS will also be absent.
5. T wave – normally conducted in the normal complexes.

TREATMENT
A pacemaker will be required if the sick sinus syndrome does not abate with the treatment of ischaemia.

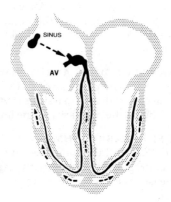

NORMAL PATHWAY

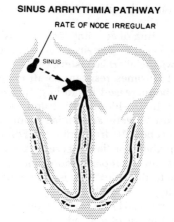

SINUS ARRHYTHMIA PATHWAY

RATE OF NODE IRREGULAR

Figure 5.32. Mechanism of sinus arrhythmia

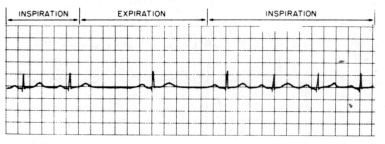

Figure 5.33. ECG of sinus arrhythmia

TRIAL ECTOPIC BEATS (AEBs)

n atrial ectopic beat (AEB) is an ectopic beat that riginates in the atria and is discharged at a rate ster than that of the sinus node. The atrial beat ccurs sooner than the next normal beat and is said to e early or premature.

AEBs constitute a very common rhythm disturb- nce and are seen in both normal and abnormal earts. They rarely cause symptoms and are believed o be of little consequence except when they occur equently, at which time they may tend to de- riorate into other more serious arrhythmias.

LTERED PHYSIOLOGY

. Beats occur *early* in the cycle; they begin in the atrium, but *outside* the sinus node where normal impulses originate (hence 'ectopic' beat).
. Since the atrial pathway is abnormal, the P wave is distorted.
. Since ventricular activation is undisturbed, the QRS is normal.

MECHANISM OF AN AEB
See Figure 5.34. The AEB begins in the atrium out- side the sinus node.

ECG OF AN AEB
See Figure 5.35.
1. AEB comes early in the cycle.
2. P wave is abnormally shaped.
3. QRS complex is normal.

TREATMENT
1. Most of the time AEBs do not need to be treated.
2. Quinidine, which is a good suppressant of atrial ectopic beats, may be used when the patient requires therapy.

PAROXYSMAL ATRIAL TACHYCARDIA (PAT)

PAT is a common dysrhythmia in young adults; it is usually found in normal hearts. There is a rapid heart rate which ranges from 140–250 beats/minute with an average of about 180 beats/minute.

NORMAL PATHWAY

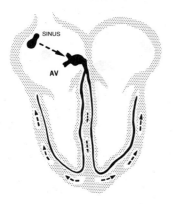

AEB PATHWAY

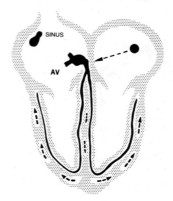

igure 5.34. Mechanism of an AEB

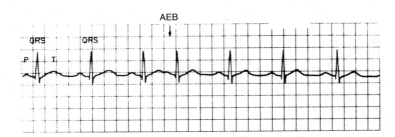

igure 5.35. ECG of an AEB

AETIOLOGY

1. Syndromes of accelerated pathways (e.g. Wolff-Parkinson-White (W-P-W) syndrome).
2. Syndrome of mitral valve prolapse.
3. Ischaemic heart disease.
4. Excessive use of alcohol, cigarettes, caffeine, drugs.

CLINICAL FEATURES

Patient will complain of a pounding or fluttering in the chest associated with shortness of breath and fainting – due to rapid heart rate.

ALTERED PHYSIOLOGY

1. Begins in an ectopic focus of the atrium outside the sinus node.
2. Its pathway over the heart is similar to that of an AEB. Thus PAT may be thought of as a rapid succession of AEBs.
3. The P wave (atrial wave) is distorted because the pathway over the atrium is abnormal. (Most of the time the rate is so fast that the P wave is buried in the previous complex and is not seen.)

4. The QRS complex (ventricular wave) is norma because the route of the cardiac impulse afte penetrating the AV node is undisturbed.

MECHANISM OF PAT

See Figure 5.36. An impulse travelling along th abnormal PAT pathway (right) produces an abnoi mal P wave and a normally shaped QRS comple (ventricular wave). Notice that the focus of the PA is the same as that of an AEB.

ECG of PAT

This is shown in Figure 5.37.
1. The rate is very rapid – over 140/minute (highe than in sinus tachycardia).
2. P waves cannot be seen since they are superim posed within the T wave of the preceding beat. I the P waves were seen they would be abnormal ii configuration.
3. The QRS complex is normal.
4. The T wave will be distorted in appearance as result of P waves being buried in them.

NORMAL PATHWAY

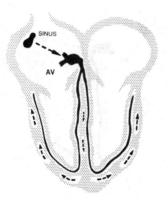

PAT PATHWAY

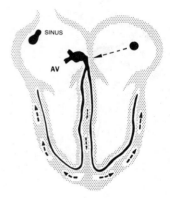

Figure 5.36. Mechanism of PAT

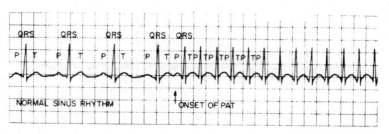

Figure 5.37. ECG of PAT

REATMENT

. Since cardiac arrest can occur with any mode of treatment for PAT, an ECG monitor should remain attached to the patient, an intravenous cannula should be inserted, and appropriate resuscitation equipment, including a defibrillator, should be at hand.

. If the patient is relatively asymptomatic and stable, with a normal blood pressure, giving a simple sedative and waiting five to ten minutes may result in spontaneous conversion of PAT.

. Start by stimulating the right carotid sinus (an area of dense nerve supply) of the carotid artery for several seconds or gagging the patient with a tongue depressor in an effort to terminate the dysrhythmia. These manoeuvres work by stimulating the vagus nerve, which puts a 'brake' on the heart (Valsalva manoeuvre).

. If the above procedure is not effective and if the blood pressure is low (many patients with PAT have a systolic pressure of about 90mmHg), a slow drip of metaraminol, intravenously, can be started.

a. Add 100mg of metaraminol to 500ml of 5 per cent glucose in water and run the intravenous infusion initially at 10 drops/minute.

b. Gradually increase the rate of the infusion until the PAT terminates, at which time the intravenous infusion should be stopped (usually a matter of seconds). (See Figure 5.38.) Verapamil or digitalis may be used in the treatment of PAT.

c. Do not raise the systolic blood pressure above 180mmHg. This drug increases the blood pressure, which in turn stimulates the vagus nerve to inhibit the ectopic focus of the atrium.

d. If the patient is already hypertensive (rare), metaraminol should not be used.

e. Some authorities do not use a vasopressor such as metaraminol because of the occasional report of a cerebrovascular accident, but this complication has usually occurred when the drug is used in bolus form. Instead of metaraminol, they prefer a fast-acting digitalis preparation which works in part by stimulating the vagal nerve.

5. In an unusual case, in which the preceding steps are ineffective or contraindicated, 1–3mg of propranolol – a sympathetic nerve blocker – may be given by intravenous infusion at a rate no greater than 1mg/minute.

6. In the extreme case when the patient is in heart failure, DC synchronized electrical shock (cardioversion) should be instituted (instead of giving propranolol).

a. Initial shock – can be 50–100 joules.

b. Electrical shock depolarizes the heart and allows the heartbeat to begin again normally at the sinus node.

ATRIAL FLUTTER

Atrial flutter is a rapid, regular 'fluttering' of the atrium.

AETIOLOGY

1. Atrial enlargement, as seen in diseases of the atrioventricular valves.
2. Myocardial infarction.
3. Heart failure.

ALTERED PHYSIOLOGY

1. P waves take on a 'sawtooth' appearance because they are coming from a focus other than the sinus node and are coming at a very rapid rate.
2. As in AEB or PAT, the impulse comes from *one* ectopic focus in the atrium, but the *atrial* rate (not the pulse or ventricular rate) is between 250 and 350/minute for atrial flutter.

The following oversimplified arbitrary rule may be used to distinguish the atrial dysrhythmias from each other:

a. Atrial rate in sinus tachycardia goes up to 140/minute.

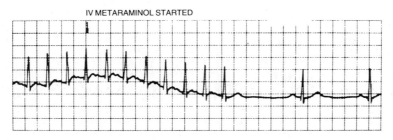

IV METARAMINOL STARTED

igure 5.38. Termination of PAT. The ECG illustrates PAT being terminated with an intravenous infusion of metaraminol

b. Atrial rate in PAT is between 140 and 250/minute.

c. Atrial rate in atrial flutter is between 250 and 350/minute.

3. Atrial flutter generally occurs in a pathological heart, as contrasted with PAT, which in many cases is associated with a normal heart.

4. Since the abnormality is above the AV node, the QRS complex (ventricular wave) is normal in configuration.

5. Since the P waves come so rapidly, the AV node cannot accept and conduct each one; therefore there is some degree of 'blockage' at the AV node.

   Example: If the atrial rate is 300, the ventricular rate (which is the same as the pulse rate) might be 150, since the AV node is not able to conduct every atrial impulse because of the excessive rapidity. In this instance, the 'block' is said to be 2:1 since there are two atrial impulses per venticular response.

6. a. The 2:1 block is the most common block in atrial flutter.

   b. This is an important feature of this rhythm; if the AV node conducted 1:1 then the outcome would be ventricular flutter, a life-threatening dysrhythmia.

7. Most cases of PAT do not exhibit a block since waves do not occur as fast as in atrial flutter. Thus in PAT all the impulses are transmitted by the AV node to the ventricles.

MECHANISM OF ATRIAL FLUTTER
See Figure 5.39. The pathways for atrial flutter are the same as for AEB and PAT, but in atrial flutter the ectopic impulse fires at a faster rate.

ECG OF ATRIAL FLUTTER
This is shown in Figure 5.40.

1. The arrows indicate the P waves generated by the fast-firing ectopic focus in the atrium.

2. Notice that not every P wave stimulates a QRS complex (ventricular wave).

3. Since the abnormality present in the heart is above the AV node, the QRS complexes that appear are normal in configuration.

TREATMENT
1. Classic initial treatment is digitalis, which partially blocks the AV node; this allows fewer P waves to pass through the ventricles and thus slows the pulse rate.

NORMAL PATHWAY

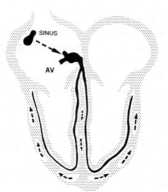

ATRIAL FLUTTER PATHWAY

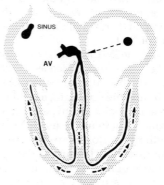

Figure 5.39. Mechanism of atrial flutter

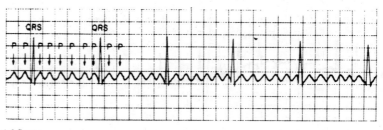

Figure 5.40. ECG of atrial flutter

2. The fast pulse rate must be slowed down (ventricular rate) because the heart is not given enough time to fill itself with blood when it is contracting rapidly; this causes the blood to dam back in the body tissues, leading to congestive failure.
3. Cardioversion:
   a. Tried when the patient is not tolerating the dysrhythmia well.
   b. Atrial flutter responds well to cardioversion at a relatively low energy (50–100 joules).

NURSING ALERT
When a patient is taking digitalis, cardioversion can be dangerous since a lethal dysrhythmia may be precipitated.

ATRIAL FIBRILLATION

Atrial fibrillation is an atrial dysrhythmia occurring at an extremely rapid and uncoordinated rate. The atria produce impulses so rapidly that the ventricles are not capable of responding to every atrial beat; therefore, only a small percentage of atrial stimuli excite the ventricles. Since the atrial rate is irregular, the ventricular rate (pulse rate) will also be irregular.

AETIOLOGY
Usually seen in patients with ischaemic heart disease.

ALTERED PHYSIOLOGY
1. Atherosclerosis leads to scarring of the atrium and thus to disruption of the normal course of the P wave (atrial wave).
2. P waves are replaced by irregular, rapid waves each of which is different in configuration from the other.
3. P waves (often called fibrillatory waves) assume different shapes because they come from different foci in the atrium. (In atrial flutter the P waves are very regular and uniform since they come from one focus.)
4. Because P waves occur at variable intervals, the QRS complexes assume an irregular rhythm, and thus the patient's pulse is irregular. (The configuration of the QRS is normal since the conduction tissue beyond the AV node has not yet become critically involved with the arteriosclerotic process.)
5. Since the P waves come so fast, all of them do not pass on to the ventricles, because of normal refraction of the AV node. Thus the atrial rate is usually much faster than the ventricular rate.

6. Occasionally, the ventricular rate is very fast because the AV node is blocking relatively fewer beats than is normal. If this is the case, atrial activity may not be seen, because the QRS complexes are so close together (since their rate is so rapid) that it is difficult to define the dysrhythmia.

Note: General rule – if *normal* QRS complexes are present at a very rapid rate, so that atrial activity cannot be seen and the rhythm is *irregular*, the probable diagnosis is atrial fibrillation.

MECHANISM OF ATRIAL FIBRILLATION
See Figure 5.41.
1. In atrial fibrillation many ectopic foci are present in the atrium (right).
2. Since each small atrial wave comes from a different focus and travels a different route, the shape of each atrial wave (P wave) is different.

ECG OF ATRIAL FIBRILLATION
See Figure 5.42.
1. Note the small, irregular fibrillating P waves (arrows).
2. As with atrial flutter, only an occasional P wave travels through the AV node to form a QRS complex, but since these complexes come at irregular intervals in atrial fibrillation, the ventricular rate is irregular.
3. Each P wave is different in shape because it comes from a different focus in the atrium.

TREATMENT
1. Depends on patient's clinical condition, cardiac rate and drug therapy.
2. For the average patient who is not critical and not on digitalis, the following treatment is common:
   a. Intravenous digoxin (0.5mg) given over a five-minute period under ECG control.
   b. After two hours, an additional 0.25–0.5mg is given, depending on the ECG and the patient's condition. (Total intravenous dose before oral maintenance therapy is 0.75–1.5mg).
3. If atrial fibrillation is an imminent, life-threatening emergency (rare):
   a. Cardioversion may be started with 100 joules.
   b. As with atrial flutter, cardioversion becomes something of a risk when the patient is taking digitalis.
   c. In contrast to atrial flutter, atrial fibrillation is more difficult to correct to normal sinus rhythm with electric countershock.

NORMAL PATHWAY

ATRIAL FIBRILLATION PATHWAY

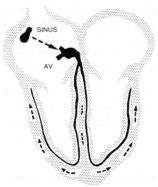
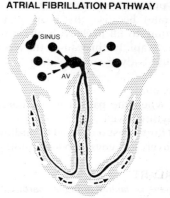

Figure 5.41. Mechanism of atrial fibrillation

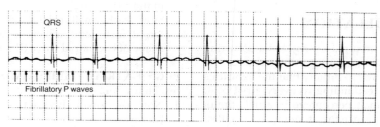

Figure 5.42. ECG of atrial fibrillation

DIGITALIS TOXICITY

Digitalis toxicity is a condition that results from excessive serum levels of digitalis. The two dysrhythmias that are most frequently associated with digitalis toxicity are ventricular bigeminy (every other beat is a ventricular ectopic) and PAT with block although any dysrhythmia may occur.

Note: Digitalis effect, in contrast to toxicity, is a characteristic pattern of S–T depression. Digitalis toxicity and digitalis effect are not synonymous.

ANALYSIS OF DIGITALIS EFFECT
1. Therapeutic levels of digitalis will frequently be manifested by ECG.
2. A 'drooping' of the S–T segment is apparent. The S–T segment depression that is manifest in myocardial ischaemia is flatter in appearance. These wave form features are sometimes not distinguishing.
3. Measurement of the Q–T interval may be helpful.
   a. The Q–T interval in digitalis effect will be shortened.
   b. The Q–T interval in digitalis toxicity will be lengthened.

ANALYSIS OF DIGITALIS TOXICITY
1. Digitalis toxicity should always be considered when the patient who has been taking the drug has a new onset of dysrhythmia, has excessive slowing of the heart rate, and complains of malaise, anorexia, and nausea and vomiting. This syndrome is frequently found in the poorly nourished population. Potassium level in the diet may be low, and hypokalaemia tends to exaggerate the effect of digitalis.
2. Digitalis may be administered concomitantly with diuretics, which may contribute to potassium loss.
3. The dysrhythmias most commonly associated with digitalis are the ventricular ectopic beats; these usually, but not always, appear as bigeminy. Multifocal ventricular ectopic beats may also occur.
4. The next most common dysrhythmia is PAT with block.

TREATMENT
1. Obtain serum levels of digitalis and potassium.
2. Discontinue digitalis until excretion can take place and administer potassium if indicated by hypokalaemia. This treatment usually resolves the problem.

3. Administer phenytoin in a single dose as prescribed; this may be done as prophylaxis for ventricular dysrhythmia.
4. In more serious situations, when the patient may be haemodynamically threatened (cardiac output is severely compromised), a pacemaker may be required until the crisis is passed.
5. Cardioversion is extremely risky because of the potential for converting this dysrhythmia to a more lethal one; it is seldom done and only because no other therapies have been of benefit.

Other drugs that may be used are verapamil to control ventricular rate and quinidine or amiodarone to restore normal rhythm.

VENTRICULAR ECTOPIC BEATS (VEBs)

Ventricular ectopic beats represent one of the most easily recognized rhythm disturbances seen on an ECG. They occur in all forms of heart disease and are seen in the majority of patients with myocardial infarction. They occur frequently in normal hearts and can be secondary to smoking, coffee or alcohol.

While not usually symptomatic, VEBs, when frequent, may cause palpitations.

ALTERED PHYSIOLOGY
1. Contractions come early in the cycle and originate in the ventricle *below* the AV node.
2. QRS configurations are wide and bizarre, since a VEB does not begin normally and therefore does not follow the true conduction path in the ventricle.

MECHANISM OF A VEB
See Figure 5.43. Since a VEB begins in the ventricle outside the AV node a bizarre ventricular QRS complex will be inscribed, with no preceding P wave.

ECG OF VEBs
See Figure 5.44. VEBs occur early in the cycle and are wider than the normal beat.

DANGER OF VEBs
VEBs can be especially dangerous when they:
1. Occur more frequently than once in 10 beats.
2. Occur in groups of two or three.
3. Land near the T wave.
4. Take on multiple configurations – this indicates

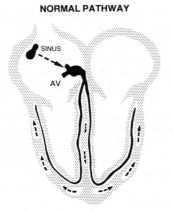

NORMAL PATHWAY

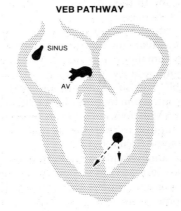

VEB PATHWAY

Figure 5.43. Mechanism of a VEB

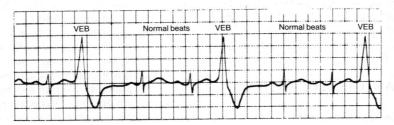

Figure 5.44. ECG of VEBs

the VEBs come from different foci, which in turn means that the ventricle is more irritable (multifocal).

TREATMENT

If a patient has an infarct, VEBs are treated vigorously since they *can precipitate ventricular fibrillation by hitting a T wave*.

1. Lignocaine can be given – VEBs are usually seen with a cardiac rate of over 60/minute; lignocaine (a cardiac muscle suppressant) is the drug of choice because VEBs are most likely to come from an irritable focus such as an infarct.
   a. Dosage: 75–100mg intravenously as a bolus over a two- to three-minute period.
   b. If effective, a continuous intravenous drip of lignocaine should be started with a delivery of 1–4mg/min.
      (i) Addition of a 50ml bottle of 2 per cent lignocaine to 1,000ml of 5 per cent glucose in water will give a concentration of 1mg of lignocaine per ml of fluid.
      (ii) Most intravenous sets are calibrated to deliver 1ml in 10 drops of fluid.
      (iii) If above concentration results in too much fluid for the patient, the amount of lignocaine in the intravenous solution should be increased.
2. If heart rate is *slow* secondary to a myocardial infarction involving the heart's normal physiological pacemaker (sinus node), VEBs may occur as a compensatory mechanism to maintain a reasonable rate so as to provide some type of cardiac contraction for pumping blood to the body tissues. (A VEB does not pump as much blood as a normal impulse from the sinus node, but it does provide some circulation.)
   a. Lignocaine would be contraindicated since it would decrease circulation by extinguishing the VEBs which are pumping needed blood.
   b. Atropine is treatment of choice in this case (since a slow rate results in VEBs).
      (i) Increases the sinus node rate, which in turn terminates the inefficient ectopic beats by replacing them with normal impulses.
      (ii) Dosage: 0.3–1.2mg intravenously.

VENTRICULAR TACHYCARDIA

Ventricular tachycardia is one of the serious complications of a myocardial infarction and can be con-

sidered as multiple (three or more), consecutive, ventricular ectopic beats that originate from an ectopic focus below the AV node in the ventricles and thus cause the complexes to be wide and bizarre in configuration.

AETIOLOGY

1. Acute myocardial infarction.
2. Metabolic acidosis.
3. Electrolyte disturbances.

DANGERS OF VENTRICULAR TACHYCARDIA

1. Leads to a reduced cardiac output (the ventricles are not being stimulated normally from the AV node, but from a focus farther down in the ventricle wall, which leads to an incomplete and inefficient contraction of the heart muscle).
2. Is a precursor of ventricular fibrillation, in which there is no cardiac output.

MECHANISM OF VENTRICULAR TACHYCARDIA

See Figure 5.45.
1. Pathway is the same as for VEBs since ventricular tachycardia can be thought of as a series of VEBs.
2. Like the VEBs, the complexes of ventricular tachycardia show a bizarre configuration.

ECG OF VENTRICULAR TACHYCARDIA

See Figure 5.46.
1. Since this dysrhythmia begins below the AV node, the atria are beating independently.
2. On the ECGs of 20 per cent of patients, when the ventricular rate is not too fast and the ventricular complexes are not too wide, P waves which are independent of the QRS complexes can be seen.
3. The rate is fast and the QRS complexes are wide. A width equivalent to 0.12 seconds (three small blocks) or more is considered abnormal for a QRS complex.

TREATMENT

1. If patient is tolerating the dysrhythmia fairly well:
   a. Give lignocaine:
      (i) 75–100mg intravenously as a bolus over a two-minute period.
      (ii) If effective, a continuous intravenous drip of lignocaine should be started (with delivery of 1–3mg/min).
      (iii) If a 50ml bottle of 2 per cent lignocaine is added to 1,000ml of 5 per cent glucose in water, 1ml will contain 1mg of lignocaine. Most intravenous sets are calibrated to deliver 1ml in 10 drops of fluid. If concen-

tration results in too much fluid for the patient, the amount of lignocaine should be increased in the intravenous solution.
b. Other drugs which may be used include:
  (i) Disopyramide.
  (ii) Mexiletine.
  (iii) Procainamide.
  (iv) Amiodarone.

NURSING ALERT

Because the heart muscle is weakened, the cardiac patient should not receive excessive fluid since this may precipitate failure.

2. Cardioversion.
  a. Used when lignocaine does not work or if patient is not tolerating the dysrhythmia well.
  b. Start with about 200 joules.
    Cardioversion is a *timed* electric shock delivered by a machine which is set so that its electrical output does not hit a T wave (synchronized) which is considered the vulnerable period on the cardiac cycle. If an electrical shock, such as that from an external source or from an electrical impulse within the heart itself (such as a VEB), hits the T wave, ventricular fibrillation

may ensue. If not terminated, ventricular fibrillation results in death.

VENTRICULAR FIBRILLATION

Ventricular fibrillation is a lethal dysrhythmia characterized by chaotic depolarization of the ventricles at rates exceeding 300/minute. Ventricular fibrillation can produce clinical death within minutes if not reversed.

AETIOLOGY
1. Acute myocardial infarction.
2. Electrical shock.
3. Ventricular ectopic beats/ventricular tachycardia.
4. Acidosis.
5. Electrolyte disturbances.

ALTERED PHYSIOLOGY
1. The heart is being stimulated simultaneously from numerous ectopic foci throughout the ventricles; therefore, there is no effective contraction of the cardiac musculature and thus loss of pulse, blood pressure, cardiac output and consciousness.

NORMAL PATHWAY

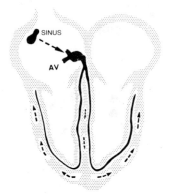

VENTRICULAR TACHYCARDIA PATHWAYS

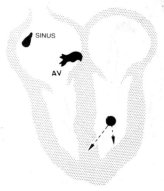

Figure 5.45. Mechanism of ventricular tachycardia

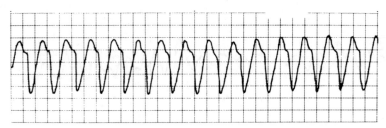

Figure 5.46. ECG of ventricular tachycardia

2. Characterized by totally irregular appearance on ECG.

MECHANISM OF VENTRICULAR FIBRILLATION
See Figure 5.47. In ventricular fibrillation the presence of multiple ectopic foci in the ventricle prohibits an effective heart beat.

ECG OF VENTRICULAR FIBRILLATION
See Figure 5.48. The complexes are completely distorted and irregular.

Note: It is extremely important to be sure that the chaotic undulations on the ECG do not represent artifacts since movement by the patient or of the monitor wires can give the same appearance. If the patient is alert or has a pulse, the rhythm does *not* represent ventricular fibrillation.

TREATMENT
See Figure 5.49. *Electrical defibrillation* at 200–400 joules. (In children, start with lower energies.)
1. If successful, the defibrillation shock stops the erratic uncoordinated electrical activity of the ventricle. After a moment the heart resumes its normal innate rhythm from the sinus node.
2. Differs from cardioversion in that timing of the defibrillation shock is not necessary since there are no T waves in ventricular fibrillation (unsynchronized).
3. Paddle placement:
   a. The centre of one paddle is applied just to the right of the upper sternum in the second interspace.
   b. The rim of the other paddle is placed just below the left nipple.
   c. Paddles should be well lubricated and in firm contact with the skin.
4. See pp. 237–240.

SUMMARY
See Figure 5.50.

ATRIOVENTRICULAR (AV) BLOCK

AV block means that the AV node is diseased and has difficulty conducting the atrial waves (P waves) into the ventricles.

NORMAL PATHWAY

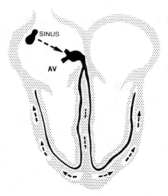

VENTRICULAR FIBRILLATION PATHWAYS

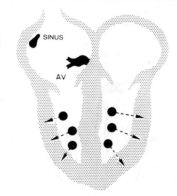

Figure 5.47. Mechanism of ventricular fibrillation

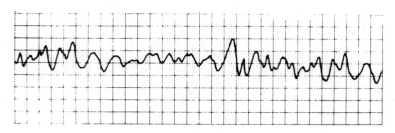

Figure 5.48. ECG of ventricular fibrillation

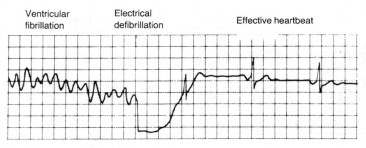

Figure 5.49. Electrical defibrillation

Figure 5.50. Emergency diagnosis and treatment of dysrhythmias

Type of dysrhythmia	Appearance of ECG	Treatment	Pathway
Normal rhythm	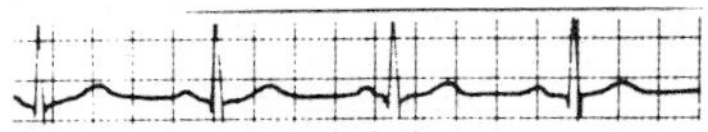	None	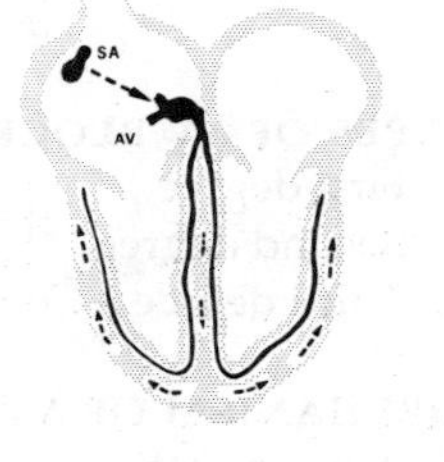
Sinus tachycardia	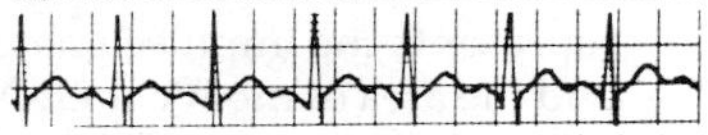	Treat cause	
Sinus bradycardia	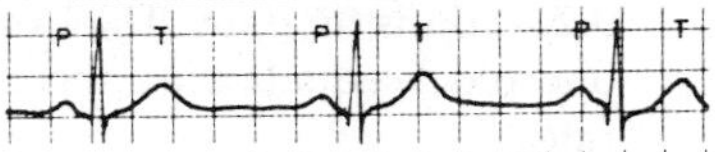	Atropine, isoprenaline hydrochloride or pacemaker when condition is pathological	
Sinus arrhythmia	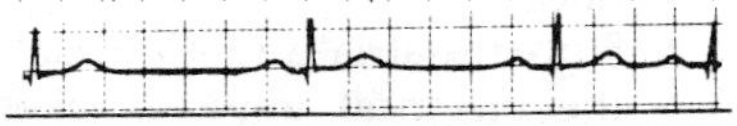	None	
AEBs	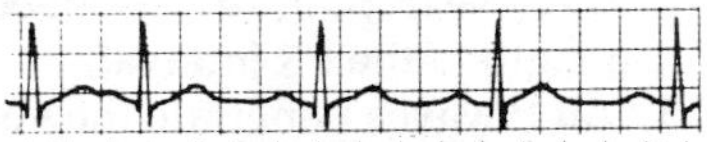	Usually none. Quinidine may be used	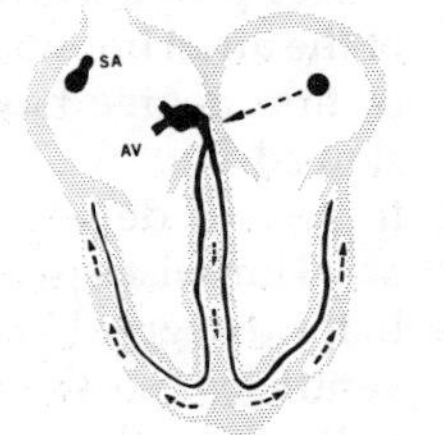
PAT	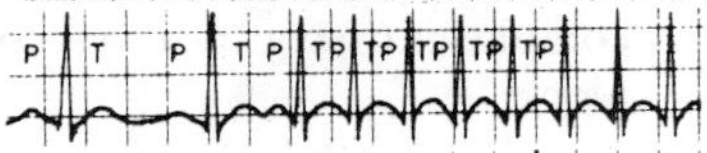	Carotid sinus pressure or metaraminol. Verapamil; digitalis	
Atrial flutter	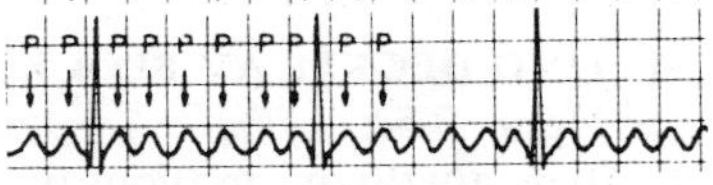	Digitalis if rate is above 100. Cardioversion* is very effective	
Atrial fibrillation	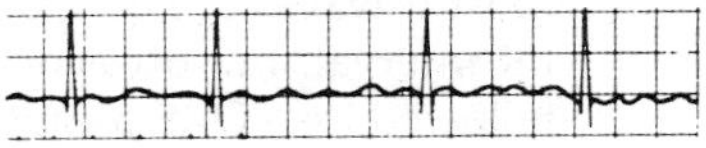	Digitalis or verapamil if rate is above 100, and if fibrillation is not caused by too much digitalis. Cardioversion* may be effective. Quinidine or amiodarone to restore rhythm	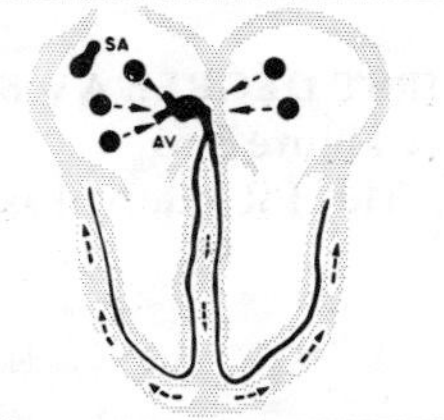
AV Blocks Second degree	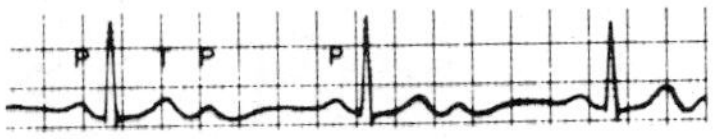	Atropine, isoprenaline hydrochloride or pacemaker	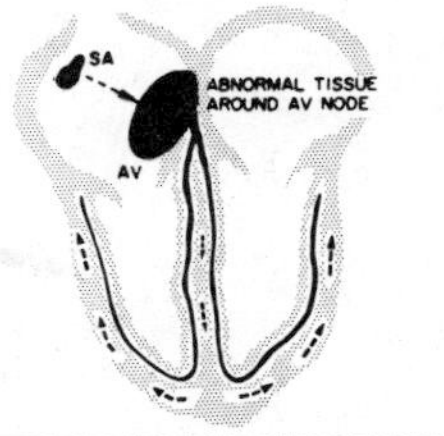
Third degree	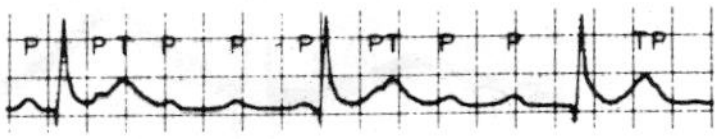	Atropine, isoprenaline hydrochloride or pacemaker	

Continued

* Cardioversion can be very dangerous when a patient has a significant level of digitalis in his bloodstream since ventricular fibrillation or other lethal dysrhythmias can be precipitated.

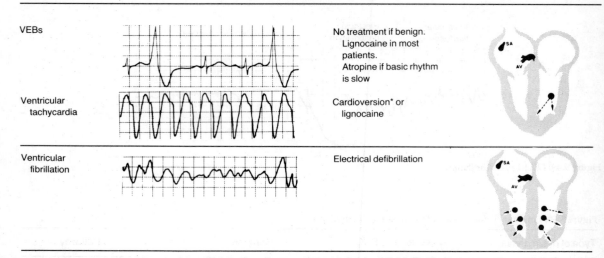

VEBs

No treatment if benign.
Lignocaine in most
patients.
Atropine if basic rhythm
is slow

Ventricular
tachycardia

Cardioversion* or
lignocaine

Ventricular
fibrillation

Electrical defibrillation

Figure 5.50. Continued

TYPES OF AV BLOCK

1. First degree ⎫
2. Second degree ⎬ Partial AV block
3. Third degree – Complete AV block

MECHANISM OF AV BLOCKS

1. Abnormal tissue around and in the AV node causes physiological blockage affecting the entry of the atrial impulse into the ventricles.
2. In first degree block – the impulses are merely slowed.
3. In second degree block – only a portion of the atrial impulses penetrate to the ventricles.
4. In third degree block – no atrial impulse enters the ventricles, so that the atria and ventricles beat independently.

FIRST DEGREE AV BLOCK

See Figure 5.51.
1. The PR interval is prolonged. (The PR interval represents the impulse going through the atrium and the area of the AV node.) It should not exceed 0.2 seconds (five small blocks on ECG paper when one block equals 0.04 seconds) at normal heart rates.
2. Since the atrial and AV nodal tissues are diseased, the electrical impulse takes a longer time to traverse its pathway (as reflected by the increased length of the PR interval).
3. All P waves penetrate the ventricles to form QRS complexes (in contrast to second and third degree block).

SECOND DEGREE AV BLOCK

See Figure 5.52.
1. There are three variations of this:
   a. Most P waves are conducted with a constant PR interval, but occasionally a P wave is not followed by a QRS complex. This is called the 'Mobitz type II' phenomenon (Figure 5.53).

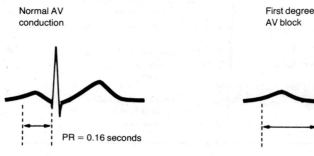

Normal AV
conduction

PR = 0.16 seconds

First degree
AV block

PR = 0.38 seconds

Figure 5.51. First degree AV block. Since the tissue around the AV node is abnormal, the impulse takes longer to traverse this area, which leads to a prolonged PR interval

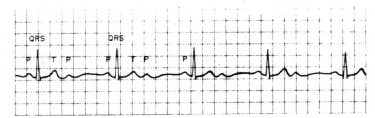

Figure 5.52. Second degree AV block. Some P waves pass through to the ventricles, but others do not

b. There is a progressive lengthening of the PR interval and then failure of conduction of a P wave followed by a conducted P wave with a short PR interval, and then a repetition of this cycle. This is called the 'Wenckebach phenomenon' (Mobitz type I) (Figure 5.54).

c. There may be alternate conducted and non-conducted P waves giving two or three times as many P waves as QRS complexes. This is called 2:1 or 3:1 block.

2. Following myocardial infarction, the Wenckebach phenomenon is usually benign, but Mobitz type II or 2:1 block may precede third degree (complete) block (Figure 5.55).

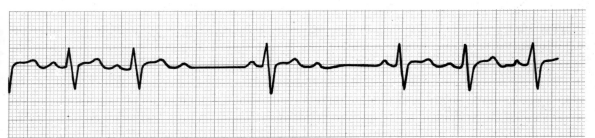

Figure 5.53. Mobitz type II second degree AV block

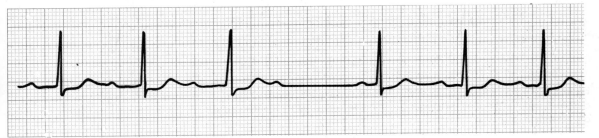

Figure 5.54. Wenckebach-type (Mobitz type I) second degree AV block

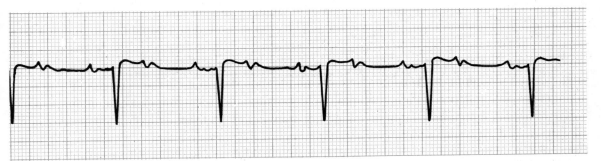

Figure 5.55. Second degree AV block (2:1 type)

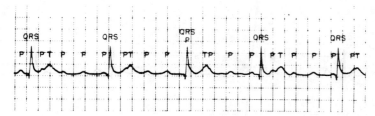

Figure 5.56. Third degree AV block. The P waves and QRS complexes are beating independently against each other

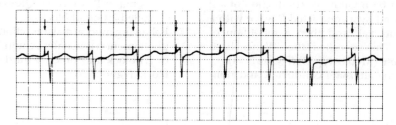

Figure 5.57. Normal pacemaker function. In this ECG each QRS complex is preceded by a small vertical line (arrows) which represents the electrical stimulus of the artificial pacemaker

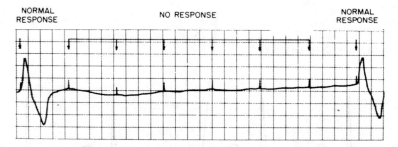

Figure 5.58. Poor pacemaker contact. Notice that the first and last pacemaker stimuli are followed by ventricular complexes and that the other pacemaker deflections failed to produce a cardiac impulse because of the lack of pacemaker contact with the heart wall

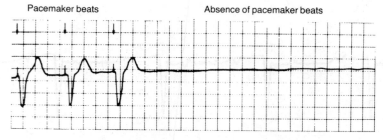

Figure 5.59. Malfunctioning pacemaker. Notice the eventual absence of pacemaker stimuli which in this case resulted in cardiac standstill. The patient had a faulty pacemaker

THIRD DEGREE AV BLOCK

1. Also called a complete AV block.
2. *No* P waves penetrate the AV node and enter the ventricles; therefore, the P waves and QRS complexes are beating *independently*.
3. P waves are seen before the QRS complexes, but the PR interval varies and there is no constant relationship of the P waves to the QRS complexes (Figure 5.56).
4. The pulse rate is usually slow since the ventricles are beating at their own inherent rhythm, which is about 35 beats/minute.

TREATMENT OF AV BLOCKS

1. First degree block:
   No treatment needed.
2. Second degree block:
   a. When certain types of second degree heart block occur in a myocardial infarction, many cardiologists insert a pacemaker which is activated when the cardiac rate falls to unacceptable levels.
   b. To increase rate while awaiting a pacemaker, atropine (0.3–1.2mg) may be given intravenously.
   c. If the rate cannot be maintained with atropine, 1mg of isoprenaline hydrochloride added to 250ml of 5 per cent glucose in water may be infused to stimulate the heart to function at an acceptable rate.

3. Third degree heart block:
   a. In myocardial infarction, third degree block is frequently treated with a pacemaker.
   b. While awaiting insertion of the pacemaker, patient may be maintained on atropine or isoprenaline hydrochloride as in second degree block.

THE ARTIFICIAL PACEMAKER

Normally functioning pacemaker

See Figure 5.57.
1. The ECG of a patient with a normally functioning ventricular artificial pacemaker shows a *vertical line* just at the beginning of the QRS complex. This represents the electrical stimulus of the artificial pacemaker.

Poorly functioning pacemakers

1. Due to lack of contact between pacing catheter and heart wall.
   a. May occur when patient performs a sudden movement.
   b. On the ECG the small vertical line denoting the pacemaker stimulus is *not* followed by a QRS complex (Figure 5.58).
2. Due to malfunctioning:
   a. Examples: wires break or disconnect from pacemaker; battery fails to function.
   b. Noted on ECG by the absence of vertical pacer lines (Figure 5.59).

GUIDELINES: SYNCHRONIZED CARDIOVERSION

Synchronized cardioversion is a *timed* electrical shock to the heart for the purpose of terminating certain dysrhythmias.

Asynchronized cardioversion is the same as defibrillation and is used principally for ventricular fibrillation.

Both types of cardioversion use the same type of electricity, but timed shock is not needed in ventricular fibrillation because there are no T waves. (Synchronized cardioversion is timed *not* to hit the T wave, since an electrical discharge during this phase of the cardiac cycle may cause ventricular fibrillation.)

OBJECTIVE

To stop the abnormal electrical activity of the heart and allow the sinus node (heart's natural pacemaker) to resume normal sinus rhythm.

CONTRAINDICATIONS

Synchronized cardioversion is relatively *contraindicated* when a patient has been taking a significant amount of *digitalis*, since more lethal dysrhythmias may ensure after electrical discharge.

EQUIPMENT

Cardioverter and ECG machine
Conduction jelly and cardiac medications
Resuscitative equipment including:

Endotracheal tubes
Laryngoscopes
Suctioning equipment
Manual breathing bag
Pacing equipment

PROCEDURE

Nursing action

1. If the procedure is elective, it is advisable to fast the patient six to 12 hours before the cardioversion.
   a. Reassure the patient and see that informed consent has been obtained.
   b. Make sure the patient has not been taking digitalis and that the serum potassium is normal.

2. Make sure intravenous line is patent.

3. Obtain a 12-lead ECG before and after cardioversion. The ECG machine leads are best left on the patient, since the ECG printout is of much better quality than that of the monitor. This fact is especially important when one is trying to dissect complicated dysrhythmias.

4. a. Allow the patient to receive oxygen before and after cardioversion.
   b. Do *not* give oxygen during the procedure.

5. Place the paddles in one of the following two positions:
   a. *Anterior–posterior position*
      One paddle – left infrascapular area
      Other paddle – upper sternum at third interspace
   b. *Anterior position*
      One paddle – just to right of sternum at second interspace
      Other paddle – just under left nipple

6. Determine if the machine's synchronization mechanism is working before applying the paddles.
   a. The discharge should hit near the peak of the R wave.

Rationale

During sedation or the procedure, the patient may vomit and aspirate if the stomach is full.

Do not use word 'shock' since this will increase the patient's apprehension.
Low potassium may precipitate postshock dysrhythmias.

An intravenous line may be necessary for medications such as lignocaine and atropine.

An ECG is taken to ensure that the patient has not had a recent myocardial infarction (either just before or after the cardioversion).

Oxygen will help prevent unwanted dysrhythmias after cardioversion.
An explosion could occur if a spark from the paddles should ignite the oxygen during the procedure.

If the electrical discharge hits the T wave, ventricular fibrillation may occur.

b. The R wave usually must be of substantial height; if it is not, adjust the gain (sensitivity) or change the lead. On many machines, the R wave must be upright before there is synchronization.

Synchronization is not used for ventricular fibrillation. (The machine will not work for *defibrillation* if the synchronization mode is on.)

7. Apply electrode paste to all of the paddle surface, but make sure there is no excess around the edges of the paddles.
   a. The paste should be rubbed into the skin very thoroughly, since this allows more electricity to penetrate the body surface.
   b. Make sure paddles are clean because surface material will interfere with the flow of electricity.
   c. Apply firm pressure to the paddle.

If there is excess paste around the paddles, the discharge may run onto the skin, causing a burn. If there is not firm contact between the paddle and skin, a burn may occur; also, electricity is lost from the heart.

8. Set dial for lowest level of electrical energy that can be expected to convert the dysrhythmia. Some dysrhythmias (such as atrial flutter) can be converted with very low energies, such as 25 joules.

Excessive energies may cause unnecessary discomfort to the patient.

9. Diazepam or a short-acting barbiturate should be given if the patient is conscious.

This helps produce amnesia concerning the cardioversion.

10. After the patient is in a light sleep from the intravenous medication and when no one is touching the bed or patient, discharge the cardioverter. If cardioversion does not occur, proceed to a higher energy level.

11. Monitor the ECG after conversion occurs. Blood pressures should be recorded about every 15 minutes until the preshock blood pressure is reached.

The patient may revert to his previous dysrhythmia after conversion.

Vascular Disorders

Vascular disorders is a term that refers to conditions of the blood vessels.

Peripheral vascular disease (PVD) refers to disease affecting the blood vessels that supply the extremities: veins, arteries and lymphatics.

NATURE OF THE DISORDER

1. Long-term. This is often discouraging to the patient: treatment may be painful and tedious; healing is slow.

2. Appears minor, but hospitalization or disability may last for months before healing takes place.

   Patient may have financial concerns and may worry about loss of job, separation from family and community responsibilities.

3. Older people are especially prone to peripheral vascular disease.

4. This condition is often compounded by other medical problems, such as diabetes.

5. If lesions heal, recurrence of the condition, with accompanying incapacity, is frequent.

THROMBUS AND EMBOLUS FORMATION

1. *Thrombus* – a blood clot which partially or completely occludes a blood vessel.
   a. Thrombosed vessel – an occluded vessel.
   b. Thrombosis – the condition of having a thrombosed vessel.
      As early as 1846, Virchow identified blood-stasis, venous wall abnormalities, and clotting abnormalities as factors promoting venous thrombosis. Remembering this triad can help with recognizing risk conditions for thromboemboli.
2. Spontaneous clotting of the blood will not usually occur unless there is damage to the intimal surface of the vessel wall.
   a. Injury by trauma.
   b. Inflammation.
   c. Degenerative changes due to arteriosclerosis.
3. Injured intima – causes platelets to collect, fibrin to form and thrombus to develop.
4. Embolus – an undissolved mass that travels in the bloodstream. It may arise due to a thromboemboli or fat emboli.
   a. *Embolism* – occurs when an embolus moving through a blood vessel arrives at a narrowing of the vessel and thus occludes it.
   b. Air embolism – a bubble of air in the bloodstream.
   c. Fat embolism – multiple droplets of fat in the bloodstream.

ISCHAEMIA

Ischaemia is lack of blood supply sufficient to meet tissue needs. This can develop as a result of:
1. Gradual occlusion of the lumen of the artery by encroachment of the thickened wall (atherosclerosis).
2. More rapid development of ischaemia due to formation of a thrombus at the atherosclerotic site.
3. Rapid occlusion of an artery when a free-flowing embolus lodges at a bifurcation or narrowing of the vessel.

MANIFESTATIONS OF VASCULAR DISORDERS

Assessment

SKIN COLOUR AND TEMPERATURE

See Table 5.8.
Objective determination of skin temperature – differences between two extremities are observed when individual is placed in a new environment; coolness of one extremity.

Coldness

1. Due to deficient blood supply to a part even though the environment is warm.
2. One extremity may be compared to another to note the difference.
3. The patient notices that the part feels uncomfortably cold.

Pallor (paleness)

1. Normally the pink hue of the skin is due to adequate superficial circulation.
2. Diminished blood supply produces paleness, or lack of colour.
3. Blanching occurs when the part is elevated about the level of the heart and the arterial pressure in that part is lower than normal.

Table 5.8   Assessment of acute arterial occlusion vs deep vein thrombosis

	Acute arterial occlusion	Deep vein thrombosis
Onset	Sudden	Gradual
Colour	Pale; later – mottled, cyanotic	Slightly cyanotic; rubescent
Skin temperature	Cold	Warm
Leg size – diameter	May be reduced from normal	Enlarged
Superficial veins	Collapsed	Appear enlarged and prominent
Arterial pulsation	Pulse deficit noted	Normal and palpable (except in marked oedema)
Effect of elevating leg	Condition worsens	Condition improves

Rubor (redness)

1. Instead of a normal rosy pink, the part may be red or reddish-blue. This is due to injury of superficial capillaries which causes them to remain dilated; it may also occur with chronic ischaemia.
2. Circulation is impaired.
3. Anoxia or coldness may be the cause of rubor.

Cyanosis (blueness)

1. Indicates that less than normal amount of oxygen is in the blood.
2. When localized, this may be due to very slow circulation in that part.

OTHER SIGNS

PAIN

1. Due to inadequate blood supply.
2. This is common, but varies with the condition. May be constant and severe.
3. When it occurs only after a certain amount of exercise it is called *intermittent claudication*. (This disappears after rest, but returns with exercise.)
4. When it occurs even at rest (rest pain), it indicates a more severe degree of ischaemia.

Necrosis

1. Loss of viability of tissue.
2. Noted first in most distal parts of the extremity.

Atrophy

1. The muscle shrinks, and there is loss of strength and joint mobility.
2. Due to chronic ischaemia.

EXERCISE TOLERANCE

This is measurement of the amount of exercise the involved part can tolerate before pain is experienced.

PULSE VOLUME

A useful method for recording peripheral pulse volume, based on a scale from zero to +4, follows:

  0 Not palpable – absent pulsations.
+1 Thready, weak, fades in and out – marked impairment of pulsations.
+2 Difficult to palpate; stronger than +1 – moderate impairment.
+3 Easily palpable, not easily obliterated with pressure – slight impairment.
+4 Strong and bounding – normal pulsations.

DIAGNOSIS OF VASCULAR CONDITIONS

See Figure 5.60.

Oscillometry

1. Degree of arterial occlusion may be measured by an oscillometer, which measures pulse volume. One extremity may be compared with the other.
2. An inflatable cuff is wrapped around the extremity and the *oscillometric index* is determined by inflating the cuff and reading the dial.
3. Normal readings (points of pressure at which circulation ceases)
   a. Lower extremity:
      (i) Midthigh   4–16mmHg
      (ii) Upper third of leg   3–12mmHg
      (iii) Above ankle   1–18mmHg
      (iv) Foot   0.2–1mmHg
   b. Upper extremity:
      (i) Upper arm   4–16mmHg
      (ii) Elbow   3–12mmHg
      (iii) Wrist   1–10mmHg
      (iv) Hand   0.2–2mmHg

Phlebography

An X-ray picture of the vascular tree after the injection of a radio-opaque dye.

1. Inform the patient that he may experience an intense burning sensation in the vessel where the solution is injected. This will last for only a few seconds.
2. Note any evidence of allergic reaction to the dye; this may occur as soon as the dye is injected or it may be delayed and occur when the patient reaches his bed.
   a. Sweating, dyspnoea, nausea, vomiting.
   b. Rapid heart rate, numbness of extremities.
   c. Hives.
   d. Treatment:
      (i) Notify doctor.
      (ii) Have adrenaline available for injection, as well as antihistamine drugs and oxygen.
3. Nursing care:
   a. Observe injection site for the following:
      (i) Signs of redness, swelling, bleeding; signs of thrombosis (loss of distal pulses). If these signs occur, notify doctor.
      (ii) Evidence of bleeding.
         Therapy:
         (a) Apply pressure dressing.
         (b) Notify doctor.
   b. Check for arterial occlusion.
      (i) Note extremity pulses; check for quality.
      (ii) Observe colour (pallor or cyanosis).
      (iii) Ask patient about sensation of pain, numbness.

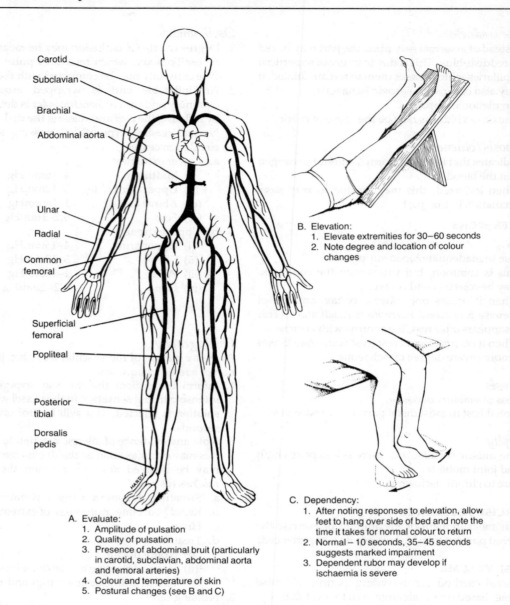

B. Elevation:
1. Elevate extremities for 30–60 seconds
2. Note degree and location of colour changes

C. Dependency:
1. After noting responses to elevation, allow feet to hang over side of bed and note the time it takes for normal colour to return
2. Normal – 10 seconds, 35–45 seconds suggests marked impairment
3. Dependent rubor may develop if ischaemia is severe

A. Evaluate:
1. Amplitude of pulsation
2. Quality of pulsation
3. Presence of abdominal bruit (particularly in carotid, subclavian, abdominal aorta and femoral arteries)
4. Colour and temperature of skin
5. Postural changes (see B and C)

Figure 5.60. Salient points in evaluating peripheral arterial insufficiency

Intermittent claudication determination

1. At rest, blood supply is adequate – but an exercised muscle may require 10 times more blood.
2. Following exercise such as walking, running or climbing stairs, a severe cramping pain or sensation of tiredness develops in those muscle areas not receiving an adequate blood supply.
3. Upon resting, pain is relieved; metabolites are carried away and normal blood-to-tissue demand ratio is restored.

4. Measurement:
   a. Walk patient up steps, counting number of steps taken before pain occurs.
   b. Use a foot-pedal device which lifts a weight when pressed.
      (i) Normally, fatigue occurs in five to ten minutes.
      (ii) The person with arterial occlusion usually complains of pain in less than a minute.

Doppler ultrasound

See Figure 5.61. A noninvasive test used to detect blood flow.

1. A beam of ultrasound is sent into the tissues through an acoustic gel on the skin. Reflected sound from moving blood cells is detected, amplified as audible sound and recorded; velocity of blood flow has a direct effect on the waveforms.
2. Usually the posterior tibial, calf, popliteal and common femoral veins are examined. Arterial flow can be detected by the pulsatile nature of the flow.
3. Signals are assessed for venous patency and valvular competence. Arterial flow is used as an indicator of patency, and the cuff pressure required to stop it indicates arterial pressure at that point.
4. Entire test takes about five to ten minutes.

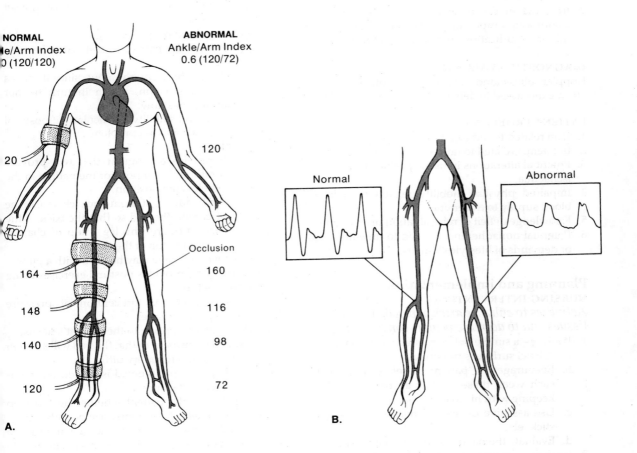

Figure 5.61. (A) The Doppler probe determines pressure over the brachial and posterior tibial or dorsalis pedis arteries. The cuff is inflated until the arterial segment disappears; the cuff is then slowly deflated until the arterial velocity signal returns at systolic pressure. NOTE: Normally, ankle pressure is equal to or slightly above arm pressure. In the presence of occlusive arterial disease (right side of diagrammed person), angle and lower leg pressures are lower by an amount proportional to the degree of circulatory impairment.

(B) Comparison of analogue wave tracings in a normal (left) and a diseased extremity (right). Note the lack of diastolic deflection and the protracted systolic components in the tracing of the abnormal extremity (from: AbuRahma *et al.* (1980) Doppler testing in peripheral vascular occlusive disease, *Surg. Gynecol. Obstet.*, Vol. 150, No. 1, p. 27)

NURSING MANAGEMENT OF PATIENTS WITH VASCULAR DISORDERS

NURSING PROCESS OVERVIEW

Assessment
CLINICAL FEATURES
1. Details concerning the signs of vascular disorders can be found in the preceding pages.
2. Included in the main list of features are skin colour and temperature, pain on walking (intermittent claudication) and exercise intolerance.

DIAGNOSTIC EVALUATION
Doppler ultrasound, oscillometry, phlebography, etc, are discussed in detail in the preceding section.

PATIENT PROBLEMS
1. Pain related to reduced blood supply.
2. Ischaemia related to impaired blood flow.
3. Potential alterations in tissue perfusion related to ischaemia.
4. Impaired physical mobility related to reduced blood supply to extremities.
5. Knowledge deficit of rehabilitation programme.
6. Potential nonadherence related to unwillingness or demands of lifestyle changes.

Planning and implementation
NURSING INTERVENTIONS
Activities to enhance arterial blood supply to tissues and to decrease venous congestion
1. *Walking* – a simple but very effective exercise.
   a. A level surface is preferred.
   b. Encourage the patient to set realistic goals; each week these goals may be extended in keeping with his tolerance.
   c. Use assistive devices as necessary – walker, stick, etc.
   d. Evaluate the patient's ability to climb stairs.
2. *Jogging* – a means of stimulating collateral blood flow not only to legs, but also to the myocardium. May be practised as long as it is comfortable and pleasurable.
3. *Buerger's exercises* – prescribed according to condition of extremities and condition of patient.
   a. Elevate extremity for a minute.
   b. Place extremities in a dependent position until cyanosis or rubor becomes maximal.

c. Lie with extremities horizontal for a minute.
d. See Buerger–Allen exercises below.
4. *Buerger–Allen exercises* – exercises by which gravity alternately fills and empties the blood vessels (Figure 5.62).
   a. Procedure:
      (i) Begin with the patient lying flat in bed. Elevate legs to above level of heart – two minutes or until blanching takes place.
      (ii) Allow legs to be dependent; exercise feet – three minutes or until legs are pink.
      (iii) Instruct the patient to lie flat – five minutes.
      (iv) Repeat a, b, and c five times; do entire set three times a day.
   b. Tolerance and proper pacing:
      (i) Advise the patient to rest when he feels pain.
      (ii) Avoid chilly environment, since it causes vasoconstriction, which in turn further diminishes flow.
      (iii) Maintain stability, particularly if postural hypotension is a problem.
   c. Comfort:
      (i) Improvise equipment that will provide comfortable support for the patient in the leg-elevated position.
      (ii) Well-padded straight-back chair can be placed on the bed so that the back of the chair supports the leg – top of chair is toward the top of the thigh.
      (iii) Overbed table may be used with a pillow.
5. *Oscillating bed* – provides postural exercises using a passive method.
   a. Aids indirectly in prevention of pressure areas – pressure sores.
   b. Prescribed according to the patient's needs.
   c. Explain to the patient that the bed will assist in relieving his circulatory difficulty.
      (i) Explain how the bed is turned on, regulated and stopped.
      (ii) Advise the patient whether he can stop for meals, treatments, rest periods, etc.
   d. Introduce motion of bed gradually in order to eliminate the possibility of headache, dizziness or nausea.
   e. Follow prescribed cycle for the individual patient.
      Cycle: Degree of angle and the length of time to be elevated
      Degree of angle and the length of time to be lowered
   f. Prevent the patient from slipping downward by providing a padded footboard.

POSITION 1
Place legs on a pillow-cushioned chair
for one minute to drain blood.

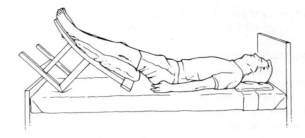

POSITION 2
Hold each of these
stretching positions for
30 seconds to enhance
blood return.

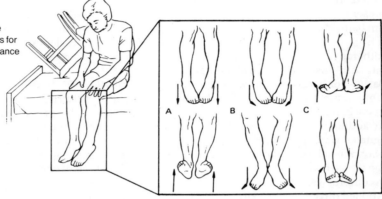

POSITION 3
Lie flat on back, with legs straight.
Hold position for one minute.

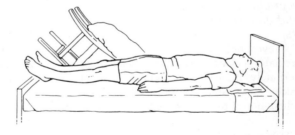

Figure 5.62. Buerger-Allen exercises. Do exercise series six times four times a day (from: Forshee, T. and Minckley, B. 1976) Lumbar sympathectomy, RN, July)

Thermotherapy to promote vasodilatation

NURSING ALERT
When heat is applied externally to an extremity – demand for circulation is increased. When applied to diseased tissues – sensations are impaired; may result in damaging burn and necrosis.

. Dry heat:
  a. Warm water bottles.

(i) Check temperature of water before filling bottle – not to exceed 49°C.
(ii) Apply cover to bottle so that it does not come in direct contact with skin.
b. Heat cradle (thermostatically controlled or regulated with electric bulbs).
  (i) Pad metal edges of cradle to prevent injury to extremities.
  (ii) Control temperature so that it will not exceed 32°C.

(iii) Ensure that bulbs are not likely to be touched by extremity (usually legs and feet).

(iv) Higher temperatures would stimulate metabolism (not desired).

(v) Reduce temperature if patient complains of pain in extremity.

c. Ultrasound (acoustic vibration with frequencies beyond human ear perception).

   (i) Useful in small areas where deeper penetration of heat is desired and where circulation needs to be stimulated.

   (ii) Application time is under 10 minutes.

   (iii) Avoid areas where metal sutures may be present.

d. Paraffin bath.

2. Moist heat:

a. Hydrotherapy.

   (i) Sitz bath – used for perineal therapy.

   (ii) Basin – for hands or feet, with prescribed temperatures and for prescribed times.

b. Whirlpool bath.

   (i) In addition to moist heat, the effect of agitated water provides hydromassage.

   (ii) May be used for one or two extremities or the whole body.

c. Warm compresses.

   (i) Applied directly to the skin.

   (ii) When hot, apply over towelling.

Pressure gradient therapy to promote vasodilatation (compression devices and garments)

1. Cuffs, sleeves, or boots.

a. Circulator – electrically produced air pressure alternately inflates and deflates a boot in which the extremity is encased. Rhythm of occlusion and release as well as pressure can be regulated to correspond to pulse.

b. Pressor sleeve or boot – a plastic tube filled with air.

   (i) Can be maintained at low pressure for several hours.

   (ii) Can be regulated to function intermittently. (Useful in lymphoedema of arm following mastectomy; see p. 721.)

2. Elastic garments.

a. Support for an extremity can be tailor-made: a unique measuring tape was devised by Jobst* so that exact 'fabric pressures' are produced with their custom-made venous pressure gradient supports.

---

* The Jobst Institute, Box 653, Toledo, OH 43694, USA

b. Method of applying supporting hose is demonstrated in Figure 5.63.

c. Any type of support hose, if applied incorrectly (such as permitting rolling at the top) can act as a tourniquet. This will produce stasis, rather than prevent it.

d. Many question the effectiveness of elastic stockings; the nurse will be guided by the preferences of the patient's doctor.

e. Elastic stockings with inflatable pneumatic bladders connected to an automatic air pump are available to help prevent deep-vein thrombi from forming in the calf and lower leg

   (i) The bladders in this device, called the *pulsatile anti-embolism system*, expand and contract and are designed to stimulate circulation.

Prevention of vasoconstriction in the vessels of the extremities

1. Impress the patient with the *dangers of smoking* especially inhaling.

2. Promote an atmosphere that is devoid of emotional tension; restrict those visitors who appear to upset the patient.

3. Advise the patient against wearing constrictive garments, such as panty girdles, garters, belts, jeans and tight stockings.

Hygienic measures and activities to increase the blood flow to the extremities

1. Maintain a warm and properly humidified environment.

2. Put on warm clothing before going out into cold air; protect hands and feet with lamb's wool lining in gloves and boots to prevent vasoconstriction.

3. Take a warm bath to offset chilling; replace vigorous rubbing of the skin after a bath with gentle patting.

4. Avoid excessive heat to extremities (using hot water bottle, electric pad, etc) – increases metabolism, so that more oxygenated blood is demanded.

5. Sleep with the head of the bed elevated about 20.3cm – if patient has pain at rest; wear bed socks to keep feet warm if necessary.

6. Walking is the best form of exercise; otherwise active or passive exercise of the extremities is recommended.

7. Use analgesic and tranquillizing medications as required to keep comfortable.

8. Take prescribed vasodilating medications eve

ut on supports early in the morning, before swelling occurs

ways begin with supports 'inside-out' . . . as they are when you receive them

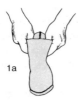

1a

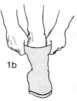

1b

Sit with feet in easy reach. Support must be 'inside-out' with its foot inverted back to heel. Seam faces down (a). rasp each side firmly and pull onto foot (b).

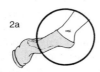

2a

2b

Pull past midpoint of heel (a), so support will not slip back. Then, reach just beyond toes and grasp fabric between gers and start pulling over foot. Pull from sides (b) never by seams.

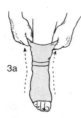

3a

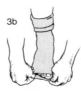

3b

Pull all the way past ankle (a). Seat heel in place. Pull foot portion of support out toward tips of toes (b) to set fabric venly on foot. Allow to settle back normally.

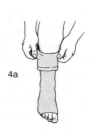

4a

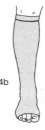

4b

Using short (5cm at a time), snappy pulls (a) pull support up to point it was measured to end (b). Smooth evenly own leg. **Never allow top to roll or turn down.**

Figure 5.63. Method of applying supporting hose. (Courtesy of Jobst)

though they may not appear to help; at times, they maintain the status quo and keep the problem from worsening.

9. Take prescribed antilipidic drugs to retard progress of concomitant atherosclerotic disease by reducing serum lipids.
10. Wear properly fitting and repaired footwear.

PATIENT EDUCATION

Teach the patient the following:

Signs and symptoms of circulatory disturbances affecting peripheral tissues

1. Pain in the extremity. (Note whether this occurs at rest, with limited activity, or with more pronounced exercise.)
2. Colour changes of the skin or nails – pallor, pinkness, rubor, cyanosis.
3. Impaired or peculiar growth of nails.
4. Shiny, taut skin.
5. Discrepancy in size of one extremity when compared to contralateral (opposite) extremity.
6. Enlarged veins or abnormal pulsations of veins.
7. Temperature variations – abnormally cold or abnormally warm.
8. Ulcerations, necrosis or gangrene.

Methods for reducing metabolic demands on the body

1. Take precautions to prevent injury and infection, particularly of the extremities.
2. Practice daily hygienic cleanliness and care of the feet: trim nails properly, avoid strong medications, utilize lamb's wool for pressure areas, wear shoes and hosiery that fit correctly.
3. Avoid exposure to cold or excessive heat.
4. Exercise within recognized limits; set up a reasonable rest plan.
5. Remain in bed if there is evidence of necrosis, ulceration, or gangrene; consult doctor.

Foot care

1. Keep the feet clean to prevent irritation and infection.
   a. Wash daily with a bland soap and warm water.
   b. Dry thoroughly, paying particular attention to areas between the toes; pat rather than rub dry.
   c. Apply lanolin or petroleum jelly to prevent drying and cracking of skin.
   d. Wear clean hose daily: woollen socks for winter, cotton for summer.

2. Avoid injury, excessive pressure or other irritant to the feet.
   a. Shoes:
      (i) Wear properly fitting shoes with comfortable heel.
      (ii) Check inside of shoe; avoid wearing shoe with protruding seams, torn lining, piercing nails, or faulty lumps.
      (iii) Wear shoes when out of bed; avoid going barefoot.
      (iv) Break in new shoes gradually; alternate with an older pair.
      (v) Leather is preferred to rubber or synthetics because the latter interfere with proper circulation of air.
      (vi) Allow wet or damp shoes to dry slowly on shoe trees to prevent misshaping.
   b. Hose:
      (i) Wear proper length and size – if too short, toes are compressed; if too long, wrinkles form and exert pressure on skin.
      (ii) Avoid seams, holes or lumpy, darned areas.
      (iii) Use bedsocks rather than hot water bottle or heating pad if feet are cold in bed.
      (iv) Use woollen or cotton hose; they absorb moisture; nylon is not as absorbent.
      (v) Avoid constricting garments – foundation garments, garters and even support hose unless they are specifically prescribed.
   c. Pedicure:
      (i) Trim toenails straight across after soaking the feet in warm water.
      (ii) Place wisps of cotton under corner of great toenail if there is a tendency toward ingrown toenails.
      (iii) Have a chiropodist cut corns and calluses; do not use corn pads or strong medications.
   d. Heat and cold:
      (i) Keep feet warm; avoid exposure to cold for long periods of time.
      (ii) Use heating devices only on advice of doctor; excessive heat can be as damaging as insufficient warmth.
      (iii) Rely on warm socks, fleece-lined boots or mitts, lightweight blankets, etc, rather than on heating extremities near a fire oven or radiator.
   e. General measures:
      (i) Care in areas where injury to feet is likely, e.g., crowded train stations, construction areas, sports shows, etc.

(ii) Prevent sunburn in the summer and avoid wading in very cold water.
3. Prevent pressure on feet; rest and exercise in moderation.
   a. Place a pillow under covers at end of bed to provide a footrest and prevent weight of top bedding from exerting pressure on toes.
   b. Avoid remaining in one position for long periods of time.
   c. Do not cross legs when sitting because of pressure on nerves and blood vessels.
   d. Elevate feet on a chair or footstool with proper support of leg; do this for about 15 minutes every two hours.
4. If damage or injury occurs to any part of foot or leg, report to doctor.
   a. Redness, swelling, irritation, blistering.
   b. Itching, burning – athlete's foot.
   c. Bruises, cuts, unusual appearance of skin.

A second opinion if lower-extremity amputation is suggested

1. Major vascular centres are reporting commendable results in vascular surgery as an alternative to amputation.
2. Various synthetic graft materials are available for very specific vascular needs.
3. Microsurgery is adding a new dimension to very fine surgical repair.

Evaluation

EXPECTED OUTCOMES

1. Demonstrates increased arterial blood supply to extremities – palpable pulses, warm extremities, reduced pain, normal colour.
2. Exhibits decreased venous congestion – reduced swelling and pain.
3. Promotes vasodilation by adhering to proper hygienic practices.
4. Has no pain; avoids practices that cause vasoconstriction/injury.
5. Attains/maintains tissue integrity; avoids injury.
6. Adheres to the rehabilitation programme.

ANTICOAGULANT THERAPY

Anticoagulant therapy is the administration of medications to achieve the following:

Objectives:

1. Disrupt the blood's natural clotting mechanism.
2. Prevent formation of a thrombus in postoperative patients.

3. Intercept the extension of a thrombus once it has formed.

TYPES OF ANTICOAGULANTS

Oral

Coumarin derivatives: dicoumarol, warfarin sodium, and warfarin potassium.
Indanedione derivatives: anisindione and phenindione.

Parenteral

Heparin sodium.

NURSING ALERT

Anticoagulants cannot dissolve a thrombus that has already formed. Precise nursing assessment is required because of the delicate balance sought between too much clotting (thrombus formation) and too little clotting (haemorrhage).

CLINICAL INDICATIONS

(Authorities disagree about the justification of long-term use of anticoagulants in various disease entities.)
1. *Venous thrombosis* – because of the danger of extension and the danger of emboli.
2. *Pulmonary embolism* – prophylactically, if patient is known to be suspect; also indicated during recovery phase to prevent further clot formation.
3. *Patient susceptible to embolism* – such as a surgical patient who has rheumatic heart disease, one who has had valve surgery.
4. *Coronary occlusion with myocardial infarction.*
5. *Cerebrovascular accident caused by emboli or cerebral thrombi* – to reduce sludging of blood: useful in prevention and treatment of strokes.

HIGHEST RISK

1. Patients whose prothrombin time has been difficult to control from the outset.
2. Men (not women) with aortic valve prostheses.
3. Patients treated with anticoagulants for more than three years.

CONTRAINDICATIONS

1. May cause spontaneous bleeding – therefore not used when there is likelihood of bleeding because of increased capillary fragility or an aneurysm.
2. Individuals with peptic ulcer and chronic ulcerative diseases are considered poor risks, because of the possibility of bleeding.
3. Should not be given following neurosurgery because of danger of haemorrhage in brain or spinal cord.

4. Liver disease may present a problem because of interference with plasma protein clotting factors.
5. Liver and kidney insufficiency diseases because of difficulty in metabolizing and eliminating them – resulting in toxicity and difficulty in responding to antidotal medication (not true of heparin).
6. Poor follow-up by patients; unless the patient cooperates by reporting for blood tests, etc, he should not be on anticoagulants.
7. Severe diabetes, infections or severe traumatic conditions are circumstances in which anticoagulant therapy may be contraindicated.

NURSING INTERVENTIONS
1. The preferred method of heparin administration is continuous infusion (using a pump) because of the low incidence of haemorrhagic complications.
2. Check patient's weight, since dosage is calculated on the basis of weight.
3. Be sure clotting profiles are obtained before treatment is initiated, to detect hidden bleeding tendencies.
4. Place pump out of reach of patient to prevent interference with its proper functioning.
   a. Check frequently to ensure that system is working properly: exact dosage, no leaks, no kinks.
5. Note that periodic coagulation tests are done; these include haematocrit and partial thromboplastin time (PTT).
6. Recognize that heparin may be given by *intermittent intravenous injection*. This may be facilitated by the use of a 'heparin-lock'.
7. *Minidose heparin* is used in certain patients preoperatively to reduce postoperative thromboembolism.
8. Since heparin may be given along with longer lasting hypoprothrombinaemic agents, for the first few days of treatment, each day's medication orders should be checked *after* reports of daily prothrombin time tests are known.
9. Have on hand the antidotes to anticoagulants being used:
   a. Heparin – protamine sulphate.
   b. Coumarin – vitamin K_1.
10. Note that the relatively long duration of action of oral anticoagulants makes it easier to maintain low prothrombin levels for long periods.
11. Observe carefully for any possible signs of bleeding and report immediately so that anticoagulant dosage may be reviewed and altered if necessary:

a. Urine – note evidence of haematuria; indanedione derivatives may turn alkaline urine a red orange colour – acidifying this urine causes this colour to disappear.
b. Stool – check for tarry colour.
c. Following tooth brushing – note any pink or bloody return.
12. Be aware of the following with regard to sensitivity to coumarin derivatives:

May be intensified by:	*May be decreased by:*
Antibiotics	Antacids
Mineral oil	Barbiturates
Quinidine	Oral contraceptives
Salicylates	Adrenal corticosteroids
Tolbutamide	

NURSING ALERT
Drug interactions can alter the effect of anticoagulants. Review with the doctor the effect of other medications the patient may be taking during anticoagulant therapy.

PATIENT EDUCATION
1. Information to be relayed to the doctor before anticoagulant therapy is initiated:
   a. What medications are currently being taken? Note that barbiturates increase metabolism of coumarin medications – therefore an increased dose of anticoagulants is in order.
   b. What treatments are being done for problems other than circulatory problems?
   c. If female, whether a pregnancy is planned or confirmed?
   d. If other treatments are anticipated, such as major dental work, haemorrhoidectomy?
2. During anticoagulant therapy:
   a. Follow instructions carefully and take medications exactly as prescribed.
   b. Take medications at the same time each day and do not stop taking them even though symptomless.
   c. Wear a bracelet or carry a card indicating that anticoagulants are being taken; include name, address, and phone number of doctor.
3. Notify the doctor:
   a. In case of accident, infection, or other significant illness that may affect blood clotting.
   b. If surgical care by another doctor or dentist is needed. Inform him that anticoagulants are being taken.
   c. If a dose of anticoagulant is forgotten. Do not take extra pills to make up for a missed dose.
   d. In case of diarrhoea, upset stomach, high fever.

4. Avoid:
   a. Taking any other medications without first checking with doctor, particularly:
      (i) Vitamins.
      (ii) Aspirin.
      (iii) Mineral oil.
      (iv) Cold medicines.
      (v) Antibiotics.
      (vi) Phenylbutazone.
   b. Excessive use of alcohol, since alcohol may affect clotting capacity; check on acceptable limits for social drinking.
   c. Participation in activities in which there is high risk of injury.
   d. Foods that may cause diarrhoea or upset stomach.
5. Be alert for these warning signs:
   a. Excessive bleeding that does not stop quickly (such as following shaving, a small cut, teeth brushing with gum injury, nose bleed).
   b. Excessive menstrual bleeding.
   c. Skin discolouration or bruises that appear suddenly.
   d. Black or bloody bowel movements; for questionable stool discolouration, use Hemoccult test tape.
   e. Blood in urine.

NURSING ALERT

Patients taking phenindione produce orange or beige coloured urine; when the urine is acidified, this colouration disappears. With true haematuria, acid does not affect colour.

   f. Faintness, dizziness, or unusual weakness.
6. A reminder:
   Later, when anticoagulant medication is stabilized, the patient must be reminded to keep prothrombin test appointments as scheduled – once a week or however often they are required.

GUIDELINES: SUBCUTANEOUS INJECTION OF HEPARIN

OBJECTIVE

When prolonged therapy is indicated, heparin may be given subcutaneously into fatty tissues (Figure 5.64).

EQUIPMENT

1 or 2ml disposable syringe
Fine sharp needle, No. 27, 1.6cm long
Skin antiseptic

CONSIDERATIONS

1. Most convenient sites are along lower abdominal fat pad – to avoid inadvertent intramuscular injection and haematoma formation.
   a. A common location site is the fatty area anterior to either iliac crest.
   b. Avoid injection sites within 5cm of the umbilicus because of possibility of entering a larger blood vessel.
2. Areas where subcutaneous layer is thin should be avoided.

PROCEDURE
Performance phase

Nursing action	Rationale
1. Sponge the area gently with alcohol. Do not rub!	Rubbing or pinching skin might initiate damage to the tissue; heparin would aggravate any bleeding.
2. Attempt to stretch skin out, using palm of left hand. Some prefer to (gently) pick up a well-defined fold of skin.	Try to empty blood vessels in local area to lessen likelihood of their being pierced by needle – with subsequent haematoma formation.

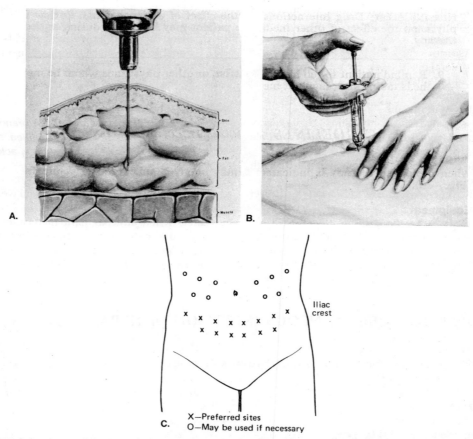

Figure 5.64. Subcutaneous injection indicating technique and sites for heparin therapy. (A) When prolonged therapy is indicated, heparin is given most conveniently subcutaneously into the fatty tissue, which is a distinct layer beneath the skin. (B) First stretch skin to empty vessels so they are less apt to be pierced by needle. Then insert the needle directly through the skin at a right angle (see A). (C) Since the site of injection of heparin must be changed each time the drug is administered, a suggested division of the abdomen into suitable areas is indicated. Do not inject into a bruised area or within 5cm of the umbilicus or any scar. (Courtesy: Wyeth Laboratories, Philadelphia, PA)

3. Holding the shaft of the syringe in dart fashion, insert needle directly through the skin at a right angle just into the subcutaneous fatty layer.

4. Move right hand into position to direct plunger.
  a. Do not move needle tip once it is inserted.
  b. Do not pull back plunger for testing.

    Aspiration in a forcible manner can damage small blood vessels and frequently lead to bleeding and haematoma formation, especially in the presence of high local concentration of heparin.

5. Firmly push plunger down as far as it will go.

    This ensures administration of total dose of heparin.

6. When injection has been made, withdraw needle gently at the same angle at which it entered, releasing skin roll upon withdrawal of needle.

    To minimize tissue damage.

7. Press an alcohol sponge to the site for a few seconds.

To minimize oozing or bleeding.

Follow-up care

Nursing action

1. *Do not rub the area. Instruct patient not to rub area.*

2. *Site of injection:*
   a. Change site of injection each time heparin is administered.
   b. A chart can be marked with time, date, and measured dosage so that rotation of sites can be ensured.

Note: Low dose heparin (5,000 units subcutaneously every eight or 12 hours) may be used to prevent deep vein thrombosis postoperatively.

Rationale

Rubbing would increase the likelihood of bleeding.

CONDITIONS OF THE VEINS

PHLEBITIS, THROMBOPHLEBITIS, PHLEBOTHROMBOSIS

Note: While the terms do not necessarily represent identical pathologies, for clinical purposes they are used interchangeably when discussing the same process.

Phlebothrombosis is the formation of a thrombus or thrombi in a vein; in general, the clotting is related to (1) stasis, (2) abnormality of the walls of the vein(s), and (3) abnormality of clotting mechanism. Deep veins of the lower extremities are most commonly involved.

Deep vein thrombosis (DVT) is the thrombosis of deep rather than superficial veins. Two serious complications are pulmonary embolism (p. 189) and postphlebitic syndrome (pp. 345–346).

Phlebitis is an inflammation of the walls of a vein.

Thrombophlebitis is a condition in which a clot forms in a vein secondary to phlebitis or because of partial obstruction of the vein.

AETIOLOGY
1. Venous stasis – following operations, childbirth or bed rest for any chronic illness.

2. Prolonged sitting or as a complication of varicose veins.
3. Injury (bruise) to a vein; may result from direct trauma to veins from intravenous injections, indwelling catheters.
4. Extension of an infection of tissues surrounding the vessel.
5. Continuous pressure of a tumour, aneurysm, heavy pregnancy.
6. Unusual activity in a person who has been sedentary.
7. Hypercoagulability associated with malignant disease, blood dyscrasias.

Basically, there are three causes: stasis, injury to a vessel wall, and hypercoagulability (or a combination of these factors).

HIGH-RISK FACTORS
1. Hip fracture.
2. Prosthetic joint replacement.
3. Malignancy.
4. Major surgery after the age of 40.
5. Acute myocardial infarction.
6. Thrombotic cerebrovascular accident.
7. Previous venous insufficiency.
8. Contraceptives (oral).

Assessment
CLINICAL FEATURES
1. For phlebothrombosis, there are no clinical signs, since there is no inflammation.

2. Slight swelling around ankle; obvious prominence of leg veins in affected leg.
3. Calf pain may be aggravated when foot is dorsiflexed with the knee flexed. Unfortunately, this is not a clear sign of early or positive thrombosis. In some patients with obvious thrombophlebitis, this sign is not present, and in other kinds of involvement (irritation of sciatic nerve roots and myositis), the sign may be positive.
4. Muscle ache – may be falsely assumed to result from wearing flat bedroom slippers postoperatively (Figure 5.65).

NURSING ASSESSMENT
1. Inspect the lower extremities by removing top bedding from foot end up to the patient's groin (remove any temperature-controlling devices such as heavy wool socks, ice bag, at least 10 minutes before clinical inspection).
2. Note symmetry or asymmetry:
   a. Measure and record leg circumferences daily (see Guidelines: Obtaining Leg Measurements to Detect Early Swelling) – mark on skin with felt-tip pen where the measuring tape is used so that the same area is measured each time.
3. Observe for evidence of venous distension or oedema, puffiness, stretched skin, hardness to touch.

4. Hand test extremities for temperature variations.
   a. The examiner's hands should be placed in cold water and then dried.
   b. Hands are then placed simultaneously on each leg – first compare ankles, then move to the calf and up to the knee.
5. Examine for signs of obstruction due to occluding thrombus – swelling, particularly in loose connective tissue of popliteal space, ankle or suprapubic area.

PATIENT PROBLEMS
1. Ischaemia and pain related to impaired circulation.
2. Possible alteration in tissue perfusion related to ischaemia.
3. Impaired physical mobility related to pathophysiological problem causing reduced blood supply to the extremities.
4. Potential nonadherence to the rehabilitation programme related to lack of understanding and nonacceptance of required lifestyle changes.

Planning and implementation
NURSING INTERVENTION
Early resolution of thrombi and prevention of sequelae
1. Avoid massaging or rubbing calf because of the

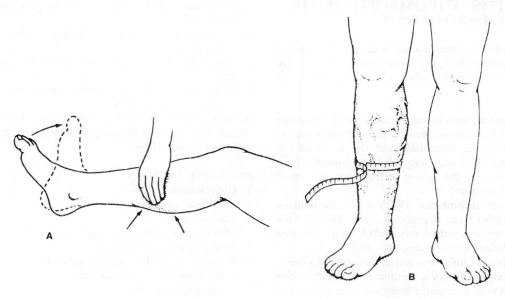

Figure 5.65. Assessment of signs and symptoms of phlebothrombosis. (A) With the knee flexed, the patient may complain of pain in the calf on dorsiflexion of foot (Homans' sign) – this was considered an unmistakable sign of early and subclinical thrombosis; it may or may not be present. Gentle compression reveals tenderness of the calf muscles (note arrow). (B) The affected leg may swell; veins are more prominent and may be palpated easily

danger of breaking up the clot, which can then circulate as an embolus.

2. Consult doctor concerning proper position of the extremity, since there may be differences of opinion.
   a. Some recommend elevation – reduces venous congestion and oedema.
   b. Others do not recommend elevation – because of the possibility of releasing emboli.
3. If prescribed, apply heat in the form of hot, wet dressings or a heat cradle to promote circulation and comfort.
4. Place the patient on anticoagulant therapy (see pp. 337–339).

NURSING ALERT
This may not be done preoperatively because of fear of increasing possibility of haemorrhage during operation. Mini-doses of heparin may be prescribed.

5. Encourage early ambulation of surgical patients – encourage leg exercises for the bedridden patient, to prevent venous stasis.
6. Suggest deep-breathing exercises that produce increased negative pressure in the thorax, which in turn assists in emptying large veins.
7. Recommend properly applied pressure gradient stockings to increase deep venous blood circulation. (Remove twice daily and check for skin changes or calf tenderness.)
8. Use electrical stimulation of calf and pneumatic compression of leg if prescribed.
9. Practise prophylactic measures for bedridden patients who are prone to develop thrombosis:
   a. Lie in bed in the slightly reversed Trendelen-burg position because it is better for the veins to be full of blood than empty.
   b. Place a footboard across the foot of the bed.
   c. Instruct the patient to press the balls of the feet against the footboard, just as if he were rising up on his toes.
   d. Then ask the patient to relax his foot.
   e. Request that the patient do this many times a day.

PATIENT EDUCATION
Teach the patient as follows.

Increase venous return from lower extremities
1. Prevent venous stasis by proper positioning in bed.
   a. Support full length of legs when they are to be elevated (Figure 5.66).
   b. Prevent bony prominence of one leg from pressing on soft tissue of other leg (in side-lying position, place a soft pillow between legs).
   c. Avoid hyperflexion at knee as in jackknife position (head up, knees up, pelvis and legs down); this promotes stasis in pelvis and extremities.
2. Initiate active exercises, *unless contraindicated*, in which case use passive exercises.
   a. If the patient is on bed rest:
      (i) Simulate walking if lying on back – five minutes every two hours.
      (ii) Simulate bicycle pedalling if lying on side – five minutes every two hours.
   b. If contraindicated, resort to passive exercises – five minutes every two hours.

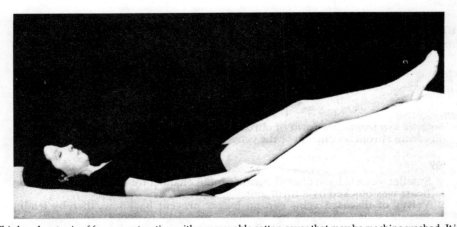

Figure 5.66. This leg elevator is of foam construction with a removable cotton cover that may be machine washed. It is clamped to the lower end of the mattress. This position is anatomically correct and provides adequate support to all parts of the leg. Oedema and stasis of the lower extremities can be controlled. (Courtesy of Jobst)

c. If permissible, have the patient sit up and move to side of bed in sitting position.

Provide a foot support (stool or chair) – dangling of feet is not desirable, since pressure may be exerted against popliteal vessels and may cause obstruction to blood flow.

d. If the patient is permitted out of bed, encourage him to walk 10 minutes each hour; otherwise, carry out passive exercises.

e. Discourage crossing of legs because compression of vessels can restrict blood flow.

Avoid further injury to damaged vessel walls

1. Promote circulation and prevent stasis by applying elastic hose. Apply elastic hose or elastic bandage from the toes up the leg; support must be consistent along entire leg.

NURSING ALERT
Elastic hose have no role in the management of the acute phase of deep venous thrombosis, but are of value once ambulation has begun. Their use will minimize or delay the development of the postphlebitic syndrome.

2. Avoid straining or any manoeuvre that increases venous pressure in the leg. Eliminate the necessity to strain at stool by providing increased fibre in the diet and administer stool softeners if necessary.

3. Also, follow Planning and Implementation – Vascular Disorders, p. 332.

Evaluation

EXPECTED OUTCOMES

1. Achieves resolution of thrombi; avoids rubbing calf; performs exercises.

2. Avoids trauma or injury to extremities; practises prescribed exercises, does not cross legs, takes stool softeners, wears proper footwear, reports injuries to leg.

GUIDELINES: OBTAINING LEG MEASUREMENTS TO DETECT EARLY SWELLING

OBJECTIVE
Obtain leg measurements for serial data compilation that may detect early swelling and thus indicate onset of thrombophlebitis.

EQUIPMENT
Flexible tape measure in centimetres
Black felt-tip pen

PROCEDURE
Preparatory phase

Nursing action
1. Instruct patient to lie in dorsal recumbent position.

Performance phase

Nursing action	Rationale
1. On admission of the patient, measure the circumference of the ankle, calf and thigh.	This will provide baseline data.
2. Obtain measurements at the widest part of the ankle, calf and thigh.	To provide a consistent anatomical place of measurement; some clinics have a predetermined starting point, such as 15 or 20cm from the knee cap.

3. Mark the leg with a black felt-tip pen. | To promote accuracy of measurements.

4. Thereafter, when measuring, place the measuring tape on the marked line.

5. Repeat measurements taken on admission the next morning before any patient activity. | Otherwise, later measurements may give a false reading because of gravitational oedema.

6. Thereafter, obtain measurements weekly unless there is evidence of swelling, in which case it is done daily. | Weekly – to detect swelling.
Daily – to monitor swelling and its response to treatment.

7. Record measurements:

Leg measurements

Date:

Time: Right   Left

Ankle _____ cm   Ankle _____ cm

Calf _____ cm   Calf _____ cm

Thigh _____ cm   Thigh _____ cm

8. Compare measurements:
   a. Check one leg with the other.

   b. Check each leg with baseline data.

Significant findings:
1.5cm (males) difference between legs or compared with baseline.
1.2cm (females) difference between legs or compared with baseline.

CHRONIC VENOUS INSUFFICIENCY (POSTPHLEBITIC SYNDROME)

Postphlebitic syndrome is a form of chronic venous stasis; it may be a residual effect of phlebitis. It results from chronic occlusion of the veins or destruction of the valves.

AETIOLOGY

1. Smaller vessels have dilated because main channel for returning blood from the leg to the heart was blocked by a thrombus.
2. Valves of diseased veins can no longer prevent backflow, thereby leading to → chronic venous stasis → swelling and oedema → superficial varicose veins.
3. Lower leg becomes discoloured because of venous stasis and pigmentation ulceration (postphlebitis).

ALTERED PHYSIOLOGY AND CLINICAL FEATURES

1. Pressure in veins at ankle is much greater than normal when leg is dependent – leads to transudation of fluid from intravascular to interstitial space.
2. Stasis, intractable induration, chronic oedema, discolouration, pain, venous congestion, ulceration, recurrent thrombosis → cellulitis.
3. The medial malleolus is the most common site.

DIAGNOSTIC EVALUATION

1. Non-invasive screening – Doppler, plethysmography (see p. 331).

TREATMENT AND NURSING MANAGEMENT

1. Best treatment is prevention of phlebitis and constant use of compression if phlebitis has occurred.
2. After this syndrome has developed, only palli-

ative and symptomatic treatment is possible because the damage is irreparable.

3. Patient education:
   Instruct the patient as follows:
   a. Wear elastic stockings to prevent oedema.
   b. Avoid sitting or standing for long periods of time.
   c. Elevate legs on a chair for five minutes every two hours.
   d. Elevate legs above level of head by lying down (two or three times daily).
   e. Raise foot of bed 15–20cm at night to allow venous drainage by gravity.
   f. Apply bland, oily lotions to prevent scaling and dryness of skin.
   g. Avoid constricting bandages.
   h. Prevent injury, bruising, scratching or other trauma to skin of leg and foot.

VARICOSE VEINS

Primary varicose veins – bilateral dilatation and elongation of saphenous veins; deeper veins are normal. As the condition progresses, because of hydrostatic pressure and vein weakness, the vein walls become distended, with asymmetrical dilatation, and some of the valves become incompetent. The process is irreversible.

INCIDENCE

This is a common venous disorder of the lower extremity; over the age of 40; 20 per cent of women and 7 per cent of men develop varicose veins.

AETIOLOGY

1. Dilatation of the vein prevents the valve cusps from meeting; this results in increased back-up pressure, which is passed into the next lower segment of the vein. The combination of vein dilatation and valve incompetence produces the varicosity (Figure 5.67).
2. Varicosities may occur elsewhere in the body (oesophageal and haemorrhoidal veins) when flow or pressure is abnormally high.
3. Predisposing factors:
   a. Hereditary weakness of vein wall or valves.
   b. Long-standing distention of veins brought about by pregnancy, obesity or prolonged standing.
   c. Old age – loss of tissue elasticity.

Assessment

CLINICAL FEATURES

1. Disfigurement due to large, discoloured, tortuous leg veins.
2. Easy leg fatigue, cramps in leg, heavy feeling, increased pain during menstruation, nocturnal muscle cramps.

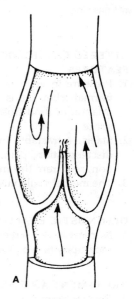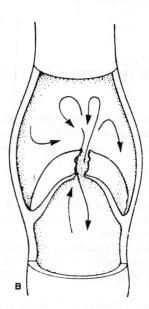

Figure 5.67. Valve incompetence develops as dilatation of a vessel prevents effective approximation of valve cusps. (A) Closed venous valve. (B) Incompetent venous valve

DIAGNOSTIC EVALUATION

1. *Trendelenburg test* – to demonstrate presence or absence of valvular incompetence of communicating veins.
   a. A tourniquet is snugly fastened around the lower extremity just above the highest noted varicosities.
   b. The patient is asked to stand with tourniquet in place.
   c. Failure of varicosities to empty suggests valvular incompetence of communicating veins distal to tourniquet.
2. *Photoplethysmography* – a non-invasive technique to observe venous flow haemodynamics by noting changes in the blood content of the skin. It can be done rapidly, is inexpensive and highly reproducible.
3. *Doppler ultrasound* – can detect accurately and rapidly the presence or absence of venous reflux in deep or superficial vessels.
4. *Venous outflow and reflux plethysmography* – able to detect deep venous occlusion.
5. *Ascending and descending venography* – an invasive technique that can also demonstrate venous occlusion and patterns of collateral flow.
   This test is expensive; it may not be required if a careful history, physical examination, and laboratory testing are done.

COMPLICATIONS

1. Leg oedema, pain from superficial thrombosis.
2. Haemorrhage due to the weakening of the vein wall and pressure upon it.
3. Skin infection and breakdown, producing ulcers (rare in primary varices).

PATIENT PROBLEMS

1. Pain related to venous insufficiency and venous stasis.
2. Oedema related to chronic venous insufficiency.
3. Potential for injury and infection of extremities related to impaired venous return.
4. Impaired physical mobility related to pain and chronic swelling.
5. Embarrassment, depression due to appearance and/or disability.

Planning and implementation

MEDICAL MANAGEMENT AND NURSING INTERVENTIONS

The patient is instructed to:
1. Avoid activities that cause venous stasis by obstructing venous flow.
   a. Wearing tight socks, tight girdle.
   b. Sitting or standing for prolonged periods of time.
   c. Crossing the legs at knees for prolonged periods while sitting (reduces circulation by 15 per cent).
2. Control excessive weight gain.
3. Wear firm elastic support as prescribed, from toe to thigh when in upright position.
   a. Put elastic stockings on in bed before getting up.
   b. Waist-high elastic support hose are available and may be useful.
4. Elevate foot of bed 15–20cm for night sleeping.
5. Avoid injuring legs.

SURGICAL MANAGEMENT AND NURSING IMPLEMENTATION

1. Indications:
   a. Progressively advancing varicosities.
   b. Stasis ulceration.
   c. Cosmetic needs.
2. Procedure: a single method or combination of methods is tailored to meet the needs of the individual:
   a. *Sclerosing injection* – not used as frequently today; may be combined with ligation or limited to treatment of isolated varicosities. The affected vessel may be sclerosed by injecting sodium tetradecyl sulphate or similar sclerosing agent. Compression bandage is then applied without interruption for six weeks; inflamed endothelial surfaces adhere by direct contact.
   b. *Multiple vein ligation.*
   c. *Ligation and stripping* of the greater and/or lesser saphenous systems. This is the most effective procedure.
   d. Some doctors are using the *laser* beam to treat varicosities.
3. Preoperative patient care:
   a. Prepare the skin at least 12 hours prior to surgery by thoroughly cleansing the lower abdomen and legs with a detergent–germicidal soap. This may be done by shower or local scrub.
   b. Hair removal may be by depilatory or shave according to surgeon's request.
   c. Have the patient prepared on the day before surgery (and after his daily skin cleansing) for the surgeon to mark his skin with a felt-tip pen (indelible).
4. Postoperative nursing care and patient support:
   a. At first, the legs are encased in pressure

bandages from the toes to the groin; this is followed by knee-level stockings for three to four weeks after surgery.

b. Elevate the legs about 30 degrees and provide adequate support for the entire leg.

c. Observe the patient for complaints of pain in specific areas of the foot or ankle; if the elastic bandage is too tight, loosen the bandage – later, have it reapplied.

d. Observe circulation to detect constriction or haemorrhage.

e. Activate the individualized therapeutic plan for the following:
   (i) Encourage ambulation according to the preoperative condition of the skin and subcutaneous tissues;
   (ii) Discourage dangling of the legs because it causes stasis of blood in the lower leg.
   (iii) Encourage the patient to walk with a normal gait; offer support if necessary; this activity should be progressive, depending on tolerance.

f. If there are significant trophic changes in the leg, due to long-term varicosities (past history), postoperative care requires more bed rest and slow ambulation; in this event, leg and foot exercises in bed are helpful.

g. Postoperatively, the leg tends to be and feel very bruised. This may be a problem in the groin, especially if the support stocking ends over a bruise.

h. Note that complaints of patchy numbness can be expected but should disappear in less than a year.

i. Recognize that varicosities may recur; therefore, conservative measures, learned preoperatively, should be continued.

j. Follow-up visits every six months are urged.

Evaluation
EXPECTED OUTCOMES
1. Reduces leg fatigue and cramps by limiting standing, avoiding restricting garments that impede leg circulation, and maintaining proper weight.
2. Recovers from surgical treatment, if indicated – demonstrates improved circulation, performs exercises and gradually ambulates as tolerated.
3. Adheres to the safeguards as taught and plans to have follow-up visits every six months.

STASIS ULCERS

Stasis ulcer is an excavation of the skin surface produced by sloughing of inflammatory necrotic tissue, usually caused by vascular insufficiency in the lower extremity.

INCIDENCE
1. Occurrence is increasing, particularly in the older age group.
2. Postphlebitic syndrome and stasis account for most leg ulcers.
3. Other causes include obstruction of one of the main veins by pregnancy or abdominal tumour, incompetency of valves of the ileofemoral vein, burns, sickle cell anaemia, neurogenic disorders.
4. Hereditary factors also play a role in the predisposition of certain individuals.

PREVENTION
1. Prevent oedema – in stasis dermatitis, pruritus and scaling pigmentation may be the only features; bed rest and a 30 degree elevation of the lower extremity may alleviate the oedema.
2. Avoid trauma.

Assessment
DIAGNOSTIC EVALUATION
1. Non-invasive screening – Doppler and plethysmography.

PATIENT PROBLEMS
1. Impaired skin integrity related to vascular insufficiency.
2. Pain related to inflamed leg ulcer.

Planning and implementation
NURSING INTERVENTIONS
Reducing inflammation
1. Elevate the leg and maintain bed rest.
2. Initiate proper cleansing routine.
   a. Handle leg very gently.
   b. Use mild soap, warm water and cotton balls.
3. Remove devitalized tissue.
   a. Flush out necrotic materials with hydrogen peroxide.
   b. Apply enzymatic ointments such as fibrinolysin and desoxyribonuclease, and proteolytic enzymes with neomycin.

Promoting healing
1. Again, elevation of the extremity is most important.
2. Participate in physiotherapy and maintain a regular exercise programme.
3. Control excess weight and provide proper vitamin and protein dietary supplements.
4. Apply gold leaf (done in some centres) directly

over ulcer site to stimulate formation of granulation tissue.

5. Use sterile saline compresses if area is inflamed or oozing.
6. Apply compression bandages to the leg (gelatin compression boot – Figure 5.68).
7. Some centres prefer moist dressings using aqueous solution of aluminium subacetate 0.25 per cent because it is inexpensive, bacteriostatic, and nonmacerating to adjacent skin.

PATIENT EDUCATION
1. Stress the importance of following explicitly the recommendations of the doctor–nurse team.
2. Explain the hazards of trying other remedies on his own at home.
3. Indicate that the treatment may be long but that patience is an important aspect.
4. Maintain healthy tissue when the ulcer is healed by continuing with the safeguards practised before, because breakdown of healthy tissue, unfortunately, frequently occurs.

Evaluation
EXPECTED OUTCOMES
1. Relates that pain is relieved.
2. Promotes healing by elevating the extremity as prescribed, participates in physiotherapy and maintains prescribed diet.
3. Controls infections by using aseptic technique when changing dressings; wears gelatin compression boot as prescribed.

CONDITIONS OF THE ARTERIES

ARTERIAL EMBOLISM

AETIOLOGY
1. Arterial emboli usually (about 85 per cent) originate from thrombi in the heart chambers.
2. Arteriosclerosis may cause roughening or ulceration of atheromatous plaques, which can lead to emboli.

CLINICAL FEATURES
May vary from:
1. The patient's being totally unaware of the event, to
2. Acute pain – severe, to
3. Loss of function – motor and sensory
   a. Paralysis of part   Due to embolic block
   b. Anaesthesia of part   or artery
   c. Pallor and coldness   Due to associated
                               vasomotor reflex

TREATMENT

Note: This is an emergency and is life-threatening; it requires immediate operative intervention if the embolus has major effect.

1. Heparin should be administered intravenously to reduce tendency of emboli to form or expand – useful in small arteries.

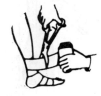
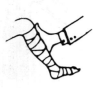
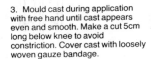

. Apply straight from can. Hold nee in slight flexion. Pad instep nd ankle with cotton wad. Start at nner ankle. Make overlapping urns. Figure-of-eight turn around nkle joint. Use firm equal ompression up to the knee.

2. If a turn does not fit snugly, nip the edges with scissors or cut bandage off and start a new turn.

3. Mould cast during application with free hand until cast appears even and smooth. Make a cut 5cm long below knee to avoid constriction. Cover cast with loosely woven gauze bandage.

4. Patient can be fully ambulatory. Boot is usually changed once a week. Remove by cutting with scissors.

Figure 5.68. Application of gelatin compression boot.

2. Protect the extremity by keeping it at or below the horizontal plane; protect leg from hard surfaces and tight or heavy overlaying bed linens.
3. Administer analgesics as prescribed for relief of pain.
4. Prepare the patient for surgery; surgical intervention (embolectomy) is essential when an embolus blocks a large artery, such as the iliac (Figure 5.69).
5. Postoperative nursing management:
   a. Encourage activity in the leg to prevent stasis – obtain specific recommendations from surgeon concerning type and duration of exercises.
   b. Administer anticoagulants with full knowledge of what to watch for.
      (i) Inspect for bleeding anywhere, including surgical wound; this may be indicative of overdose of heparin.
      (ii) Monitor vital signs.
      (iii) Recognize cardiovascular history of this patient; hence be able to assess cardiac and circulatory manifestations.

PROGNOSIS
1. Arterial embolism is a threat not only to the extremity (5 to 25 per cent possibility of amputation) but also to the patient (15 to 40 per cent mortality rate).

2. Mortality rate increases because of cardiac disease; development of gangrene also contributes to increase in number of deaths.
3. Other cardiovascular difficulties compound the problem.

OCCLUSIVE ARTERIAL DISEASE

Occlusive arterial disease is a form of arteriosclerosis in which the vascular system of the leg becomes blocked. Chronic occlusive arterial diseases occurs much more frequently than does acute (which is the sudden and complete blocking of a vessel by a thrombus or embolus).

INCIDENCE
Men are affected more than women. Parallels that of arteriosclerotic heart disease.

CLINICAL FEATURES
Symptoms appear gradually:
1. Intermittent claudication (see p. 330).
2. Coldness of extremity.
3. Colour change – pallor.
4. Decrease in size of leg.
5. Tingling, numbness of toes.
6. Later – pain, even when leg is at rest; occurs at night, requiring patient to get out of bed to walk to relieve pain.

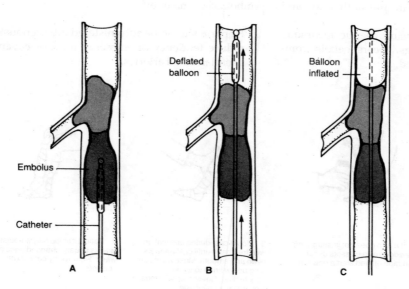

Figure 5.69. Extracting an embolus from a vessel can be done with the use of a Fogarty embolectomy catheter. (A, B) The catheter, with a soft deflated balloon near the tip, is threaded through the artery via an arteriotomy. It is passed through the embolus and its thrombus. (C) It is then inflated. (D) A steady pull downwards withdraws the embolus along with the catheter

7. Cramp-like excruciating pain in calf muscles.
8. Ulcers of toes and feet develop.

DIAGNOSTIC EVALUATION

1. Vascular physical examination, including brachial and ankle systolic pressures, before and after exercise.
2. Doppler ultrasound probe.
3. Segmental plethysmography.
4. Angiography.

TREATMENT AND NURSING MANAGEMENT
Objectives
Preserve the extremity.
Relieve the intermittent claudication.

See page 332, Nursing Management of Patients with Vascular Problems.

1. Where conservative measures clearly are not enough, constructive arterial surgery (endarterectomy, arterial bypass grafting or a combination) may be required.
2. Percutaneous transluminal angioplasty (PTA) may be used alone or with reconstructive surgery for dilatation of localized noncalcified segments of narrowed arteries.
3. Microvascular surgery may be required for small-artery occlusive disease.
4. Following any surgery, a conservative programme to manage intermittent claudication may be initiated (walking, weight reduction, no smoking, control of other conditions such as hypertension, diabetes mellitus).

VASOSPASTIC DISORDER – RAYNAUD'S PHENOMENON

Raynaud's phenomenon is a general term to describe a condition in which there is an increased or unusual sensitivity to cold or emotional factors, and it occurs primarily in the hands, rarely in the feet.

AETIOLOGY

1. Unknown; there appears to be a hereditary predisposition.
2. Vasoconstriction appears to be mediated through release of catecholamines at the neuroarteriole junction.
3. An underlying problem such as a collagen vascular disease may exist.

Assessment
CLINICAL FEATURES AND DIAGNOSTIC EVALUATION

1. Intermittent arteriolar vasoconstriction resulting in coldness, pain, pallor.
2. Occasionally, there is ulceration of the finger tips.
3. The condition occurs most commonly in females between the age of 16 and 40 years.
4. It occurs more frequently in cold climates and during winter months.
5. Involvement of the fingers appears to be asymmetric; thumbs are less often involved.
6. Characteristic colour changes: blue–white–red.
   a. Blue – cyanotic, relatively stagnant blood flow.
   b. White – blanching, dead-white appearance if spasm is severe.
   c. Red – a reactive hyperaemia upon rewarming.
7. The Allen test may provide clues to circulatory problems (Figure 5.70).

PATIENT PROBLEMS

1. Impairment of skin integrity (potential) related to the possibility of finger-tip ulceration.
2. Impaired physical mobility of hands related to intermittent arteriolar vasoconstriction.
3. Lack of knowledge related to misunderstanding about precautions necessary to minimize discomfort, as well as to avoid precipitating factors.

Planning and implementation
PATIENT EDUCATION

1. Avoid whatever provokes vasoconstriction of vessels of hands.
2. Prevent injury to hands, which can aggravate vasoconstriction and lead to ulceration.
3. Minimize exposure to cold, since this precipitates a reaction.
4. Wear warm clothing – boots, gloves, hooded jackets, when going out in cold weather.
   a. Turn heat on in car during travel.
   b. Shop in heated stores; avoid unheated buildings.
5. Avoid placing hands in cold water, the freezer or the refrigerator unless protective gloves are worn.
6. Use extra precautions to avoid injuries to fingers and hands from needle pricks, knife cuts.
7. Varying benefits are reported with such medications as reserpine, methyldopa, tolazoline and phenoxybenzamine. (See Table 5.9 for adverse effects of medications.)

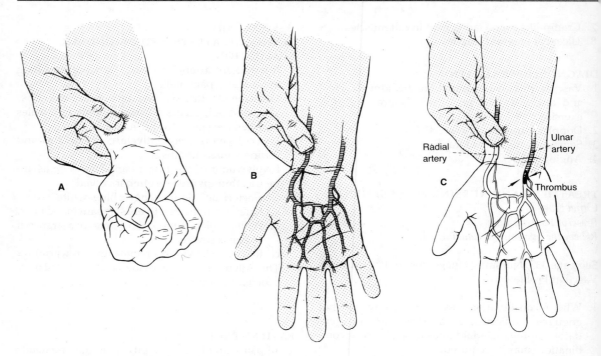

Figure 5.70. Allen test. Diagrammatic representation of the procedure (A) for determining patency of occlusion of the ulnar artery distal to the wrist. (B) The ulnar artery is patent as determined by the prompt return of colour to the skin of the hand while the radial artery is still compressed. (C) Occlusion of the ulnar artery is demonstrated by persistence of pallor as long as the radial arterial inflow is blocked by the examiner's finger. (Modified from Juergens and Fairbairn, *Arteriosclerosis obliterans, Heart Bulletin*, Vol. 8, pp. 22–4. By permission of the American Heart Association)

Table 5.9   Adverse effects of medication

Medication	Adverse effects
1. Phenoxybenzamine	Headache, tachycardia, nasal congestion, orthostatic hypotension
2. Cyclandelate	Headache, nausea, heavier than usual perspiration, vertigo, flushing, tingling
3. Tolazoline	Gastrointestinal upset, orthostatic hypotension, chilliness, tachycardia, palpitations
4. Nifedipine	None apparent

Evaluation
EXPECTED OUTCOMES
1. Avoids injury to hands.
2. Follows prescribed therapy to avoid vasoconstriction of hands – especially careful about protecting hands in cold weather.
3. Adheres to pharmacotherapy as prescribed.

DISEASES OF THE AORTA*

AORTIC ANEURYSM

Aneurysm is a distension of an artery brought about by a weakening/destruction of the media of the arterial wall. It tends to enlarge, thereby producing serious complications by compressing surrounding structures or rupturing, causing a fatal haemorrhage.

TYPES OF ANEURYSMS
Morphologically, they may be classified as follows:
1. Saccular – distension of a vessel projecting from one side.

* For aortic stenosis and aortic insufficiency, see page 280.

2. Fusiform – distension of the whole artery (i.e., entire circumference is involved).
3. Dissecting – haemorrhagic or intramural haematoma, separating the medial layers of the aortic wall.

AETIOLOGY
1. Local infection, pyogenic or fungal (mycotic aneurysm).
2. Congenital weakness of vessels.
3. Arteriosclerosis.
4. Syphilis.
5. Trauma.

ANEURYSM OF THE THORACOABDOMINAL AORTA
(Lower descending aorta and upper abdominal aorta.)

Clinical features
1. Subjective symptoms:
   a. At first no symptoms; later symptoms may come from congestive heart failure or a pulsating tumour mass in the chest.
   b. Pain and pressure symptoms:
      (i) Constant, boring pain because of pressure, or
      (ii) Intermittent and neuralgic pain because of infringement on nerves.
   c. Dyspnoea, causing pressure against trachea.
   d. Cough, often paroxysmal and brassy in sound.
   e. Hoarseness, voice weakness or complete aphonia, resulting from pressure against recurrent laryngeal nerve.
   f. Dysphagia due to impingement on oesophagus.
2. Objective signs:
   a. Oedema of chest wall – infrequent.
   b. Dilated superficial veins on chest.
   c. Cyanosis because of vein compression of chest vessels.
   d. Ipsilateral dilatation of pupils due to pressure against cervical sympathetic chain.
   e. Pulse difference in two wrists if aneurysm interferes with circulation in left subclavian artery.
   f. Abnormal pulsation may be apparent on chest wall – due to erosion of aneurysm through rib cage – in syphilis.

Management
1. The prognosis is poor for untreated patients.
2. Surgical – remove aneurysm and restore vascular continuity.

Aortic arch aneurysms are the most difficult to treat.

ABDOMINAL ANEURYSM
Clinical features
1. Many of these patients are asymptomatic; most are males (9:1) in their sixth or seventh decade.
2. Abdominal pain is most common; persistent or intermittent – often localized in middle or lower abdomen to the left of midline.
3. Low back pain.
4. Feeling of an abdominal pulsating mass.
5. Hypertension may be in evidence.

Diagnostic evaluation
1. Ordinarily the systolic blood pressure of the thigh exceeds that in the arm; in many of these patients, the opposite is true.
2. A palpable pulsating abdominal mass; fluoroscopy will reveal pulsating tumour.
3. Angioaortogram allows visualization of vessels and aneurysm.
4. Ultrasound allows visualization of vessels and aneurysm. This is the best test to confirm the presence of and check the size of abdominal aortic aneurysms. It is less expensive than other tests.
5. Computed tomography allows visualization of vessels and aneurysm.

Management
1. If untreated, the prognosis is poor.
2. Types of surgical intervention:
   a. Excision of area affected.
   b. Replacement of excised segment by a bypass (synthetic) graft.

DISSECTING ANEURYSM OF THE AORTA
1. This is a type of aneurysm in which there is a tear in the intima of the aorta; as a result of pressure, blood splits the wall and may produce a large haematoma or may continue to rip the wall.
2. Symptoms may resemble coronary occlusion; diagnosis is confirmed by aortography.
3. Prognosis is poor, but surgical removal of involved aneurysm and replacement of segment with a graft may be effective.

PERIPHERAL VESSEL ANEURYSMS
1. May involve renal artery, subclavian artery, popliteal artery (knee) or any major artery.
2. These produce a pulsating mass and may cause pain or pressure on surrounding structures.
3. Replacement grafts are used to repair these aneurysms.

HYPERTENSION

Hypertension is a disease of regulation in which the mechanisms that control arterial pressure within the 'normal range' are deranged. Predominant mechanisms are the central nervous system; the renin–angiotensin–aldosterone system; and extracellular fluid volume. Why these mechanisms fail is unknown. The basic explanation is that blood pressure is elevated when there is increased cardiac output plus peripheral vessel resistance.

NORMAL PHYSIOLOGY
1. *Normal blood pressure* (normotension) is the pressure of the blood within the systemic arterial system. It is usually considered to range from 100/60 to 140/90mmHg.
2. *Systolic pressure* represents the greatest pressure of the blood against the wall of the vessel following ventricular contraction.
3. *Diastolic pressure* represents the least pressure of the blood against the wall of the vessel following closure of the aortic valve.
4. *Pulse pressure* represents the difference between the systolic and diastolic readings – the range of pressure in the arteries.
5. The *mean arterial pressure* is the average pressure attempting to push blood through the circulatory system.
    This can be determined electronically or mathematically as well as by using an intra-arterial catheter and mercury manometer.
    a. *Mathematical determination.* (Slightly less than average of systolic and diastolic).
    Mean arterial pressure = ⅓ systolic pressure + ⅔ diastolic pressure.
        Example: for blood pressure of 130/85mmHg
        Mean arterial pressure is 100mmHg
        Kidney function requires a minimum of 70mmHg (mean arterial pressure).
6. *Basal blood pressure* is the lowest blood pressure taken in supine position after several days of hospitalization without treatment.
    Basal sitting pressure and basal standing pressure are often taken for later comparison.

FACTORS AFFECTING PRESSURE OF BLOOD
Blood volume, peripheral resistance, blood viscosity, cardiac output.

1. Blood pressure = cardiac output × total peripheral resistance.
    a. Pressure varies with exercise, emotional reaction, sleep, digestion, time of day.
    b. Such functions as renal, adrenal, vascular and neurogenic functions affect blood pressure.
2. Higher blood pressure = increased cardiac output × greater total peripheral resistance (circulatory overload).
3. Lower blood pressure = lessened cardiac output × lesser total peripheral resistance.
4. Increased diastolic pressure due to peripheral resistance indicates decrease in diameter of arterioles. These are affected by sympathetic stimulation, hereditary factors, more vasopressor hormones in the blood.
5. Increased systolic pressure indicates increased cardiac output and systolic hypertension, which is always secondary.

INCIDENCE
1. Hypertension is more common but better tolerated in women than in men.
2. Hypertensive women tend to be obese; hypertensive men do not appear to differ in size from other men.
3. There is a higher incidence in negroes.
4. It appears that a high sodium intake is related to the development of hypertension; when sodium intake is decreased, blood pressure often decreases. However, this remains controversial.
5. Increase in incidence is associated with the following risk factors;
    a. Age: between 30 and 50.
    b. Race: negroid.
    c. Hyperlipidaemia.
    d. History of smoking.
    e. The higher the blood pressure, the greater the risk.

AETIOLOGY AND THE SIGNIFICANCE OF BLOOD PRESSURE ELEVATION
1. Cause is unknown; however, there are several hypotheses:
    a. Hyperactivity of sympathetic vasoconstricting nerves.
    b. Presence of blood component which contains a vasoconstrictor that acts on smooth muscle, sensitizing it to constrictor substances.
    c. Increased cardiac output followed by arteriole constriction.
    d. Familial tendency.
2. Individual tolerance of increased blood pressure varies; however, there is a direct correlation

between increase in blood pressure and the rate at which atherosclerosis and arteriosclerosis develop.

3. Onset of hypertension occurs in the early 30s; because it is asymptomatic, it is usually untreated for at least 20 years.
4. Rising blood pressure adversely affects the brain, the heart and the kidneys.
   a. Heart – myocardial infarction, left heart failure.
   b. Kidney – nephrosclerosis, kidney failure.
   c. Brain – headache, encephalopathy, cerebral haemorrhage, cerebrovascular accident.
   d. Eye – papilloedema, swelling of optic disc.
5. Emotional stress exacerbates the problem.
6. Obesity and diabetes mellitus are associated with hypertension.

CLASSIFICATION OF HYPERTENSION

Primary or essential hypertension (approximately 90 per cent of patients with hypertension) or idiopathic hypertension

1. When the diastolic pressure is 90mmHg or higher and other causes of hypertension are absent, the condition is said to be primary hypertension.

   More specifically, when the average of three or more blood pressures taken at rest several days apart exceeds the upper limits of the following chart, an individual is considered hypertensive:

Infants	90/60mmHg
3–6 years	110/70mmHg
7–10 years	120/80mmHg
11–17 years	130/80mmHg
18–44 years	140/90mmHg
45–64 years	150/90mmHg
65 and older	160/95mmHg

2. Genetic factors contribute to this condition; patterns of the patient indicate that he is hypersensitive to internal and external stimuli.
3. Benign – the presence of hypertension for years without any symptoms.
4. Labile – intermittently elevated blood pressure levels.
5. Malignant – a sudden and severe acceleration in arterial pressure producing many symptoms and vascular damage.

Secondary hypertension

1. Occurs in approximately 5 to 10 per cent of patients with hypertension.
2. More common in men and in negroes.
3. Apparently follows other pathology.

a. *Renal pathology* which may lead to hypertension.
   (i) Congenital anomalies, pyelonephritis, renal artery obstruction, acute and chronic glomerulonephritis.
   (ii) Reduced blood flow to kidney (such as renal artery stenosis) – release of *renin*.
       (a) Renin reacts with serum protein in liver (alpha-2-globulin) → angiotensin I; this plus an enzyme → angiotensin II → leads to increased blood pressure.
       (b) Symptoms: proteinuria, polyuria, elevated blood pressure.
       (c) Therapy – endarterectomy, bypass graft, nephrectomy; blood pressure is reduced following correction of initial problem.
b. *Coarctation of aorta* (stenosis of aorta).
   (i) Blood flow to upper extremities is greater than flow to lower extremities – hypertension of upper part of body.
   (ii) Correction – removal of stenosed section of vessel; anastomosis or graft to eliminate area.
c. *Endocrine disturbance* – elevated blood pressure may be due to phaeochromocytoma.
   (i) Phaeochromocytoma – causes release of adrenaline and noradrenaline and a rise in blood pressure.
   (ii) Adrenal cortex tumours lead to an increase in aldosterone secretion and an elevated blood pressure.
   (iii) Cushing's syndrome leads to an increase in adrenocortical steroids and hypertension.
d. *Retinal changes:*
   (i) Optic disc – blurring of disc margins and contour changes.
   (ii) Papilloedema – choked disc.
   (iii) Arterial diameter lessened.
e. *Arteriosclerosis* – renal pathology.

Assessment

NURSING ALERT

The actual blood pressure reading by itself is not the sole criterion for determining the severity or urgency of the person's condition. The patient/client must be assessed in terms of what, if any, evidence there is of end organ damage. For example: a person with a blood pressure of 140/105mmHg and papilloedema is at far greater risk than one with a reading of 170/115mmHg with no evidence of papilloedema. The nurse needs to respond accordingly.

BLOOD PRESSURE DETERMINATION

Measure the blood pressure of the patient under the same conditions each time. Individuals should not have blood pressure readings taken immediately after experiencing stressful or taxing situations.

1. Place the patient in the desired position (sitting, standing, etc).
2. Support the bared arm (an unsupported arm may cause the reading to be higher and lead to a false diagnosis of hypertension). Avoid constriction of arm by a rolled sleeve.
3. Use a blood pressure cuff of the correct size (Table 5.10).
4. Record precisely the systolic and diastolic pressures:
   a. Systolic – the pressure within the pressure cuff indicated by the level of the mercury column at the moment when the first of two consecutive Korotkoff sounds is first heard (Figure 5.71).
   b. Phase 4 (first diastolic) – the pressure within the compression cuff indicated by the level of the mercury column at the moment when the

Table 5.10   Recommended bladder dimensions for blood pressure cuff

Arm circumference at midpoint* (cm)	Cuff name	Bladder width (cm)	Bladder length (cm)
17–26	Small adult	11	17
24–32	Adult	13	24
32–42	Large adult	17	32
42–50†	Thigh	20	42

* Midpoint of arm is defined as half the distance from the acromion to the olecranon.
† In people with very large limbs, the indirect blood pressure should be measured in the leg or forearm.
(Recommendations for Human Blood Pressure Determination by Sphygmomanometers, American Heart Association, 1980).

Figure 5.71. (A) Important 'rules' for accurate recording of arterial blood pressure. (B) The various phases of the Korotkoff sounds. Consult text for details. (Burch, G.E. and DePasquale, N.P. *Primer of Clinical Measurement of Blood Pressure*, C.V. Mosby, St Louis)

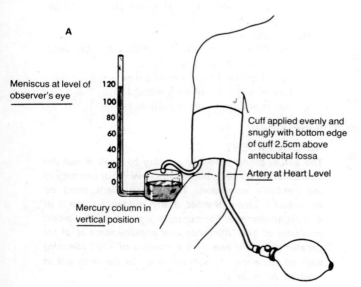

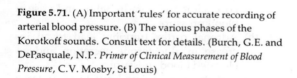

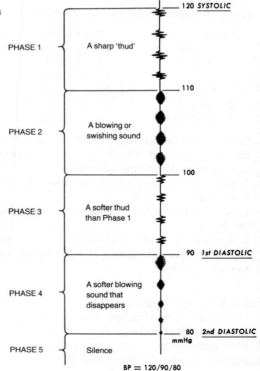

sound suddenly becomes muffled (beginning of phase 4).

c. Phase 5 (second diastolic) – the pressure within the compression cuff at the moment when the sound finally disappears (beginning of phase 5), that is, the onset of silence.

If required, document the blood pressure reading to indicate the patient's position and the arm used:

L (lying)
St (standing)
Sit (sitting)
RA (right arm)
LA (left arm)
Example: LA 152/78/68 St

Average two readings or the second and third of three readings, if procedure requires. Usually the patient's blood pressure will rise immediately and significantly when the doctor is present. Remeasurement is recommended after about 10 minutes.

Compare present reading with several previous readings to note differences and detect trends. Alert doctor if significant changes are apparent.

GENERAL DETECTION, CONFIRMATION AND REFERRAL OF PATIENTS WITH HIGH BLOOD PRESSURE*

When there is group screening and measurement of blood pressure, resources for referral, confirmation and follow-up should be provided.

1. Prior to blood pressure determination, ask the patient whether he has been or is currently under treatment for hypertension.
    a. Urge him to continue treatment even if blood pressure is normal (Table 5.11).
    b. Urge the patient to report an elevated blood pressure to his doctor.
2. Take blood pressure as described above.
3. Discuss with the patient/client:
    a. Previous treatment for high blood pressure.
    b. Numerical value of current blood pressure.
    c. Need for periodic remeasurement.
    d. Desirability of blood pressure control and the potential dangers of uncontrolled hypertension.

---

* Based on the 1984 Report of the Joint National Committee on Detection, evaluation and treatment of high blood pressure. *Arch. Intern. Med.*, May, Vol. 144, No. 5, pp. 1045–57.

Table 5.11 Drugs for parenteral treatment of hypertension

Drug	Action	Side-effects and pertinent points
Diazoxide	Orally – mildly antihypertensive Intravenously – strongly antihypertensive	Salt is restricted to prevent salt and water retention
Sodium nitroprusside	Has immediate antihypertensive effect Reduces total peripheral resistance (vasodilator) Produces a relaxation of arteriolar and venular smooth muscle	Useful in patients with hypertensive emergencies complicated by cardiac and aortic disease
Methyldopa	Effective in lowering blood pressure in 4–6 hours – effect extends 10–16 hours after injection	Sedation sometimes occurs as a result of this medication but usually wears off in a few days when a maintenance dose is established Watch for kidney toxicity
Hydralazine	Effective in treating hypertensive patients with acute glomerulonephritis Onset of action in 10–20 minutes Maximum response – 1 hour Persists – 12 hours	Monitor blood pressure every 15 minutes

e. Vital need to seek promptly and maintain anti-hypertensive therapy.

4. Referral or confirmation cut-off levels are arbitrary; they may be modified by presence of risk factors:
   a. Smoking.
   b. Hyperlipaemia.
   c. Coronary or cerebrovascular disease.
   d. Cardiac or renal failure.
   e. Diabetes.

5. The higher the blood pressure, the greater the urgency for follow-up management. (Early initial follow-up improves adherence to treatment plan.)

6. Adults with a diastolic blood pressure of 95mmHg or higher at screening or first visit should have the elevation confirmed promptly (within 1 month).
   a. Those with diastolic blood pressures of 90–95mmHg should be remeasured within three months.
   b. A diastolic blood pressure of 115mmHg or greater warrants immediate referral.

7. Adults with a systolic blood pressure over 160mmHg should have reading confirmed promptly.

   Those under the age of 35 years should have systolic elevations greater than 150mmHg confirmed.

8. *Confirmation* – to determine whether initial elevations:
   a. Remain high or require closer observation and evaluation, or
   b. Have returned to normal and require only remeasurement within one year.

Note: Two or more measurements should be taken at each visit. The diagnosis of hypertension is *confirmed* when the average of multiple blood pressure measurements made on at least two subsequent visits is 90mmHg or higher (diastolic) or when the average of multiple systolic blood pressures on two or more subsequent visits is consistently high.

DIAGNOSTIC ASSESSMENT OF PATIENT

1. Careful nursing and medical history (including family history of hypertension); note any previous history of hypertension, excessive salt intake, lipid abnormalities, cigarette smoking and history of headache, weakness, muscle cramps, palpitation, sweating.
   a. Take a complete history of all medications taken, including:
      (i) Oral contraceptives, steroids.
      (ii) Nonsteroidal, anti-inflammatory agents (NSAIDs).
      (iii) Nasal decongestants, appetite suppressants, tricyclic antidepressants.

2. Blood pressure – supine and standing; also assess vital signs and evaluate function of vital organs.

3. Physical assessment and examination.

4. Fundoscopic examination of the eye to detect vascular changes in the capillaries – note oedema, spasm, haemorrhage.

5. Careful examination of the heart; examination of peripheral pulse disparities, and evidence of oedema.

6. Listen for bruits over all peripheral arteries to determine presence of atherosclerosis; also listen for bruits in abdomen to note signs of renal arterial stenosis.

7. Chest X-ray to determine cardiac size; auscultation of lungs.

8. Neurological tests to detect cerebral damage, neurological deficits.

9. Laboratory studies:
   a. Haematocrit reading; haemoglobin.
   b. Urinalysis for blood, protein and glucose to determine renal parenchymal disease.
   c. Blood urea to determine renal excretory function.
   d. Serum potassium concentration to determine hyperaldosteronism, serum cholesterol and creatinine levels.
   e. Electrocardiogram to establish a baseline.
   f. Total and high-density lipoprotein cholesterol.

10. If the patient has:
    a. Gout or diabetes – serum glucose and uric acid need to be determined.
    b. Asthma – no beta-blockers are given.
    c. Peptic ulcer – no reserpine is given.

11. If the patient has confirmed hypertension:
    a. Is target organ involvement present?
    b. Are cardiovascular risk factors other than hypertension present?
    c. Does the patient have primary or secondary hypertension?

PATIENT PROBLEMS

1. Potential complications of underlying pathology including increased cardiac workload, kidney dysfunction, mobility impairment, weakness, lethargy, memory deficit, confusion, speech difficulties, visual defects and pain on walking.

2. Possible nonadherence to therapeutic regime

related to length of treatment and lifestyle changes.
3. Lack of knowledge – of basic problem, treatment protocols, negative effects of disease.

Planning and implementation
NURSING INTERVENTIONS
(AMBULATORY/OUTPATIENT)
Follow-up care for monitoring progress and for relieving stress
1. Measure the patient's blood pressure under the same conditions each day.
   Ask patient to get into the desired position, sitting, standing, etc, according to the preference of the doctor.
2. If elevated blood pressure can be brought down to normal range, there is very clear evidence that heart failure, strokes and renal failure can be almost completely prevented; therefore treatment should continue in spite of medication cost or inconvenience.
3. Practice supportive psychotherapy by observing the patient's reactions, appearance and personality as he relates to the professional staff, visitors, ancillary personnel, etc.
   a. Permit the patient to express his feelings; promote positive reactions; analyse negative reactions in an attempt to avoid their recurrence.
   b. Note side reactions, which can be easily missed; investigate these.
      (i) Failure to make eye contact in conversation.
      (ii) Suggestion of uneasiness, nervousness, restlessness.
      (iii) Side remarks or 'under-the-breath' comments.

Awareness of pharmacotherapeutic side-effects
See Table 5.12.
1. Assist the patient in coping with the side-effects of the therapeutic medications.
   a. Recognize that the drugs used for effective control of elevated blood pressure will very likely produce side-effects.
   b. Warn the patient of the possibility that hypotension may occur following the intake of certain drugs.
      (i) Instruct the patient to get up slowly to offset the feeling of dizziness.
      (ii) Encourage the patient to lie down immediately if he feels faint.
   c. Alert the patient to expect effects such as nasal congestion, asthenia (loss of strength), anorexia (loss of appetite), orthostatic hypotension (dizziness on changing position).
   d. Inform the patient that the goal of treatment is to control his blood pressure, reduce the possibility of complications and use the minimum number of drugs with lowest dosage necessary to accomplish this.
2. Educate the patient to be aware of toxic features and report them so that adjustments can be made in his individual pharmacotherapy.
   a. Note that dosages are individualized; therefore, they may need to be adjusted, since it is often impossible to predict reactions.
   b. Remember that certain circumstances produce vasodilatation – a hot bath, hot weather, febrile illness, consumption of alcohol.
   c. Be aware that blood pressure is decreased when circulating blood volume is reduced – dehydration, diarrhoea, haemorrhage.
   d. Suspect the presence of oedema as a reportable symptom, particularly when guanethidine is taken; these medications are less effective in the presence of oedema.

Adherence to the therapeutic regimen
1. Explain the meaning of hypertension, risk factors and their influences on the cardiovascular system; hypertension is a lifelong problem.
2. Usually, there can never be total cure, only control of essential hypertension; emphasize the consequences of uncontrolled hypertension: increased risk of stroke, heart attack.
3. Stress the fact that there may be no correlation between high blood pressure and symptoms; the patient cannot tell by the way he feels whether his blood pressure is normal or elevated.
4. Enable the patient to recognize that hypertension is chronic and requires persistent therapy and periodic evaluation, effective treatment improves life expectancy, therefore, follow-up visits to the doctor are mandatory.
5. Present a co-ordinated and complementary plan of guidance.
   a. Be available when the doctor visits the patient so that his approach and instructions to the patient are known.
   b. Inform the patient of the meaning of the various diagnostic and therapeutic activities to minimize his anxiety and to obtain his co-operation.
   c. Solicit the assistance of the patient's partner – provide information regarding the total treatment plan.

Table 5.12   Side-effects of and precautions to be taken with antihypertensive drugs

Generic name	Side-effects*	Precautions
Diuretics		
Thiazide and thiazide derivative diuretics (e.g. chlorthiazide)	Blood urea ↑, uric acid ↑, calcium ↑, serum K⁺, glucose, gastrointestinal irritation, weakness, photosensitivity, blood dyscrasias, pancreatitis†	Hypokalaemia, gout, renal insufficiency
Loop diuretics (frusemide)	Calcium ↓, Blood urea ↑, uric acid ↑, serum K⁺, photosensitivity	Hypokalaemia, gout
Potassium-sparing diuretics		
Spironolactone	Hyperkalaemia, gynaecomastia, drowsiness, hirsutism, irregular menses	Hyperkalaemia, renal failure
	Hyperkalaemia, diarrhoea, nausea	
Non-diuretics		
Rauwolfia	Drowsiness, sedation, lassitude, nasal congestion, bradycardia, depression, gastric hyperacidity, nightmares	Mental depression
Methyldopa	Orthostatic hypotension, drowsiness, depression, abnormal liver function tests, positive direct Coombs' test	Liver disease
Propranolol	Insomnia, bradycardia, bronchospasm, heart failure, sedation	Asthma, heart failure, diabetes
Hydralazine	Headache, tachycardia, palpitations, exacerbation of angina or heart failure, mesenchymal ('lupus like') reaction‡	Symptomatic coronary artery disease
Guanethidine	Orthostatic hypotension (especially in the morning), exertional weakness, bradycardia, diarrhoea, loss of ability to ejaculate	Symptomatic cardiovascular disease

* See also manufacturer's full prescribing information. Impotency may occur with any antihypertensive drug except hydralazine.

† Many side-effects, for example, blood dyscrasias and pancreatitis, are rare with diuretics.

‡ Rare with dosage under 300mg/day.

Source: Table adapted from Moser, M. *et al.* (1977) High blood pressure, *Journal of the American Medical Association*, Vol. 237, p. 260. (Copyright 1977, American Medical Association.)

    d. Be aware of the dietary plan developed for this particular patient. Is it realistic?

6. Develop a plan of instruction to be practised by the patient at home.

    a. Instruct the patient regarding proper method of taking his blood pressure at home and at work. (Some authorities recommend this practice.) Inform him of the readings that are to be reported to his doctor.

    b. Plan the patient's medication schedule so that the many medications are given at proper and convenient times; set up a daily checklist on which he can record the medication he has taken. Warn against stopping medication if he feels well – may produce 'escape hypertension'.

    c. Determine recommended dietary plans (e.g., extent of salt restriction, alcohol uptake, etc).

Lifestyle adjustments

1. Recognize the various effects of certain factors on symptoms of a patient with primary hypertension.

    a. Age, sex, occupation, race, environment, emotional response of the individual, etc.

    b. Understanding of his problem and his rapport with doctor, nurse, etc.

    c. Ability to adapt and adjust his activities in line with the prescribed therapeutic regimen.

2. Enlist the patient's co-operation in redirecting his lifestyle in keeping with the guidelines of therapy.

    a. Present an instructional pattern to fit individual requirements.

    b. Reassure the patient when encouragement is needed, the modifications required must appear meaningful to him.

HYPERTENSIVE CRISIS – INPATIENT CARE
Pharmacotherapy and nursing intervention
1. Use parenteral medications in hypertensive emergencies.
   a. Diastolic blood pressure over 150mmHg.
   b. Pulmonary oedema, cerebral haemorrhage, encephalopathy in combination with diastolic pressure over 120 or 130mmHg.
2. The patient must be hospitalized and monitored constantly.
   a. Record blood pressure frequently. Some drugs such as nitroprusside necessitate the taking of blood pressure readings every five minutes.
   b. Measure urine output accurately.
   c. Be prepared to administer vasopressors if severe hypotension develops.
   d. Administer diuretics such as frusemide and ethacrynic acid as adjuvants, when prescribed. They serve to maintain sodium diuresis when the arterial pressure falls.
   e. Administer spironolactone, when prescribed, if hypokalaemia is a problem.
3. Observe the patient for signs of cerebral nervous system complications.
   a. Note signs of confusion, irritability, lethargy, disorientation.
   b. Listen for complaints of headache, difficulty with vision; be alert for evidence of nausea or vomiting.
   c. Be prepared to offer protection to the patient if he exhibits seizures – padded bed sides, nonrestrictive garments, anticonvulsive medications.
4. Prevent those reactions or activities that will increase arterial pressure.
   a. Avoid situations that might engender feelings of anxiety, anger or annoyance in the patient. Psychological stress has a direct effect on physiological function.
   b. Prevent alterations in the ordinary functions of eating, sleeping or elimination that might lead to discomfort or annoyance – physiological disturbance may increase stress reaction.
   c. Provide rest period and maintain a pleasant, comfortable environment.
      (i) Advise the patient to rest for a short time before and after eating.
      (ii) Remind the patient to rest during the waking hours for a full hour.
   d. Serve food frequently and in small quantities rather than in three heavier meals.
      (i) Cardiac output increases with food intake.

   (ii) Blood pressure is elevated with large intake of fluids.
   (iii) Sodium intake may be restricted, depending on severity of hypertension.
5. Drug therapy:
   a. Drugs that act in a few minutes but are not satisfactory for long-term management:
      (i) Diazoxide.
      (ii) Nitroprusside.
   b. Drugs that require 30 minutes or more to obtain full effects; they can later be used orally for long-term management of hypertension:
      (i) Methyldopa.
      (ii) Hydralazine.

PATIENT EDUCATION
Instruct the patient as follows:
1. Recognize when blood pressure is above normal values.
2. Realize that long-term therapy and follow-up are essential for control.
3. Understand that an elevated blood pressure is usually asymptomatic.
4. Recognize that therapy will not cure but should control hypertension.
5. Expect that by following the suggested therapeutic regimen, the prognosis is good and normal lifestyle can be experienced.

Evaluation
EXPECTED OUTCOMES
1. Exhibits stabilized blood pressure as shown on personal daily charts and confirmed by doctors, nurses etc.
2. Corrects controllable risk factors – reduces weight, stops smoking, adheres to daily exercise programme, reduces stress.
3. Enumerates side-effects of drugs that necessitate contacting a member of the health-care team.
4. Adheres to therapeutic regimen by limiting sodium intake, exercising, conscientiously taking medications and keeping follow-up appointments.

THE LYMPHATIC SYSTEM

The lymphatic system is a network of vessels and nodes that are interrelated with the circulatory system. It removes tissue fluid from intercellular spaces and protects the body from bacterial invasion. Lymph nodes are located along the course of the lymphatic vessels and filter lymph before it is returned to the bloodstream.

Significance of lymphangiography
Radiological visualization of the lymphatic system is possible when a contrast medium is injected into a lymphatic vessel of the hands or feet.

It is a means of detecting lymph node involvement due to metastatic carcinoma, lymphoma or infection in otherwise inaccessible sites (except by surgery) such as the pelvis, retroperitoneum, deep axilla.

LYMPHANGITIS

Lymphangitis is an acute inflammation of lymphatic channels.

AETIOLOGY
Arises most commonly from a focus of infection in an extremity.

CLINICAL FEATURES
1. Displays characteristic red streaks that extend up an arm or leg from an infection that is not localized and that can lead to septicaemia.
2. Produces general symptoms – high fever, chills.
3. Produces local symptoms – local pain, tenderness, swelling along involved lymphatics.
4. Produces local lymph node symptoms – enlarged, red, tender (acute lymphadenitis).
5. Produces an abscess – necrotic, pus-producing (suppurative lymphadenitis).

TREATMENT AND NURSING MANAGEMENT
1. Administer antibiotics, since causative organisms usually are streptococci and staphylococci.
2. Treat affected part by rest, elevation and the application of hot, moist dressings.
3. Incise and drain if necrosis and abscess formation take place.

LYMPHOEDEMA

Lymphoedema is a swelling of the tissues (particularly in the dependent position), produced by an obstruction to the lymph flow in an extremity.

CLINICAL FEATURES
1. Oedema may be massive and is often firm.

2. Obstruction may be in lymph nodes, as well as in the lymphatic vessels.
   Observed in arm following radical mastectomy (see p. 721).

TREATMENT AND NURSING MANAGEMENT
1. Apply elastic bandages or stocking.
2. Keep the patient at rest, with affected part elevated; each joint higher than the preceding one.
3. Administer diuretics to control excess fluid.
4. Give antibiotics as prescribed.
5. Recommend isometric exercises with extremity elevated.
6. Suggest moderate sodium restriction in diet.
7. Advise the patient to avoid infection and trauma and to practise good hygiene to avoid superimposed infections.
8. Encourage exercise to help increase venous return.

FURTHER READING

BOOKS

Andreoli, K. *et al.* (1987) *Comprehensive Cardiac Care* (6th edn), C.V. Mosby, St Louis.

Darovic, G.O. (1987) *Hemodynamic Monitoring*, W.B. Saunders, Philadelphia.

Geddes, J.S. (1986) *The Management of the Acute Coronary Attack*. Academic Press, London.

Health Education Council (1984) *Coronary Heart Disease Prevention: Plans for Action*, Pitman, London.

Jowett, N.I. and Thompson, D.R. (1989) *Comprehensive Coronary Care*, Scutari Press, London.

Julian, D.G. (1988) *Cardiology* (6th edn), Baillière Tindall, London.

McCulloch, J., Townsend, A. and Williams, D.O. (1985) *Focus on Coronary Care*, Heinemann, London.

McGurn, W.C. (1981) *People with Cardiac Problems: Nursing Concepts*, J.B. Lippincott, Philadelphia.

Meltzer, L.E., Pinneo, R. and Kitchell, J.R. (1983) *Intensive Coronary Care: A Manual for Nurses* (4th edn), Prentice-Hall, New Jersey.

Razin, A.M. (1985) *Helping Cardiac Patients*, Jossey–Bass, San Francisco.

Safar, P. and Birchner, N.G. (1988) *Cardiopulmonary Cerebral Resuscitation: An Introduction to Resuscita-*

tion Medicine (3rd edn), W.B. Saunders, Philadelphia.

Thompson, D.R. (1982) *Cardiac Nursing*. Baillière Tindall, London.

Weeks, L.C. (1986) *Advanced Cardiovascular Nursing*, Blackwell, Boston.

Wenger, N.K. and Hellerstein, H.K. (1984) *Rehabilitation of the Coronary Patient* (2nd edn), Wiley, New York.

ARTICLES

Heart disorders

Anderson, U.K. (1987) Mitral valve prolapse: A diagnosis for primary nursing intervention, *Journal of Cardiovascular Nursing*, Vol. 1, No. 3, pp. 41–51.

Darbyshire, P. (1988) Making sense of central venous pressure monitoring, *Nursing Times*, Vol. 84, No. 7, pp. 36–8.

Hentinen, M. (1987) Teaching and adaptation of patients with myocardial infarction, *International Journal of Nursing Studies*, Vol. 23, pp. 125–38.

Jowett, N.I. and Thompson, D.R. (1988) Basic life support – The forgotten skills? *Intensive Care Nursing*, Vol. 4, pp. 9–17.

—— (1988) Advanced cardiac life support: Current perspectives, *Intensive Care Nursing*, Vol. 4, pp. 71–81.

Marrie, T.J. (1987) Infective endocarditis: A serious and changing disease, *Critical Care Nurse*, Vol. 7, No. 2, pp. 31–46.

Scrima, D.A. (1987) Infective endocarditis: Nursing considerations, *Critical Care Nurse*, Vol. 7, No. 2, pp. 47–56.

Stokes, P. and Jowett, N. (1985) Haemodynamic monitoring with the Swan–Ganz catheter, *Intensive Care Nursing*, Vol. 1, pp. 3–12.

Thompson, D.R. and Cordle, C.J. (1988) Support of wives of myocardial infarction patients, *Journal of Advanced Nursing*, Vol. 13, pp. 223–8.

Thompson, D.R. and Hopkins, S. (1987) Making sense of defibrillation, *Nursing Times*, Vol. 83, No. 49, pp. 54–5.

Ventola, C.A. (1987) Aortic and mitral valvuloplasty, *Journal of Cardiovascular Nursing*, Vol. 1, No. 3, pp. 70–4.

Watkins, L.O., Weaver, L. and Odegaard, V. (1986) Preparation for cardiac catheterization: Tailoring the content of instruction to coping style, *Heart and Lung*, Vol. 15, pp. 387–9.

Essentials of basic electrocardiography

Bailey, J.C. (1981) The electrophysiologic basis for cardiac electrical activity: Normal and abnormal, *Heart and Lung*, Vol. 10, No. 3, pp. 455–64.

Jowett, N.I., Thompson, D.R. and Bailey, S.W. (1985) Electrocardiographic monitoring I: Static monitoring, *Intensive Care Nursing*, Vol. 1, pp. 76–81.

Jowett, N.I. and Thompson, D.R. (1986) Electrocardiographic monitoring II: Ambulatory monitoring, *Intensive Care Nursing*, Vol. 1, pp. 123–9.

Purcell, J.A. and Haynes, L. (1984) Using the ECG to detect MI, *American Journal of Nursing*, Vol. 84, pp. 627–42.

Reyes, A.V. (1987) Monitoring and treating life-threatening ventricular dysrhythmias, *Nursing Clinics of North America*, Vol. 22, No. 1, pp. 61–76.

Shephard, N., Vaughan, P. and Rice, V. (1982) A guide to arrhythmia interpretation and management, *Critical Care Nurse*, Vol. 2, No. 5, pp. 58–85.

Thompson, D.R., Bailey, S.W. and Webster, R.A. (1986) Patients' views on cardiac monitoring, *Nursing Times*, Occasional paper, Vol. 82, No. 25, pp. 54–5.

Vascular disorders

Thompson, D.R. (1981) Recording patients' blood pressure: A review, *Journal of Advanced Nursing*, Vol. 6, pp. 283–90.

Venn, G. and Fox, A. (1987) Pointers to management: Leg ulcers, *Nursing Times*, Vol. 83, No. 12, pp. 49–52.

Warbinek, E. and Wyness, M.A. (1986) Designing nursing care for patients with peripheral arterial occlusive disease, Part I: Update, *Cardiovascular Nursing*, Vol. 22, No. 1, pp. 1–5.

—— (1986) Peripheral arterial occlusive disease, Part II: Nursing assessment and standard care plans, *Cardiovascular Nursing*, Vol. 22, No. 2, pp. 6–11.

6

Care of the Patient with a Blood Disorder

CELLULAR COMPONENTS OF NORMAL BLOOD

ERYTHROCYTES (RED BLOOD CELLS)

1. Comprise the vast majority of all blood cells; chiefly responsible for the colour of blood.
2. Approximately 5×10^{12} per litre of blood.
3. Normal red cell is a biconcave disc; red cell in normal blood has no nucleus.
4. Principal function is to transport oxygen – accomplished through the loose valence of an iron-containing pigment, haemoglobin, which accounts for 32–38g per decilitre of blood. Total normal concentration of haemoglobin – males 13–18g per decilitre; females 12–16.5g per decilitre.
5. Red blood cells are produced in red bone marrow, which also provides most of the blood's leucocytes and all of its platelets. Red cells of normal adults found in short and flat bones – ribs, sternum, skull, vertebrae, bones of the hands and feet, pelvis.
6. Bone marrow requires a number of nutrients,

including iron, vitamin B_{12}, folic acid and pyridoxine for normal erythropoiesis (formation of red cells).

7. Normal life expectancy of a red cell is between 115 and 130 days – then eliminated by phagocytosis in the reticuloendothelial system, predominantly in spleen and liver.

LEUCOCYTES (WHITE BLOOD CELLS)

1. Normally are present in a concentration of between 5,000 and 10,000 cells in each cubic millimetre of blood (one white cell for every 500–1,000 red cells).
2. Leucocytes have a nucleus and are capable of active movement.
3. Leucocytes are divided into three general categories: granulocytes, monocytes and lymphocytes.
4. Leucocytosis – white cell count over 10,000.
5. Leucopenia – white cell count below 5,000.
6. *Granulocytes* – leucocytes produced in the marrow.
   a. Comprise 70 per cent of all white cells.
   b. Called *granulocytes* because of the abundant granules contained in their cytoplasm, or *polymorphonuclear leucocytes* since their nuclei, when mature, are of a highly irregular, multilobed configuration.
   c. Granulocytes are divided into three subgroups according to their staining properties: eosinophils, basophils and neutrophils.
   d. The chief function of neutrophils is phagocytosis (ingestion of foreign substances and bacteria). Eosinophils and basophils mainly release histamine and heparin in response to antigen/antibody reactions.
7. *Lymphocytes* – most numerous of the *mononuclear cells*; comprise about 25 per cent of the circulating white cells.
   a. Produced in lymph nodes throughout the body and to a lesser extent in the bone marrow.
   b. Responsible for the immunological competence of an individual.
   c. Produce circulating immunglobulins (antibodies).
8. *Monocytes* – derived from components of the reticuloendothelial system (particularly spleen, liver, lymph nodes and bone marrow).
   a. Constitute a ready source of mobile phagocytes, congregating and performing their scavenging function at sites of inflammation and tissue necrosis.
   b. Account for about 5 per cent of the white cell count.

PLATELETS (THROMBOCYTES)

1. Are the smallest and most fragile of the formed elements; are small particles (devoid of nuclei) that arise as a result of budding from giant cells called *megakaryocytes* in the bone marrow.
2. Number approximately $150–400 \times 10^9$ per litre of whole blood.
3. Prime function to halt bleeding – accomplished by congregating and clumping at all sites of vascular injury and by plugging with their own substance the lumen of the bleeding vessel. As they disintegrate the tissues release factor III which initiates clot formation in their immediate vicinity, thereby checking the flow of blood through and the leakage of blood from a lacerated vessel.

COMMON PROBLEMS OF PATIENTS WITH BLOOD DISORDERS

See Table 6.1, p. 366.

BLOOD AND BONE MARROW SPECIMENS

Blood may be obtained by skin puncture (finger, toe, heel or ear-lobe) and venepuncture.

A *skin puncture* is performed when only a small amount of blood is needed (for red and white cell counts, haemoglobin and haematocrit (packed cell volume) determinations, reticulocyte counts, blood films for differential smear). However, the values for the red blood cells, haematocrit, haemoglobin and platelets are lower in capillary blood than in venous blood.

A *venepuncture* is a puncture of a vein to obtain blood and is used when larger amounts of blood are needed (preferred method).

Note: A venepuncture is performed by the doctor in the majority of cases. Nurses working in special units, e.g. intensive care, cardiac care, are trained to perform venepuncture.

Table 6.1   Common problems of patients with blood disorders

Patient problem	Nursing management and rationale
Fatigue and weakness related to effects of disease, anaemia	In order to modify lifestyle to cope: 1. Plan nursing care to preserve patient's strength 2. Allow frequent rest periods 3. Encourage ambulation activities as tolerated to prevent problems of immobility 4. Avoid disturbing activities and noise to prevent increased heart rate and cardiac output 5. Encourage optimum nutrition involving the dietician to plan a suitable diet to build up strength
Haemorrhagic tendencies related to thrombocytopenia, abnormal platelet function, blood vessel and connective tissue disease, effects of chemotherapy	In order to prevent or manage bleeding episodes: 1. Educate patient to protect self from injury 2. Avoid using articles likely to cause bruising or abrasions 3. Keep the patient at rest during bleeding episodes to lower pulse rate and blood pressure to allow clot formation 4. Apply gentle pressure to bleeding sites – five minutes if venepuncture to avoid bruising and skin damage 5. Observe for symptoms of internal bleeding 6. Give ice chips if bleeding orally to encourage vasoconstriction 7. If intramuscular infections are unavoidable, use a small gauge needle to ensure minimal puncture site 8. Observe patient for asphyxiation if bleeding from mouth or throat – ensure appropriate equipment is at hand to institute emergency treatment if necessary 9. Support the patient during transfusion therapy to detect abnormal reactions
Ulcerative lesions of the tongue, gums or mucous membranes related to susceptibility to infections; cytotoxic action of chemotherapy; bleeding gums	In order to decrease oral discomfort and increase integrity of oral mucous membranes: 1. Develop and follow a plan of care based on oral assessment 2. Avoid irritating food and beverages 3. Offer mouthwashes such as Bocasan (sodium perborate monohydrate and sodium hydrogen tartrate) to clean the gums 4. Use a soft, small headed toothbrush to clean the teeth and gums; an automatic toothbrush has been found to be effective in cleaning all parts of the mouth as the pressure is evenly exerted 5. Sugarless gum, ice chips or saliva substitute may be offered to stimulate saliva and moisturize the mouth
Dyspnoea related to reduction of oxyhaemaglobin	In order to manage the patient's symptoms: 1. Use comfort measures to alleviate shortness of breath in orthopnoeic position 2. Prevent unnecessary exertion 3. Administer oxygen when prescribed
Bone and joint pains related to proliferation of neoplastic cells; bleeding	1. Assess and plan individual care for pain control with the patient 2. Relieve pressure on painful joints and support in comfortable position 3. Provide for joint immobilization as prescribed 4. Appropriate use of heat or cold compresses in conjunction with physiotherapist.
Fever related to infection; haematological malignancy	In order to relieve the discomfort and symptoms of pyrexia: 1. Avoid potential sources of infection and detect early signs of pyrexia 2. Encourage rest to combat the extra demands made on the patient's metabolism 3. Provide cool environment without causing too rapid a reduction in body temperature, as shivering will then raise the temperature again 4. Encourage refreshing drinks to replace fluid lost from perspiration, unless contraindicated 5. Administer antipyretic drugs as prescribed

Pruritis or skin lesions related to haematological malignancy; chemotherapy

In order to monitor and protect skin integrity:
1. Advise patient to keep fingernails short to prevent scratching
2. Use soap sparingly to prevent skin reaction

Anxiety of the patient and their family related to diagnosis, treatment, procedures and prognosis

In order to provide emotional support to facilitate coping with the diagnosis and treatment of a haematological disorder:
1. Explain the nature, discomforts and the limitations of activity associated with diagnostic procedures and treatment
2. Encourage patient to verbalize feelings and listen carefully
3. Show empathetic and accepting attitude
4. Promote relaxation and comfort
5. Remember patient's individual preferences
6. Promote independence and self-care within the patient's limitations
7. Encourage the family to participate in the patient's care as desired
8. Create a comfortable atmosphere for the family's visits

Note: Patients vary in their reactions; age, sex, cultural background, social position and obligations all influence the patient's response to illness.

GUIDELINES: BONE MARROW ASPIRATION AND BIOPSY

Bone marrow aspiration or biopsy is done by trained medical staff so that specimens of bone marrow can be obtained. It is performed for the following reasons:
1. To diagnose haematological disease – enables the precursors of cells in peripheral blood to be examined and their relative number determined. Also to estimate the iron content.
2. To follow the course of disease and the patient's response to treatment.
3. To diagnose diseases other than pure haematological disorders, such as primary and metastatic tumours, infectious diseases, certain granulomas and parasitic infections.
4. To isolate bacteria and other pathogenic agents by culture or animal inoculation.

COMPLICATIONS
1. Osteomyelitis (rare).
2. Bleeding and haematoma formation in patients with bleeding disorders.
3. Puncture of vital organs if biopsy is too deep.

CONTRAINDICATIONS
Haemophilia and related haemorrhagic disorders.

EQUIPMENT
Sterile bone marrow aspiration tray
Marrow aspiration needles with guards
Sterile towels
Selection of syringes and needles
Local anaesthetic
Sterile gloves
Skin antiseptic, e.g. chlorhexidine 0.5 per cent in spirit

Laboratory equipment
  Coverslips
  Microscope slides
  Specimen bottles (plain and with heparin)
Scalpel blade and handle
Gauze swabs
Plastic dressing or plastic dressing spray

PROCEDURE FOR STERNAL ASPIRATION

Nursing action	Rationale
1. Explain procedure to the patient.	To reinforce the doctor's explanation and ensure co-operation.
2. Give light sedative if prescribed.	Usually only necessary to calm an anxious patient.
3. Help the patient into the supine position.	The correct position for sternal puncture.
4. The procedure is performed by the doctor:	
a. The skin is cleaned with antiseptic;	To minimize risk of infection.
b. Local anaesthetic is infiltrated into chosen site;	To minimize pain and ensure patient co-operation.
c. A small stab incision may be made before needle insertion;	To avoid pushing skin into the bone marrow.
d. The marrow needle with guard is inserted into the marrow cavity with a slight twisting motion;	The needle guard ensures correct positioning of the needle to avoid puncturing vital organs.
e. The guard is removed and a syringe attached;	To allow marrow to be withdrawn.
f. Warn the patient of a brief episode of sharp pain on withdrawal of marrow if no anaesthetic given;	Pain is caused by the suction.
g. A small volume of fluid is aspirated slowly. The marrow appears as whitish granular particles;	If repeated aspirations result in no marrow, it indicates that the area is not suitable for aspiration.
h. The needle is removed from the puncture site and smears are prepared by the doctor.	
5. Pressure is applied using a sterile swab until the bleeding stops.	To minimize bruising and haematoma formation. Prolonged pressure of 5 to 10 minutes is required if the patient has thrombocytopenia.
6. Cover the site with a plastic dressing and advise patient not to wash the area for 24 hours.	To prevent infection entering the puncture site.
7. Observe patient for any discomfort, continued bleeding or untoward symptoms.	Discomfort may be experienced due to bruising of the tissues. A mild analgesic may be prescribed.
8. Remove and dispose of equipment and specimens, as appropriate.	

Follow-up care
1. Give mild analgesic if needed, e.g. paracetamol tablets.
2. Observe patient for discomfort, continued bleeding and any untoward symptoms.

PROCEDURE FOR ILIAC CREST ASPIRATION/BIOPSY
Anterior approach
1. Position the patient prone or on his side. (The anterior or posterior iliac crest has the advantage of having no vital organs near the puncture site.)
2. The needle is passed into the cavity of the ilium 2cm behind and 2cm below the anterior iliac spine and perpendicular to the flat surface of the bone. (Pain is an indicator that the needle is within the marrow cavity.)

3. A small hammer may be used to tap the needle gently in place, but this is rarely necessary. (The bone of the iliac crest is harder than that of the sternum.)

Posterior approach
1. Position the patient on his side.
2. The needle is passed along an anaesthetized tract that runs behind the prominence of the posterior iliac spine and at right angles with the anterior abdominal wall.
3. Tell the patient to lie on his affected side after the procedure (this promotes haemostasis).

Follow-up care
As for sternal aspiration.

TRANSFUSION THERAPY

BLOOD
A unit of blood (drawn from a donor) consists of approximately 450ml of whole blood and 60–70ml of acid-citrate-dextrose or citrate-phosphate-dextrose, both of which are one of the anticoagulant preservative solutions.
1. Whole blood is used for acute blood loss.
2. See p. 371 for technique of administration.

BLOOD COMPONENTS
Packed red cells
Erythrocytes are separated from a unit of whole blood by centrifugation or sedimentation; about 80 per cent of the plasma is removed, leaving a haematocrit of 60–70 per cent.
1. The plasma is used for the preparation of various plasma fractions such as albumin, cryoprecipitate or gamma globulin.
2. Indicated for:
   a. Patients who need only red blood cells;
   b. Patients with severe anaemia who have relatively normal blood volume;
   c. Patients with risk of heart failure.
3. Packed cells are administered through a large bore needle at a flow rate slower than that of whole blood as it is more viscous.

Platelet transfusions
Given to patients with dangerous degrees of thrombocytopenia (decrease of platelets in circulating blood) to control or prevent bleeding.

1. Viable platelets may be supplied in the form of:
   a. Fresh blood – replaces red cells and platelets.
   b. Platelet-rich plasma – contains 80–90 per cent of original platelets.
   c. Platelet concentrates – retain nearly all original platelets in a viable state, but reduced in volume. Therefore reduced risk of circulatory overloading.
2. The use of matched platelets is more advantageous and lessens the risk of antibody formation.
3. Platelet transfusions are given in the treatment of leukaemia, aplastic anaemia and thrombocytopenia induced by chemotherapy or drugs.

Granulocyte infusions
Given to patients with severe and temporary bone marrow depression.
1. Granulocytes are harvested from a donor by continuous flow centrifugation or are trapped in nylon wool filters. (Machine used is called a cell separator.)
2. The process is complex and costly; available only at a few centres at this time.
3. One of the main limitations of granulocyte transfusion therapy is the difficulty in obtaining a therapeutic dose.

Whole plasma
Fluid portion of the blood in which corpuscles are suspended may be obtained by plasmaphoresis (the removal of plasma) whereby the red cells are separated from the plasma and returned to the donor. The advantage is that the human body takes six weeks to replace red cells whereas plasma is replaced within 12 hours. Therefore plasma can be donated as

regularly as once a month with no ill effects for the donor.

1. Clinical usefulness (used with decreasing frequency):
   a. Treatment of clotting defects – all of the plasma factors can be supplied rapidly without over-expanding the patient's blood volume.
   b. Correction of hypovolaemia due to selective loss of plasma – mainly in burned patients.
   c. Correction of hypovolaemia in acute blood loss when whole blood is not immediately available.
2. As a plasma expander for hypovolaemia or as an exogenous source of plasma albumin for hypo-albuminaemia, whole plasma has largely been replaced by pure preparations of serum albumin and other plasma fractions that are comprised largely of albumin.
3. *Freshly frozen plasma* – plasma which has been separated immediately from freshly donated blood and then promptly frozen at −30°C. Factor V (one of the accelerators of prothrombin conversion) and factor VIII (the antihaemophiliac factor) are retained by this process. Used for multiple clotting factor deficiencies such as disseminated intravascular coagulation (DIC).
4. *Factor VIII concentrate* – used in patients with haemophilia A (factor VIII deficiency – needed for blood clotting process). Cryoprecipitate contains:
   a. Factor VIII for use in the treatment of haemophilia.
   b. von Willebrand factor for use in von Willebrand's disease.
   c. Fibrinogen for use in fibrinogen deficiency.
5. Factor IX concentrate used for those suffering from Christmas disease (clotting factor IX deficiency or haemophilia B).
6. Human immunoglobulin – proteins precipitated from pools of human plasma which provide specific or nonspecific passive immunity:
   a. Specific, e.g. rhesus factor D, tetanus, herpes zoster.
   b. Nonspecific, e.g. treatment of immuno-deficiency syndromes (e.g. hypogamma-globinaemia).
7. *Human serum albumin and other albumin preparations:*
   Clinical usefulness:
   a. Combat plasma leakage and prevent haemo-concentration in burn patients;
   b. Expand blood volume in patients in hypovo-laemic shock;
   c. Elevate the circulating albumin in patients with hypoalbuminaemia.
8. Plasma replacement therapy – abnormal plasma is withdrawn and replaced by normal plasma protein fraction. Used for conditions such as:
   a. Blood hyperviscosity as a result of myeloma or macroglobinaemia;
   b. Familial hypercholesterol anaemia;
   c. Pregnant women with rhesus antibodies in their blood.

Antigens, antibodies and crossmatching

Antigens

Complex proteins on the red cell surface. Antigens may stimulate the formation of antibodies.

1. Antigens are inherited from parents:
   a. Positive – antigens present;
   b. Negative – antigens absent.
2. If an antigen is present on the red cell, the immune system recognizes it as 'self' and does not normally produce antibody.

Antibodies

Proteins circulating in the plasma, produced in response to an antigen that the individual is lacking.

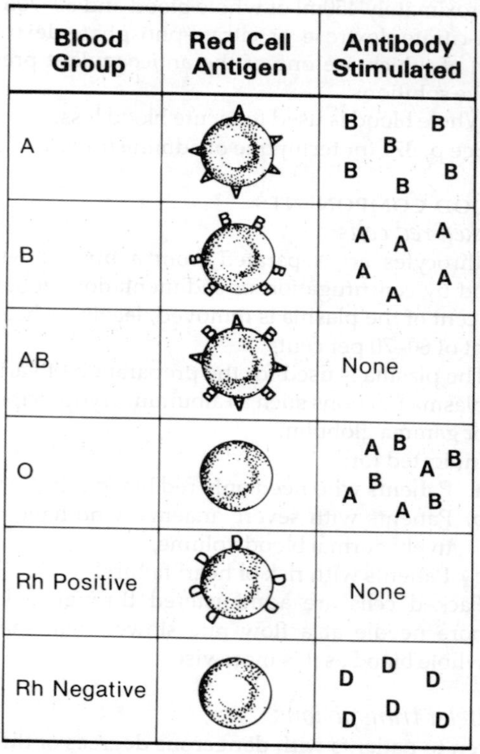

Blood Group	Red Cell Antigen	Antibody Stimulated
A		B B B B B B
B		A A A A A A
AB		None
O		A B A B B A B A B
Rh Positive		None
Rh Negative		D D D D D D

Figure 6.1. Red cell antigen activity by blood groups

1. The most potent red cell antigens are in the ABO system (Figure 6.1); they are so potent that antibody production is stimulated soon after birth by antigenically similar substances in the environment. Example: individuals lacking A antigen (blood groups B and O) make anti-A by the age of three months (naturally occurring).
2. The rhesus (Rh) system is the second most potent, but those lacking Rh antigens (Rh negative) are stimulated to produce antibody only after exposure to Rh positive red cells (transfusion or pregnancy). Such stimulated antibodies are called *alloantibodies* or atypical antibodies.

Crossmatching (compatibility testing)

Accomplished by incubating a sample of the patient's plasma with the donor's red cells to detect signs of incompatibility, which are: *agglutination* – clumping of cells; *Haemolysis* – destruction of red cells. Both are seen as the result of the interaction of antigen and antibody.

1. A compatible crossmatch between donor and recipient is necessary before a transfusion is given.

NURSING ALERT
Compatibility testing is the best available method of providing a safe transfusion, but it does not guarantee that a reaction will not occur.

2. Blood products that require crossmatch/compatibility testing prior to transfusion are those containing a significant number of red cells, such as whole blood, red blood cells and granulocytes.
3. A routine crossmatch requires one to two hours. In an emergency, an abbreviated crossmatch can be performed, or ABO compatible uncrossmatched blood can be transfused with minimal risk.

GUIDELINES: ADMINISTERING BLOOD TRANSFUSIONS

Blood transfusion is the introduction of blood into the body circulation.
1. The blood is administered via an intravenous cannula using a sterile disposable blood administration set.
2. A microaggregate blood filter may be used:
   a. To remove aggregated leucocytes and platelets accumulated during blood storage. These aggregates have been noted in the lungs following massive transfusion;
   b. To remove leucocytes and reduce the risk of febrile, nonhaemolytic transfusion reactions.

NURSING ALERT
Microaggregate filters should not be used for the transfusing of platelets or granulocytes.

PURPOSES
1. Restore circulating blood volume.
2. Replace clotting factors.
3. Improve oxygen-carrying capacity of the blood.

Nursing action	Rationale
1. The blood should be commenced if possible within 20 minutes after removing from the blood bank, and must not be warmed artificially.	Storage at 1–6°C should be maintained until just before administration. Rapid deterioration of the red blood cells can occur with uncooled blood.
2. Inspect the blood for gas bubbles and any abnormal colour or cloudiness.	Gas bubbles may indicate bacterial growth; abnormal colour or clouding may warn of haemolysis.

3. Explain the procedure to the patient.	To allay anxiety and instruct the patient to report any unusual symptoms immediately.
4. Using hospital policy, verify patient identification and check donor and recipient blood group. Check blood expiry date.	To avoid giving the wrong blood to the wrong patient which may cause a fatal reaction.
5. Infuse the blood at the prescribed rate.	The rate of transfusion depends on the patient's condition and the product transfused.
6. Record the patient's temperature, pulse, respiration and blood pressure at commencement of transfusion and then at half- to hourly intervals as requested. Observe the patient for signs of sweating, tachycardia, restlessness or loin pain.	To detect signs of possible complications of transfusion therapy: a. Acute allergic or febrile reaction; b. Septic reaction; c. Circulatory overload; d. Haemolytic reactions.
7. Record carefully the amount of blood that the patient receives and the product identification number.	It must be possible to trace each transfusion product to the original donor.
8. A diuretic may be prescribed to be given during the transfusion.	To prevent circulatory overload.

COMPLICATIONS

NURSING ALERT
Transfusion therapy (whether of whole blood or blood components) entails a number of calculated risks. Some of these potential complications cannot be prevented with absolute certainty. There is a significant incidence of morbidity and mortality associated with blood transfusion.

CIRCULATORY OVERLOADING
Due to administration of excessive volume or at a rate faster than the heart can accept. Observe for rise in venous pressure, distended neck veins, dyspnoea and cough. Râles can be heard in base of lungs with a feeling of tightness in the chest suggesting pulmonary oedema. Heart failure, if it occurs, can be irreversible and fatal.

Prevention
1. Prevent by using packed cells, proper spacing of transfusions and give at a rate which can be managed by the circulatory reserve of the patient.
2. Monitor central venous pressure of patients with heart disease.

Treatment and nursing interventions
1. Stop transfusion immediately and call the doctor.
2. Reassure the patient and sit him upright.
3. Treatment for incipient pulmonary oedema is instituted.

TRANSMISSION OF DISEASE
1. Post-transfusion hepatitis may be due to the hepatitis B virus, but there are other viruses capable of causing post-transfusion hepatitis which are considered responsible for 90 per cent of current cases. This is called 'non-A-non-B' hepatitis as the agent has not been identified.
2. Cytomegalovirus observed frequently in immunosuppressed patients.
3. Malaria is a rare complication.
4. Syphilis is extremely rarely transmitted by transfusion as the organism does not survive refrigeration temperatures for more than 72 hours.
5. Acquired immune deficiency syndrome (AIDS) transmitted by a retrovirus (HTLV-III).

Prevention
1. Screen donor carefully.
2. Reject donors with history of hepatitis or jaundice or if laboratory test is positive for hepatitis B antigen.
3. HTLV-III antibody test.

PYROGENIC (FEBRILE) REACTIONS

Usually due to presence of leucoagglutinins or platelet agglutinins in patient or to antigens in transfused blood.

Symptoms

May occur after transfusion is discontinued.
1. Sudden chilling and fever.
2. Headache.
3. Flushing; tachycardia.

Prevention

Keep blood recipients comfortably covered during transfusion. In patients who regularly have febrile reactions, yet require continued transfusions, blood products with leucocytes and platelets removed may be tried. Antipyretic or steroid drugs may also be used prophylactically.

Treatment and nursing interventions

1. Stop transfusion and notify the doctor and the blood bank (for examination of blood).
2. Check patient's temperature and for signs of shock.
3. Give an antipyretic as directed, e.g. aspirin.

BACTERIAL CONTAMINATION

Due to transfusion of bacteria or their toxins in the blood. Rare with correct storage of blood and use of disposable giving sets.

Symptoms

1. High fever (over 38.4°C).
2. Intense flushing.
3. Severe headache or substernal pain.
4. Vomiting, diarrhoea.
5. Hypotension; shock-like state with dry flushed skin.
6. Pain in abdomen and extremities.

Prevention

1. Do not allow the blood to stand unnecessarily at room temperature – accelerates growth of any contaminating organisms.
2. Do not warm containers of blood before transfusion.
3. Inspect blood for gas bubbles and change in colour before starting transfusion.

Treatment and nursing interventions

1. Stop transfusion and call the doctor.
2. Assist the doctor in obtaining cultures of donor's blood (and recipient's blood) and send the remainder of the blood to the laboratory.
3. Treat septicaemia as directed – antibiotics, intravenous fluids, fresh transfusion, steroids.

ALLERGIC REACTIONS

Blood of allergic patient may contain antibodies capable of reacting with allergens in the donor's blood.

Symptoms

1. Flushing.
2. Itching and rash.
3. Urticaria (hives).
4. Asthmatic wheezing and laryngeal oedema in full-blown anaphylactic reactions.

Prevention

1. Screen and reject all donors with known allergies.
2. Ask patient whether he has a history of allergy.
3. Prophylactic antihistamines may be given in specialized units.

Treatment and nursing interventions

1. Stop the blood and call the doctor.
2. Prepare adrenaline for administration if respiratory distress is severe.

HAEMOLYTIC REACTION AND INCOMPATIBILITY

(Most severe reaction.)
Haemolysis occurs when incompatible red cells are injected into the patient's circulating blood. It may cause oliguric renal failure and death.

Signs and symptoms

1. Chilliness; fever.
2. Loin pain due to acute tubular necrosis caused by haemolysis. This is very severe in an immediate reaction.
3. Flushing; feeling of head fullness.
4. Oppressive feeling in chest, and anxiety.
5. Distension of neck veins.
6. Tachycardia; tachypnoea.
7. Fall in blood pressure and circulatory collapse.
8. Oozing from venepuncture and haemoglobinuria.

Prevention

1. Positively identify patient and blood before transfusion is started.
2. Stay with the patient during the first 15 to 30 minutes that he is receiving the transfusion – if the transfusion is stopped early, untoward (and possibly fatal) reactions may be averted.
3. Administer blood very slowly during this period.

Treatment and nursing interventions

1. Stop the transfusion immediately – consequences are in proportion to the amount of incompatible blood given.
2. Call the doctor.
3. Assist with infusion of a diuretic to maintain urine flow, glomerular filtration and renal blood flow.
4. Maintain volume with intravenous infusions as directed if diuresis follows after the administration of a diuretic.
5. Insert indwelling urinary catheter as directed and observe urine output hourly to monitor signs of renal failure due to acute tubular necrosis.
6. Prepare patient for renal dialysis as directed.
7. Send sample of patient's blood and urine to the laboratory for the presence of haemoglobin (indicative of intravascular haemolysis) and for tests for disseminated intravascular coagulation.

A delayed haemolytic transfusion reaction may develop one to two weeks post-transfusion. These are more subtle than the immediate type and some may be asymptomatic. The cause may be due to antigen exposure during previous transfusions or pregnancy.

HYPERKALAEMIA
(Potassium excess.)

Symptoms

1. Nausea, colic, diarrhoea.
2. Muscular weakness.
3. Paraesthesia of hands, feet, tongue, face.
4. Flaccid paralysis.
5. Apprehension.
6. Slow pulse rate.
7. Cardiac arrest.

Prevention

Avoid using old blood – stored blood causes potassium levels to increase. When a massive transfusion is needed, fresh blood less than one week old should be used.

HYPOCALCAEMIA
(Calcium deficit.)
Calcium deficit can occur with administration of a large volume of citrated blood.

Signs and symptoms

1. Tingling of fingers and around the mouth.
2. Muscular cramps.
3. Hyperactive reflexes.
4. Convulsions.
5. Carpopedal spasms.
6. Laryngeal spasms.

Treatment and nursing intervention
Clamp the tubing and notify the doctor.

HAEMOSIDEROSIS
(Iron overload.)
This is a potential risk for patients who receive multiple, long-term transfusions. It is most effectively controlled through minimizing the number of transfusions given to chronically anaemic patients.

AIR EMBOLISM
May occur if blood is transfused under pressure.

Signs and symptoms

1. Chest pain.
2. Cough.
3. Dyspnoea.

Prevention

Prevent air from entering intravenous lines, especially when changing infusion sets.

Treatment and nursing interventions

1. Clamp tubing and notify doctor.
2. Position patient on his left side in a slight Trendelenburg position – to trap air in the right side of the heart.

MICROAGGREGATES IN STORED BLOOD
Microaggregates of platelets, leucocytes and fibrin are formed in stored blood. It is uncertain to what extent they form pulmonary microvascular obstruction, but it is a safe policy to use special microaggregate filters when more than five units of stored blood are to be given rapidly.

COLD BLOOD
The transfusion of large volumes of cold stored blood may lead to cardiac arrest. This may be prevented by warming the blood to 37°C by passing it through a special warming coil when transfusing rapidly.

NURSING RESPONSIBILITIES IN TRANSFUSION REACTION

1. Notify doctor and blood bank immediately when a suspected transfusion reaction has occurred.
2. Disconnect the transfusion set, but keep the intravenous line open with a dextrose or saline solution in case intravenous medication should be needed rapidly.
3. Save the blood bag and tubing; send to blood bank for repeat grouping and culture.
4. Arrange for blood to be taken for plasma haemoglobin, culture and regrouping.

5. Collect urine sample and send to laboratory for a haemoglobin determination. Save subsequent specimens of urine.

ANAEMIAS

Anaemia is a laboratory definition which implies a low red cell count and a below-normal haemoglobin or haematocrit (packed cell volume, PCV) level.

ALTERED PHYSIOLOGY
1. The appearance of anaemia reflects:
   a. Decreased production of red blood cells;
   b. Excessive red cell loss;
   c. A combination of (a) and (b), or
   d. Congenital defects in haemoglobin synthesis.
2. Marrow failure may occur as a result of drugs and chemicals, irradiation, secondary to diseases such as leukaemia, tumour invasion or from unknown causes.
3. Red cells may be lost through haemorrhage or haemolysis (increased destruction):
   a. This problem may be rooted in some red cell defect that is incompatible with normal red cell survival or is explicable on the basis of some factor extrinsic to the red cell that promotes red cell destruction.
   b. Red cell lysis occurs mainly within the phagocytic cells of the reticuloendothelial system, notably within the liver and spleen.
   c. As a byproduct of this process, bilirubin, formed from haemoglobin within the phagocyte, enters the bloodstream, and an increase in haemolysis is promptly reflected by an increase in total plasma bilirubin, causing jaundice.
4. Lack of essential constituents needed for the normal development of red cells, e.g. vitamin B_{12}, folic acid and iron, causing decreased production of red blood cells.

CLINICAL FEATURES
1. The more rapidly the anaemia develops, the more severe its symptoms, which are due to inadequate oxygen supply to the tissues:
   a. Pallor;
   b. Susceptibility to fatigue;
   c. Shortness of breath;
   d. Headache; loss of concentration; dizziness;
   e. Predisposition to angina pectoris or congestive heart failure in susceptible individuals.
2. Severity of symptoms dependent upon:
   a. The speed and degree with which the anaemia has developed;
   b. Its prior duration, i.e. its chronicity;
   c. The metabolic requirements of the particular patient;
   d. Any other disorders currently afflicting the patient, particularly cardiac conditions, etc.
   e. Special complications or concomitant features of the condition producing the anaemia.

IRON DEFICIENCY ANAEMIA

Iron deficiency anaemias are conditions in which the total body iron content is decreased below a normal level.

AETIOLOGY
Iron deficiency develops when the body's need for iron exceeds the supply.
1. Chronic blood loss – bleeding via the gastrointestinal tract, excessive bleeding from menorrhagia, multiple pregnancies.
2. Impaired gastrointestinal absorption of iron – small bowel disease, certain gastric resections.
3. Inadequate dietary sources of iron.
4. Increased iron requirements – during pregnancy, periods of rapid growth, menstruation (average of 20mg of iron lost per menstrual cycle).

DIETARY IMPLICATIONS
1. Average person ingests 10–15mg of iron daily in food iron and inorganic iron salts; less than 10 per cent of all iron ingested (including food and iron supplements) is absorbed.
2. Approximately 6mg of iron is ingested per 1,000 calories.
3. A nutritious diet should maintain normal iron balance, unless there is abnormal drain of iron (bleeding, pregnancy).
4. Food sources of iron: red meat (particularly liver); green leafy vegetables; dried fruit (apricots, prunes).
5. Ascorbic acid has been shown to enhance iron absorption.

Assessment
CLINICAL FEATURES
Reduction in haemoglobin concentration decreases the capacity of the blood to transport and deliver oxygen to the tissues. (See previous column for clinical features of anaemia.)

SPECIFIC SYMPTOMS

Some patients develop epithelial changes in chronic iron deficiency:

1. Spooning of fingernails (koilonychia);
2. Glossitis;
3. Stomatitis,
4. Dysphagia due to postcricoid webs;
5. Plummer – Vinson – Kelly – Paterson syndrome which is the association of chronic iron deficiency anaemia, dysphagia and glossitis.

Microscopic blood examination shows pale, small red blood cells (hypochromic microcytic).

Planning and implementation

TREATMENT AND NURSING INTERVENTIONS

1. Recognize and correct the underlying cause.
   a. Assist in the search for the site of chronic blood loss:
      (i) Question the patient concerning haematemesis, melaena, epistaxis, haematuria, menometrorrhagia, multiple diagnostic procedures.
      (ii) Send urine and stool specimens to lab for occult blood examination.
      (iii) Prepare patient for sigmoidoscopy, colonoscopy, barium enema, upper gastrointestinal studies.
2. Correct the haemoglobin and tissue iron deficiency with the administration of the prescribed iron preparation.

Oral iron therapy

1. Allows patient to regenerate haemoglobin. (Haematological values should return to normal in four to eight weeks.) Therapy is continued for approximately six months following the return to normal of blood values to restore iron stores.
2. Choice of iron depends on:
   a. Patient tolerance;
   b. Gastrointestinal absorption and
   c. Dosage according to estimate of haemoglobin deficiency.
3. Oral iron preparations:
   a. Ferrous sulphates (preferred);
   b. Ferrous gluconate;
   c. Ferrous fumarate.
4. Delayed-release forms of iron are not usually given. In this type of preparation the iron is released beyond the duodenum, which is the major site for iron absorption.
5. *Nursing emphasis and patient education:*
   a. Iron preparations are absorbed at all levels of the gastrointestinal tract below the stomach;

maximal absorption occurs in the duodenum and upper jejunum.
   b. Give iron immediately after meals to minimize gastric irritation; then shift to a between-meal schedule for maximum drug absorption.
   c. Educate patient to anticipate a certain amount of dyspepsia from time to time.
   d. Iron salts alter the colour of the stools; tell the patient to expect colour changes (dark green to black).
   e. Ferrous sulphate is apt to deposit on the teeth and the gums; advise patient to use frequent oral hygiene measures.
   f. The dosage of iron may be gradually increased over a few days.
   g. If gastrointestinal side-effects are troublesome, the dosage may have to be halved.
   h. Iron administration should be continued for approximately six months after haemoglobin levels return to normal – to replenish iron stores.
   i. Emphasize that the patient should take the iron faithfully.
   j. Patients should be warned that if iron tablets are taken in large numbers, they exert powerful toxic effects. Children are particularly prone to poisoning, which may be fatal.

Parenteral iron therapy

1. Parenteral iron therapy is given when:
   a. The patient is unable to tolerate iron preparations orally;
   b. The patient has severe gastrointestinal disorders;
   c. There is continuing negative iron balance while patient is taking maximum oral dose tolerated.

NURSING ALERT

Extravasation of iron medication results in painful local induration. Systemic reactions (flushing, nausea, vomiting, myalgia and fever) may occur.

2. Parenteral iron preparations:
   a. Iron dextran (Imferon);
   b. Iron sorbitol complex (Jectofer) – may cause patient's urine to turn black on standing, as about 50 per cent of iron is excreted in the urine within 24 hours.
3. Technique of parenteral iron administration:
   a. Discard needle that is used to draw medication into syringe; use a fresh needle for injection.
   b. Use a needle 5cm long – medication is injected deep into muscle.

c. Retract the skin over the muscle *laterally* before inserting needle – to prevent leakage along injection tract and staining of skin.

Patient education

1. Encourage the selection of a well-balanced diet. Adolescent girls should receive nutritional counselling.
2. Iron supplements should be given during pregnancy.

Evaluation

EXPECTED OUTCOMES

1. Patient demonstrates a return to normal haemoglobin levels.
2. Adheres to medication schedule.
3. Increases daily activities.

PERNICIOUS ANAEMIA

Pernicious anaemia is a megaloblastic anaemia* due to vitamin B_{12} deficiency caused by lack of the intrinsic factor in the gastric juice. (B_{12} deficiency is also seen in diseases of the small intestine, i.e. malabsorption, blind loop syndrome, etc.) The dietary requirement of vitamin B_{12} is only 3–10μg per day, which is readily available in a normal diet containing cereals, meat and yeast foods.

ALTERED PHYSIOLOGY

1. Pernicious anaemia is produced by a defect in the gastric mucosa; the stomach wall becomes atrophic and fails to secrete the intrinsic factor. This is thought to be due to an autoimmune response.
2. This substance normally binds with the dietary vitamin B_{12} and travels with it to the ileum, where the vitamin is absorbed. Without intrinsic factor, no orally administered B_{12} can enter the body. Vitamin B_{12} is stored in the liver for up to two years.
3. Therefore, after the body's stores of B_{12} are used up, the patient begins to show signs of the anaemia.

---

* Megaloblastic anaemias:
1. A megaloblast is a nucleated red cell with delayed and abnormal nuclear maturation.
2. The most common megaloblastic anaemias are B_{12} deficiency anaemia and folic acid deficiency.
3. Anaemias due to deficiencies of the vitamins B_{12} and folic acid show identical bone marrow and peripheral blood changes. This is because both vitamins are essential for normal deoxyribonucleic acid (DNA) synthesis.

4. Vitamin B_{12} is the extrinsic factor necessary for the maturation of red blood cells, healthy peripheral nerves and healthy tongue.

Assessment

CLINICAL FEATURES

1. Symptoms due to anaemia.
2. Symptoms due to physiological changes in gastrointestinal tract:
   a. Sore mouth with smooth red, 'beefy' tongue;
   b. Loss of appetite;
   c. Indigestion and epigastric discomfort;
   d. Recurring diarrhoea or constipation;
   e. Weight loss.
3. Symptoms due to neurological changes (occur in high percentage of untreated patients):
   a. Tingling and numbness or burning pain (paraesthesia) involving hands and feet;
   b. Loss of position sense, leading to disturbances of gait;
   c. Disturbances of bladder and bowel function;
   d. Irritability; depression;
   e. Paranoia and delirium.
4. The immature, abnormal red blood cells are destroyed earlier than the norm of 120 days, causing excess urobilinogen in the urine and a yellow tinge to the skin.

DIAGNOSTIC EVALUATION

1. Blood smear – reveals marked variation in size and shape of cells and a variable number of unusually large cells containing a normal concentration of haemoglobin.
2. Gastric analysis – the gastric juice lacks free hydrochloric acid (achlorhydria).
3. *Schilling test* – a test for vitamin B_{12} absorption, to prove that the patient cannot absorb oral vitamin B_{12} unless intrinsic factor is added.
   a. The patient is given a small dose of radioactive B_{12} in water to drink followed by a large nonradioactive intramuscular dose.
   b. When the oral vitamin is absorbed, it will be excreted in the urine; the intramuscular dose helps to flush it into the urine.
   c. A 24-hour urine specimen is collected and measured for radioactivity.
   d. If very little has been excreted, the test is repeated several days later (the 'second stage') with a capsule of oral intrinsic factor added to the oral B_{12}.
   e. If the patient has pernicious anaemia, this time much more radioactivity will be found in the 24-hour urine specimen.

4. Bone marrow aspiration – reveals megaloblastic marrow.
5. Gastroscopy – gastric mucosa appears thin and grey.
6. Low B_{12} level in the serum.

Planning and implementation

OBJECTIVES

1. Support the patient during the acute phase of his illness.
2. Give enough antianaemic factor (vitamin B_{12}) to produce a remission.
3. Help the patient accept that he must be on vitamin B_{12} maintenance for his lifetime.

TREATMENT DURING ACUTE STAGE

1. Give cyanocobalamin (vitamin B_{12}) as directed.
   a. Reticulocytes begin to increase on fourth day after therapy is started; normal haemoglobin values are obtained in approximately six weeks.
2. Give transfusion of packed cells very slowly (if prescribed).
   a. Transfusions are only given to patients whose anaemia is life-threatening (symptoms of hypoxia to heart or brain).
   b. Place the patient in a sitting position in bed. Too rapid administration of transfusion to patient with anaemia may produce acute pulmonary or cerebral oedema.
3. Support the patient with neurological involvement (see Care of the Patient with Neurogenic Bladder, Chapter 9, p. 642).

PATIENT EDUCATION

1. Impress upon the patient that vitamin B_{12} must be continued for his lifetime.
   a. Maintenance dose schedule – vitamin B_{12} intramuscularly every four weeks.
   b. Teach patient and family to give maintenance therapy. The health visitor is also involved with the therapy.
   c. Untreated pernicious anaemia is fatal.
2. Instruct the patient to report for follow-up examinations every six months – for haematocrit and physical examination.
   a. Patient may develop haematological or neurological relapse if therapy is inadequate.
   b. Patients with pernicious anaemia have a higher incidence of gastric cancer and thyroid problems; therefore, periodic stool examinations for occult blood and gastric cytology, along with thyroid function tests, should be made.
3. Following total gastrectomy (and occasionally subtotal gastrectomy) patient should receive maintenance dose of vitamin B_{12} as often as indicated – removal of gastric fundus deprives the patient of all intrinsic factor; may take as long as 10 years for clinical symptoms to appear, due to small amount of daily vitamin B_{12} required and the large body stores available for use.
4. Parenteral vitamin B_{12} therapy is preferred – greater reliability, better patient supervision, less expensive.

Evaluation

EXPECTED OUTCOMES

1. Patient begins to improve in general well-being and mental status in a few days.
2. Recent neurological changes will usually be reversed.

FOLIC ACID DEFICIENCY

Folic acid is necessary for normal red blood cell production. Folate depletion results in progressive anaemia.

CAUSES

1. Inadequate dietary intake:
   a. Common in alcoholics;
   b. Elderly individuals who live on 'tea and toast';
   c. Patients on hyperalimentation or chronic haemodialysis.
2. Impaired absorption – most absorption of folic acid takes place in upper jejunum.
3. Increased requirements – chronic haemolytic anaemias; pregnancy, etc.
4. Impaired utilization – from folic acid antagonists (methotrexate).

CLINICAL FEATURES

Symptoms of anaemia – fatigue, weakness, pallor; sore tongue, cracked lips.

DIAGNOSTIC EVALUATION

Assay of serum folate.

NURSING INTERVENTION

1. Give oral folic acid replacement as prescribed.

2. Inform the patient that a proper diet will prevent most instances of folate deficiency: green vegetables (asparagus, broccoli, spinach); yeast, liver, organ meats, some fresh fruits.

APLASTIC ANAEMIA

Aplastic anaemia is a condition of bone marrow failure which results in near absence of all blood cells (erythrocytes, leucocytes and platelets [pancytopenia]).

CAUSES
1. Idiopathic – approximately 50 per cent of aplastic anaemia cases are of unknown aetiology.
2. Chemical compounds – benzol (dry-cleaning agents) may induce permanent bone marrow damage.
3. Drugs – antibiotics (chloramphenicol), antitumour agents, antidiabetic agents, phenothiazines, antihistamines, insecticides, antidepressants, thyroid medication, heavy metals. (Almost any drug has potential.)
4. Ionizing radiation – therapeutic, industrial or laboratory accidents.
5. Viral infections – viral hepatitis, mononucleosis, etc.
6. Congenital (Fanconi's anaemia) – congenitally constituted defect in the bone marrow.

Assessment
CLINICAL FEATURES
1. Anaemia – resulting from depression of haemoglobin and rapidity of blood cell change (see p. 375, clinical features of anaemia).
2. Infections with high fever – resulting from granulocytopenia:
   a. Pharyngitis (the mucous membranes of the mouth are extremely prone to ulceration).
   b. Sepsis via gastrointestinal tract or genitourinary tract.
3. Abnormal bleeding – resulting from thrombocytopenia:
   a. Purpura; petechiae; ecchymoses;
   b. Bleeding from gums, nose, gastrointestinal and urinary tracts.

DIAGNOSTIC EVALUATION
1. Peripheral blood smear shows pancytopenia (deficiency in all the cellular elements of the blood).
2. Bone marrow aspiration – bone marrow is hypo-

plastic or aplastic; reduction of its cellular elements occurs, and there is an almost complete absence of haemopoietic activity.

PATIENT PROBLEMS
1. Ineffective coping related to anxiety about achieving a remission.
2. Potential for infection related to lack of circulating granulocytes.
3. Potential for haemorrhage related to thrombocytopenia.

Planning and implementation
NURSING INTERVENTIONS
Objectives
Bring the patient to remission.
Prolong his survival time with supportive therapy.
1. Attempt to identify and eliminate the underlying toxic agent(s) – gives marrow opportunity to recover before being damaged too severely. However, permanent damage often occurs.
   a. Question patient regarding all agents (chemicals, drugs) to which he has been exposed.
   b. Instruct patient to eliminate exposure to toxins and discontinue all unnecessary medications.
2. Support the patient undergoing bone marrow transplantation (replacement of affected bone marrow with marrow from healthy donor – preferably matched sibling). This treatment is performed at specialized centres, with variable results.
3. Treatment with antilymphocyte globulin acting as an immunosuppressive agent.

TREATMENT FOR PATIENT WHEN BONE MARROW TRANSPLANTATION IS NOT FEASIBLE
1. To relieve the symptoms of anaemia:
   a. Give packed red cell transfusions carefully – to maintain haemoglobin level compatible with patient's activities and to relieve symptoms of dyspnoea, palpitation and weakness.
   b. Provide adequate rest. Oxygen therapy may be necessary.
2. To minimize the effects and detect incidence of bleeding due to thrombocytopenia:
   a. Give transfusion of whole blood for haemorrhagic emergencies;
   b. Give platelet transfusions from histocompatible donors if possible – to arrest bleeding in patient with thrombocytopenia (haemorrhagic complications occur with platelet counts below $20,000/mm^3$);

c. Keep patient who receives multiple transfusions over a period of time under careful nursing observation – transfusion complications usually develop with these patients.
   (i) Eventually, patient may develop antibodies to minor red cell antigens and to platelet antigens so that transfusions no longer raise the counts sufficiently.
   (ii) Multiple transfusions decrease chance for successful bone marrow transplantation.
3. To minimize the risks of infection and detect early signs of infection due to leucopenia:
   a. Collect regular swabs, urine samples and gargles for evidence of infection – patients with aplastic anaemia are susceptible to infections, due to low leucocyte count.
   b. Utilize careful aseptic techniques for patients with pronounced leucopenia.
   c. Treat infections with appropriate agent.
      (i) Long-term antibiotic therapy may cause enteritis and diarrhoea from changes in intestinal flora.
      (ii) Generalized moniliasis may also occur in weakened patients taking antibiotics for prolonged periods.
4. Prepare patient for splenectomy (p. 399) if indicated – the spleen destroys large numbers of white cells and platelets; splenectomy may cause slight elevation of haemoglobin levels and decrease the transfusion requirements.
5. Anabolic steroids, e.g. prednisone, may be given to attempt to stimulate marrow regeneration and bring about remission.
6. To enable the patient to cope with possible prolonged treatment and poor prognosis, give psychological support to patient and family.

DISCHARGE PLANNING AND PATIENT EDUCATION
Instruct patient as follows:
1. Be aware of drugs that may damage the bone marrow cell.
2. When taking drugs that can produce blood dyscrasias (chloramphenicol, phenylbutazone, sulphonamides), have regular blood counts; however, aplastic anaemia may develop after drug has been discontinued.
3. During bleeding episodes, use mouthwashes instead of brushing teeth with brush.
4. Prevent minor infections. Any abrasion or wound of mucous membranes or skin is a potential site of infection.

Evaluation
EXPECTED OUTCOMES
1. Patient achieves remission of disease.
2. Avoids infection.
3. Manages bleeding episodes.
4. Copes with uncertain outcome; talks about this to health professionals.

BLOOD CELL DISORDERS

SICKLE CELL DISEASE

Sickle cell disease is a severe, chronic, haemolytic anaemia occurring in people who are homozygous for the sickle gene. Those heterozygous for the sickle gene are said to possess sickle cell trait.

AETIOLOGY
1. Genetically determined, inherited disease.
2. Each person inherits one gene from each parent which governs the synthesis of haemoglobin.
3. The gene responsible for haemoglobin S (sickle cell) is found mainly in the negroid population.

ALTERED PHYSIOLOGY
1. Sickle cell haemoglobin aggregates in low oxygen concentration conditions.
2. This distorts the membrane of the red blood cell causing the sickle or crescent shape. The cells become entangled leading to increased blood viscosity.
3. The fragile sickle cells are rapidly destroyed.
4. Anaemia results.

Assessment
POTENTIAL PROBLEMS
1. Pain related to agglutination of sickled cells within the small blood vessels.
2. Hypoxia related to increased blood viscosity and increased destruction of red blood cells.
3. Increased danger of infection related to fibrotic changes in the spleen.
4. Potential for injury related to intravenous therapy.
5. Parental guilt related to hereditary nature of the disease.
6. Knowledge deficit regarding sickle cell anaemia and its management.

Planning and implementation

OBJECTIVES

1. Increase the amount and frequency of fluid intake to dilute the blood.
2. Assist with partial exchange blood transfusion to replace the sickle cells and prevent agglutination (see p. 371).
3. Identify effective measures to alleviate pain.
4. Monitor and reduce fever of associated infection.
5. Provide emotional support.
6. See related nursing management (Table 6.1).

Evaluation

EXPECTED OUTCOMES

1. Patient achieves effective pain relief.
2. Understands the reasons for the disease and its management.
3. Avoids infection.

THALASSAEMIA MAJOR (COOLEY'S ANAEMIA)

Beta-thalassaemia (ß-thalassaemia) refers to an inherited group of blood disorders characterized by a reduction or absence of the beta-globulin chain in haemoglobin synthesis. Homozygous ß-thalassaemia is the most severe of the ß-thalassaemia syndromes and is also known as thalassaemia major or Cooley's anaemia.

AETIOLOGY

1. Genetically determined, inherited disease.
2. Autosomal-recessive pattern of inheritance. Two types of ß-thalassaemia genes produce different severities of the disease.

INCIDENCE

Most prevalent in the Mediterranean basin, Middle East, India, Pakistan, Southeast Asia, and Africa.

ALTERED PHYSIOLOGY

1. Insufficient beta-globulin synthesis allows large amounts of unstable alpha chains to accumulate.
2. The precipitates of alpha chains that form cause red blood cells to be rigid and easily destroyed, leading to severe anaemia and resultant chronic hypoxia.
3. Erythroid activity is markedly increased in an attempt to overcome the increased rate of destruction, resulting in enormous expansion of bone marrow.
4. Rapid destruction of defective red blood cells, decreased production of haemoglobin, and in-

creased absorption of dietary iron due to the body's response to anaemia result in an excess supply of available iron.
5. In response to the low level of adult haemoglobin, large concentrations of fetal haemoglobin, which does not contain beta chains, are produced.

EXPECTED OUTCOME

1. No known cure.
2. Unable to predict which severely afflicted children will follow a more favourable course.
3. Often fatal in late childhood or early adolescence.

POLYCYTHAEMIA VERA

Polycythaemia vera (erythnaemia) is a disease of unknown primary cause characterized by an increase in the number of red blood cells and in the total blood volume. The bone marrow is dark red and intensely cellular. It is characterized by leucocytosis, thrombocytosis and splenomegaly.

Secondary polycythaemia is commonly associated with hypoxia (cardiovascular and pulmonary disease), with excessive production of erythropoietin, adrenocortical steroids or androgens, or to chronic chemical exposure.

ALTERED PHYSIOLOGY

1. Increased blood volume because of increase in red cell mass.
2. Increased supply of precursor cells (to the erythroid, myeloid and megakaryocytic lines, which produce erythrocytes, granulocytes and platelets).
3. Striking increase in total blood volume; gradually increasing blood viscosity.
4. Decreased marrow iron.
5. Engorgement of all organs with blood.
6. Hyperplasia of all bone marrow elements.
7. Enlargement of spleen (sometimes).

PROGRESS OF DISEASE

1. Insidious and gradual onset – probably measured in years.
2. Clinical course of long duration – up to 20 years.
3. More frequent in males; most common during middle and later years of life.
4. Peptic ulcers are common in these patients; cerebral, gastrointestinal and nasal haemorrhages may occur at any time during the course of the disease.

Assessment
CLINICAL FEATURES
This is a multiple organ system disease.
1. Weakness and fatigue.
2. Headache, dizziness, impaired mental ability, visual disturbances.
3. Pruritus.
4. Plethoric appearance.
5. Reddish-purple hue of the face, lips, hands, feet and buccal cavity; aggravated by cold.
6. Peripheral vascular complaints.
7. Paraesthesia.
8. Splenomegaly, producing abdominal discomfort.
9. Elevated systolic blood pressure.
10. Hepatomegaly (late in course of disease).

DIAGNOSTIC EVALUATION
1. Increased red cell mass – measured by an isotopic technique.
2. Thrombocytosis; often abnormal platelet aggregation.
3. Leucocytosis.
4. Elevated granulocyte alkaline phosphatase activity.
5. Increased cellular activity of bone marrow; decreased marrow iron.
6. Low erythrocyte sedimentation rate (commonly less than 1mm per hour).

Planning and implementation
TREATMENT AND NURSING INTERVENTIONS
Objective
To reduce the red cell mass (e.g. to bring the haematocrit to within normal limits).
1. 500ml of blood removed every two to three days until haematocrit reaches desired level. Venesection may be repeated when necessary.
2. Chemotherapy:
   a. Melphalan.
   b. Chlorambucil.
   c. Busulphan.
   d. Cytosine arabinoside.
   e. See Nursing Care of the Patient Receiving Chemotherapy, Chapter 18, p. 1036.
3. Radioactive phosphorus ^{32}P, either orally or intravenously – reduces myelopoiesis (formation of bone marrow).
4. Keep patient mobile – likelihood of thrombosis increases when patient is on bed rest.
5. Evaluate and treat for complications – the clinical course of polycythaemia is determined by the development of complications.

a. Thrombotic complications – due to hypervolaemia and hyperactivity of the haematopoietic tissues. Includes deep vein thrombophlebitis, myocardial and cerebral infarction and thrombotic occlusion of the splenic, hepatic, portal and mesenteric veins.
b. Haemorrhage – bleeding occurs spontaneously from engorgement of capillary beds.
c. Gout – from overproduction of uric acid (secondary to nucleoprotein turnover of marrow cells).
d. Congestive failure – from increased blood volume and hypertension.
e. Acute leukaemia – may be a terminal complication.

PATIENT EDUCATION
1. Report at prescribed intervals for follow-up blood (haematocrit) studies.
2. Avoid taking *hot* baths/showers – worsens pruritus.

AGRANULOCYTOSIS (GRANULOCYTOPENIA)

Agranulocytosis (granulocytopenia) is an acute rare disease in which the white blood cell count drops to extremely low levels and neutropenia becomes pronounced.

CAUSE
Hypersensitivity to certain drugs or chemicals – may suppress bone marrow activity and decrease production of white blood cells. The most common drugs causing the disease are antithyroid drugs, especially thiouracil (1–2 per cent of those taking the drug), chloramphenicol, chlorpromazine and some sulphonamides.

Assessment
CLINICAL FEATURES
1. Severe infection of the throat and sometimes elsewhere due to the lack of granulocytes.
2. Profound weakness and exhaustion.

Planning and Implementation
TREATMENT AND NURSING INTERVENTIONS
1. Withdrawal of suspected drug.
2. Antibiotics.
3. The mortality rate is high. Measures to support the patient and increase comfort should be utilized.

Evaluation

EXPECTED OUTCOMES

1. The patient will express comfort.
2. No evidence of sepsis present.

LEUKAEMIAS

The leukaemias are neoplastic disorders of the blood-forming tissues (spleen, lymphatic system and bone marrow). They are characterized by widespread proliferation within the bone marrow and other blood-forming tissues of immature precursors of one of the types of leucocytes. The leukaemic process drastically reduces the production of the principle constituents of normal blood, resulting in anaemia and increased susceptibility to infection and haemorrhage.

CLASSIFICATION

Classified according to:

1. The cell line involved (lymphocytic, granulocytic or monocytic).
2. The maturity of malignant cells:
   a. Acute (immature cells);
   b. Chronic (differentiated cells).

PREDISPOSING FACTORS

Aetiology unknown: several factors are associated with increase in incidence:

1. Exposure to radiation.
2. Chemical agents – benzene.
3. Infectious agents – viruses (currently being investigated).
4. Genetic abnormalities – increased risk of leukaemia in patient with Down's syndrome.
5. Chemotherapy treatment – particularly alkylating agents.
6. Myeloproliferative disorders – polycythaemia vera, myelofibrosis (fibrosis of bone marrow).
7. Heredity – some families with incidence of leukaemia.

ACUTE LEUKAEMIA

Acute leukaemia is a rapidly progressive disease involving primitive cells or blasts. It may be lymphoblastic (lymphatic), myeloblastic (myeloid) or monoblastic (very rare).

Assessment

CLINICAL FEATURES

Produced by proliferation and infiltration of bone marrow and other organs by immature white blood cells on the lymphocytic, granulocytic or monocytic group.

1. General malaise; person tires easily; pallor from anaemia caused by depressed erythropoiesis, haemorrhage and haemolysis.
2. Persistent fever due to neutropenia (decreased production of neutrophil granulocytes which causes an increased susceptibility to infection).
3. Enlarged lymph nodes and spleen; abdominal discomfort – from local tissue invasion.
4. Bone pain, arthralgia – from expanding marrow in bone and gout of hyperuricaemia.
5. Bleeding of gums, epistaxis, petechiae, prolonged bleeding following a surgical procedure – from thrombocytopenia (lowered platelet count).
6. Tachycardia, weight loss, dyspnoea on exertion, intolerance to heat – from increased metabolism by the tumour producing more heat.
7. Leukaemia infiltration of the skin – tendency for leukaemic tissue to infiltrate other organs and tissues.
8. Cerebral haemorrhage, cranial nerve paralysis, increased intracranial pressure – from neurological complications (leukaemia cells frequently invade the central nervous system – usually in patients in long remission).
9. Pain – from infarction, particularly the spleen.

DIAGNOSTIC EVALUATION

1. Examination of the blood – total peripheral white count varies widely. There is a decreased production of neutrophil granulocytes due to a proliferation of abnormal leucocytes.
2. Bone marrow biopsy – characteristically large percentage of bone marrow's nucleated cells are immature leucocyte forms called 'blasts'.
3. Lymph node biopsy.
4. Chest X-ray – to detect mediastinal node and lung involvement.
5. Skeletal X-ray – to detect skeletal lesions.

PATIENT PROBLEMS

1. Fatigue, nausea, constipation, discomfort, related to chemotherapy.
2. Ineffective individual coping related to toxicity encountered during chemotherapy.
3. Potential development of infection related to granulocytopenia and mucosal damage.
4. Bleeding tendencies related to thrombocytopenia from leukaemia and chemotherapy.

5. Pain related to proliferation of leukaemia cells and enlargement of abdominal organs.
6. Fear related to the prognosis of the disease.

Planning and Implementation
TREATMENT
Objectives
Restore normal marrow function as quickly as possible.
Achieve complete remission.
Provide the patient with as long and as normal a life as possible.

Initial treatment in a specially equipped medical unit that treats patients with leukaemia with a team approach gives the best promise for prolonged remission.

Chemotherapy
1. The drugs are classified on the basis of their effects on cell chemistry.
2. Objective of chemotherapy – to induce remission (disappearance of all abnormal cell forms in the bone marrow and peripheral blood).

Underlying principles of chemotherapy
1. Chemotherapy inhibits growth of leukaemic cells by destroying or inactivating nucleic acids or by interfering with their synthesis; causes bone marrow depression and depresses the patient's immunological defence mechanism.
2. Drugs are usually given in combination (exert different biological effects) at high dose levels to produce greater leukaemia cell damage.
3. The treatment regimen is designed to affect cells in different phases of mitotic cycle.
4. Usually there is intensive treatment with multiple agents at the beginning of therapy to induce a remission, followed by long-term 'maintenance' therapy.
5. The nursing management of the patient with acute leukaemia includes constant assessment of the patient for effects of drug toxicity.

Some drugs used in acute leukaemia
A large number of drugs have an antileukaemia effect. The drug protocol changes as research developments are received.
1. Antimetabolites – compete with the natural metabolite, thus blocking the pathway for the synthesis of DNA or another cellular constituent (thereby blocking cell growth): methotrexate; antipurines (6-mercaptopurine); cytosine arabinoside (Ara-C).
2. Alkylating agents – may exert their anticancer effects by direct chemical interaction with the DNA of the cell (cyclophosphamide).
3. Antibiotics – inhibit synthesis of cell proteins (Adriamycin).
4. Plant alkaloids.
   Vincristine – blocks process of cell division.
5. Hormones – suppress the growth of lymphocytes: adrenal cortical steroid (prednisone).
6. Other drugs: L-asparaginase – an enzyme that breaks down asparagine, an amino acid frequently required by leukaemic cells for cell growth.

OTHER TREATMENT AVAILABLE
1. Bone marrow transplantation.
   a. High-dose chemotherapy and total body irradiation given first to destroy all residual leukaemic cells.
   b. The patient is then given intravenous infusion of allogeneic bone marrow.
   c. The patient requires excellent supportive nursing care during the three weeks following bone marrow transplantation, since he is unable to make white blood cells, red blood cells or platelets: he is transfusion-dependent and susceptible to overwhelming opportunistic infection.
2. Cranial irradiation – followed by intrathecal methotrexate (given by lumbar puncture into the subdural space) to destroy meningeal foci of leukaemic cells. This is most commonly performed as part of induction therapy for lymphocytic leukaemia.
3. Granulocyte transfusions to treat severe neutropenia may be given daily in conjunction with intravenous antibiotics. Granulocytes are obtained by cell separation techniques.

NURSING INTERVENTIONS
Constant nursing observation of patient receiving chemotherapy
See also Chapter 18, p. 1036.
1. Obtain baseline information before chemotherapy is started.
   a. Know the patient's 'normal' temperature, pulse, respiratory rate and blood pressure.
   b. Follow up the white blood cell count, differential count, haemoglobin measurements, platelet counts – to be aware of the drug's effect on the body.
   c. Follow up blood chemistry studies, electrolytes, urea nitrogen, creatinine, liver enzymes, bilirubin.
   d. Weigh the patient once or twice weekly.

e. Assist with bone marrow aspirations as directed (see p. 367).

2. *Watch for toxic manifestations during chemotherapy.*

a. Modifications of patient's chemotherapy regimen are based on laboratory and physical examinations before each course of treatment.

b. Monitor intravenous infusion of drugs – may cause local irritation in the veins; patient may complain of burning sensations during infusions of methotrexate and prednisone.
   (i) Adjust infusion flow to a slower rate.
   (ii) Change position of extremity to prevent muscular cramping.
   (iii) Patient may complain of nausea, vomiting and burning sensation along the gastrointestinal tract during or immediately after drug infusion.

c. Watch for mouth ulcers – frequently occur when patient is taking methotrexate. Offer medicated mouth rinses frequently to relieve oral discomfort.

d. Be prepared for the patient to experience loss of hair during antileukaemic treatment – alopecia occurs in high percentage of patients receiving vincristine. Encourage the patient to experiment with wigs, hair pieces, head scarfs.

e. Observe patient for footdrop, weakening hand grasp, ptosis of eyelids – vincristine may cause neuropathy.

f. Assess for constipation and abdominal pain – vincristine may produce paralytic ileus.

g. Watch for personality changes, fluid retention, hypertension, gastric ulcers and diabetes mellitus – occur with prednisone therapy.

h. Watch for other drug side-effects – diarrhoea, maculopapular rash, stomatitis, phlebitis, bone marrow depression, evidence of cardiac toxicity (tachycardia, dysrhythmias, tachypnoea, dyspnoea).

i. ECG readings may be prescribed – cardiac toxicity is associated with certain chemotherapeutic agents.

Supportive measures for patient with leukaemia or lymphoma

Underlying consideration: failure to improve is usually due to complications – infection and haemorrhage.

Objective

Control complications so that chemotherapeutic agents can demonstrate their effectiveness.

1. Eliminate the morbidity and mortality resulting from haemorrhage.

a. Major cause of haemorrhage is thrombocytopenia (decrease in platelets).

b. Risk of haemorrhage is high at platelet levels below 20×10^9 per litre (normal $250–500 \times 10^9$ per litre).

c. Prepare the patient for a transfusion of compatible platelets or pooled platelets when haemorrhage occurs. Platelet transfusion may need to be repeated two to three times weekly – average platelet half-life is three to five days.

2. To prevent and treat infection – the major morbidity and mortality associated with leukaemia; bone marrow invasion of the leukaemic cell line prevents normal production and maturation of granulocytes. Also the pathogenic organism is usually part of the patient's own flora.

a. Monitor the concentration of circulating granulocytes. Concentrations below 0.5×10^9 per litre indicate serious danger of infection.

b. Recognize infection promptly:
   (i) Monitor temperature at regular intervals – fever is major symptom of infection.
   (ii) Usual manifestations of infection are altered in patient with leukaemia.

c. Obtain cultures (for both aerobes and anaerobes) of blood, urine, sputum, spinal fluid.

d. Obtain chest X-ray.

e. Broad-spectrum antibiotics are usually given until organism is identified.

f. Watch for development of fungal infection (especially *Candida* and *Aspergillus*) – from indwelling catheters, antibiotics, immunosuppressive effects of chemotherapy and decreased resistance of patient.

3. To prevent infectious complications by control of environmental contamination.

a. Laminar air-flow room – a unidirectional air flow 'barrier' that establishes an air environment in which the infection-prone patient is free from contact with exogenous microorganisms.

b. Utilize all appropriate measures to reduce environmental contamination when special units are not available (protective isolation). Ensure correct handwashing procedure.

Other measures

1. Assist the patient to accept and participate in his therapeutic regimen.

a. Give expert physical care and support – this encourages the patient to endure much discomfort associated with treatment.

b. Help the patient to adapt to an incurable illness:
   (i) Patient may react with shock and anger when disease is first recognized; anger may be directed at health care personnel.
   (ii) Anger is a defence mechanism; patient realizes that death is inevitable; anger is also a defence against anxiety.
   (iii) Develop ability to accept and deal with this anger – important for establishing a therapeutic patient–nurse relationship.
   (iv) Allow patient and family to express their emotions.
   (v) Patient may use mechanism of denial, which may need to be supported or worked through. Different patients react in many different ways.
2. Control the pain and discomfort:
   a. Use milder analgesics when possible; change to a stronger narcotic as the patient's condition requires.
   b. Give antiemetic medication before meals – to help relieve the patient's nausea; sedatives may also be helpful.
3. Maintain oral intake between 3–4 litres daily – to prevent precipitation of uric acid crystals in the urine; overproduction of uric acid is due to the tremendous proliferation of blood cells and the destruction of these cells by antileukaemic agents.
4. Control fever – increased fluid intake, antipyretic drugs.
5. Give frequent and special mouth care – to remove dried blood, combat odour and soothe oral ulcerations.
   a. Antiseptic mouthwashes should be given to reduce susceptibility to stomatitis, oral ulceration and thrush.
   b. Soft toothbrushes should be used to prevent scratching of oral mucosa.
   c. Cleanse and lubricate the lips and nostrils – to prevent drying and cracking.
   d. Offer a soft diet if indicated – to reduce mechanical irritation to the gums.
6. Nutrition – acute leukaemia affects the general metabolism causing anorexia. A diet should be planned based on metabolic needs, especially amino acids and vitamins. Parenteral feeding may be needed if there is no response to the diet plan. Often there are taste changes for a time, therefore offer foods tempting to the patient.
7. Demonstrate continuing concern for the welfare of the patient.

PATIENT EDUCATION
1. Avoid possible sources of infection – crowds, unnecessary hospital visits, etc.
   a. Employ good, frequent handwashing practices.
   b. Report any sign of infection to doctor promptly.
   c. Report any exposure to varicella, measles, hepatitis, etc.
2. Pay careful attention to nutrition – undernourished person does not tolerate antileukaemic drugs as well as well-nourished individual.
3. Assist in central venous catheter as appropriate.
4. Monitor weight to be certain a significant amount of weight is not lost.
5. See your dentist – oral disease is frequently present; request dentist to contact your doctor before initiating dental examination.
6. Avoid rectal mucosal trauma by preventing constipation; use stool softeners, increase fluid intake, high-fibre foods; wash perineum with soap and water after each elimination.
7. Shower/bathe daily, paying attention to axillae, skin folds, groin and perineum. Use an electric shaver.
8. Use a deodorant rather than an antiperspirant (antiperspirant blocks sweat glands and may cause infection).
9. Practice oral hygiene after each meal.
10. Watch for signs of bleeding – avoid use of sharp objects, straining at stool, forceful nose blowing, products containing aspirin.
11. Use birth control pills as directed to prevent breakthrough bleeding.
12. Remember that leukaemia is a treatable disease, and that advances in treatment are continually being made; most side-effects of antileukaemic drugs are short-term and treatable.

Evaluation
EXPECTED OUTCOMES
1. Patient copes with chemotherapy; reports for treatments.
2. Remains free of infection and infectious complications.
3. Shows no evidence of bleeding; manages bleeding episodes when present.
4. Achieves relief of pain/discomfort.
5. Copes with distress; adjusts to new body image (hair loss, skin discolouration, indwelling Hickman catheter); uses support groups; verbalizes feelings and concerns.

CHRONIC LYMPHOCYTIC LEUKAEMIA

Chronic lymphocytic leukaemia is a type of leukaemia characterized by a great increase in mature lymphocytes in the circulation and in the lymphoid organs of the body. White blood cells may be in excess of 100×10^9 per litre of blood (leucocytosis). Lymphocytes may comprise 90–99 per cent of cells.

CLINICAL FEATURES

1. Insidious onset affecting older populations (mean age greater than 60 years); the disease may run a protracted, relatively asymptomatic course over a number of years.
2. Symptoms and signs are related to infiltration of lymph nodes, bone marrow, liver and spleen with lymphocytes.
   a. Gradual appearance of generalized lymph node enlargement – cervical region, axillae, groin; splenomegaly (may be painful).
   b. Anaemia, thrombocytopenia – may be due to bone marrow infiltration, to immune destruction or to hypersplenism.
   c. Weight loss, fever, enhanced susceptibility to infection.
3. Abnormalities of erythrocytes, granulocytes and platelets are common.

TREATMENT
Objective
To achieve a remission of symptoms.

Asymptomatic patient with chronic lymphocytic leukaemia
1. May not require treatment for a period of years.
2. Support the patient with optimum nutrition, rest, exercise, recreation and mental activity.

Symptomatic patient
Patient with massive adenopathy, severe anaemia, thrombocytopenia, skin involvement, recurring infections.
1. *Chemotherapy* – brings symptomatic relief; decreases size of lymph nodes and spleen:
   a. Chlorambucil;
   b. Combination drug therapy (three or four drug regimen) may be given to patients with poorly differentiated lymphocytes who are unresponsive to a single chemotherapeutic agent) – reduces white blood cell count, improves constitutional symptoms.

2. For anaemia – from blood loss; from replacement of bone marrow by leukaemia cells:
   a. Radiotherapy for local disease;
   b. Corticosteroids (prednisone);
   c. Chemotherapy;
   d. Transfusions: whole blood for haemorrhage; packed red cells when haemolysis or bone marrow failure exists.
3. For adenopathy: deep X-ray therapy for localized nodes, masses or splenomegaly.
4. For haemorrhage – may occur when severe thrombocytopenia and purpura are present or when bleeding, secondary to peptic ulcer, occurs as a complication of corticosteroid therapy. Transfusion to replace blood loss.

Planning and implementation
NURSING MANAGEMENT
See p. 384 for nursing support of patient receiving chemotherapy and p. 383 for other aspects of management of a patient with leukaemia.

CHRONIC GRANULOCYTIC LEUKAEMIA

Chronic granulocytic (myelocytic, myelogenous) leukaemia is a condition characterized by an increase in all phases of white blood cell development. It affects the granulocytes which are produced by the myeloid, or bone marrow. The condition is often associated with great enlargement of the spleen and liver. It may also occur in the acute form.

It appears most often between the ages of 35 to 50 and 60 to 70 years. It has a gradual, insidious onset. The disease runs a progressive course over several years. The Philadelphia chromosome is present in cells of bone marrow origin in over 90 per cent of patients.

CLINICAL FEATURES
1. Pallor, palpitations, dyspnoea – from anaemia.
2. Dragging sensation or enlargement of left side of abdomen – from splenic enlargement.
3. Haematological features: elevated platelet count, elevated granulocyte count; blood smear shows predominance of granulocytes at all stages of maturation.
4. Weakness, loss of weight, loss of appetite – from increased metabolic rate due to progress of disease.
5. Tenderness and pain in long bones (particularly tibia, ribs, sternum) – due to invasion by abnormal marrow.

6. Thrombocytosis – manifested clinically as thromboembolic or haemorrhagic phenomena.

TREATMENT
Objective
Achieve a remission of symptoms.

1. Chemotherapy: busulphan – will induce a complete or partial remission in majority of patients.
   a. Following initial treatment patient may be placed on long-term, low-dose maintenance therapy or high-dose therapy when evidence of disease recurs.
   b. Eventually patient will no longer respond; the acute exacerbation phase is termed myeloblastic or 'blast' crisis. The patient is then treated as for acute leukaemia (see p. 383). Other chemotherapeutic agents (second line drugs) may be used.
2. Bone marrow transplantation may be attempted during the chronic or early accelerated phase if suitable donor can be found.
3. Leucophoresis (removal of white blood cells from whole blood; red blood cells transfused back into patient) may be used for the patient who needs white blood cell count reduced rapidly.

NURSING INTERVENTIONS
1. See p. 384 for nursing support of patient receiving chemotherapy.
2. See p. 385 for other aspects of management of a patient with leukaemia.

MALIGNANT LYMPHOMAS

The lymphomas are a group of neoplastic diseases of the lymphoreticular system and include Hodgkin's disease and the non-Hodgkin's lymphomas.

1. Lymphomas are classified, according to the predominant malignant cell, as lymphocytic lymphoma (previously called lymphosarcoma), histiocytic lymphoma (previously reticulum cell sarcoma) or Hodgkin's disease.
2. These tumours usually start in lymph nodes, but can involve any lymphoid tissue in the spleen, gastrointestinal tract (tonsils, walls of stomach), liver or bone marrow.
3. They may spread to all these areas and to extra-lymphatic tissues (lung, kidneys, skin).
4. The aetiology of these diseases is unknown.

HODGKIN'S DISEASE

Hodgkin's disease is a malignant disease of unknown aetiology that originates in the lymphoid system and involves predominantly the lymph nodes. It may occur in almost any lymphoid mass of tissues: spleen, bone marrow.

ALTERED PHYSIOLOGY
1. The malignant cell of Hodgkin's disease is the 'Reed–Sternberg' cell, which is a gigantic, atypical tumour cell, morphologically unique and of uncertain lineage.
2. The different histopathological types of Hodgkin's disease are associated with varying prognoses.
3. Hodgkin's disease shows a highly predictable pattern of spread – usually via the lymphatic channels from one chain of lymph nodes to another, often to the spleen, and ultimately to extralymphatic sites. Often it is cervical lymph nodes which are first affected.
4. Hodgkin's disease may have a haematogenic spread as extra node sites involved include the gastrointestinal tract, bone marrow, skin, upper air passages and other organs.

Assessment
CLINICAL FEATURES
1. Painless enlargement of lymph nodes on one side of neck. Often painful after alcohol intake (unexplained).
2. Generalized, unexplained pruritus (itching), sweating, weight loss.
3. Progressive anaemia.
4. Slight to high fever.
5. Enlargement of lymph nodes in other regions of the body.
6. Enlargement of mediastinal and retroperitoneal lymph nodes produces pressure symptoms:
   a. Dyspnoea from pressure against the trachea.
   b. Dysphagia from pressure against the oesophagus.
   c. Laryngeal paralysis due to pressure against the recurrent laryngeal nerve.
   d. Brachial, lumbar or sacral neuralgias due to pressure on the nerve.
   e. Oedema of the extremities due to pressure on the veins.
   f. Enlargement of spleen and liver.
7. Effusions into the pleura or peritoneum.
8. Obstructive jaundice.

DIAGNOSTIC EVALUATION

The extent of the disease is determined before treatment.

1. Biopsy of lymph node(s) to identify characteristic histological features.
2. Complete blood count.
3. Chest X-ray and tomography.
4. Skeletal survey.
5. Technetium bone scan.
6. Bone marrow biopsy.
7. Liver function tests and scan.
8. Lymphangiogram:
   a. Reveals size of lymph nodes.
   b. Detects abdominal lymph node enlargements which may not be seen or felt by ordinary means.
9. Laparotomy ('staging operation') – to determine extent of disease; splenectomy (may improve blood tolerance to extensive radiotherapy and chemotherapy); open liver biopsy; biopsy of para-aortic lymph nodes. These procedures are important in determining prognosis and treatment.

PATIENT PROBLEMS

1. Discomfort related to lymph node enlargement, fever, and itching.
2. Potential for fever.
3. Alteration in breathing patterns related to tracheal pressure.
4. Alteration in nutrition related to dysphagia.
5. Potential nonadherence to treatment programme related to side-effects and length of therapy.

Planning and implementation

TREATMENT

Depends upon stage, symptoms and cell type.

Concepts

1. Radiotherapy to local field, to an extended field or to all node-bearing areas (total nodal irradiation) is the first choice of treatment in early Hodgkin's disease (without any symptoms). An important factor in treatment is the radiation dose administered.
2. Hodgkin's disease may be eradicated from any site that has received 4,000 to 4,500 rad within the space of four weeks. Megavoltage radiation techniques permit the delivery of such a dose to one or more entire lymph node chains.
3. Areas of the body in which the lymph node chains are located can tolerate doses of this magnitude without serious damage (as can the area of the spleen and the oronasopharynx); vital structures such as the lungs, liver and kidneys are protected by lead shields.
4. Radiotherapy usually given daily over a period of weeks.
5. *Complications of intensive radiotherapy:*
   a. Pneumonitis, myocardial and pericardial fibrosis, hepatitis, artificial menopause, impotence, development of second malignancy (leukaemia) – depending on site of irradiation and dose-related circumstances.
   b. Acute reactions to irradiation – dryness of mouth; loss of taste; dysphagia; nausea and vomiting; apathy and lassitude; skin redness, dry peeling in treatment fields; loss of hair at back of neck and under areas treated; reduction of white blood cells.

TREATMENT IN ADVANCED HODGKIN'S DISEASE

Objectives

Produce tumour regression and remission; relieve pressure on a vital organ (brain, bronchi, kidney).

1. Radiation alone may be used as a palliative measure, or a combination of radiotherapy and chemotherapy may be used.
2. Chemotherapy is used since Hodgkin's disease is considered a drug-responsive tumour.
   a. Multiple drug chemotherapy used (nitrogen mustard, vincristine, procarbazine and prednisone).
   b. Other combinations have also been effective.
   c. Dosage depends on patient's status and his response to treatment.
   d. Intermittent maintenance therapy may be required to keep disease under control.
   e. Toxic effects of these drugs often overlap, especially bone marrow depression.
   f. See p. 384 for discussion of patient undergoing chemotherapy.

NURSING INTERVENTIONS

1. Support the patient having toxic effects from chemotherapy.
2. Encourage the patient by saying that the therapy will end in 'a period of time' – serves as an incentive for the patient to continue with therapy.
3. Give laxatives to control constipation that accompanies chemotherapy.
4. Anticipate that patients on chemotherapy will develop leucopenia, thrombocytopenia, and anaemia.
5. Help patient cope with unpleasant side-effects of radiation.

a. Oesophagitis – bland soft foods at mild temperatures, aspirin gum (use moderately), anaesthetic lozenges, pain medication before eating if patient unable to eat.
b. Loss of taste – serve palatable meals.
c. Anorexia – encourage patient to make the effort to eat.
d. Nausea – antiemetics given to cover peak time of nausea.
e. Vomiting – reduction of radiation dose may be necessary.
f. Diarrhoea – antidiarrhoeal medication.
g. Skin reaction (sunburned/tanned appearance of treatment area) – avoid rubbing, heat, cold, application of lotions.
h. Lethargy – rest/sleep to keep energy level up; diversional activities to prevent boredom.
6. Prepare patient for surgical excision of localized lymph nodes if indicated (may be followed by radiotherapy). Surgery may also be used to alleviate complications caused by pressure or obstruction due to tumour masses.

NURSING ALERT
There is an apparent increase in second malignancies (primarily leukaemia) of patients who are long-term survivors of Hodgkin's disease, especially in those who have received combination chemotherapy as well as radiotherapy.

PATIENT EDUCATION
The control of the disease requires continuing observation by the patient.
1. Report fever or any sign of infection (skin redness, tenderness, lesions, cough) immediately, since the disease and its treatment make one susceptible to infection. Herpes zoster occurs frequently; may become generalized in immunosuppressed patients.
2. Use humidifier/throat lozenges for dry throat and to control desire to cough.
3. Express feelings and anxieties; seek supportive people and groups:
a. Depression and fear are normal reactions to diagnosis, treatment and stress of uncertain outcome.
b. Expect to feel fatigued up to a year after therapy.
c. Remain active and employed (if possible); seek to enjoy the present.
4. Expect some degree of hair loss if taking vincristine or nitrogen mustard; almost always reversible after therapy is completed.
5. Avoid taking alcohol, narcotics, antihistamines, tranquillizers or sympathomimetic agents when taking procarbazine.
6. Report for follow-up.

Evaluation
EXPECTED OUTCOMES
1. Patient is free of symptoms.
2. Adheres to therapeutic programme.
3. Achieves a cure/remission.

LYMPHOCYTIC LYMPHOMA (NON-HODGKIN'S LYMPHOMAS)

Lymphocytic lymphoma is a malignant growth of lymphocytes in lymphoid tissue characterized by progressive generalized lymphadenopathy and splenomegaly, often progressing to involvement of one or more non-lymphoid organ systems. Marrow damage, manifested by anaemia and thrombocytopenia, and immune dysfunction, with heightened susceptibility to bacterial and fungal infections, are also evident in these patients.

CLINICAL FEATURES
1. Prominent generalized lymphadenopathy.
2. Fatigue – attributable primarily to anaemia from impaired erythropoiesis and haemolysis.
3. Malaise, anorexia, weight loss.
4. Fever and sweating.
5. Abdominal distension – due to enlargement of spleen.

CLINICAL EVALUATION
1. Bone scan.
2. Reticuloendothelial (liver, spleen) scan.
3. Intravenous pyelogram.
4. Retroperitoneal lymphography.
5. Bone marrow biopsy.
6. Liver biopsy.
7. Laparotomy.

TREATMENT AND NURSING INTERVENTIONS
Objective
Induce a remission.
1. Give chemotherapy as directed.
a. Combination drug therapy used (cyclophosphamide, vincristine, prednisone) – in different dosages and schedules.
b. See p. 384 for nursing management of the patient having chemotherapy.
2. Prepare the patient for radiation – may be helpful in palliation.

3. Be on the alert for complications.
   a. Infection – by bacteria, viruses, fungi; due to deficiencies of cellular immunity.
   b. Anaemia – from bone marrow invasion, haemorrhage, chemotherapy, hypersplenism, failure of bone marrow, haemolysis.
   c. Spinal cord compression – from lymphomatous infiltration.
   d. Hyperuricaemia.
4. See also discussion of the care of patients with Hodgkin's disease (above).

MYCOSIS FUNGOIDES

Mycosis fungoides is a cutaneous lymphoma that may progress to involve the lymph nodes and other internal organs. The late stage of the disease closely resembles malignant lymphoma.

Assessment
CLINICAL FEATURES
1. Generalized severe itching – may last for several years.
2. Erythematous, urticarial, eczematous or psoriasis-like lesions – there are exacerbations and remissions of these eruptions.
3. Ulcerating and necrotic tumours of the skin – lesions become indurated and more fungoidal until they are mushroom-like growth (scarlet or purplish in colour), varying in size from 1–5cm; the body may be covered with these lesions.
4. Patient usually dies from systemic lymphoma.

DIAGNOSTIC EVALUATION
Biopsy of skin lesion – gives distinctive diagnostic pattern of mycosis fungoides.

PATIENT PROBLEMS
1. Alteration in comfort (generalized itching, burning in affected areas of skin, pain) related to lymphomatous skin lesions.
2. Ineffective coping related to body image problems and general discomforts of the disease.

Planning and implementation
TREATMENT
Objectives
Bring about a remission; enable the patient to cope with body image problems and the general discomforts of the disease.
1. Radiation is applied by electron beam – gives very little skin penetration and permits total body irradiation without visceral damage; used primarily when there is no evidence of systemic involvement.

2. Chemotherapy – to arrest the disease.
   a. Topical therapy (for cutaneous manifestations):
      (i) Nitrogen mustard used as topical therapy – effective in certain stages of the disease.
      (ii) Allergic contact hypersensitivity to the mustard may develop.
      (iii) Other agents used include topical fluocinolone acetonide (under plastic occlusive dressings).
   b. Intralesional injections of triamcinolone or nitrogen mustard may be tried.
   c. Systemic chemotherapy is carried out when internal organs are involved to prevent progressive growth and dissemination of disease.
      (i) Single agent chemotherapy protocol may be used.
      (ii) Antimetabolites, cytotoxic antibiotics and corticosteroids may be used.
      (iii) See p. 384 for management of patient receiving chemotherapy.
3. Radiotherapy (electron beam therapy) – for patients with widespread mycosis fungoides.

NURSING INTERVENTIONS
1. Watch for evidence of infection (major cause of death, particularly septicaemia, bacterial pneumonia).
2. Support the patient who has painful ulcerative lesions.
   a. Place bed cradle over patient when he is unable to tolerate the weight of the bed clothing on his skin lesions.
   b. Apply bacteriostatic ointment (as prescribed) to lesions as a prophylaxis against infection and to promote comfort by excluding air from open nerve endings.
   c. Give analgesics for pain.
   d. Handle the patient with care:
      (i) Give the patient time to move slowly.
      (ii) Use two health care personnel to lift and turn the patient.
      (iii) Use distraction techniques when nursing care causes pain.
      (iv) Watch for development of contractures and pressure sores.
   e. Keep up nutritional status, since the patient loses protein and fluid from body surface.
3. Assist the patient to cope with foul odour from bacterial growth in lesions:
   a. Wash hands before and after patient contact to reduce bacterial spread.
   b. Continue with excellent skin care to keep bacterial levels low.

c. Use whirlpool therapy to aid in skin cleansing and debridement.

See p. 389 for discussion of the nursing management of patients with Hodgkin's disease.

PATIENT EDUCATION

1. Emphasize the importance of personal hygiene and skin care:
   a. Daily bathing with a mild superfatted soap and medicated bath oil.
   b. Application of prescribed creams/ointments.
2. Discuss modifications that may need to be made in lifestyle (role changes, sexual relations); psychotherapy may be helpful, especially for patient in terminal phase of illness.
3. Avoid using perfumes and aftershave lotion.
4. Wear nonrestrictive cotton clothing.
5. Report to the doctor any flare-up skin condition, fever, signs and symptoms of systemic illness; hospitalization is usually necessary.

Evaluation
EXPECTED OUTCOMES

1. Patient gains some relief from pain and discomfort.
2. Demonstrates coping ability in relation to body image.

MULTIPLE MYELOMA

Multiple myeloma (plasma cell myeloma; plasmocytoma; myelomatosis) is a malignant disease of the plasma cell that infiltrates bone and soft tissues. The cause is not known. It is a disease of older people and is not classified as a lymphoma.

ALTERED PHYSIOLOGY

1. The malignant cell is the plasma cell; neoplastic proliferation takes place mainly in the bone marrow. (The plasma cell is derived from B-lymphocytes and produces immunoglobulin [antibodies]).
2. The bones most commonly affected are the vertebrae, skull, ribs, sternum, pelvis, upper ends of humerus.
3. The malignant plasma cells usually produce abnormal amounts of an immunoglobulin or parts of an immunoglobulin protein (Bence Jones protein) that can usually be detected in urine by immunoelectrophoresis.
4. There is a constant threat of hypercalcaemia, hypercalciuria and hyperuricaemia due to skeletal destruction, because myeloma cells stimulate osteoclasts.

5. Increased loss of bone substance leads to collapse of vertebral bodies, rib fractures, etc.

Assessment
CLINICAL FEATURES

1. Constant severe bone pain, especially on movement – marrow is infiltrated with plasma cells and there are destructive bone lesions.
   a. Low back pain – the most characteristic symptom.
   b. Skeletal lesions – producing swelling, tenderness, pain and *pathological fractures*.
2. Anaemia – due to malignancy and/or replacement of marrow with neoplastic plasma cells. May be associated with thrombocytopenia and granulopenia – causes increased susceptibility to infection and abnormal bleeding.
3. Marked weight loss.
4. Symptoms of renal failure – may be due to precipitation of the immunoglobulin in the tubules or to pyelonephritis, hypercalcaemia, increased uric acid, infiltration of the kidney with plasma cells (myeloma kidney), renal vein thrombosis.
5. Bleeding tendencies.
6. Nausea, vomiting, constipation, lethargy (late stage), due to hypercalcaemia.

DIAGNOSTIC EVALUATION

1. Abnormalities present in basic haemogram – anaemia, elevated sedimentation rate, leucopenia with diminished granulocytes; decreased platelets.
2. Malignant plasma cells produce abnormal globulins which appear in serum electrophoresis as a paraprotein 'spike' – fragments of these globulins are excreted in urine as Bence Jones proteins.
3. Bone marrow biopsy – may show evidence of increased number of abnormal plasma cells in the marrow.
4. Bony lesions may appear on X-ray; numerous areas of localized bone destruction may be visible; demineralization of skeleton (osteoporosis) may occur.
5. Radioactive technetium bone scans – involved areas show increased uptake of technetium.

PATIENT PROBLEMS

1. Bone pain related to bone erosion and possible pathological fractures.
2. Potential for complications related to plasma cell proliferation.
3. Fatigue related to anaemia.
4. Weight loss related to disease process.
5. Potential for injury related to frailty of bones.

6. Coping difficulties related to change in lifestyle and body image.

Planning and implementation
TREATMENT AND NURSING INTERVENTIONS
Objectives
Decrease the tumour mass.
Control pain.

Decrease tumour mass and relieve bone pain
1. Give the appropriate chemotherapy (foundation of treatment):
   a. Combination drug therapy appears more effective than single dose therapy in most patients.
   b. Melphalan, prednisone, cyclophosphamide are some of the agents currently being given.
   c. See p. 385 for supportive care of patient receiving chemotherapy.
2. Support patient receiving radiotherapy – given for relief of pain from large lesions (especially from nerve compression and fracture) and for reducing size of extraskeletal plasma cell tumours.

Give attentive and supportive care
1. Keep the patient mobile unless lesion in spine produces danger of cord compression – prevents further bone resorption and hypercalcaemia.
   a. Avoid total immobilization.
   b. *Watch for pathological fractures* – may occur when patient turns, is placed on bedpan, transferred to a stretcher.
   c. Avoid excessive lifting and straining. Handle patient with smooth, unhurried movements.
   d. Use analgesics, supportive splints and back brace for patient with pathology of spine.
   e. Local irradiation may be employed to achieve mobilization.
   f. Assist patient to *walk* as much as possible.
2. Evaluate for spinal cord compression – from invasion of canal by neoplastic tissue. Watch for bladder distension (spinal cord compression).
   a. Radiation therapy – to prevent paraplegia.
   b. Laminectomy for decompression – for cord compression or vertebral fractures.
3. Watch for recurrent infections – patient has impaired capacity for antibody production.
   a. Record temperature frequently – patients on steroids may not have overt symptoms of infection. Observe for apathy, lethargy.
   b. Observe for symptoms of urinary tract infection and bronchopneumonia.

c. Take cultures from skin lesions, blood, sputum and urine as indicated.
4. Observe the patient for signs and symptoms of renal insufficiency – from precipitation of Bence Jones protein in renal tubules, leading to tubular obstruction and dilatation and uraemia; or from pyelonephritis, hypercalcaemia (which may result from bony destruction and immobilization), amyloidosis, hyperuricaemia, myeloma kidney.
   a. Encourage free fluids – to prevent protein precipitation and to minimize hypercalcaemia.
   b. Give allopurinol as ordered – to control hyperuricaemia.
   c. Watch for symptoms of haemorrhagic cystitis in patient taking Cytoxan; maintain on high dose free fluids.
   d. Give prednisone as prescribed by doctor – may be used in management of hypercalcaemia.
   e. Avoid dehydration – can precipitate acute renal failure; intravenous fluids may be necessary.

NURSING ALERT
Patients with multiple myeloma should not be put on fasting regimens for diagnostic tests, since dehydrating procedures can precipitate acute renal failure.

5. Treat concomitant anaemia – occurs in most patients.
   a. Give packed red cell transfusions for patients with severe anaemia.
   b. Administer chemotherapy, steroid hormones and androgens – to stimulate erythropoiesis; may improve anaemia.
   c. Determine methods to conserve patient's energy; note this on nursing care plan.
6. Be aware of the complications:
   a. Infection – from decrease in normal circulating antibodies due to proliferation of abnormal plasma cells which produce ineffective globulins; extensive bone marrow involvement causes leucopenia; chemotherapy and radiotherapy also cause marrow depression; steroid hormones increase susceptibility to opportunistic infection.
   b. *Neurological complications:*
      (i) Paraplegia – from collapse of supporting structures, from infiltration of nerve roots or from cord compression of plasma cell tumours.
   c. Bone complications – pathological fractures.
   d. Haematological complications:
      (i) Renal failure – from plugging of renal tubules by proteinaceous casts.

(ii) Renal stones from hypercalcaemia – due to bone destruction and increased bone resorption.

(iii) Infiltration of kidney from plasma cells, etc.

(iv) Hypercalciuria – excessive bone destruction creates increased excretion of calcium in urine.

(v) Hyperuricaemia – may produce renal failure.

e. Multiple primary neoplasms may occur – disordered immune surveillance may make patient susceptible to multiple tumour development.

PATIENT EDUCATION AND EMOTIONAL SUPPORT

1. Instruct the patient about proper body mechanics and avoiding heavy lifting.
2. Make the patient aware of potentially nephrotoxic factors such as *dehydration* or drugs.
3. Instruct the patient to wear a back brace as prescribed and to use muscle-strengthening exercises to maintain performance status.
4. Report the presence of fever, bone pain, bleeding or neurological complications; report for regular follow-up.
5. Support the patient emotionally and demonstrate continuing interest:
   a. Reinforce the patient's understanding of treatment and its possible side-effects.
   b. Take a positive approach emphasizing the benefits of therapy.
   c. Emphasize the patient's strengths:
      (i) Share and work through the patient's anxieties.
      (ii) Explore precisely what the patient fears.
      (iii) Allow the patient to talk about his problems. Give *specific* help (for pain, breathlessness, depression, etc).
      (iv) Anticipate the patient's anxieties after leaving the hospital.
6. Use diet supplement during periods of anorexia.

Evaluation

EXPECTED OUTCOMES

1. Patient reports relief of disabling bone pain; increases activities.
2. Demonstrates minimal/no complications; shows reduction of tumour cell mass by laboratory evaluation; achieves reversal of symptoms.
3. Demonstrates improved results of blood studies – haemoglobin, platelet count, white blood cell count.

4. Increases weight and has good appetite.
5. Becomes more alert and is able to cope with life changes.

BLEEDING DISORDERS

VASCULAR PURPURAS

The term purpura refers to extravasation (escape) of blood into the skin and mucous membranes. Purpuric lesions may occur spontaneously as an isolated phenomenon or as an accompaniment of obvious disease.

TYPES OF PURPURA

1. *Petechiae* – small pinpoint haemorrhages under the skin.
2. *Ecchymoses* – escape of blood into tissues, producing a large bruise.
3. Petechiae and ecchymoses may occur as the result of vascular rupture, permitting the leakage of blood into the subcutaneous tissue of the mucous membranes.
4. *Symptomatic or secondary purpura* – certain types of bloodstream infections (e.g. meningococcaemia and infective endocarditis) exhibit this phenomenon due to damage to the vascular walls by the infectious agent.
5. Severe arterial hypertension – may cause the patient to bruise easily; Valsalva manoeuvre may cause petechiae.
6. *Anaphylactoid purpura* – generally regarded as an allergic disorder in which there are various skin lesions (purpuric and otherwise) and episodes of arthritis, abdominal pain, haematuria, gastrointestinal haemorrhages and fever.
   a. Attacks last several weeks and recur for years.
   b. Steroid therapy is often effective.
7. *Familial haemorrhagic telangiectasia* – a hereditary disorder manifested by an abnormal tendency to bleed and bruise.
   a. Precise nature of defect is obscure.
   b. Condition does not respond to any proved method of treatment.
8. *Toxic purpura* – a condition observed after exposure to certain drugs and poisons.
9. *Vitamin C deficiency* – a vascular purpura.
10. Senile purpura.

11. Collagen and vascular disease.
12. Steroid purpura.

THROMBOCYTOPENIA

Thrombocytopenia is a decrease in the circulating platelet count, which may result in bleeding or haemorrhage.

ALTERED PHYSIOLOGY AND CAUSES

1. Decreased platelet production (infiltrative diseases of bone marrow, leukaemia, myelosuppressive therapy, other tumours, myelofibrosis, radiotherapy, drug effect, aplastic anaemia, etc).
2. Increased platelet destruction (infection, immune thrombocytopenic purpura, disseminated intravascular coagulation, drug-induced, etc).
3. Abnormal distribution or sequestration – hypersplenism.
4. Loss of platelets from body (extracorporeal circulation, dilution due to blood loss and multiple blood transfusions).

IDIOPATHIC AUTOIMMUNE THROMBOCYTOPENIC PURPURA

Immune thrombocytopenic purpura is a group of bleeding disorders due to immune destruction of platelets. Antiplatelet antibodies are produced for unknown reasons, so that the platelet life span is markedly shortened. Antibody-coated platelets are removed from the circulation by reticuloendothelial cells of the spleen and liver.

Assessment
CLINICAL FEATURES
1. May be acute or chronic.
2. Bleeding – mild to severe (thrombocytopenia is not usually accompanied by bleeding unless the platelet count falls below 20×10^9 per litre of blood).
   a. Skin lesions – small red haemorrhages; do not blanch on pressure.
   b. Purpuric lesions may occur in vital organ (brain).
   c. Bleeding may occur from nose, mouth, genitourinary tract.

LABORATORY FEATURES
1. Platelets may be absent or only slightly decreased in number; abnormalities may be seen in platelet size or morphological appearance.

2. Increased levels of immunoglobulins (IgG) or complement components on the platelet surface.
3. Bone marrow examination – bone marrow megakaryocytes are increased in number.

Planning and implementation
TREATMENT AND NURSING INTERVENTIONS
Objectives
Search for possible causes of bleeding; treat patient during spontaneous bleeding episodes.
1. Corticosteroids (prednisone) – may produce improvement by reducing bleeding (by affecting blood vessels, resulting in decreased capillary fragility; by elevating the level of circulating platelets; or by suppression of phagocytic cells of reticuloendothelial system).
2. Prepare the patient for a splenectomy (p. 399). Splenectomy may bring about improvement by elevating the platelet levels and by removing major site of platelet breakdown.
3. Immunosuppressive therapy – used for patients who do not respond to corticosteroids or splenectomy: azathioprine, cyclophosphamide, vincristine, etc.
4. Support the patient receiving transfusions.
   a. Transfusions of fresh whole blood (blood collected within 24 hours) – fresh blood is a source of platelets as well as plasma-clotting factors. Given to enhance haemostasis during bleeding episodes, to restore circulating blood volume and to correct anaemia.
   b. Transfusions of platelets (in form of platelet concentrates, platelet-rich plasma, fresh whole blood). Used in treating patients with thrombocytopenia secondary to bone marrow suppression caused by drugs (chemotherapy) or an idiopathic thrombocytopenic purpura.
5. Utilize other measures to help the patient with haemorrhagic tendencies (Table 6.1).

PATIENT EDUCATION
Instruct the patient as follows:
1. Employ self-monitoring for infectious complications if you are on long-term steroid therapy.
2. Avoid aspirin or aspirin-containing products.
3. Avoid potential sources of accidents; protect yourself from injury.

Evaluation
EXPECTED OUTCOMES
1. No further bleeding or bruising.
2. Early detection and treatment of infection.

CLOTTING DEFECTS

DISSEMINATED INTRAVASCULAR COAGULATION (DIC)

Disseminated intravascular coagulation is the formation of microthrombi in the capillaries and small vessels with consequent consumption of coagulation factors, especially fibrinogen and platelets, causing bleeding tendency.

1. Disseminated intravascular coagulation is a complication of many illnesses; often fatal.
   a. Infections.
   b. Obstetrical complications.
   c. Malignancies.
   d. Massive tissue injuries (burns)
   e. Vascular and circulatory complications
   f. Anaphylaxis.
   g. Haemolytic transfusion reactions.
2. Haemorrhagic tendency is the consequence of the acute activation of the clotting mechanism of the blood – results in intravascular consumption of the plasma clotting factors.
3. Clotting factors are consumed more quickly than they can be replenished by the liver.

Assessment

CLINICAL FEATURES
1. Diffuse bleeding – skin and mucous membranes.
2. Ecchymoses; petechiae.
3. Bleeding from gastrointestinal and urinary tracts.
4. Prolonged bleeding from venepuncture.
5. Signs and symptoms of acute renal failure.

DIAGNOSTIC EVALUATION
1. Coagulation screening tests – prolonged.
2. Thrombocytopenia.
3. Hypofibrinogenaemia.
4. Deficiencies in prothrombin factors V and VIII and elevated levels of fibrin degradation products.

Planning and implementation

TREATMENT
1. Removal and treatment of precipitating cause.
2. Antibiotics to treat overwhelming infection.
3. Supportive measures (fluid replacement, oxygenation, maintenance of blood pressure and urine output) – to restore circulating blood volume and deliver oxygen to ischaemic tissues.
4. Replacement therapy for serious haemorrhagic features (transfusions of red cells, platelet concentrates, and, if indicated by very low fibrinogen level, cryoprecipitate).
5. Heparin may be given to prevent fibrin formation to enable clotting factors to be replaced. It must be used with caution as haemorrhage may be aggravated.

NURSING INTERVENTIONS
1. See Table 6.1 for care of patient with haemorrhagic tendencies.
2. Carry out ongoing nursing assessment for occult bleeding and thromboembolic occlusion from formation of thrombi in multiple body sites.
   a. Look for bleeding from suture line, and oozing of blood from intravenous sites.
   b. Assess colour of skin and mucosa, petechiae, cold mottled hands and feet, gingival bleeding, nose-bleeding, bleeding/jaundice of conjunctivae and sclerae, haemoptysis.
   c. Monitor for vascular occlusion, which produces circulatory obstruction and organ hypoperfusion.
      (i) Kidneys – monitor for urine volume and haematuria.
      (ii) Skin – petechiae, purpura, ecchymoses – reflect bleeding into skin.
      (iii) Lungs (interstitial haemorrhage) – monitor for dyspnoea, respiratory distress, haemoptysis, cyanosis.
      (iv) Central nervous system (cerebral thromboemboli/dysfunction) – assess level of responsiveness, orientation, sensory and motor dysfunction, convulsions and coma.
3. Ask about bone and joint pain; changes in vision (retinal haemorrhage).
4. Evaluate cardiopulmonary function; assess for tachypnoea, orthopnoea, tachycardia, palpitations, orthostatic hypotension – reflect inadequacy of tissue oxygenation and/or fall in blood volume.

Evaluation

EXPECTED OUTCOMES
1. Absence of bleeding.
2. Demonstrates tissue and organ perfusion.
3. Absence of dyspnoea.
4. Maintains adequate urine output.

HAEMOPHILIA

Haemophilia is an inherited, congenital blood dyscrasia which is characterized by a disturbance of blood clotting factors. It appears in males but is transmitted by females.

ALTERED PHYSIOLOGY

1. Haemophilia results from the absence or malfunction of any one of the blood clotting factors from the plasma.
2. These blood clotting factors are necessary for the formation of prothrombin activator, which acts as a catalyst in the conversion of prothrombin to thrombin.
   a. The rate of formation of thrombin from prothrombin is almost directly proportional to the amount of prothrombin activator available.
   b. The rapidity of the clotting process is proportional to the amount of thrombin formed.
3. The most common types of haemophilia and the clotting factors involved are shown in Table 6.2.

Table 6.2   Types of haemophilia and the clotting factors involved

Type of haemophilia	Clotting factor
Haemophilia A (classic haemophilia)	Factor VIII (antihaemophilic globulin)
Haemophilia B (Christmas disease)	Factor IX (plasma thromboplastin component)
Haemophilia C	Factor XI (plasma thromboplastin antecedent)

POTENTIAL PROBLEMS

1. Danger of shock or exsanguination related to inability of blood to clot.
2. Potential for injury from blood replacement therapy.
3. Pain related to bleeding into joints.
4. Anxiety and coping difficulty related to the need for frequent transfusions.
5. Activity intolerance related to painful joints.
6. Maternal guilt related to hereditary nature of the disease.
7. Parental overprotection related to fear of injury.
8. Lack of knowledge regarding haemophilia and its management.
9. With the advent of the spread of acquired immunodeficiency syndrome (AIDS) through infected blood products, haemophiliacs are at risk of developing the virus which causes this disease. (see Chapter 17 on communicable diseases – AIDS). The risk is greater for haemophiliacs who are being treated regularly with factor VIII or factor IX because these concentrates are manufactured from huge numbers of plasma donations. A high percentage of haemophiliacs are now anti-HTLV III positive, of whom 1 to 5 per cent are thought to be at risk of developing overt AIDS.

PREVENTION OF VIRUS TRANSMISSION

1. Heat treatment to 68°C for 22 hours of clotting factor concentrate has been found to reduce the potential for transmission of the AIDS virus. Therefore, heat-treated concentrates are used in preference to those that have not been treated. Unfortunately, 15 per cent of the clotting activity of factor VIII, is lost when heat treated. This makes it more expensive due to loss of yield. Advances are being made towards the production of synthetic factor VIII.
2. Fresh frozen plasma may be used to treat minor bleeds in haemophilia B.
3. In mild haemophilia A or von Willebrand's disease, the alternative is DDAVP (desmopressin), a vasopressin analogue.

PATIENT EDUCATION

1. It is important that treatment for haemophiliac bleeds is continued. Premature death is more likely from haemophilia than from AIDS.
2. Advice may be given to the haemophiliac to reduce or change certain activities to lessen bleeding episodes.
3. Provide information on the spread of AIDS.
4. Provide facilities for confidential counselling for haemophiliacs and their families.

The impact of AIDS has had a profound effect on haemophiliacs who have previously learnt to lead a normal life with an already debilitating disease. Their need for psychosocial support is greatly increased to help them cope with future prospects of contracting AIDS and the possibility of death from this disease.

TREATMENT AND NURSING INTERVENTIONS
Objectives

1. Control the bleeding (see Table 6.1 for nursing care). Administer plasma or therapeutic concentrate as directed – see section on blood components, p. 369.
2. Alleviate painful joints (see Table 6.1).
3. Maintain a safe environment during hospital admission to prevent further haemorrhage.
4. Provide emotional support. Further information and support from: The Haemophilia Society, PO Box 9, 16 Trinity Street, London SE1 1DE.

VON WILLEBRAND'S DISEASE

Von Willebrand's disease is a common bleeding disorder with either autosomal dominant or recessive inheritance, which is due to an abnormality of the factor VIII complex. There are several genetic variants.

CLINICAL FEATURES
1. Epistaxis; gingival oozing; easy bruising.
2. Gastrointestinal bleeding.
3. Menorrhagia.
4. Prolonged bleeding from cuts.
5. Postoperative bleeding.

LABORATORY EVALUATION
1. Prolonged bleeding time.
2. Immunological tests of subcomponents of the factor VIII macromolecular complex.

NURSING INTERVENTIONS
1. Infusions of cryoprecipitate – correct the defects of von Willebrand's disease. May be repeated every 12 hours until bleeding stops or postoperative period stabilizes.
2. See Table 6.1 for nursing management of the patient who is bleeding.

ACQUIRED DEFECTS IN COAGULATION

Acquired defects in coagulation may be associated with many conditions, including:
1. Vitamin K deficiency.
2. Administration of coumarin–indanedione anticoagulant drugs.
3. Heparin therapy.
4. Diseases of the liver.
5. Disseminated intravascular coagulation.
6. Uraemia.
7. Transfusion-induced clotting factor deficiency.
8. Chronic renal failure.
9. Certain antibiotics – inhibit coagulation factors.

VITAMIN K DEFICIENCY
Vitamin K deficiency produces a characteristic abnormality of blood clotting mechanisms.

General considerations
1. Vitamin K is obtained partly from diet and partly from bacterial action in the intestinal tract.
   a. Foods high in vitamin K – leafy vegetables (spinach, cauliflower, cabbage, kale, dandelion greens).
   b. Vitamin K is not absorbed in the absence of bile salts.

Causes
1. Interference with flow of bile salts into gastrointestinal tract – obstructive jaundice, biliary fistula.
2. Impaired intestinal absorption (sprue, steatorrhoea, gastrocolic fistula, regional enteritis).
3. Extensive surgical resection of small bowel.
4. Dietary deprivation.
5. Therapy with broad spectrum antibiotics.

Clinical features
1. Ecchymoses.
2. Epistaxis.
3. Gingival bleeding.
4. Haematuria.
5. Haematemesis and melaena.
6. Menorrhagia.
7. Operative and postoperative bleeding.

Treatment
1. Administer vitamin K via oral, subcutaneous or intramuscular route – bleeding will cease in three to four hours, clotting activity rises and a normal prothrombin level may be obtained in 12 to 14 hours.
   a. Phytomenadione – used in neonates.
   b. Menadiol sodium disphosphate – used for malabsorption syndromes.
2. Administer whole blood or component therapy for severe bleeding.

BLEEDING DUE TO INGESTION OF COUMARIN–INDANEDIONE ANTICOAGULANT DRUGS
Causes
Bleeding may develop from long-term use of coumarin or indanedione anticoagulant drugs that are used in the treatment of thromboembolic disorders.

NURSING ALERT
Laboratory determinations of the anticoagulant status should be carried out on patients taking anticoagulant drugs who have had a change in physical condition or have had other drugs suddenly introduced or withdrawn. The anticoagulant dosage must be adjusted appropriately in these circumstances.

Clinical features

1. Bleeding in gastrointestinal tract or central nervous system.
2. Ecchymoses.
3. Haematomas.
4. Epistaxis.
5. Haematuria.
6. Vaginal bleeding.

Treatment

1. Administer vitamin K subcutaneously or intramuscularly – will reverse the effects of the drugs.
2. Nursing precautions – pain, swelling and tenderness occasionally occur at site of subcutaneous or intramuscular injection.
3. Patient may be resistant to further anticoagulant therapy for a few days after vitamin K is given.
4. Concentrates of vitamin K-dependent factors, factors II, VII, IX and X may be given in emergencies, even though this may increase the risk of hepatitis in some patients.

HEPARIN THERAPY AS A CAUSE OF BLEEDING

Heparin therapy is given for thromboembolic disorders.

Causes of bleeding

1. Secondary to anticoagulant effect.
2. Overdosage of heparin.
3. Trauma (avoid intramuscular injections).
4. Surgery.

Complications

1. Cerebral haemorrhage.
2. Haemoptysis.
3. Bleeding from pre-existing gastrointestinal lesions and from sites of surgery or trauma.

Treatment

1. Stop heparin therapy immediately.
2. Give protamine sulphate as directed – neutralizes the action of heparin.

SURGICAL INTERVENTION

SPLENECTOMY

Splenectomy is removal of the spleen. It is useful in severe forms of autoimmune diseases.

INDICATIONS FOR SPLENECTOMY

1. Bleeding from trauma/rupture of the spleen:
   a. History of injury;
   b. Persistent abdominal pain;
   c. Abdominal rigidity, rebound tenderness, shock.
2. Staging procedure for lymphomas.
3. Primary haematological problems:
   a. Hypersplenism (sequestration and premature destruction of red and white blood cells and of platelets by an enlarged spleen);
   b. Autoimmune haemolytic anaemia, immune thrombocytopenia and/or immune neutropenia. Spleen is the major clearance site for antibody and/or complement-coated blood cells.

UNDERLYING CONSIDERATION

New approaches are being tried following trauma to conserve splenic tissue, since the spleen has a vital role in host defence.

NURSING INTERVENTIONS

Preoperative care

1. Coagulation studies are performed.
   a. Platelet donor packs and fresh frozen plasma must be available.
   b. Administer vitamin K for abnormalities of prothrombin time, as directed.
   c. Prepare for transfusion of packed red cells or fresh whole blood if patient has significant anaemia.
2. Assist with preoperative physiotherapy – to reduce incidence of pulmonary complications; patient may be debilitated from haematological disease, from immunosuppressants, etc.
3. Preoperative preparation for patient with rupture of spleen:
   a. Administer whole blood if rupture of spleen has occurred.
   b. Empty stomach contents with nasogastric tube – to prevent aspiration.
   c. Check patient for pneumothorax/haemothorax – thoracotomy tube may be in place before anaesthesia is started.

Postoperative care

1. See p. 466, general aspects of nursing management following abdominal surgery.
2. Watch for the development of complications – related to location of spleen, the reason for its removal and sequelae of splenectomy.
   a. Infection – especially in children.

b. Thrombocytopenia – if patient had thrombocytopenia before splenectomy, the condition may become extreme after splenectomy.

c. Persistent or recurrent haemorrhage.

d. Thrombosis – may follow a few days after splenectomy; platelet count of three to five times normal values may occur; this postoperative physiological thrombocytosis may be conducive to thromboembolic complications.

   (i) Abdominal discomfort and fever may be caused by thrombi lodging in branches of portal system.

   (ii) Mesenteric thrombosis – watch for postprandial cramping, abdominal pain; small bowel resection is indicated.

e. Atelectasis of left lower lobe with pneumonia; pleural effusion – operations on left upper quadrant predispose to limited diaphragmatic movement.

f. Subphrenic abscess – observe for persistent fever.

FURTHER READING

BOOKS

Aronstam, A. (1985) *Haemophilic Bleeding: Early Management at Home*, Baillière Tindall, Eastbourne.

Faulkner, A. (1985) *Nursing – A Creative Approach*, Baillière Tindall, Eastbourne.

Hoffbrand, A.V. and Pettit, J.E. (1984) *Essential Haematology* (2nd edn), Blackwell Scientific, Oxford.

Hughes-Jones, N.C. (1984) *Lecture Notes on Haematology* (4th edn), Blackwell Scientific Publications, Oxford.

Jones, P. (1985) *AIDS and the Blood: A Practical Guide*, Newcastle Haemophilia Reference Centre, Newcastle on Tyne.

Jones, P. (ed.) (1986) *Proceedings of the AIDS Conference 1986*, Intercept, Newcastle on Tyne.

Priestman, T.J. (1981) *Cancer Begins to Yield*, Farmitalia Carlo Erba, Barnet.

The Royal Marsden Hospital (1988) *Manual of Clinical Nursing Procedures* (2nd ed), Harper and Row, London.

Tiffany, R. (1981) *Cancer Nursing Update*, Baillière Tindall, London.

Tiffany, R. (ed.) (1987) *Oncology for Nurses and Health Care Professionals*, Vols 1 and 2, Harper and Row, London.

Weatherall, D.J. (ed.) (1983) *The Thalassaemias*, Churchill Livingstone, Edinburgh.

ARTICLES

Anaemia

Booram-Ogeer, S.B. and Alvarez-Clarke, J. M. (1985) Sickle cell anaemia, *Nursing*, Vol. 2, No. 40, pp. 1196–7.

Kirk, S.A. (1987) Sickle cell disease and health education, *Midwife*, Health Visitor and Community Nurse, Vol. 23, No. 5, pp. 200, 204, 206.

Lubkin, I. (1982) Evaluating iron deficiency anaemia, *Nurse Practitioner*, Vol. 7, No. 9, pp. 34–6, 38.

Nicolle, L.S. (1984) Anaemia of chronic disorders, *Nurse Practitioner*, Vol. 9, No. 11, pp. 19–20, 22.

Bleeding disorders

Harris, A. (1983) Nursing care study – idiopathic thrombocytopaenic purpura, *Nursing Times*, Vol. 79, 21 Sept., pp. 50–3.

Clotting defects

Cartlidge, J. (1984) Haemophilia, *Nursing Mirror*, Vol. 158, No. 7, Clinical forum I–VIII.

Flavell, G. (1982) Disabilities and how to live with them: haemophilia, *Lancet*, Vol. 1, 10 April, pp. 845–6.

Raw, A.Y. (1982) Home therapy for patients with haemophilia and Christmas disease, *Nursing Times*, Vol. 78, 14 April, pp. 615–16.

Thorne, T. (1984) Disseminated intravascular coagulation, *Nursing Times*, Vol. 80, 10 October, pp. 46–7.

Haematology

Brandt, J.T. (1985) Current concepts of coagulation, *Clinical Obstetrics and Gynaecology*, Vol. 28, No. 1, pp. 3–14.

Goodwin, S.A. (1985) Drug-induced coagulation alterations, *Critical Care Quarterly*, Vol. 7, No. 4, pp. 1–18.

Symposium on Haematology (1982) A field guide to the bleeding disorders for the general practitioner, *Practitioner*, Vol. 226, pp. 23–94.

Leukaemia

Barker, S.M. (1980) Blood cell products in the supportive care of patients with acute leukaemia, *Nursing Times*, Vol. 79, No. 3, 79(3), pp. 152–4.

Campbell, J.B. (1983) The leukaemias – definition, treatment and nursing care, *Nursing Clinics of North America*, Vol. 18, No. 3, pp. 523–41.

Lakhani, A.K. (1987) Current management of acute leukaemia, *Nursing*, Vol. 3, No. 20, pp. 755–8.

Thomson, L. (1979) Cancer chemotherapy – guide for nurses, *Nursing Times*, Supplement, 21 June.

Malignant lymphomas

Shackelford, P. (1985) Multiple myeloma, *Orthopaedic Nursing*, Vol. 4, No. 5, pp. 61–4.

Nursing care

Allbright, A. (1984) Oral care for the cancer chemotherapy patient, *Nursing Times*, 23 May, pp. 40–2.

Wallace, J. and Freeman, P.A. (1978) Mouthcare in patients with blood dyscrasias, *Nursing Times*, Vol. 74, 1 June, pp. 921–2.

Thalassaemia

Sawley, L. (1983) Clinical thalassaemia: a shift to the north, *Nursing Mirror*, Vol. 157, 14 Dec., pp. 38–9.

Transfusion therapy

Contreras, M. and Barbara, J. (1985) Acquired immune deficiency syndrome and blood transfusion, *Journal of Hospital Infection*, Vol. 6, Supplement C, pp. 27–34.

Davis, K.G. (1985) The blood story: Part III – The storage and administration of blood and blood products, *The Australian Nurses Journal*, Vol. 15, No. 5, pp. 40–3, 59.

— (1986) The blood story: Part IV – Adverse reactions to blood transfusion, *The Australian Nurses Journal*, Vol. 15, No. 6, pp. 40–3.

Nicholson, E. (1988) Autologous blood transfusion, *Nursing Times*, Vol. 84, No. 2, pp. 33–5.

7

Care of the Patient with a Gastrointestinal Disorder

MOUTH CONDITIONS

NURSING ASSESSMENT FOR EFFECTIVE MOUTH CARE
Psychosocial significance
1. The person's comfort, good nutrition, and general well-being are promoted by maintaining clean and well-cared-for teeth and gums.
2. Personal attractiveness is enhanced.
3. Participation in community dental health programmes promotes prevention, early detection and correction of dental problems.

Self-care goals
1. Reduce bacterial count and prevent tissue infection by removing food and rinsing the mouth.
2. Prevent dental caries when plaque is removed periodically by the dentist.
3. Emphasize importance of regular periodic dental examination to maintain good mouth health.
4. Maintain healthy mouth structures by tooth brushing, flossing between teeth and massaging gums (see Figure 7.1).

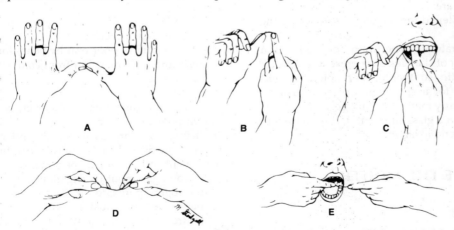

Figure 7.1. Flossing technique. (A) Wrap floss on middle fingers. (B) Thumb to the outside for upper teeth. (C) Flossing between upper back teeth. (D) Holding floss for lower teeth. (E) Flossing between lower back teeth. (From: *Effective Oral Hygiene*. Developed by USAF School of Aerospace Medicine, Brooks Air Force Base, TX. Published by the American Academy of Periodontology, Chicago)

5. Promote proper nutrition, since dentition and mouth tissue tone are directly affected.
6. Encourage topical application of fluoride, as well as fluoridation of water, since this chemical significantly reduces dental caries.
7. Recognize that fatigue, emotional upsets and injury lower resistance of dental tissue to infection.
8. Examine soft tissues of the mouth frequently for evidences of irritation, unusual growths, discolouration, encrustation and leucoplakia, since abnormal manifestations may herald malignancy and early detection may achieve early correction.

Causes of trauma to oral structures

1. *Mechanical* – stiff-bristled toothbrush, hot pipe stem, ill-fitting dentures, carious or broken teeth, grinding of teeth, cheek and lower lip biting.
2. *Thermal* – smoking, hot liquids, hot foods.
3. *Chemical* – sucking hard sweets, using full-strength antiseptic mouthwashes, chewing or smoking tobacco, drinking alcoholic beverages, chewing, sucking mouth lozenges, using breath sweeteners, drinking citrus juices, drug reactions.
4. *Bacterial* – poor oral and nutritional attention that permits food to collect.
5. *Irradiation* – exposure to sun, ultraviolet rays, caesium and X-rays.
6. *Nutritional* – improper dietary habits.
7. Metabolic disorders, blood dyscrasias.

Oral cell smear for cytological examination

1. Grasp the tongue with a 10×10cm gauze square and gently move the tongue to expose the questionable area.
2. Using a moistened tongue depressor, scrape the area or lesion.
3. If a hyperkeratotic (hypertrophy of the stratum cornium layer of skin) lesion is present, scrape off surface keratin so that deeper epithelial cells are available for a specimen (these are usually involved in early malignant change).
4. Smear cells on a glass slide, immerse carefully in alcohol and send to laboratory.

LESIONS OF THE MOUTH

LEUCOPLAKIA
See p. 407.

See p. 407.

LICHEN PLANUS
Lichen planus consists of minute white papules, which form a reticular or plaque pattern; it is often difficult to differentiate from leucoplakia. This condition may be related to a dermatological problem.

1. Aetiology – unknown.
2. Assessment:
   a. Usually asymptomatic;
   b. Some complain of burning sensations, a metallic taste or pain;
   c. May last for weeks or years; if erosive, it is longer-lasting.
3. Management:
   a. Asymptomatic – no treatment;
   b. Topical steroids, topical anaesthetics and perhaps intralesional steroids.

GINGIVITIS
Also called inflammation of gums.

1. The most common infection of oral tissues.
2. Clinical features:
   a. Inflammation and slight swelling of superficial gingivae and interdental papillae;
   b. With continued neglect may advance to chronic degenerative gingivitis and eventually to periodontal disease.
3. Nursing management:
   a. Conscientious mouth hygiene;
   b. Periodic professional dental cleaning.

ACUTE ULCERATIVE GINGIVITIS
Also called Vincent's gingivitis.

1. Pseudomembranous painful ulceration affecting gums, inner dental papillae, mouth mucosa, tonsils and pharynx, especially in young adults and adolescents.
2. *Aetiology:*
   a. Thought to be caused by both a spirochaete and a fusiform bacillus.
   b. May be due to poor oral hygiene, low tissue resistance and infection from complex micro-organisms.
3. Clinical features:
   a. Painful bleeding gums, mild fever, swelling of lymph nodes of neck.
   b. If infection spreads to tonsils and pharynx, swallowing and talking may be painful.
4. Treatment and nursing management:
   a. Encourage mouth irrigations with dilute hydrogen peroxide or 2 per cent sodium perborate (to combat anaerobic spirochaetes) to treat infection, control fetid breath and provide comfort.
   b. Administer antibiotics as prescribed to curb infection; give analgesics for pain and discomfort.

c. Offer soft foods and liquids to reduce gum trauma.

d. Instruct the patient to avoid highly seasoned foods, alcoholic beverages and smoking, all of which irritate infected oral tissues.

e. Teach the patient the importance of regular eating habits and sufficient rest.

CONDITIONS OF THE SALIVARY GLANDS

SALIVARY CALCULUS (SIALOLITHIASIS)

1. Salivary stones may form in the submaxillary gland following glandular infection or ductal structure due to trauma or inflammation.
2. Salivary stones are usually mostly calcium oxalate.
   a. Stones found in the gland are irregularly lobulated.
   b. Stones found in the duct are small and oval in shape.
3. Diagnostic evaluation – sialogram (X-ray with contrast medium).
4. Clinical features:
   a. None unless there is an infection.
   b. If calculus obstructs gland, the following conditions may occur:
      (i) Sudden, local pain, which is suddenly relieved by a gush of saliva.
      (ii) Gland is swollen and tender.
      (iii) Stone may be palpable.
      (iv) Stone is visible with X-ray studies.
5. Treatment:
   a. Surgical extraction of stone.
   b. Gland may have to be removed if condition occurs repeatedly.

MAXILLOFACIAL FRACTURES

Fractures of the maxillofacial area usually include injury to the soft tissues and may occur as a result of a fall or if patient has been hit by a fist or a flying object.

IMMEDIATE ASSESSMENT AND MANAGEMENT

1. Determine whether there is obstruction to the airway.
   a. Remove any obstruction from pharynx, such as broken teeth, dentures, blood clots or broken bits of bone.
   b. Determine whether tongue has been displaced posteriorly; if so, insert index finger and pull tongue forward.
   c. Prepare for emergency tracheostomy if airway is obstructed.
2. Control haemorrhage by direct pressure on vessels supplying the area. Prepare for fluid replacement.
3. Assess vital signs and note extent and involvement of other parts of the head and body.
4. Ascertain localization of pain to determine nerve injury.
5. Administer analgesics to relieve pain and anxiety but not to depress respirations.
6. Reassure the patient that he is being given the best possible care.

MANDIBULAR FRACTURES

1. Two-thirds of significant facial fractures are of the mandible.
2. Most mandibular fractures can be treated with closed reduction and intermaxillary fixation.
3. Open reduction is preferred for certain patients:
   a. Aged, senile, edentulous and debilitated;
   b. Children and those who cannot tolerate intermaxillary fixation;
   c. Professional athletes;
   d. Patients who are psychotic or have a history of seizures;
   e. The diabetic person with special nutritional needs.

Assessment

CLINICAL FEATURES

1. Malocclusion, asymmetry, abnormal mobility and crepitus (grating sound with movement).
2. Tissue injury; note extent and involvement.

TREATMENT

Mandibular fractures are reduced first; maxillary fractures follow in positioning.

Lower jaw is held tightly against upper jaw by cross-wires or rubber bands placed around arch bars wired to the teeth (intermaxillary fixation).

PATIENT PROBLEMS

1. Ineffective airway clearance related to malposition of mandible or jaw, and tissue oedema related to injury.
2. Pain in lower face area and referred areas related to injury to tissues and fracture of mandible (maxilla).
3. Impaired verbal communication related to oedema, pain and fracture of jaw and subsequent intermaxillary fixation.

4. Alteration in nutrition related to limited or absent function of jaw (fracture) that interferes with normal eating.
5. Potential for mouth infection related to inter-maxillary fixation and poor access to mouth for cleaning.

Planning and implementation
NURSING INTERVENTIONS
Preoperative preparation
1. Determine priorities for fracture reduction:
   a. Irrigate laceration with copious amounts of normal physiological saline.
   b. Prepare for debridement and suturing of lacerations.
   c. Apply sterile pressure dressings to control swelling, prevent tension on stitches and maintain an area that is as clean as possible to minimize or prevent infection.
   d. Administer tetanus prophylaxis as prescribed. Give antibiotics as prescribed.
2. Prepare the patient for X-rays to determine method of reducing and immobilizing fractures.

Postoperative care
(Management of patient with intermaxillary fixation.)
1. Immediately position patient on his side with head slightly elevated to facilitate breathing and for ease of suctioning.
2. Note wire cutter or scissors in obvious place.
   a. These cutters or scissors are to cut wires or rubber bands in the event the patient vomits; this will prevent aspiration.
   b. After the patient emerges from anaesthesia, scissors or cutters must still be kept nearby for emergency use.
3. Suction and drainage of stomach contents as required to lessen danger of aspiration.
   a. Connect nasogastric suction to low-pressure suction.
   b. If vomiting is anticipated, administer anti-emetic medications as prescribed.
   c. Insert small catheter into nasopharyngeal area for suctioning if a nasogastric catheter has not been inserted during surgery.
   d. Aspirate oral cavity; this is facilitated by inserting a spatula to move cheek away from teeth.
   e. Insert oral catheter behind third molar (or where a tooth may be missing) to aspirate within the oropharynx.
4. Modify care as the patient emerges from anaesthesia.

a. Remind the patient that his jaw is wired but that he can breathe and swallow.
b. Provide a means of communication such as a pad and pencil, 'magic slate' (or chalk and chalkboard) or signal system.
c. Elevate the head of the bed for comfort and to facilitate breathing.
d. Administer parenteral intravenous fluids as prescribed until nourishment can be taken by mouth.
e. Administer medications to control pain and restlessness, as well as to prevent nausea and infection.

Nutritional considerations
Maintain adequate nutritional levels to promote healing:
1. Provide privacy for the patient to eat, since he might be sensitive to his appearance and to the noisy sounds he makes as he tries to eat and drink.
2. Provide a straw if the patient can manage it; the patient may suck soft foods from a teaspoon.
3. Serve food attractively and arrange an environment that is as pleasant as possible (music, television, view from window) to encourage nutritional intake.

Prevention of infection
Promote a climate to prevent complications and to promote recovery:
1. Apply lubricant to the lips to prevent drying and cracking.
2. Provide frequent and careful attention to the mouth.
   a. Irrigate the mouth with tap water or normal saline after each feeding; use a syringe or irrigating set under low pressure.
   b. Swab the area between teeth and cheek by using a spatula to retract the cheek. Provide light with a torch.

PATIENT EDUCATION
Set up a plan of instruction so that the patient will be able to manage at home even with the jaw wired.
1. Encourage exercise and proper diet to promote general good health and tissue healing, and to prevent constipation.
2. Develop a plan that is convenient for the patient to follow in maintaining oral cleanliness.
3. Work with the patient's family, if required, in determining interesting pursuits to counterbalance any worries he might have about appearance or other problems.

4. Remind the patient of follow-up visits to his doctor.
5. Prepare the patient for possible reconstructive or orthodontic work if this is required.

Evaluation

EXPECTED OUTCOMES

1. Patient is able to breathe easily; oedema subsides once jaw has been positioned.
2. Has no pain in the face – demonstrates fracture is healing.
3. Able to communicate in an understandable manner.
4. Receives adequate nourishment through a straw and via teaspoon.
5. Demonstrates proper mouth hygiene – utilizes mouth rinses after feedings; swabs the area between his teeth and cheeks every morning and evening.

PREMALIGNANT MOUTH LESIONS

LEUCOPLAKIA BUCCALIS
('Smoker's patch'.)

1. Characterized by the appearance of one or more small, often crinkled, pearly patches on the mucous membrane of tongue or mouth.
2. Due to the keratinization of the mucosa and sclerosis of the underlying tissues.
3. Patient education:
   a. If there are no symptoms other than appearance, emphasize importance of careful oral hygiene:
      (i) Recommend dental care and gingival treatment.
      (ii) Advise the patient to avoid alcohol, tobacco, coffee and tea.
      (iii) Suggest mouth rinses of half-strength milk of magnesia after meals and at bedtime.
      (iv) Encourage increased vitamin intake, particularly of vitamin C.
   b. If in addition to appearance of white patches there is pain, induration and ulceration, do the following:
      (i) Suggest biopsy to rule out cancer.
      (ii) Follow above regimen (3a).

MALIGNANT MOUTH LESIONS

INCIDENCE

1. Malignant neoplasms of the lip, oral cavity and pharynx newly diagnosed in 1983 amounted to 1,681 cases in England and Wales.
2. Males are afflicted nearly twice as often as females.
3. Evidence suggests that the risk of cancer in the heavy smoker and drinker may be as much as 15 times greater than in those who neither smoke nor drink.

PREVENTIVE MEASURES

1. Eliminate causes of chronic irritation.
2. Practice good oral hygiene.
3. Obtain proper dental care – remove or repair jagged, carious and infected teeth.
4. Reduce or eliminate smoking and smokeless tobacco (chewing tobacco); also eliminate pipe smoking if it irritates the lip.
5. Restrict or eliminate ingestion of highly spiced foods and reduce alcohol consumption.
6. If sexually transmitted disease is suspected, seek treatment (see p. 986).

TREATMENT

1. Selection of treatment depends on size of lesion and how extensively surrounding tissues are involved.
2. Small lesions can be removed by wide excision or can be treated with radiotherapy or interstitial irradiation.
3. Large lesions may be excised widely or treated by external irradiation followed by radical neck dissection (see p. 410).
4. Advanced cancer, p. 1046.
   a. Radiotherapy can be palliative, providing it has not been given previously.
   b. Extensive surgical resection may be feasible but is done only with patient's full understanding that cure is not achievable.
   c. Intra-arterial chemotherapy has been done, but only with limited success. A brief regression in tumour size may be achieved.

Assessment

CLINICAL FEATURES

1. For precancerous mouth lesions – leucoplakia buccalis, keratosis labialis:
   a. Pearly patches – one or two small, thin, often crinkled areas on mucous membranes of the tongue, mouth or both, due to:
      (i) Keratinization of mucosa;
      (ii) Sclerosis of underlying tissue.
   b. Later, most of tongue and mouth may become covered:
      (i) Creamy white, thick, fissured mucous membrane;

(ii) Sometimes desquamates, leaving a beefy-red base.

2. For cancerous lesions:
   a. White patch area, sore spot or ulcer on lips, gums, or mouth, which fails to heal;
   b. Swelling, numbness or loss of feeling in the part;
   c. An asymmetric, firm nodal enlargement or mass;
   d. Erythroplakia – red plaques or well-defined velvety red patches, often with tiny areas of ulceration.

NURSING HISTORY

1. Determine amount of patient discomfort, such as tenderness (where?), pain (type?), bleeding (where and when?), oozing or discharge?
2. Difficulty speaking? Eating? With what particular kinds of food?
3. Any referred pain? To where? Other parts of face, ear, head?

DIAGNOSTIC EVALUATION

1. X-ray of head and neck to determine involvement.
2. Cytological examination of sputum (see p. 104).
3. Biopsy of suspected tissue.

PATIENT PROBLEMS

1. Alteration in comfort (pain) related to malignant infiltration of oral tissues.
2. Nutritional deficit related to inadequate fluid and food intake; caused by pain and difficulty in chewing and swallowing, excess salivation.
3. Impaired verbal communication related to a tendency to inhibit movement of jaw and mouth because of painful lesions.
4. Disturbance in self-concept related to changes occurring in facial image and contour.
5. Fear and anxiety related to misinformation, suspected poor prognosis and altered (post-operative) function.

Planning and implementation
NURSING INTERVENTIONS
Preoperative preparation
1. Provide optimal mouth care.
   a. Proper care of teeth because they are essential to mastication.
      (i) Stress regular dental care.
      (ii) Promote good nutrition.
   b. Mouth cleanliness to reduce incidence of infectious disease such as mumps and surgical parotitis.

   (i) Brush teeth frequently.
   (ii) Use oxygen-releasing and antiseptic mouth-rinsing solutions.
   (iii) Apply lipsalve or vaseline to dry and cracking lips.
   (iv) Remove dentures and clean them frequently.
   c. Adequate fluid intake, particularly in debilitated patients who are prone to mouth infections.
   d. Stimulation of flow of saliva.
      (i) Offer chewing gum.
      (ii) Encourage the patient to suck lemon drops, a fresh lemon or orange slices.
      (iii) Administer antibiotics as prescribed to assist in control of infection.

Postoperative care
1. Maintain a patent airway.
   a. Recognize that the patient may have an airway, endotracheal tube or tracheostomy to facilitate air exchange.
   b. Observe the patient closely for signs of respiratory embarrassment, such as changes in vital signs, dyspnoea and restlessness.
   c. Place the patient in a prone position, or in a supine position with head turned to side, or laterally; position should facilitate drainage and prevent aspiration.
   d. Suction as required; precautions are necessary to avoid injury to suture line and sensitive tissues.
   e. When the patient has regained consciousness, elevate head of bed for comfort, to facilitate deep breathing and coughing up of secretions, and to lessen oedema.
2. Monitor for bleeding.
   a. Take frequent vital sign readings.
   b. Observe tissues and dressings for evidence of oozing or bleeding.
   c. Inspect back of neck for accumulation of bloodstaining; observe patient for frequent swallowing.
3. Check pressure dressings that are used to control oedema.
   a. Note whether dressings are hindering respirations.
   b. Observe surrounding tissues to determine whether dressings are constricting blood circulation.
   c. If portable suction is used, pressure dressings may not be applied.
4. Control pain so that respirations are not depressed. Employ nursing measures to make the

patient comfortable so that narcotics for pain relief are not used unless absolutely required.

Improved nutritional intake

1. Maintain nutritional and electrolyte levels. Following intravenous therapy, administer tube feedings by nasogastric tube or gastrostomy (see pp. 434 and 447).
2. Feeding problems may be handled in the following ways:
   a. Use straws, teaspoon, feeders, etc.
   b. Provide food that is soft, liquid and nonirritating – not too hot or cold or highly seasoned.
   c. Serve small, frequent meals attractively.
3. Allow the patient to have his meals in privacy if he so desires.
4. Keep mouth clean for comfort and to assist in healing process.
   a. Mouth irrigations, using normal saline, diluted hydrogen peroxide, sodium bicarbonate or alkaline mouthwashes.
   b. Gentle lavaging, using a catheter between cheek and teeth to loosen mucus.
   c. Power spray to clean inaccessible spaces.
   d. Vaporizer to provide moisture to traumatized tissue and to discourage crusting.
5. Excessive salivation and mouth odours may be handled as follows:
   a. Insert gauze wick in corner of mouth; place basin conveniently to catch drippings.
   b. Use small rubber catheter and suction.
   c. Encourage use of mouthwashes, particularly oxidizing agents such as half-strength hydrogen peroxide.
   d. Use power spray, if available.

Improvement in communication techniques

1. During preoperative period, prepare for postoperative communication, since the patient may not be able to talk for a few days after surgery. Practise lip reading, hand signals, magic slate, eye-blink codes and flash cards (words or pictures).
2. Supply pad and pencil, magic slate, signal system (eye blinks or hand), so that the patient can express his needs and thoughts. Note that if the patient usually wears glasses to read and write, he may not be able to put his glasses on because of dressings, skin flaps, etc.
3. Refer the patient to a speech therapist if the services of this specialist are indicated.

Psychosocial adjustment

1. Promote optimal physical condition and psychological adjustment.

a. Assess the patient's reaction to his condition.
   (i) Evaluate the patient's apprehension and offer emotional support.
   (ii) Correct any misinformation.
   (iii) Determine therapeutic plan of care for the patient's rehabilitation.
2. Recognize that face and neck surgery can be disfiguring and the patient often is embarrassed, withdrawn, and depressed.
3. Encourage the patient's family and friends to visit so that he is aware others care for him.
4. Assist the patient in caring for his personal appearance.
5. Observe closely for indications of the patient's needs, which may be communicated in other ways.
6. Be consistent with emotional support.
7. Provide an environment conducive to the patient's recovery.
   a. Maintain proper humidification and aeration of room.
   b. Prevent odours by removing soiled dressings; use effective and pleasant deodorizers.
   c. Inform the patient that his general throat discomfort is due to endotracheal anaesthesia and will improve in a few days.
8. Prepare the patient for convalescence and extended care at home.
   a. Provide detailed instructions to the patient and/or a member of his family.
   b. If suctioning is required, instruct as to method, type of equipment, and where it can be obtained.
   c. Emphasize adequate nutrition – proper consistency, proper seasoning and right temperature. Suggest commercial baby foods or the use of a blender if available.
   d. Repeat the details of good mouth care and cleanliness of dressings.
   e. Review signs of obstruction, haemorrhage, infection and depression and what to do about them if they are evident.

Evaluation

EXPECTED OUTCOMES

1. Emerges from surgical treatment and radiotherapy with minimal problems.
2. Maintains satisfactory nutritional status; controls mouth odours; utilizes a power spray and dilute hydrogen peroxide.
3. Demonstrates proficiency in speaking clearly; when mouth is sore, uses a magic slate.
4. Displays interest in personal appearance as manifested by attention to shaving daily and request-

ing the services of a barber, or applying make-up; looks forward to visits from family members.
5. Voices optimism about the immediate future.

HEAD AND NECK MALIGNANCY

Head and neck cancer refers to a group of malignant tumours that may occur at any one of a number of anatomical sites in the upper digestive tract.

INCIDENCE
1. Usually occurs in individuals in their sixth or seventh decade; ratio of males to females is 3:1.

Assessment
POSSIBLE CLINICAL FEATURES
1. Pain, dysphagia, dysphonia, difficulty in breathing, hoarseness.
2. Haemoptysis, excessive salivation, loosening of teeth, dentures no longer fitting.
3. Earache, nasal bleeding, infection.
4. Neck swelling, weight loss.

DIAGNOSTIC EVALUATION
1. Close scrutiny of head and neck structures during physical examination; neurological examination of cranial nerves.
2. Examination of mouth by family dentist may disclose problems.
3. Use of nasal speculum, laryngoscope and endoscope is necessary.
4. Biopsy and histological examination of suspicious areas.
5. X-ray of head and chest, tomogram, CAT scan, magnetic resonance imaging.

TREATMENT
Goal: remove all lymph-node-bearing tissue on the involved side of the neck.
1. Removal of all tissue under the skin from the ramus of the jaw down to the clavicle; from midline back to the angle of the jaw. This includes sternocleidomastoid muscle, other smaller muscles, jugular vein in the neck.
   Concomitant surgery – tracheostomy (see p. 146).
2. In some cases, surgical reconstruction is performed, utilizing a pectoral flap from the chest. In other cases, a very conservative functional neck dissection is done.

3. Radiotherapy is often performed following surgery.

PATIENT PROBLEMS
1. Ineffective airway clearance related to obstruction by tumour or oedema of tissues.
2. Difficult swallowing related to impingement on oropharyngeal cavity by tumour pressure or extension, or oedema.
3. Possible haemorrhage related to surgical procedure.
4. Infections related to difficulty in cleansing affected area because of inaccessibility or acute sensitivity of tissues.
5. Weight loss related to growth of malignancy.
6. Lack of knowledge of the effects of alcohol and tobacco abuse.
7. Social isolation and ineffective coping related to sensitivity about possible disfigurement, odour, tubes and equipment.

Planning and implementation
NURSING INTERVENTIONS
Preoperative preparation
Preoperative care including diagnostic evaluation – see specific related condition, such as cancer of the mouth, p. 407, cancer of the oesophagus, p. 422, etc.

Postoperative care – immediate
1. Ensure effective breathing and oxygen exchange:
   a. Place the patient in upright position.
   b. Observe for signs of respiratory embarrassment, such as dyspnoea, cyanosis and oedema.
   c. Provide supplemental oxygen by face mask if necessary; if tracheostomy is present, provide oxygen by collar or T-piece.
   d. Auscultate for decreased breath sounds, wheezing, rhonchi.

Prevention of complications of haemorrhage and infection
1. Evaluate vital signs that may suggest haemorrhage or onset of infection.
2. Note condition of dressings to detect early signs of haemorrhage.
3. Be aware of principal causes of sudden haemorrhage following surgery:
   a. Loose ligature around a large vessel.
   b. Sudden distension of tied-off blood vessel followed by rupture.
   c. Slipping of ligature that may occur in violent coughing spasm.
   d. Rupture of a vessel due to trauma during surgery.

e. Rupture of a vessel weakened by erosion, tumour or slough.

f. Sloughing associated with secondary infection.

4. Institute immediate care if haemorrhage occurs:

a. Pressure over the common carotid and internal jugular vessels in the neck may be life-saving.

b. Have someone notify the operating room immediately.

c. Treat the patient for shock.

d. Prepare the patient for surgical intervention to repair vessel defect.

  (i) Correct fluid and blood loss with proper replacement.

  (ii) Initiate postoperative monitoring programme until vital signs remain consistently normal.

Improved swallowing and coughing

1. Observe for throat irritation – oedema, clearing of throat.

2. Note how the patient accepts liquids – refusal may mean difficulty in swallowing, which in turn may be indicative of superior laryngeal nerve damage.

3. Encourage the patient's intake of fluids in order to 'thin' secretions.

4. Encourage coughing to remove secretions.

5. Allow the patient to assume sitting position to bring up secretions (the nurse should support his neck with her hands).

6. Suction secretions if the patient is unable to bring them up himself.

Improved wound healing

1. Reinforce pressure dressings from time to time to assist in obliterating dead spaces and providing immobilization.

2. Observe dressings for evidence of haemorrhage and constriction which may affect respiration.

3. If portable suction (Redivac) is used, approximately 80–120ml of serosanguineous secretions are drawn off during the first postoperative day; this diminishes with each day.

4. Apply Opsite or other antiseptic plastic spray to protect the wound.

5. Cleanse skin area around drain exit using sterile saline or half-strength hydrogen peroxide.

Improved communication ability

1. Inform the patient that temporary hoarseness can be expected with extensive neck surgery and tracheostomy.

2. Encourage the patient to write messages for first few days; if writing is a problem, it may be due to denervation of the trapezius muscle.

3. Recognize that for this patient to nod 'yes' or 'no' may be difficult because of the neck dissection.

4. Place call bell and other articles within the patient's reach.

5. Recognize the need for support and encouragement, since this patient often is depressed and frustrated even during limited communication.

Psychosocial adjustment

1. Respect the patient's desire for privacy during treatments, dressing change and feedings.

2. Inform the patient's visitors of his appearance before they see him so that their expressions do not cause him to be upset.

3. Provide frequent aeration of the room and utilize deodorants to prevent unpleasant odours.

4. Observe for lower facial paralysis, since this may indicate facial nerve injury.

5. Watch the shoulder dysfunction, which may follow resection of spinal accessory nerves. See section on rehabilitation exercises below.

a. Utilize postoperative muscle exercises and muscle re-education.

b. Work with the patient to obtain good functional range of motion.

6. Consult with the surgeon and patient in decisions on future cosmetic surgery or in use of a prosthetic device.

7. Encourage the patient to verbalize his concerns and feelings.

a. Consult the doctor to determine the nature and extent of explanation and prognosis he has given to the patient.

b. Encourage the patient to seek confirmation of his personal philosophy and religious beliefs because this may provide answers for him.

c. Accentuate the positive.

d. Encourage the patient to participate in his plan of care.

e. Recognize that a great effort has to be made in behaviour modification to change a lifestyle that included alcohol consumption and cigarette smoking. It is difficult to do.

Provisions for family adjustments

1. Collaborate with the doctor in informing the family of the nature and extent of the patient's disease and surgery.

2. Help them to understand that without surgery, the patient's condition would be worse.

3. Prepare them for the patient's postoperative appearance; how this will be done depends on the

strengths and coping mechanisms of the family and the individual circumstances.

4. If there is difficulty with a partner or person close to the patient in accepting his appearance, refer the person to the doctor, social worker, psychiatrist or whatever resource seems advisable.

REHABILITATION EXERCISES FOLLOWING HEAD AND NECK SURGERY

Exercises are recommended when the neck incision is sufficiently healed in as much as the patient may experience limited range of shoulder motion, as well as neck and shoulder discomfort.

Goal: Regain maximum shoulder function, as well as head and neck motion, following surgery.

1. Perform exercises morning and evening. At first, exercises are done only once; then the number is increased by one each day until each exercise is done 10 times.
2. Following each exercise, the patient is instructed to relax.
3. For neck:
   a. Gently rotate head to each side as far as possible.
   b. Tilt head to the right side as far as possible; repeat for left side.
   c. Drop chin to chest and then raise chin as high as possible.
4. For shoulder:
   a. Standing beside bed, place hand from unoperated side on bed for support.
   b. Gradually swing arm on operated side up and back as far as is comfortable for the patient.
   c. Each day, work toward finishing a complete circle.

Evaluation

EXPECTED OUTCOMES

1. Breathes easily following surgery, with subsequent drainage of neck area and reduction of oedema.
2. Demonstrates ability to swallow fluids and soft foods.
3. Exhibits no sensitive areas, puffiness of tissue or temperature elevation that would suggest infection.
4. Maintains weight with no additional loss; relates that nutritional intake has been increased.
5. Makes resolutions to reduce and possibly abolish intake of alcohol; smoking fewer cigarettes each day and plans to join a smoking cessation group.
6. Demonstrates increasing sociability.

CONDITIONS OF THE OESOPHAGUS

DIAGNOSTIC EVALUATION OF THE OESOPHAGUS

Nursing assessment

During the taking of the nursing history, ask the following questions:

1. What problems or discomfort do you have when you eat? Do you have pain? Where? Any pain along oesophagus noted about five seconds after swallowing? Is there food sticking in your throat or chest? Are you nauseated? How long does the discomfort last? Is it daily or intermittent?
2. How is your appetite? Are there any signs of anorexia (loss of appetite)? Weight loss? Indigestion?
3. Do you have to restrict the kinds of food you eat as determined by size or consistency (meat for example, as determined by seasoning, or as determined by spiciness or acidity (citrus fruits)? Do you have to limit food because of temperature (hot or cold)?
4. Do you experience any nausea, heartburn (pyrosis), difficulty swallowing (dysphagia), regurgitation, reflux, or vomiting? Have you noticed bad breath (halitosis) or a disagreeable taste in your mouth?
5. Does the position of your body (bending, stooping, lying down) affect the problem? Do you lie flat when sleeping or do you have the head of the bed elevated? Does assuming a particular position help or make the problem worse?
6. Do you have any gas formation? Belching? Early satiety?
7. How has your weight been (stable, increasing or decreasing)?
8. What relieves the discomfort?
9. Do you find food or saliva on your pillow in the morning on awakening?
10. How are your teeth? Do you have difficulty chewing?

Upper gastrointestinal radiography

(See p. 436.)

Oesophageal endoscopy

This is the direct visualization of the entire mucosa of the oesophagus utilizing a rigid oesophagoscope or a flexible oesophagogastroduodenoscope to detect inflammation, ulceration, masses (tumours) or varices, and to obtain specimens for cytological studies or biopsy.

NURSING ALERT
For all endoscopies, bougienage and pneumatic dilatation procedures, have the following ready: oropharyngeal suction and emergency cardiopulmonary resuscitation equipment.

Nursing management and patient instruction
1. Give the patient nothing by mouth for six hours prior to test. This is done to decrease the possibility of aspiration and to be sure the oesophagus is clear of particles that would block visibility.
2. Explain the procedure to the patient before it is done, and explain the steps during the examination.
3. Administer diazepam (Valium) as a relaxant and pethidine as a narcotic as prescribed.
4. Spray the throat with local anaesthetic (lignocaine spray) to dull the effects of passing the oesophagoscope and to reduce retching.
5. If the oesophagus is dilated (fluid-filled oesophagus was seen on X-ray), first pass tube and then evacuate and irrigate oesophagus.
6. If a rigid scope is used, position the patient on his back. During insertion of oesophagoscope, his neck is hyperextended and his head is tilted back and supported.
7. The flexible oesophagofibroscope is passed with the patient sitting; the examination is then completed with the patient lying on his left side.

Following endoscopy
1. Withhold fluid and foods until the patient's swallowing reflex has returned (about two hours). Test the patient's swallowing with sips of water before foods or fluids are given.
2. Offer anaesthetic lozenges or normal saline gargles for throat discomfort.
3. Observe the patient for 24 hours for symptoms such as bleeding, dysphagia, fever and neck pain (cervical area) that are suggestive of perforation. Check also for substernal or epigastric pain (thoracic area); shoulder pain, dyspnoea, abdominal pain (diaphragmatic area) and subcutaneous emphysema.

Oesophageal biopsy and exfoliative cytology
1. Biopsy of tissue may be taken during oesophagoscopy: prepare tisue for laboratory examination.

2. Cytology:
   a. Usually an overnight fast is required (no food or fluids).
   b. A No. 12 or No. 16 French nasogastric tube is passed to the cardio-oesophageal junction (45cm).
   c. Residual contents are aspirated.
   d. Physiological saline (50ml) or Ringer's lactate solution is forcefully instilled with a syringe and is immediately aspirated below the cardia; this procedure is repeated at various levels of the oesophagus (5cm intervals from 45 to 25cm from incisor teeth).
   e. Aspirated contents are collected in separate containers surrounded by ice; when all specimens are collected, they are to be taken *immediately* to the laboratory for analysis (must be centrifuged and pallet spread on slide as soon as possible after aspiration).

OESOPHAGEAL TRAUMA

Oesophageal trauma is injury to the oesophagus caused by external or internal insult.
1. Externally – stab or bullet wounds, crush injuries, etc.
2. Internally – swallowed foreign bodies (i.e. metal objects, fishbones, false teeth, poison – acid burn).

TREATMENT AND NURSING MANAGEMENT
Goals: institute emergency life-saving treatment; restore continuity of oesophagus; facilitate healing and prevent infection and constriction.
1. Assess condition of the patient to determine his physiological needs.
2. Maintain open airway. Often, difficulty in respiration is due to oedema of the throat or a collection of mucus in the pharynx.
3. Control haemorrhage if present.
4. Treat for pain and shock. (Shock may be due to haemorrhage, impairment of cardiorespiratory function.)
5. Provide high fluid intake; may require parenteral therapy.
6. For external wound:
   a. Initiate emergency first-aid wound care and prepare for surgery.
   b. Maintain feeding through nasogastric tube.
7. For internal chemical damage, give specific antidote. If caustic or organic solvent was swallowed, do NOT try to induce vomiting. (See also Swallowed Poisons, p. 1088.)

a. A gastrostomy may be performed, either as a temporary or a permanent means of feeding the patient (see p. 446.)
b. Resulting strictures may be relieved by dilating the narrow oesophagus with bougies. (See Guidelines: Oesophageal Dilatation, p. 420.)
c. Reconstructive surgery may be necessary to create a new passageway for food between pharynx and stomach.
8. For swallowed foreign bodies.
a. When foreign body is made of metal, such as safety pins, needles, nails and other similar objects, it is not considered safe to allow object to make its way through the gastrointestinal tract.
b. These usually can be removed with the aid of an oesophagoscope. A large-bore, rigid oesophagoscope is best.
c. A skilled operator is required; magnets can be used on the end of a retrieving instrument passed through the oesophagoscope.

OESOPHAGITIS

Oesophagitis is an acute or chronic inflammation of the oesophagus. Severity of symptoms may be unrelated to the degree of inflammation seen at endoscopy.

CAUSATIVE FACTORS
1. Reflux of hydrochloric acid; gastric or duodenal contents (most common).
2. Fungal – *Candida*.
3. Chemical – acid, ammonia, aerosols.
4. Physical – alcohol, excessively hot liquids.
5. Trauma – swallowing foreign body. Medications (pills, capsules; see Nursing Alert below).
6. Reflux oesophagitis due to incompetent lower oesophageal sphincter; condition appears to have no relationship to hiatal hernia.
7. Malignancy associated with achalasia.
8. Prolonged nasogastric intubation.
9. Following gastric or duodenal surgery.
10. Repeated vomiting (common in alcoholics).
11. Bending, stooping, coughing and straining at stool.

NURSING ALERT
When administering any solid medication (pills, capsules), have the individual sit or stand and follow drug with at least 100ml liquid. Otherwise, the patient should have liquid medication.

CLINICAL FEATURES
(Sudden or gradual in onset.)
1. Hot burning pain (heartburn or burning sensation) behind xiphoid or sternum → spreading to throat, jaw, arms and back.
2. Pain with belching or regurgitation of acidic or bitter fluid (reflux).
3. Symptoms aggravated by bending over.
4. Symptoms may be precipitated by increases in intra-abdominal pressure, such as when the patient bends over, lifts heavy objects or has to strain to pass stool or urine (constipation or prostatism).
5. Dysphagia – worse at onset of meal. Food 'sticking' in throat or chest – produced by spasm, oedema or narrow lumen. While swallowing bolus of food, the patient may require 'washing down' of food with liquids.
6. Pain on drinking citrus liquids, alcohol or hot or cold fluids. Coffee often aggravates the pain.
7. Bleeding – acute or chronic; melaena or haematemesis also occurs.

DIAGNOSTIC EVALUATION
(For all oesophageal disorders.)
1. Cineradiographic oesophagograms.
2. Oesophagoscopy (see p. 412) with cytology and biopsy may differentiate oesophagitis from carcinoma.
3. Oesophageal manometry.
4. Acid perfusion test.
5. Gastro-oesophageal scintiscanning.

MEDICAL AND NURSING MANAGEMENT
Nutritional considerations
1. Institute a feeding regimen similar to that for gastric ulcer (see p. 442).
a. Frequent feedings, progressing to five meals – bland, low residue – no bedtime feedings.
b. Avoid foods high in residue, very hot foods, spices, alcohol, tobacco and coffee (even decaffeinated).
c. Avoid salicylates, phenylbutazone (Butazolidin), and anticholinergics.
d. Do not give food within two hours of retiring to avoid nocturnal reflux.
e. Chew food well and eat slowly.
f. Pain may be relieved by standing or walking, but aggravated in recumbent position.

NURSING ALERT
Milk actually is contraindicated for ulcer or oesophagitis because of high calcium content, which stimulates gastric acid secretion.

Relief of pain

1. Administer antacids, especially at bedtime – administer cimetidine if prescribed to reduce gastric secretions.
2. Place 15–20cm bed blocks at head of bed. Be sure to remove wheels from bed.
3. Provide adequate mouth care and recommend appropriate dental attention.
4. Administer cholinergic agents.
5. Promote a relaxing environment during meal times.
6. Avoid constricting abdominal garments.
7. Suggest a weight-reduction programme if the patient is overweight.

Surgical treatment

Dilatation therapy or surgery if necessary:

1. Dilatation therapy may be initiated for strictures; this is done several times weekly at first, then on a monthly basis.
2. Surgery is indicated when conservative measures fail:
   a. Combined with vagotomy–pyloroplasty if associated with gastroduodenal ulcer.
   b. Stricture may need to be resected, and an oesophagogastrostomy may be required.

NURSING ALERT

Anticholinergics are contraindicated because they may further impair competence of lower oesophageal sphincter and interfere with cleansing action of oesophageal peristalsis.

ACHALASIA

Achalasia refers to a benign spasm of the lower oesophageal sphincter, often with marked dilatation of the oesophagus. It is a neuromuscular disorder due to absent or defective nerves (of the myenteric plexus) going to the involuntary muscles in the oesophagus.

CLINICAL FEATURES

1. Difficulty in swallowing both liquids *and* solids, substernal pressure, fullness and regurgitation, often heartburn appears.
2. Halitosis and inability to belch may be noticed.
3. Secondary pulmonary complications due to spill-over of oesophageal contents (aspiration pneumonia).
4. Loss of peristaltic activity and failure of oesophageal sphincter to relax during swallowing process (detected by X-ray or manometry) may occur.

5. Emotional upsets, sudden shock or dietary indiscretion may aggravate this disorder.
6. Weight loss is eventually noticed in as much as the patient has a decreased intake in order to avoid discomfort; eventually this can lead to emaciation.
7. Increased risk of oesophageal carcinoma (8–10 per cent) and suppurative lung disease.
8. The patient may also have carcinoma at cardia invading oesophagus, simulating achalasia.

DIAGNOSTIC EVALUATION

1. Cineradiography of oesophagus with barium; this reveals weak or absent peristaltic waves and failure of sphincter relaxation.
2. Oesophagoscopy with cytological studies and biopsy.
3. Oesophageal manometry with perfused open-tip catheters and injection of methacholine.

NURSING ASSESSMENT

1. Determine what the patient can and cannot swallow.
2. Note location and kind of pain.
3. Determine how relief is obtained.
4. Ascertain what aggravates the problem.

TREATMENT AND NURSING MANAGEMENT

Goals:

1. Enlarge the passageway so that contents pass more readily from oesophagus to stomach.
2. Pneumatic bag dilatation.
3. Surgical oesophagomyotomy.

Nursing management – medical therapy or minor surgical therapy

1. Direct patient to eat slowly, chew food thoroughly and arch his back while swallowing to provide relief.
2. Suggest that the patient sleep with his head elevated to avoid reflux or aspiration.
3. Provide a bland diet and tell the patient to avoid alcohol, as well as spicy, very hot and very cold foods, in order to minimize symptoms.
4. Administer pharmacological agents such as bethanechol chloride to increase lower oesophageal sphincter tone, as prescribed.

NURSING ALERT

Anticholinergic drugs are contraindicated for achalasia because they further decrease oesophageal peristalsis.

5. If medication fails, pneumatic dilatation is tried.

Nursing management – major surgical therapy
(Used only if pneumatic dilatation fails.)
1. Oesophagomyotomy – a division of muscular fibres enclosing the narrowed oesophagus that permits mucosa to pouch out through the divided area in muscle layers.
2. Cardiomyotomy – when above operation is extended to include cardiac end of stomach.
3. Incisional approach determines nature of post-operative care; thus, an incision through chest implies nursing care similar to that given to a patient with a thoracotomy (see p. 208).

DIFFUSE SPASM OF OESOPHAGUS

Diffuse oesophageal spasm is a motor disorder of the oesophagus. It is common in old age and may be an early stage of achalasia (see p. 415).

CLINICAL FEATURES
1. Pain on swallowing, dysphagia, chest or back pain.
2. Diffuse spasm may be associated with achalasia, obstruction of the cardia by tumour, precipitation by reflux acid.

TREATMENT AND NURSING MANAGEMENT
Conservative
1. Administer sedatives for pain.
2. Avoid food and beverages that precipitate symptoms.
3. Eliminate source of tension as a precipitating factor producing stress during meal times.

Later, if necessary
Pneumatic dilatation will be indicated if manometric studies reveal increased lower oesophageal sphincter pressure (provided that gastro-oesophageal reflux is not part of the problem).

See guidelines
1. Feeding the Patient with Dysphagia (see below).
2. Teaching a Patient with Dysphagia How to Swallow, p. 418.
3. Oesophageal Dilatation, p. 420.

GUIDELINES: FEEDING THE PATIENT WITH DYSPHAGIA

Dysphagia – difficulty or discomfort in swallowing; a bolus of food becomes impeded in its movement between the mouth and stomach.

CAUSATIVE FACTORS
1. Circulatory disturbances of brain (stroke, brain stem vascular accidents).
2. Cranial nerve disturbances.
3. Trauma to neck.
4. Radiotherapy/surgery for head and neck tumours.
5. Presence of tumours, inflammation.
6. Disturbances of laryngeal sphincter.
7. Psychological pathology.

CLINICAL FEATURES
1. Patient complains of a sticking sensation behind sternum; relief is obtained by:
   a. Retching;
   b. Drinking liquids to dislodge bolus.
2. Upper or thoracic oesophageal discomfort noted in three to five seconds after attempting to swallow.
3. Lower thoracic discomfort noted in 5 to 15 seconds.

NURSING ASSESSMENT
1. Determine whether dysphagia occurs only with solid food. Does it occur with soft foods? Liquids? Warm liquids or cold liquids? Saliva? Does it vary?

2. Has the patient lost weight? Evidence of cachexia?
3. Is hoarseness present? If so, it may be indicative of laryngeal lesion.
4. How long has the patient experienced this discomfort?
5. Did painful swallowing precede dysphagia? How long? Heartburn? How long? Hiccough?
6. Regurgitation – bringing up of undigested food or gastric acid into the mouth. Has this occurred?
7. In general, determine the patient's eating habits and their relevance to this problem.

PROCEDURE

Nursing action	**Rationale**
1. Make a preliminary assessment of the patient's problem (see above, Assessment). a. Determine the swallowing limitation.	By individualizing the approach, a more effective plan to meet particular needs will be achieved.
2. Prepare environment so that it will be well ventilated, uncluttered and cheerful without distractions.	This will make the patient's feeding experience more pleasant and easier.
3. Place the patient in an upright sitting position (90 degrees) for about 20 minutes before and after feeding. a. Provide adequate support and comfort.	This will provide time to adjust to this position, thereby eliminating postural change disturbances during feeding.

4. Explain what you plan to do; sit rather than stand, and encourage conversation. Face patient and proceed in an unhurried manner.
  a. Encourage eating; allow time for chewing.
  b. Remove tray when the patient is finished.
	This procedure will more likely secure co-operation.
	
	Proceed slowly and give patient time to swallow. Unclean or used tray may be psychologically distressing and may interfere with digestion.

5. If food is difficult to manage, begin with liquids; if he continues to have trouble:
  a. Place tip of irrigation syringe in the back of the mouth cavity on the better side; gently squeeze bulb.
  b. When he is ready, allow the patient to squeeze bulb himself.
  c. Frequent small feedings are offered initially.
	Proceed slowly and give the patient time to swallow.
	
	Aim to involve the patient in his own care.
	
	Liquidized or commercially prepared liquid formula supplements are available.

6. If the patient has difficulty chewing:
  a. Manipulate jaw in an upward and downward motion.
  b. Encourage the patient to close his lips after food is in his mouth, keep lips closed until the food is swallowed.
  c. If the patient does not swallow as soon as he should but appears to retain food in his mouth, place thumb on his chin and press downward toward his chest.
	This not only stimulates jaw but will actually stimulate act of chewing.
	It may be necessary to manually close the patient's lips, using your thumb and index finger. When lips are closed, the swallowing reflex is stimulated.
	This manoeuvre moves his larynx superiorly and anteriorly, thereby facilitating swallowing.

7. In spoon-feeding, when one mouthful is swallowed, remove spoon at once. If the patient drools, wipe his mouth before the next mouthful is presented.

The patient is more comfortable without the sensation of food trickling down his chin.

Feeding the patient with an affected side of the mouth (facial paralysis, hemiplegia, hemilaryngectomy)

Nursing action

1. Turn the patient to his unaffected side.

2. Place food on the strong side of mouth rather than in the middle to the mouth.

3. Encourage the patient to form a bolus by moving his tongue around inside of mouth.

Rationale

This provides better head and neck support.

Permits food to be managed more effectively.

This assists in placing food in a proper position for swallowing, rather than permitting food to collect near cheek.

FOLLOW-UP CARE

Nursing action

1. Record the amount of intake, the patient's taste and food preferences, his progress and any special tactics that were effective in helping him.

2. Encourage family members to participate in the patient's feeding programme.

Rationale

Progress notes will assist in moving the patient towards self-care.

GUIDELINES: TEACHING A PATIENT WITH DYSPHAGIA HOW TO SWALLOW

PURPOSE
To assist the patient who has difficulty swallowing after injury/surgical correction of the oropharyngeal or upper oesophagus, neurological deficit, stroke.

EQUIPMENT
Baby bottle with nipple
Rubber glove for instructor's hand

PROCEDURE

Nursing action

1. Explain to the patient that you plan to work with him in developing the sensation of swallowing.

Rationale

The patient's co-operation, concentration and directed participation are essential to the success of this learning experience.

2. Demonstrate first how the lips pucker as you draw inward in sucking your gloved finger.

The patient's observation will assist him in imitating this action.

3. Wash your gloved hand and then put your gloved finger in the patient's mouth. When the patient demonstrates good sucking ability, proceed to the next step.

4. The teacher redemonstrates the sucking manoeuvre with one hand while placing the other hand on her throat to feel the motions caused by sucking and swallowing.

It becomes apparent that after sucking, a need to move whatever is in the mouth causes the complex swallowing process to be initiated.

5. Ask the patient to duplicate these motions.

It may help to have the patient place his hand on the neck of the demonstrator to grasp the mechanisms of swallowing.

6. The swallowing function can be further stimulated as follows:
   a. Have the patient suck on a fresh lemon (if permissible), or use lemon glycerin swabs in his mouth.
   b. If the sucking reflex is intact, a straw may be effective in initiating swallowing as he sucks on it. The straw may need to be placed further inside the mouth or patient's head may have to be tilted.
   c. Place a cup at corner of the lips and tilt slightly so that the patient can take liquid slowly. Encourage the patient to move toward cup.

This will stimulate salivation reflexes.

This offers the patient more control as he moves forward; swallowing reflex occurs more easily.

7. Use a baby bottle if it appears that it might help.

Recognize the psychological effect this might have – will patient feel he is regressing?

Special food considerations for the patient with dysphagia

1. Avoid milk and milk products, since they stimulate production of thick saliva, which is difficult to swallow.
2. Serve liquids that are close to room temperature rather than cold or hot.
3. Diluted fruit juices are more palatable than concentrated juices.
4. Provide textured foods rather than foods that are too smooth (i.e. chopped cooked vegetables rather than pureed vegetables, baked rather than mashed potatoes).
5. Avoid strong-flavoured foods, acids or bitter-tasting foods – except lemon juice added to food.

GUIDELINES: OESOPHAGEAL DILATATION (BOUGIENAGE)

PURPOSE
To dilate the cardio-oesophageal sphincter so that food may pass from the oesophagus into the stomach.

EQUIPMENT
Water-soluble lubricant
Bougies – flexible, woven silk-tipped or rubber, of various sizes
Dilators of the doctor's preference

PROCEDURE
Preparatory phase
1. Cleanse dilators with povidone-iodine (Betadine) to prevent infection and bacteraemia.
2. Explain the procedure to the patient and indicate why it is necessary for him to fast and drink no fluids for 12 hours beforehand.
3. Administer sedative or narcotic as prescribed to allay apprehension and assist the patient in relaxation.
4. Have the patient in a sitting position in a chair or in bed elevated 30 to 45 degrees.
5. Place a cover bib-fashion around the patient's chest and over his shoulders to protect his clothing.
6. Provide the patient with a vomit bowl; have suction equipment (oropharyngeal) available.
7. Remove dentures if present.

Performance phase

Nursing action	Rationale
1. Spray the patient's throat with a local anaesthetic if prescribed (gargle may be preferred).	The spray or gargle will desensitize local tissues.
2. Lubricate bougie with water-soluble lubricant (some bougies are weighted with mercury); remove excess lubricant.	Lubrication reduces friction between the mucous membrane and tube. Excess lubricant may be aspirated.
3. Assist the doctor as he passes the tube and first dilator. Support the patient's head and encourage him to swallow.	The more relaxed the patient, the easier the bougie will descend to the cardiac sphincter.
4. Progressively larger bougies are passed until pain occurs. (For achalasia, a pneumatic or hydrostatic balloon is used with fluoroscopy.)	Sizes are increased to dilate the stricture progressively. By increasing the pressure of the balloon under fluoroscopy, the sphincter may be gradually dilated.

Note: If bougies do not pass the stricture, it will be necessary to pass a guide wire through the stricture via oesophagoscope. The scope is then removed, and metallic olive dilators are passed down the guide wire, progressively increasing in size.

Follow-up phase

Nursing action	Rationale
1. Have the patient rest in bed following procedure.	Observe for 24 hours for evidence of oesophageal perforation.
a. Give nothing by mouth for an hour after dilatation.	Nil by mouth to prevent aspiration.
b. Check pulse and temperature at least hourly for six hours.	Elevated pulse and temperature, plus chest pain and evidence of subcutaneous emphysema may indicate presence of air in the mediastinum.
c. Be attentive to complaints of chest pain.	It may be necessary to have X-ray verification.
d. Observe upper chest for signs of subcutaneous emphysema. Should any of the above abnormal signs occur, notify doctor.	

OESOPHAGEAL DIVERTICULUM

An oesophageal diverticulum is an outpouching of the wall, usually in the cervical posterior side.

TYPES
1. Pharyngo-oesophageal (pulsion) – also called Zenker's diverticulum; upper end of oesophagus through cricopharyngeal muscle.
2. Midoesophageal (traction) – near tracheal bifurcation.
3. Epiphrenic (traction–pulsion) – lower third of oesophagus.

CLINICAL FEATURES
Pharyngo-oesophageal
1. Difficulty in swallowing, fullness in neck, a feeling that food stops before it reaches the stomach and regurgitation of undigested food.
2. Belching, gurgling or nocturnal coughing brought about by diverticulum becoming filled with food or liquid, which is regurgitated and may irritate the trachea.
3. Halitosis and foul taste in mouth caused by decomposing of food in a pouch (diverticulum).
4. Hoarseness, asthma and pneumonitis may be the only signs in the very elderly.
5. Weight loss due to nutritional depletion.

Midoesophageal
Generally no symptoms.

Epiphrenic
1. At times associated with achalasia or diffuse oesophageal spasm (see p. 415).

2. No symptoms at first, but condition eventually may cause dysphagia, pain and pulmonary complications.

DIAGNOSTIC EVALUATION
1. X-rays using barium should be taken.
2. Oesophagoscopy is risky, because of danger of perforation of diverticulum, which may lead to mediastinitis.

TREATMENT
Surgery is usually recommended as soon as the diagnosis is made to prevent further nutritional deficit and complications.

Pharyngo-oesophageal
Usually a transverse cervical diverticulectomy and myotomy are done. Some surgeons use myotomy alone, and others do a diverticulopexy.
1. Caution is taken to avoid injury to common carotid artery and internal jugular vein.
2. Sac is dissected free and then excised flush with oesophageal wall.
3. If transthoracic approach is used, nursing management is similar to that described for chest operations (see p. 206).

Midoesophageal
Therapy is usually not required because of absence of symptoms and rareness of complications.

Epiphrenic
Underlying primary condition must be treated.

NURSING MANAGEMENT

1. Immediate postoperative care is as described on p. 208.
2. If a nasogastric tube is in place, institute nasogastric feedings utilizing fluids.
   a. Irrigate tube carefully with water following each feeding.
   b. Record kind and amount of irrigating fluid.
3. Prepare the patient the morning after surgery for X-ray following ingestion of diatrizoate meglumine (Gastrografin) and diatrizoate sodium solution, or barium, to detect any leakage at mucosal closure site.
4. If no leakage occurs, liquid diet is started, with diet increased to regular in the next 72 hours.
5. Drains are shortened on third to fourth day.
6. Discharge when comfortable and able to resume activities.
7. If leakage occurs (rare), drains are left in place, and the patient will be maintained on parenteral feedings until repeat X-rays show adequate healing and closure.

OESOPHAGEAL VARICES

See p. 518.

OESOPHAGEAL PERFORATION

Oesophageal perforation is an acute surgical emergency in which the oesophagus is punctured by a swallowed foreign object (e.g. dental prosthesis, open safety pin), by gunshot, which results in trauma, or by an oesophagoscope or stiff tube.

CLINICAL FEATURES
1. Chest pain, usually substernal – may be mild or severe.
2. Temperature elevation occurring within 24 hours.
3. Abdominal pain and tenderness, and epigastric muscle spasm.
4. Subcutaneous emphysema and crepitus of neck, face and chest wall – noted in cervical and thoracic oesophageal perforations.

DIAGNOSTIC EVALUATION
1. History of recent oesophageal trauma.
2. Chest film to look for air in mediastinum.
3. Oesophagogram.

SURGICAL TREATMENT AND NURSING MEASURES
1. Utilize emergency resuscitative procedures.
2. Prepare for surgical intervention (may not be needed if diagnosed and treated early).
3. Administer parenteral fluids and antibiotics as prescribed.
4. Pass nasogastric suction tubing to minimize pleural or mediastinal contamination. Give nothing by mouth.

CANCER OF THE OESOPHAGUS

INCIDENCE
1. Benign tumours and sarcomas of oesophagus are unusual, except for leiomyomas.
2. About 80 per cent of cancers of the oesophagus involve men who are usually older than 60.
3. Middle third of oesophagus is most involved, with the lower third next most frequent.
4. Carcinoma of oesophagus is responsible for 2 per cent to 4 per cent of all cancer deaths.
   a. Usually this is a geriatric patient who also has pulmonary and cardiovascular disorders.
   b. Proximity of lesion to vital body structures (e.g. heart and lungs); lymph-node spread is easy and rapid.
   c. Before significant symptoms occur, the tumour may already have invaded surrounding structures.

RISK FACTORS
Causative factors have not been proved; the condition is associated with achalasia.
1. Chronic trauma – excessive use of alcohol, tobacco, spicy foods, hot liquid (tea) ingestion.
2. Geographical – certain areas of Iran, Kenya, Honan Province in China, India and Zimbabwe show a higher incidence.
3. Oral and pharyngeal cancer – probably related to smoking.
4. Genetic predisposition – nonwhite male population.
5. Nitrosamines.
6. Sodium hydroxide ingestion.

CLINICAL FEATURES
1. Progressively increasing difficulty in swallowing (dysphagia). At first, only solid foods give trouble; then, as growth progresses and obstruction becomes more complete, even liquids pass with difficulty into the stomach.
2. Pain on swallowing.
3. Possible haemorrhage – usually only occult bleeding.
4. Progressive loss of weight and strength due to starvation.

5. Later symptoms – vague substernal pain, hiccough, respiratory difficulty, foul breath, regurgitation of food and saliva.

DIAGNOSTIC EVALUATION
1. Barium swallow; air contrast studies of oesophagus. A piece of bread or a marshmallow coated with barium may serve as a radiopaque bolus to locate the lesion.
2. Cineradiography.
3. Endoscopy – inspection and photography.
4. Biopsy.
5. Computed tomography may be helpful in delineating the extent of the tumour, as well as in identifying presence of adjacent tissue invasion.

TREATMENT
1. The wide variety of treatments available reflects the overall poor results from any one approach. Palliation is usually the goal.
   a. Radiation alone; radiation with surgery.
   b. Surgery and chemotherapy.
   c. Chemotherapy alone.
   d. Surgical removal of the involved segment.
2. Lesions in middle and upper third, in particular, are not often suitable for excision.
   a. Irradiation is the preferred form of therapy.
   b. Some hospitals report success with insertion of a prosthetic tube (Celestin or other plastic) through the mouth to bridge the involved area and to facilitate swallowing. This insertion may be done after dilatation of tumour-bearing portions of the oesophagus.
3. Lesions of middle and lower oesophagus are excised if there is no evidence of local or distant metastases.
   a. The portion of oesophagus containing the tumour is removed.
   b. Continuity of gastrointestinal tract is restored by bringing the stomach (or a tube in stomach, or a segment of colon) into the chest and implanting proximal end of oesophagus into it. Some hospitals prefer a side-to-side oesophagogastrostomy.
   c. Chest drainage of pleural cavity is carried out (see p. 204).
4. Gastrostomy is not recommended, since it provides little palliation and does not restore the swallowing mechanism. It is used only as a temporary measure.

NURSING MANAGEMENT
Preoperative
1. Preoperative preparation includes promoting the nutritional status with a diet high in calories, vitamins and protein. This may have to be by mouth, intravenous infusion or hyperalimentation.
2. To avoid aspiration, a recumbent position is recommended for feeding.
3. A nasogastric tube may be inserted prior to surgery.

Postoperative
1. With Celestin tube (or other tube replacement), swallowing may be easier if small sips of water are offered at first.
2. Food is usually not given for several days and then in small quantities, leading to a soft diet.
3. Remind the patient to remain in the upright position after eating to promote digestion.
4. Monitor the patient for tube leakage; this may be manifested early by low-grade fever, fluid in the pleural space or elevated pulse.

Nursing principles for pre- and postoperative management are similar to those given for radical neck dissection (p. 410) and thoracic surgery (p. 206).

GASTROINTESTINAL CONDITIONS

NUTRITIONAL ASSESSMENT
1. Interviewing is a convenient method of determining a patient's eating habits.
2. Determine the following factors, which are influential in affecting the patient's attitudes toward foods:
   a. Cultural heritage, religion, family background;
   b. Socioeconomic status, education, current situation, effect of food fads and superstitions.
3. Observation (Table 7.1).

Questionnaire for nutritional assessment

Adults
Background information:
Name, age, sex, family, and occupational roles, general health status, dietary restrictions (past or present).

Table 7.1   Physical signs indicative of nutritional status

Body area	Signs of good nutrition	Signs of poor nutrition
Hair	Shiny, lustrous; firm, healthy scalp	Dull and dry, brittle, depigmented, easily plucked
Face	Skin colour uniform; healthy appearance	Skin dark over cheeks and under eyes, skin flaky, face swollen
Eyes	Bright, clear, moist	Eye membranes pale, dry (xerophthalmia); Bitot's spots, increased vascularity, cornea soft (keratomalacia)
Lips	Good colour (pink), smooth	Swollen and puffy (cheilosis), angular lesion at corners of mouth (angular fissures)
Tongue	Deep red in appearance, surface papillae present	Smooth appearance, swollen, beefy red, sores, atrophic papillae
Teeth	Straight, no crowding, no cavities, bright	Cavities, mottled appearance (fluorosis), malpositioned
Gums	Firm, good colour (pink)	Spongy, bleed easily, marginal redness, recession
Glands	No enlargement of the thyroid	Thyroid enlargement (simple goitre)
Skin	Smooth, good colour, moist	Rough, dry, flaky, swollen, pale, pigmented; lack of fat under skin
Nails	Firm, pink	Spoon-shaped, ridged
Skeleton	Good posture, no malformation	Poor posture, beading of ribs, bowed legs or knock knees
Muscles	Well developed, firm	Flaccid, poor tone, wasted, underdeveloped
Extremities	No tenderness	Weak and tender; presence of oedema
Abdomen	Flat	Swollen
Nervous system	Normal reflexes	Decrease in or loss of ankle and knee reflexes

Food purchase and preparation:
Who purchases and prepares food?
What factors influence kinds of foods purchased?
Is budgeting a matter of concern when buying food?
Where is food purchased?
How often do you shop?
What facilities are available for food storage and preparation?
What foods are served most frequently?
Do you have 'meals-on-wheels'?

Relationship of food to lifestyle:
Food likes and dislikes.
Favourite foods when growing up.
Special family foods for celebrations.
Atmosphere at meal times.
Foods your body needs.
Food supplements (vitamins, minerals).
Sources of information about nutrition.
Eating away from home – frequency and location.

Adolescents
What is nutritious? Foods body needs?
Where are meals eaten? When is food eaten?
How much snacking?

4. Anthropometric measurements (of body size and composition) – necessary for assessment of nutritional status and for diet planning.

MAJOR MANIFESTATIONS OF GASTROINTESTINAL DISTURBANCE

ANOREXIA, NAUSEA AND VOMITING

NORMAL PHYSIOLOGY
Appetite
A desire for food, or an agreeable attitude toward ingesting food, often specific kinds of food.
1. The frontal and parietal areas of the cerebrum, but especially the hypothalamus, are known to be associated with appetite.
2. Desire for food is acutely associated with increased rates of gastric hydrochloric acid secretion, with gastric hyperaemia and hypermotility.

Hunger

A strong sensation or urge to eat following a period of fasting.
1. Hunger is temporarily associated with rhythmic contractions of the stomach.
2. The precise mechanisms by which hunger is produced are unknown; it is related to a low blood sugar level.

Satiety

A condition following consumption of an amount of food sufficient to meet present requirements; a feeling that one has had enough to eat.

ANOREXIA

Lack of appetite for food; lack of interest in all food.
1. Associated with a disinterest in consumption of even those foods that one ordinarily likes to eat.
2. Associated with decreased secretion of gastric hydrochloric acid.
3. Possible causes:
    a. Unpleasant or upsetting experiences;
    b. Apprehension, fear and anxiety;
    c. Excitement, both pleasurable and undesirable;
    d. Systemic and local diseases, such as hepatic failure and uraemia.

DYSPEPSIA (INDIGESTION)

Painful, difficult or disturbed digestion. The person suffers from several of a group of symptoms – nausea, regurgitation, vomiting, heartburn, bloating and stomach discomfort.

NAUSEA

A most unpleasant sensation usually associated with a distinct revulsion toward the ingestion of food; it may or may not precede vomiting.
1. Very often, anorexia is succeeded by nausea and vomiting. However, either of these states may occur without the others.
2. Associated with decreased motor activity of the stomach, pallor of gastric mucosa and contraction of proximal duodenum.
3. Frequently associated with evidence of diffuse autonomic discharge – profuse watery salivation, sudden drenching perspiration, tachycardia.
4. Many patients find it difficult to describe:
    a. Vague unpleasantness in epigastrium;
    b. Distressing feelings in the throat;
    c. Vague unpleasantness spread diffusely in abdomen (must be distinguished from mild visceral abdominal pain).

VOMITING

Sudden forceful expulsion of stomach contents through the mouth.
1. Vomiting centre is located in the medulla.
2. May or may not be preceded by nausea and retching.
3. Exaggerated and often extreme vasomotor activities may immediately precede and accompany the vomiting act; watery salivation, sweating, pulse rate change, vasoconstriction and pallor.
4. Tachycardia prior to vomiting becomes bradycardia during process.
5. Incited by neuromuscular 'reverse peristalsis' or mechanical obstruction.

NURSING MANAGEMENT

1. Observe the preliminary symptoms.
    a. The patient is often lightheaded, weak and dizzy.
    b. Irregularity of respiration before and during vomiting.
    c. Blood pressure may fall before and then fluctuate during vomiting.
2. Observe character and quantity of expectorated material.
    a. Note whether it has an odour, is sour-smelling or is odourless.
    b. Is it liquid, containing mucus or pus, or food particles?
    c. Describe its colour, taste and consistency (Table 7.2).

Table 7.2 Nature of vomitus

Colour/taste/ consistency	Possible source
Yellowish or greenish	May contain bile Medication – senna
Bright red (arterial)	Haemorrhage, peptic ulcer
Dark red (venous)	Haemorrhage, oesophageal or gastric varices
'Coffee grounds'	Digested blood from slowly bleeding gastric or duodenal ulcer
Undigested food	Gastric tumour? Ulcer obstruction?
'Bitter' taste	Bile
'Sour' or 'acid'	Gastric contents
Faecal components	Intestinal obstruction

3. Be aware of progression of events when there is a diminution of intake and output – weight loss, dehydration, fluid and electrolyte imbalance:
   a. Skin becomes dry and loses elasticity;
   b. Poor mouth hygiene leading to halitosis.
4. Recognize progression of events that might lead to shock, tachycardia, hypotension, oliguria.

DISTURBANCES ASSOCIATED WITH ANOREXIA, NAUSEA, AND VOMITING
Psychological and neurological factors
1. Life situations that evoke subjective manifestations of fear, frustration, depression and anxiety may be associated with these symptoms.
2. Anorexia is commonly a manifestation of a depressed state, which can lead to a profound impairment of food intake and possibly anorexia nervosa.
3. Nausea and vomiting:
   a. Frequently occurs during or shortly after meals.
   b. Often unaccompanied by nausea and retching.
   c. Frequently does not empty stomach.
   d. After vomiting, patient may desire to continue to eat.
   e. No recurrence of vomiting occurs.
   f. Accompanying migraine headache:
      (i) Hypoxaemia affecting the vomiting centre;
      (ii) Vascular changes;
      (iii) Associated visual disturbances.
   g. Caused by unusual stimulation of labyrinth of the ear.
   h. Projectile type associated with increasing intracranial pressure:
      (i) Commonly not preceded by nausea;
      (ii) May indicate meningitis, internal hydrocephalus, space-occupying lesion, cerebellar lesions.
   i. Associated with vertigo.

Associated with gastrointestinal and biliary conditions
1. Systemic diseases (e.g. liver failure, uraemia).
2. Gastritis (alcohol, viruses, bacteria or poisons).
3. Pyloric or intestinal obstruction.
4. Cholecystitis, pancreatitis or peptic ulcer.
5. Mechanical obstruction in gastrointestinal tract.

Drugs and toxic agents
1. Pharmacological effect:
   a. Medullary chemoreceptor zone may be stimulated.
   b. Direct effect on gastrointestinal organs brought about by mercury.
   c. Stimulation of hypothalamus nuclei brought about by alcohol, apomorphine, histamine, adrenaline.
2. Mucosal damage of upper gastrointestinal tract caused by mercury, ammonium chloride, copper sulphate, aminophylline, alcohol, aspirin.

Other factors
1. Febrile illness.
2. Chronic renal failure (see p. 614).
3. Motion sickness.
4. Ménière's disease (see p. 880).
5. Hepatocellular disease.

NURSING INTERVENTIONS
1. Observe and assess status of the patient when he experiences anorexia, nausea and vomiting. Note the general effect of these symptoms on the patient:
   a. Food and fluid intake.
   b. Balance between intake and output.
   c. Effect on body weight, indicating malnutrition.
   d. Character and amount of vomitus – measure and record.
   e. Effect on the patient's activity – malaise or apathy.
   f. Changes in the patient's skin colour and elasticity and in mucous membranes.
   g. Note other fluid losses – perspiration, faeces, urine, fluid and electrolyte balance – which may result in dehydration.
2. Improve psychological desire for food in order to overcome anorexia, nausea and vomiting.
   a. Determine the patient's eating habits, cultural preferences, etc.
   b. Include the patient's family in soliciting information.
   c. Encourage adequate rest before, during and after his meal; allay anxiety.
   d. Prepare the patient for his meals by being certain that he has had good oral hygiene, is comfortable and has clean bedding and clothing.
   e. Promote the patient's physical comfort so that he may enjoy his food and not be distracted by discomfort during or after his meal.
   f. Protect the patient's environment from noise, foul odours, confusion, too many visitors, etc.
   g. Serve food with attractive appearance and in appropriate quantity.

h. Be sure that food is served at proper temperature.
3. If the patient is nauseated but does not vomit:
   a. Reduce environmental stimuli:
      (i) Visual – other 'sick' patients; soiled dressings;
      (ii) Olfactory – drainage bottle;
      (iii) Sensory – colostomy; cauterization; bedpan;
      (iv) Auditory – noise.
   b. Encourage rest and deep breathing.
   c. Cater to the patient's preferences in food.
   d. Limit size of servings.
   e. Remove meal tray as soon as the patient is finished.
   f. If he does vomit, carefully observe vomitus and remove promptly; clean area and patient if necessary and offer mouthwash.
4. Provide opportunity for the patient to express his feelings.
   a. Keep channels of communication open.
   b. Provide time to allow patient to talk.
5. Correlate administration of medication with needs of the patient.
   a. If the patient has pain, analgesics may be administered.
   b. If the patient is tired and exhausted, sedatives may be prescribed.
   c. If the patient appears tense and worried, tranquillizers may be indicated.
   d. Specific antiemetic agents.
6. If secondary to intestinal obstruction, nasogastric suction or the insertion of a Miller–Abbott tube is indicated.

ANOREXIA NERVOSA AND BULIMIA
Anorexia nervosa is voluntary refusal to eat, usually occurring in a female between the ages of 12 and 18 years.

Bulimia nervosa is extreme overeating and subsequent attempts to rid the body of food by self-induced vomiting and laxative abuse.

CONSTIPATION AND DIARRHOEA

CONSTIPATION
Constipation is a decrease in the frequency, volume or ease of stool passage.
Obstipation is absence of intestinal output (no stool).
1. Constipation is usually caused by altered routine in dietary and activity patterns; by drugs such as morphine, codeine and atropine; by mechanical obstruction or surgery; by psychological factors resulting from restricted use of toilet facilities; and by old age. It may also occur as a result of chronic, strong laxative abuse.
2. Manifestations of constipation include changes in colour, consistency and ease of expulsion of stools, which may be darker, harder and difficult or painful to pass.

DIARRHOEA
Diarrhoea is an increase in frequency, fluidity and/or volume of stools.
1. It is a leading cause of death in developing countries, where sanitation is poor and dietary deficiency widespread.
2. Acute diarrhoea can be a serious problem in elderly and debilitated persons.
3. Chronic diarrhoea is associated with malabsorption, malnutrition, anaemia and increased susceptibility to other diseases.

Assessment
PATIENT PROBLEMS
1. Determine whether onset was sudden or gradual.
2. Find out how long the patient has had diarrhoea – days? weeks? months?
3. Describe the character, consistency and appearance of stools. Note that colour changes are produced by presence of abnormal constituents.
   a. 'Tarry' stools – may indicate digested blood that usually originates in upper gastrointestinal tract.
   b. Bloody stools – may indicate haemorrhage, usually from lower gastrointestinal tract.
   c. Blood streaking on stool surface or on toilet paper – may indicate haemorrhoid or fissure.
   d. Pale, pasty (clay-coloured) stools – indicate totally obstructed biliary tract.
   e. Foamy, foul-smelling stools – indicates malabsorption or malabsorption syndrome.
   f. Other colour changes due to food or medication ingested indicates dietary excesses or effect of medication.
4. Learn when the bouts of diarrhoea occur – in the daytime only, after meals, either day or night?
5. Determine whether diarrhoea is associated with cramping or abdominal pain, fever, chills, nausea, weakness, travel exposure, etc.
6. Is pain in rectum or anus experienced at the time stools are passed? May be indicative of tumour, inflammation, haemorrhoids or anal fissure.
7. Has the patient had any change in dietary habits, meals eaten away from home, etc?

NURSING ALERT

Alteration in bowel habits (such as constipation, then diarrhoea, then constipation, then diarrhoea) may mean partial obstruction.

8. Determine degree of dehydration. Look for signs of dehydration – weakness, postural hypotension, tachycardia, mucosal dryness, lethargy, poor skin elasticity.
9. Expect the need for laboratory evaluation – serum electrolytes, creatinine, haemoglobin, serum albumin, blood gases and pH, stool cultures and stool examination for ova and parasites.

Planning and implementation
NURSING MANAGEMENT
Constipation and diarrhoea

1. Disturbances in elimination produce psychological discomfort; conversely psychological deviation can produce elimination disturbances.
2. Assist the patient in overcoming correctable problems by:
   a. Affording privacy;
   b. Helping the patient approach near-normal position during evacuation, as much as possible;
   c. Providing comfort measures such as warmed bedpan;
   d. Providing sufficient time and a schedule as close to the patient's own as possible.

Constipation

1. Correct dietary habits to include adequate fluids, fresh fruits and vegetables, whole-grain cereal, bread.
   a. Dried fruits such as prunes, apricots; figs, bran are high in fibre.
   b. Cut back on highly processed foods (sweets) and foods high in fat.
2. Suggest a small glass of prune juice or lemon juice in warm water each morning.
3. If possible, encourage the patient to participate in active daily exercise – brisk walking, swimming.
4. Encourage a regular time for evacuation each day.
5. Avoid taking laxatives if at all possible. If necessary, suggest a bulk-forming laxative, such as Metamucil, that does not irritate the bowel. One to two heaped teaspoonfuls in a glass of water, once or twice daily, followed by a second glass of water.
6. Do not expect to have a bowel movement every day or even every other day.

Diarrhoea

1. Consider hospitalization if diarrhoea continues unresolved and there is significant dehydration.
2. Perform rectal examination to check for a faecal impaction (common in the elderly, in psychiatric patients and in patients with neurological disorders). If found, manually disimpact (see p. 499). Then give enemas.
3. Remove such causative factors as stress and food until cause is determined.
4. Encourage patient to take fluids such as juices, soups and broths; avoid milk, fruits and extreme roughage.
5. Prepare for fluid therapy administration if dehydration is suspected.
6. General measures:
   a. Have required bathroom facilities readily available.
   b. Pay particular attention to proper hand and body hygiene, since diarrhoea may be infectious.
   c. Use talcum powder or emollients to prevent skin excoriation.
   d. Provide dry and clean bed linen and clothing.
   e. Prepare for fluid therapy and electrolyte replacement if dehydration is suspected. Administer prescribed medications.
      (i) Kaolin mixture (Kaopectate) – acts as an absorbent to bind gas and bacteria.
      (ii) Diphenoxylate (Lomotil) – decreases intestinal motility by acting on gastrointestinal smooth muscle (contraindicated when aetiological agent is *Shigella* or invasive bowel disease).
      (iii) Opiates – act to decrease bowel motility.

GASTROINTESTINAL PROBLEMS IN THE ELDERLY

TYPES OF PROBLEM
Aberration of taste

1. May be related to chronic smoking and frequent intake of hot beverages, causing thermal injury to taste buds.
2. Reduced capacity for drinking and eating.
3. Overindulgence can cause bloating and belching.
4. Greater reliance on antacids.

Lactose intolerance

1. Symptoms produced are bloating, gas and diarrhoea which develop from one to three hours after taking milk, cream or ice cream.

Use of sweeteners in foods and beverages

1. Symptoms produced are bloating, flatulence and diarrhoea.
2. Cause is fermentation of the nondigestible sweetener by colonic bacteria.

Belching and flatus

1. Probably due to swallowed air.
2. May also be caused by methane and hydrogen produced by bacterial fermentation from indigestible carbohydrates from certain fruits and vegetables.
3. Odoriferous gases may also be produced by bacterial fermentation in colon. Thought to result from incomplete digestion of wheat, barley, rye, oats, corn and potatoes.

Indigestion and heartburn

1. Often due to rich or greasy foods in combination with alcohol.
2. May be caused by carbonated beverages, tea or coffee.
3. Excessive relaxation of lower oesophageal sphincter may be caused by foods rich in fat or chocolate, as well as foods containing carminatives (onions, peppermint).

Hiatus hernia

1. When lower oesophageal sphincter mechanism becomes impaired, the problem often is aggravated in the presence of hiatus hernia.
   Symptoms:
   a. Fullness in upper abdomen, heartburn, regurgitation.
   b. Usually, eating less, taking antacids and not reclining after eating will alleviate symptoms.

Oesophageal spasm

1. Symptoms – episodic, intermittent difficulty in swallowing while eating or drinking.
2. Pain under sternum may be caused by hot/cold beverages.
3. On occasion, a large piece of meat is swallowed too quickly, followed by retching and the urge to vomit.
4. Encourage complete chewing and eating slowly.

Diverticulosis

1. Occurs as a result of inherent weakness in colon wall; pressures within colon increase with colonic contractions.
2. Those with irritable bowel are prone to develop diverticulosis.
3. Maintain a high-fibre diet to increase bulk content of stool.

Cholelithiasis

1. Usually associated with females who have borne children.
2. A high-calorie diet seems related to increasing amounts of biliary cholesterol.
3. Only about 25 per cent of patients who develop symptoms (abdominal pain, jaundice) require therapy.

Other conditions

1. Incidence of gastric and duodenal ulcer increases in middle years.
2. Colitis and ileitis become less common.
3. Gastrointestinal cancers (stomach, pancreas, colon) increase in frequency after age 40.
4. Alcohol-related cirrhosis of liver increases.

PATIENT EDUCATION

1. Practice moderation in eating and alcohol consumption.
2. Alcohol-induced damage requires an average daily intake of 150g of alcohol for several years. This can be reached with the following daily intake:
   a. Ninety-proof whisky – 250ml (four strong drinks).
   b. Wine – 700ml bottle contains 100g of alcohol.
   c. Beer – six-pack of 350ml cans or bottles contains 120g of alcohol.
3. Daily dietary calories to be regulated in three meals with foods from vegetables, fruits, starches, grains, protein and dairy products.
4. Vitamin supplements are probably unnecessary.
5. Augment diet with fibre supplements – this appears to reduce incidence of diverticula and haemorrhoids.
6. Do not ignore these signs: change in bowel habits, unusual pain, weight loss, bleeding or jaundice.

INTUBATION AND DIAGNOSTIC STUDIES FOR GASTRODUODENAL CONDITIONS

GUIDELINES: NASOGASTRIC INTUBATION – LEVIN TUBE (SHORT TUBE)

GOALS
1. Remove fluid and gas from the gastrointestinal tract (decompression).
2. Prevent or relieve nausea and vomiting.
3. Determine the amount of pressure and motor activity in the gastrointestinal tract (diagnostic studies).
4. Treat patients with mechanical obstruction and bleeding within the upper gastrointestinal tract.
5. Administer medications and feeding (gavage) directly into the gastrointestinal tract.
6. Obtain a specimen of gastric contents for laboratory studies (when pyloric or intestinal obstruction is suspected).

EQUIPMENT
Nasogastric tube – usually Levin (rubber or plastic, No. 12 to 18 French) – preferably disposable (plastic tubes are less irritating than rubber)
Water-soluble lubricant
Clamp for tubing
Towel, tissues and vomit bowl

Glass of water and straw, or perhaps ice chips
Adhesive tape (hypoallergenic) 1.25cm and 2.5cm
Irrigating set with 20ml syringe
Stethoscope
Penlight

FOLLOW-UP EQUIPMENT
Decongestant spray
Mouth hygiene materials

PROCEDURE
Preparatory phase
1. Explain procedure to the patient and tell him how mouth breathing, panting and swallowing can help in passing the tube.
2. Have the patient in an upright position; place a towel across his chest.
3. Determine with the patient what sign he might use, such as raising his index finger, to indicate 'wait a few moments' because of retching or discomfort.
4. Remove dentures; place vomit bowl and tissues within the patient's reach.
5. Place rubber tubing in ice-chilled water, making tubing firmer. Plastic tubing may already be firm enough; if too stiff, dip in warm water.
6. Mark distance tube is to be passed by measuring as indicated in Figure 7.2. This will ensure the passage of the tubing into the stomach.

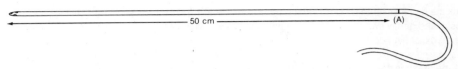

1. Mark the nasogastric tube at a point 50cm from the distal tip; call this point (A)

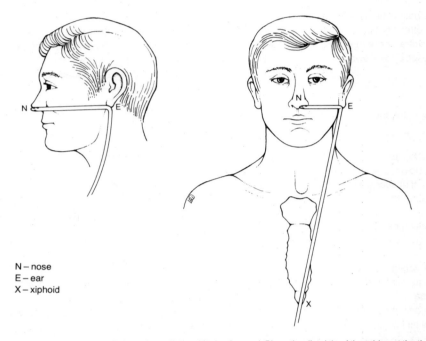

N – nose
E – ear
X – xiphoid

2. Have the patient sit in a neutral position with head facing forward. Place the distal tip of the tubing at the tip of the patient's nose (N); extend tube to the tragus (tip) of his ear (E), and then extend the tube straight down to the tip of his xiphoid (X). Mark this point (B) on the tubing

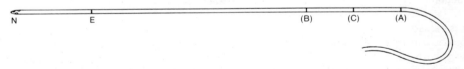

3. To locate point (C) on the tube, find the midpoint between points (A) and (B). The nasogastric tube is passed to point (C) to ensure optimum placement in the stomach

Figure 7.2. Steps 1, 2 and 3 indicate how far a nasogastric tube is passed for optimal placement in the stomach (Hanson, R.L. (1979) Predictive criteria for length of nasogastric tube insertion for tube feeding, *Journal of Parenteral Enteral Nutrition*, May/June, Vol. 3, No. 3, pp. 160–3)

Performance phase

Nursing action	**Rationale**
1. Lubricate tube for about 15–20cm with thin coat of water-soluble jelly.	Lubrication reduces friction between mucous membrane and tube.

Nursing action	Rationale
2. Tilt back the patient's head before inserting tube into nostril and gently pass tube into the posterior nasopharynx, aiming downward and backward.	Passage of tube is facilitated by following the natural contours of the body.
3. When tube reaches the pharynx, the patient may retch; allow him to rest for a few moments.	Swallowing reflex is triggered by the presence of the tube.
4. Have the patient hold his head in a partially flexed position: offer him several sips of water sucked through a straw or permit him to suck on ice chips. Advance tube as he swallows.	Flexed head position makes swallowing easier and the tube less likely to enter trachea. Swallowing facilitates passage of tube. Actually, once the tube passes the cricopharyngeal sphincter into the oesophagus, it can be slowly and steadily advanced, even if the patient does not swallow.
5. Continue to advance tube gently each time patient swallows.	
6. If obstruction appears to prevent tube from passing, do *not* use force. Rotating tube gently may help. If unsuccessful, remove tube and try other nostril.	Avoid discomfort and trauma to patient.
7. If there are signs of distress such as gasping, coughing or cyanosis, immediately remove tube.	
8. To check whether the Levin tube is in the stomach: a. Aspirate contents of stomach with a 20ml syringe. b. Place a stethoscope over epigastrium; inject 5ml of air into Levin tube.	Aspirated stomach contents would indicate that the tube is in the stomach. Air can be detected by a 'whooshing' sound entering stomach rather than the bronchus.
9. Adjust tubing after these tests to proper position in the stomach.	

Nursing action	Rationale
After tube is passed: 1. Anchor tube with hypoallergenic tape. a. Using 5cm hypoallergenic tape, split lengthwise and only halfway; attach unsplit end of tape to nose and cross split ends around tubing.	Prevent the patient's vision from being disturbed; prevent tubing from rubbing against nasal mucosa.
2. Anchor the tubing to the patient's gown.	To permit mobility of patient.
3. Clamp the tube until the purpose for inserting the tube is about to take place.	

NURSING ALERT
All enteric tubes must be irrigated at regular intervals with small volumes of fluid to ensure patency.

4. Administer oral hygiene frequently. Cleanse tubing at nostril. Utilize a decongestant spray, if necessary.	To promote patient comfort.
5. Apply cream or lipsalve to lips and nostril to prevent encrustation.	To keep tissue soft.
6. If tube is to be in place for prolonged periods (beyond 12 hours), keep head of patient elevated at least 30 degrees.	To minimize gastro-oesophageal reflux.
7. Rotate tubing daily or more frequently.	To prevent adherence to mucosa.

Follow-up phase

Before removing nasogastric tubing:
1. Be certain that gastric drainage is not excessive in volume nor from the small bowel.
2. Ensure, by auscultation, that audible peristalsis is present.
3. Determine whether the patient is passing flatus so that abdomen is not distended.

NURSING ALERT
Recognize the potential for complications when intubation is prolonged – nasal erosion sinusitis, oesophagitis and gastric ulceration. Pulmonary complications may occur postoperatively in patients with nasogastric intubation because of interference with coughing and clearing of the pharynx (Figure 7.3).

Nursing action	**Rationale**
Removing nasogastric tubing:	
1. Place a towel across the patient's chest and inform him that the tube is to be withdrawn.	No doubt the patient will be happy to have progressed to this stage.
2. Rotate tubing and inject about 10ml of saline before clamping tubing.	This will ensure its mobility. Tubing is clamped to prevent drainage within tube from being aspirated.
3. Instruct the patient to take a deep breath and exhale slowly.	Slow exhalation will relax the pharynx and facilitate withdrawal of tubing.
4. Slowly but evenly withdraw tubing and cover it with a towel as it emerges.	Covering the tubing should dispel the momentary feeling of nausea.
5. Provide the patient with materials for oral care and lubricant for nasal dryness.	Mouthwash and a nasal lubricant will be appreciated by the patient.
6. Document time of tube removal and the patient's reaction.	
7. Continue to monitor the patient for signs of gastrointestinal difficulties; changes in vital signs may suggest infection (Figure 7.3).	Recurrence of nausea or vomiting may require reinsertion of nasogastric tube.

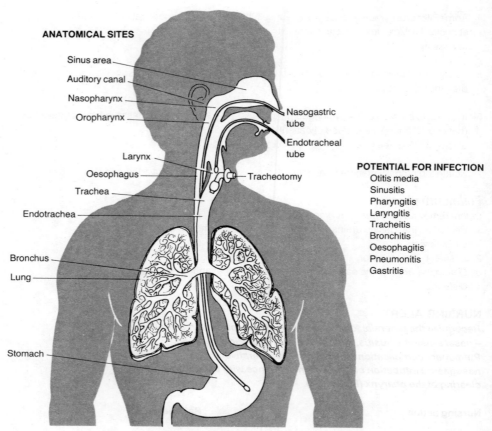

ANATOMICAL SITES

Sinus area
Auditory canal
Nasopharynx
Oropharynx
Nasogastric tube
Endotracheal tube
Larynx
Oesophagus
Trachea
Tracheotomy
Endotrachea
Bronchus
Lung
Stomach

POTENTIAL FOR INFECTION
Otitis media
Sinusitis
Pharyngitis
Laryngitis
Tracheitis
Bronchitis
Oesophagitis
Pneumonitis
Gastritis

Figure 7.3. All along the upper respiratory tract and upper digestive system there is the potential for abnormal areas of colonization (infection) when various tubes are in place (e.g. tracheostomy, nasogastric or endotracheal tube). In addition, there is the potential for aspiration of secretions that may cause bronchitis and/or pneumonitis

GUIDELINES: GASTRIC ANALYSIS (ASPIRATION OF STOMACH CONTENTS VIA NASOGASTRIC TUBE)

GOALS
1. Determine secretory activity of the gastric mucosa because of diagnostic significance.
2. Study the secretory component, hydrochloric acid.
3. Analyse gastric contents in patients suspected of having pyloric or intestinal obstruction.
4. Remove poisons.

EQUIPMENT
Rubber or plastic tube, No. 12–18 French, depending upon patient's size
Tube clamp; drape or towel; vomit bowl and tissues
Syringe, 50ml or low-pressure intermittent suction apparatus
Water-soluble lubricant
Bowl of chipped ice for rubber tubing
Specimen containers

PROCEDURE
Preparatory phase

Nursing action

1. Instruct the patient to take no food or fluids and not to smoke for eight to ten hours prior to analysis.

2. Withhold anticholinergics, antacids, alcohol, cimetidine and adrenergic blockers, and any other medications as prescribed.

3. Explain procedure to the patient; cover his upper body with a cover to protect his clothing and provide a vomit bowl for spittle and vomit.

4. Instruct the patient to sit in a back-supporting chair or to assume upright position in bed with neck flexed, leaning forward from the waist.

5. Establish with the patient a signal system to indicate when he wishes to rest for a few minutes.

6. If dentures or bridges are present, they should be removed.

7. Chill tubing in ice water to make it firmer; if plastic tubing is too stiff, dip in warm water.

Rationale

An accurate sampling of stomach contents is ensured.

To permit normal emptying of the stomach and remove suppressive effect on gastric secretion.

Patient's understanding of how to breathe through his mouth with occasional swallowing will assist in passing the tube.

Gravity and this anatomical position will facilitate tubes passing into oesophagus. If neck is hyperextended, tube is more likely to enter trachea.

Greater patient co-operation is obtained.

Dislodging of dentures could occur, with risk of asphyxiation.

A manageable tube that droops naturally and is neither too stiff nor too limp is the objective.

Performance phase
Pass the nasogastric tube (see Guidelines, p. 430).

Nursing action

1. Verify that the tube is in the stomach (for absolute assurance of tube position, fluoroscopic verification is required). Tip of the tube should be at least 50cm down from nose. When syringing air in and out, gurgling over stomach is audible with stethoscope.

2. Place the patient semi-recumbent in left lateral position.

3. Aspirate fasting stomach contents completely; then measure and record. If abnormal, notify doctor before proceeding.

4. When tubing is properly positioned in the stomach, allow the patient to rest for 20 to 30 minutes and continuously aspirate contents. This procedure allows the patient to attain a basal state and to adjust to the tube in his throat.

5. See below for types of analyses.

Rationale

Blue litmus turns pink in the presence of acid.

Normal – clear and watery; often contains green or yellow bile.
Abnormal – see Nursing Alert (below).

Production of hydrochloric acid may be inhibited by the irritation of the tubing and by anxiety.

NURSING ALERT

In gastric analysis, note the following:
1. *Residual of 100ml or more, including undigested food particles, may be indicative of gastric stasis or pyloric obstruction.*
2. *Faecal odour – suggests neoplasm or gastric fistula, intestinal obstruction.*
3. *Blood – indicates ulcerating lesion. Streaks of blood – suggest trauma from tubing.*

TYPES OF GASTRIC ANALYSIS

Basal analysis

A test to determine nature of secretions in the absence of stimuli.
1. For 12 hours preceding test – no food; for eight hours preceding test – no fluids or smoking.
2. Obtain specimens as follows:
   a. First specimen – label 'residual';
   b. Second specimen (30 minutes later) – label as to amount and time of collection;
   c. Then four additional specimens must be collected at 15-minute intervals – label as to amount and time of collection. Continuous or frequent aspiration is required (manually or with suction apparatus) to avoid losses through pylorus.
3. Normal ranges:
   Female: 0.2–3.8mEq/hour
   Male: 1–5mEq/hour

Stimulation analysis

(Betazole hydrochloride or pentagastrin) usually performed following basal study.
1. Test of gastric secretion following injection of a stimulant:
   a. Collect fasting specimen of gastric contents.
   b. Administer betazole hydrochloride (Histalog) or pentagastrin.
   c. Collect specimens every 15 minutes for 90 minutes, or longer if doctor desires.
2. Significance:
   a. In presence of gastric ulcer visualized radiologically or endoscopically, the absence of any acid after stimulation (pH never falls below 6.0) suggests that ulcer is malignant and that surgical treatment is indicated.

   Note: In absence of an ulcer, achlorhydria does *not* have the same significance (present in 40 per cent of adults over age 60 without ulcer or cancer).

   b. In presence of a duodenal ulcer, basal output is greater than 20mEq/hour peak or maximal acid output greater than 50mEq/hour. A basal/maximal ratio greater than 0.6 should strongly suggest Zollinger–Ellison syndrome.
   c. Otherwise, acid outputs, either basally or after stimulation, are of no diagnostic significance in peptic ulcer disease.

Hypoglycaemic analysis (Hollander test), or 'insulin gastric analysis'

A test that shows the vagal stimulation of parietal cells following a blood sugar drop to a hypoglycaemic level of less than 50mg/100ml. (Hypoglycaemia stimulates the secretory activity of the vagus nerve: if the nerve is divided, secretion will not occur. This test may be done postsurgically to determine effectiveness of vagotomy.)
1. Collect fasting specimen of gastric contents; label 'residual'.
2. Collect specimens every 15 minutes for one hour; label 'basal secretion'.
3. Administer prescribed insulin intravenously (calculated according to body weight).
4. Collect gastric specimens every 15 minutes for next two hours. Concomitantly, collect blood specimens every 15 minutes for determination of blood sugar. Measure, note characteristics and record.

NURSING ALERT

Observe the patient for signs of hypoglycaemia – weakness, vertigo, tremors, perspiration, convulsions, unconsciousness. Have 50 per cent glucose ready for intravenous administration if blood glucose level drops too low.

RADIOGRAPHY

X-rays of the gastrointestinal tract (upper gastrointestinal series)

1. The entire gastrointestinal tract can be delineated by X-rays following the introduction of barium

sulphate as the contrast medium. This procedure may be combined with cineradiography.
2. Barium is a tasteless, odourless, completely insoluble powder:
   a. It can be ingested in an aqueous suspension for upper gastrointestinal tract study (upper gastrointestinal series), micronization of particles, as well as chocolate or strawberry flavouring, makes it more palatable.
   b. Effervescent fluids may also be administered to obtain air-contrast studies.
   c. Follow serially through small bowel over next four to six hours.
3. The fasting patient is required to swallow barium under direct fluoroscopic examination.
   a. Oesophagus:
      (i) Patency, calibre, and motility noted – may indicate anatomical and functional derangement.
      (ii) Abnormally enlarged right atrium noted – indicates impingement on oesophagus.
      (iii) Oesophageal varices noted – usually indicates liver cirrhosis.
   b. Stomach:
      (i) Motility and thickness of gastric wall noted.
      (ii) Spasms, ulcerations, malignant infiltrates and anatomical abnormalities noted.

NURSING ALERT
If the patient stands when drinking barium, transit time may be too rapid through the oesophagus; if this is a problem, consider supine position with the head somewhat elevated.

   (iii) Pressure from outside of stomach detected.
   (iv) Patency of pyloric valve observed.
   c. Small intestine:
      Barium swallow or a continuous infusion of a thin barium sulphate suspension via duodenal tube may be done to visualize jejunum and ileum.
4. During fluoroscopic examination, X-rays or video tapes are taken for permanent records.

Implementation
NURSING MANAGEMENT AND PATIENT EDUCATION
A careful nursing history may suggest that a patient is at high risk for reactions to contrast medium (Table 7.3).

Table 7.3   Reactions to radiographic contrast material and their management

Reaction	Incidence	Features	Medical and nursing management
Vasomotor	Up to 50 per cent of patients	Mild flushing Warmth Tingling sensations Slight giddiness Metallic taste Nausea	Because these features are mild and transient, treatment or pre-X-ray medication is not required

Anaphylactoid	Up to 4 per cent of people with history of allergy, hay fever or bronchial asthma	Sneezing
		Chest tightness
		Wheezing
		Angioedema
		Bronchoconstriction
		Hypotension
		Compensatory tachycardia
			Check pulse frequently
			Vasopressors
			Intravenous fluids
			Oxygen
			Antihistamines
			Steroids
			Pretreatment medication may help:
			    Steroids (oral prednisone) three times prior to X-ray
			    Antihistamine (Benadryl) one hour before examination

Vagus		Apprehension Restlessness Hypotension Bradycardia – 50 beats/minute or less	Atropine – high doses Intravenous fluids Monitor pulse rate, since this indicates response to atropine Pretreatment – some recommend atropine

NURSING ALERT
For patients receiving radiographic contrast agents intravenously – observe closely for a delayed reaction during the next 30 to 60 minutes.

1. The patient is to be on a low-residue diet for preceding two to three days and is to receive nothing by mouth after midnight prior to the test.
2. During this interim, the patient is to receive no purgative, however mild, and no other medication unless specifically prescribed.
3. The patient remains in a fasting state until the last X-ray is taken.
4. Barium from prior barium enema must be fully evacuated before gastrointestinal series, or it will interfere with visualization of stomach and upper intestine. Cleansing enema is of particular value here.
5. Since this test takes five to six hours, and much time is spent waiting, encourage the patient to take some reading material with him.

Lower gastrointestinal series
See p. 460.

UPPER GASTROINTESTINAL ENDOSCOPY
Upper gastrointestinal endoscopy is the direct visualization of the gastric mucosa through a lighted endoscope (gastroscope). Endoscopes are flexible scopes equipped with a fibreoptic lens through which coloured photographs or motion pictures can be taken.

Primary diagnostic gastrointestinal endoscopy (PRIDGE) is a rapid, accurate, and safe method of examining the upper gastrointestinal tract in selected patients and is an excellent initial examination.

Nursing interventions
1. Explain the following to the patient:
   a. What is about to happen.
   b. That he must fast before the examination to prevent aspiration of gastric contents and to permit complete visualization of the stomach.
   c. That dentures must be removed to facilitate passing the scope and to prevent injury.
   d. That a sedative or tranquillizer may be given to help him to relax.
   e. That a topical anaesthetic may be used for local comfort and to prevent retching.
   f. That air will be pumped into the stomach during the procedure to permit visualization of the stomach.
2. Following a gastric examination:

a. Check the swallowing reflex before offering food or fluids.
   (i) Tickle the back of the patient's throat with a tongue depressor or cotton swab; usually two to four hours after the examination, the reflex functions return to normal.
   (ii) If fluids are handled normally, the patient may then be offered food.
   b. Check for signs of perforation – abdominal pain, subcutaneous emphysema, dyspnoea, cyanosis, back pain, temperature elevation, hydrothorax, rigid abdomen.
   c. Offer throat lozenges or warm saline gargles to relieve throat soreness.
   d. Inform the patient that because of air pumped into the stomach he may pass gas by belching or passing flatus.

Gastric biopsy
Obtaining a piece of gastric mucosa can be done through a gastroscope during endoscopy. Forceps extended through the scope may be used to bite tissue, or tissue may be obtained via suction as it pulls mucosa to excising blades within the scope. Tissue in one area may be representative of tissue in all sections of the stomach; however, by looking through the scope, the doctor can be discriminating in selection of specific tissue.

Nursing management is similar to that for gastric endoscopy (see above).

COMPUTED TOMOGRAPHY (CT SCAN) AND ULTRASONOGRAPHY (ULTRASOUND)
Computed tomography
This is accomplished using a scanner that operates by detecting X-rays from a finely focused beam that rotates around a patient. The subtle differences in X-ray absorption by various tissues are then assembled by a computer and displayed on a screen as a radiological image.
1. It provides precise anatomical and pathological information for a wide array of intra-abdominal and other conditions.
2. Abscesses can be drained using CT as a guide for catheter placement (obviating the need for surgery).
3. By exactly noting the full extent (staging) of a malignancy, surgical intervention can be more precise.
4. In abdominal trauma, multiple organ involvement can be noted by CT, thereby reducing number of diagnostic tests.
5. Invasive vascular techniques may be reduced utilizing a CT scanner.

Ultrasonography

This is the focusing of a beam of high-frequency sound waves over an abdominal organ. This creates waves that vary with changes in tissue density (see also Biliary Conditions, p. 523.)

GASTRODUODENAL CONDITIONS AND MANAGEMENT

GASTROINTESTINAL BLEEDING

Bleeding is a symptom of a digestive or vascular problem or problems. It may be obvious in vomit or stool, or it may be *occult* (hidden).

AETIOLOGY AND CAUSATIVE FACTORS

1. Trauma anywhere along the gastrointestinal tract.
2. Erosion of a blood vessel due to an ulcer, benign tumour or malignancy.
3. Rupture of an enlarged vein, such as a varicosity (oesophageal varices, haemorrhoid).
4. Inflammation such as oesophagitis, caused by acid or bile, gastritis, small intestine (Crohn's disease), polyps.
5. Irritation of mucous membrane due to certain drugs – alcohol, aspirin, aspirin-containing compounds, other drugs.
6. Infection, such as intestinal (ulcerative colitis).
7. Diverticulosis.

CLINICAL FEATURES

1. Signs of blood:
   a. Bright red – vomited from high in oesophagus; from rectum or distal colon (coating stool).
   b. Mixed with dark red – higher up in colon and small intestine; mixed with stool.
   c. Shades of black ('coffee ground') – oesophagus, stomach and duodenum; vomitus from these areas.
2. Symptoms of massive bleeding:
   a. Weakness, dizziness, faintness, short of breath, crampy abdominal pain, diarrhoea;
   b. Rapid pulse, drop in blood pressure, shock;
   c. Pale appearance, fatigue, lethargy.

DIAGNOSTIC EVALUATION

1. It is not difficult to diagnose bleeding, but it may be a problem to locate source of bleeding.

2. History – change in bowel pattern, presence of pain or tenderness, recent intake of food and what kind (red beetroot?).
3. Complete blood count; occult test of stool.
4. Endoscopy.
5. Radioactive scanning.

TREATMENT

1. Depends on cause and whether bleeding is acute or chronic:
   a. If aspirin, eliminate aspirin and treat bleeding.
   b. If ulcer, an anti-ulcer drug is prescribed, along with lifestyle change and dietary change.
   c. If cancer, tumour to be removed (see Mouth Cancer, p. 405, Oesophageal Cancer, p. 422, Gastric Cancer, p. 445, Colon Cancer, p. 490).
2. May require skilled endoscopist with a well-prepared diagnostic team.
   a. Intravenous lines and oxygen therapy equipment to be available.
   b. If life-threatening bleeding occurs, treat shock, administer blood replacement:
      (i) Equipment – large-bore irrigation tube, Pitressin, irrigating equipment of doctor's preference.
      (ii) Cardiac monitor, pulse/blood pressure monitor.
      (iii) Surgery if conservative measures fail.
3. Electrocoagulation and photocoagulation (laser) may be the treatment of choice.
   a. Postlaser treatment requires careful monitoring for bleeding recurrence, nasogastric intubation, dependent drainage.

PEPTIC ULCER

A peptic ulcer is an excavation found in the mucosal wall of the oesophagus, the stomach, the pylorus or the duodenum because of the erosion of a circumscribed area of its mucous membrane. Basically, the problem is too much secretion of hydrochloric acid in relation to the degree of protection afforded by both mucus secretion and the neutralization of gastric acid by duodenal, biliary and pancreatic fluid.

PREDISPOSING FACTORS

1. Emotional stress – anxiety, anger, resentment.
2. Intake of methylxanthines (tea, coffee, cola, chocolate) and cigarette smoking are associated with increased risk of ulcer development.
3. Drugs (salicylates, aspirin, reserpine, phenylbutazone, aminophylline, and others) may be irritating to the mucous lining of the stomach, pylorus and duodenum.

4. Genetic susceptibility.
5. A combination of the above factors.

INCIDENCE

1. Duodenal ulcer is found most frequently in the 25 to 40 age-group and in males four times more than in females.
2. Gastric ulcer occurs most frequently in the 40 to 55 age-group and in males 2.5 times more often than in females.
3. Duodenal ulcers occur 10 times more frequently than gastric ulcers (Figure 7.4).
4. Peptic ulcer occurs 2–2.5 times more frequently among siblings with ulcers as among the general population.
5. Duodenal ulcer occurs more frequently in patients with type O blood.

ALTERED PHYSIOLOGY

(Duodenal ulcer)

1. Increased mass of gastric mucosa and more parietal and peptic cells.
2. Increased sensitivity of gastrin (peptide hormone secreted by gastric antrum stimulates gastric secretion).
3. Increased vagal stimulation, which in turn releases gastrin.
4. Increased release of gastrin in response to a meal.
5. More rapid gastric emptying.
6. Increased acid load to duodenum.

Figure 7.4. The stomach is divided on the basis of its physiological functions into two main portions. The proximal two-thirds, the fundic gland area, acts as a receptacle for ingested food and secretes acid and pepsin. The distal third, the pyloric gland area, mixes and propels food into the duodenum and produces the hormone gastrin. 'Peptic' lesions may occur in the oesophagus (oesophagitis), stomach (gastritis) or duodenum (duodenitis). Note peptic ulcer sites and common inflammatory sites

Assessment

CLINICAL FEATURES

Underlying observations

1. Peptic ulcers are more likely to be in the duodenum than in the stomach (ratio of 10:1).
2. A peptic ulcer occurs only in the areas of the gastrointestinal tract that are exposed to hydrochloric acid and pepsin (see Figure 7.4).
3. A small percentage of patients will have no symptoms and will first be diagnosed during a bleeding episode (more common in teenagers).

Pain

1. Types:
   a. Pain or discomfort – quality usually not well described; may be sharply localized in midepigastrium. Description may be 'hunger-like', burning, gnawing.
   b. Pyrosis (heartburn, substernal burning) is associated with peptic ulcer in many patients.
   c. Pain may radiate to the back if the duodenal ulcer has begun to penetrate the pancreas.
2. Time of occurrence:
   a. Pain is worse when stomach is empty – usually half to two hours after meals; it may waken the patient in early morning hours (12 to 3 a.m.).
   b. Pain is seldom present when the patient first wakens, because gastric secretion is lowest at this time.

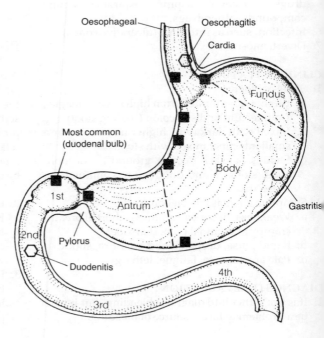

Sites of peptic lesions

Common inflammatory sites

c. Periodicity occurs in clusters – the patient may have trouble for days to weeks, then experience long symptom-free intervals.
3. Relief – obtained by ingesting food or taking antacids; if truly effective, this occurs within five to ten minutes.

Belching
Belching is due to increased air swallowing. (This is a nonspecific symptom and is most common in people with *no* organic gastrointestinal disease.)

Nausea and vomiting
Reflex vomiting occurs in 10 to 20 per cent of patients, with some retching; it is associated with ulcer pain and also is seen with duodenal obstruction in chronic ulcer disease, when it usually occurs with or just after evening meal.

DIAGNOSTIC EVALUATION
1. Observation, nursing history and assessment include the following:
   a. Determine location of pain, whether it is localized, whether it radiates, how long it lasts and when it occurs.
   b. Find out if pain is relieved by food, alkalis, vomiting.
   c. Determine eating patterns – regularity, type of food, conditions for eating, such as relaxed atmosphere, standing at 'fast food' counter, while driving a lorry, etc.
   d. Learn if there is a history of tension, problematic situations, fears or anxiety.
   e. Determine whether the patient ingested drug irritants.
   f. Determine whether the patient smokes or consumes alcohol.
2. Fibreoptic panendoscopy, which permits visualization of entire stomach and proximal duodenum, is most accurate.
3. Upper gastrointestinal series (see p. 436).
4. Gastric secretory studies (p. 436) are of value mainly to check for possible Zollinger–Ellison syndrome.
5. Stool specimen to detect occult blood, which indicates bleeding.

PATIENT PROBLEMS
1. Pain and epigastric distress related to gastric hyperactivity, mucosal erosion.
2. Fear and anxiety related to possibility of developing a complication (haemorrhage, perforation).
3. Ineffective rest/activity pattern related to type A personality or lack of understanding.

4. Knowledge deficit related to misunderstanding of biological, dietary and pharmaceutical limitations.
5. Potential for development of complications.

MEDICAL MANAGEMENT
1. The patient is advised to reduce stressful activities and to provide for rest and relaxation; sedation/tranquillizers may be prescribed.
2. Antacids, anticholinergics and ulcer-healing medications may be prescribed as required.
3. Fluid, electrolyte, and blood needs are monitored; intravenous replacement is prescribed.
4. Dietary intake may consist of frequent, small feedings – soft, bland foods at first, then diet as tolerated.
5. Vital signs and clinical features are monitored for progress.

Planning and implementation
NURSING INTERVENTIONS
Relief of pain and discomfort
1. Administer antacid medications to neutralize hydrochloric acid and relieve pain.
   a. Liquid antacids are more effective than tablets.
   b. Increasing aluminium in antacids leads to constipation; increasing magnesium leads to diarrhoea.
   c. Antacids are given one hour after meals, at bedtime and during the night as required for pain.
   d. Look for antacids that effectively neutralize stomach acid, leave low sodium content, require about 5ml to swallow at a time, and are least expensive.
   e. Antacids with calcium may produce hypercalcaemia.
2. Administer anticholinergic drugs to suppress gastric secretions and delay gastric emptying. This is most useful at night.
   a. Anticholinergics are contraindicated in patients with glaucoma, urinary retention, gastric retention and possibly arrhythmia.
   b. Encourage hydration to minimize side-effects of anticholinergic medications.
3. If ulcer problems persist after first being treated with antacids, it may be necessary to administer cimetidine (Tagamet).
   a. Cimetidine (Tagamet) owes its effectiveness to its H_2-receptor blocking action in inhibiting gastric acid secretion; to its potency (superior to that of cholinergics); and to its failure to produce acute side-effects.
   b. Cimetidine is administered with meals be-

cause it is rapidly absorbed and its blood concentration peaks about 75 minutes after ingestion.

c. Between 60 and 90 per cent of patients with duodenal ulcers heal within four weeks.

d. About 85 per cent of patients with duodenal ulcers suffer acute episodes, which can be managed effectively without surgery.

e. During short-term therapy, side-effects are most unusual.

f. Symptoms of misuse of cimetidine should be noted: diarrhoea, dizziness, gynaecomastia, decreased sperm count, hallucinations, bradycardia.

g. Cimetidine is effective only in preventing bleeding from starting, not in stopping bleeding once it has started.

Dietary considerations

1. Eliminate foods that the patient says cause him pain or distress; otherwise the diet is unrestricted.

2. Offer regular milk, since the fat in milk decreases secretion. (Skimmed milk is usually not given, because the calcium in milk increases secretion.)

3. Give small servings to decrease distention and release of gastrin.

4. Provide frequent feedings to neutralize gastric secretions and to dilute stomach contents.

5. Advise the patient to avoid coffee and other caffeinated beverages and cola drinks.

6. Advise the patient to avoid hot or cold foods and fluids, to chew food thoroughly, and to eat in a leisurely fashion.

Modification in lifestyle to promote physical and mental rest

1. Encourage bed rest to reduce physical activity and to separate patient from usual environment.

2. Offer sedatives or tranquillizers to lessen the response to stimuli and to promote relaxation and sleep.

3. Provide frequent feedings, antacids, and other medications given on time.

4. Inform visitors to avoid upsetting conversation.

5. Emphasize the need to avoid anxiety-producing situations.

6. Alert the patient to the irritating effects on the gastric mucosa of certain drugs – especially aspirin and aspirin-containing drugs such as Alka-Seltzer.

7. Review the reasons for smaller meals and mid-meal snacks.

8. Suggest that he cut down on smoking; suggest switching from coffee and cola to caffeine-free beverages such as ginger ale, 7-Up.

Prevention of complications

1. Prevent complications by following therapeutic regimen.

2. Treat epigastric or 'warning' pain by taking an antacid.

3. Renew the taking of anti-ulcer medication if indiscretions have been 'unavoidable' – limited rest because of studying for tests, excess socializing with alcohol consumption, etc.

4. Practice coping measures to reduce stress.

5. Rest and notify doctor if black, tarry stool is noted; prepare for possible hospital admission.

PATIENT EDUCATION

1. Modify lifestyle to incorporate health practices that will prevent recurrences of ulcer pain, bleeding and distress.

2. Plan for rest periods and avoidance of stressful situations.

3. Chew food thoroughly and eat in leisurely manner on a regular schedule.

4. Avoid large meals, since they tend to overstimulate acid secretion.

5. Avoid irritating substances such as alcohol, coffee, cola, highly spiced foods, tart fresh fruits and rich pastries.

6. Avoid specific foods that cause this particular patient distress.

7. Assume responsibility for rejecting ulcerogenic drugs – aspirin, steroids.

8. Monitor one's practices – avoid fatigue, recognize signs of potential problems (mid-epigastric pain), walk away from stress-producing situations, reinstitute anti-ulcer medication if necessary.

Evaluation
EXPECTED OUTCOMES

1. Obtains relief from discomfort and pain of duodenal ulcer by following therapeutic regimen.

2. Reviews activity schedule and allocates time for rest periods to offset fatigue and tension.

3. Describes the therapeutic regimen to be followed to prevent recurrence of ulcers – such as avoiding caffeine, heavily spiced and fried food, stressful stiuations, irritating drugs (such as aspirin).

4. Lists signs that indicate potential complications and what to do about them, such as treating epigastric pain with an antacid and avoiding intake of aspirin or indomethacin.

COMPLICATIONS OF PEPTIC ULCER

Haemorrhage → shock
Perforation → peritonitis
Pyloric obstruction → dehydration
Intractability → incapacitation → surgery

Haemorrhage

1. Experienced by 15 to 25 per cent of patients with duodenal ulcer; accounts for 40 per cent of deaths from peptic ulcer.
2. Features:
   a. Giddiness, faintness, breathlessness with slight exertion.
   b. Tachycardia, sweating and coldness of extremities.
   c. Black, tarry stool (melaena) – test for occult blood.
   d. Vomiting of blood (haematemesis).
3. Medical and nursing interventions
   a. Encourage bed rest and check vital signs frequently.
   b. Give medication for restlessness or pain, but be on alert for shock.
   c. Employ nasogastric suction to empty stomach of clots and to monitor rate of bleeding.
   d. Give whole blood or blood component therapy to keep circulating blood volume at a safe level. (This is not needed if haematocrit is greater than 30 and vital signs are stable, with no orthostatic drop in blood pressure or rise in pulse.)
   e. Note colour, consistency and volume of stools and vomitus.
   f. Provide treatment if the patient goes into oligaemic shock (see p. 63).

Perforation

1. Clinical features:
   a. Severe upper abdominal pain, persisting and increasing in intensity and often spreading from upper to lower abdomen.
   b. Vomiting suddenly.
   c. Referring of pain to top of shoulders (phrenic nerve irritation).
   d. Abdomen – extremely tender and rigid.
   e. X-ray of abdomen – 50 per cent to 75 per cent free air visible.
   f. Shock.
   g. Patient lying still in bed, afraid to move; pain increased by the patient's coughing or jostling the bed.
2. Surgical intervention:
   a. Repair fluid deficit.
   b. Close perforation; plication of ulcers is per-

formed (see Postoperative Care, p. 445) if chronic symptoms preceded perforation.

Pyloric obstruction

1. Aetiology – area around pyloric sphincter becomes narrowed from spasm, oedema or scar tissue formed when ulcer alternately heals and breaks down. Inflammation, muscle spasm or oedema may cause a temporary obstruction.
2. Assessment and major manifestations – nausea, vomiting of retained food, constipation, weight loss, cramping, epigastric pain after meals.
3. Medical and nursing intervention:
   a. Gastric decompression and intravenous fluids.
   b. Later, test emptying with fluid load and then with solid bolus.
   c. Surgery may follow if clinical course is prolonged and obstruction is unrelieved.

Intractability

The failure of medical management to accomplish healing of the ulcer – usually a calloused posterior ulcer that penetrates into the pancreas.

1. Features – pain continues without adequate relief from milk or antacid.
2. Surgical intervention:
   a. Vagotomy and gastrojejunostomy or pyloroplasty – to abolish cephalic phase of secretion.
   b. Vagotomy and hemigastrectomy – to abolish cephalic and gastric phase of secretion.
   c. Gastric resection – to abolish acid-secreting parietal cells.

SURGICAL TREATMENT

Surgery is required in only about 15 to 20 per cent of ulcer patients; operation is individualized, based on patient's age, ability to withstand procedure, preoperative nutritional status and particular indications.

Goal:

Relieve complications:

1. Perforation (described above)
2. Haemorrhage (described above)
3. Pyloric obstruction (described above)
4. Intractability (described above).

Treat the tendency to ulcer formation.

Types of gastric operations

1. Gastrojejunostomy and vagotomy (Figure 7.5) – the jejunum is anastomosed to the stomach to provide a second outlet of gastric contents. The severed vagus nerve reduces secretions and

movements of the stomach (90 per cent good results).

2. Partial gastrectomy and vagotomy (Figure 7.6) – the resected portion includes a small cuff of duodenum, the pylorus, and the antrum (about one half of the stomach). The stump of the duodenum is closed by suture, and the side of the jejunum is anastomosed to the cut end of the stomach.

3. Subtotal gastrectomy (Figure 7.7) – the resected portion includes a small cuff of the duodenum, the pylorus, and from two-thirds to three-quarters of the stomach. The duodenum or side of the jejunum is anastomosed to the remaining portion of the stomach.

4. Vagotomy and pyloroplasty (Figure 7.8) – a longitudinal incision is made in the pylorus, and it is closed transversely to permit the muscle to relax and to establish an enlarged outlet. This compensates for the impaired gastric emptying produced by vagotomy.

Nursing management
(See p. 445, for management of the patient undergoing a gastric resection.)

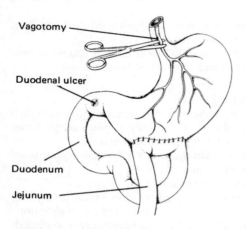

Figure 7.5. Gastrojejunostomy and vagotomy

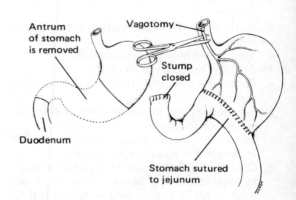

Figure 7.6. Partial gastrectomy (polya type) and vagotomy

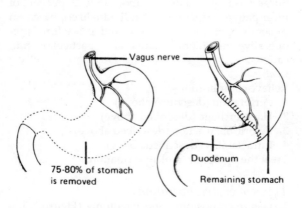

Figure 7.7. Subtotal gastrectomy. It is also possible to do the Billroth II procedure by suturing the gastric stump to the side of the jejunum

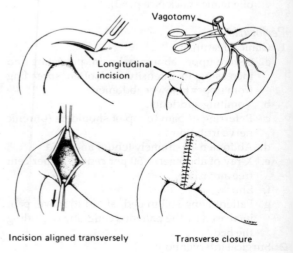

Figure 7.8. Vagotomy and pyloroplasty

GASTRIC CANCER

Cancer of the stomach accounted for 11,553 newly diagnosed cases in England and Wales in 1983; 7,060 were males with the highest number of cases in the 65–79 age group.

CLINICAL FEATURES
Early features
(Most often patient presents with same symptoms as gastric ulcer; later, on evaluation, the lesion is found to be malignant.)
1. Progressive loss of appetite.
2. Noticeable change in, or appearance of, gastro-intestinal symptoms – gastric fullness (early satiety), dyspepsia lasting more than four weeks.
3. Blood (usually occult) in the stools.
4. Vomiting, which may indicate pyloric obstruction or cardiac-orifice obstruction.
5. Occasionally, vomiting that has a 'coffee-ground' appearance because of slow leaks of blood from ulceration of the cancer.

Later features
1. Pain is a late symptom, often induced by eating and relieved by vomiting.
2. Weight loss, loss of strength, anaemia, metastasis (usually to liver), haemorrhage, obstruction.

DIAGNOSTIC EVALUATION
1. Nursing history – weight loss and loss of strength over several months.
2. Cytological examination of gastric juice, which may show cancer cells.
3. Palpable, unusual abdominal mass.
4. Suspicion of metastasis by palpable lymph nodes – surface of liver, skin at umbilicus, supraclavicular nodes, etc.
5. Gastric analysis – absence of acid after maximal stimulation (Histalog, gastrin) indicates that ulcer is malignant.
6. X-rays, fluoroscopy and gastroscopy also cytological studies and biopsy-fibroscopy.
7. Stool examination and tests for occult blood may be indicated.
8. Ultrasonography and computed tomography may be required. These are usually reserved for questionable diagnoses, since they are more costly tests.

TREATMENT
1. The only successful treatment of gastric cancer is surgical removal.
2. If tumour is localized to stomach and can be removed chances are still poor that the patient can be cured.
3. If tumour has spread beyond the area that can be excised surgically, cure cannot be accomplished. Palliative surgery such as subtotal gastrectomy with or without gastroenterostomy may be performed to maintain continuity of the gastro-intestinal tract. Surgery may be combined with chemotherapy to provide palliation and prolong life.

GASTRIC RESECTION

Gastric resection is the surgical removal of part of the stomach.

TREATMENT AND NURSING MANAGEMENT
Promote comfort and wound healing by relieving the patient of pain and discomfort
1. Frequently turn the patient and encourage deep-breathing to prevent vascular and pulmonary complications.
2. Institute nasogastric suction to remove fluids and gas in the stomach.
3. Provide conscientious mouth care to prevent mouth dryness and ulceration.
4. Administer parenteral antibiotics to prevent infection, as prescribed.
5. See that the patient has nothing by mouth until prescribed (to promote gastric wound healing).

Meet nutritional needs of the patient
1. Give intravenous fluids to prevent shock and to provide adequate fluid and electrolytes.
2. Give fluids by mouth when audible bowel signs are present.
3. Increase fluids according to the patient's tolerance.
4. Offer a diet with vitamin supplements when the patient's condition permits.
5. Give protein–vitamin supplements to foster wound repair and tissue building.
6. Avoid high-carbohydrate foods, such as milk, that may trigger 'dumping syndrome'.

Anticipate complications in order to prevent them
1. Shock and haemorrhage:
   a. Evaluate status of blood pressure, pulse and respiration.

b. Observe the patient for evidence of apathy, apprehension, air hunger, pallor or clammy skin.

c. Check the dressings and drainage bottle frequently for evidence of bleeding.

d. Administer fluid and blood as prescribed.

2. Cardiopulmonary complications:

a. Encourage the patient to cough and take deep breaths to produce ventilatory exchange and enhance circulation.

b. Assist the patient to turn and move, thereby mobilizing secretions.

c. Promote ambulation as prescribed to increase respiratory exchange.

3. Thrombosis and embolism:

a. Initiate a plan of self-care activities to promote circulation.

b. Encourage early ambulation to stimulate circulation.

c. Prevent venous stasis by use of elastic stockings if indicated.

d. Check for tight dressings that might restrict circulation.

4. 'Dumping syndrome' – a complex reaction, which may occur because of excessively rapid emptying of gastric contents.

Features – nausea, weakness, perspiration, palpitation, some syncope and possibly diarrhoea. Instruct the patient as follows:

a. Eat small, frequent meals rather than three large meals.

b. Suggest a diet high in protein and fat and low in carbohydrates, and avoid meals high in sugars, milk, chocolate, salt.

c. Reduce fluids with meals but take them between meals.

d. Take anticholinergic medication before meals (if prescribed) to lessen gastrointestinal activity.

e. Relax when eating; eat slowly and regularly.

f. Take a rest after meals.

5. Phytobezoar formation (formation of a gastric ball composed of vegetable matter):

a. Avoid fibrous foods such as citrus fruits (skins and seeds), because they tend to form phytobezoars.

(i) Following a gastric resection, the remaining gastric tissue is not able to disintegrate and digest fibrous foods.

(ii) This undigested fibre congeals to form masses that become coated by mucous secretions of the stomach.

b. Stress the importance of adequate mastication.

PATIENT EDUCATION

(Adjustment to self-care and return to the community.)

1. Emphasize the importance of coping with stressful situations.

2. Review nutritional requirements and regimen with the patient (Table 7.4).

3. Stress the importance of vitamin B_{12} supplements.

4. Encourage follow-up visits with the doctor.

5. Recommend annual blood studies and medical check-ups for any evidence of pernicious anaemia or other problems.

6. See 'dumping syndrome', in previous column.

Table 7.4   Diet guidelines following gastric surgery*

Food usually well tolerated

Meat, fish, poultry, eggs, cheese, refined breads and cereals (unsweetened)

Unsweetened canned fruits and juices

Cooked mild vegetables, including potatoes

Fats and oils

Foods to add as tolerance improves

Sweetened canned fruits*

Whole grains

Foods that often cause symptoms of dumping*

Sugar, sweets, syrup, sweetened desserts (cake, biscuits, pie, pudding, ice cream)

Foods and beverages to avoid

Cold high-carbohydrate items such as milkshakes, fruit ice

Coffee and tea (unless allowed by doctor)

Special considerations

Begin with *very* small portions; eat five to six times daily

Take most liquids between rather than with meals

Milk – include in early stages unless poorly tolerated

Fresh fruits and vegetables – gradually include after two to three weeks; chew thoroughly

---

* Add gradually to diet if desired unless bothered by symptoms of dumping or unless weight loss is a desirable goal. (Suitor, C.W. and Crowley, M.F. (1984) *Nutrition* (2nd edn), J.B. Lippincott, Philadelphia)

GASTROSTOMY

A gastrostomy is an opening into the stomach performed for the purpose of administering food and fluids when a complete obstruction of the oesophagus exists. The obstruction may be due to scartissue contracture such as may result from acid burn or a carcinomatous growth. A gastrostomy may also be done occasionally in the unconscious or debilitated patient for prolonged nutritional support.

PREOPERATIVE PATIENT CARE
1. Explain the nature of the problem and the recommended treatment to the patient; use simple line drawings for clarification.
2. Achieve adequate fluid, electrolyte, and nutritional balance by administering the required foods and fluids.
3. Immediate preoperative care is similar to that described on page 45.

SURGERY
1. Frequently performed under local anaesthesia.

2. The anterior gastric wall is incised through a left rectus incision.
3. A tube is inserted and held in place in the stomach wall with several purse-string sutures. The tube may be a rubber tube or a Foley catheter inflated with 5–8ml of water or air and pulled taut to the abdominal wall.
4. The skin is closed close to the tube to prevent leakage.
5. The tube is clamped at all times except for feedings.

GUIDELINES: ASSISTING THE PATIENT WITH GASTROSTOMY FEEDINGS

PURPOSE
To provide a means of alimentation when the oral route is inaccessible.

TYPES OF FEEDINGS
1. Powdered feedings that are easily liquified are commercially available.
2. Avoid milk in excess in lactate-deficient patients.

PROCEDURE
Preparatory phase
1. Food blender is very useful in preparing a normal diet; blended food is physiologically more acceptable, since fibre and residue content are retained and good bowel function is promoted.
2. Prepare a tray containing a funnel, tubing and adapter, and water at room temperature.
3. Pour feed into a graduated container; warm to 37.8°C in a basin of water.
4. Begin feeding the patient when peristalsis has returned.
5. Place the patient in upright position unless contraindicated.
6. Place a half-sheet or bath towel over upper half of patient; fold top bedding down to cover the patient from the waist downward. This permits a space for gastrostomy tube exposure.

Performance phase

Nursing action	Rationale
1. Connect funnel to tubing and connecting tube.	
2. Uncover opening of gastrostomy (or jejunostomy) tube and insert connecting tube.	Provides a receptacle for feeding that will lead into gastrostomy tube.
3. Pour feeding into tilted funnel, unclamp tubing and allow fluid to flow into the stomach by gravity.	Tilting the funnel allows air bubbles to escape; when tubing is unclamped, air bubbles will not enter stomach.

| 4. Regulate flow by raising or lowering receptacle. | Raising increases pressure; lowering decreases pressure. |

NURSING ALERT
Force should not be used nor should feeding be given directly from the refrigerator; such action would cause abdominal discomfort to the patient. If there appears to be an obstruction, stop feeding and report the problem.

5. After each feeding, the tube is irrigated with water (room temperature) and clamped.	A water flush prevents the tube from clogging and assists in keeping it clean.
6. Apply a small dressing over the tube opening, using a rubber band to keep it in place.	This keeps the tube opening clean for the next feeding.
7. Twist a thin strip of adhesive around tube and attach firmly to abdomen, or coil the tubing on a dressing.	Prevents the tubing from being accidentally pulled out of the stomach.
8. Cover tubing with a dressing and apply a firm bandage to hold in place.	Provides maximum mobility for the patient.

TUBE FEEDING (GASTRIC GAVAGE)

Gastric gavage is the introduction of liquid feedings directly into the stomach.

PURPOSE
1. Effective in persons who have difficulty swallowing (dysphagia), prolonged unconsciousness or anorexia.
2. Useful when there is oral or oesophageal obstruction or trauma.
3. Life-saving in one who is debilitated or who has had surgery on some part of the gastrointestinal tract that does not permit normal ingestion of food.

AVENUES
These vary with the patient and circumstances (Figure 7.9).
1. Nasogastric – orogastric – see Guidelines, p. 430.
2. Oesophagotomy – a stoma (temporary or permanent) may be created at one of several sites along the oesophagus.
   a. The feeding tube is introduced through the skin directly into the oesophagus.
   b. The tube is usually removed between meals, making this method easy to manage.

3. Gastrostomy – see p. 446 and Guidelines, p. 447.
4. Jejunostomy – an abdominal stoma is constructed providing direct access to the jejunum.
   a. This is advantageous when the stomach must be bypassed.
   b. Disadvantages are the high incidence of diarrhoea and dumping syndrome.

FEEDING ELEMENTS
1. Formulae may be prepared or purchased commercially – 'elemental' diets.
2. Doctor orders type, amount and frequency.

FEEDING METHODS
1. Gravity – a funnel or large syringe (minus bulb) is used as the receptacle for feedings. The rate of flow is affected by raising or lowering receptacle.
2. Drip-regulated:
   a. A Murphy drip is connected by tubing to a receptacle (Kelly flask), which hangs on an intravenous pole.
   b. From the other end of the Murphy drip, tubing is connected to the feeding tube.
   c. The rate of flow of liquid can be adjusted.
   d. Requires thorough cleaning or may be disposable. Consider cost.
3. Motor pump – feeding is delivered at a preset rate.

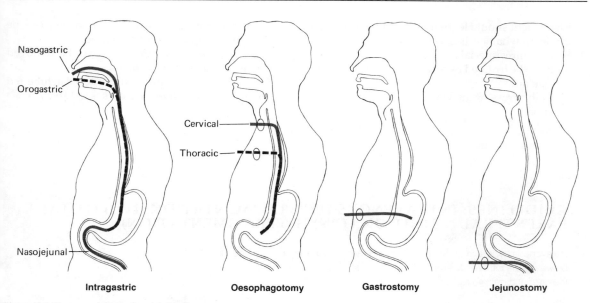

Figure 7.9. Types and sites of gastric feeding

Intragastric (nasogastric): A tube is passed through the nose or mouth into the stomach and secured in place. (A tube passed through the mouth is more correctly called an orogastric tube. This is ordinarily inserted at meal times and removed following the meal.) Intragastric tube preferred for short-term tube feeding; easily inserted by doctor or nurse, remains in place between feedings. (Some clients are taught to insert their own tube; they may remove the tube between meals.) Variations include nasopharyngeal and nasojejunal feeding tubes

Oesophagotomy: A temporary or permanent opening (stoma) is constructed at one of several sites to allow a tube to be introduced through the skin into the oesophagus. Feeding tube is usually removed between meals. Advantages – dependable for long-term feeding, allows concealment of apparatus, easy to handle

Gastrostomy: A temporary or permanent stoma is constructed, allowing food to be introduced through the skin directly into the stomach. Preferred for long-term tube feeding of children and for long-term feeding of adults when use of oesophagus is contraindicated. Disadvantages – partial undressing necessary at meal times, skin care may pose problems

Jejunostomy: A stoma is constructed to give direct access to the jejunum. This method of feeding may be used when the stomach must be bypassed. Disadvantages – high incidence of dumping syndrome and diarrhoea; adequate nutrient intake difficult to maintain (Suitor, C.W. and Crowley, M.F. (1984) *Nutrition. Principles and Application in Health Promotion,* J.B. Lippincott, Philadelphia, p. 391)

CONTINUOUS NURSING ASSESSMENT

1. Recognize that even though some nutritional deficits are corrected, other problems may arise, such as fluid deficit, electrolyte imbalance, diarrhoea, oesophageal reflux.
2. Cleanse all containers and tubing thoroughly; formulae and feedings make excellent media for bacterial growth.
3. Aspirate the tubing prior to feeding to verify that the tube is in place.
4. Avoid air bubbles in the system, which could cause distention.
5. Provide oral and nasal hygiene before and after orogastric and nasogastric feedings for comfort and to prevent infection.
6. Follow last amount of each feeding with water to flush tubing for cleansing and to promote fluid balance.
7. Monitor the patient for signs of fluid and electrolyte imbalance.
8. Record amount of feeding and water; indicate the patient's participation and acceptance.
9. See Table 7.5 regarding problems that may be encountered and examples of corrective measures.

PATIENT EDUCATION

1. Since the tube should be changed every two or three days, the patient may be taught how to do it. (The tube should be clean but not necessarily sterile.)

2. The patient should learn how to feed himself. (He can learn what foods may be taken.)
3. Skin requires special care.
   a. It can be irritated by action of gastric juices that leak out.
   b. Daily dressing of wound averts skin maceration.

   c. Bland ointment, such as zinc oxide, can be applied to area around the tube.
4. After several weeks, the tube may be removed and inserted only for feedings.
5. For problems that may be encountered in tube-fed clients and corrective measures, see Table 7.5.

GUIDELINES: INTRAVENOUS HYPERALIMENTATION (IVH) (TOTAL PARENTERAL NUTRITION (TPN) HYPERALIMENTATION)

Intravenous hyperalimentation (IVH) is a means of providing body nutrients by way of the intravenous route when it is impossible or inadvisable to use the normal digestive routes.

PHYSIOLOGICAL BASIS
1. The intravenous route has heretofore not provided adequate nutrition; caloric and nitrogen deficiencies occurred.
2. Because of nutritional deficiencies, the process of *gluconeogenesis* takes place; this is the body's conversion of protein to carbohydrate.
3. Approximately 1,500 calories/day are required by the average adult postoperative patient to prevent body protein from being utilized.
4. Body needs are increased when the patient has a hypermetabolic disease, a fever or injury – these needs may require up to 10,000 calories daily.
5. To meet the fluid volume necessary to provide so many additional calories would exceed fluid tolerance and lead to pulmonary oedema or congestive heart failure.
6. This process (IVH) provides desired calories in concentration directly into the intravenous system, which rapidly dilutes incoming nutrients to satisfactory levels of body tolerance.
   a. Hypertonic glucose → fulfils caloric requirement → permits amino acids to be released for protein synthesis (not energy).
   b. Potassium → provides proper electrolyte balance → transports glucose and amino acids across cell membranes.
   c. Calcium, magnesium and sodium chloride → meet cell requirements as determined by serum electrolyte needs.
   d. Other trace elements whose function is not known may be deficient in IVH, since they are not included.

CLINICAL INDICATIONS
1. As a substitute for oral or nasogastric intubation when these are not effective, undesirable, or even hazardous. Use IVH under the following conditions:
   a. Chronic vomiting;
   b. Cancer, chemotherapy or radiotherapy;
   c. Cerebrovascular accident;
   d. Anorexia nervosa.

Table 7.5   Potential problems in tube-fed clients and examples of corrective measures

Factors to assess	Possible causes of problems	Corrective measures
Gastrointestinal function		
Vomiting	Feeding too soon after intubation	Allow patient time to relax and rest after tube is inserted
	Improper location of tip of feeding tube	Qualified health professional should reposition tube
	Rapid rate of infusion	Administer slowly
	Excessive volume	
	Air	Be sure tube feeding container does not run dry before feeding is completed
	Formula	Check with doctor regarding number and size of feedings
	Position of patient	Position on right side for 30 minutes following feeding
Applies to both vomiting and diarrhoea	Food infection or poisoning	Check sanitation of formula and equipment
	Anxiety	Explain procedures; provide reassurance and other needed types of support; provide privacy
Diarrhoea	Rapid rate of infusion	Administer slowly – very slowly if formula is cold
	High osmolarity of formula or high concentration of formula	Adapt the patient to formula gradually
	Lactose intolerance	Contact doctor regarding change of formula
Constipation	Lack of fibre	Contact doctor regarding:
	Inadequate fluid intake	Change in formula
		Laxatives
		Increasing fluid
Fluid and electrolyte balance		
Dehydration	Rapid infusion of carbohydrate → hyperglycaemia → osmotic diuresis → dehydration	Administer slowly; exogenous insulin is sometimes needed
	Excess protein and electrolytes in formula	Change formula and/or increase fluid according to doctor's requests
	Inadequate fluid intake	
Oedema	Excessive sodium in formula	Check with doctor about change in formula
Nutritional adequacy		
Undernutrition (gradual weight loss)	Inadequate number of calories to meet energy requirements	Check to see if the patient is receiving prescribed amount of formula. Estimate the patient's calorie intake
		Check with doctor regarding increasing the volume, concentration or number of feedings given
Overnutrition (gradual, undesirable gain of weight)	Excessive caloric intake	Check with doctor regarding decreasing the volume, concentration or number of feedings given
Undernutrition (inadequate intake of protein and/or micronutrients leading to biochemical or clinical signs of deficiency)	Amount of standard formula needed to maintain weight is too low to meet requirements for essential nutrients	Check with doctor regarding providing appropriate nutrient supplements

(Suitor, C.W. and Crowley, M.F. (1984) *Nutrition* (2nd edn), J.B. Lippincott, Philadelphia)

2. As a supplement for patients demonstrating large nitrogen losses (e.g. burn patients, those with metastatic cancer and those who are receiving radiation and chemotherapy).
3. As a means of putting the gastrointestinal tract at rest.
   a. When there is evidence of gastrointestinal fistula;
   b. With severe and extensive inflammatory bowel disease;
   c. Following major intestinal resection;
   d. Instances of intestinal obstruction.

EQUIPMENT

Skin antiseptic
Sterile drapes and gloves
20ml syringe
No. 14 (5cm) needle
No. 16 gauge 20cm radio-opaque catheter

Connecting tubing and adapters
250ml container of 50% dextrose
3 × 3 dressing – adhesive for occlusive dressing
Suture material

PROCEDURE – FOR SUBCLAVIAN VEIN CATHETERIZATION
Preparatory phase – nurse

Nursing action/doctor's action	Rationale
1. Explain the procedure to the patient and why it is important for him not to touch the area where the catheter is inserted.	To provide reassurance; to prevent dislodging and contaminating catheter.
2. Tell the patient that he will probably be ambulatory during the extended time of therapy.	In the absence of other conditions requiring bed rest, ambulation is possible.
3. Place patient in head-low position.	This position permits dilatation of neck and shoulder vessels, which makes catheter entry easier and prevents air embolus.
4. Suggest that the patient turn his face away from the area selected.	To prevent contamination of TPN site.
5. Support the patient in proper position to permit hyperextension of shoulder.	This position can be facilitated by placing a rolled sheet or towel vertically along spinal column.
6. Use depilatory or shave area if necessary.	To reduce probability of contamination to the barest minimum.
7. Instruct the patient to be still during insertion of catheter.	To prevent the possibility of dislodging of catheter and perforation of subclavian vein.

Performance phase (doctor)

Doctor's action	Rationale
1. Prepare area with antiseptic and place sterile cover in proper position.	To prevent infection.

2. Inject local anaesthesia to skin and underlying tissues.

To promote comfort of patient and prevent patient movement.

3. Using a no. 14 (5cm) needle with syringe, insert needle beneath the clavicle and into subclavian vein.

Subclavian vein is selected because it leads into the superior vena cava, which has a large volume of blood flow, and provides rapid dilution of hypertonic solution.

4. Instruct the patient to perform Valsalva manoeuvre.

By the patient's bearing down with mouth closed, positive pressure is produced when syringe and needle are replaced by catheter.

5. Detach syringe and insert a no. 16 gauge 20cm radio-opaque catheter through the needle into the vein; withdraw needle.

This permits the more flexible catheter to remain in position during subsequent feedings.

6. Attach Intra-Cath to tubing from a bag of 50 per cent dextrose in water.

To keep tube patent between feedings and to provide calories.

7. Prepare the patient for X-ray.

To ensure that tip of catheter is in proper location.

NURSING ALERT AND PRIORITIES OF CARE
Patients receiving hyperalimentation are particularly susceptible to catheter-related infections. To minimize these complications:
1. Solutions are to be prepared under a laminar flow hood.
2. Solutions are prepared fresh daily and refrigerated until used.
Maintain sterility during entire IVH procedure to prevent sepsis.
Maintain consistent infusion rate, which is calculated on a 24-hour basis.
Monitor patient carefully – including vital signs.
Record data accurately.
Provide emotional support to the patient.

Follow-up phase

Nursing action

Rationale

1. Remind the patient not to touch dressings.

Permit the patient to turn in bed or to ambulate, but caution him against handling dressings, which would cause contamination.

2. Check infusion rate every 30 minutes. Adjust infusion rate to not more than 10 per cent of the original rate if too fast or too slow.

If too rapid → hypermolar diuresis occurs → excess sugar is excreted → intractable seizures occur → coma → death.
If too slow → inadequate nutritional intake.

3. Weigh the patient daily and keep accurate intake and output records.

Accurate comparison of daily weight change is noted.

4. Check vital signs every four hours.

Note temperature rise, which could signify a complication.

5. Change dressings every 48 to 72 hours and as required.

Strict aseptic technique must be followed.

6. Intravenous tubing and filters must be changed daily.

Procedure is done by a nurse especially trained to do this.

7. Encourage diversional therapy and activity during extended therapy.

This distracts the patient from the procedure and promotes assimilation of nutrients.

GUIDELINES: INTRAVENOUS FAT EMULSION

Intravenous fat emulsion is a form of essential fatty acids that can be administered to the patient intravenously when these essential nutrients are needed and cannot be acquired in any other way. Lipid emulsions (10 and 20 per cent) may be 'fed' onto the hyperalimentation solution and administered by this central line.

CHIEF ADVANTAGE
A concentrated amount of essential fatty acids and calories can be supplied in a relatively small volume of liquid.

CLINICAL INDICATIONS
Treatment or prevention of essential fatty acid deficiencies that may be due to:
1. Severe nutritional disorders and inability to take nourishment by mouth.
2. Malignancies, burns, ulcerative colitis, severe renal disorders, nonfunctional gastrointestinal tracts.
3. Extended semiconsciousness or unconsciousness.
4. Specific preoperative and postoperative patients in whom it is necessary to increase caloric intake.
5. Essential fatty acid deficiencies – characterized by sparse hair growth, eczematous scaly skin lesions, thrombocytopenia, and poor wound healing.

ACTION
1. Lipid emulsion is introduced into the blood; protein in the blood acts as emulsifier (lipid–protein complex).
2. The lipid–protein complex carries nutrients to the liver, adipose tissue, etc., where they are degraded, synthesized, stored, mobilized and oxidized for energy.
3. It is delivered with amino acid dextrose solution in order not to deplete the patient's protein resources.

EQUIPMENT
Amino acid dextrose solution
Fat emulsion
Y-type nonphthalate administration set:
    Vented line for fat emulsion
    Nonvented line (with filter) for amino acid dextrose solution

NURSING ALERT
Use the administration set as recommended by the manufacturer, since some plastics in combination with lipids cause leaching of diethylhexyl phthalate.

PROCEDURE
Preparatory phase

Nursing action	Rationale
1. Do not shake emulsion flask.	Agitation of emulsion may cause fat globules to aggregate.
2. Inspect flask of fat emulsion.	Look for signs of altered stability: Inconsistency in texture and colour; Separation of oil.
3. Connect tubing to emulsion flask and clear tubing of all air (do not use the pump to prime tubing but use gravity only).	Air in system may cause an air embolus in the patient.
4. Connect intravenous tubing to Y-tube connection closest to insertion site; insert tubing primed with intravenous fat emulsion directly into this site.	This reduces length of time emulsion comes in contact with substances that may affect its stability.
5. Do not use in-line filters.	Particles are too large to go through a filter.
6. If infusion is to be administered by gravity drip, hang fat emulsion flask higher than flask of amino acid solution.	This will prevent backflow of fat emulsion (less density) into other amino acid flask (higher density).*
7. Explain procedure to the patient; tell him that the milk-white solution is unlike other solutions he has received intravenously. Remind him that he is not to leave the unit while this emulsion is running.	Patient will have a better understanding of the reason for more frequent vital signs and other observations.
8. Document the patient's vital signs.	These will be used as a baseline comparison for later evaluation.

Performance phase

Nursing action	Rationale
1. Start flow rate at 1ml/minute for first 30 minutes; monitor vital signs every 10 minutes during this time.	Provides opportunity to assess patient for chills, fever, headache, dizziness, sleepiness, allergic reactions, back pain, chest pain, nausea, vomiting, pressure over eyes, etc.

* Pennington and Richards (1983) Three-litre bags containing Intralipid for parenteral nutrition (letter), *Journal of Parenteral/Enteral Nutrition*, Vol. 7, No. 3, p. 304 (suggest combining Intralipid in parenteral nutrition formulations).

2. If untoward signs occur, stop infusion and notify doctor.

3. If problems occur, doctor may prescribe heparin.

    Heparin will hasten clearing of lipids from the patient's plasma.

4. If no complications occur, infusion rate may be increased – a good gauge is to administer 500ml in four to six hours.

    Continue constant observation; monitor vital signs hourly.

5. At conclusion of infusion, detach emulsion flask and attach flask of 5 per cent dextrose as per doctor's request.

    Dextrose flushes out remaining fat emulsion from tubing.

Follow-up phase

Nursing action

Rationale

1. When dextrose has run in, clamp tubing securely until next lipid emulsion is to be given. If this is final treatment, disconnect as with any intravenous treatment.

2. Continue to be alert for delayed adverse reactions.

    Fat overload syndrome manifestations – headache, low-grade fever, nausea, abdominal pain, irritability.*

3. Record the nature of lipid emulsion given, amount, time, patient reactions, time of termination of procedure.

    Include documentation of vital signs.

4. Doctor will request periodic serum triglyceride levels and liver function studies.

    These will provide indicators of the patient's ability to metabolize and clear the emulsion from the bloodstream.

5. Monitor the patient for effectiveness of this treatment. Observe for changes in his clinical status.

    This would determine effectiveness in treating an essential fatty acid deficiency.

GUIDELINES: DUODENAL DRAINAGE

PURPOSES

1. To detect abnormal constituents of bile, pancreatic juice, or duodenal fluid.
2. To assist in diagnosis of cholelithiasis (gallstones), choledocholithiasis (common duct stones), pancreatitis and pancreatic carcinoma.
3. To assist in diagnosing gallbladder problems if X-rays prove inadequate.
4. To assist in parasitological studies, especially in detection of *Giardia intestinalis*.

---

* This may be indicative of splenomegaly, hepatomegaly, hyperlipaemia, thrombocytopenia, jaundice, gastroduodenal ulcer.

EQUIPMENT

Rehfuss' tube (metal tip) with markings: 45, 60, 65, 70
    and 90cm (or rubber tubing with mercury-weighted
    bag)
Clamp for tubing
Towel and vomit bowl
Glass of water; straw
Container for specimen

30g of magnesium sulphate in 50ml of water
Optional: Clear plastic tubing (7.5cm) to use as a
             sleeve over rubber tubing; this can be
             slipped over tubing and kept near
             patient's teeth to prevent biting of rubber
             tubing

PROCEDURE
Preparatory phase

Nursing action	Rationale
1. Explain procedure to the patient and tell him how to breathe through mouth and swallow.	This can help in passing the tube.
2. Have the patient in a chair or upright position in bed, with neck flexed; place a towel across his chest.	This position will facilitate passing of tube utilizing gravity.
3. Determine with the patient what sign he might use to indicate retching or discomfort.	Such as raising his index finger to indicate 'wait a few moments'.
4. Remove dentures.	To prevent their becoming dislodged during procedure and even obstructing airway.

Performance phase (by the doctor assisted by nurse)

Nursing action	Rationale
1. Ask the patient to open his mouth and breathe through it.	Mouth-breathing facilitates the relaxation process.
2. Place the tube's metal tip or the tubing with the mercury bag on the back of the tongue.	Proper positioning of the tip encourages and promotes swallowing.
3. Ask the patient to close his mouth (without biting the tubing) and swallow.	
4. Permit the patient to drink water through a straw as he swallows tubing until the 45cm mark is reached. It is even better to have him suck on ice chips.	Water aids in lubricating and swallowing. However, avoid administering more than 100ml in volume.
5. Instruct the patient to sit in chair or on edge of bed and to lean forward with elbows on his knees. The tube is slowly advanced to the 60cm mark.	These are all manoeuvres that have been found helpful in permitting the tube to pass through.

6. Next have the patient curl up on his *right* side with hips on a pillow and shoulders low. Advance tube to the 70cm mark.

The tube tip should be in the second portion of the duodenum (Figure 7.10). Check to see if bile can be aspirated and if the pH is greater than 7.0.

7. The patient is then rolled over on his back for five minutes.

8. Drainage procedure may now take place with the patient in right lateral position. The following are ways of testing to see if tube is in duodenum:
   a. Aspirate gently – inspect fluid; instil 30ml water.
   b. Instil 30ml air rapidly and aspirate immediately; if as much as 5ml can be recovered, the tip is probably in the stomach.
   c. Use a stethoscope to locate tube's tip as air is slowly injected through tubing by syringe.

Record colour, amount and consistency of bile, as well as duration of flow (normal – clear, golden brown). Usually no air can be recovered from the duodenum.

A bubbling sound is substantially louder than elsewhere. The spot should be small and well to the right of the midline. If bubbling can be heard over an area as large as the hand, the tip is in the stomach.

   d. To be absolutely sure of position of tube, check position fluoroscopically.

9. Anchor tube by using plastic guard.

To prevent the patient biting the rubber tube.

10. Collect specimens as directed by gravity drainage or by low-pressure intermittent suction with container on floor. If the tube is determined to be in the duodenum, an appropriate stimulant is injected and collection begins.
    a. Administer magnesium sulphate solution to stimulate relaxation of sphincter of Oddi and contraction of gallbladder.
    b. Administer secretin or secretin-CCK if directed to stimulate pancreatic secretion. Measure volume, bicarbonate concentration and amylase content.

Done if gallbladder function is to be evaluated.

Done if pancreatic function is to be evaluated.

Follow-up phase

Nursing action

Rationale

1. At conclusion of test, slowly withdraw tubing.

Rapid withdrawal may be injurious to mucous lining because of metal tip; teeth also may be injured by metal tip.

2. Offer toothbrush and paste or mouthwash.

To freshen mouth.

3. Record test and patient's reaction.

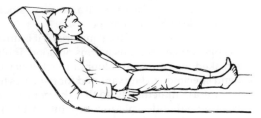

1. With patient in sitting position pass tube to 45cm mark.

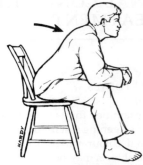

2. Have patient sit up (this may be in bed or in a chair), leaning forward, sway back, with elbows on knees. Slowly advance tube to 60cm mark.

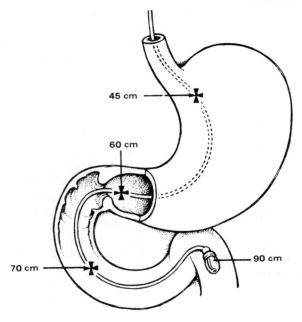

45 cm

60 cm

70 cm

90 cm

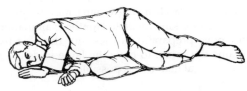

3. Then have patient curl up on right side with hips on a pillow and shoulder low. Tube is advanced to 70cm mark.

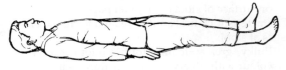

4. Turn patient on back for a few minutes.

5. Now turn patient to the right lateral position for collection of drainage. (Same as 3.)

Figure 7.10. Positions to be assumed by the patient in passing a duodenal drainage tube. Note on the central diagram how the tubing is advanced by each position change

INTESTINAL CONDITIONS AND TREATMENT

DIAGNOSTIC STUDIES

Stool specimen

1. The stool is examined for its amount, consistency and colour; a screening test for occult blood is also done. Normal colour varies from light to dark brown. Special tests may be made for faecal urobilinogen, fat, nitrogen, parasites, food residue and other substances.
2. Various foods affect stool colour:
   a. Meat protein – dark brown;
   b. Spinach – green;
   c. Beetroot – red;
   d. Cocoa – dark red or brown;
   e. Liquorice – black.
3. Various medications affect stool colour:
   a. Phenylbutazone (Butazolidin) – black;
   b. Oxyphenbutazone (Tanderil) – black; phenazopyridine (Pyridium) – orange–black;
   c. Aluminium hydroxide – grey–white;
   d. Viprynium embonate – red–orange;
   e. Bismuth compounds – black;
   f. Senna laxatives – yellow–green;
   g. Haematinics (iron salts) – black;
   h. Barium – white.
4. Haemoglobin and bleeding affect the stool in the following way:
   a. Considerable quantities of haemoglobin – occult blood (not visible to naked eye); use 'Haemoccult Stool' testing packet;
   b. Upper gastrointestinal bleeding – tarry black (melaena);
   c. Lower gastrointestinal bleeding – bright red blood;
   d. Lower rectal or anal bleeding – blood streaking on surface of stool or on toilet paper.
5. Characteristic clinical entities related to characteristics of stool:
   a. Bulky, greasy, foamy, foul in odour, grey in colour with silvery sheen – steatorrhoea;
   b. Light grey 'clay-coloured' (due to absence of 'acholic' bile pigments) – biliary obstruction;
   c. Mucus or pus visible – chronic ulcerative colitis, shigellosis;
   d. Small, dry, rocky-hard masses – constipation, obstipation, faecal obstruction;
   e. Marble-sized stool pellets – spastic colon syndrome.

Nursing management

1. Use a spatula to place a small amount of stool in a disposable waxed container.
2. Save a sample of any faecal material if it is unusual in appearance, contains worms or blood, is blood-streaked, has unusual colour or much mucus.
3. Send specimen to be examined for parasites to the laboratory immediately so that the parasites may be observed under microscope while viable, fresh and warm.
4. Test for occult blood or to confirm grossly visible melaena or blood.

Radiography of the colon – barium enema

The fasting patient receives a rectal installation of a barium sulphate suspension, which is viewed in the fluoroscope and then filmed. If the patient is adequately prepared, fluoroscope will reveal:
1. Colon – contour of entire colon is visible;
2. Caecum and appendix – contour and motility observed.

Note: Air may be induced to give air contrast studies.

Nursing management and patient instruction

1. Explain to the patient:
   a. What the X-ray procedure involves;
   b. That proper preparation provides a more accurate view of the tract;
   c. That it is important to retain the barium so that all surfaces of the tract are coated with opaque solution.
2. Two days before the examination, the patient may be given a minimal-residue diet.
3. The day before the examination, some doctors limit food intake to liquids; others advise liquids for the evening meal only.
4. The day before the examination, an aperient may be prescribed.
5. The evening before and on the morning of the examination, a cleansing enema may be given. Food and fluids are restricted for the examination.
6. The above preparation varies, but the objective remains the same: to have the large intestine as clear of faecal material as possible.

NURSING ALERT

Use nursing judgment regarding the administration of purgatives or enemata in the presence of acute abdominal pain or obstruction. For the patient with ulcerative colitis, purgatives or cleansing enemas may be too rigorous, and can possibly cause bleeding.

7. Administer an oil-retention enema or an aperient following the barium enema to completely evacuate the barium.

8. Encourage the patient to eat following the examination, since he has been fasting and is undoubtedly hungry.

Visualization measures

1. Two visualization measures are sigmoidoscopy and colonoscopy.

2. The details of these two procedures are presented in the Guidelines on pp. 462 and 464.

GUIDELINES: NASOINTESTINAL INTUBATION (LONG TUBE)

PURPOSES

1. To remove fluid and flatus from the intestinal tract (decompression).
2. To assess gastrointestinal bleeding.

EQUIPMENT

(Choice made by doctor)

1. Type of tube

   Single-lumen tube: Harris, Cantor

   Distal end has a small rubber bag weighted with mercury; suction openings are proximal to bag.

   Some single-lumen tubes use air to inflate balloon or have a metal bulb at distal end.

   Double-lumen tube: Miller–Abbott

   a. One outlet is for drainage.

   b. The other outlet is for filling the small rubber bag near the distal end.

2. Tube selection:

   a. Miller–Abbott tube is used in presence of mechanical bowel obstruction with hyperactive bowel sounds.

   b. Other tubes are used for adynamic ileus (absent bowel sounds).

PROCEDURE

Preparatory and performance phases

NURSING ALERT

All tubes and endoscopes should be pretested routinely for patency and function before passage.

Doctor's action – nurse-assisted	Rationale
1. Similar to passing a short nasogastric tube (p. 430). Exception: Miller–Abbott. Carry out the procedure as follows:	
a. Pretest the bag volume; the proper amount of air will fill the bag to just less than full distended (slightly compressible).	This will ensure that the bag is not leaky.
b. Place 1ml mercury in the bag after it is in the stomach.	This helps to pass tubing through the pylorus.
c. After duodenum has been entered, instil 20–50ml air in bag according to pretested volume; place other opening on suction.	This position checked by X-ray. Air-filled bag acts as a bolus and is carried distally by peristatic action as suction evacuates retained air and fluid just ahead of bag.

2. After the tubing enters the stomach, it passes by peristalsis and gravity into the small intestine.
   a. Change position from upright to a position in which the patient is leaning forward.

3. Upon X-ray confirmation that the tubing is past the pylorus, permit the patient to ambulate.

This will assist in advancing the tubing to and through the pylorus; tilting to the right is helpful.

Passing the tube through the pylorus and into the duodenum under fluoroscopic guidance allows the entire procedure to be completed in less than 15 minutes with little patient discomfort.

Nursing action

4. At specified time intervals, advance tubing 5–10cm.

5. Tubing may be taped to the face, and suction may be applied when the tubing tip has reached its destination.

6. Measure drainage; record its characteristics every eight hours.

Rationale

Doctor may prescribe or suggest these times.

NURSING ALERT
If drainage is clear and up to 3,000ml obtained/day, there is complete intestinal obstruction. If drainage is yellow with a faecal odour, the patient may have an obstruction of the small intestine.

Follow-up phase

Nursing action

1. Similar to short nasogastric tube.

2. Exception: in removing tubing, patient may feel tube resistance and become nauseated.

3. As tubing is drawn through posterior nasopharynx, have the patient open his mouth so that balloon or bag can be grasped with a clamp. Withdraw remaining tubing through the nose.

4. If tubing has advanced beyond the ileocaecal valve, the doctor may release it so that it can pass through the gastrointestinal tract. Peristalsis aids in passing the tubing.

Rationale

See page 430.

Due to action of sphincters through which the tube is withdrawn.

This permits balloon or bag to be removed through the mouth.

After distal tube has been retrieved at the rectum, the proximal end can be released at the nose.

GUIDELINES: SIGMOIDOSCOPY

A sigmoidoscopy is the viewing of the lumen of the sigmoid and rectum by means of a sigmoidoscope, a tubular instrument that can be illuminated.

EQUIPMENT

Disposable enema – used at least one hour before the sigmoidoscopy

Water-soluble lubricant

Sigmoidoscope – a two-part instrument (obturator and cannula); and a long, thin metal tube with light bulb at one end

Glass eyepiece to fit on scope during insufflation of air

Inflation bulb

Long applicator sticks (cotton)

Disposable gloves for preliminary digital examination

PROCEDURE

Preparatory phase

1. An hour before the sigmoidoscopy, a disposable enema may be administered by the nurse (or by the patient himself).
2. The enema is retained for five minutes before being evacuated.
3. Some doctors request that the patient be on a light diet the evening before and the breakfast before the examination. Others prefer an aperient the evening prior to the examination.

Performance phase

Nursing action	Rationale
1. Have the patient assume the knee–chest or Sims' lateral position.	The position used depends on doctor's preference, patient condition, and nature of examining table (or bed).
a. Knee–chest position:	The position permits the sigmoid to hang forward, diminishing the angle at the rectosigmoid junction.
(i) Knees are spread comfortably apart;	
(ii) Thighs are perpendicular to table;	
(iii) Feet are extended over the edge;	
(iv) Head is turned sideways to right (head shares pillow with chest);	
(v) Left arm is flexed to side of chest;	
(vi) Right arm may rest above head.	
b. Sims' lateral position:	Used for elderly, ill, or arthritic patients or those who are reluctant to assume the knee–chest position.
(i) Place patient on left side with left leg partially flexed at hip and knees; right leg should be fully flexed;	
(ii) Pelvis to be perpendicular to table.	
2. Drape the patient so that only the perineum is visible.	A disposable large sheet with a circular opening is practical.
3. Check scope lights after connecting cord to battery.	
4. Doctor first examines anal and perianal region. Digital examination indicates the direction of the anal canal, its patency and the presence of any abnormality.	The purpose is to note inflammation, fistula and ulceration. Digital examination also promotes anal relaxation and helps to lubricate orifice.

Nursing action	Rationale
5. Warm sigmoidoscope in tap water or sterilizer to slightly above body temperature; lubricate tip of scope.	A cold scope would cause discomfort and promote contraction rather than relaxation of perianal muscles. Water-soluble lubricant permits easier passage of scope.
6. Doctor spreads buttocks and anal margins with left hand and inserts instrument with right hand (or vice versa).	Keep instrument out of view of patient.
7. Nurse encourages relaxation and explains each step in advance.	Reassuring patient promotes relaxation.
8. Doctor may use a glass eyepiece over viewing end of scope; an insufflation bulb and tubing are attached. He may proceed to pump a small quantity of air into the bowel.	The purpose of inflating lower bowel with air is to expand the area viewed so that vision is not obstructed by mucosal folds.
9. The nurse should relay to the doctor expressions or complaints of pain by the patient.	Tenderness and pain may be experienced by the patient with a history of abdominal surgery; procedure may have to be terminated in order not to risk perforation.
10. As the scope advances, it may be necessary to attach suction to remove secretions, exudate, blood or excreta.	Connect tubing to suction equipment and turn to lowest degree at first.

Follow-up phase

Nursing action	Rationale
1. Upon withdrawal of scope, assist patient in gradually assuming a relaxed position.	Wipe the perineal area to prevent soilage of garments and to promote comfort.
2. If disposable scope is used, rinse scope and discard in proper receptacle. Reusable scopes are throughly cleaned in soap and water.	Sterilizable parts are sterilized before scope is stored.
3. Record the procedure and the reaction of the patient.	

GUIDELINES: COLONOSCOPY

Colonoscopy is the direct visual inspection of the large intestine by means of the colonoscope.

PURPOSES
1. As a diagnostic aid to view and assess the status of the large intestine (Figure 7.11).
2. As an operative instrument to remove polyps, to obtain tissue for biopsy and to remove foreign bodies.

Figure 7.11. Technique of colonoscopy. The patient is turned from one side to the other to take advantage of gravity as the scope is being advanced. Insert shows path of flexible scope from rectum through sigmoid colon and descending, transverse, and ascending colon. If the doctor wishes to check scope position with fluoroscopy, he should don a lead apron

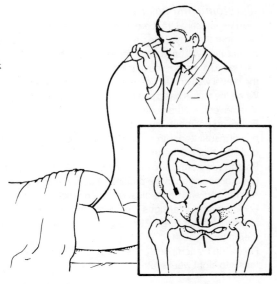

EQUIPMENT

Complete colonoscope, possibly with sidearm second observer scope
Water-soluble lubricant
Suction apparatus
Air-insufflating equipment
Snares
Drapes
Fluoroscope

The colonoscope:
The colonoscope is an instrument consisting of a flexible 4mm glass bundle (containing about 250,000 glass fibres).
1. There is a lens at both ends equipped to focus and magnify.
2. Light is transmitted from an external source by way of a fibreoptic bundle to the tip of the scope; an image is transmitted regardless of the looping and twisting of the flexible bundle.
3. Accessory channels provide for:
    a. Suction of fluid, blood and mucus;
    b. Insufflation of air or water;
    c. Biopsy.
4. There are two kinds of colonoscopes:
    a. To visualize left side of colon – 105cm;
    b. To visualize entire colon – 165–185cm.

PROCEDURE
Preparatory phase
1. Explain procedure to patient; his understanding and co-operation will promote his relaxation and facilitate his comfort during examination.
2. Limit the patient's intake to liquids for 24 to 48 hours prior to the procedure (as directed by the endoscopist).
3. Serve the patient an aperient as prescribed, in the evening for two days before the examination.
4. Give tap water or saline enemas approximately three hours prior to the colonoscopy until the returns are clear.

Polypectomy and postcare

1. Prepare intestinal tract meticulously; if there is any faecal matter in the field near the polyp, the procedure will be postponed and bowel preparation will have to be repeated.
2. Skill is required to remove the optimum amount of polyp, to avoid burning the bowel wall and to prevent cutting the base too close to the bowel wall.
3. When the tissue has been cut by cauterization, the snare-cautery device is removed and the polyp tissue is withdrawn by suction.
4. Following polypectomy, the colonoscope may be reinserted, the inner bowel insufflated with air and the operated area carefully examined for possible haemorrhage.
5. Postpolypectomy care depends on size of the polyps removed and the general condition of the patient. Usually the ambulatory patient can be discharged with no medication and no dietary restriction.
6. For inpatients, vital signs are checked for several hours, full liquid diet is given the day of surgery and soft, low-residue diet is given for two weeks thereafter.
7. Follow-up by complete colonoscopic examination usually is scheduled for six to eight weeks later.

NURSING ALERT

If polypectomy is done through sigmoidoscope or colonoscope, barium enema should not be done until seven to ten days thereafter because of risk of perforation at the polypectomy site.

MANAGEMENT OF THE PATIENT UNDERGOING MAJOR INTESTINAL SURGERY

NURSING PROCESS OVERVIEW

PATIENT PROBLEMS

1. Alteration in bowel elimination related to surgical intervention.
2. Impairment of skin integrity related to surgical wound and possible stoma placement.
3. Possible infection related to surgical wound.
4. Alteration in nutrition related to dietary modification following surgery.
5. Lack of knowledge of special care and function of possible ileostomy or colostomy.

Planning and implementation

PREOPERATIVE NURSING INTERVENTIONS

Physical preparation

1. Administer parenteral therapy to correct fluid and electrolyte imbalance as prescribed.
2. Correct nutritional deficiencies – protein supplements, between-meal feedings.
3. Provide blood replacement to overcome losses sustained by bleeding, infection, and neoplasm.
4. Assist with diagnostic studies as they relate to the evaluation of the cardiopulmonary, hepatorenal bodily functions.
5. Give the patient psychological support as he encounters the stresses of accepting the diagnosis, surgery and possibly a colostomy.
6. Insert an indwelling urinary catheter immediately prior to the patient's going to the operating room.
7. Oversee general personal cleanliness to minimize skin and wound infection postoperatively.

Preoperative measures to prevent infection

1. Administer antibiotic agents to suppress aerobic colon microflora. Combinations of kanamycin or neomycin with tetracycline, erythromycin or lincomycin.
   Note: Evidence that administration of antibiotic agents is preferable to a good intestinal cleansing is lacking.
2. Reduce content of colon:
   a. Give low-residue diet and, when required, change to liquid diet.

b. Offer laxatives as prescribed. Saline purgative may be preferred.

c. Administer enemas or colonic irrigations.

3. Decompress gastrointestinal tract by means of indwelling gastrointestinal tube to control distension and vomiting, if necessary. (Miller–Abbott or Cantor tube, see p. 461).

POSTOPERATIVE NURSING INTERVENTIONS
Nutritional requirements

1. Utilize intravenous catheter of intravenous therapy is to continue several days. Observe tissue for infiltration of fluid.
2. Maintain meticulous mouth hygiene while the patient is on parenteral therapy.

Nasogastric decompression and increased comfort

1. Observe and record quality and quantity of aspirated material.
2. Lubricate nostrils with water-soluble lubricant.
3. Humidify room to prevent dryness of mucous membranes.
4. Turn the patient frequently to minimize discomfort.
5. Remove tube (when required) upon reestablishment of peristalsis (determined by auscultation, passage of flatus rectally).
6. Administer analgesics according to needs.
7. Promote restfulness with appropriate nursing measures prior to giving sedation or hypnotics.

Prevention of complications

1. Evaluate vital signs and recognize patterns of development that may suggest haemorrhage, infection, shock, obstruction, etc.
2. Stress preventive measures, such as turning frequently, maintaining fluid balance, encouraging coughing, emphasizing cleanliness and movement of legs.

Convalescence and follow-up care

1. Encourage the patient to express concerns and questions. (See Colostomy and Ileostomy Management if these are pertinent, pp. 495 and 475.)
2. Encourage ambulation and self-care activities.
3. Stimulate appetite by promoting those measures that will make the patient want to eat what he should eat.
4. Help patient set goals toward which he can progress.
5. Emphasize the importance of follow-up visits to evaluate healing process, general physical and psychological adjustment.

Evaluation
EXPECTED OUTCOMES

1. Regains normal pattern of elimination or learns to accommodate any intestinal diversion surgery such as colostomy or ileostomy.
2. Recovers from surgery with proper wound healing and no signs of infection.
3. Modifies diet if need be in accordance with after-effects of surgery (colostomy, ileostomy).
4. Demonstrates ability to carry out stoma care if diversional surgery was performed.

APPENDICITIS

Acute appendicitis is an inflammation of the appendix due to an infection. It is almost always a surgical problem.

INCIDENCE

1. Occurs most frequently in young adults but may occur in any age-group.
2. Incidence of appendicitis has been decreasing during the past decade.

CLINICAL FEATURES

1. Begins with a progressively severe abdominal pain, beginning in midabdomen (periumbilical) and moving to right lower quadrant after six to twelve hours.
2. An effective early assessment of the patient for acute appendicitis is to have him rise on his toes and then drop down on his heels with a thump or to have him cough. If he has an acute inflammation, he will feel localized pain in the inflamed area.
3. Within a few hours, the acute tenderness becomes localized in the right lower quadrant (McBurney's point).
4. Anorexia, slight or moderate temperature elevation, mild change in bowel habit (usually constipation), and perhaps nausea and vomiting occur.

Note: If these clinical features occur in any person, encourage him to see a doctor immediately. There is a tendency in the ageing person to ignore aches and pains and to delay seeing a doctor. Consequently, mortality in elderly persons with inflammatory bowel lesions is as high as 20 per cent.

DIAGNOSTIC EVALUATION

1. Physical examination, noting especially location and localization of pain, rebound tenderness, etc.
2. Blood studies, with particular attention to white

blood cell count; urinalysis. A white blood cell count reveals a moderate leucocytosis.
3. Careful history to rule out other possibilities.
4. In some hospitals, when appendicitis is difficult to diagnose, laparoscopy may be utilized.

TREATMENT AND NURSING MANAGEMENT
Palliative preoperative care
1. Place the patient in a comfortable position to relieve abdominal pain and tension – usually upright position.
2. See that the patient takes nothing by mouth – to decrease peristalsis and to allow stomach to empty before going to surgery. Note time and nature of last meal.
3. Place ice bag to right lower quadrant – *never heat* because of the possibility of causing a rupture of appendix and peritonitis.
4. Do not administer an aperient – may cause rupture.
5. Evaluate vital signs frequently – to assess progression of infection.
6. When diagnosis of acute appendicitis is made, administer antibiotics, as directed.
Note: If there is evidence that perforation has occurred recently and a generalized peritonitis has developed, operative urgency is increased (see below).

Operative care
1. If diagnosis of acute appendicitis is established, a simple appendectomy is performed.
2. Because the patient will obtain relief from pain, he usually accepts surgery very willingly which affords a smooth recovery.
3. Anaesthetic may be general or spinal.
4. Incision may be McBurney, muscle-splitting or grid-iron or right rectus.

Postoperative care
See also p. 58.
1. Without drainage:
   a. Following recovery from anaesthetic, an upright position is maintained, analgesic is given every three or four hours as needed, and fluids and food are given as tolerated.
   b. Stitches removed between the fifth and seventh day.
2. With drainage – treat same as for peritonitis (see below).

PERITONITIS

Peritonitis is an inflammation of the peritoneal cavity.

AETIOLOGY
Peritonitis indicates transgression of peritoneum by trauma (blunt or penetrating) or inflammatory or neoplastic disease. The point of origin may be the gastrointestinal tract, the ovaries, the uterus or extraperitoneal organs (i.e. inflammation of the kidney).

Primary peritonitis – acute, diffuse
1. Occurs primarily in young females; often due to pathogenic bacteria (streptococci, pneumococci, gonococci) introduced through uterine tubes or through haematogenous spread.
2. In patients with nephrosis or cirrhosis, the offending organism is most often *E. coli*.

Secondary peritonitis
1. Commonly seen in surgical patients; caused by appendicitis, peptic ulceration, biliary tract disease, colonic inflammation.
2. May occur following gunshot wound, stab wounds and motor vehicle accidents.

Postoperative
1. Theoretically preventable.
2. Noted following poor preoperative preparation – inadequate nutrition and fluid and blood replacement and technical problems.
3. May occur in compromised patients who are diabetic, have malignancy or are taking steroids.

ALTERED PHYSIOLOGY
1. Any irritant, such as blood, bile or pancreatic enzymes, causes an exudation of plasma-like, protein-rich fluid – 'internal burn'.
2. Secondary peritonitis often presents mixed flora, which include *E. coli*, as well as the enterococci, *Clostridium*, *Klebsiella*, *Pseudomonas* and *Bacteroides*.
3. If there is failure to seal the source of contamination (i.e. perforation along gastrointestinal tract), peritonitis will become progressively worse.
4. When offended, the surface of the peritoneal cavity begins to exude a plasma-like fluid. This process can account for losses of as much as 5 litres/day.
5. Paralytic ileus is usual, with fluid loss into dilated intestinal loops and stomach.

6. Individual is compromised because of fluid loss, abdominal distention with respiratory embarrassment; nutrients are not absorbed, leading to progressive rapid catabolism.

Assessment

CLINICAL FEATURES

(Dependent on location and extension of inflammation.)

1. Initially, local type of abdominal pain tends to become constant, diffuse and more intense.
2. Abdomen becomes extremely tender, and muscles become rigid; rebound tenderness and ileus may be present; patient lies very still, usually with legs drawn up.
3. Nausea and vomiting often occur; peristalsis diminishes; anorexia is present.
4. Elevation of temperature and pulse as well as leucocyte count.
5. Fever and thirst occur.
6. Percussion – resonance and tympany due to paralytic ileus; loss of liver dullness may indicate free air in abdomen.
7. Auscultation – decreased bowel sounds.

DIAGNOSTIC EVALUATION

1. Blood studies – to show leucocytosis (leucopenia, if severe).
2. Urinalysis – may indicate urinary tract problems as primary source.
3. Peritoneal aspiration – to demonstrate blood, pus, bile, bacteria (gram-staining), amylase.
4. X-ray of abdomen – may indicate free air in abdomen under diaphragm; of thorax – to rule out unexpected pneumonia.

PATIENT PROBLEMS

1. Increasing abdominal pain related to the spread of an infection.
2. Generalized discomfort (malaise, nausea, vomiting, abdominal pain, elevated temperature, thirst) related to elevated temperature, paralytic ileus, fluid loss and other effects of infection.
3. Anxiety concerning spread of infection and possible death.

MEDICAL TREATMENT

1. If localized:
   a. If acutely inflamed appendix – an appendectomy is necessary.
   b. If ruptured duodenal ulcer – ulcer closed or plicated.
   c. Resection of diseased bowel; decompression (gastrostomy, colostomy, ileostomy).

2. If not localized, the patient is acutely ill, and surgery is not performed until after distension and electrolyte and fluid problems are treated.

Planning and implementation

NURSING INTERVENTIONS

General prevention measures

1. Encourage the individual who has early signs and symptoms of appendicitis to see his doctor.
2. Instruct the patient to avoid taking a laxative or applying heat to abdomen when abdominal pain of unknown cause is experienced.
3. Practice meticulous aseptic technique during abdominal surgery.

Ongoing assessment

1. Monitor central venous pressure if *in situ* (see p. 221).
2. Record urinary output hourly.
3. Note and record blood pressure every other hour.
4. Check vital signs frequently.
5. The doctor will obtain baseline and take frequent analyses of haematocrit, blood gases and electrolytes.

Prevention of infection and promotion of comfort

1. Give nothing by mouth – to reduce peristalsis; ensure meticulous oral hygiene.
2. Provide fluids by vein to establish adequate fluid level and to promote adequate urinary output.
3. Record accurately intake and output, including the measurement of vomit.
4. Administer antibiotics as prescribed.
5. Observe and describe symptoms accurately – pain and tenderness have a tendency to shift and must be reported precisely.
6. Reassure the patient and gain his confidence because he usually realizes the seriousness of his condition.

Prevention of complications

1. Following recovery from anaesthetic, place the patient in upright position to facilitate drainage.
2. Administer fluids by vein, since nothing is given by mouth initially.
3. Prevent nausea, vomiting, and distention by use of nasogastric suction; institute proper nursing measures for nasal and oral comfort.
4. Reduce parenteral fluids and give oral food and fluids when the following occur:
   a. Temperature and pulse return to normal.
   b. Abdomen becomes soft.

c. Peristaltic sounds return (determined by abdominal auscultation).

d. Flatus is passed and patient has bowel movements.

5. Be alert for possibility of complications – *report immediately*:

a. Burst abdomen – 'It feels as if something just gave way.'

b. Abscess formation – an area of abdomen is tender or painful, and fever increases.

Evaluation
EXPECTED OUTCOMES

1. Reports little or no pain or discomfort – is out of bed and has no complaints of physical discomfort.

2. Recovers from surgery with little or no complications – is not nauseated; has no abdominal pain, has normal vital signs.

3. Demonstrates lessening of anxiety.

ABDOMINAL HERNIA

A hernia is a protrusion of viscus through the wall of the cavity in which it is normally contained. It is often called a 'rupture'.

INCIDENCE

1. Occurs three times more frequently in men than women; may occur at any age.

2. Results from congenital or acquired weakness of the abdominal wall.

3. Tends to increase in size and occurrence with increase of intra-abdominal pressure brought about by coughing, straining or pressure from a nearby tumour.

CLASSIFICATION
According to area

1. Inguinal:

a. In male – due to weakness in abdominal wall where spermatic cord emerges; enters inguinal canal and then scrotum.

b. In female – due to weakness in abdominal wall where round ligament is located; enters inguinal canal and then labia.

(i) Direct inguinal:
Medial-to-deep epigastric artery;
Majority are acquired.

(ii) Indirect inguinal:
Lateral-to-deep epigastric artery;
Majority are congenital.

2. Femoral:

a. Occurs most often in women.

b. Located below Poupart's ligament (below groin).

3. Umbilical:

a. Results from failure of umbilical orifice to close.

b. Occurs most often in obese women and children and in patients with cirrhosis and ascites.

4. Ventral or incisional:

a. Due to weakness in abdominal wall.

b. May occur following impaired healing of incision because of drainage, infection, etc.

According to severity

1. *Reducible* – the protruding mass can be replaced in abdomen.

2. *Irreducible* – the protruding mass cannot be moved back into abdomen.

3. *Incarcerated* – an irreducible hernia in which the intestinal flow is completely obstructed.

4. *Strangulated* – an irreducible hernia in which the blood and intestinal flow are completely obstructed. Symptoms – pain, vomiting, swelling of hernial sac, fever, lower abdominal signs of peritoneal irritation.

TREATMENT
Mechanical
(Reducible hernia only.)

A *truss* is an appliance having a pad that is held snugly in the hernial orifice.

1. Does not cure a hernia – it prevents abdominal contents from entering hernial sac.

2. May be used in treatment of hernia in adults when, because of disease or age, it is inadvisable to perform surgery. In general, surgical treatment is preferred.

Surgical

Surgical treatment is recommended to correct the hernia before a strangulation occurs, in which case an emergency situation ensues.

1. Hernial sac is dissected free.

2. Contents of sac are replaced in abdominal cavity.

3. Neck of sac is ligated.

4. Muscle and fascial layers are sewed together firmly to prevent a recurrence. If this is not possible, synthetic mesh may be sutured over area.

5. Strangulated hernia requires resection of ischaemic bowel in addition to hernia repair.

NURSING MANAGEMENT
Preoperative

1. If hernia is strangulated, emergency conditions prevail (see Intestinal Obstruction, p. 488).

2. If surgery is elective, the patient is usually in good physical condition.
3. Use depilatory or shave suprapubic region and anterior surface of upper thigh.
4. Observe for upper respiratory infection – if present, surgery will be postponed because coughing or sneezing postoperatively may break the sutures.
5. Surgery may be done with patient admitted to the hospital or it may be performed in the day surgery ward.

Postoperative

1. Take the following measures for scrotal oedema or swelling:
   a. Bed rest.
   b. Ice pack and scrotal suspensory for support.
2. Observe for urinary retention.
3. Ambulate patient in a day or two, or sooner if permissible.

Patient education

1. Athletics and extremes of exertion are not permitted for eight to twelve weeks postoperatively.

ULCERATIVE COLITIS

Ulcerative colitis is an inflammatory disease of the mucosa and less frequently, the submucosa, of the colon and rectum. Occasionally it involves the distal ileum as well.

AETIOLOGY AND INCIDENCE

1. Unknown (idiopathic); however, there are several unproven possibilities:
   a. Emotional response alters blood supply to colon mucosa, but there is question as to whether stress is a cause or effect of the disease process.
   b. Unidentifiable organisms cause pathology.
   c. A combination of causative factors – infection, stress, allergy, autoimmunity.
2. Most common in young adulthood and middle life; almost equal between sexes (slightly more in females); more prevalent among Jewish people; highest in third and fourth decades, familial incidence.

Assessment
CLINICAL MANIFESTATIONS

1. Diarrhoea (may be bloody), tenesmus (painful straining), sense of urgency and cramping.
2. Multiple crypt abscesses of intestinal mucosa that may become necrotic and lead to ulceration.

3. Increased bowel sounds; abdomen may appear flat but as condition continues, abdomen may become distended.
4. There often is weight loss, fever, dehydration, hypokalaemia, anorexia, nausea and vomiting, iron deficiency anaemia and cachexia.

Note: See differences between regional enteritis and ulcerative colitis, in Table 7.6, p. 476.

5. May appear depressed and show difficulty in getting along with others.

CLINICAL FEATURES

1. Involvement extends proximally from rectum and is mainly of left colon.
2. The disease usually begins in the rectum and sigmoid and spreads upward, eventually involving the entire colon. Anal area may be excoriated and reddened; left lower abdomen may be tender on palpation.
3. There is a tendency for the patient to experience remissions and exacerbations.
4. Very high frequency of secondary and often multiple colon cancer.
5. It is a serious disease accompanied by systemic complications (see Complications below) and high mortality rate.

DIAGNOSTIC EVALUATION

1. Stool examination to rule out bacillary or amoebic dysentery.
2. Sigmoidoscopy; proctoscopy to reveal petechiae, hyperaemia, and ulcerations.
3. Barium enema X-ray.

NURSING ALERT
If disease is in acute stage, aperient may be contraindicated because it may cause exacerbation and lead to toxic megacolon.

4. Review of nursing history for patterns of fatigue and overwork, tension, family problems.
5. Assessment of behavioural features indicative of emotional concerns.
6. Assessment of food habits that may have a bearing on triggering symptoms (milk intake may be a problem).
7. Careful clinical assessment to rule out diverticulitis, cancer, etc.
8. Complete blood studies if they appear to be warranted.
9. Faecal analysis if blood and mucus are evident.

COMPLICATIONS

1. Skin ulcers.
2. Arthritis.
3. Malnutrition.
4. Anaemia.
5. Abscess formation.
6. Stricture, and fistula.
7. Erythema nodosum.
8. Amyloidosis.
9. Electrolyte imbalance.
10. Malignancy (colonic cancer).
11. Toxic megacolon.
12. Ankylosing spondylitis.

PATIENT PROBLEMS

1. Alteration in comfort (cramp-like pain in lower abdomen, especially prior to defaecation) related to disease process.
2. Inadequate nutrition and alteration in fluid and electrolyte balance related to effects of diarrhoea, nausea and vomiting.
3. Diarrhoea, dehydration, anorexia related to course of disease.
4. Impaired mobility related to fatigue, anorexia and anaemia.
5. Compromised coping related to fatigue, feeling of helplessness and lack of support systems (friends and family).

Note: There is no cure for ulcerative colitis because the cause is unknown; the prime goal is to control the disease to achieve patient comfort and improve the quality of life. This can be done by:

1. Initiating early, effective management of exacerbations.
2. Prolonging remissions with appropriate therapy.
3. Subjecting the patient to surgery only when judiciously necessary.

Planning and implementation

NURSING INTERVENTIONS

Comfort measures to rest and relax the intestinal tract

1. It may be necessary to reduce or eliminate food and fluid and then to resort to parenteral feeding or to low-residue diets.
2. Give sedatives and tranquillizers not only to provide general rest but also to allow peristalsis to slow down and afford rest to the inflamed bowel.
3. Be aware of the possibility of pressure sores in this patient because of malnourishment and enforced inactivity, especially if he is thin. Cleanse the skin gently after each (or every other) bowel move-

ment. Apply a protective emollient such as petroleum jelly, karaya gel.
4. Administer tincture of belladonna, atropine or diphenoxylate (Lomotil), as prescribed, to lessen intestinal motility. Sulphasalazine (Salazopyrin) is effective for antidiarrhoeal effect even though it is an antibiotic. Some patients experience side-effects (epigastric distress, headache, dizziness); discontinue medication for two to three days and gradually introduce it again.
5. Relieve painful rectal spasms (produced by frequent diarrhoeal stools) with Anodesyn suppositories.
6. Report any evidence of sudden abdominal distension, since it may indicate toxic megacolon.
7. Reduce physical activity to a minimum or provide frequent rest periods.
8. Provide commode or bathroom next to bed, since urgency of movements may be a problem.

Interventions to combat infection and toxicity

1. Give sulpha drugs as prescribed – nonabsorbable sulphasalazine (Salazopyrin) may be prescribed as an oral medication.
2. Administer corticosteroids as prescribed – the type depends on the condition of patient; mode of administration may be oral, intravenous or rectal. Rectal administration may be in the form of hydrocortisone-retention enemas.
3. Provide conscientious skin care because excoriation is common following severe diarrhoea.
4. For severe proctitis, nightly instillations of steroids as prescribed (dissolved in tap water, or as suppositories) may produce a remission of symptoms. Belladonna suppositories also may help.

Nutritional and fluid requirements

1. If the patient is acutely ill, maintain him on parenteral replacement of vitamins, fluids and electrolytes (potassium is very important).
2. When resuming oral fluids and foods, select those that are nonirritating to the mucosa (mechanically, thermally and chemically).
3. Consider a milk-free diet, since studies have shown that fewer relapses occur on a milk-free diet; the incidence of lactase deficiency is more frequent in patients having attacks than in those in remission.
4. Provide a well-balanced, low-residue, high-protein diet to correct malnutrition.
5. Determine which foods agree with this patient and which do not. Modify diet plan accordingly.

6. Supplemental vitamin therapy, including vitamin C, B complex and K.
7. Avoid cold fluids because they increase intestinal motility.
8. Administer appropriate electrolytes, which have been lost in diarrhoeal bouts, especially potassium.
9. Administer diphenoxylate (Lomotil) as prescribed for symptomatic relief of diarrhoea.
10. Prohibit smoking because it also increases intestinal motility.

NURSING ALERT

Since opiates may precipitate toxic megacolon, use only for brief periods, if at all, in acutely ill patients.

11. Administer prescribed therapy to correct existing anaemia.
12. Carefully note fluid intake and output and character of bowel movements.
13. Weigh the patient frequently and record weight; rapid increase or decrease may relate to fluid imbalance.

Coping and psychological adjustment
1. Offer psychological support.
2. Educate the patient to accept and learn to live with this chronic disease. This is done on a long-range basis, and the patient should participate in the evaluation and planning of his care.
3. Plan all aspects of the patient's care in conference so that a team effort promotes the nursing process and ensures continuity of care, communication and periodic evaluation.
4. Indicate by actions and expressions that you, the nurse, are responsible for and care for him. An effective nurse–patient relationship enables him to satisfy his dependency needs.
5. Solicit the assistance of the family in helping to understand the patient; assist the family in understanding the patient.
6. If the patient is to have an ileostomy, before surgery it is helpful to have the patient visited by someone who has had a similar operation and has made a good adjustment. After surgery, these people can also help with management problems.

Note: Impotence occurs in males rather frequently after a colectomy because of damage to pudendal nerves.

Prevention of complications
1. Observe for signs of colonic perforation and haemorrhage.

2. Assess carefully the patient's behaviour and all his complaints.

SURGICAL TREATMENT AND NURSING MANAGEMENT
Indications and contemplated surgery
1. Approximately 20 per cent of patients with ulcerative colitis require surgical intervention.
2. Recommended when no improvement occurs through conservative means – evidenced by impending perforation, actual perforation, deteriorating clinical course after 24 to 48 hours of maximum medical regimen, severe haemorrhage, or persistent colonic dilatation for longer than one week.
3. Total proctocolectomy and permanent ileostomy are frequently used. Becoming more popular is an ileoanal abdominal colectomy with mucosal proctectomy and construction of an ileoanal reservoir (see p. 485).

Preoperative physical and psychological preparation
1. Institute an intensive programme of fluid, blood and protein replacement.
2. Administer chemotherapy and antibiotics to reduce intestinal organisms.
3. Recognize psychological needs of this patient:
   a. Fear, anxiety and discouragement accompany diarrhoea.
   b. Hypersensitivity may be evident.
   c. Let the patient know that his complaints are understood.
4. Encourage the patient to talk; listen to what he says is bothering him.
5. Answer his questions about the permanent ileostomy he is about to have.

Postoperative care including ileostomy management
(See Management of Patient having Major Intestinal Surgery, p. 466.)
(See Conditions – Caring for a Patient with an Ileostomy, p. 475.)

PATIENT EDUCATION
1. It is important to involve the patient in understanding chronic ulcerative colitis and each component of care prescribed; he should be made to feel that he is sharing responsibility for maintaining his health.
2. This patient needs encouragement and support postoperatively even though surgery is considered curative; there may be problems with skin

care; there may also be aesthetic difficulties, surgical revisions.
3. When early indications of relapse are noted, such as bleeding or increased diarrhoea, the patient should report these findings early so that steroid treatment may be initiated.
4. Monitoring of the patient's condition should continue when new symptoms develop and on a regular annual basis.
5. Let the patient know that he has a valuable resource person, the stomatherapist, and that he should not hesitate to call this person about his ileostomy problems.

Evaluation
EXPECTED OUTCOMES
1. Reports a lessening of pain; functions well without analgesics.
2. Demonstrates improved food and fluid intake; avoids roughage intake.
3. Tolerates moderate activity, such as short walks or visits, without becoming fatigued.
4. Shows improved psychological outlook; appears to enjoy visits from friends and family.

REGIONAL ENTERITIS (CROHN'S DISEASE, GRANULOMATOUS COLITIS, TRANSMURAL COLITIS)

Regional enteritis is a chronic inflammatory disease of the small intestine, usually affecting the terminal ileum at the region just before the ileum joins the colon. The aetiology is unknown.

INCIDENCE
1. Affects both sexes equally.
2. Appears more often in Jewish people of Eastern European origin.
3. A familial tendency exists.
4. May occur at any age, but occurs mostly in those between 15 and 35 years of age.

CLINICAL FEATURES
1. Intestinal tissue thickens first by oedema and later by formation of scar tissues and granulomas.
2. At times, 'skip lesions' occur with normal intestine in between.
3. This condition interferes with the ability of the intestine to transport the contents of upper intestine through the constricted lumen; this causes cramp pains after meals.
4. Inflammation and ulcers form in the lining membrane, producing a constant irritating discharge.

5. In some patients, the inflamed intestine may perforate and form intra-abdominal and anal abscesses.

Assessment
CLINICAL FEATURES
These are characterized by exacerbations and remissions – may be abrupt or insidious:
1. Cramp after meals; this causes the patient to eat in small amounts or even to avoid eating, which then results in malnutrition, weight loss and possibly anaemia (hypochromic or macrocytic).
2. Chronic diarrhoea due to irritating discharge may occur; usual consistency is soft or semi-liquid.
3. Milk products and chemically or mechanically irritating food may aggravate the problem.
4. Melaena and malabsorption syndrome may occur; occult blood may appear in stool.
5. Low-grade fever occurs if abscesses are present.
6. Lymphadenitis occurs in mesenteric nodes.
7. Abdominal tenderness, especially in right lower quadrant.

DIAGNOSTIC EVALUATION
1. Regional enteritis may simulate acute appendicitis.
2. Upper gastrointestinal barium studies – classic 'string sign' is noted at terminal ileum that suggests a constriction of a segment of intestine.
3. Barium enema to permit visualization of lesions of large intestine and terminal ileum.
4. Proctosigmoidoscopy to note ulceration.

CLINICAL COMPLICATIONS
1. Stricture and fistulae formation (ischiorectal, perianal – even to bladder or vagina).
2. Haemorrhage, bowel perforation, mechanical intestinal obstruction.
3. Incidence of colorectal cancer is higher in these patients.

PATIENT PROBLEMS
1. Reduced nutritional intake related to postprandial pain.
2. Abdominal pain related to the inflammatory disease of the small intestine.
3. Ineffective coping mechanisms related to feelings of dejection and embarrassment.
4. Knowledge deficit related to insufficient information about regional enteritis.

Planning and implementation

NURSING INTERVENTIONS

Promotion of comfort, adequate nutrition and fluid intake

1. Administer a diet low in residue, fibre and fat, and high in calories, protein and carbohydrates, with vitamin supplements (especially vitamin K). Prepare for hyperalimentation if the patient is debilitated.
2. Provide iron medications if anaemia is present.
3. Treat pain and diarrhoea symptomatically; encourage the patient to rest.

Prevention of transmission of pathogenic organisms

1. Practise conscientious handwashing before and after patient care.
2. Dispose of soiled linen according to hospital policy.
3. Maintain good hygienic practices and instruct the patient in this regard.

Drug therapy

1. Consider antibiotics and sulphonamides such as sulphasalazine for control of inflammatory process.
2. Some hospitals treat this patient with sulpha-salazine, steroids, prednisone.
3. If the patient does not respond to conservative medical treatment, surgery may be necessary to relieve segmental obstruction.
   a. Surgery is determined specifically for each patient.
   b. The involved segment may be resected with anastomosis; bypass procedures may be done.
4. Unfortunately, recurrence of the disease is possible following surgery.

Psychosocial considerations

1. The nurse can offer understanding, concern and help in encouraging this person, who is often dejected, debilitated, embarrassed about frequent and malodorous stools, and even fearful of eating.

Evaluation

EXPECTED OUTCOMES

1. Achieves relief of pain after several days of dietary, drugs and psychological therapy.
2. Maintains proper nutritional intake and adequate fluid intake.
3. Verbalizes improved mental attitude toward ways to live with the disease and methods for socializing with others.
4. Demonstrates an understanding of the need for lifestyle changes.

See Table 7.6 for differences between regional enteritis and ulcerative colitis.

ILEOSTOMY

An ileostomy is an opening in the ileum for the purpose of treating intractable granulomatous or ulcerative colitis or of diverting intestinal contents in colon cancer, familial polyposis, congenital defects or trauma. The opening (stoma) is brought out through the abdominal wall, usually the lower right section of the abdomen. This stoma becomes the outlet for discharge of intestinal contents.

IMPLICATIONS FOR THE PATIENT

(See also Colostomy for Preoperative and Postoperative Nursing Management, p. 492).

1. Some patients welcome the ileostomy, since it means the removal of a longstanding incapacitating disease process; in general, however, many patients experience psychological problems that are often overwhelming. Preoperative counselling by the medical and nursing team, as well as by a trained visitor from the local ostomy association, is most helpful.
2. The patient appreciates that now he has the prospect of enjoying a normal diet, instead of the low-residue diet to which he was restricted. Ethnic groups and patient on special diets will need help from the dietician.
3. The patient wears a soft vinyl or rubber pouch with an open-end bottom; a clamp fitted on the bottom of the pouch permits emptying. He empties the pouch four to five times a day, usually when he goes to the bathroom to urinate.
4. The ileostomate requires instruction – first from the nurse in the hospital or stoma therapist and then from the community nurse.
5. Appliances may be reusable or disposable. They are held in place in several ways – cement, double-faced adhesive discs, karaya rings.
6. Waterproof tape is effective in anchoring the appliance when the patient showers or swims.
7. At first the discharge will be liquid, but later the small intestine will begin to take on its water-absorbing function to permit a more semi-solid, pasty discharge.

Table 7.6   Differences between regional enteritis and ulcerative colitis

	Regional enteritis	Ulcerative colitis
Pathology:		
Early	Transmural thickening	Mucosal ulceration
Later	Deep, penetrating granulomas	Mucosal minute ulcerations
Involvement:		
Rectum	Approximately 50 per cent	Over 90 per cent
Right colon	Frequently	Occasionally
Small intestine	Yes	Usually not
Disease distribution	**Segmental**	**Continuous**
Clinical features:		
Bleeding	Generally no, but may occur	Common
Perianal disease	Common	Rare
Fistula	Common	Rare
Perforation	Common	Rare
Disease course	**Slowly progressive**	**Remissions and relapses**
X-ray – barium studies:		
Stricture	Common	Rare
Distribution	Segmental	Continuous
Associated with malignancy	Not common	Common

8. Because the discharge is rich in enzymes, it may cause skin irritation; therefore optimal skin care becomes a top priority consideration for the patient. Cleanse the skin thoroughly with mild soap and water; rinse well. Take baths or showers as soon after surgery as possible. Dry area thoroughly. For elderly patients, soap may be too drying for the skin; however, oil-based soaps may prevent adhesives from adhering.

GUIDELINES: CHANGING AN ILEOSTOMY APPLIANCE

GOALS
1. Prevent leakage (bag is usually changed every two to four days).
2. Permit examination of skin around stoma.
3. Assist in controlling odour if this presents a problem.

TIME
1. Early in morning, before breakfast or two to four hours after a meal, when the bowel is least active.
2. Immediately, if patient is complaining of burning or itching underneath the disc or has pain around the stoma.

EQUIPMENT

Duplicate ileostomy appliance with or without belt
   (Figure 7.12); pouch-closing device
Soap, water and washcloth
Appropriate skin barrier (karaya powder, karaya paste
   and/or karaya ring, Stomahesive, ReliaSeal, Skin
   Prep or other)

Gauze
Small bowl
Tape (hypoallergenic)

PROCEDURE
Preparatory phase

Nursing action	**Rationale**
1. Have the patient assume a relaxed position. Provide privacy.	Encourage patient participation and understanding so that eventually he will be able to change appliance himself.
2. Explain details of this activity to the patient.	Encourage questions.
3. Expose ileostomy area; remove ileostomy belt (if worn).	
4. Position lamp; wash hands.	

Performance phase

Nursing action	**Rationale**
1. To remove appliance:	
a. Sit or stand in a comfortable position.	Have the patient sit on toilet or on a chair facing toilet. If standing, face toilet.
b. Fill a container with prescribed solvent, then fill medicine dropper with solvent; apply a few drops of solvent between disc of appliance and skin. *Do not pull off appliance.*	As solvent works, pouch loosens and pulling is unnecessary. Solvent is often unnecessary when skin cement is not used. Pouch can be removed by gently pushing skin away from adhesive.
c. If adhesive residue builds up on skin, use very small amount of adhesive remover on gauze.	Do not use acetone, ether or benzene because they are irritating to skin.
2. To cleanse skin	
a. Remove any excess karaya with dry toilet tissue.	During this time, a gauze dressing or pieces of tissue may be used to cover the stoma to absorb excess drainage while skin is being cleaned.
b. Wash skin gently with soft cloth moistened with *tepid* water and mild soap, or bathe before putting on clean appliance.	The patient may shower before removing appliance. Micropore or waterproof tape applied to sides of disc will keep it secure while bathing.
c. Rinse and dry skin thoroughly after cleansing.	Moisture or soap residue will interfere with appliance adhesion.

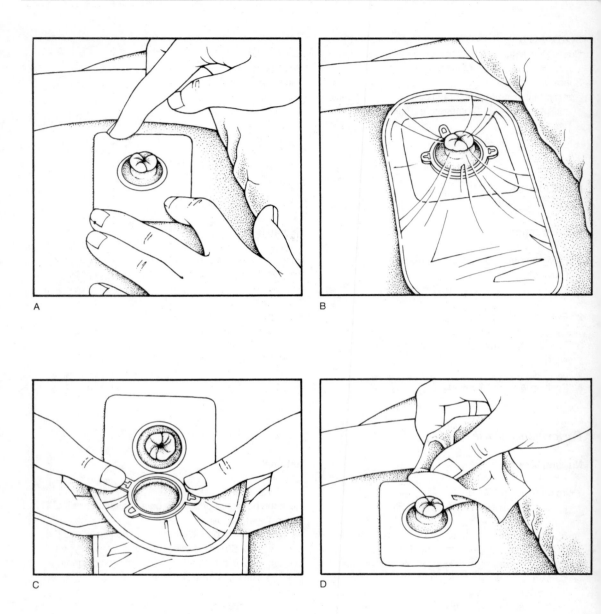

Figure 7.12. Ileostomy care. (A) A Stomahesive wafer with flange can be applied directly to the peristomal area after it has been thoroughly cleaned and dried. (B) An opaque or transparent drainable pouch is positioned at desired angle over stoma. (C) Pouch may be removed without removing wafer. (D) Stoma may be assessed without removing wafer (adapted by permission from ConvaTec, a Division of E.R. Squibb & Sons)

3. To put on appliance if no skin irritation:
   a. An appropriate skin barrier should be applied to peristomal skin before the pouch is applied.

   Stomahesive (Figure 7.12) or karaya preparation (powder, paste, or rings) may be used. Many disposable pouches have a built-in skin barrier. **Note:** Do not confuse with tincture of benzoin compound, which is too irritating.

   b. It is optional to apply tincture of benzoin or one of the many specially formulated skin preparations to help protect peristomal skin.

   c. Remove cover from adherent surface of disc of disposable plastic pouch and apply directly to skin.

   Be sure skin is thoroughly dry.

   d. Press firmly in place for 30 seconds.

   To ensure adherence.

4. To put on appliance if there is skin irritation:
   a. Cleanse skin thoroughly but gently; pat dry.

   To remove debris.

   b. (i) An effective measure is to apply a wafer of Stomahesive, which is available in 10 × 10cm and 20 × 20cm pieces. The stomal opening should be cut the same size as the stoma; use a cutting guide (supplied with Stomahesive). The wafer is applied directly to the skin.

   The steroid preparation (Kenalog) helps decrease inflammation. The antifungal (nystatin) treats those types of infections that are common around stomas. A prescription is required for both medications. Stomahesive is a substance that facilitates healing of excoriated skin. It adheres well even to 'weepy', irritated skin.

   (ii) A second alternative is to moisten a karaya gum washer and apply when it is tacky. If skin is 'weepy', karaya powder may be applied first and any excess dusted off gently.

   Karaya also facilitates skin healing. Tackiness promotes adherence.

   c. The pouch is then applied to the treated skin.

   This will allow skin to heal while appliance is in place.

5. Check the pouch bottom for closure; use rubber band or clip provided.

   Proper closure controls leakage.

Follow-up phase

Nursing action

Rationale

1. Dispose of waste materials

2. Clean reusable ileostomy pouch by washing in soap and water.

   Preserves life of appliance and controls odour.

3. Soak pouch in deodorant solution and hang to dry.

   Deodorizing agents should be effective but not destructive to rubber or vinyl.

NUTRITIONAL MANAGEMENT OF THE ILEOSTOMATE

Nutritional needs of the patient with an ileostomy are similar to those of a healthy individual. With adequate diet, additional vitamins or food supplements are unnecessary.

PATIENT EDUCATION

Discharge from hospital for patient with ileostomy or colostomy.

Clothing

1. A girdle is permissible – a size larger is recommended to accommodate the pouch.
2. Swim suits (even two-piece) can be worn; men prefer boxer-styled trunks; women may prefer a swim suit with a skirt.
3. For swimming, a rubber belt is preferred to elastic cloth which sometimes loses elasticity when wet.

Medications

1. The ileostomate should not have laxatives, irrigations, enteric-coated or time-release capsules.

Travel

1. Travel by plane or any other vehicle is not contraindicated.
2. If travelling by plane, it is suggested that patient carry his ostomy kit with him (in the event that there is a delay in retrieving baggage).
3. Colostomates who irrigate should use only water suitable for drinking.
4. Ileostomates should bring along a suitable anti-diarrhoeal medication.

Sports

1. All kinds of sports may be participated in, as reported by ostomates – tennis, water surfing, skin diving, water skiing, ice skating, horseback riding.

2. Problems may arise if the ileostomate participate in contact sports such as football, ice hockey.

Sexual functioning

1. Approximately 10 to 20 per cent of male ileostomates experience impaired sexual function; in many individuals this is only temporary.
2. Male colostomates vary from being fully potent to impotent.
3. Most males who have urinary surgery for malignancy as adults are impotent – may be candidates for penile implant.
4. In many instances, potency is regained, but this may take up to two years.

Pregnancy

1. An ostomy is not a contraindication to a successful pregnancy.
2. Careful medical supervision during pregnancy is required for a female ileostomate. The ostomy opening may change in size (stretch) as the pregnancy continues; thereafter, changes in the size of the appliance opening may be required. Change in abdominal contour may necessitate the use of a very flexible appliance or faceplate.

Sleeping

1. Almost any position of comfort can be assumed if the pouch is fitted properly.
2. Sleeping on the stomach is comfortable when a small cushion is placed under the hip on the side of the stoma.

Obstruction or blockage

1. Know signs and symptoms; notify stoma therapist or surgeon if necessary.

See Table 7.7 for the problems encountered by the patient with an ileostomy.

GUIDELINES: CONTINENT ILEOSTOMY (KOCK POUCH)

A continent ileostomy is the surgical creation of a pouch of small intestine that can act as an internal receptacle for faecal discharge; a nipple valve is constructed at the outlet to permit drainage from the abdomen. This kind of ileostomy may be done initially for selected patients when they present for an ileostomy, or it may be constructed from the conventional ileostomy (Figure 7.13).

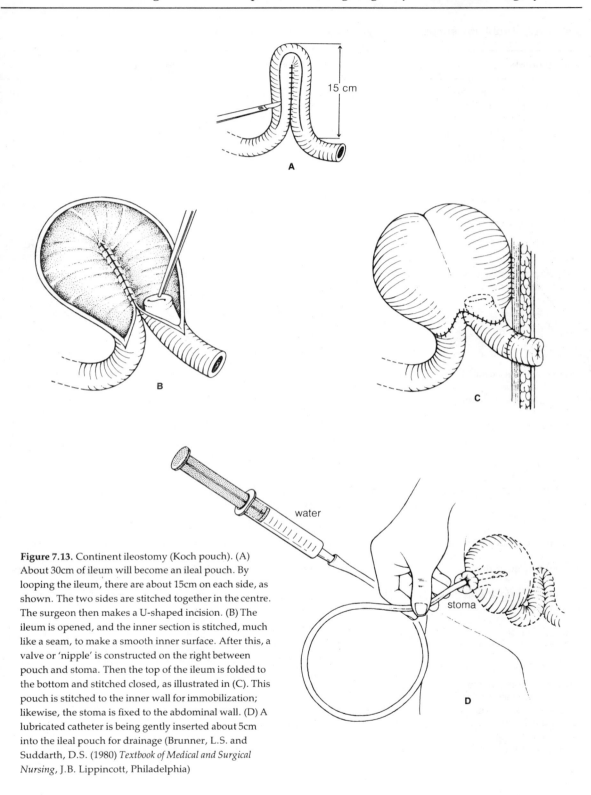

Figure 7.13. Continent ileostomy (Koch pouch). (A) About 30cm of ileum will become an ileal pouch. By looping the ileum, there are about 15cm on each side, as shown. The two sides are stitched together in the centre. The surgeon then makes a U-shaped incision. (B) The ileum is opened, and the inner section is stitched, much like a seam, to make a smooth inner surface. After this, a valve or 'nipple' is constructed on the right between pouch and stoma. Then the top of the ileum is folded to the bottom and stitched closed, as illustrated in (C). This pouch is stitched to the inner wall for immobilization; likewise, the stoma is fixed to the abdominal wall. (D) A lubricated catheter is being gently inserted about 5cm into the ileal pouch for drainage (Brunner, L.S. and Suddarth, D.S. (1980) *Textbook of Medical and Surgical Nursing*, J.B. Lippincott, Philadelphia)

Table 7.7   Problems encountered by the patient with an ileostomy

Patient problems	Interventions, prevention and management
Negative nutritional balance during or immediately after surgery	Offer diet high in calories and protein, and additional vitamin and mineral supplements.
Fluid and electrolyte depletion related to vomiting, diarrhoea and excessive perspiration	Avoid salt tablets, which may act as a purgative. Supplement fluids with beverages containing electrolytes and glucose
Inadequate absorption of nutrients	Continue diet high in protein with vitamin and mineral supplements; fat restriction may be necessary
	Consider use of elemental diets (diet preparations already broken down to simple, easily digested forms) until ileum adapts to new shortened length (e.g. Vivonex [Eaton], Clinifeed [Roussel])
Weight loss or gain	Weigh and record weight daily. Explain to the patient that ileostomy will continue to function even if oral intake is limited and that adequate nutritional intake is essential for healing to occur. Dietary supplements are appropriate (Isocal, Flexical [Mead-Johnson])
Loss of specific absorptive site for vitamin B_{12} and bile salts related to resection of terminal ileus	Blood is checked for B_{12} levels. Give replacements by injection, as prescribed
	Restrict fat, since the patient may not be able to digest and absorb fats because of bile salt deficiency. This must be monitored carefully because on a fat-restricted diet the patient may lose weight and be unable to absorb fat-soluble vitamins: A, D, E, and K. Also, with bile salt deficiency, this patient may be more susceptible to formation of gallstones
Excessively watery effluent	Restrict fibrous foods: wholegrain bread and cereals, fresh fruit skins, fresh vegetables, beans, corn, and nuts.
Excessively dry effluent	Increase salt intake. Note: *increased intake of water does not increase effluent because excess water is excreted in urine*
Stomal obstruction	Restrict fibrous foods; be alert to offenders such as celery, cabbage, nuts and sweetcorn. Instruct the patient to chew food thoroughly.
Skin excoriation, related to:	
1. Irritating intestinal effluent	Evaluate for proper fit of appliance
2. Materials used to hold appliance in place	Karaya protects skin – it comes as powder, paste, rings and sheets
3. Allergies	Good substitutes for karaya are Stomahesive (Squibb) or ReliaSeal (Davol). An appropriate skin barrier should always be used between skin and appliance
4. Fungal or bacterial growth	Avoid products to which the patient may be sensitive. Patch test any new or suspect problems on patient's inner arm
5. Belt applied too tightly	If large areas of skin are involved or ulcerated, avoid rubber cement-type adhesive
6. Poor stoma location – peristomal skin folds or scars	Severe problems due to poor stoma location necessitate surgical revision
Minor stomal bleeding, related to irritation This may occur following wiping the stoma	Mucosa is friable and easily injured. However, when handled gently, these tissues heal readily because of the rich blood supply
Prolapsed stoma, related to an oversized opening resulting from:	
1. Excessive bowel shrinkage	Remove appliance. Observe bowel for signs of compromised circulation (pale or dark colour)
2. Abdominal pressure due to coughing	Apply cold pads or packs to control oedema
3. Failure of opposing layers of bowel to adhere in the turnback suture procedure	Notify surgeon. He will manually replace bowel into abdomen (medical treatment) or suggest surgical correction

Odour related to:

1. A reusable appliance that is not changed frequently enough or not cleaned properly
2. An appliance that is not odour-proof
3. Certain foods: onions, cabbage, eggs, fish
4. Obstruction or dysfunction of ostomy
5. Certain medications; vitamins, penicillin, oestrogens

Be meticulous in cleaning procedure
Alternate reusable pouches; when not in use, allow pouch to hang in fresh air (not sun)
If using disposable pouches, select odour-proof materials
Change medications when one is found to be odour-producing
Use oral deodorants: chlorophyll derivatives, bismuth subcarbonate or bismuth subgallate
Insert deodorizer in appliance: charcoal, Nilodor or baking soda
Encourage foods such as spinach and parsley that act on the intestinal tract as deodorizers

Expulsion of intestinal flatus, related to lack of sphincter control. Because of this the patient often feels everyone around him is aware of gas passage

Limit gas-producing foods such as beans, cabbage, onions, beer
Try to avoid air-swallowing, which may occur during smoking, talking, eating, emotional upset

Potential for obstruction
This is suggested by the following signs:
1. Abdominal cramping, distension
2. Malodour, along with liquid projectile effluent
3. Vomiting
4. Signs of dehydration

Obstruction or stenosis may be due to oedema or lymphatic blockage
More commonly, it is due to food blockage brought about by poor chewing habits and high-cellulose foods
Nursing intervention:
1. Remove appliance
2. Have the patient lie down in bed and apply hot compresses to abdomen, or have the patient relax in bath of warm water
3. Offer hot tea drinks. If this does not help within two to three hours, check with surgeon; it may be necessary to gently irrigate the ileostomy (doctor prescribed) with a small volume of saline

Obstruction due to adhesions or volvulus
Potential for kidney stones, related to:
1. Dehydration – increases formation of urate crystals because of loss of bicarbonate in intestine
2. Increased absorption of oxalates after ileal resection – oxalate stones form

This may require surgical correction

Increase patient's fluid intake
If stones are urate crystals, sodium bicarbonate may be required to alkalinize urine
If stones are calcium, ascorbic acid may be prescribed to acidify urine

Diarrhoea
Observe whether there is an increase in the number of times the patient needs to empty pouch
Normal output is about 750ml/day: check for food poisoning, mechanical obstruction, stomal stenosis
Assess for signs of dehydration

Electrolyte imbalance may easily occur. Treat with clear liquids and antidiarrhoeal medications
Water, salts and fluids can be replaced with commercial preparations
Another suggestion is to alternate a cup of salted broth and a cup of sweetened tea each hour
Water-absorbing drugs (hydrophilic colloids) such as Metamucil powder are sometimes effective
If diarrhoea does not resolve in 24 hours, the patient should seek medical care. Intravenous fluids and electrolytic therapy may be necessary

Medication difficulties
1. Drug action can be affected by the absence of the colon and altered transit time through small intestine
2. Suggest taking uncoated tablets or liquids for oral medication
3. Have the patient check effluent to be sure pills are not being passed undissolved
4. Do not use time-release tablets or sustained-release capsules
5. Administer vitamin B_{12} subcutaneously if distal ileum has been removed

1. The various functions of the small and large bowel are interrupted or absent.

2. Coated tablets may pass undissolved through bowel into ileostomy appliance
3. If they do pass undissolved, thereafter crush them and take them with water
4. They may not be absorbed

5. The terminal ileum is where the absorptive site for B_{12} is located

PREOPERATIVE MANAGEMENT
This is essentially the same as for the patient having a traditional ileostomy.

POSTOPERATIVE MANAGEMENT
1. A catheter will extend from the stoma and be attached to closed suction; drainage will be maintained about 10 days.
2. Catheter irrigation is done usually every two hours with a 20–30ml saline to ensure patency; return flow is by gravity.
3. Nasogastric suction is used to relieve pressure on suture line by preventing a buildup of gastric contents.
4. Parenteral fluids are administered for four to five days; thereafter, clear liquids and diet as tolerated.
5. Monitor for nausea and abdominal distension.
6. Pain medication is given as required; early ambulation is encouraged.
7. In about 10 to 14 days, the catheter is removed from the stoma and the patient participates in the management of his ileostomy.

EQUIPMENT
Catheter
Water-soluble lubricant
Gauze squares

Syringe
Irrigating solution in a bowl, receiving basin

Nursing action	Rationale
1. Lubricate catheter and gently insert about 5cm.	Resistance may be felt at valve or 'nipple'.
2. If much resistance, fill syringe with 20ml air or water and inject through catheter – gently exert pressure on catheter.	This will permit catheter to enter pouch.
3. Place end of catheter in drainage basin (below level of stoma); later this can be done at lavatory bowl.	Gravity facilitates drainage. Drainage may include flatus as well as effluent.
4. Following drainage, remove catheter. Wash area around stoma; dry and apply absorbent pad. Fasten with hypoallergenic tape.	Entire procedure requires about five to ten minutes. At first, irrigation is done every two hours, then gradually extended to three times daily. If faeces are not too thick, drainage through catheter may occur successfully without irrigation.

OSTOMY ASSOCIATIONS/PATIENT WELFARE GROUPS/ADVICE

Colostomy Welfare Group (CWG)
38–39 Eccleston Square
London SW1V 1PB (Tel: 01 828 5175)

The Urostomy Association (UA)
'Buckland'
Beaumont Place
Danbury, Essex (Tel: 024 541 5294)

Ileostomy Association (IA) of Great Britain and Ireland
Amblehurst House
Chobham, Woking
Surrey (Tel: 09905 8277)

Abbott Stoma Advisory Service
Abbott Laboratories Ltd
Queensborough, Kent (Tel: 0795 663371, ext. 3358)

Squibb Surgicare Ltd
Squibb House
141–149 Staines Road
Hounslow TW3 3JA

ILEOANAL ABDOMINAL COLECTOMY WITH MUCOSAL PROCTECTOMY AND CONSTRUCTION OF AN ILEOANAL RESERVOIR

PATIENT SCREENING
Eliminate patients:
1. With Crohn's disease;
2. Acutely ill with ulcerative colitis;
3. Who are nutritionally depleted and steroid-dependent;
4. With frequent episodes of diarrhoea.

SURGICAL INTERVENTION
This may be performed in two stages (first performing a temporary ileostomy); or two teams may work together doing the abdominal and perineal surgery.

The S-shaped reservoir is one type; a J-shaped or side-to-side reservoir may be done.

POSTOPERATIVE MANAGEMENT
1. General postoperative abdominal care is applicable (see p. 58).
2. Assess for potential complications – partial obstruction of small intestine, pelvic sepsis due to leakage from reservoir.
3. Diarrhoea, which frequently occurs with permanent ileostomy, is eliminated with this procedure.
4. Long-term follow-up studies need to be done for proper evaluation, since this procedure has been done only relatively recently.

DIVERTICULOSIS AND DIVERTICULITIS

A diverticulum is a pouch or saccular dilatation leading out from a tube or main cavity (Figure 7.14).

Diverticulitis is an inflammation of diverticula. Diverticulosis is the condition in which an individual has multiple diverticula.

PREDISPOSING FACTORS
1. Weakening and degeneration of muscular wall of the intestine, causing herniation of the lining mucous membrane through a muscle at site of artery penetration.
2. Increased mechanical pressure due to abnormal high-pressure contractions of sigmoid colon in response to neurohumoral stimuli.
3. Chronic overdistention of the large bowel.
4. Probably congenital predisposition.

INCIDENCE
1. Diverticulosis usually occurs in about 10 per cent of individuals over 40 years of age and nearly 50 per cent of people over the age of 60; only a small percentage develop diverticulitis.
2. The condition is most common in the sigmoid colon.
3. Small-bowel diverticula are unusual, but when they occur they are often multiple. They may act as areas of stasis and bacterial overgrowth, leading to malabsorption of fat and vitamin B_{12}.

ALTERED PHYSIOLOGY
(Colon diverticulosis and diverticulitis.)
Constipation from spastic colon syndrome often precedes the development of diverticulosis by many years.
1. Following local inflammation of the diverticula, there may be narrowing of the colon with fibrotic stricture, which then leads to narrowed stools, cramps and increasing constipation.
2. With the development of granulation tissue, occult bleeding may occur, producing iron

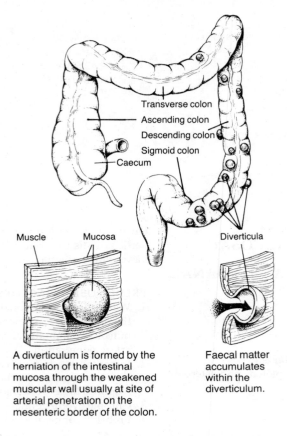

Transverse colon

Ascending colon

Descending colon

Sigmoid colon

Caecum

Muscle   Mucosa   Diverticula

A diverticulum is formed by the
herniation of the intestinal
mucosa through the weakened
muscular wall usually at site of
arterial penetration on the
mesenteric border of the colon.

Faecal matter
accumulates
within the
diverticulum.

Figure 7.14. Diverticula are most common in the sigmoid colon; they diminish in number and size as the colon approaches the caecum. Diverticula are rarely found in the rectum

deficiency anaemia; fatigue and weakness are then evident. However, massive bleeding is more common.

3. Abscess development causes a tender palpable mass; fever and leucocytosis also occur.
4. If the diverticulum perforates, local abscess or peritonitis results; peritonitis causes rigidity, abdominal pain, loss of bowel sounds and eventually shock.
5. Uninflamed or minimally inflamed diverticula may erode adjacent arterial branches, causing acute massive rectal bleeding.

Assessment
CLINICAL FEATURES
General clinical signs
1. May occur in acute attacks or may persist as a long, drawn-out smouldering infection.
2. Tends to spread into surrounding bowel wall, increasing the irritability and spasticity of the colon.
3. When infections are severe, perforation of the colon can occur, leading to peritonitis.
4. When infection is less acute but slowly progressive, extensive scarring and abscess formation involving the bowel wall may occur, with the possibility of lower bowel obstruction. Sometimes, fistulae form with the bladder, the adjacent small bowel, the vagina or even the skin.
5. Sepsis may spread via portal vein to liver, causing liver abscesses.

Specific clinical signs
1. Diverticulosis:
   a. Bowel irregularity, constipation, and diarrhoea.
   b. Sudden massive haemorrhage (occurs in 10 to 20 per cent of patients).

2. Milder forms of diverticulitis:
   a. Bouts of soreness, mild lower abdominal cramps.
   b. Bowel irregularity, constipation and diarrhoea.
3. Moderately severe acute diverticulitis:
   a. Crampy pain in lower left quadrant of abdomen.
   b. Low-grade fever, chills, leucocytosis.

DIAGNOSTIC EVALUATION
1. Sigmoidoscopy; possibly colonoscopy.
2. Fluoroscopy and X-ray with barium enema.

PATIENT PROBLEMS
1. Intestinal discomfort, diarrhoea or constipation related to bowel irregularity.
2. Alteration in nutrition related to uncertainty as to appropriate diet to follow.
3. Anxiety related to concern about the possibility of malignancy.
4. Lack of knowledge related to lack of understanding of the relation between diet and diverticulosis.

Planning and implementation
NURSING INTERVENTIONS
Provide rest for the intestinal tract and alleviate constipation
1. During acute episode, maintain fluid and nutritional requirements with intravenous therapy, as directed. Give nothing by mouth.
2. Maintain antibiotic therapy as prescribed to reduce infection.
3. For pain, pethidine is the analgesic of choice because it is less spasmogenic than other analgesics.
4. When indicated, employ stool-softeners such as docusate sodium (Dioctyl).
5. Administer bulk additives to counteract tendency toward constipation; a frequently prescribed smooth bulk laxative is psyllium hydrophilic mucilloid (Metamucil).
6. Warm-oil-retention enemas may be prescribed to treat inflammation locally by softening faecal mass.

NURSING ALERT
Ordinary enemas and laxatives may be harmful and should not be used.

Note: In some patients, an increase in mass results in an increase in symptoms.

7. Check with doctor as to type of diet to be followed. Some authorities prefer fibre content in the diet rather than a low-residue diet. With increased fibre more bulk is added to give the stool proper consistency. With a low-residue diet, the colon may work harder to propel contents, thereby producing high pressure on the intestinal wall, which in turn promotes diverticula formation.

SURGICAL TREATMENT
1. If there is little response to medical treatment, or if complications such as haemorrhage, obstruction or perforation occur, surgery is necessary.
2. Preparation for surgery:
   a. Low-residue diet or nothing by mouth.
   b. Antibiotics, systemic and intestinal surface-acting, to reduce bowel bacterial flora, diminish bulk of stool and soften faecal mass for easier movement.
   c. Cleansing enemas may be prescribed.
3. Resection of segment of intestine involved with diverticula, reuniting (anastomosing) two ends to maintain continuity.
4. Temporary colostomy is sometimes performed to divert faecal stream (see p. 493), with continuity restored in later second-stage procedure.

PATIENT EDUCATION
Objective
Prevent recurrence of diverticular disease.
1. Maintain a diet that is high in soft residue and low in sugar; obtain lists of these foods in order to be familiar with proper dietary control; how well the intestinal tract functions in great measure depends on proper food intake.
2. Bran products will add bulk to the stool and can be taken with milk or sprinkled over cereal.
3. Establish regular bowel habits to promote regular and complete evacuation; mineral oil can be used nightly if necessary, but dependence on it should be discouraged.
4. Have the patient continue periodic medical supervision and follow-up; report problems and untoward symptoms.

Evaluation
EXPECTED OUTCOMES
1. The patient reports near-normal bowel function; no diarrhoea or constipation.
2. Consumes a prescribed diet and can relate what foods to include or avoid.
3. Expresses relief that diagnostic studies revealed no malignancy.
4. Delineates the general nature of diverticulosis and can list what helps or aggravates the condition.

INTESTINAL OBSTRUCTION

Intestinal obstruction is an interruption in the normal flow of intestinal contents along the intestinal tract.

The block may occur in the small or large intestine, may be complete or incomplete, may be mechanical or paralytic, and may or may not compromise the vascular supply. Obstruction most frequently occurs in the very young and the very old.

TYPES OF OBSTRUCTION

1. Mechanical – a physical block to passage of intestinal contents without disturbing blood supply of bowel.
   a. Location:
      (i) Extrinsic (e.g. adhesion, hernia, intussusception);
      (ii) Intrinsic (e.g. haematoma, tumour);
      (iii) Intraluminal (e.g. foreign body, faecal or barium impaction, polyp).
   b. Clinical pattern:
      (i) High small-bowel (jejunal) or low small-bowel (ileal) occurs four times more frequently than colonic obstruction.
2. Paralytic (adynamic, neurogenic) ileus:
   Peristalsis is ineffective (diminished motor activity perhaps because of toxic or traumatic disturbance of the autonomic nervous system); there is no physical obstruction and no interrupted blood supply.
3. Strangulation:
   Obstruction also compromises blood supply, leading to gangrene of the intestine.

CAUSES

1. Mechanical (extramural):
   a. Adhesions – postoperative;
   b. Hernia;
   c. Malignancy;
   d. Volvulus (loop of intestine that has twisted).
2. Mechanical (intramural);
   a. Carcinoma;
   b. Haematoma;
   c. Intussusception (telescoping of intestine);
   d. Stricture or stenosis (scarring).
3. Paralytic:
   a. Spinal cord injuries, vertebral fractures;
   b. Postoperatively after any abdominal surgery;
   c. Peritonitis, pneumonia;
   d. Wound (breakdown) dehiscence;
   e. Gastrointestinal tract surgery.

Note: .
1. In postoperative patients, approximately 90 per cent of mechanical obstructions are due to adhesions.
2. In nonsurgical patients, hernia (most often inguinal) is the most common cause of mechanical obstruction.

ALTERED PHYSIOLOGY

1. Disturbed physiological responses as a result of mechanical small-intestine obstruction results in increased peristalsis, distension by fluid and gas and increased bacterial growth proximal to obstruction. The intestine empties distally.
2. Increased secretions into the intestine are associated with diminution in the bowel's absorptive capacity.
3. The accumulation of gases, secretions and oral intake above the obstruction causes increasing intraluminal pressure.
4. Venous pressure in the affected area increases, and circulatory stasis and oedema result.
5. Bowel necrosis may occur because of anoxia and compression of the terminal branches of the mesenteric artery.
6. Bacteria and toxins pass across the intestinal membranes into the abdominal cavity, thereby leading to peritonitis.
7. 'Closed-loop' obstruction is a condition in which the intestinal segment is occluded at both ends preventing either the downward passage or the regurgitation of intestinal contents.

Assessment
CLINICAL FEATURES

Fever, peritoneal irritation, increased white blood cell count, toxicity and shock may develop with all types of intestinal obstruction.

1. Simple mechanical – high small bowel:
   Colic (cramps) mid-to-upper abdomen, some distension, early bilious vomiting, increased bowel sounds (high-pitched tinkling heard at brief intervals), minimal diffuse tenderness.
2. Simple mechanical – low small-bowel:
   Significant colic (cramps) midabdominal, considerable distension, vomiting (slight or absent), later faeculent, increased bowel sounds and 'hush' sounds, minimal diffuse tenderness.
3. Simple mechanical – colon:
   Cramps (mid-to-lower abdomen), later-appearing distension, then vomiting may develop (faeculent), increase in bowel sounds, minimal diffuse tenderness.
4. Partial chronic mechanical obstruction – may

occur with granulomatous bowel (Crohn's) disease. Symptoms are cramping abdominal pain, mild distension and diarrhoea.

5. Strangulation:
Symptoms are initially those of mechanical obstruction but later progress rapidly: pain is severe, continuous and localized. There is moderate distension, persistent vomiting, usually decreased bowel sounds and marked localized tenderness. Stools or vomitus become melaenous or bloody, or contain occult blood.

6. Paralytic ileus:
Gaseous distension is prominent; abdomen is tense; pain is dull, continuous and diffuse; obstipation (intractable constipation) is rarely complete, since small amounts of flatus may be passed; peristalsis is usually depressed, and bowel sounds are infrequent or absent; vomiting occurs only after eating (vomiting may later become faecal).

NURSING ASSESSMENT

NURSING ALERT
Because of loss of water, sodium and chloride, signs of dehydration become evident – intense thirst, drowsiness, general malaise, aching; tongue becomes parched, face appears pinched, abdomen becomes distended. Shock may result (pulse increasingly rapid and weak, temperature and blood pressure lowered, skin pale, cold, clammy) ending in death.

1. In the nursing history, describe accurately the nature and location of the patient's pain, the presence of distension, the absence of flatus or defaecation.
2. The overview of symptoms is important in differentiating intestinal obstruction from other more benign conditions.
3. Monitor and record vital signs (including blood pressure) every four hours.
4. Elderly patients with poor bowel tonus who often remain in the recumbent position for extended periods are likely to experience air-fluid lock syndrome, which is described below:
   a. Fluid collects in dependent bowel loops.
   b. Peristalsis is too weak to push fluid 'uphill'.
   c. Obstruction occurs primarily in the large bowel.
   d. Management consists simply of alternately turning the patient from supine to prone position every 10 minutes until enough flatus is passed to decompress the abdomen. A rectal tube may help.

5. Measure and record accurately all intake and output.
6. Save any stool that may be passed; this is to be tested for occult blood.
7. Anticipate doctor's request for urinalysis, haemoglobin determination and blood cell counts.
8. Frequently, determine the patient's level of consciousness; decreasing responsiveness may offer a clue to an increasing electrolyte imbalance.
9. Observe for evidence of postural hypotension as patient is moved from a recumbent position to an upright position; this may suggest circulatory insufficiency.
10. Compare the patient's state of orientation with his admission status; a lessening awareness of his environment may suggest he is going into shock.

PATIENT PROBLEMS
1. Alteration in bowel elimination related to an obstruction, whatever the cause.
2. Abdominal pain (colicky, continuous, sometimes severe and localized) related to distensions/ strangulation of a segment of intestine.
3. Respiratory impairment related to abdominal distension that interferes with proper lung expansion.
4. Compromised fluid balance related to impaired fluid intake, fluid lost by vomiting and diarrhoea resulting from an intestinal obstruction; potential for hypovolaemia.
5. Alteration in nutritional status related to intestinal obstruction, which prevents normal food intake.
6. Anxiety and fear of death related to life-threatening symptoms of intestinal obstruction.

Planning and implementation
NURSING INTERVENTIONS
Relief of pain
1. Administer prescribed analgesics.
2. The doctor may institute long-tube decompression of intestine proximal to block (p. 461); this can be passed more effectively with the patient lying on his right side; begin decompression to remove gas and fluid.
3. Provide supportive care during nasoenteral intubation, since this will help in relieving discomfort.

Relief of anxiety and fears
1. Recognize the patient's concern and initiate

measures to secure his co-operation and confidence in the staff.
2. Ascertain the patient's specific anxieties and provide him with therapeutic responses.

Fluid therapy
1. The doctor will correct fluid imbalance by initiating the following:
   a. Na^+, K^+, blood component therapy.
   b. Ringer's lactate to correct interstitial fluid deficit.
   c. Dextrose/water to correct intracellular fluid deficit.
2. Minimize those factors that would enhance gastric secretions in order to prevent fluid loss (via nasogastric suction); avoid conversation about enticing meals and eliminate meals being served within his range of seeing or smelling.

Ongoing assessment to monitor progress
1. Prevent infarction by carefully assessing the patient's status; if pain increases in intensity, localizes or becomes continuous, it may herald strangulation.
2. Detect early signs of peritonitis, such as rigidity and tenderness, in an effort to minimize this complication.
3. Recognize that giving an enema may distort an X-ray picture by introducing gas into the tract distal to the obstruction. An enema may make a partial obstruction worse; hence it is contraindicated.

SURGICAL CORRECTION
Preoperative nursing interventions
1. Undertake measures to prepare the patient for surgery, since most problems of mechanical obstruction require surgical correction.
2. Complete small-bowel obstruction and colon obstruction require an operation for relief. When tube suction therapy does not help after 12 hours, surgery is indicated.
   a. *Resection* of obstructing lesion and end-to-end anastomosis is done when no evidence of peritonitis and only minimal oedema exist; this requires a proximal colostomy to decompress new anastomosis.
   b. Resection of all necrotic intestine is necessary.
   c. A tube *enterostomy* may be done by introducing a catheter into distended bowel; the other end of catheter is brought out through the abdominal wall via a separate incision. This is a palliative measure.

d. A *loop colostomy* is done when relief is sought by drawing a proximal loop or segment of colon up to the skin surface and opening it as a colostomy; the distal portion of colon is treated later.

Postoperative nursing care
1. To meet fluid, electrolyte and nutritional needs, administer prescribed amounts of fluids; keep accurate intake and output records.
2. For an enterostomy, connect tube to drainage bottle at side of bed; expect considerable amount of faecal drainage during the first 12 to 15 hours (500–1,000ml).
   a. Observe frequently the patency of drainage equipment.
   b. If there is difficulty with drainage, it may be necessary to inject 15ml of warm saline into the enterostomy tube every two to four hours, with approval of doctor.
   c. Protect skin around enterostomy tube with a skin barrier such as Stomahesive or karaya preparations.
3. Follow additional postoperative management described in Major Intestinal Surgery, p. 466.

Evaluation
EXPECTED OUTCOMES
1. Demonstrates relief of bowel obstruction – passes flatus, has first bowel movement.
2. Demonstrates improved breathing ability.
3. Takes food and fluid orally.
4. Exhibits no vomiting or diarrhoea.
5. Experiences minimal pain.
6. Appears relaxed and reports he is 'feeling better'.

CANCER OF THE COLON

INCIDENCE
1. Cancer of the colon and rectum accounted for 24,112 newly diagnosed cases in England and Wales in 1983.
2. Males are affected slightly more often than females.
3. The highest incidence occurs in patients in the 60–79 age group.

AETIOLOGY AND RISK FACTORS
1. Familial polyposis (numerous pedunculated growths arising from mucosa and extending into lumen of intestine).
2. Chronic ulcerative colitis – definite risk of colon

cancer (up to 20 per cent after 20 years of age with active disease).

3. Diverticulosis and cancer may be found together and simulate each other – no definite evidence that the presence of diverticula is significant in the development of cancer.

4. Cancer of the colon occurs much more frequently in developed countries and rarely in under-developed countries. The increased incidence of colon cancer in developed countries is probably related to the relatively lower fibre content of diet in these areas.

5. Unabsorbable fibre deficit appears to be related to intestinal transit time, stool bulk and consistency.

6. The effect of diet on the colon bacterial flora is a factor possibly contributing to cancer.

RISK REDUCTION

Studies (Burkitt, 1979) indicate that high risk populations should:

1. Double daily intake of starch and fibre.
2. Reduce sugar and salt intake by one-half.
3. Reduce dietary fat by one-third.

Assessment

CLINICAL FEATURES

1. Distribution of cancer in the colon is shown in Figure 7.15.
2. Most common symptoms:
   a. Blood in stools (usually occult) – causing anaemia.

b. Partial obstruction – causing constipation alternating with diarrhoea, lower abdominal pains (crampy), distension.

c. Additional signs – progressive weakness, anorexia, weight loss, shortness of breath, anginal pain, anaemia.

DIAGNOSTIC EVALUATION

1. Digital rectal examination – half of all colon and rectal cancers are found this way.
2. Endoscopy (fibreoptic sigmoidoscopy/colon-oscopy) – two-thirds of all colon and rectal cancer can be seen and biopsied via proctoscope alone.
3. Stool examination for blood – often reveals evidence of carcinoma when the patient is otherwise asymptomatic.
4. Blood haemoglobin determination for anaemia.
5. Barium enema – especially significant in unexplained abdominal mass. Napkin-ring-type outline clearly indicates obstruction and possible tumour.
6. Intravenous pyelography and possible cystoscopy may be indicated to assess whether malignancy has spread locally to involve ureter or bladder.

TREATMENT
Diagnosis
This is confirmed by:

1. Removing rectosigmoid polyps through sigmoidoscope for histological study.

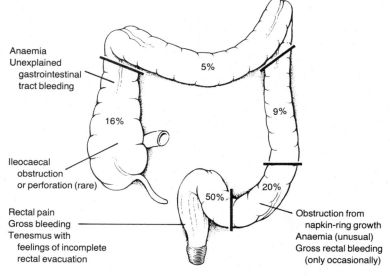

Figure 7.15. Distribution of the incidence of cancer in the colon

Anaemia
Unexplained
gastrointestinal
tract bleeding

5%

9%

16%

Ileocaecal
obstruction
or perforation (rare)

50%   20%

Rectal pain
Gross bleeding
Tenesmus with
feelings of incomplete
rectal evacuation

Obstruction from
napkin-ring growth
Anaemia (unusual)
Gross rectal bleeding
(only occasionally)

2. Removing polyps above rectosigmoid by colonoscopy or laparotomy (if other symptoms are present) to verify diagnosis.

Surgical therapeutic plan

1. Recommend total colectomy for patient with familial history of polyposis or prolonged, universal, chronically active colitis, even before cancer is confirmed.
2. Most common operative procedures:
   a. Wide segmental resection of colon and mesentery with anastomosis, or;
   b. Abdominoperineal resection with colostomy (if lesion is in rectum). See Colostomy below.
   c. Even more extensive surgery involving removal of other organs if cancer has spread – such as to the bladder, uterus, small intestine, groin, etc.
   d. If cancer is extensive and it may not be in the patient's best interest to do radical surgery, palliative treatment may be done using radiotherapy (combined surgery and preoperative radiotherapy is being done in several hospitals).
3. Colostomy. This is a temporary or permanent opening of the colon through the abdominal wall. The placement of the colostomy will influence the nature of the discharge (Figure 7.16). The stoma is that part of the colon that is brought above the abdominal wall in a colostomy and becomes the outlet for discharge of intestinal contents. Purposes are as follows:
   a. It may be part of an abdominoperineal resection for cure or palliation of cancer.
   b. It may be palliative when unresectable malignancy is present.
   c. It can be a temporary measure to protect an anastomosis, such as after abdominal trauma.
   d. It may be temporary to divert faecal stream during radiotherapy or other treatment.

PATIENT PROBLEMS

1. Nutritional deficit and weight loss related to malignant tumour.
2. Pain/discomfort related to spread of malignancy, inflammation and possible obstruction of intestinal tract.
3. Worry and fear related to anaesthesia, results of surgery and potential for complications.

Planning and implementation

PREOPERATIVE NURSING INTERVENTIONS
When colostomy is not anticipated

1. Meet the patient's nutritional needs by serving a high-calorie, low-residue diet for several days prior to surgery, if condition permits.
2. Observe and record fluid losses, such as may be sustained by vomiting and diarrhoea.
3. Maintain hydration by assisting with intravenous

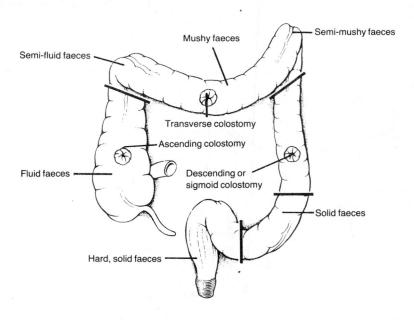

Figure 7.16. Placement of colostomies and the nature of the discharge at these sites

infusion, and observing and recording urinary output.

4. Reduce bacterial count of colon by mechanical cleansing and administering antibiotics as prescribed – orally and systemically. Whatever the choice, it should be effective against the full spectrum of aerobic and anaerobic faecal microbes. The degree of obstruction, acuteness, inflammation – all have a bearing on the nature of antibiotics administration.

5. Assist the patient during nasoenteral intubation for decompression of intestinal tract.

In preparation for colostomy

1. Determine the nature of anticipated surgery; the colostomy must be positioned where the patient can see and care for it (this is determined by the surgeon or stomatherapist).
   a. The colostomy should not be placed in the laparotomy incision.
   b. It should be placed where it will not interfere with proper fitting and comfortable wearing of an appliance – away from iliac crest, costal margin, umbilicus, scars, deep folds.

2. Make specific plans for the patient's understanding and acceptance of a colostomy.
   a. Collaborate with the surgeon in ascertaining the nature of communication and information exchanged between surgeon and patient, including initial patient contact, in-hospital experience, plans for rehabilitation.
   b. Reinforce the patient's hope for a future that will be manageable and will lead to independent functioning.
   c. If possible, show the patient the intended appliance and have him try it on.
   d. Arrange a preoperative visit by a trained visitor from the local colostomy association.
   e. Develop a plan with the stoma therapist and patient to include short-term and long-term goals. Provide the patient with literature and information according to his level of understanding. Take care not to overwhelm the patient with too much information.

3. Preparation for surgery – follow usual preoperative procedures and modify to meet individual needs.

POSTOPERATIVE NURSING INTERVENTIONS
See also General Postoperative Care, p. 58.

Initial care of the colostomy

1. Apply a temporary plastic colostomy bag to control odours and soiling. Tactfully try to have the patient look at his colostomy, and encourage him to participate in caring for it. Psychosocial skills and understanding are required. Evaluate learning readiness; never force independence.

2. Often the recognition of a bowel movement occurs when the patient's pouch or dressing is checked; for others, it may be the awareness of the escape of flatus or the contact of stool on the skin.

3. For some there is an awareness of motility, which enables them to get to the bathroom in time for discharging stool into the toilet.

4. Frequency and number of movements vary from person to person.

5. Regulation is enhanced when there is systematic planning, balanced meals eaten at regular intervals, and a regular time for irrigation and evacuation.

6. If directed by surgeon, irrigate when the immediate postoperative period is past and bowel function has resumed (usually fifth or sixth day) (See Guidelines, p. 495). This procedure is not so common in the UK.

7. Utilize the treatment time of irrigating the colostomy as the learning time for the patient to begin to master the art of managing his colostomy independently. Recognize that some patients are learning to control their colostomy without irrigation.

8. Although irrigation is widely used, recognize that there are some people who cannot control the colostomy this way (i.e. the patient with an 'irritable' colon or unpredictable bowel movements). Also, because of the nature of the contents in various parts of the colon, only colostomies in the descending or sigmoid colon can be expected to be controlled by irrigation. Ascending and transverse colostomies have outputs that are too frequent and too liquid to facilitate control.

9. Irrigations for most people are done every other day.

10. The cone-tip is excellent to prevent insertion of a catheter into insensitive mucosa with risk of perforating the bowel wall. The cone-tip is plugged into the stoma for about 2.5cm and permits irrigation without perforation or leakage.

DISCHARGE PLANNING/PATIENT EDUCATION
See also Patient education (discharge from hospital), p. 480.
See also Irrigation of Colostomy, p. 495.

Skin care
1. One group of effective skin barriers is made of karaya gum. Karaya is available in powder form, discs or rings, which can be placed on excoriated peristomal skin (i.e. new skin can grow under them). Karaya paste and rings are excellent for preventing skin irritation immediately around the stoma.
2. Hypoallergenic skin shields include Stomahesive (Squibb). These tend to deteriorate less quickly than the karaya washers and often can be worn in areas where there are creases and wrinkles.
   a. Stomahesive can be used as 10 × 10cm sheets or can be cut into washer size. Stomahesive adheres well on weepy, irritated skin and allows healing to occur.
3. Coverings over the stoma may be a disposable pouch, gauze, facial tissue covered with petroleum jelly, cling film, or stoma wipes over a dressing. Hypoallergenic tape may be used.
4. For peristomal excoriation, corticosteroid aerosol sprays or nystatin powders are useful when used sparingly.
5. For allergic reactions, try other products until a compatible one is found; antacid suspensions are found to be practical for some patients.

Odour control
1. Avoid foods known to cause odours – for example, onions, members of the cabbage family, eggs, fish and beans.
2. Note that faecal odours are lessened with yoghurt, cranberry juice and buttermilk.
3. Odours can be controlled by using odour-absorbing powder, aspirin tablet or vanilla essence in the bag.

Control of gas
1. Most gas is due to swallowed air (often taken in while chewing gum), highly spiced foods and carbonated beverages, including beer.
2. Avoid gas-forming foods: beans, cabbage family, onions, radishes, cucumbers and highly seasoned foods.

Diet
1. Avoid overeating and eating irregularly; chew food well.
2. Individualize the diet so that it is balanced and will not cause diarrhoea and constipation. A daily diary is effective in determining what foods cause difficulty and can then be eliminated from the diet.

3. Note that fruits, fruit juices and tomatoes may cause frequent bowel movements. Beer may be a laxative, as well as a gas-producer.

Enhanced lifestyle
1. There may be some impairment of sexual function and potency; fortunately, this impairment is temporary in most cases. Male colostomates vary in degree of potency from full potency to complete impotence. Some patients take up to two years to regain potency.
2. A colostomy in a woman does not preclude a successful pregnancy; close medical care is required.
3. There is no contraindication to any form of travel, including horseback riding.
4. Participation in any type of sport is possible.
5. Showering is possible with or without the appliance.
6. Girdles, swimming trunks and tights may all be worn, provided there is neither discomfort nor too much constriction.
7. Promote the patient's acceptance of the colostomy by building up self-esteem; encourage the family to assist the patient during the period of adjustment.
8. Be aware that patients of ethnic origins may have cultural or religious reasons that make acceptance of a colostomy difficult.
9. Contact the community nurse, who will serve as a liaison among hospital, surgeon and home as a follow-up when the patient continues to adjust to the colostomy at home.
10. Inform the patient about the Colostomy Welfare Group and enrol him in a local group so that he may obtain information and exchange ideas with other colostomates.
11. Provide the patient with literature, addresses and telephone numbers of the organizations listed on p. 484.

Evaluation
EXPECTED OUTCOMES
1. Exhibits weight gain trend and improved nutritional status as demonstrated by adequate dietary intake.
2. Has no pain and minimal discomfort following surgery for removal of colon cancer.
3. Is adjusting to changed lifestyle following surgery; no evidence of complications.
4. Demonstrates ability to care for colostomy.

GUIDELINES: IRRIGATING A COLOSTOMY

PURPOSES
1. Empty the colon of its contents: faeces, gas, mucus.
2. Cleanse the lower intestinal tract.
3. Establish a regular pattern of evacuation so that normal, everyday activities may be pursued.

EQUIPMENT

Reservoir for irrigating fluids; enema bag, irrigating can

Irrigating fluid: 500–1,500ml lukewarm tap water or other solution if prescribed by doctor

Tubing, connecting tubes and clamp; preferable clamp – one that can be operated with one hand

Irrigating tip: soft rubber catheter – No. 22 or No. 24 with some type of shield to prevent backflow of

irrigating solution (or soft rubber or plastic cone irrigating tip)

Irrigating sleeve or sheath; self-adhering (adhesive) or held in place with a belt (a plastic or rubber sheet can be used as a trough in place of a sheath)

Newspaper or plastic bag: to collect soiled dressings and disposable pouch

Toilet tissues and water-soluble lubricant

PROCEDURE
Preparatory phase
1. Select a suitable time, preferably after a meal, so that this hour fits into the patient's posthospital pattern of activity. Irrigation should be done at the same time each day.
2. Hang irrigating reservoir with solution 45 to 50cm above stoma (shoulder height with patient seated).
3. Have the patient sit in front of toilet commode on chair or on commode itself.
4. Remove dressings or pouch and place in bag.

Performance phase

Nursing action	Rationale
1. Apply irrigating sleeve or sheath to stoma. Place end in commode.	Helps control odour and splashing. Allows faeces and water to flow directly into commode.
2. Allow some of solution to flow through tubing and catheter/cone.	To release air bubbles in the equipment so that air is not introduced into the colon, which would cause cramp pains.
3. Lubricate catheter/cone and gently insert into stoma. Insert catheter no more than 8cm. Hold shield/cone gently, but firmly, against stoma to prevent backflow of water.	These steps are necessary to prevent intestinal perforation.
4. If catheter does not advance easily, allow water to flow slowly while advancing catheter. *NEVER FORCE CATHETER.*	Slow rate of flow helps relax bowel and facilitates passage of catheter.

5. Allow fluid to enter colon slowly. If cramp occurs, clamp off tubing and allow the patient to rest before progressing. Water should flow in over a 5- to 10-minute period.

Painful cramps are usually caused by too-rapid flow or too much solution: 500ml is usually sufficient for initial postoperative irrigation; volume may be increased with subsequent irrigations to 1,000 or 1,500ml, to produce effective results.

6. Hold shield/cone in place 10 seconds after water has been instilled, then gently remove.

7. Allow 10 to 15 minutes for most of return, then dry bottom of sleeve/sheath and attach it to top, or apply appropriate clamp to bottom of sleeve.

Most of water, faeces and flatus will be expelled in 10 to 15 minutes.

8. Leave sleeve/sheath in place about 20 minutes while patient gets up and moves around.

Ambulation stimulates peristalsis and completion of irrigation return.

Follow-up phase

Nursing action

Rationale

1. Cleanse area with mild soap and water; pat dry.

Cleanliness and dryness will provide the patient with hours of comfort.

2. Apply a karaya preparation or other peristomal skin barrier; replace colostomy dressing or pouch.

The patient should use pouch until colostomy is sufficiently controlled. Karaya will protect skin from irritation.

3. Clean equipment with soap and water; dry before storing in well-ventilated area.

This will control odour and prolong life of equipment.

ANORECTAL CONDITIONS AND TREATMENTS

NURSING PROCESS OVERVIEW

Assessment
NURSING HISTORY
1. Observe the stool for evidence of bleeding. Is stool mixed or coated with blood?
2. Determine presence of pain during and after evacuation. Is there associated abdominal pain? How long does it last?
3. When recording, describe the problem in the patient's words.
4. Note presence of a discharge. Is it purulent, bloody?

PATIENT PROBLEMS
1. Pain in rectal region related to pathology, infection or surgery.
2. Alteration in bowel elimination related to discomfort during defaecation.
3. Psychosocial and diversional activity deficit related to discomfort.
4. Self-care deficits (hygiene, toileting) related to difficulty in seeing or reaching anal area.
5. Lack of knowledge about how to keep rectal area clean and reasons why this is important.

Planning and implementation
PREOPERATIVE NURSING INTERVENTIONS
1. Be an understanding and concerned listener when this patient relates problems of a personal nature.
2. Ensure and respect the patient's privacy when

attending to personal hygiene, examinations and treatments.
3. Do not minimize complaints of discomfort.

POSTOPERATIVE NURSING INTERVENTIONS
Comfort and wound healing
1. Be gentle in changing dressings, shaving, irrigating or administering perineal care.
2. Use petroleum gauze (tulle gras) in protecting edges of wounds (e.g. following incision and drainage of ischiorectal abscess, excision of pilonidal sinus) to prevent crusting and the dressings from sticking to wound.
3. Provide baths when recommended; adjust temperature of solution and provide a comfortable position for the patient.
4. Use caution in applying analgesic or anaesthetic ointments, since this often leads to secondary skin rashes from allergy.
5. Keep the perineal area clean to minimize or eliminate infection; presence of E. coli demands meticulous cleanliness to prevent infection and promote healing.
6. Change the patient's position from side to side to prevent added discomfort of pressure areas; use air ring if appropriate.
7. Prevent constipation by proper attention to diet needs of patient; give mild aperient only as prescribed; use stool softeners.
8. Encourage voluntary voiding of urine to avoid catheterization; this may be facilitated by getting patient out of bed.
9. Observe vital signs and dressings for evidence of haemorrhage, particularly following haemorrhoidectomy.
10. Daily rectal sphincter dilatation may be needed to relieve pain from spasm, to ensure granulation of incisional wounds from the bottom out, and to prevent postoperative stricture.

HAEMORRHOIDS

Haemorrhoids are varicosities in the lower rectum or anus resulting from congestion in the veins of the haemorrhoidal plexus; external haemorrhoids appear outside the external sphincter, whereas internal haemorrhoids appear above the internal sphincter. When blood within the haemorrhoids becomes clotted and infected, the haemorrhoids are referred to as thrombosed.

PREDISPOSING FACTORS
1. Pregnancy.
2. Straining at stool.
3. Chronic constipation.
4. Prolonged sitting.
5. Anal infection.
6. Hereditary factor.
7. Portal hypertension (cirrhosis).

CLINICAL FEATURES
1. Sensation of incomplete faecal evacuation.
2. Protrusion.
3. Constipation.
4. Bleeding during defaecation.
5. Infection or ulceration.
6. Pain noted more in external haemorrhoids.
7. Mucus discharge.
8. Cosmetic deformity.

DIAGNOSTIC EVALUATION
1. History and visualization by external examination and the use of an anoscope or proctoscope.
2. Barium enema also should be performed, since haemorrhoids are often warning signs of more serious colonic lesions, which may be the actual source of observed rectal bleeding.

TREATMENT AND NURSING INTERVENTION
Haemorrhoids appear to be normal; asymptomatic haemorrhoids require no treatment.

Medical
1. Patient should adhere to a low-roughage, high-fibre diet to keep stool soft. Some authorities suggest a diet that includes 30g miller's bran per day or replacing white bread with whole wheat.
2. Bowel habits should be regulated with nonirritating stool softeners (e.g. milk of magnesia) to keep stools soft.
3. Frequent hot baths.
4. Insertion of soothing anal suppository two to three times daily.
5. Application of witch ·hazel compresses for comfort.
6. Control of itching by placement of a cotton gauze in folded soft tissue between the buttocks against the anus to absorb moisture.
7. Do not use topical anaesthetics on haemorrhoids or fissures, since they often produce hypersensitivity (allergic) perianal skin rashes with severe itching.
8. If haemorrhoids are prolapsed and the patient is unable to reduce them himself, the nurse may have to reduce them manually:

a. Apply cold compresses to anal area.

b. Gently apply anaesthetic ointment with a gloved finger.

c. Very gently manipulate haemorrhoids back through rectal sphincter.

d. Apply an anaesthetic ointment on a dressing to rectal area.

9. Surgery may be indicated when the following conditions exist:

a. Prolonged bleeding.

b. Disabling pain.

c. Intolerable itching.

d. General unrelieved discomfort.

Surgical

1. Barron ligation with a rubber band is considered 'ideal' treatment.

a. A large anoscope is used; the apex of the internal haemorrhoid is grasped and drawn through a double-sleeved cylinder.

b. An elastic band is loaded on the inner cylinder and released by a trigger device so that the band encircles the base of the haemorrhoid.

c. After a period of time, the haemorrhoid sloughs away.

2. Cryodestruction – freezing of haemorrhoids. It is claimed to be less painful; some patients have a foul-smelling discharge for about a week to 10 days following cryosurgery.

3. Dilatation – forced dilatation of the anal canal and lower rectum under general anaesthesia is another advocated treatment. This procedure is not advocated for patients whose main complaints are prolapse or incontinence. It also is not recommended for ageing patients with weak sphincters.

4. Incision and removal of clot from acutely thrombosed haemorrhoid.

5. Excision of haemorrhoids includes the following procedures:

a. Dilatation of rectal sphincter.

b. Ligation and excision of haemorrhoid under local or spinal anaesthesia.

c. Insertion of drainage tube to permit escape of flatus and blood.

d. Postoperative dilatation with metal dilator.

PATIENT EDUCATION

(To prepare patient for posthospital convalescence.)

1. Instruct the patient on perianal hygiene to minimize the possibility of infection; avoid rubbing area with toilet tissue; instead, pat the area dry.

2. Apply wet dressings to relieve oedema.

3. Advise the patient regarding the effect of diet on stool formation; plant fibres of leafy vegetables and the roughage of bran flakes, wholegrains and wholewheat bread add roughage to the diet to form cellulose. Cellulose absorbs water, swells and softens stool, thereby stimulating peristalsis and aiding in intestinal elimination. Encourage the patient to eat fresh fruits, fruit juice and fresh vegetables except for seeds, skins, sweetcorn and nuts.

4. Avoid aperient so that stool is formed rather than being soft or liquid.

5. Recommend hot baths or hot compresses to relieve painful sphincter spasm.

6. Suggest adequate fluid intake and daily exercise to prevent constipation; encourage the patient to have a regular time each day for having a bowel movement.

7. Stool softeners are often given until good bowel habits are established.

a. 'Wetting agents' contain dioctyl sodium sulphosuccinate, a substance that penetrates, moistens and softens hard, dry stool.

b. 'Bulk producers' such as psyllium and agar preparations absorb water, add bulk and add moisture to stool.

c. Mineral oil tends to destroy oil-soluble vitamins A, D, E and K and interferes with absorption of calcium and phosphorus. It should be given at least three hours after the evening meal. (Do not give mineral oil to elderly patients because of possible aspiration pneumonia.)

8. Administer enemas only when absolutely necessary; rectal suppositories may be helpful.

Evaluation

EXPECTED OUTCOMES

1. Describes the dietary modification to be practised to ensure regular and moderately soft stool.

2. Experiences decreased discomfort in rectal area.

3. Is mobile and active as a result of decrease or elimination of pain and discomfort.

4. Practices hygienic health measures and uses special comfort cushion when sitting.

5. Increases social contacts.

6. States explicitly how to clean perineal area after defaecation/voiding.

See Table 7.8 for descriptions of perineal abscess, fistula in ano and fissure in ano.

Table 7.8 Perianal abscess / fistula in ano / fissure in ano

Condition	Description	Management
Perianal abscess	Localized infection in fatty tissue near rectum; pain increases Condition should raise suspicion of granulomatous bowel disease	Incision and drainage
Fistula in ano	Abnormal opening from the skin near the anus that winds tortuously into the anal canal Because it is an infectious area, pus leaks outward Condition should raise suspicion of granulomatous bowel disease	1. Surgical identification of the path of a fistula 2. Fistulotomy or partial sphincterotomy
Fissure in ano	Longitudinal ulcer (a crack that does not heal in the anal canal) frequently associated with constipation, as well as excruciating pain and blood-streaking on defaecation	1. Stool softener (dioctyl sodium sulphosuccinate) 2. If failure to heal with nonoperative therapy, dilatation of anal sphincter and sphincterotomy or fissurotomy

GUIDELINES: MANUAL REMOVAL OF FAECAL IMPACTION

A faecal impaction is the retention of hardened faeces in the rectum or lower sigmoid.

CLINICAL FEATURES AND OCCURRENCE
1. The patient may say he is constipated; often he has a desire to defaecate but is unable to do so.
2. Diarrhoea or liquid faecal seepage may occur around the obstructing impaction.
3. The patient may complain of rectal pain.
4. This condition may occur in elderly people following chronic constipation, insufficient hydration or ingestion of fibrous foods.
5. Orthopaedic patients who have been in traction or in body casts may develop an impaction.
6. Occasionally, impaction occurs in patients following rectal surgery or when barium has not been adequately removed following radiological examination.
7. Impaction is also common in patients with neurological or psychotic disorders.

PURPOSE OF FAECAL DISIMPACTION
Remove hardened faeces in the rectum or lower sigmoid.

EQUIPMENT
Clean (not necessarily sterile) rubber or plastic glove
Water-soluble lubricant
Bedpan
Plastic or rubber sheet with cloth protection
Soap, water, washcloth

PROCEDURE
Preparatory phase

Nursing action	Rationale
1. Explain procedure to the patient.	
2. Position the patient on left side with upper knee flexed.	To permit access to rectum and lower sigmoid.
3. Drape the patient and place protecting pad under buttocks.	To prevent chilling and undue exposure.
4. Place bedpan in a convenient place.	To serve as receptacle.
5. Put on glove and lubricate index finger generously (some prefer the middle finger because it is longer).	

Performance phase
See Figure 7.17.

Nursing action	Rationale
1. Insert gloved finger *gently* into rectum until impaction is felt.	This stimulation may increase peristalsis.

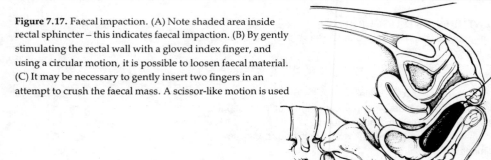

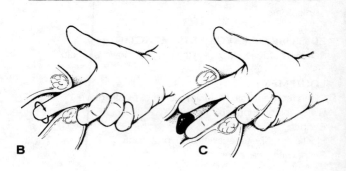

Figure 7.17. Faecal impaction. (A) Note shaded area inside rectal sphincter – this indicates faecal impaction. (B) By gently stimulating the rectal wall with a gloved index finger, and using a circular motion, it is possible to loosen faecal material. (C) It may be necessary to gently insert two fingers in an attempt to crush the faecal mass. A scissor-like motion is used

Faecal mass

2. *Gently* remove or break faecal material within reach and deposit in bedpan; work finger around and into mass to break it up if possible.

The emphasis is on *gentleness*, since this may be painful.

3. Gently stimulate rectal sphincter by making a circular motion once or twice.

This may stimulate peristalsis and relax the sphincter.

4. If step 3 does not result in removal of the impaction, it may be necessary to *gently* insert the middle and index finger and attempt to break up the mass by a scissorlike movement of the fingers. Repeat steps 2 or 4 until all easily reachable faecal masses are removed.

Greater leverage is afforded, and the mass may be more easily broken.

5. Note any bleeding or pain; observe the patient for shortness of breath or perspiration.

Should any of these responses occur, stop the procedure.

Follow-up phase

Nursing action

Rationale

1. Gently wash and dry the rectal area; make the patient comfortable and encourage him to rest.

Drying the area prevents skin excoriation and promotes comfort.

2. Note bedpan contents and then empty.

3. Record colour, consistency and odour of stool.

These characteristics may provide clues to the nature of the problem.

4. Plan health instruction measures in an effort to prevent a recurrence. Explore nutritional and fluid needs of the patient; determine activity level and encourage suitable exercises to promote adequate elimination.

Investigate the possibility of using stool softeners; suggest periodic use of Klyx enema.

CONDITIONS OF THE HEPATIC AND BILIARY SYSTEM

FEATURES OF DISORDERS OF THE LIVER

PATHOPHYSIOLOGY

Disorders of the liver result from direct damage to the liver cells (hepatocytes) or indirectly as a result of alterations in bile or blood flow through the liver.

AETIOLOGY

1. Viral infections and the effects of toxins may lead to hepatocellular dysfunction.
2. Chronic alcohol consumption, along with malnutrition, may cause toxic liver damage (cirrhosis).
3. Impairment of liver function may occur when flow of bile into the intestine is impeded (i.e. obstruction of the biliary tract by gallstones or a tumour).

GENERAL ASSESSMENT, WHICH MAY INDICATE LIVER DYSFUNCTION
Physical assessment of liver
1. Begin by placing the left hand under the patient's

back at the level of the eleventh or twelfth rib. The liver border, if felt, should be firm and smooth. Place the right hand, with fingers angled and slightly facing the costal margin, just below the percussed lower border of the liver.

2. During palpation with the right hand, press upward with the left hand to move the liver anteriorly (to facilitate palpation).

3. Have the patient inspire, and on expiration press the fingers of the right hand inward. On deep inspiration by the patient do not change the position of the right hand, feel for the liver edge moving over the fingers. If nothing is felt on inspiration, palpate more deeply, then on each subsequent inspiration, move the finger upward toward the costal margin. With each new position of the fingers, have the patient breathe deeply and feel for the liver.

CLINICAL FEATURES
Altered skin integrity related to jaundice and oedema
Jaundice is present when all tissues, including the sclerae and skin, assume a yellow or greenish-yellow tinge because of an increased concentration of bilirubin. (See p. 506 for types of jaundice.) Oedema occurs when the liver is no longer able to synthesize adequate amounts of albumin. These changes impair normal skin integrity.

1. Normal bilirubin concentration in blood is 2–17mmol/l of blood.
2. Clinical jaundice is detected if circulating bilirubin exceeds two to three times the normal.
3. Normal albumin level is 3.5–5g/dl.
4. An albumin level below 3g/dl, with an increased serum globulin level occurs with liver disease.

Bleeding tendencies related to altered clotting mechanisms and portal hypertension
1. Because of blood coagulation defects, gastrointestinal haemorrhage, bleeding gums, blood in urine, rectal bleeding and tarry stool, may occur.
2. Minor skin trauma may produce bruising (ecchymosis).
3. Following all types of intramuscular and intravenous injections and arterial punctures, it is necessary to apply pressure for longer than usual and to observe for haematoma.

Altered fluid and electrolyte balance
1. Tissue oedema and intra-abdominal fluid (ascites) are manifestations of sodium and water retention, combined with potassium excretion.
2. Hypoproteinaemia, iron-decreased hepatic synthesis and disturbed kidney function also contribute to fluid retention.

Altered mental and neurological states related to deterioration of liver function
1. Pyridoxine deficiency can result in nervous irritability and convulsive seizures.
2. Thiamine deficiency may lead to polyneuritis and Wernicke–Korsakoff psychosis.
3. Failure to metabolize ammonia arriving from intestine in portal venous system and impaired metabolism of sedative drugs produce range of symptoms from irritability and confusion to stupor, somnolence and coma.

DIAGNOSTIC EVALUATION OF LIVER DISEASE

LIVER DIAGNOSTIC STUDIES
See Table 7.9.

Table 7.9   Liver diagnostic studies

Test and purpose	Normal	Clinical and nursing significance
Bile formation and secretion		
1. *Serum bilirubin (van den Bergh reaction)* Measures bilirubin in the blood; this determines the ability of the liver to take up, conjugate and excrete bilirubin. Bilirubin is a product of the breakdown of haemoglobin:		
a. Direct (conjugated) – soluble in water	<5mmol/l	Abnormal in biliary and liver disease causing jaundice clinically
b. Total serum bilirubin	2–17mmol/l	Abnormal in haemolysis and in functional disorders of uptake or conjugation

2. *Urine bilirubin*
   Not normally found in urine, but if direct serum bilirubin is elevated, some spills into urine

None

Mahogany-coloured urine; when specimen is shaken, yellow tint to foam can be observed. Confirm with Ictotest tablet or Dipstick
If phenazopyridine (Pyridium) is being taken, there may be a false-positive bilirubin result (mark laboratory slip if this medication is being taken)

3. *Urobilinogen*
   Formed in small intestine by action of bacteria on bilirubin. Related to amount of bilirubin excreted into bile

Urine urobilinogen up to 0–6.7mmol/l
Faecal urobilinogen 50–504mmol/l

Urine specimen is collected over two-hour period after lunch. Place specimen in dark brown container and send it to laboratory immediately to prevent decomposition
If the patient is receiving antibiotics, mark laboratory slip to this effect, since production of urobilinogen can be falsely reduced

Protein studies
1. *Albumin and globulin measurement*
   Is of greater significance than total protein measurement.

   a. Albumin – produced by liver cells

   3.5–5g/dl

   b. Globulin – produced in lymph nodes, spleen and bone marrow and Kupffer's cells of liver

   0.5–1.5g/dl

   c. Total serum protein

   60–80g/l

As one increases, the other decreases; hence,

Albumin ↓ cirrhosis
          chronic hepatitis
Globulin ↑ cirrhosis
          chronic obstructive
            jaundice
          viral hepatitis

2. *Prothrombin time (PT)*
   Prothrombin and other clotting factors are manufactured in the liver; its rate is influenced by the supply of vitamin K

10–14 seconds

Prothrombin time may be prolonged in liver disease, in which case it will not return to normal with vitamin K. It may also be prolonged in malabsorption of fat and fat-soluble vitamins, in which case it will not return to normal with vitamin K

Fat metabolism
1. *Cholesterol*
   It is possible to measure lipid metabolism by determining serum cholesterol levels

3.6–5.7mmol/l (fasting) (depends on age and diet)

Serum cholesterol level is decreased in parenchymal liver disease.
Serum lipid level is increased in biliary obstruction

Liver detoxification
1. *Serum alkaline phosphatase*
   Since bile disposes this enzyme, any impairment of liver cell excretory function will cause an elevation. In cholestasis or obstruction, increased synthesis of enzyme causes very high levels in blood

Varies with method: 1.5–4.0 Bodansky units, 21–100dl

Abnormalities: The level is elevated to more than three times normal in obstructive jaundice, intrahepatic cholestasis, liver metastasis, or granulomas. Also elevated in osteoblastic diseases, Paget's disease and hyperparathyroidism
Continued

Table 7.9   Continued

Test and purpose	Normal	Clinical and nursing significance
Enzyme production		
Transaminase (SGOT) (aspartate aminotransferase or AST)	5–15IU/l	An elevation in these enzymes indicates liver cell damage
Transaminase (SGPT) (alanine aminotransferase or ALT)	5–30IU/l	**Note:** Opiates may also cause a rise in SGOT and SGPT
		Aspirin may cause an increase or decrease in SGOT and SGPT
Other 'liver profile' tests		
GGT (gamma glutamyl transpeptidase)		
Bile acids radioimmunoassay are replacing bromsulphalein (BSP) tests		

Normal values vary considerably from one laboratory to another according to conditions under which enzyme estimates are performed. All figures are approximate and vary from centre to centre.

GUIDELINES: ASSISTING WITH LIVER BIOPSY

Liver biopsy is the sampling of liver tissue by needle aspiration.

PURPOSE
Establish a diagnosis of liver disease by histological study of liver tissue.

EQUIPMENT
Sterile aspiration syringe and biopsy needle (Silverman)
Local anaesthetic
Skin antiseptics, sterile fenestrated towel, gloves
Glass slides, specimen bottles containing fixative and/or test tubes

PROCEDURE
Preparatory phase
1. See that consent form is signed.
2. Verify that the patient has had prothrombin tests and blood typing by checking the chart.
3. Determine availability of compatible blood, since these patients often have clotting defects.
4. Determine and record patient's pulse, respiration, arterial pressure and prothrombin time immediately before the biopsy in order to have a baseline of comparison with the postbiopsy condition of the patient.
5. Explain the steps of this procedure to the patient to reduce his concerns and gain his co-operation.

Performance phase

Nursing action	**Rationale**
1. Place the patient flat in bed with right arm under head and face turned left.	
2. Expose the upper abdomen in readiness for skin disinfection and local anaesthetic injection.	For optimal exposure and comfort of patient, the right hypochondriac region is treated as a surgical area, to minimize danger of infection.
3. Doctor will determine biopsy site – one interspace below upper border of liver dullness, 2cm behind anterior axillary line.	
4. Doctor anaesthetizes the skin, intercostal tissues and liver capsule with local anaesthetic.	To promote local comfort.
5. Doctor introduces biopsy needle into intercostal tissues but not into liver.	To prevent tearing of diaphragm or liver.
6. Instruct the patient to inhale and exhale deeply three or four times, then to exhale and hold his breath.	Holding one's breath immobilizes the chest wall and diaphragm; this helps to prevent the needle from tearing the diaphragm or the liver.
7. The doctor rapidly introduces biopsy needle into the liver, aspirates tissue and withdraws.	
8. As soon as needle is withdrawn, inform the patient to resume normal breathing.	Actual insertion and withdrawal of needle takes about 10 seconds.

Follow-up phase

Nursing action	**Rationale**
1. Following biopsy, assist the patient to turn on his right side, place a pillow under his lower rib cage and instruct him to remain in this position for several hours.	Compressing the liver against the chest wall near the biopsy site reduces the possibility of bleeding.
2. Determine and record the patient's pulse and respiratory rates and his blood pressure at frequent intervals until they stabilize. Observe biopsy site for bleeding or drainage.	The nurse needs to be aware of the possible complications of liver biopsy; haemorrhage and bile peritonitis. Anticipatory nursing includes early recognition of symptoms.
3. Recognize that an increasing pulse and decreasing blood pressure may be indicative of haemorrhage; note any indication of pain.	

JAUNDICE

Jaundice is a symptom of dysfunction or disease and not a disease itself. Dysfunction of several body organs or systems may be implicated when jaundice occurs.

HAEMOLYTIC JAUNDICE

Haemolytic jaundice is attributable to an abnormally high concentration of bilirubin in blood exceeding the capacity of liver cells to excrete it. This form is also referred to as prehepatic jaundice; liver function is usually normal.

1. Most common cause is massive haemolysis seen in haemolytic transfusion reactions, hereditary spherocytosis, autoimmune haemolytic anaemia, erythroblastosis fetalis and other haemolytic disorders.
2. Bilirubin in the blood is unconjugated (indirect reacting).
3. In faeces and urine, urobilinogen is increased; urine is free of bilirubin.
4. Prolonged jaundice leads to formation of 'pigment stones' in gallbladder.
5. Extremely severe jaundice (unconjugated bilirubin elevated: causes brain stem damage in neonates).

HEPATOCELLULAR JAUNDICE

Hepatocellular or hepatic jaundice is due to an inability of diseased liver cells to clear the normal amount of bilirubin from the blood.

Causes

1. Infection – hepatitis A, hepatitis B or hepatitis non-A, non-B.
2. Drug or chemical toxicity – carbon tetrachloride, chloroform, phosphorus, arsenicals, ethanol, halothane, isoniazid, mushroom poisoning.

Clinical features

1. Mildly or severely ill patient.
2. Lack of appetite, nausea, loss of vigour and strength, weight loss.
3. Elevated aspartate aminotransferase (AST, transaminase or SGOT) and alanine aminotransferase (ALT, SGPT) – two enzymes that are liberated with cellular necrosis.
4. Rise in bromsulphalein (BSP) and bilirubin. Alkaline phosphatase mildly elevated.
5. Abnormal serum proteins in prolonged illness; prothrombin time increased.
6. Headache and chills possible in infectious condition.

7. Bile acids radioimmunoassay are replacing BSP tests.

POSTHEPATIC OR OBSTRUCTIVE JAUNDICE (CHOLESTATIC JAUNDICE)

Causes

1. Extrahepatic obstruction – blockage of bile ducts by gallstone(s), tumour(s), an inflammatory process or an enlarged pancreas pressing on the duct.
2. Intrahepatic cholestasis – caused by injury to bile canaliculi or blockage of intrahepatic ducts due to tumours or granulomas. Certain drugs may cause this, for example, 'cholepulmonarystatic' agents: phenothiazine derivatives, perphenazine (Fentazin), sulphonamides, tolbutamide (Pramidex) and other antidiabetic drugs, thiouracil and aminobenzoic acid (previously named para-aminobenzoic acid [PABA]).

CLINICAL FEATURES

Because of damming-back of bile, it is reabsorbed by blood. The following responses may be noted:

1. Jaundice of skin and sclerae.
2. Deep orange-coloured urine.
3. White or clay-coloured stools.
4. Itchy skin and dyspepsia due to impaired bile acid excretion.
5. SGOT and SGPT (AST and ALT) rise only moderately.
6. Bilirubin and BSP are increased.
7. Alkaline phosphatase is strikingly elevated.
8. Cholesterol is elevated.

Assessment

PATIENT PROBLEMS

Although the clinical features and treatment depend on the type and outcome of the dysfunction, the patient with jaundice is likely to experience the following problems:

1. Altered skin integrity related to pruritis.
2. Altered self-esteem related to change in appearance.
3. Bleeding tendencies related to altered clotting mechanism and portal hypertension.
4. Altered fluid and electrolyte balance related to fluid deficit.
5. Altered mental and neurological status related to deterioration of liver function.

Planning and implementation

NURSING INTERVENTIONS

Relief of pruritus and maintenance of skin integrity

1. Use starch or baking soda baths, soothing lotions such as calamine.

2. Administer antihistamines, tranquillizers and sedatives, if prescribed.
3. Administer cholestyramine (Questran) to promote faecal excretion of bile salts to decrease itching.
4. Assist the patient in reducing the strong tendency to scratch his skin:
   a. Encourage activities to divert the patient's attention.
   b. Keep nails trimmed and clean.
   c. Avoid excessive top bedding.
   d. Give soothing massages, particularly at night in preparing the patient for sleep, since this is a time when he is especially likely to scratch.
   e. Provide clean white gloves to use at night if the patient scratches during sleep.

Increase in self-esteem
1. Encourage the patient to discuss his concerns; accept the patient's concerns without minimizing them.
2. Instruct staff and the patient's visitors to avoid remarks or behaviours that indicate rejection or fear of the patient's altered appearance.
3. Explain cause of jaundice and altered appearance.
4. Reinforce the fact that change in appearance is usually temporary.
5. Place the patient's bed in a position where he cannot look at himself in a mirror.

Evaluation
EXPECTED OUTCOMES
1. Demonstrates improved skin integrity – does not scratch or complain of itching; no signs of excoriation or infection of skin.
2. Demonstrates improved self-esteem by verbalizing own reactions to altered appearance and by interacting with others.

HEPATITIS

Hepatitis is a diffuse inflammation of the liver parenchyma.

AETIOLOGY
Hepatitis is usually caused by one or more viruses; however, a less common form is toxic or drug-induced hepatitis.

TYPES OF HEPATITIS
1. Hepatitis A virus; HAV, infectious hepatitis, short-incubation hepatitis.
2. Hepatitis B virus; HBV, serum hepatitis, homologous serum hepatitis, long-incubation hepatitis.
3. Hepatitis non-A non-B; NANB.

Features of HAV, HBV, and NANB hepatitis are summarized in Table 7.10.

SIGNIFICANCE
1. Community health – concern with ease of disease transmission and morbidity.
2. Socioeconomic – prolonged loss of time from school and employment.

TREATMENT
1. Management is devoted largely to treatment of symptoms and support of the patient during the acute and convalescent phases.
2. Treatment consists of nutritional support and moderate restriction of activity, depending on the severity of the patient's fatigue, anorexia and abdominal discomfort.
3. The patient is monitored closely for deterioration of liver function or the occurrence of complications.

GENERAL PREVENTIVE MEASURES
1. Stress importance of proper public and home sanitation.
2. Recognize merits of conscientious surveillance in the proper and safe preparation and dispensation of food.
3. Promote effective health supervision in schools, dormitories and holiday camps.
4. Initiate and support health education programmes.
5. Identify individuals or groups of individuals at high risk.
6. Encourage administration of appropriate immune globulin or vaccine when indicated.
7. Protect self through use of appropriate measures and precautions (gloves, etc.) when indicated in care of patients with known or suspected hepatitis.
8. Instruct the patient and family members about transmission and prevention of transmission.

Assessment
DIAGNOSTIC EVALUATION
1. SGPT (or ALT) levels rise one to two weeks before clinical jaundice appears.
2. The presence of HAV/immunoglobulin M (IgM) indicates antibody to hepatitis A virus and an acute stage of hepatitis A infection.

Table 7.10 Brief summary of hepatitis

	Hepatitis A virus (HAV)	Hepatitis B virus (HBV)	Non-A, non-B hepatitis virus (NANBH)
Other names	Type A hepatitis, infectious or epidemic hepatitis	Type B hepatitis, serum hepatitis	Hepatitis 'C'; 'D'; type C
Epidemiology			
Cause	Hepatitis A virus	Hepatitis B virus	Another virus; more than one virus
Method of transmission	Faecal–oral; poor sanitation Person-to-person Waterborne, foodborne – shellfish Rarely, if at all, by blood transfusion	Parenterally or by intimate contact with carriers or those with acute disease; male homosexuals. Vertical transmission from mothers to babies Contaminated instruments, syringes, needles (e.g. ear-piercing and acupuncture); renal dialysis*	Transfusion of blood or blood products Personnel in renal transplant and dialysis units Parenteral drug abusers Blood transfusion products Institutions with long-term residents* Male homosexuals
Source of virus/antigen	Blood, faeces, saliva	Blood Saliva Semen, vaginal secretions	Appears to be bloodborne Sexual contact
Distribution by age	Young adults (15–29) and middle-aged who have escaped childhood infection	Affects all ages, but mostly young adults	Same as HBV
Incubation period	3–5 weeks Mean, 30 days	2–5 months Mean, 90 days	Variable; 2–6 months Mean, 50 days
Occurrence	Worldwide	Worldwide	Worldwide Accounts for 20 per cent of sporadic cases
Antibody	Anti-HAV Present in convalescent sera and immune serum globulin (ISG)	Anti-HB$_c$ (core antigen) Anti-HB$_s$ (surface antigen)	
Immunity	Homologous	Homologous	
Severity	Most anicteric and asymptomatic	More severe than HAV	Wide spectrum of severity resembling HAV or HBV. Often prolonged illness – months May progress to chronic hepatitis*
Nature of disease			
Signs and symptoms	May occur with or without symptoms; flu-like illness Preicteric phase: headache, malaise, fatigue, anorexia, lassitude, fever Icteric phase: Dark urine, scleral icterus, jaundice, liver tenderness, and perhaps enlargement	May occur without symptoms 1,000IU/litre serum transaminase level May develop antibodies to virus Similar to HAV, but more severe Fever and respiratory symptoms rare, but may have arthralgias, rash	Similar to HBV Less severe and anicteric
Diagnosis and method	Elevated serum transaminase Complement fixation rate Radioimmunoassay	Check serum for HB$_s$Ag, HB$_e$Ag, anti-HB$_c$ in absence of anti-HB$_s$ (obtainable as panel)	Diagnosed by excluding HAV and HBV

		Elevated serum transaminase Radioimmunoassay – haemagglutination	
Severity	Usually mild Fatality rate 0–1 per cent	Variable, may be severe Fatality rate varies, 1–10 per cent	Variable, usually mild Fatality rate 1–2 per cent
Specific treatment	Adequate fluids, rest, nutrition Avoid alcohol; use drugs with caution	Same as HAV In research, vaccine antiviral chemotherapy to eliminate chronic HBV carrier state (being tested)	Same as HAV
Prevention	Good sanitation Proper personal hygiene Effective sterilization procedures Careful screening of food handlers Immune serum globulin (ISG) given within a few days of exposure	Specific hepatitis B immune globulin (HBIG) probably useful after exposure by ingestion, inoculation or splash involving hepatitis B surface antigen (HB$_s$Ag) Hepatitis B vaccine recommended for pre-exposure immunization of those at high risk	Mandatory screening of blood donors: 1. for HB$_s$Ag, 20 per cent 2. for non-A, non-B, 80 per cent

* Probably the same for HBV and NANBH, recent intensive research suggests.

3. The presence of hepatitis B antigen (HB$_s$Ag) is detected in individuals who have hepatitis B. The antigen can be detected before the onset of symptoms.
4. The absence of markers for hepatitis A or B leads to the diagnosis of non-A, non-B hepatitis, hepatic toxicity or some other viral infection.

PATIENT PROBLEMS
1. Alteration in nutritional status related to anorexia, nausea and vomiting.
2. Impaired skin integrity related to pruritus.
3. Activity intolerance related to fatigue and generalized malaise.
4. Abdominal pain related to tender, enlarged liver.

Planning and implementation
NURSING INTERVENTIONS
Improved nutritional status
1. Provide balanced meals consistent with the patient's food preferences.
2. Provide pleasant environment for meals.
3. Encourage the patient to eat in a sitting position to decrease abdominal tenderness and feeling of fullness.
4. Provide frequent, small meals if anorexia is severe.
5. Instruct the patient about the importance of a balanced diet and the need to avoid alcohol during illness.

Relief of pruritus and improvement in skin integrity
See p. 506.

Increase in ability to carry out activities
1. Encourage the patient to limit activity when fatigued.
2. Assist the patient in planning periods of rest and activity when symptoms begin to subside.
3. Encourage gradual resumption of activities and mild exercise during recovery.

Decrease in abdominal pain/tenderness
1. Assess and record presence or absence of abdominal pain or tenderness, hepatomegaly and splenomegaly.
2. Encourage the patient to maintain bed rest or restricted activities if abdominal pain or tenderness is present.
3. Administer analgesics as prescribed.
4. Notify the doctor of sudden occurrence of or increase in pain or tenderness.

Evaluation
EXPECTED OUTCOMES
1. Maintains adequate nutritional intake, avoids alcohol during illness, maintains weight and identifies features of a balanced diet.
2. Reports decrease in anorexia, nausea and vomiting.
3. Demonstrates improved skin integrity – intact

skin with no evidence of excoriation for infection; decreased scratching, no pruritus.

4. Exhibits increased ability to carry out desired activities and allows sufficient periods for rest and relaxation.
5. Reports a decrease or absence of abdominal pain and tenderness; restricts activities if pain recurs; participates in planned activities when free of pain; takes prescribed analgesics if necessary.

TYPE A HEPATITIS (HAV)

EPIDEMIOLOGY
1. HAV is probably a ribonucleic acid (RNA) virus of the enterovirus family.
2. Mode of transmission:
   a. Faecal–oral route.
   b. Poor sanitation; person-to-person (epidemic-type prevalent in camps and overcrowded residences).
   c. Contaminated food, milk, polluted water or shellfish.
   d. Sexual contact.
   e. Blood transfusion (rarely).
3. Incubation: three to seven weeks; average, four weeks.
4. Occurrence:
   a. Worldwide.
   b. Usually in children and young adults.
5. Mortality – 0.3 per cent develop fulminating disease, which has a mortality rate of 75 to 80 per cent.

ASSESSMENT AND CLINICAL FEATURES
1. Preicteric phase (prior to period of jaundice):
   a. Most patients are anicteric and symptomless. Highly contagious during preicteric phase.
   b. Initial symptoms – headache, fatigue, anorexia, fever, flu-like upper respiratory infection.
2. Icteric phase – jaundice, dark urine, vague epigastric symptoms, anorexia, flatulence. When jaundice reaches its peak, symptoms tend to subside. Liver is tender and perhaps enlarged.

NURSING MANAGEMENT
1. Promote rest during acute or symptomatic stage.
2. Encourage an adequate diet. The patient may have severe anorexia, which may hinder ordinary efforts to promote an adequate dietary intake.
3. Utilize appropriate measures to minimize spread of the disease.

PREVENTIVE MEASURES AND PATIENT EDUCATION
1. Encourage optimum sanitation practices.
2. Instruct the patient to practice good personal hygiene.
3. Employ proper safeguards to prevent use of blood and its components from infected donors.
4. Screen food handlers carefully.
5. Practise safe preparation and serving of food.
6. Administer immunoglobulin intramuscularly or subcutaneously within a few days of exposure.
7. Use disposable needles and syringes; dispose of these carefully.
8. Wear gloves when handling bedpans and faecal-contaminated linens.

TYPE B HEPATITIS (HBV)

Hepatitis B virus is a double-shelled particle containing deoxyribonucleic acid (DNA).

EPIDEMIOLOGY
1. Causative agent – this particle is composed of:
   a. Antigenic material in an outer coat – hepatitis B surface antigen (HB_sAg).
   b. Antigenic material in an inner coat – hepatitis B core antigen (HB_cAg).
   c. An independent protein circulating in the blood – HB_eAg.
2. Antibody – each antigen elicits a specific antibody:
   a. Anti-HB_s (produced early after hepatitis B infection). Its presence indicates immunity. Therefore, it is present if the patient has received hepatitis B vaccine.
   b. Anti-HB_c (noted late in acute phase or in convalescence).
   c. Anti-HB_e (noted later in convalescence).
3. Significance:
   a. HB_sAg – may be detected transiently in blood of 80 to 90 per cent of infected people, may be noted in blood for months and years, indicating that the patient has acute or chronic hepatitis B or is a carrier.
   b. HB_cAg – found only in liver cells, not serum.
   c. HB_eAg – if absent, the patient is an asymptomatic carrier. If present, it indicates highly infectious period of acute, active hepatitis. If it persists, indicates progression to chronic state.
4. Modes of transmission (percutaneous or permucosal routes):
   a. Oral – via saliva (i.e. mother to child via breast feeding).

b. Parenterally, or by intimate contact with carriers. (Susceptible persons are surgeons, clinical laboratory workers, nurses, physiotherapists.)

c. Male homosexuals.

d. Blood, saliva, semen, vaginal secretions.

e. Via needles used for acupuncture or ear-piercing.

5. Incubation – two to five months.

6. Occurrence – affects all ages but mostly young adults; worldwide.

ASSESSMENT AND CLINICAL FEATURES

1. Resembles hepatitis A clinically.

2. Symptoms insidious and variable.

3. Arthralgias and rashes may be observed; fever and respiratory symptoms are rare.

4. Jaundice may or may not be present.

5. Anorexia, abdominal pain, generalized malaise may be noted.

TREATMENT AND NURSING MANAGEMENT

1. Provide adequate fluids, nutrition and bed rest.

2. Administer alkalis, antiemetics if these agents are required to control dyspepsia and malaise.

3. Recognize that recovery and convalescence are slow and prolonged, sometimes taking three to four months; provide psychosocial support and diversional activities.

PREVENTIVE MEASURES AND PATIENT EDUCATION

1. Screening of blood donors to exclude carriers.

2. Caution in giving care to patients with known or suspected HBV. Use gloves when starting intravenous infusions or handling blood-contaminated articles from patients with known or suspected hepatitis.

3. Hepatitis B vaccine is recommended for those individuals at high risk for hepatitis B.

4. Hepatitis B immunoglobulin (HBIG) should be administered within 72 hours to those exposed directly to hepatitis B virus by accidental needle stick or splashing with blood products of patients with HBV.

5. Transfuse a patient only when justified.

6. Use blood substitutes when feasible.

7. Use disposable needles and syringes; dispose of these carefully.

8. Instruct *all* patients who have received a blood transfusion to refrain from donating blood for six months. This is necessary because of the long incubation period of hepatitis B.

HEPATITIS NON-A NON-B

This type of hepatitis is a viral infection that at present does not have an identified agent or antigenic markers. Therefore, it is diagnosed by excluding HAV and HBV.

EPIDEMIOLOGY

1. Over 80 per cent of post-transfusion hepatitis fall into this category.

2. Mode of transmission:

   a. Associated with blood transfusions.

   b. Personnel in renal dialysis units.

   c. Parenteral drug abusers.

   d. Appears to be bloodborne.

3. Incubation – two to six months.

4. Occurrence – same as hepatitis B.

ASSESSMENT AND CLINICAL FEATURES

Same as that of hepatitis B; less severe and anicteric.

TREATMENT AND NURSING MANAGEMENT

(Similar to that for hepatitis B.)

1. Non-A non-B hepatitis waxes and wanes over many months. There is probably a chronic carrier state.

2. Gamma globulin significantly reduces the incidence of this type of hepatitis and also that of chronic active liver disease.

PREVENTIVE MEASURES AND PATIENT TEACHING

Same as that for hepatitis B, although there is no vaccine available for protection against non-A non-B hepatitis.

HEPATIC CIRRHOSIS

Cirrhosis of the liver is a chronic disease in which there has been diffuse destruction of parenchymal cells followed by liver cell regeneration and an increase in connective tissue. These processes result in disorganization of the lobular architecture and obstruction of the hepatic venous and sinusoidal channels, causing portal hypertension.

CLASSIFICATION OF HEPATIC CIRRHOSIS

1. Alcoholic cirrhosis (micronodular):

   a. Fibrosis – mainly around central veins and portal areas.

   b. Most commonly due to chronic alcoholism and malnutrition.

2. Postnecrotic (macronodular):
   a. Broad bands of scar tissue – due to collapse of necrotic lobules and confluence of portal areas.
   b. Due to previous acute viral hepatitis or drug-induced massive hepatic necrosis.
3. Biliary:
   a. Scarring around bile ducts and lobes of liver.
   b. Results from chronic biliary obstruction (with or without infection).
   c. Much more rare than alcoholic and postnecrotic cirrhosis.

AETIOLOGY

1. Cirrhosis of the liver is characterized by repeated occurrences of death of the liver cells, replacement with scar tissue, and regeneration of liver cells.
2. Onset is insidious; it may be developing and progressing over many years.
3. Major causes are excessive consumption of alcohol with nutritional deficiencies and chronic viral hepatitis.
4. Twice as many men as women are affected; the age-group most often affected is from 40 to 60 years.

PATHOPHYSIOLOGY

1. Early in disease – gastrointestinal disturbances, fever and liver enlargement due to deposits of fats in the liver cells; as tissue is replaced, scars contract and become smaller, the surface becomes rough and has a hobnail appearance.
2. Anorexia, weight loss, weakness and fatigue occur; jaundice and fever may be present in the active stage. There are signs of portal hypertension and oestrogen–androgen imbalance.
3. Later – chronic failure of liver function and obstruction of portal circulation.
   a. Obstruction of portal circulation, causing portal hypertension with congestion of spleen, pancreas, and gastrointestinal tract.
      (i) Chronic dyspepsia, change in bowel habits – diarrhoea, constipation.
      (ii) Oesophageal varices, dilated cutaneous veins around the umbilicus, internal haemorrhoids, ascites, splenomegaly, pancytopenia and caput medusae.
   b. Chronic failure of liver function:
      (i) Plasma albumin is reduced, thereby leading to oedema and contributing to ascites.
      (ii) Weakness increases, leading to depression, wasting, delirium, coma and eventually death.
      (iii) Oestrogen–androgen imbalance, causing spider angiomata and palmar erythema, amenorrhea develops in females; testicular and prostatic atrophy, gynaecomastia, loss of libido and impotence develop in males.
      (iv) Bleeding tendencies may be evident.

TREATMENT

Medical management is directed toward minimizing further deterioration of liver function, correction of nutritional deficiencies and fluid and electrolyte imbalances and relief of the patient's symptoms.

1. Prevent further damage to the liver by withdrawing toxic substances, alcohol, and drugs.
2. Offer supportive care of the patient.
3. Maintain adequate nutritional levels.
   a. Provide protein within ability of liver to handle it. Normal nutritious diet with vitamin supplements, especially B, C and K, and folate.
   b. Eliminate alcohol consumption.
4. Restrict salt intake when fluid retention occurs.
5. Protect the patient from infections and toxic agents.
6. Treat ascites with diuretics gently and only when acute activity of liver damage has subsided. (Potassium-sparing diuretics are frequently prescribed.)
   a. Although rarely the treatment of choice, portacaval shunt may be tried to control ascites; however, operative mortality is high.
   b. Abdominal paracentesis is to be avoided if possible (if necessary, see Procedure, p. 514).
   c. Peritoneovenous shunt may be performed; this is used only in patients with 'intractable' ascites, circulatory failure of cirrhosis or abdominal hernia with severe ascites.
      (i) Complications: coagulopathy (bleeding) – requires monitoring of clotting factors; shunt malfunction.
7. Treat hepatic coma as necessary (see p. 516).
8. Provide multivitamin supplements and thiamine to compensate for liver's inability to store or activate them and folic acid to correct folic acid deficiency anaemia.

Assessment

DIAGNOSTIC EVALUATION

1. Liver biopsy – high risk of massive bleeding in presence of clotting defects (see p. 504 for precautions).
2. Oesophagoscopy.
3. Barium-contrast oesophagography (only about 50 per cent accurate) to check for oesophageal varices.

4. Radioisotopic liver scans – increased splenic and vertebral uptake of radioactive technetium (^{99}Tc) colloid.
5. Paracentesis to examine ascitic fluid, for cell count, for protein content and for bacterial count.

PATIENT PROBLEMS
1. Potential bleeding related to altered clotting mechanism and portal hypertension.
2. Altered nutritional status related to inadequate dietary intake, anorexia and gastrointestinal distress.
3. Altered skin integrity related to oedema, jaundice and altered immune response.
4. Activity intolerance related to fatigue, muscle wasting and general disability.

Planning and implementation
NURSING INTERVENTIONS
Decrease in the risk of bleeding
1. Anticipate manifestations of haemorrhage, such as ecchymosis, petechiae and epistaxis; and initiate preventive measures.
2. Maintain a safe environment to prevent injury.
3. Avoid trauma such as forceful nose blowing, use of hard toothbrush, large-gauge needles for injection.
4. Apply prolonged pressure after arterial and venous punctures, and all injections.
5. Note and report signs of haematemesis and melaena.
   a. Assess for anxiety, weakness, restlessness and epigastric fullness as possibly heralding haemorrhage.
   b. Take and record vital signs frequently.
   c. Administer vitamin C as prescribed.
   d. Observe each stool for colour, consistency and amount. Test for occult blood.
   e. Record nature, amount and time of vomiting.

Improvement in nutritional status
1. Evaluate nutritional status and needs.
2. Assist the patient in overcoming anorexia, weight loss and fatigue.
   a. Encourage him to eat all meals and supplementary feedings by serving them with eye-catching appeal, in small servings and in small, frequent meals.
   b. Recognize the effect of aesthetic factors – control odours, disturbing conversations, unpleasant situations.
   c. Eliminate alcohol but encourage high caloric intake.
   d. Give supplementary vitamins (A, B complex, C and K) and folate.

e. Conserve the patient's energy so that total food intake is not expended to replace energy requirements.
f. Provide special mouth care if the patient has bleeding from gums.
g. Offer small, frequent meals rather than three large meals.
h. Consider the patient's preferences in food.
i. If the patient is severely anorexic or nauseated and eating poorly, tube feeding may be necessary; include milk and starch hydrolysate. Do not increase dietary protein if serum ammonia level is increased.
j. Give pancreatin (if diarrhoea and steatorrhoea are present) to permit better tolerance of diet.
3. Monitor intake and output accurately; weigh carefully.
4. Adjust nutritional offerings if the patient has ascites or oedema.
   a. Restrict sodium intake to 200 to 500mg daily (less than 10mEq daily).
   b. Maintain caloric and vitamin intake; give protein as tolerated.
   c. Avoid table salt, salty foods, salted margarine and butter, as well as all ordinary frozen and canned foods, mouthwash, baking soda and all other products containing large quantities of salt.
   d. Use 'salt' substitutes such as lemon juice, oregano, thyme to enhance flavour; commercial salt substitute should be approved by doctor.
   e. Encourage use of powdered low-sodium milk and milk products.
   f. If water accumulation is not controlled on above regimen, resort to the following:
      (i) Limit sodium allowance to 200mg daily.
      (ii) Restrict fluids if serum sodium is low.
      (iii) Administer oral diuretics – hydrochlorothiazide (HydroSaluric), frusemide (Lasix), as directed.
      (iv) Administer spironolactone (Aldactone) if prescribed – this is an aldosterone-blocking agent used to reinforce the actions of diuretics and prevent undue potassium loss.
      (v) Promote slow diuresis to avoid renal failure.
   g. Measure and record abdominal girth daily.

Improvement in skin integrity
1. Observe skin and control pruritus.
   a. Provide good skin care; bathe without soap; apply soothing lotions.

b. Keep the patient's fingernails short to prevent him from scratching his skin.

c. Administer medications as prescribed for pruritus; be alert for side-effects of nausea, diarrhoea or constipation and vitamin K depletion, which leads to bleeding.

2. Turn the patient frequently to prevent pressure sores.

3. Avoid trauma to skin through gentle handling and prevention of falls.

4. Encourage intake of foods high in vitamin C.

Promotion of rest and balanced activities

1. Promote rest during acute episodes to decrease demands on the liver.

2. Limit visitors.

3. Encourage the patient to limit activity when fatigued.

4. Assist the patient in planning activities to limit exertion.

5. Encourage gradual resumption of activities.

PATIENT EDUCATION

Instruct the patient regarding precautions and regimen to follow upon discharge from the hospital.

1. Stress the necessity of giving up alcohol completely; urge acceptance of skilful assistance from psychiatrist, Alcoholics Anonymous or the alcohol treatment unit in the hospital.

2. Provide written dietary instructions, emphasizing the restriction of sodium (and protein, if necessary).

3. Emphasize the significance of rest, a sensible lifestyle and an adequate, well-balanced diet.

4. Involve the person closest to the patient (usually spouse) because recovery often is not easy and relapses are common; a close, trusted helper can help patient over the rough spots.

Evaluation
EXPECTED OUTCOMES

1. Experiences decreased risk of bleeding:
   a. No episodes of haemorrhage or frank bleeding (absence of melaena, haematemesis and epistaxis; no petechiae, haematoma formation or ecchymosis).
   b. Minimizes risk of trauma (blows nose gently, uses soft toothbrush, avoids straining during defaecation, avoids falls by following safety measures).

2. Increases nutritional intake – consumes diet based on specific nutritional and vitamin needs; eliminates alcohol from diet; gains weight without increased oedema or ascites.

3. Skin intact, with no evidence of excoriation or infection; decreased scratching; normal skin elasticity without oedema:
   a. Applies soothing lotions to skin to avoid itching.
   b. Changes position frequently to relieve pressure and avoids trauma to skin.

4. Demonstrates increased activity tolerance with periods of rest and relaxation as needed; shows increased strength and sense of well-being; carries out own self-care as capable; plans activities to avoid undue exertion.

GUIDELINES: ASSISTING WITH ABDOMINAL PARACENTESIS

Paracentesis is the withdrawal of fluid from the abdominal or peritoneal cavity.

PURPOSES

1. Withdraw fluid for diagnostic examination.
2. Remove ascitic fluid when large accumulation of fluid causes severe symptoms and is resistant to other therapy.
3. Prepare for other procedures (peritoneal dialysis, ascitic fluid reinfusion, surgery, etc).

DANGER AND COMPLICATIONS

1. In chronic liver disease, paracentesis may precipitate hepatic coma.
2. Shock and hypovolaemia can occur if fluid from general circulation shifts to abdomen to replace withdrawn fluid; this can be minimized if no more than 1 litre of paracentesis fluid is withdrawn, or if lost fluid is replaced by parenteral administration of salt-poor human albumin.

EQUIPMENT
Sterile paracentesis tray and gloves
Procaine hydrochloride 1 per cent
Sheet/blanket to cover patient
Collection bottle (vacuum bottle)
Skin preparation tray with antiseptic
Specimen bottles and laboratory forms

PROCEDURE
Preparatory phase

Nursing action	Rationale
1. Explain procedure to the patient.	This may reduce the patient's fear and anxiety.
2. Record the patient's vital signs.	Provides baseline values for later comparison.
3. Have the patient void urine before treatment is begun. See that consent form has been signed.	This will lessen the danger of accidentally piercing the bladder with the needle or trocar.
4. Position the patient in upright position with back, arms and feet supported (sitting on the side of the bed is a frequently used position).	The patient is more comfortable, and a steady position can be maintained.
5. Drape the patient with sheet, exposing abdomen.	Minimizes exposure of patient and keeps him warm.

Performance phase

Nursing action	Rationale
1. Assist doctor in preparing skin with antiseptic solution.	This is considered a minor surgical procedure, requiring aseptic precautions.
2. Open sterile tray and package of sterile gloves; provide anaesthetic solution.	
3. Have collection bottle and tubing available.	
4. Assess pulse and respiratory status frequently during procedure; watch for pallor, cyanosis or syncope (faintness).	Preliminary indications of shock must be watched for. Keep emergency stimulants available.
5. Doctor administers local anaesthesia and introduces no. 20 needle or trocar.	
6. Needle or trocar is connected to tubing and vacuum bottle or syringe; fluid is drained from peritoneal cavity.	Drainage is usually limited to 1–2 litres to relieve acute symptoms and minimize risk of hypovolaemia and shock.
7. Apply dressing when needle is withdrawn.	Elasticized adhesive patch is effective, serving as waterproof adhering dressing.

Follow-up phase

Nursing action	Rationale
1. Assist the patient to be comfortable after treatment.	
2. Record amount and kind of fluid removed, number of specimens sent to laboratory, the patient's condition through treatment.	
3. Check blood pressure and vital signs every half hour for two hours, every hour for four hours, and every four hours for 24 hours.	Close observation will detect poor circulatory adjustment and possible development of shock.
4. Usually, a dressing is sufficient; however, if the trocar wound appears large, the doctor may close the incision with sutures.	
5. Watch for leakage or scrotal oedema after paracentesis.	If seen, notify doctor at once.

HEPATIC COMA/HEPATIC ENCEPHALOPATHY

TWO MAJOR TYPES
1. Fulminant – due to acute massive liver cell necrosis, usually in previously healthy liver. Mortality in adults is 50 to 60 per cent, but it is lower in younger age-groups.
2. Subacute – due to acute metabolic insult in a cirrhotic patient with borderline compensation of hepatic function. Mortality is 10 to 20 per cent. It is usually reversible if the precipitating cause is withdrawn (see below).

CAUSES
1. Incomplete metabolism of nitrogenous compounds by the diseased liver – manifestation of profound liver failure.
2. Biochemical abnormalities responsible are not known; however, significant accumulation of nitrogenous substances, particularly ammonia, in the blood is believed to be highly suspect.
3. Shunting of portal blood that contains ammonia and other bacterial metabolites of protein around the damaged liver.

PRECIPITATING FACTORS
1. Progressive hepatocellular diseases not associated with any acute irritation of the liver.
2. Increased sources of ammonia in the blood; high-protein diet, gastrointestinal bleeding, following administration of ammonium chloride, thiazides.
3. Infections, paracentesis, acute alcoholism, hypotension, shock, general anaesthesia, minor surgery, hypokalaemia, alkalosis, administration of sedatives or narcotics.
4. Portacaval shunts, especially if protein in the diet is not restricted postoperatively.

PATHOPHYSIOLOGY
Cellular changes
1. Disruption of enzymatic function in liver cells, muscle and brain.
2. Failure of liver cells to detoxify the ammonia (by converting it to urea).
3. Accumulation of sympathomimetic amines (false neurotransmitters) from abnormal metabolism of aromatic amino acids.

Sources of ammonia
It comes from the bloodstream as a result of the following:
1. Its absorption from the *gastrointestinal tract* (largest source). Enzymatic and bacterial digestion of ingested protein and of urea passing from blood into the gastrointestinal tract increases blood ammonia.

Increases result from:
a. Gastrointestinal bleeding.
b. High-protein diet.
c. Ingestion of ammonium salts (diuretic – ammonium chloride).
d. Bacterial overgrowth in small bowel (infection).
e. Uraemia.
2. Its production by metabolizing *kidney* tissue (deamination of various amino acids, especially glutamine). Increases with:
a. Diuretics (steroids, chlorothiazide).
b. Restriction of dietary sodium (hyponatraemia).
c. Potassium depletion (hypokalaemia).
d. Alkalosis.
3. Its liberation from contracting *muscle* cells. Increases during exercise.

TREATMENT/MANAGEMENT
Precipitating causes
These are identified and treated if possible.
Nitrogen load and ammonia production and absorption from gastrointestinal tract are decreased.
1. Arrest gastrointestinal bleeding and reduce intestinal nitrogen.
a. If there is upper gastrointestinal bleeding, constant gastric aspiration may be required.
b. If bleeding has ceased, administer aperient or enema to clear blood from intestine.
c. Cancel requests for ammonium products, sedatives, tranquillizers and narcotics.
d. Greatly reduce dietary protein – if patient begins to improve, gradually increase protein intake; provide sufficient calories in absorbable form (i.e. intravenous glucose or lipid emulsion).
e. Cleanse the intestinal tract of nitrogenous substrates by administering prescribed purgatives such as magnesium citrate or sorbitol, or enemas.
f. Administer oral lactulose, if prescribed, to reduce intestinal absorption of ammonia.
g. Give neomycin, a nonabsorbable antibiotic, if prescribed, to suppress urea-splitting enteric bacteria.
h. Administer lactulose to reduce blood ammonia if neomycin is contraindicated.
i. Reduce and eliminate all unnecessary sedatives and analgesics. Administer only those specifically prescribed.
j. Weigh the patient daily and keep an accurate intake and output record; record frequency and characteristics of faeces.

Prevention and treatment of complications
Underlying liver disease is treated if possible.
1. Correct pre-existing complicating diseases – cardiovascular, renal and pulmonary.
2. Treat any infections, including respiratory infections, since these can become severe in this patient.
3. Administer antacids to reduce gastric acid and to protect against peptic ulceration. Prophylactic use of intravenous cimetidine to keep gastric pH above 5.0 is helpful.
4. Monitor blood glucose as directed every eight hours or whenever level of consciousness deteriorates; administer intravenous glucose, as prescribed.
5. Monitor status of hydration and correct any electrolyte, acid–base, or fluid imbalance, as prescribed.

Supportive therapy
1. The doctor will correct electrolyte abnormalities, especially hypokalaemia.
2. Provide adequate nutrition.

Assessment
CLINICAL FEATURES
There are five stages:
1. Minor mental aberrations – the patient is slightly confused, untidy, and displaying inappropriate behaviour and defective abstract thinking.
2. Motor disturbance – coarse or 'flapping' tremor (*asterixis*), especially of hands, hyperreflexia.
3. Progression to gross disturbances of consciousness – somnolence or stupor, hepatic encephalopathy.
4. Complete disorientation to time and place; eventual coma.
5. Decerebrate rigidity, hypoventilation → apnoea.

PATIENT PROBLEMS
1. Risk of bleeding.
2. Impaired skin integrity.
3. Altered nutritional status related to inadequate dietary intake, anorexia and gastrointestinal distress.
4. Impaired thought processes related to rising blood ammonia levels.
5. Impaired ability to carry out activities of daily living related to deterioration of neurological function and rising blood ammonia levels.

Planning and implementation
NURSING INTERVENTIONS
Improvement in neurological status and thought processes

1. Evaluate neurological function:
   a. Assess the patient's neurological status (i.e. his ability to do handwriting and perform simple arithmetic calculations). Keep daily record and note differences.
   b. Observe and record the extent and magnitude of characteristic tremor.
   c. Note and record state of consciousness, including slight drowsiness, slight confusion, drowsy, confused or disoriented.
   d. Note response to painful stimuli.
   e. When the patient does not respond, note sucking and grasping abilities; check corneal reflex.
2. Recognize signs of increasing stupor, notify doctor and initiate nursing measures as follows:
   a. Be alert for evidence of mental changes, lethargy, hallucinations.
   b. Avoid giving the patient narcotics and barbiturates.
   c. Restrict dietary protein; offer small high-calorie feedings frequently.
   d. Protect the patient by keeping him in bed; pad side rails.
   e. Arouse the patient at intervals; orient to time, place and person.
   f. Limit visitors.
   g. Provide constant nursing surveillance and emphasize sensitivity to the patient's changes and needs.
3. Remove factors that precipitate hepatic coma.
   a. Administer intestinal antibiotics (neomycin) as prescribed to reduce serum ammonia absorption from gastrointestinal tract.
   b. Administer medications with caution.
   c. Promote bowel evacuation to reduce intestinal nitrogen load.
   d. Prevent complications that increase metabolic rate and severity of hepatic coma (e.g. infection, sepsis, aspiration, hypovolaemia).

Promotion of rest and activity as indicated

1. Eliminate unnecessary stimuli to promote rest when indicated.
   a. Group nursing activities together to minimize disruption of the patient's rest.
   b. Limit visitors.
   c. Eliminate or reduce environmental noise and light.
2. Assist the patient in planning periods of rest and activity when symptoms begin to subside.
3. Encourage gradual resumption of activities during recovery.

Evaluation
EXPECTED OUTCOMES

1. Demonstrates improved thought processes – identifies time, place, person correctly; initiates conversation and responds appropriately to others' conversations; shows no signs of hallucinating or periods of confusion.
2. Shows improved mental status – performs simple arithmetic calculations, responds normally to painful (and other) stimuli.
3. Demonstrates return of normal neurological reflexes and responses.
4. Participates in appropriate schedule of rest and activity – carries out own hygiene and self-care activities as capable, reports increased strength and well-being; gradually resumes mild activities.

BLEEDING OESOPHAGEAL VARICES

Oesophageal varices are dilated tortuous veins found in the submucosa of the lower oesophagus; they may extend up in the oesophagus and down into the stomach.

PATHOPHYSIOLOGY

1. Increasing portal vein obstruction – venous blood returning to right atrium from intestinal tract and spleen seeks new pathways, through enlarging collateral oesophageal veins.
2. Usually no symptoms are produced by dilated veins unless mucosa becomes ulcerated.
3. Haematemesis and melaena, plus a history of alcoholism, tend to suggest oesophageal varices; however, bleeding may result from associated gastritis or duodenal ulcer in 25 per cent of patients with varices.
4. The strain of coughing or vomiting may precipitate variceal rupture, haemorrhage, and death.
5. Irritation of vessels by gastro-oesophageal reflux may cause oesophagitis, oesophageal rupture, haemorrhage and death.
6. Has a high mortality rate due to further deterioration of liver function (hepatic coma) and complications (e.g. aspiration pneumonia, sepsis, renal failure).

AETIOLOGY

1. Nearly always due to portal hypertension, which

may result from obstruction of the portal venous circulation and cirrhosis of the liver.
2. Abnormalities of the circulation in splenic vein or superior vena cava.

TREATMENT
Control of haemorrhage
1. Purpose:
   a. To lessen transfusion requirements.
   b. To reduce large amounts of blood in gastro-intestinal tract.
   c. To avoid hepatic coma.
2. Methods:
   a. Administer vasopressin systemically to reduce portal pressure and to initiate haemostasis. Intra-arterial infusion into the superior mesenteric artery may be used after angiography, but offers no definitive advantage.
   b. Ice-water lavage of stomach (gastric hypothermia) may temporarily control bleeding.
   c. Aspirate blood from the stomach.
   d. Oesophageal tamponade – pressure is exerted on the cardiac portion of the stomach and against the bleeding varices by a double balloon tamponade (Sengstaken–Blakemore tube).
   e. Treat bleeding by complete rest of the oesophagus (parenteral feedings); avoid straining and vomiting and continue gastric suction.
   f. Initiate vitamin K therapy; administer multiple blood transfusions.
   g. Avoid sedation, since it may lead to coma.
   h. Administer saline aperient (magnesium citrate) plus enemata to remove blood, as prescribed.

Injection sclerotherapy
This method of controlling bleeding from oesophageal varices has been used recently to treat patients who are poor surgical risks.
1. A sclerosing agent is injected through a fibreoptic endoscope into the bleeding varices to promote thrombosis and sclerosis.
2. May be used as prophylactic measure to treat varices before bleeding has occurred.
3. The patient may require repeated treatments if bleeding recurs.
4. The patient must be observed after treatment for bleeding, perforation of the oesophagus and aspiration pneumonia.

Surgical intervention
If bleeding of oesophageal varices is not controlled by conservative measures, surgical procedures may be employed:
1. Surgical procedures:
   a. Direct ligation of varices.
   b. Surgical bypass (portacaval anastomosis) – by shunting portal blood into the vena cava, pressure in the portal system is reduced.
   c. Splenorenal shunt – a shunt is made between the splenic vein and the left renal vein; this is done when the portal vein cannot be used because of thrombosis or for other reasons.
2. Evaluation of surgery:
   a. Varying degrees of success are reported with shunting procedures.
   b. The success depends mainly on the condition of the patient; it is used as an emergency procedure following bleeding. Most common use is to prevent recurrence after the patient recovers from an initial variceal bleed.
   c. Complications are acute hepatic failure and chronic portal systemic encephalopathy.
   d. Postoperative care is similar to postabdominal surgery complicated by care required for a patient with severe cirrhotic liver.

Assessment
CLINICAL FEATURES
1. Blood loss may be sudden and massive; frank haemorrhage from upper gastrointestinal tract may occur.
2. Haematemesis, melaena or rectal bleeding (bright red blood).
3. May develop signs of hypovolaemia and shock.
4. Should be suspected in all patients with signs of portal hypertension (e.g. ascites, dilated abdominal veins) or any occurrence of upper gastrointestinal haemorrhage.

DIAGNOSTIC EVALUATION
1. The patient's history, physical examination and neurological examination will assist in identifying any evidence of hepatic encephalopathy.
2. Fibreoptic endoscopy may be used if bleeding is controlled. It is essential to exclude other causes of bleeding.
3. If bleeding is massive, arteriography or umbilical venous catheterization to visualize portal collaterals; by placement of a catheter in the portal vein via recanalized umbilical vein, direct venous pressure and portovenography can be done in 75 per cent of patients.
4. Splenoportography can be effective when studied as a series of X-ray plates or done as segmental X-rays; extensive collateral circulation of oesophageal vessels may be indicative of varices.

5. Portal vein pressure above 150mm of water is abnormal; this can be measured in the operating room by introducing a needle into spleen or via umbilical vein catheter.
6. Liver function tests, include bromsulphalein retention, serum transaminase, bilirubin, serum proteins, alkaline phosphatase, serum ammonia levels.

PATIENT PROBLEMS
1. The patient who experiences bleeding oesophageal varices has severe liver disease and, as a result, is subject to the problems encountered in cirrhosis and hepatic coma (see p. 516 for discussion). In addition, this critically ill patient experiences the following problems:
2. Potential hypovolaemia related to blood loss.
3. Potential impaired gas exchange related to asphyxiation and aspiration pneumonia.
4. Increased risk of bleeding related to erosion of gastric and oesophageal mucosa, portal hypertension and abnormal clotting mechanism.
5. Fear related to possibility of massive haemorrhage and possibly impending death.

Planning and implementation
NURSING INTERVENTIONS
Maintaining adequate fluid volume
1. Assess for signs of potential hypovolaemia:
   a. Monitor blood pressure; arterial catheter may be inserted to monitor blood pressure directly. Use central venous pressure monitoring for fluid replacement.
   b. Assess urinary output; indwelling catheter may be required.
   c. Check blood gases to assess oxygenation of blood. An endotracheal tube may be inserted to protect, control and manage the patient's airway.
2. Initiate measures to overcome blood loss, as directed:
   a. Replace blood with *fresh* whole blood.
      (i) Ammonia content is lower than in stored blood.
      (ii) Coagulation effect is greater, particularly if the patient has severe liver disease.
   b. Administer vitamin K intramuscularly as prescribed.

Improving gas exchange
1. Assess respirations and blood gases frequently.
2. Note and report occurrence of signs of obstructed airway or ruptured oesophagus from Sengstaken–Blakemore tube (e.g. changes in skin colour, respirations, breath sounds, level of consciousness, presence of chest pain, vital signs, etc).
3. Check location and inflation of balloons of Sengstaken–Blakemore tube frequently.
4. Have scissors readily available. Cut tubing and remove Sengstaken–Blakemore tube immediately if the patient develops acute respiratory distress.
5. Keep head of bed elevated to avoid gastric regurgitation and aspiration of gastric contents.

Reducing fear and apprehension
1. Explain all procedures to the patient.
2. Remain with patient; place call bell within patient's reach.
3. Maintain close surveillance of the patient.
4. Avoid discussing the patient's condition or unrelated matters in the patient's vicinity.
5. Provide alternate means of communication if tubes or other equipment interfere with patient's ability to talk.
6. Use touch and other tactile stimuli to provide reassurance to patient.
7. Use protective restraints to prevent dislodging of Sengstaken–Blakemore tube in confused, combative patient.
8. Aspirate the patient's airway if indicated.

Reducing the risk of bleeding
1. Observe the patient for straining, retching or vomiting; these increase pressure in portal system and increase risk of further bleeding.
2. Note and report signs of haematemesis and melaena. Check all gastrointestinal secretions and faeces for occult and frank blood.
3. Observe for signs of hypovolaemia and shock.
4. Remove blood from gastrointestinal tract to reduce possibility of hepatic encephalopathy (hepatic coma).
5. Perform wash out with iced saline if bleeding recurs, as directed.
6. Have extra Sengstaken–Blakemore tube available for reinsertion if bleeding occurs or recurs.
7. When bleeding has ceased, introduce non-irritating, soothing foods and fluids gradually.
8. Reinforce need for the patient to avoid alcohol.

Evaluation
EXPECTED OUTCOMES
1. Experiences decreased risk of bleeding – no episodes of straining, retching or vomiting; no haematemesis or melaena; blood-free gastrointestinal secretions and stools; no recurrence of bleeding, hypovolaemia or shock.
2. Demonstrates improved gas exchange – normal

respiratory rate and pattern, normal breath sounds, adequate blood gases; absence of chest pain, dyspnoea, or shortness of breath; appropriate cough, clear sputum.

3. Demonstrates lessening of fear and apprehension.
4. Uses alternate means of communication when necessary.

GUIDELINES: USING THE SENGSTAKEN–BLAKEMORE TUBE TO CONTROL OESOPHAGEAL BLEEDING

PURPOSES
1. Exert pressure on the cardiac portion of the stomach and against bleeding varices by a double balloon tamponade.
2. Reduce transfusion requirements.
3. Prevent blood accumulation in the gastrointestinal tract, which could precipitate hepatic coma.

EQUIPMENT
Sengstaken–Blakemore tube
Basin with cracked ice
Clamp for tubing

Towel and vomit bowl
Glass of water and straw
Torch

PROCEDURE
See Figure 7.18.

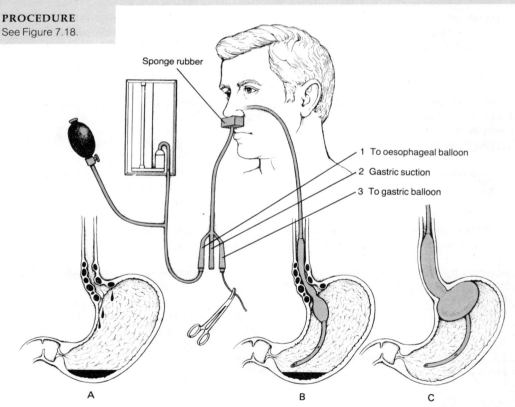

Sponge rubber

1 To oesophageal balloon
2 Gastric suction
3 To gastric balloon

A   B   C

Figure 7.18. Oesophageal varices and their treatment by a compressing balloon tube (Sengstaken–Blakemore). (A) Dilated veins of the lower oesophagus. (B) The tube is in place in the stomach and the lower oesophagus but is not inflated. (C) Inflation of the tube and compression of the veins, which can be obtained by inflation of the balloon. In some instances it may be necessary to pass an additional tube through the other nostril to aspirate secretions

Preparatory phase

1. Provide nursing support by reassuring the patient that this procedure will help to control his bleeding.
2. Explain procedure to the patient and tell him how breathing through the mouth and swallowing can help in passing the tube.
3. Elevate head of bed slightly unless the patient is in shock.

Performance phase

Nursing action	**Rationale**
1. Check balloons by trial inflation to detect leaks.	This is best done under water because it is easier to see escaping air bubbles.
2. Chill the tube, then lubricate it before doctor passes it via mouth or nose (preferable).	Chilling will make the tube more firm and lubrication will lessen friction.
3. After the tube has entered the stomach, wash out stomach and aspirate all clots.	
4. After obtaining an X-ray of the lower chest and upper abdomen to check position of the balloon, it is fully inflated (200–250ml) of air and then pulled back gently.	This is to exert force against cardia. The triple-lumen tube provides two channels to inflate compression balloons, one in the stomach and one in the oesophagus. Balloons are inflated using a manometer to measure pressure to 25 or 30mmHg.
5. Traction is placed on tubing where it enters the patient's nose. Then the oesophageal bag is inflated to 35–40mmHg. This is tied with double ties to prevent leakage (Figure 7.18).	This keeps balloons in position and assists in exerting proper pressure.
6. Gastric suction may be attached to the third outlet of the catheter.	By using suction and irrigating the tubing hourly, it is possible to tell how well the bleeding is controlled by the appearance of the drainage.
7. A second nasogastric (Levin) tube is passed into the lower oesophagus.	To aspirate saliva and to check for bleeding *above* the oesophageal balloon.
8. Deflate oesophageal balloon for five minutes at eight- or 12-hour intervals. Do not deflate gastric balloon under traction.	To prevent erosion and necrosis of the oesophagus or stomach. If the gastric balloon is deflated or ruptures while traction on the tube is applied, the inflated oesophageal balloon will be pulled upward and obstruct the patient's airway.
9. Pressure on tubes and traction is released in two to four days.	If bleeding remains controlled, the tubing is removed in 24 hours.

NURSING RESPONSIBILITIES

1. Maintain *constant* vigilance while balloons are inflated in the patient.
2. Keep balloon pressures at required level to control bleeding. (Haemostats are utilized as clamps.)

3. Observe and record vital signs frequently – bleeding, shock, etc.
4. Be alert for chest pain – may indicate injury or rupture of oesophagus.
5. Irrigate suction tube as prescribed; observe and record nature and colour of aspirated material.
6. Keep head of bed elevated to avoid gastric regurgitation and to diminish nausea and a sensation of retching.
7. Maintain nutritional and electrolyte levels parenterally.
8. Maintain nasogastric suction to aspirate saliva through an accessory nasogastric tube.
9. Note nature of breathing; if counterweight pulls the tube into oropharynx, the patient may be asphyxiated.

NURSING ALERT
*Keep a pair of scissors taped to the head of the bed. In the event of acute respiratory distress, **use the scissors to cut across tubing (to deflate both balloons) and remove tubing.***

Note: This procedure should be reserved for patients who are known, without a doubt, to be bleeding from oesophageal varices, and in whom all forms of conservative therapy have failed.

Chief hazard: Vomiting with an inflated oesophageal balloon tamponade in place, which results in massive pulmonary aspiration. Manage this problem by inserting a nasogastric tube in the free nostril to drain the oesophagus above the oesophageal balloon, thereby preventing aspiration.

DISEASES OF THE BILIARY (GALLBLADDER) SYSTEM

INCIDENCE
. Fifteen per cent of the population in the UK have formed gallstones by the time they die.
. Women develop the disease more frequently than men. Under 40 years, the ratio is 3:1; over 80 years it is 3:2.
. The majority of patients are not fair, fat and forty. They can occur at any age and are not associated with skin colour.
. Postmenopausal women on oestrogen therapy are at greater risk for gallbladder disease; likewise, women on birth control pills are at greater risk than non-users of these pills.
. Malabsorption of bile salts in patients with gastrointestinal disease or T-tube fistula or those who have had ileal resection increases the risk of gallstones and gallbladder disease.

PATHOPHYSIOLOGY
. Ninety-five per cent of patients with acute cholecystitis have gallstones; however, a majority with gallstones have no pain and are unaware of the presence of stones.
2. There are two types of gallstones: those composed of pigment and those composed of cholesterol.
3. Pigment stones form when unconjugated pigments in the bile precipitate to form stones, which must be removed surgically.
4. Cholesterol stones account for most gallbladder disease; these stones form in the presence of cholesterol-saturated bile, which is low in bile acid synthesis.
5. Cholesterol-saturated bile acts as an irritant and produces inflammatory changes in the gallbladder.

TYPES OF GALLBLADDER DISEASE
('Chole' – gallbladder.)
1. Cholecystitis – inflammation of the gallbladder.
2. Cholelithiasis – stones in the gallbladder.
3. Choledocholithiasis – stones in the common duct.

DIAGNOSTIC EVALUATION OF BILIARY CONDITIONS
Overall assessment of the patient should include

detection of associated disease processes (cardio-vascular, pulmonary, and renal); diabetes status; and realization of increased surgical risk if patient is over age 65.

Flat plate of abdomen
Used to visualize the 25 per cent of stones that are radio-opaque.

Cholecystogram
Used to visualize the shape and position of the gallbladder.

Note: This test is effective only if the liver cells are functioning properly and are capable of excreting the radio-opaque contrast medium into the bile.

1. Purpose:
   a. Detect gallstones.
   b. Estimate ability of gallbladder to fill, concentrate its contents, contract and empty in a normal manner.
2. Method:
   a. Because gallstones are usually radiolucent, it is necessary to fill the gallbladder with a radio-opaque contrast medium, which permits stones to show up as clear areas.
   b. Iodide-containing contrast medium is excreted into bile by the liver and concentrated in the gallbladder. *Caution:* prior to administration of iodide, determine whether patient is sensitive to iodine.
      (i) Orally:
         (a) Contrast media may be given by mouth (e.g. Telepaque).
         (b) Iodide preparation is usually given in oral doses of 3.6g approximately 10 to 12 hours before X-ray. If there is no visualization the next morning, repeat dose of 3.6g the following evening.
         (c) Administer nothing by mouth from the time of iodide administration to the time of X-ray to prevent contraction of gallbladder and expulsion of contrast medium.
      (ii) Intravenously: intravenous cholecystogram involves giving an iodide preparation (e.g. Cholografin) about 10 minutes before X-ray.
3. Patient preparation:
   a. At least one hour after the evening meal, the patient takes the prescribed tablets or capsules of iodide preparation by mouth.
   b. These tablets are taken one at a time at three- to five-minute intervals with at least 250ml of water.
   c. From this time until bedtime, nothing is taken by mouth except water; from midnight on water is also excluded. (If nausea, vomiting or diarrhoea occurs, notify doctor; test may be postponed.)
   d. No laxatives are given during this time; however, a saline enema may be required on the morning of the X-ray.
   e. Breakfast is withheld, and the patient goes to X-ray.
   f. Right upper abdominal quadrant is X-rayed.
   g. The patient is fed a fatty meal containing cream, butter or eggs to test contractility of the gallbladder.
   h. X-ray examination is repeated at intervals until gallbladder has expelled contrast medium.

NURSING ALERT
Cholecystogram is ineffective in the jaundiced patient since the liver cells in this situation cannot transport contrast medium to the biliary tract.

Cholangiogram
Contrast medium is injected directly into biliary tree
1. Advantages:
   a. Procedure is best way to visualize biliary tree in the patient after cholecystectomy.
   b. All components of the biliary tree can be observed – hepatic ducts within liver, common hepatic duct and cystic duct, but the gall bladder is often not well visualized.
2. Clinical usefulness:
   a. In differentiating hepatocellular jaundice from jaundice due to biliary obstruction.
   b. In locating stones within bile ducts.
   c. In detecting and diagnosing cancer of the biliary system.
   d. In investigating gastrointestinal symptoms of patients who had cholecystectomy.
3. Patient preparation:
   a. The patient is dehydrated by restricting his fluid intake.
   b. Enema is given early in morning of test.
   c. A sedative is given at least one hour before the X-ray.
   d. Contrast medium (e.g. Cholografin sodium) is injected either intravenously (results not as conclusive) or directly into the common duct.
      (i) Operatively; this can be done during surgery.
      (ii) Postoperatively, by injecting contrast medium into the common duct drain.

(iii) Via retrograde endoscopic cannulation of duct via duodenum.

e. Following the X-ray, regardless of method of contrast medium injection, as much as possible of the contrast medium and bile is aspirated to prevent leakage into the peritoneal cavity, thus avoiding a possible bile peritonitis.

Note: Operative cholangiogram may be done during gallbladder surgery in the operating room.

Ultrasound examination (echogram)

B scanner and transducer: this test can be used to demonstrate gallbladder distension, bile duct distension and calculi.

Liver scan

1. In the jaundiced patient, this scan may show evidence of hepatocellular disease or metastatic lesions.
2. With radioactive rose bengal, which is excreted by the liver-like gallbladder dyes, obstructive pathology of the biliary tree may be revealed.

Endoscopic retrograde cholangiopancreatography (ERCP)

See Guidelines, below.

GUIDELINES: ENDOSCOPIC RETROGRADE CHOLANGIOPANCREATOGRAPHY (ERCP)

A fibreoptic endoscope (a side-viewing instrument) is placed in the descending duodenum so that the ampulla of Vater can be located and cannulated (Figure 7.19).

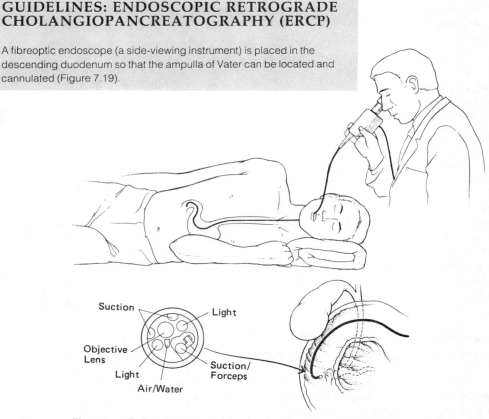

Figure 7.19. Endoscopic retrograde cholangiopancreatography (ERCP). The patient is moved from left lateral to prone position as the flexible scope is passed. The circle on the left shows the tip of the scope; the objective lens is the viewing section assisted by two side lights. Air or water may be directed to an area, and suction is available. If a biopsy is to be taken, a separate channel is available. The lower right diagram shows the scope nearing the ampulla of Vater; the scope is in the duodenum; the gallbladder is the topmost sac – note the biliary and common bile ducts

In this examination, both the common and pancreatic ducts may be injected with contrast media to visualize the hepatobiliary tree and pancreatic ducts radiologically.

The doctor is able to diagnose abnormalities of the ductal system, detect disease processes and obtain direct secretory information, as well as cells for cytological examination.

INDICATIONS

1. Biliary disease.
2. Pancreatic disease.
3. To diagnose:
   a. Cancer of the papilla.
   b. Obstructive jaundice.
   c. Calculus disease, pre- and postcholecystectomy.
   d. Carcinoma of biliary ducts.
   e. Carcinoma of pancreas.
   f. Pancreatitis.

CONTRAINDICATIONS

1. Acute cardiorespiratory disease.
2. Acute recent attack of pancreatitis (within three weeks) because of risk of inducing another attack.
3. Stricture or obstruction of oesophagus or duodenum.
4. Acute cholangitis.

EQUIPMENT

A side-viewing duodenoscope (to be sterilized after use with suspected infectious patients)
Sterilized cannula
This duodenoscope is 125cm long and 1cm in diameter. Visual fields are oriented 90 degrees to its long axis. It includes a channel through which a cannula or biopsy forceps can be passed under direct vision.

CONSIDERATIONS

1. ERCP is not a simple endoscopic procedure; it must be done by a skilful, well-trained doctor.
2. There are certain risks, described below:
   a. After ERCP, a very small percentage of patients develop clinical pancreatitis, which may last one to three days.
   b. The patient may retain contrast material injected proximal to an obstructed duct; this may result in cholangitis or pancreatitis. Such a patient should be given broadspectrum antibiotics; surgical drainage may be indicated.
   c. A very few patients are sensitive to iodinated compounds.
   d. The more experienced the team in performing ERCPs, the fewer the complications and the better the success rate.

PROCEDURE

Preparatory phase

Nursing action	Doctor's role	Rationale
1. Be sure that consent form is signed and noted on the patient's chart.	Obtain informed consent..	
2. Remind the patient to take nothing by mouth after midnight.	Collaborate with nurse in patient preparation.	Limited intake produces a basal condition with reduced body secretions; this permits better visualization of tissues.
3. Explain contemplated examination to patient; discuss possibilities of after-effects.		
4. Determine the patient's sensitivity to iodine (or fish, which contains iodine) or any other medication.		A few patients are sensitive to iodine preparations (Hypaquesodium).
5. Take and record vital signs.		This information becomes a baseline for later comparison.
6. Offer the patient 3ml of tetracaine (Pontocaine) to be used as a gargle and swallow.		Tetracaine is an oropharyngeal topical anaesthetic.
7. Intravenous infusion may be started, for administration of medications.	Start an intravenous infusion with normal saline.	This becomes the avenue for direct intravenous medications such as diazepam (Valium) and meperidine (Demerol) to promote relaxation prior to insertion of duodenoscope.
8. Instruct the patient to remove dentures; a mouthpiece is inserted.		To facilitate insertion of scope.

Performance phase

Nursing action	Doctor's role	Rationale
1. Place the patient in left lateral position.	Scope is passed through the patient's mouth into oesophagus and stomach.	Anatomy is carefully examined as the scope advances.
2. Administer intravenous medication, which may include Demerol, Valium, atropine or glucagon.	Gently advance tip through pyloric ring into duodenal bulb and into descending duodenum.	Atropine will produce a hypotonic duodenum and relaxed sphincter at ampulla of Vater; secretion will be reduced.

3. Minimal air insufflation used to search for the ampulla of Vater.		Unless this is obstructed by tumour it can usually be identified with careful search.
4. Place the patient in prone position. (This provides the radiologist with a better position for fluoroscopy and radiography.)	Administer glucagon.	Glucagon is given to further reduce duodenal motility.
5. Prepare a special radio-opaque Teflon cannulation tube by filling it with contrast medium (to eliminate air).	When cannulation tubing is in correct position, contrast medium is slowly injected: 3–5ml for pancreatic ductal system; 15–20ml for biliary ductal system.	Cannulation tube is passed through biopsy channel of scope. Contrast medium is warmed to body temperature. Tube is advanced under fluoroscopy. X-ray pictures are taken while patient is in prone position following injection of contrast medium.
6. Upon completion of film-taking, turn patient to lateral position. Draw blood sample for serum amylase determination. Use suction to remove oropharyngeal secretions.	Keep scope and cannula in place and patient in prone position until films are completed. If films are satisfactory, scope is carefully removed.	Await return and reading of films.

Follow-up phase

Nursing action	**Rationale**
1. Check vital signs every four hours. Notify family as to when the patient will return.	Postcannulation patient may experience a temperature rise, chills, abdominal pain. Report these responses to doctor.
2. In the absence of complications, permit the patient to eat in two to four hours (light diet); permit a full diet the next day.	A mild rise in serum amylase is observed in a high percentage of patients.
3. Watch for palpitations related to atropine sulphate injection. Also watch for respiratory depression and transient hypotension.	Some patients experience mild to severe epigastric pain, nausea and vomiting. These discomforts are usually transitory.

CHRONIC CHOLECYSTITIS WITH CHOLELITHIASIS

ASSESSMENT AND CLINICAL FEATURES
1. History of episodic, usually colicky epigastric or right upper quadrant pain, often associated with nausea and vomiting.
2. Jaundice due to choledocholithiasis.

TREATMENT
1. Surgery is advised if gallstones are present with typical pain attacks and/or jaundice. Whether asymptomatic stones should be removed surgically is still open to debate.

In the older patient, the risk of surgery must be evaluated in relation to other disease conditions present.

Chenodeoxycholic acid (Chendol) can decrease the size of existing stones, dissolve small ones and prevent new stones from forming.

a. The major adverse effects appear to be mild diarrhoea and cramps and SGOT elevation; with dose regulation these disappear.

b. Stones may recur; therefore, long-term therapy may be required.

c. Useful only in treatment or prevention of stones composed chiefly of cholesterol.

d. Should be used with caution in patients at risk from elevated serum cholesterol levels.

e. Indicated in patients at high risk from gall-bladder surgery because of systemic disease or age.

ACUTE CHOLECYSTITIS

CLINICAL FEATURES

. Right upper quadrant pain, fever, nausea and vomiting.

. The condition may occur at any age, but it is most common in patients over the age of 50.

. The chief hazard is perforation with local or generalized peritonitis.

TREATMENT

. Provide hospitalization, bed rest, withholding of oral fluids and insertion of nasogastric tube with suction.

. Administer intravenous fluids as directed to correct electrolyte imbalance, to maintain adequate urinary output and to provide nutritional needs.

3. Administer medication for pain and antibiotics for infection control, as prescribed.

. Prepare patient for laboratory studies, chest X-ray, ECG, and possibly intravenous cholangiogram.

5. Record vital signs every four hours.

6. Evaluate and prepare the patient for surgery, if indicated. (Most patients achieve remission with rest, intravenous fluids, nasogastric suction, analgesia and antibiotic administration. Surgery is usually delayed until the acute symptoms subside; however, deterioration of the patient's condition mandates surgical intervention.)

NONSURGICAL MANAGEMENT

PATIENT PROBLEMS

1. Pain and discomfort related to obstruction of biliary system and inflammation and obstruction of the gallbladder.

2. Altered nutritional status related to dietary intolerance and medical therapy (withholding of food and fluids and nasogastric suctioning).

3. Impaired skin integrity related to jaundice (a rare occurrence).

Planning and implementation

NURSING INTERVENTIONS

Relief of pain and increase in comfort level

1. Assess level, location and severity of pain.

2. Administer pethidine as prescribed for pain relief.

3. Avoid use of morphine sulphate, which is thought to increase spasm of the sphincter of Oddi and thus increase pain.

4. Assist the patient to assume position of comfort.

5. Assess and record response to pain medication.

6. Assist the patient to cough and breathe deeply to avoid respiratory complications secondary to upper abdominal pain.

Improved nutritional status

1. Maintain intravenous infusion and withhold oral fluids during acute episode of cholecystitis.

2. Introduce foods and fluids gradually after acute symptoms subside.

3. Provide high protein and carbohydrate diet that is low in fat content.

4. Instruct the patient to avoid foods that may initiate pain and gas-forming foods.

Evaluation

EXPECTED OUTCOMES

1. Demonstrates decreased pain and abdominal distention – normal respiratory rate and pattern; reports increased comfort, uses analgesics as prescribed.

2. Maintains adequate dietary intake – consumes diet low in fat, high in protein and carbohydrates during recovery period, and identifies food to be avoided.

3. Indicates fewer episodes of nausea, vomiting, food intolerance, and abdominal discomfort after meals.

SURGICAL MANAGEMENT

TYPES OF GALLBLADDER SURGERY
Cholecystostomy
Simple opening of gallbladder to remove stones, bile or pus; a tube is then sutured into the gallbladder for drainage.

Note: When the patient returns to the recovery unit, this drainage tube is connected to a drainage bag.

Cholecystectomy
Removal of the gallbladder after ligation of the cystic duct and vessels; done in most situations of acute or chronic cholecystitis. A drain (Penrose type) may be inserted in the gallbladder bed to permit drainage into dressings.

Choledochostomy
An opening into the common duct to remove obstructing stones; a drainage T-tube is inserted into the duct and is connected to a drainage bag. Usually a cholecystectomy is done at this time because the gallbladder often contains stones also.

PREOPERATIVE NURSING MANAGEMENT
1. Diagnostic evaluation:
   a. Gallbladder X-rays (p. 524).
   b. Chest X-ray.
   c. Examination of urine and stool.
   d. Blood studies including liver function tests (see p. 502).
2. Vitamin K and fresh blood may be administered to correct a low prothrombin level.
3. Supplements of protein hydrolysate may be required to maintain proper nutrition, to aid in wound healing and to prevent liver damage.
4. An operative consent form is obtained after the operative procedure is described to the patient.
5. Adequate instruction regarding immediate postoperative requirements such as turning, deep-breathing and use of incentive spirometry to prevent hypostatic pneumonia, a common postoperative complication.

PATIENT PROBLEMS
1. Pain and discomfort related to surgical procedure.
2. Altered respiratory pattern and potential for inadequate gas exchange related to the high surgical incision and its effects on breathing.
3. Nutritional alterations related to dietary restrictions.
4. Potential complications from biliary drainage.

Planning and implementation
NURSING INTERVENTIONS
Improvement in gas exchange and prevention of respiratory complications
To prevent respiratory complications, which are common in obese patients and in those having upper abdominal incisions.
1. Encourage the patient to take 10 deep breaths hourly and to turn frequently.
2. Administer analgesics as prescribed to permit the patient to take deep breaths comfortably (may be painful otherwise).
3. Splint abdominal incision with hands or pillow when the patient coughs.
4. Place the patient in an upright position to facilitate lung expansion.
5. Activate and ambulate as early as permissible.
6. Since he may still have a drainage bag, place it in a below-the-waist pocket or fasten so that it is at a desired level.

Prevention of complications from biliary drainage
To promote drainage from T-tube or cholecystostomy tube until normal flow of bile is established.
1. Place the patient in semi-recumbent and later upright position, as tolerated, to facilitate drainage.
2. Connect drainage tube to drainage bag at side of bed; observe for kinking, twisting and blockage of tubes.
3. Check postoperative orders regarding positioning of drainage bag; often, the bag or tubing is elevated so that bile drains through the apparatus only if pressure develops in the system. This is done to prevent total bile loss and to promote normal bile flow through the common bile duct.
4. Allow enough tubing leeway to permit the patient to be turned without dislodging tubes.
5. Observe, describe and record amount and character of drainage frequently.
6. After five or six days of drainage, the T-tube may be clamped one hour before and after each meal to allow bile to flow into duodenum to aid in digestion. (Done with doctor's permission.)
7. T-tube drain may be removed in 10 days. Cholecystostomy tube is removed in six weeks to six months. Drainage tube from gallbladder bed may be removed in 24 hours.
8. Observe colour changes in skin (and mucus membranes in patients with dark pigmentated skin), sclerae and stool, which will indicate whether bile pigment is disappearing from blood and draining again into the duodenum.

a. Note colour and consistency of all stools; chart an accurate description.

b. Send specimens of urine and stool to the laboratory at frequent intervals for examination of bile pigments.

c. Observe skin and sclerae for yellowish colour, which would indicate bile-flow obstruction.

9. Protect skin around incision site from bile seepage.

a. Change the outer dressings frequently to provide for absorption of drainage.

b. Apply skin pastes of zinc oxide to prevent the bile drainage from attacking and digesting the skin (if necessary).

PATIENT EDUCATION
Objective
Stress elements in posthospital care that will assist the patient in his convalescence.

1. It is not unusual after cholecystectomy for the patient to have 'looseness of the bowel', consisting of one to three movements a day. This diminishes over a period of a few weeks to several months; within a year, the bowel habit is normal.

2. Usually there are no dietary instructions except to maintain a nutritious diet and to restrict fats for four to six weeks. (Otherwise, flatulence may occur.) Thereafter, adequate bile will be released into the digestive tract to emulsify fats and permit their digestion.

3. Review medications and their purpose – vitamins, anticholinergics, antispasmodics.

4. Be aware of reportable symptoms – jaundice, dark urine, pale-coloured stools, pruritus, pain or fever.

5. Emphasize the importance of follow-up visits to the doctor.

Evaluation
EXPECTED OUTCOMES
1. Is free of respiratory complications – normal respiratory rate and pattern, no fever, full respiratory excursion with normal breath sounds, effective cough.

2. Is free of complications related to biliary drainage – no fever, no abdominal pain, normal vital signs, no drainage around tubes, normal colour of skin, sclerae, urine and stool.

3. Maintains skin integrity – area around tube or drainage tube is intact and free of excoriation.

4. Identifies signs and symptoms of complications to be reported.

CONDITIONS OF THE PANCREAS*

ACUTE PANCREATITIS

Acute pancreatitis is an inflammation of the pancreas brought about by the digestion of this organ by enzymes, particularly trypsin, an enzyme that it produces.

AETIOLOGY
1. Autodigestion of the pancreas by its own enzymes, although the exact mechanism is unknown.

2. Alcohol causes secretory and, eventually, structural changes in the pancreas; excessive alcohol intake is the most common cause.

3. Also associated with gallstones, which block ampulla of Vater, causing reflux of bile into pancreatic duct and activation of pancreatic enzymes in the pancreas itself.

4. Less commonly associated with mumps, bacterial disease, blunt trauma to the abdomen, use of oral contraceptives and congenital hyperlipidaemias.

PATHOPHYSIOLOGY
1. There is a broad spectrum of pathological changes in acute pancreatitis, ranging from oedema and inflammation of the pancreas to necrosis and haemorrhage.

2. Pancreatic enzymes, normally activated in the gastrointestinal tract following dietary stimulation, are activated in the pancreas in acute pancreatitis and begin to digest the pancreas itself.

3. Kinins are activated, altering the permeability of cell membranes and producing loss of protein-rich fluid into the tissues and peritoneal cavity, and hypovolaemia.

TREATMENT
1. Medical management is focused on alleviation of symptoms and support of the patient to prevent hypovolaemia, shock and death.

2. Includes medications and gastric suction to relieve pain and decrease stimulation of pancreatic enzymes, and fluid maintenance to prevent hypovolaemia and shock.

---

* For discussion of diabetes mellitus, see pp. 556–71.

3. Surgical intervention:
    a. There is considerable disagreement about the place of surgery in treating acute pancreatitis. It is considered only if all other therapy has failed.
    b. Laparotomy may reveal an alternate problem, which can be corrected:
        (i) Tense gallbladder – cholecystostomy.
        (ii) Stones in ductal system – establish common duct patency.
        (iii) Necrotic material and fluid removed by peritoneal lavage.

Assessment
CLINICAL FEATURES
Acute interstitial or oedematous pancreatitis
1. Pancreatic oedema and escape of enzyme into nearby tissues and peritoneal cavity.
2. Fat necrosis of omentum caused by pancreatic lipase.
3. Increase in peritoneal fluid.
4. Abdominal and back pain.
5. Nausea, vomiting; fever.
6. Tenderness across upper abdomen – often minimal.
7. Elevated blood lipase and amylase.
8. May be self-limiting if intense medical and nursing supportive care is provided.

Acute haemorrhagic pancreatitis
1. A more advanced, severe form of acute pancreatitis with mortality rate greater than 30 per cent.
2. Enzymatic digestion of gland more widespread.
3. Tissue becomes necrotic – blood escapes into pancreas and retroperitoneally, producing bloody ascites.
4. Severe abdominal and back pain; tenderness is often present in epigastrium, but rigidity is often absent.
5. Symptoms similar to acute interstitial pancreatitis, only more severe.
6. Blood lipase and amylase are elevated.
7. Respiratory distress may occur.
8. With severe pancreatitis, there is often psychic disturbance manifested in restlessness, hallucinations, coarse tremor.
9. Severe leakage of exudate from plasma into peritoneum (large third-space loss).
10. Shock, due to activation of kinins.
11. Hypokalaemic alkalosis and hypocalcaemia usually present.
12. Pancreatic cysts and abscesses are late complications.

DIAGNOSTIC EVALUATION
1. Determination of serum amylase. If serum amylase is elevated, and there is clinical evidence, pancreatitis is likely.
2. An elevated serum lipase level may also be present and persists longer than elevation of amylase levels.
3. Ultrasonography and computed tomography (CT) scan may be indicated to identify pancreatic cysts or pseudocysts in acute pancreatitis.

PATIENT PROBLEMS
1. Pain and discomfort related to oedema and inflammation of the pancreas and to peritoneal irritation.
2. Potential alteration in gas exchange related to immobility, pain and pulmonary infiltrates.
3. Altered fluid and nutritional intake related to vomiting, long-standing malnutrition, gastric intubation, sepsis, fluid shifts and paralytic ileus.

Planning and implementation
NURSING INTERVENTIONS
Relief of pain and discomfort
1. Relieve discomfort and pain to control restlessness, which increases body metabolism, causing stimulation of enzyme secretions.
    a. Give pethidine, as prescribed; this is preferred because it depresses the central nervous system. (Opiates, on the other hand, may produce spasm of biliary–pancreatic ducts.)
    b. Encourage the patient to assume comfortable position.
2. Remove stimulus to secretion of pancreatic enzymes.
    a. Give nothing by mouth, to eliminate chief stimulus to enzyme secretion.
    b. Offer anticholinergic medications as prescribed to assist in reducing pancreatic secretions by suppressing vagal mechanisms.
    c. Initiate nasogastric suction to remove hydrochloric acid from stomach, thus preventing release of secretin; adynamic ileus is also treated.
        (i) Record colour and nature of gastric secretions.
        (ii) Measure secretions at periodic intervals.
    d. Maintain the comfort of the intubated patient.
        (i) Assist the patient in cleansing and refreshing mouth care.
        (ii) Apply lubricant to external nares to prevent irritation of mucous membrane and skin.
        (iii) Alternate side-positioning to prevent

oesophageal and gastric irritation by tube.

(iv) Provide cool-mist vapour therapy to increase humidity and control drying of mucous membrane.

Improvement in gas exchange

1. Monitor blood gases to detect early signs of respiratory failure.
2. Perform pulmonary assessment frequently to observe for changes in respiratory status (anticholinergic medications, given to decrease pancreatic secretions, also predispose the patient to respiratory complications by drying the mucous membranes of the respiratory tract).
3. Position the patient in semi-upright position to decrease pressure on the diaphragm from the distended abdomen and to allow full respiratory excursion.
4. Turn the patient frequently to prevent pulmonary–vascular complications.
5. Teach and assist the patient to cough and take deep breaths.
6. Decrease oxygen requirements by keeping the patient's body metabolism low.
   a. Administer oxygen therapy if breathing is laboured.
   b. Keep the patient in bed to control overexertion.
   c. Turn on air-conditioning to keep body heat under control.

Adequate fluid and nutritional intake

1. Maintain the patient's fluid volume and prevent hypovolaemia.
   a. Maintain surveillance of vital signs.
   b. Monitor haematocrit (if it rises in first 24 to 48 hours, volume replacement was inadequate).
   c. Monitor central venous pressure (keep to 8–10cm of water above baseline).
   d. Monitor urinary output (keep to 50–100ml/h).
   e. Provide blood, balanced electrolytes to maintain blood volume; limit solutions containing glucose because this patient is often hyperglycaemic.
   f. Monitor blood sugar every four hours; administer intravenous insulin to keep blood sugar levels under 200mg/100ml, as prescribed.
   g. If marked hyperglycaemia occurs, give insulin in small doses (soluble insulin at six-hour intervals) rather than long-acting insulin, as prescribed.
2. Provide fluids and medications to correct deficiencies and prevent complications.

   a. Give parenteral fluids – electrolytes and blood to meet body's nutritional needs, replace losses and combat shock. Keep accurate intake and output record.
   b. Administer antibiotics as prescribed to ward off secondary infection or abscess formation. (Use of antibiotics remains controversial.)
   c. Monitor serum calcium; it may be necessary to administer calcium gluconate if calcium level falls low enough to produce symptoms.
3. Control nausea and vomiting.
   a. Administer antiemetics as prescribed.
   b. Maintain gastric suction and monitor closely.
4. Instruct the patient about normal, adequate nutrition and importance of avoiding alcohol during recovery.
   a. Provide diet high in carbohydrate, low in fat, proteins and stimulants.
   b. Instruct the patient to avoid alcohol and heavy meals.

PATIENT EDUCATION AND DISCHARGE PLANNING

Manage recovery phase and offer guidelines to the patient to prevent future attacks of pancreatitis.

1. When the patient's condition permits, offer the following:
   a. Small amounts of fat-free liquids.
   b. Anticholinergics, parenterally or orally.
   c. Nonabsorbable antacids hourly.
2. Instruct the patient as follows:
   a. Gradually resume normal diet.
   b. Alcohol use and excessive use of coffee are prohibited, since they increase pancreatic secretion.
3. Urge follow-up visits with doctor. (Biliary tract studies and surveillance may uncover the cause of the pancreatitis.)

Evaluation

EXPECTED OUTCOMES

1. Experiences relief of pain and discomfort – indicates less discomfort, describes self as feeling better, ambulates and participates in mild forms of activity without complaints of pain.
2. Shows no signs of respiratory complications – normal blood gases, normal respiratory rate and pattern, normal breath sounds, adequate cough and frequent deep breaths, adequate fluid intake to liquify secretions.
3. Attains adequate fluid and nutritional intake – regular body weight without increase in ascites or oedema; normal blood glucose levels and urine glucose levels; eating prescribed diet; no complaints of gastric distress, vomiting or nausea.

CHRONIC PANCREATITIS

Chronic pancreatitis is a chronic fibrosis and calcification of the pancreas with obstruction of its ducts and destruction of its secreting acinar cells.

INCIDENCE
1. Occurs most often in men between 45 and 60 years.
2. Follows repeated attacks of acute interstitial pancreatitis.
3. Usually occurs in patients having a history of prolonged use of alcohol.
4. Gallstones, hyperparathyroidism and hyperlipidaemia are occasionally associated with chronic pancreatitis.

PATHOPHYSIOLOGY
1. Alcohol exerts direct toxic effect on cells of the pancreas; the likelihood of chronic pancreatitis is increased by genetic predisposition.
2. Alcohol may also stimulate pancreatic secretion at the same time it induces spasm of the sphincter of Oddi, causing pain.
3. Repeated episodes of acute pancreatitis and alcohol ingestion produces fibrosis, cyst formation and distortion of pancreatic tissue.

CLINICAL FEATURES
1. Recurrent episodes of severe upper abdominal and back pain (morphine often does not relieve pain), vomiting and low-grade fever. Drug addiction is often a secondary problem.
2. Protein and fat digestion is disturbed because of deficient pancreatic secretion.
3. Steatorrhoea – stools that are frequent, frothy and foul-smelling with high fat content because of faulty fat digestion.
4. Later formation of calcium stones in the duct as calcification develops.
5. Weight loss.
6. Jaundice may occur because of constriction of common bile duct as it passes through head of pancreas.

DIAGNOSTIC EVALUATION
1. Determine whether levels of serum amylase and lipase are elevated. Levels often are not elevated in chronic pancreatitis.
2. Examine stool to measure faecal fat and trypsin content.
3. Arteriography and X-ray may show fibrous tissue and calcification.
4. Diabetes or abnormal glucose tolerance may be detectable.

TREATMENT AND NURSING MANAGEMENT
1. The treatment measures indicated depend on the nature and severity of the patient's symptoms, which may be similar to those of acute pancreatitis.
   a. The patient is often drug dependent because of recurring episodes of severe pain requiring careful assessment and management of pain.
   b. The long-term nature of chronic pancreatitis often results in an acutely ill patient who is malnourished, emaciated and at risk of multiple complications.
   c. The patient is frequently a poor surgical risk.
2. Offer the patient bland, low-fat diet in six feedings daily.
3. Give antacids and anticholinergic medication to reduce acid, which would stimulate the release of secretin and enhance pancreatic activity.
4. Pancreatic insufficiency is controlled by giving medication containing amylase, lipase and trypsin (Pancreatin). Medication may need to be administered with antacids or bicarbonates.

Note: Steatorrhoea should be present before enzyme replacement therapy is initiated.

5. Since these patients often develop diabetes, be alert for symptoms such as polydipsia, polyuria, weakness, polyphagia (excessive eating) or weight loss and report these to the doctor.
6. The use of alcohol should be discouraged, since this will aggravate the pancreatitis; treatment of alcoholism must be done if this is a problem, as it usually is.
7. If hyperparathyroidism or hyperlipaemia is diagnosed, these certainly must be treated.
8. Surgical aspects are similar to those of biliary tract surgery (see p. 530).
9. Nature of surgery is determined by identifying the cause; surgery usually fails if alcoholism or drug addiction persists.
   a. With gallbladder disease – biliary tract surgery to explore common bile duct, choledocholectomy (removing stones in duct) and cholecystectomy (removing gallbladder).
   b. Sphincteroplasty or sphincterotomy may be done to divide sphincter of Oddi to improve drainage of common bile duct, or;
   c. Selective or generalized drainage of dilated ducts via pancreaticojejunostomy.
   d. Pancreatectomy may be done when pancreas is severely diseased or when persistent pain is a major problem.

PSEUDOCYSTS AND PANCREATIC ABSCESSES

Pseudocysts of the pancreas are collections of inflammatory fluid walled off by fibrous tissue in the pancreas, usually resulting from local necrosis at the time of acute pancreatitis.

CLINICAL FEATURES AND DIAGNOSIS

1. Cysts may attain considerable size; they develop rapidly or slowly (within 72 hours or over several weeks or months).
2. Because they occur in the posterior peritoneum, they may exert pressure against the stomach or colon, which is visible on barium studies.
3. Persistent elevation of amylase (serum or urine) is the most common finding. Pain and vomiting may occur.
4. Leucocytosis and fever are common but are usually mild with pseudocysts; these responses are more striking with abscess formation.
5. Sonography has been found useful in confirming the diagnosis.

TREATMENT

1. Pseudocysts may occasionally subside spontaneously.
2. Symptoms of secondary infection may require surgery for drainage.
3. Drainage may be established into gastrointestinal tract (internal) or through skin surface (external); this latter method is controversial because it presents the risk of the patient developing pancreatic fistulae.

NURSING MANAGEMENT

1. Should external drainage be done, recognize the irritating qualities of the pancreatic enzyme; meticulous skin care is required.
2. Maintain adequate drainage, avoiding tube dislodgment.

PANCREATIC CANCER

Cancer may arise in the head, body or tail of the pancreas; insulin-secreting pancreatic islet cells may or may not be involved.

TREATMENT

Surgical only. Although surgical cures are possible, five-year survival is about 25 per cent. Tumour is removed if it has not invaded important surrounding structures.

1. Whipple resection – removal of head (and sometimes neck) of pancreas; removal of adjacent stomach, distal portion of common duct and duodenum. Patient has severe malabsorption afterwards.
2. If Whipple procedure cannot be done, jaundice may be relieved by diverting bile from gallbladder into the jejunum (cholecystojejunostomy). If duodenum is invaded, gastrojejunostomy should be done to bypass duodenal obstruction.
3. For cancer of the body and tail of the pancreas, distal pancreatectomy and splenectomy are the most commonly employed procedures.
4. Total pancreatectomy – en bloc resection of the common bile duct, stomach, duodenum, pancreas and spleen.

Assessment

CLINICAL FEATURES

The 'big three' are *weight loss*, *pain* and *jaundice*.

1. Initial symptoms of cancer of the pancreas are often vague, thereby accounting for a reported four to nine months' delay from onset of symptoms to diagnosis.
2. Disease usually occurs in older men; alcoholism may be a contributing cause.
3. Weight loss, anorexia, dyspepsia, nausea, some bowel disturbance and occasionally chills and fever develop.
4. Intermittent, dull-to-severe, vague, epigastric or back pain, often aggravated by eating or associated with fullness and bloating after meals.
   a. Right upper quadrant pain suggests involvement of the head of the pancreas.
   b. Left upper quadrant pain suggests involvement of the body or tail of the pancreas.
   c. Pain often radiates to the back or is exclusively in back.
   d. Pain is often worse at night, aggravated in recumbent position and relieved by lying with legs drawn up or by walking bent over.
   e. Fear of eating may take place.
5. The patient may experience depression and lethargy, combined with a feeling of anxiety and premonition of serious illness.
6. Obstruction of the common bile duct produces jaundice, clay-coloured stools, dark urine and itching (due to cancer of the head of pancreas). Differentiation must be made between jaundice from biliary obstruction (due to a stone in the common duct) and jaundice from hepatic metastases.

DIAGNOSTIC EVALUATION

1. Blood studies, including serum bilirubin, alkaline phosphatase, SGOT and prothrombin time.
2. Secretin studies and radiological procedures, gallbladder studies and possibly fibreoptic duodenoscopy with cannulation of papilla and pancreatic ductography, or transhepatic cholangiography.
3. Scanning – radioactive selenomethionine (^{75}Se); note that frequent false-positive findings occur.
4. Angiography.
5. Ultrasonography.
6. Computed tomography.

PATIENT PROBLEMS

1. Altered nutritional status related to anorexia and increased gastrointestinal disturbances after eating.
2. Pain and discomfort related to tumour involvement of the pancreas.
3. Impaired skin integrity related to jaundice and debilitation.
4. Altered self-concept related to change in role function.
5. Inability to cope related to depression over diagnosis of cancer.

Planning and implementation

NURSING INTERVENTIONS

Appropriate fluid and nutrient intake to meet body needs

1. Because of the patient's poor nutritional state, it is a challenge to maintain adequate calorie levels. A bland, low-fat diet is recommended, plus whatever he can tolerate without overeating.
2. Medium-chain triglycerides are better tolerated, since they cause less fat excretion.
3. Alcohol to be avoided.
4. Anticholinergics used.
5. Provide small, frequent meals.
6. Determine and provide foods preferred by the patient.
7. Provide supplements of high-calorie foods between meals.
8. Encourage the patient to drink adequate fluids to prevent complications (e.g. urinary tract infection, etc).

Relief of pain and promotion of comfort

1. Administer analgesic medication for pain as prescribed.
2. Assist the patient to assume comfortable positions.
3. Assess quality, severity and location of the patient's pain.
4. Assess and record the patient's response to analgesia.
5. Provide additional means of pain relief (e.g. distraction, massage, etc).

Improved skin integrity

1. Assist the patient to change position frequently to prevent pressure sores.
2. Massage bony prominences frequently.
3. Note appearance of reddened areas of skin.
4. Apply sheepskin or foam rubber to bed; or special mattress to relieve pressure on the skin.
5. Provide soothing lotions and baths to alleviate pruritus and scratching.
6. Administer medications prescribed for pruritus.
7. Keep the patient's fingernails short to prevent scratching of skin.
8. Avoid trauma to skin through gentle handling and prevention of falls.

Promotion of coping abilities

1. Assist the patient in recognizing and verbalizing feelings and reactions to current situation.
2. Identify tasks and activities that the patient can accomplish.
3. Assist the patient in identifying his own priorities of tasks.
4. Assist the patient in planning achievable goals and activities.
5. Assist the patient in confronting his future with dignity (e.g. major surgical procedure, persistent pain, increasing disability or impending death).

Evaluation

EXPECTED OUTCOMES

1. Maintains adequate fluid and nutritional intake – good appetite; meals are consumed when delivered; weight is maintained without oedema; urine output is normal.
2. Achieves pain relief or increased comfort via drugs.
3. Maintains skin integrity – no redness, breakdown, excoriation or infection; normal skin elasticity, no complaints of pruritus; uses precautions to prevent trauma.
4. Demonstrates improved coping abilities – verbalizes feelings and participates in own care.

FURTHER READING

BOOKS

Bokey, E.L. and Shell, R. (1985) *Stomal Therapy: A Guide for Nurses, Practitioners and Patients*, Pergamon, Sydney.

Bouchier, I. (1982) *Gastroenterology* (3rd edn), Concise Medical Textbook Series, Baillière, Eastbourne.

Brunt, P.W., Losowsky, M.S. and Read, A.E. (1984) *The Liver and Biliary System*, Heinemann, London.

Burkitt, D. (1979) *Don't Forget Fibre in Your Diet*, Martin Dunitz, London.

Elcoat, C. (1986) *Stoma Care Nursing*, Baillière Tindall, London.

Elias, E. and Hawkins, C. (1985) *Lecture Notes on Gastroenterology*, Blackwell, Oxford.

Grant, A. and Todd, E. (1982) *Enteral and Parenteral Nutrition, A Clinical Handbook*, Blackwell Scientific, Oxford.

Jones, P.F., Brunt, P.W., Mowat, N. and Ashley, G. (1985) *Gastroenterology*, Heinemann, London.

Langman, M.J.S. (1982) *A Concise Textbook of Gastroenterology*, Churchill Livingstone, London.

Moghissi, K. and Boore, J. (1982) *Parenteral and Enteral Nutrition for Nurses*, Heinemann, London.

Royal College of Nursing (1981) *Stoma Care: A Team Approach*, RCN, London.

Schindler, M. (1981) *Living with a Colostomy*, Thorsons, Wellingborough.

Sherlock, S. (1985) *Diseases of the Liver and Biliary System* (7th edn), Blackwell, Oxford.

Sykes, M. (1981) *Aspects of Gastroenterology for Nurses*, Pitman Medical, London.

Thompson, R. (1985) *Lecture Notes on the Liver*, Blackwell, Oxford.

ARTICLES

Cancer

Bennett, M. (1985) As normal a life as possible (community care study of patient with a squamous carcinoma of the mouth), *Community Outlook*, Vol. 81, No. 7, pp. 35, 37–8.

Harvey, J. (1985) Staff of life (nutritional support for cancer patients), *Nursing Mirror*, Vol. 161, p. 24.

Nichols, S. (1985) Research: gut feelings that don't add up (large bowel cancer), *Nursing Mirror*, Vol. 161, pp. 22–3.

Northover, J. (1984) Colorectal cancer – today and tomorrow, *The Practitioner*, Vol. 228, pp. 569–72.

Phillips, R. (1984) Oesophago-gastric cancer: helping the patient swallow, *Geriatric Medicine*, Vol. 14, No. 2, pp. 83–5.

Gastroenterology

Bateson, M.C. (1984) Progress in gallstone disease, *British Medical Journal*, Vol. 289, November, pp. 1163–4.

Brooks, S.L. (1984) Disturbances of bowel function, *Nursing Add On*, Vol. 2, October, pp. 870, 872–3, 875–6.

Clark, C.G. (1986) Advances in the treatment of peptic ulcer, *The Practitioner*, Vol. 230, March, pp. 283–8.

Datta, P. (1984) Diagnosing obstructive jaundice, *Nursing Mirror*, Vol. 159, 19 September, pp. 33–4.

Dewar, B.J. (1985) Management of oesophageal varices, *Nursing Times*, Vol. 81, 5 June, pp. 32–5.

Docherty, C. (1985) Acute pancreatitis (care study), *Nursing Mirror*, Vol. 160, 19 June, pp. 48–51.

Fuller, J.H.S. (1984) Ano-rectal bleeding, *The Practitioner*, Vol. 228, September, pp. 825–6, 828.

Gillespie, I. (1986) Bleeding oesophageal varices, *British Medical Journal*, Vol. 292, 7 June, pp. 1479–80.

Heaton, K.W. (1984) The sweet road to gall stones, *British Medical Journal*, Vol. 288, April, pp. 1103–4.

Milne, B., Joachim, G. and Miedhardt, J. (1986) A stress management programme for inflammatory bowel disease patients, *Journal of Advanced Nursing*, Vol. 11, No. 5, September, pp. 561–7.

Morris, J.S. (1984) Ascites, *British Medical Journal*, Vol. 289, 28 July, p. 209.

Silvester, G.A. (1984) Investigation of the gastrointestinal tract, *Nursing Add On*, Vol. 2, October, pp. 896–7.

Smith, S. and Wright, P. (1984) Constipation (nursing research in this area), *Nursing Times*, Vol. 80, 30 May, pp. 64–7.

Stoker, F. (1985) Cirrhosis of the liver, *Nursing Mirror*, Vol. 160, No. 26, June, pp. 29–31.

Hepatitis

Alexander, G. and Williams, R. (1986) Antiviral treatment in chronic infection with hepatitis B virus, *British Medical Journal*, Vol. 292, 5 April, pp. 915–17.

Hegarty, J. and Williams, R. (1985) Chronic hepatitis in the 1980s, *British Medical Journal*, Vol. 290, 23 March pp. 877–8.

Ho-Yen, D.O. Grossman, M.N. and Walker, E. (1985). Nursing knowledge of hepatitis B infection, *Journal of Advanced Nursing*, Vol. 10, March, pp. 169–72.

Sutherland, G. (1986) Update on viral hepatitis, *The Practitioner*, Vol. 230, March, pp. 237–46.

Zuckerman, A.J. (1984) Who should be immunized against hepatitis B? *British Medical Journal*, Vol. 289, 10 November, pp. 1243–4.

— (1985) New hepatitis B vaccines, *British Medical Journal*, Vol. 290, 16 February, pp. 492–6.

Liver and biliary system

Hall, J. (1984) Liver transplantation 1: patient selection and surgery, *Nursing Times*, Vol. 80, 3 October, pp. 28–31.

— (1984) Liver transplantation 1: postoperative care, *Nursing Times*, Vol. 80, 10 October, pp. 59–62.

Hegarty, J. and Williams, R. (1984) Liver biopsy: techniques, clinical applications and complications, *British Medical Journal*, Vol. 288, 28 April, pp. 1254–6.

Parenteral

Davidson, L. (1986) Dressing subclavian catheters (a study into the quality of a selection of catheter dressings), *Nursing Times*, Vol. 82, 12 February, p. 40.

Dewar, B.J. (1986) Total parenteral nutrition at home, *Nursing Times*, Vol. 82, 9 July, pp. 35, 37–8.

Holloway, H. (1985) Nutrition 2 – short-term parenteral feeding (use of parenteral nutrition postoperatively for a patient with a prolonged paralytic ileus), *Nursing Mirror*, Vol. 161, 20 February, pp. 42–3.

Holmes, S. (1984) Total parenteral nutrition, *Senior Nurse*, Vol. 1, 1 August, pp. 10–13.

Pascoe, D.A. (1986) Total parenteral nutrition, *Nursing Add On*, Vol. 3, No. 8, August, pp. 286–92.

Stoma care

Allen, S. (1984) Stoma management, *Nursing Add On*, Vol. 2, October, pp. 877–81.

Black, P. (1985) Stoma care 1. Selecting a site, *Nursing Mirror*, Vol. 161, 28 August, pp. 22–4.

— (1985) Stoma care 2. The right appliance, *Nursing Mirror*, Vol. 161, 4 September, pp. 34–5.

— (1985) Stoma care 3. Drugs and diet, *Nursing Mirror*, Vol. 161, 11 September, pp. 26, 28.

— (1985) Stoma care 4. Rehabilitation and problem-solving, *Nursing Mirror*, Vol. 161, 18 September, pp. 34–6.

Breckman, B. (1986) Success by stages (counselling the stoma patient – a case history sample), *Senior Nurse*, Vol. 5, No. 3, September, pp. 14–16.

Cunningham, S.C. (1984) The cosmetics of stoma care, *Nursing Add On*, Vol. 2, October, pp. 890, 892, 895.

Fryer, S. and Jones, H. (1985) Colostomy care, *Nursing Times*, Vol. 81, 13 February, pp. 31–2, 34–5, 38.

Murphy, M. (1984) Stoma care, going home (problems after discharge), *Senior Nurse*, Vol. 1, 5 September, pp. 20–1.

Pringle, W. (1984) Colostomy irrigation, *Nursing Mirror*, Vol. 159, No. 8, 5 September, pp. 29–31.

Rossiter, M.C. (1984) Diverting the flow (bowel conditions requiring stoma), *Nursing Add On*, Vol. 2, October, pp. 882–5.

Salter, M. (1986) Quality above quantity (the care of patients with advanced cancer who face stoma surgery), *Senior Nurse*, Vol. 5, No. 3, September, pp. 12–13.

Snow, B. (1984) Ileostomy – sexual problems and self-image, *Nursing Add On*, Vol. 2, October, pp. 888–9.

Stewart, E. and Cotton, B. (1986) Leaking stoma bags: nursing action, *Professional Nurse*, Vol. 1, January, pp. 105–6.

— (1986) The essential anatomy and physiology of a stoma, *Professional Nurse*, Vol. 1, February, pp. 129–31.

Stewart, L. (1984) Stoma care: preoperative preparation of the patient, *Nursing Add On*, Vol. 2, October, pp. 886–7.

8

Care of the Patient with a Metabolic or Endocrine Disorder

THE THYROID GLAND AND TESTS OF THYROID FUNCTION

PHYSIOLOGY

1. The thyroid gland affects the rate at which all tissues metabolize.
   a. Speed of chemical reactions.
   b. Volume of oxygen consumed.
   c. Amount of heat produced.
2. The stimulating effect is through the production and distribution of two hormones:
   a. Levothyroxine (T_4) – contains four iodine atoms; maintains body's metabolism in a steady state; it is believed that T_4 serves as a precursor of T_3.
   b. Tri-iodothyronine (T_3) – contains three iodine atoms; is approximately five times as potent as thyroxine; has a more rapid metabolic action and utilization than thyroxine. Most conversion of T_4 to T_3 occurs at the cellular level in the periphery. Some T_3 is produced in the thyroid gland.

DIAGNOSTIC EVALUATION

Radio-iodine (^{131}I) (^{99m}Tc)

1. ^{131}I *uptake:*
   a. A solution of sodium iodide-131 is administered to the patient orally or by intravenous injection.
   b. After a prescribed interval (anywhere from two to 48 hours, but frequently by 24 hours), measurements are taken with a scintillator of radioactive counts per minute that are detected above the isthmus of the thyroid gland.
   c. Normal thyroid will remove 15 to 50 per cent of the iodine from the bloodstream.
   d. Hyperthyroidism may result in the removal of as much as 90 per cent of the iodine from the bloodstream.
2. *Thyroidal iodide clearance:*
   a. Radio-iodine clearance test measures the amount of circulating blood that is completely cleared of iodide per unit of time.
   b. Radio-iodine is injected intravenously; radioactivity over the thyroid gland is measured continuously for 30 to 60 minutes – total amount of ^{131}I concentrated in the gland per minute is computed.
   c. Also, plasma ^{131}I content is measured in samples of blood collected 45 to 70 minutes after injection; these values are averaged.

   d. Thyroid ^{131}I divided by the mean plasma ^{131}I equals thyroid clearance, i.e. millilitres of plasma cleared of iodide per minute.
   e. Normal, 25ml/minute; hyperthyroidism, 250ml/minute; hypothyroidism, 1.6ml/minute.
3. ^{131}I *excretion:*
   a. Urinary output of radio-iodine is measured during six-hour and 24-hour periods after ingestion.
   b. Normal, 40 to 80 per cent of ingested iodine in 24-hours; hyperthyroidism, less than 40 per cent; hypothyroidism, greater than 80 per cent.
4. *Thyroid 'scan' ^{131}I:*
   a. Patient ingests sodium iodide-131 and is scanned the next day; if medium is given intravenously, patient may be scanned within 30 to 60 minutes.
   b. Patient is supine; the detector head of the scintillation camera with a pinhole colimeter is centred over the patient's neck.
   c. The thyroid images from the oscilloscope of the camera are recorded on film; colour adds dimension.
   d. A decrease in ^{132}I uptake in a particular area of the thyroid is considered suggestive of malignancy.
5. *Thyroid 'scan' ^{99m}Tc:*
   a. Patient is given an intravenous injection of sodium pertechnetate.
   b. A scintillator electromechanically maps the activity in the scanned area to produce a scintogram.
   c. This simple procedure facilitates the diagnosis of goitrous changes, cold and hot nodules, cystic degeneration and thyroid malignancy.
6. *Tri-iodothyronine (T_3) suppression test:*
   a. 24-hour radioactive uptake is measured.
   b. Patient is given T_3 for seven days.
   c. 24-hour radioactive uptake is measured again.
   d. Normal: suppression to a radioactive iodine uptake below 20 per cent at 24 hours (half original value). Graves' disease: no suppression.

NURSING ALERT

The use of radioactive substances is contraindicated in pregnancy. During pregnancy, thyroid testing is limited to blood testing.

Thyroid tests must be scheduled carefully so that thyroid-blocking contrast agents for other X-rays, diagnostic tests and medications do not interfere with interpretation of tests of thyroid function.

Serum thyroxine (T₄)

1. It is a direct measurement of the concentration of total thyroxine in the blood; a good index of thyroid function when thyroxine-binding globulin (TBG) is normal.
2. Normal values: 4.5–11.5μg.
3. Normally elevated in pregnancy and with oestrogen therapy.
4. Used to diagnose hypofunction and hyperfunction of thyroid and to guide and evaluate therapy.

Serum tri-iodothyronine (T₃)

1. Directly measures concentration of tri-iodothyronine in the blood; T₃ is much less stable than T₄ and occurs in minute quantities in the active form.
2. Useful to rule out T₃ thyrotoxicosis, hypofunction and hyperfunction of the thyroid, to determine thyroid gland status, and to evaluate effects of thyroid replacement therapy.
3. Normal values: 110–130ng.
4. When the T₃ level is low, the patient is usually hypothyroid.

T₃ Resin uptake

1. Is an indirect measure of thyroid function based on the available protein-binding sites in a serum sample that can bind to radioactive T₃.
2. The radioactive tri-iodothyronine is added to the serum sample in the test tube.
3. The effect of oestrogen and pregnancy is to produce an increase in binding sites, causing a lowered percentage of binding by the available thyroid hormones.
4. Rates:
   a. Normal binding: 25 to 35 per cent.
   b. High T₃ is associated with hyperthyroidism.
   c. Low T₃ is associated with hypothyroidism.
5. This test is often used in conjunction with serum thyroxine (T₄).
6. Results may be altered if this patient has been taking oestrogens, androgens, salicylates or phenytoin.

Thyrotropin-releasing hormone (TRH)

1. Prior to TRH injection, a blood specimen is drawn.
2. Doctor injects into venous system 0.2mg synthetic TRH; blood specimen for TSH (thyroid-stimulating hormone) is drawn.
3. Blood specimens are drawn at 15, 30, 45, 60, 90 and 120 minutes.

Thyrotropin radioimmunoassay (TSH)

1. Useful in differentiating between thyroid disorders due to disease of the thyroid gland itself and disorders due to disease of the pituitary or hypothalamus.
2. In patients with primary hypothyroidism, TSH levels are elevated. In secondary hypothyroidism (failure of the pituitary gland), TSH levels are low.
3. In patients with hyperthyroidism, TSH levels are low.
4. Blood sample is analysed by radioimmunoassay.

DISORDERS OF THE THYROID GLAND

HYPOTHYROIDISM

Hypothyroidism may be classified as primary, secondary or tertiary. *Primary hypothyroidism* is a condition resulting from the inability of the thyroid gland to secrete a sufficient amount of hormone. *Secondary hypothyroidism* is caused by a failure of the pituitary gland to secrete an adequate amount of TSH (thyroid-stimulating hormone). *Tertiary hypothyroidism* results from failure of the hypothalamus to release thyroid-releasing hormone (TRH).

Cretinism is a severe form of hypothyroidism resulting from deficiency of thyroid function during fetal life or shortly after birth. The mother has usually had deficiency of thyroid hormone function during pregnancy.

AETIOLOGY

1. Primary hypothyroidism is the most common form of this condition and is generally due to:
   a. Removal, destruction or suppression of all or some of the thyroid tissue by thyroidectomy;
   b. Use of radioactive iodine;
   c. Overtreatment with anti-thyroid drugs.
2. Hypothyroidism may also be idiopathic in origin or a result of chronic immunological dysfunction, as in Hashimoto's thyroiditis.

PATHOPHYSIOLOGY

1. Inadequate secretion of thyroid hormone leads to a general slowing of all physical and mental processes.

2. There is a general depression of most cellular enzyme systems and oxidative processes.
3. The metabolic activity of all cells of the body decreases, reducing oxygen consumption, decreasing oxidation of nutrients for energy and producing less body heat.
4. The signs and symptoms of the disorder range from vague, nonspecific complaints that make diagnosis difficult, to severe symptoms that may be life-threatening if unrecognized and untreated.

Assessment
CLINICAL FEATURES
1. Fatigue and lethargy.
2. Temperature and pulse become subnormal; unable to tolerate cold and desires increase in room temperature.
3. Complains of cold hands and feet.
4. Menorrhagia or amenorrhoea; may have difficulty conceiving or experiences spontaneous abortion.
5. Mental processes become dulled; develops loss of memory.
6. Gains weight.
7. Hair thins and falls out; skin becomes thickened and dry.
8. Develops severe constipation.
9. Neurological signs develop (polyneuropathy, cerebellar ataxia); muscle aches or weakness, clumsiness.
10. Facial expression becomes solid and mask-like; later, facial bloating and pallor develop.
11. In severe hypothyroidism, hypotension, unresponsiveness, bradycardia, hypoventilation, hyponatraemia, (possibly) convulsions, hypothermia, cerebral hypoxia and myxoedema may occur.
12. Accelerated atherosclerosis and coronary artery disease may occur because of deposits of mucopolysaccharides in myocardium.
13. Increased susceptibility to all hypnotic and sedative drugs and anaesthetic agents.
14. Has a mortality rate of 50 per cent.

DIAGNOSTIC EVALUATION
1. T_3 and T_4 levels are low.
2. Thyroid-stimulating hormone levels are elevated in primary hypothyroidism.
3. Elevation of serum cholesterol.
4. ECG – sinus bradycardia, low-voltage of QRS complexes, and flat or inverted T waves.
5. Prolonged deep tendon reflex response, especially ankle jerk.

6. The patient's past medical history may reveal previous treatment with radioactive iodine.
7. Complete physical examination may reveal subtle signs of hypothyroidism or a general suppression and depression of organs and systems.

PATIENT PROBLEMS
The patient with severe hypothyroidism experiences multiple systemic problems, including:
1. Potential alteration in cardiac output related to decreased metabolic rate, decreased cardiac conduction, elevated cholesterol levels, atherosclerosis and coronary artery disease.
2. Activity intolerance related to lethargy and fatigue, depressed neuromuscular status.
3. Alterations in fluid and nutritional status related to decreased metabolic rate, poor appetite and depressed gastrointestinal function.

Planning and implementation
TREATMENT
Approach
1. The medical management depends on the severity of the patient's symptoms and may necessitate replacement therapy in mild cases or life-saving support and treatment for the patient with severe hypothyroidism and myxoedema coma.
2. As the patient's thyroid hormone levels are gradually returned to normal, the patient is also monitored closely to prevent complications resulting from sudden increases in metabolic rate and oxygen requirements.

Objective of medical management
To restore a normal metabolic state (euthyroid) as rapidly and safely as possible.
1. Administer thyroid hormone once a day.
   a. Because tri-iodothyronine acts more quickly than thyroxine, give this initially; if the patient is unconscious, give via stomach tube.
   b. Administer liothyronine sodium parenterally (until consciousness is restored) to restore thyroxine level; continue daily.
   c. Later, continue the patient on oral thyroid hormone therapy.
   d. Recognize that with rapid administration of thyroid hormone, plasma thyroxine levels may initiate adrenal insufficiency – hence, steroid therapy may be initiated.
2. Monitor the patient carefully to anticipate such effects of treatment as:
   a. Diuresis, decreased puffiness;
   b. Improved reflexes and muscle tone;

c. Accelerated pulse rate;

d. A slightly higher level of total serum thyroxine.

3. Monitor ECG tracings to detect arrhythmias and deterioration of cardiovascular status.

4. Provide assisted ventilation if needed to combat hypoventilation.

NURSING INTERVENTIONS
Improved cardiac output

1. Control factors that increase metabolic rate and threaten cardiovascular status:

a. Monitor vital signs frequently to detect changes in the patient's cardiovascular status and ability to respond to stress.

b. Prevent and treat factors that increase metabolic rate (infection, stress, trauma).

c. Prevent chilling to avoid increasing metabolic rate, which, in turn, places strain on the heart. Provide bed socks, bed jacket, warm environment.

d. Even though hypothermia exists, do not apply external heat, since the resulting increased oxygen requirements and decreased peripheral vascular tone may compound the existing cardiac failure.

e. Administer fluids cautiously even though hyponatraemia is present.

f. Give glucose in concentrated amounts to prevent fluid overload if hypoglycaemia is in evidence.

2. Administer all drugs with caution before and after thyroid replacement begins.

a. Before treatment with thyroid hormone, the patient is susceptible to the effects of sedatives, narcotics, anaesthetics and other medications.

b. After thyroid replacement is initiated, the thyroid hormones may increase the effects of digitalis and anticoagulants.

3. Report occurrence of angina, and the signs and symptoms of myocardial infarction and cardiac failure.

4. Instruct the patient how and when to take medications.

5. Instruct the patient about signs and symptoms to insufficient and excessive medication.

Increased activity tolerance and a balance of rest and activity

1. Limit visitors during acute stage to prevent excessive stimulation.

2. Carry out activities, hygiene and care for the patient during acute stage of illness.

3. Prevent pulmonary complications of immobility during acute stage by turning, and encouraging the patient to cough and take deep breaths.

4. Encourage very gradual resumption of activities as severe symptoms begin to subside and the patient begins to improve.

5. Assist the patient in planning activities to limit exertion and provide ample periods of rest.

6. Identify for the patient signs and symptoms indicating excessive exertion.

7. Provide good skin care to prevent skin breakdown secondary to immobility.

a. Apply lubricant to the skin, since it is usually dry and scaly.

b. Observe for pressure areas and initiate measures to stimulate circulation to these areas.

Improved fluid and nutritional status

1. Administer prescribed foods and fluids cautiously during acute stage.

2. Offer oral fluids and food gradually and carefully.

3. Assess the patient's dietary preferences.

4. Serve attractive, low-calorie meals; this patient is usually overweight, although his appetite is poor.

5. Offer fluids frequently and include dietary fibre to prevent constipation.

6. Assess return and gradual increase of gastrointestinal function (return of bowel sounds, absence of abdominal distention, occurrence and frequency of bowel movements).

7. Administer prescribed stool softeners if necessary.

8. Discourage straining at stool because of increased strain on the heart.

Evaluation
EXPECTED OUTCOMES

1. Experiences/demonstrates improved cardiac status and output – normal blood pressure and pulse rate; normal ECG tracing (normal amplitude and return of normal T wave).

2. Avoids factors and events that increase metabolic rate (trauma, respiratory or other infections, stressful situations).

3. Reports absence of chest pain, dyspnoea or palpitations.

4. Reports increased sense of warmth to a comfortable level (decreased sensitivity or intolerance to cold).

5. Identifies appropriate schedule of medications and takes medications as prescribed.

6. Identifies signs and symptoms of hypothyroid-

ism and hyperthyroidism that should be reported.

7. Demonstrates increased activity tolerance:
   a. Plans activities and exercise to allow adequate periods of rest and relaxation.
   b. Ceases activities as signs and symptoms of cardiac dysfunction develop.
   c. Reports increased strength and well-being; decreased fatigue and lethargy.
   d. Participates in own care and hygiene.

8. Takes measures to prevent respiratory complications and skin breakdown – turns frequently when in bed; coughs and takes deep breaths.

9. Reports absence of respiratory complications or infections.

10. Demonstrates adequate fluid and nutritional intake:
    a. Identifies foods encouraged in diet; consumes low-calorie meals.
    b. Avoids foods restricted in diet.
    c. Reports loss of weight and absence of oedema.
    d. Drinks adequate fluids daily.

11. Reports return of normal bowel function and decrease in gastrointestinal disturbances and constipation.

HYPERTHYROIDISM

Hyperthyroidism (diffuse toxic goitre) is excessive activity of the thyroid gland.

INCIDENCE
More common in women than in men; occurs in about 2 per cent of the female population.

TYPES
1. Graves' disease (most prevalent) – diffuse hyperfunction of the thyroid gland associated with ophthalmopathy; most common in younger women; may subside spontaneously.
2. Toxic nodular goitre (single or multiple) – more common in older females with pre-existing goitre; will continue to be overactive unless eradicated or kept under suppressive therapy.

AETIOLOGY
1. Unknown; immunological origin is likely.
2. Possible causes:
   a. Thyroid-stimulating antibody (TSA$_b$; formerly LATS – long-acting thyroid stimulator) correlates very closely with the clinical course of Graves' disease.
   b. TSA$_b$, an immunoglobulin found in the blood of patients with Graves' disease, is capable of reacting with the receptor for TSH on the thyroid plasma membrane and stimulating glandular function.
   c. May appear after an emotional shock, infection or emotional stress.
   d. Genetic predisposition, female sex.
   e. B and T lymphocytes (immunological factors) have been implicated.

PATHOPHYSIOLOGY
1. Hyperthyroidism is characterized by hypertrophy and hyperplasia of the thyroid gland, which is accompanied by increased vascularity and blood flow and enlargement of the gland.
2. A hypermetabolic condition results from the excessive secretion of thyroid hormone, resulting in exaggeration of all metabolic processes.
3. The majority of cases of hyperthyroidism are thought to be due to an autoimmune reaction in which circulating autoantibodies mimic the action of TSH and increase the secretion of thyroid hormone.
4. Most of the clinical features result from increased metabolic rate, excessive heat production, increased neuromuscular and cardiovascular activity, and hyperactivity of the sympathetic nervous system.
5. Hyperthyroidism ranges from a mild increase in metabolic rate to the severe hyperactivity known as thyrotoxicosis, thyroid storm or thyroid crisis.
6. A patient with mild hyperthyroidism is not usually admitted to the hospital unless admitted for another problem and the hyperthyroidism is initially unsuspected.
7. The patient with severe thyrotoxicosis or thyroid crisis, however, is admitted to control the hypermetabolic state, prevent cardiac failure or prepare for surgery.

Assessment
CLINICAL FEATURES
1. Single or multiple adenomas.
2. Nervousness, emotional hyperexcitability, irritability, apprehension.
3. Difficulty in sitting quietly.
4. Rapid pulse, at rest as well as on exertion (ranges between 90 and 160); palpitation is evident.
5. Low heat tolerance; profuse perspiration; flushed skin (warm, soft, moist).
6. Fine tremor of hands; change in bowel habits – constipation or diarrhoea.

7. Bulging eyes (exophthalmos) – startled expression.
8. Increased appetite – progressive weight loss.
9. Muscle fatigue and weakness; amenorrhoea.
10. Atrial fibrillation possible. (Cardiac decompensation is common in elderly patients.)

DIAGNOSTIC EVALUATION
1. Serum thyroxine } if elevated – hyper-
2. T_3 resin uptake } thyroidism is suspected.
3. Complete physical examination reveals a hypermetabolic state.
4. A bruit or thrill over the thyroid can often be detected because of the increased blood flow.
5. Thyroid gland may be palpable on examination.

CLINICAL COURSE
1. Mild, characterized by remissions and exacerbations.
2. In rare instances, it may progress relentlessly – leading to emaciation, extreme nervousness, delirium, disorientation and eventual death.

PATIENT PROBLEMS
The patient problems encountered in hyperthyroidism depend on the severity of the disorder and occur in varying degrees. In general, the patient could be expected to experience:
1. Alterations in fluid, electrolyte and nutritional balance related to hypermetabolic state, increased fluid and calorie requirement, and fluid loss through diaphoresis.
2. Potential impaired skin integrity related to extreme diaphoresis, pyrexia, excessive restlessness, movement and tremor, and rapid weight loss.
3. Altered thought processes related to insomnia, decreased attention span and irritability.
4. Apprehension and anxiety related to concern about upcoming surgery.

Planning and implementation
MEDICAL MANAGEMENT/TREATMENT
Immediate treatment
For severe hyperthyroidism or thyroid storm.

Restoring and maintaining vital functions
1. Admit patient to hospital if thyroid storm or other complications, such as heart failure, are imminent.
2. Sedatives such as phenobarbital or tranquillizers such as chlordiazepoxide (Librium) are given to combat nervousness, hyperactivity and irritability.

3. Temperature may be lowered by tepid sponging, fanning or salicylates.
4. Phenothiazines in large doses may be prescribed for hyperpyrexia, but watch for hypotension.
5. Administer fluids, electrolytes and vasopressor agents, as prescribed, to treat dehydration, electrolyte imbalance and hypotension.
6. Administer prescribed digitalis if heart failure or atrial fibrillation occurs.
7. Give propranolol as prescribed for sinus tachycardia and other supraventricular arrhythmias.
8. Give steroids as prescribed because of possibility of a relative adrenal insufficiency state.
9. Sustain nutritional requirements with prescribed glucose administered intravenously; administer vitamin B, as prescribed. Guard against infection; treat if infection is likely.
10. Give prescribed vitamin supplements to offset demands of appetite which may continue after hyperthyroidism is controlled.

Controlling synthesis and release of thyroid hormone
1. Administer sodium iodide intravenously as prescribed – inhibits release of hormone from thyroid.
2. Give carbinazole or propylthiouracil orally or by nasogastric tube to prevent accumulation of hormone stores.

Diminishing metabolic effects of thyroid agents and reversing peripheral effects of hyperthyroidism
Administer propranolol, reserpine or guanethidine, as prescribed.

OTHER FORMS OF TREATMENT
1. General considerations:
   a. Types of treatment – pharmacology, radiotherapy and surgery.
   b. Treatment depends on causes, age of patient, severity of disease and complications.
2. *According to causes:*
   a. Remission of hyperthyroidism (Graves' disease) occurs spontaneously within one to two years; however, relapse can be expected in half of the patients.
   All three forms of therapy are appropriate.
   b. Nodular toxic goitre – excessive amounts of thyroid hormone secreted. Surgery or radioiodine is preferred.
   c. Thyroid carcinoma. Surgery or radiotherapy.

3. *According to age of patient:*
   a. Radio-iodine therapy may be used in all patients, regardless of age, when other forms of therapy are contraindicated.
   b. Use radio-iodine in older patients for whom surgery is contraindicated.
   c. Radio-iodine therapy is contraindicated in pregnancy and in women of childbearing age.
4. *According to severity:*
   Administer drug therapy before proceeding with radio-iodine or surgery.
5. *According to patient preference:*
   a. Radio-iodine or surgery is suggested to patient who does not take medication regularly.
   b. Surgery is recommended to those who prefer it.

PHARMACOTHERAPY – DRUGS THAT INHIBIT HORMONE FORMATION
Objective
Bring the metabolic rate to normal as soon as possible and maintain it at this level.

Anticipated results
1. Diagnosis can be confirmed if patient responds to antithyroid therapy.
2. Autonomic nervous system is brought into balance and patient is more comfortable.
3. Opportunity is provided for getting to know the patient.

Antithyroid drugs
1. Most commonly used.
2. Act by interfering with the formation of thyroid hormone.
3. Administered orally.
   a. Detectable in blood in 15 minutes.
   b. 80 per cent absorbed within two hours.
   c. Because half-life is short, must be given every 6–8 hours.
4. Preparations:
   Propylthiouracil; carbinazole.
5. Assessment and duration of treatment determined by clinical criteria.
   a. Observe clinical course – thyroid gland usually gets smaller.
   b. Measure T_4 and T_3 uptake to determine adequacy of dose.
   c. Continue treatment for one to two years; if euthyroidism cannot be maintained without therapy, then another form of therapy (i.e. radioactive iodine (RAI) or surgery) should be recommended.

d. Gradually withdraw therapy to prevent exacerbation.
e. For relapses, recommend radio-iodine or surgery.
6. Toxicity:
   a. Agranulocytosis is a most serious toxic condition, occurring with a sudden onset – therefore, patient should be informed of this possibility and urged to report any signs of infection such as fever, sore throat, upper respiratory infection.
   b. Skin rashes, fever, urticaria, granulocytopenia, inflammation of the salivary glands are other possible side-effects.
   c. Substitute an alternate drug if there are toxic features.

PHARMACOTHERAPY – DRUGS THAT CONTROL PERIPHERAL SYMPTOMS OF HYPERTHYROIDISM
Propranolol (Inderal)
1. Acts as a beta-adrenoceptor blocking agent.
2. Abolishes tachycardia, tremor, excess sweating, nervousness.
3. Controls hyperthyroid symptoms until antithyroid drugs or radio-iodine can take effect.

RADIOACTIVE IODINE
1. Action:
   a. Limits secretion of thyroid hormone by damaging and destroying thyroid tissue.
   b. Controls dosage so that hypothyroidism does not occur.
2. Considerations in use:
   a. Radiation thyroiditis, a transient exacerbation of hyperthyroidism, may occur as a result of leakage of thyroid hormone into the circulation from damaged follicles.
   b. Iodide should not be given prior to radio-iodine since it interferes with the uptake of [131]I.
   c. Vigilance is required during treatment to detect occurrence of hypothyroidism.

PSYCHOTHERAPY
1. Greater emphasis is being placed on the effect that psychogenic factors have on the severity of this disease.
2. A determination needs to be made in caring for each patient about whether psychotherapy would be of value in preventing exacerbations.
3. The patient and family may require psychological support because of the disturbance caused by the irritability and outbursts related to the patient's hypermetabolic state.

SURGERY

Subtotal thyroidectomy

Effective in treating hyperthyroidism; involves removal of most of the thyroid gland.

Preparation for surgery

1. Patient must be euthyroid at time of surgery.
2. Antithyroid drugs are given to control hyperthyroidism.
3. Iodine is given to increase firmness of thyroid gland and reduce its vascularity.

NURSING ALERT

Observe patient for evidence of iodine toxicity – swelling of buccal mucosa, excessive salivation, coryza, skin eruptions. If these occur, discontinue iodides.

Complications

1. Damage to recurrent laryngeal nerve may occur (1 to 4 per cent).
   a. Unilateral damage – results in minimal voice change.
   b. Bilateral damage – serious airway obstruction develops.
2. Hypothyroidism:
   Occurs in 5 per cent of patients in first postoperative year; increases at rate of 2 to 3 per cent/year.
3. Hypoparathyroidism:
   a. About 4 per cent occurrence.
   b. Usually is mild and transient.
   c. Requires calcium supplements intravenously and orally when more severe.

Nursing management

See p. 550.

NURSING INTERVENTIONS

Improved fluid, electrolyte and nutritional intake

1. Assess the patient's fluid, electrolyte and nutritional requirements.
2. Determine the patient's food and fluid preferences.
3. Provide high-calorie foods and fluids consistent with the patient's requirements.
4. Provide a quiet, calm environment at meals.
5. Restrict stimulants (tea, coffee, alcohol).
6. Explain rationale of requirements and restrictions to patient.
7. Encourage/permit the patient to eat alone if embarrassed or otherwise disturbed by voracious appetite.

8. Maintain intravenous infusion if indicated to maintain fluid, nutritional and electrolyte balance.
9. Monitor fluid and nutritional status by weighing the patient daily and keeping accurate intake and output records.
10. Monitor vital signs to detect changes in fluid volume status.
11. Assess skin elasticity, mucous membranes and neck veins for signs of increased or decreased fluid volume.

Improved skin integrity

1. Assess skin frequently to detect perspiration.
2. Bathe frequently with cool water; change bedsheets when damp.
3. Provide cool environment to prevent pyrexia; use fans or air conditioning.
4. Use hypothermia unit, antipyretics, cool water, ice packs to reduce body temperature; avoid shivering.
5. Protect and massage bony prominences while less mobile.

Promotion of normal thought processes

1. Explain procedures to patient in an unhurried, calm manner.
2. Limit visitors; avoid stimulating conversations or television programmes.
3. Reduce stressors in the environment; reduce noise and lights.
4. Promote sleep and relaxation through use of prescribed medications, massage and relaxation exercises; draw the blinds for nap times.
5. Minimize disruption of the patient's sleep or rest by clustering nursing activities.
6. Employ safety measures to reduce risk of trauma or falls; maintain bed in low position.
7. Encourage the patient to express concerns and fears about illness, treatment and possible surgery.
8. Be selective in placing a suitable neighbour with the patient (preferably one who is convalescing).
9. Gain the patient's confidence and attempt to uncover anything that might cause aggravation or unhappiness; if a disturbance exists, it could thwart treatment efforts.

Evaluation

EXPECTED OUTCOMES

1. Achieves adequate fluid, electrolyte and nutritional intake.

2. Maintains normal fluid and electrolyte balance as measured by serum electrolyte levels and vital signs.
3. Demonstrates normal skin elasticity, moist mucous membranes and normal neck vein distention.
4. Reports and records balance of urine output and fluid intake.
5. Demonstrates skin integrity – skin is dry, cool and intact without reddened, excoriated or infected areas.
6. Reports improved tolerance to heat or warmth; normal rectal temperature.
7. Demonstrates improved thought processes:
   a. Maintains concentration, follows conversation and responds appropriately.
   b. Expresses concerns and fears about illness, treatment and possible surgery.
   c. Interacts with family members and visitors.
8. Uses medications as prescribed and relaxation techniques to promote sleep and relaxation.
9. Reports increased sense of well-being, decreased fatigue and lethargy.

EXOPHTHALMOS IN HYPERTHYROIDISM

Exophthalmos is abnormal protrusion of the eyeball, probably due to an autoimmune phenomenon.

TREATMENT
Objective
Protect eyes from irritation.

Mild
1. Recommend wearing sunglasses.
2. Instil prescribed methylcellulose eyedrops 0.5 to 1 per cent for comfort.
3. Advise the patient to elevate his head while sleeping to improve drainage.

Rapidly progressive or severe (chemosis, conjunctivitis, proptosis, visual impairment)
1. Tarsorrhaphy (suturing eyelids together) may be required – to extend lid when proptosis is so marked that lid does not close during sleep.
2. Administer prescribed corticosteroids in high doses to help arrest rapid progression of exophthalmos; with improvement, reduce dose.

Orbital decompression procedures
1. Decompression of orbit into ethmoid sinus and maxillary antrum.
2. Removal of lateral orbital wall.
3. Decompression of orbit into cranial cavity.

THYROID CRISIS

Thyroid crisis is characterized by tachycardia, vasomotor activity, agitation and, at times, delirium and heart failure. It is assumed to result from an increase in thyroid hormone.

PREDISPOSING FACTORS
1. Decompensation of hyperthyroid state occurs spontaneously.
2. May be precipitated by infection (pneumonia, appendicitis, pharyngitis, cystitis); surgical procedures (thyroidectomy, caesarean section, appendicectomy); minor procedures (dental extractions, forceps delivery); insulin reaction; pulmonary embolism; palpation of thyroid gland; and even fear.
3. Crisis may also be precipitated by inadequate surgical preoperative preparation (unrecognized hyperthyroidism).

CLINICAL FEATURES
1. Hyperpyrexia, diarrhoea, dehydration, tachycardia, dysrhythmias (Figure 8.1).
2. Coma, leading to shock and death.

OBJECTIVES OF TREATMENT AND NURSING MANAGEMENT
Control synthesis and release of thyroid hormone
1. Administer prescribed sodium iodide intravenously – inhibits release of hormone from thyroid.
2. Give prescribed propylthiouracil orally or by nasogastric tube to prevent accumulation of hormone stores.

Diminish metabolic effects of thyroid agents and reverse peripheral effects of hyperthyroidism
Administer propranolol, reserpine or guanethidine, as prescribed.

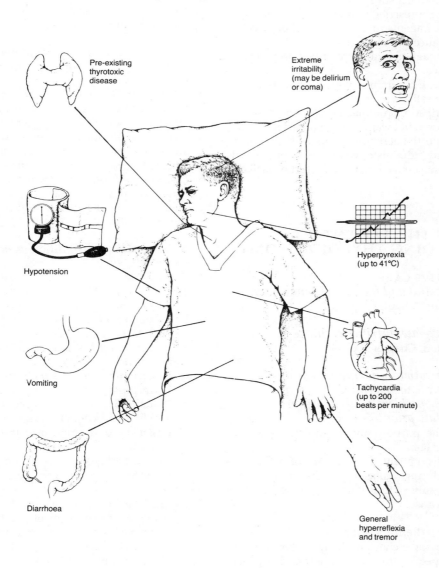

Figure 8.1. Thyrotoxic crisis. Any rise in temperature and pulse rate without discernible cause in a thyrotoxic patient should be considered a thyroid crisis. (From: *Hospital Medicine*, Vol. 3, No. 39, 1967, by permission. Copyright 1967 Hospital Publications Inc.)

Restore and maintain vital functions

1. Give prescribed steroids because of possibility of a relative adrenal insufficiency state.
2. Administer prescribed fluids, electrolytes and vasopressor agents to treat dehydration, electrolyte imbalance and hypotension.
3. Control agitation with prescribed intravenous barbiturates.
4. Lower the temperature with electric fans and prescribed salicylates.
5. Try prescribed phenothiazines in large doses for hyperpyrexia, but watch for hypotension.
6. Sustain nutritional requirements with glucose intravenously; administer vitamin B, as prescribed.
7. Guard against infection; treat if infection is likely.

CARE OF THE PATIENT UNDERGOING THYROIDECTOMY

PREOPERATIVE CARE

Provide a restful and therapeutic environment
(See discussion, Chapter 3, p. 45.)

Promote adequate nutritional intake
(See discussion, Chapter 3, p. 49.)

Support the patient undergoing various diagnostic tests to determine nature of the endocrine problem or to ensure an euthyroid state prior to surgery

1. Explain the purpose and requirements of each prescribed test.
2. Inform the patient and visitors of safeguards required during radioisotope tests.
3. Explain results of tests if unclear to the patient or questions arise.

Prepare the patient for surgery

1. Shave the upper chest, neck, up to chin edge.
2. Make a special effort to ensure that this patient has a good night's rest preceding surgery.
3. Explain to the patient that speaking is to be minimized immediately postoperatively and that oxygen may be administered to facilitate breathing.
4. Tell the patient that postoperatively, fluids may be given intravenously to maintain fluid, electrolyte and nutritional needs; glucose may also be given intravenously in the hours before the administration of anaesthesia.
5. Proceed with usual preoperative preparation.

POSTOPERATIVE CARE

Provide optimum immediate postoperative care in order to avoid complications

1. Move the patient carefully; provide adequate support to the head, so that no tension is placed on the sutures.
2. Place the patient in an upright position with the head elevated and supported by pillows; avoid flexion of neck.
3. Administer oxygen for a few hours if breathing is laboured; check the infusion for prescribed flow rate and smooth flow into patient.
4. Avoid administration of adrenaline, noradrenaline, anticholinergic (atropine) because of patient's sensitivity to these drugs.
5. Discontinue antithyroid drugs as a metabolic rate closer to normal is attained (to continue such medication might cause a hypometabolism – hypothyroidism).

Assess the patient's condition as he emerges from anaesthesia

1. *Damage of laryngeal nerve:*
   a. Observe for hoarseness or 'whispery' voice suggesting possible nerve damage.
   b. Recognize that a bilateral flaccid paralysis may lead to cord paralysis → closure of glottis – suffocation, months after operation.
2. *Haemorrhage:*
   a. Be alert for this possibility between 12 to 24 hours postoperatively.
   b. Watch for signs of irregular breathing, swelling and choking – signs pointing to the possibility of haemorrhage and tracheal compression.
   c. Keep a tracheostomy set in the patient's room for 48 hours for emergency use.
3. *Tetany:*
   a. The likelihood that tetany may develop depends on the number of parathyroid glands that have been removed or disturbed:
      (i) No clinical tetany.
      (ii) Tetany mild and transient.
      (iii) Tetany within 24 hours and worsening within the next 24 hours.
   b. Progression of signs:
      (i) *First* – tingling of toes and fingers and around the mouth; apprehension.
      (ii) *Second* – positive Chvostek's sign (tapping the cheek over the facial nerve causes twitch of the lip or facial muscles).
      (iii) *Third* – Trousseau's sign (carpopedal spasm induced by occluding circulation in the arm with a blood pressure cuff).

MEDICAL AND NURSING MANAGEMENT

1. Position patient for optimal ventilation; pillow may be removed to prevent head from bending forward and compressing trachea.
2. Position patient to prevent injury if a convulsion occurs; do not use restraints since they only aggravate patient and may result in muscle strain or fractures.
3. Have equipment available to treat respiratory difficulties; provide tracheostomy and cardiac arrest equipment.
4. Determine calcium levels: if in 48 hours levels are low (normal range 2.25–2.55mmol/l) replacement of calcium (gluconate, lactate) is done intravenously.
5. Exert caution in intravenous administration of calcium to the patient who has renal disease or who is receiving digitalis preparations.

OTHER THYROID-RELATED CONDITIONS

PHYSIOLOGICAL GOITRE

Slight enlargement of the thyroid gland.

INCIDENCE
Affects girls at or soon after onset of puberty.

CAUSE
Unknown. Generally thought to happen at the time when whole endocrine system is coming into full function. In some women the thyroid gland enlarges slightly seven to ten days before menstrual period.

SUBACUTE THYROIDITIS

Thyroiditis is inflammation of the thyroid gland.

INCIDENCE
Affects younger women predominantly.

CLINICAL FEATURES
1. Pain, swelling, thyroid tenderness which lasts weeks or months, then disappears.

2. Pain referred to the ear, making swallowing difficult and uncomfortable.
3. Fever, malaise, chills.
4. Irritability, nervousness, insomnia and weight loss.

TREATMENT
1. Patient may be placed on thyroid medications to maintain a normal level of circulating thyroid hormone.
2. Steroids may be administered in active inflammatory stage.

HASHIMOTO'S THYROIDITIS (CHRONIC THYROIDITIS)

Hashimoto's thyroiditis is a progressive disease of the thyroid gland caused by infiltration of lymphocytes and resulting in progressive destruction of the parenchyma and hypothyroidism.

CAUSE
Unknown. Believed to be autoimmune disease, genetically transmitted and perhaps related to Graves' disease.

INCIDENCE
1. Predominantly affects women (95 per cent) in their 40s and 50s.
2. Possibly the most common cause of adult hyperthyroidism.
3. Appears to be increasing since it was described in 1912.

CLINICAL FEATURES
1. Marked by slowly developing firm enlargement of the thyroid gland.
2. Usually no gross nodules.
3. Basal metabolic rate usually low.

DIAGNOSTIC EVALUATION
1. Twenty-four-hour radioactive iodine (RAI) uptake.
2. Thyroid scan.
3. Resin T_3 uptake determination.
4. Thyroid needle biopsy.
5. T_3 and T_4 usually become subnormal as the disease progresses.

TREATMENT

1. Patient should be placed on thyroid medications to maintain a normal level of circulating thyroid hormone; this is done to suppress production of thyrotropin, to prevent enlargement of the thyroid and/or to maintain a euthyroid state.
2. Firm nodular thyroid enlargement may at times be associated with tracheal compression, cough, hoarseness. Resection of isthmus can produce relief of symptoms.

CANCER OF THE THYROID

INCIDENCE

1. It has been estimated that of the thyroid lumps, which occur in 40,000 out of one million people in any one year, only 25 will be cancerous; this is a relatively rare disease.
2. It occurs twice as frequently in females as in males and more frequently in whites than in blacks; incidence increases with age.
3. It appears well established that an association exists between external radiation to the head and neck in infancy and childhood, and subsequent development of thyroid carcinoma. (Between 1940 and 1960 radiotherapy was often given to shrink enlarged tonsil and adenoid tissue, to treat acne or to reduce an enlarged thymus.)
   It is advised that these individuals should:
   a. Consult a doctor.
   b. Submit to surgical thyroidectomy or take thyroid hormones if abnormalities of the gland are present.
   c. Continue with annual check-ups if all is normal.

TYPES

1. Papillary and well-differentiated adenocarcinoma.
   a. Growth is slow and spread is confined to lymph nodes that surround thyroid area.
   b. Cure rate is excellent after removal of involved areas.
2. Rapidly growing, widely metastasizing type.
   a. Occurs predominantly in middle-aged and elderly persons.
   b. Brief encouraging response may occur with X-ray irradiation.
   c. Progression of disease is rapid; high mortality rate.

DIAGNOSTIC EVALUATION

1. History and physical examination are important.
2. Needle biopsy is recommended only for the very skilled performer and for the experienced pathologist.
3. Surgical exploration.

TREATMENT

1. Surgical removal is extensive, as required.
2. Thyroid replacement.
   a. Thyroid hormone is administered to suppress secretion of TSH.
   b. Such treatment is continued indefinitely and requires annual checkups.
3. For unresectable cancer, patient is referred to a thyroid specialist for consideration of treatment with chemotherapy or radiotherapy.

THE PARATHYROID GLANDS

The parathyroid glands are small, bean-sized structures embedded in the posterior section of the thyroid gland.

FUNCTIONS

1. Produce, store and secrete parathormone.
2. Increase plasma calcium ions by action on:
   a. The kidney – to decrease elimination of calcium ions in the urine.
   b. The gastrointestinal tract – to increase absorption of calcium ions from chyme.
   c. Bone – to increase its contributions of calcium ions to the plasma.

DISORDERS OF THE PARATHYROID GLANDS

HYPERPARATHYROIDISM

Hyperparathyroidism is overactivity of the parathyroids.

CAUSE

1. An overgrowth or hypertrophy of parathyroid glands, as a primary disorder of the parathyroid glands or as a secondary condition occurring with renal failure as a result of renal retention of phosphorus.
2. Carcinoma of the parathyroid or secretion of parathyroid hormone by ectopic tissue in malignancy may produce features of hyperparathyroidism.

Assessment

CLINICAL FEATURES

1. Decalcification of bones.
   a. Skeletal pain, backache, pain on weight-bearing, pathological fractures, deformities, formation of bony cysts.
   b. Formation of bone tumours – overgrowth of osteoclasts.
2. Formation of calcium-containing stones in the kidneys.
3. Depression of neuromuscular apparatus.
   a. The patient may trip, drop objects, show general fatigue and experience blurring of the mind.
   b. Cardiac dysrhythmias, hypertension and cardiac standstill may result.

DIAGNOSTIC EVALUATION

1. Persistently elevated serum calcium (normal range 2.25–2.55mmol/l; test must be taken three times to determine consistency of results).
2. Exclusion of all other causes of hypercalcaemia – malignancy, vitamin D excess, multiple myeloma, sarcoidosis, milk-alkali syndrome, drugs such as thiazides, Cushing's disease, hyperthyroidism.
3. Skeletal changes – revealed by X-ray.
4. Diagnosis often extremely difficult (complications may occur before this condition is diagnosed).
5. Cineradiography will disclose parathyroid tumours more readily than X-ray.
6. Serum calcium and alkaline phosphatase levels are elevated and serum phosphorus levels are decreased with increased parathyroid activity.
7. Parathyroid hormone (PTH) levels are increased with hyperactivity of the parathyroid glands.

COMPLICATIONS

1. Kidney disturbances:
   a. Formation of renal stones.
   b. Calcification of kidney parenchyma.
   c. Renal shutdown.
2. Gastrointestinal complications: ulceration of upper gastrointestinal tract (stomach, duodenum) leading to haemorrhage and perforation.
3. Skeletal problems:
   a. Simple demineralization.
   b. Cysts and fibrosis of marrow – leading to fractures.
   c. Collapse of vertebral bodies and fractures of the ribs.

PATIENT PROBLEMS

1. Alterations in fluid and electrolyte balance related to effects of elevated serum calcium levels.
2. Potential alteration of urinary elimination related to renal calculi and calcium deposits in the kidneys.
3. Alterations in musculoskeletal status related to abnormal bone formation, weakness, bone pain and pathological fractures.
4. Potential complications of surgery and hypocalcaemia.

Planning and implementation

NURSING INTERVENTIONS

Establishment of normal fluid and electrolyte balance to prevent or counteract life-threatening effects of hypercalcaemia

1. Assess fluid intake and output.
2. Provide adequate hydration – administer water, glucose and electrolytes by mouth or intravenously, as prescribed.

NURSING ALERT

A low specific gravity for urine does not necessarily mean adequate hydration.

3. Avoid calcium and alkalis in the diet to prevent stone formation and renal calcification. Daily serum calcium and urea estimations are taken.
4. Administer prescribed diuretic – frusemide (Lasix).
5. Prevent or promptly treat dehydration; report vomiting or other sources of fluid loss promptly.

NURSING ALERT

Thiazide diuretics should not be used in the patient with hyperparathyroidism since they decrease the renal excretion of calcium, thereby causing hypercalcaemia.

6. Administer phosphate therapy as prescribed to control hypercalcaemia. Daily serum calcium, urea and electrolyte estimations are taken.
   a. A rising serum calcium level may indicate increasing dehydration – impending crisis.

b. A falling serum calcium indicates dehydration is being corrected.

Improved urinary elimination

1. Assess urinary output; strain all urine to observe for kidney stones (renal calculi).
2. Increase fluid intake to 3,000ml/day to maintain hydration and prevent precipitation of calcium and formation of stones.
3. Provide diet low in calcium; eliminate milk and milk products.
4. Instruct the patient about dietary recommendations.
5. Observe the patient for signs of urinary tract infection, haematuria and renal colic.
6. Instruct the patient to avoid medications containing calcium (some antacids).

Normal musculoskeletal function

1. Assist the patient in hygiene and activities if bone pain is severe or if the patient experiences musculoskeletal weakness.
2. Protect the patient from falls or injury.
3. Turn the patient cautiously and handle extremities gently to avoid fractures.
4. Administer analgesia as prescribed.
5. Assess level of pain and the patient's response to analgesia.
6. Encourage the patient to participate in mild exercise gradually as symptoms subside.
7. Instruct and demonstrate correct body mechanics to reduce strain, backache and injury.
8. Ensure early diagnosis and treatment of fractures:
   a. Treatment for vertebral body fractures (see p. 830).
   b. Treatment for rib fractures, p. 198.
   c. Fixation of other long bones.
   d. Continued hydration of the patient.
   e. Earliest mobilization of fracture areas.

Postoperative recovery without complications or manifestations of hypocalcaemia

1. See p. 550 as postoperative care is similar to that after thyroidectomy.
2. Recognize that the patient will retain some fluid postoperatively.
   a. This will be manifested by a low urinary output.
   b. Therefore, avoid overhydration for first day or two.
3. Avoid giving calcium until the patient's calcium level is determined.
4. Evaluate signs and symptoms of hypocalcemia and onset of tetany.

a. Observe calcium levels – if well below normal and if decline continues into the second week, the skeletal system is absorbing calcium. If some involvement was noted preoperatively (elevated alkaline phosphatase level), calcium should be administered.
b. Administer prescribed calcium – usually lactate or gluconate. When gastrointestinal tract cannot absorb large amount, administer intramuscularly as gluconate, or intravenously in emergency situation.
c. Give prescribed vitamin D to increase absorption of calcium.

5. Reassure the patient about skeletal recovery.
   a. Bone pain diminishes fairly quickly.
   b. Cysts, bone tumours and osteoporosis resolve themselves.
   c. Fractures are cared for by usual orthopaedic procedures.

Evaluation
EXPECTED OUTCOMES

1. Achieves/maintains adequate fluid and electrolyte balance:
   a. Balance of urine output and fluid intake.
   b. Normal skin elasticity, moist mucous membranes and no thirst.
   c. Normal calcium levels and electrolyte levels.
   d. No ECG changes; normal sinus rhythm.
2. Maintains high fluid intake with low calcium intake and uses phosphate therapy as prescribed.
3. Uses prescribed diuretics.
4. Attains/maintains improved urinary elimination:
   a. Adequate urine output without signs of kidney stones.
   b. Urine is acidic (low pH), dilute and clear.
   c. No signs and symptoms of urinary tract infection, haematuria or renal colic.
   d. Normal kidney function as indicated by normal serum creatinine and electrolyte levels.
5. Achieves normal musculoskeletal function:
   a. Decreased bone and joint pain.
   b. Increased strength and well-being.
   c. Analgesia taken as prescribed.
   d. Mild exercise as musculoskeletal symptoms subside.
   e. Uses correct body mechanics to move, turn and carry out activities.
6. Recovers from surgery without complications or manifestations of hypocalcaemia.
   a. Normal fluid balance postoperatively without manifestations of hypervolaemia (distended neck veins).

b. Normal calcium balance as indicated by normal serum calcium levels.

c. No manifestations of hypocalcaemia and tetany.

d. No numbness and tingling in extremities or around mouth (circumoral paraesthesias).

7. Uses calcium and vitamin D if indicated and prescribed.

HYPOPARATHYROIDISM

Hypoparathyroidism results from a deficiency of parathyroid hormone and is characterized by hypo-calcaemia and neuromuscular hyperexcitability.

CAUSES

1. Decrease in gland function (idiopathic hypoparathyroidism).
2. Surgical or radiation trauma to parathyroid glands.
3. Malignancy or metastasis from a cancer to the parathyroid glands.
4. Resistance to parathyroid hormone action.

PATHOPHYSIOLOGY

1. With inadequate parathyroid hormone (PTH) secretion, there is decreased resorption of calcium from the renal tubules, decreased absorption of calcium in the gastrointestinal tract and decreased resorption of calcium from bone.
2. Blood calcium falls to a low level, causing symptoms of muscular hyperirritability, uncontrolled spasms and hypocalcaemic tetany.
3. In response to decreased serum calcium levels and in the absence of parathyroid hormone, there is a rise in serum phosphate level and decreased phosphate excretion by the kidneys.
4. If onset of hypocalcaemia is acute, the major concerns are laryngeal spasm, acute airway obstruction, and cardiovascular failure.
5. Long-term effects of persistent hypoparathyroidism include calcium deposits in tissues.

Assessment
CLINICAL FEATURES

1. Due to deficiency of parathormone:
   a. Accumulation of phosphorus in blood.
   b. Decrease in amount of blood calcium.
2. Tetany:
   a. General muscular hypertonia; attempts at voluntary movement result in tremors and spasmodic or unco-ordinated movements; fingers assume classic position.
   b. Chvostek's sign – a spasm of facial muscles that occurs when muscles or branches of facial nerve are tapped.
   c. Trousseau's sign – carpopedal spasm induced by occluding circulation in the arm with a blood pressure cuff.
   d. Reduced blood calcium level – to a low level (normal range 2.25–2.55 mmol/l).
   e. Laryngeal spasm.
3. Anxiety and apprehension are very marked.
4. Renal colic is often present if the patient has had stones; pre-existing stones loosen and fall down into the ureter.

PATIENT PROBLEMS

1. Altered electrolyte balance related to decreased serum calcium level.
2. Anxiety related to impending sense of disaster.
3. Altered urinary elimination related to presence of kidney stones.
4. Pain related to passage of kidney stones.

Planning and implementation
TREATMENT AND NURSING MANAGEMENT

1. Administer calcium, as prescribed.
   a. A syringe and an ampule of a calcium solution are to be kept at the bedside at all times.
   b. Most rapidly effective calcium solution is ionized calcium chloride (10 per cent).
   c. For rapid use to relieve severe tetany, infuse every 10 minutes.
      (i) Administer ionized calcium chloride (10 per cent) slowly. It is highly irritating, stings and causes thrombosis; patient experiences unpleasant burning flush of skin and, more particularly, of the tongue. Too rapid calcium administration may cause cardiac arrest.
      (ii) Give prescribed calcium intravenously; calcium carbohydrate combination may also be used – gluconate or heptonate (10 per cent) are not irritating.
   d. Continue a slow drip of prescribed intravenous saline containing calcium gluconate until control of tetany is ensured; then switch to intramuscular or oral administration of calcium.
   e. Later, add prescribed vitamin D to calcium intake – increases absorption of calcium and also induces a high level of calcium in the bloodstream.
2. Control anxiety:
   a. It is difficult to reassure this patient since he has a strong feeling of impending disaster.

b. Administration of intravenous calcium seems to bring about rapid relief of anxiety.

3. Relieve renal colic: stone may have to be removed cystoscopically or by surgery.

4. Monitor for hypercalciuria. Recommend periodic 24-hour urinary calcium determinations.

5. Monitor blood calcium periodically; variations in vitamin D may affect calcium levels.

6. Inform the patient about symptoms of hypo-calcaemia and hypercalcaemia; should these occur, he is to notify his doctor.

NURSING INTERVENTIONS
Establishment of normal electrolyte balance

1. Assess neuromuscular status in patients at risk for hypocalcaemia (patients in the immediate post-operative period following thyroidectomy, para-thyroidectomy, radical neck dissection).

2. Check for positive Trousseau's or Chvostek's sign.

3. Assess respiratory status frequently in post-operative recovery phase.

4. Place airway and tracheostomy set at patient's bedside.

5. Report indications of respiratory distress, laryngeal stridor, or cardiovascular failure.

6. Instruct the patient about signs and symptoms of hypocalcaemia and hypercalcaemia that should be reported.

7. Use caution in administering other drugs to the patient with hypocalcaemia.
   a. The hypocalcaemic patient is insensitive to digoxin; as hypocalcaemia is reversed, the patient may rapidly develop digitalis toxicity.
   b. Cimetidine (Tagamet) interferes with normal parathyroid function, especially in the patient with renal failure, which increases the risk of hypocalcaemia.

Evaluation
EXPECTED OUTCOMES

1. Demonstrates normal neuromuscular status without evidence of tremor or neuromuscular excitability.

2. Demonstrates negative Trousseau's and Chvostek's signs.

3. Demonstrates and reports absence of respiratory distress; respiratory rate and pattern normal.

4. Demonstrates normal serum calcium and phosphorus levels.

5. Identifies symptoms of respiratory distress and cardiovascular changes that should be reported.

6. Demonstrates absence of seizures.

7. Identifies reportable signs of symptoms of hypo-calcaemia and hypercalcaemia.

8. Uses calcium salts and consumes high-calcium diet if prescribed.

9. Identifies importance of avoiding other medications unless checking first with nurse or doctor.

DIABETES MELLITUS (PANCREATIC DISORDERS)

Diabetes mellitus is a disease characterized by abnormalities of the endocrine secretions of the pancreas resulting in disordered metabolism of carbohydrate, fat and protein and, in time, structural abnormalities in a variety of tissues.

ALTERED PHYSIOLOGY

1. Insulin reduces the release of glucose from the liver of both inhibiting glycogenolysis and gluconeogenesis.

2. Insulin also promotes the storage of glycogen in the liver, the utilization of glucose in the muscles and the storage of fat in adipose tissue by enhancing the transport of glucose across the cell wall. In nondiabetics, the rate of insulin-release from the pancreas is proportional to the amount of glucose in the blood.

3. In diabetes, insulin is not proportional to blood sugar levels because of several possible factors:
   a. Insufficient numbers of islet cells (juvenile diabetes).
   b. Delayed or insufficient release (adult-onset diabetes).
   c. Excessive inactivation by chemical inhibitors of 'binders' in the circulation and at the cell membrane.

4. Glucose in the blood comes from ingested carbohydrates or from conversion of amino acids and fatty acids to glucose by the liver (gluconeogenesis). An elevated fasting blood glucose level in diabetes reflects the presence of decreased utilization of glucose and increased gluconeogenesis. If the concentration of glucose in the blood is sufficiently high, the kidney does not reabsorb all of the filtered glucose; glucose then appears in the urine (glycosuria).

5. With increased gluconeogenesis (in part under the control of the adrenocortical hormones), protein and fats are mobilized rather than stored or

deposited in the cells. Persistently elevated levels of fats in the blood may damage blood vessels.

6. When there is a deficiency of insulin, muscles cannot utilize glucose, and free fatty acids are mobilized from adipose tissue cells and broken down by the liver into ketone bodies for energy.
7. Diabetic ketoacidosis is characterized by excessive amounts of ketone bodies in the blood.
8. Patients with diabetic ketoacidosis exhibit hyperventilation and the loss of sodium, potassium, chloride and water from the body.
9. The net metabolic result of diabetes mellitus is loss of fat stores, liver glycogen, cellular protein, electrolytes and water.
10. The sequelae of long-term diabetes lead to involvement of large vessels in the brain, heart, kidneys and extremities and of the small vessels in the eyes and kidneys, and to neuropathy. The mechanism is not precisely determined.

TYPES OF DIABETES
Differ in prognosis, treatment, causative mechanisms.

Growth-onset or juvenile type
1. Patient usually lacks insulin and requires exogenous insulin therapy.
2. Onset abrupt.
3. Stable or labile.
4. Usually begins in childhood, but may occur at any age.
5. Patient more prone to ketoacidosis and is *dependent upon insulin.*

Maturity-onset (adult diabetes)
1. Usually occurs after the age of 40; about three-quarters of adult-onset patients are obese.
2. Patient usually retains a capacity for endogenous insulin production.
3. Patient not usually ketosis-prone.
4. Usually stable.

Secondary or nonhereditary
1. Damage to or removal of pancreatic islet tissue – tumours of pancreas, surgical removal of pancreas, pancreatitis.
2. Several drugs, chemicals, hormones and genetic syndromes are associated with decreased insulin activity and hyperglycaemia.

INCIDENCE
1. Approximately 5 per cent of the world population

has diabetes mellitus – it is estimated that 25 per cent of people are carriers.
2. About 2 per cent of British population has diabetes.
3. One-third of all patients have a known relative with the disease.

INDIVIDUALS AT RISK
1. Relatives of known diabetics (heredity).
2. Overweight individuals.
3. Mothers of large babies or those who have had an abnormal obstetrical history.
4. People with early onset of arteriosclerosis:
   a. Premenopausal women with myocardial infarction.
   b. Men having myocardial infarctions before the age of 40.
5. People with frequent or chronic infections (gallbladder disease, pyelonephritis, pancreatitis).
6. Patients exhibiting temporary reduction in glucose tolerance during stress (myocardial infarction, infection, trauma, surgery).
7. Patients developing glucose intolerance during drug therapy (thiazides, glucocorticoids, ovulatory suppressants).
8. People with retinopathy, nephropathy, neuropathy or other vascular manifestations.

CLINICAL FEATURES
Growth-onset or juvenile diabetes
1. May occur in adults as well as children.
2. Abrupt onset – weight loss, weakness, polyuria (excessive excretion of urine), polydipsia (excessive thirst), polyphagia (excessive ingestion of food). (Polyphagia may be shortlived as the metabolic imbalance worsens.)
3. The insulin deficiency causes hyperglycaemia, which in turn causes glycosuria, osmotic diuresis and the loss of water and electrolytes.
4. Increased gluconeogenesis from the mobilization of protein and fat stores results in weight loss and muscle wasting.
5. Patient prone to develop ketosis – may be brought into hospital with acidosis or in coma.

Maturity-onset
1. Early adult diabetes exhibits postprandial hypoglycaemia.
2. Insidious onset – fatigue, tendency to be drowsy after a meal, irritability, nocturia, pruritus (especially of vulva in the female), poorly healing skin wounds, blurring of vision, loss of weight, muscle cramps.

3. Symptoms may be absent in mild cases.
4. Stress (surgery, febrile illness, etc.) will induce hyperglycaemia.

CLINICAL COURSE

1. Intensity of diabetes mellitus, as measured by blood sugar levels, tends to wax and wane – depends on patient's general state of health, life stresses, dietary control, weight control, physical activity and other factors.
2. Lifelong care is mandatory – poorly controlled diabetes leads to accelerated development of neuropathy, nephropathy, retinopathy, generalized atherosclerosis and decreased resistance to infection. *The threat of complications always exists.*
3. Meticulous control of diabetes may postpone but does not necessarily prevent the development of complications.

DIAGNOSTIC EVALUATION

1. Suspiciousness of diabetes mellitus (signs and symptoms; family history).
2. *Urine testing for glucose (sugar):*
   a. Negative finding does not always rule out diabetes.
   b. Instruct patient to micturate and discard urine.
   c. Micturate 30 to 45 minutes later and check this specimen; the second urine specimen gives an indication of the blood sugar at the *time of testing.*
3. *Postprandial blood glucose:*
   a. Blood sample taken two hours after a high carbohydrate meal (75–100g).
   b. Values over 10mmol/l (150mg/100ml) of blood are dignostic of diabetes.
      Values under 6.7mmol/l (100mg/100ml) rule out diabetes.
      Values within this range indicate a glucose tolerance test should be done.
4. *Glucose tolerance test* (most sensitive test):
   a. Blood samples are drawn after an overnight fast.
   b. Glucose load (50–100g) is given (usually in form of a carbonated sugar beverage).
   c. Specimens of blood for glucose determination are taken one, two and three hours after glucose ingestion.
      (i) Patient fasts for eight hours prior to test.
      (ii) During test the patient is to avoid exercise, emotional stress, tobacco or any oral intake except water.
5. The following glucose tolerance curve is considered within the upper limits of normal:

Serum glucose		True blood glucose	
Fasting value 7.0mmol/l	(125mg/100ml)	6.0mmol/l (110mg/100ml)	
1-hour value of 10.5mmol/l	(190mg/100ml)	9.0mmol/l (170mg/100ml)	
2-hour value of 8.0mmol/l	(140mg/100ml)	6.5mmol/l (120mg/100ml)	
3-hour value of 7.0mmol/l	(125mg/100ml)	6.0mmol/l (110mg/100ml)	

TREATMENT AND NURSING MANAGEMENT

Treatment will correct biochemical and metabolic abnormalities, attain and maintain the ideal body weight, and postpone the progression of the complications of diabetes by maintaining the plasma glucose level as close to normal as possible. *Every new patient requires intensive and extensive education in order to learn to eat properly, take prescribed insulin or oral agents, test blood and urine, and exercise adequately. Reinforcement of diabetes education at every opportunity is an important part of the nursing management of the patient with diabetes mellitus.*

DIETARY MANAGEMENT
Objective
The purpose of dietary management is to attain or maintain ideal body weight and ensure normal growth.

1. The meal plan is designed to contain adequate calories, protein, vitamins and minerals. Most adults require 30 calories/kg of ideal body weight.
   a. This may be increased to 35–40 calories/kg for children or adults who are extremely active.
   b. This may be reduced to 15–25 calories/kg for obese patients and sedentary adults.
2. For most patients the meal plan is calculated to give protein 0.5–1.2g/kg (12 to 20 per cent of total calories) and carbohydrates 2–4g/kg (55 to 60 per cent of total calories).
3. Fat is added to make up the difference and varies from 0.5–1.5g/kg to give 20 to 30 per cent of the total calories. Saturated fats are decreased and polysaturated fats increased as much as possible.

4. An effort is made to use high-fibre food and add more fibre to the meal plan in order to lower glucose absorption. High fibre levels should be added gradually. Intake (40g) should be maintained daily because of possible fluctuations in blood glucose levels. High fibre content may cause abdominal fullness, nausea, vomiting, increased flatulence, increased bowel movements and vitamin/mineral deficiencies.

5. Use of complex rather than simple carbohydrates should be used because of their effect on glycaemia. Not all complex carbohydrates produce the same degree of glycaemia response. The effect depends not just on the food itself, but how it is prepared, when it is eaten, what it is eaten with, when the last meal was eaten and what it contained, as well as the physiology of the person eating it.

6. The menu should be varied according to the patient's ethnic and cultural background, lifestyle, food preferences, exercise routine and eating habits. The emphasis should be on what is allowed rather than on what is forbidden. The meal plan should be adapted to the diabetic, not the diabetic to the meal plan.

7. When insulin is taken, special consideration must be given to ensure adequate carbohydrate intake to correspond to the time when insulin is most effective and less carbohydrate when insulin is least effective.

8. Obese diabetics should be on a strict weight-control programme. Many will have a normal plasma glucose after they lose weight. (Remember that obese patients have an excessive amount of circulating insulin but are insulin-resistant because of obesity.)

9. The British Diabetic Association has prepared a very comprehensive exchange list to add variety to meal planning. (British Diabetic Association, 10 Queen Anne Street, London W1M 0BD; tel: 01 323 1531.)

10. Each individual patient must be taught how to measure the correct portions at each meal and how to exchange one item for another on the list.

11. Routine blood glucose testing before each meal and at bedtime is necessary during initial control, in unstable patients and during illness. Well-controlled, stabilized patients may be followed with fewer tests daily (see p. 565).

EXERCISE

1. Exercise promotes metabolism and utilization of carbohydrates and thus diminishes insulin requirements of the body.

2. Exercise enhances the effects of insulin and helps regulate blood glucose levels.

3. Encourage the patient to engage in *daily* exercise.

INSULIN THERAPY

1. Insulin is the active principle of secretion of beta cells in the islets of Langerhans. It is given to persons who do not have adequate endogenous insulin.

2. Physiological effect of insulin – lowers the blood sugar by facilitating the uptake and utilization of glucose by muscle and fat cells by decreasing release of glucose from the liver.

3. One or more insulin injections each day is usually required by:
   a. People whose diabetes is characterized by polydipsia, polyuria, weight loss and ketonuria.
   b. Hyperglycaemic pregnant patients.
   c. Patients with acute infections, febrile illness; those undergoing major surgery, or those with acutely decompensated diabetes. These may include those patients who are normally controlled on diet alone or diet and tablets.

NURSING ALERT

There is a narrow margin between the therapeutic and toxic (hypoglycaemic) effects of insulin. Exercise, illness and emotional stress can alter needs for insulin.

INSULIN PREPARATIONS

1. Insulin is extracted from the pancreas of slaughtered pigs and cows or is produced synthetically by amino acid substitution or by recombinant deoxyribonucleic acid (DNA) techniques in bacteria. The latter two insulin production techniques result in an insulin identical in amino acid sequence to human insulin.

2. Indications for human insulin use include newly diagnosed insulin-dependent diabetes, diabetics using insulin temporarily (e.g. surgery, pregnancy), insulin allergy and insulin resistance because of the likelihood of producing few if any insulin antibodies.

3. The available preparations vary in onset of action, time of peak effect, and duration of action (Table 8.1). It is important to know the action curve for each type of insulin in order to treat the patient properly.

4. Insulin is prescribed in units. U-100 insulin contains 100 units per millilitre.

Table 8.1　Insulin preparations

Agent	Duration of action
Short-acting insulin Insulin injection (soluble) Neutral insulin injection	These have a relatively rapid action and when injected subcutaneously, their effect is maximal in two to four hours and last up to 12 hours
Intermediate-acting insulin Biphasic insulin injection Insulin zinc suspension Isophane insulin injection (NPH)	These are usually given twice daily, producing much smoother blood glucose control than twice daily soluble insulin. They may be combined with soluble insulin
Long-acting insulin Insulin zinc suspension (mixed) Insulin zinc suspension (crystalline) Protamine zinc insulin (PZI) injection	Peak activity occurs about six hours after injection and its action lasts up to 24 hours

Insulin syringes and needles

1. The insulin syringe is a British standard 1ml or 2ml.
2. Needles are numbered according to diameter; the higher the number the thinner the needle.
3. No. 26G, 27G, 27.5G or 28G × 1.2cm needles are usually used either with a separate syringe or as a syringe–needle combination.

Regulation of insulin dosage

1. The dosage of insulin is adjusted according to the presence (or absence) of glycosuria; the degree in which it is present; and its time of appearance in relation to insulin injections and meals. The dosage of insulin is also adjusted according to determinations of blood glucose levels.
2. In the absence of complications, treatment may be started with 10 to 20 units of Lente or Isophane insulin (NPH) given subcutaneously before breakfast.
   a. Dosage is increased as indicated by patient's response to the previous dose until glycosuria is absent and the blood sugar before each meal is normal.
   b. During initial regulation and when insulin requirements are changing rapidly, supplemental injections of soluble insulin may be given before each meal, depending on results of urine testing and response of patient.
3. Instruct the patient to test his urine for sugar before each meal and at bedtime while insulin is being regulated (use the second of two specimens micturated 30 minutes apart for greater accuracy) or blood glucose may be estimated.
4. Ask the patient to keep a record of results in a notebook – to facilitate subsequent insulin adjustments.

Insulin administration

See p. 567.

HYPOGLYCAEMIA AS A COMPLICATION OF INSULIN TREATMENT

1. Hypoglycaemic reaction is an abnormally low level of glucose (sugar) in the blood; likely to occur when for any reason the blood sugar falls below 2.5mmol/l (50mg/100ml) of blood; it may occur at a higher level if glucose has fallen rapidly.
2. Hypoglycaemia occurs as a result of too much insulin, not enough food (delayed or missed meal) and/or unusual vigorous activity.
3. Reactions begin five to 20 minutes following injection of regular insulin but not for several hours after NPH insulin – majority of attacks occur in morning and in early evening.

Signs and symptoms

1. Sweating, tremor, pallor, tachycardia, palpitation, nervousness – from release of adrenalin from the central nervous system when the blood glucose falls rapidly.
2. Headache, lightheadedness, confusion, emotional changes, memory lapses, numbness of lips and tongue, slurred speech, lack of co-ordination, staggering gait, double vision, drowsiness, convulsions, coma – from depression of the central nervous system when the blood glucose level falls slowly.

NURSING ALERT

Patients with longstanding diabetes complicated by autonomic neuropathy may develop hypoglycaemia without warning, as well as patients taking certain beta-blockers. Severe and prolonged hypoglycaemia may cause brain damage and death. Any abnormal behaviour in a patient taking insulin should be considered as resulting from hypoglycaemia until proven otherwise.

Treatment

1. Give some form of glucose orally if patient is conscious – orange juice, sweets, sugar lump.
2. Give prescribed glucagon (subcutaneously or intramuscularly) if patient cannot take anything by mouth – causes glycogenolysis in the liver, which raises blood glucose level.
3. Give patient orange juice or milk as soon as he regains consciousness – glucose level may fall faster than the transient rise produced by glucagon.
4. If patient is unconscious for period of time:
   a. Give prescribed 50 per cent glucose solution intravenously – to restore normal blood glucose level quickly.
   b. Follow this with intravenous infusion of 5 to 10 per cent glucose solution in water, as prescribed.
   c. Administer mannitol to combat cerebral oedema if necessary – cerebral function may be compromised when patient has low level of blood glucose.
5. Once rapidly absorbed carbohydrate is given, give a feeding with protein or fat.

Preventing hypoglycaemic reactions due to insulin

Instruct the patient as follows:

1. Prevent hypoglycaemia with uniformity and timing of diet, insulin and daily exercise.
2. Recognize the early symptoms of hypoglycaemia – hunger, nausea, faintness, sweating, headache, rapid heart rate, double vision, inability to concentrate.
3. Take between-meal and bedtime snacks – to distribute the carbohydrate load over period of maximum insulin effect.
4. Test the urine so that changing insulin requirements can be anticipated.
5. Check urine for glucose before and after unusual physical exertion and consume extra food if needed.
6. Carry rapidly absorbed carbohydrate (sugar/ sweets) and take at first warning of a reaction.
7. Carry an identification card or wear an identi-fication bracelet – hypoglycaemic symptoms can imitate intoxication with alcohol or drugs.
   a. Card – British Diabetic Association, 10 Queen Anne Street, London W1M 0BD.
   b. Identification bracelet – Medic Alert Foundation, 9 Hanover Street, London W1R 9HF.

OTHER COMPLICATIONS OF INSULIN THERAPY

Insulin allergy

1. Local reaction associated with stinging, redness and induration at injection site.
2. The reaction may be immediate (within an hour) or delayed (within six to 24 hours).
3. These reactions usually occur at beginning stages of therapy and do not last longer than a few weeks.
4. If local reactions continue, the more highly purified crystalline insulin or pork or human insulin may be tried.
5. Patients with severe insulin resistance or hypersensitivity should be referred to a hospital for antibody testing and regulation of insulin therapy.

Insulin lipodystrophy

1. Two forms of lipodystrophy:
   a. Hypertrophy (bumps that may progress to thickened patches in the skin) at site of injection.
   b. Reinforce patient teaching about changing sites of insulin injection so that same site will not be used more than once in one month (see Figure 8.3, p. 570).
2. Fatty atrophy (sunken areas at site of injection):
   a. Incidence higher in girls and older patients.
   b. The newer, highly purified forms of insulin appear to have a lower incidence of fat atrophy.

Insulin oedema

1. Characterized by generalized retention of fluid.
2. Usually appears with sudden restoration of diabetic control in a patient with uncontrolled diabetes over a period of time.

Insulin resistance

Term applied to a patient whose insulin requirement is at least 200 units daily over a period of weeks to months in the absence of infection.

ORAL HYPOGLYCAEMIC AGENTS

1. Oral hypoglycaemic agents (Table 8.2) may be given to maturity-onset nonketotic diabetics who

Table 8.2   Oral Hypoglycaemic agents

Agent	Duration of action
Sulphonylurea group – stimulates release of insulin from the pancreatic beta cells: these drugs depend on a functioning pancreas	
Tolbutamide (Rastinon)	6–12 hours
Chlorpropamide (Diabinese)	Up to 60 hours
Glibenclamide (Daonil, Euglocon)	12–24 hours
Tolazamide (Tolanase)	12–24 hours
Biguanides – act in a different way from the sulphonylureas. They are effective only in the presence of functioning pancreatic islet cells, and inhibit glucose absorption from the intestine and glucose oxidation. They should not be regarded as interchangeable with sulphonylureas	
Metformin (Glucophage)	8–12 hours

cannot be treated by diet alone and who are unable or unwilling to take insulin (aged, infirm, blind, unable to follow a diet).

2. Serious questions have been raised about the effectiveness and safety of long-term use of oral hypoglycaemic agents – increase in cardiovascular mortality during treatment with sulphonylureas.
3. Patient should be placed on an effective dietary and weight control programme before trying oral hypoglycaemia agents.
4. Insulin is preferable to oral agents if dietary treatment fails to control diabetes.
5. Insulin is *required* when infection, trauma, major surgery or gangrene are present since these conditions usually produce temporary insulin resistance.
6. Side-effects of sulphonylureas – nausea and skin rash.
7. Side-effects of biguanides – anorexia, nausea, vomiting, diarrhoea, loss of weight.

COMPLICATIONS OF DIABETES

KETOACIDOSIS AND COMA

Ketoacidosis is caused by the absence or by an inadequate amount of insulin. This lack results in decreased utilization of carbohydrate and increased breakdown of fat and protein and, consequently, in dehydration and loss of sodium, potassium, chloride and bicarbonate. The number of ketone bodies (organic acids) increases as a result of rapid breakdown of fat.

PRECIPITATING CAUSES
1. Failure to take insulin, insufficient insulin intake or resistance to insulin.
2. Infections (respiratory tract, urinary, gastrointestinal or skin).
3. Physiological stresses – pregnancy, injury, shock, surgery emotional stress – make available insulin less effective.

CLINICAL FEATURES
Early features
1. Polyuria, thirst, malaise, drowsiness.
2. Abdominal pain.
3. Headache, weakness, shortness of breath.
4. Fever.
5. Hot, dry skin.

Later features
1. Kussmaul breathing – very deep but not laboured respiratory movements; a symptom of profound acidosis.
2. Sweetish odour of breath – due to acetone.
3. Lowered blood pressure.
4. Drowsiness; coma.

LABORATORY TESTS
Blood
1. Blood glucose elevated.
2. Serum bicarbonate decreased.
3. Blood pH decreased.
4. Blood urea increased.
5. Plasma ketone is strongly positive.

Urine
Strongly positive for sugar, ketones; also contains protein.

TREATMENT AND NURSING MANAGEMENT
Objective
Restore carbohydrate utilization and correct electrolyte imbalance.
1. Secure blood and urine samples immediately.
   a. Insert indwelling catheter in comatose patient to obtain urine specimens at prescribed times.
   b. Obtain full blood count, blood glucose, urea and serum, electrolytes and blood pH.
2. Carry out rapid physical examination.
   a. Look for evidence of infection.

b. Look specifically at vital signs, state of hydration, skin colour, cardiac status.
3. Start intravenous infusion of isotonic saline, as prescribed to establish urine flow and improve hydration and circulation.
4. Simultaneously administer insulin (intravenous or subcutaneous route), as prescribed.
   a. A continuous infusion of small amounts of insulin may be given or a low, medium or high dose regime may be administered.
   b. Subsequent insulin is given depending on the response to the previous dose, changes in the blood and urine chemistry, and condition of the patient.
   c. If intravenous insulin is given, administer it in intravenous tubing.
5. Carry out frequent determinations of blood glucose, serum ketone, serum bicarbonate and serum potassium; use other tests as needed.
6. Administer potassium as prescribed – hyperkalaemia may occur owing to rapid migration of potassium ions into the cells.
7. Give prescribed glucose infusion to prevent hypoglycaemia when blood glucose reaches desired level, since carbohydrate metabolism will be accelerated by insulin and blood glucose will begin to decrease.
8. Treat for circulatory collapse if present – diabetic patients in ketoacidosis may also be hypovolaemic.
   a. Give intravenous fluids, plasma expanders and vasopressors as prescribed.
   b. Elevate the lower extremities.
9. Prepare for gastric lavage – to relieve vomiting or acute dilatation of stomach.
10. Obtain serial electrocardiogram tracings – used to determine potassium need.
11. Keep a flow sheet giving patient's vital signs, urine test, blood chemistries, mental state and treatment.
12. Prevent the recurrence of diabetic ketoacidosis; *the precipitating cause of coma should be determined.*
    a. Avoid and treat infection.
    b. Make insulin and dietary adjustments during the period of illness.
    c. Teach and reteach the fundamentals of insulin administration, urine testing and home management (see pp. 567–70).

INFECTION

UNDERLYING CONSIDERATIONS
1. Infections are more serious in the diabetic for the following reasons:

a. Resistance to infection is decreased because of hyperglycaemia.
b. Diabetes becomes temporarily more severe.
c. Insulin deficiency may impair ability of granulocytes to carry out a number of vital functions.
d. Several important steps in normal host defence are impaired in poorly controlled diabetic patient.
e. May precipitate ketoacidosis.
2. Infection increases the need for insulin.

TYPES OF INFECTION
1. Infections of urinary tract – probably from increased frequency of catheterization; aggravated by incomplete emptying of bladder due to bladder paresis that may result from diabetic neuropathy.
2. Gram-negative bacteraemia.
3. Furunculosis and other staphylococcal infections.
4. Tuberculosis – diabetics more susceptible to tuberculosis than the general population.
5. Fungal infections.
   a. Candidiasis:
      (i) Due to *Candida albicans* normally found on skin, oral cavity, gastrointestinal tract and vagina.
      (ii) Local infection of these areas (particularly vagina and skin) may occur in poorly controlled diabetes.
6. Yeast infections – *Monilia* infections of intertriginous (where folds of skin rub together) areas.
7. Gas gangrene – by nonclostridial organisms (*Aerobacter* or other coliform organisms) which are part of normal faecal flora; lower extremities usual site for these infections, which often lead to gangrene and amputation.

TREATMENT
1. The dosage of insulin is increased – due to elevation of blood glucose and the inability of leucocytes to effectively destroy bacteria.
2. Test the urine for sugar and acetone frequently and carry out frequent blood glucose determinations – to ascertain and compensate for rapidly changing insulin requirements.
3. Carry out cultures so that appropriate antibiotic may be given.

LONG-TERM COMPLICATIONS OF DIABETES

UNDERLYING CONSIDERATIONS
1. Diabetes is the most common cause of blindness in people aged between 35 and 64 years; heart

attacks and strokes may also be related to diabetes. The majority of amputations performed for gangrene are the result of diabetes; diabetic nephropathy and neuropathic complications are significant factors.

2. The life expectancy among people with diabetes is approximately one-third less than that of the general population.
3. Current clinical and experimental data demonstrate that optimal regulation of glucose levels should be achieved, since microvascular complications occur less frequently when blood glucose concentrations are reduced.

VASCULAR COMPLICATIONS

1. The specific pathological lesion (microangiopathy) of longstanding diabetes is characterized by thickening of the capillary basement membrane in every organ.
2. The prevalence of microangiopathy parallels the duration and rate of progression of diabetes; it is probably associated with poor control.
3. Intracapillary glomerulosclerosis (Kimmelstiel–Wilson syndrome) is the specific renal disease of diabetes and is related to the thickening of the capillary basement membrane in the glomeruli.
4. Microangiopathy of the vessels supplying the skin, peripheral nerves and walls of large arteries may be a factor in skin diseases, diabetic neuropathy and the increased prevalence of atherosclerosis.
5. Major vessel occlusion (macroangiopathy) due to atherosclerosis causes strokes, myocardial infarction, intermittent claudication and gangrene; often occurs before the diabetes is recognized.

DIABETIC RETINOPATHY

Diabetic retinopathy is a progressive impairment of retinal circulation that causes vitreous haemorrhage and sudden loss of vision.

1. Incidence and severity of retinopathy are generally proportional to the duration of the disease; half of the people who have diabetes of more than 10 years' duration will have some evidence of retinopathy.
2. Impaired vision (and blindness) are caused by haemorrhages into the vitreous, formation of scar tissue and detachment of retina.
3. Treatment:
   a. Photocoagulation – produced when a narrow, intensive beam of light is directed into the eye and focused on the retina; the absorption of light produces heat which coagulates the treated vessel and prevents it from bleeding.

(i) Used when there are localized areas of newly formed blood vessels and proliferative retinopathy, to prevent the events that lead to blindness.
(ii) Photocoagulation must be done when proliferative changes first occur.

   b. Patient education: patient should have yearly funduscopy (examination of the fundus of the eye) by an ophthalmologist.

DIABETIC NEUROPATHY

Diabetic neuropathy affects the peripheral and autonomic nervous system and produces a wide variety of syndromes.

1. Cinical features:
   a. Peripheral neuropathy – pain (dull, aching, burning, lancinating, or crushing), paraesthesias (sensations of tingling or burning or coldness and numbness).
   b. Involvement of autonomic nervous system – orthostatic hypotension, sexual impotency, retrograde ejaculation, pupillary changes, abnormal sweating, bladder paralysis, nocturnal diarrhoea.
2. Assessment of the feet of diabetic patients:
   (The complications of neuropathy and vascular disease are most evident in the feet. Most amputations, other than those occurring from trauma, occur in diabetics.)
   a. Watch for lesions of the feet that do not heal.
   b. Compare the skin colour of both feet and ankles. A blue-grey colour is caused by diminution of the blood supply.
   c. Change the position of the extremity and note the colour change. Pallor on elevation and dusky cyanosis on dependency indicate vascular insufficiency.
   d. Feel the temperature of the skin with the back of your hand and notice decreased temperature.
   e. Examine the toenails. Thick, ridged nails suggest circulatory impairment or fungus infection.
   f. Look for athlete's foot between the toes (epidermophytosis), and fungus infection of the nails (onychomycosis). Fungal infection is more serious in the diabetic and requires treatment.
   g. Look for calluses, corns, blisters, cracks and abrasions; look between the toes and on the soles of the feet.
   h. Palpate the dorsalis pedis and posterior tibial arterial pulses; absence of a discernible pulse

or diminution of the pulses indicate athero-sclerosis.

CARE OF THE DIABETIC PATIENT UNDERGOING SURGERY

UNDERLYING CONSIDERATIONS
The diabetic patient must be followed very closely at the time of surgery because of the incidence of gener-alized vascular disease, diabetic neuropathy, de-creased resistance to infection and changing insulin requirements due to stress and infection.
1. Surgical stress may increase hyperglycaemia be-cause of increased secretion of adrenaline and glucocorticoids.
2. Infection may cause insulin antagonism.
3. Diabetic ketoacidosis may simulate an acute surgical abdomen.
4. Metabolic stress of anaesthesia also accentuates problems of hyperglycaemia and ketosis.
5. Surgical trauma produces further metabolic de-rangements, depending on degree and duration of surgery.

TREATMENT AND NURSING MANAGEMENT
Objective
Achieve the best nutritional balance and best possible metabolic control of diabetes preoperatively.

Preoperative preparation
1. Essential evaluation studies are done preoper-atively – urinalysis for sugar and acetone, blood sugar levels, blood urea and other essential tests.
2. Give an adequate diet; the insulin dose may be reduced the day before surgery.

Day of surgery
1. A fasting blood glucose is drawn and an in-travenous infusion of 1,000ml of 5 per cent glu-cose may be given over a four-hour period for each meal that is missed.
2. The patient is usually given one-half to three-quarters his usual dose of insulin.

Postoperative management
1. Maintain nutrition with intravenous glucose until patient is able to tolerate food by mouth.
2. Give insulin as directed. The usual dose of in-termediate-acting insulin is started the day after surgery, and supplemental regular insulin may be given on a sliding scale according to blood glucose tests.

PRINCIPLES OF PATIENT EDUCATION FOR DIABETES MELLITUS

The person with diabetes mellitus must accept a major role in the management of his disease. His education must be amplified, reinforced and updated continuously, since diabetes is a life-long disease.

Objective
Maintain the best possible control of diabetes.

PATIENT'S OBJECTIVES
Become familiar with diabetes and how it affects the body
1. Visit the doctor or specialist nurse on a regular basis.
2. Study and review available literature from reput-able sources.
3. Secure booklets and pamphlets from the British Diabetic Association, 10 Queen Anne Street, London, W1M 0BD.
4. Attend available classes.

Maintain health at an optimal level
1. Maintain a consistent daily routine.
2. Get adequate rest and sleep.
3. Exercise regularly and consistently.
   a. Avoid 'spurts' of arduous exercise before meals.
   b. Exercise 1½ hours after meals.
   c. Keep some form of carbohydrate (sugar or sweets) available during exercise periods.
4. Seek employment with regular hours.
5. Have an annual test for tuberculosis.

Follow the prescribed dietary regimen
1. Eat three or more regular meals each day.
2. Become thoroughly familiar with the carbo-hydrate exchange lists.
3. Avoid concentrated carbohydrates.
4. Keep weight at optimal level; correct body weight.
5. If taking insulin, eat extra calories when unusual physical activity is anticipated.
6. Eat a bedtime snack when taking insulin (if per-missible).

Be aware of the degree of diabetes control
1. Test blood for sugar.

2. Test blood before each meal and at bedtime while control is being attained or during periods of illness.
3. Test urine when blood sugar levels are high.
4. Keep a daily record of blood sugar tests (date, hour, value).
5. Test only freshly voided urine.
6. Take the record of blood tests to doctor at appointed times.
7. Know that acetone in the urine indicates need for *more insulin*.
8. Protect all urine-testing and blood-testing equipment from light, moisture and heat (to prevent false interpretation due to deterioration of test materials).
9. Monitor blood glucose when insulin requirements vary and during illness.
   a. Capillary blood is obtained from finger puncture and spread on enzyme strip.
   b. Reaction may be quantitated visually or with the use of a metre.

Become familiar with all aspects of insulin usage
(See opposite page for guidelines for teaching self-injection of insulin.)
1. Know when the prescribed insulin is having its peak action.
2. Adjust insulin dosage according to urine and blood sugar tests as prescribed.
3. Rotate the sites of insulin injections in a systematic manner.
4. Keep the syringe and needle in one particular place.
5. Keep a reserve supply of insulin in the refrigerator.
   a. Keep bottle in current use at *room temperature*.
   b. Avoid injecting cold insulin because it may contribute to tissue reaction.
6. Have an extra insulin syringe available.
7. Know the conditions that produce insulin reactions:
   a. Omission of a meal.
   b. Unaccustomed or strenuous exercise.
   c. Too much insulin.
8. Know the symptoms of an insulin reaction:
   a. Any unfamiliar or peculiar sensation.
   b. Hunger, perspiration, palpitation, tachycardia, weakness, tremor, pallor.
9. Know how to combat an impending insulin reaction:
   a. Eat carbohydrates (sugar, sweets) when symptoms first occur.
   b. Test blood sugar.

c. Carry extra carbohydrate at all times (sugar lumps, sweets).
d. Eat extra carbohydrate before strenuous exercise and during periods of prolonged exercise, or reduce insulin dosage.
e. Eat a snack at bedtime.
10. Keep a check-off system to ensure taking insulin.
11. Carry diabetic identification card or wear identification bracelet.

Take prescribed oral hypoglycaemic medication
1. Adhere faithfully to the prescribed diet.
2. Test urine or blood sugar daily.
3. Take the medication *exactly* as directed.

Appreciate the importance of proper foot care to prevent infection, ischaemia and neuropathy which may lead to amputation and death
1. Inspect the feet carefully and routinely for calluses, corns, blisters, abrasions, redness and nail abnormalities.
   a. Use a small mirror to check bottom of each foot.
   b. Use a magnifying glass under good light if eyesight is poor, or ask someone else to check feet.
2. Bathe the feet daily in warm (never hot) water.
   a. Do not soak the feet for prolonged periods.
   b. Dry feet carefully, especially between the toes.
3. Massage the feet with a lubricating lotion, except between the toes.
4. Prevent moisture between the toes to avert maceration of the skin.
   a. Insert sheepskin between overlapping toes.
   b. Use powder in the web spaces, especially if feet perspire.
5. Wear well-fitting, noncompressive shoes and socks – long enough, wide enough, soft, supple and low-heeled.
   a. Buy shoes in the afternoon – feet are larger in the afternoon than in the morning.
   b. Have each foot measured before buying shoes – feet enlarge with age.
   c. Have the measurement taken while standing, since foot is larger in the standing position.
   d. Do not 'break in' shoes all at one time.
   e. Avoid working in bedroom slippers or other casual footwear.
6. Go to a chiropodist on a regular basis if corns, calluses and ingrown toenails are present.
   a. Cut toenails straight across to prevent ingrown toenails.

7. Avoid heat, chemicals and injuries to the feet – do not go barefoot or expose feet to hot water bottles, heating pads, caustic solutions, etc.
8. If an injury occurs to the foot:
   a. Wash the area with mild soap and water.
   b. Cover with a dry sterile dressing *without* adhesive.
   c. Consult the doctor.

Maintain diabetic control during periods of illness

1. Call doctor immediately when any unusual symptoms become evident; *do not allow diabetes to get out of control*.
2. Make dietary adjustments during illness according to doctor's directions.
3. Continue taking insulin; doctor may increase dosage during illness.
4. Test blood for sugar and urine for acetone more frequently; keep records; monitor blood glucose.
5. Know the conditions that bring about diabetic acidosis:
   a. Nausea and vomiting.
   b. Failure to increase insulin when urine sugar is increasing.
   c. Failure to take insulin.
   d. Dietary excesses.
   e. Infections.
   f. Stress.
   g. Menstrual periods.
6. Know how to combat impending diabetic acidosis:
   a. Examine blood for sugar and urine for acetone and report results to doctor.
   b. Take additional insulin as advised by doctor.
   c. Go to bed and keep warm.
   d. Alert someone to be in attendance.
   e. Drink a glass of liquid hourly if possible.

Follow other health directives

1. Avoid tobacco – nicotine constricts blood vessels, causing reduction in blood flow to feet.
2. Report excessive itching – may indicate elevated blood sugar.
3. Take only medications prescribed by doctor – many drugs enhance effect on insulin and oral antidiabetic agents.

GUIDELINES: TEACHING SELF-INJECTION OF INSULIN

UNDERLYING CONSIDERATIONS

1. Insulin injection should be taught as soon as the need for insulin treatment has been established.
2. A member of the patient's family should also be taught how to administer insulin.
3. An optimistic approach will offer the patient encouragement.
4. Teach insulin injection *first* since this is the patient's major concern; then include loading the syringe and sterilizing equipment as the patient is able to grasp these concepts.

EQUIPMENT

Prescribed bottle of insulin
Insulin syringe and needles (may be disposable), usually bought by patient
Carrying case
Industrial methylated spirit

PROCEDURE

Teaching action	Rationale
1. Give the patient the prepared syringe containing the prescribed dose of insulin.	
2. Instruct the patient to hold the syringe as he would a pencil.	

3. Show the patient how to spread the skin taut on the anterior thigh (Figure 8.2a), *or* Form a skin fold by picking up subcutaneous tissue between the thumb and forefinger if the patient is thin (Figure 8.2b).

Either of the techniques ensures that the needle tip is inserted into subcutaneous tissue and outside the muscle. Avoid pressing the skin *tightly* between the fingers since this is a common cause of local induration and infection.

4. Select areas of upper arms, thighs, flanks and upper buttocks or abdomen for injection after patient becomes proficient with needle insertion (Figure 8.2a).

The skin is loose and there is more subcutaneous fat in these areas. The skin of the abdominal wall is a good site for women who develop atrophy of subcutaneous fat at sites of insulin injection.

5. Assist the patient to insert needle with a quick thrust to the hub at a right angle to the skin surface (Figure 8.2c).

The insulin is injected into deep subcutaneous tissue.

6. Instruct the patient to release the skin fold.

7. Gently withdraw the needle. Wipe area with paper tissue if necessary.

This manoeuvre prevents painful pulling of the skin as the needle is withdrawn.

8. Put syringe and needle into carrying case. Carrying case is half-filled with industrial methylated spirit which is changed weekly.

9. Remove all traces of spirit before loading syringe, by pushing plunger back and forth. Spirit may alter the effect of insulin and is also irritating when introduced under the skin.

10. Develop a systematic plan for insulin administration; e.g. rotation of sites in a clockwise fashion (Figure 8.3).

Systematic rotation of sites will keep the skin supple, will favour uniform absorption of insulin and will prevent scar formation.

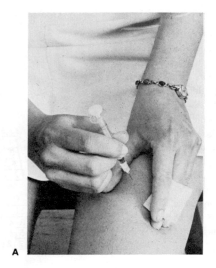

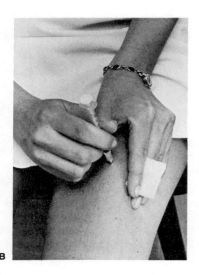

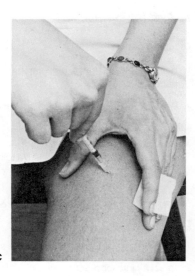

Figure 8.2. Self-injection of insulin. (A) The insulin syringe is held perpendicular to the stretched skin before the needle is thrust into the subcutaneous tissues. (B) Alternative method: if the patient has only a thin layer of subcutaneous fat, a fold of skin is pinched between the fingers to keep the needle from penetrating into the muscle. (C) With thumb on top of plunger, insulin is smoothly and quickly injected

Figure 8.3. Setting up a rotation circle. The right arm is marked A, the right side of the abdomen is B and the right thigh is C. The left side of the body, going upwards, is marked D, E and F, anti-clockwise. Each of these areas can be marked as a rectangle and divided into eight squares more than 2.5cm on each side. These squares are numbered starting from the upper and outside corner (number 1) to the lowest corner (number 8). All even numbers are towards the body. If the patient takes the number 1 square and injects into it at each of the six sites from A to F, it will take him six days to reach area A again. He then takes square number 2 and injects each time on the squares so numbered in areas A to F, and so on. This provides 48 different places for an injection (6×8). At one injection daily, it will take 48 days, or seven weeks, to cover each of the squares (from: A. D. A. *Forecast – the Diabetics' Own Magazine*, Vol. 4, January 1951; courtesy, Becton, Dickenson)

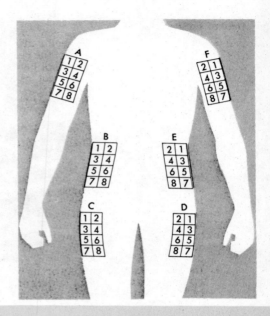

To load the syringe

Teaching action	Rationale
1. Roll the bottle of insulin between the palms of the hands.	The rolling action mixes the insulin.
2. Wipe off the top of the insulin vial with an alcohol swab.	
3. Inject approximately the same volume of air into the insulin vial as the volume of insulin to be withdrawn.	Air is injected into the vial to keep its contents under slight positive pressure and to make it easier to withdrawn the insulin.

To fill a syringe with long-acting and short-acting insulin

Teaching action

1. Wipe off the vial tops with an alcohol swab.

2. Inject air into long-acting insulin first; withdraw needle

3. Inject air into short-acting insulin bottle and withdraw prescribed amount of insulin.

4. Then withdraw prescribed amount of insulin from long-acting insulin bottle.

Insulin pumps

Insulin can be given by continuous subcutaneous infusion using soluble insulin in an infusion pump. This provides continuous basal insulin infusion with preprandial boosts. Its chief benefit is the considerable improvement in the quality of life enjoyed by some patients. The disadvantages are the bulkiness of equipment and mechanical failure. Patients must be well motivated and able to monitor their own blood glucose. There is a selection of injection aids available for the visually handicapped diabetic.

RAPID METHODS OF URINE TESTING FOR GLUCOSE (SUGAR), KETONES (ACETONE) AND BLOOD GLUCOSE

UNDERLYING CONSIDERATIONS

1. In diabetes, sugar may appear in the urine when the level of glucose in the blood rises above 9mmol/l (160mg/100ml); as patients grow older the renal threshold tends to rise above 9mmol/l (160mg/100ml).
2. Urinary sugar (glycosuria) may appear when:
   a. Treatment is inadequate.
   b. Patient is not following his prescribed diet.
   c. Exercise is inadequate.
   d. Infection is present.
3. Incorrect test results may occur because:
   a. Deteriorated reagent tablets or reagent strips are used.
   b. The directions are not followed accurately.
   c. Certain medications affect results; can give false positive or negative results.

INSTRUCTIONS TO THE PATIENT

Use the second-micturition technique to collect the urine specimen.
1. Micturate and discard the urine.
2. Drink several glasses of liquid.
3. Micturate into a clean container 30 to 45 minutes later – the second specimen reflects the status of glucose spillover into the urine more accurately.
4. Test this specimen.

TESTS FOR GLUCOSE (SUGAR)

1. Clinitest* (uses a reagent tablet).
2. Diastix* (reagent strip).
Tests for acetone (ketone bodies).
1. Acetest* (reagent tablets).
2. Ketostix * (reagent strip).
Combined ketone–glucose reagent strip.
1. Keto-Diastix*.

---

* Clinitest, Diastix, Acetest, Ketostix, Keto-Diastix and Dextrostix are products of Ames Company, Division of Miles Laboratories, Inc., Stoke Poges, Slough SL2 4LY.

RAPID METHODS OF BLOOD TESTING FOR GLUCOSE

Normal blood glucose level between 3–7mmol/l and no greater than 10mmol/l after a meal. Patient is taught to use a lancet to obtain blood from finger tip.

Dextrostix*

1. Compare test area on strip closely with 'o' block on colour chart. If reagent area on strip does not closely match the 'o' block discard strip.
2. Freely apply a large drop of capillary or venous blood sufficient to cover entire reagent area on printed side of strip.
3. Wait exactly 60 seconds (use sweep second hand or stop watch for timing).
4. Quickly wash off blood (within one or two seconds) with a sharp stream of water using a wash bottle.
5. Read result within one or two seconds after washing. Hold the strip close to the colour chart. Interpolate if necessary.

BM test

1. Drop blood onto BM test strip; after one minute wipe excess blood.
2. After two minutes match colour with chart.
3. When more than 13.3mmol/l (240mg/100ml), compare colours after three minutes.

A selection of glucose meters is available for the patient to use at home, e.g. Glucocheck, Hypocount, Ames Eyetone Meter.

THE ADRENAL GLANDS

Medulla

1. Is not necessary to maintain life but enables a person to cope with stress.
2. Secretes two hormones:
   a. Adrenaline:
      (i) Acts on alpha and beta receptors.
      (ii) Increases contractility and excitability of heart muscle, leading to increased cardiac output.

(iii) Facilitates blood flow to muscles, brain and viscera.

(iv) Enhances blood sugar – by stimulating conversion of glycogen to glucose in liver.

(v) Inhibits smooth muscle contraction.

b. Noradrenaline:

(i) Acts primarily on alpha receptors.

(ii) Increases peripheral vascular resistance leading to increases in diastolic and systolic blood pressure.

Cortex

1. Is essential to life.
2. Secretes adrenocortical hormones – synthesized from cholesterol.
   a. Glucocorticoids: cortisone and hydrocortisone:
      (i) Enhance protein catabolism and inhibit protein synthesis.
      (ii) Antagonize action of insulin.
      (iii) Increase synthesis of glucose by liver.
      (iv) Influence defence mechanism of body and its reaction to stress.
      (v) Influence emotional reaction.
   b. Mineralocorticoids:
      (i) Aldosterone – supplied by adrenal cortex.
      (ii) Desoxycorticosterone – usually not present in significant amounts.
      (iii) Regulate reabsorption of sodium cation.
      (iv) Regulate excretion of potassium cation by renal tubules.
   c. Sex hormones.

DISORDERS OF THE ADRENAL GLANDS

PHAEOCHROMOCYTOMA

Phaeochromocytoma is a neoplasm associated with hyperfunction of the adrenal medulla.

CLINICAL FEATURES

1. Variable symptoms depend upon whether the tumour secretes adrenaline or noradrenaline. Symptoms are often triggered by allergic reactions, physical exertion, emotional upset; they can also occur without identifiable stimulus.
2. Hypertension may be paroxysmal or chronic. Chronic form may be difficult to differentiate from 'essential hypertension'.
3. Tachycardia, excessive perspiration, tremor, pallor or face flushing, nervousness and hyperglycaemia.
4. Polyuria, nausea, vomiting, diarrhoea and abdominal pain, paraesthesia in extremities.

DIAGNOSTIC EVALUATION

1. If there is sympathetic overactivity along with marked elevation of blood pressure, phaeochromocytoma is strongly suspected.
2. Administration of certain drugs produces certain changes in arterial pressure.
3. Intravenous pyelogram (IVP) or computerized tomography (CT scan) may help in identifying the location of the tumour.
4. Tests:
   a. Vanillylmandelic acid (VMA) determination in urine.
   b. Normal urinary value: VMA up to 35mmol/24 hours (0.7–6.8mg/24 hours).

TREATMENT AND NURSING MANAGEMENT
Objective
Remove the cause.

Preoperative preparation

1. This requires effective control of blood pressure and blood volume. Often may take one or two weeks.
2. To accomplish blood pressure control, administer prescribed alpha-adrenergic blocking agents such as phentolamine (Rogitine) or phenoxybenzamine hydrochloride (Dibenyline) to inhibit the effects of catecholamines.
3. Catecholamine synthesis inhibitors may also be used.
4. Propranolol is helpful in controlling cardiac dysrhythmias, if present.

Postoperative care

See also p. 576. Of particular concern is the evaluation and documentation of 24-hour urine specimens. The patient is considered surgically cured when 24-hour urine specimens are evaluated as 'normal' when tested for previously 'abnormal' substances.

CUSHING'S SYNDROME

Cushing's syndrome is a disease produced by hyperactivity of the adrenal cortex.

AETIOLOGY

1. Cushing's syndrome results mainly from the hypersecretion of cortisol and corticosterone.

2. The disorder may be caused by:
   a. A neoplasm of the adrenal cortex: adenoma or carcinoma.
   b. Hyperplasia of both glands due to over-stimulation of the adrenal cortex by adreno-corticotrophic hormone (ACTH).
   c. Pituitary tumours.
   d. Tumours elsewhere in body producing excess ACTH.

DIAGNOSTIC EVALUATION
1. Excessive plasma cortisol levels.
2. An increase in blood sugar – diabetes.
3. A decrease in concentration of potassium in the blood.
4. A reduction in the number of blood eosinophils.
5. Elevation in the urine level of 17-hydroxy-corticoids and 17-ketogenic steroids.
6. Elevation of plasma ACTH in patients with pituitary tumours.

CLINICAL FEATURES
In children
1. Precocious puberty.
2. Affected growth rate.

Females
Cushing's syndrome occurs ten times more frequently in females than in males.
1. 'Virilism' or masculinization.
   a. Hirsutism – excessive growth of hair on the face and midline of trunk.
   b. Breasts – atrophy.
   c. Clitoris – enlarges.
   d. Voice – masculine.
2. In utero – possible hermaphrodite.
3. Menses – irregular and scanty; libido lost.

Adult ('central type obesity')
1. 'Buffalo hump' in neck and supraclavicular area.
2. Heavy trunk; thin extremities.
3. Skin – fragile and thin; striae and ecchymosis, acne.
4. Face – rounded, plethoric, oily.
5. Muscles – wasted due to excessive catabolism.
6. Osteoporosis – characteristic kyphosis, backache.
7. Mental disturbances – mood changes, psychosis.
8. Increased suspectibility to infections.
9. Hypertension oedema.

OBJECTIVES OF TREATMENT AND NURSING MANAGEMENT
Establish the diagnosis
1. Overnight dexamethasone suppression test.

a. Dexamethasone is administered orally the night before in the amount equivalent to amount of cortisol normally produced by the patient in a day.
b. Dexamethasone will normally suppress ACTH secretion and stop cortisol production.
c. The next day, blood studies will be done; patients with Cushing's syndrome will not show suppression below a certain level.
2. If above test does not rule out the possibility of Cushing's syndrome, specific urinary excretion tests are performed with dexamethasone suppression.
3. Additional tests are done to determine whether the problem is due to hyperplasia or adreno-cortical tumour.
4. Explain to the patient the necessity for the many blood and urine studies.
5. Recognize the need for accurately recording intake of food and fluid as well as output of urine.
6. Record all pertinent observations that may assist the doctor in making the diagnosis.

Consider medical treatment in patients unable to face surgery (e.g. myocardial infarction)
1. The doctor may prescribe:
   a. Mitotane, an agent toxic to the adrenal cortex (DDT derivative) – 'medical adrenalectomy'; serious side-effects accompany this drug.
   b. Metyrapone (Metopirone) to inhibit steroid biosynthesis; this is used for temporary control.

Encourage the patient to eat the prescribed diet
1. Explain to the patient that his diet (low sodium and high potassium) is as significant to his treatment as his medications.
   a. Foods high in potassium – meats, fish, most vegetables and fruits, legumes.
   b. Foods low in sodium – cereal, fruits, squash, potatoes, lettuce, honey, unsalted butter.

Be aware of the psychological manifestations of this syndrome
1. Identify those situations which are disturbing to the patient; record these on the nursing care plan as situations to be avoided.
2. Be alert for evidence of depression; in some instances this has progressed to suicide; therefore, mood changes are most important.
3. Report when depression continues after surgery.
4. Understand the emotional stress in female patients who manifest masculinization tendencies.

5. Reassure the patient who has benign adenoma or hyperplasia that, with proper treatment, evidence of masculinization can be reversed.
6. Note that weakness is a frustrating experience in a patient who previously has been active.

Remove the cause via surgery
1. Tumour (adrenal or pituitary) – should be removed or treated with irradiation.
2. Hyperplasia of adrenals – calls for an adrenalectomy.

Administer replacement therapy postoperatively
This is a lifelong corticosteroid maintenance therapeutic programme.
1. Adrenalectomy patients require replacement therapy with the following:
   a. A glucocorticoid – cortisone.
   b. A mineralocorticoid – fludrocortisone (Florinef).
   c. Extra salt.
2. Following pituitary irradiation or hypophysectomy, patients may require adrenal replacement plus thyroid and gonadal replacement therapy.
3. Protein anabolic steroids may facilitate protein replacement; potassium stores are usually depleted rapidly and may require replacement.

ADDISON'S DISEASE

Addison's disease is a condition due to deficiency of the adrenal glands.

CAUSE
A deficiency of cortical hormones due to:
1. Destruction of adrenal cortex.
2. Atrophy – following prolonged steroid therapy or secondary to pituitary deficiency.

Assessment
CLINICAL FEATURES
Due to (1) disturbance of sodium and potassium metabolism and (2) depletion of sodium and water – urine loss, severe chronic dehydration.
1. Muscular weakness, fatigue, weight loss.
2. Gastrointestinal problems – anorexia, nausea, vomiting, diarrhoea, constipation, abdominal pain.
3. Low blood pressure, low blood sugar, low basal metabolic rate, low blood sodium.

4. High potassium.
5. After a while, symptoms worsen and the patient is forced to go to bed.
   a. Skin colour changes to tan, bronze or brown – diffuse or patchy, freckling.
   b. Mucous membranes also discolour – bluish black or grey.
   c. Mental changes occur – depression, irritability, anxiety, apprehension.
6. Normal responses to stress are lacking.

DIAGNOSTIC EVALUATION
Blood studies
1. Hypoglycaemia – decrease in sugar concentration.
2. Hyponatraemia – decrease in sodium concentration.
3. Hyperkalaemia – increase in potassium concentration.
4. Lymphoid hyperplasia.
5. Low fasting plasma cortisol levels.

Urine studies
A 24-hour specimen for 17-ketosteroids, 17-hydroxycorticoids and 17-ketogenic steroids is needed – all values decreased.

Injection of a potent pituitary adrenocorticotropic hormone to artificially stimulate adrenals
1. Normal response – normal rise in plasma cortisol and urinary 17-ketosteroids.
2. In Addison's disease:
   a. Decrease in circulating eosinophils.
   b. Increase in uric and excretion is about four hours.
   c. No rise in plasma cortisol and urinary 17-ketosteroids.

PATIENT PROBLEMS
1. Altered fluid and electrolyte balance related to renal losses of sodium and water and renal retention of potassium, gastrointestinal losses of fluid and electrolytes, and inadequate dietary intake.
2. Inadequate physiological response to stressors related to decreased secretion of glucocorticoids and aldosterone.
3. Activity intolerance related to fatigue.
4. Anorexia, nausea, vomiting, diarrhoea related to effects of endocrine imbalance.

Planning and implementation
TREATMENT AND NURSING MANAGEMENT
1. Attempt to restore normal electrolyte balance.
   a. Administer high sodium, low potassium diet and fluids.
   b. Give prescribed hydrocortisone (17-hydroxycorticosterone).
      (i) Addisonian crisis – inject hydrocortisone 21-sodium succinate (Solu-Cortef) or hydrocortisone phosphate, 50–100mg intravenously and follow with an infusion of Solu-Cortef intravenously over eight hours.
      (ii) Long-term basis – hydrocortisone in doses of 20–30mg plus deoxycortone (DOCA) or Florinef.
2. Detect early signs of Addisonian crisis:
   a. Nausea, vomiting, cyanosis.
   b. Sudden drop in blood pressure.
   c. Very high temperature.
3. Recognize that circulatory collapse may result from the following:
   a. Overexertion.
   b. Exposure to cold.
   c. Acute infection.
   d. Decrease in salt intake.
   e. Excessive diarrhoea.
4. Be on guard for later signs of Addisonian crisis.
   a. Fall in systolic pressure to 40–50mmHg.
   b. Weak pulse and cold clammy skin.
5. Initiate prescribed treatment immediately.
   a. Administer prescribed blood transfusions to replace blood volume.
   b. Administer intravenous infusion of sodium chloride solution to replace sodium ions.
   c. Give hydrocortisone, as prescribed.
6. Assess vital signs frequently for deviation:
   a. Monitor vital signs and blood pressure; a drop in blood pressure may suggest impending crisis.
   b. Record the temperature hourly since an elevation may easily be precipitated.
7. Observe carefully the emotional state of the patient:
   a. Encourage rest periods to avoid overexertion.
   b. Control the temperature of the room to avoid sharp deviations in patient's temperature.
   c. Maintain a quiet, peaceful environment; avoid loud talking and noisy radios.
8. Record conscientiously the salt intake and urine output. Inform the patient's family as well as all nursing staff who come in contact with this patient that all urine must be saved for a 24-hour urine specimen.

9. Give total nursing care:
   a. Do not allow the patient who is in adrenal crisis to do anything for himself.
   b. Assist him in moving and turning, in feeding and in providing mouth care.
   c. Limit conversation to what is essential to his care.
10. Protect the patient from infection:
    a. Control his contacts so that infectious organisms are not transmitted.
    b. Protect him from draughts, dampness, etc.
11. Be familiar with the nature of hormonal replacement required by the individual patient.
    a. Some require cortisol.
    b. Other patients require additional electrolyte-type medications to maintain homeostasis.
    c. Note whether there is an effect on fluid retention – weigh patient frequently and record weight.

PATIENT EDUCATION
1. Instruct the patient about the necessity for long-term therapy for adrenocortical insufficiency and medical follow-up.
   a. Inform the patient that therapy must be continued for the rest of his life.
   b. Emphasize the importance of taking more hormones when the patient is under stress.
   c. Suggest that the patient carry an identification card on which are indicated the type of medication he is receiving and the telephone number of his doctor.
2. Instruct the patient about features of excessive use of medications and reportable symptoms.

Evaluation
EXPECTED OUTCOMES
1. Demonstrates adequate circulatory status by normal vital signs.
2. Maintains balance of fluid intake and output; maintains weight at normal level without signs and symptoms of fluid overload.
3. Demonstrates normal skin elasticity and moist mucous membranes.
4. Demonstrates normal serum sodium and potassium levels.
5. Consumes foods high in sodium and with normal potassium content.
6. Uses glucocorticoids and mineralocorticoids as prescribed.
7. Demonstrates normal response to stressful situations as evidenced by normal vital signs.
8. Plans rest and activity to avoid overexertion.
9. Identifies actions to take to avoid factors that

may precipitate Addisonian crisis (infection, extremes of temperature, etc).

10. Carries identification card with information about condition, and emergency treatment with him at all times.

PRIMARY ALDOSTERONISM

Primary aldosteronism is a disorder caused by hypersecretion of the adrenal cortex.

DIAGNOSTIC EVALUATION AND CLINICAL FEATURES

1. A profound decline in blood levels of potassium (hypokalaemia) and hydrogen ions (alkalosis) – results in muscle weakness and inability of kidneys to acidify or concentrate urine, leading to excess volume of urine (polyuria).
   a. Increase in pH.
   b. Increase in CO_2-combining power.
2. A decline in hydrogen ions (alkalosis) – results in tetany, paraesthesias.
3. An elevation in blood sodium (hypernatraemia) – results in excessive thirst (polydipsia) and arterial hypertension.
4. Hypertension.

TREATMENT
Removal of adrenal tumour – adrenalectomy (see below).

SECONDARY ALDOSTERONISM
Management is dependent on treatment of the underlying disorder.

CARE OF THE PATIENT HAVING AN ADRENALECTOMY

PREOPERATIVE CARE
1. Correct hyperglycaemia by proper diet and insulin.
2. Administer high-protein diet to correct protein deficiency.
3. See Chapter 3, Care of the Surgical Patient – care of patient is similar to that for general surgery of abdomen.

POSTOPERATIVE CARE
1. Similar to that for an abdominal operation.
2. Will require administration of hydrocortisone or similar compounds in large amounts; this should begin prior to surgery. If bilateral adrenalectomy is performed, lifetime replacement is necessary.

3. For removal of phaechromocytoma:
   a. Because of manipulation of tumour during surgery, there may be extreme fluctuations of blood pressure.
   b. Upon ligation of vessels from tumour an abrupt fall of blood pressure may result. Large amounts of adrenaline are given intravenously.

NURSING ALERT
Be prepared to monitor blood pressure frequently for 24 to 48 hours and alter the dose of vasopressor intravenous medications in order to stabilize the blood pressure.

4. Monitor vital signs, including blood pressure and central venous pressure, up to 48 hours – to detect early changes which may lead to cardiovascular collapse.
5. Anticipate stressful situations for the patient and avoid them; provide rest periods, anticipate his needs, provide comfort measures.

STEROID THERAPY*

CLASSIFICATION OF STEROIDS
By major metabolic effects on body.
1. Mineralocorticoids.
   a. Concerned with sodium and water retention and potassium excretion.
   b. Example – aldosterone and 11-desoxy-corticosterone.
2. Glucocorticoids.
   a. Concerned with metabolic effects, including carbohydrate metabolism.
   b. Example – cortisol.
3. Sex hormones.
   a. Important when secreted in large amounts or when the growth of hormone-sensitive cancers is stimulated.
   b. Examples:
      (i) Androgens – dehydroepiandrosterone, testosterone;
      (ii) Oestrogens – oestradiol;
      (iii) Progestins – progesterone.

EFFECTS OF GLUCOCORTICOIDS (CORTICOSTEROIDS, STEROIDS)
1. Antagonize action of insulin – promote gluconeogenesis, which provides glucose.

---

* Source acknowledgement: Melick, M.E. (1977) Nursing intervention for patients receiving corticosteroid therapy, in Kintzel (ed.) *Advanced Concepts in Nursing* (2nd edn), J.B. Lippincott, Philadelphia.

2. Increase breakdown of protein (inhibit protein synthesis).
3. Increase breakdown of fatty acids.
4. Suppress inflammation, inhibit scar formation, block allergic responses.
5. Decrease number of circulating eosinophils and leucocytes; decrease size of lymphatic tissue.
6. Exert a permissive action (allow full expression of effects of another hormone) on all effects caused by catecholamines.
7. Exert a permissive action on functioning of central nervous system.
8. Inhibit release of adrenocorticotropin.

IN SUMMARY: Glucocorticoids give an organism the capacity to resist all types of noxious stimuli and environmental change.

USES OF STEROIDS
1. Physiologically – to correct deficiencies or malfunction of a particular endocrine organ or system, e.g. Addison's disease.
2. Diagnostically – to determine proper functioning of the endocrine system.
3. Pharmacologically – to treat the following:
   a. Rheumatoid arthritis.
   b. Acute rheumatic fever.
   c. Blood conditions.
      (i) Idiopathic thrombocytopenic purpura.
      (ii) Leukaemia.
      (iii) Haemolytic anaemia.
   d. Allergic conditions – bronchial asthma, allergic rhinitis.
   e. Dermatological problems – drug rashes, atopic dermatitis.
   f. Ocular diseases – conjunctivitis, uveitis.
   g. Collagen diseases – lupus erythematosus, polyarteritis nodosa.
   h. Gastrointestinal problems – ulcerative colitis.
   i. Organ-transplant recipients – as an immuno-suppressive.
   j. Neurological – cerebral oedema.
   k. Other conditions – gout, multiple sclerosis.
4. Emergency conditions:
   a. Status asthmaticus.
   b. Acute adrenal insufficiency.
   c. Anaphylactic reaction (only after adrenaline has been given).

PREPARING THE PATIENT TO RECEIVE STEROID THERAPY
1. A thorough physical examination and medical history is required.
2. Determine contraindications for such therapy:

   a. Peptic ulcer
   b. Diabetes mellitus.
   c. Viral infections.
3. A tuberculin test is taken to determine need for antituberculin drugs. If this is not done prior to steroid therapy, the patient's hypersensitivity to tuberculin may be suppressed.
4. The patient's own level of steroid secretion is assessed if possible.
5. Explain the nature of the therapy, what is required of the patient, how long he is to be on steroid medications, what adverse signs to watch for, etc.

CHOICE OF STEROID AND METHOD OF ADMINISTRATION
1. Determined on an individual basis by the doctor.
2. May be given for local effects or systemic effects.
3. May be given by a wide variety of methods: orally, parenterally, sublingually, rectally, by inhalation or by direct application to skin or mucous membrane.
4. Combinations of steroids with other drugs should be avoided.
5. To help avoid steroid side-effects, alternate-day therapy should be used if at all possible; this is not always feasible.
6. Sometimes steroids are given in extremely high doses, then sharply reduced; if patient has been taking steroids for a while, doses must be tapered off gradually.

POTENTIAL SIDE-EFFECTS OF STEROID THERAPY (See Table 8.3)
Classification
1. Mineralocorticoid.
   a. Sodium and water retention.
      Oedema, weight gain, elevated blood pressure.
   b. Potassium depletion.
      Weakness, tiredness, alkalosis.
2. Glucocorticoid.
   a. Masking of infections.
   b. Osteoporosis.
   c. Steroid diabetes.
   d. Exacerbation of tuberculosis.

Control or avoidance of side-effects
1. Mineralocorticoid – triamcinolone or newer synthetic steroids are used. (Some of the newer synthetics cause less sodium retention but have other side-effects).
2. Glucocorticoid – difficult to separate anti-inflammatory effects from sodium-retaining effects.

Table 8.3   Potential side-effects of steroid therapy

Acceptable and expected side effects

Nature of effect	Medical action
Facial mooning (Cushing's syndrome)	May be minimized by restricted calorie intake
Weight gain	Restrict calorie intake; may require a change in steroid medication; may require a diuretic
Oedema	May require diuretics and potassium
Potassium loss	Prescribe diuretics and potassium
	May require addition of a fluorinated synthetic
Acne	Administer potassium supplement as prescribed
	Treat with topical medications
Increase frequency and nocturia	Check for evidence of genitourinary infection or diabetes mellitus; urinalysis
Insomnia, headache, fatigue, euphoria	
Glycosuria leucocytosis	Treat symptomatically

Undesirable and unacceptable side-effects

Nature of effect	Medical action
Allergic reaction to ACTH or steroid	Withdraw drug promptly
	Substitute steroid or synthetic ACTH
Cardiovascular system effect:	
Hypertension	Suggest reduction in dosage of steroids
Thromboembolic complications	
Arteritis	
Infection	Suggest antibiotic medications as indicated
Eye complications:	
Glaucoma	
Corneal lesions	Refer to ophthalmologist
Subcapsular cataract	
Musculoskeletal effects:	
Osteoporosis	Suggest sex hormones – synthetic oestrogens and/or androgens
Pathological fractures	
Growth suppression	
Myopathies	Suggest calcium supplement
Central nervous system:	
Seizures	Refer to neurologist
Neuritis	
Psychotic reactions	
Adrenal insufficiency (after steroid withdrawal) manifested by peripheral circulatory collapse – in upright position	Administer hydrocortisone promptly (intravenously)
	The following day give steroid replacement

Advice for patients on long-term steroids

1. Recognize that steroids are valuable and useful medications but if taken longer than two weeks, they may produce certain side-effects.
2. 'Acceptable' side-effects may include weight gain (perhaps due to water retention), acne, headaches, fatigue and increased urinary frequency (see above).
3. 'Unacceptable' side-effects which are to be reported to the doctor: dizziness when rising from chair or bed (postural hypotension indicative of adrenal insufficiency), nausea, vomiting, thirst, abdominal pain or pain of any type (see above).
4. Additional side-effects which are reportable are: convulsive seizures, feelings of depression or nervousness or development of an infection (see above).
5. If the patient has a fall or is in a road traffic

accident, his condition may precipitate adrenal failure. He requires an immediate injection of hydrocortisone phosphate. (Long-term patients should wear an identification bracelet and carry hydrocortisone.)

6. See doctor on a regular follow-up basis.

NURSING MANAGEMENT OF PATIENTS RECEIVING STEROID THERAPY

1. Know the routes by which steroids are given.
   a. Ascertain advantages of the method chosen for the particular patient.
   b. Determine what is expected of the medication in a particular situation.
   c. Be informed about side-effects and untoward manifestations.
   d. **Note:**
      (i) Local application of steroid medications to the skin (to a large area, over a prolonged period, using occlusive dressings) leads to adrenal suppression.
      (ii) Local administration to the eye over a prolonged period leads to increased eye pressure, corneal ulceration.
   e. Recognize that it is necessary to understand pharmacological action of a particular steroid before planning the scheduled doses. Be aware of the following:
      (i) How frequently it can be given.
      (ii) How late in the day it may be administered.
      (iii) Whether every other day is sufficient, etc.

   Patients on intermittent therapy have few side-effects.
2. Be aware of the problems encountered during periods when steroids are being withdrawn or lowered in dosage.
   a. Associate symptoms of tiredness, muscular weakness and lethargy with drug withdrawal.
   b. Report any stress situations during this time, such as surgery, a family crisis, etc.
   c. Instruct the patient why it may be necessary to save all urine for 24 hours (for determination of 11-hydroxycorticosteroid level).
3. Monitor carefully the patient who is on intravenous corticosteroid therapy.
   a. Determine the flow rate of fluids necessary to give a precise amount of medication.
   b. Observe the tissues, catheter site, flow rate, fluid level and patient's response at frequent intervals to be sure the system is functioning well.
   c. Note signs and symptoms indicative of adrenal crisis – restlessness, weakness, headache, nausea, vomiting, diarrhoea and falling blood pressure.

PATIENT EDUCATION

1. Be sure the patient or a responsible member of his family knows that he is taking a steroid medication; explain why he is receiving it and what effects are desired.
2. The patient must also know what complications can occur, how to prevent them and what to do should they occur.
3. Inform patient of the need for him to tell any doctor, dentist or nurse in his future contacts that he is on steroid therapy.
4. Be sure he knows that steroids are unique drugs prescribed in a dosage specific for him and that no one else should use his medications.

GUIDELINES: THE PATIENT RECEIVING STEROID THERAPY – CLINICAL ASSESSMENT, SURVEILLANCE AND PATIENT EDUCATION

Objective
Detect early signs of side-effects from steroid therapy.

Infection control

Nursing action	Rationale
1. Encourage patient to avoid crowds and the possibility of exposure to infection.	Because steroids may affect the circulating blood – resulting in decreased eosinophils and lymphocytes, increased red cells and increased incidence of thrombophlebitis and infection.

2. Utilize exercise schedules to prevent stasis.

3. Be aware that cardinal symptoms of inflammation may be masked.

4. Instruct everyone coming in contact with this patient to wash hands thoroughly and practise meticulous asepsis.

Diet and metabolism considerations

Nursing action	Rationale
1. Determine whether the patient needs assistance in dietary control.	Because steroids may cause weight gain and an increase in appetite.
2. Administer a high-protein, high-carbohydrate diet.	Because steroids affect protein metabolism, there may be negative nitrogen balance.
3. Encourage patient to take steroids with milk or food.	Because steroids cause an increase in secretion of gastric hydrochloric acid and have an inhibiting effect on secretion of mucus in the stomach, they may aggravate an existing peptic ulcer.
4. Be on guard for early evidence of gastric haemorrhage such as melaena, blood in vomitus.	
5. Check urine for evidence of glucose.	Because steroids precipitate gluconeogenesis and insulin antagonism, which results in hyperglycaemia, glycosuria, decreased carbohydrate tolerance.

Possible bone complications

Nursing action	Rationale
1. Be on the alert for the possibility of pathological fractures. Stress safety measures to prevent injury.	Because steroids affect the musculoskeletal system, causing potassium depletion and muscular weakness. (Steroids cause increased output of calcium and phosphorus, which leads to osteoporosis.)
2. Administer a diet high in calcium and protein.	
3. Recommend a programme of activities of daily living, normal range of movement for the bedridden.	

Electrolyte disturbance

Nursing action	Rationale
1. Restrict sodium intake and increase potassium intake. a. Lemon juice is high in potassium and low in sodium. b. Avoid saline as a diluent in preparing injectable medications.	Because mineralocorticoid differs from other steroids, resulting in sodium retention and potassium depletion: oedema, weight gain.

2. Check blood pressure frequently and weigh patient daily.

3. Observe for evidence of oedema.

Behavioural reactions

Nursing action

1. Watch for convulsive seizures (especially in children).

2. Avoid overstimulating situations.

3. Recognize and report any mood deviating from the usual behaviour patterns.

4. Report unusual behaviour, haunting dreams, withdrawal or suicidal tendencies.

Rationale

Because steroids may alter behaviour patterns, increase excitability and affect the central nervous system.

Stress reactions

Nursing action

1. Recommend that the patient carry at all times an identification card indicating that he is on steroid therapy and including the name of his doctor and hospital and instructions for emergency care.

2. Advice patient to avoid extremes of temperature, as well as infections and upsetting situations.

Rationale

Because steroids affect the hypothalmic–pituitary–adrenal system, this in turn affects the individual's ability to respond to stress.

Safety measures

Nursing action

1. Instruct the patient to avoid injury; stress safety precautions.

2. Observe daily the healing process of wounds, particularly surgical wounds, in order to recognize the potential for wound dehiscence.

Rationale

Because steroids interfere with fibroblasts and granulation tissue, there is altered response to injury, resulting in impaired growth and delayed healing.

THE PITUITARY

The pituitary gland is called the master gland of the endocrine system because it controls hormone pro-duction of the other endocrine glands. It lies in the sella turcica at the base of the brain and is connected to the hypothalamus by the hypophyseal (pituitary) stalk.

1. *Anterior lobe* – produces at least seven hormones, six of which primarily affect the other endocrine glands and also control the posterior lobe.

2. *Posterior lobe* – believed to be responsible for storage of the antidiuretic, oxytocic and vasopressor hormones produced in the hypothalamus.

DISORDERS OF THE PITUITARY

HYPERPITUITARISM

Hyperpituitarism results from an excessive amount of growth hormone secreted by the pituitary gland.

PREDISPOSING FACTORS
1. Overactivity of the eosinophilic portion of the anterior lobe of the pituitary.
2. Effects of a benign adenoma (tumour).

TYPES OF HYPERPITUITARISM
Gigantism
Hyperfunction of the pituitary, causing a generalized increase in size, particularly in the long bones of children before the epiphyseal lines close.

Acromegaly
1. Excessive secretion of growth hormone after epiphyseal closure, causing a chronic disease characterized by enlargement of bone, cartilage and soft tissues of the body.
2. Causes:
   a. Increase in size and function of a portion of the anterior lobe of the pituitary gland.
   b. Eosinophilic tumour of the pituitary gland.

HYPOPITUITARISM (SIMMONDS' DISEASE, PITUITARY CACHEXIA)

Hypopituitarism is pituitary insufficiency resulting from destruction of the anterior lobe of the pituitary gland.

Panhypopituitarism (Simmonds' disease) is total absence of all pituitary secretions.

CLINICAL FEATURES
1. Extreme weight loss.
2. Atrophy of all organs.
3. Loss of hair.
4. Impotence; amenorrhoea.
5. Hypometabolism; hypoglycaemia.
6. Coma; death.

CAUSE
Total destruction of the anterior lobe of the pituitary by trauma, tumour, haemorrhage.

DIABETES INSIPIDUS

Diabetes insipidus is a disorder of water metabolism caused by deficiency of vasopressin, the antidiuretic hormone (ADH) secreted by the posterior pituitary.

AETIOLOGY
1. Primary cause is unknown.
2. Secondary causes – head trauma, neoplasm, surgical removal or irradiation of pituitary gland.

CLINICAL FEATURES
1. Marked polyuria – daily output of 5–25 litres of very dilute urine; appearance of urine like that of water, with a specific gravity of 1.001–1.005.
2. Polydipsia (intense thirst); 4–40 litres of fluid daily; patient has a craving for cold water.

DIAGNOSTIC EVALUATION
Fluid deprivation test.

Objective
Restrict water intake and observe changes in urine volume and concentration.
1. Fluids withheld for eight to 12 hours or until 3 per cent of body weight is lost.
2. Plasma and urine osmolality studies are determined at beginning, during and end of test – inability to increase specific gravity and osmolality of urine is characteristic of diabetes insipidus.

TREATMENT AND NURSING MANAGEMENT
Objectives
Replace vasopressin (usually a lifelong therapeutic programme).
Search for and correct underlying intracranial pathology.
1. Give prescribed antidiuretic hormone, vasopressin tannate (Pitressin tannate) – reduces urinary volume for 24 to 48 hours.
   a. Warm vial – medication is in oil and warming makes administration easier.
   b. Shake bottle vigorously before administering drug – active hormone settles to the bottom of the oil.
   c. Give in evening – maximum results obtained during sleep – or
2. Give prescribed vasopressin by topical application to the nasal mucosa (lypressin nasal spray [Syntopressin]) – drug absorbed through the nasal mucosa into the blood.

a. Nasal insufflation administered by one or two sprays in each nostril as directed.

b. Watch for chronic rhinopharyngitis.

3. Administer prescribed chlorpropamide (Diabinese) – reduces urine volume.

a. May be used as an antidiuretic in *mild* cases to potentiate action of vasopressin.

b. Warn the patient of possible hypoglycaemic reactions.

4. Weigh patient frequently.

5. Support the patient undergoing studies for a cranial lesion (see Chapter 16, Care of the Patient with a Neurological Disorder).

PITUITARY TUMOURS

TYPES OF PITUITARY TUMOUR

1. *Chromophobe adenoma* – tumour of the anterior pituitary gland of adults.

a. Comprises 90 per cent of pituitary tumours; produces no hormones but can destroy rest of pituitary gland.

b. Produces failing vision, optic atrophy, bilateral hemianopia, enlargement of sella turcica and endocrine disturbances.

2. *Eosinophilic adenoma* – endocrine secretion of tumour produces gigantism in children and acromegaly in adults.

3. *Basophilic adenoma* – gives rise to so-called Cushing's syndrome with features largely attributable to hyperadrenalism – masculinization and amenorrhoea in females, girdle obesity, hypertension, osteoporosis and polycythaemia.

HYPOPHYSECTOMY

Hypophysectomy is removal of the pituitary gland.

INDICATIONS

1. Primary neoplasms (tumours) of the pituitary gland.

2. Diabetic retinopathy.

a. Used to halt progress of haemorrhagic diabetic retinopathy and to prevent blindness.

b. Also reduces insulin requirements.

3. Palliative measure for relief of bone pain secondary to metastasis of malignant lesions of breast and prostate; alters hormonal milieu of body to create a hormonal environment hostile to continued growth of neoplasm.

METHODS OF PITUITARY ABLATION (REMOVAL)

1. Extirpative hypophysectomy – done by transfrontal, subcranial or transsphenoidal approaches.

2. Hypophyseal stalk section.

3. Implantation of radioactive yttrium.

4. Radiation X-ray – proton irradiation from a cyclotron.

5. Destruction with cryosurgery (freezing).

TREATMENT AND NURSING MANAGEMENT

The absence of the pituitary gland alters the function of many parts of the body.

1. The patient may need substitution therapy with adrenal steroids (hydrocortisone) and thyroid hormone.

2. Menstruation ceases and infertility occurs almost always after total or nearly total ablation (removal).

3. See p. 582 for treatment of diabetes insipidus.

4. See Chapter 16, Care of the Patient with a Neurological Disorder, for nursing management of the patient undergoing intracranial surgery, p. 931.

DISORDERS OF PURINE METABOLISM

GOUT

Gout is a disease caused by excessive accumulation of uric acid in the blood and eventual deposition of uric acid crystals in various tissues.

1. *Uric acid* – end produce of purine metabolism.

2. *Hyperuricaemia* – persistent elevation of urates in the blood.

3. *Tophi* – deposits of urates in the tissues about the joints or on the ear; development of tophi related to duration of disease, degree of hyperuricaemia and renal function status.

UNDERLYING CONSIDERATIONS

1. Hereditary factor present – mode of genetic transmission not established.

2. Males are predominantly affected; peak incidence between 30 and 50 years.

3. Potential inciting agents – rich food, overindulgence in alcohol, physical and emotional stress, acute infection – may contribute to temporary disorganization of homeostatic mechanisms

of body as well as bring about factors that alter uric acid level in body.

TYPES OF GOUT

1. *Primary* – basic problem appears to be a genetic defect in purine metabolism.
2. *Secondary* – hyperuricaemia is produced by increasing breakdown of nucleic acids in certain diseases (such as blood dyscrasias) or because of interference with renal excretion.

May be precipitated by prolonged ingestion of diuretic agents, trauma, treatment of myeloproliferative diseases.

CLINICAL FEATURES

1. Sudden onset of severe pain in one or more peripheral joints – may be accompanied by intense inflammation, swelling and tenderness.
   a. First joint of great toe is susceptible; later, other joints of foot are affected.
   b. Joints of feet, ankles, knees, wrist and elbow commonly affected.
2. Fever 38.3–39.4°C.
3. Attacks involving the same joints tend to recur; variable lengths of time between attacks.

DIAGNOSTIC EVALUATION

1. Sudden attack of severe pain in one or more peripheral joints in a previously healthy male.
2. Therapeutic response to full course of colchicine.
3. Elevation of serum uric acid.
4. Identification of uric acid crystals in synovial fluid – obtained by arthrocentesis (aspiration of fluid from a joint cavity).
5. Elevated erythrocyte sedimentation rate (ESR) and white blood count – in acute attack.
6. X-ray findings – presence of tophi and radiographic evidence of urate deposits in bone (late manifestations).
7. Other diagnostic features:
   a. Positive family history for gout.
   b. Unexplained proteinuria and hypertension.
   c. Passage of renal stones.
   d. Patient taking thiazide for non-gouty conditions.

TREATMENT AND NURSING MANAGEMENT
Objectives
Relieve acute discomfort.
Prevent the development of chronic gouty arthritis, renal calculi and renal damage.

Acute attack of gout
1. Colchicine given *early* in attack – suppresses in-flammatory manifestations of acute gout; useful in establishing diagnosis since it gives dramatic relief if patient has gout.
   a. An initial dose of colchicine is given and is followed by doses every two to three hours until the pain disappears and gastrointestinal symptoms develop (nausea, vomiting, abdominal cramping, diarrhoea).
   b. Colchicine produces diarrhoea – stop drug temporarily until diarrhoea subsides. Give prescribed medication to relieve diarrhoea.
   c. A maintenance dose of colchicine is given as soon as diarrhoea stops as a prophylactic agent against recurrent gouty arthritis.
   d. Colchicine may be given before and after surgery to patients with gout – reduces the incidence of acute attacks of gouty arthritis precipitated by operative procedures.
2. Alternative forms of therapy:
   a. Phenylbutazone (Butazolidin) or oxyphenbutazone or indomethacin (Indocid) are other drugs given during the acute stage of gout – these drugs reduce the fever and have an anti-inflammatory effect.
   b. Give these drugs as prescribed with meals or with milk since they are ulcerogenic.
3. Give prescribed analgesic for severe pain until specific drug is effective.
4. Encourage the patient to stay on bed rest for 24 hours after acute attack – early ambulation may precipitate a recurrence.
5. Advise the patient to avoid high purine foods (Table 8.4).
6. Encourage large fluid intake to maintain a high 24-hour urinary volume – urinary urate excretion increases 24 hours after introduction of uricosuric drugs and may lead to stone formation.

Chronic gouty arthritis
1. Give prescribed drug (uricosuric agent) – acts on renal tubule to inhibit urate reabsorption and thereby increases urinary excretion of urate and lowers the serum urate level; prevents formation of new tophi and reduces size of those already present. *Purines* are derived from ingested food and from the breakdown of body proteins. Purines are also synthesized in the liver. A low purine diet is seldom used but it is advocated that patients with high blood uric acid levels avoid foods highest in purine content and also avoid alcohol.
   a. Probenecid (Benemid).
      Side-effects – headache, gastrointestinal disturbances, skin rash.

Table 8.4   Low purine diet.* Purines are derived from ingested food and from the breakdown of body proteins; they are also synthesized in the liver. A low-purine diet is seldom used but it is advocated that patients with high blood uric acid levels avoid foods highest in purine content and also avoid alcohol.

Foods highest in purines	Foods high in purines	Foods lowest in purines
Sweetbreads	Meat	Fruits
Anchovies	Poultry	Vegetables (except those listed)
Sardines in oil	Fish	Most breads, cereals and cereal products
Liver (calf, beef)	Lobster, crabs, oysters	Milk
Kidneys	Meat soups and broth	Cheese
Meat extracts	Beans, dried	Eggs
Gravy	Peas, dried	Fish roe
	Lentils, dried	Nuts
	Spinach	Fats
	Oatmeal	Sugars, syrups, sweets
	Wheatgerm and bran	Gelatin
		Milk and fruit desserts
		Vegetable and cream soups

* Foods listed from Church, C.F. and Church, H.N. (1975) *Food Values of Portions Commonly Used* (12th edn), J.B. Lippincott, Philadelphia.

   b. Sulphinpyrazone (Anturan).
     Side-effects – gastrointestinal disturbances (including peptic ulcer), skin rash, haematological side-effects.
   c. Give after meals or with antacids if there are gastric side-effects.
2. Or give prescribed allopurinol (Zyloric), a xanthine oxidase inhibitor – interferes with final stages of conversion of the products of purine metabolism to uric acid (inhibits formation of uric acid). Dosage based on serum urate determinations.
3. Encourage large fluid intake to maintain a high 24-hour urinary volume – urinary urate excretion increases 24 hours after introduction of uricosuric drugs and may lead to stone formation.
   a. Maintain an alkaline urine in patients with a history of stone formation.
   b. Give prescribed sodium bicarbonate or citrate solutions.

PATIENT EDUCATION
Instruct the patient as follows:
1. Take colchicine as prescribed as a prophylactic measure against acute attack.
2. Take uricosuric agent (see above) or allopurinol – to prevent further deposition of uric acid in joints. Colchicine and uricosuric agents may be given in combination for indefinite periods of time.

3. Avoid specific foods (or alcohol) known to precipitate an attack (see Table 8.4).
4. Maintain a high fluid intake to maintain high urinary volume – minimizes urate precipitation in urinary tract.
5. Avoid fasting (to lose weight or when on alcoholic spree) – fasting has been found to increase the serum uric acid level.
6. Avoid crash diets – rapid reduction of weight may increase the serum uric acid level; slow weight reduction reduces the serum urate level without inducing an acute attack.
7. Recognize the warnings of an impending attack. Start therapy promptly.

FURTHER READING

BOOKS

Anderson, J.W. (reprinted 1983) *Diabetes. A Practical New Guide to Healthy Living*, Martin Dunitz, London.

Anthony, G. *et al.* (1985) *The Patient with an Endocrine Disorder*, Harper and Row, London.

Baylis, R.I.S. (1982) *Thyroid Disease: The Facts*, Oxford University Press.

Bloom, A. (1982) *Diabetes Explained* (4th edn), MTP Press, Lancaster.

Kinson, J. and Nattrass, M. (1984) *Caring for the Diabetic Patient*, Churchill Livingstone, Edinburgh.

Laycock, J. and Wise, P. (1983) *Essential Endocrinology* (2nd edn), Oxford University Press.

Lewis, J.G. (1984) *The Endocrine System*, Churchill Livingstone, Edinburgh.

Sonksen, P., Fox, C. and Judd, S. (1985) *The Diabetes Reference Book*, Harper and Row, London.

ARTICLES

Adrenal gland

Editorial (1983) Clinical insight: Cushing's syndrome, *Nursing Mirror*, Vol. 157, No. 4, p. 105.

O'Daniel, L.G. (1983) The adrenal gland and the use of cortisone in the management of patients with Addison's disease and Cushing's syndrome, *American Association of Nurse Anaesthetists*, Vol. 51, No. 1, pp. 31–7.

O'Donnell-O'Toole, S. (1985) Adrenoleukodystrophy – a fatal disorder with new opportunities for prevention and treatment, *Journal of Neurosurgical Nursing*, Vol. 17, No. 1, pp. 53–60.

Waide, R. and Ladson, I. (1986) All we could do was to help him live with dignity (patient with adrenoleukodystrophy, an hereditary degenerative disease of the adrenal glands and nervous system), *RN*, September, pp. 55–7, 59.

Diabetes

Armstrong, N. (1983) Critical elements of diabetes education in the workplace, *Occupational Health Nursing*, Vol. 30, No. 12, pp. 19–24.

Bateup, L. (1985) Helping a patient understand diabetes, *Nursing Times*, Vol. 82, No. 12, pp. 46–9.

Craddock, S. (1985) Highlights of change, *British Journal of Nursing*, Vol. 5, No. 6, pp. 10–12.

Devlin, R. (1986) Injecting confidence, *Community Outlook, Nursing Times*, Vol. 82, No. 2, pp. 15–17.

Dinsdale, C. and Cochrane, W. (1986) The changing face of treatment for diabetes, *Nursing Times*, Vol. 82, No. 7, pp. 46–9.

Fow, S.M. (1983) Home blood glucose monitoring in children with insulin-dependent diabetes mellitus, *Pediatric Nursing*, Vol. 9, No. 6, pp. 439–42.

Frost, C.J. and Caiger, P. (1984) Diabetes in childhood: management update, *Midwife, Health Visitor, Community Nurse*, Vol. 20, No. 5, pp. 148, 150, 152, 156.

Gill, G. (1985) Community care of diabetics, *Primary Health Care*, Vol. 3, No. 5, pp. 10–12.

Ginsburg, J. and Fink, R.S. (1983) Diabetes mellitus. *Nursing*, Vol. 2, No. 13, pp. 369–70, 374–8.

Hilton, A. (1986) Nursing practice. Monitoring blood glucose levels, *Nursing Times*, Vol. 82, No. 18, pp. 55–6.

Ho, E. (1984) Diabetes mellitus in pregnancy, *Nursing Mirror*, Vol. 158, No. 8, pp. 37–8.

Hutchinson, A. and Pooley, J. (1985) Diabetic control in adolescents, *Nursing Mirror*, Vol. 161, No. 30, pp. 26–7.

Medows, S. and Trewick, A. (1984) Diabetes 1: insulin without tears (use of insulin pump), *Nursing Times*, Vol. 80, No. 34, pp. 40–2.

Noakes, B. (1984) Diabetes 3: helping diabetics help themselves (work of the British Diabetic Association), *Nursing Times*, Vol. 80, No. 36, 46, 48.

Robinson, G.E. (1985) Diabetes in pregnancy, *Midwife, Health Visitor and Community Nurse*, Vol. 21, No. 6, pp. 196–7, 200.

Shuldham, C. (1985) Diabetic ketoacidosis – an endocrine emergency, *Nursing*, Vol. 2, No. 42, pp. 1246–9.

Thurston, R. and Beattie, C. (1984) Diabetes 2: foot lesions in diabetics, *Nursing Times*, Vol. 80, No. 34, pp. 44–6, 48–50.

Tredger, J. (1983) Trends in the dietary management of diabetics, *Nursing*, Vol. 2, No. 14, pp. 395–6.

Overview

Harris, G. (1983) The endocrine system, *Nursing*, Vol. 2, No. 13, pp. 359–60, 362.

Maxwell, M. (1983) The endocrine system, *Nursing Mirror*, Vol. 157, No. 5, pp. 23–8.

Pituitary

Volner, J.S. (1983) Endocrine dysfunction associated with pituitary surgery, *Journal of Neurosurgical Nursing*, Vol. 15, No. 6, pp. 325–31.

Disorders of the thyroid gland

Coody, D. (1984) Congenital hypothyroidism, *Pediatric Nursing*, Vol. 10, No. 5, pp. 342–5.

Editorial (1983) Clinical insight: Graves' disease (hyperthyroidism), *Nursing Mirror*, Vol. 157, No. 27, p. 101.

Gever, L.N. (1984) Understanding and teaching thyroid hormone therapy, *Nursing*, Vol. 14, No. 8, p. 4.

Payne, N.R. (1986) Emergency care of the patients with myxodema coma, *Journal of Emergency Nursing*, Vol. 12, No. 6, pp. 343–7.

Ryan, A. (1986) Thyroidectomy, *Irish Nursing Forum*, Vol. 3, No. 1, Spring, pp. 10–12.

Vogal, P. (1986) Lithium and the thyroid, *Journal of Psychosocial Nursing and Mental Health Services*, Vol. 24, No. 2, pp. 9–14.

9

Care of the Patient with a Renal or Genitourinary Disorder

ASSESSMENT OF UROLOGICAL FUNCTION

PATIENT HISTORY

Seek the following information related to urinary and renal function:

1. What is the patient's chief concern? Why is he seeking help?
2. What is (are) the patient's present and past occupation(s)? (Look for occupational hazards related to the urinary tract – contact with chemicals, plastics, pitch, tar, rubber.)
3. What is the patient's smoking history?
4. What is the past history, especially in relation to urinary problems?
5. Is there any family history of renal disease?
6. What childhood diseases did the patient have?
7. Is there a history of urinary infections?
8. Did enuresis continue beyond the usual age (past three years of age)?
9. Are there any voiding of urine disorders?
   a. Dysuria? When does it occur? Where is it felt? Initial or terminal dysuria?
   b. Hesitancy? Straining? Pain during or after urination?
   c. Changes in colour of urine? Diminished urine output?
   d. Incontinence? Stress incontinence? Urgency incontinence?
   e. Any history of haematuria?
   f. How often does the patient get up to void urine during the night? How much urine is passed?
10. Is pain present? Location? Character? Radiation? Duration? Related to voiding? What brings it on? What relieves it?
11. Has the patient had fever? Chills? Passage of stones?
12. Any history of genital lesions or sexually transmitted diseases?
13. For the female patient:
    What is the number of children? Their ages? Any forceps deliveries? Catheterizations? When? Any signs of vaginal discharge? Vaginal/vulvar itch or irritation?
14. Does the patient have diabetes mellitus? Hypertension? Allergies?
15. Has the patient ever been hospitalized with a urinary tract infection? Urinary tract infection before the age of 12? Ever cystoscoped? Catheterized with an indwelling catheter? Kidney X-ray procedures?

CLINICAL FEATURES OF URINARY DYSFUNCTION

CHANGES IN MICTURITION (VOIDING)

1. Haematuria (red blood cells in urine):
   a. Haematuria is considered a serious sign and requires assessment.
   b. Colour of bloody urine dependent on pH of urine and amount of blood present:
      (i) Acid urine is dark, smoky colour.
      (ii) Alkaline urine is red colour.
   c. Haematuria may be due to systemic cause such as blood dyscrasias, anticoagulant therapy, neoplasms, trauma, extreme exercise.
   d. Painless haematuria may indicate neoplasm in the urinary tract.
   e. Haematuria from renal colic (stones in kidney).
   f. Bloody spotting reveals bleeding from urethra, bladder neoplasms.
   g. Haematuria also seen in renal tuberculosis, polycystic disease of kidneys, septic pyelonephritis, thrombosis and embolism involving renal artery or vein.
2. Proteinuria (albuminuria):
   a. Normal urine does not contain persistent protein in significant quantities.
   b. Proteinuria characteristically seen in all forms of acute and chronic renal disease (more characteristic of glomerulonephritis than pyelonephritis).
      (i) The protein is mainly albumin, but globulin is also present.
      (ii) Albumin and globulin escape through damaged glomerular capillaries in a greater amount than can be reabsorbed by the tubules, or damaged tubules fail to reabsorb normal amount filtered.
   c. Proteinuria occurs in systemic diseases where there are varying degrees of renal anoxia, as in cardiac decompensation, diabetic glomerulosclerosis.
   d. Mild proteinuria may occur from other sources – urethritis, prostatitis, cystitis.
3. Dysuria (painful or difficult voiding) – seen in a wide variety of pathological conditions.

4. Frequency – voiding of urine occurs more often than usual, when compared with the patient's usual pattern (or with a generally accepted norm of once every three to six hours).
   a. Determine if habits governing fluid intake have been altered; it is essential to know normal voiding pattern in order to assess frequency.
   b. Increasing frequency can result from a variety of conditions – such as infection and diseases of urinary tract, metabolic disease, hypertension, medications (diuretics).
5. Urgency (strong desire to urinate) – due to inflammatory lesions in bladder, prostate or urethra, acute bacterial infections, chronic prostatitis in men and chronic posterior urethrotrigonitis in women.
6. Burning upon urination – seen in urethral irritation or bladder infections.
7. Pneumaturia (passage of gas in urine during voiding) – caused by fistulous connection between bowel and bladder, rectosigmoid cancer, regional ileitis, sigmoid diverticulitis (most common) and gas-forming urinary tract infections.
8. Strangury (slow and painful urination); only small amounts of urine voided; blood staining may be noted – seen in severe cystitis.
9. Hesitancy (undue delay and difficulty in initiating voiding) – may indicate compression of urethra, outlet obstruction, neurogenic bladder.
10. Nocturia (excessive urination at night) – suggests decreased renal concentrating ability or heart failure, diabetes mellitus, poor bladder emptying.
11. Urinary incontinence (involuntary loss of urine) – may be due to injury to external urinary sphincter, acquired neurogenic disease, severe urgency, etc.
12. Stress incontinence (intermittent leakage of urine due to sudden strain) – indicates weakness of sphincteric mechanism.
13. Polyuria (large volume of urine voided in given time) – demonstrated in diabetes mellitus, diabetes insipidus.
14. Oliguria (small volume of urine; output between 100–500ml/24 hours) – may result from acute renal failure, shock, dehydration, fluid–ion imbalance.
15. Anuria (absence of urine in the bladder; output less than 50ml/24 hours) – indicates serious renal dysfunction requiring immediate medical intervention.
16. Enuresis (involuntary voiding during sleep) – may be physiological up to the age of three years; thereafter, may be functional or symptomatic of obstructive disease (usually of lower urinary tract).

URINARY TRACT PAIN
1. Genitourinary pain is not always present in renal disease, but is generally seen in the more acute conditions.
2. Pain of renal disease is caused by sudden distension of the renal capsule; severity is related to how quickly the distension develops.
3. Kidney pain – may be felt as a dull ache in costovertebral angle; may spread to umbilicus.
4. Ureteral pain – felt in the back and radiates to the abdomen, upper thighs, testes or labia.
5. Flank pain (side area between ribs and ilium) – radiates to lower abdomen or epigastrium and often is associated with nausea, vomiting and paralytic ileus; most commonly secondary to a renal lesion (stone, tumour or infection).
6. Bladder pain (low abdominal pain or pain over suprapubic area) – may be due to bladder infection or overdistended bladder.
7. Urethral pain from irritation of bladder neck, from foreign body in canal, or from urethritis due to infection or trauma.
8. Pain in scrotal area from inflammatory swelling of epididymis or testicle, or torsion of the testicle.
9. Testicular pain due to injury, mumps orchitis, torsion of spermatic cord.
10. Perineal or rectal discomfort from acute prostatitis, prostatic abscess.
11. Back and leg pain from cancer of prostate with metastases to pelvic bones.
12. Pain in glans penis is usually from prostatitis; penile shaft pain is from urethral problems.

RELATED GASTROINTESTINAL SYMPTOMS
Gastrointestinal symptoms related to urological conditions include nausea, vomiting, diarrhoea, abdominal discomfort, paralytic ileus and gastrointestinal haemorrhage with uraemia.

DIAGNOSTIC TESTS

RADIOLOGICAL TECHNIQUES
X-rays
Flat plate, X-ray of kidney, ureters, bladder is used to delineate size, shape and position of kidneys, but includes organs up to the level of symphysis pubis.
1. Gives a baseline reference for subsequent films.
2. Reveals any deviations, such as stones, hydro-

nephrosis, cysts, tumours or kidney displacement by abnormalities in the surrounding tissues.

Computed tomography
This provides a cross-sectional view of kidney and urinary tract to detect the presence and extent of urological disease; a computer measures small changes in X-ray absorption and magnifies the differences from tissue to tissue so a display can be made and read. No preparation needed; non-invasive.

Nephrotomogram
Body section X-rays which bring into focus the different layers of the kidney and the diffuse structures in that layer; carried out also as part of intravenous pyelogram study.

Excretory urography
Intravenous urogram [IVU] or intravenous pyelogram [IVP] – introduction (IV) of a radio-opaque contrast medium, which concentrates in the urine and thus facilitates visualization of the kidneys, ureter and bladder. The contrast medium is cleared from the bloodstream by renal excretion.
1. Excretory urography is used in the following:
   a. Initial investigation of any suspected urological problem, especially in diagnosis of lesions in kidneys and ureters.
   b. To provide a rough estimate of renal function.
2. Patient preparation:
   a. See that the patient is not overhydrated – will dilute contrast material and thus cause inadequate visualization (except in patients with myeloma).
   b. Remove obstructing intestinal content, if possible, to minimize intestinal gas; enema not usually given, since it may increase gas in the gastrointestinal tract.
   c. It is customary to take no liquids for eight to ten hours before this test, although good films are often obtained in the hydrated patient.

NURSING ALERT
Elderly patients with poor renal reserve or those with multiple myeloma may not tolerate dehydrating procedures and should be given water to drink. People with uncontrolled diabetes may be sensitive to fluid restriction.

   d. Give laxative the night before the test to eliminate faeces and gas in the intestinal tract.
   e. Ascertain if the patient has history of allergies – to find the high-risk patient.
   See p. 784.

Retrograde pyelography
Injection of opaque material through ureteral catheters, which have been passed up ureters into renal pelvis by means of cystoscopic manipulation. The opaque solution is introduced by gravity or syringe.
1. Retrograde pyelography usually done when nonfunctioning kidney is suspected or if the patient is allergic to intravenous contrast material.
2. Performed with decreasing frequency because of improvement of IVP techniques.

Renal angiography
Visualization of renal arterial supply. Contrast medium is injected through a catheter (which is placed under fluoroscope control) via the femoral and iliac arteries into the aorta or renal artery.
1. Angiography assesses blood flow dynamics, demonstrates abnormal vasculature and differentiates renal cysts from renal tumours.
2. *Nursing responsibilities before procedure:*
   a. Give aperient or enema as prescribed to eliminate faecal material and gas from colon and to ensure unobstructed radiographs.
   b. Prepare proposed injection sites – groin (for femoral approach) or axilla (for axillary approach).
   c. Locate and mark peripheral pulses to facilitate postprocedure nursing assessment.
   d. Inform the patient what to expect during procedure:
      (i) Procedure is done under local anaesthesia; the patient will probably be given preoperative medication.
      (ii) The procedure may take from 30 minutes to two hours.
      (iii) There may be a transient feeling of heat along the course of the vessel upon injection of contrast material.
3. *Nursing responsibilities following procedure:*
   a. Take vital signs until stabilized; take blood pressure readings on opposite arm if axillary artery was punctured.
   b. Assess puncture site for swelling and development of haematoma.
   c. Palpate peripheral pulses (radial, femoral, dorsalis pedis).
   d. Note colour and temperature of involved extremity, comparing it with the uninvolved extremity.
   e. Apply cold compresses to puncture site – to decrease oedema and pain.

Radionuclide techniques
These are non-invasive procedures that do not inter-

fere with normal physiological processes and require no specific patient preparation.
1. Radioactive isotopes are injected intravenously.
2. Studies obtained with a scintillation camera placed posterior to the kidney with the patient in a supine, prone or sitting position.
3. The resultant image (scan) indicates the distribution of the radioactive isotopes within the kidney.

Ultrasonic scan (echogram, sonography)

Scanning by ultrasound is a non-invasive technique for investigation of renal disease. The kidneys produce a characteristic ultrasonic pattern, making abnormalities readily identifiable. Also used in assessing retroperitoneal disease and in staging malignancies of urinary tract bladder and prostate. Non-invasive test; no special patient preparation is necessary.

UROLOGICAL ENDOSCOPIC PROCEDURES

Cystoscopic examination

Involves direct visualization of the urethra, prostatic urethra and bladder by means of a tubular, lighted, telescopic lens.
1. *Uses:*
   a. To inspect bladder wall directly for tumour, stone or ulcer and to inspect urethra, especially the prostatic urethra prior to surgery.
   b. To allow insertion of catheters into the ureters to obtain a separate specimen from each kidney and evaluate renal function separately.
   c. To see configuration and position of ureteral orifices.
   d. To remove calculi from urethra, bladder and ureter.
   e. To treat lesions of bladder, urethra and prostate.
2. *Patient preparation:*
   a. Preparation depends on type of anaesthesia to be used (general or local).
   b. Give information about the examination, prescribed oral fluids and preoperative medication.
3. *Nursing support following procedure:*
   a. Expect the patient to have some burning upon voiding of blood-tinged urine and urinary frequency from trauma to mucous membrane.
   b. Watch patients with prostatic hypertrophy for urinary retention due to oedema from instrumentation.
   c. If the patient complains of pain, give warm baths.
   d. Use indwelling catheter if urinary retention persists.

4. *Complications following cystoscopy:*
   (More apt to occur in patients with obstructive pathology.)
   a. Urinary retention
   b. Urinary tract haemorrhage
   c. Infection within prostate or bladder

Renal and ureteral brush biopsy

Introduction of catheter followed by a biopsy brush, which is passed through the catheter; suspected lesion is brushed back and forth to obtain cells and surface tissue fragments for histology.

Renal endoscopy, nephroscopy

Introduction of fibreoptic scope into the renal pelvis during an open renal operation (pyelotomy) or percutaneously to view interior of renal pelvis, remove calculi, biopsy small lesions and diagnose renal haematuria and selected renal tumours.

NEEDLE BIOPSY OF KIDNEY

Needle biopsy of the kidney is performed by percutaneous needle biopsy through renal tissue (Figure 9.1) or by open biopsy through a small flank incision. It is useful in evaluating the course of renal disease and in securing specimens for electron and immunofluorescent microscopy.

Prebiopsy management

1. Coagulation studies are carried out to identify the patient at risk for postbiopsy bleeding; serum creatinine and urinalysis are done.
2. The patient may be placed on a fasting regimen for three hours before the procedure. An intravenous line may be established.
3. Secure and save a voided specimen of urine before biopsy – for comparison with postbiopsy specimen.
4. Instruct the patient that he may be asked to hold his breath (to stop movement of the kidney) while the biopsy needle is inserted.

Postbiopsy nursing management
Objective

Observe the patient for evidences of bleeding.
1. Keep the patient supine as long as directed.
2. Take the vital signs every five to fifteen minutes for first hour, and then with decreasing frequency if stable to assess for haemorrhage, which is a major complication.
   a. Watch for rise or fall in blood pressure, anorexia, vomiting or development of a dull, aching discomfort in abdomen.
   b. Assess for flank pain (usually represents

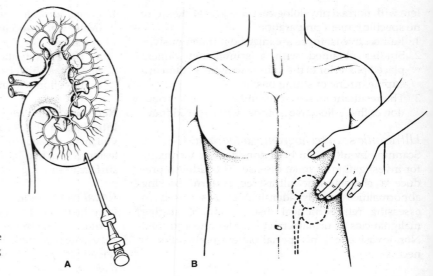

Figure 9.1. (A) Percutaneous needle biopsy of the kidney. (B) Examining for enlarging haematoma

A   B

bleeding into the muscle) or colicky pain (clot in the ureter).
c. Assess for backache, shoulder pain or dysuria.
d. Persistent bleeding may be suspected when there is an enlarging haematoma, which is palpable (Figure 9.1).
e. If perirenal bleeding develops, avoid palpating or manipulating the abdomen after the first examination has determined that a haematoma exists.
3. Measure each specimen of urine and inspect for bleeding. Compare samples with each other and with prebiopsy specimen.
4. Assess for any patient complaints, especially frequency and urgency.
5. Keep the fluid level at 3,000ml daily if tolerated, unless the patient has renal insufficiency.
6. A haematocrit and haemoglobin study may be done within eight hours to assess for anaemia.
7. Prepare for transfusion and surgical intervention for control of haemorrhage, which may necessitate surgical drainage or nephrectomy (removal of kidney).

Discharge planning and patient education
Instruct the patient as follows:
1. Avoid strenuous activity, strenuous sports and heavy lifting for at least two weeks.
2. Notify doctor if any of the following occur: flank pain, haematuria, light-headedness and fainting, rapid pulse or any other signs and symptoms of bleeding.
3. Report for follow-up one to two months after biopsy; the patient is checked for hypertension, and the biopsy area is auscultated for any murmur.

URODYNAMIC STUDIES
Urodynamic studies provide physiological and structural tests to evaluate bladder and urethral function by measuring the (1) rate of urine flow, (2) bladder pressures during voiding and at rest, (3) internal urethral resistance, and (4) bladder contraction and relaxation.

Uroflowmetry (flow rate)
This is a record of the volume of urine passing through the urethra per unit of time (ml/second).

Cystometrogram
Indications for this investigation include persistent enuresis, severe frequency/urgency of micturition and minor incontinence. A cystometrogram measures the function of the bladder muscle (detrusor) by filling the bladder and monitoring the pressure at increasing volumes. To avoid changes in bladder pressure due to changes in abdominal pressure rather than increased volume, the rectal pressure is monitored simultaneously and subtracted from the total bladder pressure. Modern multi-channel electronic recorders have replaced manometers.
1. Prior to filling, the patient voids urine and a catheter is passed and the residual urine measured.
2. A catheter-tipped transducer is introduced alongside the urethral filling catheter.

3. During filling the following is noted:
   a. First sensation of bladder filling (normal approximately 150–200ml).
   b. Strong desire to void (normal approximately 300–350ml).
   c. Maximum capacity (normal approximately 400–500ml).
   d. Uninhibited bladder muscle activity (normally none).
4. At the end of filling the catheter is removed and the patient voids.
5. Measurements are made of:
   a. Urinary flow rate.
   b. Voided volume.
   c. Voiding pressure.
   d. Calculated residual volume.

Urethral pressure profile

This is a graphic recording of the pressure within the urethra at each point along its length. Gas and fluid are instilled through a catheter that is withdrawn while pressures along the urethral wall are obtained.

Cystourethrogram

This is visualization of urethra and bladder either by retrograde injection or by voiding of contrast material.
1. Bladder is filled with radio-opaque medium, and the patient then voids urine while rapid spot films are taken.
2. With the image intensifier, the presence or absence of vesicoureteral reflux and/or congenital abnormalities in the lower urinary tract can be demonstrated. Also used to investigate difficulty in bladder emptying and incontinence.

Electromyography

Uses placement of electrodes into the anus or insertion of fine needle probes through the perineum into the periurethral or perianal musculature.

TESTS OF RENAL FUNCTION

1. Renal function tests are used to determine the effectiveness of the kidneys' excretory functioning, to assess the severity of kidney disease and to follow the patient's progress.
2. Renal function may be within normal limits until about 50 per cent of renal function has been lost.

3. Best results are obtained by combining a number of clinical tests. Table 9.1 lists the more common tests of renal function.

URINE EXAMINATION

FACTORS AFFECTING COMPOSITION OF URINE
1. Nutritional status.
2. Metabolic processes.
3. Status of kidney function.

AMOUNT
1. 1,200 to 1,500ml/24 hours; less than 500ml is considered oliguria.
2. Day volume two to three times more than night volume.

APPEARANCE
1. Normal urine is clear.
2. Turbid (cloudy) urine is not always pathological. Normal urine may develop turbidity on refrigeration or from standing at room temperature; bacteria ferments urine quickly at room temperature.
3. Abnormally cloudy urine – due to pus, blood, epithelial cells, bacteria, fat, colloidal particles, phosphate, urates.

ODOUR
1. Normal – faint aromatic odour.
2. Characteristic odours produced by ingestion of asparagus, thymol.
3. Cloudy urine with ammonia odour – urea-splitting bacteria such as *Proteus*, causing urinary tract infections.
4. Offensive odour – bacterial action in presence of pus.

COLOUR
1. Colour shows degree of concentration and depends on amount of urine voided.
2. Normal urine is clear yellow or amber because of the pigment urochrome.
3. Colour varies with specific gravity:
   a. Dilute urine is straw-coloured.
   b. Concentrated urine is highly coloured, a sign of insufficient fluid intake.
4. Abnormally coloured urine:
   a. Turbid or smoky coloured – may be from haematuria, spermatozoa, prostatic fluid, fat droplets, chyle.
   b. Red or red-brown – due to blood pigments,

Table 9.1   Tests of renal function

1. There is no single test of renal function; renal function is variable from time to time
2. The rate of change of renal function is more important than the result of a single test

Test	Purpose/rationale	Test protocol

Renal concentration test
  Specific gravity
  Refractive index
  Osmolality of urine
	Assesses the ability to concentrate solutes in the urine
	Concentration ability is lost early in kidney disease; hence, this test detects early defects in renal function
		Fluids may be withheld 12–24 hours to assess the concentrating ability of the tubules under controlled conditions. Specific gravity measurements of urine are taken at specific times to determine urine concentration

Phenolsulfonphthalein excretion test (PSP)	A diagnostic agent (phenolsulfonphthalein) is given to determine the functional capacity of the kidney. (PSP test can also be used as a measure to assess residual urine.) Delayed excretion is seen in renal disease, cardiac failure, primary vascular disease	Encourage fluids 1–1½ hours before the test Phenolsulfonphthalein is given intravenously: 1. Record exact time dye is administered 2. Collect urine in 15 minutes, 30 minutes and one hour
Creatinine clearance* (endogenous creatinine clearance)	Provides a reasonable approximation of rate of glomerular filtration Measures volume of blood cleared of creatinine in one minute. Most sensitive indication of early renal disease Useful to follow progress of the patient's renal status	Collect all urine over 24-hour period Draw one sample of blood within the period
Serum creatinine	A test of renal function reflecting the balance between production and filtration by renal glomerulus Most sensitive test of renal function	Do test on blood serum
Serum urea nitrogen (blood urea nitrogen [BUN])	Serves as index of renal excretory capacity Serum urea nitrogen is dependent on the body's urea production and on urine flow (urea is the nitrogenous end-product of protein metabolism) Affected by protein intake, tissue breakdown	Do test on blood serum

* Clearance is the amount of blood cleansed of a constituent per unit of time.

porphyria, transfusion reaction, bleeding lesions in urogenital tract, some drugs.
c. Yellow-brown or green-brown – may reveal obstructive lesion of bile duct system or obstructive jaundice.
d. Orange-red or orange-brown – from urobilin or from Pyridium (phenazopyridine hydrochloride), a urinary antiseptic.

e. Dark brown or black – due to malignant melanoma, leukaemia.

REACTION (pH)
1. Reflects the ability of kidney to maintain normal hydrogen ion concentration in plasma and extracellular fluid; indicates acidity or alkalinity of urine.

2. The pH should be measured in fresh urine, since the breakdown of urine to ammonia causes urine to become alkaline.
3. Normal pH is around 6 (acid); may normally vary from 4.6 and 7.5.
4. Urine acidity or alkalinity has relatively little clinical significance unless the patient is on special diet or therapeutic programme or is being treated for renal calculus disease.
5. Alkaline urine is often cloudy because of phosphate crystals.

SPECIFIC GRAVITY

1. Reflects the kidney's ability to concentrate or dilute urine; may reflect degree of hydration or dehydration.
2. Normal specific gravity ranges from 1.005 to 1.025.
3. Specific gravity is fixed at 1.010 in chronic renal failure.
4. In a person eating a normal diet, inability to concentrate or dilute urine indicates disease.

OSMOLALITY

1. Osmolality is an indication of the amount of osmotically active particles in urine (specifically, it is the number of particles per unit volume of *water*). It is similar to specific gravity, but is considered a more precise test; it is also easy to do – only 1–2ml of urine are required.
2. The unit of osmotic measure is the *osmole*.
   Average values:
   a. Females: 300–1,090mOsmol/kg.
   b. Males: 390–1,090mOsmol/kg.

ABNORMAL URINE CONSTITUENTS

1. *Proteinuria* (albuminuria) – characteristically seen in all forms of acute and chronic renal disease.
   a. Normal urine does not have persistent protein in significant quantities.
   b. Proteinuria also occurs in systemic diseases where there are varying degrees of renal anoxia, cardiac decompensation, diabetic glomerulosclerosis, etc.
2. *Glycosuria* – glucose in the urine; seen most frequently in diabetes mellitus.
3. *Ketonuria* – the presence of ketone bodies (acetone, acetoacetic acid and beta-hydroxybutyric acid). Ketonuria indicates incomplete fat metabol-

ism (diabetic ketoacidosis), dehydration, starvation; also seen after aspirin ingestion.
4. *Haematuria* – red blood cells in the urine.
5. *Pyuria* – white blood cells in the urine.
6. *Bacteriuria* – bacteria in the urine.
7. *Crystalluria* – excretion of crystals in the urine.

DIPSTICK TESTS (REAGENT TESTS)
Strips that have been impregnated with chemicals are dipped quickly in urine and 'read' as a means of testing urine.
1. When dipped in urine, the chemicals react with abnormal substances in the urine by changing colour.
2. Some dipsticks can test for only one substance, whereas others can test several substances simultaneously.

BASIC PRINCIPLES FOR COLLECTING URINE SPECIMENS
1. The first morning urine specimen is most concentrated and more likely to reveal abnormalities.
2. Urine should not be left standing at room temperature, since it becomes alkaline because of contamination of urea-splitting bacteria from the environment.
3. All specimens should be refrigerated as soon as possible after they are voided.
4. Microscopic examination should be done within half an hour after collection – standing causes dissolution of cellular elements and casts, and bacterial overgrowth unless obtained by sterile methods.
5. Urine specimens should be collected from the patient by means of the clean-catch midstream technique using a wide-mouth container (see below and Figure 9.2).
6. Collection of 24-hour specimen:
   a. Ensure that the patient understands the procedure. *All* urine must be collected within a 24-hour period via clean-catch technique.
   b. Have the patient empty the bladder at specified time (e.g. 08.00). *Discard urine*.
   c. Collect all urine voided during the next 24 hours.
   d. Collect last specimen at 08.00 on following day (or 24 hours after collection was started).
   e. Keep collected urine in the refrigerator in a clean bottle; a suitable preservative/stabilizer may be required.
   f. Start with an empty bladder and finish with an empty bladder.

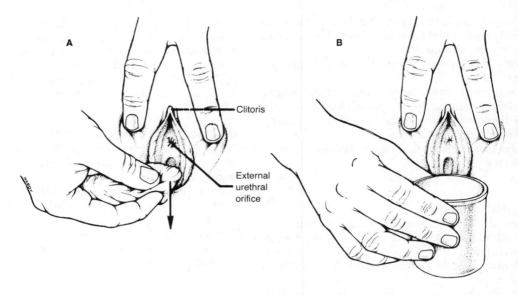

Figure 9.2. Obtaining a clean-catch midstream urine specimen in the female. (A) Instruct the patient to hold the labia apart and wash from high up front towards the back with gauze soaked in soap. (B) The collection cup is held so that it does not touch the body, and the sample is obtained only while the patient is voiding with the labia held apart

GUIDELINES: TECHNIQUE FOR OBTAINING CLEAN-CATCH MIDSTREAM URINE SPECIMEN

A clean-catch midstream specimen is the best clinically effective method of securing a voided specimen of urine for urinalysis. It is not a simple procedure and requires patient education and active assistance of the female patient.

EQUIPMENT
Antiseptic solution or liquid soap solution
Sterile water
4 × 4 gauze squares
Disposable gloves for nurse assisting female patient
Sterile specimen container

PROCEDURE
Male patient

Nursing action	Rationale
1. Instruct the patient to expose glans and cleanse area around meatus. Wash area with mild antiseptic solution or liquid soap. *Rinse thoroughly.*	The urethral orifice is colonized by bacteria. Urine readily becomes contaminated during voiding. Rinse antiseptic solution or soap solution thoroughly because these agents can inhibit bacterial growth in a urine culture.

2. Allow the initial urinary flow to escape.

The first portion of urine washes out the urethra and contains debris.

3. Collect the midstream urine specimen in a sterile container.

4. Avoid collecting the last few drops of urine.

Prostatic secretions may be introduced into urine at the end of the urinary stream.

5. Send specimen to laboratory immediately.

Female patient

Nursing action

Rationale

1. Ask the patient to separate her labia to expose the urethral orifice.
   If no one is available to assist the patient, she may sit backwards on the toilet seat facing the water tank or sit on (straddle) the wide part of the bedpan.

Keeping the labia separated prevents labial or vaginal contamination of the urine specimen. By straddling the toilet seat/bedpan, the patient's labia are spread apart for cleansing.

2. Cleanse the area around the urinary meatus with gauze soaked with antiseptic/soap solution. Rinse thoroughly.
   a. Wipe the perineum from the front to the back.
   b. Do not use swabs more than once.

The urethral orifice is colonized by bacteria. Urine readily becomes contaminated during voiding.

3. While the patient keeps the labia separated (Figure 9.2), instruct her to pass urine forcibly.

This helps wash away urethral contaminants.

4. Allow initial urinary flow to drain into bedpan (toilet) and then catch the midstream specimen in a sterile container, making sure that the container does not come in contact with the genitalia.

The first portion of urine washes out the urethra. Have the patient remove the container from the stream while she is still voiding.

5. Send the specimen to the laboratory immediately.

Too long an interval between collection and analysis produces unreliable results.

CATHETERIZATION

GUIDELINES: CATHETERIZATION OF THE URINARY BLADDER

PURPOSES
1. Relieve acute or chronic urinary retention.
2. For preoperative and postoperative urinary drainage.
3. Determine amount of residual urine after voiding urine.

EQUIPMENT

Sterile gloves
Disposable sterile catheter set with single-use packet of lubricant
Antiseptic solution for periurethral cleansing (sterile)
Gloves, drape, gauze squares
Sterile container for culture
Sheet for draping
Standing lamp (preferred) or flashlight

SELECTION OF CATHETER SIZE

Use the smallest sized catheter capable of providing adequate drainage
(Figure 9.3). Catheters are manufactured in two lengths for male and female
patients. The female ones are shorter.

PROCEDURE

Female patient

Preparatory phase

Nursing action	**Rationale**
1. Put the patient at ease.	The patient will feel reassured if the procedure is explained and if she is handled gently and considerately.

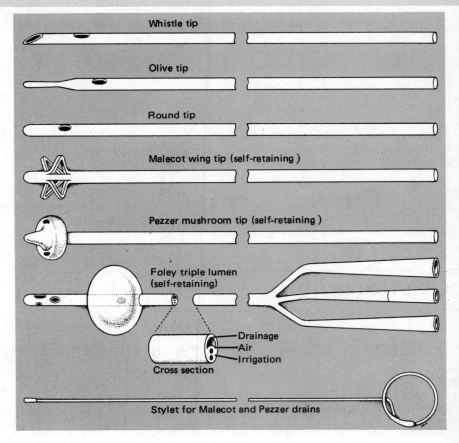

Whistle tip

Olive tip

Round tip

Malecot wing tip (self-retaining)

Pezzer mushroom tip (self-retaining)

Foley triple lumen
(self-retaining)

Drainage
Air
Irrigation
Cross section

Stylet for Malecot and Pezzer drains

Figure 9.3.
Types of catheter

2. Open catheter tray using aseptic technique. Place waste receptacle in accessible place.

Catheterization requires the same aseptic precautions as a surgical procedure.

3. Direct light for visualization of genital area.

4. Place the patient in a supine position with knees bent, hips flexed, and feet resting on bed about 0.6m apart. Drape the patient.

5. Position moisture-proof pad under the patient's buttocks.

6. Wash hands. Put on sterile gloves.

Performance phase

Nursing action

Rationale

1. Separate labia minora so that urethral meatus is visualized; one hand maintains separation of the labia until catheterization is finished.

This manoeuvre helps prevent labial contamination of the catheter (Figure 9.4).

2. Cleanse around the urethral meatus with cetrimide.
   a. Manipulate cleansing gauze with forceps, cleansing with downward strokes from anterior to posterior.
   b. Dispose of gauze after each use.
   c. If the patient is sensitive to iodine, benzalkonium chloride or other cleansing agent is used.

Micro-organisms inhabiting the distal urethra may be introduced into the bladder during or immediately after catheter insertion. Inadequate preparation of the urethral meatus is a major cause of infection.

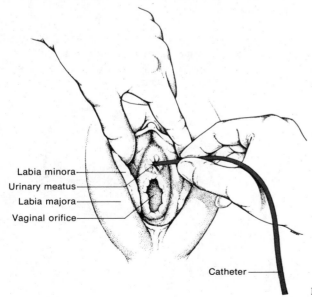

Labia minora
Urinary meatus
Labia majora
Vaginal orifice

Catheter

Figure 9.4. Catheterization of urinary bladder in female

3. Introduce well-lubricated catheter 5–7.5cm into urethral meatus using strict aseptic technique.
    a. Avoid contaminating surface of catheter.
    b. Ensure that catheter is not too large or too tight at urethral meatus.

A well-lubricated catheter reduces friction and trauma to the meatus. The female urethra is a relatively short canal, measuring 3–4cm in length.
Too large a catheter may cause painful distension of the meatus.

4. Pinch off catheter and remove gently when urine ceases to flow.

Pinching off the catheter prevents air from entering the bladder as the catheter is removed.

Follow-up phase
1. Dry area; make patient comfortable.
2. Measure urine and dispose of equipment.
3. Send specimen to laboratory as indicated.
4. Record time, procedure, amount and appearance of urine.

Male patient

Nursing action

Rationale

1. Carry out all of 'preparatory phase' as for female patient except:

2. Place the patient in supine position with legs extended. Place the moisture-proof pad across upper thighs.

3. Position the perineal drape.

4. Lubricate the catheter well.

A well-lubricated catheter prevents urethral trauma (decreasing the opportunity for bacterial invasion).

5. Wash off glans penis around urinary meatus with cetrimide using forceps to hold cleansing gauze. Keep the foreskin retracted. Maintain sterility of right hand.

Cleanse urethral meatus from tip to foreskin with downward stroke on one side. Discard sponge. Repeat as required.

6. Grasp shaft of penis (with left hand) raising it almost straight up (Figure 9.5). Maintain grasp on penis until procedure is ended.

This manoeuvre straightens the penile urethra and facilitates catheterization. Maintaining a grasp of the penis prevents contamination and retraction of penis.

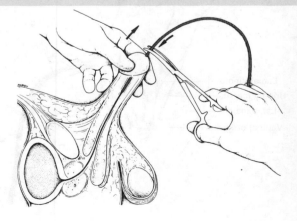

Figure 9.5. Technique for catheterization in male

7. Using sterile gloves or forceps, insert catheter into the urethra; advance catheter 15–25cm until urine flows.	The male urethra is a canal extending from the bladder to the end of the glans penis. The length varies within wide limits; the average length is about 21cm.
8. If resistance is felt at the external sphincter, slightly increase the traction on the penis and apply steady, gentle pressure on the catheter. Ask patient to strain gently (as if passing urine) to help relax sphincter.	Some resistance may be due to spasm of external sphincter. Inability to pass the catheter may mean that a urethral stricture or other forms of urethral pathology exist. The urethra may have to be dilated with sounds by a urologist.
9. When urine begins to flow, advance the catheter another 2.5cm.	Advancing the catheter ensures its position in the bladder.
10. Reduce (or reposition) the foreskin.	Paraphimosis (retraction and constriction of the foreskin behind the glans penis), secondary to catheterization, may occur if the foreskin is not reduced.

Follow-up phase
Same as for female patient.

GUIDELINES: MANAGEMENT OF THE PATIENT WITH AN INDWELLING (SELF-RETAINING) CATHETER AND CLOSED DRAINAGE SYSTEM

PURPOSES
1. Empty urine from the bladder following bladder, prostate or vaginal surgery.
2. Relieve urinary tract obstruction.
3. Permit urinary drainage in patients with neurogenic bladder dysfunction/urinary retention.
4. Determine accurate measurement of urinary drainage in critically ill patients.

EQUIPMENT
Completely closed system of urinary drainage (Figure 9.6)
Catheter tray with triple-lumen catheter
Antibacterial solution for cleansing
Gauze squares
Single-use packet of lubricant

PROCEDURE
General considerations

Nursing action	Rationale
1. Catheterize the patient (p. 597), using a catheter that is preferably preconnected to a closed drainage system.	A closed drainage system is one that is closed to outside air.

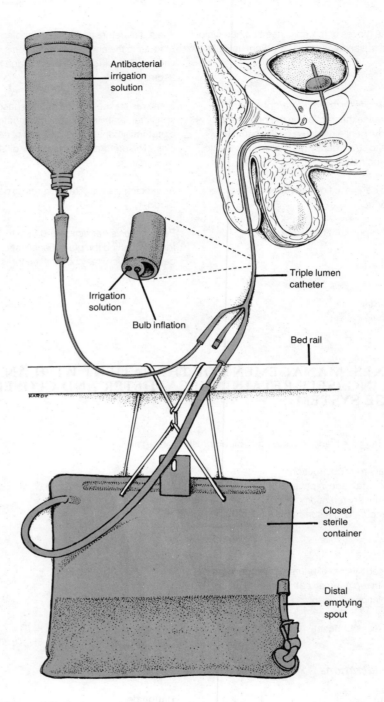

Figure 9.6. Closed sterile drainage system

a. Advance catheter almost to its bifurcation (for male patient).

This prevents the balloon from becoming trapped in the urethra.

b. Inflate the balloon according to manufacturer's directions. Be sure catheter is draining properly before inflating balloon, then withdraw catheter slightly.

Inadvertent inflation of the balloon within the urethra is painful and causes urethral trauma.

2. Secure the indwelling catheter.

Properly securing the catheter prevents catheter movement and traction on the urethra.

a. Female: tape the catheter and drainage tubing to the thigh.
Male: tape the catheter to the lower abdomen and the tubing to the shaved thigh (Figure 9.7).

This smooths out urethral curve and eliminates pressure on the urethra at the penoscrotal junction, which can eventually lead to the formation of a urethrocutaneous fistula.

b. Allow some slack of the tubing to accommodate the patient's movements.

c. Keep the tubing over the patient's leg.

This tubing position helps prevent kinking or forming loops of stagnant urine.

Care of the indwelling catheter

Nursing action

Rationale

1. Cleanse around the area where catheter enters urethral meatus (meatal–catheter junction) with soap and water during the daily bath to remove debris.

Suppurative drainage and encrustation occur at the end of any tube. Infectious organisms can migrate to the bladder along the outside of any indwelling catheter.

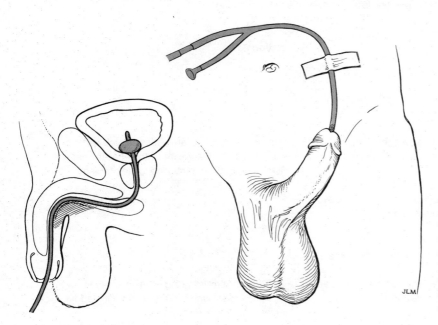

Figure 9.7. In the male patient, the indwelling catheter is taped to the abdomen to straighten the angulation of the penoscrotal junction, thus reducing pressure exerted by the catheter on the urethra

2. Avoid using powders and sprays on the perineal area.

This helps prevent infection.

3. Avoid pulling on the catheter during cleansing.

This action may introduce new organisms into the urethra.

To obtain urine for culture

Nursing action

Rationale

1. Clamp the drainage tubing below the aspiration (sampling) port for a *few minutes* to allow urine to collect.

Avoid separating catheter and connecting tube. Disconnection of the catheter and tubing is a major cause of urinary tract infection.

2. Cleanse the aspiration port with 70 per cent alcohol.

3. Insert a sterile No. 25 gauge needle (attached to a sterile syringe) into the aspiration port or hub of the catheter.

Avoid inserting needle into the shaft of the catheter because this may cause balloon deflation.

4. Aspirate a small volume of urine for culture.

5. Remove needle from syringe and release urine carefully into sterile specimen container.

6. *Unclamp the drainage tube.*

To irrigate the catheter

Note: This is not done unless obstruction is anticipated (bleeding following bladder/prostate surgery).

Nursing action

Rationale

1. Wash hands. Don gloves.

2. Using aseptic technique, pour sterile irrigating solution into sterile container.

3. Cleanse around catheter/drainage tubing connection with sterile gauze pads soaked in cetrimide.

If frequent irrigations are necessary to keep the catheter open, change the catheter as the catheter itself is probably contributing to the problem.

4. Disconnect catheter from drainage tubing. Cover tubing with a sterile cap or drainage-tubing adapter bag (sleeve).

5. Place a sterile drainage basin under the catheter.

6. Irrigate catheter using a large volume syringe and prescribed amount of sterile irrigant.

Instil about 30ml irrigating solution at a time. Avoid instilling the solution forcibly to prevent bladder irritation and spasms.

7. Remove syringe and place end of catheter over drainage basin, allowing returning fluid to drain into basin.

This provides gravitational flow.

8. Repeat irrigation procedure until fluid is clear or according to doctor's directives.

9. Disinfect the distal end of the catheter and end of drainage tubing; reconnect the catheter and tubing. Remove gloves. Wash hands.

10. Document type and amount of irrigating solution, colour and character of returning fluid, presence of sediment/blood clots and patient's reaction.

Use irrigating equipment once and then discard.

Changing the catheter

Nursing action

Rationale

Change catheter according to the needs of the patient.

An indwelling catheter should *not* be changed at arbitrarily fixed intervals.

Principles of care when managing a closed drainage system

Nursing action

Rationale

1. Wash hands immediately before and after handling any part of the system. Wear clean disposable gloves when handling the drainage system.

Hands are the major route of transmission of gram-negative bacteria.

2. Maintain unobstructed urine flow.

   a. Keep the drainage bag below the level of the bladder.
   b. Urine should not be allowed to collect in the tubing, since a free flow of urine must be maintained to prevent infection.

Urine flow must be downhill. Avoid excessively long tubing.
Raising the bag will cause reflux of contaminated urine from the bag into the patient's bladder.
Improper drainage occurs when the tubing is kinked or twisted, allowing pools of drainage to collect in the loops of tubing.

3. To empty the drainage bag:

   a. Wash hands; don gloves.

   b. Disinfect spigot. Empty the bag in a separate collecting receptacle for each patient. Disinfect spigot again.
   c. Avoid letting the drainage bag touch the floor.
   d. Change the drainage bag if contamination occurs, if the urine flow becomes obstructed or if the connecting junctions start to leak.

Ensure that no part of the drainage system comes into contact with the floor.
Empty the bag at regular intervals, taking care to see that the drainage valve/spout is not contaminated.
Each patient should have his own collecting receptacle that is labelled with his name and kept in the bathroom, not on the floor.

Measures to prevent cross-contamination

Nursing action	Rationale
1. Wash hands before and after handling the catheter/drainage system and between patients.	Many urinary tract infections are due to extrinsically acquired organisms transmitted by cross-contamination.
2. Assign only one patient with an indwelling catheter to a room. If this is not possible, separate the infected patient with an indwelling catheter from an uninfected patient.	There appears to be a greater risk of microbial transmission between catheterized patients.
3. Know the patients at risk.	Female, elderly, debilitated and critically ill patients, those in the postpartum state and patients with obstructed or neurologically impaired bladders are at risk from infection.

PATIENT EDUCATION (SELF-CARE OF CATHETER AT HOME)
1. Wash hands before and after handling the catheter.
2. Wash around urinary opening and then up the catheter with soap and water daily, taking care to avoid pulling on the catheter during cleansing.
3. Drink eight to 12 glasses of fluids daily; increase fluid intake if urine becomes dark and concentrated.
4. Wipe all connecting junctions with alcohol before changing from leg-bag drainage to overnight bottle drainage.
5. Call doctor/nurse if fever, cloudy, bloody or odoriferous urine develops.

GUIDELINES: ASSISTING THE PATIENT UNDERGOING SUPRAPUBIC DRAINAGE (CYSTOSTOMY)

Suprapubic bladder drainage is a method of establishing drainage from the bladder by inserting a catheter or tube through the suprapubic area into the bladder by either a stab incision or puncture with a needle or trocar.

PURPOSES
1. Drain the bladder via a tube placed in the bladder through the suprapubic area.
2. Divert the flow of urine from the urethra.
3. Obtain a urine specimen for culture.

CLINICAL USEFULNESS
1. When urethral route is impassable – urethral stricture, injuries.
2. Following gynaecological operations – vaginal hysterectomy, vaginal repair.
3. Following bladder surgery.
4. Pelvic fractures.

EQUIPMENT
Sterile suprapubic drainage system package (disposable)
Antiseptic for suprapubic skin preparation
Local anaesthetic agent if needed

PROCEDURE
Preparatory phase

Nursing action	Rationale
1. Place the patient in a supine position with one pillow under head.	
2. Expose the abdomen.	

Performance phase (by doctor)

Nursing action	Rationale
1. The bladder is distended with 300–500ml of sterile saline via an urethral catheter, which is removed, or the patient is given fluids (oral or intravenously) before the procedure.	Distension of the bladder makes it easier to locate by the suprapubic route.
2. The suprapubic area is surgically prepared. After the skin is dried, the needle entry point is located.	The needle entry point is approximately 5cm above the symphysis.
3. The procedure may be performed in several ways:	
a. By open operation (incision of the bladder)	
b. By puncture with a trocar/cannula assembly	
(i) The trocar/cannula is passed in a slightly caudal direction.)	Entrance into the bladder is usually felt and can be verified by reflux of urine through a hole in the trocar/cannula.
(ii) After the bladder has been entered, the trocar is removed, leaving the outer cannula in place.	Usually, a three-way stopcock is attached to the proximal end of the catheter and connected to a siphon drainage system.
(iii) The catheter is threaded through the cannula and well into the bladder (Figure 9.8A).	
(iv) The cannula is slowly withdrawn, leaving the catheter in position.	
(v) The catheter is secured with sutures, tape, or a body-seal system (Figure 9.8B).	Aseptic technique is employed in the area around the cystostomy tube.
(vi) Cover the area around the catheter with a sterile dressing.	
(vii) Attach the drainage tubing to a closed sterile system.	
c. By needle puncture into bladder to secure a specimen for culture.	Avoid 'forcing fluids' before a urine culture is obtained, since this will produce a low density of organisms.

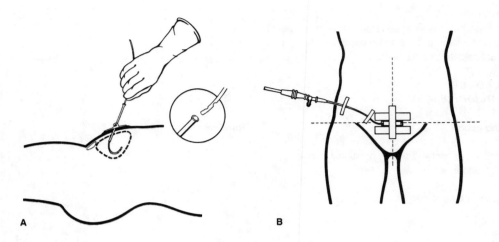

Figure 9.8. (A) Introduction of suprapubic catheter. (B) The body seal and catheter are taped to the abdomen (courtesy of Dow Corning Corporation)

4. Secure drainage tubing to lateral abdomen with tape (Figure 9.8B).	Prevents undue tension on the catheter.
5. If the catheter is not draining properly, withdraw the catheter 2.5cm at a time until urine begins to flow. Do not dislodge catheter from bladder.	
6. The drainage is maintained continuously for several days.	

7. If a 'trial of voiding' is requested, the catheter is clamped for four hours.
  a. Have the patient attempt to void urine while the catheter is clamped.
  b. After the patient voids urine, unclamp the catheter and measure residual urine.
  c. Usually, if the amount of residual urine is less than 100ml on two separate occasions (morning and afternoon), the catheter may be removed.
  d. If the patient complains of pain or discomfort, or if the residual urine is over the prescribed amount, the catheter is usually left open.
	Usually, patients will void urine earlier after surgery with suprapubic drainage than with indwelling catheters.

8. The catheter is removed as directed and a sterile dressing is placed over the site.	Suprapubic drainage is considered more comfortable than an indwelling urethral catheter; it allows greater patient mobility, and there is less risk of bladder infection.

RENAL DISORDERS

URINARY RETENTION

Urinary retention is the inability to urinate despite a desire to do so. Retention may be acute or chronic. Chronic retention will often lead to overflow incontinence or residual urine (urine that remains in the bladder after voiding).

AETIOLOGY
Males
1. Benign prostatic hyperplasia.
2. Stricture of urethra, calculus or foreign body in urethra, urethritis, tumour.
3. Phimosis.

Females
1. Urethral obstruction secondary to stricture, stones, vaginal cysts, carcinoma, oedema.
2. Retroverted gravid uterus.

Either male or female
1. Following any operation, particularly on anal or perineal region – due to reflex spasm of sphincters.
2. Trauma.
3. Neurogenic bladder dysfunction – spinal cord tumour, trauma, herniated intervertebral disc, multiple sclerosis.
4. Certain drugs (anticholinergics, antihistamines).
5. Faecal impaction.
6. Psychogenic urinary retention.

CLINICAL FEATURES
See Figure 9.9.
1. History of no voiding of urine or frequent passing of small amounts of urine without relief.
2. Progressive slowing of urinary stream; hesitancy.
3. Lower abdominal discomfort and distress; severe pain. The patient may have little or no discomfort if bladder distends slowly.
4. Smooth, firm, oval-shaped mass that is palpable over bladder area.
5. Dullness to percussion above symphysis pubis (residual urine below 130ml is not usually percussible).
6. Visualization of a rounded swelling arising out of the pelvis.
7. Urine-stained clothing.

TREATMENT AND NURSING MANAGEMENT
Objective
The patient empties his bladder completely.
1. Use nursing measures to help patient void urine:
   a. Transport the patient to bathroom (or bedside commode) or allow to stand beside bed if possible – many patients are unable to void while lying in bed.
   b. Use warmth to relax sphincters – bath, warm compresses to perineum, warm shower.
   c. Give hot tea to drink.
   d. Have patient listen to sound of running water, place hands in warm water.
   e. Administer bethanechol chloride (Myotonine chloride) only if directed.
   f. Give psychological reassurance and support.
2. Give prescribed analgesic medication post-operatively.
   a. Voiding may be difficult because of pain in the incisional area, especially in anterior vaginal operations.
   b. Sphincter spasm is generally present in patients with acute urinary retention.
3. Decompress bladder before overdistension occurs – bladder mucosa that has been stretched from urinary retention is readily infected.
   a. Utilize indwelling catheter and closed drainage.
      (i) It may be advisable to decompress the bladder gradually if the patient is elderly or hypertensive or has diminished renal reserve, or if retention of large amounts of urine has persisted for several weeks.
      (ii) Call urologist if unable to pass catheter easily; he will use special instruments (or operation may be necessary).
      (iii) Blood pressure may fluctuate and renal function decline the first few days after bladder drainage is instituted.
   b. Suprapubic cystostomy may be required if it is impossible to pass urethral catheter (p. 606).
4. Assist in determining the underlying cause.
   a. Doctor will carry out blood urea nitrogen (BUN) tests and other renal function tests.
   b. Assist in carrying out diagnostic tests if obstructive uropathy (pathological change in urinary tract from obstruction) is suspected.

NURSING ASSESSMENT FOR FLUID AND ELECTROLYTE IMBALANCE

For the signs and symptoms which tend to occur in patients with renal disease see Table 9.2.

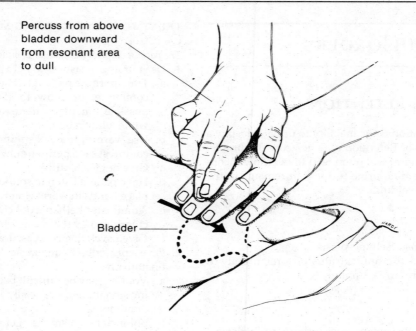

Percuss from above
bladder downward
from resonant area
to dull

Bladder

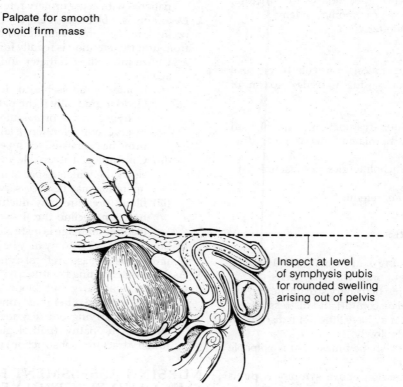

Palpate for smooth
ovoid firm mass

Inspect at level
of symphysis pubis
for rounded swelling
arising out of pelvis

Figure 9.9. Nursing assessment for urinary retention

Table 9.2   Signs and symptoms which occur with fluid and electrolyte imbalance

Signs and symptoms	Possible indication
Acute weight loss (in excess of 5 per cent), drop in body temperature, dry skin and mucous membranes, longitudinal wrinkles or furrows of tongue, oliguria or anuria	Volume deficit of extracellular fluid
Abdominal cramps, apprehension, convulsions, finger-printing on sternum, oliguria or anuria	Sodium deficit of extracellular fluid
Dry, sticky mucous membranes, flushed skin, oliguria or anuria, thirst, rough and dry tongue	Sodium excess of extracellular fluid
Anorexia, gaseous distension of intestines, silent intestinal ileus, weakness, soft, flabby muscles	Potassium deficit of extracellular fluid
Diarrhoea, intestinal colic, irritability, nausea	Potassium excess of extracellular fluid
Abdominal cramps, carpopedal spasm, muscle cramps, tetany, tingling of ends of fingers	Calcium deficit of extracellular fluid
Deep bone pain, flank pain and muscle hypotonicity	Calcium excess of extracellular fluid
Deep, rapid breathing (Kussmaul), shortness of breath on exertion, stupor, weakness	Primary base bicarbonate deficit of extracellular fluid
Depressed respiration, muscle hypertonicity, tetany	Primary base bicarbonate excess of extracellular fluid
Chronic weight loss, emotional depression, pallor, ready fatigue, soft, flabby muscles	Protein deficit of extracellular fluid
Positive Chvostek's sign, convulsions, disorientation, hyperactive deep reflexes, tremor	Magnesium deficit of extracellular fluid

NURSING INTERVENTIONS

1. Observe the clinical course of the patient; record the data collected.
2. Keep an accurate intake and output record.
3. Check the vital signs every four hours. Weigh the patient daily.
4. Support the patient having repeated blood examinations for the surveillance of electrolyte balance.

ACUTE RENAL FAILURE

Acute renal failure is a sudden decline in renal function caused by failure of the renal circulation or by glomerular or tubular damage. The substances normally eliminated in the urine accumulate in the body fluids as a result of impaired renal excretion and lead to a disruption in homeostatic, endocrine, and metabolic functions. Renal failure is a disease affecting the entire body.

PRECIPITATING FACTORS

1. Reduction in renal blood flow – volume depletion, hypotension, shock, trauma, burns, haemorrhage.
2. Sepsis.
3. Dehydration; trauma.
4. Obstructive lesions – vascular lesions, bladder outlet obstruction, calculi.
5. Nephrotoxic drugs.
6. Multiple blood transfusions and mismatched blood.
7. Cardiopulmonary bypass.
8. Surgery of aorta, renal vessels, biliary tree.
9. Extensive surgery in the elderly.

PREVENTIVE MEASURES

1. Initiate adequate hydration before, during and after operative procedures.
2. Avoid exposure to various nephrotoxins. Be aware that the majority of drugs or their metabolites are excreted by the kidneys.
3. Avoid chronic analgesic abuse – causes interstitial nephritis and papillary necrosis.
4. Prevent and treat shock with blood and fluid replacement. Prevent prolonged periods of hypotension.
5. Monitor urinary output and central venous pressure hourly in critically ill patients to detect onset of renal failure at the earliest moment.
6. Schedule diagnostic studies requiring dehydration so that there are 'rest days', especially for the older person who may not have adequate renal reserve.
7. Avoid infections, which may produce progressive renal damage.
8. Pay special attention to draining wounds, burns, etc, which can lead to sepsis.
9. To avoid infection, give meticulous care to patients with indwelling catheters and intravenous lines.
10. Take every precaution to ensure that the right person receives the right blood – to avoid severe transfusion reactions, which can precipitate renal complications.

Assessment

CLINICAL PHASES AND CLINICAL FEATURES

Period of oliguria (urine volume less than 400ml/24 hours).

1. However, there can be a decrease in renal function with increasing nitrogen retention even when the patient is excreting more than two to three litres of urine daily – called high output failure.
2. Accompanied by rise in serum concentration of elements usually excreted by kidney (urea, creatinine, uric acid, organic acids and the intracellular cations – potassium and magnesium).
3. Clinical features – scant, bloody urine, lethargy, nausea, vomiting, diarrhoea, dryness of skin and mucous membranes.
   a. Central nervous system (CNS) manifestations – drowsiness, headache, muscle twitching and convulsions.
   b. Period of oliguria lasts approximately ten days to three weeks.

Period of diuresis

Gradually increasing urinary output, which doubles daily until relatively fixed volume is attained – glomerular filtration has started to recover, but renal function is still abnormal. With dialysis, the diuretic phase may not occur.

Period of recovery

Signals the improvement of renal function and may take from three to twelve months; usually there is a permanent partial loss of some glomerular filtration rate and concentrating ability.

DIAGNOSTIC EVALUATION

1. Urinalysis – reveals proteinuria, haematuria, casts.
2. Rising blood urea nitrogen and serum creatinine concentrations.
3. Abnormalities in fluid and electrolyte homeostasis.

PATIENT PROBLEMS

1. Alteration in urinary elimination related to impaired renal function.
2. Retention of metabolic wastes related to impaired renal function.
3. Fluid and electrolyte imbalance.
4. Potential for complications (infection, gastrointestinal and central nervous system complications) related to build-up of toxic wastes in system.

Planning and implementation

NURSING INTERVENTIONS

Restoration of normal homeostasis to allow repair of renal tissue

1. Assist in removing the cause of renal failure if possible.
2. Implement prescribed treatment for underlying condition.
3. Prepare for peritoneal dialysis or haemodialysis to prevent metabolic deterioration (see p. 612 and p. 622).
   a. Dialysis produces a more sustained correction of biochemical abnormalities.
   b. Allows for liberalization of fluid, protein, and sodium intake; helps wound healing; diminishes bleeding tendencies and predisposition to infection.

Establishment of fluid and electrolyte balance

1. The doctor will carry out biochemical and urinary

studies. (Electrolyte administration is guided by serial measurements of central venous pressure, serum and urine electrolyte concentrations, fluid losses and the clinical status of the patient.)

   a. Record these parameters on a flowchart to indicate rate and trend of biochemical improvement/deterioration.

   b. Weigh the patient daily to provide an index of fluid balance – expected weight loss 0.25–0.5kg daily.

   c. Monitor the urinary output and urine specific gravity. Measure and record intake and output (include urine, gastric suction, stools, wound drainage, perspiration, etc).

   d. Observe fluid excess by assessing the patient's clinical status – dyspnoea, tachycardia, distended neck veins, crackles, peripheral oedema, pulmonary oedema.

2. Give only enough fluids to replace losses during oliguric phase (usually 400–500ml/24 hours, plus measured fluid losses associated with gastrointestinal drainage, fever, surgical drainage or other routes).

3. Measure and replace sodium losses, especially if large losses occur from the gastrointestinal tract via suction, vomiting or diarrhoea as directed.

   a. The doctor will monitor arterial blood gases and institute ventilatory measures if severe acidosis is present and respiratory problems develop.

   b. Prepare for sodium bicarbonate therapy or dialysis if necessary.

4. Control potassium balance (protein catabolism causes release of cellular potassium into body fluids, resulting in serious potassium intoxication).

   a. Sources of potassium are diet, tissue breakdown, blood in the gastrointestinal tract, blood transfusion, other sources (intravenous infusions, potassium penicillin) and extracellular shift in response to metabolic acidosis.

   b. The doctor will assess for hyperkalaemia (potassium intoxication) by monitoring serum potassium levels (potassium value above 6.0mEq/litre correlated with ECG changes (peaked T waves) and patient assessment.

   c. Give ion exchange resins – sodium polystyrene sulphonate (Resonium A), if directed; provides for more prolonged correction of elevated potassium.

     (i) Orally (laxative may be given concurrently to avoid faecal impaction), or

     (ii) By retention enema, since the colon is the principal site for potassium exchange.

     (a) Use catheter with balloon to facilitate retention if necessary.

     (b) Assist the patient to retain the resin 30 to 45 minutes to remove the potassium.

    (iii) Sorbitol (induces water loss in gastrointestinal tract) may be given orally.

   d. Intravenous glucose and insulin or calcium gluconate sometimes used as emergency (and temporary) measure for potassium intoxication; causes potassium to enter cells.

   e. Give sodium bicarbonate as directed – promotes elevation of plasma pH; when available sodium ions are provided, there is a migration of potassium into the cell and a lowering of potassium in the plasma; this is short-term therapy and is used along with other, long-term measures.

   f. Watch for cardiac dysrhythmias (cardiac arrest) and congestive heart failure from hyperkalaemia, electrolyte imbalance and/or fluid overload.

5. Assess for an increase in serum phosphate concentrations (hyperphosphataemia) – occurs because of failure of glomerular filtration. Give phosphate-binding antacid (aluminium hydroxide), as prescribed, to keep phosphate from being absorbed into bloodstream and to help prevent a continuing rise in serum phosphate levels.

Sufficient nutritional intake to preserve protein stores of the body until renal function returns

1. Limit dietary protein during oliguric phase to minimize accumulation of toxic end-products, etc, that result from digestion and metabolism of dietary protein.

   a. Offer high-carbohydrate feedings, since carbohydrates have a greater protein-sparing power.

   b. Restrict foods and fluids containing potassium and phosphorus (bananas, citrus fruits/juices, coffee).

   c. Restrict sodium intake as directed.

   d. Prepare for hyperalimentation (see p. 450) when adequate nutrition cannot be taken through the gastrointestinal tract.

Prevention of complications

1. Watch for signs and symptoms of dehydration or hypovolaemia – regulating capacity of kidneys is usually still inadequate.

2. Monitor for reduction in body weight, poor skin

elasticity, dryness of mucous membranes, hypotension, tachycardia.
3. Prevent and forestall the following if possible:
   a. Infection.
   b. Gastrointestinal complications (bleeding; sepsis).
   c. Central nervous system complications (drowsiness to acute psychoses, delirium, and coma).
   d. Metabolic acidosis.
   e. Circulatory overload (dyspnoea, orthopnoea, pulmonary congestion, pulmonary oedema).
   f. Hypertension, hypertensive crisis, convulsions.
   g. Neurological complications – abnormalities of mental status.

Evaluation
EXPECTED OUTCOMES
1. Patient excretes metabolic wastes; is in acid–base equilibrium.
2. Patient attains fluid and electrolyte balance.
3. Patient is free of complications.

CHRONIC RENAL FAILURE

Chronic renal failure is a progressive deterioration of renal function, which ends fatally in uraemia (an excess of urea and other nitrogenous wastes in the blood) and its complications unless dialysis or a kidney transplant is performed.

REVERSIBLE CAUSES
1. Urinary tract obstruction and infection.
2. Infectious diseases, which cause increased catabolism with retention of metabolites and hyperkalaemia.
3. Hypertension.
4. Metabolic disease.
5. Nephrotoxic (poisonous to kidney cells) agents.
6. Dehydration.

STAGES OF CHRONIC RENAL FAILURE
Decreased renal reserve → renal insufficiency → renal failure → uraemia.

Assessment
CLINICAL FEATURES
1. Gastrointestinal manifestations – anorexia, nausea, vomiting, hiccoughs, ulceration of gastrointestinal tract and haemorrhage.
2. Cardiopulmonary features – hypertension, fibrinous pericarditis, pleuritis.
3. Neuromuscular disturbances – fatigue, sleep disorders, headache, lethargy, muscular irritability, peripheral neuropathy, seizures, coma.
4. Fluid and electrolyte disturbances.
5. Metabolic and endocrine alterations – glucose intolerance, hyperlipidaemia, sex hormone disturbances.
6. Personality changes – emotional dullness, lability with impatient, demanding behaviour.
7. Dermatological disturbances – pallor, hyperpigmentation, pruritus, ecchymoses, uraemic frost.
8. Anaemia.

DIAGNOSTIC EVALUATION
1. Anaemia (a characteristic sign).
2. Elevated serum creatinine.
3. Elevated serum phosphorus.
4. Decreased serum calcium.
5. Low serum proteins, especially albumin.
6. Usually, low CO_2 and acidosis (low blood pH).

PATIENT PROBLEMS
1. Alteration in urinary elimination related to disturbance of renal function.
2. Electrolyte abnormalities related to biochemical derangements due to renal failure.
3. Acute fluid volume deficit or overhydration related to impaired concentrating and diluting mechanisms of the kidneys.
4. Potential for complications of every organ system related to biochemical and physiological disturbances from progressive destruction of neurons.
5. Alteration in thought processes (shortened attention span, diminished cognitive ability, irritability, personality changes) related to altered central nervous system function and declining renal function.
6. Potential alteration in skin integrity related to itching and hyperpigmentation.
7. Powerlessness and ineffective coping related to restrictions imposed by disease and treatment.
8. Potential for non-adherence with the therapeutic regimen related to feelings of hopelessness.

Planning and implementation
NURSING INTERVENTIONS
Maintenance of homeostasis and conservation of renal function as long as possible
1. Detect and treat reversible causes of chronic renal failure (see Reversible Causes, previous column).

2. Offer diet according to blood chemistry levels and clinical status of the patient, as directed.
   a. Regulate protein intake according to impairment of renal function, since metabolites that accumulate in the blood derive almost entirely from protein catabolism.
      (i) Protein should be of high biological value, rich in essential amino acids (dairy products, eggs, meat), so that the patient does not rely on tissue catabolism for essential amino acids.
      (ii) Low-protein diet may be supplemented with essential amino acids and vitamins.
      (iii) As renal function declines, protein intake may be restricted proportionately.
      (iv) Protein will be increased if the patient is on a dialysis programme to allow for loss of amino acids occurring during dialysis.
   b. Ensure high calorie intake – essential to spare protein for its own work, to provide energy and to prevent wasting. Encourage intake of hard sweets, jellies, flavoured carbohydrate powders.

Achieving fluid and electrolyte balance

1. Weigh the patient daily to assess fluid overload or depletion – weight should not increase or decrease more than 0.45kg per day.
2. Treat acidosis if the patient is symptomatic; acidosis commonly appears in chronic renal failure.
   a. Assess the patient for stupor, deep, rapid breathing of Kussmaul type, shortness of breath on exertion, weakness, unconsciousness.
   b. Replace bicarbonate stores by infusion or oral administration of sodium bicarbonate, as directed.
3. Adjust sodium requirements as required (determined by serum and urine measurements and daily weights) – patients with chronic renal diseases cannot tolerate severe restriction or marked excess in sodium intake.
4. Restrict dietary potassium and administer potassium-binding agents, as directed if decreasing renal function results in hyperkalaemia.
5. The following measures may or may not be employed:
   a. Decrease phosphorus intake (restrict meat, milk, legumes, carbonated beverages) – phosphate retention contributes to development of secondary hyperparathyroidism and development of uraemic bone disease (renal osteodystrophy).
   b. Reduce elevated levels of phosphorus with phosphate-binding agents (aluminium hydroxide compounds), since they bind phosphorus in the intestinal tract.
      (i) Phosphate binders cause constipation, which *cannot* be managed with the usual interventions.
      (ii) Employ stool softeners and bulk laxatives (Metamucil).
      (iii) Avoid laxatives and aperients which cause electrolyte toxicities (compounds containing magnesium or phosphorus).

Adjustment of fluid intake to maintain adequate urinary volume and to avoid dehydration

1. Fluid restriction is not usually initiated until renal function is quite low.
2. Fluid allowance should be distributed throughout the day.
3. Avoid restricting fluids for prolonged periods for laboratory and radiological examinations, since dehydrating procedures are hazardous to those patients who cannot produce concentrated urine.
4. Restrict salt and water intake if there is evidence of extracellular excess (congestive heart failure, pulmonary oedema, hypertension).

Prevention of complications

1. Treat associated cardiac conditions with digitalis, diuretics and antidysrhythmic agents to reverse congestive heart failure and to improve renal haemodynamics.
   a. Patient with chronic renal failure may also have a variety of other conditions – hypertension, neuropathy, bone disease infection, anaemia – that require drug therapy.
   b. Patients with renal failure have increased sensitivity to drugs because of impaired metabolism and renal excretion.

NURSING ALERT
Patients with impaired renal function may require major adjustments of common therapeutic agents. Give medications with caution.

2. Monitor blood pressure. Hypertension increases rate of renal deterioration and adversely affects the vascular system.
3. Observe for other complications:
   a. Anaemia – has many causes and is invariably found in patients with advanced renal failure.
   b. Renal osteodystrophy – uraemia is associated

with abnormal calcium metabolism, which causes bone pathology.
c. Infection.
d. Paraesthesiae – neurological abnormalities (dysarthria, muscle twitching, tremulousness, disorientation, stupor, seizures, coma).
e. Hyperkalaemia.

Prevention or reduction of cognitive distortions
1. Speak to the patient in simple orienting statements, using repetition when necessary.
2. Maintain predictable routine and keep change to a minimum.
3. Correct cognitive distortions.
4. Anticipate psychiatric intervention for acute changes in personality and cognition.

Maintenance of skin integrity
1. Use measures to produce vasoconstriction; cool environment, removal of excessive bedding.
2. Provide tepid, cooling baths or cool wet dressings – gradual evaporation of water from dressings cools skin and relieves pruritus.
3. Eliminate irritants; apply emollient lotions.

Preparation for dialysis or kidney transplant
1. Offer hope tempered by reality.
2. Advent of chronic dialysis and renal transplantation have revolutionized treatment and prognosis of patient with chronic renal failure (see Dialysis, below, and Renal Transplantation, p. 626).

Evaluation
EXPECTED OUTCOMES
1. Patient maintains homeostasis.
2. Patient attains improved electrolyte measurements.
3. Patient attains adequate fluid balance.

4. Patient is free of 'new' complications.
5. Patient is oriented to time, place and person.
6. Patient achieves some relief of itching.
7. Patient verbalizes interest in dialysis/renal transplantation.

DIALYSIS

Dialysis refers to the diffusion of solute molecules through a semipermeable membrane, passing from the side of higher concentration to that of lower concentration. The purpose of dialysis is to maintain the life and well-being of the patient until kidney function is restored. It is a substitute for some kidney excretory functions but does not replace the kidneys' endocrine and metabolic functions.

METHODS
1. Peritoneal dialysis:
   a. Intermittent peritoneal dialysis (short-term [see below] or chronic).
   b. Continuous ambulatory peritoneal dialysis (CAPD) (see p. 622).
   c. Continuous peritoneal dialysis – uses automated peritoneal dialysis machine overnight with prolonged dwell time during day.
      (i) The patient is connected to dialysis machine every evening, receiving three to five exchanges during the night. In the morning, after infusing fresh dialysate, the catheter is capped.
      (ii) Permits freedom for exchanges during day.
2. Haemodialysis (see p. 622).

GUIDELINES: ASSISTING THE PATIENT UNDERGOING (ACUTE) PERITONEAL DIALYSIS*

Peritoneal dialysis is a substitute for kidney function during renal failure. The peritoneum acts as a dialysing membrane, and dialysate is delivered into the peritoneal cavity.

PURPOSES
1. Aid in the removal of toxic substances and metabolic wastes.

* Automated closed-system peritoneal cycling machines are available.

2. Establish electrolyte balance.
3. Remove excessive body fluid.
4. Assist in regulating the fluid balance of the body.
5. Control blood pressure.
6. Control severe, intractable heart failure when diuretics no longer promote elimination of water and sodium.

EQUIPMENT

Dialysis administration set (disposable, closed system)
Peritoneal dialysis solution as requested
Supplemental drugs as requested
Local anaesthesia
Central venous pressure monitoring equipment
Electrocardiograph
Suture set
Sterile gloves
Skin antiseptic

PROCEDURE

Nursing action	Rationale
1. Prepare the patient emotionally and physically for the procedure.	Nursing support is offered by examining procedure mechanics, providing opportunities for the patient to ask questions, allowing him to verbalize his feelings and giving expert physical care.
2. See that the consent form has been signed.	
3. Weigh the patient before dialysis and every 24 hours thereafter.	The weight at the beginning of the procedure serves as a baseline of information. Daily weight is helpful in assessing the state of hydration.
4. Take temperature, pulse, respiration and blood pressure readings prior to dialysis.	Measurement of vital signs at the beginning of dialysis is necessary for comparing subsequent changes in vital signs.
5. Have the patient empty his bladder.	If the bladder is empty, there is less likelihood of perforating it when the trocar is introduced into the peritoneum.
6. Assist with insertion of central venous pressure (CVP) catheter; ECG monitoring may also be employed.	CVP measurements may be carried out to assess fluid volume changes. Cardiac dysrhythmias may occur because of serum potassium changes and vagal stimulation.
7. Flush the tubing with dialysis solution.	The tubing is flushed to prevent air from entering the peritoneal cavity. Air causes abdominal discomfort and drainage difficulties.
8. Make the patient comfortable in a supine position.	

Performance phase (by the doctor)

Action

Rationale

The following is a brief summary of the method of insertion of a temporary peritoneal catheter (*done under strict asepsis*).

1. The abdomen is prepared surgically, and the skin and subcutaneous tissues are infiltrated with a local anaesthetic.

   Surgical preparation of the skin minimizes or eliminates surface bacteria and decreases the possibility of wound contamination and infection.

2. A small midline stab wound is made 3–5cm below the umbilicus.

3. The trocar is inserted through the incision with the stylet in place, or a thin stylet cannula may be inserted percutaneously.

4. The patient is requested to raise his head from the pillow after the trocar is introduced.

   This manoeuvre tightens the abdominal muscles and permits easier penetration of the trocar without danger of injury to the intra-abdominal organs.

5. When the peritoneum is punctured, the trocar is directed toward the left side of the pelvis. The stylet is removed, and the catheter is inserted through the trocar and manoeuvred into position.
   a. Dialysis fluid is allowed to run through the catheter while it is being positioned.

   This prevents the omentum from adhering to the catheter, impeding its advancement or occluding its opening.

6. After the trocar is removed, the skin may be closed with a purse-string suture. (This is not always done.) A sterile dressing is placed around the catheter.

   The catheter is attached to the skin to prevent loss of the catheter in the abdomen.

7. Attach the catheter connector to the administration set, which has been previously connected to the container of dialysis solution (warmed to body temperature, 37°C.)

   The solution is warmed to body temperature for patient comfort and to prevent abdominal pain. Heating also causes dilatation of the peritoneal vessels and increases urea clearance.

8. Drugs (heparin, potassium, antibiotic) are added in advance.

   The addition of heparin prevents fibrin clots from occluding the catheter. Potassium chloride may be added on request unless patient has hyperkalaemia. Antibiotics are added for the treatment of peritonitis.

9. Allow the dialysing solution to flow unrestricted into the peritoneal cavity (usually takes five to ten minutes for completion). If the patient experiences pain, slow down the infusion.

   The inflow solution should flow in a steady stream. If the fluid flows in too slowly, the catheter may need to be repositioned, since its tip may be buried in the omentum, or it may be occluded by a blood clot. Flushing may help.

10. Allow the fluid to remain in the peritoneal cavity for the prescribed time period (15 minutes to four hours). Prepare the next exchange while the fluid is in the peritoneal cavity.

In order for potassium, urea and other waste materials to be removed, the solution must remain in the peritoneal cavity for the prescribed time (dwell or equilibration time). The maximum concentration gradient takes place in the first five to ten minutes for small molecules, such as urea and creatinine.

11. Unclamp the outflow tube. Drainage should take approximately 10 to 30 minutes, although the time varies with each patient.

The abdomen is drained by a siphon effect through the closed system. Gravity drainage should occur fairly rapidly, and steady streams of fluid should be observed entering the drainage container. The drainage is usually straw-coloured.

12. If the fluid is not draining properly, move the patient from side to side to facilitate the removal of peritoneal drainage. The head of the bed may also be elevated. Ascertain if the catheter is patent. Check for closed clamp, kinked tubing or air lock. *Never push the catheter in.*

If the drainage stops, or starts to drip before the dialysing fluid has run out, the catheter tip may be buried in the omentum. Rotating the patient may be helpful (or it may be necessary for the doctor to reposition the catheter). Pushing in the catheter introduces bacteria into the peritoneal cavity.

13. When the outflow drainage ceases to run, clamp off the drainage tube and infuse the next exchange, using strict aseptic technique.

Performance phase (by the nurse)

Nursing action

Rationale

1. Take blood pressure and pulse every 15 minutes during the first exchange and every hour thereafter. Monitor the heart rate for signs of dysrhythmia.

A drop in blood pressure may indicate excessive fluid loss from glucose concentrations of the dialysing solutions. Changes in the vital signs may indicate impending shock or overhydration.

2. Take the patient's temperature every four hours (especially after catheter removal).

An infection is more apt to become evident after dialysis has been discontinued.

3. The procedure is repeated until the blood chemistry levels improve. The usual duration for short-term dialysis is 36–48 hours. Depending on the patient's condition, he will receive 24–48 exchanges.

The duration of dialysis depends on the severity of the condition and on the size and weight of the patient.

4. Keep an exact record of the patient's fluid balance during the treatment.
   a. Know the status of the patient's loss or gain of fluid at the end of each exchange. Check dressing for leakage and weigh on gram scale if significant.
   b. The fluid balance should be about even or should show slight fluid loss or gain, depending on the patient's fluid status.

Complications (circulatory collapse, hypotension, shock, and death) may occur if the patient loses too much fluid through peritoneal drainage. Large fluid losses around the catheter may not be noted unless the dressings are checked carefully.

5. Make patient comfortable during dialysis.
   a. Provide frequent back care and pressure area care.
   b. Have the patient turn from side to side.
   c. Elevate head of bed at intervals.
   d. Allow the patient to sit in chair for brief periods if condition permits (only with surgically implanted catheter; with trocar, patient is usually on bed rest).

The dialysis period is lengthy, and the patient becomes fatigued.

6. Observe for the following:
   a. Respiratory difficulty.
      (i) Slow the inflow rate.
      (ii) Make sure tubing is not kinked.
      (iii) Prevent air from entering peritoneum by keeping drip chamber of tubing three-quarters full of fluid.
      (iv) Elevate head of bed; encourage coughing and breathing exercises.
      (v) Turn patient from side to side.

This is caused by pressure from the fluid in the peritoneal cavity and the upward displacement of the diaphragm – producing shallow respirations. In severe respiratory difficulty, the fluid from the peritoneal cavity should be drained immediately and the doctor notified.

   b. Abdominal pain.
      (i) Encourage the patient to move about.

Pain may be caused by the dialysing solution not being at body temperature, incomplete drainage of the solution, chemical irritation, pressure by the catheter, peritonitis, or air pressing on the diaphragm, causing referred shoulder pain.

   c. Leakage.
      (i) Change the dressings frequently, being careful not to dislodge the catheter.
      (ii) Use sterile plastic drapes to prevent contamination.

Leakage around the catheter predisposes the patient to peritonitis.

7. Keep accurate records.
   a. Exact time of beginning and end of each exchange: starting and finishing time of drainage.
   b. Amount of solution infused and recovered.
   c. Fluid balance.
   d. Number of exchanges.
   e. Medications added to dialysing solution.
   f. Pre- and postdialysis weight, plus daily weight.
   g. Level of responsiveness at beginning, throughout, and at end of treatment.
   h. Assessment of vital signs and patient's condition.

Complications

Nursing action

Rationale

1. Peritonitis:
   a. Watch for nausea and vomiting, anorexia, abdominal pain, tenderness, rigidity and cloudy dialysate drainage.

Peritonitis is the most common complication. Antibiotics may be added to dialysate and also given systemically.

b. Send specimen of dialysate for white blood cell count and full set of cultures.

2. Bleeding:
    a. A haematocrit of the drainage fluid may be taken to determine the amount of bleeding.

A small amount of bleeding around the catheter is not significant if it does not persist. During the first few exchanges, blood-tinged fluid from subcutaneous bleeding is not uncommon. Small amounts of heparin may be added to inflow solution to prevent the catheter from becoming clogged.

3. Low serum albumin level.

Small amounts of albumin are lost with each exchange, resulting in a lowered serum albumin level. Oedema may occur, with possible hypotension.

4. Constipation.

Inactivity, altered nutrition, phosphate binders and the presence of fluid in the abdomen tend to cause constipation.

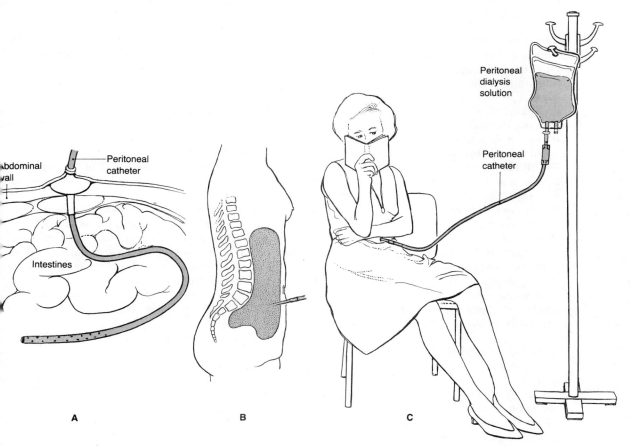

Figure 9.10. Continuous ambulatory peritoneal dialysis (CAPD). (A) The peritoneal catheter is implanted through the abdominal wall. (B) Fluid infusing into the peritoneal cavity. (C) The patient allows for the prescribed dwell time and then drains the peritoneal cavity by gravity

CONTINUOUS AMBULATORY PERITONEAL DIALYSIS (CAPD)

Continuous ambulatory peritoneal dialysis is a practical self-dialysis method that involves almost constant peritoneal contact with a dialysis solution for patients with end-stage renal disease (see Figure 9.10).

1. A permanent indwelling catheter is implanted into the peritoneum; the internal cuff on the catheter becomes embedded by fibrous ingrowth, which stabilizes it and minimizes leakage.
2. A connecting tube is attached to the external end of the peritoneal catheter, and the distal end of the tube is inserted into a sterile plastic bag of dialysate solution.
3. The dialysate bag is raised to shoulder level and infused by gravity into the peritoneal cavity.
4. Then the plastic bag attached to the connecting tube is folded and placed in a pouch at the waist, under the patient's clothing.
5. At the end of the dwell time (approximately four hours) the bag is removed from the pouch, unfolded, and placed near the floor to allow the dialysate to drain by gravity over a 20- to 40-minute period.
6. After the dialysate is drained, a fresh bag of dialysate solution is attached under aseptic conditions, and the procedure is repeated.
7. The patient performs four to five exchanges daily, seven days a week with an overnight dwell time allowing uninterrupted sleep; most patients become unaware of fluid in the peritoneal cavity.
8. Advantages:
   a. Physical and psychological freedom and independence.
   b. Free dietary intake; improvement of nutritional status.
   c. Relatively simple and easy to use.
   d. Satisfactory biochemical control of uraemia.
   e. Least expensive form of dialysis therapy.
   f. Eliminates need for complicated machines/dialysers.
9. Complications:
   a. Peritonitis and damage to peritoneal membrane.
   b. Pain (decreases with repeated treatments).
   c. Orthostatic hypotension.
10. Patient education:
    a. The use of CAPD as a long-term treatment depends on prevention of recurring peritonitis.

   (i) Use strict sterile techniques while caring for catheter.
   (ii) Report signs and symptoms of peritonitis – cloudy peritoneal fluid, abdominal pain or tenderness, malaise, fever.
   (iii) Send sample of peritoneal fluid to laboratory for culture and stain.
   (iv) Expect some type of treatment with intraperitoneal antibiotics at home or in hospital.
    b. Do not omit bag changes – this will cause inadequate control of renal failure.
    c. Some weight gain may accompany CAPD; the dialysate fluid contains a significant amount of dextrose, which adds calories to daily intake.

HAEMODIALYSIS

Haemodialysis is a process of cleansing the blood of accumulated waste products. It is used for patients with end-stage renal failure or for acutely ill patients who require short-term dialysis.

UNDERLYING PRINCIPLES

1. Heparinized blood passes down a concentration gradient through a semipermeable membrane by dialysis to the dialysate fluid.
2. The dialysate is composed of all of the important electrolytes in their ideal extracellular concentrations.
3. Through the process of diffusion, the blood components equilibrate with those in the dialysate. By appropriate adjustment of the dialysate bath composition, noxious substances (urea, creatinine, uric acid, phosphate and other metabolites) are transferred from the blood into the dialysate so that they can be discarded. Small pores of the membrane hold back desirable blood components.
4. Excess water is removed from the blood (ultrafiltration).
5. The body's buffer system is maintained by the addition and diffusion of acetate from the dialysate into the patient; it is metabolized to form bicarbonate.
6. Purified blood is returned to the body through one of the patient's veins.
7. At the end of the treatment, most poisonous wastes have been removed, electrolyte and water balances have been restored, and the buffer system has been replenished.

REQUIREMENTS FOR HAEMODIALYSIS
1. Access to the patient's circulation.
2. Dialyser with semipermeable membrane.
3. Appropriate dialysate bath.
4. Time – approximately four hours, three times weekly, for a total of 12 hours.
5. Place – home (if feasible) or at a renal dialysis centre.

METHODS OF ACCESS TO THE PATIENT'S CIRCULATION
1. Arteriovenous fistula (AVF) – creation of a vascular communication by suturing a vein directly to an artery.
   a. Usually, radial artery and cephalic vein are anastomosed in nondominant arm; vessels in leg may also be used.
   b. Following the procedure, the superficial venous system of the arm dilates.
   c. By means of two large-bore needles inserted into the dilated venous system, blood may be obtained and passed through the dialyser. The arterial end is used for arterial flow and the distal end for reinfusion of dialysed blood.
   d. Healing of AVF requires several weeks; an external shunt (see below) is used in the interim.
   e. Problems:
      (i) Infection; thrombosis; aneurysm formation.
      (ii) Disadvantage of being injected with large-bore needles before each dialysis treatment.
      (iii) Average life expectancy of fistula – five years.
2. Prosthetic arteriovenous fistula – vascular prosthesis (bovine; human umbilical vein; polytetrafluoroethylene [PTFE]).
3. External arteriovenous shunt (cannula):
   a. Teflon–Silastic cannula sewn into radial artery and a forearm vein (or placed in leg). The two are connected by a Teflon bridge.
   b. During dialysis, the bridge is removed and the arterial and venous ends are connected to the flow lines of the artificial kidney.
   c. Currently used while AVF is healing.
   d. Problems:
      (i) Clotting and infection; chronic erosion of the skin.
      (ii) Limited shunt life – must be surgically revised every few months.
      (iii) Dislodgement with haemorrhage.
      (iv) Visible reminder to the patient of his disability.
4. Direct cannulation of vessels (femoral or subclavian vein).

ARTIFICIAL KIDNEYS (DIALYSERS)
Many varieties of artificial kidneys have been described, but most conform to one of the following types:
1. Coil dialyser.
2. Flat plate or parallel flow dialyser.
3. Hollow-fibre kidney.

MONITORING DURING DIALYSIS
The management of the patient on a dialyser is a complex subject beyond the scope of this discussion. The reader is referred to the written protocol for the machine being used.

NURSING ALERT
Nurses attending patients undergoing haemodialysis are at risk of acquiring hepatitis B.

DIETARY MANAGEMENT OF THE PATIENT ON LONG-TERM HAEMODIALYSIS
1. The individual patient's dietary regimen is adjusted according to the extent of his residual renal function to avoid wide fluctuation in body chemistry.
2. Dietary management involves restriction or adjustment of protein, sodium, potassium and/or fluid intake.
   a. Protein – protein of highest biological quality is given to prevent poor protein utilization, to maintain positive nitrogen balance and replace amino acids lost during each dialysis.
      (i) Usually 1–1.2g of protein/kg body weight is given; additional supplement given when stress situations (bleeding, infection) occur.
      (ii) Calories (35kcal/kg body weight) are supplied from carbohydrates and fats to provide energy and to spare tissue breakdown.
   b. Sodium:
      (i) The patient may not excrete the necessary amount of sodium to maintain balance.
      (ii) Observe for fluid overload – hypertension, oedema.
      (iii) Or the patient may be a 'salt loser', unable to conserve salt; he thus loses large amounts of sodium in the urine and will require sodium replacement by drugs and dietary means.
   c. Potassium – a mineral found in the body cells.
      (i) Ability to eliminate excessive amounts of

potassium is decreased in chronic renal failure.

(ii) Accumulation of potassium in body can be toxic to heart and cause serious dysrhythmias.

(iii) Potassium is found in practically all foods – fruit juices, salt substitutes, bananas, chocolate, and baked potatoes are rich sources of potassium.

d. Fluid limitations:

(i) Fluid is restricted according to output; usually between 500 and 800ml, depending on renal function, losses, activity, environmental temperature.

(ii) The patient should be able to adjust his fluid intake according to the weight he has gained between dialysis treatments.

(iii) Lemon drops are satisfactory to use as thirst quenchers.

e. Calcium and phosphorus intake may have to be adjusted.

NUTRITION – PATIENT EDUCATION

Instruct the patient as follows:

1. Avoid eating frequently in places where salt-free cooking cannot be obtained consistently.
2. Read food labels carefully; avoid commercially prepared foods that have added sodium.
3. Avoid 'salt substitutes' – may contain potassium chloride, which should be avoided.
4. Eat fresh vegetables and fruits within dietary prescription.

PHARMACOLOGICAL MANAGEMENT

1. Phosphate-binding gels (aluminium hydroxide):
   a. Phosphorus tends to accumulate, resulting in hyperparathyroidism and osteodystrophy.
   b. These medications bind phosphate in the intestine and may help maintain proper calcium and phosphorus levels in the blood.
2. Potassium-binders – bind potassium in intestine to prevent dangerous elevations in blood.
3. Multivitamins – necessary because of significant nutrient losses during dialysis (especially of ascorbic acid and folic acid).

HEALTH PROBLEMS OF PATIENTS ON LONG-TERM HAEMODIALYSIS

Although haemodialysis can prolong life indefinitely, it does not completely control uraemia or halt the natural course of the underlying kidney disease. There are various abnormalities, syndromes, discomforts and long-term metabolic complications associated with haemodialysis.

1. Arteriosclerotic cardiovascular disease – leading cause of death and major factor limiting long-term survival.
   a. Disturbances of lipid metabolism (hypertriglyceridaemia) appear to be accentuated by haemodialysis.
   b. Congestive heart failure, coronary heart disease with anginal pain, stroke, peripheral vascular insufficiency may incapacitate the patient.
2. Intercurrent infection – patient has reduced resistance to infection.
   a. Exposure of blood to blood products and foreign material – may cause infection and gram-negative and gram-positive bacteraemia.
   b. Local infection of shunt site and in fistulas.
   c. Haemodialysis-associated hepatitis.
   d. Immunosuppression – facilitates opportunistic infection.
3. Anaemia and fatigue – may be caused by accelerated red cell loss (from haemolysis and bleeding) and impaired erythropoietin production.
   a. Sleeplessness, fatigue and malaise may be persistent.
   b. Diminution of physical and emotional well-being – lack of energy, drive, loss of interest.
4. Intractable pruritus (itching).
5. Bleeding:
   a. Bleeding from heparin rebound.
   b. Gastrointestinal bleeding.
   c. Subdural haematoma.
   d. Haemorrhagic pericarditis.
   e. Menorrhagia.
6. Hypertension.
7. Bone problems:
   a. Renal osteodystrophy (leading to bone pain and fractures) – pathogenesis obscure, but excessive parathyroid hormone secretion and vitamin D resistance may be causal factors.
   b. Aseptic necrosis of hip.
   c. Vascular calcification.
8. Chronic ascites – may be due to fluid overload associated with congestive heart failure, malnutrition (hypoalbuminaemia) and inadequate dialysis.
9. Disequilibrium syndrome – from rapid fluid and electrolyte changes, may produce increased intracranial pressure, hypertension, headache, vomiting, convulsions, coma and psychiatric problems.
10. Dialysis dementia – progressive, irreversible and fatal neurological syndrome thought to be due to aluminium intoxication (from aluminium-

containing dialysate fluid) or prolonged oral administration of aluminium hydroxide.

PSYCHOSOCIAL PROBLEMS

Long-term haemodialysis has unpredictable and uneven results. The impact of renal disease and the stresses of dialysis can be destructive to the ego and can place patients and families under severe mental and emotional stress.

1. Depression – an expected occurrence; most common psychological feature seen in patients on haemodialysis. Depression occurs from multiple causes – losses of bodily functions, working capability, and sexual drive; impotence, other physical complications, chronic illness, feelings of deprivation from diet and fluid restriction, limited capacity to compete, fear of death and dying, unpredictable medical status.
2. Dependence–independence conflict:
   a. Although the patient is dependent on the dialysis machine, personnel and treatment regimen, he is at the same time encouraged to be independent, work and lead a 'normal' life.
   b. Dependence may create aggressive feelings that cannot be expressed.
   c. The patient may repress hostility toward medical and nursing staff.
   d. The highly dependent patient may 'enjoy' haemodialysis.
3. Anxiety – a normal reaction to stress and threat.
   a. The patient is anxious because of constant changes in his clinical status and unpredictability of his health.
   b. The patient may use denial, fantasy, repression, rejection, etc, as defence mechanisms to deal with anxiety.
   c. Try to clarify the nature of the patient's anxiety before attempts at reassurance.
4. Suicidal behaviour – usually an act that stems from depression – suicide rate is more than 100 times that of general population.
   a. Allow the patient to express his feelings about self-destruction.
   b. Point out the patient's positive coping mechanisms and emphasize his capabilities.
   c. Psychiatric referral may be necessary.
5. Denial – a common response to a shift in health status:
   a. Denial may be protective and useful to a certain extent – may protect the patient from emotional decompensation (denial has both adaptive and maladaptive functions).
   b. Failure of this defence may lead to depression.

6. Stress from dietary restrictions – patient may 'act out' conflicts by binges of overeating/drinking.
7. Sexual dysfunctions – diminished interest and ability due to biological, pharmacological, and psychological reasons.

IMPACT OF DIALYSIS ON FAMILY

1. Altered family lifestyle:
   a. Social activities may be curtailed because of the large amount of time spent on dialysis.
   b. Close confinement to home (if the patient is on home dialysis) may create conflicts, frustration and depression in some families.
   c. Role changes – traditional roles altered.
   d. The patient and family may impose unnecessary limitations on their own activities.
2. Decreasing sexual activity may lead to marital problems.
3. Feelings of resentment (revealed or hidden) – due to personal sacrifices made by family.
4. Feeling that patient is a 'marginal' person with limited life expectancy can be transmitted to the patient.
5. Developmental/social problems of family members.
6. Difficulties in communication between the patient and partner – difficult to express anger, negative feelings and fear of death.
   a. Fear that expressed anger will cause something to happen to the patient.
   b. Expressions of anger may be displaced or covered up by anxiety.

PATIENT EDUCATION

1. Encourage the patient to assume the management and control of his therapeutic regimen.
   a. Determine the patient's own value system and ego strengths; use these to help him adapt to a different lifestyle.
   b. Emphasize the patient's capabilities.
   c. Teach the patient about his condition and treatment in 'small doses'.
   d. Discourage the patient's image of himself as 'sick'.
   e. Help the patient develop a sense of independence from the machine.
   f. Encourage the patient to interact with his surroundings during dialysis.
2. Encourage the patient to set realistic goals.
   a. Work activities should be introduced gradually – returning to work may not be a realistic goal for some patients.
   b. Modify attitudes in direction of permissiveness in area of productivity.

3. Encourage the patient to express his angry feelings (pain, discomfort, frustration) – helps to reduce level of emotional tension and will help prevent depression.
4. Let family have an opportunity (away from the patient) to express their feelings of anger, helplessness, etc.
   a. Help family to accept their negative feelings.
   b. Teach family what is involved in chronic haemodialysis.
5. Organizations helpful to patients on chronic dialysis: British Kidney Patient Association, Bordon, Hants (tel: 04203 2022/1).

RENAL/UROLOGICAL SURGERY

KIDNEY TRANSPLANTATION

Kidney transplantation is the transplantation of a kidney from a living donor or human cadaver donor to a recipient with end-stage renal failure who requires support from dialysis in order to maintain life.

Kidney transplants from well-matched related living donors are more successful than those from cadaver donors.

TRANSPLANTATION PROCEDURE
1. The donor kidney is transplanted retroperitoneally in either iliac fossa.
2. The ureter of the newly transplanted kidney is transplanted into the bladder or anastomosed to the ureter of the recipient.

POTENTIAL PROBLEMS
1. Infection – leading cause of death after transplant.
2. Renal graft failure and renal graft rejection. Except when the donor is a twin, the immunological defence of the recipient tends to reject (and destroy) a foreign substance, e.g. the kidney graft.
3. Possibility of recurrence of original disease in the graft (e.g. rapidly progressive glomerulonephritis).
4. Death from complications.

PROCEDURES DONE BEFORE TRANSPLANTATION
1. Bilateral nephrectomy – for uncontrolled hypertension (renin variety), for removal of potential source of infection, if present, and for patients with obstructed kidneys or vesicoureteral reflux, rapidly progressive glomerulonephritis, polycystic renal disease.
2. Immunosuppressive drugs given in order to minimize or overcome body's defence mechanism:
   a. Azathioprine (Imuran) and prednisone administration is usually begun 48 hours preoperatively for a scheduled transplant patient.
3. Donor-specific blood transfusion may be given – appears to improve graft survival.
4. Haemodialysis (see p. 622) is usually done 24 hours preoperatively.
5. Use of a skin depilatory cream is preferable to shaving (see p. 52, Chapter 3). Otherwise preoperative shaving is done in ᴛ̲ᴇ operating room as scratches and nicks from shaving provide opportunity for bacterial colonization.

Assessment
DIAGNOSTIC EVALUATION
This is in addition to the usual preoperative preparation.
1. Tissue typing done to determine histocompatibility of donor and recipient.
2. Antibody screening for red and white cell antibodies.
3. Blood counts, chemistries, coagulation profiles, liver function tests, required cultures, ECG, state of hydration, blood pressure, temperature, pulse, respiration and weight are corrected and documented.

PATIENT PROBLEMS
1. Potential for infection.
2. Fear related to threat of rejection and loss of kidney.
3. Disturbance in self-image (moon face, acne, hirsutism, etc) related to steroid medications.
4. Potential for complications.
5. See Patient Problems, Chronic Renal Failure, p. 614.

Planning and implementation
POSTOPERATIVE NURSING INTERVENTIONS
Monitoring for threatened rejection
1. Watch for signs of rejection – progressive enlargement, pain and tenderness of graft, elevated blood pressure, diminished urine volume, increased serum creatinine, weight gain, apprehension and fever.
   a. Acute rejection is common and usually reversible; often occurs in first weeks or months following transplant.

b. If rejection is inevitable or when excessive immunosuppression is required, transplanted kidney is removed.

c. The patient is placed back on maintenance dialysis; he will require understanding and supportive emotional care.

2. Assist with various test systems used to monitor graft recipient immune status; tissue injury monitoring may be predictive of a rejection episode.

3. Give prescribed combinations of immunosuppressive agents: azathioprine, corticosteroids, cyclosporine.

4. Be aware of complications of immunosuppressive protocols – infection or incomplete control of rejection.

Prevention of infection

1. Monitor and protect the patient from infection – kidney recipient is susceptible to faulty healing and infection because of both immunosuppressive therapy, which suppresses the immune response, and complications of renal failure.

a. Infection may be masked or confused with symptoms of rejection since impaired renal function and fever are evidences of both infection and rejection.

b. Immunosuppressive drugs render the transplant recipient more vulnerable to infection, permitting opportunistic infections to occur (fungal, viral, bacterial infections).

2. Carry out protective isolation as required; health team members and family may wear masks until immunosuppressive drug dosages are lowered.

3. Give aseptic care to wounds and puncture sites (central venous pressure and intravenous lines, draining sites, etc).

a. Wound healing may be delayed because of effects of renal disease and immunosuppressive drugs.

b. Change dressings promptly if drainage is present – drainage is an excellent culture medium for bacteria.

c. Carry out bacteriological testing of urine and all exit wounds. Catheter and drain tips are cultured on removal.

(i) Before removing catheter, disinfect skin around entry site of catheter (or drain). Remove.

(ii) Using aseptic technique, cut off tip of catheter or drain and place in sterile container for laboratory culture.

4. Monitor vascular access to haemodialysis to ensure patency and watch for evidence of infection.

5. Give oral nystatin mouthwash – to prevent mucosal candidiasis (fungal colonization occurs secondarily to steroid and antibiotic administration).

6. Give regular skin hygiene.

Maintenance of fluid and electrolyte balance

After kidney transplant, the following may occur:

1. A few donor kidneys function immediately after grafting.

a. May produce large quantities of dilute urine (10 to 15 litres in first 24 hours) – due partly to tubular dysfunction or overhydrated state found in some dialysed patients.
Give intravenous fluid replacement to balance losses as directed.

b. Cadaver kidney (because of period of ischaemia following donor's death) may undergo tubular necrosis and not function for two to three weeks. This is common in early postoperative period. Restrict fluid intake – usually approximately 600ml per 24 hours, plus amount of fluid losses from drainage, etc.

c. Or kidney may produce amounts of urine varying from extremes of no urine to large volumes of urine.

2. Monitor central venous pressure, ECG, and skin temperature frequently to guard against occult blood volume depletion and electrolyte imbalance.

a. Central venous pressure readings observed and recorded hourly or more frequently as necessary.

b. Avoid using dialysis access extremity for intravenous lines, intra-arterial monitoring or restraints.

3. Monitor output from indwelling catheter, which has been connected to a closed drainage system.

a. Measure urine every 30 minutes to one hour.

b. Irrigate catheter only on direct request.

c. Palpate bladder to detect presence of distension.

d. Instruct the patient to void urine frequently after catheter removal to avoid over-distension of the bladder and breakdown of anastomosis.

4. Monitor serum and urine electrolytes to determine the patient's chemical balance.

a. Anticipate adjustment of fluid replacement.

b. Give intravenous fluids according to urine volume and serum electrolyte levels; as directed serum and urine chemistries are measured at specified intervals.

c. Notify doctor immediately if dysrhythmias or other cardiac symptoms develop.

5. Prepare for haemodialysis in postoperative

period until transplanted kidney is functioning well.

Prevention of complications

1. Acute renal failure – from ischaemia, renal artery thrombosis, hyperacute rejection.
2. Gastrointestinal complications:
   a. Gastrointestinal ulceration and bleeding; perforation; sepsis.
      (i) Steroids mask symptoms of ulceration.
      (ii) Gastrointestinal haemorrhage associated with high mortality rate.
      (iii) Give antacids frequently as directed until steroid doses are lowered – as a means of protection against gastrointestinal ulceration.
   b. Fungal colonization of gastrointestinal tract – occurs secondarily to steroid and antibiotic administration.
   c. Faecal impaction – decrease in colonic motility may occur from steroid effect.
3. Other late complications; some may be the cause of death.
   a. Infection, diabetes, gastrointestinal bleeding, thrombosis, osteoporosis, psychosis, disorders of calcium metabolism, cushingoid face, glaucoma, cataracts, acne – from prolonged steroid administration.
   b. Bone marrow depression – from immunosuppressive therapy.
   c. Vascular complications – haemorrhage and thrombosis.
   d. Grafted ureter – stricture, fistula (also fistula of bladder).
   e. Viral hepatitis; liver failure.
   f. Hypertension – from renal artery stenosis in allograft, from steroids, from renovascular disease.
   g. Cardiovascular complications – myocardial infarction; stroke.
   h. Bone complications – aseptic necrosis due to secondary hyperparathyroidism.
   i. Suicide.
   j. Cancer – people on long-term immunosuppressive therapy develop cancer more frequently than does the general population.

Psychosocial support

1. Be aware of the stresses associated with renal transplantation – difficulty in planning for uncertain future, fear of organ rejection, problems associated with immunosuppressants and steroids.
2. Keep the patient informed of his progress, proposed treatment plans, and short and long-term goals.
3. Observe for changes in behaviour, altered thought and feeling processes.
4. See p. 625 for other aspects of psychological support.

PATIENT EDUCATION

1. The hospitalization period for a kidney transplant may be prolonged.
2. The patient receives individualized instruction about the following:
   a. Diet.
   b. Medications (immunosuppressive drugs, antacids, vitamins, iron).
      (i) Review medications in detail, including colour identification of pills, dose schedules, side-effects and the necessity for taking the medication.
   c. Fluids.
   d. Daily weight.
   e. Daily measurement of urine.
   f. Management of intake and output.
   g. Stool test for occult blood twice weekly.
   h. Prevention of infection.
   i. Resumption of activity; exercise.
3. Instruct the patient to report to the doctor immediately if any of the following occur:
   a. Decrease in urinary output.
   b. Weight gain (detectable oedema means excess fluid).
   c. Malaise.
   d. Fever.
   e. Graft swelling and tenderness.
   f. Changes in blood pressure readings.
   g. Respiratory distress.
   h. Anxiety, depression, changes in eating, drinking or other habit patterns.
4. Advise the patient to avoid strenuous contact sports after surgery.
5. The patient should know that follow-up care after transplantation is a lifelong necessity.
6. Encourage the patient to become active in renal self-help group:
   British Kidney Patients Association, Bordon Hants (Tel: 04203 2022/1).

Evaluation

EXPECTED OUTCOMES

1. Patient is free of infection.
2. Patient shows no signs of rejection or renal failure.

3. Patient copes with fear of graft rejection – communicates feelings and concerns; takes responsibility for health monitoring.
4. Patient adapts to changes in self-concept and appearance.

NURSING MANAGEMENT OF THE PATIENT UNDERGOING RENAL/UROLOGICAL SURGERY

NURSING PROCESS OVERVIEW

Preoperative assessment
Note: Surgical approaches to the kidney predispose the patient to respiratory complications and paralytic ileus.

1. Support the patient undergoing diagnostic examination of the urinary tract.
2. Determine history of patient's ability to engage in physical activity without distress. Observe for dyspnoea, productive cough, other cardiac symptoms.
3. An electrocardiogram is usually performed on all patients over 50. The preoperative cardiogram also serves as a baseline reference in event of postoperative cardiopulmonary complications.
4. Secure a chest X-ray.
5. The doctor will carry out pulmonary function studies and blood gas analysis in patients with impaired respiratory function.
6. Assess status of vascular system of lower extremities (especially varicosities).
   a. Elevate the patient's leg and apply elastic stockings to minimize stasis in superficial veins.
   b. Encourage patients to do leg exercises.
7. Inquire if the patient has any bleeding tendencies.
8. Assess fluid and electrolyte status.
   a. Weigh the patient daily to determine status of fluid balance.
   b. Assess status of mucous membranes and skin elasticity; maintain the haematocrit at optimal level.
   c. Measure and record intake and output as an index of hydration.

PREOPERATIVE NURSING INTERVENTIONS
1. Encourage liberal intake of fluids to promote excretion of waste products before surgery and to ensure that the patient is well-hydrated.
2. Give antibiotic therapy as directed; kidney infection may be present preoperatively.
3. Teach the patient deep-breathing exercises and an effective cough routine.
4. Encourage the patient to express his feelings and concerns about impending surgery.
   a. Keep in mind that most patients entering hospital with urological conditions have pain, fever, haematuria, difficulty in voiding urine, etc.
   b. Obtain the patient's confidence by establishing a relationship of trust and by giving gentle and considerate care.
   c. Increase the patient's understanding of what to expect during both preoperative and postoperative periods.
   d. Assess for alertness, appetite and general well-being of the patient.
   e. Avoid physical inactivity.
   f. Give preoperative medications as prescribed to allay worry and fear.
5. See p. 45 for general preoperative preparation.

PATIENT PROBLEMS
1. Potential for complications related to the site of incision and nature of surgery.
2. Pain and discomfort related to the surgical procedure(s) and presence of drainage tubes/catheters.
3. Anxiety related to uncertainty of surgical outcome.

Planning and implementation
NURSING INTERVENTIONS
Prevention of complications
1. Employ frequent and close observation of blood pressure, pulse and respiration in order to recognize haemorrhage (and shock) – the chief danger after renal surgery.
   a. Watch for pain, blood loss from drain site, mass over flank, shock.
   b. Prepare for reoperation; see management of haemorrhage, p. 66
2. Assess for pulmonary complications; postoperative atelectasis, p. 67, pneumothorax, p. 197, and pneumonia, p. 171.
3. Be alert for symptoms of postoperative ileus (fairly common following renal surgery).
   a. Assess for abdominal distension, pain and lack of intestinal peristalsis (determined by stethoscope auscultation).
   b. Avoid oral intake for patient until active bowel

sounds are heard (auscultation) or passage of flatus is noted.

c. Give adequate and appropriate fluid and electrolyte replacement intravenously as directed.

d. Assist with decompression via nasogastric tube for relief of abdominal distension (p. 430). See p. 488 for treatment of paralytic ileus.

e. Keep record of fluid status.

4. Monitor for thromboembolic episodes.

a. Employ early ambulation as an aid in preventing thromboembolic episodes and improving patient endurance.

Note: Ambulation is contraindicated in prostatic patients with bleeding and with some types of reconstructive surgery.

b. Encourage the patient to do leg exercises in bed.

5. Watch for elevation of temperature and monitor the drainage tube sites and urine output for evidences of infection.

Relief of pain and discomfort

1. Give postoperative sedation and pain control on an individual basis to aid respiratory movements and to permit coughing, since incision is close to diaphragm.

a. Administer analgesics at regular intervals – to help the patient perform deep breathing and coughing more effectively.

b. Use moist heat, massage and analgesics for muscular aches and pain resulting from position on operating table.

c. Assess for pain similar to renal colic – caused by passage of clotted blood down the ureter; requires adequate doses of analgesics for relief.

d. Encourage coughing after each deep breath to loosen secretions.

Management of drainage tubes and catheters

1. Make certain that drainage tubes are functioning, since almost all urological patients have drains, tubes or catheters.

a. Make sure indwelling catheter is dependent and draining.

(i) Tape tubing to thigh to relieve traction on bladder. In supine male patient, tape catheter to lower abdomen. In women, anchor catheter to thigh, allowing enough slack for movement.

(ii) Give meticulous catheter care.

b. Change dressings as indicated when the patient has profuse drainage.

c. Employ care with the patient with nephrostomy tube drainage (insertion of tube directly into kidney for temporary or permanent urinary diversion). It is attached to closed gravity drainage or to a urostomy appliance. A self-retaining U-tube or circular nephrostomy tube may be used.

(i) Purpose of nephrostomy drainage:

(a) To provide drainage from kidney after surgery.

(b) To conserve and permit physiological restoration of renal tissue that has been traumatized by obstruction.

(c) To provide drainage when ureter is no longer functioning.

(ii) Evaluate for bleeding from nephrostomy site (main complication of nephrostomy).

(iii) Ensure that the nephrostomy tube is draining freely – plugging of the tube causes pain, trauma, bursting of suture lines and infection.

(a) Call doctor *immediately* if tube is inadvertently dislodged.

(b) Do not clamp the nephrostomy tube.

(c) Irrigate nephrostomy tube only by direct doctor request. Use 10ml warm sterile saline solution – to avoid mechanical damage to kidney or infection from pyelorenal backflow.

(d) Encourage adequate fluid intake – to produce effective mechanical flushing and to dilute urinary elements that cause calculus formation.

(e) If there is a nephrostomy tube in each kidney, keep separate output records for each nephrostomy tube.

2. Assess the patient with indwelling ureteral catheter (utilized to permit drainage from affected kidney).

a. Ureteral catheters are inserted through a cystoscope and left in place for a period of time; they are taped to the indwelling urethral catheter to hold them in place.

b. Tape catheter to thigh to reduce pulling on catheter.

c. Make notation on nursing care plan that catheter is a *ureteral* catheter.

d. Do not irrigate a ureteral catheter; this is done by the urologist.

3. Watch for complications from ureteral catheter; infection (from foreign body in genitourinary

tract), bleeding or clot obstruction within the catheter, dislodgement of the catheter.

PATIENT EDUCATION

1. Teach the patient/family about care of catheters/tubes and management of dressings if the patient is to return home with indwelling tubes.
2. Continue a liberal intake of fluids.
3. Take frequent short rest periods and increase activities gradually.
4. Avoid straining or lifting heavy objects until permitted by doctor.

Evaluation

EXPECTED OUTCOMES

1. Patient remains free of complications.
2. Patient achieves relief of pain and discomfort; requests pain medication; moves freely.
3. Patient discusses fears; makes post-discharge plans.

INFECTIONS OF THE URINARY TRACT

A urinary tract infection (UTI) is caused by the presence of pathogenic micro-organisms in the urinary tract with or without signs and symptoms. Infection may predominate at the bladder (cystitis), urethra (urethritis), prostate (prostatitis), or kidney (pyelonephritis). Unfortunately, noninfectious conditions may generate symptoms that mimic those of urinary tract infection.

Bacteriuria refers to the presence of bacteria in the urine (10^5 bacteria/ml of urine or greater generally indicates infection).

In *asymptomatic bacteriuria*, organisms are found in urine, but the patient has no symptoms.

Recurrent urinary tract infections may indicate the following:

1. Relapse – recurrence of bacteriuria with same infecting micro-organism.
2. Reinfection – recurrence of bacteriuria with a micro-organism different from that of the original infection (i.e., a 'new' infection).

NURSING ALERT

Infections in any part of the urinary tract may persist for months or years without symptoms and eventually cause serious kidney damage.

PREDISPOSING FACTORS

1. Urinary stasis and obstruction (ureteral stenosis, stone, tumour) – slowing of urinary flow causes kidney to be more susceptible to bacterial infection.
2. Increasing intraluminal pressure or overdistended bladder.
3. Reflux:
   a. Urethrovesical reflux – flowing back of urine from urethra into bladder.
   b. Vesicoureteral reflux (ureterovesical reflux) – flowing back of urine from bladder into one or both ureters.
4. Faecal soiling of urethral meatus.
5. Instrumentation – catheter, cystoscope.
6. Metabolic disorders (diabetes mellitus) and diseases of blood vessels (arteriosclerosis) may diminish blood supply to organs of urinary tract.
7. Neurological abnormalities (neurogenic bladder dysfunction).
8. Renal disease increases susceptibility of kidney to infection.

PATHWAYS OF INFECTION WITHIN URINARY TRACT

Bacteria invade and spread within tract by the ascending (most common), bloodstream and/or lymphatic pathways.

1. Urethra – from ascending bacteria.
2. Bladder – from bacteria ascending from urethra (or, less commonly, descending from kidney).
3. Kidney – from ureterovesical reflux (incompetence of ureterovesical valve, which allows urine to regurgitate into ureters, usually at time of voiding); blood-borne.
4. Prostate – from ascending urethral flora.
5. Epididymis – from infected prostate.
6. Testis – from bacteria via the bloodstream.

LOWER URINARY TRACT INFECTION (CYSTITIS, ACUTE URETHRAL SYNDROME)

Cystitis is an inflammation of the urinary bladder; it is usually a superficial infection that does not extend to the bladder mucosa.

Acute urethral syndrome is symptomatic urinary tract infection in women whose urine is either sterile or contains less than 10^5 bacteria/ml.

AETIOLOGY

1. Ascending infection after entry via the urinary meatus.

a. Women seem to be more apt to develop acute cystitis because of shorter length of urethra, anatomic proximity to vagina, periurethral glands and rectum (faecal contamination), and the mechanical effect of coitus.

b. Women with recurrent urinary tract infections often have Gram-negative organisms at the vaginal introitus; there may be some defect of the mucosa of the urethra, vagina or external genitalia of these patients that allows enteric organisms to invade the bladder.

c. Poor/abnormal voiding patterns cause decrease in blood supply to bladder.

d. Acute infection in women most often from organisms of the patient's own intestinal flora (*Escherichia coli*).

2. In males, obstructive abnormalities (strictures, prostatism) – most frequent cause.

3. Upper urinary tract disease may occasionally cause recurrent bladder infection.

Assessment

CLINICAL FEATURES

1. Frequency, urgency, burning and pain on urination.
2. Nocturia.
3. Bearing-down sensation in region of bladder; suprapubic pain.
4. Changes in composition of urine (bacteria and red blood cells).

DIAGNOSTIC EVALUATION

Urine culture is done to detect presence of bacteria and for antibiotic susceptibility testing.

PATIENT PROBLEMS

1. Urinary frequency and dysuria related to presence of bacterial infection.
2. Potential for recurrence of infection.

Planning and implementation

NURSING INTERVENTIONS

Eradicating the causative pathogen

1. Obtain uncontaminated urine specimen for smears, culture and antibiotic sensitivity studies to determine pathogen so that the appropriate drug may be selected.

2. Give prescribed antibiotics, since urinary infections usually respond to drugs that are excreted in the urine in high concentrations; a potentially effective drug should rapidly sterilize the urine and thus relieve the patient's symptoms.

   a. For uncomplicated infection:

      (i) Single-dose antibiotics (co-trimoxazole, Septrin, Bactrim).

      (ii) Side-effects are nausea, diarrhoea, drug-related rash and vaginal candidiasis.

   b. For acute urethral syndrome:

      (i) Antibiotics for 10 days.

      (ii) Repeat urine culture after seven to 10 days to ensure elimination of infection.

   c. For recurrent infections with closely spaced episodes:

      (i) The patient may require treatment for six months or more.

      (ii) Patients with recurring infections should have periodic urine cultures, since most recurrences are new infections with different organisms; relapses may occur with same organism.

3. Maintain an appropriate urine pH – efficacy of certain antibiotics is affected by the reaction (pH) of the urine. Sodium bicarbonate alkalinizes urine; ascorbic acid acidifies urine.

Increasing the body's normal defence mechanisms

1. Encourage the patient to drink fluids sufficient to promote renal blood flow and to flush out bacteria in urinary tract.

2. Encourage the patient to void urine frequently (every two to three hours) and to empty bladder completely, since this enhances bacterial clearance, reduces urine stasis and prevents reinfection. Infrequent voiding overstretches the bladder wall, leading to hypoxia of bladder mucosa, which is then susceptible to bacterial invasion.

3. Promote patient comfort.

   a. Give analgesics and antispasmodics.

   b. Encourage bed rest during the acute phase.

PATIENT EDUCATION

1. Encourage the patient to have follow-up urine studies to determine if there is resolution of infection or if asymptomatic infection is present; there is a marked tendency for infection to recur.

2. For women with repeated urinary tract infections, give the following instructions:

   a. Reduce vaginal introital concentration of pathogens by hygienic measures.

      (i) Wash in shower or while standing in bath – bacteria in bath water may gain entrance into urethra.

      (ii) Cleanse around the perineum and urethral meatus after each bowel movement, with front to back cleansing to minimize faecal contamination of periurethral area.

b. Drink liberal amounts of fluid to flush out bacteria.

c. Avoid irritants – coffee, tea, alcohol, cola drinks.

d. Void urine every two to three hours during day and completely empty bladder.

e. In certain women, sexual intercourse is the initiating event for the development of bacteriuria – urethral massage associated with intercourse facilitates entry of micro-organisms into the bladder.
   (i) Void urine before and immediately after sexual intercourse.
   (ii) A single dose of an oral antibiotic agent may be prescribed following sexual intercourse.

f. Avoid external irritants such as bubble baths and perfumed vaginal cleansers or deodorants.

g. An antibacterial vaginal suppository may be prescribed to reduce concentration of bacteria in introitus.

h. Patients with persistent bacteria may require long-term antibiotic therapy to prevent colonization of periurethral area and recurrence of urinary tract infection.
   (i) Take the drug last thing at night after emptying bladder to ensure adequate concentration of drug during overnight period, since low rates of urine flow and infrequent bladder emptying predispose to multiplication of bacteria.

3. Instruct patients who have had urinary tract infections during pregnancy to have follow-up studies.

4. Teach the patient that bacteriuria in young girls (under five years) increases the risk of developing a urinary tract infection as an adult.

Evaluation

EXPECTED OUTCOMES

1. Patient is free of urinary frequency, dysuria and bacteriuria.
2. Patient demonstrates no evidence of recurrence.

BACTERIAL PYELONEPHRITIS

Bacterial pyelonephritis is an acute inflammatory renal disease caused by bacteria.

CAUSES

1. Enteric bacteria (*E. coli*).

2. Secondary to vesicoureteral reflux (incompetence of ureterovesical valve, which allows urine to regurgitate into ureters, usually at time of voiding).
3. Urinary obstruction/infection.
4. Trauma.
5. Blood-borne infection.
6. Renal disease.
7. Pregnancy.
8. Metabolic disorders.

CLINICAL FEATURES

Flank pain; tenderness in the costovertebral angle, dysuria, fever, urgency, and frequency.

DIAGNOSTIC EVALUATION

1. Identification of antibody-coated bacteria in urine; bacteria invading kidney induce an antibody response that coats the bacteria – differentiates renal infection from bladder infection.
2. Identification of pyuria, bacteriuria and casts in urinary sediment.
3. Other radiological/urinary tests, as directed.

NURSING INTERVENTIONS
Eradication of bacteria from the urinary tract

1. Assist with carrying out intravenous urogram and other diagnostic tests – relief of obstructions is essential to save kidney from rapid destruction.
2. Obtain urine specimen (under aseptic conditions) for culture and sensitivity studies, since choice of drug is based on sensitivity studies.
3. Give organism-specific antibiotic as prescribed. Antibacterial agent is maintained in urine for a long enough period to prevent reseeding of residual foci of infection.
   a. Acute pyelonephritis usually caused by *E. coli*, which is sensitive to many antibiotics.
   b. A minimum of 14 days of treatment with an appropriate antibiotic is needed for bacteriuria of renal origin.
      (i) The patient is admitted to hospital if he is toxic and cannot tolerate oral antibiotics; bacteraemia is common.
      (ii) Parenteral antibiotics may be necessary.
4. Obtain urine for repeated cultures to determine the patient's response to treatment, to search for secondary organisms and to determine clinical and microbiological resolution of infection.

For the patient with chronic or recurring infections: preservation of renal function

1. Employ continuous treatment with urine-sterilizing agents after initial antibiotic treatment has been employed.

2. Advise the patient to continue this regimen for months to years until (a) there is no evidence of inflammation, (b) causative factors have been treated or controlled, and (c) there is evidence of stability of renal function.
3. Emphasize to the patient that serial urine cultures and evaluation studies must be done for an indefinite period of time.
4. Encourage the patient to have blood counts and serum creatinine determinations if he is on long-term therapy.

GENITOURINARY TUBERCULOSIS

Genitourinary tuberculosis is caused by the organism *Mycobacterium tuberculosis* and is usually disseminated from the lungs via the bloodstream to one or both of the kidneys and to other organs of the genitourinary tract.

CLINICAL FEATURES
1. Haematuria (microscopic or gross).
2. Bladder irritation – burning on urination, frequency, nocturia.
3. Features from infection of prostate and epididymis.
4. Slight afternoon fever, loss of weight, anorexia.

DIAGNOSTIC EVALUATION
1. Urine culture for tubercle bacilli (smears of urinary sediment also stained for acid-fast bacilli).
2. Excretory urogram – to reveal renal and ureteral lesions.
3. Cystoscopic examination – to determine extent of bladder involvement, for biopsy purposes and for ureteral catheterization of each kidney to determine if one or both kidneys are affected.

NURSING ALERT
A search for tuberculosis elsewhere in the body must be conducted when tuberculosis of the kidney or urinary tract is found. Be alert for patient who has had previous contact with tuberculosis.

MANAGEMENT
1. Combination of the following drugs usually given: rifampicin, isoniazid, ethambutol.
   a. Multiple drug regimen appears to delay the emergence of resistant organisms.
   b. Many centres are using short-term chemotherapy for initial treatment of genitourinary tuberculosis.
2. Surgical intervention may be necessary to prevent obstructive problems and to remove severely infected organ. However, emphasis is on medical treatment.

PATIENT EDUCATION
Instruct the patient as follows:
1. Follow-up examinations, including periodic urine examinations and excretory urograms are necessary to detect reactivation of disease.
2. Report for cystoscopic examination as directed to detect ureteral stricture formation, which is a complication of genitourinary tuberculosis.
3. Adhere to medication regimen.
4. Maintain good health practices since genitourinary tuberculosis is a manifestation of a systemic disease.

ACUTE GLOMERULONEPHRITIS

Acute glomerulonephritis refers to a group of kidney diseases in which there is an inflammatory reaction in the glomeruli. It is not an infection of the kidney *per se*, but rather the result of untoward side-effects of the defence mechanisms of the body. It is thought to involve an antigen–antibody reaction, which produces damage to the glomeruli, the filtering bed of the kidney.

ALTERED PHYSIOLOGY
Cellular proliferation, infiltration of glomerulus by leucocytes → glomerular trapping of circulating immune complexes → thickening of glomerular filtration membrane → scarring and loss of filtering surface → renal failure.

Assessment
CLINICAL FEATURES
1. The disease may be so mild that it is discovered accidentally through a routine urinalysis.
2. History of preceding pharyngitis or tonsillitis with fever (two to three weeks previously); majority of cases caused by streptococci.
3. Dark or smoky urine; oliguria.
4. Facial oedema; oedema of extremities.
5. Fatigue and anorexia.
6. Hypertension (mild, moderate, or severe); headache.
7. Tenderness over costovertebral angle.
8. Anaemia from loss of red blood cells into the urine.

DIAGNOSTIC EVALUATION

1. Urinalysis – haematuria (microscopic or gross), proteinuria (500mg–3g/day), red cell casts, white cells, renal epithelial cells and various casts in the sediment.
2. Blood – elevated blood urea nitrogen and serum creatinine levels, low total serum protein level, increased antistreptolysin titre (from reaction to streptococcal organism).
3. Needle biopsy of the kidney reveals obstruction of glomerular capillaries from proliferation of endothelial cells.

CLINICAL COURSE

1. Diuresis usually starts one to two weeks after onset of symptoms.
   a. Renal clearances and blood urea concentration return to normal.
   b. Oedema decreases and hypertension lessens.
   c. Microscopic proteinuria or haematuria may persist for many months.
2. Recovery is usual in children and young adults; in an older person, the disease may progress to chronic glomerulonephritis.

PATIENT PROBLEMS

1. Altered urinary elimination patterns.
2. Severe protein loss related to glomerular damage.
3. Fluid imbalance.
4. Potential for renal failure.
5. Fatigue and anorexia related to underlying disease.

Planning and implementation
NURSING INTERVENTIONS
Promotion of kidney function

1. Encourage bed rest during the acute phase until the urine clears and blood urea, creatinine and blood pressure normalize. (Rest also facilitates diuresis.)
2. Restrict dietary protein moderately if there is oliguria and the urea is elevated.
   a. Give carbohydrates liberally to provide energy and reduce catabolism of protein.
   b. Restrict protein more drastically if acute renal failure develops (see p. 611).
   c. Restrict sodium intake in presence of oedema or signs of congestive heart failure.
3. Measure and record intake and output.
4. Give fluids according to the patient's fluid losses (urine, respiration, faeces) and daily body weight.

Prevention of complications

1. Recognize and treat any intercurrent infections promptly.
2. Watch for symptoms of renal failure – nausea, fatigue, vomiting, diminished urinary output (see p. 612).
3. Evaluate the patient for:
   a. Hypertensive encephalopathy.
   b. Cardiac failure and pulmonary oedema.
4. Dialysis may be considered if uraemia and fluid retention cannot be controlled.

PATIENT EDUCATION
Instruct the patient as follows:

1. Explain that the patient must have follow-up evaluations of blood pressure, urinary protein and blood urea nitrogen concentrations to determine if there is exacerbation of disease activity.
2. Treat any infection promptly.
3. Call doctor if symptoms of renal failure occur.

Evaluation
EXPECTED OUTCOMES

1. Patient shows no signs of proteinuria.
2. Patient achieves stabilization of renal function – normal urine/blood evaluations; normal blood pressure.

NEPHROTIC SYNDROME

Nephrotic syndrome is a clinical disorder characterized by (1) marked proteinuria, (2) hypoalbuminaemia, (3) oedema, and (4) hyperlipidaemia as a consequence of excessive leakage of plasma proteins into the urine because of increased permeability of the glomerular capillary membrane to protein.

AETIOLOGY
In any condition that seriously damages the glomerular capillary membrane, any of the following aetiologies are possible.

1. Chronic glomerulonephritis.
2. Diabetes mellitus with intercapillary glomerulosclerosis.
3. Amyloidosis of kidney.
4. Systemic lupus erythematosus (SLE).
5. Renal vein thrombosis.
6. Secondary to malignancy (older adults).

Assessment
CLINICAL FEATURES

1. Insidious onset of oedema; easily pitting oedema.
2. Marked proteinuria – leads to negative nitrogen balance.
3. Extensive depletion of body proteins (hypoalbuminaemia) from extensive urinary protein losses.

4. Hyperlipidaemia – may lead to accelerated atherosclerosis.

DIAGNOSTIC EVALUATION

1. Needle biopsy of kidney – for histological examination of renal tissue to confirm diagnosis.
2. Serum electrolyte evaluations (protein, albumin, etc).
3. Triglyceride profile – to evaluate degree of hyperlipidaemia.
4. Urinary tests – for microscopic haematuria, proteinuria, red blood cells, white blood cells, casts, fat bodies.
5. Renal function tests.

PATIENT PROBLEMS

1. Oedema related to renal retention of salt and water.
2. Potential for infection.
3. See also Acute Glomerulonephritis (p. 634).

Planning and implementation
MEDICAL MANAGEMENT

1. Sodium restriction.
2. Diuretics, if renal insufficiency is not severe.
3. Steroids (prednisone) – to reduce oedema and proteinuria.
4. Immunosuppressive agents – may be effective when nephrosis is associated with autoimmune disease.

NURSING INTERVENTIONS

1. Keep on bed rest for a few days to mobilize oedema.
2. Utilize dietary treatment to replace protein losses.
   a. High protein diet to replenish wasted tissues and restore body proteins.
   b. Mild to moderate sodium restriction to control severe oedema.
   c. High calorie diet (25–50cal/kg body weight/day)
3. Protect patient from infection – thought to be due to loss of serum immunoglobulins into the urine.
4. Evaluate for thromboembolism (renal vein thrombosis, pulmonary emboli, thrombophlebitis) – increased incidence in patients with nephrotic syndrome.
5. See p. 634 for nursing the patient with acute glomerulonephritis, and p. 614 for care of the patient with chronic renal failure.

Evaluation
EXPECTED OUTCOMES

1. Patient is free of oedema.
2. Patient shows no signs of proteinuria or infection.
3. Patient adheres to diet to replace protein loss.
4. Patient is free of complications.

HYDRONEPHROSIS

Hydronephrosis is distension of the pelvis and calyces by urine due to obstruction of the ureter.

CAUSES

1. Congenital causes – stenosis of ureteropelvic junction, urethral valves.
2. Progressive changes in bladder, ureters and kidneys from obstruction anywhere in urinary tract:
   a. Obstruction from enlarged prostate.
   b. Obstructing calculus.
   c. Malignant lesion (cancer of prostate, bladder or cervix).
   d. Obstruction of ureter – from calculus, stricture, etc.
3. Neurogenic causes.
4. Vesicoureteral reflux.

ALTERED PHYSIOLOGY

Interference with passage of urine from kidney → chronic infection → increasing pressure → distension of renal pelvis and calyces → decreased renal blood flow → atrophy of renal parenchyma (as one kidney undergoes gradual destruction, the contralateral kidney gradually enlarges [compensatory hypertrophy]) → impairment of renal function.

Assessment
CLINICAL FEATURES

1. Often asymptomatic and insidious onset.
2. Aching in flank and back (present with acute obstruction).
3. Bladder irritability – fever and dysuria if infection is present.
4. Gastrointestinal disturbances.
5. Chills, fever, tenderness, pyuria – from infection.
6. Haematuria – hydronephrotic kidney may bleed from congestion.
7. Uraemia – if condition is advanced.

DIAGNOSTIC EVALUATION

Complete urographic survey.

PATIENT PROBLEMS

1. Alteration in urinary elimination (reduced urinary output, haematuria) related to obstruction of ureters.

2. Pain and discomfort related to obstruction of urinary flow.
3. Potential for infection.

Planning and implementation
NURSING INTERVENTIONS
1. Relieve obstruction, etc.
   Urine may have to be diverted by nephrostomy or other types of diversion.
   a. Ureteral catheter may be inserted by urologist to decompress kidney if the patient is having severe flank pain.
   b. See p. 630 for care of the patient having a nephrostomy.
2. Give antibiotic as directed to eradicate infection, since residual urine in calyces produces infection and pyelonephritis.
3. Prepare for surgical intervention to correct obstruction (see p. 629).
   a. Removal of obstructive lesions (calculus, tumour, obstruction of ureter).
   b. Operations to improve drainage of kidney; plastic reconstruction procedures.
   c. Nephrectomy – if one kidney is severely damaged.

PATIENT EDUCATION
Report for urinalysis follow-up every two to three weeks and excretory urography as directed to determine if satisfactory progress is being made.

Evaluation
EXPECTED OUTCOMES
1. Patient demonstrates normal urinary output without signs of haematuria.
2. Patient is free of infection.

UROLITHIASIS

Urolithiasis refers to the presence of stones in the urinary system. Stones are formed in the urinary tract by the deposit of crystalline substances (calcium phosphate, oxalate, uric acid) excreted in the urine. They may be found anywhere in the urinary system and vary in size from mere granular deposits (called sand or gravel), to bladder stones the size of an orange.

FACTORS FAVOURING STONE FORMATION
1. Obstruction and urinary stasis facilitating precipitation of salts from the urine.
2. Infection – particularly of urea-splitting organisms (*Proteus vulgaris*).
3. Dehydration and urine concentration – encourages precipitation of solids.
4. Immobilization – produces slowing of renal drainage and altered calcium metabolism.
5. Metabolic disorders:
   a. Hypercalcaemia (abnormally high concentration of blood calcium compounds) and hypercalciuria (abnormally large amounts of calcium in urine) from dissolution of bone, excessive ingestion or excessive absorption of calcium from gastrointestinal tract or faulty renal reabsorption of calcium.
   b. Hyperparathyroidism.
   c. Excessive intake of vitamin D.
   d. Excessive intake of milk and alkali.
   e. Myeloproliferative disorders (leukaemia, polycythaemia vera) and chemotherapy for cancer – patients excrete increased amounts of uric acid.
6. Excessive excretion of uric acid.
7. Vitamin deficiency (especially vitamin A).
8. Foreign bodies in urinary tract.
9. High intake of protein, calcium, excessive consumption of tea and fruit juices.
10. Small bowel disease or small bowel surgery.
11. Heredity – plays a part in calcium oxalate stones (most common type), cystine and uric acid stones.
12. Idiopathic – no cause can be found.

CLINICAL FEATURES
1. The problem occurs predominantly in the third to fifth decade, affecting men more than women.
2. The majority of stones are composed of calcium oxalate with or without uric acid or (rarely) cystine.
3. Infection and obstruction may cause destruction of renal tissue and subsequent loss of a kidney.
4. Most renal stones migrate downward (causing severe, colicky pain) and are discovered in the lower ureter.
5. People who have had two stones tend to have recurrences.

MEDICAL MANAGEMENT
(Dictated by size, shape, position and likely chemical composition of stone[s].)
Specific therapy – regimen depends on stone type/metabolic abnormality.
1. *Calcium stones* (calcium oxalate and calcium phosphate; most prevalent):
   a. Moderate dietary intake of calcium and phosphorus; restrict oxalate-containing beverages (cola, tea).

b. Administer drugs, depending on classification of hypercalciuria – orthophosphates, thiazides, magnesium oxide, sodium cellulose phosphate, potassium citrate.

c. Round-the-clock intake of fluid to maintain a high urine flow rate.

2. *Uric acid stones* (develop in highly acidic and concentrated urine):
   a. Alkalinize the urine to enhance urate solubility.
   b. Limit protein and purine intake; encourage high fluid intake.
   c. Administer allopurinol to lower serum and urinary acid levels and inhibit uric acid synthesis.
   d. Amenable to dissolution techniques.

3. *Cystine stones* (rare):
   a. Increase fluid intake; exclude excess dietary animal protein.
   b. Administer penicillamine – decreases stone formation and sometimes results in stone dissolution.

4. *Struvite stones* (infection-related stones) – associated with urinary tract infections with urea-splitting bacteria (*Proteus* species, *Klebsiella*, *Pseudomonas, Staphylococcus*). May occur as a large staghorn calculi and cause significant renal damage from infection and obstruction.
   a. Acidify urine.
   b. Given appropriate antibiotic therapy – patient may be given continuous antibiotic therapy to keep urine sterile if surgery is not possible.
   c. Stone dissolution may be an alternative to surgery for selected patients.

INTERVENTIONAL PROCEDURES

Percutaneous stone removal procedures

See Figure 9.11.

1. *Percutaneous nephrostomy/nephrolithotomy* (radiological placement of tube into collection system of kidney). Under fluoroscopic or ultrasound guidance, needle is advanced into collecting system; guide wire is advanced into kidney pelvis (or ureter). On the following day, dilators are passed over guide wire for dilatation, tract is established through the renal parenchyma, and catheter placed in renal pelvis.
   a. After 24 hours, endoscope is passed down through established tract to visualize interior of collecting system.
   b. Small stones may be retrieved through forceps, snared with a basket extractor under vision, or washed out.
   c. Larger or impacted stones require fragmentation (by ultrasound, electrohydraulic shock waves, or lasers).
   d. Offers shorter hospital stay, less patient morbidity and earlier return to employment.

Surgical procedures

1. *Pyelolithotomy* – removal of stones from kidney pelvis.
   Coagulum pyelolithotomy – intraoperative injection of certain coagulation factors into the renal pelvis, producing a coagulum that entraps the stones and expedites their removal (Figure 9.12).

2. *Nephrolithotomy* – incision into kidney for removal of stone.

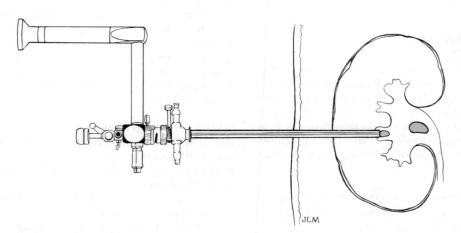

Figure 9.11. A percutaneous nephrostomy tract permits access to the collecting system of the kidney for removal of kidney stones under direct vision via a nephroscope

3. *Nephrectomy* – removal of kidney; indicated when kidney is extensively and irreparably damaged and is no longer a functioning organ; partial nephrectomy is sometimes done.
4. *Ureterolithotomy* – removal of stone in ureter.
5. *Cystolithotomy* – removal of stone from bladder.

Stone destruction (by energy in various wave forms)

This allows endoscopic removal of stones too large to pass.
1. Percutaneous nephrolithotomy (ultrasonic lithotripsy) – introduction of an ultrasonic probe through a nephrostomy tube to shatter the stone into fragments.
   a. The portion of the stone in contact with vibrating tip of probe is reduced to dust/small fragments, which are continuously removed by suction.
   b. Remaining stone fragments are retrieved by forceps or stone basket (residual calculi may present a problem).
2. Extracorporeal shock-wave lithotripsy (ESWL) (electrohydraulic lithotripsy) – disintegration of stone by creating an electrical discharge in a fluid.
   a. The patient is placed in tank of water through which are propagated shock waves that break up the stone.
   b. Considered investigational.

3. Stone disruption by laser impulse (investigational).

Assessment
CLINICAL FEATURES
Dependent on presence of obstruction, infection, oedema.
1. Stones blocking flow of urine produce symptoms of urinary tract infection – chills, fever, dysuria.
2. Renal stones – produce an increase in hydrostatic pressure and distension of the renal pelvis and proximal ureter, causing:
   a. Pain in renal area – radiates anteriorly and downward toward bladder in female and toward testicle in male.
   b. Renal colic – acute pain with tenderness over loin; nausea and vomiting.
3. Ureteral stones:
   a. Acute colicky pain, referring down the thigh and to genitalia (ureteral colic).
   b. Frequent desire to void, but little urine is passed.
4. Gastrointestinal symptoms:
   a. Due to renal-intestinal reflexes and anatomical relation of kidneys to stomach, pancreas, colon, etc.
   b. Include nausea, vomiting, diarrhoea, abdominal discomfort.

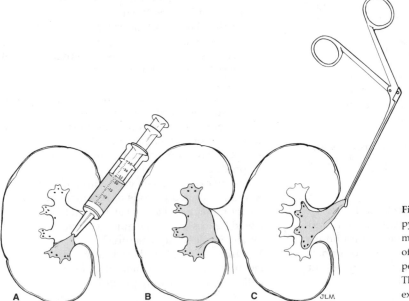

Figure 9.12. The procedure, coagulum pyelolithotomy, is useful for removal of multiple kidney stones. (A) Components of coagulum are instilled into the renal pelvis (B) to produce a jelly-like clot. (C) The stones are entrapped in the clot and extracted with forceps

DIAGNOSTIC EVALUATION

1. Intravenous urography.
2. Laboratory screening studies – complete blood count, urinalysis/culture, serum chemistry survey; 24-hour urine study for calcium, phosphorus, uric acid, creatinine, sodium oxalate.

PATIENT PROBLEMS

1. Pain and discomfort related to location/migration of stone(s).
2. Alteration in urinary elimination related to blockage of urine flow by stones.
3. Potential for infection and obstruction related to obstruction of urine flow.
4. Nausea, vomiting, diarrhoea related to intestinal reaction to urinary disturbance.
5. Potential for stone recurrence.

Planning and implementation

NURSING INTERVENTIONS

Relief of pain

1. Initiate treatment for renal and ureteral colic; relieve pain until its cause can be removed – administration of morphine or pethidine hydrochloride, hot baths or moist heat applied to flank areas.
2. Strain all urine through gauze for stone analysis – crystallographic studies and X-ray diffraction are useful in obtaining data about the amount and distribution of chemical components of the stone.
3. Give specific therapy as directed – regimen depends on stone type (see Management, p. 637).
4. Maintain proper urine reaction (pH); give appropriate drugs to acidify or alkalinize urine (depending on stone type).
   a. Phosphate, oxalate and carbonate stones form in alkaline urine.
      Drugs used to acidify urine include ammonium chloride and methenamine mandelate (mandelamine) and vitamin C.
   b. Uric acid, urate and cystine stones form in acid urine.
      Drugs used for alkalinizing the urine include potassium acetate or citrate, sodium bicarbonate.

Prevention of infection and obstruction

1. Encourage the patient to maintain a high round-the-clock fluid intake (250–300ml of fluid hourly when awake) to reduce concentration of urinary crystalloids and to ensure a high urinary output; also lowers specific gravity of urine.
2. Treat infection (if present) with appropriate drugs

– infection may accelerate stone growth and be difficult to eradicate.
3. Correct obstructive process to prevent impairment of tubular function, atrophy of nephrons, reduced renal blood flow and increased susceptibility to infection.
4. Treat and correct metabolic problems (hyperparathyroidism, renal tubular acidosis).
5. Prepare for surgical intervention if the patient's condition indicates that the stone:
   a. Is too large to pass, or
   b. Is producing obstruction, unremitting pain, infection that does not respond to treatment, or is causing progressive renal damage

Prevention of stone recurrence

1. Employ principles of diet therapy if stone composition is known – to control urine pH, supply proper vitamins, and eliminate stone-forming substances.
2. See Patient Education (below).

PATIENT EDUCATION

Instruct the patient as follows:
1. Maintain a high fluid intake over a 24-hour period, since stones form more readily in concentrated urine.
   a. Drink enough fluids to achieve a urinary volume of 2,000–3,000ml or more/24 hours.
   b. Drink larger amounts during periods of strenuous exercise, if you perspire freely.
   c. Take fluids in evening to guarantee a high urine flow during the night.
   d. Set the alarm clock in order to drink water in middle of night.
   e. Avoid sudden increases in environmental temperatures that may cause a drop in urinary volume.
   f. Increase fluid intake when engaging in activities that produce excessive perspiration.
2. For patients who form stones because of excessive absorption of dietary calcium:
   a. Stay on low-calcium diet; avoid dairy products.
   b. Avoid excessive salt and vitamin C intake.
3. Avoid prolonged periods of recumbency – slows renal drainage and alters calcium metabolism.
4. Avoid excessive ingestion of vitamins and minerals, especially vitamin D.
5. Test urine pH with a pH indicator if urine pH is a factor in causing particular type of stone.
6. Follow a healthy eating pattern.
   a. Avoid excessive sugar and animal protein,

which can cause changes in chemical composition of urine.

b. Increase consumption of fibre.

Evaluation

EXPECTED OUTCOMES

1. Patient achieves relief of pain/discomfort; passes stone.
2. Patient is free of infection and obstruction; excretes clear urine without burning or discomfort.
3. Patient participates in educational programme to avoid stone recurrence.

RENAL TUMOURS

GENERAL CONSIDERATIONS

1. All renal tumours should be considered malignant until proved otherwise.
2. Renal cell carcinoma is the most common malignant renal tumour; occurs more frequently in males and metastasizes early to the lungs, bone, liver, brain and contralateral kidney.

CLINICAL FEATURES

1. Many renal tumours produce no symptoms and are discovered on routine physical examination as a palpable abdominal mass.
2. Classic triad (late symptoms):
   a. Haematuria (intermittent, microscopic or gross) – may be initial, terminal, or total, depending on location of tumour.
   b. Pain – from distension of renal capsule, invasion of surrounding structures.
   c. Palpable mass in flank.
3. Low-grade fever, anaemia, weight loss – systemic effects common to most tumours.
4. Gastrointestinal symptoms – due to reflex action or encroachment on intraperitoneal organs.

DIAGNOSTIC EVALUATION

1. Plain film of abdomen – often shows kidney enlargement.
2. Intravenous urography – usually initial screening procedure.
3. Cystoscopic examination – for visualization of tumour by retrograde pyelography.
4. Assessment of urinary lactic dehydrogenase activity; this enzyme may be elevated in carcinoma of the kidney, bladder, prostate, in infection, etc.
5. Ultrasonography – helpful in differentiating renal cyst from renal tumour.
6. Renal angiogram.
7. Computed tomography – used in assessing solid renal masses and to detect invasion of perirenal structures; contributes to staging of renal cell carcinoma.

MANAGEMENT

Objective

Eradicate the tumour and prevent metastasis.

(The following treatment options may be done singly or in combination.)

1. Radical nephrectomy (en bloc removal of kidney, perirenal fat, adrenal gland, fascia and possibly regional lymph nodes.
2. Chemotherapy.
3. Hormonal therapy (progesterone) may exert an anti-tumour effect.
4. Interferons (glycoproteins produced by human cells in response to viral infections/other inducers) – have anti-tumour effects; can induce regression of metastatic tumours.
5. Immunotherapy – to stimulate host's own immune system.
6. Renal artery embolization – for the patient with metastatic renal cancer:
   a. Catheter is advanced into renal artery.
   b. Embolizing material (Gelfoam, steel coils, blood clot) is injected into artery and carried with arterial blood flow to occlude the tumour vessels.
   c. Procedure usually followed by nephrectomy.
   d. Tumour embolization decreases tumour vascularity, relieves pain and bleeding, and may slow tumour growth, thus allowing time for chemotherapy to achieve greater effect on neoplastic cells; may stimulate host immune response and enhance prognosis.
   e. Monitor and treat postinfarction syndrome – severe abdominal pain, nausea, vomiting, diarrhoea, fever.
   f. Complications – arterial obstruction, bleeding, diminution of renal function.
7. Symptomatic management to promote comfort:
   a. Radiation of skeletal lesions.
   b. Internal fixation for large-bone lesions.
   c. Nutritional support.
   d. Psychological support.

PATIENT EDUCATION

Have a yearly physical examination and X-ray examination of chest.

INJURIES TO THE KIDNEY

Trauma to abdomen, flank or back may produce renal injury. Suspicion is high in a patient with multiple injuries.

TYPES OF INJURIES

1. Contusion.
2. Laceration.
3. Rupture.
4. Renal pedicle injury.

MAJOR PROBLEMS FOLLOWING KIDNEY TRAUMA

1. Control of haemorrhage – may be persistent or recurring.
2. Injuries to other organs.
3. Late complications are significant.

CLINICAL FEATURES

1. Haematuria – amount shows no correlation with extent of injury.
2. Pain – costovertebral, flank, upper abdomen.
3. Nausea, vomiting, abdominal rigidity – from ileus (seen when there is retroperitoneal bleeding).
4. Shock – from severe/multiple injuries.

DIAGNOSTIC EVALUATION

1. History of injury – determine if injury was caused by blunt or penetrating trauma (stab/gunshot wounds).
2. Serial urine studies for haematuria.
3. Plain film of abdomen – to determine presence of other fractures (pelvis, ribs, transverse processes of lumbar vertebrae).
4. Excretory urography (intravenous pyelogram) – to define extent of injury to involved kidney and function of contralateral kidney.
5. Renal angiography – to assess vascular integrity, outline renal parenchyma.

TREATMENT AND NURSING MANAGEMENT
Prevention of haemorrhage and infection

NURSING ALERT
Excessive bleeding may occur several days after renal injury. Perirenal abscess or infection may occur two to four weeks following injury.

1. Place the patient on bed rest to minimize bleeding.
2. Monitor blood pressure and pulse – to assess for bleeding and impending shock; perirenal haemorrhage may cause rapid exsanguination.
3. Save, inspect and compare each urine specimen – to follow the course and degree of haematuria.
4. The doctor will carry out serial haematocrit and haemoglobin determinations – to assess degree of anaemia, since progressive anaemia indicates haemorrhage.
5. Evaluate the patient frequently during the first few days following injury.
    a. Assess for flank and abdominal pain, muscle spasm, and swelling over flank – suggests renal haemorrhage and extravasation.
    b. Outline original mass with marking pencil for future comparisons.
    c. Examine renal area for development of bruising and/or swelling.
    d. Watch for any *sudden* change in the patient's condition. This may indicate haemorrhage, which require surgical intervention.
6. Avoid narcotic analgesia – may mask accompanying abdominal symptoms.
7. Give antibiotics as directed to discourage infection – from perirenal haematoma and/or urinoma (cyst containing urine).
8. Maintain urinary drainage.

Restoration or maintenance of renal function
1. Monitor for complications – haemorrhage, infection, stone formation, thrombosis of major/minor arteries of kidneys, eventually leading to hypertension, loss of renal function.
2. Prepare for surgical exploration if the patient has penetrating injury (laceration, rupture, pedicle injury), palpable mass and tenderness in flank or shock.

PATIENT EDUCATION

1. Activity should be restricted for about one month following trauma to minimize incidence of delayed/secondary bleeding.
2. Encourage the patient to have follow-up examinations after discharge – to detect late-developing complications (post-traumatic hypertension, decreasing renal function).

BLADDER DISORDERS

NEUROGENIC BLADDER

Neurogenic bladder refers to a bladder disturbance due to dysfunctions related to lack of neural control of voiding of urine.

NORMAL PHYSIOLOGY

1. Normal bladder action depends on intact sensory and motor nerve supply.
2. The bladder fills to approximately 300–500ml – triggers an emptying reflex.
3. This reflex initiates a contraction of the musculature inside the bladder wall, which forces urine out through the urethra until the bladder is empty.

CAUSES

1. Spinal cord injury; spinal tumour; herniated intervertebral disc.
2. Disease – multiple sclerosis, diabetes mellitus, syphilis.
3. Certain congenital anomalies (spina bifida, myelomeningocele).
4. Infection.

TYPES OF NEUROGENIC BLADDER

Spastic (reflex or automatic)

1. A bladder disorder caused by any lesion of the cord above the voiding reflex arc (upper motor neurone lesion); most common type.
2. There is loss of conscious sensations and cerebral motor control.
3. The patient has reduced bladder capacity and marked hypertrophy of bladder wall.
4. Bladder behaves in reflex fashion with minimal or no controlling influence to regulate its activity (spontaneous uncontrolled voidings).

Flaccid (atonic, nonreflex or autonomous)

1. A bladder disorder caused by a lower motor neurone lesion.
2. Bladder continues to fill until it becomes greatly distended – bladder musculature does not contract forcefully at any time.
3. When pressure reaches a breakthrough point, small amounts of urine dribble from urethra as bladder continues to fill (overflow incontinence).
4. Sensory loss may accompany flaccid bladder; the patient is not aware of discomfort.
5. Extensive distension causes damage to bladder musculature, infection of stagnant urine and infection of kidneys by back pressure of urine.

Mixed (spastic/flaccid)

1. Generally associated with injuries occurring at the conus–cauda equina junctions.
2. Leads to a combination of upper motor neurone/ lower motor neurone dysfunction.

COMPLICATIONS

1. *Infection* – from stasis of urine and subsequent catheterization.
2. *Hydronephrosis* – hypertrophy of bladder wall leads ultimately to vesicoureteral reflux.
3. *Urolithiasis* – from demineralization of bone from bed rest; urinary stasis and infection.
4. *Renal failure* – major cause of death of patients with neurological impairment of the bladder.

Assessment

DIAGNOSTIC EVALUATION

1. Measurement of residual urine volume.
2. Measurement of fluid intake and urinary output.
3. Evaluation of urine (colour, odour, concentration, pH, protein content, specific gravity).
4. Assessment of sensory awareness (bladder fullness) and motor control.
5. Urodynamic studies (see p. 592).

PATIENT PROBLEMS

1. Alteration in patterns of urinary elimination (partial or complete, temporary or permanent loss of control of bladder function) related to lack of neural control of bladder.
2. Disturbance in self-image (social isolation, lack of self-esteem) related to potential/actual loss of bladder control.
3. Potential for infection and renal failure related to urinary retention.

Planning and implementation

NURSING INTERVENTIONS FOR INITIAL PHASE

Catheterization to reduce bladder distension

Following spinal cord injury, the syndrome of spinal shock is reflected in the bladder; sensation is not perceived, and the bladder usually cannot contract and empty itself. The bladder must be decompressed by either intermittent or continuous catheterization.

1. Intermittent catheterization (preferred):
   a. Bladder catheterized at designated intervals (four, six or eight hours) with a small-calibre catheter; this intermittent emptying approximates physiological function; circumvents complications usually seen with indwelling catheter.
      (i) Hourly fluid intake and output record is kept to assess individual output patterns.
      (ii) Catheterization technique requires strict asepsis and skilled personnel.
      (iii) Patients with upper extremity function may be taught to catheterize themselves.

2. Continuous catheterization:
   a. Bladder is catheterized using continuous drainage and irrigation system (p. 601) to avoid overdistension and risk of contracture from being constantly empty.
      (i) Tape catheter to abdomen (male) to remove sharp angulation and pressure at penoscrotal angle.
      (ii) Maintain a high fluid intake.

Assist with evaluation studies

(As soon as the patient's condition permits.) To assess for bladder and bladder neck problems. Do initial studies to provide a baseline against which later changes can be measured.

1. Serial studies of blood urea, serum creatinine, creatinine clearance – to determine status of renal function – are taken.
2. Cystogram – to determine presence of vesico-ureteral reflux.
3. Urethrogram – for presence of urethral complications.
4. Intravenous urogram – to outline upper urinary tract.
5. Pressure and flow studies.
6. Cystoscopy – to assess for loss of muscle fibres and elastic tissues; gives opportunity for biopsy.

NURSING INTERVENTIONS FOR CHRONIC PHASE

Each person with neurogenic bladder disease has a particular type of problem(s); it is difficult to assess what the rehabilitation potential and eventual urological disability may be.

Establishing an effective spontaneous reflex voiding

1. Encourage the patient to drink a measured amount of fluid from 08.00 to 20.00 hours; no fluids (except sips) taken after 20.00 hours to avoid bladder overdistension.
2. At specified time, the patient attempts to void by using pressure over bladder or stimulates reflex voiding by abdominal tapping or digital stretch of anal sphincter to trigger the bladder.
3. Estimate residual urine by comparing intake and output; palpate and percuss over bladder.
4. Palpate the bladder at repeated intervals to determine if bladder is being emptied.
5. Immediately following voiding attempt, catheterize the patient to determine urine residual.
   a. Measure all urine, voided and catheterized.
   b. Avoid *overdistension* of bladder.
   c. Caution patient to be alert for any sign that his

bladder is full – perspiration, coldness of hands or feet, feelings of anxiety, etc.

6. *Intervals between catheterizations.*
   Catheterization intervals are lengthened and programme is moved forward as less and less urine is retained; catheterization checks are usually discontinued when the volume of residual urine is at an acceptable level compatible with urine sterility and radiological normalcy of the upper urinary tract.
7. Encourage liberal fluid intake – to reduce urinary bacterial count, reduce stasis, decrease the concentration of calcium in urine and minimize the precipitation of urinary crystals and stone formation.
8. Keep the patient as mobile as possible – to reduce incidence of calculosis (presence of calculi).
   a. Turn, move, and exercise the patient.
   b. Get the patient up on tilt table or in wheelchair as soon as possible.
   c. Give low-calcium diet – to prevent calculosis.

NURSING INTERVENTION FOR FLACCID BLADDER

Establishing complete and regular emptying of bladder

1. The patient may be placed on bladder routine (outlined above); the fluid intake and output are adjusted to prevent bladder overdistension. The patient may be given orally administered doses of parasympathomimetic drugs (bethanechol chloride) to facilitate detrusor contraction.
2. *Or,* if no reflex or only a partial reflex can be induced, the patient is maintained on intermittent catheterization until he develops spontaneous reflex voiding; or surgical intervention may be required.
   a. Male patient – may use condom collecting device if bladder empties well and no residual remains.
   b. Female patient – may use pads, waterproof pants; or urinary diversion procedure may be required.
3. Electrical stimulation – application of electrical stimulation to bladder or reflex voiding centre in spinal cord.

SURGICAL INTERVENTION

Surgical intervention may be carried out to correct bladder neck contractures, correct vesicoureteral reflux, or prepare urinary diversion procedures. However, intermittent self-catheterization is now seen as being preferable to surgical intervention, and in some cases ileal conduits are being reversed.

Operations performed are:

1. Tubeless cystostomy (continent vesicostomy) – a tube is formed from the bladder wall and brought to the abdominal surface: an external valve is created by intrassusception of the proximal portion of the tube into the bladder; the procedure appears useful in patients with neurogenic bladder.
   a. Bladder emptied by intermittent transabdominal catheterization.
   b. Urinary collection device not necessary.
   c. Complications – bladder stone formation, stricture of cutaneous stoma, incontinence (urinary flooding of vesicostomy).
2. Ileal conduit (see p. 650).

PATIENT EDUCATION

1. Instruct the patient to do vaginal and pelvic floor exercises to strengthen periurethal tissue.
   a. Tighten the rectum and vaginal vault.
   b. Hold the contraction while counting slowly to six and then relax.
   c. Continue relaxing and tightening for a five-minute period.
   d. Perform these exercises several times a day, even one- to two-hourly, over a six- to eight-week period – success or failure of exercise programme is then evaluated.
2. Bladder rehabilitation may take weeks to months and results are not obvious for some time. Encouragement to motivate the patient to continue is essential.
3. The patient with chronic problems should have kidney function tests and intravenous urograms annually.

Evaluation
EXPECTED OUTCOMES

1. Patient achieves bladder control – no signs of overdistension, fever, concentrated cloudy or odoriferous urine.
2. Patient assumes responsibility for bladder care and regulates fluid intake.

GUIDELINES: INTERMITTENT SELF-CATHETERIZATION – CLEAN (NONSTERILE) TECHNIQUE

Intermittent self-catheterization is the periodic drainage of urine from the bladder by the patient via catheterization; it is necessitated by temporary or permanent inability to empty the bladder (vesical dysfunction, neurogenic disease, obstructive uropathy, decompensated bladder).

UNDERLYING CONSIDERATIONS

1. Intermittent catheterization is the treatment of choice following spinal cord injury. It is done under aseptic conditions by qualified health professionals until the patient is able to catheterize himself. After discharge from the hospital, the patient is able to use a 'clean' (nonsterile) technique.
2. The patient should be medically followed at regular intervals to prevent complications – reflux, hydronephrosis, external sphincter spasm, infection.
3. Advantages of self-catheterization: better patient acceptance; promotes independence; fewer complications; permits more normal sexual relations.
4. Goal: to decrease morbidity associated with long-term use of indwelling catheter and to achieve a catheter-free status, if possible.

EQUIPMENT
No. 14 Fr. catheter (several to be kept in reserve); lubricant
Mirror (female patient)
Shallow pan
Irrigation tip syringe
Clear plastic bag or case – for carrying catheter

PROCEDURE

Action (by patient)

	Rationale
1. The patient must understand the importance of frequent catheterization and emptying of bladder at prescribed time regardless of circumstances.	An overdistended bladder slows the circulation of blood through the bladder walls and weakens its resistance to infection.
2. Try to void before catheterizing self using reflex triggering mechanisms – pressure on abdomen, thigh stroking, etc.	This may help to develop voluntary voiding without catheterization.
3. Wash hands with soap and water.	Do not forgo catheterization if soap and water are not available.

Action by female patient

1. Position mirror in line of vision with urinary meatus. Assume modified dorsal recumbent position with feet on bed, legs flexed and knees apart; later, the patient may sit on toilet seat if physical condition permits.	This position helps to expose the urethral meatus.
a. The nurse points out the location of the clitoris, urethral meatus and vaginal outlet (in the mirror). Once the technique is mastered, the mirror is usually dispensed with.	The patient is taught to confirm the position of the clitoris, urethral meatus and vaginal outlet by palpation so that eventually a mirror will not be necessary.
b. Expose the urinary meatus and cleanse.	
2. Lubricate the catheter with water or water-soluble jelly. Hold the catheter 7.5cm from its tip and insert it 5–7.5cm in a downward and backward direction into the urethra. Allow urine to flow into a shallow pan/toilet or into a disposable plastic urine bag.	
3. Remove catheter when urine stops flowing.	Measure or estimate volume of residual urine.

Action by male patient

1. Assume sitting position until technique is learned.	
2. Lubricate the catheter.	A well-lubricated catheter is particularly necessary in the male to avoid traumatic urethritis.
3. Retract foreskin of penis with one hand; then grasp penis and hold it at right angle to body.	This manoeuvre straightens the urethra and facilitates ease of catheter insertion.
4. Insert the catheter 15–25cm until urine begins to flow.	
5. Then advance catheter about 2.5cm and allow urine to flow into shallow pan/toilet. When urine stops flowing, remove catheter.	Measure or estimate volume of residual urine.

Follow-up phase

Action	Rationale
1. Wash catheter in warm, soapy water. Rinse.	
2. Wrap catheter in clean towel/paper towel.	The catheter may be carried in a clean plastic bag or case. The emphasis should be on availability and cleanliness.

URINARY INCONTINENCE

DEFINITION

Involuntary urine loss which is sufficient to cause social or hygiene problems. The patient may present with the initial problem to the gynaecologist, the urologist or the geriatrician.

AETIOLOGY

Apart from congenital causes, urethral urinary incontinence is usually due to either sphincter weakness or bladder instability, and the causes will differ between the sexes.

Assessment

SPHINCTER WEAKNESS

1. Typical causes in the female are obesity, parity, menopause and neuropathic disorders. For the male, post-prostatectomy, pelvic fracture and/or urethral injuries and neuropathic disorders are the most common.
2. The major symptom is stress incontinence which is most noticeable when the patient coughs or strains.

DIAGNOSTIC EVALUATION

1. A specimen of urine is taken for culture and sensitivity.
2. An intravenous urogram is performed.
3. Urodynamic studies, such as:
   a. Urethral pressure profile.
   b. Cystometrogram.
   c. Micturating cystourethrogram (MCU).
4. Assessment of urine loss by the amount of protection the patient finds necessary to use.

Planning and implementation

TREATMENT AND NURSING INTERVENTION

1. Minor incontinence in women may improve with:
   a. Reduction of weight loss – of at least 30kg.
   b. Pelvic floor exercises.
   c. A Hodge or ring pessary.
   d. Drugs if the patient is post-menopausal, e.g. combination of ephedrine and oestrogen.
2. Surgical treatment is indicated in men with post-prostatecomy sphincter weakness if the incontinence does not improve spontaneously within six months.
3. Significant treatment for women is necessary if a severe degree of incontinence is diagnosed, for example:
   a. Anterior colporrhaphy (see Chapter 10, p. 694).
   b. Teflon injections round the bladder neck.
   c. Suprapubic repair – Marshall–Marchetti–Krantz operation or Burch colposuspension.
   d. Sling operations – this involves placing a sling of the rectus sheath muscle or synthetic material around the bladder neck.
   e. Implantable sphincters – usually used when standard surgical procedures have failed.

Assessment

BLADDER INSTABILITY

This is treated by drugs and/or bladder training.

1. Examples of the drugs used are:
   a. Propantheline hydrochloride (Probanthine).
   b. Emepronium bromide (Cetiprin).
   c. Flavoxate hydrochloride (Urispas).
   (Side-effects include a dry mouth and constipation.)
2. Bladder training is designed to re-educate the bladder. (See implementation, Chapter 3, p. 15.)

Planning and implementation

NURSING INTERVENTION

1. Careful recording day and night of periods of incontinence often reveals a 'pattern' from which nursing intervention can be planned.
2. Remember that a large number of patients with quite severe incontinence are within the 40 to 50 year range. Incontinence produces depression and exhaustion, and the woman feels activities

are limited and she becomes socially isolated. She therefore needs much support, reassurance and encouragement.

3. The appropriateness of toilet facilities have an important bearing on the degree of incontinence and the achievement of continence.
4. Patient mobility in getting to the toilet in time and then manual dexterity to remove outer garments in time must also be assessed.
5. Give advice on skin care, wash and dry the area carefully, apply barrier creams if the skin becomes red and sore.
6. Most districts have appointed an incontinence adviser who will help assess and plan an individual programme, as well as giving advice on the incontinence aids available.
7. Indwelling catheters may be used for either sex. With bladder instability, some leakage will occur around the catheter due to the lack of contraction. A larger size catheter should not be inserted to solve the problem as this will not stop the leakage and lead only to enlarging the urethra and bladder neck.
8. Actual appliances available are really suitable only for men and the condom type is the most effective.

Evaluation

EXPECTED OUTCOMES
1. Patient regains continence and there is no skin excoriation.
2. Patient feels he can participate in normal activities.

INJURIES TO THE BLADDER (AND URETHRA)

TYPES OF BLADDER INJURIES
1. Contusion of bladder.
2. Intraperitoneal rupture
3. Extraperitoneal rupture } or combination of both.
4. Injury to urethra.

TYPES OF URETHRAL INJURIES
1. Contusion.
2. Partial or complete rupture.

PROBLEMS ASSOCIATED WITH BLADDER INJURY
1. Injuries to the bladder and urethra are commonly associated with pelvic fractures and multiple trauma. Certain surgical procedures (hysterectomy, surgery of lower colon and rectum) also carry a risk to the bladder.
2. With injury, there is a rise in intravesical (within bladder) pressure, which produces extravasation of urine into the peritoneal cavity or perivesical space.
3. Rupture of the bladder requires immediate treatment.

CLINICAL FEATURES
1. Failure to void urine.
2. Haematuria; presence of blood at urinary meatus.
3. Shock and haemorrhage – pallor, rapid and increasing pulse rate.
4. Suprapubic pain and soreness.
5. Rigid abdomen – indicates intraperitoneal rupture.
6. Swelling/discoloration of penis, scrotum and anterior perineum.

DIAGNOSTIC EVALUATION
1. Retrograde urethrogram – to detect any rupture of urethra. *Do first* (before catheterization).
2. Cystogram – to detect and localize perforation/rupture of bladder.
3. Plain film of abdomen – may show associated pelvic fracture.
4. Intravenous urogram – to survey the kidneys for injury.

TREATMENT AND NURSING MANAGEMENT
1. Treat for shock and haemorrhage.
2. Carry out retrograde urethrography in suspected injuries involving lower urinary tract.
3. Catheterize the patient only after urethrogram is done.
   a. Indwelling catheter serves as a means of continuous urinary drainage.
   b. Catheter also serves as a splint to urethra if urethra has been injured, but it may complete a partial rupture if urethral injury is not recognized with a urethrogram.
4. Prepare for surgical intervention for bladder rupture:
   a. Extravasated blood and urine will be drained and urine diverted with suprapubic cystostomy and indwelling catheter.
   b. Bladder tears will be sutured; urethral repairs may be postponed.
5. Observe drainage systems after surgery.
   a. Suprapubic cystostomy drainage – until healing of bladder is complete.

b. Indwelling urethral catheter drainage – to divert urine drainage and permit suprapubic incision to heal.

c. Perivesical areas drained with Penrose drain (will be brought out through suprapubic incision).

For urethral injury (treatment is controversial)

1. Assist with cystostomy drainage (p. 606) – to provide urine drainage until reconstructive surgery is done.
2. Treatment method determined by level of urethral injury and its effect on bladder continence.

PATIENT EDUCATION

Urethral stricture, incontinence and impotence may follow urethral injury.

CANCER OF THE BLADDER

AETIOLOGY

It appears that multiple agents are responsible for the development of cancer of the bladder. The specific aetiology is unknown.

1. Cigarette smoking.
2. Prolonged exposure to aromatic amines or their metabolites – generally dyes manufactured by the chemical industry and used by other industries.
3. Causal relationship may exist between excessive coffee drinking and consumption of excessive amounts of analgesics and bladder cancer.
4. Chronic infection and irritation.
5. Bladder schistosomiasis (rare in UK).
6. Secondary metastasis from prostate (males), lower gynaecological tract (females) and colon and rectum in both sexes.

NURSING ALERT

High-risk people should have annual cytological examinations of the urine.

CLINICAL FEATURES

1. Bladder cancer is a highly malignant condition; it occurs three times more frequently in males, particularly after the fifth decade.
2. Large numbers of these tumours occur in the lateral and posterior bladder wall and near the trigone.

3. Metastases appear in vesical, hypogastric, common iliac and lumbar lymph nodes; in liver, lungs, vertebrae, pelvis.
4. Recurrences may occur years after last known tumour is treated.
5. Small bladder tumours are seeded from tumours of renal pelvis.

CLINICAL MANIFESTATIONS

1. Painless haematuria, either gross or microscopic – most characteristic sign.
2. Dysuria, frequency, urgency – symptoms of bladder irritability.
3. Flank pain, chills, fever – from progressive tumour growth, infiltration of bladder wall, ureteral obstruction and bladder infection.
4. Pelvic or back pain – from distant metastasis.
5. Leg oedema – from invasion of pelvic lymph nodes.

DIAGNOSTIC EVALUATION

1. Intravenous urography (IVU) – to rule out ureteral obstruction or presence of renal pelvic tumour.
2. Cystourethroscopy – for visualization and biopsy of lesion.
3. Bimanual examination of pelvis – to determine degree of mobility, fixation of tumour and degree of extravesical extension.
4. Retrograde pyelography – to define presence/absence of upper urinary tract pathology.
5. Computed tomography (CT scan) and ultra-sonography – to assess disease status and measure tumour responsiveness.
6. Cytological study of fresh urinary sediment to assess for malignant transitional cells shed from tumour.
7. Chest X-ray and bone scan – to demonstrate distant metastases.

MANAGEMENT
Underlying rationale

1. There is no single effective method of treatment. The surgical procedure of choice depends on the characteristics of the tumour and whether or not bladder wall infiltration and local or distant metastasis has occurred. The patient's age and physical, mental and emotional status are considered.
2. The patient is usually considered incurable if gross extension of the tumour beyond the bladder wall has occurred; in such cases, adjuvant modalities such as radiotherapy and chemotherapy may be somewhat palliative.

Types of treatment

1. Surgery:
   a. Transurethral resection – for superficial tumours; usually combined with intravesical chemotherapy (see below).
   b. Cystectomy (removal of bladder) or radical cystectomy for invasive or poorly differentiated tumours; may be combined with radiotherapy but is now rarely used.
   c. Urinary diversion procedures (see below) to relieve frequency and haemorrhage in patients with inoperable disease.
   d. Hydrostatic pressure therapy – placement of water-filled balloon within the bladder to produce tumour necrosis by reducing blood circulation in the bladder wall (Helmstein's procedure).
2. Radiotherapy – may be internal or external.
3. Chemotherapy:
   a. Topical chemotherapy – places a high concentration of drug in contact with neoplastic cells.
   b. Systemic chemotherapy.
4. Combinations of surgery, radiotherapy and chemotherapy.

NURSING INTERVENTIONS

1. Emphasize the positive aspects of the treatment to the patient.
2. See nursing management of the patient undergoing chemotherapy (p. 1036), radiotherapy (p. 1039) and urinary diversion, below.
3. Support the patient undergoing intravesical chemotherapy (instillation of antineoplastic agent into the bladder, allowing a high concentration of drug to come into contact with the tumour with minimal systemic toxicity).
   a. Instruct the patient as follows:
      (i) Do not take fluids during instillation period (about two hours) to prevent excessive diuresis and to promote retention of drug in the bladder.
      (ii) Change position every half an hour during instillation.
      (iii) Wash hands and perineal area after voiding the medication to prevent contact dermatitis.
      (iv) Void frequently after procedure to avoid chemical cystitis from residual drug in the bladder.
      (v) Drink fluids liberally after procedure is completed.
   b. Monitor the patient for allergic reaction during instillation period.
   c. Monitor the patient for signs and symptoms of urinary infection.

URINARY DIVERSION

Urinary diversion refers to diverting the urinary stream from the bladder so that it exits via a new avenue. There are a large number of operative procedures.

Assessment

CLINICAL CONDITIONS REQUIRING URINARY DIVERSION

1. Malignancy of bladder or ureters; pelvic malignancy.
2. Congenital abnormality of lower urinary tract.
3. Stricture and trauma to ureters and urethra.
4. Neurogenic bladder.
5. Severe ureteral and renal damage due to vesicoureteral reflux or chronic infection.
6. Injuries.

METHODS OF URINARY DIVERSION

See Figure 9.13.
The most common methods of urinary diversion are:

1. *Ileal conduit* – transplanting the ureters to an isolated section of the terminal ileum and bringing one end to the abdominal wall as an ileostomy. The ureter may also be transplanted into the transverse colon (colon conduit) or proximal jejunum (jejunal conduit).
2. *Ureterosigmoidostomy* – implantation of the ureter(s) into the sigmoid, thereby allowing urine to flow through the colon and out of the rectum.
3. *Cutaneous ureterostomy* – bringing the detached ureters through the abdominal wall and attaching them to an opening in the skin.
4. *Suprapubic cystostomy* (vesicostomy) – draining the bladder through an abdominal wound.
5. *Nephrostomy* – inserting a catheter via an incision into the flank or by percutaneous catheter placement into the kidney.

PATIENT PROBLEMS

1. Disturbances in body image related to change in toileting habits, presence of external stoma and collecting device, fear of urine leakage.
2. Fear (of recurring disease, sexual impotency) related to diagnosis of genitourinary cancer.
3. Potential for morbidity and complications related to nature of surgery and tumour effects.

Planning and implementation
PREOPERATIVE NURSING INTERVENTIONS
Preoperative assessment to correct physiological abnormalities

1. For the patient undergoing renal surgery, see p. 629 for general aspects of preoperative care.
2. Pay careful attention to cardiopulmonary status, since the patient is probably older and undergoing a lengthy, complex procedure.
3. Prepare the patient for sigmoidoscopy and barium enema if ureterosigmoidostomy is to be performed.
   a. Enemas are given (increasing in amount of fluid) to help develop sphincter control.
   b. Assess the patient's ability to retain enema as a means of evaluating adequacy of rectal sphincter.
4. Prepare the bowel for surgical intervention to minimize faecal stasis and postoperative ileus.
   a. Give clear liquids.
   b. Administer antibiotics (neomycin) as prescribed – for bowel disinfection to reduce pathogenic bacterial flora, since bowel contents frequently spill with transsection of intestine.
   c. Give enemas as directed for mechanical cleansing of lower bowel.
5. Employ adequate hydration procedures, including intravenous infusions, to ensure urine flow during surgery and to prevent hypovolaemia during the prolonged operative procedure.
6. Reinforce the surgeon's explanations of the surgical procedures.

   a. The stoma site is planned preoperatively with the patient standing, sitting and lying – to place the stoma away from bony prominences, skin creases and scars, and where the patient can see it.
   b. Apply several types of skin adhesives or cement to abdomen preoperatively to determine contact allergies and to facilitate management of ostomy appliance postoperatively.
   c. Have the patient wear the intended appliance preoperatively.
7. Assist with enteral or intravenous hyperalimentation – to give nutritional support, minimize toxicity, promote healing and improve response to treatment.
8. Assist the patient undergoing nasogastric intubation before surgery (p. 430).

Enhancing coping abilities to adapt to altered body state

1. Encourage the patient to express his feelings about his situation; reflect and amplify the patient's insights and judgements.
2. Help the patient talk about his support network.
3. Include the family in caring for the patient; allow for verbalization of fear and anxiety.
4. Encourage membership in a self-help group (Urostomy Association) and visits by an ostomy association visitor.
5. Help the patient and family gain a positive attitude and hope.

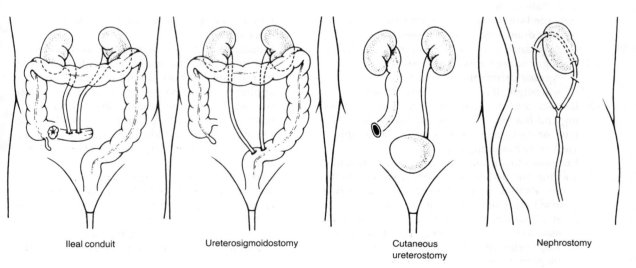

Ileal conduit   Ureterosigmoidostomy   Cutaneous ureterostomy   Nephrostomy

Figure 9.13. Methods of urinary diversion

POSTOPERATIVE NURSING INTERVENTIONS

1. See p. 466 for nursing management of patient following intestinal surgery, and p. 629 for nursing management of the patient following urological surgery.
2. Watch for any abnormal signs and symptoms (wound infections, leaking at anastomosis site, peritonitis, paralytic ileus, intestinal obstruction, stenosis of stoma). These operations are extremely taxing, and patients have little or no reserve.
3. Ensure adequate circulating volume with intravenous fluids and blood as directed.
4. Keep nasogastric tube in place until the patient passes gas via rectum.
5. Monitor total parenteral nutrition (p. 450) if the patient is unable to return to oral feeding.
6. Accept the patient's depression, which usually follows any surgery that interferes with body integrity.
   a. Accept the patient's irritability and lack of motivation to learn.
   b. Give extra support until the patient can cope with his situation.
   c. Counsel the patient to take one day at a time.

NURSING INTERVENTIONS FOLLOWING ILEAL CONDUIT

1. The patient wears a transparent disposable urinary drainage bag cemented to the abdominal wall until oedema subsides and stoma shrinks to normal size. (Some patients prefer using disposable bags thereafter.)
2. The patient with an ileal conduit wears a cemented-on appliance day and night. The ileal bladder drains urine (but not faeces) constantly.
   a. Appliance is connected to a drainage tube and bag; urinary volume is recorded hourly.
   b. Appliance remains in place as long as it is watertight; it is changed as necessary.
3. Inspect stoma for congestion and cyanosis, bleeding and friability of stomal mucosa – during first few postoperative weeks, the stoma appears swollen and oedematous.
4. Examine skin around stoma for signs of irritation, alkaline encrustation with peristomal dermatitis (from alkaline urine coming in contact with exposed skin), and wound infections.
   a. Alkaline urine is usually a result of bacteria; assess for odorous, cloudy-appearing urine.
   b. Keep urine pH below 6.5; test the urine dribbling from the stoma with pH indicator.
   c. Ascorbic acid may be given to acidify urine.

d. Encourage high fluid intake – to flush ileal conduit and prevent mucus from congealing.

PATIENT EDUCATION FOR STOMA CARE
Appliance
The urinary appliance may consist of one or two pieces and may be disposable, semidisposable, or reusable (choice determined by location of stoma, patient activity, body build).
1. Reusable appliance – has a faceplate that is attached to the body with cement or adhesive.
2. Semidisposable appliance – has a reusable faceplate to which disposable pouches are attached.
3. Disposable appliance – discarded after each change.

Determining stoma size (for ordering correct ostomy appliance)
1. The stoma will shrink considerably as oedema subsides, and the opening is recalibrated every three to six weeks for the first few months postoperatively.
2. Measure the widest part of the stoma with a ruler. The inside diameter of the faceplate should not be more than 1.5 to 3.1mm larger than the diameter of the stoma.
3. The patient is taught to dilate stoma himself with a finger in a plastic glove (usually weekly).

Changing the appliance (every five to seven days)
1. Change appliance early in morning, before taking fluids.
2. Assemble all equipment needed for the type used.
3. Prepare the appliance according to the manufacturer's directives.
4. Moisten the edge of the faceplate with adhesive solvent or soap and water and gently remove it by pushing the skin down and away from the appliance. Adhesive solvent is not used if skin barriers (ReliaSeal or Stomahesive) are used.
5. Instruct the patient to bend over quickly and remain in that position for a minute to allow conduit to empty before the skin is washed and dried.
6. Clean all cement from the skin with adhesive solvent; use a soft cloth. Wash skin with non-cream-based soap and water. Pat dry. *The skin must be dry or appliance will not adhere.*
   a. Inspect skin for signs of irritation.
   b. Keep the skin free from direct contact with urine.
   c. A gauze or tissue wick may be applied over

the stoma to absorb urine while the appliance is being changed.

7. Centre the appliance directly over the stoma and apply it carefully. Apply gentle pressure around appliance for secure adherence and to remove air bubbles and creases.
8. Apply hypoallergenic tape in a picture-frame effect around the pouch.
9. The skin under the appliance may be dusted with pure talcum powder and a cotton cover used to absorb perspiration and eliminate warmth from the pouch.
10. The use of a belt is optional, but follow manufacturer's directions, since an ill-fitting belt can cause abrasion of the stoma.

Odour control
1. Instruct the patient to avoid foods and medication that produce strong odours.
2. Drink liberal amounts of fluids to flush the conduit free of mucus and reduce possibility of urinary infection.
3. Introduce a few drops of liquid deodorizer or diluted white vinegar through the drain spout into the bottom of the pouch with a syringe or eye dropper.

Managing the ostomy appliance
1. Empty the appliance when it is one-third to one-half full to prevent weight of urine from loosening adhesive seal – urinary ostomy appliances are closed with a drain valve (spigot) for periodic emptying.
2. Some patients prefer wearing a leg bag attached with an adapter to the drainage apparatus.
3. Attach outlet on appliance to a collecting bottle with plastic tubing for night-time drainage; have at least 1.5m of tubing to allow patient to turn in bed. The tubing may be threaded down the pyjama leg to prevent kinking.
4. Position the drainage bottle lower than the level of the bed – to enhance flow by gravity.

Securing a urine specimen for culture from an ileal conduit
1. Open catheter set.
2. Remove the bag from the stoma. Place a 10 × 10cm gauze sponge over the stoma to absorb the urine.
3. Don sterile gloves.
4. Using sterile surgical forceps and cotton wool swabs, cleanse the area around the stoma from the centre outward.
5. Insert a catheter 5cm into the stoma and wait for the urine flow.

Cleaning and deodorizing the appliance
1. Clean faceplate with solvent and remove all adhesive; rinse in clear water.
2. Clean appliance with a brush and detergent solution, rinse and soak in a solution of water and white vinegar, washing soda solution, a few drops of bleach, or any commercial deodorizing solution.
3. After soaking (five to ten minutes) hang it up to air-dry away from direct sunlight.
4. Discard equipment that can no longer be cleaned adequately.

General patient instructions
1. Urinary stoma care is not difficult or complicated and should be regarded as part of personal grooming and dressing routine.
2. The stoma is normally red in colour; it may protrude or be flush with the skin. It may bleed if it is bumped or rubbed. Report to your doctor if it continues bleeding for several hours.
3. Mucus shreds in the urine are normal following an ileal conduit operation.
4. Choose an appliance that fits your needs. Successful urinary ostomy requires a well-fitting appliance, meticulous skin care and control of urinary odour.
5. Always carry spare pouches and cement in a small case in handbag or pocket.
6. The wearing time of an appliance varies. Experiment with your appliance; usually an appliance may be worn five to seven days. See above for changing, cleaning and management of appliance.
7. Before changing to a new skin adhesive, apply a test patch to the other side of the abdomen or forearm.
8. Wear cotton (rather than nylon) underwear. Avoid a heavy girdle because it may cause chafing of the stoma and leakage from pressure on the pouch.
9. Avoid heavy lifting for six weeks. Sexual activities, driving the car, returning to work, etc, may be resumed when energy level increases.
10. Make arrangements to see stoma therapist/appliance officer for appliances, deodorizers, skin barriers and other new products.
11. Call your doctor for instructions if skin problems develop or if one or more of the following symptoms of kidney complications occur: fever, chills,

pain, change in colour of urine (cloudy, bloody), diminishing urine output.

12. Contact local ostomy association for visits, reassurance and practical information from ostomy visitor.

13. For further information:
Urostomy Association
Buckland
Beaumont Park
Danbury Essex CM3 4DE
(Tel. 024 541 4294)

NURSING INTERVENTIONS FOLLOWING URETEROSIGMOIDOSTOMY

1. Patient will have rectal tube (or mushroom catheter) draining urine postoperatively – to ensure drainage and prevent reflux of urine into ureters and kidneys.
   a. Tape the tube to the buttocks.
   b. If the tube must be removed for defaecation, reinsert the tube approximately 10cm into rectum to prevent trauma to site of ureteral anastomosis.
2. Give special skin care around anus to prevent skin erythema and excoriation.
3. Following removal of the tube, the patient voids through his rectum.
   a. Encourage the patient to empty rectum every two to three hours (or more often) to keep rectal pressure low and to minimize the absorption of urinary constituents from the colon.
   b. In time, the patient will be able to differentiate between the sensation to void and the urge to defaecate.
   c. Reinsert the tube (catheter) at night (attached to drainage bottle) to permit uninterrupted sleep.
   d. Do not give enemas or aperients.
   e. If irrigations are requested, avoid using force because of danger of introducing an infection into newly implanted ureters.
4. Evaluate for electrolyte imbalance and acidosis – potassium and magnesium imbalances may occur from presence of urine in the bowel, which stimulates diarrhoea.
   a. Maintain fluid and electrolyte balance in immediate postoperative period by serum chemical determinations and intravenous infusions.
   b. Low-chloride diet supplemented with sodium potassium citrate – to prevent acidosis.

5. Patient education:
   a. Give specific diet instructions when the patient can tolerate oral intake.
      (i) Avoid gas-forming foods, since flatus can cause stress incontinence, socially embarrassing offensive odour and discomfort.
      (ii) Watch for air swallowing (chewing gum, smoking, carbonated beverages) to avoid gas.
      (iii) Reduce salt intake to prevent hyperchloraemic acidosis.
      (iv) Increase potassium intake through medication and foods, since potassium may be lost in acidosis.
   b. Take prophylactic antibiotics as directed – pyelonephritis (due to reflux of bacteria from colon) can occur in some patients.
   c. Report for frequent follow-up studies (incidence of carcinoma of colon is significant); watch for changes in bowel patterns.

NURSING INTERVENTIONS FOLLOWING OTHER DIVERSIONARY PROCEDURES
Following cutaneous ureterostomy
1. A urinary appliance is fitted immediately following surgery and is worn at all times.
2. Ureteral dilatation with sterile catheter is performed at regular intervals to ensure patency and prevent ureteral stricture.
3. See p. 652, nursing considerations for patient having ileal conduit – for general aspects of care.

Following cystostomy (temporary)
1. Usually done on the patient with an obstruction below bladder (prostatic obstruction) when it is not possible to insert urethral catheter.
2. Encourage liberal amounts of fluid to avoid encrustation around catheter.
3. See also p. 606

Following nephrostomy (temporary)
1. May be performed rapidly under local anaesthesia when other procedures are not technically possible.
2. See p. 629 for care of the patient.

Evaluation
EXPECTED OUTCOMES
1. Adapts to change in body image – takes responsibility for care of stoma and appliance.
2. Discusses fears and feelings.
3. Is free of complications – excretes urine freely; maintains healthy appearing stoma and skin; has no signs of wound or urinary infection.

PROBLEMS AFFECTING THE URETHRA

URETHRITIS

Urethritis is inflammation of the urethra.

AETIOLOGY
1. Nongonococcal urethritis – urethritis not caused by gonococcus. However, a large number of cases are sexually transmitted by:
   a. *Chlamydia* – a virus-like intracellular bacterium.
   b. *Trichomonas vaginalis*.
   c. *Herpes simplex* virus.
   d. *Candida*.
   e. *Ureaplasma urealyticum*.
   f. Mycoplasms.
   g. Unknown organisms.
2. Nonsexually transmitted:
   a. Bacterial urethritis – may be associated with urinary tract infection.
   b. From trauma – secondary to passage of urethral sounds, repeated cystoscopy, indwelling catheter.
3. These agents can cause either mucosal urogenital tract infection (urethritis, cervicitis) or spread contiguously or haematogenously to produce epididymitis, endometritis, pelvic inflammatory disease (PID) or disseminated gonococcal infection.
4. Reiter's syndrome – urethritis, conjunctivitis, arthritis of unknown aetiology.

CLINICAL FEATURES
1. Itching and burning around area of urethra.
2. Dysuria and frequency.
3. Urethral discharge; may be scant or profuse; thin, clear or mucoid; or thick and purulent.
4. Penile pain.

DIAGNOSTIC EVALUATION
1. Study of stained urethral smear.
2. Culture for gonorrhoea.
3. Blood test for syphilis.
4. History and physical findings (interview to elicit past history of gonorrhoea).

TREATMENT
1. Antibiotics (tetracyclines are usually effective for nongonococcal urethritis).

2. Metronidazole (Flagyl) may be administered for *Trichomonas* infection.
3. Treatment of associated prostatitis (see p. 657).

NURSING MANAGEMENT
1. Encourage the patient to stay on the antibiotic regimen for the prescribed time period.
2. Advise the patient to temporarily discontinue sexual activity and ingestion of alcohol – these activities may prolong the acute phase of urethritis.
3. Urge treatment for sexual partner – in event of treatment failure and recurrence.
4. Support and reassure patient – nongonococcal urethritis is usually self-limiting and is not a serious health threat.

URETHRITIS FROM GONORRHOEA

AETIOLOGY
1. *Neisseria gonorrhoeae* – the specific organism.
2. Transmitted through sexual contact.
3. More and more asymptomatic carriers are being recognized.

CLINICAL FEATURES
Male
1. Inflammation of meatal orifice; burning on urination; *may be asymptomatic*.
2. Urethral discharge – scant and serous to thick, yellowish pus (four to ten days or longer after sexual exposure).

Female
1. Purulent urethral discharge.
2. • Frequency, urgency, nocturia.
3. Red, swollen urinary meatus.
4. Pelvic infection accompanied by abdominal pain.
5. Often is asymptomatic.

COMPLICATIONS (LOCAL)
1. Male – periurethritis, prostatitis, epididymitis, urethral stricture, sterility due to vasoepididymal duct obstruction.
2. Female – pelvic infection, abscess of greater vestibular glands (Bartholin's glands), urethral stricture.

TREATMENT AND PATIENT EDUCATION
1. See p. 986 for treatment of gonorrhoea.
2. Instruct the patient to avoid sexual activity with untreated previous sexual partners until they have been treated and examined to prevent reinfection.

3. Emphasize that the patient must return in four to seven days to assess results and determine if there is need for further treatment and tests.
4. Urge the patient to have any sexual contacts present themselves for treatment.

URETHRAL STRICTURE

Urethral stricture is a narrowing of the lumen and loss of distensibility of the urethra caused by scar tissue formation and contraction.

AETIOLOGY
1. Urethral injury:
   a. Urethral instrumentation – transurethral surgical procedures, indwelling catheters, cystoscopic procedures.
   b. Straddle injuries, automobile accidents, pelvic fractures, direct trauma to urethra.
2. Untreated gonorrhoeal urethritis.
3. Congenital abnormalities.

CLINICAL FEATURES
1. Diminution in force and size of urinary stream.
2. Urinary infection and retention – dysuria and urgency.
3. Symptoms of complication from stricture – back pressure produces cystitis, prostatitis, pyelonephritis, etc.

DIAGNOSTIC EVALUATION
1. Urethrogram and voiding cystogram – to locate site and degree of stricture.
2. Elevated white blood cell count, pus and bacteria in urine – if urinary tract infection present.
3. Passing of catheter or sounds (bougies) – to determine the diameter and location of urethral narrowings.
4. Residual urine measurement.

PREVENTION
1. Treat urethral infections promptly.
2. Utilize utmost care in urethral instrumentation (catheterization, etc).
3. Avoid prolonged urethral catheter drainage.

TREATMENT
1. Dilatation of urethra with urethral sounds.
   a. Sounds of increasing size are used.
   b. Sounds are passed at lengthening intervals (two weeks, one month, three months) for an indefinite period, depending on how long the strictured lumen is patent.
   c. Hot baths and non-narcotic analgesics – to control pain after instrumentation.
   d. Antibiotics may be given several days after dilatation – lessens discomfort and minimizes infectious reaction.
2. Surgical excision, urethroplasty or suprapubic cystostomy may be necessary for severe strictures.

CONDITIONS OF THE PROSTATE

BENIGN PROSTATIC HYPERPLASIA (HYPERTROPHY)

Benign prostatic hyperplasia is enlargement of the prostate. The aetiology is uncertain but is presumably related to endocrine changes associated with ageing that initiate hyperplasia of both glandular and cellular tissue of the prostate.

CLINICAL FEATURES
1. In early or gradual prostatic enlargement may be no symptoms, since the bladder can compensate for increased peripheral resistance.
2. Obstructive symptoms – hesitancy, diminution in size and force of urinary stream, postvoiding dribbling, sensation of incomplete emptying of the bladder.
3. Symptoms of recurring urinary infection and stasis – frequency, nocturia, chills, fever.
4. Renal symptoms (prolonged obstruction) – ureteral dilatation, hydronephrosis, renal infection, azotaemia, uraemia.

DIAGNOSTIC EVALUATION
1. Rectal examination – allows rough estimate of size of gland.
2. Cystourethroscopy – to inspect urethra and bladder and evaluate prostatic size.
3. Catheterization after voiding – to determine amount of residual urine.
4. Excretory urogram – to document upper urinary tract obstruction.
5. Serum creatinine and blood urea – to assess renal function.

MANAGEMENT
(The plan of treatment depends on the cause, the

severity of obstruction, and the condition of the patient.)

1. Conservative treatment if no symptoms of urinary impairment – intermittent catheterization, urethral dilatation, prostatic massage – to relieve symptoms of acute obstruction.
2. Prepare the patient for surgery (enucleation or removal of hyperplastic prostatic tissue) when obstructive symptoms occur. See p. 660 for nursing management of the patient having a prostatectomy.
3. Cystostomy drainage of bladder – for the poor-risk patient or one acutely ill with retention, uraemia, etc.

PATIENT EDUCATION

1. Surgical procedures for benign enlargement usually do not result in impotence, but may cause retrograde ejaculation (passing back of fluid into the bladder during sexual intercourse).
2. See p. 662.

PROSTATITIS

Prostatitis is an inflammation of the prostate gland.

CLASSIFICATION

Bacterial prostatitis (acute or chronic), nonbacterial prostatitis, prostatodynia.

AETIOLOGY (BACTERIAL PROSTATITIS)

1. Bacterial invasion of prostate:
   a. From haematogenous (bloodstream) origin (tonsils, gastrointestinal tract, genitourinary tract).
   b. From ascent of bacteria from urethra.
   c. Secondary to urethritis.
2. Descending infection from kidneys.

CLINICAL FEATURES

(From infection and local inflammation.)

1. Sudden chills and fever (moderate to high fever).
2. Bladder irritability – frequency, dysuria, urgency, haematuria.
3. Pain in perineum, rectum, lower back, lower abdomen, and penile head.

DIAGNOSTIC EVALUATION

1. Culture and sensitivity tests of urethral and prostatic fluid and urine.
   a. The pathogens in each specimen are identified by collection of divided urine specimens and expressed prostatic fluid (obtained by prostatic massage).

   b. The pH of the prostatic fluid is usually elevated.
2. Rectal examination – frequently reveals exquisitely tender, painful, swollen prostate, warm to the touch.

TREATMENT

Acute bacterial prostatitis

Antibiotic therapy (10 to 14 days) based on drug-sensitivity studies of the organisms.

Chronic bacterial prostatitis

1. Specific therapy (doxycycline, trimethoprim) – chronic bacterial prostatitis is difficult to cure because many antibacterial agents diffuse poorly into prostatic fluid.
   a. Prolonged therapy (three to six months) may be necessary to effect a cure.
   b. Chlamydia now frequently identified as sole pathogen or may be present with other common bacterial uropathogens.

Nonbacterial prostatitis

1. Most common type; aetiology obscure.
2. Therapy is directed toward control of symptoms and is individualized to meet specific needs; acute symptoms may be controlled with anticholinergic or anti-inflammatory drugs, hot baths, etc.

Prostatodynia

The patient has symptoms of urinary irritation but no evidence of bacteria or inflamed prostatic fluid or tissue. Treatment is symptomatic.

NURSING MANAGEMENT

1. Give supportive care.
   a. Bed rest – to relieve perineal and suprapubic pain.
   b. Hot baths – to promote muscular relaxation of pelvic floor and reduce potential for urinary retention.
   c. Antipyretics, analgesics, stool softeners, as necessary.
2. Watch for urinary retention – due to oedema of prostatic tissue; suprapubic catheter may be required.
3. Monitor for persistence of fever, perineal pain or difficulty in voiding – may indicate presence of prostatic abscess, which may require surgical drainage.
4. Be aware of other complications – urinary retention (from swelling of gland), recurring urinary tract infection, relapsing infection, epididymitis, bacteraemia, septicaemia.

PATIENT EDUCATION

Instruct the patient as follows:

1. Take antibiotic for the full time period.
2. Use hot baths (10 to 20 minutes) several times daily.
3. Drink fluids to satisfy thirst, but avoid 'forcing fluids', since an effective level of drug must be maintained in the urine.
4. Avoid food and drinks that have diuretic action or are prostatic irritants and increase prostatic secretions (alcohol, coffee, tea, chocolate, cola, spices).
5. Avoid sexual arousal/intercourse during period of acute inflammation; sexual intercourse may be beneficial in the treatment of chronic prostatitis; chronic prostatic infection is *not* sexually transmissible.
6. Be assured that the causative agent of prostatitis is not the type that causes venereal disease. (This may be an unspoken fear.)
7. Avoid sitting for long periods of time.
8. Prolonged follow-up is necessary, since recurrence of prostatitis due to the same or different organisms can occur.

CANCER OF THE PROSTATE

Cancer of the prostate is a malignant tumour of the prostate gland. It arises from the parenchyma of the prostate, usually in the most posterior part; therefore most prostatic cancers are palpable on rectal examination. An endocrine base is thought to be the cause but the precise changes have not been identified.

1. Cancer of the prostate is the most common carcinoma in men over 65 years of age.
2. It can spread by local extension, by lymphatics or via the bloodstream.
3. Prostatic cancer is potentially curable at an early stage; however, the majority of patients present with obstructive symptoms or metastatic lesions.

TNM CLASSIFICATION

Staging of cancer of the prostate is classified as follows:

T_0 incidental, impalpable carcinoma;
T_1 palpable nodule not deforming the gland;
T_2 palpable nodule deforming the gland;
T_3 capsule involvement;
T_4 involvement of adjacent organs.

NURSING ALERT

Annual rectal examination of males over 40 is important for early diagnosis of prostatic cancer.

MEDICAL AND SURGICAL MANAGEMENT

Curative (depends on stage)

1. Radiotherapy:
   a. Megavoltage radiotherapy (cobalt, high-energy linear accelerator) – delivers tumorcidal doses to prostate without undue damage to normal structures.
      (i) Some degree of proctitis, diarrhoea and dysuria may be seen toward end of treatment.
      (ii) Impotence may occur.
   b. Interstitial implantation of ^{125}I radioactive seeds in the prostate combined with bilateral pelvic lymphadenectomy.
2. Surgical interventions:
   a. Transurethral resection or open enucleation of prostate – for patients with obstructive symptoms who do not respond to radiotherapy or hormonal manipulation.

Palliative

1. Radiotherapy for palliation and to relieve bone pain from metastases (bone metastases are almost always multiple).
2. Hormonal manipulation – the aim of hormonal treatment is to suppress or eliminate the main sources of androgen production (most prostatic cancers are androgen dependent) and thereby to alleviate symptoms and retard progress of disease.
   a. Bilateral orchidectomy (removal of testes) – removes major source of androgen production, since 95 per cent of circulating plasma testosterone originates from testes. Or,
   b. Oestrogen therapy (diethylstilboestrol) – thought to inhibit the gonadotropins (responsible for testicular androgenic activity), thus removing androgenic hormone upon which the tumour growth depends.
      (i) Therapy with oestrogens leads to cardiovascular side-effects and gynaecomastia (soreness and enlargement of breasts).
      (ii) Synthetic gonadotropin-releasing hormone agonist (leuprolide acetate) – acts by inhibiting production of testosterone (investigational).
   c. Orchidectomy (removal of the testes) – lowers plasma testosterone, resulting in removing the testicular stimulus required for continued prostatic growth.

d. Both orchidectomy and oestrogen administration may be used in treatment of metastatic prostatic cancer.

e. Although not yet widely used in the UK, the anti-androgen cyproterone acetate (Cyprostat) is currently being evaluated for effectiveness in treating metastatic prostatic cancer.

3. Chemotherapy (singly or in combination) appears to be beneficial in advanced prostatic cancer, e.g. cyclophosphamide, methotrexate or estramustine.

4. Treatment of bone pain:
a. After hormonal therapy is established, chemotherapy, systemic bone-seeking radioactive materials or radiotherapy may be used.
b. Prevent pathological fractures.

Assessment

CLINICAL FEATURES

1. Symptoms due to obstruction of urinary flow
a. Hesitancy and straining on voiding, frequency, nocturia.
b. Diminution in size and force of urinary stream.
2. Symptoms due to metastases:
a. Pain in lumbosacral area radiating to hips and down legs (from bone metastases).
b. Perineal and rectal discomfort.
c. Anaemia, weight loss, weakness, nausea, oliguria (from uraemia).
d. Haematuria – from urethral or bladder invasion, or both.

DIAGNOSTIC EVALUATION

1. Digital rectal examination – reveals 'stony hard', fixed gland if lesion is advanced (there are indurated lumps without fixation if condition is found earlier).
2. Prostatic biopsy.
3. Cystoscopy – helps evaluate local extent of disease.
4. Radioimmunoassay for prostatic acid phosphatase – levels frequently become elevated with progression of disease.
5. Radionuclide bone scan – to detect metastases.
6. Skeletal X-rays – to reveal osteoblastic metastases.
7. Excretory urogram – to demonstrate changes from ureteral obstruction.
8. Lymphangiography – to determine the presence and extent of lymph node involvement.
9. Pelvic lymphadenectomy and biopsy – for staging and to determine spread to lymph nodes.

PATIENT PROBLEMS

1. Urinary dysfunction (frequency, nocturia, incontinence, haematuria) related to prostate tumour and sequelae of surgical intervention.
2. Potential for sexual dysfunction related to radical surgery and external radiotherapy.
3. Weight loss, fatigue, activity intolerance related to effects of cancer.

Planning and implementation

NURSING INTERVENTIONS

Relief from symptoms of urinary dysfunction

1. Support the patient undergoing radiotherapy (see p. 1039) and prostatic surgery.
2. See nursing management of the patient with pain (p. 1048), and care of the patient with late-stage cancer (p. 1046).
3. Monitor catheter drainage (see p. 597; either via suprapubic or urethral) when maintaining patency of the urethral passage becomes difficult.

Sexual rehabilitation

1. Be aware that the patient may be in ill health and suffering from pain, weight loss and the effects of endocrine therapy or chemotherapy; in this event, the patient may not be much concerned with sexuality.
2. Give the patient permission to communicate his concerns and sexual needs.
3. Understand the stages (shock and denial, mourning, resolution) the patient goes through concerning sexual dysfunction.
4. Expect some patient feelings of depression, anxiety, anger and regression.
5. Help the patient to use positive coping strategies (sexual counselling, learning other options of sexual expression, consideration of penile implant).

PATIENT EDUCATION

Be alert for neurological changes in lower extremities (prostatic cancer can lead to paraplegia); but this is a rare complication.

Evaluation

EXPECTED OUTCOMES

1. Patient achieves relief of urinary dysfunction.
2. Patient verbalizes coping strategies in dealing with fears, sexual dysfunction and anxiety.

MANAGEMENT OF THE PATIENT UNDERGOING PROSTATIC SURGERY

SURGICAL PROCEDURES

Four approaches for prostatectomy

1. Transurethral removal of prostatic tissue by an instrument introduced through urethra.
2. Open surgical removal of prostate (procedures used are named for area of incision):
   a. Perineal.
   b. Retropubic.
   c. Suprapubic.

Factors influencing choice of surgical approach

1. Size of gland and severity of obstruction.
2. Age and condition of the patient.
3. Presence of associated disease(s).

PREOPERATIVE MANAGEMENT

Establishing optimal kidney function

1. Maintain adequate bladder drainage via indwelling catheter or suprapubic cystostomy – renal function usually improves with re-establishment of drainage.
   a. Introduce indwelling catheter if the patient has continuing retention, if residual urine is more than 75–100ml, or if renal function has been impaired by back pressure of urine into the upper tract.
   b. Utilize cystostomy if the patient cannot tolerate urethral catheter.
   c. Give antibiotics (according to culture and sensitivity tests) – to combat and control infection, as prescribed.
   d. Watch the patient closely after drainage is instituted – blood pressure fluctuates and renal function may decline first few days after drainage is established.
   e. Ensure adequate hydration – the patient is frequently dehydrated from self-limitation of fluids because of frequency.
      (i) Encourage fluid intake of 2,500–3,000ml daily (if cardiac reserve is adequate) – to help in overcoming azotaemia.
      (ii) Weigh the patient daily and monitor fluid intake and output.
      (iii) Give intravenous fluids according to need as indicated by clinical status and serum electrolyte determinations.
2. Carry out prescribed renal function studies – to determine if there is renal impairment from prostatic back pressure and to evaluate renal reserve.

Ensuring optimal preoperative condition

1. The doctor will carry out complete haematological investigation – to ascertain specific clotting defects, since haemorrhage is a major postoperative complication.
2. Correct nutritional deficiencies, hypoproteinaemia, vitamin deficiencies and anaemia.
3. Give cardiac supporting drugs when indicated – helps alleviate renal symptoms.
4. Prepare the patient with pulmonary emphysema with antibacterial agent, tracheobronchial cleansing and incentive spirometry. The patient should stop smoking at least two days before surgery.
5. Teach active leg exercises; apply graded anti-embolism stockings to prevent deep vein thrombosis.
6. Type and cross match for blood transfusion(s).

POSTOPERATIVE PATIENT PROBLEMS

1. Potential complications (haemorrhage, urinary infection, urethral stricture) related to the surgical procedure.
2. Urinary elimination dysfunction related to problems with indwelling catheter, bladder spasms and the nature of the surgery.
3. Pain and discomfort related to bladder spasms and surgical procedure.
4. Anxiety concerning incontinence and sexual function.
5. Knowledge deficit of postoperative self-care and after-effects of surgery.

Planning and implementation

NURSING INTERVENTIONS

Prevention of complications

1. Assess for shock and haemorrhage.
   a. Watch for evidence of haemorrhage in drainage bag, on dressings and at incision site.
   b. Take blood pressure, pulse and respiration as frequently as clinical condition indicates. Compare with preoperative vital sign readings to assess degree of hypotension present.
      (i) Observe for cold, sweating skin, pallor, restlessness, fall in blood pressure, increasing pulse rate.
      (ii) Apply manual traction on the urethral catheter as directed to help stop bleeding; release traction intermittently and reassess the bleeding.
      (iii) Prepare for surgical intervention if bleeding persists (suturing of bleeders or transurethral coagulation of bleeders).
   c. Give blood transfusion as indicated.

2. Monitor for other postoperative complications.
   a. Urinary infection, septic shock, urethritis (from catheter), urinary fistula.
   b. Epididymitis.
   c. Late complications – urethral stricture, internal meatal stenosis.

Establishing adequate drainage of the bladder

1. Utilize a closed sterile gravity system of drainage – three-way system is useful in controlling bleeding; irrigating system keeps clots from forming (does not correct the *cause* of bleeding).
2. Watch drainage for evidence of increased bleeding – bright red urine indicates arterial bleeding; dark red urine suggests venous bleeding.
3. Irrigate bladder (amount and time prescribed by urologist) to avoid clot formation in the bladder.
   a. Frequency of bladder irrigation determined by amount of bleeding.
   b. Irrigation is adjusted to keep urine a light pink to straw colour, free of clots, and transparent in appearance.
   c. Irrigate catheter *gently* if it is occluded – catheter opening may be obstructed by blood clot, tissue remnant, or by being in contact with the bladder wall.
      (i) Rotate catheter to move drainage eye of catheter away from bladder wall/clot.
      (ii) Irrigate catheter with small amount of sterile fluid; too much force or fluid may damage recently operated area.
      (iii) Apply *gentle* suction; strong suction on a recently occluded vessel can cause bleeding.
      (iv) Avoid overdistending bladder – may produce secondary haemorrhage by stretching the coagulated vessels in the prostatic capsule.
4. Maintain an input and output record, including the amount of fluid used for irrigation.
5. Tape the drainage tubing (not the catheter) to shaved inner thigh – to prevent traction on bladder. (However, traction on the catheter by the urologist may control bleeding.)
6. Tape cystostomy catheter to lateral abdomen.
7. Note time and amount of each voiding after removal of catheter.
   a. May be urinary leakage around wound several days after removal of cathether in perineal, suprapubic, and retropubic surgery.
   b. Cystostomy tube may be removed before or after removal of urethral catheter.

Relief of pain and discomfort

1. Keep the patient quiet and comfortable during *immediate* postoperative period to prevent episodes of bleeding. When a patient experiences pain following prostatectomy, it may cause him to strain (from bladder irritability); this causes pelvic vein engorgement and promotes venous haemorrhage and clot formation.
2. Use tranquillizers, sedatives, antispasmodics, and appropriate analgesics for pain control.
   a. Elderly patients do not usually tolerate barbiturates.
   b. Take blood pressure before administering tranquillizers and analgesics.
   c. Give pain medication before irrigation if bladder spasms are severe.
3. Explain again to the patient the purpose of the catheter.
   a. Tell the patient that the urge to void urine is caused by the presence of the catheter and bladder spasm (painful contractions of muscles of bladder wall and neck).
      (i) Watch catheter tubing; a column of urine moving between pain episodes or when patient coughs may indicate bladder spasms.
      (ii) A frequent cause of spasm is the catheter touching (and stimulating) the posterior bladder wall.
      (iii) Gently draw catheter back toward external meatus; adjust catheter so that only its tip projects into the bladder.
   b. Give antispasmodics (propantheline bromide) as directed.
   c. Encourage him to refrain from pulling on catheter – will cause bleeding, clots, plugging of catheter, and distension.
   d. Tape catheter to lower abdomen to prevent pressure on penoscrotal junction.
   e. Wash urethral meatus adjacent to catheter with soap and water; rinse and apply an antibacterial ointment as directed.
4. Be alert for blockage of urinary drainage tube by kinking, mucous plugs, and blood clots.
5. Give antibiotics as directed – to promote urinary antisepsis.
6. Avoid rectal instrumentation (thermometers, rectal tubes, enemas) following prostatic surgery. Because the rectum is close to the prostatic fossa, instrumentation may be dangerous until healing has taken place.
7. Help the patient to ambulate as quickly as possible; avoid sitting for prolonged periods, since this increases intra-abdominal pressure and also the

possibility of bleeding.
8. Promote the comfort of the patient with perineal sutures.
   a. Wash perineum with surgical soap as directed.
   b. Assist the patient with bath as directed – to promote healing.

DISCHARGE PLANNING AND PATIENT EDUCATION
Instruct the patient as follows.

Urinary control
1. After the catheter is removed, there may be some burning on urination and/or frequent desire to void urine. These symptoms will disappear in a few weeks.
2. Expect urinary dribbling for a period of time (especially after catheter removal). Urinary incontinence may follow any type of prostatic surgery.
3. Exercises to gain urinary control.
   a. Pelvic floor exercises:
      (i) Tense the perineal muscles by pressing the buttocks together. Hold this position as long as possible; relax.
      (ii) Perform this exercise 10 to 20 times each hour.
      (iii) Continue with perineal exercises until full urinary control is gained.
   b. When starting to void:
      (i) Shut off the stream for a few seconds.
      (ii) Continue with full voiding.
      (iii) Continue this exercise with each urination until control improves; may take many weeks.
4. Urinate as soon as the first desire to do so is felt.
5. The urine may be cloudy for several weeks after surgery. As the prostate area heals, the cloudiness will disappear.
6. Avoid long car journeys, which increase tendency to bleed.
7. Avoid alcohol, which increases urinary burning.
8. Drink adequate fluids (eight glasses/day), since dehydration increases tendency for clot obstruction.
9. Do not take anticholinergics and diuretics unless by direct prescription of the doctor.

Sexual functioning
1. Prostatectomy does not usually cause impotence – penile erection depends on intact spinal cord, intact autonomic nerves to penis, normal erectile tissue/adequate blood supply and psychological well-being; a simple prostatectomy does not affect these factors.

   a. Total prostatectomy (removal of entire prostatic contents and capsule) results in impotence, since the nerves and muscular tissue surrounding the capsule (which have a function in penile erection) have been severed.
   b. Penile prosthesis (inflatable, semi-rigid and flexible types) may be surgically implanted – used to make the penis rigid for sexual intercourse.
2. In most instances sexual activity may be resumed in six to eight weeks; this is the time required for healing of the prostatic fossa to take place.
3. Do not be alarmed if no fluid appears on ejaculation; following ejaculation, the fluid goes into the bladder and is voided at the next urination.
   a. This does not reduce the level of sexual performance or satisfaction.
   b. The urine voided after intercourse may have a milky appearance.

Other considerations
1. Avoid straining and strenuous exercises.
2. Report to the doctor any bleeding or a decrease in the size of the urinary stream.

Evaluation
EXPECTED OUTCOMES
1. Patient shows no signs of complications – no evidence of haemorrhage or infection.
2. Patient achieves bladder drainage; no clots; urine becoming clear.
3. Patient reports diminished discomfort and pain; taking minimal amount of analgesics.
4. Patient expresses feelings about urinary control and sexual functioning; performing perineal exercises; gaining urinary control.

HYDROCELE

Hydrocele is a collection of fluid generally in the tunica vaginalis of the testicle, although it may also occur within the spermatic cord.

CAUSES
Caused by defective or inadequate reabsorption of normally produced hydrocele fluid.
1. Secondary to local injury, including hernia operation.
2. Secondary to infection.
3. Following epididymitis or orchitis.
4. As a complication of tumour of testicle.
5. In oedematous states such as congestive heart failure, cirrhosis of the liver.
6. Idiopathic.

CLINICAL FEATURES
1. Enlargement of the scrotum.
2. Usually painless until fluid accumulation is large enough to cause pressure.
3. Transmits light when transilluminated.

TREATMENT
1. No treatment is required unless complications are present.
   a. Circulatory complications involving testicle.
   b. Painful large hydrocele, which is uncomfortable and cosmetically unacceptable to the patient.
2. Surgical intervention – hydrocelectomy (excision of tunica vaginalis of testis) for removal of fluid and control of swelling.
   a. Periodic aspiration of hydrocele fluid in poor-risk patient.
   b. Open operation for eversion or removal of hydrocele sac.
3. See below, Postoperative Nursing Support (Varicocele).
4. Complication – formation of a haematoma in the loose tissues of the scrotum.

VARICOCELE

Varicocele is a mass of varicose veins in the scrotum, usually part of the spermatic cord.

CLINICAL FEATURES
1. Subfertility may occur with varicocele – may suppress spermatogenesis due to vascular and temperature changes or more likely to reflux of left adrenal corticosteroids to both testes because of intercommunication of their venous circulations.
2. A dragging sensation in the scrotum is usually the patient's chief complaint.
3. Varicocele on the right may indicate retro-peritoneal tumour.

DIAGNOSTIC EVALUATION
Palpation of intrascrotal mass (with patient in upright position) that disappears in a short time after he has been lying down.

MANAGEMENT
1. Scrotal support to relieve discomfort.
2. Surgical intervention – ligation and excision of veins (varicocelectomy).

POSTOPERATIVE NURSING SUPPORT
1. Apply ice bag for first few hours postoperatively to relieve oedema.
2. Apply scrotal support for comfort.

TUMOURS OF THE TESTIS

The aetiology of testicular tumours is unknown, but cryptorchidism, infections and genetic and endocrine factors appear to play a role in their development.

CLINICAL FEATURES
1. Tumours of the testis are usually malignant; they occur primarily in men between the ages of 20 and 40.
2. Most testicular tumours metastasize early to the periaortic and pericaval lymph nodes, lungs and liver.
3. A patient with a history of one testis tumour is more apt to develop another than is the random patient to develop a first testis tumour.
4. Testicular germ cell tumours are now considered curable.

CLINICAL MANIFESTATIONS
1. Mass in scrotum; painless enlargement of the testis, accompanied by feeling of heaviness in scrotum.
2. Pain in the testis (if patient has epididymitis or bleeding into tumour).
3. Gynaecomastia (enlargement of the breasts) from elaboration of chorionic gonadotropins from testicular tumour.
4. Symptoms of metastases:
   a. Left supraclavicular or abdominal mass.
   b. Abdominal pain.
   c. Cough (lung metastases).

DIAGNOSTIC EVALUATION
1. Testicular tumour markers – radioimmunoassay of human chorionic gonadotropins (hCG) and alphafetoprotein (AFP) – serological and cellular markers used for diagnosis, detection of early recurrence, staging and monitoring treatment.
2. Intravenous urogram to evaluate presence of enlarged lymph nodes as manifested by ureteral displacement.

3. Chest film to seek pulmonary or mediastinal metastases.
4. Lymphangiography – to assess extent of lymphatic spread of tumour.
5. Computed tomography – to identify lesions in retroperitoneum and to follow the patient's course during/after treatment.
6. Ultrasound examination – non-invasive method of identifying scrotal masses.

TREATMENT
1. *Surgery* – orchidectomy (removal of testis and its tunica and spermatic cord):
   a. Usually done through an inguinal incision.
   b. Retroperitoneal lymphadenectomy usually performed after orchidectomy.
      (i) Orchidectomy (unilateral) usually has no adverse effects on sexual potency or fertility. Gel-filled prosthesis can be implanted at time of orchidectomy or electively thereafter to offset absence of one testis.
      (ii) Possible postoperative complication is ejaculation without emission (loss of ejaculation due to interruption of sympathetic ganglia at L2–L4 level, since they are in close proximity to involved nodes). Patient will not be fertile, but normal libido and orgasm will be unimpaired.
2. *Radiotherapy* to lymphatic drainage pathways is used in most patients with testicular cancer; may be curative or palliative, depending on circumstances. Treatment of choice for seminoma.
3. *Chemotherapy* – used in the treatment of primary tumour and regional lymphatic metastases and in managing distant metastatic disease; usually given in combination.
   a. Vinblastine, actinomycin-D, bleomycin, and etoposide (Vepesid) – induce a high percentage of durable complete remissions (metastatic testicular cancer is potentially curable).
   b. These regimens are toxic and require intensive therapeutic support, and a high degree of patient commitment and cooperation.
   c. May be used as adjuvant to surgery and/or radiotherapy in advanced disease.

NURSING INTERVENTIONS
1. See p. 629 for care of the patient following surgery, p. 1039 for care of the patient undergoing radiotherapy, and p. 1036 for care of the patient undergoing chemotherapy.
2. Teach the patient that one testis is expendable.
3. Make it clear that an orchidectomy will not diminish potency, fertility or virility.
4. Give the adolescent male or younger patient the opportunity to discuss depositing sperm in sperm bank, particularly if he is to receive radiotherapy. (However, he may be ineligible for sperm-banking because of disease-impaired sperm production.)
5. Inform the patient of the following:
   a. Genital cancer is not 'punishment' for real/imagined sexual activity.
   b. Radiotherapy to the abdomen will cause no change in sexual performance but may diminish semen volume.
   c. Refer the patient to social worker as required; frequent hospitalization may be necessary with interruption of work/personal life.

PATIENT EDUCATION
Instruct the patient as follows:
1. Follow-up evaluation includes chest films, excretory urography and radioimmunoassay of human chorionic gonadotropin and alpha-fetoprotein, examination of lymph nodes – to monitor success of therapy and to detect recurrence of malignancy.
2. Carry out periodic self-examinations of the testes (see Guidelines, below).

GUIDELINES: SELF-EXAMINATION FOR TESTICULAR TUMOUR

1. The testis is easily accessible for self-examination. Most tumours are palpable and can be detected by self-examination.
2. The hormonally active years (20 to 40) are the tumour-prone years.

PROCEDURE

Action by patient	Rationale
1. Examine for testicular tumour periodically, preferably while showering/bathing.	Detection of abnormalities is more readily accomplished after or during a warm shower or bath, when the scrotum wall is relaxed.
2. Use both hands to palpate (feel). Carefully examine all scrotal contents.	A small lump (nodule) can slip away from one hand. You can feel differences in weight between the testicles by using both hands.
3. Locate the epididymis; this is the cord-like structure at the back of the testis.	It is important to know what the epididymis feels like so you will not confuse it with an abnormality.
4. The spermatic cord (and vas) extends upward from the epididymis.	
5. Feel each testis between the thumb and first two fingers of each hand.	The testes lie freely in the scrotum, are oval shaped, and measure 4–5cm in length, 3cm in width, and about 2cm in thickness.
6. Note size, shape, abnormal tenderness.	An abnormality may be felt as a firm area on the front or side of the testicle.
7. Stand in front of mirror and look for changes in size/shape of scrotum.	Tumours or cystic masses tend to involve only one side.

EPIDIDYMITIS

Epididymitis is an infection of the epididymis that usually descends from an infected prostate or urinary tract.

CAUSES
1. Prostatic infection (most common cause); complication of infected urine containing pyogenic bacteria.
2. Trauma; urethral stricture.
3. Postoperative epididymitis – complication of prostatectomy and urethral catheterization.
4. Specific causes – gonorrhoea, syphilis, tuberculosis, *Chlamydia trachomatis* infection, *Ureaplasma urealyticum* infection.

CLINICAL FEATURES
1. Localized scrotal pain and tenderness.
2. Oedema, redness and tenderness of scrotum.
3. Chills and fever.
4. Pyuria and bacteriuria.

DIAGNOSTIC EVALUATION
1. Examination of initial and midstream urine sample for pyuria.
2. Elevated white blood count (may be as high as 20,000–30,000/ml^3).
3. Epididymal aspiration.
4. Staining of urethral discharge if preceded by urethritis (either nonspecific or gonorrhoeal); usually no discharge is present with epididymitis.

TREATMENT AND NURSING MANAGEMENT
1. Give specific antibiotic therapy until all evidence of acute inflammatory reaction has subsided.
2. Encourage bed rest during the acute phase.
3. Apply scrotal support for enlarged testicle (scrotal bridge; rolled towel under scrotum) – to relieve oedema and discomfort, to improve venous

drainage, and to take the tension off the cord. A cotton-lined athletic supporter may promote comfort.
4. Assist with infiltration of spermatic cord with local anaesthetic agent (procaine hydrochloride) – for pain relief if patient is seen within 24 hours after onset.
5. Give analgesics for pain relief – this gives pain relief while more specific therapy begins to work.
6. Apply intermittent cold compresses to scrotum during initial period – for pain relief.
7. Use local heat or bath later – to hasten resolution of inflammatory process.
8. Offer stool softeners.
9. Observe for possible abscess formation.

PATIENT EDUCATION
Instruct the patient as follows:
1. Avoid straining (lifting, defaecation) and sexual excitement until infection is under control.
2. It may take four weeks or longer for epididymis to return to normal.
3. Sex partners of patients with chlamydial urethritis or epididymitis should be examined and treated.
4. Reassure the patient that sexual performance should not be affected after the inflammation has subsided.

VASECTOMY

Vasectomy is the ligation and transection of a section of the vas deferens; a bilateral vasectomy is a sterilization procedure for males.

CLINICAL INDICATIONS
1. Performed as a sterilization procedure.
2. Performed if the patient has recurrent acute epididymitis (see above).

UNDERLYING CONSIDERATIONS
1. A vasectomy interrupts the transportation of the sperm. This procedure has no effect on sexual potency, erection, ejaculation or production of male hormones.
2. Seminal fluid is mostly manufactured in the seminal vesicles and prostate, which are unaffected by vasectomy.
   a. There will be no noticeable decrease in the amount of ejaculated fluid; the sperm accounts for less than 5 per cent of the volume. The sperm cells are reabsorbed into the body.
   b. Psychological problems have been noted in an occasional patient following this procedure.

3. A vasectomy can be done on an outpatient basis with local anaesthesia.
4. A legal consent form must be obtained, usually from the patient and his partner.
5. The patient should be advised that he will be sterile but that potency will not be altered following a bilateral vasectomy. Rarely is there a spontaneous re-anastomosis resulting in pregnancy.
6. A vasectomy may not be reversible and should be considered permanent; microsurgical techniques are being used for vasectomy reversal (vasovasotomy); success rates are promising.

COMPLICATIONS
1. Sperm granuloma – due to extravasation of sperm.
2. Infection; scrotal abscess.
3. Recanalization of vas deferens (very rare).
4. Bleeding and haematoma.

TREATMENT AND NURSING INTERVENTIONS
1. Place patient on bed rest for several hours.
2. Apply ice bags intermittently to the scrotum for several hours after surgery to reduce swelling and relieve discomfort.
3. Reassure the patient that discoloration of scrotal skin, swelling, and oedema are to be expected.
4. Advise the patient to wear scrotal support for added comfort and support.

PATIENT EDUCATION
Instruct the patient as follows:
1. The primary function of the testicle(s) is the production of hormones and of sperm. A vasectomy will not interfere with these functions, but it will interrupt the descent of sperm from the testicle to the ejaculatory ducts.
2. Rest for 48 hours after surgery to prevent discomfort.
3. Avoid strenuous activities for several days.
4. Sexual intercourse may be resumed as desired.
5. Contraceptives should be used until the sperm stored distal to the point of interruption of the vas is evacuated (two negative semen specimens one month apart). *The patient is still fertile for a variable period of time after vasectomy.*
6. Absence of sperm must be demonstrated microscopically; laboratory tests confirm that no sperm are present in the seminal fluid.
7. A vasectomy does not prevent venereal disease.

CONDITIONS AFFECTING THE PENIS

INFECTIONS

1. Chancre – venereal ulceration caused by *Treponema pallidum* (see Syphilis, p. 988).
2. Chancroid – a sexually transmitted disease caused by *Haemophilus ducreyi*; usually one or several penile ulcers are present, as well as enlarged lymph nodes.
3. Genital herpes (herpes simplex virus [HSV]) – a sexually transmitted disease that produces multiple bilaterally distributed vesicles on or near the penis.
4. Gonorrhoea – see p. 986.

CLINICAL FEATURES
Ulceration of the penis should be suspected as being venereal in origin until proved otherwise.

DIAGNOSTIC EVALUATION
1. Dark field microscopic examination of smear for spirochaetes.
2. Serological (blood) test for syphilis.

TREATMENT
Varies greatly, depending on the cause of ulceration.

OTHER CONDITIONS

PHIMOSIS
A condition in which the foreskin is constricted so that it cannot be retracted over the glans. The treatment is circumcision.

PARAPHIMOSIS
A condition in which the foreskin is retracted behind the glans, and because of narrowness and subsequent oedema, cannot be reduced back to its normal position.

PRIAPISM
An uncontrolled persistent erection of the penis occurring from neural or vascular causes, including sickle cell thrombosis, spinal cord tumours and tumour invasion of the penis or its vessels. This condition is considered a urological emergency. Treatment includes bed rest, sedation and/or surgery.

CARCINOMA OF THE PENIS
Carcinoma of the penis occurs in the skin of the penis; appears as a painless, wart-like growth or ulcer on the glans or coronal sulcus under the prepuce. Treatment is radiotherapy or surgical intervention.

CIRCUMCISION

Circumcision is the excision of the foreskin (prepuce) of the glans penis.

CLINICAL INDICATIONS
1. Usually done in infancy for hygienic purposes.
2. In adults – phimosis; paraphimosis; recurrent infection of the glans and foreskin; personal desire of the patient.
3. Circumcision is thought to be a preventive measure against carcinoma of the penis.

POSTOPERATIVE NURSING MANAGEMENT
1. Watch for bleeding.
2. Change Vaseline gauze dressing as directed.
3. Give analgesia as the patient's condition indicates; circumcision can be quite painful in the adult male.

CONTACT ADDRESSES

British Kidney Patient Association
Bordon
Hants
Tel: 04203 2022/1

Urostomy Association
Buckland
Beaumont Park
Danbury
Essex CH3 4DE
Tel: 024 541 4294

FURTHER READING

BOOKS

Asscher, A.N. and Moffat, D.B. (1983) *Nephro-Urology*, Heinemann, London.

Association of Continence Advisers (1985) *Directory of Aids To Toiletting* (3rd edn), Association of Continence Advisers, London.

Atkins, R.C., Thomson, N.M. and Farrell, P.C. (1981) *Peritoneal Dialysis*, Churchill Livingstone, Edinburgh.

Brown, C.B. (1985) *Manual of Renal Disease*, Churchill Livingstone, Edinburgh.

Cameron, S. (1981) *Kianey Disease: The Facts*, Oxford University Press, Oxford.

Davison, A.M. (1981) *A Synopsis of Renal Diseases*, John Wright, Bristol.

Evans, D.B. and Henderson, R.G. (1985) *Lecture Notes on Nephrology*, Blackwell Scientific Publications, Oxford.

Feneley, R.C.L. and Blannin, J.P. (1984) *Incontinence*, Churchill Livingstone, Edinburgh.

Gabriel, R. (1982) *A Patient's Guide to Dialysis and Transplantation* (2nd edn), MTP, Lancaster.

James, J. (1984) *Handbook of Urology*, Harper & Row, London.

Kilmartin, A. (1980) *Understanding Cystitis*, Pan, London.

King's Fund (1983) *Action on Incontinence*, Report of a Working Group, Project Paper, No. 43, Kings Fund, London.

Mandelstrom, D. (1986) *Incontinence and Its Management* (2nd edn), Croom Helm, London.

Mitchell, J.P. (1981) *Endoscopic Operative Urology*, John Wright, Bristol.

Norton, C. (1986). *Nursing for Incontinence*, Beaconsfield Publishers, England.

Scott, R. *et al.* (1982) *Urology Illustrated* (2nd edn), Churchill Livingstone, Edinburgh.

Slade, N. and Gillespie, W.A. (1985) *The Urinary Tract and the Catheter: Infection and Other Problems*, Wiley, Chichester.

Whitfield, H.N. (1985) *Urology* (Pocket Consultant Series), Blackwell Scientific Publications, Oxford.

Winder, E. and Faber, S. (1982) *Renal Nursing*, Macmillan, London.

ARTICLES
Incontinence
Blannin, J.P. (1984) Assessment of an incontinence patient, *Nursing*, Vol. 2, September, pp. 863–5.

Cunningham, R.J. (1984) Second opinion: a woman with stress incontinence, *Modern Medicine*, Vol. 29, May, pp. 16, 18–21.

Gooch, J. (1986) Care of the urinary incontinent patient, *Professional Nurse*, Vol. 1, August, pp. 298–300.

Harrison, S. (1984) Re-education of the pelvic floor muscles, *Nursing Times*, Vol. 80, 4 April, Incontinence Supplement, pp. 29–30.

Norton, C. (1984) The promotion of continence, *Nursing Times*, Vol. 80, 4 April, Incontinence Supplement, pp. 4, 6, 8, 10.
— (1986) Continence. Promoting research, *Nursing Times*, Vol. 82, 9 April, p. 55.

Tattersall, A. (1985) Continence: getting the whole picture. A holistic approach to continence promotion, *Nursing Times*, Vol. 81, 3 April, pp. 55, 57–8.

Webb, C. (1984) Promoting continence: How would you feel? The effects of incontinence on sexuality, *Community Outlook*, February, pp. 45–6.

Renal disorders and transplantation
British Transplantation Society (1986) Recommendations on the use of living kidney donors in the United Kingdom, *British Medical Journal*, Vol. 293, July, pp. 257–8.

Coles, G.A. (1985) Is peritoneal dialysis a good, long-term treatment? *British Medical Journal*, Vol. 290, 20 April, pp. 1164–6.

Donnelly, P.F. *et al.* (1985) Continuous ambulatory peritoneal dialysis and renal transplantation: a five-year experience, *British Medical Journal*, Vol. 291, 12 October, pp. 1001–04.

Goodinson, S. (1984) Renal function: an overview, *Nursing*, Vol. 2, September, pp. 843, 845–6, 848, 851–2.

Goodinson, S. and Holmes, S. (1985) Acute renal failure: aetiology and emergency treatment, *Nursing*, Vol. 2, October, pp. 1254–7.

Holmes, S. (1984) The nutritional management of renal disease, *Nursing*, Vol. 2, September, pp. 860–2.

Leigh, J. (1985) Acute renal failure, *Nursing*, Vol. 2, October, pp. 1258–9.

Morgan, A. and Burden, R. (1986) Effect of continuous ambulatory peritoneal dialysis on a British renal unit, *British Medical Journal*, Vol. 293, October, pp. 935–7.

Newton, G. (1984) Peritoneal dialysis, *Nursing Mirror*, Vol. 158, No. 12, pp. 35–7.

Phillips, K. (1986) Psychological effects of chronic renal failure, *Nursing Times*, Vol. 82, 28 May, pp. 56–7.

Ward, E. (1986) Dialysis or death? Doctors should stop covering up for an inadequate health service, *Journal of Medical Ethics*, Vol. 12, June, pp. 61–3.

Williams, A.J. (1984) End-stage renal failure: coping with the demand, *Health Trends*, Vol. 16, No. 1, pp. 1–3.

Workman, B. (1984) Nephrotic syndrome, *Nursing Times*, Vol. 80, 13 June, pp. 32–6.

Urology

Barnes, K.E. (1986) Long-term catheter management: minimizing the problem of premature replacement due to balloon deflation, *Journal of Advanced Nursing*, Vol. 11, May, pp. 303–7.

Clark, N. and O'Connell, P. (1984) Prostatectomy: a guide to answering your patient's unspoken questions, *Nursing*, Vol. 84, No. 14, pp. 48–51.

Crummy, V. (1985) Hospital-acquired urinary tract infection, *Nursing Times*, Vol. 81, 5 June, *Journal of Infection Control Nursing Supplement*, pp. 7, 9, 11–12.

Editorial (1985) Treatment trends: prostate cancer, *Journal of District Nursing*, Vol. 2, June, pp. 18, 33.

Gooch, J. (1986) Catheter care, *Professional Nurse*, Vol. 1, May, pp. 207–8.

Gould, D. (1985) Management of indwelling urethral catheters: a report on research, *Nursing Mirror*, Vol. 161, 4 September, pp. 17–18, 20.

Granise, C.A. (1984) Indwelling catheter care: a run-through, *Nursing*, Vol. 84, No. 14, pp. 26–7.

Jacques, L. *et al.* (1986) Effects of short-term catheterisation, *Nursing Times*, Vol. 82, 18 June, pp. 59, 61–2.

Johnson, A. (1986) Urinary tract infection, *Nursing*, Vol. 3, March, pp. 102–5.

Kennedy, A. (1984) Catheter concepts (research into the development of a new indwelling urethral catheter), *Nursing Mirror*, Vol. 159, October, pp. 42–4, 46.

— (1984) Trial of a new bladder washout system (the Uro-Trainer system), *Nursing Times*, Vol. 80, 14 November, pp. 48–51.

Latham, E. and Marden, W. (1986) Percutaneous nephrolithotripsy, *Nursing Times*, Vol. 82, 18 June, pp. 65–6.

McConnell, E. (1985) Assessing the bladder, *Nursing*, Vol. 85, No. 15, pp. 44–6.

Mitchell, J.P. (1984) Management of chronic urinary retention, *British Medical Journal*, Vol. 289, September, pp. 515–6.

Winder, A. (1986) Intermittent self-catheterisation, *Professional Nurse*, Vol. 2, No. 2, p. 58.

10

Care of the Patient with a Gynaecological or Breast Disorder

Care of the Patient with a Gynaecological Disorder

OVULATION AND MENSTRUATION

Ovulation refers to the expulsion of an ovum from the ovary 14 days before the onset of the next menstrual period.

As the endometrium is being shed, the process of repair and regrowth starts again – preparing once more for the reception of a fertilized ovum.

1. If conception does not occur, the ovum dies; tissue lining the endometrial cavity, which has become thickened and congested, becomes haemorrhagic.
2. Tissue lining the uterus, blood cells and breakdown products slough off and are discharged through the cervix into the vagina.
3. This cyclic process is called menstruation (Table 10.1).

Table 10.1 Menstruation

Characteristics	Range	Average
Menarche (onset)	9–17 years of age	12.5 years of age
Cycle length	24–32 days	29 days
Flow – duration	1–8 days	3–5 days
Flow – amount	10–75ml	35ml
Menopause – onset	45–55 years of age	47–50 years of age

DISTURBANCES OF MENSTRUATION

A relationship with feedback mechanism exists between the hormonal secretions of the ovary, adrenal, thyroid, and pituitary glands. An increase or decrease in the activity of one or more glands can cause a disturbance in menstruation.

DYSMENORRHOEA

Dysmenorrhoea is painful menstruation.

OCCURRENCE
Common in unmarried women and women who have not borne children.

TYPES
1. Primary – due to unknown factors; thought to be intrinsic to uterus; extrinsic pathology such as polyp and fibroids may be a factor. May involve emotional and psychological factors.
2. Secondary – due to factors such as endometriosis, pelvic infection or intrauterine device.

SYMPTOMS
1. Pain may be due to uterine spasm caused by a narrowing of the cervical canal (exaggerated uterine contractility).
2. Pain – colicky, cyclic, nagging, dull ache; usually in lower abdomen, may radiate down back of legs. May be severe enough to require bed rest for a day or two.
3. Severe dysmenorrhoea may be experienced – with chills, headache, diarrhoea, nausea, vomiting and syncope.

AETIOLOGY

1. Endocrine:
   Some investigators believe there is a relation between release of prostaglandin from the endometrium and the symptoms of dysmenorrhoea; this has not been proved.
2. Anatomical:
   a. Some discomfort results from the passing of a cervical sound or from dilatation of the cervix; a pathological growth could produce the same symptoms.
   b. An infantile or small uterus may contribute to dysmenorrhoea, but this has not been proved.
3. Constitutional:
   Chronic illnesses and general debilitation seem to be associated with a high incidence of dysmenorrhoea (anaemia, fatigue, diabetes, tuberculosis).
4. Psychogenic:
   Most studies indicate that strong underlying psychological factors cause dysmenorrhoea. Parental instruction and a healthy emotional environment for the growing young girl, in a setting where realistic family relations are cultivated, almost preclude primary dysmenorrhoea.

TREATMENT AND NURSING MANAGEMENT

Since there is no single treatment for dysmenorrhoea, a three-pronged approach seems best to relieve symptoms: combine therapies as they relate to constitutional, hormonal, and psychological factors.

1. Be selective, according to needs of individual and severity of problem.
   a. Proper psychological preparation of girls for menarche.
   b. Good posture; use special exercises to improve posture and correct weak musculature and imbalance.
2. Since emotional make-up may accentuate discomfort, psychotherapy or pharmacotherapy may be necessary.
3. Complete physical examination to rule out other physical abnormalities.
4. Instructions to patient:
   a. Usual activity is possible – should be encouraged.
   b. Mild analgesics for discomfort are permissible, – e.g. aspirin, paracetamol.
   c. Avoid use of habit-forming drugs such as narcotics and alcohol.
5. Dysmenorrhoea can usually be eliminated by low-dose oral contraceptives which block ovulation.
6. Regular exercises (as well as physical activity) are recommended.
7. Administration of a prostaglandin inhibitor such as ibuprofen (Brufen), mefenamic acid (Ponstan) or naproxen sodium (Synflex) are recommended in relieving primary dysmenorrhoea.
   a. Medications are to be taken with water; milk may be used if the medication causes an upset stomach.
   b. If medication causes drowsiness or sleepiness, do not drive a car or operate machinery.
8. Psychological counselling may also benefit some individuals.

PREMENSTRUAL TENSION SYNDROME (PMT)

Premenstrual tension syndrome (PMT) is a condition related to neuroendocrine events within the hypothalamus–pituitary axis that modulate neurotransmitter function.

1. It differs from dysmenorrhoea in that it has no relation to ovulation.
2. Some women accept these symptoms as normal.
3. When symptoms are severe, medical relief is sought.

CLINICAL FEATURES

1. Symptoms may begin 10 days or more prior to menstrual flow onset; they diminish one or two days after menses begin.
2. Oedema, breast swelling, abdominal distension – transitory because of increase in water content in tissues.
3. Behavioural – irritability, sleep disturbance, lethargy, depression.
4. Neurological – headache, vertigo, paraesthesia of hands or feet.
5. Respiratory – colds, hoarseness, allergies (asthma) usually worse.
6. Miscellaneous – palpitation, backache, skin problems, eye complaints.

TREATMENT AND NURSING INTERVENTIONS

1. Many forms of therapy have been tried, but research fails to support consistent success.
2. Medications prescribed – progesterone (injection, suppository), oral contraceptives, diuretics, monamine oxidase inhibitors (MAOIs).
3. Placebo/tranquillizers may be helpful.
4. Encourage women with PMT to explore ways and means to avoid stress in the premenstruum; relaxation techniques may be helpful.
5. Restrict sodium intake and limit use of caffeine, tobacco and alcohol.

6. Try a modified hypoglycaemic diet with small, frequent meals; this often alleviates irritability.
7. Suggest contacting a premenstrual tension centre for supportive services and access to recent research-based treatment recommendations.
8. Give address of self-help group, e.g.
National Association for Premenstrual Tension
23 Upper Park Road
Kingston upon Thames
Surrey KT2 52B

AMENORRHOEA

Amenorrhoea is absence of menstrual flow.

PRIMARY
When a girl is 16 or 17 and has not menstruated.
1. May be caused by embryonic maldevelopment.
2. Treatment is according to aetiology.

SECONDARY
Menstruation has begun (initial menarche) but stops.
1. Criteria:
   a. No bleeding for six months after having regular cyclic bleeding.
   b. No bleeding for 12 months after a history of irregular bleeding.
2. Causes:
   a. Normal pregnancy and lactation.
   b. Psychogenic (minor emotional upsets). Hypothalamic disturbances (autonomic nervous system) may also be the cause (e.g. anorexia nervosa).
   c. Constitutional:
      Any disturbance of metabolism and nutrition (e.g. diabetes, tuberculosis, obesity).
   d. Exercise-related – rigorous involvement.
3. Assessment:
   a. Progesterone challenge test:
      (i) Positive – if bleeding (or even 'spotting'); anovulation is most likely;
      (ii) Negative – no bleeding occurs; indication of end organ failure. Other tests are indicated.
4. Treatment – directed at cause – constitutional therapy, psychotherapy, hormone therapy, surgery.

OLIGOMENORRHOEA

Oligomenorrhoea is markedly diminished menstrual flow – nearing amenorrhoea.

MENORRHAGIA

Menorrhagia is excessive bleeding during regular menstruation.

CAUSES
1. Endocrine disturbances.
2. Inflammatory diseases; benign or malignant pelvic tumours.
3. Emotional stress.

TREATMENT
1. Search for underlying cause.
2. Correct blood deficiency.

METRORRHAGIA

Metrorrhagia is bleeding from the uterus between regular menstrual periods. It is significant because it is usually a symptom of some disease – often cancer or benign tumours of uterus.

POLYMENORRHOEA

Polymenorrhoea is frequent menstruation occurring at intervals of less than three weeks.

MENOPAUSE

Menopause is the stage of female life when there is physiological cessation of the menses along with progressive ovarian failure.
   Climacteric is the transition period (perimenopausal period: premenopause, menopause and postmenopause) during which the woman's reproductive function gradually diminishes and disappears. It usually occurs between the ages of 49 and 55 years (mean, 51.4).

CLINICAL FEATURES
1. The monthly menstrual flow becomes smaller in amount, then becomes irregular, and finally ceases.
2. Hot or warm flushes and other vascular disturbances may be in evidence and are of endocrinological origin.
3. Additional physical signs:
   a. Manifestations of atrophy – sagging structures, atrophic vaginitis.

b. Evidence of stress incontinence on occasion.
c. Skin dryness; weight gain.
d. Calcium deficiency (which may lead to osteoporotic changes).
4. Psychological features:
   a. Dizziness, weakness, nervousness, insomnia.
   b. Headaches; inability to concentrate.
   c. A feeling of being unneeded.
   d. Fear of growing old; depression.

TREATMENT AND NURSING INTERVENTIONS

1. Most women respond favourably to a regimen of education and modification of lifestyle. Adherence to habits that promote good health is desirable. In the past, this time in a woman's life was regarded as the onset of old age; a realistic and helpful approach is to realize that the menopausal woman can expect to live another 30 or 35 years.
2. Mild sedatives and tranquillizers may be required by some to relieve nervousness and tension.
3. For persistent or severe hot flushes, it may be necessary to resort to oestrogen therapy: Premarin or ethinyloestradiol (Lynoral). Close medical supervision is required.
4. Continued use of oestrogens to prevent widespread degenerative changes continues to be controversial. Also long-term use of oestrogens may be linked with cancer.
   a. Indications for oestrogen replacement therapy include psychomotor complaints, urogenital atrophy, prevention of osteoporosis and prevention of coronary heart disease.
   b. Future research needs to be directed toward identifying postmenopausal women at risk for osteoporosis and/or coronary heart disease.
   c. Oestrogen replacement should not be withheld from women who need it (less than one-quarter of menopausal women). Indiscriminate use of oestrogens is strongly discouraged.

PATIENT EDUCATION

1. 'Change of life' is not abnormal nor need it be limiting.
2. Sex life is by no means terminated; in many instances, it is enhanced.
3. Avoid overfatigue and stressful situations, since these exaggerate minor problems.
4. Encourage a nutritious diet and keep weight under control.
5. Develop outside interests that help to absorb anxieties and lessen tension.
6. Continue to exercise and develop self-fulfilling and enriching activities.

7. Recognize that the expected life span after menopause is 30 to 35 years.
8. To alleviate vaginal dryness and pain on intercourse (due to oestrogen deficiency), it is safer to use a water-based lubricant (K-Y Jelly) than an oestrogen cream. Topical oestrogens produce systemic effects; therefore it cannot be assumed that their action has limited local effects.

DIAGNOSTIC STUDIES FOR GYNAECOLOGICAL CONDITIONS

PELVIC EXAMINATION

A pelvic examination is an inspection of the external genitalia for signs of inflammation, swelling, bleeding, discharge or local skin and epithelial changes. A speculum is inserted to permit the examiner to visualize the vagina and cervix.

(For Guidelines: Vaginal Examination by the Nurse, see p. 676.)

Patient preparation

1. Provide psychological support – the patient needs reassurance, understanding, and skilful consideration of her emotional as well as physical problems.
2. Instruct the patient to avoid douching, if this is practised, for 24 hours before examination; cellular deposits might wash away.
3. Encourage the patient to void urine and evacuate the bowels before examination – provides more relaxation of perineal tissues.
4. Advise the patient to remove sufficient clothing to permit adequate exposure of genitalia and allow for examination of the abdomen.
5. Avoid undue exposure of the patient.

Positioning of patient (best done on an examining table but can be achieved on a bed)

1. *Lithotomy* – knees and hips flexed; heels resting on foot rests. Drape sheet diagonally over the patient so that corner may be grasped and pulled upward to expose perineal area.
2. *Sims position* – the patient lies on one side, usually the left, with the left arm behind her back. The right (uppermost) thigh and knee are flexed as much as possible; left leg is partially flexed.

3. *Knee–chest* – the patient kneels on a table with feet extending over the end.
   a. Separate the patient's knees and maintain thighs at right angles to the table.
   b. Turn the patient's head to one side and allow face and chest to rest on a soft pillow.
   c. The patient's arms may grasp sides of table.
4. *Semi-sitting* – the patient is placed in a position similar to the lithotomy position with the exception that instead of lying supine, she is in a semi-sitting position. Advantages:
   a. Greater patient comfort physically.
   b. Enhanced eye and spoken communication.
   c. Easier bimanual examination for examiner.
   d. With hand-held mirror, the patient is able to see anatomy, lesions, etc.
   e. More effective patient teaching concerning anatomy, pathology, contraceptive information, etc.

Procedure for examining the pelvis

1. A speculum is inserted so that the vaginal tissues and condition of cervix can be visualized.
2. *Cytology smear* (cervical smear, Papanicolaou, or Pap) is best made by scraping cervix directly (see Figure 10.1).
3. *Bimanual examination* – by inserting one or two gloved fingers of the left hand in the vagina and palpating the abdomen with the right hand, it is possible to further examine the uterus.
4. *Rectal examination* – to detect abnormalities of contour, motility and placement of adjacent structures and tissues.

Nursing intervention and support

1. Attend and support the patient by encouraging her to relax, by holding her hand, etc.
2. Focus the light and uncover examining tray with speculum, swabs, cytology necessities, etc.

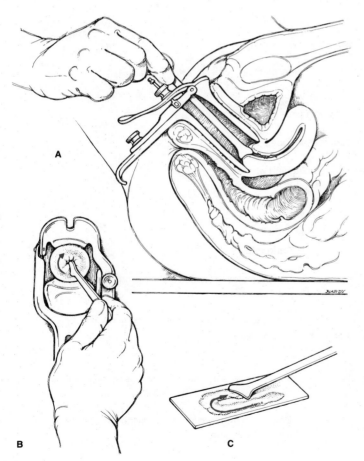

Figure 10.1. Cervical scrape of secretions for cytology is obtained by using a wooden Ayre spatula. (A) Speculum in place: the Ayre spatula is inserted so that the longer end is placed snugly in the os. (B) A representative sample of secretions is obtained by rotating the spatula. (C) Cervical secretions are smeared gently on a glass slide in a single circular motion. The slide is placed in the appropriate fixative. Using a cotton-tipped applicator, also obtain a smear from the floor of the vagina below the cervix, and preserve in the same manner

3. Assist doctor by providing gloves, lubricant, etc.
4. At conclusion of examination, wipe discharge from the patient before assisting her from the table.
5. Allow time for the older patient to adjust to sitting position before helping her off the table.
6. Answer any questions the patient may have; elaborate on doctor's instructions.
7. Assist the patient with dressing if necessary.

GUIDELINES: VAGINAL EXAMINATION BY THE NURSE

PURPOSES
1. Inspect the vaginal canal and cervix.
2. Obtain tissue specimen for cervical cytology and other tests.

EQUIPMENT
Perineal drape
Vaginal specula
Water-soluble lubricant
Sterile gloves
Long swab sticks
Cervical smear equipment
Adequate lighting

PROCEDURE

Preparatory phase

1. Have the patient void urine before assistant positions her on examination couch.
2. Position the patient on couch (slip may be kept on, but other clothing from waist to knees is removed).
   a. Use semi-sitting position.
   b. Make the patient as comfortable as possible with a small pillow under her head.
   c. Drape the patient to permit minimal exposure (but adequate for examiner).
3. Encourage the patient to relax; tell her what you are doing and what she may feel.
4. Adjust light for maximum focus.

Performance phase

Nursing action	Rationale
1. Be gentle and take your time; don sterile gloves; lubricate fingers.	This promotes relaxation of the patient, making the procedure easier for both.
2. Observe external genitalia for apparent abnormalities, gently separate labia and continue visual inspection.	Note any evidence of irritation, infection or abnormalities.
3. To encourage relaxation in the patient, gently place the tip of one or two fingers into introitus.	Say to the patient, 'Tighten your muscles and squeeze my fingers – try hard – then relax.'
4. Identify cervix manually and depress the perineum downward with your fingers.	Downward pressure is away from the more sensitive anterior structures.

5. Gently insert warm speculum horizontally, passing it over your fingers and aiming it toward the cervix.

If it is preferred not to initially insert gloved fingers, the speculum is introduced vertically using a downward pressure; after entering the vestibule, the speculum is slowly rotated to the horizontal position.

6. Slowly open the speculum and lock into position. With slow manipulation, the speculum can be turned to permit visualization of the vaginal walls.

Walls normally are pink and moist. A pale white secretion may be noted.

7. Inspect the cervix, which should be pink. Normally, the os is a dent, unless the woman has had children, in which case a slit is noted.

If woman is taking an oral contraceptive, the cervix may be deep pink to red. A thread coming out of the cervix would suggest presence of an intrauterine device (IUD).

8. If a cervical smear is to be done, follow procedure in Figure 10.1.

9. When removing speculum, hold it open until cervix is cleared, then withdraw speculum, allowing it to close.

By the time speculum is completely withdrawn, it will be closed.

10. For palpation (bimanual examination), see p. 675.

Follow-up phase

Nursing action

Rationale

1. Gently wipe the perineal area with soft tissue or gauze, using firm strokes from the pubic area back to beyond the rectum.

This will remove secretions and liquid lubricant.

2. Instruct assistant in carefully helping the patient to remove feet from stirrups (if used).

Both feet must be removed at the same time to reduce strain.

3. Elevate the lower third of the examining table to receive legs. Keep the patient covered with a sheet.

This permits the patient to assume dorsal recumbent position.

4. Assist the patient in sliding toward head end of table; provide a wide-based stool for her to step on as she gets off table.

Do not rush the patient as she is getting off the table, since sudden shifting from recumbent to sitting position may cause a feeling of dizziness.

5. Assist the patient in dressing (closing zippers, etc) if necessary. Answer any queries she may have.

OTHER DIAGNOSTIC TESTS

CYTOLOGY TEST FOR CANCER (CERVICAL SMEAR)

Cervical cancer kills approximately 2,000 women each year in the UK and yet is preventable by regular screening. Screening for cervical cancer has been undertaken by GPs, family planning clinics and genitourinary clinics, but only recently has a national screening programme been proposed for all women. The aim of screening by cervical cytology is to detect cancer in its premalignant phase, which can occur several years before frank malignancy develops. Thus the importance of careful follow-up of positive smears.

Procedure
See Figure 10.1.
1. Examination and interpretation of cytological smear is done by the pathologist.
2. Classification of cytological findings (after cervical smear):
    Grade 1 – normal smear.
    Grade 2 – inflammatory smear.
    Grade 3 – dyskaryosis (abnormal nuclei demanding further investigation).
    Grade 4 – a few malignant cells.
    Grade 5 – large numbers of malignant cells; frank malignancy.
3. If a patient has an abnormal smear, explain to her that this is not conclusive but requires additional investigation such as cone biopsy of the cervix and curettage.
4. The League of Nations classification of *clinical* stages of cancer of the cervix was devised so that results of treatment from different centres all over the world might be compared, as follows:
    Stage 0 – Intraepithelial carcinoma (carcinoma *in situ*). The growth remains within the epithelial layer.
    Stage 1 – Cancer clinically limited to the cervix.
    Stage 2 – The growth has spread to the vagina but only to the upper two-thirds or into the parametrium, but not to the pelvic wall.
    Stage 3 – The growth has spread to the lower one-third of the vagina or into the parametrium as far as the lateral pelvic wall.
    Stage 4 – The growth has metastasized beyond the pelvis or has involved the bladder or the rectum.
(**Note:** These are clinical classifications, and 20 per cent of Stage 1 cases are found at operation to have metastases in the lymph glands.)

CERVICAL BIOPSY AND CAUTERIZATION
Purpose
Remove cervical tissue for laboratory study.

Patient preparation
1. To be done preferably at a time when cervix is least vascular (usually a week after the end of the menstrual flow).
2. Explain the nature of the procedure to the patient.

3. Place the patient in lithotomy position and drape her properly.
4. Explain to the patient that no anaesthesia is required, since the cervix does not have pain receptors.

Procedure
1. After the speculum is positioned in the vagina and the cervix properly exposed, the surgeon, under colposcopic guidance, uses biopsy forceps to obtain fragments of cervical tissues.
2. Tissue is preserved in 10 per cent formalin, labelled and sent to the laboratory.
3. If bleeding occurs, suturing and packing may be necessary.

Aftercare of patient
1. A brief rest after the procedure is usually necessary before the patient leaves.
2. Discharge instructions/health education – instruct the patient as follows:
    a. Avoid heavy lifting for 24 hours.
    b. Packing will remain in place for 12 to 24 hours, depending on doctor's preference.
    c. There may be some bleeding; however, more than that of a normal period must be reported to the doctor.
    d. Obtain doctor's instructions regarding sexual relations.

UTEROTUBAL INSUFFLATION
Carbon dioxide is injected under pressure through a special cannula into the cervical canal. If one or both tubes are patent, the gas will pass through the uterine tubes into the peritoneal cavity.
1. The patient is prepared as for a vaginal examination.
2. A speculum is positioned in the vagina.
3. Special cannula is passed through intrauterine canal; cervix is held tightly with a tenaculum against a rubber stopper to prevent gas leakage.
4. Tubing is connected to a machine that measures and records pressure.

Findings
1. Normal – if pressure is below 180mmHg, and gas is heard (with a stethoscope) passing through the tubes.
2. Partial obstruction – 180–200mmHg.
3. Complete obstruction – 200mmHg and above.

CULDOSCOPY
A culdoscopy is an uncommon operative, diagnostic procedure in which an incision is made into the

posterior vaginal cul-de-sac so that a culdoscope can be inserted for the purpose of visualizing the uterus, tubes, broad ligaments, uterosacral ligaments, rectal wall, sigmoid and even the small intestines.

1. The patient is prepared as for any vaginal operation.
2. Anaesthesia may be local, general or regional.
3. The knee–chest position is best for a culdoscopy.
4. Following the examination, the scope is withdrawn and sutures placed; the patient is returned to her ward.

HYSTEROSCOPY

Hysteroscopy is the endoscopic visualization of the uterine cavity by means of a hysteroscope.

1. Earlier attempts were usually unsuccessful because uterine bleeding obscured the view.
2. Today, fibreoptic lighting and the distension of the uterine cavity with dextran solution permits optimal visualization.

Indications

Primarily to complement other diagnostic procedures, chiefly the staging of endometrial cancer.

1. Problem of infertility.
2. When the cause of uterine bleeding is unknown.
3. To view lesions that can be photographed and, in some instances, removed.
4. To diagnose and manage intrauterine adhesions.
5. For transuterine tubal sterilization.

Contraindications

1. Pelvic infection.
2. Recurrent upper genital tract infection.
3. Uterine perforation.
4. Pregnancy, because of possible disturbance of pregnancy and risk of infection.

Patient preparation and examination

1. Administer the prescribed sedative and mild tranquillizer prior to the examination. Explanation is similar to that for dilatation and curettage (D&C).

2. Place the patient in the lithotomy position as for a D&C.
3. Cleanse the perineum and vagina immediately prior to sterile draping.
4. The examiner performs a bimanual palpation of the uterus.
5. Inject local anaesthesia into the cervix, which is positioned with a tenaculum forceps.
6. Insert sounds into the cervical canal for dilatation prior to insertion of endoscope.
7. With endoscope in place, slowly infuse endometrial cavity with a concentrated solution of dextran.
8. Uterine walls are visualized with a 30 degree oblique lens rather than with the 180 degree system.

Follow-up

1. Following removal of instruments, the patient is encouraged to rest.
2. The patient may be discharged later the same day.

X-RAY STUDIES – HYSTEROSALPINGOGRAM

A hysterosalpingogram is an X-ray study of the uterus and uterine tubes following the injection of a contrast medium.

Purpose

1. Study sterility problems.
2. Determine extent of tubal patency.
3. Note the presence of pathology in the uterine cavity.

Procedure

1. The patient is placed in lithotomy position on a fluoroscopic X-ray table.
2. The bivalve speculum is introduced to expose cervix.
3. Contrast medium is injected into uterine cavity.
4. X-rays are taken to determine configuration of pelvic area.

GUIDELINES: COLPOSCOPY

Colposcopy is a stereoscopic examination of the cervix using a binocular instrument with strong light illumination.

PURPOSES

1. Determine distribution of abnormal squamous epithelium.
2. Pinpoint areas from which biopsy tissue can be taken.

INDICATIONS
1. Following atypical vaginal or cervical cytology (in cervical smear).
2. When suspicious cervical lesions are present.
3. Previous treatment for dysplasia or cancer of the cervix.
(*Advantage:* Colposcopy may spare the patient a conization or D&C.)

PROCEDURE
Preparatory phase
1. Identical to that for preparation of patient having pelvic examination (see p. 674).
2. Additional explanation may be required so that the patient will know what to expect.

Performance phase

Doctor's action	Rationale
1. Use a long cotton applicator stick to dry cervix.	This will clear away mucus and other secretions.
2. Swab cervix with saline, using long cotton applicator.	Moistening of cervical epithelium allows vascular patterns and squamous columnar junction to be visualized.
3. Examine tissue with colposcope, utilizing green filter illuminator.	
4. Paint cervix with 3 per cent acetic acid.	This acts as a mucolytic agent and accentuates epithelial topography.
5. Note colposcopic patterns – particularly the transformation area (where columnar epithelium is replaced by squamous epithelium).	Acetic acid tends to draw moisture from tissues of high nuclear density – this accounts for colour changes in the cervical epithelium.
6. Biopsy (using fine biopsy forceps) any questionable area; endocervical curettage should also be done.	Since the cervical os has few nerve endings, the patient will experience minimal discomfort.
7. If bleeding occurs, direct pressure or application of silver nitrate stick will usually stop it.	Measures to prevent or control bleeding.
8. Insert a vaginal tampon following examination.	To absorb discharge; may be removed after five to six hours.

Follow-up phase
Similar to that following pelvic examination, see p. 675.

DILATATION AND CURETTAGE (D&C)

Dilatation and curettage is a widening of the cervical canal with a dilator and the scraping of the uterine canal with a curette. The cervix is scraped first without dilatation.

Goals
1. Control abnormal uterine bleeding.

2. Secure endometrial and endocervical tissue for tissue study.
3. Serve as a therapeutic measure for incomplete abortion.

NURSING MANAGEMENT

Preoperative care

1. Inform the patient of the nature of the operation to be done (usually done by a gynaecologist).
2. Ascertain what the patient has been told about postoperative discomfort and drainage following the dilatation and curettage.
3. Answer questions the patient has about the procedure and aftercare.
4. Request the patient to void urine.

Postoperative care

1. Check that perineal pad is in place with a sanitary belt.
2. Replace each perineal pad with a sterile pad as required during the time packing is in place.
3. Report excessive bleeding.
4. Recommend bed rest for the remainder of the day, with bathroom privileges.
5. Offer mild analgesics for low back pain and pelvic discomfort.
6. Offer meals as desired.

CONDITIONS OF THE EXTERNAL GENITALIA AND VAGINA

PRURITUS (ITCHING) AND CONTACT DERMATITIS (VULVA)

ASSESSMENT

Nursing history and physical examination. Itching is often more acute at night; aggravated by warmth and scratching.

CAUSATIVE FACTORS

1. Faulty perineal hygiene followed by itching.
2. Itching causes scratching, which presents an open lesion subject to many irritants:
   a. Vaginal discharge, skin secretions, menstrual discharge.
   b. Urine, faeces.

3. Mechanical irritation:
   a. Close-fitting, synthetic fabrics.
4. Chemical irritation:
   a. Laundry detergent (washed clothing not completely rinsed).
   b. Vaginal sprays, deodorants, perfumes.
5. Chronic infections, such as:
   a. Trichomonas, gonorrhoea, monilia;
   b. Systemic – diabetes mellitus.
6. Allergy or sensitivity reactions.

PATIENT EDUCATION

1. Cleanliness must be scrupulous.
   a. Use cotton gauze squares that have been moistened in a warm, bland soap solution.
   b. Always wipe from front to back.
   c. Pat dry.
   d. Dust lightly with non-irritating powder (starch).
2. Do not use sprays, perfumed soaps or topical anaesthetic agents – they may compound the problem.
3. Replace synthetic-fabric undergarments with loose cotton underclothing.
4. Avoid wearing tight garments over the cotton undergarments.
5. Take medication if prescribed.
   a. Utilize cool compresses.
   b. Apply soothing lotions and ointments (hydrocortisone) if recommended.
6. Control allergies if this is a cause.
7. Control glycosuria and incontinence.

VULVITIS AND ABSCESS OF BARTHOLIN'S GLAND

Vulvitis is an inflammation of the vulva; the cause may be infection, possibly caused by uncleanliness. Common offending organisms are *Escherichia coli*, staphylococcus, streptococcus, gonococcus and *Trichomonas vaginalis*.

Inflammation of the Bartholin's glands by similar organisms also occurs. The ducts of the Bartholin's glands open on each side, just posterior to the vaginal orifice. A Bartholin's cyst may occur when the duct of the gland has become fibrosed from chronic or repeated infection or when it has been damaged by an episiotomy or perineal repair.

CLINICAL FEATURES

1. Burning pain, which is worse with intercourse.
2. Red and oedematous tissue with profuse purulent exudate.

3. Acute throbbing pain and swelling between labia, indicating vulvovaginal abscess (infection of Bartholin's glands).
4. When the acute infection subsides, the problem tends to become chronic.

TREATMENT AND NURSING INTERVENTIONS

1. Advise the patient to remain in bed; administer analgesics for the relief of pain.
2. Employ thermotherapy in the form of hot packs and baths for comfort.
3. Administer broad-spectrum antibacterial agents to combat infection, as prescribed.
4. Prepare the patient for incision and drainage of the abscess, which will afford immediate relief.
5. Marsupialization (creation of a pouch), with or without biopsy, is indicated when there are painful recurrences or obstruction at introitus.
   a. Ice packs are applied intermittently for 24 hours to reduce oedema and provide comfort.
   b. Thereafter, warm baths are comforting.

GUIDELINES: VAGINAL IRRIGATION

PURPOSES

1. Cleanse or disinfect the vagina and adjacent tissues.
2. Soothe inflamed tissue.

EQUIPMENT

Sterile reservoir for irrigating fluid – can or bag.
Sterile irrigating fluid as prescribed (1,000–4,000ml) at 40.5°–43.3°C
Tubing, connecting tubes, and clamp (sterile)
Irrigating vaginal nozzle (sterile)
Bedpan
Plastic sheet with cloth protection
Sterile cotton wool swabs, cleansing solution
Sterile disposable gloves

PROCEDURE

See Figure 10.2.

Preparatory phase

Nursing action	Rationale
1. Have the patient void urine before beginning irrigation.	A full bladder would prevent adequate distension of vagina by solution.
2. Place the patient in dorsal recumbent position.	To permit gravity to assist in allowing fluid to reach distal areas of vagina.
3. Drape the patient.	To prevent chilling and undue exposure.
4. Arrange irrigating receptacle at a level just above the patient's hips (not more than 0.66m above hips) so that fluid flows easily but gently.	The higher the fluid source, the greater the pressure.

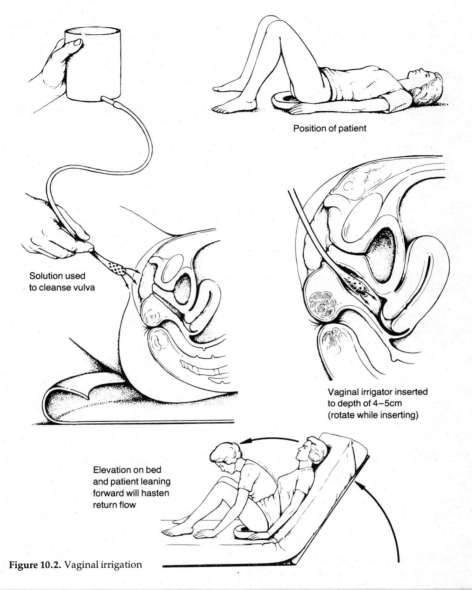

Position of patient

Solution used
to cleanse vulva

Vaginal irrigator inserted
to depth of 4–5cm
(rotate while inserting)

Elevation on bed
and patient leaning
forward will hasten
return flow

Figure 10.2. Vaginal irrigation

Performance phase

Nursing action	**Rationale**
1. Cleanse vulva by separating labia and allowing solution to flow over area; if insufficient, use cotton wool swabs saturated in soap solution, cleanse from front towards anal area.	Materials found around vaginal meatus may be introduced into vagina and cervix. This is to be avoided.
2. Allow some solution to flow through tubing and out over nozzle to lubricate it.	Moisture provides lubrication and less resistance when one surface is moved against another.

3. Insert nozzle gently into vagina in a downward and backward direction.

When the patient is in a dorsal recumbent position, the natural anatomical position of the vagina is in the downward-backward direction.

4. Rotate nozzle gently in the vagina during inflow.

All surfaces are irrigated when nozzle is rotated.

5. Clamp tubing when solution is almost all used, remove nozzle and permit the patient to sit on bedpan for return flow.

Gravity will assist in allowing return flow to drain from vagina tract.

Follow-up phase

Nursing action

Rationale

1. Wipe the patient dry, using cotton wool swabs in a front-to-back direction.

Drying the area prevents skin excoriation and promotes comfort.

2. Remove bedpan from the patient and apply sterile perineal pad.

3. Cleanse equipment with soap and water, dry before storing in well-ventilated area.

This will prolong life of equipment.

GUIDELINES: VULVAL IRRIGATION AND PERINEAL CARE

PURPOSE
Cleanse the perineal area after urination or a bowel movement in order to minimize infection.

EQUIPMENT
Sterile pitcher with irrigating fluid (300–500ml) 40.5°–43.3°C
Sterile sponge forceps (or sterile disposable gloves) and cotton gauze
Bedpan
Plastic sheet with cloth protection
Paper bag for cotton gauze disposal

PROCEDURE
See Figure 10.3.

Preparatory phase
1. Place patient in dorsal recumbent position with knees flexed and separated.
2. Place protecting sheet under patient.

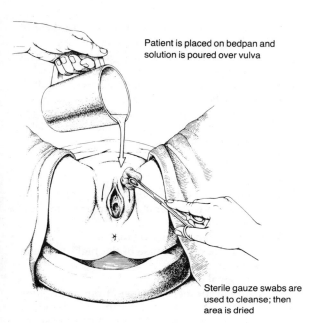

Patient is placed on bedpan and solution is poured over vulva

Sterile gauze swabs are used to cleanse; then area is dried

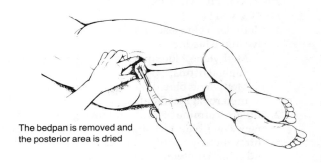

Figure 10.3. Perineal care

The bedpan is removed and the posterior area is dried

Performance phase

Nursing action

1. Pour warmed irrigating solution gently over vulva from a sterile pitcher.

2. Cleanse perineal area with cotton gauze held in a sponge holder or gloved hand, use a top-down direction and discard each sponge in a plastic or paper bag after one use.

3. Dry perineal area using dry cotton gauze in same fashion as for cleansing.

Rationale

Materials will be flushed from perineal area into bedpan.

Friction facilitates cleansing process and the removal of soil.

Cleansing from front to back assists in preventing intestinal organisms from entering vaginal area.

Follow-up phase

Nursing action

1. Apply sterile perineal pad.

Rationale

To maintain cleanliness and provide comfort for patient.

VAGINAL FISTULA

A fistula is an abnormal, tortuous opening between two internal hollow organs, or between an internal hollow organ and the exterior of the body.

Ureterovaginal fistula is an opening between the ureter and vagina.

Vesicovaginal fistula is an opening between the bladder and vagina.

Rectovaginal fistula is an opening between the rectum and vagina.

CAUSES

Vaginal fistula may result from:
1. Obstetric injury.
2. Pelvic surgery (hysterectomy or vaginal reconstructive procedures are most common).

3. Extension of carcinoma or a complication of treatment for carcinoma.

CLINICAL FEATURES
1. Patient with vesicovaginal fistula will experience continuous trickling of urine into vagina.
2. Patient with rectovaginal fistula will experience faecal incontinence and flatus passed through vagina, a distressing condition.

DIAGNOSTIC AIDS IN LOCATING FISTULA SITE
1. Methylene blue test – following instillation of this dye in the bladder:
   a. Methylene blue appears in vagina in vesicovaginal fistula.
   b. Methylene blue does not appear in vagina in ureterovaginal fistula.
2. Indigo carmine test – following a negative methylene blue test, indigo carmine is injected intravenously. If dye appears in vagina, this indicates a ureteral fistula.
3. Intravenous pyelogram – (see p. 590) a valuable test for determining presence of hydroureter or hydronephrosis, and position or location of the fistula.
4. Cystoscopy – performed to determine number and location of fistulae.

TREATMENT
1. In rare cases, a fistula will heal without surgical intervention.
2. Fistulae recognized at time of delivery should be corrected immediately.
3. Treatment of postoperative fistulae is delayed, sometimes for two or three months, to allow for treatment of inflammation.
4. Surgery is recommended if tissues are healthy.

NURSING INTERVENTIONS
Promotion of healing
1. Maintain cleanliness by encouraging frequent, soothing baths and deodorizing douches.
2. Obtain help from the incontinence adviser regarding the selection of appropriate aids.
3. Provide optimal skin care to prevent excoriation; bland creams or a light dusting of starch powder may be soothing.
4. Recognize value of meeting psychosocial needs, such as feminine morale boosters (attractive hairdo, nail polish, perfume, new bed jacket, etc); encourage visitors, diversion, recreation, activities, etc.

Preoperative
1. Maintain adequate nutrition; increase intake of vitamins and protein content of meals.
2. Promote local cleanliness by vaginal flushing and rectal enemas.
3. Administer chemotherapeutic agents to reduce pathogenic flora in intestine, as prescribed.
4. If the patient is postmenopausal, oral oestrogen may be given to promote healthier, more viable tissue in the operative area.

Postoperative
1. Rectovaginal fistula:
   a. Limit bowel activity by keeping patient on clear fluids for several days; progress to a low residue, then a full diet.
   b. Give warm perineal irrigations.
   c. Encourage rest because of the high degree of debilitation.
2. Vesicovaginal fistula:
   a. Maintain proper drainage from indwelling catheter – otherwise, pressure may build up and be exerted against newly sutured tissues.
   b. Employ gentleness in administering bladder or vaginal irrigations because of tenderness of the operative site.
   c. Pay particular attention to urinary output.

VAGINAL INFECTIONS

NORMAL VAGINAL CONDITION
1. The vaginal secretions are acid (pH 3.5–4.5); acidity is produced by the conversion of cellular glycogen to lactic acid by Döderlein's bacilli, which normally inhabit the vagina.
2. When oestrogen production is low (before menarche and after menopause) the epithelium is inactive; the cells contain no glycogen; lactobacilli (Döderlein's bacilli) are absent, and the pH is between 6 and 7.
3. *Leucorrhoea* is a whitish vaginal discharge; it is considered normal to have a slight discharge at the time of ovulation or just before menstruation.

KINDS OF VAGINITIS
See Table 10.2.

Assessment
HISTORY AND PHYSICAL EXAMINATION
1. Health history including questions specific to the condition:
   a. Nature of discharge: Cheese-like, frothy, pus-like, thick or thin, scant? When was it first

noticed? Character, colour, odour? Other symptoms: dysuria, itching, dyspareunia?

b. Menstrual history: Age at menarche, menopause; length of cycles, duration and amount of flow, dysmenorrhoea, amenorrhoea, dysfunctional bleeding?

c. Disease history: Presence of diabetes mellitus in patient or family? Other debilitating diseases? Control of these? Previous vaginal infections? Sexually transmitted diseases?

d. Pregnancy history?

e. Sexual history: Partner(s), how active sexually? Its nature? Urogenital infections in partner? Nature of contraceptives?

f. Medications being taken: Purpose?

g. Vaginal hygiene: Use of douches, deodorants, sprays, ointments; type of tampons, bubble bath, shower/bath, nature of clothing (tight-fitting)?

h. Concerns, stresses, anxieties, any questions?

2. Physical examination, including vaginal examination.

Table 10.2   Kinds of vaginitis

Description	Features	Treatment
Simple vaginitis		
An inflammation of the vagina, with discharge; this may be due to invading organisms, irritation, poor hygiene. Urethritis often accompanies vaginitis because of the proximity of the urethra to the vagina. Predisposing factors: *Trichomonas vaginalis, Candida* or *Monilia, Gardnerella vaginalis, Pediculosis pubis*, contact allergens, excessive perspiration, poor hygiene, foreign bodies (tampons, condoms, diaphragms that have been left in too long)	1. Increased vaginal discharge with itching, redness, burning and oedema. 2. Voiding and defaecation aggravate the above symptoms.	1. Enhance the natural vaginal flora by administering a weak acid douche, 15ml of vinegar to 1,000ml water. 2. Stimulate the growth of lactobacilli (Döderlein's bacilli) by administering beta-lactose vaginal suppository; this dissolves with body heat, and the sugar then acts. 3. Foster cleanliness by meticulous care after voiding urine and defaecation. 4. Control infection by initiating chemotherapy: insert medication into vagina via applicator or by using a chemotherapeutic cream locally as prescribed.
Gardnerella vaginitis		
An inflammation of the vagina heretofore referred to as 'nonspecific vaginitis', since it is not caused by *Trichomonas, Candida* or gonorrhoea. It is considered a sexually transmitted disease.	1. Vaginal discharge with odour. 2. Itching and burning may suggest concomitant organisms present. 3. It is benign in that when the discharge is wiped away, underlying tissue is healthy and pink. 4. Vaginal pH is between 5.0 and 5.5.	1. Metronidazole (Flagyl) taken three times daily for seven days. 2. Alcohol intake should be avoided during Flagyl treatment to avoid nausea and vertigo. 3. Treating partners with Flagyl is not recommended unless the condition is recurrent.
Trichomonas vaginalis		
A condition produced by a protozoan that infects the vagina and that is evident as a bubbly, greenish-yellow, irritating leucorrhoea and as red, speckled ('strawberry') punctate haemorrhages on the cervix.	1. Caused by a pear-shaped mobile flagellate that thrives in an alkaline medium. 2. *Trichomonas vaginalis* is persistent and resistant. 3. Vulvar oedema, dysuria and hyperaemia occur secondary to irritation of discharge. 4. Remissions may occur; the organism meanwhile remains inaccessible to treatment in the urinary tract. 5. The male may carry the organism in his urogenital tract and reinfect his partner.	1. Destroy infective protozoa by taking metronidazole (Flagyl) for 10 days (orally). *Note: Flagyl is contraindicated in the first trimester of pregnancy.* 2. Prevent reinfection by treating male concurrently with Flagyl.

Table 10.2   Continued

Description	Features	Treatment
Candida albicans A fungal infection caused by *Candida albicans*. Incidence – several factors have been found to be significantly associated with the incidence of *Candida albicans*: 1. Drug addiction. 2. Obesity. 3. Pregnancy. 4. Antibiotic therapy. 5. Diabetes mellitus. 6. Oral contraceptives. 7. Frequent douching. 8. Chronic debilitative diseases. Characteristics: 1. *Candida albicans* is a normal inhabitant of the intestinal tract and therefore a frequent contaminant of the vagina. 2. Since this fungus thrives in an environment rich in carbohydrates, it is seen commonly in patients with poorly controlled diabetes. 3. This infection is observed in patients who have been on antibiotic or steroid therapy for a while (reduces natural protective organisms in vagina).	1. Vaginal discharge is thick and irritating; white or yellow patchy, cheese-like particles adhere to vaginal walls. 2. Itching is common; dyspareunia, frequency and dysuria. 3. Appearance of vulva and vagina varies from normal to that of an acute inflammation.	1. Eradicate the fungus by applying miconazole nitrate (Gyno-Daktarin or Monistat) vaginal cream, one application daily at bedtime for seven days; and clotrimazole (Canestan) one applicator-full intravaginally nightly for one week. 2. Treat the symptomatic or uncircumcised partner by applying antifungal cream under the foreskin nightly for 7 nights.
Atrophic (postmenopausal) vaginitis This is a common postmenopausal occurrence. Because of atrophy of vaginal mucosa, the woman is prone to postmenopausal dyspareunia (painful intercourse due to a tight vagina).	Vesicovaginal itching, burning, dyspareunia, and vulvar irritation. **NURSING ALERT** *In the postmenopausal woman, if vaginal bleeding occurs, encourage the patient to see her doctor immediately, because cancer may be suspected.*	Since this is a manifestation of general body oestrogenic depletion, the patient should be treated with oral, water-soluble, natural, conjugated oestrogen (Premarin). The condition reverses itself under treatment, which must be maintained. If infection is also present, this is treated. Oestrogenic or cortisone vaginal cream may be prescribed.

DIAGNOSTIC TESTS

1. Laboratory tests, including wet smear for microscopic examination:
   a. Saline slide – discharge mixed with saline; useful in detecting *Gardnerella* and *Trichomonas*.
   b. Potassium hydroxide (KOH) – discharge mixed with 10 per cent KOH; useful in detecting *C. albicans*. If fishy odour is noted, suspect *Gardnerella*.
2. Culture – significant when purulent discharge is present; used to detect gonorrhoea.
3. Vaginal pH:
   a. Normal pH – 4.0–4.5;
   b. *Gardnerella* – 5.0–5.5;
   c. *Trichomonas* – 5.5+.

4. Cervical smear.

PATIENT PROBLEMS
(For vaginal infections.)
1. Discomfort and pain related to abnormal discharge.
2. Irritation of vaginal mucous membrane and perineum related to infection and invasion of pathogenic organisms.
3. Lack of knowledge about adequate vaginal hygiene.
4. Fear related to possible acquisition of an 'incurable' sexually transmitted disease.
5. Potential for altered pH and growth of pathogens related to excess carbohydrate intake.
6. Sexual dysfunction related to discomfort and abnormal discharge.

Planning and implementation
NURSING INTERVENTIONS
Relief of pain and correction of abnormal discharge
1. Reduce local irritation and discomfort by applying prescribed medication to affected area as recommended.
2. Foster cleanliness by meticulous care after voiding urine and defaecation.
3. Initiate antibiotics as prescribed to control infectious organisms.

Treatment regimen for abnormal vaginal condition
1. Explain why the perineal area must be clean before applying prescribed ointments, etc.
2. Demonstrate how medication is applied locally, depending on its nature (ointment, suppository or tubeful of vaginal cream).
3. Stress the importance of following the recommended interval for taking medication.
4. Emphasize the importance of keeping follow-up appointments.

Practice of proper hygienic vaginal care
1. Encourage correct procedure of wiping from front to back following urination and/or defaecation.
2. Suggest a daily shower rather than bathing, since the latter may cause reinfection of the genital area.
3. Discuss the problem of irritation of tissues that results when tight-fitting garments are worn.
4. Explain the importance of changing sanitary pads and tampons frequently.

Coping abilities to overcome fear of 'incurable illness'
1. Discuss the nature of the infecting organisms and

its preference for the 'warm, dark, undisturbed' cavity (vagina).
2. Explain the effect of prescribed local or systemic medication on the offending organism.

Modification of dietary intake of carbohydrates
1. Explain the effect of a high-carbohydrate diet on maintaining an optimal pH in the vaginal vault to prevent growth of undesirable organisms.
2. Describe what foods (that the patient enjoys) should be eliminated.
3. Suggest alternate kinds of equally satisfying goods.

Promotion of satisfactory sexual relations with partner
1. Recommend that the partner be checked medically if he has a discharge or other symptoms suggestive of an infection.
2. Discuss interim sexual habits that can be enjoyed without intercourse.

PATIENT EDUCATION
1. Avoid irritating douches, bubble bath and deodorant sprays.
2. Following urination and defaecation, wipe from front to back.
3. Wear comfortable fitting undergarments; white cotton is safer than other fabrics during the treatment period.
4. Avoid intercourse during active infection of vagina.
5. Encourage partner to seek treatment if he has a discharge or infection.
6. Vaginal infections increase with multiple sex partners.
7. Recommend partner wear a condom if intercourse is resumed before treatment is completed.

Evaluation
EXPECTED OUTCOMES
1. Patient enjoys relief of pain and absence of abnormal discharge.
2. Patient accepts treatment regimen and can describe what is to be done if there is a recurrence of the problem.
3. Patient recites the proper practice for maintaining adequate vaginal hygiene.
4. Patient demonstrates lessening of fear; can discuss difference between malignancy and vaginal infection.
5. Patient prepares a dietary plan to show how carbohydrate intake is reduced.
6. Patient indicates to what extent sexual relations may be resumed.

HERPES VIRUS TYPE 2 INFECTION (HERPES GENITALIS, HERPES SIMPLEX VIRUS [HSV])

Herpes genitalis is a viral infection that causes herpetic lesions on the cervix, vagina and external genitalia; it is primarily acquired by sexual transmission.
1. In 1982, 14,836 cases of genital herpes were seen in genitourinary departments in the UK.
2. It is the sixth most common disease seen in sexually transmitted disease clinics.
3. American figures far exceed those in the UK.

HEALTH IMPLICATIONS
1. Babies delivered vaginally may become infected with the virus; there is significant fetal morbidity and mortality. In early pregnancy, there is increased incidence of spontaneous abortion.
2. Incidence of cervical cancer is higher in women who have had genital herpes.

Assessment
HISTORY, NURSING AND MEDICAL
1. A sexual history is taken to reveal frequency and types of sexual activity and kinds of discomforts noted.
2. Urogenital history to suggest nature of problems – pruritus, burning, tenderness, urinary symptoms and unusual discharge.
3. Psychosocial concerns – stigmas, fears, misinformation.

CLINICAL FEATURES
1. Herpes genitalis is manifested within three to seven days and is most prevalent in young adults.
2. Multiple vesicles appear on the vulva; surrounding area is inflamed and oedematous.
3. Itching may be intense and even painful; scratching may further aggravate the problem.
4. Lesions appear on the vulva, and in most patients, the cervix is also involved; it, too, may be inflamed and oedematous, and bleeds easily when touched. Lesions may develop into painful ulcers.
5. A profuse watery discharge may be present.
6. Fever, malaise and headache may accompany the acute flare-up.
7. A sensation of burning may develop along with dysuria.
8. Within one to four weeks, the sores disappear; however, the virus remains in the body, and recurrences are common with leucorrhoea, abnormal bleeding, vaginal pain and dyspareunia.

DIAGNOSTIC EVALUATION
1. Usually can be made by inspection.
2. To determine true causative agent, cell cultures are taken; one to three days required for results.
3. Cervical smear – if herpes infection is present, multinucleated giant cells are noted.
4. Tzanck smear:
   a. Scrapings from base of a vesicle are obtained.
   b. If herpetic, multinucleated giant cells containing viral inclusion bodies are noted.
   c. **Note**: Other herpetic disease such as 'shingles' or chickenpox will also yield positive findings.
5. Immunofluorescence.

PATIENT PROBLEMS
1. Pain and discomfort related to herpetic lesions/ulcers of the genitalia.
2. Distorted self-image related to the 'stigma' of having genital herpes, and possibly a feeling of being betrayed by the partner.
3. Sexual dysfunction and social isolation related to the effects of a sexually transmitted condition, including guilt and embarrassment.
4. Lesions and ulcer of the genitalia.
5. Lack of knowledge of the nature of genital herpes.
6. Urinary retention in severe cases.

Planning and implementation
TREATMENT
1. Acyclovir (Zovirax) ointment reduces pain and shortens time the herpetic patient can infect others.
2. Oral acyclovir (investigational) given in capsule form interferes with the reproductive process of the virus, thereby reducing recurrences. Recommended for those who have had repeated recurrences.
3. Support and understanding are part of the therapeutic regimen.

NURSING INTERVENTIONS
Healing of genital tissue with relief of pain and discomfort
1. Recommend that the patient take the prescribed analgesics and apply the proper topical medications.
2. Take baths three times a day to increase blood supply to the genital area and facilitate tissue healing.
3. Keep genital area dry; remind the patient to wear fresh, clean, loose-fitting undergarments daily.
4. Apply acyclovir ointment as prescribed.
5. Take drying agents and antibiotics if prescribed.
6. Avoid sexual relations during healing process.

Coping strategies and psychological support

1. Encourage the patient to verbalize whatever psychological disturbance she is experiencing.
2. Ensure the patient of the confidentiality of information.
3. Suggest that the patient join a support group such as The Herpes Association, c/o Spare Rib Ltd, 27 Clerkenwell Close, London EC1.
4. Reiterate that when she is feeling better physically, her feelings about self and others will improve.
5. Advise the patient to tell new partner that she has been/is a victim of herpes.
   a. During active stages of disease, suggest sexual abstinence.
   b. Consider developing noncoital aspects of sexual relationship.
   c. When symptom-free, recommend use of lambskin condom for male.

PATIENT EDUCATION

1. Provide information about the management of the infection; sexual activity should be avoided until the infection is cleared; recognize that this person is a potential transmitter of the disease.
2. Encourage the patient to describe the nature of the condition and what can be done to avoid/treat it.
3. Assist the patient in recognizing precipitating factors.
4. Review the necessary hygienic measures that discourage infection.
   a. Health-spa bathers can place clean, dry towels on seats to avoid inadvertently picking up herpes virus.
   b. Towel sharing should be avoided.

Evaluation

EXPECTED OUTCOMES

1. Patient is pain-free with an absence of discomfort and no draining lesions.
2. Patient is at ease while verbalizing the impact such a disease can have on one emotionally and mentally.
3. Patient demonstrates clean, healed, normal genital tissue; reports no burning sensation on urination and no unusual vaginal discharge.
4. Patient describes a new lifestyle that is optimistic, wholesome, and knowledgeable with regard to sexual encounters with partner(s).
5. Patient recalls essential information about the nature of herpes genitalis and lists adequate health measures to manage any future situation.

ACQUIRED IMMUNODEFICIENCY SYNDROME (AIDS)

See section in Chapter 17 on Communicable Diseases (p. 1011).

TOXIC SHOCK SYNDROME (TSS)

Toxic shock syndrome (TSS) is a condition caused by a bacterial toxic (*Staphylococcus aureus*) in the bloodstream; it can be life-threatening. This condition, first identified in 1975, came to public attention in 1980 because of increased incidence.

1. Over 90 per cent of patients are women under 30 years of age.
2. The disorder is almost always associated with menstruation; women using high-absorbency tampons are at greatest risk.
3. Research studies suggest that magnesium-absorbing fibres in tampons may account for lower levels of magnesium in the body; this contributes to providing an ideal condition for toxin production by the bacteria.
4. TSS has been observed in nonmenstruating individuals with conditions such as cellulitis, surgical wound infection, vaginal infections and subcutaneous abscesses.

CLINICAL FEATURES

1. Sudden onset of high fever >39°C.
2. Vomiting and profuse, watery diarrhoea.
3. Rapid progression to hypotension and shock within 72 hours of onset.
4. Mucous membrane hyperaemia.
5. Sometimes, sore throat, headache and myalgia are experienced.
6. Rash (similar to sunburn) that develops one to two weeks after onset of illness and is followed by desquamation, particularly of the palms and soles.

DIAGNOSTIC EVALUATION

1. Determine whether the female patient has used tampons recently.
2. Doctor will take blood and urine samples and throat cultures, and where appropriate, cerebrospinal fluid, vaginal and/or cervical specimens.
3. Blood and urine studies will be undertaken.
4. Rule out other illnesses – sepsis, etc.
5. Determine whether there is a history of recent skin infection.

TREATMENT AND NURSING INTERVENTIONS

1. Fluid replacement is instituted to replace fluid and electrolyte deficits.
2. Medications to raise the blood pressure are given, as prescribed.
3. Because of the need to administer large fluid volumes, oedema becomes a problem, and even respiratory distress syndrome may result. This can be managed with endotracheal intubation and continuous positive airway pressure.
4. Administer antibiotics to control infection, as prescribed.
   a. Patients at risk but having only mild symptoms – cloxacillin (Orben), cephalexin (Keflex).
   b. These are given for 10 days to two weeks.
   c. For severely ill – anti-staphylococci methicillin (Celbenin).
5. The use of antibiotics, switching to sanitary towels and avoidance of using tampons for the next three menstrual cycles will reduce recurrence significantly.
6. The use of steroid therapy is still controversial.
7. After a bout of toxic shock syndrome, recommend close follow-up with pelvic examination and repeat cultures.

PATIENT EDUCATION

1. Until more definitive research provides answers to this puzzling problem, women are advised to:
   a. Alternate use of pads with tampons.
   b. Be alert to the symptoms of toxic shock syndrome.
   c. Change tampons frequently and not wear one longer than eight hours; four hours is maximum for heavy discharge times.
   d. Be careful of vaginal abrasions that can be caused by some applicators.
   e. Avoid using super-absorbent tampons.
2. Since the risk is low (1/1,000 over age 30, 4/1,000 under age 30), it seems unwarranted to recommend that the use of tampons be discontinued.

CANCER OF THE VULVA

INCIDENCE

1. Most common in elderly women; cancer of the vulva represents 3–4 per cent of all malignancies of the female reproductive system.
2. Women seem reluctant to seek medical attention in early phases when ulcer is small and on the skin surface; they tend to delay until the ulcer becomes infected and painful.

Assessment
CLINICAL FEATURES

1. In orderly progression, symptoms are severe vulvar pruritus, reddened, pigmented, whitish or slightly elevated lesions with ulceration.
2. Frequent site:
   a. Labia majora – mid or anterior portion.
   b. Clitoris.
   c. Encroachment upon urethra in larger lesions.
3. Less frequent sites – fourchette and posterior labial areas.
4. As disease progresses, tissues become oedematous, and lymphadenopathy is apparent.
5. Secondary infection is responsible for foul-smelling discharge.

DIAGNOSTIC EVALUATION

1. A biopsy is taken after procaine is injected. The entire lesion, when it is small, may be excised; but final treatment is reserved until laboratory studies are completed.
2. Superficial lymph nodes on both sides are palpated for metastasis.
3. Pelvic examination is necessary to determine the extent of the cancer (clinical stage) and to rule out other pelvic neoplastic disease.

PREOPERATIVE PREPARATION
Physical preparation

1. Shave or prepare a wide area to include perineal, pubic and inguinal areas.
2. Cleanse vulva thoroughly two or three days prior to surgery by using baths twice daily.
3. Evacuate the intestinal tract before surgery to provide the advantage of no bowel movements for two to three days postoperatively.
4. Adhere to protocol for preoperative care as described on p. 45.

Psychosocial support

1. Have the patient describe what her understanding is regarding her problem.
2. Emphasize the positive outcomes of the prescribed treatment plan; reinforce what the surgeon has discussed with her.
3. Answer her questions tactfully; utilize available resources for those questions about which assistance is needed.
4. Encourage her to talk about her concerns regarding fear of mutilation and loss of sexual function.

POSTOPERATIVE PATIENT PROBLEMS

1. Pain and discomfort related to nature of the surgery.

2. Potential postoperative complications – infection, abdominal distension, bowel and bladder problems.
3. Inadequate coping, poor self-image, related to fear of effects of surgery on sexual functioning.

Planning and implementation
TREATMENT
This depends on type and extent of malignancy:
1. Basal cell carcinoma requires superficial hemivulvectomy.
2. Carcinoma *in situ* (noninvasive carcinoma) is treated by simple vulvectomy.
3. Invasive carcinoma calls for a radical vulvectomy and bilateral lymph node resection.
4. Early radical vulvectomy with complete node dissection is curative. If the lesion is large and treatment late, cures are unlikely.

NURSING INTERVENTIONS
1. Maintain proper drainage and compression of tissues, connect drains to suction.
2. Promote comfort; place patient in semi-recumbent position with knees slightly elevated with a pillow to lessen tension on sutures.
3. Minimize postoperative complications; mobilize the patient on the day of surgery.
4. Prevent infection of wound and bladder, clean the wound daily with warm sterile solutions as prescribed (dilute hydrogen peroxide, saline, antibacterial solution) and follow with a warm water spray. Later, after the stitches are removed, a heat lamp to the vulva for five minutes twice a day may be required.
5. Facilitate wound healing; some surgeons prefer dry heat such as that provided by a heating lamp until the stitches are removed; this is followed by perineal packing or soaking.
6. Prevent straining on defaecation and wound contamination; offer a low-residue diet.
7. Prevent bladder infection, give meticulous care to the vagina and urethral orifice.
8. Promote tissue repair, baths of pHisoHex solution may be prescribed after the tenth day.
9. Encourage social adjustment, maintain a relationship conducive to allowing the patient to voice her concerns.

Evaluation
EXPECTED OUTCOMES
1. Patient is free of discomfort following surgery.
2. Absence of complications.
3. Patient adjusts to altered physical status; discusses lifestyle changes.

4. Patient understands and can relate what to watch for regarding future problems:
   a. Possible metastasis.
   b. Adhesions.
   c. Other complications.

PROBLEMS RESULTING FROM RELAXED PELVIC MUSCLES

CYSTOCELE AND URETHROCELE

Cystocele is a downward displacement (protrusion) of the bladder into the vagina.

Urethrocele is a downward displacement of the urethra into the vagina. This condition is often referred to as a cysto-urethrocele. The downward displacement of the bladder neck is one of the major causes of genuine stress incontinence.

AETIOLOGY
1. Associated with obstetrical trauma to fascia, muscle and ligaments during childbirth (results in poor support).
2. Often becomes apparent years later, when genital atrophy associated with ageing occurs – usually starts around menopause.

CLINICAL FEATURES
No early symptoms.
1. Later, fatigue and pelvic pressure – 'like sitting on a ball'.
2. Urinary symptoms – urgency, frequency, incontinence.
3. Aggravated with vigorous activity such as coughing, sneezing – relieved by resting or lying down.

PREVENTION
Medical
1. Pelvic floor exercises are useful and may prove beneficial in some women.
   a. Conscious contraction of the pelvic floor or levator ani muscles.
   b. This can be done many times during the day, as one sits, stands or lies in bed.
2. Voluntarily stopping the flow of urine during micturition is a good exercise.
3. Oestrogen therapy after menopause may be of some effectiveness.

4. A vaginal pessary may be used temporarily. Prolonged use may lead to pressure necrosis and vaginal ulceration.

Surgical

Performed when cystocele is large and interferes with proper bladder functioning – anterior vaginal colporrhaphy. This is often combined with vaginal hysterectomy and posterior colpoperineorrhaphy.

RECTOCELE/ENTEROCELE

Rectocele is displacement (protrusion) of the rectum into the vagina. Enterocele is displacement of intestine into vagina.

AETIOLOGY

Similar to cystocele; however, posterior vaginal wall is weakened in a rectocele.

CLINICAL FEATURES

1. Disturbance of bowel function – constipation.
2. A 'bearing down' feeling – as though the 'pelvic organs were going to fall out'.
3. Difficulty in faecal evacuation; some patients state that 'they must put their fingers in the vagina to push the mass up' so that defaecation can take place.
4. Symptoms disappear in the recumbent position.
5. Incontinence of gas and faeces (in patients with a complete tear between rectum and vagina).

TREATMENT

Surgery is carried out only when rectocele becomes so large that faecal evacuation is impaired or difficult. Posterior colpoplasty (perineorrhaphy) – repair of posterior vaginal wall.

NURSING INTERVENTIONS

Preoperative care

1. Promote rest, particularly in a patient who has been working hard.
2. Suggest semi-recumbent position in bed to lessen oedema and congestion.
3. Recognize that this problem often occurs in older women.
4. Prepare intestinal tract by administering an aperient and enema.

Postoperative care

1. Encourage voiding of urine every four to eight hours to reduce pressure so that no more than 150ml will accumulate in bladder – catheterization or use of an indwelling catheter may be required.
2. Administer perineal care to the patient after each voiding of urine and defaecation.
3. Employ a heat lamp to help dry the incision line and enhance the healing process.
4. Utilize available sprays for anaesthetic and antiseptic effects.
5. Apply an ice pack locally to relieve congestion and discomfort.
6. Administer analgesics as prescribed for relief of pain.

MALPOSITION OF THE UTERUS

When the uterus is in a normal position, the cervix lies in the axis of the vagina with the corpus inclined forward on the bladder. Twenty-five per cent of women have, to some degree, the reverse position (retroversion).

RETROVERSION AND RETROFLEXION

In retroversion, the cervix remains in the normal axis, but body is directed to hollow of the sacrum.

In retroflexion, angulation of the corpus on the cervix is extreme.

Clinical features

1. There may be none.
2. With significant uterine displacement, e.g. due to some underlying pathology, pelvic pain, backache, menstrual aberration, possibly infertility.

Treatment

1. A pessary may be required to temporarily treat symptoms.
2. Uterine suspension may be done as part of a surgical procedure.

PROLAPSE AND PROCIDENTIA

Uterine prolapse is a herniation of the uterus through the pelvic floor with a resultant protrusion into the vagina (prolapse) and at times even beyond the introitus (procidentia).

Prolapse

1. First degree – cervix, without straining or traction, is at the introitus (spread the labia and it is visible).
2. Second degree – the cervix extends over the perineum.
3. Third degree – the entire uterus (or most of it) protrudes.

Procidentia

The uterus, vaginal vault, rectum and bladder (and in some cases the posterior fornix) protrude.

Factors aggravating the condition

1. Obstetrical trauma.
2. Overstretching of the musculofascial supports.
3. Standing, straining, coughing, lifting a heavy object.

Treatment

1. A vaginal pessary may be used temporarily or for palliation.
2. Surgical correction is recommended treatment. This usually is a vaginal hysterectomy – combined with anterior and posterior repair.

TUMOURS OF THE UTERUS

INCIDENCE AND THE IMPORTANCE OF PATIENT EDUCATION

1. In the UK, malignant tumours of the uterus are the second commonest tumour in women and are responsible for about 3,000 deaths in women in England and Wales every year.
2. The death rate for uterine cancer has been showing some decline; this is attributed to the unremitting education of women, which stresses the importance of annual check-ups, including the cervical smear.
3. Nurses need to seek out the reasons why millions of women have not had cervical smears – lack of information, no transportation, inconvenient schedules of clinics, fear of results and general lack of motivation.

CANCER OF THE CERVIX

AETIOLOGY

1. It is most common between the ages of 45 and 55, but it can occur at any age.
2. Early cancer of the cervix is usually asymptomatic; it is almost always curable in its pre-invasive stage.
3. Early sexual activity and multiple sexual partners appear to be related to the incidence of this cancer.
4. Viral and chronic infections, as well as erosions of the cervix, appear to be significant in the development of cancer.
5. Incidence of cancer of the cervix is higher in groups with low socioeconomic status; occurs more often in black women than in white.
6. In developing countries, cancer of the cervix is the most frequent malignancy among females.

CLINICAL FEATURES

1. There are no symptoms of early cervical carcinoma.
2. Initial symptoms of carcinoma of the cervix:
   a. Post-traumatic bleeding (coitus);
   b. Irregular vaginal bleeding or spotting – between periods (metrorrhagia) or after the menopause; at first it may be very slight, but as disease progresses, bleeding becomes more constant;
   c. Leucorrhoea – increases in amount, becomes dark and foul-smelling because of necrosis and infection of tumour mass. This is a late feature.
3. With advanced cancer, there is excruciating pain in back and legs, relieved only by large doses of narcotics.
4. Later, extreme emaciation and anaemia; occasionally there is irregular fever due to secondary infection, peritonitis, and abscesses in ulcerating mass.

DIAGNOSTIC EVALUATION

1. Physical, including pelvic examination, plus a complete history are done initially.
2. Laboratory studies include cytology smear, routine blood examinations, plus fasting blood sugar to detect diabetes, total plasma proteins for nutritional status evaluation and bleeding and clotting times.
3. Colposcopy, biopsy (cone and punch) and proctosigmoidoscopic examination are essential diagnostic aids.
4. X-ray studies should include chest X-ray, intravenous pyelogram, barium enema, and bone scan.
5. Electrocardiogram.

TREATMENT

1. Hysterectomy (see p. 698) – depending on stage of lesion:
   a. Cervical amputation, wide conization, cryosurgery are alternatives to hysterectomy, but there is less assurance of complete removal of the lesion.
2. Invasive carcinoma:
   a. Treatment is individualized, depending on the

stage of the disease, age of the patient and general physical condition.

PATIENT EDUCATION AND FOLLOW-UP EMPHASIS

Regardless of the treatment, the nurse must emphasize the necessity of follow-up visits for this patient, since they will be required for the rest of her life:

1. To determine the patient's response to treatment.
2. To detect spread of cancer (metastasis);
3. To take regular cytological smears.
4. To maintain the best health possible.

NURSING CARE OF THE PATIENT RECEIVING RADIOTHERAPY OF THE UTERUS AND CERVIX

RADIOTHERAPY

See also p. 1039.

1. Caesium-137, radioactive cobalt is introduced into the cervical canal and vagina for a prescribed time, caesium is placed in tubes designed to filter out most alpha and beta rays while allowing gamma rays to penetrate into the tumour.
2. Such therapy may be supplemented by external beam radiation (supervoltage X-ray, cobalt-60 or linear accelerator sources) directed over the pelvis in an effort to eliminate cancer spread via lymphatic system; energy may be delivered via anterior or posterior portals over lower abdomen or back, or by means of rotational therapy permitting more uniform exposure of pelvis.
3. Therapy is individualized according to stage of disease and the patient's response to and tolerance of radiation.

PATIENT PREPARATION FOR CAESIUM IMPLANTATION

1. The doctor explains to the patient the reason why such therapy is advocated; nurse can amplify or answer any questions the patient may later raise. Insertions are often done prior to surgery.
2. Prepare the patient for various preliminary tests (may be done on an outpatient basis) – blood studies, biopsies (endometrial and cervical), chest X-ray, electrocardiogram.
3. Be available for questions and conversation with the patient regarding any phase of the preliminary studies or treatment.
4. Following admission to the hospital, prepare the patient for surgery and, in addition, prepare the intestinal tract by two glycerine suppositories and the vaginal tract by a cleansing douche (if directed).

CAESIUM APPLICATION

After-loading technique using an applicator.

1. In theatre, the central tube and ovoids are positioned (without caesium).
2. Upon recovery from anaesthesia, X-rays are taken in various positions in the X-ray department.
3. The radiotherapist then inserts caesium into pre-positioned apparatus.

NURSING MANAGEMENT

NURSING ALERT
It is imperative to keep the radiation applicator in the uterine canal and to prevent its changing position. Adjust all nursing measures to meet this.

While caesium is in place

1. Maintain the patient on a low-residue diet to prevent bowel movements, which might dislodge apparatus.
2. Inspect catheter frequently to ensure straight drainage – a distended bladder may cause severe radiation burns.
3. Observe for symptoms of radiation sickness – nausea, vomiting, elevated temperature.
4. Encourage the patient to eat by offering a variety of small rather than large servings and present meals attractively to offset poor appetite.
5. Offer citrus fruit juices because vitamin C is essential in tissue repair.
6. The patient must lie on her back; head of bed may be elevated 30 degrees.
7. Provide back care but spend a minimum amount of time at the bedside.
8. Relieve the patient of anxiety and fear by utilizing wisely the contact time with the patient – engage in profitable conversation about her interests and health problems.

Caesium removal

1. Notify radiotherapy department when it is time to remove caesium.
2. Provide sterile gloves, long forceps and a large waste basin.
3. Note on the chart the number of tubes applied so that this number is accounted for on removal.
4. Practise radium precautions in handling and returning caesium to the radiotherapy department.
5. A catheter specimen is taken prior to removal of catheter.

Post-irradiation patient care

1. Keep the patient's skin (exposed to radiation) dry; avoid use of soap since it irritates.

2. Apply a soothing, nonmedicated powder such as starch to relieve itching and discomfort.
3. For erythematous areas, apply a bland ointment (hydrocortisone) to relieve irritation.
4. Nausea or vomiting may occur with large doses of radiation.

NURSING ALERT

Do not tell the patient nausea and vomiting may occur since the power of suggestion may initiate these symptoms.

5. Observe for any symptoms that might suggest radiation reaction to the intestine – diarrhoea, tenesmus; report these if they occur.
6. Tell the patient the importance of regular follow-up visits to her doctor for the first six months – to assess effects of radiation on tumour.
   a. Cytological smears are taken; if positive, surgery may be indicated.
   b. If cytology smear is negative and tissue looks satisfactory, follow-up visits after six months may be further apart.

NURSING ALERT

Recognize that 5–8 per cent of women who are followed for the treatment of a particular cancer may develop other primary cancers. Therefore, such follow-up visits are essential even though the woman is symptomless.

CANCER OF THE CORPUS UTERI

INCIDENCE
1. Carcinoma of the body and carcinoma of the cervix of the uterus is accountable for 2,000 deaths per year and this has remained the same for the last five years.
2. Endometrial cancer is most common in women past 50 (peaks at age 60).
3. Seventy-five per cent of women with cancer of the corpus uteri are postmenopausal.
4. Often this malignancy occurs when the patient is also affected by obesity, hypertensive cardio-vascular disease and diabetes.
5. Prolonged oestrogen exposure is thought to increase the risk of cancer.

CLINICAL FEATURES
1. Postmenopausal bleeding is the commonest early sign.
2. Irregular bleeding may occur in menopausal women and this should be fully investigated.
3. Pain is not a symptom until the late stages.

4. Anaemia may result if there is considerable bleeding.

DIAGNOSTIC EVALUATION
1. Determine source of bleeding; even if it is coming from the cervical canal, it could be caused by a condition other than carcinoma. (If a tampon is inserted in the vagina overnight, the place where blood is noted on the dressing may offer a clue to bleeding source [i.e. near the string could suggest bladder source, but near the tip of the tampon would suggest cervix as source]).
2. Endometrial biopsy – positive test result indicates cancer, whereas a negative test result does not necessarily exclude carcinoma.
3. Dilatation and curettage is the most effective and accurate diagnostic aid.

TREATMENT
1. Hysterectomy (p. 698) – depending on stage of lesion.
2. Radiotherapy (p. 696) – depending on stage of lesion.

MYOMA OF THE UTERUS

Myomas are benign tumours of the uterus (they are also called fibromyomas, 'fibroids' and leiomyomas).

INCIDENCE AND CHARACTERISTICS
1. Such tumours are uncommon before the age of 30.
2. Myomas rarely develop after menopause; tumours that developed earlier may regress slightly after menopause – but the significant ones do not disappear.
3. Incidence is higher in black women than in white.
4. These tumours tend to be of dense musculo-fibrous structure; they are encapsulated and tend to form small or large nodules.

CLINICAL FEATURES
1. Small myomas do not cause symptoms.
2. After myomas (or myomata) grow, the first indication of the presence of a tumour is a palpable mass.
3. Excessive or prolonged menstruation is usually the chief symptom (with little or no change in the menstrual interval); intermenstrual or post-menopausal bleeding may also occur.
4. Pain comes from pressure on adjacent organs. As myomas grow, there may be a sensation of weight – a heavy feeling.

5. Secondary symptoms may be a feeling of lassitude, general weakness, anaemia and lower abdominal discomfort.

DIAGNOSTIC MEASURES
1. These are done primarily to rule out cancer – cytology, dilatation and curettage, cervical biopsy.
2. Diagnosis is made by abdominal and bimanual palpation.

TREATMENT
1. If the patient is of childbearing age and desires children, treatment is conservative.
   a. If small tumour – myomectomy.
   b. If large tumour – hysterectomy.
   c. Ovaries are preserved.
2. For medical and nursing management, see next column.

HYSTERECTOMY

Hysterectomy is the surgical removal of the uterus.

POSSIBLE INDICATIONS
1. Malignant and nonmalignant growth on uterus, cervix and adnexa that should be removed.
2. Control of uterine bleeding and/or haemorrhage.
3. Severe (life-threatening) pelvic infection.
4. Correction of problems associated with pelvic floor relaxation – cystocele, rectocele.
5. Treatment of endometriosis when conservative measures have failed.
6. Irreparable rupture or perforation of uterus.

QUALIFYING CONSIDERATIONS
1. Woman's age.
2. Woman's desire to have children.
3. Possible effectiveness of alternative treatment.
4. Degree of dysfunction.
5. Woman's willingness to endure dysfunction in order to retain her uterus.

TYPES OF ABDOMINAL HYSTERECTOMY
(Approximately 70 per cent performed abdominally.)
1. *Subtotal hysterectomy* – corpus of uterus is removed, but cervical stump remains.
2. *Total hysterectomy* – entire uterus is removed, including cervix; tubes and ovaries remain.

3. *Total hysterectomy with bilateral salpingo-oophorectomy* – entire uterus, tubes and ovaries are removed.

VAGINAL HYSTERECTOMY
1. Repair of utero-vaginal prolapse (urinary stress incontinence, cystocele/rectocele) is more easily managed vaginally than abdominally.
2. High-risk patients, very obese patients or those unable to withstand prolonged anaesthesia.

Advantages
1. Less likelihood of paralytic ileus, postoperative pain and intestinal adhesions.
2. Less chance of pulmonary complications and thrombophlebitis.
3. Wound dehiscence possibility is less; shorter hospitalization.
4. No abdominal scar.

Disadvantages
1. More limited surgical field; inability to examine intrapelvic and intra-abdominal organs.
2. May be increased risk of bleeding and post-operative infection.
3. Contraindicated where pathology of uterus and adnexa suspected. Large fibroids cannot be removed in this way.

Assessment
POSTOPERATIVE PATIENT PROBLEMS
1. Potential bladder problems related to proximity of bladder to surgical site.
2. Pain and discomfort related to surgical procedure and abdominal distension.
3. Potential complications following surgery.
4. Fear and anxiety related to fear of cancer, loss of reproductive function and sexual concerns.

Planning and implementation
NURSING INTERVENTIONS
Resolution of bladder problems
1. Monitor and record intake and output; administer parenteral fluids as prescribed.
2. Insert an indwelling catheter, if prescribed, because oedema or nerve trauma may cause temporary bladder atony.
3. Remove catheter as soon as feasible (as directed).
4. Catheterize the patient if no catheter is in place and the patient has not voided urine after eight hours, or is uncomfortable.
5. Determine whether there is residual urine; catheterize the patient after each voiding; otherwise, bladder infection may develop.

Relief of pain, discomfort and abdominal distension

1. Fluids and food may be restricted until peristalsis has resumed.
2. Auscultate abdomen for bowel sounds to determine onset of peristalsis.
   a. Apply heat to the abdomen and insert a rectal tube to relieve abdominal flatus.
   b. Permit the patient to sit on edge of bed with feet supported and to get out of bed and walk.
   c. Serve additional fluids and soft diet as peristalsis returns.
3. A nasogastric tube may be inserted if necessary.

Prevention of complications

1. Assist the patient in turning every two hours and encourage her to take deep breaths.
2. Avoid upright position and pressure under the knees, which might cause stasis and pooling of the blood.
3. Assess dressings or vaginal pad for amount and nature of discharge.
4. Assess legs for positive Homans' sign (tenderness, pain in calf upon dorsiflexion of foot).
5. Observe legs for the presence of varicosities; promote circulation with special leg exercises.
6. Apply antiembolic stockings as a precautionary measure to promote peripheral circulation. These should be applied before the operation and worn throughout stay in hospital.
7. Attempt to counteract effects resulting from removal of a large tumour or unusual blood loss.
   a. Administer high-protein diet with iron supplement to combat anaemia.
   b. Recommend a girdle following removal of a large tumour to provide support for relaxed abdominal muscles.

Reduction in fear and anxiety

1. Patient may have deep-seated fears that cancer or a sexually transmitted disease may be discovered.
2. There may be a conflict between recommended medical treatment and her personal religious beliefs.
3. Concerns may be raised regarding the possibility that all phases of her reproductive process may be disturbed.
4. She may be disappointed, particularly if she never had children.
5. The patient may feel that she will no longer be able to fulfil her role and needs as a woman.
6. Depression and heightened emotional sensitivity to people and situations may have to be assessed.
7. The complexity of problems that are a mixture of physical, emotional and social factors needs to be considered by the nurse as she assists this patient.
8. Questions arise about how a hysterectomy will affect the patient's participation in sexual activities.
9. The relationship of this woman to her partner and family should be determined.

PATIENT EDUCATION/DISCHARGE PLANNING

1. A total hysterectomy produces a surgical menopause (if the ovaries were also removed).
2. Explain to the patient the importance of hormonal replacement (prescribed) if she has had a total hysterectomy with oophorectomy/salpingectomy. Routine replacement is controversial and is contraindicated if surgery is done for malignancy.
3. Advise her against sitting too long at one time, as in driving long distances, because of the possibility of pooling of blood in the pelvis and of thromboembolism.
4. Suggest that the patient delay driving a car until the third postoperative week, since even pressing the brake pedal may initiate slight discomfort in the lower abdomen.
5. Tell the patient to expect a 'tired feeling' for the first few days at home and, therefore, not to plan too many activities for the first week.
6. Assist her in planning a flexible schedule so that she will be able to perform most of her usual household activities within a month; within two months, she will feel her 'normal' self.
7. Stress that the patient should assume employment outside the home only when her doctor indicates; this will depend on the type of work, etc. Advice will usually be given on this at the follow-up, six weeks after surgery.
8. Tell the patient not to feel discouraged if at times during convalescence she experiences depression, feels like crying, and seems unusually nervous. This is common, but will not last.
9. Remind her to ask her doctor regarding resumption of various preferred physical activities; note that some of the most strenuous tasks are hanging clothes on a line and using the vacuum cleaner. These tasks should be delayed for several weeks. The patient should not lift heavy objects for at least six weeks. Advise about sitting down to do tasks like ironing, preparing vegetables etc.
10. Determine what the doctor has told the patient regarding resumption of intercourse; reinforce this and explain that too-enthusiastic genital sex may injure the incision site and produce bleed-

ing. In other words, she is to proceed carefully at first. Suggest coital position variation. Usually sexual relations, douching or use of tampons is discouraged for four to six weeks, unless otherwise specified by the doctor.

11. Showers are permitted, but bathing is deferred until the doctor indicates that tissues are sufficiently healed.

12. Emphasize the importance of keeping follow-up appointments. Temperature elevation over 37.8°C, heavy vaginal bleeding, drainage and foul odour of discharge are reportable. Seek advice from GP in the first instance.

13. Give advice regarding self-help groups, e.g. Hysterectomy Support Group, Ravendell, Warren Way, Lower Geswell, Wirral L60 9HO.

Evaluation
EXPECTED OUTCOMES
1. Patient reports no difficulties with urinary control or output.
2. Patient asserts that pain is gone; discomfort is lessening each day postoperatively.
3. Patient recognizes the signs that suggest possible complications; none noted.
4. Patient presents an optimistic outlook regarding general state of health, reproduction and sexual activity.

ENDOMETRIOSIS

Endometriosis is a disease characterized by displaced groups of cells (resembling the cells that line the uterus) growing aberrantly in the pelvic cavity outside of the uterus.

INCIDENCE
1. Frequency of occurrence is about 25–30 per cent in white women.
2. It is rarely encountered in black women.
3. Usually this condition becomes evident in the third or fourth decade of a woman's life.

CHARACTERISTICS
1. Pelvic endometriosis attacks many areas. Order of frequency is the ovary, ureterosacral ligaments, the cul-de-sac, ureterovesical peritoneum, cervix, umbilicus, laparotomy scars, hernial sacs and appendix.

2. Misplaced endometrium responds to ovarian hormonal stimulation and even depends on this for survival.
   a. When the uterus goes through the process of menstruation, this misplaced tissue also bleeds; because there is no outlet for accumulated blood, pain and adhesions result.
   b. At surgery, concealed bleeding is in evidence because lesions are brown or blue-black.
   c. Ovarian cysts in which such bleeding has occurred are referred to as 'chocolate cysts', but all such cysts are not indicative of endometriosis.

AETIOLOGY
1. Embryonic tissue remnants may cover pelvic peritoneum and ovaries and may differentiate as a result of hormonal stimulation.
2. Such tissue may be spread via lymphatic or venous channels.
3. Endometrial tissue, during surgery, may accidentally be transferred by way of instruments (uncommon).

CLINICAL FEATURES
1. Persistent infertility in an otherwise healthy, married woman.
2. Lower abdominal and pelvic pain or discomfort, rectal pain, increasing dyspareunia (painful intercourse) and abnormal uterine bleeding and haematuria.
3. Symptoms are more acute during menstruation and subside after menstruation.
4. When a cyst ruptures, symptoms mimic acute appendicitis or ruptured ectopic pregnancy – an acute abdomen is apparent.

DIAGNOSTIC EVALUATION
1. Manual rectal and pelvic examinations reveal fixed, tender nodular structures, ovarian abnormalities and the uterus fixed by restraining adhesions.
2. X-ray studies, such as barium enema, may demonstrate constrictions suggestive of endometriosis.
3. Laparoscopy is an effective diagnostic aid because tissue can be visualized.

TREATMENT
1. If the patient is pain-free and does not desire pregnancy, no treatment is prescribed.
2. For discomfort, analgesics/antiprostaglandin drugs are prescribed for dysmenorrhoea.
3. Endocrine therapy utilizing hormones to produce

pseudopregnancy (such as danazol [Danol]) may be prescribed. A combination-type oral contraceptive may be used – with the least amount of oestrogen necessary to suppress ovulation and the maximum amount of progestogen to induce a decidual reaction in the implants.

4. Surgical intervention may be required – laparoscopic surgery, laparotomy, laser surgery or more radical definitive surgery, such as hysterectomy, bilateral salpingo-oophorectomy.

NURSING INTERVENTIONS
Relief of discomfort
1. Administer hormonal therapy as prescribed – oestrogen–progestogen, 'pseudopregnancy'.
2. Explain to the patient why such medications as these are prescribed.
3. Prepare the patient for surgery when indicated; this is directed toward the resection of cysts and lysis of adhesions. Perhaps other, more involved, surgery may be indicated.
4. Describe why radical surgery may be necessary.
5. Tell the patient that menopause also improves or cures endometriosis; this is only of value to the older patient.

Psychosocial considerations
1. Include the patient in the treatment plans so that she knows why a particular method of treatment has been selected and how her role is a vital one in its success.
2. Encourage the patient to express her concerns; false ideas often emerge – such as, 'Perhaps I have endometriosis because I used tampons'.
3. Monitor the reaction of the patient to the various treatments prescribed.
4. Encourage the patient to continue the therapeutic drug programme even though she is beginning to feel little discomfort.
5. Give advice on self-help groups, e.g. Endometriosis Self-Help Group, 65 Holmdene Avenue, Herne Hill, London SE22 9LD.

OVARIAN CANCER

Ovarian cancer is high-risk cancer of the ovary.

INCIDENCE
Cancer of the ovary is the leading cause of death from gynaecological cancer; it is the third most frequent gynaecological cancer.

CLINICAL FEATURES
1. Earliest features – insidious and vague:
   a. Some abdominal discomfort.
   b. Indigestion.
   c. Flatulence.
   d. Slight anorexia.
2. These gastrointestinal symptoms may be due to an acid reaction of the peritoneal fluid in ovarian cancer.
3. Advanced cancer – abdominal swelling, pain and a mass in the abdomen.

DIAGNOSTIC EVALUATION
1. Because of the high-risk nature of ovarian cancer, it is important that every effort be made to diagnose the condition early.
2. The nurse should recognize those conditions in a woman that collectively place her in a high-risk category. Individuals at high risk include women who are:
   a. Infertile.
   b. Anovulatory.
   c. Nulliparous.
   d. Habitual aborters.
3. If only *one* of the above conditions is present, along with *three* of the following symptoms, the patient should be labelled as 'high risk'.
   a. Increasing premenstrual tension.
   b. Irregular menses.
   c. Menorrhagia with breast tenderness.
   d. An early menopause.
4. Six-monthly gynaecological examination and cervical cytology.
5. Investigate any ovarian enlargement by laparoscopy or laparotomy. This is particularly true of postmenopausal women whose ovaries should not be palpable.

TREATMENT
1. Surgical removal of diseased area – extensiveness depends on the malignancy.
2. Treatment may be oophorectomy, hysterectomy, bilateral salpingo-oophorectomy, omentectomy, appendectomy.
3. Treatment may be surgery first, radiotherapy and chemotherapy, and finally immunotherapy. The effectiveness of combination therapy is being studied.
4. Chemotherapy is usually used following surgery.

PELVIC INFECTION

All structures in the pelvic cavity can become infected (referred to as pelvic inflammatory disease). Two types can be roughly distinguished according to the site of the infection and its spread.

AETIOLOGY
Nongonococcal infections
Chlamydia trachomatis is a genital tract infection in women that is similar to gonorrhoea; the incidence is increasing.
1. This condition may occur with or without a gonorrhoeal infection.
2. It may be mild enough to be ignored or severe enough to cause symptoms. Mucopurulent cervical exudate with erythema, oedema and congestion; in addition, there may be friability (easily crumbled) of the cervix.

Gonococcal and mixed infection
1. Gonococcal infection originates in the urethra, cervix and/or rectum.
2. If reinfection does occur following proper treatment, the disease is self-limiting.
3. Most frequently, women are reinfected, and the secondary invaders (streptococcus, staphylococcus, *Escherichia coli*, etc.) take over. Accordingly, as a rule, what started as a self-limiting salpingitis becomes a chronic process. The disease is spread by way of the uterine canal into the tube and through the fimbria.
4. As a rule, the endometritis resulting from gonorrhoea is short-lived.
5. The largest group of infections are created by pelvic cellulitis (i.e. endometritis from a complication of pregnancy or an intrauterine device).
6. Here all the cervical and vaginal pathogens are offenders. They spread by way of the lymphatics and blood vessels.
7. Cellulitis tends to be unilateral, whereas gonorrhoea is a bilateral process.
8. Tuberculous endometritis – uncommon in the UK – is a likely cause of infertility.

RISK FACTORS
1. Higher occurrence in sexually active women; especially if they or their mates or partners have more than one sexual partner.
2. The use of an intrauterine contraceptive device (IUD).

Assessment
CLINICAL FEATURES
1. Abdominal pain, nausea and vomiting, temperature elevation, malaise.
2. Leucocytosis.
3. Malodorous, purulent vaginal discharge.

DIAGNOSTIC EVALUATION
1. Nursing history, pelvic and physical examination.
2. Culture of endocervix.
3. Laparoscopy.

PATIENT PROBLEMS
1. Pain and discomfort related to presence of pelvic infection.
2. Potential for spread of infection.
3. Potential for complications.

Planning and implementation
NURSING INTERVENTIONS
Control of discomfort and improvement in fluid and nutritional status
1. Provide prescribed analgesics to control abdominal discomfort.
2. Support patient nutritionally. Review principles of nutrition with patient.
3. Recognize the depressing nature of the disease and that the patient needs support and understanding, particularly when she has discomfort and vague symptoms.
4. Apply heat to the abdomen externally and warm douches vaginally as prescribed to improve circulation.

Control of infection
1. Administer appropriate antibiotics as prescribed:
   a. Nongonococcal (chlamydiae) – tetracycline regimen.
   b. Gonococcal – penicillin G, ampicillin, spectinomycin.
2. Place the patient in a semi-upright position to facilitate drainage.
3. Avoid use of tampons.
4. Instruct the patient to protect herself and others from reinfection by careful handwashing and proper hygienic measures.
5. Document the patient's progress. Record vital signs, patient responses (physical and mental) to therapy, and nature and amount of vaginal discharge.
6. Control spread of infection by the following safeguards:

a. Handle perineal pads with extreme precautions:
   (i) Use an instrument or gloves.
   (ii) Deposit pad in paper bag for proper disposal.
b. Wash hands carefully before and after patient contacts.
c. Disinfect utensils, bedpans, toilet seats and linen. Adopt procedure appropriate for specific organism.
7. Encourage use of barrier methods of contraception (condom, diaphragm with foam or jelly, birth control pills) after completion of treatment.

Prevention of complications from untreated or recurrent infection
1. Chronic pelvic discomfort; disease becomes rampant.
2. Sterility occurs because of closing of uterine tubes with scar tissue.
3. Ectopic pregnancy is possible if fertilized egg is unable to pass stricture.
4. Inflammatory masses may develop, eventually requiring removal of uterus, tubes and ovaries.

Evaluation
EXPECTED OUTCOMES
1. Absence of discomfort.
2. No evidence of infection.
3. Patient relates what signs and symptoms are reportable that may suggest the development of a complication(s).

FERTILITY CONTROL

BASIC PRINCIPLES
1. The nurse should be familiar with the application, advantages and disadvantages of the various methods of contraception available.
2. The most effective method is the one a woman selects for herself and will use consistently.
3. Women are entitled to contraceptive advice as part of good health care without the burden of moral judgement.

CONTRACEPTIVE METHODS
Note: Failure rate (pregnancy) is determined by the experience of 100 women for one year and is expressed as *pregnancies per 100 woman years*.

Periodic abstinence
Abstention from sexual intercourse during the fertile period of each cycle.
1. This depends on:
   a. Identification of fertile period – usually about 14 days before next menstrual period.
   b. Abstaining for about seven to 18 days.

Natural family planning
1. Cervical mucus method – abstain when mucus is present and also during menstruation.
2. Symptothermal method – based on rise in basal body temperature, as well as changes in cervical mucus.

Coitus interruptus
This is the withdrawal of the penis from the vagina when ejaculation is imminent.
1. Indications – effective when mechanical devices are unavailable.
2. Contraindications:
   a. When male is not able to exert self-control.
   b. Ineffective when premature ejaculation occurs – this is true of almost 50 per cent of males.
3. Undesirable effects:
   a. Failure rate is between 35 and 40 per cent.
   b. Psychological ill-effects for both male and female.
   c. Subsequent prostatitis has been substantiated.

Condom
Application of a rubber sheath worn over the penis by the male during coitus.
1. Procedure for use and precautions:
   a. Place condom over erect penis.
   b. Leave a dead space at the tip of the condom (from which air has been expelled) to allow room for ejaculate.
   c. Lubricate (spermicidal) exterior of condom – as an added precaution.
   d. Avoid leaving condom in vagina during withdrawal; this is facilitated by grasping ring around top of condom at time of withdrawal.
2. Advantages:
   a. Inexpensive and easy to use; available without a prescription.
   b. Protects against pregnancy and offers some protection against sexually transmitted diseases.
   c. May lessen premature ejaculation.
   d. Ensures male's involvement in the contraceptive process.
3. Disadvantages:
   a. May dull sensation somewhat for male and female.

b. Requires an erect penis for application.
c. Condom may tear or rupture and thus be ineffective.
d. May cause a contact dermatitis.
4. Failure rate (pregnancy): varies from 15 to 35 (various authorities) undesired pregnancies per 100 woman years.

Note: If condom ruptures, the female should see her gynaecologist immediately to obtain 'morning-after pill' (high oestrogen) for pregnancy interception.

Diaphragm

A rubber, dome-shaped device with a flexible wire rim, which is inserted in the vagina to fit snugly behind the pubic bone and over the cervix into the posterior fornix. It is used to prevent sperm from reaching the cervical os. Spermicidal jelly is often used on both sides of the diaphragm.
1. Indications – preferred by women who:
   a. Object to a device *in utero*.
   b. Object to hormonal or chemical contraceptives.
   c. Do not object to insertion of the diaphragm immediately prior to intercourse.
2. Procedure for insertion and follow-up:
   a. Bimanual pelvic examination and cytology smear are preliminary to measurement for a diaphragm.
   b. Measure depth of vagina; select largest diaphragm that can be retained comfortably; if too small, the device will be displaced during intercourse.
   c. Teach the patient how to insert diaphragm behind lower edge of pubic bone; use spermicidal jelly or cream for additional contraceptive action.
   d. Instruct her to retain diaphragm for six to eight hours after intercourse.
   e. Remind the patient of the need for follow-up appointment with GP or family planning clinic.
   f. Inform the patient that a larger diaphragm may be necessary after a pregnancy.
3. Failure rate (pregnancy): 15 undesired pregnancies per 100 woman years of using diaphragm.

Vaginal foam

This is a spermicidal cushioning foam that is available in cream, gel, aerosol or tablet form. All except the tablet are effective immediately – tablets require five to ten minutes to dissolve.

1. Advantages:
   a. Requires little instruction; a favourite method with lower socioeconomic groups.
   b. May be used to advantage with coitus interruptus.
2. Disadvantage: higher failure rate than other contraceptive methods.
3. Failure rate (pregnancy): between 35 and 45 per 100 woman years.

Intrauterine device (IUD)

The IUD is a device made of metal or plastic that fits inside the uterus; it may be in the shape of a spiral, loop, shield or ring.

NURSING ALERT
It is now apparent that the IUD may be more dangerous than anticipated. Endometritis, ovarian abscesses, ruptured uteri and their consequences have resulted in pelvic surgery.

1. Indications:
   a. When hormonal medications appear to be contraindicated.
   b. When motivation and other resources are lacking; as a last resort.
2. Contraindications:
   a. Inflammation or infection of cervix, uterus or uterine tubes.
   b. Objections on the part of the woman to a foreign device in her uterus.
   c. Severe dysmenorrhoea.
3. Advantages:
   a. Effectiveness listed as 97 to 99 per cent.
   b. Convenient; permits spontaneity of intercourse.
4. Disadvantages:
   a. Increased dysmenorrhoea and amount of menstrual flow.
   b. Some discomfort with insertion of IUD.
   c. Increased risk of pelvic inflammatory disease.
   d. In prolonged use (over three years without IUD having been removed) there is increasing risk of pelvic actinomycosis.
5. Procedure for insertion:
   a. Nursing history is obtained to determine contraceptive history and pertinent health information such as abnormal vaginal bleeding, pelvic infections, past surgery on reproductive organs, pregnancy history, nature of menses, presence of other diseases.

b. Client is counselled:
   (i) Pre-insertion:
       What you should know about the IUD.
       Use-effectiveness.
       What you should tell your doctor/clinic.
       Adverse reactions.
   (ii) Post-insertion:
       Description of the IUD.
       Directions for use.
       Side-effects.
       Warnings.
       Special warning about pregnancy with an
       IUD in place.
c. A pelvic examination and a cervical smear is
   done.
d. Calibre of interior of the uterus is determined
   by means of sounding.
e. Insertion of IUD with the aid of a plastic in-
   serter at time of menstruation is done by a
   doctor (or one specifically trained). Menstruation ensures dilatation of cervix and that the
   patient is not pregnant.
f. A nylon string attached to the IUD dangles
   from the cervix and can be detected during
   vaginal examination.

NURSING ALERT

If the patient is pregnant when an IUD is inserted, she
may suffer septic abortion and possibly fatal septi-
caemic shock; hence the wisdom of having the device
inserted during menstruation.

6. Patient education:
   a. Inform the patient how to check for IUD nylon
      string.
   b. Instruct the patient to avoid intercourse for
      five days (time to permit IUD to induce en-
      dometrial changes).
   c. Recommend follow-up visits as directed.
   d. Suggest that the patient promptly seek assist-
      ance if any of the following occurs:
        (i) Unusually heavy or prolonged bleeding.
       (ii) Bleeding between periods.
      (iii) Pain; unusual vaginal discharge.
       (iv) Infection signs – chills/fever.
        (v) Inability to locate string.
       (vi) Signs of pregnancy.
      (vii) Suspected or obvious expulsion of IUD.
     (viii) IUD sometimes 'migrates' into peri-
            toneal cavity.
   e. Provide the patient with a wallet card showing
      IUD insertion date, clinic and emergency tele-
      phone numbers.
   f. Suggest that the woman consult her doctor as

to how long her particular IUD can be worn
before being removed.

Hormonal control – the 'Pill'

1. Basis of operation of oral contraceptives: oral
   synthetic preparations of oestrogens and progesterone are used. It is believed that in the
   presence of sufficient amounts of these synthetic
   compounds, the hypothalamus fails to secrete the
   usual luteinizing hormone (LH) releasing factor
   and its stimulating product LH, which normally
   occurs about 12 to 14 days after the onset of
   the monthly menstrual cycle and is essential to
   ovulation.
2. Indications:
   a. For those who want a highly effective con-
      traceptive with no special preparation im-
      mediately before intercourse.
   b. For women who will conscientiously adhere to
      a daily plan of pill-taking.
3. Methods:
   a. Combined steroid therapy – a pill with an
      oestrogen and progestogen usually taken 20
      days during each month, beginning on the
      fifth day after the onset of menstruation.
   b. Microprogestational therapy – low dosage of
      progestational drug given continuously:
        (i) Androgens – 19-carbon compounds.
       (ii) Progesterone – 21-carbon compounds.
      (iii) Oestrogens – ethinyloestradiol.
4. Protective effects:
   a. Minimizes menstrual blood loss.
   b. Decreases dysmenorrhoea.
   c. Decreased incidence of first attacks of rheuma-
      toid arthritis.
   d. Lower incidence of pelvic infection.
   e. Appears to have protective effect against
      ovarian and endometrial cancer.
5. Risk factors and possible contraindications:

NURSING ALERT

Cigarette smoking increases risk of serious cardio-
vascular side-effects from oral contraceptives. Women
who use the Pill should be strongly advised not to
smoke.

   a. Women over 40 years of age.
   b. History of migraine, hypertension, epilepsy.
   c. Leiomyomas of the uterus.
   d. Past history of cardiovascular disease.
   e. Known or suspected breast carcinoma.
   f. Known or suspected oestrogen dependent
      neoplasia of uterus (endometrium or cervix).
   g. Liver disease or impaired liver function.

h. Known or suspected pregnancy.
i. Genital bleeding – undiagnosed.
j. Obesity, diabetes mellitus and hyper-cholesterolaemia.

6. Management:
   a. Monitored carefully with physical examin-ation and cervical smear at least annually.
   b. The lowest effective dose of oestrogen and progesterone (compatible with low failure rate and needs of individual patient) is used.

7. Disadvantages:
   a. Interference with laboratory diagnostic pro-cedures; sedimentation rate, thyroid test for protein-bound iodine or thyroxine, cervical smears, and biopsy.
   b. Oral contraceptive use may be associated with an increased risk of cervical carcinoma.

8. Side-effects: occur in approximately 1 to 3 per cent of women on low-dose pill.

9. Failure rate (pregnancy): combined – less than one pregnancy per 100 woman years.

Topical spermicide

Chemically active substance that incapacitates sper-matozoa; when used properly, it is estimated to be 95 per cent effective, and even when used improperly, it is considered about 85 per cent effective. Sponges are available made of disposable, polyurethane im-pregnated with a spermicide.

1. To use:
   a. Moisten sponge with water; fold between thumb and forefinger.
   b. Insert with concave side over the cervix.
   c. Upper walls of vagina hold sponge in place.
   d. A flat polyester ribbon serves as a 'handle' for removal.
   e. A spermicide kills sperm on contact; sponge blocks path of sperm and absorbs them.
   f. May be worn up to 30 hours; leave in place for six hours after intercourse, then discard.

2. Advantages:
   a. One size fits all; it is comfortable and easy to use.
   b. No prescription required.
   c. As effective as diaphragm.

3. Disadvantages:
   a. Some find it expensive.
   b. Others believe the effectiveness rate is too low.

Other contraceptives

Depo-Provera (injectable depot progesterone, med-roxyprogesterone) for long-acting contraception – investigational.

STERILIZATION PROCEDURES

Indications

1. The patient's desire:
   a. Socioeconomic reasons.
   b. Therapeutic reasons to prevent a pregnancy that might endanger the mother's life.

2. Legal considerations:
   a. Laws much less rigid than those governing therapeutic abortion.
   b. Written consent required from a legally re-sponsible and informed person.

3. Incidence and indications:
   a. Increasing numbers are performed annually.
   b. Done for multiparity, two or more previous caesarean sections, hypertensive cardio-vascular disease.
   c. Done for other reasons – vaginal plastic pro-cedures, for inheritable life-threatening disease.

Tubal sterilization

1. Types:
   a. Tubal ligation with or without resection.
   b. Tubal ligation with or without crushing.
   c. Tubal transection and burying of stumps.
   d. Cornual resection.
   e. Cornual occlusion utilizing cautery.

2. Approaches:
   a. Abdominal – if done during another surgical procedure.
   b. After a caesarean section.
   c. Virtually all sterilizations in the UK are done by laparoscopy.

3. Evaluation:
   a. There are advantages and disadvantages to each of the above – the individual situation must be considered.
   b. Reversible methods of tubal occlusion or semi-permanent sterilization using metal clips or chemical injections are still investigational.

4. Laparoscopy:
   a. A procedure in which coagulation and trans-section of the isthmic tubal segments are done through a laparoscope (an electrical current is passed for three to five seconds to cut and coagulate tube).
   b. The procedure is considered rapid, safe, and effective.
   c. Effectiveness – no adverse effects occur in sex relations, menstrual function or outward bodily appearance.
   d. Hazards:
      (i) Pulmonary embolism, haemorrhage, in-fection.

(ii) Tubal pregnancy.

(iii) Some women are disturbed emotionally by procedure; however, 90 per cent of patients who request this have no subsequent regret.

Vasectomy
See p. 666.

Abortion
See p. 708.

GYNAECOLOGICAL EMERGENCIES

These include:
1. Ectopic pregnancy.
2. Hydatidiform mole.
3. Abortion.
4. Rape.

Patients are usually admitted from the accident and emergency department or surgical outpatients

ECTOPIC PREGNANCY

This is an extrauterine pregnancy and the commonest site is in the fallopian tubes and therefore is often referred to as a tubal pregnancy.

INCIDENCE
This is variable, but occurs in approximately one in every 300 pregnancies in the UK.

AETIOLOGY
The ovum is usually fertilized in the fallopian tube and reaches the uterus in about five days. Anything which delays this passage will result in a tubal pregnancy, namely:
1. Salpingitis (destruction to tubal cilia or structure).
2. Tuberculous salpingitis.
3. Congenital malformation of fallopian tubes.
4. Endometriosis.
5. Contralateral implantation (ovum fertilized in one tube carried to the other).

The embryo cannot grow beyond a certain size in the tube. The trophoblast gradually erodes the tubal wall and blood vessels and bleeding eventually occurs. The pregnancy is terminated as follows by:

1. Absorption.
2. Tubal mole – embryo dies in the tube, some bleeding occurs and it is retained in the tube.
3. Pelvic haematocele – bleeding is more extensive and collects in the pelvic cavity.
4. Tubal rupture – the most dramatic and familiar presentation. The tube does not rupture but erosion of an artery occurs resulting in intraperitoneal haemorrhage.
5. Secondary abdominal pregnancy – the embryo is expelled completely into the peritoneal cavity. Occasionally the pregnancy does continue to full term.

Assessment
CLINICAL FEATURES
1. Amenorrhoea for about six weeks and early signs of pregnancy.
2. Pain – cramp-like and colicky in nature.
3. Bleeding – less than a normal period and dark brown in colour.
4. Abdominal tenderness over tubal point. Diagnosis is usually made on clinical findings.

PATIENT PROBLEMS/NURSING ASSESSMENT
1. The patient's condition may vary from mildly unwell to a deep state of shock, depending on blood loss and will need urgent surgery. Observe pulse, blood pressure, colour and evidence of air hunger.
2. The doctor will take blood for cross-matching.
3. The patient will be frightened due to the sudden onset of her condition and lack of knowledge regarding what has happened.
4. She will be disappointed at the outcome of her pregnancy.
5. Assess when she last ate and drank.

Planning and implementation
TREATMENT AND NURSING INTERVENTION
1. Give nothing by mouth and prepare the patient for the operating theatre.
2. Prepare equipment to give intravenous fluids and a blood transfusion.
3. Reassure the patient by a careful explanation regarding what has happened and the nature of the operation.
4. Contact husband/partner and explain situation as appropriate.
5. A laporotomy is performed and the affected tube is generally removed.
6. Postoperative care is as for any abdominal operation (see Chapter 3).

Evaluation

EXPECTED OUTCOMES

1. Pulse and blood pressure are within normal limits and vaginal loss minimal.
2. Patient understands that she has a higher-than-average risk of having another ectopic pregnancy.
3. Only the affected tube has been removed, therefore she is not infertile.
4. Husband/partner is supportive in understanding the disappointment over lost pregnancy.

HYDATIDIFORM MOLE (VESICULAR MOLE)

AETIOLOGY

This is a benign tumour of the chorionic villi. The villi degenerate and form a mole which varies in size. They are potentially malignant.

Assessment

CLINICAL FEATURES

1. Amenorrhoea followed by continuous or intermittent bleeding.
2. Early symptoms of pregnancy, e.g. breast changes and vomiting which may be severe.
3. Enlarged uterus – feels 'boggy' on palpation.
4. No fetal parts will be felt, and this confirmed on X-ray/scan.
5. Painful uterine contractions.
6. High gonadotrophin levels in blood or urine.

Planning and implementation

TREATMENT AND NURSING INTERVENTION

This depends on the patient's condition.

1. If the mole is being expelled by good uterine contractions, no intervention is needed. Ergometrine is given to minimize bleeding. Blood is taken for cross-matching in case of haemorrhage.
2. If poor uterine contraction, oxytocin may be used. After the mass is expelled, curettage is done at five days to ensure uterus is clear.
3. In the case of a woman who does not desire further children or in cases of intraperitoneal haemorrhage with perforating moles a hysterectomy is performed.

Evaluation

EXPECTED OUTCOME

1. The patient is aware of the reason for the follow-up tests – usually for two years.
2. The patient and her husband/partner have seen the doctor and have information regarding the possibility of malignancy.
3. They understand that another pregnancy should not be considered until they are told that it is safe (usually one year).
4. The contraceptive pill or an IUD must not be used.
5. The patient is aware that if malignancy does occur there is a high chance of cure with prompt, efficient treatment.

CHORIOCARCINOMA

1. Choriocarcinoma is rare, but can be a consequence of hydatidiform mole in 50 per cent of cases.
2. Histological examination following spontaneous delivery of a hydatidiform mole is recommended for early detection.
3. Choriocarcinoma spreads rapidly via the bloodstream, but use of cytotoxic drugs (e.g. methotrexate) have had good results.

ABORTION

Abortion is defined as the expulsion of the products of conception before the 28th week of pregnancy. Abortion is usually classified into:

1. Spontaneous (or a miscarriage).
2. Induced.

SPONTANEOUS ABORTION

AETIOLOGY

Approximately 15 per cent of pregnancies may terminate in spontaneous abortion and these may be due to fetal or maternal causes. Fetal causes are due to abnormalities in the developing embryo and is the highest cause of abortion; many have chromosomal abnormalities. It may also be due to defective implantation in the endometrium. Maternal causes include systemic disease, infection, disorders of the uterus, incompetent cervix or psychological stress.

CLINICAL MANIFESTATIONS

1. The patient presents with slight uterine bleeding signs of pregnancy, slight backache and there may be uterine contractions.
2. The cervix is closed.
3. At this stage the abortion is considered 'threatened'.

TREATMENT AND NURSING INTERVENTION

1. Bed rest in a quiet area of the ward until bleeding ceases.
2. Give sedation as prescribed, e.g. diazepam.
3. Ensure patient passes urine frequently and give mild aperient to prevent constipation.
4. Keep anything passed per vaginum for inspection to assess blood loss.
5. Give full explanation to patient and partner.
6. A pregnancy test should be done before discharge.
   If this treatment does not succeed then the abortion becomes 'inevitable' and may be complete or incomplete.

INEVITABLE ABORTION

CLINICAL MANIFESTATIONS

1. Bright red blood loss from the vagina, which becomes heavy.
2. Pain in the abdomen due to uterine contractions.
3. The cervix becomes dilated.
4. Shock may become apparent.
5. Expulsion of part (incomplete) or all (complete) products of conception.

TREATMENT AND NURSING INTERVENTION

Treatment of inevitable, complete or incomplete abortion follows the same principles:

1. Prevent shock by maintaining circulatory blood volume. This may be intravenous infusion initially followed by a blood transfusion.
2. Give analgesics as prescribed, e.g. morphia or pethidine.
3. Evacuation of retained products under general anaesthetic.
4. Give intramuscular ergometrine as prescribed to ensure uterus is well contracted.

MISSED ABORTION

This is when the pregnancy has started but the fetus has died and has not been expelled. There may be a small haemorrhage into the amniotic sac which eventually forms a clot or 'carneous mole'. The symptoms are those of pregnancy which gradually regresses and a dark brown discharge may appear. The pregnancy test becomes negative. Treatment is by evacuation of the uterus.

INDUCED ABORTION (THERAPUTIC OR TERMINATION OF PREGNANCY)

The 1967 Abortion Act states that abortion is permissible provided two doctors agree on one of the following:

1. Continuation of the pregnancy would involve a greater risk to the life of the pregnant woman than if the pregnancy was terminated.
2. Continuation of pregnancy would cause greater risk of injury to the mental or physical health of the woman, than if it was terminated.
3. Continuation of the pregnancy would cause risk of injury to the physical or mental health of any existing children.
4. There was a substantial risk that if the child was born it would suffer from mental or physical abnormality as to be seriously handicapped.

Since the Act was passed, the number of requests/operations for termination of pregnancy has increased. However, the number of maternal deaths from abortion and the number of prosecutions for criminal abortion have declined greatly.

TREATMENT AND NURSING ASSESSMENT

1. Be nonjudgemental in caring for this patient and be aware of the reasons for termination.
2. The patient should have had access to a counsellor when first seeking the termination. The counsellor should be aware of the social, cultural and religious background of the patient.
3. Observe for verbal and nonverbal clues which might indicate the patient has doubts regarding the termination. Inform the doctor.
4. Prepare the patient as for dilatation and curettage (D&C).

SEPTIC ABORTION

This can occur following any abortion but is more common following an abortion performed illegally.

CLINICAL FEATURES

1. Pyrexia and tachycardia.
2. Unpleasant pinkish vaginal discharge.
3. Signs and symptoms of bacteriogenic shock.
4. Infection may spread to fallopian tubes and myometrium and consequently into the peritoneum, causing peritonitis.

The most common causative organisms are:
1. *Clostridium welchii* (mortality rate as high as 30 per cent).
2. *Streptococci*.
3. *Staphylococci*.
4. *Escherichia coli*.

TREATMENT AND NURSING INTERVENTION
1. Take a high vaginal swab to identify causative organism.
2. Give antibiotics as prescribed, e.g. amoxycillin, metronidazole.
3. Monitor for signs of shock, e.g. subnormal temperature, reduced urine output, drop in blood pressure.
4. Encourage clear fluids to drink and perform regular mouth care.
5. Tepid sponge and change bedclothes frequently.
6. Evacuation of retained products if necessary.

RAPE

Rape is classified as the entry of the penis beyond the labia majora without consent of the woman or girl involved. Sexual assault is synonymous with indecent assault and refers to all sexual activity other than actual rape against the victim's will.
1. Statutory rape – with a female under the age of 16 years, i.e. age of consent.
2. Forcible rape – over the age of consent, but forcibly against her will.

Most rape victims are in the 16 to 35 age group, but it can happen to young girls and old women. It can happen any time of the night or day, and in half the cases the rapist is known to the victim. The nurse may find herself involved in a number of ways:
1. She may be a victim herself.
2. She may be on duty in the accident and emergency department when someone is admitted having been raped or sexually assaulted.
3. She may be approached by a victim who needs help but is reluctant to go to the hospital or tell the police.

NURSING INTERVENTION
1. Have a calm, caring, unbiased approach to the situation.
2. Obtain consent of parents, prior to examination if patient under 16, or from legal guardian if the patient is under care or is mentally subnormal.
3. Examination will include:
   a. History taking.
   b. Physical examination.
   c. Internal examination.
   d. Collection of specimens.
4. Provide a private room for the examination, if possible, with facilities afterwards for washing. Bathing and changing before reporting the crime will inevitably mean much evidence is lost.
5. Encourage patient to answer questions, help position patient, be gentle and unhurried.
6. Do not leave patient alone with a male nurse and ensure a nurse is in attendance at all times.
7. The emotional trauma of rape gives rise to certain fears:
   a. Rejection – by husband or boyfriend once he discovers she has been raped.
   b. Pregnancy – if no contraceptive precautions were taken.
   c. Venereal disease – could well become a reality.
   d. Agoraphobic – fears about going out again, especially when alone.
   e. Home – if she becomes a victim in her own home.
   f. Frigidity – can she ever trust men again or have a physical relationship again?

PATIENT EDUCATION
1. Violation of the body without consent gives the patient a sense of bereavement. Patient should be aware of the stages of grief she may display.
2. Patient is aware of support mechanisms available, e.g. religions, counselling GP or local Rape Crisis Centre.
3. Patient is aware of the symptoms of venereal disease and knows she should contact her GP or special clinic if necessary.
4. Psychosexual counselling is also available if necessary.

Care of the Patient with a Breast Disorder

ASSESSMENT AND DIAGNOSTIC EVALUATION

Figure 10.4. Breast self-examination (courtesy American Cancer Society)

BREAST SELF-EXAMINATION

CLINICAL VALUE

1. Experience has verified that more than 90 per cent of breast cancers are found by women themselves.
2. When women discover lumps in their breasts at a very early stage, surgery can save 70 to 80 per cent of proved cases.

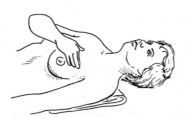

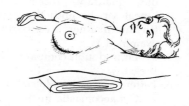

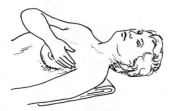

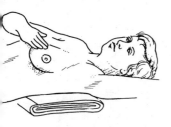

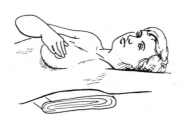

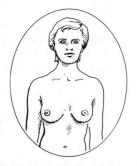

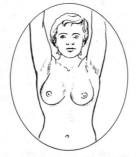

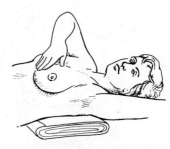

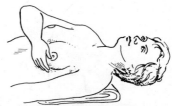

Careful examination of the breasts before a mirror symmetry in size and shape, noting any puckering impling of the skin or retraction of the nipple.

2. Arms raised over head, again studying the breasts in the mirror for the same signs.

3. Reclining on bed with flat pillow or folded bath towel under the shoulder on the same side as breast to be examined.

To examine the inner half of the breast, the arm is ed over the head. Beginning at the breastbone and, series of steps, the inner half of the breast is ated.

5. The area over the nipple is carefully palpated with the flat part of the fingers.

6. Examination of the lower inner half of the breast is completed.

With arm down at side, self examination of breasts inues by carefully feeling the tissues which extend e armpit.

8. The upper outer quadrant of the breast is examined with the flat part of the fingers.

9. The lower outer quadrant of the breast is examined in successive stages with flat part of the fingers.

PATIENT EDUCATION

1. Encourage women to examine their breasts once a month, just after the menstrual period, because breasts are less engorged at this time and a tumour is easier to detect, and at regular monthly intervals after the cessation of menses (Figure 10.4).
2. The breast can be examined in the sitting or standing position, noting in a mirror any contour changes, asymmetry, nipple discharge or eczematoid scaling around the nipple.
3. Then the breast is examined in the supine position with the breast spread out on the chest wall; use the flattened, more sensitive surface of the fingers to gently knead breast tissue in the search of abnormalities.
4. Since most of the lesions occur in the upper outer quadrant (Figure 10.5B), an effective pattern to follow is to start the examination in the upper outer quadrant, proceed around the breast, and repeat (at the end) the upper outer quadrant. (In this manner, five-fourths of the breast are examined.)
5. When in doubt, compare findings with opposite breast.
6. Differences in the adolescent (11 to 18 years):
   a. Gynaecomastia in the male occurs in one of three young men; these signs regress in one or two years.
   b. Thelarche (breast development in young female) commonly occurs unilaterally.
   c. The areola enlarges and forms a contour separate from the rest of the breast; the areola later becomes part of the normal contour.

SUGGESTIONS FOR PATIENTS WHO FIND SELF-EXAMINATION DIFFICULT OR IMPOSSIBLE TO DO

1. Determine the problem:
   a. If the patient complains of tenderness, gentle self-examination may be more effective and less painful than examination by someone else.
   b. For the woman who has cysts or lumps, recommend professional examination annually and instruct her in detecting changes from one month to the next.
   c. If the patient has large, pendulous breasts, encourage her to lie on her back and perform self-examination slowly and in a specific pattern or order.
2. Recommend other diagnostic aids periodically, e.g. mammography (see below) as condition indicates.

COMMUNITY PATIENT EDUCATION

1. Development of national screening projects (Forrest Report, 1986).

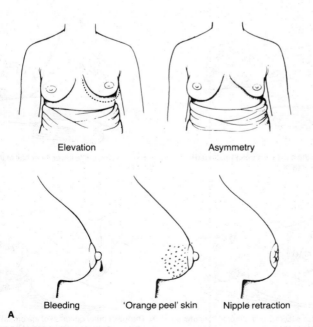

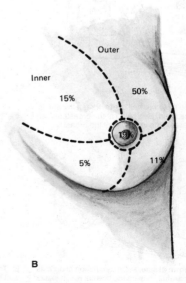

Figure 10.5. (A) Signs of cancer of the breast. (B) Distribution of carcinomas in different areas of breast

2. Well women clinics.
3. Family planning clinics.
4. Breast self-examination, although this or clinical

examination is not considered effective on its own.

5. Help to create healthy psychological attitudes.

GUIDELINES: EXAMINATION OF THE BREAST BY THE NURSE

PURPOSES
1. Detect abnormalities in the breasts.
2. Teach a woman how to perform breast self-examination.

EQUIPMENT
A good lamp and privacy.

PROCEDURE
Preparatory phase and superficial examination

Nursing action	Rationale
1. Have the woman strip to her waist and sit comfortably, facing the examiner.	This provides an opportunity to observe breasts visually for lack of symmetry and for gross signs such as redness, irritated nipple, dimpling, orange-peel skin.
2. Wash your hands under warm water and dry them; powder if they feel sticky.	The breast is sensitive to cold.

Examination

Nursing action	Rationale
1. Palpate supraclavicular area.	Note whether lymph nodes are enlarged, fixed, movable or difficult to locate.
2. Palpate axillary nodes; hold the woman's forearm in your left palm while you check nodes with your right fingertips. Repeat on other side.	Same as above.
3. Instruct the patient to lie down with her right arm under her head. Place a small pillow under the right shoulder.	This will spread breast tissue evenly over chest wall.
4. With the flattened surface of two or three fingers, gently palpate breast tissue, beginning at the upper outer quadrant. a. Proceed in an orderly pattern around the breast and repeat the first quarter examined. b. Repeat procedure for other breast.	The sensitive fingers, proceeding in a kneading fashion, can detect thickened, lumpy tissue between the patient's skin and chest wall. Since the majority of breast lesions are in the upper outer quadrant, this segment is double checked.
5. Recognize that there is a prolongation of the axillary extension of normal breast tissue, which may extend high into axilla.	This is normal if symmetrical and abnormal if asymmetrical.

6. Check the areolar area for crustiness, nipple discharge, signs of infection.

Prepare to collect a discharge specimen for cytology if indicated (see Figure. 10.6).

7. Record findings and report abnormalities to the doctor.

8. Instruct the patient in performing self-examination on her own (see Figure 10.4). Encourage her to ask any questions; provide her with appropriate literature.

Some 95 per cent of women discover their own abnormalities.

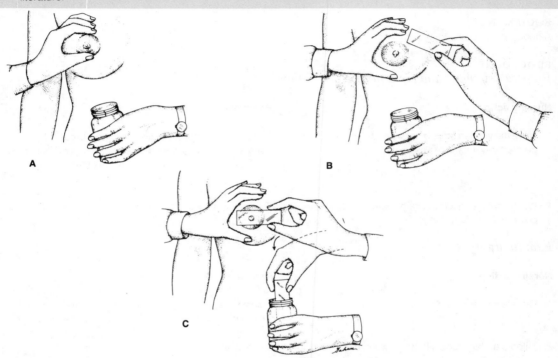

Figure 10.6. Obtaining nipple discharge specimen for cytologic examination. (1) Wash nipple gently with cotton gauze; pat dry. (2) Gently strip duct and express fluid only until a small, pea-sized drop appears on nipple. (3) Obtain assistance of patient in holding container of fixative solution near breast to receive the prepared slide. (4) Stabilize breast with fingers and thumb of one hand (A). (5) Gently place one end of slide on nipple (B); rapidly draw slide across nipple and immediately drop into fixative solution (C). (6) This may be repeated to secure additional specimens if necessary. **Note:** Positive results are significant. Negative results may be 'false-negatives'. This test is never used alone but in conjunction with other diagnostic texts

DIAGNOSTIC TESTS

MAMMOGRAPHY (X-RAY)

1. Modern mammography equipment provides excellent imaging. Contrast medium radiography rarely needed.

2. Views taken on location of suspicious areas and breast density.
3. Both breasts are examined for comparison.
4. Density of breast tissue products less satisfactory imaging in premenopausal women.
5. In women over 50, more accurate than clinical examination.
6. Small, difficult-to-locate lesions, deep in breast sometimes injected with dye under radiographic

control – just before operation. Helps surgeon locate lesion.

ULTRASONOGRAPHY
Sensitive to differentiating a solid from a cystic lesion.
1. Can detect hidden lesions.
2. Painless and non-invasive.

COMPUTED TOMOGRAPHY
1. May be useful in detecting cancer in small, dense breasts, which are difficult to examine by mammography.
2. It is unsuitable for routine screening and diagnostic studies. In summary, none of the techniques described above are used as a substitute for mammography. None of the above techniques eliminates the need for surgical biopsy or breast aspiration if clinically indicated.

BIOPSY
Aspiration (needle)
Purpose: this is a simple, rapid and accurate procedure to detect breast cancer.
1. Tumour or cyst is immobilized between two fingers to stabilize it during needle insertion (Figure 10.7).
2. Gently create a vacuum in syringe by pulling back and forth on plunger; allow pressure to equalize before withdrawing needle.
3. Spread needle contents on glass slide; further spread specimen with a second glass slide held at an angle.

Note: Positive results are significant. Negative results are ignored; other clinical evaluations must be done.

Open biopsy
A specimen of tissue is obtained in the operating theatre and sent to the laboratory for frozen section, which is then stained and examined under the microscope. This provides a quick diagnosis. It is preferable not to proceed to a mastectomy immediately, but rather delay so that the type of operation may be discussed fully with the patient.

Excisional
Following an incision into the breast, the entire lump is removed for microscopic study.

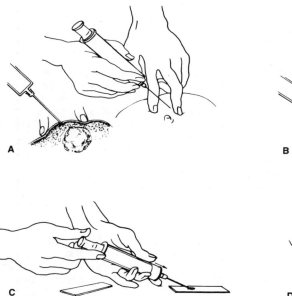
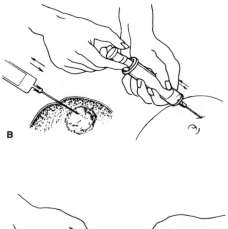
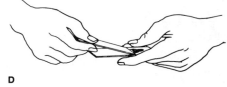

Figure 10.7. Needle biopsy. (A) Tumour is immobilized with two fingers before the needle is inserted. (B) A vacuum is created by withdrawing the plunger slowly but forcefully several times. Before the needle is removed, the pressure is allowed to equalize. (C) Contents of needle are placed on glass slide. (D) The smear is spread forwards gently with a glass slide inclined at an angle of about 35°, with an up-and-down movement (Zajdela, A. The value of aspiration cytology in the diagnosis of breast cancer, *Cancer*, 35)

Oestrogen-receptor and progesterone-receptor assay
A test of tumour tissue to determine whether or not the cancer cells have receptor sites. If such sites are present, the patient is more likely to respond to hormonal manipulation.

CONDITIONS OF THE NIPPLE

FISSURES AND BLEEDING

See below.

Table 10.3 Fissures and bleeding

	Fissure of nipple	Bleeding from nipple
Assessment and clinical features	A *fissure* of the nipple is a longitudinal type of ulcer that occasionally develops in the breast of a nursing mother: nipple appears sore and irritated; bleeding from nipple.	Bloody discharge – usually on edge of areola.
Causes	1. Lack of preparation of nipples in prenatal period. 2. Condition aggravated by sucking infant.	1. Most commonly due to wart-like papilloma in one of larger collecting ducts at edge of areola. 2. Occasionally a malignancy is responsible (see Figure 10.6, cytology examination).
Patient education	1. Keep nipple clean by washing and drying after each nursing period. 2. In prenatal period, wash, dry and lubricate nipples in preparation for nursing.	
Treatment and nursing interventions	1. Wash nipples with sterile saline solution. 2. Use artificial nipple for nursing. 3. If above does not initiate healing process, stop nursing and use breast pump.	1. Surgery for palpable mass. a. Duct is identified. b. Papilloma is excised (or a wedge of breast from area producing the bleeding is excised if no gross papilloma is identified) through a small periareolar incision – send for laboratory analysis. c. Sterile dressings applied. 2. If no palpable mass, mammography and xerography.

INFLAMMATION OF THE BREAST

ACUTE MASTITIS AND MAMMARY ABSCESS

See below.

Table 10.4   Acute mastitis and mammary abscess

	Acute mastitis	Mammary abscess
Incidence	May occur at beginning or end of lactation.	Often follows acute mastitis.
Source of infection	1. Hands of patient. 2. Personnel caring for the patient. 3. Infection from baby. 4. Blood-borne.	Same.
Assessment and clinical features	1. Infection attacks duct, causing stagnation of milk in lobules. 2. Dull pain occurs in the area affected. 3. Breast feels doughy and tough. 4. May also have a discharging nipple.	1. Area is very sensitive, appears dusky red. 2. Pus may be expressed from nipple (see Figure 10.6, nipple discharge for cytology). 3. Mass is palpable.
Treatment and nursing interventions	1. Have the patient stop breast-feeding. 2. Apply heat or cold (depending on stage of infection). 3. Administer antibiotics as prescribed. 4. Give progesterone to relieve congestion. 5. Have the patient wear firm breast support. 6. Encourage the patient to practice meticulous personal hygiene.	1. Administer antibiotics and chemotherapy as prescribed. 2. Incise and drain. 3. Apply hot, wet dressings to increase drainage and hasten resolution.

FIBROCYSTIC DISEASE

Fibrocystic disease is mammary dysplasia characterized by increased formation of fibrous tissue, hyperplasia of the epithelial cells of the ducts and breast glands and dilatation of the ducts. It is related to the cyclic stimulation of the breast by oestrogen, but represents a departure from the normal stimulation and regression pattern of this process.

INCIDENCE
1. The most common lesion of the female breast; three to four times more prevalent than cancer.
2. Overgrowth of fibrous tissue around ducts; dilatation of the ducts to form cysts; epithelial hyperplasia of the ducts.
3. Occurs usually in women between 35 and 50 years and is endocrine-related.

CLINICAL FEATURES
1. The patient complains of an uncomfortable feeling in the breast.
2. Cysts or lumps are usually firm, single or multiple, smooth, round masses; bilateral.
3. They are tender on palpation or pressure and slightly mobile.

4. Pain may be of the 'shooting' type and may be aggravated by congestion before a menstrual period.

TREATMENT AND NURSING INTERVENTIONS
1. Aspiration:
   a. The patient is placed in supine position. Under aseptic precautions, skin area is cleansed with a skin antiseptic.
   b. Local anaesthesia is given.
   c. The doctor immobilizes cyst with thumb and index finger of one hand.
   d. Using a 20ml syringe and No. 16 or 18 gauge needle, the cyst is penetrated and aspirated.
2. Excision: if cyst refills within a week on two, excisional biopsy is usually performed.
3. The nurse emphasizes the importance of frequent re-examinations.
   a. Individuals with fibrocystic disease have an increased incidence of subsequent malignancy.
   b. Self-examination is difficult in the markedly fibrotic breast.
4. Avoidance of methylxanthines (coffee, tea, cola and chocolate) tends to resolve these cysts.

Note: The palpable changes of fibrocystic disease may mask an underlying cancer.

TUMOURS OF THE BREAST

FIBROADENOMATA

CLINICAL FEATURES
1. Firm, round, movable, benign tumours of the breast.
2. Appear in breasts of girls in their late teens or early twenties.
3. No pain or tenderness.

TREATMENT
Removal through a small incision.

PROGNOSIS
No malignant potential.

CANCER OF THE BREAST

Major changes in approaches and treatment have developed in the last five years. It is now recognized to be a chronic systemic disease and therefore systemic treatment is now carried out at an early stage. Statistically, radical surgery has not improved survival.

INCIDENCE
1. Breast cancer is the leading cause of cancer incidence and death in woman in the UK, with 24,000 new cases and 15,000 deaths each year.
2. One in 12 women in the UK develops breast cancer.
3. Despite all efforts to date, the breast cancer death rate continues to rise in the UK.
4. Screening by mammography have demonstrated that early detection and treatment can reduce mortality – particularly in the 50 to 65 age group.

RISK FACTORS IN BREAST CANCER
Major risk factors
See also Table 10.5.
1. Sex – 99 per cent occur in females.
2. Age – more than 85 per cent of women with breast cancer are over the age of 45.
3. Genetics – women whose mothers and sisters have had breast cancer are twice as likely to develop cancer.
4. Parity – decreased risk threefold to fourfold if first birth is before 18 years of age. Decrease in risk continues, but at a declining rate up to age 25 for first parity. Increased risks in unmarried women, infertile women, women with fewer than three children, and women who have first child after 34.
5. If breast cancer appears in one breast, the likelihood of cancer in the other breast is greater.
6. Benign cystic breast is considered to be a precursor to cancer; likelihood of cancer is about four times greater in women who have cystic disease.
7. Severely constipated women (two or fewer bowel movements a week) demonstrate a fourfold increase in risk of breast cancer.

Prominent risk factors
1. Prolonged total menstrual activity. Increased incidence under the following circumstances:
   a. When menarche occurs before 12 years of age.

Table 10.5 Major risk factors – breast cancer

Characteristic	Risk	
	High	Low
Sex – female	High	
Age		
Early 40s	Yes	No
45–55 (past menopause)	Yes	No
Genetics – women whose mother and sisters had breast cancer are twice as likely to develop cancer	Yes	No
Race	Caucasian	Oriental
Menarche	Early	Late
Parity	Nulliparous	Parous
Unmarried	Higher	Lower
Infertile	Higher	Lower
Women who have had first child after 34	Yes	No
Menopause		
Natural	Late	Early
Artificial	No	Yes
History of severe constipation (two or fewer bowel movements/week)	Yes	No

b. In those with 30 or more years' menstrual activity.
c. When menopause occurs after 55.
2. Other organ cancers such as ovary, colon, endometrium.
3. Wet-type cerumen (earwax) – genetic predisposition.

Possible risk factors
1. Heavy radiation exposure.
2. Immunodeficiency.
3. Exogenous oestrogen administration.
4. Excessive intake of dietary fat.

TREATMENT
Objectives
1. Preserve the life of the woman.
2. Achieve permanent local control of the disease.
3. Minimize the possibility of recurrence.
4. Provide the best cosmetic result.
These may be accomplished by surgical removal of the cancer. Radiotherapy, chemotherapy and immunotherapy are other treatment methods that may be employed independently or in combination with surgery for the purpose of helping to cure, control growth, alleviate pain and/or prevent recurrence.

Prognosis
1. When malignancy is confined to breast: five-year survival – 80 per cent.
2. When malignancy has spread to axilla: five-year survival – 55 per cent.

Types of surgical intervention
1. 'Lumpectomy' (tumorectomy) – removal of circumscribed area around and including tumour.
2. Partial mastectomy (wide local excision) – removal of the tumour plus 2–3cm wedge of normal tissue surrounding the tumour.
3. Simple mastectomy – removal of breast only, and sometimes axillary lymph node sampling.
4. Extended simple mastectomy – removal of breast, axillary tail and axillary lymph node clearance.
5. Modified radical – entire breast is removed, as is the pectoralis minor muscle; some or most of axillary lymph nodes are removed.
6. Total mastectomy – entire breast is removed, but pectoralis muscles left intact; most or all of axillary lymph nodes are left intact.
7. Classical radical mastectomy (Halsted) – removal of breast and underlying muscles down to chest wall; also removal of nodules and lymphatics of axilla. This is rarely performed nowadays.

Radiation
1. Radiation is effective in damaging and preventing cell reproduction. Cancer cells are especially susceptible to radiation.
2. Utilization in breast cancer:
   a. As adjuvant therapy with surgery.
   b. To shrink a large tumour to operable size.
   c. To alleviate pain caused by metastasis.
   d. As primary therapy.
3. Method – following tumour and lymph node excision, a series of external radiation treatments are begun:
   a. Usually four to five treatments a week for four to five weeks (a total of approximately 5,000 rads).
   b. Radiation directed to chest wall, remaining lymph nodes.
   c. Side-effects – mild fatigue; later, skin will look and feel sunburned and eventually the breast becomes more firm.
   d. A 'booster' or second phase of treatment may be given:

(i) electron beam, or

(ii) radioactive implant.

Adjuvant therapy

This is therapy used to supplement surgery or primary radiotherapy.

1. Local or regional adjuvant therapy – radiotherapy. Value is controversial.

2. Systemic adjuvant therapy – this includes chemotherapy, hormonal therapy or immunotherapy.

Assessment

CLINICAL FEATURES

See also Figure 10.5.

1. Early signs are insidious.

2. A nontender lump appears in the breast, most frequently in the upper outer quadrant; it may be movable and isolated.

3. Pain usually is absent except in the late stages.
   A recent study indicated that 13 per cent of patients described pain as a primary symptom; 7 per cent indicated that it was the first clue that led them to probe and examine the breast. Pain was described as a 'hurt' or 'funny feeling' rather than acute or sharp.

4. Retraction or dimpling of the skin over the mass may be noted.

5. On mirror examination, asymmetry may be observed – the affected breast appears more elevated than the other.

6. Nipple retraction or nipple bleeding may be apparent.

7. Later, the nodule becomes more fixed to the chest wall.

8. Nodular axillary masses may appear.

9. Ulceration appears in late stages.

Table 10.6 shows the international TNM classification.

PATIENT PROBLEMS

1. Anxiety and fear related to possibility of mutilation, disturbance of patient's marriage and death.

2. Impairment in skin integrity related to breast surgery, wound drainage and radiation.

3. Lack of knowledge related to inadequate information of preoperative and postoperative care and the many support services available.

4. Grieving about lost femininity and a coveted body part as well as alteration in self-image related to breast removal for cancer.

5. Potential physical and sexual dysfunction related to loss of a breast.

Table 10.6　International TNM classification

T	Tumour
T_1	2cm diameter or less; no fixation or tethering
T_2	2–5cm diameter (or less than 2cm) with tethering or nipple retraction
T_3	5–10cm diameter (or less than 5cm) with infiltration ulceration, or peau d'orange over the tumour, or deep fixation
T_4	Any tumour with infiltration or ulceration wider than its diameter
	Tumour longer than 10cm
N	Nodes
N_0	No palpable axillary nodes
N_1	Mobile palpable axillary nodes
N_2	Fixed axillary nodes
N_3	Palpable supraclavicular nodes; oedema of the arm
M	Metastases
M_0	No evidence of distant metastases
M_1	Distant metastases

Planning and implementation

PREOPERATIVE NURSING INTERVENTIONS

Psychosocial preoperative preparation

1. Begin emotional support when the patient is told that biopsy and hospitalization may be required.

2. Dispel fear by:
   a. Listening to the patient's concerns and dispelling misconceptions.
   b. Collaborating with doctor on a unified approach to informing the patient.
   c. Emphasizing successful programme of rehabilitation, use of prosthesis and possibly reconstruction.
   d. Having a patient who made a satisfactory postoperative adjustment visit present patient.
   e. Soliciting support of the husband and/or significant others.
   f. Providing encouragement and reassurance.

3. Minimize delay before operation.
   Determine physical, nutritional and emotional needs.

4. Include the patient's husband/partner by keeping him informed of the treatment plan and its progress.

5. Administer hypnotic to block the patient's concerns.

6. Relay any positive verified information related to the successful removal of all tumours, limited spread, etc; this can accelerate recovery.

7. Support the surgeon's plan to remove malig-

nancy, minimize disfigurement and prevent spread of cancer cells.
8. Work with the patient in preparation for anaesthesia and surgery; describe each activity to the patient.

Note: Protocols for preoperative and postoperative care are given in detail on pp. 45–60.

POSTOPERATIVE NURSING INTERVENTIONS
General care
1. See Chapter 3 for detailed discussion of postoperative care.
2. Upon the patient's return from the recovery room, promote comfort and rest; administer analgesics for pain.
3. Encourage fluid and nutritional support as tolerated and desired.
4. Position the patient comfortably in semi-recumbent position; if arm is free, elevate on a pillow; the most distal part (hand) is placed higher to permit gravity to aid in removal of fluid via lymphatics and venous pathways.
5. Check dressings for undue constriction, signs of haematoma, haemorrhage, etc; ensure that portable suction or other drainage devices are operating properly.

Exercises and ambulation
1. Encourage mobility of arm on the affected side as recommended by the surgeon, to prevent such complications as lymphoedema and 'shoulder shrugging' helps to prevent frozen shoulder:
   a. Initiate bed exercises after 24 hours, such as wrist and elbow flexion and extension, hourly.
   b. Encourage the patient to use her arm in self-care: washing face, applying lipstick, combing hair.
   c. See Table 10.7 for activities to be resumed eventually.
2. Ambulate the patient early, as determined by the individual patient.
3. Need to support breast. Brassiere is usually worn as soon as drainage tube is removed.

Other treatment methods
1. Radiotherapy:
   a. Primary treatment when surgery has been ruled out by advanced age, inoperable condition, other complications.
   b. Adjuvant therapy to surgery.
   c. To reduce tumour size; as palliation for pain. When radiotherapy is used, follow principles of care, p, 1039.

2. Chemotherapy – also see p. 1036:
   a. Used as adjunct therapy to surgery and/or radiotherapy.
   b. Usually various combinations of drugs are preferred.
   c. Four major types of drugs are alkylating, antimetabolite, antibiotic, and mitotic inhibitor.
3. Immunotherapy (unproved). Theory is that immunological response could destroy invading cancer cells while sparing normal cells.

Coping measures
1. Permit the patient to view incision line when psychologically appropriate; get her to help in keeping the wound clean; have her use a mirror if necessary to view the area adequately; instruct her in the proper technique to use in applying dressings and fixing them properly.
2. Familiarize the patient with appropriate literature:
   a. Combine this with visits by helpful people who have had successful mastectomy rehabilitation.
   b. Acquaint the patient with prosthetic possibilities as determined feasible by the surgeon.
   c. Suggest clothing adjustments and possibilities.
3. Encourage the patient to 'talk out' and express her feelings – provide support, including psycho-spiritual if required.
4. Assist the patient in addressing psychosocial adjustment problems, including sexual problems; include her husband or important others as required.

COMPLICATION: LYMPHOEDEMA OF THE ARM
Lymphoedema is an obstruction of the lymph flow in the arm on the operated side, producing a chronic swelling of the part, particularly if it is in a dependent position. Lymphoedema is due to lymph node removal and compression of axillary vein by tumour or scar. This is seen less these days with the advent of less radical surgery.

Prevention
1. Exercises should be done.
2. The affected arm should be massaged for three or four months postoperatively to increase circulation and lessen oedema.
3. The affected arm is elevated frequently to prevent dependent oedema.
4. The arm and operative site is kept scrupulously clean to prevent infection.
5. Nonconstrictive clothing is worn to permit adequate circulation.

Treatment

1. May include a diuretic.
2. An intermittent compression unit with press-urized sleeve may be used to force fluid back into venous system.

PATIENT EDUCATION

1. Talk to and listen to patient; encourage questions and provide helpful answers.
2. Prepare the husband for his role in providing the necessary emotional support.
3. Initiate active exercise on the affected side 24 hours postoperatively for hand and elbow. Check with doctor on extent of exercise for each individual patient. Exercises will increase daily, and the patient will do more of her own activities, such as hair combing, teeth brushing, etc.

Note: Be cautious in exercising the shoulder during the first week after surgery. Excessive abduction of the arm at the shoulder can lift skin flaps from chest wall and increase serous formation.

   a. Exercise should not be painful.
   b. Bilateral activity is emphasized.
   c. Proper posture should be maintained.
   d. If the patient has had a skin graft or if the skin was approximated under tension, exercises will be limited.

4. Care of wound:
   a. Explain how the wound will gradually change.
   b. Note that the newly healed wound may have less sensation due to severed nerves.
   c. Bathe gently and blot carefully to dry.
   d. Recognize signs of infection – pain, tender-

Table 10.7   Exercises for rehabilitation of the patient following surgery of the breast

Exercise	Equivalent daily activities

1. Stand erect
  Lean forward from waist
  Allow arms to hang
  Swing arms from side to side together: then in opposite direction
  Next: swing arms from front to back together; then in opposite direction
	Broom sweeping
	Vacuum cleaning
	Mopping floor
	Pulling out and pushing in drawers
	Weaving
	Playing golf

2. Stand erect facing wall with palms of hand flat against wall; arms extended
  Relax arms and shoulders and allow upper part of body to lean forward against hands
  Push away to original position; repeat
	Pushing self out of bath
	Kneading bread
	Breast stroke – swimming
	Sawing or cutting types of crafts

3. Stand erect facing wall with palms of hands flat against wall Climb the wall with the fingers; descend, repeat	Raising windows Washing windows Hanging clothes on line Reaching to an upper shelf
4. Stand erect and clasp hands at small of back; raise hands; lower; repeat Clasp hands back of neck; reach downward; upward; repeat	Fastening brassiere Buttoning blouse or dress Pulling up a dress zipper Fastening beads Washing the back

5. Toss a rope over the shower curtain rod
  Hold the ends of the rope (knotted) in each hand and raise arms sideways
  Using a seesaw motion and with arms outstretched slide the rope up and down over the rod
	Drying the back with a bath towel
	Raising and lowering a window blind
	Closing and opening window drapes

6. Flex and extend each finger in turn	Sewing, knitting, crocheting Typing, painting, playing piano or other musical instrument

ness, redness, swelling; if these are present, report to doctor.

e. Massage gently the healed incision with lanolin or baby oil to encourage circulation and increase skin elasticity. This is initiated with surgeon's approval.

5. Use of prosthesis – advice is usually given by the breast counsellor or the appliance officer.

a. Soft fibre-filled prosthesis with a cotton backing are most commonly used for the first six weeks following operation.

b. Silicone prosthesis with polyurethane 'skin' can be washed with soap and water, and worn when swimming in chlorinated or salt water.

IMPORTANCE OF FOLLOW-UP VISIT

1. Incision healing evaluated.
2. Rehabilitative effort assessed.
3. Effectiveness of prosthesis determined.
4. Patient's psychosocial adjustment evaluated.
5. Possible recurrence detected.

Evaluation
EXPECTED OUTCOMES

1. Patient accepts diagnosis of breast cancer and adjusts positively.
2. Patient experiences acceptable wound closure and adapts to rehabilitation programme.
3. Patient utilizes various support services as required, e.g. The Mastectomy Association of Great Britain, 26 Harrison Street, London WC1H 8JG.
4. Patient moves through the grieving process and exhibits a satisfactorily optimistic outlook.
5. Patient adjusts to physical and sexual dysfunction and proceeds with positive alternate plans.

BREAST RECONSTRUCTION

Reconstruction of the breast takes place by using prosthetic implants or fashioning a flap from the patient's own tissues; an areola–nipple reconstruction may also be performed.

PREVALENCE AND INDICATIONS

1. The possibility of breast reconstruction is receiving more attention for several reasons:
   a. Breast surgery is less radical.
   b. Recent advances in plastic surgery.
   c. Greater acceptance of cosmetic surgery.
2. Reconstruction is performed usually three months to a year after a mastectomy; there is no maximum time limit.
3. Reconstruction may be inadvisable for women under the following circumstances:

a. Presence of large tumours or extensive nodular involvement; recent history of breast abscess or history of diffuse, painful cystic mastitis.
b. Presence of other diseases that might impair the healing process.
c. Marked obesity.
d. Advanced age.

IMPLANTS

Flexible silicone sacs filled with silicone gel (greater firmness) or saline solution (lesser firmness). Some can be subtly adjusted by injection of additional saline solution (Figure 10.8).

1. This prosthesis can be inserted through a small incision at the submammary crease and positioned underneath breast skin.
2. The tightness of the skin often determines the size of the implant; this may require alteration of the remaining breast to match the reconstructed breast.

Patient education

1. The patient is instructed to keep her elbow close to her side for several days to a week.
2. Full use of the patient's arm is achieved in about a

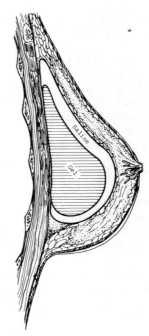

Figure 10.8. The placement of a mammary implant – in this case, one featuring a sealed inner gel implant surrounded by an inflatable outer saline implant (courtesy American Heyer-Schulte Corporation, Goleta, CA, 1980)

month; however, strenuous arm use in tennis, golf or swimming may be delayed.
3. A well-fitted brassiere worn day and night 'for three months may assist the breast(s) in taking on the desired shape.
4. Instruct the patient to report thinning or discoloration of skin over the implant area.
5. The patient is instructed in how to distinguish the prosthesis from normal or abnormal breast tissue during self-examination for breast cancer.

FLAP GRAFT
This is the transfer of skin, sometimes muscle, from another part of the body, usually in stages, to the mastectomy site (see Grafts, p. 773). It is used when the chest skin is insufficient or too thin (e.g. post-radiotherapy) to allow a prosthesis to be implanted beneath it.

AREOLA–NIPPLE RECONSTRUCTION
The nipple and areola are saved during mastectomy and banked (suturing to a temporary site, usually thigh or abdomen) until the breast reconstruction is done.
1. If banking is not possible, tissue from the other breast, labia or ear lobe may be grafted.

RECURRENT OR METASTATIC BREAST CANCER

ENDOCRINE MANIPULATION
Theory and objective
Malignant tumour cells depend on hormonal function in the host; deprivation of hormones reduces tumour's growth. Currently, tumour removed at operation is tested for oestrogen receptors. If positive, the use of hormonal therapy or ablation can be carried out on a more rational basis than heretofore, with an anticipated good response.

Ablative procedures
1. Bilateral salpingo-oophorectomy:
   a. This is often the initial treatment of choice for premenopausal patients with metastatic breast cancer.
   b. Remission lasts from three months to several years (median – one year).
   c. If signs of reactivation of tumour growth occur, further endocrine therapy may be done.

Hormones
1. Oestrogens:
   The introduction of hormone antagonist drugs has now largely been replaced by the use of oestrogens in postmenopausal women. Tamoxifen is the first drug of choice. It is highly effective with very few side-effects.
   a. Administered orally – a single dose daily (premenopausal for one year; post-menopausal for two to five years).
   b. Causes tumour to regress in six to seven months. It is effective in 50 per cent of all patients, and is effective in 66 per cent of women who are oestrogen receptor-positive.
   c. Incidence of side-effects is very low. Hypocalcaemia occurs transiently where bony metastases is being treated.
2. Aminoglutethimide (Orimeten):
   This drug blocks the conversion of androgen to oestrogen but also inhibits adrenal steroid production, so steroid replacement is necessary.
   a. Administered with hydrocortisone.
   b. Best responses in women with metastases to bone and soft tissues.
   c. Side-effects – lethargy, unstable gait, dizziness, transient rash.

Cytotoxic chemotherapy
Alkylating agents: 5-fluorouracil, methotrexate, vincristine. None of these drugs cause complete hair loss (temporary). There will be need for the patient to be provided with psychological support. Wigs are also available under the NHS.
1. Remission lasts about six months (in 20 per cent of patients).
2. Five-drug combination can boost remission rate to about nine months (in 65 per cent of patients) – 5-fluorouracil, methotrexate, vincristine, cyclophosphamide, prednisone.
3. Recommended for patients who have metastasis to liver or lungs and are poor surgical risks for endocrine ablative surgery.
4. Recommended for premenopausal patients who are not benefiting from oophorectomy or hypophysectomy.
5. Doxorubicin hydrochloride (Adriamycin) usually used when five-drug chemotherapy fails.

CONTACT ADDRESSES

Endometriosis Self-Help Group
65 Holmdene Avenue
Herne Hill
London SE2X 9LD
Tel: 01 737 4764

The Herpes Association
c/o Spare Rib Ltd
27 Clerkenwell Close
London EC1

Hysterectomy Support Group
Raven Dell
Warren Way
Lower Heswell
Wirral
Merseyside L60 9HO
Tel: 051 342 3167

London Rape Crisis Centre
PO Box 69
London WC1X 9NJ
Tel: 01 837 1600
(Centres are in all major towns and cities)

The Mastectomy Association of Great Britain
26 Harrison Street
Off Gray's Inn Road
London WC1H 8JG
Tel: 01 837 0908

National Association for Premenstrual Tension
C/O 23 Upper Park Road
Kingston Upon Thames
Surrey KT2 5LB

FURTHER READING

BOOKS

Barnes, J. (1983) *Lecture Notes on Gynaecology*, Blackwell Scientific, Oxford.

Chamberlain, G. and Dewhurst, J. (1986) *A Practice of Obstetrics and Gynaecology* (2nd edn), Pitman, London.

Clayton, S.G. and Newton, J.R. (1983) *A Pocket Gynaecology*, Churchill Livingstone, Edinburgh.

Clayton, S., Lewis, T.L.T. and Pinker, G.D. (1985) *Gynaecology by Ten Teachers* (14th edn), Arnold, London.

Dunn, B. and Rossler, S. (1985) *Nursing Care of Women: A Gynaecological Perspective*, Harper & Row, London.

Faulder, C. (1982) *Breast Cancer – A Guide to Early Detection and Treatment* (2nd edn), Virago, London.

Harvey Kemble, J.V. and Lamb, B.E. (1984) *Plastic Surgery and Burns Nursing*, Chapter 8, The thorax and breast, Baillière Tindall, London.

Health Education Council *Living with the Loss of a Breast*: A booklet for Mastectomy Patients, HEC, London.

Hull, M.G.R., Joyce, D.N. and Turner, G. (1986) *Undergraduate Obstetrics and Gynaecology* (2nd edn), John Wright, Bristol.

King's Fund Centre (1986) *Treatment of Primary Breast Cancer – Consensus Statement*, 2nd King's Fund Forum.

Ledward, R.S. (1984) *Drug Treatment in Gynaecology*, Butterworths, London.

Llewellyn-Jones, D. (1982) *Everywoman: A Gynaecological Guide for Life* (3rd edn), Faber & Faber, London.

— (1983) *The A-Z of Women's Health*, Oxford University Press, Oxford.

Mackenzie, R. (1984) *Menopause: A Practical Self-help Guide for Women*, Sheldon, London.

Marks Maran, D.J. and Pope, B. (1985) *Breast Cancer: Nursing and Counselling*, Blackwell Scientific, Oxford.

Reynolds, M. (1984) *Gynaecological Nursing*, Blackwell Scientific, Oxford.

Simons, W. (1985) *Learning to Care in the Gynaecological Ward*, Hodder & Stoughton, London.

Webb, C. (1986) *Women's Health: Midwifery and Gynaecological Nursing*, Hodder & Stoughton, London.

ARTICLES

Abortion

Hulme, H. (1983) Therapeutic abortion and nursing care, *Nursing Times*, Vol. 79, No. 41, pp. 54–60.

Jacob, F. (1981) Abortion counselling, *Maternal and Child Health*, Vol. 16, No. 9, pp. 338–41.

Savage, W. (1982) Abortions, methods and sequelae, *British Journal of Hospital Medicine*, Vol. 28, No. 4, pp. 364–82.

Breast

Burn, I. (1984) The diagnosis and treatment of early breast cancer, *The Practitioner*, Vol. 228, June, pp. 563–7.

Cox, E. (1984) Breast cancer 1 – practice: psychological aspects, *Nursing Mirror*, Vol. 159, 14 November, pp. 18–19.

Dewar, J. and Kerr, G. (1985) Value of routine follow-up of women treated for early carcinoma of the breast, *British Medical Journal*, Vol. 291, 23 November, pp. 1464–7.

Faculty of Community Medicine (1987) Guidelines for Health Promotion No. 10. Screening for Breast Cancer.

Fallowfield, L.J. *et al.* (1986) Effects of breast conservation on psychological morbidity associated with diagnosis and treatment of early breast cancer, *British Medical Journal*, Vol. 293, 22 November, pp. 1331–4.

Faulkner, A. (1985) Mastectomy. Reclaiming a body image, *Community Outlook*, May, pp. 11, 13.

Forrest, Prof. Sir P. (1986) *Breast Cancer Screening*, Report to the Health Ministers, HMSO, London.

Gavin, A. (1985) Patience first (the role of the breast specialist nurse), *Senior Nurse*, Vol. 2, 13 February, pp. 16–18.

Gazet, J.C. *et al.* (1985) Survey of treatment of primary breast cancer in Great Britain, *British Medical Journal*, Vol. 290, 15 June, pp. 1793–5.

Harwood, D. (1983) Breast self-examination by NHS staff, *Nursing Times*, Vol. 79, No. 14, pp. 27–9.

Hopkins, M.B. (1986) Information seeking and adaptational outcomes in women receiving chemotherapy for breast cancer, *Cancer Nursing*, Vol. 9, No. 5, October, pp. 256–62.

Howell, A. and Ribeiro, G. (1985) Management of advanced carcinoma of the breast, *The Practitioner*, Vol. 229, March, pp. 255–6, 258–62.

Hughson, A. *et al.* (1986) Psychological impact of adjuvant chemotherapy in the first two years after mastectomy, *British Medical Journal*, Vol. 293, 15 November, pp. 1268–71.

Hutcheson, H.A. (1986) TAIF: new option for breast reconstruction, *Nursing 86*, Vol. 16, No. 2, February, pp. 52–3.

Jones, J. (1984) Breast cancer 2 – primary radiotherapy (nursing care study), *Nursing Mirror*, Vol. 159, 21 November, pp. 34, 36.

Lyall, J. (1986) Counting the cost of screening (for breast cancer), *Health Service Journal*, 20 November, p. 1506.

Marks, M. (1985) Breast self-examination, *The Practitioner*, Vol. 229, March, pp. 255–6, 258–62.

Pendleton, L. and Smith, A. (1986) Provision of breast prostheses, *Nursing Times*, Vol. 82, 4 June, pp. 37–9.

Pike, M.C. and Chilvers, C. (1985) Oral contraceptives and breast cancer: the current controversy, *Journal of the Royal Society of Health*, Vol. 105, February, pp. 5–10.

Rowden, R. (1983) Talking about taboos (the RCN breast cancer forum which has now been set up), *Nursing Times*, Vol. 79, No. 14, p. 12.

Spittle, M.F. (1985) Radiotherapy in the management of breast cancer, *The Practitioner*, Vol. 229, March, pp. 247–8, 250, 253.

Tarrier, N. (1984) Coping after a mastectomy, *Nursing Mirror*, Vol. 158, No. 2, pp. 29–30.

Taylor, A. (1984) Breast cancer 1: Clinical medical treatment, *Nursing Mirror*, Vol. 159, 14 November, pp. 16–17.

Tierney, J. (1984) Breast cancer 1 – 'Breast off!', *Nursing Mirror*, Vol. 159, 14 November, pp. 20–22.

Tierney, J. and Murrell, D. (1985) The Mastectomy Association, *The Practitioner*, Vol. 229, March, pp. 265–7.

Wing, M. (1984) Breast cancer 2 – Practice healing the image, *Nursing Mirror*, Vol. 159, 21 November, pp. 30–32.

Youssef, M.A. (1984) Crisis intervention: a group therapy approach for hospitalized breast cancer patients, *Journal of Advanced Nursing*, Vol. 9, May, pp. 307–13.

Cervical cancer

Brown, S. *et al.* (1984) Social class, sexual habits and cancer of the cervix, *Community Medicine*, Vol. 6, November, pp. 281–6.

Chamberlain, J. (1984) Failures of the cervical cytology screening programme, *British Medical Journal*, Vol. 289, 6 October, pp. 853–4.

Davison, R. (1984) Cervical cancer 5 – Health education, *Nursing Mirror*, Vol. 159, 31 October, pp. 32–3.

Goodman, M. (1984) Caring for laser vulvectomy patients, *Nursing Mirror*, Vol. 159, 1 August, Clinical Forum suppl., pp. i–iii, vi–vii.

Hill, G. (1984) Cervical cancer 4 – The nurse's role, *Nursing Mirror*, Vol. 159, 24 October, pp. 26–8.

Hunter, R. (1984) Cervical cancer 3 – Treatment techniques, *Nursing Mirror*, Vol. 159, 17 October, pp. 44–7.

Imperial Cancer Research Fund Co-ordinating Committee on Cervical Screening (1984) Organisation of a programme for cervical cancer screening, *British Medical Journal*, Vol. 289, 6 October, pp. 894–5.

International Agency for Research on Cancer Working Group on Evaluation of Cervical Cancer Screening Programmes (1986) Screening for squamous cervical cancer: duration of low risk after negative results of cervical cytology and its implication for screening policies, *British Medical Journal*, Vol. 293, 13 September, pp. 659–64.

Philip, G. (1984) Cervical screening – letting the patient know, *Community Medicine*, Vol. 6, November, pp. 287–90.

Tindall, V. (1984) Cervical cancer 1 – Pathology and research, *Nursing Mirror*, Vol. 159, 3 October, pp. 16–18.

Walker, G. *et al.* (1984) General practice audit: cervical cytology recall, *Modern Medicine*, Vol. 29, April, pp. 20–22.

WHO (1985) Collaborative Study of Neoplasia and Steroid Contraceptives: invasive cervical cancer and combined contraceptives, *British Medical Journal*, Vol. 290, 30 March, pp. 961–4.

Yule, R. (1984) Cervical cancer 2 – Screening for prevention, *Nursing Mirror*, Vol. 159, 10 October, pp. 37–9.

Gynaecology

Blackwell, A. (1985) Vaginal discharge, *The Practitioner*, Vol. 229, November, pp. 987–90, 992–5.

Crawford, M. and Pettit, D. (1986) Hydatidiform mole and choriocarcinoma, *Nursing Times*, Vol. 82, No. 49, 3 December, pp. 38–9.

— (1986) Treatment schedules for hydatidiform mole and choriocarcinoma, *Nursing Times*, Vol. 82, No. 50, 10 December, pp. 40–2.

Gould, D. (1985) The myth of the menopause, *Nursing Mirror*, Vol. 160, 5 June, pp. 25–7.

Howarth, P. (1985) Clinical Revision Series 12. Uterovaginal prolapse, *Nursing Mirror*, Vol. 161, 24 July, pp. 46–7.

Hunter, L. (1985) Easing the tension (PMT), *Nursing Times*, Vol. 81, 16 January, pp. 40–43.

Mindel, A. and Allason-Jones, E. (1987) Herpes infection in gynaecology, *The Practitioner*, Vol. 231, No. 8, January, pp. 96–8.

Robert, A. (1985) Helping Edith to cope (hysterectomy and colposuspension – nursing care), *Nursing Times*, Vol. 81, 12 June, pp. 40–41.

Schmid-Heinisch, R. (1985) Health education. Fair to middling (health education for women after the menopause), *Nursing Mirror*, Vol. 161, 23 October, p. 29.

Webb, C. (1985) Gynaecological nursing: a compromising situation, *Journal of Advanced Nursing*, Vol. 10, January, pp. 47–54.

Webb, C. and Wilson-Barnett, J. (1983) Hysterectomy: dispelling the myth – 1, *Nursing Times*, Vol. 79, Occasional Paper 30, 23 November, pp. 52–4.

— (1983) Hysterectomy: dispelling the myth – 2, *Nursing Times*, Vol. 79, Occasional Paper 31, 30 November, pp. 44–6.

Wright, S. (1985) Patient's page: conspiracy of silence (hysterectomy), *Nursing Mirror*, Vol. 160, 15 May, pp. 47–8.

11

Care of the Patient with a Skin Disorder or Burn

Care of the Patient with a Skin Disorder

NURSING PROCESS OVERVIEW

PSYCHOLOGICAL CONSIDERATIONS

1. Patients with dermatological problems can see and feel their problems and are more disturbed by their complaints than many patients with other conditions.
2. Skin eruptions evoke feelings of shame, disgust, avoidance, withdrawal and anger that compound the problems of management of patients with skin conditions.
3. Irritation is frequently a feature of skin disease and produces loss of sleep, anxiety and depression, which in turn reinforce discomfort and fatigue.
4. Cosmetic needs constitute the underlying motive that brings the patient to treatment.
5. Nursing support requires understanding, unending patience and continuing encouragement for these patients.

Assessment

1. Be aware that many systemic conditions may be accompanied by dermatological features.
2. The skin may be a portal of entry for locally invasive disseminated infection.

HISTORY

1. Obtain a dermatological history.
   a. How long has the patient had the skin condition?
   b. Has it occurred previously?
   c. Were there any other symptoms besides the rash?
   d. What site was first affected?
   e. What did the rash/lesion look like when it first appeared?
   f. How did it spread?
   g. What is the distribution of the lesion – symmetrical, linear, circular?
   h. Are there itching, burning, tingling or crawling sensations? Loss of sensation?
   i. Is it worse at a particular time?
   j. Does the patient have any idea how it started?
   k. Is there a history of hay fever, asthma, urticaria? (These problems are associated with eczema.)
   l. Was the appearance of the eruption related to the intake of food?
   m. Was there a relationship between a specific event and the outbreak of the rash/lesion?
   n. What medications, creams, ointments, lotions have been applied to the lesion? This has to include over-the-counter medications.
   o. What is the patient's occupation?
   p. What is in his immediate environment (plants, animals) that might be precipitating the problem?
   q. Ask if there is anything else the patient wishes to talk about in regard to this problem.
2. Describe the dermatosis (abnormal condition of the skin) clearly and in detail.
   a. What is (are) the colour(s) of the lesion?
   b. Is there redness, heat, pain or swelling?
   c. How large an area is involved; where is it?
   d. Is the eruption macular, papular, scaling, oozing, discrete, confluent?

EXAMINATION OF THE SKIN

1. Ask the patient to undress; the entire skin must be examined.
2. Have good lighting available. Use a hand magnifying lens to inspect for fine detail (altered skin markings, loss of skin lines, etc).
3. Inspect the skin in an orderly sequence: hair, scalp, nails, buccal mucosa, skin surface.
4. Assess the general appearance of the skin, observing temperature, moisture, dryness, skin texture (rough or smooth).
5. Look at the distribution, arrangement and grouping of the rash/lesions. Compare the left and right sides of the body.
6. Note the shape, border, colour, texture and surface of the lesion.

7. Palpate the shape, border, texture and surface of the lesion.
8. Use a metric ruler to measure the size of lesions – to compare extension of lesions from baseline measurements.

ASSESSMENT OF PATIENTS WITH DARK OR BLACK SKIN

1. Healthy dark skin has a reddish undertone; buccal mucosa, tongue, lips and nails normally appear pink.
2. Lightening, darkening or blotching of the skin are very noticeable and can cause emotional distress.
   a. Hyperpigmentation of the mouth is normal in some individuals.
   b. Some black people have pigmented streaks on nails; usually normal.
3. The degree of pigmentation of the black-skinned patient may affect the appearance of a lesion; lesions may be black, purple or grey (instead of tan or red colour that is seen in the white-skinned patient).
4. Certain procedures (freezing, topical peeling and drying agents, or diseases) can cause hypopigmentation (loss or decrease in skin colour) or hyperpigmentation (increase in colour). These changes are more apparent in dark-skinned patients.

EXAMINATION OF DARK OR BLACK SKIN

1. Have good lighting; look in mouth and nail beds as well as entire skin area.
2. Palpate all suspicious areas.
3. For rash:
   a. Ask the patient if he has an area of itching.
   b. Stretch the skin gently to decrease the reddish tone and make the rash stand out.
   c. Palpate by running fingertips lightly over the skin – to feel the differences in skin temperature and to feel the borders of the rash.
   d. Palpate the lymph nodes; take the patient's temperature.
4. For erythema:
   a. Inspect for a purplish–greyish cast of skin.
   b. Palpate for increase in warmth and for signs of smoothness (oedema) or hardness – to detect possible infection.
5. For cyanosis:
   a. Look for a grey cast of the skin.
   b. Inspect areas around the mouth, lips, over cheek bones and earlobes.
   c. Evaluate for the usual signs of shock (see p. 63).

6. Describe and document the dermatosis clearly and in detail.
   a. What is (are) the colour(s) of the lesion?
   b. Is there redness, heat, pain, or swelling?
   c. How large an area is involved; where is it?
   d. Is the eruption macular, papular, scaling, oozing, discrete, confluent?
   e. What is the distribution of the lesion – symmetrical, linear, circular?

DESCRIPTION OF SKIN LESIONS
Primary lesions (initial lesions)

1. Macule – flat discoloration of the skin; of various sizes, shapes and colours.
2. Papule – a solid, raised lesion.
3. Nodule – a raised lesion that is larger and deeper than a papule.
4. Vesicle – a small collection of fluid in or under the epidermis.
5. Bulla – a large vesicle or blister.
6. Pustule – an elevation of the skin that contains pus; may form as a result of purulent changes in a vesicle.
7. Wheal – transient elevation of the skin caused by oedema of the dermis and surrounding capillary dilatation.
8. Plaque – a patch on the skin or mucous membrane.
9. Cyst – a tumour that contains semi-solid or liquid material in a membranous sac.

Secondary lesions (changes that take place in primary lesions and possibly modify them)

1. Scales – heaped-up horny layer of dead epidermis; may develop as a result of inflammatory changes.
2. Crusts – a covering formed by the drying of serum, blood or pus on the skin.
3. Excoriations – linear scratch marks or traumatized area of skin. May be self-produced.
4. Fissure – a crack in the skin, usually from marked drying and longstanding inflammation.
5. Erosion – lesion formed by loss of epidermis from mucous membranes or skin.
6. Ulcer – lesion formed by local destruction of the epidermis and part or all of the underlying dermis.
7. Lichenification – thickening of skin accompanied by accentuation of skin markings.
8. Scar – a fibrotic change in the skin following a destructive process.
9. Atrophy – loss of substance.

SELECTED DERMATOLOGICAL DIAGNOSTIC TESTS

1. Wood's light examination – a special long-wave ultraviolet light produced by a Wood's lamp induces visible fluorescence in certain skin lesions; best seen in a darkened room.
2. Skin biopsy – performed to obtain tissues for examination.
3. Patch testing:
   a. Used to document contact sensitivity or allergy.
   b. Suspected allergens are placed on normal skin beneath patches of tape.
   c. Patches are removed and the skin under the patches is examined at specified intervals.
4. Fungal scraping – scales from a lesion are scraped with a scalpel and placed on a glass slide, covered with potassium hydroxide (KOH), and examined.
5. Tzanck smear:
   a. Used for cytological evaluation of blistering diseases of the skin.
   b. Suspected vesicle or pustule is opened, and contents applied to a glass slide and examined after staining.
6. Clinical photographs – reveal nature and extent of skin condition and show progress or improvement from treatment.

PATIENT PROBLEMS

1. Potential alteration in skin integrity related to change in barrier function of skin.
2. Potential nonadherence to treatment regimen related to length of treatment or the lifestyle adjustments required.
3. Lack of knowledge of underlying cause of ailment and methods of treating.
4. Potential for infection related to entry of organisms through break in skin.
5. Potential fluid and electrolyte imbalance related to loss of tissue fluids and serum from denuded skin.
6. Pain and discomfort related to irritated nerve endings in open lesions.
7. Disturbance in self-awareness related to unsightly skin appearance.
8. Ineffective coping related to emotional drain of dealing with painful, unsightly skin condition.

Planning and implementation
NURSING INTERVENTIONS
Reduction in pain and discomfort and pruritus
1. Examine area of involvement:
   a. Attempt to discover the cause of discomfort.

b. Record observations in detail, using descriptive terminology.
   c. Be aware that *sudden* onset of a generalized rash may indicate a drug allergy.
2. Advise the patient to employ measures that produce vasoconstriction:
   a. Maintain cool, humid environment – itching is aggravated by heat, chemicals and physical irritants.
   b. Eliminate irritants and strong and perfumed soaps.
   c. Reduce excess clothing or bedding.
   d. Provide tepid, cooling baths or cool, wet dressings – gradual evaporation of water from dressings cools the skin and relieves pruritus.
3. Treat dryness (xerosis) as prescribed.

NURSING ALERT
Xerosis (dry skin) is a common skin problem of the elderly, resulting from diminished sebaceous secretion and a slower rate of perspiration.

   a. Keep humidity above 40 per cent; use a humidifier.
   b. Avoid excessive bathing and excessive exposure to soaps, solvents, etc.
   c. Apply emollient to moist skin frequently, especially after baths or compresses.
4. Apply prescribed lotions or ointments.
5. Supply analgesic and antipruritic medications as prescribed.
6. Administer tranquillizing agents or sedatives as prescribed and as necessary.
7. Instruct the patient to refrain from self-medication with salves or lotions that are commercially advertised.

Reduction in inflammation
1. Instruct the patient clearly and in detail to ensure that treatments are carried out as prescribed.
2. Apply continuous or intermittent wet dressings as prescribed to reduce intensity of inflammation.
3. Remove crusts and scales before applying topical medications.
4. Use topical medications containing corticosteroids as prescribed and as indicated.
   a. Observe lesion periodically for changes in response to therapy.
   b. Instruct the patient about possible ill-effects of long-term use of potent topical steroids.

Removal of crust formation and management of oozing

1. Provide tub baths and wet dressings to loosen exudates and scales.
2. Remove medications with mineral oil before reapplying fresh medication.
3. Use mildly astringent solutions to precipitate proteins and decrease oozing.
4. Supply a high-protein diet if oozing is voluminous and serum loss is substantial.
5. Administer antibiotics as prescribed and indicated.

Protection of skin from trauma and infection

1. Protect healthy skin from maceration when applying wet dressings.
2. Remove moisture from skin by blotting gently and avoiding friction.
3. Guard carefully against risk of thermal injury from excessively hot wet dressings.
4. Advise the patient to use sun-screening agents to prevent actinic damage (chemical changes from ultraviolet light).

Coping mechanisms to deal with skin condition

1. Help the patient to accept the prolonged treatment that some skin conditions require.
2. Listen empathetically to expressions of grief about changes in body image.
3. Assist the anxious patient to improve his insight and to identify and cope with his problems.
4. Mobilize the patient's support systems.
5. Advise the patient of available cosmetic measures to conceal disfiguring conditions.

Evaluation

EXPECTED OUTCOMES

1. Patient obtains relief of itching and pain – states that itching is relieved; no excoriation or scratch marks; no complaints of discomfort; skin begins to regain healthy appearance.
2. Patient follows treatment as prescribed and understands rationale for measures taken – carries out the prescribed baths, application of lotions and wet dressings; dries skin carefully after washing; takes medication if prescribed.
3. Patient avoids infection or adheres to treatment if infection occurs; takes care to avoid trauma or maceration to skin; applies antibiotic ointments or takes antibiotic medication as prescribed.
4. Patient demonstrates an improved self-image and coping abilities – appears less self-conscious; is not afraid to socialize or be seen by others; uses concealing and highlighting techniques to enhance appearance.

SKIN TREATMENTS

OPEN WET DRESSINGS

Purposes

1. Cleanse skin of exudates, crusts, scales – thus making a cleaner and drier surface.
2. Reduce inflammation by producing vasoconstriction – thus decreasing vasodilatation and the local blood flow present in inflammation.
3. Maintain drainage of infected areas.

Clinical uses

1. Vesicular, bullous, pustular and ulcerative disorders.
2. Acute inflammatory conditions.
3. Erosions.
4. Exudative, crusted surfaces. (See Table 11.1.)

BATHS

Baths are useful for applying medications to large areas of the skin, removing crusts, scales and old medications, and relieving inflammation and itching. See Table 11.2.

TOPICAL MEDICATIONS

See Table 11.3.

Patient education

1. Use topical medication *only* as directed.
2. Wash hands thoroughly before applying.
3. Avoid reapplying prescribed topical agent at frequent intervals to improve appearance or for cosmetic purposes; may cause further irritation or impede healing.
4. Do not use over-the-counter hydrocortisone preparations indiscriminately because chronic abuse can produce steroid rosacea and thinning of the skin.

DRESSINGS FOR SKIN CONDITIONS

Occlusive dressing

An airtight plastic film is applied to cover medicated skin (usually corticosteroid) (Figure 11.1).

1. Enhances absorption of topically applied medication.
2. Increases penetration of corticosteroids into the skin, thus enhancing anti-inflammatory effect.
3. Produces moisture retention; prevents medication from evaporating.

Table 11.1   Open wet dressings

Solution and material	Desired effect	Nursing action
Solution Cool tapwater Normal saline Burow's solution (aluminium acetate solution) Magnesium sulphate Potassium permanganate	Effective in treating oozing dermatosis or swollen, infected dermatitis (furunculitis, cellulitis)	Keep dressing cool or at room temperature Moisten compress to the point of slight dripping Compresses may be remoistened with asepto syringe
Material Soft towelling Napkins Soft cotton sheeting	Relieves inflammation, burning and itching Has cooling effect Useful for removing crusts Cleansing and soothing	Add ice cubes to solution if coolness is desired Apply for 15 minutes every two to three hours unless otherwise indicated Keep patient warm if extensive areas are to be compressed Do not treat more than a third of the body at one time Discard dressing material daily *Caution*: Avoid burns

Table 11.2   Types of bath

Bath solution and medication	Desired effect	Nursing action
Water	Same effects as wet dressings	Fill the bath half full – 120 litres
Saline	Used for widely disseminated lesions	
Colloidal-Oatmeal or Aveeno	Antipruritic and drying	Keep the water at a comfortable temperature (approximately 36°C)
Sodium bicarbonate	Cooling	Do not allow the water to cool excessively
Starch		Use a bath mat – *medications may cause bath to be slippery*
Medicated tars (follow package directions) Polytar emollient, psoriderm bath emulsion, liquor picis carbonis	Tar baths are used for psoriasis and chronic eczematous conditions	Apply a lubricating agent to wet skin after bath if emollient action is desired – increases hydration Dry by blotting with a towel
Bath oils Oilatum emollient, emulsifying ointment	Bath oils are used for antipruritic and emollient actions Used for acute and subacute eczematous eruptions	Keep room warm to minimize temperature fluctuations Encourage patient to wear light, loose clothing after the bath
Antiseptics Potassium permanganate, hexachlorophane Antifungal Sterzac	Used for infected lesions and when mild antiseptic action is required	

Table 11.3   Topical medications

Type of medication	Desired effect	Nursing action
Lotions Liquid vehicles for carrying medication; act by evaporation	Lubricate Cool through water evaporation May be protective, antiparasitic, antifungal, antipruritic; may act as sunscreen	May be applied with cotton gauze or soft paintbrush
Ointments and creams Have greasy, nongreasy or penetrating base depending on nature of lesion and drug applied	Lubricate Protect the skin Serve as vehicle for medications Retard water loss Used in chronic or localized skin conditions Cause vasoconstriction; reduce blood flow to skin	Apply ointments with a wooden tongue depressor Creams are rubbed into the skin by hand Teach patient to apply his own ointment or cream Ointments may have to be covered with a dressing to prevent soiling of clothing.
Gels Semi-solid emulsions that become liquid when applied to skin	Dries as a thin greaseless, nonocclusive, nonstaining film; some topical steroids are prescribed in gel form	See corticosteroid agents below
Topical adrenocorticosteroid agents (many preparations available)	Have anti-inflammatory action	Apply to localized area requiring medication Use only a small amount Use with occlusive dressing as directed – enhances penetration Nurse should wear gloves when applying steroids to prevent absorption through her skin
Powders (usually with a talc, zinc oxide, bentonite or cornstarch base)	Act as hygroscopic agents (take up moisture) Increase evaporation; absorb perspiration Reduce friction	Dispense with shaker top Avoid accumulating powder in intertriginous areas
Pastes Suspension of powder in a greasy base, usually soft paraffin	Serve as a vehicle for medication, e.g. dithranol in Lassar's paste	Apply thickly with a spatula Apply dithranol only to affected areas Dust with powder Cover with tubular gauze Remove old paste with liquid paraffin
Intralesional therapy Injection with a tuberculin syringe of sterile suspension of medication (usually suspension of corticosteroid) into or just below a lesion	Has anti-inflammatory action	Be aware that local atrophy may result Check patient for anaphylactoid reaction which may occur
Systemic medications Adrenocorticosteroids Antibiotics Antihistamines Sedatives and tranquillizers Analgesics Antineoplastics		

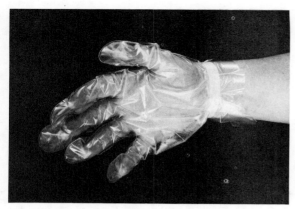

Figure 11.1a. A plastic glove may be used for occlusion treatment of the hands. Seal

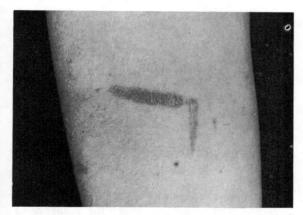

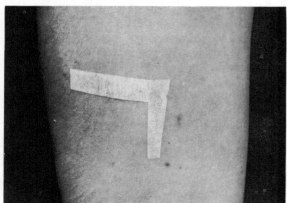

Figure 11.1b and c. Plastic surgical tape containing corticosteroid in the adhesive layer can be cut to size and applied to individual lesions (courtesy Department of Medical Illustration, The Institute of Dermatology, London)

NURSING ALERT

Prolonged use of occlusive dressings may cause skin atrophy, striae, telangiectasia, folliculitis, nonhealing ulceration, erythema or systemic absorption of corticosteroids. Dressings should be removed for 8 out of 24 hours, to prevent some of these complications.

Plastic surgical tape containing corticosteroid is also available and can be cut to size.

Other dressings

1. Fingers and toes – tubular gauze or, when required, bigger gauze or cotton dressings held in place with tubular gauze (Tubinette, Tube-gauze).
2. Hands – disposable polyethylene gloves, sealed at wrists; cotton gloves.
3. Feet – cotton socks or disposable plastic bags; tubular gauze socks.
4. Extremities (arms and legs) – cotton cloth covered with tubular material.
5. Groin, perineum – disposable nappies; cotton cloth folded in nappy fashion; napkin, tubular gauze pants.
6. Axillae – cotton cloth taped in place or held by cotton bandage or tubular gauze.
7. Trunk – cotton or light flannel pyjamas or tubular gauze suit.
8. Scalp – turban or plastic shower cap or tubular gauze cap.
9. Whole body – a suit is made of the various sizes of tubular gauze.
10. Face – mask made from gauze with holes cut out for eyes, nose and mouth.

SEBORRHOEIC DERMATOSES

Dermatoses refers to abnormal skin conditions. Seborrhoea is excessive production of sebum (secretion of sebaceous glands) in those areas where glands are normally found in large numbers (face, scalp, scrotum).

Seborrhoeic dermatitis is a chronic inflammatory disease of the skin with a predilection for areas that are well supplied with sebaceous glands or that lie between folds of skin where the bacterial count is high.

CLINICAL FEATURES

1. Characteristic lesion (remarkably varied):
   a. Dry, moist or greasy scales.
   b. Crusted pinkish-yellow or yellowish patches of varying shapes and sizes.

c. Possible erythema (redness), fissuring (cracking) and secondary infection.
d. Dry, flaky desquamation on scalp with profuse amount of fine, powdery scales (dandruff).
2. Sites: scalp (dandruff), eyebrows, eyelids, nasolabial crease, lips, ears, axillae, under breast, groin, gluteal crease.
3. Seborrhoeic dermatitis is associated with genetic predisposition; hormones, nutrition, infection and emotional stress influence its course.
4. There is a tendency to lifelong recurrences lasting for weeks, months or years.

TREATMENT AND NURSING MANAGEMENT
Objective
Control the disorder (no known cure at this time) and allow the skin to repair itself.
1. Advise patient to remove external irritants and avoid excess heat and perspiration – rubbing and scratching will prolong the disorder.
2. Suggest local remedies.
   a. For scalp – to control dandruff.
      (i) Give the hair an initial cleansing shampoo to remove accumulated scale.
      (ii) Use shampoo with zinc pyrithione suspension (Head and Shoulders or ZP11); leave shampoo on scalp 10 minutes; rinse thoroughly.
      (iii) Shampoos containing tar are also effective, especially in controlling itching.
      (iv) Shampoo daily or once or twice weekly, depending on condition of the scalp.
      (v) Other shampoos based on detergents, selenium sulphide or antibiotic agents are often effective.
      CAUTION: Observe precautions on container.
   b. Seborrhoeic dermatitis of the body and face.
      (i) May respond to a topically applied corticosteroid cream.
      (ii) Use with extreme caution on the eyelids, since it can induce glaucoma in predisposed individuals.
      (iii) Prolonged use of fluorinated steroids on face can produce an acne-like eruption. Prolonged use in intertriginous areas can produce striae and atrophy. Therefore, plain hydrocortisone is used.
3. Systemic steroids are given on rare occasions for severe and acute seborrhoeic dermatitis.
4. Use antibacterial measures if exudation and crusting occur.
   a. Systemic antibiotic may be required to prevent infection spreading.
   b. Topical antibiotics (cream or lotion) may be applied.
5. Watch for occurrence of secondary candidiasis (yeast infection) that may occur in body creases or folds.
   a. Advise patient to cleanse intertriginous areas carefully; ensure maximum aeration of skin.
   b. Patient with coincidental candidiasis should be investigated for diabetes mellitus.

PATIENT EDUCATION
1. Advise the patient to avoid aggravating systemic factors – overwork, lack of sleep, infection, emotional stress.
2. Seborrheic dermatitis may be made worse by conditions that increase perspiration.
3. Sunlight may be beneficial.
4. Seborrheic dermatitis does recur, and treatment should be recommenced.
5. Encourage patient to eat a well-balanced diet.

ACNE VULGARIS

Acne vulgaris is a chronic disorder of the sebaceous (oil) glands, characterized by the presence of comedones (blackheads), whiteheads, papules, pustules, nodules and cysts. It usually begins at puberty (or earlier) and usually clears by 30 years of age.

PREDISPOSING FACTORS
1. Genetic predisposition – strong genetic overtones.
2. Hormonal changes of adolescence – sebaceous glands start to enlarge under the influence of adrenal hormones; there is increased seborrhoea.
3. In adults – can occur postpartum or related to use of oral contraceptive drugs.
4. Can be aggravated by anxiety, stress, emotional tension.

ALTERED PHYSIOLOGY
Stimulation of androgenic hormones → increase in amount and thickness of oil secretion → to colonization by bacteria of lipids arising in sebaceous glands → obstruction of sebaceous glands by blackheads (comedones) → disruption of the follicular epithelium, allowing discharge of the follicular contents in the dermis → inflammatory reaction → papules → pustules → nodules → cysts.

TREATMENT AND NURSING MANAGEMENT
The overall objectives of treatment and nursing management are to:

1. Reduce colonization by *Corynebacterium acnes* bacteria.
2. Prevent follicular obstruction.
3. Reduce inflammation and combat secondary infection.
4. Minimize scarring.
5. Eliminate factors that may predispose to acne.

The therapeutic regimen is tailored to the individual patient's needs.

Prevent obstruction of the oil glands

1. Wash face gently three times daily with mild soap and water – to remove surface oil. Mild abrasive soaps and drying preparations may be used for mild involvement (mainly comedones).
2. Shampoo scalp nightly or twice weekly with medicated shampoo.
3. Use bath brush if back is involved.

Topical agents for more severe involvement
Objective
Clear keratin plugs from follicular ducts.

1. Topical vitamin A acid, tretinoin (Retin-A) – speeds up the cellular turnover, which forces out the comedones; produces a clinical improvement in patients with comedonal acne. Instructions to patient:
   a. Apply vitamin A acid to thoroughly dry skin. Wet skin enhances penetration and increases the potential for irritation.
   b. Apply Retin-A as tolerated (available as gel, cream, liquid). Some individuals tolerate applications daily; others only every two or three days.
   c. Warn the patient that the symptoms may worsen during the early weeks of treatment due to action of medication on previously unseen comedones; there is possibility of some erythema and peeling. Improvement may take four to eight weeks.
   d. Be cautious during first few weeks about exposure to sun (including sun-lamps) – anti-keratinizing effect of tretinoin makes patient more sensitive to sunburn.
   e. Avoid other irritants, such as strong and perfumed soaps.
   f. Read the product information brochure.
2. Topical benzoyl peroxide, in gel base (PanOxyl) – exerts an antibacterial effect and is useful for inflammatory acne.
   a. Apply sparingly once daily and adjust to needs of patient thereafter.
   b. May dry the skin and produce some peeling.
3. Topical antibiotic – recent developments have shown some success with the use of clindamycin 50 per cent in industrial methylated spirit.
   a. Apply sparingly once or twice daily after washing.
   b. Apply to the acne-affected areas as one would an astringent or aftershave lotion.

Systemic therapy
Systemic antibiotics
Appear to reduce fatty acids on skin surface; thought to suppress anaerobic lipase-producing bacteria (*C. acnes*) in the skin with reduction of the inflammation-inciting free fatty acids of sebum; useful when patient does not respond to topical therapy.

1. Tetracycline, minocycline or erythromycin is given and adjusted according to therapeutic response (250–500mg daily).
2. Long-term, low-dose antibiotic may be given (usually at least three to six months).
3. May take several weeks for effect of antibiotics to show.
4. Instruct the patient to take tetracycline at least one hour before or two hours after mealtimes; avoid taking any dairy products (milk, ice cream) within two hours before or after taking medication – tetracycline is poorly absorbed with food.
5. Side-effects of tetracycline include photosensitivity, nausea, diarrhoea, superinfection and candidiasis. (Vaginitis in women; cutaneous infection in either sex, but more often in men.) Should not be taken during pregnancy.

Retinoid therapy
Oral retinoids (isotretinoin), synthetic derivatives, are being used to treat severe, recalcitrant, nodular–cystic acne that is unresponsive to conventional therapy; appears to have an inhibitory effect on sebum production and sebaceous gland secretion.

1. Adverse effects, comparable to hypervitaminosis (mucocutaneous and systemic), are frequently encountered.
   a. Mucocutaneous effects – cheilitis, facial dermatitis, dry nose and mouth, dry eyes, conjunctivitis, pruritus, epistaxis.
   b. Systemic effects – headache, thirst, arthralgia, fatigue, elevation of triglyceride and cholesterol levels, and lowering of high-density lipoproteins.
   c. Headache is a serious symptom. It may be associated with increased intracranial pressure, papilloedema, projectile vomiting and other signs of pseudotumour cerebri. Persistent headache should be evaluated by the doctor.

2. Patient education for those receiving retinoid therapy:
   a. Have careful monitoring of lipid status.
   b. Women of childbearing potential should be counselled about risks to fetus and advised to use an effective form of contraception. Some doctors advocate pregnancy tests before beginning drug therapy in women of childbearing age.
   c. Avoid vitamin supplements containing vitamin A because of possible additive toxic effects.

Oestrogen therapy
Usually in form of oral contraceptive that combines an oestrogenic and a progestational agent.
1. Oestrogens may be given to antagonize androgens – counteracts production of sebum.
2. Usually reserved for young women with severe cystic acne.

Acne surgery
1. Comedo extraction (see below).
2. Incision and drainage of cysts – may be required in large, fluctuant, nodular-cystic lesions.
3. Intralesional injection of corticosteroids (triamcinolone acetonide). Diluted steroid suspension is injected using a small syringe with a needle to distend the cyst – leads to rapid resolution.
4. Cryosurgery (freezing with liquid nitrogen) – for indurated lesions and cysts.

5. Dermabrasion – surgical planing of the skin.
   Note: Carries risk of causing hyperpigmentation.

PATIENT EDUCATION
1. Keep hands away from face.
2. Do not squeeze pimples or blackheads – squeezing the skin makes acne worse. The majority of blackheads are pushed down into the skin by squeezing. This may cause the follicle to be ruptured.
3. Acne is not caused by dirt and cannot be washed away; it is a chemical imbalance that causes the oil in the skin to form blackheads.
4. Acne is *not* related to sexual activity.
5. Eat a healthy diet; eliminate any food that you feel worsens your acne.
6. Keep hair off the face; wash hair daily if necessary.
7. Avoid friction and trauma:
   a. Do not prop your hands against your face.
   b. Avoid overzealous washing of face, rubbing the face, pressure from tight collars/helmets.
8. Avoid cosmetics (including cleansing creams) – contain chemicals that can aggravate acne.
9. Avoid perspiration around the face.
10. Be able to talk over your problems with an understanding person – acne may become a source of power struggle between teenager and parent.
11. Continue treatment even though your skin clears.

GUIDELINES: COMEDO EXTRACTION*

A comedo (blackhead) is a mass composed of lipids and keratin that forms a solid plug in a dilated follicular opening (pore).

UNDERLYING CONSIDERATIONS
1. Blackheads are approximately 4mm deep and cannot be washed away.
2. Comedones are considered end-stage lesions and their removal is only of temporary benefit. However, their removal is necessary in some patients.

EQUIPMENT
Light
Magnifying loupe
Alcohol and sponges
Comedo extractor

* This procedure must be performed with skill by a prepared person.

PROCEDURE

Nursing action	Rationale
1. Apply warm compresses to face for a few minutes.	Facilitates emptying of the lesions.
2. Wipe off the site with an alcohol sponge.	For antisepsis.
3. Gently express the contents of the lesion through the hole of the comedo extractor.	Overly vigorous attempts to express comedones may result in an increased inflammatory response.
4. Wipe off the site with a fresh alcohol sponge.	

BACTERIAL INFECTIONS

FURUNCLES

A furuncle, or boil, is an acute inflammation arising deep within one or more hair follicles. Furunculosis refers to multiple or recurrent lesions. A stye is a furuncle that forms on eyelid margin.

CLINICAL FEATURES
1. Initial occurrence – usually begins around a hair follicle.
2. Sites of predilection – back of neck, axillae, buttocks.
3. Causative factors – irritation, pressure, friction, excessive perspiration, shaving of axillae (in people with lowered resistance).
4. Symptoms – tenderness, pain and surrounding cellulitis; after furuncle localizes, the centre becomes boggy and fluctuant and a soft yellow or white head appears on the surface.

NURSING ALERT
Every person with boils should be checked for diabetes mellitus.

TREATMENT AND NURSING MANAGEMENT
1. Protect area from irritation, squeezing and trauma.
2. Apply hot wet compresses – to increase vascularization and hasten resolution.
3. Cleanse surrounding skin with antibacterial soap.
4. Apply antibacterial ointment as prescribed to surrounding skin – to prevent spillage and seeding of the bacteria when furuncle ruptures or is incised.
5. Prepare for surgical drainage when furuncle has become localized and shows fluctuation (wavelike motion upon palpation); furuncle may rupture spontaneously.
6. Systemic antibiotic therapy is given (selected by sensitivity study) if spreading still occurs or if area of involvement poses a risk of complications.

NURSING ALERT
Take special precautions with boil on face, since the skin area drains directly into the cranial venous sinuses. There is danger of cavernous sinus thrombosis.
1. *Place patient with boils on nose, lip, groin, perineal or perianal region on bed rest.*
2. *Course of systemic antibiotic therapy is given – to control spread of infection.*

PATIENT EDUCATION
Instruct the patient as follows:
1. Keep draining lesion covered with a dressing.
2. Wash hands thoroughly after caring for lesion.
3. Wrap soiled dressings in paper and burn.
4. Discard razor blades after each use; keep razor in alcohol between shaves.
5. Bathe with bacteriostatic soap.

CARBUNCLES

A carbuncle is an abscess of the skin and subcutaneous tissues – an extension of a furuncle invading multiple follicles; usually caused by staphylococcal infection.

CLINICAL FEATURES
1. Seen most frequently within the thick, fibrous, inelastic skin of the back of the neck and upper back.

2. More apt to occur in older and debilitated persons; especially frequent in diabetics.

NURSING ALERT
Every patient with a carbuncle should be suspected of having diabetes until it is disproved.

3. Symptoms:
   a. Fever, leucocytosis, extreme pain and prostration.
   b. Bacteraemia is common because the extensive inflammation makes it difficult to completely wall off the infection, so that absorption of toxins takes place; extension of infection to bloodstream may take place.

TREATMENT AND NURSING MANAGEMENT
1. Administer antibiotic (based on sensitivity studies) – antibiotic is continued until infective process is controlled.
2. Determine whether there is an underlying disease condition (diabetes, haematological disease, etc).
3. Prepare for surgical incision and drainage when definite fluctuance occurs. (Local surgical incision is usually necessary.)
4. Symptomatic treatments (infusions, tepid sponges, etc) are used for the toxic patient.

IMPETIGO

Impetigo (impetigo contagiosa) is a superficial infection of the skin caused by streptococci, staphylococci or multiple bacteria. Bullous impetigo is a superficial infection of the skin caused by *Staphylococcus aureus*, characterized by the formation of bullae from the original vesicles.

CLINICAL FEATURES
1. Lesion appears as discrete, thin-walled vesicle that ruptures and becomes covered with a loosely adherent, honey-yellow crust.
2. Crusts are easily removed and reveal smooth, red, moist surface on which new crusts soon develop.
3. Areas affected – exposed parts of body (face, hands, neck and extremities).
4. Impetigo is a contagious disease. It is seen in all ages, but is particularly common among undernourished children living in poor hygienic conditions.
5. Sources of infection – children's pets, dirty fingernails, other children, adults, barber shops, beauty parlours, swimming pools.

6. May be secondary to pediculosis capitis, scabies, herpes simplex, insect bites, poison ivy, eczema.

TREATMENT AND NURSING MANAGEMENT
1. Give a prescribed systemic antibiotic (benzathine penicillin, erythromycin, oral penicillin). Glomerulonephritis is a complication of impetigo, depending on strain of streptococcus found. However, this therapy has not been proved to prevent nephritis.
2. Give penicillinase-resistant penicillin for staphylococci that may be penicillin-resistant.
3. Wash lesions with anti-bacterial soap or treat with warm, moist compresses to remove the loci of bacterial growth and to give topical medication an opportunity to reach the infected site.
4. Apply a prescribed topical antibiotic cream (neomycin, bacitracin, polymyxin B) after crust removal.
5. Wear gloves while treating patient.

PATIENT EDUCATION
1. The patient and family should bathe at least once daily with bacteriostatic soap as recommended.
2. The child with impetigo should be observed for at least seven weeks for signs of acute glomerulonephritis.
3. Keep infected child away from other children.
4. Dispose of tissues and materials that come in contact with lesions.
5. Encourage good hygienic practices to prevent spread of disease from one skin area to another and from one person to another.

MYCOTIC (FUNGAL) INFECTIONS

Fungi are plant-like organisms that feed on organic matter; they are responsible for a variety of common skin infections. The mycoses affecting primarily the skin may be divided into three groups: dermatophyte (*Trichophyton*, *Epidermophyton* and *Microsporum* genera), candida (*Candida albicans*) and *Malassezia furfur*.

TINEA PEDIS (ATHLETE'S FOOT) OR RINGWORM OF THE FEET

Tinea pedis (athlete's foot) is a superficial fungal infection which may manifest itself as an acute, inflammatory, vesicular process or as a chronic rash involving the soles of the feet and the interdigital web spaces.

CLINICAL FEATURES
1. Tinea pedis is the most common fungal infection.
2. Causes intense itching and burning.
3. Lymphangitis and cellulitis may occur when bacterial superinfection is present.

DIAGNOSTIC EVALUATION
1. Direct examination of scrapings (skin, nails, hair).
2. Isolation of the organism in culture.

TREATMENT
1. Use soaks (potassium permanganate, Burow's solution, saline) to remove scales, crusts, debris and residual medications; also for mild antiseptic effect.
2. Apply fungistatic creams or lotions as prescribed such as tolnaftate (Tinactin), miconazole (Daktarin) or clotrimazole (Canesten) to involved skin.
3. Continue with topical therapy for several weeks – there is a high rate of recurrence.
4. Systemic antifungal agent (griseofulvin) (500mg daily) is given if indicated.

PREVENTIVE MEASURES AND PATIENT EDUCATION
Instruct the patient to keep feet dry – moisture encourages the growth of fungi.
1. Dry carefully between the toes.
2. Alternate shoes – to permit adequate drying of shoes between wearings.
3. Change socks frequently.
4. Wear light cotton socks or stockings with cotton feet – synthetic material does not absorb perspiration as well as cotton.
5. Wear perforated shoes if feet perspire excessively – to permit aeration of feet.
6. Foot powder can be applied twice daily – to keep feet dry.
7. Use clogs in community pools, showers, etc.
8. Use small pieces of cotton between toes at night – to absorb moisture.

TINEA CAPITIS (RINGWORM OF THE SCALP)

Tinea capitis (ringworm of the scalp) is a fungal disease of the scalp.

CLINICAL FEATURES
1. Lesions appear as round, grey, scaly bald patches on the scalp.
2. Sometimes boggy swelling (kerion) occurs in an area of involvement; this may be followed by scarring.
3. Tinea capitis is contagious; usually occurs in prepubertal children.

TREATMENT AND PATIENT EDUCATION
1. Griseofulvin, a fungistatic and fungicidal antibiotic, is given. Take medication with or just after a meal. The presence of fat aids in absorption of the drug.
2. Instruct the patient as follows:
   a. Shampoo scalp two or three times weekly.
   b. Apply topical antifungal preparation as directed – to reduce dissemination of organisms.
   c. Each person should have his own comb and brush. Avoid exchanging headgear.
   d. All infected members of family and all household pets should be treated.

TINEA CORPORIS OR TINEA CIRCINATA

Tinea corporis or tinea circinata is ringworm of the body.

CLINICAL FEATURES
1. Appearance – rings of vesicles with central clearing; appear in clusters.
2. Lesions usually appear on exposed areas of body; may extend to scalp, hair or nails.
3. An infected pet is a common source of infection.
4. Ringworm of the body causes intense itching.

TREATMENT
1. Apply topical antifungal medication as prescribed to small areas (Tinaderm, Daktarin, Canesten).
2. Griseofulvin may be used in very extensive cases. Side-effects include photosensitivity, skin rashes, headache, nausea, etc.

PATIENT EDUCATION
Instruct the patient as follows:
1. Wear clean cotton clothing next to the skin.
2. Use a clean towel daily; dry thoroughly all areas and skin folds that retain moisture.

TINEA CRURIS

Tinea cruris is a superficial fungal infection of the groin, which may extend to the inner thighs and buttock area and is commonly associated with tinea pedis.

CLINICAL FEATURES

1. Appears as a dull-red to red-brown eruption of the upper thighs; then advances outward from the crural (thigh) creases and extends to form circular plaques with elevated scaly or vesicular borders. Itching is usually present.
2. Seen most frequently in joggers, obese individuals and those wearing tight underclothing.

TREATMENT

1. Topical therapy (miconazole cream or lotion; clotrimazole cream and lotion).
2. Griseofulvin (orally) for extensive eruption.
3. Treat concomitant tinea pedis to minimize reinfection.

PATIENT EDUCATION

1. Avoid excessive washing/scrubbing.
2. Avoid nylon underclothing, tight-fitting underwear and prolonged wearing of a wet bathing suit.
3. Wear cotton underwear.

PARASITIC SKIN DISEASES

Three varieties of lice infest man; their itching bites are the cause of many skin problems. Lice bite the skin to obtain blood, which they feed on. They leave their eggs and excrement on the skin and are passed from person to person.

PEDICULOSIS CAPITIS

Pediculosis capitis is an infestation of the scalp by the head louse, *Pediculus humanus* var. *capitis* (Figure 11.2a).

CLINICAL FEATURES

1. Appearance – minute white nits (eggs) (Figure 11.2b) attached to hair shaft in series: usually on scalp and hair at back of head and behind ears.

2. Most often found in children and people with long hair.
3. The bite of the insect causes intense itching, and the resulting scratching may lead to complications such as impetigo, furuncles and enlarged cervical lymph nodes.
4. May be transmitted by direct physical contact or contact with infested combs, brushes, wigs, hats and bedding.

TREATMENT AND NURSING MANAGEMENT

1. Instruct the patient as follows:
   a. Use a shampoo containing gamma benzene hexachloride (Lorexane, Quellada) or malathion 0.5 per cent lotion (Prioderm), as directed.
   b. Shampoo the scalp usually at least four minutes with this preparation; rinse thoroughly.
   c. Comb hair with a fine-tooth metal comb – to remove remaining nits.
   d. Disinfect comb and brushes with Lorexane or Prioderm shampoo; sterilize all washable fomites.
   e. Repeat in 24 hours if necessary.
2. Treat all family members and close contacts.
3. Treat complications – severe pruritus, pyoderma (pus-forming infection of the skin) and dermatitis – with antipruritics, systemic antibiotics and topical corticosteroids.

PATIENT EDUCATION

1. Head lice infestation may happen to anyone; it is not a sign of being dirty.
2. Treatment should be started immediately, since the condition spreads rapidly.
3. Control of school epidemics may be helped by having all of the students shampoo their hair on the same night.

PEDICULOSIS CORPORIS

Pediculosis corporis is an infestation of the body by the body louse, *P. humanus* var. *corporis* (Figure 11.2c and d).

CLINICAL FEATURES

1. The body louse lives chiefly in the seams of undergarments and other clothing, to which it clings.
2. Its bite causes characteristic minute haemorrhagic points.
   a. Widespread excoriations may appear on the back and shoulders.

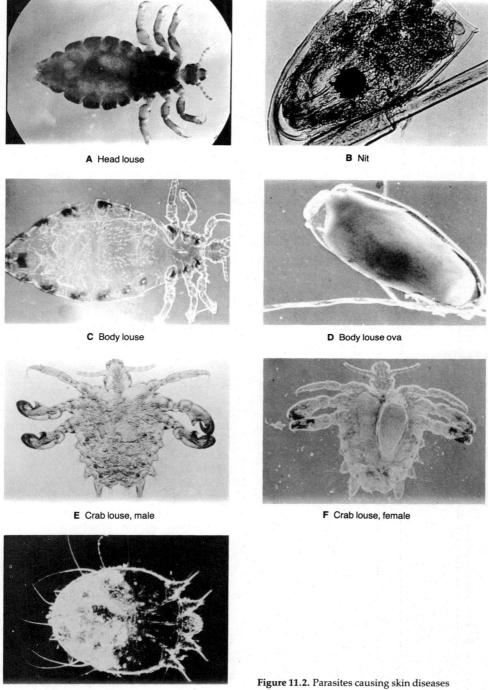

A Head louse

B Nit

C Body louse

D Body louse ova

E Crab louse, male

F Crab louse, female

G Scabies

Figure 11.2. Parasites causing skin diseases (courtesy Reed and Carnrick Research Institute)

b. May produce secondary lesions – hyperaemia, parallel linear scratches and hyperpigmentation in persistent cases.

3. Areas of skin involved are those that come in closest contact with the undergarments (neck, trunk, thighs).

4. The lice may be seen in the seams of clothing. They move to the skin for blood feedings and then return to the clothing.

TREATMENT AND NURSING MANAGEMENT

1. Instruct the patient as follows:
   a. Bathe with soap and water.
   b. Apply gamma benzene hexachloride (Lorexane, Quellada) cream or lotion to trunk and extremities – leave medication on skin 24 hours.
   c. Eliminate parasites and nits from clothing, bedding and sleeping bags. Launder, dry clean, press with hot iron.

2. Examine and treat all family members and contacts.

3. Treat pruritus, secondary bacterial infections and dermatitis.

NURSING ALERT

Body lice are vectors for rickettsial disease, epidemic typhus, relapsing fever, trench fever. The causative organism may be in the gastrointestinal tract of the insect and excreted on the skin surface.

PEDICULOSIS PUBIS

Pediculosis pubis is an infestation by *Phthirus pubis* (crab louse) (Figures 11.2e and f); it is chiefly transmitted by sexual contact and is generally localized to the genital region.

CLINICAL FEATURES

1. Chief symptom is itching.

2. Reddish brown 'dust' (formed from the excretion of the insects) may be found on the underclothing.

3. Lice may infest hairs of chest, axillary hair, beard and eyelashes.

4. Grey-blue macules (1–3cm in diameter) may be seen on the trunk, thighs and axillae as a result of the action of the insects' saliva on bilirubin – converts it to biliverdin.

MANAGEMENT AND PATIENT EDUCATION

1. Instruct the patient as follows:
   a. Bathe with soap and water.

b. Apply gamma benzene hexachloride (Lorexane, Quellada) cream or lotion or malathion 0.5 per cent (Prioderm) to areas of involvement.
   (i) Leave on for the specified time.
   (ii) Treat again in 4–7 days for heavy infestations.
   (iii) Do not apply Lorexane or Quellada to eyebrows.
       (a) Remove nits manually from eyebrows or eyelashes with cotton-tipped applicator or toothpick.
       (b) Apply yellow oxide of mercury or physostigmine ophthalmic ointment before removing nits.
   c. Machine wash all clothing and bedding in a hot wash.

2. Treat all sexual contacts and family members.

3. Screen patient for coexisting venereal disease.

4. Treat secondary bacterial infection, itching and dermatitis.

5. Be sure to follow directions; do not misuse product. Persistent itching is not uncommon even after infestation has been controlled effectively.

SCABIES

Scabies is an infestation of the skin by *Sarcoptes scabiei* (itch mite) (Figure 11.2g). Scabies is transmitted by close personal contact.

CLINICAL FEATURES

1. Primary lesion:
   a. Adult female burrows into superficial layer of skin after fertilization has occurred on skin surface; burrows are short, wavy, brownish or blackish thread-like lesions.
   b. She extends the burrow, laying two or three eggs daily for up to two months, and then dies; larvae hatch in two or three days and migrate to skin surface where they reach maturity in two to three weeks.
   c. Male mites die shortly after mating.

2. Ask patient where itch is most severe at the time you are examining him; look for burrows with a magnifying glass (may or may not see them).

3. Sites – between fingers, on flexor surfaces of wrists and palms, around nipples, in axillary folds, under pendulous breasts, in or near groin or gluteal fold, penis, scrotum.

4. Secondary lesions include vesicles, papules, pustules, excoriations and crusts; bacterial super-

infection of eczematization may complicate the picture.

5. Symptoms – intense itching, more pronounced at night; usually occurs one month after initial infection.
6. The disease may be found in poor persons living under substandard hygienic conditions, but is also found in very clean individuals.
   a. Promoted by close physical contact.
   b. However, infestations are not dependent on sexual activity, since the mites frequently involve the fingers – hand contact may produce infection.
   c. Infestations with mites may also result from contact with dogs, cats and small animals.

TREATMENT AND PATIENT EDUCATION
Instruct patient as follows:

1. Take a warm bath or shower if necessary to remove scaling debris from the crusts. Ensure that the skin is thoroughly dry. Wet skin enhances the absorption of the scabicide and can cause increased irritation and sensitivity.
2. Apply a scabicide such as gamma benzene hexachloride (Quellada lotion) or crotamiton (Eurax cream and lotion) at bedtime.
   a. Apply emulsion all over the body including between fingers and toes and the soles of the feet. Leave out no part except the head and face.
   b. Allow time for the emulsion to dry and repeat the application at once. When this has dried, go to bed.
   c. Leave the medication on for the specified time then take a bath or shower to remove it.
   d. Put on freshly laundered or dry cleaned clothes and change all bed linen, underclothes and night clothes.
   e. A bland ointment may be applied to the skin after completion of treatment.
   f. Treatment should only be repeated on doctor's instructions and not within three weeks.
   g. Benzylbenzoate, malathion (Prioderm) and carbaryl are also used.
3. All family members and close contacts should be treated simultaneously, whether they are infected or not, to eliminate the mites.
4. All used linen must be washed. The cuffs of all coats worn during the previous three weeks must be ironed. Gloves must be washed or laid aside for three weeks. Blankets and other bed linen need not be treated provided that sheets are used.
5. Advise patient that he may be uncomfortable for some weeks – the treatment solution is irritating to the skin and pruritus may remain for a time. Calamine cream will help to relieve itching.

GUIDELINES: SKIN SCRAPING FOR SCABIES

PURPOSE
Demonstrate the mite *Sarcoptes scabiei* (or ova or faeces) in skin scrapings removed from burrows or papules (Figure 11.3).

EQUIPMENT
Hand lens
Mineral oil in dropper bottle
Scalpel and scalpel blade, No. 15
Glass slide/coverslip
Microscope

PROCEDURE
Preparatory phase

Nursing action	Rationale
1. Place a small drop of oil in the middle of a glass slide.	

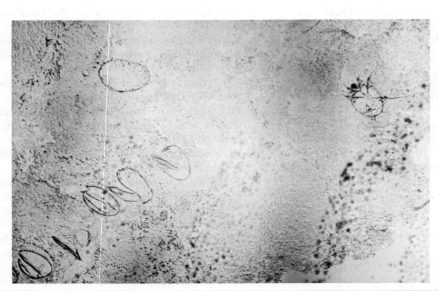

Figure 11.3. Scabies; scraping from a burrow. (Lower left) Hatched eggs. (Upper left) Intact egg. (Upper right) Newly hatched organism (courtesy Mervyn L. Elgart, MD)

Performance phase

Nursing action	**Rationale**
1. Inspect for the burrows of *Sarcoptes scabiei* on webs of fingers, lower abdomen, pubic and axillary areas, legs, arms.	The female scabies mite, ova, and faecal deposits may be found in burrows on the skin.
2. Apply a small amount of mineral oil on unexcoriated burrows or papule.	The mineral oil causes the mite to float and enhances visualization.
3. Scrape the involved skin with the scalpel blade.	
4. Transfer the scrapings to the prepared glass slide and apply coverslip; or pick out the mite with a disposable needle and transfer it to a glass slide.	To avoid air bubble.
5. Examine the slide with a scanning lens of the microscope.	Look for the mites, eggs, and faecal pellets (which outnumber living organisms).

BEDBUG INFESTATION

Two species of bedbugs, *Cimex lectularius* and *C. hemipterus* invade human habitations. These are nocturnal blood-sucking insects.

CLINICAL FEATURES
1. Appearance – bites tend to be grouped in a straight line and consist of haemorrhagic spots associated with papular or wheal-like lesions; there may be a tiny red point marking the original site of the bite.
2. Sites – buttocks, back and extremities are most frequently bitten – patient experiences itching and burning; urticaria (hives) may accompany the lesions.
3. Secondary infection and pyoderma may occur.

PATIENT EDUCATION
1. Direct patient to apply lotions containing menthol and phenol to local areas of bites. Antihistamines may be prescribed for intense itching (e.g. Piriton).
2. Advise patient to eliminate insect by vacuum cleaning and then spraying in crevices of furniture, walls, floors, mattresses and beds.

INFLAMMATORY DERMATOSES

HERPES ZOSTER

Herpes zoster (shingles) is an inflammatory condition in which the virus produces a painful vesicular eruption along the distribution of the nerves from one or more posterior ganglia.

AETIOLOGY
Virus appears to be identical with the causative agent of varicella (chickenpox); herpes zoster may be a reactivation of the latent varicella virus and reflects a lowered immunity.

CLINICAL FEATURES
1. Malaise and gastrointestinal disturbances may precede the eruption.
2. Vesicles appear within 12 to 24 hours.
   a. Characteristic patches of grouped vesicles on erythematous and oedematous skin.
   b. Early vesicles contain serum – they appear purulent and rupture, forming crusts.
   c. Some vesicles dry up without scarring.
3. Eruption appears posteriorly and progresses to the anterior and peripheral distribution of the nerves from one or more posterior ganglia.
4. Eruption usually accompanied or preceded by itching, tenderness and pain, which may radiate over entire region supplied by the nerves. Inflammation is usually unilateral, involving the thoracic, cervical or cranial nerves in a band-like configuration.
5. Clinical course varies from one to three weeks; healing time varies between seven and 26 days.
6. The disease is considered infectious only for the first two or three days and only to those with immunosuppression or to those who have not previously had varicella.
7. There is a greater tendency towards complications and sequelae in the older patient.

NURSING ALERT
Varicella zoster virus may be a life-threatening condition to the patient who is immunosuppressed or is receiving cytotoxic therapy.

DIAGNOSTIC EVALUATION
Culture of varicella zoster virus from lesions or detection by fluorescent antibody techniques.

TREATMENT AND NURSING MANAGEMENT
Objectives
Make the patient comfortable.
Reduce or avoid complications (infection, paralysis, scarring, postherpetic neuralgia).

1. The lesions usually clear spontaneously in healthy adults.
2. Place immunosuppressed patient or patients with disseminated disease on strict isolation.
3. Control the pain – controlling the pain may reduce incidence of postherpetic neuralgia.
   a. Give analgesics – aspirin, codeine, dextropropoxyphene, propoxyphene hydrochloride (Distalgesic) – to control pain and promote rest.
   b. Give sedatives – to control nervousness associated with neuralgia and itching.
   c. Give antihistamines – to control itching.
4. The following treatment regimen may be given.
   a. Apply local treatment to skin lesions.
      (i) Apply cool wet dressings to pruritic lesions.
      (ii) Apply topical idoxuridine (5 per cent) in dimethyl sulphoxide (Herpid) to individual lesions.
   b. Treat secondary bacterial infection of skin lesions – culture and sensitivity studies will indicate appropriate antibiotic.
   c. For the immunocompromised patient:
      (i) Antiviral drugs:
         (a) Acyclovir – prevents progressive cutaneous dissemination and development of visceral zoster; reduces pain, prevents new lesion formation, and heals skin faster.
         (b) Vidarabine – reduces severity of acute pain, new vesicle formation, cutaneous dissemination, and visceral complications if given early.
      (ii) Interferons (broadspectrum antiviral proteins) – act directly to induce other antiviral enzymes to modulate host response (investigational).
   d. Systemic corticosteroids may be given to the elderly to prevent postherpetic neuralgia – usually initial high dose gradually tailed off over two to five weeks.
   e. Support the patient undergoing diagnostic studies to investigate the possibility of underlying disease.

NURSING ALERT
Herpes zoster may indicate the presence of serious internal disease, especially in people past middle age (Hodgkin's disease, leukaemia, malignancy).

5. Watch for complications:
   a. Persistent pain (neuralgia) of affected nerve following healing, especially in the elderly.
   b. Ophthalmic herpes zoster – pain in the orbit radiating up over the forehead; constant, boring pain.
      (i) Pain particularly severe in elderly following ophthalmic herpes zoster.
      (ii) Patients with ophthalmic herpes zoster should be examined by ophthalmologist to avoid serious ocular complications.
   c. Facial nerve paralysis.
   d. Encephalitis.
6. Treatment of severe postherpetic pain: procaine or alcohol injection to nerve ganglia.

PATIENT EDUCATION

1. Shingles is a viral infection of the nerves; 'nervousness' does not cause shingles.
2. Do not open blisters.

CONTACT DERMATITIS

Contact dermatitis (dermatitis venenata) is a common inflammatory, often eczematous, condition caused by a skin reaction due to contact with a variety of irritating or allergenic materials. There is damage to the epidermis by repeated physical and chemical insults.

1. *Primary irritant contact dermatitis* is a nonallergic reaction caused by exposure to an irritating substance.
2. *Allergic contact dermatitis* results from exposure of sensitized individuals to contact allergens.

CAUSES

1. Plants.
2. Cosmetics.
3. Soaps, detergents and scouring compounds.
4. Industrial chemicals.
5. Hair dye, nickel, rubber, chemicals.

PREDISPOSING FACTORS

1. Extremes of heat and cold.
2. Frequent immersion in soap and water.
3. Pre-existing skin disease.

CLINICAL FEATURES

1. Skin eruptions begin at point of contact with causative agent.
2. Itching, burning, erythema, vesiculation and eczema.
3. Weeping, crusting, drying, fissuring and peeling.

4. Thickening of skin and pigmentation changes, if repeated reactions occur or if there is continual scratching by patient.
5. Secondary bacterial invasion may occur – prevention of normal sweating produces vesicles, itching and inflammation.

TREATMENT
Objective
Protect and rest the involved skin.

1. Inspect the entire body for a distribution pattern – helps differentiate between allergic contact dermatitis and the irritant type.
2. Obtain a detailed history, including the site of the initial eruption.
3. Instruct the patient as follows:
   a. Identify and remove the offending irritant.
      (i) Avoid the use of soap until healing occurs.
      (ii) Avoid exposing skin to the causative agent after recovery.
      (iii) Wear lined rubber gloves while working, if hands are involved.
   b. Topical treatment:
      (i) Use bland, unmedicated lotion for small patches of erythema.
      (ii) Use cool, wet dressings for small areas of acute, vesicular dermatitis – for soothing and to help stop oozing.
      (iii) Cleanse away softened crusts and other debris.
      (iv) Apply a thin layer of cream or ointment containing one of the steroids, as directed – usually not as beneficial when blisters are present, although some authorities feel it is helpful in these instances if used more frequently; i.e. at least five times daily.
      (v) Use medicated baths at room temperature (p. 732) for larger areas of dermatosis.
4. Give sedatives and antihistamines if necessary to relieve itching and burning.
5. Give systemic antibiotics if secondary bacterial infection is present – purulent exudate and systemic symptoms (fever, lymphadenopathy, etc).
6. Administer short course of systemic steroids if a more widespread and disabling condition is involved – can shorten the course of a severe disease; allays inflammation.
7. See also the patient with a dermatosis, p. 729.

PATIENT EDUCATION
Instruct the patient as follows:

1. Avoid heat, soap, rubbing – all these are external irritants.
2. Avoid topical medications except when specifically prescribed.
3. Wash thoroughly immediately after exposure to antigens.
4. Do not touch uninvolved body areas with involved areas.

PATCH TESTING

Patch testing is the method used for diagnosis of allergic contact dermatitis.

EQUIPMENT
Patch testing strips, A1-Test or Finn chambers
Adhesive tape if A1-Test is used
Substances to be applied (usually a standard battery as well as substances indicated by patient's history)
Skin marker

METHOD
1. Strips are prepared with substances to be tested.
2. Patient is informed of procedure.
3. The prepared strips are fixed to normal skin – usually on the back.
4. Patches are marked with a skin marker to indicate position and order of test substances.
5. Patches are removed after 48 hours and results of any reaction recorded.
6. Skin marks are renewed.
7. Reactions are recorded again after a further 48 hours.
8. Patients who have positive reactions are advised on how to avoid future contact with the substances responsible.

NONINFECTIOUS INFLAMMATORY DERMATOSES

ECZEMA

Eczema is one of the most common abnormal skin conditions. (The terms eczema and dermatitis are often used synonymously.)

CLINICAL FEATURES

1. Characteristics:
   a. Epidermis becomes erythematous and thickened followed by a vesicular eruption.
   b. When the vesicles rupture, the serous exudate dries and forms a crust.
   c. Skin becomes scaly and may be thickened in patches of varying shapes and sizes.
   d. Itching can be severe, causing the patient to scratch and lichenification can develop.

2. Types:
   a. Atopic eczema.
      (i) Chronic fluctuating disease.
      (ii) May occur at any age.
      (iii) Genetically determined disorder; there may be a family history of eczema, asthma or hay fever.
      (iv) Distribution of the lesions may vary considerably.
      (v) Common symptom is itching.
      Forms:
      (i) Infantile eczema.
      (ii) Atopic eczema of childhood.
      (iii) Adolescent and adult atopic eczema.
         (a) May follow childhood eczema or may occur at the first manifestation of atopic eczema.
         (b) Affects the limbs, flexures, face and may spread to the neck and trunk.
         (c) The total skin surface may be affected in severe cases.
   b. Nummular eczema.
      (i) Appears as well-defined round or oval coin-like patches of eczema.
      (ii) Common sites are the calves, shins, forearms, backs of fingers and hands.
      (iii) Itching is usually severe, as in atopic eczema.
   c. Pompholyx (eczema of thick skin, e.g. of the hands and feet).
      (i) Occurs on the sides and palms of the fingers and hands and the sides and soles of the toes and feet.
      (ii) The thick horny layer at these sites inhibits rupture of vesicles – thus the vesicles may remain for days looking like whitish grains in the skin.
      (iii) Seborrhoeic eczema (seborrhoeic dermatitis) (see p. 735).
      (iv) Contact dermatitis (see p. 748).

TREATMENT AND NURSING MANAGEMENT

1. Advise patient to remove any known irritants. Patch test any suspect patient to confirm any contact dermatitis.
2. Topical therapy to be used regularly.
   a. Apply moisturizing cream (e.g. Boots E45) liberally and frequently during day and after washing to all dry or inflamed areas.
   b. Use oilatum emollient in bath.
   c. Emulsifying ointment should be used instead of soap.
   d. Moisturizer and emulsifying ointment should be used even after eczema has cleared to help prevent skin becoming dry and a recurrence of the eczema.
3. Steroid therapy:
   a. Topical corticosteroids (hydrocortisone, Benovate, Dermovate, Haelan, Synalar) should be used only when prescribed and only on the affected areas. Nurse must wear gloves to apply topical steroids.
   b. More potent preparations (Betnovate, Dermovate) should never be used on the face.
   c. Systemic corticosteroid therapy (prednisone) may be used in acute exacerbations.
4. Antibiotic therapy is given for secondary infection.
   a. Systemic antibiotics are given as prescribed.
   b. Topical antibiotics may be prescribed.
5. Baths (see p. 732):
   a. Antiseptic baths are given for infected eczema.
   b. Bath oils are used for emollient and anti-pruritic effect.
6. Open wet dressings are applied as prescribed (see p. 732).
7. Systemic therapy:
   a. Antihistamines (Piriton) are given as prescribed to relieve itching.
   b. Sedatives may be prescribed to help patient sleep and prevent scratching.
8. Diet therapy:
   a. Review the patient's history for any indication of allergies.
   b. Avoid substances that have a high potential for sensitization. Foods such as milk, eggs, wheat cereal, chocolate, orange juice and those containing artificial colourings should be avoided.
   c. Monitor the patient's reactions carefully when an elimination diet is prescribed.
      (i) A trial diet may be composed of: milk substitute, rice cereal, two fruits, two vegetables, beef, aqueous vitamins, no egg products.
      (ii) A new food is added to the diet every three to five days, during which time the response to that food is observed.
      (iii) An allergic response occurring during this three- to five-day period indicates sensitivity to that food; that particular food is then eliminated from the diet.
      (iv) If no response is apparent, that food is added to the diet.
      (v) Steps (ii) to (iv) are repeated until the food allergen is determined.

PATIENT EDUCATION

1. Advise patient on importance of continuing moisturizing therapy.
2. Advise the patient to avoid aggravating factors and any other known allergen: woollen clothing, blankets, rubber etc.
3. Help patient with chronic condition in planning his own management.
4. Reassure and support patient and family in coping with long-term problems.
5. Advise patient of the existence of the National Eczema Society, Tavistock House North, Tavistock Square, London WC1.

PSORIASIS

Psoriasis is a chronic, proliferative, inflammatory dermatosis of unknown aetiology appearing as an eruption of dry, red patches of all sizes, sharply defined against the normal skin and covered with heavy, dry, silvery scales (Figure 11.4). In time the patches can coalesce, forming extensive irregularly shaped patches.

CLINICAL FEATURES

1. In psoriasis, the rate of production of the epidermis of the skin is about nine times faster than normal; this abnormal process does not allow for formation of normal protective layers of skin.
2. There appears to be a hereditary biochemical defect that causes an overproduction of keratin; there is also thought to be a hormonal influence.
3. Onset is usually before the age of 20, but all age groups are affected.
4. Psoriasis may be coupled with polyarthritis and cause crippling disability.
5. Sites (bilateral symmetry):
   a. Bony prominences (knees, elbows, sacrum), scalp, external ears, genitalia, perianal area, nails and dorsa of hands.

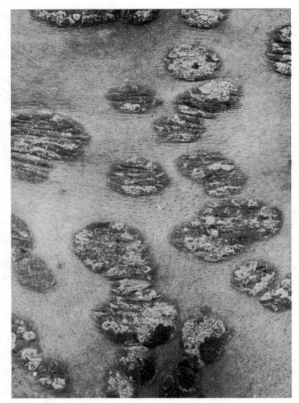

Figure 11.4. Psoriasis of the back (courtesy Department of Medical Illustration, The Institute of Dermatology, London)

b. Psoriasis of the ears – scaling and dryness.
c. Psoriasis of palms and soles – vesicular and pustular pruritic lesions.
d. Psoriasis of nails – thickening, discoloration, crumbling beneath free edges; pitting of nails.
e. Psoriasis between skin folds – smooth, shiny red lesions, easily fissured.

6. The disease may range from being a cosmetic source of annoyance affecting small areas, to one involving most of the skin. In severe cases psoriasis may be physically disabling. Psoriasis sufferers require a high level of psychological and emotional support to enable them to cope with their condition. Psoriasis may be life-ruining – physically, emotionally and economically.

TREATMENT AND NURSING MANAGEMENT
Objective
Reduce scaling and any itching; the goal is control since no cure is known.
1. Instruct patient to take daily bath – to help soak off scales.

a. Gently remove excess scales with a soft brush while bathing.
b. Apply prescribed ointment after removal of scales.
2. Topical therapy (includes corticosteroids, coal tar, dithranol, salicylic acid, etc).
a. Corticosteroids:
   (i) Apply wet dressings to irritated areas of psoriasis.
   (ii) Apply corticosteroid preparations – as prescribed.
   (iii) Hold dressings in place with occlusive film (traps heat and moisture, softens scaly plaques and enhances transepidermal penetration).
       (a) Occlusive dressings over the entire body may be held in place with polythene pyjama suit or a large plastic bag with holes cut out for the head and arms; another bag may be used for the legs; extremities (arms) may be wrapped in plastic film. Total body occlusion is rarely used and should only be done under strict medical supervision.
       Caution the patient not to smoke while wrapped in these dressings.
       (b) In patients being treated at home, hands can be wrapped in gloves, the feet in plastic bags and the hair covered by a shower cap.
b. Dithranol preparations (a distillate of crude coal tar).
   (i) Useful for especially thick and resistant psoriatic plaques.
   (ii) Instruct patient to apply dithranol medication to affected areas only; do not apply to normal skin, face or flexures.
   (iii) Dithranol should always be applied with a spatula – *never* with the hands. Wash hands thoroughly after application – medication can produce a chemical conjunctivitis.
c. Coal tar preparations (ointments/baths) – retard and inhibit the rapid growth of psoriatic tissue.
   (i) Coal tar is applied for a period of time; may then be removed; this treatment can be followed by carefully graded doses of ultraviolet radiation, after performing ultraviolet test.
   (ii) Begin ultraviolet radiation with low dose (10 seconds) and build up dosage time gradually.

(iii) Ultraviolet may produce mild redness and slight desquamation.
3. Systemic medications:
a. Methotrexate – folic acid antagonist may be used in patients with extensive psoriasis that is resistant to all other forms of treatment. It is taken in a small weekly dose.
  (i) Liver biopsy may be done before initiation of treatment.
  (ii) Patient should avoid alcohol intake while on methotrexate – increases possibility of liver damage.
  (iii) Laboratory studies should be conducted to ensure adequate function of hepatic, haematopoietic and renal systems; these parameters should be monitored before the course of drug treatment is started.
  (iv) Methotrexate is a potent abortive or teratogenic agent and is used with extreme caution in women of childbearing age.
b. Hydroxyurea – inhibits cell replication by affecting deoxyribonucleic acid (DNA) synthesis.
4. Phototherapy. Regular exposure to sunlight or ultraviolet light – B therapy as prescribed by the doctor may be sufficient to control psoriasis for some patients.
5. Photochemotherapy (PUVA therapy):
a. Oral psoralen tablets (methoxsalen or 8-MOP, a photosensitizing chemical) followed by exposure to long-wave ultraviolet light (UVA) – in the presence of ultraviolet light, methoxsalen binds to DNA and leads to temporary inhibition of DNA synthesis (inhibits abnormally rapid multiplication of cells).
b. Long-term concerns include skin cancer, cataracts, ageing effect and systemic effects on other organs.
c. Methoxsalen capsules taken with milk or food two hours before scheduled UVA exposure in a UVA irradiation chamber; exposure is determined by the patient's skin type.
d. An average of 25 treatments given two or three times per week is required for clearing; maintenance treatments are usually necessary.
e. Patient education:
  (i) Since PUVA treatment produces photosensitization, the patient is sensitive to sunlight the entire day of treatment; he must wear protective clothing and use a sunscreen on the face and exposed areas of the body.
  (ii) Grey- or green-tinted glasses must be worn for a 24-hour period following ingestion of methoxsalen for exposure to direct or indirect sunlight outdoors or through a window – to prevent irreversible binding of methoxsalen to the proteins and DNA components of the lens.
  (iii) Initial blood tests and urinalysis are done, and eye examinations are required at specified times.
  (iv) PUVA may cause irreversible or slowly reversible clinical and histological skin changes; loss of elasticity; irreversible solar damage; carcinogenesis.

PATIENT EDUCATION
1. Psoriasis is thought to have multifactorial aetiology, involving genetic, environmental and systemic considerations.
2. Psoriasis is a disease of the entire skin, but it is not infectious or contagious.
3. Be aware of factors that may precipitate flare-ups.
a. Know inciting factors – illness, certain drugs (propranolol, lithium, etc).
b. Develop insight and determine what life events may worsen the condition.
4. Avoid injury to the skin (patches of psoriasis bleed after minor trauma).
a. Keep skin, especially on the hands, as pliable and soft as possible by applying appropriate creams.
b. Wear heavy gloves when doing gardening, etc.
c. Report to doctor if severe injury to skin has occurred; injection of intralesional steroids may prevent untoward response.
5. Consider learning stress-reduction techniques.
6. Find another person with psoriasis to exchange ideas.
7. Learn to live with psoriasis and accept that it is a chronic disease, often requiring continuous therapy; treatment can be time-consuming and expensive.
8. Encourage patients to develop a skin care plan to help them maintain and carry out their own treatments.
9. If possible, the patient should try to schedule exposure to sunlight on a regular basis. Avoid sunburn, since it can cause a generalized inflammation.
10. Advise patient of the Psoriasis Association, 7 Milton Street, Northampton NN2 7JG.

EXFOLIATIVE DERMATITIS (GENERALIZED ERYTHRODERMA)

Exfoliative dermatitis is a serious condition characterized by progressive inflammation in which erythema and scaling often occur in a more or less generalized distribution. It may be associated with chills, fever, prostration, severe toxicity and an itchy scaling of the skin.

CLINICAL FEATURES
Systemic effects
Exfoliative dermatitis has a marked effect on the entire body.
1. There is a profound loss of stratum corneum (outermost layer of the skin) – causes capillary leakage, hypoproteinaemia and negative nitrogen balance.
2. Iron loss from the skin produces anaemia.

Appearance
1. Starts acutely as either a patchy or generalized erythematous eruption (Figure 11.5) accompanied by fever, malaise and occasionally gastro-intestinal symptoms.
2. The skin colour changes from pink to dark red; then after a week the characteristic exfoliation (scaling) begins, usually in the form of thin flakes which leave the underlying skin smooth and red, new scales forming as the older ones exfoliate (cast off).
3. Hair loss and nail shedding may accompany the disorder.

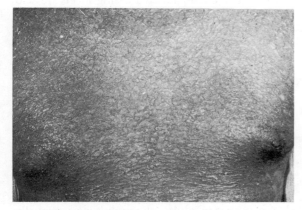

Figure 11.5. Exfoliative dermatitis of chest (courtesy Department of Medical Illustration, The Institute of Dermatology, London)

Multiplicity of causes
1. May arise as a primary condition.
2. May follow a previous skin condition (eczema, psoriasis) that had become generalized.
3. May appear as a part of the lymphoma group of diseases and may precede the appearance of lymphoma or leukaemia.
4. Also appears as a severe reaction to a wide number of drugs, including penicillin, phenyl-butazone and phenytoin (Epanutin).

TREATMENT AND NURSING MANAGEMENT
Objectives
Maintain fluid and electrolyte balance.
Prevent intercurrent or cutaneous infection.
1. Hospitalize the patient and place him on bed rest. Maintain comfortable room temperature – patient does not have normal thermoregulatory control owing to temperature fluctuations from vaso-dilation and evaporative water loss.
2. Maintain fluid and electrolyte balance – considerable water and protein loss from skin surface.
3. Give systemic corticosteroids as prescribed – for anti-inflammatory action; may be a life-saving procedure.
4. Apply compresses and soothing baths – to treat acute extensive dermatitis.
5. Maintain nursing surveillance for intercurrent or cutaneous infection; the erythematous, moist skin is receptive to infection and becomes colonized with pathogenic organisms which produce more inflammation. Antibiotics are given if infection is present; selected by culture and sensitivity.
6. Watch for symptoms of heart failure – hyperaemia and increased cutaneous blood flow can produce a cardiac failure of high-output origin.

PATIENT EDUCATION
Advise patient to avoid all irritants, particularly drugs.

PEMPHIGUS

Pemphigus is a serious autoimmune disease of the skin and mucous membranes characterized by the appearance of blisters (bullae) of various sizes on apparently normal skin and mucous membranes (mouth, vagina) (Figure 11.6). The cause is unknown.

Familial benign chronic pemphigus (Hailey-Hailey disease) is a familial type of pemphigus appearing in adult life affecting particularly the axillae and groin. There are other variants of the disease.

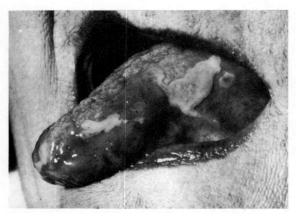

Figure 11.6. Pemphigus lesions of the tongue (courtesy Department of Medical Illustration, The Institute of Dermatology, London)

CLINICAL FEATURES

1. Appearance:
   a. Asymptomatic large bullae appear on apparently normal skin and mucous membranes.
   b. The bullae enlarge and rupture, forming painful raw and denuded areas.
   c. Bullae and erosions occur on the skin, mouth and vagina; large areas of skin may be denuded.
   d. Bacterial superinfection is common.
2. An offensive odour emanates from the bullae.
3. Positive Nikolsky's sign – production of a blister upon rubbing adjacent normal skin.

DIAGNOSTIC EVALUATION

1. Laboratory evaluation.
2. Immunofluorescent studies of skin and serum.
3. Skin biopsies of blisters or margins of erosion.

TREATMENT AND NURSING MANAGEMENT

Objectives

Bring the disease under control as rapidly as possible.

Prevent loss of serum and development of secondary infection.

Promote re-epithelialization of skin.

1. Administer corticosteroids (prednisone) in large doses, as prescribed – to control the disease.
   a. High dosage level is maintained until remission is apparent.
   b. Dosage is reduced to minimum daily maintenance dose as soon as possible.
   c. Give medication with or immediately after a meal; may be accompanied by an antacid as prophylaxis against gastric complications.

2. Take fluid measurements of body weight, blood pressure; test urine for glucose. Record fluid balance (input and output).
3. Give immunosuppressive agents (methotrexate; cyclophosphamide) as prescribed – may be given to help control the disease and reduce the maintenance dose of corticosteroids.
4. Assess patient for evidence of local and systemic infection – bullae are susceptible to infection, and septicaemia may follow.
5. Evaluate for fluid and electrolyte imbalance – extensive denudation of the skin leads to fluid and electrolyte imbalance.
   a. Give soft, high-protein, high-calorie diet – patients with painful oral involvement have difficulty maintaining nutrition.
   b. Administer saline infusions as directed – significant loss of tissue fluids and therefore of sodium chloride occur through the skin.
   c. Encourage patient to maintain adequate fluid intake.
6. Give blood or component therapy (packed red cells, plasma, etc) as necessary – large amount of protein and blood lost through denuded skin; nursing management is similar to that of patient with an extensive burn (see p. 769).
7. Administer cool wet dressings and/or baths – patients with large areas of blistering have a characteristic odour that is lessened when secondary infection is under control.
8. Foam-padded nonadherent dressings which have been smeared liberally with a prescribed bland emollient (emulsifying ointment) reduce the patient's discomfort, help maintain body temperature and shorten the time taken to carry out dressings on these patients. The non-adherent, foam-padded dressing sheets are held in place with a soft tubular gauze to suit.
9. Give meticulous oral hygiene – lesions and painful erosions in the mouth are common.
10. Usually associated with serious underlying medical condition, e.g. systemic lupus erythematosus. Some authorities suggest that cancer may be associated with pemphigus.

TOXIC EPIDERMAL NECROLYSIS (TEN)

Toxic epidermal necrolysis (TEN) is a severe, potentially fatal skin disease most commonly related to drug exposure in adults, although it is occasionally induced by staphylococcus. The drugs most commonly implicated are the sulphonamides, phenytoin, allopurinol, phenylbutazone, salicylates, penicillins and barbiturates.

CLINICAL FEATURES
1. Fever.
2. Erythema, involving much of skin surface.
3. Appearance of large, flaccid bullae.
4. Wide, sheet-like peeling and denudation of the skin – appearance is that of a second-degree burn with a moist, blistered and tender surface (Figure 11.7).
5. Skin necrosis; ulcerations of lips and oral pharynx.
6. Positive Nikolsky's sign (desquamation of skin in sheets upon light digital pressure).

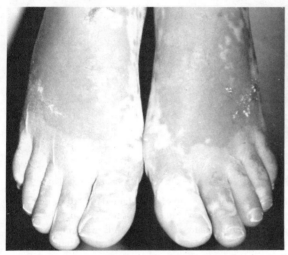

Figure 11.7. Toxic epidermal necrolysis, showing denudation of the skin of the feet (courtesy Melvyn L. Elgart, MD)

DIAGNOSTIC EVALUATION
Microscopic examination of skin biopsy specimens obtained from lesions; may be done as a frozen section because prompt diagnosis is important.

TREATMENT AND NURSING MANAGEMENT
Fluid and electrolyte balance
1. Transfer the patient to unit (burn unit) equipped to handle long-term management of extensive dermal loss – the principles of *burn wound management* with its associated haemodynamic problems apply to this condition (see p. 769).
2. Stop all administration of nonessential drugs immediately.
3. Start intravenous (IV) fluid resuscitation in volumes required to maintain urine output of 50ml/hour; start on oral fluid intake when the patient demonstrates tolerance.
4. Monitor serum electrolytes and osmolarity.
5. Keep room warm.

Avoidance of infectious complications
1. Use strict isolation precautions (as with a second-degree burn) and wear a mask and sterile gloves.
2. Take cultures of nasopharynx, eyes, ears, blood, urine, skin and unruptured bullae as directed to determine presence of pathogenic organisms.
3. Monitor IV sites for infection, which may result in septicaemia.
4. Give parenteral steroids as directed – may be given in an attempt to abort skin necrosis and denudation.
5. Administer antibiotics as directed.
6. Apply warm compresses of aqueous silver nitrate *gently* to raw areas to reduce bacterial population.
7. Employ meticulous oral hygiene.
8. Use extreme care in handling the patient, since skin fragility is a problem.
   a. Place the patient on a turning frame.
   b. Secure services of several health care personnel to support an extremity evenly when the patient moves – to reduce trauma and shearing of the superficial epidermis.
   c. Use indwelling arterial line with pressure transducer giving a constant readout of blood and pulse; avoid using a cuff sphygmomanometer because of skin trauma.
   d. Give analgesics for the patient experiencing pain from raw areas.

Nutritional balance
1. Consider parenteral nutrition because the patient may have perioral lesions.
2. Monitor nutritional status, with measurement of nitrogen excretion because this provides a guide to adequacy of protein intake; collect urine for assay of nitrogen excretion.

ULCERS AND TUMOURS OF THE SKIN

ULCERS OF THE SKIN

Ulceration is a superficial loss of surface tissue due to death of cells.

CAUSES

Ulcers of the skin usually arise from infection or an interference with the blood supply.

1. Infection as cause of skin ulcers.
   a. Usually develop from an infection with anaerobic streptococci or from combination of infections (haemolytic streptococci and staphylococci).
   b. Tend to progress peripherally – characterized by an overhanging edge.
2. Deficient circulation as cause of skin ulcers.

TUMOURS OF THE SKIN

CYSTS

Epidermal cysts are common, slow-growing, firm, elevated tumours consisting of a mass of epidermal cells; frequently found on the back.

Sebaceous cysts are rounded tumours of variable size caused by retention of the excretion in the sebaceous follicles; also referred to as *wens*.

BENIGN TUMOURS

Verrucae (warts)

Common, benign skin tumours caused by a virus.

1. Many times warts do not need treatment, since they tend to disappear spontaneously.
2. Treatment:
   a. Freezing with liquid nitrogen – this has a somewhat destructive action, although it tends to spare the epidermis (Figures 11.8a and b).
   b. Area may be treated locally with salicylic acid plasters, or paint, formalin 3 per cent or podophyllin. In some cases curettage and electrocautery may be used.

Angiomas (birthmarks)

Benign vascular tumours involving the skin and subcutaneous tissues.

1. May occur as flat, violet-red patches (portwine angiomas) or as raised, bright-red nodular lesions (strawberry angiomas). Strawberry angiomas may involute spontaneously.
2. Portwine angiomas usually persist indefinitely.

Pigmented naevi (moles)

Common skin tumours of various sizes and shapes ranging from yellowish to brown to black.

1. May be flat macular lesions or elevated papules or nodules that occasionally contain hair.
2. Majority of pigmented naevi are harmless; however, in rare cases malignant changes supervene

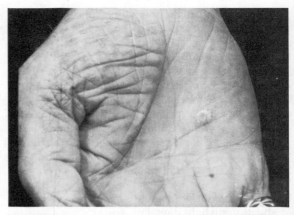

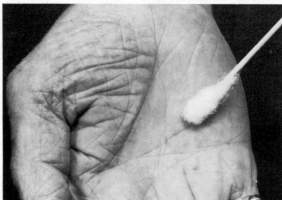

Figures 11.8a and b. Wart of palm. Liquid nitrogen is delivered to the wart by a cotton applicator. It should be applied repeatedly until the freezing part extends to 1–2mm around the tissue (courtesy Department of Medical Illustration, The Institute of Dermatology, London)

and a melanoma develops at the site of the naevus.

3. Treatment:
   a. Naevi at sites subject to repeated irritation from clothing and so on should be removed – for comfort.
   b. Naevi that show change in size or colour, or which bleed, should be removed – to determine if malignancy has occurred.
   c. Excised naevi should be examined histologically.

Keloids

Benign overgrowths of fibrous tissue at site of scar or trauma.

1. More prevalent among black-skinned races.
2. Usually asymptomatic – may cause disfigurement and cosmetic concern.

3. Treatment – topical corticosteroids (Haelan), intralesional injection with corticosteroids, or radiotherapy.

Actinic keratoses

Premalignant skin lesions appearing as rough, scaly patches with underlying erythema.
1. Develop in chronic sun-exposed areas of the body.
2. Many available treatments; liquid nitrogen cryo-surgery, or curettage, or biopsy.

CANCER OF THE SKIN

CLINICAL FEATURES
1. Skin cancer has a greater incidence than cancer of any other organ.
2. There is a 95 per cent cure rate due to early diagnosis, the slow progression of most skin cancers and the effective methods of treatment available.

CAUSES
1. Exposure to sun over a period of time (outdoor workers).
2. Texture of skin and its pigment content – people with ruddy or light complexions seem to develop skin cancer more frequently than those with coarser or darker skin.
3. Exposure to irradiation (history of X-ray treatment for benign skin lesions).
4. Exposure to certain chemical agents (arsenic, nitrates, tar and pitch, oils and paraffins).
5. Cancer of skin may develop on scars of severe burns 20 to 40 years later.

NURSING ASSESSMENT
Look for:
1. Chronic sunburn.
2. Actinic damage – pigment change, splotches, wrinkling, leathery complexion.
3. Precancerous lesions (keratosis; leucoplakia).
4. Change in a skin lesion.

NURSING ALERT
Any skin lesion that changes in size or colour, bleeds, ulcerates or becomes infected may be skin cancer.

DIAGNOSTIC EVALUATION
1. Biopsy.
2. Histological evaluation.

TYPES OF SKIN CANCER
Basal cell carcinoma or rodent ulcer
1. Most common skin cancer; higher incidence in regions where population is subjected to intense and extensive exposure to sun.
2. Lesions are small nodules with a rolled, pearly, translucent border with telangiectasia (dilation of end blood vessels), crusting and occasionally ulceration (Figure 11.9).
3. These tumours may be pigmented, multiple, superficial or cystic.
   a. Basal cell carcinoma is chiefly caused by prolonged skin exposure to irritants.
   b. Characterized by invasion and erosion of continuous tissues – rarely metastasizes.
   c. Lesions appear most frequently on face, between hairline and upper lip.

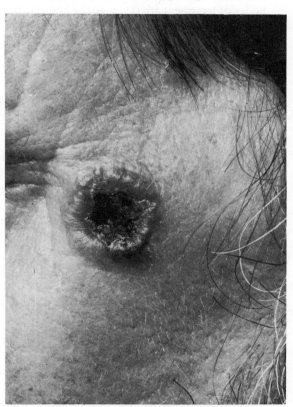

Figure 11.9. Basal cell carcinoma on temple (courtesy Department of Medical Illustration, The Institute of Dermatology, London)

Squamous cell carcinoma
1. A malignancy that arises on sun-exposed areas of skin and mucous membrane and is considered a truly invasive carcinoma.

2. Appears as an infiltrated, plaque-like or nodular, rapid-growing tumour.
3. May be preceded by leucoplakia (premalignant lesion of mucous membrane), actinic keratoses, scarred or ulcerated lesions.
4. Seen most commonly on lower lip, tongue, head, neck and dorsa of hands.
5. Requires more aggressive approach (wider margin of normal skin included in excision) – greater chance of metastases from squamous cell carcinoma and significantly lower cure rate.

TREATMENT

1. Method of treatment depends on tumour location; cell type (location and depth); history of previous treatment; and whether or not it is invasive and if metastatic nodes are present. Usual modes of treatment are (1) curettage and electrocautery, (2) surgical excision, and (3) radiotherapy.
2. *Curettage followed by electrocautery* – usually done on small tumours (less than 1–2cm):
   a. Curettage – excision of skin tumour by scraping with a curette; electrocautery is used to achieve haemostasis and to destroy any viable malignant cells in margins or in base of wound.
   b. This form of treatment takes advantage of the fact that the tumour in each instance is softer than the surrounding skin and can be outlined by curette, which 'feels' the extent of the tumour.
   c. Tumour is removed and the base cauterized; process repeated a number of times.
3. *Surgical excision:*
   a. Wide surgical excision – adequacy of excision verified by microscopic study of sections of the specimen.
   b. Histological study of excised tissue allows determination of whether or not margins are free of tumour.
   c. Skin grafting may be necessary.
4. *Radiotherapy* – usually done for cancer of eyelid, tip of nose, in or near vital structures (facial nerve) where tissue sparing is difficult with other forms of treatment; used for extensive malignancies when the goal is palliation or when other medical conditions contraindicate other forms of therapy.
   a. Explain to patient that he may experience skin reddening and swelling about the time of the third treatment; may progress to blistering.
   b. Stress importance of follow-up care – there is always the possibility of recurrence or a new primary lesion.

c. Caution the patient against exposure to the sun.
5. *Cryosurgery* – deep freezing to selectively destroy tumour tissue.
   a. Liquid nitrogen is applied by cryospray or cryoprobe technique.
   b. Site thaws naturally and then becomes gelatinous and heals spontaneously.
6. *Microcontrolled surgery* – fresh tissue is sequentially excised in layers and immediate microscopic examination of each tissue layer is made. More extensive carcinomas are examined with a fixed tissue technique (chemosurgery). Useful for recurrent skin cancers, since surgical excision is guided by microscopic study.
7. *Topical chemotherapy* – application of topical antitumour agent (fluorouracil) to destroy cancer cells.

PATIENT EDUCATION

Most skin cancer can be prevented by avoidance of and protection from excessive direct exposure to sun. Susceptible patients should show any suspect lesions to their doctor.

Instruct the patient as follows:

1. Avoid unnecessary exposure to the sun, especially during times when ultraviolet radiation is most intense (10.00 to 14.00 hours).
2. Wear appropriate protective clothing (e.g. broad-brimmed hat, long-sleeved garments).
3. Use shading devices (e.g. umbrella).
4. Apply a protective sunscreen with recommended sun protection factor if an activity requires a long period of exposure.
   a. Sun protection factor (SPF) ranges from 2 (minimal protection) to 15 (ultra- or super-protection).
   b. Specific SPF number is selected according to skin sensitivity ('burns easily' to 'never burns'). Use a sunscreen with SPF 15 *routinely.* Apply evenly to all exposed areas of body.
   c. Sunscreen selected should not come off easily; those which contain 5 per cent para-aminobenzoic acid in 55 to 70 per cent alcohol do not come off easily.
   d. Periodically reapply more sunscreen, especially after swimming/bathing.
   e. Protect your lips – use darker shades of lipstick or ultraviolet-absorbing lip salve.
5. Watch for indications of potential malignancy in moles (e.g. change in colour, increase in size, ulceration, bleeding or serous exudation).
6. Follow-up after treatment of squamous cell cancer and malignant melanoma should be carried out

for the patient's lifetime and should include palpation of adjacent lymph nodes.

MALIGNANT MELANOMA

Malignant melanoma is a malignant tumour of the skin (Figure 11.10) which occurs in three forms: lentigo-maligna melanoma, superficial spreading melanoma and nodular melanoma. It has a higher mortality rate than other forms of skin cancer.

CLASSIFICATION
Lentigo-maligna melanoma
1. Slowly evolving pigment lesions; occur on exposed skin surfaces of elderly.
2. First appears as tan, flat lesion – in time undergoes change in size and colour.

Superficial spreading melanoma
1. Occurs anywhere on body; usually affects middle-aged people.
2. Tends to be circular with portion of its outline irregular (either protruding or indenting).
3. Has combination of colours – hues of tan, brown and black admixed with grey, bluish-black or white.
4. May be dull pink-rose colour in a small area within the lesion.

Nodular melanoma
1. Spherical blueberry-like nodule with relatively smooth surface and relatively uniform blue-black colour.
2. May be polypoidal, with smooth surface of rose-grey or black colour; may be present as elevated, irregular plaque.

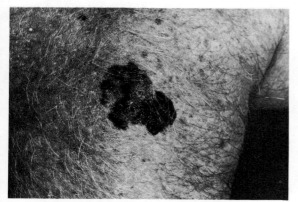

Figure 11.10. Malignant melanoma on upper arm (courtesy Department of Medical Illustration, The Institute of Dermatology, London)

CLINICAL FEATURES
1. Signs that suggest malignant change:
   a. Variegated colour:
      (i) Colours that may indicate malignancy in a brown or black lesion are shades of red, white and blue; shades of blue are considered ominous.
      (ii) White areas within a pigmented lesion are suspicious.
      (iii) Some malignant melanomas are not variegated but are uniformly coloured (bluish-black, bluish-grey, bluish-red).
   b. Irregular border – look for angular indentation or notch present in the border of a malignant melanoma.
   c. Irregular surface:
      (i) Look for uneven elevations of the surface; irregular topography may be palpable or visible.
      (ii) Some nodular melanomas have a smooth surface.
2. Common sites of melanoma – skin of back, legs, between toes, and on feet, face, scalp, fingernails, back of hands.
3. In the black race, melanomas are most apt to occur on less pigmented sites – palms, soles, subungual areas and mucous membranes.

DIAGNOSTIC EVALUATION
1. Any change or alteration in size or colour; symptoms such as itching, oozing, bleeding.
2. Biopsy – excision of suspicious mole from both raised and invasive areas and from flat, non-invasive area.
3. Prognosis – survival is related to depth of dermal invasion of malignant melanocytes in the primary lesion; melanoma is curable only when confined to primary site.

TREATMENT
The therapeutic approach depends on the depth of the lesion.
1. Radical surgery – wide excision with possible regional node dissection, usually followed by plastic repair or skin grafting.
2. Regional isolation perfusion; specific area is isolated by mechanically controlling its arterial inflow and venous outflow. This allows high concentration of cytotoxic drugs to be delivered to cancer-bearing sites.
3. Chemotherapy.
4. Grenz ray therapy for lentigo-maligna melanoma.

PATIENT EDUCATION

1. Educate people to observe their moles and to report moles that *change* colours, enlarge or become raised or thicker.
2. Treatment should be initiated immediately.

SYSTEMIC DISEASES WITH SKIN MANIFESTATIONS

LUPUS ERYTHEMATOSUS

Systemic lupus erythematosus is an inflammatory disease of unknown origin involving the vascular and connective tissues of many organs (primarily skin, joints, kidneys and serous membranes) with resultant multiple local and systemic symptoms.

Discoid lupus erythematosus is a chronic eruption of the skin which, although often disfiguring, does not pose a threat to life.

CLINICAL FEATURES

1. Aetiology is not understood – evidence indicates that it is an autoimmune disease.
2. Appears to be familial in nature. Family studies suggest a genetically determined predisposition to autoimmune disease but that other factors (e.g. sunlight, pregnancy, some drugs) are needed to precipitate or exacerbate the disease.
3. Most frequently found in young women with signs and symptoms referable to the joints and skin.
4. May be drug-induced (procainamide; hydralazine).
5. Is characterized by remissions and exacerbations.

CLINICAL MANIFESTATIONS

1. Vary greatly, since they can affect every organ system; mimic many other diseases.
2. Weakness, malaise, weight loss.
3. *Skin manifestations:*
   a. Malar rash, alopecia, dermal vasculitis, Raynaud's phenomenon, purpura.
   b. Possible skin rash with butterfly distribution over bridge of nose and malar bone prominences (butterfly distribution).
   c. Similar lesions over neck, chest, upper and lower extremities – may become pruritic and scaly.
   d. Broken-off hair ('lupus hair').
4. Generalized lymphadenopathy.

5. Long-continued low grade fever.
6. Arthritis and arthralgia.
7. Cardiac involvement (pericarditis, myocarditis, pleural effusion).
8. Renal involvement (proteinuria, haematuria, renal insufficiency and failure).
9. Central nervous system involvement (convulsive disorders, abnormalities in mental function and cranial nerves, depression, emotional lability, neurosis).

DIAGNOSTIC EVALUATION

Many laboratory abnormalities may be found.
1. Positive lupus erythematosus cell test.
2. Immunological abnormalities present in most people with systemic lupus erythematosus.
   a. Antinuclear antibody test positive – high titres of antibody to nuclear antigens.
   b. DNA-binding test.
   c. Serum complement fixation test – decreased complement titres in patients with renal disease.
   d. Increased gamma globulins.
3. Urine – may reveal proteinuria and cellular casts.
4. Cerebrospinal fluid examination – may have elevated protein concentration and mononuclear cells.
5. Blood evaluation – shows evidence of anaemia, leukopenia, thrombocytopenia.
6. Abnormal renal function tests.

TREATMENT

No known cure at this time.

Objective

Control the disease by suppressing inflammation and relieving symptoms.
1. Treat intercurrent illness – exacerbations of systemic lupus erythematosus may follow infection, drug administration, emotional stress, surgical procedures.
2. Other forms of treatment – selection depends on nature and severity of disease.
   a. Corticosteroids (prednisone) – used for suppressing inflammation and thus relieving symptoms.
      (i) Observe patient carefully – may be difficult to distinguish between drug effects and those of SLE.
      (ii) See p. 576 for side-effects of steroids.
   b. Salicylates – for musculoskeletal pain; will also lower temperature. Patient should take salicylates on a regular schedule so that adequate blood levels are maintained.

c. Antimalarials (chloroquine) – to control the skin and joint manifestations. Patient should be examined by ophthalmologist at least twice yearly – retinal degeneration resulting in visual impairment may be a problem.

d. Immunosuppressive agents (cyclophosphamide; azathioprine) – to suppress manifestations of systemic lupus erythematosus. Usually reserved for patients who are unresponsive to steroids or who develop unacceptable side-effects from steroids.

e. Plasmapheresis – to remove immune complexes. Further trials and experience needed to assess this treatment.

3. Treat the patient as each problem arises (depending on the organ system involved and its physiological consequences) – nephritis, renal failure, congestive heart failure, central nervous system lupus, etc.

4. Give continuing emotional support. Psychiatric treatment may be indicated for debilitating depression, etc.

5. Be aware that some patients do not react favourably to immunization procedures.

6. Watch for development of complications – uraemia, central nervous system disorders, malignancies, infection (namely 'opportunist' bacterial pathogens), acute abdominal catastrophes.

PATIENT EDUCATION

Instruct the patient as follows:

1. Avoid whatever you know may aggravate the condition.

2. Avoid undue exposure to sunlight – can produce exacerbations and worsen dermal lesions.

3. Use a sunscreening agent when exposure to sun is necessary.

4. Avoid sensitizing drugs (penicillin; sulphonamides) and avoid using hair sprays and hair colouring agents.

5. Avoid taking contraceptive pills – anovulatory drugs may precipitate lupus syndrome in susceptible person.

6. Try to avoid (and cope with) stress – emotional turmoil may precipitate a flare-up.

7. Obtain more rest.

8. Eat a well-balanced diet.

9. The makeup 'Cover-Mark' or Keromask may conceal facial lesions and scarring (of discoid lupus erythematosus).

10. Report to the doctor immediately any worsening of symptoms – fever, cough, skin rash, increasing joint pain, etc.

POLYARTERITIS NODOSA

Polyarteritis nodosa is a disease of unknown cause characterized by inflammation and necrosis of medium-sized and small vessels, especially arteries, which results in altered function of the organ system in which the arterial supply has been impaired.

CLINICAL FEATURES

1. The walls of the vessels are involved; spotty inflammation causes changes in circulation and tissue damage.

2. Clinical manifestations vary according to organ(s) involved and amount of necrosis produced by obstructing vascular lesion.

   a. Prolonged fever; myalgia and arthralgia; renal involvement; gastrointestinal manifestations (abdominal pain, nausea, vomiting, diarrhoea); cardiovascular manifestations (coronary insufficiency, myocardial infarction); palpable nodules along the arterial trunks – may occur.

   b. Ocular manifestations (retinal exudates and haemorrhages) are fairly common.

   c. Skin lesions are usually in the form of painful nodules that may ulcerate.

      (i) Subcutaneous nodules vary in size and may be located in any part of the body.

      (ii) Overlying skin may be reddened or ulcerated.

      (iii) Purpuric papules may be present.

3. Polyarteritis is apt to run a course of a few years' duration; recovery is unpredictable – death may ensue from renal decompensation, congestive cardiac failure, etc.

TREATMENT

Treatment is similar to that of systemic lupus erythematosus.

Objective

To give the patient symptomatic and supportive care.

1. A search is made for any offending drug that may precipitate the disease.

2. Corticosteroids (prednisone) – given to control symptoms and to prevent progression of disease.

   a. Large doses may be given initially; patient is observed for evidence of disease regression.

   b. See Chapter 8, p. 576, for management of patient having steroid therapy.

3. In severe cases immunosuppressive drugs (cyclophosphamide; azathioprine) may be given in combination with corticosteroids, or plasma exchange may be necessary.

4. Watch for and treat intercurrent infections.

5. Advise patient to avoid drugs that may exacerbate symptoms.

SCLERODERMA (PROGRESSIVE SYSTEMIC SCLEROSIS)

Scleroderma (progressive systemic sclerosis) is a disease of unknown aetiology in which there is chronic hardening or shrinking of the connective tissue throughout the body. It is characterized by vascular abnormalities (sclerosis of the blood vessels), fibrosis of the skin, atrophy of smooth muscle and loss of visceral function.

CLINICAL FEATURES
1. The disease starts insidiously on face and hands; skin acquires a tense, wrinkle-free, bound-down appearance (cannot be picked up from adjacent structures).
   a. Wrinkles and lines are obliterated.
   b. Skin is dry – sweat secretion over involved area is suppressed.
   c. Face appears mask-like, immobile and expressionless; mouth becomes rigid.
   d. Condition spreads slowly; extremities become stiff and immobile; the fingers semiflexed, immobile and useless; the hands claw-like.
2. Detectable clinical changes may occur in the internal organs.
   a. Heart becomes fibrotic – causing dyspnoea and other symptoms.
   b. Oesophagus is hardened, with disruption of normal oesophageal peristalsis – gastro-oesophageal reflux, with heartburn and dysphagia.
   c. Lungs are scarred – impeding respiration.
   d. Intestines become hardened – digestive disturbances.
   e. Progressive renal failure may occur. Proteinuria and hypertension are bad prognostic signs.
   f. Variety of other disturbances develop, including Raynaud's phenomenon and arthritis.

TREATMENT
Methods of treatment may include:
1. Steroid therapy for anti-inflammatory effect. Care should be taken as steroids may make the hypertension dramatically worse.
2. Salicylate therapy – to relieve joint stiffness.
3. Physical therapy – helpful in preventing joint contractures and in maintaining joint mobility.
4. Surgical procedures (as in surgery for arthritis) – for hand deformities.
5. Vasoactive drugs, anti-inflammatory and anti-fibrotic agents – may be helpful for Raynaud's phenomenon.
6. Operative control of gastro-oesophageal reflux (reconstruction of oesophago-gastric junction) may be considered for reflux oesophagitis.
7. Cardiac, pulmonary and renal involvement are treated symptomatically.
8. The skin is kept lubricated with a bland cream (e.g. E45 cream).

PATIENT EDUCATION
Instruct the patient as follows:
1. Keep warm; take warm hand baths/paraffin dips for hand involvement.
2. For gastrointestinal disturbances:
   a. Chew well and eat slowly to allow oesophagus time to empty by gravity, since there is disruption of normal oesophageal peristalsis.
   b. Elevate head of bed on blocks.
   c. Take antacids between meals and before bedtime.

Care of the Burn Patient

BURNS

Burns are wounds caused by excessive exposure to four categories of agents: thermal, electrical, chemical and radioactive.

INCIDENCE
1. Over 150,000 burn injuries occur annually in England and Wales.
2. Approximately 15,000 burn victims require hospitalization each year in this country.
3. Nearly 800 people die from burns each year in England and Wales.

4. Most burn accidents occur in the home and are caused primarily by carelessness or ignorance.
5. Authorities estimate that at least 75 per cent of all burns could be prevented.
6. The nurse is in a strategic position for teaching burn prevention and for promoting legislation for safety practices.
7. Of burn victims, 30 per cent are children.

SEVERITY

Severity of burn injury is related to:
1. Depth.
2. Extent (percentage of body surface burned) (Figure 11.11).
3. Age (the elderly and the very young have a poorer prognosis).
4. Parts of body burned.
5. Past medical history.
6. Concomitant injuries and illnesses.
7. Presence of inhalation injury.

PATHOPHYSIOLOGY
Burn injury

Burn injury usually results from energy transfer from a heat source to the body. It can occur by direct conduction or electromagnetic radiation. Many factors alter the response of body tissues to these sources of heat:
1. Conductivity of local tissues – nerves and blood vessels conduct heat with greatest ease, whereas bone is most resistant.
2. Peripheral circulation.
3. Surface pigmentation; presence of insulating material or clothing.
4. Water content of tissue.

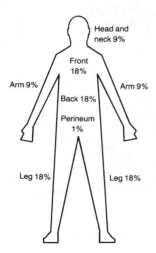

Figure 11.11. The Wallace 'Rule of Nine' chart

Inhalation injury

Carbon monoxide poisoning, smoke toxicity, upper airway trauma and restrictive defects are the four major types of pulmonary injury associated with burn injury.
1. Carbon monoxide (CO) is a colourless, odourless, tasteless, and nonirritating gas produced from incomplete combustion of carbon-containing materials.
2. Affinity of haemoglobin for CO is 200 times greater than for oxygen.
3. Toxicity will depend on concentration of CO in inspired air and the length of time of exposure.
4. Inhalation of hot, dry air (148.9°C or higher) appears not to have much effect on the lower respiratory tract because a sudden closing of the glottis and reflex apnoea occur.
5. From fire in a closed space, most particles of soot are filtered through upper airway, but because they may be superheated they may cause direct damage to mucosa.
6. Sulphur dioxide (SO_2) and nitrous oxide (N_2O) (toxic agents) most likely are clinging to soot; in the presence of water, they form corrosive acids and alkalies that are extremely toxic.
7. Toxic fumes from burning plastic are more dangerous than smoke; noxious gases include hydrogen cyanide, hydrochloric acid, sulphuric acid, halogens, and perhaps phosgene.
8. Upper airway obstruction may occur during the first 48 hours postburn due to pharyngeal and laryngeal oedema resulting from superficial burn of the upper airway. Oedema of the neck may also decrease tracheal patency.
9. Restrictive pulmonary complications can occur because of the tourniquet effect of oedema seen with circumferential chest burns. Lung compliance and alveolar gas exchange can also be decreased because of pulmonary oedema.

LOCAL EFFECTS OF BURNS
1. The depth of injury is directly related to the temperature of the burning agent and the duration of contact with body tissue.
2. A full-thickness burn may occur in as little as one second of exposure at 70°C.
   a. *Partial-thickness* burn injuries involve the epidermis and upper portions of the dermis. Some of the dermal appendages remain, from which the wound can spontaneously re-epithelialize.
   b. In *full-thickness injuries*, all layers of the skin and sometimes underlying tissues are de-

stroyed. Grafting usually is required to close the wound (Figure 11.12).

3. Physiological reaction:
   a. When skin is burned, adjacent intact vessels dilate.
   b. Platelets and leucocytes begin to adhere to the vascular endothelium as an early event in the inflammatory process.
   c. Increased capillary permeability produces wound oedema.
   d. An influx of polymorphonuclear leucocytes and monocytes occurs at the injury site.
   e. Eventually, new capillaries, immature fibroblasts and newly formed collagen fibrils appear within the wound. This supports the regenerating epithelium or forms a granulating tissue bed to accept a skin graft.

SYSTEMIC CHANGES IN MAJOR BURNS
Fluid shifts
1. In addition to changes in the local burned area, there are alterations and disruptions in the vascular and other systems of the body.
2. The water vapour barrier for the body is the outermost layer of epidermis. When it is rendered nonfunctioning, severe systemic reactions from fluid losses can occur.
3. Blanching of the skin following burn injury is caused by contraction of skin capillaries; redness occurs when arterioles and capillaries dilate.
4. Fluid volume deficit is directly proportional to extent and depth of burn injury.
5. Capillary permeability increases, permitting fluid and protein to move from vascular to interstitial spaces (oedema results). Protein-rich fluid is lost in blisters of the burned tissues, as well as by weeping of second-degree wounds and surface of full-thickness wounds. With reduced vascular volume, the patient will go into shock if untreated.
6. Vascular fluid loss occurs rapidly and peaks at 12 hours postburn.
7. Capillary permeability returns to near normal in about 48 hours – but protein lost in interstitial spaces remains there for several weeks, before returning to the vascular system.
   a. When fluid mobilizes (moves from interstitial spaces back to vascular compartment) patients with good cardiac and renal function will diurese.
   b. Observe carefully for fluid overload and pulmonary oedema; patient requires decreased fluid intake, frequent observation of vital signs, central venous pressure and urine output.
8. Red cell mass is also diminished, because of

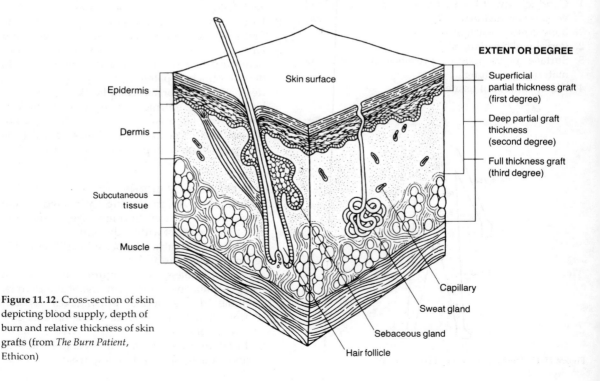

Skin surface

Epidermis

Dermis

Subcutaneous tissue

Muscle

EXTENT OR DEGREE

Superficial partial thickness graft (first degree)

Deep partial graft thickness (second degree)

Full thickness graft (third degree)

Capillary

Sweat gland

Sebaceous gland

Hair follicle

Figure 11.12. Cross-section of skin depicting blood supply, depth of burn and relative thickness of skin grafts (from *The Burn Patient*, Ethicon)

thrombosis sludging, and red cell death from thermal injury; as fluid escapes from capillary walls, blood concentrates, and the flow is sluggish – haematocrit rises.

9. Capillary stasis may cause ischaemia and even necrosis.
10. The body attempts to compensate for losses of plasma volume (Table 11.4).
    a. Constriction of vessels.
    b. Withdrawal of fluid from undamaged extra-cellular space.
    c. Patient is thirsty. (Oral fluids are not given until bowel sounds are heard.)

Table 11.4   Fluid loss

	Amount per hour per square metre of body surface
Normal unburned individual	15–20ml
Average adult with a flame burn of 40 per cent of his body	100ml

Haemodynamics

1. Lessened circulating blood volume results in decreased cardiac output initially and increased pulse rate.
2. There is a decreased stroke volume, as well as a marked rise in peripheral resistance (due to constriction of arterioles and increased haemoviscosity).
3. This results in inadequate tissue perfusion, which may in turn cause acidosis, renal failure and irreversible burn shock.
4. A burn injury often upsets the acid–base balance; therefore, careful monitoring of arterial blood gases, serum electrolytes, and urine volume is needed for proper fluid therapy; this will allow replacement of fluid loss and prevent dilatation and paralytic ileus.

Metabolic demands

1. Immediately following an extensive burn, there is a breakdown of cells (catabolism), resulting in a marked outpouring of potassium and nitrogen.
2. Healing a large surface area requires much energy; glucose is the primary metabolic fuel.
3. Because total body glucose stores are limited and

liver and muscle glycogen is exhausted within the first few days postburn, hepatic glucose synthesis increases.

4. When adequately treated, an extensively burned patient will probably increase his weight the first three or four days, because of collection of fluid in the interstitial spaces; thereafter, weight loss will be progressive, at the rate of about 2.2kg a day in a young adult, for about a month, depending on nutritional support. *Adequate nutritional therapy can reduce this loss to no more than 5 to 10 per cent of preburn body weight before weight stabilizes.*
5. In spite of all nutritional support, it is almost impossible to counteract a negative nitrogen balance; the sooner a burn wound is closed, the more rapidly a positive nitrogen balance is reached.
6. The postburn adult may require 4,000 to 6,000 calories a day; high calories, high protein may be given orally and in some instances by intravenous hyperalimentation or by nasogastric feeding along with normal meals and snacks.

Renal activity

1. Glomerular filtration may be decreased in extensive injury.
2. Without resuscitation or with delay, decreased renal blood flow may lead to high output or oliguric renal failure and decreased creatinine clearance.
3. Haemoglobin and myoglobin, present in the urine of patients with deep muscle damage, often associated with electrical injury, may cause acute tubular necrosis and calls for a greater amount of initial fluid therapy and osmotic diuresis.

Pulmonary changes

1. Hyperventilation and increased oxygen consumption are associated with major burns.
2. The majority of deaths from fire are due to smoke inhalation. See p. 763 for discussion of inhalation injury.
3. Fluid resuscitation may cause pulmonary oedema, contributing to decreased alveolar exchange.
4. Initial respiratory alkalosis resulting from hyperventilation may change to respiratory acidosis associated with pulmonary insufficiency as a result of major burn trauma.

Haematological changes

1. Thrombocytopenia, abnormal platelet function, depressed fibrinogen levels, inhibition of fibri-

nolysis and a deficit in several plasma clotting factors occurs postburn.

2. Anaemia results from the direct effect of destruction of erythrocytes due to burn injury, reduced life span of surviving red cells, overt or (more commonly) occult blood loss from duodenal or gastric ulcers, and blood loss during diagnostic and therapeutic procedures.

Immunological activity

1. The loss of the skin barrier and presence of eschar favour bacterial growth.
2. Granulation tissue, richly vascular, resists bacteria.
3. Abnormal inflammatory response after burn injury causes a decreased delivery of antibodies, white blood cells and oxygen to the injured area.
4. Hypoxia, acidosis and thrombosis of vessels in the wound area impair host resistance to pathogenic bacteria.
5. Several major immunoglobulins, complement and serum albumin are decreased soon after the burn occurs.
6. Depressed cellular immunity is reflected by lymphocytopenia, impaired delayed skin sensitivity, decreased allograft rejection potential, depletion of thymus-dependent lymphoid tissue and increased susceptibility to fungi, viruses and gram-negative organisms.
7. Burn wound sepsis:
   a. Following colonization of the burn wound surface by bacteria, subeschar and intrafollicular colonization develop. Intraeschar and subeschar colonization may progress to invasion of subadjacent, nonburned, previously viable tissue.
   b. A bacterial count of 10/g of tissue as determined by burn wound biopsy indicates burn wound sepsis.
8. Seeding of bacteria from the wound may give rise to systemic septicaemia.

Gastrointestinal changes

1. As a result of sympathetic nervous system response to trauma, peristalsis decreases and gastric distention, nausea, vomiting and paralytic ileus may occur.
2. Ischaemia of the gastric mucosa and other aetiological factors put the burn patient at risk for duodenal and gastric ulcer manifested by occult bleeding, and, in some cases, life-threatening haemorrhage.

ASSESSMENT OF BURNS

OBTAIN BRIEF HISTORY
1. Previous state of health.
2. Allergies.
3. Tetanus immunization status.
4. Height and weight of patient (pre- and postburn).
5. Vital signs.

EMERGENCY FIRST-AID MEASURES
See also Chapter 20 on emergency nursing.

NURSING ALERT
*Grease, ointment or antiseptic solutions should **not** be applied to any burn as a first-aid measure.*

1. Immediately stop the burning process.
2. When clothes catch fire, have victim fall to floor or ground and roll him in a carpet or blanket – if available within 1 or 2m; otherwise drop, roll and beat out flames with anything (including hands as last resort).
   a. Running would fan flames.
   b. Standing would force him to breathe flames and smoke, cause his hair to be ignited or cause facial disfigurement.
   c. After fire is extinguished, soak hot clothing with cold water.
3. Apply cold to the burn – immerse in cold water for 10 minutes, intermittently (if pain present, repeat up to three times) or apply towels soaked in cold water – this relieves pain and reduces tissue oedema and damage.
4. Cover burn as quickly as possible with sterile dressings or any clean cloth – to prevent further wound contamination.
   a. Bacterial contamination is minimized.
   b. Pain is decreased by preventing air from contacting injured surface.
5. Irrigate chemical burns immediately – continue irrigating for 10 to 15 minutes.
   a. Flush eyes, if affected, with clean, cool water.
   b. Consult doctor.
6. Allow victim to lie down while awaiting transportation to accident department.
   a. Do not remove clothing unless instructed by the doctor.
   b. Cover victim with a blanket to prevent loss of body heat.

c. Place ice bottles or ice strategically to reduce pain. (Do not do this if burn is large – patient may become hypothermic and go into shock.)

7. Determine best disposition of the patient depending upon severity of burns using the Wallace 'rule of nine' (see Figure 11.11) and triage criteria.
   a. Critically burned person should be moved to a well-equipped burns unit that has a medical and nursing staff experienced in burn care.
   b. Moderately burned person may be taken to a district hospital. This includes victims with:
      (i) Partial-thickness burns – 10 per cent (adults) or 5 per cent (children) of body surface.
      (ii) Full-thickness – more than 5 per cent of body surface.
   c. Minimally burned person may be treated in a GP's surgery or hospital outpatient department. This includes victims with:
      (i) Partial-thickness burns – less than 5 per cent.
      (ii) Full-thickness – less than 2 per cent.

Table 11.5 shows how burn injuries are assessed (see also Figure 11.12).

OTHER FACTORS TO ASSESS

1. Causative agent – hot water, chemical, petrol, flame, etc.
2. Duration of exposure.
3. Circumstances of injury, including whether in closed or open space.
4. Age.
5. Initial treatment, including first aid.
6. Pre-existing medical problems – heart disease, diabetes, ulcers, alcoholism, chronic obstructive airway disease, epilepsy, psychosis.
7. Current medications.

Table 11.5   Assessment of burn injury

Extent or degree	Assessment of extent	Reparative process
Superficial partial thickness (first degree)	Pink to red: slight oedema, which subsides quickly Pain may last up to 48 hours; relieved by cooling	In about five days, epidermis peels, heals spontaneously Itching and pink skin persist for about a week
Deep partial thickness (second degree)	*Superficial:* Pink or red; blisters form (vesicles); weeping, oedematous, elastic. Superficial layers of skin are destroyed; wound moist and painful. *Deep dermal:* Mottled white and red; oedematous reddened areas blanch on pressure May be yellowish but soft and elastic – may or may not be sensitive to touch; sensitive to cold air Hair does not pull out easily	No scarring Heals spontaneously if it does not become infected within ten days to two weeks Takes several weeks to heal Scarring may occur
Full thickness (third degree)	Destruction of epithelial cells – epidermis and dermis destroyed Reddened areas do not blanch with pressure Not painful; inelastic; coloration varies from waxy white to brown; leathery devitalized tissue is called *eschar*	Eschar must be removed. Granulation tissue forms to nearest epithelium from wound margins or support graft For areas larger than 7–8cm, grafting is required Expect scarring and loss of skin function
Fourth degree	Destruction of epithelium, fat, muscles and bone	Area requires debridement, formation of granulation tissue and grafting

8. Concomitant injuries (e.g. from fall or explosion).
9. Evidence of inhalation injury (p. 763).
10. Allergies.
11. Tetanus immunization status.
12. Height and weight.
13. Take photograph of burned area (with patient permission) for medical record of extent of burn, if directed.

PATIENT PROBLEMS

1. Impaired gas exchange related to carbon monoxide poisoning, upper airway obstruction, smoke inhalation and/or oedema of lung parenchyma.
2. Impaired ventilation related to circumferential oedema of chest.
3. Decreased cardiac output related to fluid changes and hypovolaemic shock.
4. Inadequate tissue perfusion related to peripheral burn-wound oedema, generalized oedema, and circumferential full-thickness burn.
5. Fluid volume deficit related to increased capillary permeability and evaporative fluid loss from burn wound.
6. Potential for fluid volume excess related to fluid mobilization three to five days postburn.
7. Impaired skin integrity related to burn injury and surgical interventions (donor sites).
8. Altered urinary elimination related to indwelling catheter.
9. Hypothermia related to loss of skin and microcirculatory regulation.
10. Potential for infection related to loss of skin barrier and altered immune response.
11. Impaired physical mobility related to oedema, pain, skin and joint contractures.
12. Ineffective rest–activity pattern related to burn wound discomfort and treatment priorities.
13. Activity intolerance related to long periods of immobility.
14. Alterations in nutrition – less than body requirements – related to hypermetabolic response to burn injury.
15. Alteration in gastric function related to stress response.
16. Alteration in comfort (skin tightness, dryness and itching) related to loss of skin lubricants, wound contraction in healing, altered nerve function.
17. Pain related to injured nerves in burn wound.
18. Ineffective individual coping related to fear and anxiety.
19. Knowledge deficit related to inexperience with burn injury and subsequent related health care needs.
20. Self-care deficit related to functional sequelae of burn injury.
21. Disturbance in self-concept related to altered body image.
22. Anticipatory/dysfunctional grieving related to biological, psychological, and social losses resulting from burn injury.

ASSESSMENT FOR INHALATION INJURY

1. If victim was burned in closed area, there should be a high index of suspicion that smoke inhalation has occurred (Figure 11.13).
2. Assess all patients in closed space fires for presence of symptoms of carbon monoxide poisoning: headache, visual changes, confusion, irritability, decreased judgement, nausea, ataxia, collapse (Table 11.6).
3. Question the patient about types of things that burned in this room – type of carpet, vinyl articles, synthetics.
4. Observe for upper body burns, erythema or blistering of lips, buccal mucosa or pharynx, singed nares hair, soot in oropharynx, dark grey or black sputum.
5. Listen for hoarseness and crackles.
6. Obtain blood gases and carboxyhaemoglobin levels.
7. Prepare the patient for bronchoscopy to confirm

Table 11.6 Signs and symptoms of toxicity from carbon monoxide

CO blood level (per cent)	Manifestations
0–10	None Smokers may normally have 10 per cent CO level
10–20	Headache, visual disturbance, angina in patients with cardiovascular disease, slowed mental function
20–40	Tight feeling in head, rapid fatigue from muscular effort, decreased muscular coordination, confusion, irritability, ataxia, nausea, vomiting, increased pulse rate, decreased blood pressure, dysrhythmias
40–60	Pulmonary and cardiac dysfunction, collapse, coma, convulsions
Over 60	Often fatal

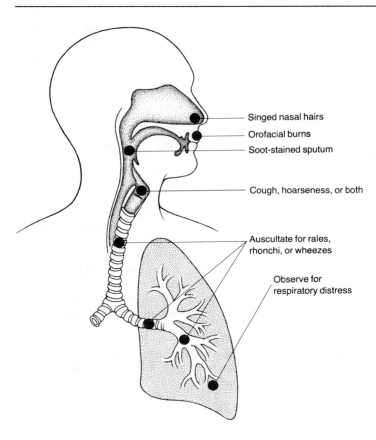

Singed nasal hairs

Orofacial burns

Soot-stained sputum

Cough, hoarseness, or both

Auscultate for rales, rhonchi, or wheezes

Observe for respiratory distress

Figure 11.13. In the nursing history, determine whether the victim was in a closed area during the fire and whether he lost consciousness. If any of the above physical findings are noted in addition to the nursing history data, the victim should be taken to a burns centre for further assessment. Baseline arterial blood gas measurements (to detect hypoxaemia) should be taken immediately upon admission

presence of mucosal erythema, haemorrhage, ulceration, oedema, carbonaceous particles.

8. Obtain chest X-ray for baseline data.

METHODS OF TREATING BURNS

OVERVIEW

1. Treatment of burn injury includes haemodynamic stabilization, metabolic support, wound debridement, use of topical antibacterial therapy and skin grafting and wound closure.

2. Prevention and treatment of complications, including infection and pulmonary damage and rehabilitation, are also of major importance.

INTRAVENOUS THERAPY AND METABOLIC SUPPORT

HAEMODYNAMIC STABILIZATION; PREVENTION OF BURN SHOCK
Intravenous fluid therapy

1. Immediate intravenous fluid resuscitation is indicated for:
   a. Adults with burns over greater than 15 per cent of body surface area.
   b. Children with burns involving more than 10 per cent of body surface area.
   c. Patients with electrical injury, the elderly or anyone with cardiac or pulmonary disease and compromised response to burn injury.

2. The goal is to give sufficient fluid to allow perfusion of vital organs without overhydrating the patient and risking later complications and circulatory overload.

3. Generally, a colloid solution is used: weight (kg) × surface area burn (percentage) × 2/3 = no. of ml of colloid in each period. First, second and third

periods each last four hours; fourth and fifth periods each last six hours; sixth and seventh each last 12 hours.

4. Use formula as a guide only: patient parameters, including urine output, vital signs, central venous pressure and haematocrit are the best indicators of fluid requirements and response.
5. A large-bore central venous catheter is recommended for large-volume replacement.
6. Fluids may be titrated to achieve a urine output of 30–50ml/hour (0.5ml/kg/hour) in an adult and 1ml/kg/hour in a child.
7. An indwelling urinary catheter is needed to monitor response to fluid therapy.
8. Weigh the patient on admission and then daily.
9. Elevate extremities.
10. Monitor peripheral pulses.
11. Administer humidified oxygen.

METABOLIC SUPPORT

1. Initially, give the patient restricted fluids (adult up to 100ml water hourly).
2. Reduce metabolic stress by allaying pain, fear and anxiety and maintaining a warm environment.
3. Nutritional management must be aggressive to combat acute nutritional deficiency and weight loss; a positive nitrogen balance should be the goal throughout the postburn course.
4. When bowel sounds return, advance diet as tolerated.
5. Offer more solid food after two or three days postburn as tolerance for food improves.
   a. Build up daily caloric intake to match daily caloric expenditure.
   b. Provide 3g protein/kg body weight; 20 per cent of needed calories in form of fats; remainder in carbohydrates.
6. When calorie requirements cannot be met by oral and fine bore nasogastric tube feeds, it may rarely be necessary to initiate intravenous hyperalimentation, e.g. amino acids, carbohydrates and fat emulsions.
7. Provide potassium and vitamin supplements.

WOUND CARE

There are three basic methods of wound care used in the treatment of burns.

Exposed (open)

This method is usually confined to areas of the body which are difficult to dress, e.g. face and ears, and these are left exposed to the air. Exudate needs to be removed frequently, using sterile saline. The dry wound inhibits bacterial growth, but also delays healing, and the patient must be nursed in a single room to prevent wound contamination. This method has largely been replaced by the semi-open or closed methods.

Semi-open

The wound is covered with a topical, antiseptic agent or biological dressing (see p. 771) with a few layers of gauze to hold it in place.

Closed

Bactigras tulle (Vaseline gauze), silver sulphadiazine or silver nitrate is applied, and this is covered with many layers of gauze and wool. Dressings are changed daily or on alternate days. The disadvantages of this method is that the wound is kept warm and moist and, therefore, encourages bacterial proliferation. Dressing changes may be uncomfortable for the patient and time-consuming for the nurse.

NURSING ALERT

Infection of the burn wound remains a serious complication until the wound has healed or has been successfully skin-grafted.

PREVENTION OF INFECTION

1. Be aware of micro-organisms being introduced to the wound by:
   a. The patient's own flora.
   b. The attendant's flora.
   c. Fomites (see also p. 69).
2. Frequent monitoring of the wound surface by bacteriological swabbing is imperative.
3. Cap, gown and mask should be worn by attendant.
4. No burn wound should be touched by the attendant's hands unless absolutely necessary, and then only with sterile gloves.
5. Dress wounds using the 'no-touch' technique with sterile instruments.

WOUND CLEANSING AND DEBRIDEMENT

1. Bacterial swabs are sent for culture and sensitivity from the burned areas before the first dressings are applied.
2. Clean wounds with chlorhexidine solution (0.05 per cent) or cetrimide (1 per cent).
3. Debridement with scissors is gently carried out, using an aseptic technique (e.g. remove dead epithelium and blisters).
4. Circumferential burns of the limb or chest are divided with a sterile scalpel (by the surgeon) to

prevent them constricting blood flow or interfering with respiration (escharotomy). It may be necessary to make multiple longitudinal incisions to reduce pressure adequately.

5. Dressings of tullegras impregnated with chlorhexidine (Bactigras) or silver sulphadiazine are applied and covered with gauze.
6. Special attention needs to be paid to burns of the hands. Hands should be bandaged with the metacarpophalangeal joints flexed at 90°, the interphalangeal joints straight and wrist extended. This reduces joint stiffness and facilitates mobility. Alternatively, hands may be mobilized immediately in clean polythene bags containing silver sulphadiazine.
7. Unless there are signs of infection or exudate soaks through, dressings should not be changed more than two to three times per week (see also p. 772).
8. Rest of the burn area is essential, e.g. sling, foot stool. Patients with burns on the back are more easily nursed on a low-air-loss bed or air-fluidized bed, so as to avoid pressure on damaged areas.
9. Eschar is lifted off with forceps and scissors after seven to ten days.
10. Failure of the burn to heal within 10 to 14 days (i.e. usually a full-thickness burn) will require immediate grafting (see p. 780).

Bathing

Many burns units consider that the dangers of cross-infection from baths outweigh their advantages as a method of wound cleansing. Their use is therefore limited to those patients with healed wounds who require hydrotherapy to encourage joint mobilization.

TOPICAL ANTIBIOTICS

Topical medications are used to cover burn areas and to reduce the number of organisms.

1. They are applied directly to the burn area as ointments, creams or solutions, or they may be incorporated in single-layer dressings that do not stick to the wound but permit drainage (Figure 11.14).
2. On top of the fine mesh gauze are placed bulky dry dressings to permit drainage to enter dressing but not come through.
3. Usually, these dressings are held in place by a single layer of stretch bandage or by net tube dressings.
4. When the patient is lying in bed, fluffy absorbent dressings or pads are placed on the bed where the burn area will make contact.

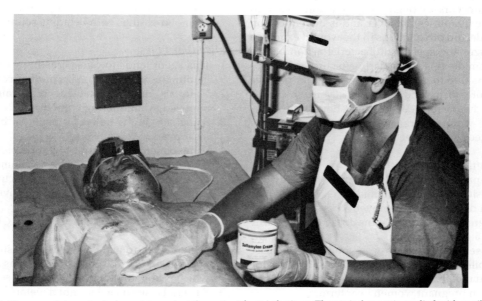

Figure 11.14. Nurse applying a topical agent to protect the patient from infections. The topical agent is applied with sterile gloves. A nasogastric tube is inserted to prevent abdominal distension and for the administration of antacids to prevent Curling's ulcers (courtesy US Army Institute of Surgical Research, Fort Sam Houston, Texas)

5. Desired characteristics in a topical antibiotic:
   a. Demonstrate action against Gram-negative aerobic intestinal bacteria *Pseudomonas aeruginosa* and *Staphylococcus aureus*.
   b. Ability to diffuse through the wound and penetrate the eschar.
   c. Nontoxic and noninjurious to body tissue.
   d. Inexpensive, pleasant to use, odourless or has pleasant odour; will not stain skin or clothing.
   e. Will not cause resistant strains of pathogenic organisms to develop.
6. To date there is no 'ideal' topical antibiotic.

SILVER SULPHADIAZINE 1 PER CENT (FLAMAZINE)
In a hydrophilic (readily absorbing moisture) water-soluble cream base.

Advantages and mode of action
1. Chlorides of the body are not readily precipitated, as with silver nitrate. Therefore, no electrolyte abnormality occurs and no acidosis develops.
2. Applied as a cream with sterile spatula or sterile gloves.
3. Little pain experienced with application of cream.
4. Viscous dressings are easily and painlessly removed.
5. Silver sulphadiazine is odourless; absorption of silver is minimal, and toxicity is rare.
6. Action occurs by oligodynamic action (active in minute quantities) of silver and is dependent on chloride and other anions in the wound exudate.
7. It utilizes the special antibacterial action of sulphonamide; it is particularly effective against infections due to gram-negative and gram-positive microorganisms and to *Candida albicans*.
8. It can be bactericidal up to 48 hours; however, when wounds are not clean, dressings are changed two or three times daily.

Disadvantages
1. Some patients develop a skin rash, probably due to sensitivity to sulphonamides.
2. When dressings are removed, they often have a grey-green appearance – this does not necessarily mean a gross infection.
3. Because sulpha drugs are known to increase possibility of kernicterus, silver sulphadiazine should not be used in infants in the first month of life or in pregnant women near term.
4. If topical proteolytic enzymes are used in debriding, silver sulphadiazine may inactivate them.
5. Lately it has been suggested that with protracted

use, gram-negative bacilli, particularly Enterobacteriaceae, can become highly resistant.
6. Because isolated incidences of leucopenia have occurred following use of Flamazine, it is suggested that blood counts be monitored carefully.

Mode of application
1. Silver sulphadiazine can be applied directly to the burn wound, spread thinly (2–4mm), and left exposed; wound should be so covered that no part is visible.
2. Some surgeons prefer that after ointment or cream is applied, it should be covered with a single layer of mesh gauze; others apply ointment to gauze and then apply the medicated gauze to the burn. Cover with stockinette or stretch gauze.
3. Reapply as it rubs off (remove all old cream before applying new); if occlusive dressings are used, change every 48 hours.

POVIDONE-IODINE OINTMENT 10 PER CENT AND BETADINE SOLUTION
Advantages
1. This agent appears to be effective against a wide variety of Gram-negative and Gram-positive organisms as well as yeasts, fungi and viruses.
2. It can be applied as an ointment (similar to Sulfamylon), the solution can be sprayed on, or it can be incorporated into mesh-gauze dressings.
3. The dressings are usually changed every six hours; remove outer dressings and rewet inner layer of dressings with Betadine solution.

Disadvantages
1. This agent tends to cause crusting – this may be helpful in some situations, a hindrance in others.
2. Materials may be stained, but stain can be removed by laundering immediately.
3. Some stinging is noted by patients, but it soon disappears.
4. Some patients are allergic to iodine preparations. Although povidone-iodine is recommended for moderate and major burns, more documentation is needed to recommend it for extensive burns.

CHLORHEXIDINE 0.05 PER CENT (BACTIGRAS)
Advantages
1. Bactericidal to a wide range of organisms.
2. Is incorporated into Vaseline gauze as a dressing which is nonadherent to the wound.
3. Bacterial resistance does not develop.

Disadvantages
1. Very rarely skin reactions have been reported.

SILVER NITRATE (0.5 PER CENT) SOLUTION

(Silver nitrate is being used less because of its disadvantages.)

Advantages and mode of action

1. Silver nitrate is a bacterostatic chemical and is effective in reducing colonization.
   a. Above 1 per cent concentration produces tissue necrosis.
   b. Below 0.5 per cent solution is ineffective as an antiseptic.
2. Cap, gown and mask are not required.
3. An effective method for treating large numbers of burns; is relatively inexpensive.
4. Several layers of four-ply gauze dressings *must be thoroughly wet every two to four hours with silver nitrate solution* to be effective. It is held close to the wound by stretch bandage or net tube dressings.
5. Silver nitrate can be used over grafted areas and donor sites, as well as burn surfaces.
6. Bacterial flora with which it is principally effective are Gram-negative.

Disadvantages

1. Since silver nitrate solution penetrates only 1–2mm of burn eschar, only surface contaminants can be controlled.
2. The wound must be completely free of oil or grease for silver nitrate solution to be effective.
3. Hyponatraemia (loss of sodium ions), hypokalaemia (loss of potassium ions) and hypochloraemia (loss of chlorine ions) may occur. (For this reason, it should not be used for children.)
4. Frequent blood samples are required to determine sodium, potassium and calcium ion levels.
5. It is necessary to replace electrolytes that are lost.
6. Methaemoglobinaemia (a modified form of oxyhaemoglobin) may be caused by the reduction of nitrates to nitrites, resulting in cyanosis.
7. Silver nitrate turns black in sunlight.

SKIN GRAFTING

(See also p. 780 for definitions of grafts and more detail of treatment.)

HOMOGRAFTS AND HETEROGRAFTS

DONOR CRITERIA

1. Skin colour unimportant, since it is only a temporary graft.
2. Donor should be an adult free of infection.

PURPOSE AND BENEFITS

1. Decreases heat, fluid and protein losses.
2. Reduces bacterial proliferation.
3. Closes wound temporarily; enhances production and protection of granulation tissue.
4. Protects exposed neurovascular and muscle tissue as well as tendons.
5. Reduces pain and facilitates patient comfort.
6. Acts as a test-graft to determine when granulating wounds will accept autograft successfully.
7. Provides an effective donor-site dressing.

CLINICAL PROCEDURE

1. Devitalized tissue is first removed surgically.
2. Skin graft is applied directly (epidermis side up) to the denuded area; it may be trimmed to adhere to wound contour. Before applying, it may be dipped in saline solution.
3. Grafts are usually left exposed except when applied to circumferential wounds; stretch gauze is applied to prevent adherence to and malpositioning by bed sheets.
4. The first skin graft dressing may have to be changed in 24 hours to permit more intimate adherence to granulating wound bed.
5. Thereafter, grafts may be left in place two to five days between changes; inspect wound daily to detect early signs of suppuration.
6. After good skin graft adherence is achieved, the wound is ready for autografting.

WOUND CLOSURE

1. Skin grafting is usually required or preferred with full-thickness burns greater than 2cm in diameter or in deep partial-thickness wounds.
2. Following gradual eschar removal and development of a base of granulating tissue, or in the presence of viable tissue following excision, grafts of the patient's own skin (autografts) are applied.
3. Sheet grafts or meshed grafts, providing wider expansion from donor sites, may be used.
4. Blood flow is established by the third or fourth day, and by the seventh to tenth day postgrafting, vascular continuity and wound closure have been established.

5. Many partial-thickness burn wounds will heal spontaneously within a few weeks, provided they are protected from infection (see the following).

PREVENTION AND TREATMENT OF COMPLICATIONS

Primary causes of morbidity and mortality in burn victims are those related to infection and pulmonary problems.

1. Topical antibacterial agents help to retard the proliferation of pathogenic organisms until wound closure occurs spontaneously or through surgical intervention.
2. Broadspectrum antibiotics may be necessary to treat systemic Gram-positive and Gram-negative infections and sometimes fungal infection.
3. Critical diagnostic parameters include observing for signs of burn-wound sepsis, including quantitative and qualitative wound biopsy and observing for signs of systemic septicaemia and taking blood for cultures.

Planning and implementation

NURSING INTERVENTIONS

Establishing adequate tissue oxygenation and respiratory function

1. Provide humidified 100 per cent oxygen until carbon monoxide level is known. (CAUTION: Adjust oxygen flow rate for patient with chronic obstructive airway disease as prescribed.)
2. Assess for signs of hypoxaemia and differentiate this from pain.
3. Note history of injury; suspect respiratory injury if burn occurred in an enclosed space.
4. Observe for erythema or blistering of buccal mucosa, singed nares, burns of lips, face, or neck, increasing hoarseness.
5. Monitor respiratory rate, depth, rhythm, cough.
6. Auscultate chest and note breath sounds.
7. Note character and amount of respiratory secretions. Report carbonaceous sputum, tracheal tissue.
8. Observe for signs of inadequate ventilation and include monitoring of arterial blood gases.
9. Provide mechanical ventilation, continuous positive airway pressure or positive end-expiratory pressure if requested.
10. Keep intubation equipment at bedside and be alert for signs of respiratory obstruction.
11. In mild inhalation injury:
    a. Provide humidification of inspired air.
    b. Encourage coughing and deep breathing.
    c. Maintain pulmonary toilet.
12. In moderate to severe inhalation injury:

a. Initiate more frequent bronchial suctioning.
b. Monitor vital signs, urinary output, and blood gases.
c. Administer bronchodilators, if prescribed.
d. For additional respiratory problems, it may be necessary to have patient intubated and placed on mechanical ventilation.

Maintaining adequate tidal volume and unrestricted chest movement

1. Observe rate and quality of breathing; if progressively more rapid and shallow, notify doctor.
2. Assess tidal volume; report decreasing volume to doctor.
3. Encourage deep-breathing and incentive spirometry (or hyperinflation with Ambu-bag for artificial airway) hourly.
4. Place patient in upright position to permit maximal chest expansion.
5. Ensure that chest dressings are not constricting.
6. Document and report respiratory changes, including dyspnoea, shortness of breath.
7. Prepare the patient for escharotomy and assist surgeon as indicated.

Restoration of normal haemodynamic status with slightly elevated cardiac output

1. Position the patient to increase venous return.
2. Give digoxin per surgeon's request.
3. Give fluids as prescribed.
4. Monitor vital signs, including apical pulse, respirations, central venous pressure, pulmonary artery pressures and urine output, at least hourly.
5. Determine cardiac output as requested.
6. Monitor level of consciousness.
7. Document all observations and particularly note trends in vital-sign changes.

Maintaining adequate circulation to all areas, including extremities

1. Monitor peripheral pulses hourly.
2. Elevate extremities.
3. Remove all constricting jewellery and clothing. Loosen dressings if necessary.
4. Prepare the patient for escharotomy (surgical procedure to relieve constricting effect of oedematous circumferential burns and permit adequate circulation to underlying tissues).
5. Monitor signs of adequate tissue perfusion, including renal status; appraise mental reactions and responses.

Maintaining fluid and electrolyte balance within a normal range

1. Titrate fluid intake as prescribed.
2. Maintain accurate intake and output records.
3. Weigh the patient daily.
4. Provide potassium replacement after fluid resuscitation is completed.
5. Be alert to signs of fluid overload and congestive heart failure during period of fluid mobilization, three to five days postburn.

Re-establishing skin integrity

1. Cleanse wounds as directed with cetrimide 1 per cent or chlorhexidine 0.05 per cent.
2. Debride eschar using scissors and forceps. Limit time to 20 minutes; stop if there is pain or bleeding.
3. Apply topical antibiotic agents as directed (see p. 771).
4. Dress wounds with coarse mesh gauze for new wounds requiring debridement; use fine-mesh gauze on granulating and healing wounds.
5. For grafted areas, use extreme caution in removing dressings; observe for serous or sanguineous blisters or purulent drainage; report to surgeon. Redress grafted areas as directed.
6. Observe all wounds daily and document wound status on the patient's record.
7. Promote healing of donor sites by:
   a. Preventing contamination of donor sites that are clean wounds.
   b. Opening to air for drying 24 hours postoperatively if gauze or impregnated gauze dressing is used.
   c. Following surgeon's or manufacturer's instructions for care of sites dressed with synthetic materials.
   d. Allowing dressing to peel off spontaneously.
   e. Cleansing healing donor site with mild soap and water once dressings are removed; lubricating site twice daily when healed.

Avoiding bladder infection

1. Maintain closed urinary drainage system.
2. Ensure a patent urinary catheter.
3. Observe colour, quality, amount of urine every hour.
4. Empty drainage bag frequently.
5. Provide catheter-care.
6. Encourage removal of catheter and use of urinal, bedpan, or commode as soon as frequent urine-output determinations are not required.

Maintaining normal or only slightly elevated body temperature

1. Be efficient in care; do not expose wounds unnecessarily.
2. Maintain high room temperature (25–28°C).
3. Use heat lamps, radiant warmers, space blankets to keep the patient warm.
4. Provide a dry top layer for wet dressings to reduce evaporative heat loss.
5. Warm wound cleansing and dressing solutions to body temperature.
6. Use dry dressings and blankets in transporting patient outside of hospital.

Avoiding wound or systemic infection

1. Wash hands before and after all patient contact with antibacterial cleansing agent.
2. Use barrier garments – isolation gown or plastic apron – for all care requiring contact with the patient or the patient's bed.
3. Be sure nurse covers hair and wears mask when wounds are exposed or when performing a sterile procedure.
4. Use clean examination gloves for all care involving patient contact.
5. Maintain proper concentration of topical antibacterial agents used in wound care.
6. Be alert for reservoirs of infection and sources of cross-contamination in equipment, assignment of personnel, etc.
7. Check history of tetanus immunization and provide passive and/or active range tetanus prophylaxis as prescribed.
8. Change intravenous lines every 24 to 48 hours; change intravenous tubing every 24 to 48 hours.
9. Administer antibiotics as prescribed and be alert for toxic effects and incompatibilities.
10. Assess wounds daily for local signs of infection – swelling and redness around wound edges, purulent drainage, discoloration, loss of grafts, etc.
11. Be alert for early signs of septicaemia, including changes in mental state, tachycardia and decreased peristalsis, as well as later signs, such as increased pulse, decreased blood pressure, increased or decreased urine output, facial flushing, increased temperature, malaise; report promptly to doctor.
12. Promote optimal personal hygiene for the patient, including daily cleansing of unburned areas, meticulous care of teeth and mouth, shampooing of hair every other day, shaving of hair in or near burned areas, meticulous care of intravenous and urinary catheter sites.

13. Inspect skin carefully for signs of pressure and breakdown.
14. Observe for and report signs of thrombo-phlebitis or catheter-induced infections.
15. Prevent atelectasis and pneumonia through therapy, postural drainage, meticulous pulmon-ary technique and, if indicated, tracheostomy care.

Enhancing range of joint motion and ability to perform activities of daily living

1. Obtain consultation from physiotherapist and occupational therapists.
2. Assist the patient with prescribed exercise regimen, passive and active range-of-motion exercises, ambulation (Figure 11.15).
3. Maintain splints in proper position as prescribed by physiotherapist; remove splints regularly and observe for signs of skin irritation before re-applying.
4. Position the patient to decrease oedema and avoid flexion of burned joints.
5. Coordinate pain management and other care to allow optimal effort during periods of physical exercise.
6. Encourage independence in activities that afford motion of burned joints.
7. Initiate passive and active range-of-motion and breathing exercises during early postburn period.
8. Plan with physiotherapist, occupational and re-spiratory therapists for a conditioning regimen that gradually increases energy expenditure and tolerance for activity.
9. Coordinate plan for rest, nutritional intake and pain minimization to maximize physical and mental energy available for increasing activities.
10. Contract with the patient to assist him to meet goals for type and level of activity desired.
11. Act as advocate for the patient's need for rest by coordinating the patient's therapeutic and social activities and prioritizing interventions and visits.
12. Assess preburn sleep pattern and determine what helps the patient achieve relaxation and sleep; implement to the extent possible.
13. Provide sleep medication as prescribed.

Augmenting nutritional intake

1. Weigh the patient daily with dressings removed.
2. Obtain consultation from dietitian for calculation of nutritional needs based on age, weight, height and burn size.
3. Administer vitamins and mineral supplements as prescribed.
4. Minimize metabolic stress by allaying fears, pain

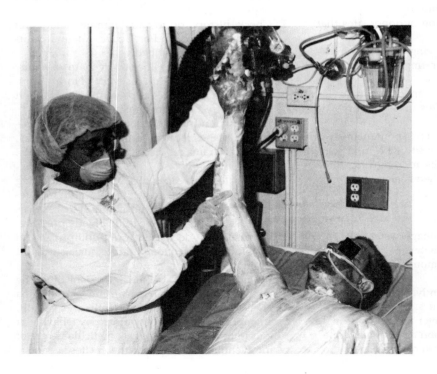

Figure 11.15. The patient is put through full range-of-motion exercises at least twice daily to prevent contractures (courtesy US Army Institute of Surgical Research, Fort Sam Houston, Texas)

and anxiety and by maintaining a warm environmental temperature.

5. When bowel sounds return, administer oral fluids slowly, so that patient tolerance can be observed. If there are no problems, advance diet to the patient's usual diet, as tolerated.
6. Provide nasogastric tube feedings as prescribed, using caution to prevent aspiration by checking tube placement prior to each feeding and checking amount of gastric aspirate.
7. Administer intravenous hyperalimentation and fat emulsions prescribed with usual nursing precautions.
8. Keep record of caloric intake.
9. Encourage the patient to feed self.
10. Supplement meals with between-meal high-protein, high-caloric snacks, including appropriate foods brought from home.

Resumption of normal gastric motility and function

1. Keep on restricted fluids until bowel sounds resume (100ml hourly).
2. Assess bowel sounds every two to four hours while acutely ill. (Decreased peristalsis may be an early sign of septicaemia.)
3. Decompress stomach with nasogastric tube on low intermittent suction until bowel sounds resume.
4. Check amount and pH of gastric drainage or aspirate and report as requested.
5. Administer antacids as prescribed.
6. Heed complaints of nausea while intubated by checking for abdominal distension, tube placement.
7. Provide mouth care every four hours while intubated.
8. Test stools for occult bleeding.

Reducing pain and enhancing relaxation

1. Assess the patient for pain periodically.
2. Teach relaxation, imagery, breathing exercises or other techniques to help the patient cope with pain.
3. Determine previous experience with pain, the patient's response and coping mechanisms.
4. Offer analgesics prior to wound care or before particularly painful treatments.
5. Change the patient's position when possible, supporting extremities with pillows.
6. Reduce anxiety by explanations of procedures.

Care of concomitant illnesses and injuries

1. Obtain complete nursing database, including history of events surrounding the burn injury, past health/illness, physical assessment and laboratory results.
2. Observe for fractures, spinal, head or internal organ damage in victims of electrical burns, explosions, or history of falling or jumping from a fire.
3. Obtain ophthalmological consultation if face is burned.
4. Observe for signs and symptoms of chronic illness heightened by stress of burn injury.
5. Implement appropriate independent and dependent nursing activities related to above findings.

Promoting an understanding of consequences of burn injury, required therapy and rationale

1. Develop an individualized teaching plan that includes explanations of pathophysiological changes resulting from burn injury, both immediate and long-term, treatments and rationale.
2. Include aspects of care provided by all burn team members.
3. Periodically 'test' the patient's understanding.
4. Provide time for and encouragement of questions related to care, both in hospital and projected home setting.

Enhancing coping strategies

1. Assess the patient's coping mechanisms from past history and current behaviour.
2. Provide opportunities for the patient to express his thoughts and feelings, and fears and anxieties regarding his injury.
3. Explore with the patient alternative mechanisms for coping with the burn injury and its consequences.
4. Assure the patient of the normality of his responses and the effect that time and healing will likely have on his current concerns.
5. Interpret patient behaviour to concerned family and significant others.
6. Respect current coping mechanisms and remove them only when an appropriate alternative can be provided.
7. Support family and friends' communications and visits if this is noted to help the patient.
8. Assess need for psychiatric nursing consultation/medical (psychiatric) intervention.
9. Offer antianxiety medications as prescribed.
10. Assist the patient to adapt to altered body image or lifestyle resulting from burn injury.
    a. Gather data on the patient's preburn self-image and lifestyle.
    b. When the patient is ready, encourage him to

express his concerns regarding changes in self-image or lifestyle that may result from burn injury.

   c. Be honest, but positive, in responding to the patient and family.

   d. Positively reinforce appropriate, effective coping mechanisms.

   e. Utilize hospital and community resources, including psychologists, counsellors, teachers, clergy and significant others to provide support for the patient.

11. Assist the patient to resolve grief related to burn injury in an appropriate manner.

   a. Recognize the patient's need to grieve over losses related to the burn injury.

   b. Support the patient and significant others through the grieving process, recognizing that each individual may move through this at a different pace.

   c. Differentiate between normal depression following traumatic injury and depression that requires medication or psychiatric intervention.

   d. Arrange for the patient to talk with other patients who have had a similar injury and are progressing satisfactorily.

   e. Help the patient set short-term goals and reflect on progress in small steps.

PATIENT EDUCATION

Health education is closely related to the rehabilitation of the burn patient as he prepares to return to a productive place in society. Functional and cosmetic reconstruction is accomplished, and the patient attempts to integrate a new self-concept into social realities. Broadly viewed, patient education focuses on biological, psychological and social parameters.

1. Assist the patient in transition from dependence on the health team to independence by helping him develop methods of communicating his needs and functioning abilities to others.

2. Guide the patient in thinking positively about himself. Promote ability to redirect others' attention from the scarred body to the self within.

3. Demonstrate and explain wound care procedures to be continued after discharge:

   a. Wash hands.

   b. Cleanse small open wounds with mild soap in bath or shower.

   c. Rinse well with tap water.

   d. Pat dry with clean towel.

   e. Apply prescribed topical agent and/or dressing.

4. Observe for local signs of wound infection:

   a. Increased redness of normal skin around burn area.

   b. Increased cloudy yellow pus or drainage.

   c. Increased pain, foul odour in burn area.

   d. Elevated body temperature.

5. Instruct the patient in measures to lubricate and enhance comfort of healing skin:

   a. Cleanse skin with mild soap and rinse well daily.

   b. Apply lubricant such as cocoa butter or Nivea to healed areas twice daily.

   c. Wear clean, white underwear and clothing free of irritating dyes.

   d. Take antipruritics as prescribed.

   e. Stay in a cool environment if itching occurs.

   f. Protect skin from further trauma, including sunburn (use sunblock containing PABA).

6. Develop a schedule to incorporate exercise regimen as prescribed by physiotherapist:

   a. Assist the patient and family to practise exercises.

   b. Suggest scheduling exercises immediately after wound cleansing and application of topical agent, since skin may be more pliable and less sensitive to stretching then.

7. Instruct the patient in use and care of splints and pressure garments:

   a. Cleanse with mild soap and rinse well daily.

   b. Keep away from heat; dry garment by laying it flat on towels.

   c. Wear garment on schedule prescribed by therapist.

   d. Pad open wounds with light dressing under splints or pressure garments.

   e. Observe for signs of skin breakdown.

   f. Wear/bring splints and pressure garments to follow-up visits to be checked for proper fit.

8. Acquaint patient and family with resources, including support groups for recovering burn victims, family group meetings in burn centre, community resources as required.

9. Review with the patient and family common emotional responses during convalescence (depression, withdrawal, grieving, dreaming, anxiety, guilt, excessive sensitivity, emotional lability, insomnia, fear of future) and discuss usual temporary nature of these and effective coping mechanisms.

10. Arrange for return visit for follow-up care and home health-care services, as needed in interim.

11. Provide written instruction regarding all care required on discharge.

Evaluation

EXPECTED OUTCOMES

1. Achieves normal respiratory function (e.g. $CO < 10$, arterial blood gases within normal limits, respiratory rate 12–20).
2. Achieves normal cardiovascular function (e.g. pulse 60–100, peripheral tissues adequately perfused).
3. Maintains fluid and electrolyte parameters in healthy balance.
4. Demonstrates adequate wound healing – small open wound areas are clean.
5. Skin is soft, comfortable; scars flat.
6. Has normal urinary elimination.
7. Demonstrates normal body temperature.
8. Is free of pathogenic organisms.
9. Achieves normal range of motion and can perform activities of daily living with necessary endurance.
10. Achieves positive nitrogen balance; regains optimal weight.
11. Regains normal integrity and function of gastro-intestinal system.
12. Reports minimal pain in burn area and joints; explains use of analgesics and other pain-reduction techniques.
13. Uses appropriate coping mechanisms to deal with stress of burn injury and its sequelae.
14. Adapts to losses and alterations in body image and to lifestyle resulting from the burn injury.
15. Explains rationale of required self-care related to burn injury. Demonstrates ability to carry out wound and skin care, exercises, splint and pressure garment application.

CARE OF THE PATIENT UNDERGOING PLASTIC RECONSTRUCTIVE SURGERY

Reconstructive surgery (plastic surgery) is performed to repair extravisceral defects and malformations, both congenital and acquired, and to restore function as well as prevent further loss of function.

Aesthetic surgery (cosmetic surgery) involves reconstruction of the cutaneous tissues around the neck and face; done to restore function, correct defects and remove the marks of time (Table 11.7).

Table 11.7 Common cosmetic operations

Operation	Purpose	Surgery	Postoperative expectations
Rhinoplasty (nose)	To improve the shape of the nose in relation to the rest of the face	1–1½ hours; excess bone or cartilage is removed; nose is reshaped	Nasal splint; soft intranasal packing
Chin augmentation	To improve the profile, as is necessary with a receding chin	Incision approach is within the mouth; inorganic (silicone) implant is positioned	Healing complete in one week
Rhytidoplasty (face-lifting)	To remove excess skin due to elastosis and to tighten remaining skin	Incision is anterior and posterior to the ear	Improvement lasts up to 10 years
Glabellar rhytidoplasty	To remove two vertical furrows between eyebrows	Dermabrasion	
Otoplasty (ear)	To correct deformed, flattened or protruding ears	1–1½ hours; silicone or plastic implant may be used	Ear bandaged for one week; protection during sleep required for three weeks
Blepharoplasty (eyelid)	To remove wrinkles and bulges caused by herniation of fat, ageing or inheritance	1–1½ hours; two incisions, one on upper lid and one on lower lid	Antibiotic ointment applied around eyes and lids; individual eye dressings are applied; swelling and discoloration subside in about 10 days

SKIN GRAFTING

DEFINITIONS

1. *Skin graft* – a section of skin tissue that is separated from its blood supply and transferred as a free section of tissue to the recipient site.
2. *Skin flap* – a section of skin tissue used to cover or fill a defect; it is lifted from its bed but still has partial attachment by a pedicle from which it receives its blood supply until healing takes place in its new location. Flaps are used to cover defects in which there is poor vascularity; for reconstruction of eyelids, ears, nose, and cheeks.
3. *Autograft* – transfers or transplants from one person to the same individual.
4. *Homograft* – transfer or transplants between two individuals of same species.
5. *Isografts* – grafts between identical twins.
6. *Heterografts* – grafts between two animals of different species (e.g. rabbit to mouse, pig to man).
7. *Split-thickness skin graft* (Thiersch's graft) – graft of approximately one-half the thickness of skin, which is removed by a knife or dermatome; deeper layers of dermis are left behind. (Used for coverage and closure of skin defects.)
8. *Full-thickness skin graft* – contains the epidermis and all of the dermis.
   a. Used frequently for reconstruction of facial defects, for it neither contracts nor develops unsightly pigmentation.
   b. Grafts may be further subdivided into thin and thick:
      (i) Thin (0.25–0.5mm) – used to resurface contaminated granulations or recipient sites in which blood supply is jeopardized.
      (ii) Thick (0.75–1mm) – used where durability is the important factor.
9. *Pinch graft* – a small piece of skin graft obtained by elevating the skin with a needle or forceps and cutting it off with scissors or knife.
10. *Take* – refers to the appearance of the graft between the third and fifth day after transfer, signifying that the vascular connections have developed between the recipient bed and the transplant.

CAUSES OF GRAFT FAILURE

1. Avascular bed.
2. Haematoma or seroma under the graft.
3. Infection.
4. Movement of the graft on its bed.

Planning and implementation

PREOPERATIVE NURSING INTERVENTIONS

Establishing optimal grafting procedure

1. Prepare the patient psychologically.
   a. Attempt to establish the reasons why the patient seeks surgery.
      (i) The patient's attitudes toward his disfigurement; his motivations for seeking surgery and his assessment of how his disfigurement has influenced his life; and his psychosocial relationships are taken into consideration before surgery is considered.
      (ii) Desirable to have unimpaired body image and realistic acceptance of surgical limitations.
      (iii) Poor candidate for aesthetic surgery is one who has delusions concerning his deformity, unhealthy psychological responses and unrealistic expectations of results.
   b. Explain the limitations of the contemplated procedure, the possibility of complications and the unpredictability of the result (responsibility of the surgeon).
2. Assess for nutritional status.
   a. Increase protein intake as directed – to facilitate healing.
   b. Note haemoglobin level and clotting time – these levels can affect healing process.
3. Prepare donor and recipient sites for surgical excision.
4. Inform the patient of what to expect postoperatively.
   a. Appearance of the wound – redness, distortion, swelling and unattractive suture lines are characteristics that will change with time.
   b. Pressure dressings, immobilization devices, etc.

POSTOPERATIVE NURSING INTERVENTIONS

Care of recipient site

1. Inspect graft under dressing daily, using a good light – to be sure that oedema, blistering or haematoma has not formed and is not jeopardizing success of graft.
   a. Carefully tease dressing away from wound – changing dressing may cause avulsion (tearing away) of recent graft around margin of wound.
   b. Nick graft to evacuate blood clots.
      (i) Fluid may be rolled out of graft with cotton-tipped applicator or by aspirating with needle and syringe.

(ii) Seromas or haematomas may impede healing.

2. Apply mittens to the patient if he is inadvertently scratching the graft during sleep – to protect graft and donor site from inadvertent scratching.

3. Apply wet dressings to infected graft as directed.

4. Use antibiotic therapy for the patient with infected graft. Utilize sensitivity testing to identify organism.

5. Elevate grafted extremity for seven to ten days.
   a. Immobilize part – movement of body areas beneath graft may predispose to loss of graft.
   b. Apply cast or immobilizing bandages to restrict all regional movements of the extremity.
   c. Begin ambulation activities very gradually.

Care of the donor site

1. The donor site is usually covered with a layer of nonadherent Vaseline gauze and held in place with a gauze dressing with cotton to absorb blood and serum from the wound.
   a. The outer dressings may be removed to the first layer if infected.
   b. Vaseline gauze is not disturbed until it separates spontaneously (about ten days).
2. Apply dressing as directed e.g. chlorhexidine tullegras, if donor site becomes infected.
3. Lubricate donor site with lanolin or cocoa butter after healing – to keep it soft and pliable.
4. Donor sites heal by re-epithelialization; healing should be complete in two weeks' time.

PATIENT EDUCATION

1. Inform the patient of the changing hues of the graft – to help him accept his situation.
   a. Free graft is at first pale, then pink and red – it then fades and appears similar to neighbouring skin.
   b. Full-thickness grafts may remain deeply red for months.
   c. Anticipate skin scaling in full-thickness grafts.
   d. Teach the patient that the graft is vulnerable to sun; avoid overexposure to the sun.
2. Instruct the patient to apply a thin coating of mineral oil or lanolin on wound after the second or third week – to remove superficial crusts, moisten the graft and stimulate circulation to the wound area.

Evaluation
EXPECTED OUTCOMES
1. Skin-grafted area healing in a desirable manner – absence of inflammatory signs such as puffiness, redness, tenderness.

2. Patient moves body part where graft has taken place with caution to avoid breaking down newly healed tissue.

3. Patient indicates signs that would suggest wound disruption by infection, trauma, extremes in temperature – tells what he should do under these conditions.

4. Patient appears pleased with results and verbalizes this feeling.

DERMABRASION

Dermabrasion is surgical planing of the superficial portion of the skin.

CLINICAL INDICATIONS

1. Done on selected patients with facial disfigurements from scars due to acne, trauma, naevi, chickenpox or smallpox, benign tumours, tattoos.
2. To smooth and improve colour of transplanted or grafted skin.

TREATMENT AND NURSING MANAGEMENT
Preoperative
1. Wash the part to be treated with pHisoHex for several days before surgery.
2. Administer adequate preoperative sedation as prescribed.

Operative
The epidermis and some superficial dermis are removed, but enough of the dermis is preserved to allow re-epithelialization of the dermabraded areas.
1. The patient is anaesthetized.
2. The superficial layer of skin is removed by an abrasive machine (Dermabrader) or by sandpapering.
3. Copious saline irrigations are carried out during and after the planing procedure.
4. At the conclusion of surgical planing:
   a. The surgeon may apply a layer of Vaseline gauze, followed by fluffed gauze and a pressure dressing.
   b. Another method is to apply a thick paste of thrombin (mixture of thrombin powder and saline) to the abraded areas. This controls bleeding and oozing, which dries to form a protective eschar.
   c. The wound is left undressed.

Postoperative
1. The wound may be gently cleaned with saline.
2. Within 48 hours an eschar forms as the serum

dries; this can be aided by using a hair dryer. These crusts are shed in seven to ten days.

3. The eschar separates spontaneously after 10 to 14 days, leaving exposed pink epithelium which eventually fades (four to nine months).

PATIENT EDUCATION

1. In the later stages of healing, cold cream may be applied; these aid in the removal of crusts. These should never be removed forcibly because this would injure new epithelium and delay healing.
2. Advise the patient to avoid exposure to direct or reflected sunlight for six months. Suggest applying an effective sun-screening cream to the affected area; reapply frequently and use for about three months postoperatively.
3. Should hyperpigmentation occur, it may regress in three to 18 months. Hypopigmentation occurs occasionally but also regresses. Meanwhile, effective cover-up cosmetics are recommended.

CHEMICAL PEEL

Chemical peel (chemosurgery, chemabrasion, chemical face-lifting) is the application of a cauterant (caustic material) to the skin for the purpose of superficially destroying epidermis and upper levels of dermis.

1. Phenol combined with other agents and trichloracetic acid are the agents commonly used.
2. *Salabrasion* is a combination of chemical and mechanical action occasionally used for tattoo removal.
3. Chemical planing is painful; meticulous care is required over a period of time. It is not corrective surgery but may supplement it. It should be done by a skilled plastic surgeon.

FURTHER READING

BOOKS

Burns and reconstructive surgery

Artz, C.P., Moncrief, J.A. and Pruitt, B. (1979) *Burns: A Team Approach*, W.B. Saunders, Philadelphia.

Cason, J.S. (1981) *Treatment of Burns*, Chapman and Hall, London.

Collyer, H. (1984) *Facial Disfigurement – Successful Rehabilitation*, Macmillan, London.

Dickinson, D.S. (1983) *Nursing and the Management of Burns* (5th edn), Faber and Faber, London.

Hummel, R.P. (ed.) (1982) *Clinical Burn Therapy*, John Wright, Bristol.

Kemble, J.V.H. and Lamb, B.E. (1984) *Plastic Surgical and Burns Nursing*, Baillière Tindall, London.
— (1987) *Practical Burns Management*, Croom Helm, London.

Skin disorders

Cronin, E. (1980) *Contact Dermatitis*, Churchill Livingstone, Edinburgh.

Fregert, S. (1981) *Manual of Contact Dermatitis* (2nd edn), Munksgaard, Copenhagen.

Fry, L., Wojnarowska, F. and Shahrad, P. (1981) *Illustrated Encyclopedia of Dermatology*, MTP Press, London.

Hughes, G.R.V. (1985) *Lupus: A Guide for Patients*, Rheumatology Department, St Thomas' Hospital, London.

Malten, K.E., Nater, J.P. and Venketel, W.G. (1976) *Patch-Testing Guidelines*, Dekker and van de Vegt, Nijmegen.

Marks, R. (1981) *Psoriasis*, Martin Dunitz, London.
— (1984) *Acne*, Martin Dunitz, London.

McKie, R. (1983) *Eczema and Dermatitis*, Martin Dunitz, London.

Meneghini, C. and Bonifazi, E. (1986) *An Atlas of Paediatric Dermatology*, Martin Dunitz, London.

Murray, D. (1981) *The Anti-Acne Book*, Arlington Pocket Books, London.

Orton, C. (1981) *Learning to Live with Skin Disorders*, Souvenir Press, London.

Rook, A., Wilkinson, D.S. and Ebling, A. (1979) *A Textbook of Dermatology* (3rd edn), Blackwell Scientific, Oxford.

Wilkinson, D.A. (1977) *Nursing and Management of Skin Diseases* (4th edn), Faber and Faber, London.

ARTICLES

Burns and reconstructive surgery

Abshagen, D. (1984) Topical agents in minor burn injuries, *Journal of Emergency Nursing*, Vol. 10, p. 325.

Bingham, H.G., Krischler, J.P., Shuster, J.J. and Engelman, I.A. (1980) Effects of nutrition on length of stay and survival for burned patients, *Burns*, Vol. 7, p. 252.

Dossing, M. and Sorensen, B. (1975) Freeze-dried and non-freeze-dried allografts on excised burns, *Burns*, Vol. 2, p. 36.

Gaston, S.F. and Schumann, O.L. (1980) Inhalation injury; smoke inhalation, *American Journal of Nursing*, Vol. 1, pp. 94–7.

Gray, D.T. *et al.* (1982) Early surgical excision versus conventional therapy in patients with 20% to 40% burns, *American Journal of Surgery*, Vol. 144, No. 1, pp. 76–80.

Hurt, R.A. (1985) More than skin deep; guidelines on caring for the burn patient, *Nursing 85*, Vol. 15, No. 6, pp. 52–7.

Jeffcott, M. (1981) Management of burns, *Journal of Clinical Nursing*, Vol. 26, pp. 1126–7.

Kenner, C. and Manning, S. (1980) Emergency care of the burned patient, *Critical Care Update*, Vol. 10, p. 24.

Lawrence, J.C. (1981) Burns: causes, management and consequences, *Journal of Clinical Nursing*, Vol. 26, pp. 1123–5.

Martin, V. (1981) Preventing hypertropic scarring: a burning issue, *Nursing Mirror*, Vol. 153, pp. 32–3.

Surveyor, J.A. and Clougherty, D.M. (1983) Burn scars: fighting the effects, *American Journal of Nursing*, Vol. 5, pp. 746–51.

Contact dermatitis

Armstrong-Esther, C.A. (1981) Skin and hypersensitivity, *Nursing*, Vol. 26, pp. 1152–6.

Stone, L.A. (1983) Contact dermatitis, *Nursing*, Vol. 2, No. 9, p. 252–3.

Treadgold, A. (1983) Patch testing for contact dermatitis, *Nursing*, Vol. 2, No. 9, pp. 255–8.

Dermatological surgery

Deener, D. (1980) Plastic surgery: result – a lip to be kissed with relish, *Nursing Mirror*, Vol. 151: pp. 30–33.

Herrick, M. (1983) Surgery in dermatology, *Nursing*, Vol. 2, No. 10, pp. 272–3.

Martin, V. (1981) Preventing hypertropic scarring: a burning issue, *Nursing Mirror*, Vol. 153, pp. 32–3.

General

Chaplain, S. (1981) Skin problems in the community, *Nursing*, Vol. 26, pp. 116–8.

Greenhow, M.M. (1983) Topical treatments – a simple guide, *Nursing*, Vol. 2, No. 10, pp. 281–4.

Lovell, C.R. (1983) The skin and systemic disease, *Nursing*, Vol. 2, No. 10, pp. 277–9.

Millard, L.D. (1983) Dermatology in pigmented skin, *Nursing*, Vol. 2, No. 10, pp. 274–6.

Ryan, T.J. (1981) The handicap of skin diseases, *Nursing*, Vol. 26, pp. 1144–5.

Sidhanee, A.C. (1983) Structure and function of the skin, *Nursing*, Vol. 2, No. 9, pp. 239–42.

Stoughton, R.D. (1979) Topical antibiotics for acne vulgaris, *Archives of Dermatology*, Vol. 115, pp. 486–9.

Tring, F.C. (1981) Warts and their treatment, *Nursing Times*, Vol. 77, pp. 1415–7.

Infectious disorders

Maunder, J.W. (1981) Clinical and laboratory trials employing carbaryl against the human head-louse, *Pediculosis humanus capitis* (de Gear), *Clinical and Experimental Dermatology*, Vol. 6, pp. 605–12.

Mohlnycky, N. (1983) Parasitic skin infections, *Nursing*, Vol. 2, No. 9, pp. 246–8.

Stone, L.A. (1983) Infections of the skin, *Nursing*, Vol. 2, No. 10, pp. 285–7.

Psoriasis

Amann, L.P. (1981) The management of psoriasis, *Nursing*, Vol. 26, pp. 1123–5.

Marks, R. (1986) Psoriasis and its treatment with etretinate, *Retinoids Today and Tomorrow*, Vol. 2, pp. 4–6.

Runne, V. and Kunze, J. (1982) Short duration ('minutes') therapy with dithranol for psoriasis: a new outpatient regimen, *British Journal of Dermatology*, Vol. 106, pp. 135–9.

12

Care of the Patient with an Allergy Problem

ALLERGIC REACTIONS

DEFINITIONS

1. *Antigen* – a substance that, when repeatedly in contact with the body, stimulates production of a counteracting substance, a globulin 'antibody'.
2. *Antibody* – a globulin produced by the lymphoid cells as a result of stimulation of these cells by an antigen; the antibody is capable of combining with the antigen in a very specific manner.
3. *Immunity* – a state of increased resistance to a particular substance.
   a. *Active immunization* – resistance brought about by the injection of an antigenic substance (e.g. tetanus toxoid).
   b. *Passive immunization* – resistance brought about by the transfer of antibody-containing serum from an immunized donor to a normal recipient (e.g. tetanus antitoxin).
4. *Allergic reactions* – resulting from the interaction between an allergen and an antibody with subsequent release of mediators responsible for the local and/or systemic inflammatory reactions.

PHARMACOLOGICAL MEDIATORS OF IMMEDIATE HYPERSENSITIVITY REACTIONS

1. Histamine – released from tissue mast cells by the interaction of an antigen and its corresponding antibody.
   a. Causes contraction of smooth muscle of bronchioles, uterus, intestines.
   b. Dilates and causes increased permeability of capillaries of skin and mucous membrane.
   c. Produces itching of skin and mucous membrane.
   d. Stimulates secretion of nasal, lacrimal, salivary and gastrointestinal glands.
   e. Lowers blood pressure.
2. SRS-A – slow reacting substance of anaphylaxis now referred to as a leukotriene. A lipidopeptide with powerful constricting action on bronchial smooth muscle. Probably a very important mediator in asthma.
3. Bradykinin – acts chiefly by increasing capillary permeability and contractility of smooth muscle.
There are many other mediators.

IMMUNOGLOBULINS

Antibodies that are formed by plasma cells (which are derived from lymphocytes) in response to an immunogenic stimulus comprise a group of serum proteins called immunoglobulins.

1. The abbreviation for immunoglubulin is Ig.
2. Antibodies combine with antigens in a 'lock and key style'.
3. There are five classes of immunoglobulins:
   a. IgM (gamma 'M') – a macromolecule; tends to stay in bloodstream and is primarily engaged in defence in intravascular compartment.
   b. IgG (gamma 'G') – most abundant. Readily diffuses into tissue spaces and crosses the placenta. Assists in combating infection.
   c. IgA (gamma 'A') – circulates in the blood, but its role here is uncertain; it is prominent in external secretions (saliva, tears) where it provides a primary defence mechanism.
   d. IgD – function has not yet been determined.
   e. IgE (gamma 'E') – responsible for most of the 'immediate types' of allergic reactions.

HYPERSENSITIVITY REACTIONS

Hypersensitivity is said to exist when the body reacts adversely against substances in the environment which elicit no response from most people. This may, or may not, be due to antibody–allergen interaction.

Antibody–allergen interactions consist of (a) those that are protective and beneficial to the body ('immunity'), and (b) those that are not always protective and beneficial to the body. They may cause tissue damage resulting in discomfort to the patient ('allergy').

TYPES OF ALLERGEN

1. Inhaled allergens:
   a. Plant pollens – grasses, shrubs, trees, flowers and weeds.
   b. Animal – dander, urinary proteins.
   c. Moulds (spores).
   d. Faeces of the house dust mite *Dermatophagoides pteronyssinus* and *Dermatophagoides farinae*.
   e. Occupational allergens – isocyanates, flour, grain and its contaminants, acid anhydrides (epoxy resins), colophony (pine tree resin), complex salts of platinum, enzyme detergents, wood dusts, drugs, laboratory animals. This list is under constant review.
2. Ingested allergens – cow's milk, fish, nuts, shellfish, and certain fruits. Rarely a cause of respiratory reactions.
3. Contact allergens – contact dermatitis:
   a. Nickel, chromium, formaldehyde.

DELAYED HYPERSENSITIVITY

1. Term for a reaction that reaches its peak 24 to 48 hours after an antigen is injected intradermally into a sensitized individual.
2. The reaction usually consists of erythema and induration.
3. Delayed hypersensitivity is mediated by sensitized 'T' (thymus-dependent) lymphocytes (not by immunoglobulins).
4. Example: tuberculin skin test.

TESTS FOR ALLERGY

GUIDELINES: SKIN TESTING

Skin testing consists of the introduction of an allergen into or on the skin surface of the person to determine hypersensitivity. This may be performed by a nurse under the supervision of a doctor.

PURPOSE

1. Assisting in the diagnosis of allergy.
2. Confirming the need for hyposensitization when the history is suggestive (increasingly rarely).

METHOD

1. Skin prick test – a drop of allergen is applied to the skin then a needle is used to prick the surface of the skin through the drop.

　　a.　Advantage: little risk of a general constitutional reaction.
　　b.　Disadvantage: risk of misinterpretation if the allergens are not correctly standardized.
　　c.　Depends on normal skin response to histamine. For that reason a solution of histamine should be used as a positive control.
2.　Intradermal – injection of a small amount of allergen into the superficial layers of the skin.
　　a.　Advantage: slightly more accurate than prick test method.
　　b.　Disadvantage: more dilute solutions of allergen are required.
　　c.　There is a serious risk of systemic reactions.
3.　Patch test – application of test material to the skin surface. Skin is immediately covered with small gauze dressing (or gauze part of a sticking plaster).
　　a.　Advantage: effective in cases involving contact hypersensitivity to topically applied substances, e.g. nickel, chromium, primula.
　　b.　Disadvantage: not as accurate as other methods.

SITES FOR SKIN PRICK TESTING OR INTRACUTANEOUS TESTING

1.　Volar or anterior surface of the upper third of the forearm approximately 10cm below the bend of the elbow.
2.　The back, below top of the scapula, avoiding the spine. A useful site for children.

PROCEDURE

1.　Place tests approximately 5cm apart (to prevent results of one test from coalescing with those of another).
2.　Avoid hairy area (will interfere with interpreting the results).
3.　Avoid areas near bone or tendons or areas without adequate subcutaneous tissue.

PREPARATION OF PATIENT

1.　Explain to patient what is being done and why.
2.　Provide adequate lighting.

SKIN PRICK TEST

TECHNIQUE

1. Mark each site where a skin test is to be performed using a biro or felt-tip pen. They should be spaced about 5cm apart (spacing is required to prevent the coalescing of one reaction with another).
2. Place a drop of glycerine-saline and at another site a drop of histamine solution on the skin (the glycerine-saline acts as a negative control, the histamine as a positive control).
3. Place a drop of each allergen to be tested at the other marked sites then with a separate needle for each test very gently prick the surface of the skin through each drop. (A separate needle is essential to eliminate the possibility of false positive recordings.)

4. When all the tests have been performed blot the whole area dry using absorbent paper tissues taking care not to smear the solutions.
5. Cover the arm, if possible, instructing the patient not to scratch the sites if they itch and wait 15 to 20 minutes before reading the results.
6. Record type of allergen used and the results in the following manner:
　　–　No weal or flare.
　　+　Weal absent or slight. Erythema no more than 3mm diameter.
　　++　Weal not more than 3mm diameter. Erythema not more than 5mm.
　　+++　Weal between 3mm and 5mm diameter, with erythema.
　　++++　Any larger reaction.
7. If a permanent record of weal size is required the

weal is drawn around using a fine-tipped biro. Sellotape is pressed over the drawn area. It is lifted off and placed on a blank piece of paper recording the date of testing and the allergen used. The weal can then be measured by recording the widest diameter horizontally and vertically and then dividing the sum by two.

INTRADERMAL TEST

1. Limit number of intradermal tests to no more than 20.
2. Use sterile tuberculin syringe with graduation of one-hundredths of a millilitre.
3. Use a hypodermic needle, size 25g × 16mm.
4. Use a separate syringe and needle (preferably disposable) for each antigen.

TECHNIQUE
1. Eject all air from syringe and needle. (Air injected will affect reading.)
2. Hold forearm with one hand and use thumb to stretch skin.
3. Hold syringe between thumb and forefinger and place plunger against heel of hand.
4. Position bevel upwards and place needle and syringe almost parallel along long axis of arm (with bevel upwards, needle can penetrate superficial layer of skin and allergen can be deposited directly under skin surface).
5. Depress needle into arm and advance until bevel just disappears into the epidermis.
6. Contract hand and advance plunger, injecting amount necessary to raise a bleb of approximately 3mm (0.01–0.05ml).
7. Remove needle (transient bleeding is usually of no significance). Wait 15 to 20 minutes before reading results.
8. Record type of allergen used and the results as for skin prick testing.

INTERPRETATIONS OF SKIN PRICK TESTING AND INTRACUTANEOUS SKIN TESTING METHODS
1. Positive:
   a. Indicates IgE antibody response to previous contact with antigen.
   b. False positive reactions may occur with non-specific histamine liberators sometimes present in certain allergen extracts, e.g. fish, shellfish.
2. Negative:
   a. Indicates antibodies have not been formed against the antigen.

b. Patient is not reacting normally to histamine.
3. Suppressed reaction – may occur if the patient:
   a. Is on antihistamines.
   b. Feels faint or is cold.

PATCH TEST

TECHNIQUE
Apply test material directly to skin for purpose of producing a small area of allergic dermatitis, e.g. nickel, chromium, primula, plant oils, hair tonic, shaving cream. Either leave the area exposed or cover with a small lint dressing and adhesive or use a sticking plaster.

REACTION
1. Remove patch after 48 hours.
2. It is important to wait for 20 to 30 minutes to allow any unrelated reaction to subside. A true allergic reaction will persist for several days.
3. Observe reaction and describe:
   + Erythema.
   ++ Erythema, papules.
   +++ Erythema, papules, vesicles.
   ++++ Erythema, papules, vesicles and severe oedema.
4. Positive reactions often show an increase in severity in next 24 hours. It is important that the site is re-examined in 72 hours.
5. Record nature of sensitizing agents and reactions.

HYPOSENSITIZATION

1. This form of therapy consists of injections of dilute allergenic extracts of such substances as pollens, dusts, mould spores and insect venom.
2. It is thought that as amounts of injected substances are gradually increased, the body builds up a supply of blocking antibodies (mainly immunoglobulin G type–IgG). This is a theory which is yet to be proven.
3. When the patient comes into contact with allergens that previously caused allergic reactions, it may be that the blocking antibodies combine with the allergens in a way that reduces or prevents symptoms.

ANAPHYLAXIS

NURSING ALERT

With injection of allergenic extracts for the purpose of hyposensitization, the risk of systemic reaction is always present. Current recommendations by the Committee on Safety of Medicines reads: 'Such treatment should only be carried out where facilities for full cardiopulmonary resuscitation are immediately available, and patients should be kept under medical observation for at least two hours after treatment.'

EARLY MANIFESTATIONS
1. Feeling of uneasiness or apprehension, weakness, perspiration, sneezing or nasal pruritus.
2. Generalized pruritus, urticaria, angioedema.
3. Dyspnoea, wheezing, dysphagia, vomiting, abdominal pain.
4. Pulse – may be rapid, weak, irregular or unobtainable.
5. Syncope or shock – may follow rapidly.
6. Possible urgency, faecal and urinary incontinence, convulsions and coma.

TREATMENT
Administer adrenaline – the pharmacological antagonist of the action of chemical mediators on smooth muscle and other effector cells.

Immediate
Always have an emergency tray of drugs readily available.
1. Inject 0.3ml of 1:1,000 adrenaline subcutaneously into upper arm; gently massage site of injection.
2. Have hydrocortisone ready for injection.
3. Have antihistamine ready for injection.
4. Aminophylline ready when bronchospasm is a feature of the reaction.

If reaction is not reversed by adrenaline
1. Vasopressors or volume expanders for hypotension.
2. Oxygen and tracheotomy pack for laryngeal obstruction.
3. Equipment necessary for performing cardiopulmonary resuscitation.

Further observations
1. Evaluation of patient reaction and response to treatment.
2. Repeat adrenaline, if necessary.
3. Monitor blood pressure/pulse at regular intervals.
4. Assess pulmonary function.

RESPIRATORY HYPERSENSITIVITY

ALLERGIC RHINO-CONJUNCTIVITIS

May be seasonal 'hay fever' caused by grass, tree, weed and flower pollens or mould spores, and/or perennial and induced by the faeces of the house dust mite, animal dander and urinary proteins, mould spores and some occupational agents. The body reacts by releasing histamine and other pharmacological agents which produce the symptoms.

CLINICAL FEATURES
1. Rhinitis – nasal itch, watering, blockage and sneezing.
2. Conjunctivitis – red, burning, itching and watering.

SENSITIVITY TESTS
Skin tests confirm patient's hypersensitivity to causative allergen.

TREATMENT
1. Avoid causative allergen if possible.
2. Use antihistamines.
3. Local disodium cromoglycate or local corticosteroids when antihistamines are ineffective or cause too many side-effects.
4. Hyposensitization, when appropriate.

BRONCHIAL ASTHMA

Bronchial asthma manifests itself clinically by intermittent episodes of wheezing and dyspnoea; it is always associated with bronchial hyperresponsiveness and allergies are often an important cause. Bronchial asthma differs from other causes of wheeze in that it is reversible either with time or as a result of treatment.

INCIDENCE
Asthma affects approximately 3 to 4 per cent of the population and represents about 25 per cent of chronic diseases of childhood.

PATHOPHYSIOLOGY
1. Allergen–antibody reaction.

a. Susceptible individuals form abnormally large amounts of IgE when exposed to certain allergens.
b. This immunoglobulin (IgE) fixes itself to the mast cells of the bronchial mucosa.
c. When the individual is exposed to the appropriate allergen, it combines with cell-bound IgE molecules, causing the mast cell to degranulate and release chemical mediators.
d. These chemical mediators, primarily histamine and leukotrienes (formerly known as SRS-A, slow reacting substance of anaphylaxis) are thought to produce bronchospasm.
2. Infections, i.e. common cold, sinusitis.
3. Autonomic nerves probably stimulated by non-specific triggers, e.g. exercise, cold air, smoke, laughter, fumes, coughing.

CLINICAL FEATURES
1. Can be symptom-free periods between attacks (episodic asthma).
2. During an attack of asthma, the amount of airway obstruction determines the degree of severity of symptoms.
   a. During early or mild episodes – cough or mild chest tightness.
   b. As asthmatic episodes become more severe – wheezing, coughing, shortness of breath.
   c. Dyspnoea may become apparent, inspiratory wheezing and use of accessory respiratory muscles.
   d. As severity of attack increases, the patient becomes more anxious, restless and apprehensive.
   e. A fatigue state may follow – respirations are less laboured and there is less audible wheezing.
   f. This may lead to respiratory failure with hypercapnia, respiratory acidosis and hypoxaemia.

DIAGNOSTIC EVALUATION
1. Generalized rhonchi on auscultation.
2. Obstruction to airflow as shown by spirometry.
3. Reversal of obstruction after administration of a bronchodilator.
4. Sputum eosinophilia.

CLASSIFICATION
Extrinsic bronchial asthma
1. Cause:
   a. Hypersensitivity reaction to inhalent allergens (IgE-mediated).
2. Diagnosis:

a. Correlation with exposure to aeroallergens (and less commonly ingestants).
b. Positive skin tests.
3. Major inhalent allergens, e.g. house dust mite, pollens, animal dander, mould spores.
4. Other inhalent allergens are the occupational agents (see p. 785).
5. Prognosis: favourable, with avoidance or reduction of exposure to allergens responsible for the symptoms. Good response to bronchodilators and specific treatment.

Intrinsic bronchial asthma
1. Cause:
   a. Unknown. Skin tests to common allergens are usually negative (non-IgE-mediated).
   b. Viral respiratory tract infections. Known to increase bronchial responsiveness.
2. Occurrence: after age 35, more common in women.
3. Prognosis:
   a. Remission is variable.
   b. Control may be difficult.

Aspirin-induced asthma (ASA sensitive)
A type of intrinsic asthma induced by ingestion of aspirin and related compounds.
1. Clinical features spread over a period of time have been described as a 'triad':
   a. Bronchial asthma.
   b. Nasal polyposis.
   c. Severe reactions to aspirin.
2. Onset of symptoms after aspirin ingestion (20 minutes to 2 hours).
   a. Watery rhinorrhoea, followed by marked flushing of upper part of body.
   b. Nausea, vomiting.
   c. Wheezing, dyspnoea and cyanosis.

PRECIPITATING FACTORS
Any one of these may trigger an asthmatic attack in someone with bronchial asthma.
1. Strong odours (fumes): turpentine, paints, chemicals, sprays, heavily scented flowers, perfumes, tobacco smoke.
2. Cold air; sudden barometric changes.
3. Air pollutants.
4. Emotion-triggering situations.

Popular misconceptions in asthma
1. That there are exclusive causes of asthma.
2. That most people grow out of asthma.
3. Longstanding asthma leads to permanent damage to the lungs or heart.

4. The dangers of aerosols.
5. Asthma is never fatal.

MEDICAL AND NURSING THERAPEUTIC MANAGEMENT
Objective
Achieve sufficient control of symptoms to prevent physical and psychological incapacitation.
1. Treatment must be individualized.
2. Therapy includes concern not only for the physical condition of the person but also for his psychosocial situation and his environment.
3. There is no cure for asthma, but present-day treatment regimes can improve and control the disease.

PATIENT EDUCATION
In order to prevent further attacks:
1. Avoid causative allergens when possible.
2. Avoid any medication that may aggravate asthma.
3. Hyposensitization – increasingly thought to be inappropriate for treating asthma.

TREATMENT
Environmental control
1. Control the environment as much as possible to reduce exposure to relevant allergens.
   a. In bedroom carry out regular vacuum cleaning and damp dusting, remove feather pillows and dust collecting articles.
   b. Exclude house pets, to eliminate dander.
   c. Exclude plants, to eliminate mould spores.
   d. When an occupational agent has been found to be responsible, control of the working environment may be possible by the installation of an efficient air extraction system, enclosing or modifying the process and encouraging good working practice. Some people will have to ask for relocation or seek a job change. Occupational asthma is now a prescribed disease in the UK and patients should claim for compensation through their local Social Security office. Relocation or job change can cause emotional stress and financial hardship.

ACUTE SEVERE ASTHMA (STATUS ASTHMATICUS)

Acute severe asthma is severe bronchial asthma in which the patient has failed to respond to his usual medication. This is a medical emergency and requires rapid therapeutic measures.

CONTRIBUTING FACTORS
1. Infection.
2. Dehydration.
3. Overuse of sedation.
4. Inadequate education of the patient.
5. Inadequate treatment.

CLINICAL FEATURES
1. Severe dyspnoea with wheeze, but in the late stage no wheeze may be audible.
2. Hypoxia causes changes in the central nervous system: fatigue, headache, irritability, dizziness, impaired mental functioning.
3. With continued carbon dioxide retention: muscle twitching, somnolence, flapping tremor.
4. Tachycardia, elevated blood pressure.
5. At very low oxygen levels and high carbon dioxide levels, sudden hypotension may occur.
6. Heart failure.

TREATMENT AND MANAGEMENT
Requires team effort – chest doctor, anaesthetist, physiotherapist and intensive care nursing.
1. Careful monitoring of pH, Pco_2, Po_2, repeatedly, in order to evaluate serially the changes in gas exchange and the patient's response to therapy.

Note: In early acute severe asthma, a low Po_2 is followed by increased respiratory effort; this leads to low Pco_2 (hyperventilation). Then follow fatigue, reduced ventilation and increasing Pco_2.

NURSING ALERT
In acute severe asthma the return to a normal or increasing Pco_2 does not necessarily mean the asthmatic patient is improving – it may mean a fatigue state which develops just before the patient slips into respiratory failure.

2. Correction of derangement of blood gases (hypoxaemia) and haemoconcentration by providing adequate hydration orally and intravenously and use of humidified oxygen.
3. Rapid mobilization and removal of bronchial and bronchiolar secretions with chest physiotherapy and, in rare circumstances, by bronchoscopy and suction.
4. Reverse bronchoconstriction.
   a. Nebulized bronchodilators.
   b. Intravenous theophyllines (must be given cautiously if patient is currently on oral theophylline treatment).
   c. Intravenous or oral corticosteroids.
5. Monitoring of airway calibre with regular peak flow measurements.

6. Suitable treatment of any accompanying infection.

Note: These patients must never be sedated.

OTHER ALLERGIC CONDITIONS

ATOPIC DERMATITIS (ATOPIC ECZEMA)

Largely a disease of children. Characterized by extreme itching. It is often chronic and relapsing and occurs almost characteristically in the flexures of the elbows and behind the knees. Although the patients develop IgE antibody to common inhalent allergens, it is not considered to be a truly allergic disease. There is disagreement as to whether food is a primary or contributory factor in the development and course of this disease.

PATIENT EDUCATION
1. Avoid skin irritants, e.g. wool, wool alcohols and lanolin in medications, certain soaps and detergents.
2. Avoid skin dryness, itching and infection.
3. Avoid hot, humid and cold, dry atmospheres.
4. Use skin moisturizers.
5. Antihistamines at night can reduce itching and scratching.
6. Education in correct use of topical steroids.
7. Antibiotics if associated with infection.

URTICARIA (HIVES, NETTLE RASH)

Characterized by itching weals. Histamine is the main mediator. May be caused by food allergy, food additives, insect stings, drugs, transfusion reactions. The cause of chronic urticaria may be malignancy but in the majority of cases the cause is unknown.

PATIENT EDUCATION
1. Avoid causative factors if possible.
2. Elimination diet may be tried, but is seldom helpful.
3. If caused by acetylsalicylic acid, a diet without preservatives, dyes or naturally occurring salicylic acid should be tried.
4. Antihistamines.

ANGIOEDEMA

Often occurs with urticaria and appears as large, diffuse swellings which are tender rather than itchy and can involve the larynx, mouth and pharynx. When the larynx is involved it can be a life-threatening situation. Angioedema can be allergic, idiopathic and hereditary.

PATIENT EDUCATION
1. As for urticaria.

See Table 12.1 for immediate food hypersensitivity reactions.

Table 12.1 Immediate food hypersensitivity reactions*

Immunological reactions	
Generalized reactions	**Some causes**
Anaphylaxis	Nuts, e.g. almond, brazil
Angioedema	Egg white, peanuts, shellfish
Skin reactions	Tomatoes, sea foods,
Urticaria ('hives', 'nettle rash')	strawberries, nuts, apples, food additives, e.g. tartrazine
Respiratory reactions	Dairy products, all of the
Sneezing, runny nose, runny eyes (hay fever)	above, including food preservatives and flavour
Wheeze, cough, tight chest (asthma)	enhancers, e.g. benzoates, sodium metabisulphate
Gastrointestinal reactions	
Vomiting, diarrhoea, colic	Egg, wheat, shellfish
Neurological reactions	
Migraine	Various foods

* Immunological food/additive reactions classically occur within 20 minutes to two hours following ingestion. The number of people affected is small. However, no large-scale, scientifically based, double-blind study has been done in order to establish the true number of those affected.
Exclusion diets, with the very gradual reintroduction of foods thought to be responsible need to be done under strict medical supervision.
Other immunological reactions may be involved, e.g. IgG and IgM in coeliac disease.
Food toxicity, food aversion and food intolerance should not be confused with the true immunological reactions.

PATIENT EDUCATION FOR ALLERGY

OBJECTIVES

1. Assist the patient in recognizing the importance of avoiding offending antigens whenever possible.
2. Make sure that the patient understands how the medication he is taking acts, and therefore why it is important that they be taken strictly as instructed.

See Table 12.2 for drugs used in the treatment of allergic diseases.

ADMINISTRATION OF MEDICATIONS

1. Warn patients that it is dangerous to drive or use machinery during the first few days of antihistamine therapy since these medications often cause drowsiness. If drowsiness persists either the dosage or type of drug used will need to be changed.
2. Nasal decongestants should not be used repeatedly. They have an unpleasant rebound effect which means that addiction for the sake of relief is a common feature.
3. Inhaled disodium cromoglycate (either in powder form for asthma, liquid form for nose, liquid form for eyes or inhaled steroids, because they are thought to stabilize mast cells, must be taken prophylactically. For that reason, if treatment is prescribed to be taken four times a day this must be adhered to even if the patient is feeling unwell.
4. Inhaled bronchodilators have a recommended dose which should not be exceeded. Patients should be advised that if they do need to take more than the prescribed dose they either need more treatment or current treatment is not being effective, in which case they need to consult their doctor.

Table 12.2   Drugs uses in the treatment of allergic diseases

Drug	Action	Side-effects
1. Bronchodilators: a. Selective adrenergic drugs, e.g. salbutamol (Ventolin), terbutaline (Bricanyl), rimiterol (Pulmodil), fenoterol (Berotec), pirbuterol (Exirel)	Bronchodilation. Given by aerosol and side-effects are few Orally because blood levels have to be adequate to be effective, may cause side-effects May be given intravenously, as an infusion or as a wet aerosol	Tremor, tachycardia
b. Catecholamines, e.g., orciprenaline (Alupent) adrenaline (Medihaler-epi) isoprenaline (Medihaler-iso) Adrenaline	Stimulate alpha- and beta-adrenergic receptors of autonomic nervous system It has short duration of action Given as subcutaneous injection – a 1:1,000 (1mg/ml) solution is used and 0.3ml injected at ½-hourly intervals	Anxiety, tremor, palpitation, tachycardia and dysrhythmia (therefore infrequently used)
c. Atropine-like, e.g. ipratropium bromide (Atrovent)	Blocks cholinergic receptor sites Bronchodilation is of slow onset, but lasts longer than adrenaline or isoprenaline	Dryness of mouth Urinary retention Contraindication: in narrow angle glaucoma
2. Xanthines, e.g. theophylline (Ronaphyllin, Nuelin), aminophylline (Phyllocontin)	Bronchodilator and vasodilator Given orally, the measurement of drug concentration levels in the serum is necessary to ensure that it is within 'therapeutic range' Given intravenously, it is of established value in the treatment of severe attacks of asthma. Plasma concentrations should be monitored, particularly if patients have been taking oral xanthine preparations	May cause severe gastric irritation, nausea, vomiting, cardiac dysrythmias, epilepsy

3. Sodium cromoglycate bronchial inhalation (Intal), for nasal inhalation (Lomusol) and for the eyes (Opticrom)	Sodium cromoglycate inhibits the release from sensitized cells of mediators of the allergic reaction	Occasional irritation of the throat and trachea may occur when taking Intal in powder form
4. Antihistamines Ethanolamines (e.g. Dramamine) Alkylamines (e.g. Piriton) Phenothiazines (e.g. Phenergan, Vallergan)	Antagonizes the main actions of histamine in the body, probably by occupying the receptor sites in the effector cells to the exclusion of histamine; they do not prevent the production of histamine	Sedation with the inability to concentrate, lassitude, hypotension, muscular weakness. Sedative effects, when they occur, may diminish after a few days Other side-effects include gastrointestinal disturbances, headaches, blurred vision, tinnitus, elation or depression, dryness of the mouth, difficulty in micturition
Astemizole (Hismanal) Terfenadine (Triludan)	May have some advantages over other antihistamines because they only penetrate the blood–brain barrier to a slight extent and therefore cause less sedation	Weight gain occasionally with Hismanal
5. Corticosteroids a. Systemic, e.g. prednisone prednisolone, hydrocortisone	No clear idea how these drugs benefit asthmatics. Thought to influence the responsiveness of bronchial-adrenoreceptors and thus modifying bronchomotor tone May also inhibit prostaglandin biosynthesis	High doses given for long periods cause weight gain, fluid retention, diabetes mellitus, hypertension osteoporosis, proximal myopathy, hypokalaemia, easy bruising of skin, adrenal suppression, growth retardation in children, may mask some signs of infection Abrupt withdrawal of oral corticosteroids may precipitate acute adrenal insufficiency
b. Topical, e.g. beclomethasone dipropionate (Beconase, Becotide, Becloforte), budesonide (Pulmicort), betamethasone valerate (Bextasol)	As above Beclomethasone dipropionate is rapidly destroyed in the gut and therefore causes no side-effects due to lack of systemic absorption	Inhaled steroids have been known to cause pharyngeal thrush and hoarseness of the voice Beconase may cause epistaxis

5. If taking oral corticosteroids, it is important that the patient carries a steroid card detailing current dosage and that if there is a need to increase the dosage due to infection or at time of an operation, this be done under medical supervision. Similarly if the dosage is being reduced it must be done under supervision.

6. Slow-release theophyllines must be taken at recommended times and the dose may need to vary depending on blood levels. Other factors may influence blood levels, such as the influence of other drugs and smoking. Emergency administration of theophyllines must not be given to patients on oral theophylline treatment without the knowledge of the blood levels because of severe toxic reactions associated with overdosage.

As with all drugs, these must be kept out of the reach of children.

FURTHER READING

BOOKS

Bernard, J., Gee, L., Keith, W., Morgan, C. and Brooks, Stuart M. (1984) Airway diseases. In

Occupational Lung Diseases, pp. 189–99, Raven Press, New York.

Lane, D.J. and Storr, A. (1979) *Asthma: The Facts*, Oxford University Press, Oxford.

Mygind, N. (1986) *Essential Allergy. An Illustrated Text for Students and Specialists*, Blackwell Scientific Publications, Oxford.

ARTICLES

Allergy tests

Lessof, M.H., Buisseret, P.D., Merrett J., Merrett T.G. and Wraith, D.G. (1980) Assessing the value of skin prick tests, *Clinical Allergy*, Vol. 10, pp. 115–20.

Asthma

Ayres, J., Barnes, G., Hek, G. and Carswell, F. (1986) Asthma: Blowing away the myths, *Nursing Times Community Outlook*, July, pp. 18–23.

Boyd, G. (1980) Allergic bronchial asthma – some problems in diagnosis and management, *Clinical Allergy*, Vol. 10, pp. 497–501.

Cooper, P.J., Darbyshire, J., Nunn, A.J. and Warner, J.O. (1984) A controlled trial of oral hyposensitization in pollen asthma and rhinitis in children, *Clinical Allergy*, Vol. 14, pp. 541–50.

Editorial (1980) Occupational asthma, *Thorax*, Vol. 35, pp. 241–5.

— (1981) Compensating occupational asthma, *Thorax*, Vol. 36, pp. 881–4.

— (1985) Prognosis in occupational asthma, *Thorax*, Vol. 40, pp. 241–3.

— (1986) Bronchial asthma and the environment, *The Lancet*, Vol. 2, pp. 786–7.

Grant, I.W.B. (1986) Does immunotherapy have a role in the treatment of asthma? *Clinical Allergy*, Vol. 16, pp. 7–16.

Jenkins, P.F., Mullins, J., Davies, B.H. and Williams, D.A. (1981) The possible role of aero-allergens in the epidemic of asthma deaths, *Clinical Allergy*, Vol. 11, pp. 611–20.

Levy, M. and Bell, L. (1985) Night cough – is it asthma? *Maternal and Child Health*, Vol. 10, No. 12, December, pp. 376–82.

Lewis, G.M. (1985) Nebulisers in the home – a blessing or a danger? (for asthmatic children) *Maternal and Child Health*, Vol. 10, No. 11, November, pp. 326–30.

Littlewood, J. (1984) Asthma – a support group, *Nursing Times*, Vol. 80, 1 August, pp. 40–2.

Milner, A.D. (1982) Childhood asthma: treatment and severity, *British Medical Journal*, Vol. 285, No. 6336, pp. 155–6.

Reed, S., Diggle, S., Cushley, M.J., Sleet, R.A. and Tattersfield, A.E. (1985) Assessment and management of asthma in an accident and emergency department, *Thorax*, Vol. 40, pp. 897–902.

Stellman, J.L., Spicer, J.E. and Cayton, R.M. (1982) Morbidity from chronic asthma, *Thorax*, Vol. 37, pp. 218–21.

Food hypersensitivity

Carter, C.M., Egger, J. and Soothill, J.F. (1985) A dietary management of severe childhood migraine, *Human Nutrition: Applied Nutrition*, Vol. 39A, No. 4, pp. 294–303.

David, T. (1985) Intolerant babies, *Nursing Times Community Outlook*, March, pp. 22–8.

Editorial (1986) Adverse reactions to food and food additives, *Journal of Allergy and Clinical Immunology*, Vol. 78, No. 1, Part 2, July.

Haddington, E. (1980) Diet and migraine, *Journal of Human Nutrition*, Vol. 34, pp. 175–80.

Joint report of the Royal College of Physicians and the British Nutrition Foundation (1984) Food intolerance and food aversion, *Journal of the Royal College of Physicans of London*, Vol. 18, No. 2.

Jung, R. (1983) Food allergic disease, *Hospital Update*, 1 March, pp. 811–8.

Lessof, M.H., Wraith, D.G., Merrett, T.G., Merrett, J. and Buisseret, P.D. (1980) Food allergy and intolerance in 100 patients – local and systemic effects, *Quarterly Journal of Medicine*, New Series XLIV, No. 195, pp. 259–71.

Lindsay, M. (1982) Food allergy or food allergic disease? *Nursing Times*, 19 May, Vol. 78, pp. 830–2.

Reinann, H.J., Ring, J., Ultsch, B. and Wendt, P. (1985) Intragastral provocation under endoscopic control (IPEC) in food allergy: mast cell and histamine changes in gastric mucosa, *Clinical Allergy*, Vol. 15, pp. 195–202.

Soothill, J.F. (1984) Food allergy – the state of the art. *Midwife, Health Visitor and the Community Nurse*, Vol. 20, No. 8, August, pp. 274–8.

Warner, J.O. (1980) Food allergy in fully breast-fed infants, *Clinical Allergy*, Vol. 10, pp. 133–6.

— (1985) Intolerance and food allergy, *Maternal and Child Health*, Vol. 10, No. 2, February, pp. 40–6.

Urticaria

Editorial (1982) Chronic urticaria, *British Medical Journal*, Vol. 283, No. 6295, pp. 805–6.

Gibson, A. and Clancy, R. (1980) Management of chronic idiopathic urticaria by the identification and exclusion of dietary factors, *Clinical Allergy*, Vol. 10, pp. 699–704.

13

Care of the Patient with a Musculoskeletal Disorder

SPECIFIC PROBLEMS ASSOCIATED WITH MUSCULOSKELETAL DISORDERS

NURSING PROCESS OVERVIEW

Assessment
GENERAL OBSERVATION
Information on ability to move, existence of discomfort and gross abnormalities, and presence of involuntary movement.
1. Observe gait and intentional movement for coordination and speed.
2. Note posture and body positions.
3. Identify use of assistive devices – sticks, frames, walker, prosthesis, etc.

NURSING HISTORY INFORMATION
The patient supplies information on primary problem, indicating impact of problem on lifestyle.
1. Information concerning chief complaint (e.g., onset of problem, how the patient has been coping with the problem).
2. Ask the patient to describe symptoms such as pain, stiffness, cramps and area affected.
3. Identify concurrent health problems, health maintenance practices (including medications) and allergies.
4. Note impact of musculoskeletal disorder on lifestyle, family interactions, family's economics, etc.
5. Assess the patient's perceptions and expectations related to health problems.
6. Estimate the patient's ability to learn (i.e., note language barriers).

PHYSICAL ASSESSMENT
General condition and functional abilities secured through inspection, palpation and measurement.

Skeletal component
1. Note deviations from normal structure – bony deformities, length discrepancies, alignment, amputations.
2. Identify abnormal movement and crepitus (grating sensation) as found with fractures and in arthritis.

Joint component
1. Identify swelling that may be due to inflammation or effusion.

2. Note deformity associated with contractures or dislocations.
3. Evaluate stability which may be altered.
4. Estimate ROM (range of movement), both actively and passively.

Muscle component
1. Inspect for size and contour of muscles.
2. Assess coordination of movement.
3. Palpate for muscle tone.
4. Estimate strength through cursory evaluation (i.e., handshake) or scaled criteria (i.e., 0 = no palpable contraction, to 5 = normal range of motion against gravity with full resistance).
5. Measure girth to note increases due to swelling or bleeding into muscle or decreases due to atrophy (difference of more than 1cm is significant).
6. Identify abnormal clonus (rhythmic contraction and relaxation) or *fasciculation* (contractions of isolated muscle fibres).

Neurovascular component
1. Assess circulatory status of involved extremities by noting skin colour and temperature, peripheral pulses, capillary refill response, pain.
2. Assess neurological status of involved extremities by the patient's ability to move distal muscles and description of sensation (e.g. paraesthesia).
3. Test reflexes of extremities.
4. Note hair distribution and nail condition.

Skin component
1. Inspect traumatic injuries (e.g. cuts, bruises, etc).
2. Assess chronic conditions (e.g. eczema, stasis ulcers, etc).

Subjective component
Elicit information from patient concerning presence of pain, tenderness, abnormal sensation or tightness during physical examination.

DIAGNOSTIC EVALUATION
Radiological and imaging studies
1. X-rays:
   a. Of bone – to determine bone density, texture, erosion, changes in bone relationships.
   b. Of cortex – to detect any widening, narrowing, irregularity.
   c. Of medullary cavity – to detect any alteration in density.
   d. Of involved joint – to show fluid, irregularity, spur formation, narrowing, changes in joint contour.
2. Tomogram – special X-ray technique for detailed view of specific plane of bone.

3. Computed tomogram – to identify tumours of the soft tissues or injuries to ligaments or tendons; to identify location/extent of fractures in difficult-to-define areas; to identify disc herniation.
4. Bone scan – parenteral injection of bone-seeking radiopharmaceutical; concentration of isotope uptake revealed in primary skeletal disease (osteosarcoma), metastatic bone disease, inflammatory skeletal disease (osteomyelitis); fracture.
5. Arthrogram – injection of radio-opaque substance or air into joint cavity to outline soft tissue structures (e.g. meniscus) and contour of joint.
6. Myelogram – injection of contrast medium into subarachnoid space at lumbar spine to determine level of disc herniation or site of tumour; see p. 915.
7. Discogram – injection of small amount of contrast medium into lumbar disc to visualize disc space.

Joint examinations
1. Arthrocentesis – insertion of needle into joint and aspiration of synovial fluid for purposes of examination.
2. Arthroscopy – endoscopic procedure that allows direct visualization of a joint, especially the knee. May be combined with arthrography.
   Technique
   a. Under local or general anaesthesia, a large-bore needle is inserted into the suprapatellar pouch, and the joint is distended with saline.
   b. An arthroscope is introduced and the knee joint visualized, including the synovium, articular surfaces and menisci.
   c. Patient may be advised to limit his activities for several days following the procedure, which is relatively painless.

Muscle and nerve studies
Differentiate nerve root compression, muscle disease (dystrophy, myositis, etc.), peripheral neuropathies, central nervous system – anterior horn cell neuropathies, neuromuscular junction problems.
1. Electromyography (EMG) – measures electrical potential generated by the muscle during relaxation and contraction.
2. Nerve conduction velocities (NCVs) – measures the rate of potential generation along specific nerves (speed of impulse conduction).

Laboratory studies
Baseline haematology, serum chemistry and urinalysis provide information on the general health of the patient. Few laboratory studies are specific for orthopaedic conditions.

1. Clotting factors – evaluation prior to orthopaedic surgery desirable; person with haemophilia prone to specific orthopaedic problems; assessed in prophylactic and therapeutic anticoagulant regimens.
2. Calcitonin – bone metabolism.
3. Calcium – osteomalacia, parathyroid function.
4. Creatine – trauma to muscle.
5. Creatine phosphokinase (CPK) – skeletal muscle disease.
6. Parathyroid hormone (PTH) – bone metabolism.
7. Hyperkalaemia – trauma with massive tissue damage.
8. Phosphatase, alkaline – bone metabolism (osteoblastic activity), bone tumours, Paget's disease.
9. Phosphorus, inorganic – parathyroid problems.
10. Thyroid studies – bone metabolism.
11. Transaminase (SGPT) – skeletal muscle disease.
12. Vitamin D $(1,25(OH)2D_3)$ – bone metabolism.
13. Urine: Bence–Jones protein – multiple myeloma.
14. Urine: calcium – bone metabolism; parathyroid function.
15. Urine: creatinine – muscular atrophy.
16. Urine: phosphorus – rickets.

Special studies
Bone biopsy, densitometry, total body calcium, etc.

PATIENT PROBLEMS
(Associated with musculoskeletal conditions.)
1. Pain related to muscular or skeletal dysfunction.
2. Impaired mobility related to limitations imposed by underlying condition and treatment modalities such as casts, traction or bed rest.
3. Ineffective coping related to enforced immobility and altered lifestyle.
4. Potential for injury (neuromuscular compromise such as compartment syndrome) related to constrictive dressings, crush injuries, ischaemic swelling following arterial injury.
5. Potential impairment of circulation and nerve function related to increased tissue pressure.

Planning and implementation
NURSING INTERVENTIONS
Relief of pain
1. Secure information concerning pain.
   a. Have the patient describe the pain, location, characteristics (dull, sharp, continuous, throbbing, boring, radiating, aching).
   b. Ask the patient what causes the pain; makes the pain worse; relieves the pain.
   c. Evaluate the patient for proper body alignment, pressure from equipment (casts, traction, splints, appliances).

d. Recall pathophysiology related to different types of musculoskeletal pain.
  (i) Soreness and aching – muscular discomfort.
  (ii) Associated with weather changes – chronic arthritic discomfort.
  (iii) Associated with movement – joint sprain or muscle strain.
  (iv) Sharp and piercing – fracture pain, muscle spasm.
  (v) Steady, increasing pain – osteomyelitis, tumour, vascular complication.
  (vi) Radiating pain – pressure on nerve root.
  (vii) Boring, night pain – bone pathology.
2. Initiate activities to prevent or modify pain:
  a. Assist the patient with pain-reduction techniques – cutaneous stimulation, distraction, guided imagery, transcutaneous electrical nerve stimulation (TENS), biofeedback, etc.
  b. Position the patient in correct alignment.
  c. Move the patient slowly and steadily, providing adequate support to painful structure, and help of additional personnel as needed.
  d. Elevate painful extremity above the level of the heart.
  e. Apply heat or cold treatments as prescribed.
  f. Modify environment to facilitate rest and relaxation.
3. Administer medications as indicated and encourage use of less potent drugs as severity of discomfort decreases.
4. Encourage the patient to become an active participant in rehabilitative plans.

Establishing maximum physical mobility within limits of musculoskeletal problem and therapeutic regimen
1. Assess degree of physical mobility present:
  a. Identify use of mobility aids.
  b. Note ability to reposition self and ability to transfer from one place to another.
  c. Determine availability of assistants to facilitate mobility.
  d. Assess body systems (e.g. respiratory, gastro-intestinal) for responses to limited activity.
  e. Evaluate short-term and long-term effects of chosen treatments on mobility.
2. Identify true extent of imposed physical immobility.
3. Develop exercise regimen within prescribed physical activity limits.
4. Encourage weight-bearing and walking activities when possible.
5. Establish range-of-movement and isometric exer-cise (e.g. quadriceps sets) plan in preparation for resumption of ambulation.
6. Encourage movement of all uninvolved bodily parts.
7. Teach proper and safe use of mobilization aids.

Avoiding neuromuscular compromise and ensuring optimum circulation, tissue perfusion, and nerve function
1. Assess for clinical features of neuromuscular compromise:
  a. Complaint of deep, throbbing pain with persistent pressure sensation.
  b. Abnormal sensory evaluation (e.g. paraes-thesia, hyperaesthesia, loss of sensation).
  c. Pain with stretch of involved muscle.
  d. Tight, tense muscle mass on palpation.
  e. Elevation of tissue pressure indicated by direct needle measurement (above 30mmHg).
  f. Paresis or weakness.

NURSING ALERT
Pulse and capillary refill may be present with inadequate tissue perfusion and can contribute to a false sense of security concerning impending compartment syndrome.

2. Elevate injured extremity above heart level, if possible, to minimize oedema.
3. Apply ice pack to fresh injury if prescribed to control bleeding and swelling.
4. Inform the patient that frequent neurovascular assessments will be performed.
5. Have the patient move fingers or toes distal to injury.
6. Have the patient describe sensations in injured extremity.
7. Assess colour, temperature, capillary refill and pulses of involved extremity.
8. Notify doctor immediately of compromised neurovascular status.
9. Release constrictive devices (e.g. bivalve cast).
10. If no improvement when external devices are released, a decompression fasciotomy (incision of tissue surrounding muscle) *will be anticipated*.
11. Give patient education concerning preoperative and postoperative care.
12. Teach the patient to recognize and report increasing pain, tingling and numbness.

Strengthening coping abilities
1. Nursing assessment:
  a. Assess the patient and family for reactive

behaviours of denial, anger, bargaining, depression, acceptance.
b. Identify social isolation behaviours.
c. Note expressions of diminished self-worth and self-concept.
d. Assess degree of independence in self-care activities.
e. Identify anxious behaviours.
2. Promote gradual acceptance of disabilities due to musculoskeletal problem.
a. Assist the patient to recognize the impact of the musculoskeletal problem.
b. Support the patient through the phases of acceptance.
c. Recognize that the patient and family may be at different phases of coping/acceptance process.
d. Accept the patient's behaviours as expressions of the coping process.
e. Encourage the patient to focus on current abilities (instead of losses).
3. Reduce anxiety related to impact of musculoskeletal problem on lifestyle.
a. Explore the patient's understanding of musculoskeletal problem and its therapeutic regimen.
b. Identify areas for additional teaching.
c. Clarify misconceptions.
d. Encourage the patient to participate actively in planning and implementation of therapeutic regimen.
e. Facilitate acceptance of abilities by the patient and family.
f. Assist the patient to identify stress-producing situations.
4. Minimize social isolation related to hospitalization and decreased mobility.
a. Plan frequent periods of interaction with the patient.
b. Encourage contacts with family and friends.
c. Facilitate visits with children and other family members when feasible.
d. Involve the patient in personal and therapeutic decision-making processes.
e. Develop supportive relationships.
5. Initiate measures to cope with altered self-concept related to modified life role.
a. Identify activities within treatment regimen where the patient can establish control.
b. Provide genuine praise for self-care abilities.
c. Encourage the patient to make own decisions within scheduled therapeutic regimen.
d. Assist family in use of the patient's contributions to solve home problems.

e. Promote feelings of independence.
6. Counter-reduction in self-care related to musculoskeletal problem or treatment.
a. Assess residual abilities and utilize these in development of self-care regimens.
b. Encourage the patient to assist in own care to fullest ability.
c. Modify activities to facilitate maximum independence.
d. Maximize time allotted for accomplishment of self-care activities.
e. Integrate change, occupational therapy, and other therapeutic approaches into nursing care activities.

Evaluation
EXPECTED OUTCOMES
1. Achieves pain relief:
a. Participates in pain-reduction activities by elevating extremity, use of pain-reduction treatment, accepting assistance in pain-producing situations.
b. Decreases use of medications in the management of discomfort.
2. Increases participation in rehabilitative activities by self-care activities, mobilization activities, planning for continuing care needs.
3. Maintains adequate circulation and nerve function:
a. Minimal discomfort, normal sensations and normal movement of fingers or toes of involved extremity.
b. No extremity contracture or evidence of loss of function of extremity due to compromised circulation.
4. Moves unaffected joints and extremities.
5. Utilizes mobilization aids safely and effectively.
6. Participates in rehabilitation programme.
7. Remains free of immobility complications.
8. States modifications in lifestyle necessary to accommodate musculoskeletal disability.

MUSCULOSKELETAL TRAUMA

CONTUSIONS

A contusion is an injury to the soft tissue produced by a blunt force, blow, kick or fall.

CLINICAL FEATURES

1. Haemorrhage into injured part (bruising) – from rupture of small blood vessels; also associated with fractures.
2. Pain, swelling and discoloration.

NURSING INTERVENTIONS

Relief of discomfort

1. Elevate the affected part.
2. Apply cold compresses for the first 24 hours (20 to 30 minutes at a time) – to produce vasoconstriction, decrease oedema and reduce discomfort.
3. Apply heat to affected area after 24 hours (20 to 30 minutes at a time) four times a day – to promote circulation and absorption.
4. Apply pressure bandage – to control bleeding and swelling.
5. Assess neurovascular status of contused extremity every hour to every four hours as the patient's condition indicates.

Activity schedule

1. Encourage range of movements of all joints.
2. Assist with activities as needed.
3. Teach the patient to avoid excessive exercise of injured part.
4. Teach the patient to avoid re-injury.

STRAINS AND SPRAINS

A *strain* is a microscopic tearing of the muscle caused by excessive force, stretching, or overuse.

A sprain is an injury to ligamentous structure surrounding a joint; it is usually caused by a wrench or twist resulting in a decrease in the joint stability.

CLINICAL FEATURES

Strains

There is usually haemorrhage into the muscle, swelling, tenderness and pain, with isometric contraction of the muscle.

Sprains

1. Rapid swelling – due to extravasation of blood within tissues.
2. Pain upon passive movement of joint.
3. Increasing pain during first few hours due to continued swelling.
4. X-ray of area reveals no bone injury.

NURSING INTERVENTIONS

Relief of discomfort

1. Apply cold compresses (or ice bag) for 15 to 20

minutes intermittently for 12 to 36 hours – vaso-constricting effects of cold retard extravasation of blood and lymph (oedema) and suppress pain.
2. After 24 hours, apply mild heat (15 to 30 minutes, four times daily) – to promote absorption.
3. Instruct the patient on use of pain medication as prescribed.

Immobilization of injured part to allow for healing

1. Splint and immobilize injured part.
2. Elevate injured extremity to minimize swelling.
3. Use elastic compressive dressing to support weakened joint structures and to control oedema.
4. Severe sprains may require surgical repair and/or cast immobilization.

Resumption of self-care activities

1. Assist the patient in use of self-care and mobility aids to maintain independence within activity restrictions.
2. Participate in patient teaching on need to rest injured part for about a month to allow for healing.
3. Teach the patient to resume activities gradually.

JOINT DISLOCATIONS

A dislocation of a joint is a condition in which the articular surfaces of the bones forming the joint are no longer in contact (bones are 'out of joint'). This is a medical emergency because of associated disruption of surrounding blood and nerve supplies.

CLASSIFICATION

1. Congenital (hip most often affected).
2. Pathological or spontaneous – from disease of articular or periarticular structures.
3. Traumatic – from injury.

CLINICAL FEATURES

1. Pain.
2. Deformity.
3. Change in the length of the extremity.
4. Loss of normal movement.
5. X-ray confirmation of dislocation without associated fracture.

TREATMENT AND NURSING MANAGEMENT

1. Immobilize part while the patient is transported to the accident and emergency department, X-ray department or clinical unit.
2. Reduction of dislocation (bring displaced parts

into normal position) as soon as possible; usually performed under anaesthesia.
3. Stabilize reduction until joint structures are healed.
4. Monitor for development of sequelae (unstable joint, aseptic necrosis of bone, circulatory or nerve impairment).

NURSING INTERVENTIONS
Promoting comfort
1. Check patient's consent for surgery has been obtained if reduction of dislocation is to be undertaken by anaesthesia.
2. Give medication to relieve discomfort.
3. Immobilize reduced joint.

Resumption of self-care activities
1. Assist the patient with activities of daily living as needed.
2. Initiate health teaching concerning need to comply with activity limitations, rehabilitation therapies, and long-term monitoring for sequelae.

KNEE INJURIES

CAUSES
1. Severe stresses are applied to the knee during many sport activities (e.g. soccer, skiing, running).
2. Injury to knee structures occur during rapid position changes involving flexing and twisting of the joint.
3. Torn cartilage (meniscus) causes pain, tenderness, joint effusion, clicking sensations and decreased range of movement.
4. Knee ligaments may be torn, resulting in pain and joint instability. The patellar tendon may rupture.

MANAGEMENT
1. Arthroscopic meniscectomy: removal of cartilage fragments through operating arthroscope inserted through a small incision into the knee joint.
2. Open meniscectomy: direct surgical approach to knee joint structures for repair of disrupted structures.
3. Ligament injuries: treated with immobilization (i.e. elastic bandage, splint, cast) or suturing of ligament, depending on severity of injury.
4. Rupture of tendon: must be sutured and immobilized during healing.

PATIENT EDUCATION
1. Elevate leg to minimize swelling.

2. Quadriceps setting exercises and straight leg raising.
3. Weight-bearing and exercise programme as prescribed.

FRACTURES

A fracture is a break in the continuity of bone. Although the bone is the part most directly affected, other structures may be involved, resulting in soft tissue oedema, haemorrhage into muscles and joints, joint dislocations, ruptured tendons, severed nerves, damaged blood vessels and injury to body organs.

AETIOLOGY
A fracture occurs when the stress placed on the bone is more than the bone can absorb. When a fracture occurs through an area of diseased bone (osteoporosis, bone cyst, bony metastasis) it is considered a *pathological fracture*.

CLASSIFICATION OF FRACTURES
See Figure 13.1.

General classification
1. Complete – a fracture involving the entire cross section of the bone; usually displaced.
2. Incomplete – a fracture involving only a portion of the cross-section of bone; usually undisplaced.
3. Open – there is communication between the fracture and the skin (formerly called compound fracture).
4. Closed – the fracture does not communicate with outside area (formerly called simple fracture).

Specific types of fracture
See Figure 13.1.
1. Greenstick – a fracture in which one side of a bone is broken and the other side is bent.
2. Transverse – the fracture is straight across the bone.
3. Oblique – a fracture occurring at an angle across the bone (less stable than transverse).
4. Spiral – a fracture twisting around the shaft of the bone.
5. Comminuted – a fracture in which bone has splintered into several fragments.
6. Complicated – where a nerve, tendon, blood vessel or organ may be damaged by the fracture.
7. Depressed – a fracture in which fragment(s) are in-driven (seen frequently in fractures of skull and facial bones).

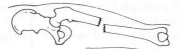

Simple (closed) fracture:
No open wound

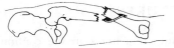

Compound (open) fracture – Wound in
skin communicates with fracture

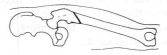

Extracapsular fracture – Bone broken
outside joint

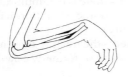

Intracapsular fracture – Bone broken
inside joint

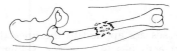

Comminuted fracture – Bone
splintered into fragments

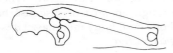

Greenstick fracture – Bone broken,
bent but still securely hinged at one
side

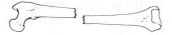

Longitudinal fracture – Break runs
parallel with bone

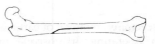

Transverse fracture – Break runs
across bone

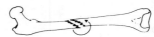

Oblique fracture – Break runs in
slanting direction on bone

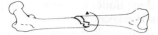
Spiral fracture – Break coils around
bone

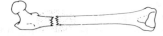
Pathological fracture – Break is at site
of bone disease

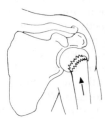

Impacted fracture – Bone broken and
wedged into other break

Fracture dislocation – Break
complicated by bone out of joint

Depressed fracture – Broken skull
bone driven inward

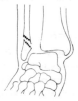

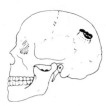

Figure 13.1. Types of fracture (from: *Nursing Care of the Patient in the O. R.* Somerville, New Jersey, Ethicon Inc.)

8. Impacted – a fracture in which the fractured bone has been compressed by another bone(s) (seen in vertebral fractures).
9. Pathological – a fracture that occurs through an area of diseased bone (bone cyst, Paget's disease, bony metastasis).
10. Avulsion – fragment of bone pulled off by ligament or tendon and its attachment.
11. Fracture dislocation – a fracture complicated by the bone being out of the joint.
12. Other – described according to anatomical location – epiphyseal, supracondylar, mid-shaft, intra-articular.

FRACTURE TREATMENT

There is no one solution in the management of fractures. Consideration is given to the severity of the fracture, damage to soft tissues, the age and condition of the patient and economic factors before a specific form of treatment is selected.

Objectives

1. Regain and maintain correct position and alignment.
2. Regain the function of the involved part.
3. Return the patient to his usual activities in the shortest time and at the least expense.

Process

1. *Reduction* – setting the bone; refers to restoration of the fracture fragments into anatomical position and alignment.
2. *Immobilization* – maintains reduction until bone healing occurs.
3. *Rehabilitation* – regaining normal function of the affected part.

Methods

1. *Closed reduction* – bony fragments are brought into *apposition* (ends in contact) by manipulation and manual traction – restores alignment.

a. May be done under anaesthesia for pain relief and muscle relaxation.

b. Cast or splint applied to immobilize extremity and maintain reduction (see Casts, p. 807).

2. *Traction* – force applied to accomplish and maintain reduction and alignment (see Traction, p. 815).

   a. Frequently used for fractures of long bones.

   b. Techniques:

   (i) Skin traction – force applied to the skin using foam rubber, extensions, etc.

   (ii) Skeletal traction – force applied to the bony skeleton directly using wires, pins, or tongs placed into or through the bone.

3. *Open reduction with internal fixation* – operative intervention to achieve reduction, alignment and stabilization (see Orthopaedic Surgery, Special Nursing Considerations, p. 835).

   a. Bone fragments are directly visualized.

   b. Internal fixation devices (metal pins, wires, screws, plates, nails, rods) may be used to hold bone fragments in position until solid bone healing occurs (may be removed when bone is healed).

   c. After closure of the wound, splints or casts may be used for additional stabilization and support.

4. *Endoprosthetic replacement* – replacement of a fracture fragment with an implanted metal device; utilized when fracture disrupts nutrition of the bone or treatment of choice is bony replacement.

5. *External fixation device* – stabilization of complex and open fracture with use of a metal frame and pin system; permits active treatment of injured soft tissue.

   a. Wound may be left open (delayed primary wound closure).

   b. Repair of damage to blood vessels, soft tissue, muscles, nerves, and tendons as indicated.

   c. Reconstructive surgery may be necessary.

   (See External Fixation for Complicated Fractures, p. 820.)

NURSING PROCESS OVERVIEW (THE PATIENT WITH A FRACTURE)

Assessment

CLINICAL FEATURES

1. Physical findings implicating fracture include:

   a. Pain at site of injury.

   b. Swelling.

   c. Tenderness.

   d. False movement and crepitus (grating sensation).

   e. Deformity.

   f. Loss of function.

   g. Bruising.

   h. Paraesthesia.

2. X-ray and other imaging techniques demonstrating fracture.

3. Signs and symptoms of shock:

   a. Bone is very vascular; following trauma, large amounts of blood escape from circulating blood into soft tissues or through open wounds (especially in femoral and pelvic fractures).

   b. May be fatal within a few hours after injury.

4. Overt haemorrhage and covert blood loss (bleeding into the tissues) – note haemoglobin and haematocrit.

5. *Fat embolism syndrome* – embolization of marrow or tissue fat or lipids with platelets and circulating free fatty acids within the pulmonary capillaries; pulmonary capillary leak may result, producing respiratory distress and central nervous system dysfunction.

   a. Onset may occur within 48 hours after injury.

NURSING ALERT

Have a high degree of suspicion of fat embolism syndrome in patients with multiple fractures, and fractures of long bones and pelvis. Hypoxaemia is an early feature and is detected by arterial blood gas analysis.

   b. Assess patient for:

   (i) Respiratory distress – tachypnoea, dyspnoea, hypoxaemia, crackles, wheezing, acute pulmonary oedema. Lung filters and traps embolic material, producing disturbed ventilation, perfusion and interstitial pneumonitis.

   (ii) Mental disturbances – irritability, restlessness, confusion, disorientation, stupor and coma – effects of systemic embolization and severe hypoxaemia (may be first sign).

   (iii) Fever.

   (iv) Petechiae – in buccal membranes, conjunctival sacs, on the hard palate, retina, chest and anterior axillary folds – from occlusion of capillaries by fat and fibrin platelet particulate substances.

6. Neurovascular status – watch for neurovascular impairment in all patients with fractures – pain, decreased circulation, decreased sensation and decreased motor activity.

PATIENT PROBLEMS

1. Pain related to fractured bone, soft tissue injury and swelling, and muscle spasm.
2. Inadequate tissue perfusion related to swelling of injured part and disrupted fluid circulation.
3. Self-care deficits related to fracture immobility and therapeutic treatments.
4. Potential systemic problems (e.g. shock, fat emboli) related to injury and postinjury sequelae.
5. Potential local fracture problems (i.e. compartment syndrome, non-union, infection) related to disruption of healing sequence.
6. Ineffective coping and social isolation related to fracture event and ramifications.

Planning and implementation
NURSING INTERVENTIONS
Relief of discomfort

1. See pain related to musculoskeletal conditions, p. 797.
2. Immobilize bone fragments – movement of fragments causes pain.
3. Support splinted fracture above and below fracture when repositioning or moving the patient.
4. Reposition patient with slow and steady movement; use additional personnel as needed.

Reduction in swelling associated with the injury

1. Elevate injured extremity.
2. Apply ice pack to injury if prescribed.
3. Assess neurovascular status of injured extremity.

Promotion of self-care activities within the limits of fracture treatment

1. Assist the patient with hygiene and nutrition activities as needed.
2. Encourage independence within immobility limits.
3. Modify activities to facilitate maximum independence.
4. Allow time for the patient to accomplish task.
5. Teach technique for safe use of mobility and other aids.

Prevention of systemic problems (e.g. shock [haemorrhagic or neurogenic]; fat emboli; pulmonary emboli)

1. Monitor vital signs.
2. Maintain arterial blood pressure – administer fluids/blood as needed.
3. Review laboratory reports for abnormal values.
4. Observe for signs and symptoms of fat embolism.
   a. Evaluate mental status.

b. Maintain satisfactory pulmonary gas exchange and support the respiratory system.
   (i) Draw arterial blood for gas analysis – arterial hypoxia is present with fat emboli; cannot always be recognized clinically.
   (ii) Administer oxygen as indicated by results of blood gas analysis (respiratory failure is the most common cause of death).
   (iii) Assist with endotracheal intubation (for airway control); controlled volume ventilation and positive end-expiratory pressure (PEEP) – to obtain maximum aeration of lungs.
   (iv) Administer steroids – to block chemical inflammation caused by free fatty acids; decreases endothelial damage (controversial).
   (v) See treatment of respiratory failure and insufficiency, p. 98.
5. Assess for development of:
   a. Thromboembolism (particularly of fractures of lower extremities).
   b. Infection – all open fractures are considered contaminated. (See also gas gangrene, p. 1004, and tetanus, p. 1005).
   c. Disseminated intravascular coagulation (DIC) – a group of bleeding disorders with diverse causes (see p. 396).

Prevention of neurovascular and healing problems

1. See neurovascular compromise, p. 798.

NURSING ALERT

Monitoring the neurovascular integrity of the injured extremity is essential. Development of compartment syndrome (increased tissue pressure causing anoxia) – leads to permanent loss of function in six to eight hours. This situation must be identified and managed promptly.

2. Support the patient if healing does not occur as projected because of inadequate immobilization, interposed tissue between bone fragments or infection.
   a. Delayed union – signifies that a specific fracture has not healed in the time considered average for this type of fracture.
   b. Nonunion – failure of the ends of a fractured bone to unite (and union not expected to occur).
   c. Avascular necrosis of bone – may occur when the bone loses its blood supply following frac-

ture of dislocation (notably in the hip) or in certain diseases.

   d. Malunion.

Prevention of infection

1. Minimize chance of infection of wound, soft tissue and bone.
2. Cleanse, debride and irrigate the wound as soon as possible – to minimize chance of infection.
   a. Take swabs for culture and sensitivity of wound.
3. Protect the patient from tetanus.
   a. Determine the patient's status of immunization for tetanus.
   b. See p. 1005 for protocol of administration.
   c. Give antibiotics as directed (usually intravenous antibiotics are started quickly) – to avoid and treat serious infection; many open fractures are contaminated with bacteria at the time of admission.
4. Observe and record the patient's temperature at regular intervals – for septic complications.

Adjustment of lifestyle and responsibilities to accommodate limitations imposed by fracture

See psychological and social problems associated with musculoskeletal problems, p. 798.

PATIENT EDUCATION

1. Explain basis for fracture treatment and need for patient participation in therapeutic regimen.
2. Instruct the patient to actively exercises joints above and below the immobilized fracture at frequent intervals.
   a. Isometric exercises of muscles covered by cast – start exercises as soon as possible after cast application.
   b. Increase isometric exercises as fracture stabilizes.
3. After removal of immobilizing device (e.g. cast, splint), have the patient start active exercises and continue with isometric exercises.
4. Instruct the patient on exercises to strengthen upper extremity muscles if crutch walking is planned.
5. Instruct the patient in methods of safe ambulation – frames, crutches, walking stick.
6. Emphasize instructions concerning amount of weight-bearing that will be permitted on fractured extremity.
7. Discuss prevention of recurrent fractures – safety considerations; avoidance of fatigue; proper footwear.
8. Discharge teaching – follow-up medical super-

vision; symptoms needing attention (e.g. numbness, decreased function, increased pain, elevated temperature); medication teaching.

Evaluation

EXPECTED OUTCOMES

1. Patient achieves relief of discomforts related to fracture; elevates fractured extremity and uses pain-relief techniques.
2. Patient experiences minimal swelling of injured part; applies ice pack as prescribed to fresh injury and demonstrates intact neurovascular status.
3. Patient achieves self-care within limits of therapeutic regimen; participates in hygiene and nutritional care; uses assistive devices safely.
4. Patient is free of potential systemic problems; maintains normal vital signs and laboratory values.
5. Patient shows no signs of potential local fracture problems; intact neurovascular status and fracture healing within anticipated period for particular type of fracture.
6. Patient demonstrates psychological adjustment to impact of therapeutic regimen on lifestyle; actively participates in therapeutic–rehabilitation programme.

CASTS

A cast is an immobilizing device consisting of layers of plaster bandages, fibreglass or resin impregnated bandages. Plaster of paris is manufactured from an inorganic material – anhydrous calcium sulphate (gypsum). The new splinting materials require a slightly different technique in application.

OBJECTIVES

1. Immobilize and hold bone fragments in reduction.
2. Apply uniform compression of soft tissues.
3. Permit early weight-bearing activities.
4. Correct chronic deformities with wedging or special hinges or by serial cast changes.
5. Support and stabilize weak joints.

TYPES OF CAST

See Figure 13.2.

1. *Below elbow cast* – extends from below the elbow to the proximal palmar crease.

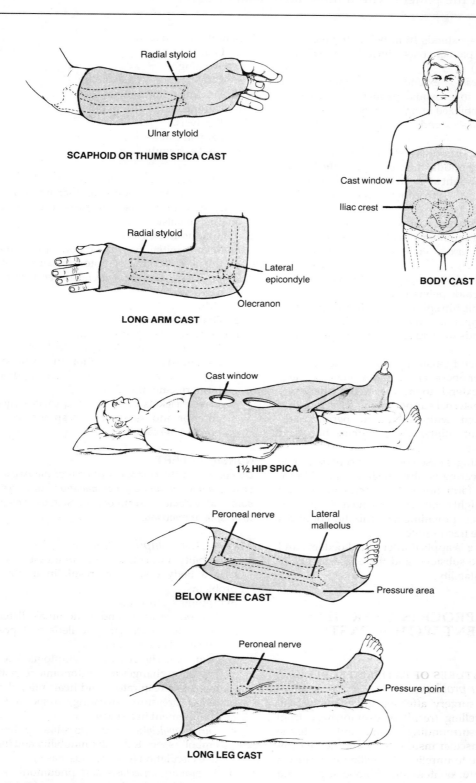

SCAPHOID OR THUMB SPICA CAST
Radial styloid
Ulnar styloid

LONG ARM CAST
Radial styloid
Lateral epicondyle
Olecranon

BODY CAST
Cast window
Iliac crest

1½ HIP SPICA
Cast window

BELOW KNEE CAST
Peroneal nerve
Lateral malleolus
Pressure area

LONG LEG CAST
Peroneal nerve
Pressure point

Figure 13.2. Pressure areas in different types of cast

2. *Scaphoid cast* – extends from below the elbow to the proximal palmar crease, including the thumb (thumb spica).
3. *Above elbow cast* – extends from upper level of axillary fold to proximal palmar crease; elbow usually immobilized at right angle.
4. *Below knee cast* – extends from below knee to base of toes.
5. *Long leg (above knee) cast* – extends from junction of the upper and middle third of thigh to the base of toes; foot is at right angle in a neutral position.
6. *Spica or body cast* – incorporates the trunk and an extremity.
   a. *Shoulder spica cast* – a body jacket that encloses trunk and shoulder and elbow.
   b. *Hip spica cast* – encloses trunk and lower extremity.
      (i) Single hip spica – extends from nipple line to include pelvis and one thigh.
      (ii) Double hip spica extends from nipple line or upper abdomen to include pelvis and extends to include both thighs and lower legs.
      (iii) One-and-a-half hip spica – extends from upper abdomen, includes one entire leg, and extends to the knee of the other.
7. *Cast-brace* – external support about a fracture that is constructed with hinges to permit early movement of joints, early mobilization and independence.
   a. Cast-bracing is based on the concept that some weight-bearing is physiological and will promote the formation of bone and contain fluid within a tight compartment which compresses soft tissues, providing a distribution of forces across the fracture site.
   b. Cast-brace is applied after initial oedema and pain have subsided and there is evidence of fracture stability.

NURSING PROCESS OVERVIEW (THE PATIENT WITH A CAST)

Assessment
CLINICAL FEATURES OF PATIENT PROBLEMS
Neurovascular problems
1. Trauma or surgery affecting an extremity will produce swelling (result of haemorrhage from bone and surrounding tissue and of tissue oedema). Vascular insufficiency and nerve compression due to unrelieved swelling can cause a reduction in or obliteration of blood supply and peripheral nerve damage to an extremity.

2. Symptoms and signs:
   a. Pain.
   b. Swelling.
   c. Discoloration – pale or blue.
   d. Tingling or numbness.
   e. Diminished or absent pulse.
   f. Paralysis.
   g. Pain on extension.
   h. Cool extremity.

Necrosis, pressure sores and nerve palsies
1. Pressure of cast on neurovascular structures and bony structures causes necrosis, pressure sores and nerve palsies.
2. Symptoms and signs:
   a. Severe initial pain over bony prominences; this is a warning symptom of an impending pressure sore. *Pain decreases when ulceration occurs.*
   b. Odour.
   c. Drainage on cast.
3. Pressure sites (see Figure 13.2):
   a. *Lower extremity* – heel, malleoli, dorsum of foot, head of fibula, anterior surface of patella.
   b. *Upper extremity* – medial epicondyle of humerus, ulnar styloid.
   c. Plaster jackets or body spica casts – sacrum, anterior and superior iliac spines, vertebral borders of scapulae.

NURSING ALERT
Do not ignore the complaint of pain of the patient in a cast. Suspect circulatory complications or a pressure sore. Notify doctor if symptoms persist. Cast may have to be split or removed.

Multisystem complications
1. Immobility and confinement in a cast – particularly a body cast – can result in multisystem problems.
2. Symptoms/signs/causes:
   a. *Nausea, vomiting* and abdominal distension associated with paralytic ileus and possible intestinal obstruction.
   b. *Acute anxiety* reaction symptoms (i.e. behavioural changes and autonomic responses – increased respiratory and heart rate, elevated blood pressure, sweating) associated with confinement in a space.
   c. *Thrombophlebitis* and possible pulmonary emboli associated with immobility and ineffective circulation (e.g. venous stasis).
   d. *Respiratory atelectasis* and pneumonia associated with ineffective respiratory effort.

e. *Renal and bladder calculi* associated with urinary stasis, low fluid intake, and calcium excretion associated with immobility.

f. *Anorexia and constipation* associated with decreased activity.

g. *Psychological reaction* (e.g. depression) associated with immobility, dependence, and loss of control.

Planning and implementation
NURSING INTERVENTIONS
Maintaining adequate tissue perfusion

1. Elevate the extremity on cloth-covered pillow above the level of the heart. Keep the heel off the mattress.
2. Avoid resting cast on hard surfaces or sharp edges that can cause denting or flattening of the cast and consequent pressure sores.
3. Handle moist cast with palms of hands.
4. Turn the patient every two hours while cast dries.
5. Spica or body cast:
   a. Place a bedboard under the mattress – prevents sagging of bed from pressure of cast.
   b. Support the curves of the cast with cloth-covered flexible pillows – prevents cracking and flat spots while cast is drying.
      (i) Place three pillows crosswise on bed for body cast.
      (ii) Place one pillow crosswise at the waist and two pillows lengthwise for affected leg for spica cast. If both legs are involved, use two additional pillows.
6. If symptoms of neurovascular compromise occur:
   a. Bivalve the cast: split cast on each side over its full length into two halves.
   b. Cut the underlying padding – blood-soaked padding may shrink and cause constriction of circulation.
   c. Spread cast sufficiently to relieve constriction.
7. If symptoms of pressure area occur, cast may be 'windowed' (hole cut in it) so that the skin at the pain point can be examined and treated. The window must be replaced so that the tissue does not swell and cause additional pressure problems at window edge.

Countering immobility side-effects

1. Monitor for development of symptoms associated with paralytic ileus. If symptoms occur:
   a. Place the patient prone to relieve pressure symptoms.
   b. Remove the cast from the patient if necessary.
   c. Employ nasogastric suction.

d. Maintain normal electrolyte balance by intravenous replacement of fluid.
Surgical intervention (duodenojejunostomy) may be necessary when conservative measures fail to relieve duodenal obstruction.

2. Encourage the patient to verbalize fears and concerns. Facilitate active participation in decision-making. Encourage family support.
3. *Be alert for evidences of thromboembolic complications.* Individuals at high risk (increased age, previous thromboembolism, obesity, congestive heart failure, cancer of pancreas or lung, trauma) may require prophylaxis against thromboembolism.
   a. Encourage the patient to move about as normally as possible.
   b. Do prescribed exercises faithfully.
   c. Have the patient exercise the parts of the body that are not immobilized by the cast at regular and frequent intervals.
   d. Turn the patient.
4. Encourage deep-breathing exercises and coughing at regular intervals.
5. Encourage the patient to drink liberal quantities of fluid – to avoid urinary calculi.
6. Encourage balanced nutritional intake. Assess the patient's food preferences. Serve small meals. Provide natural bowel stimulants (e.g. fibre). Monitor bowels and utilize a bowel programme if necessary.
7. Facilitate patient participation in care planning and activities. Encourage mobility within limits of therapeutic regimen.

SPECIFIC CARE FOR PATIENT IN SPICA/BODY CAST

1. Keep the cast level by elevating the lumbar sacral area with a small pillow when the head of the bed is elevated or when the patient is placed on the bedpan.
2. Protect the toes from the pressure of the bedding.
3. Encourage the patient to maintain physiological position by:
   a. Using the overhead trapeze (monkey pole).
   b. Placing good foot flat on bed and pushing down while lifting himself up on the trapeze.
   c. Avoiding twisting movements.
   d. Avoiding positions that produce pressure on groin, back, chest and abdomen.
4. Provide hygienic care of the patient:
   a. Cover perineum with a towel and apply spray (lacquer-type) to perineal area of cast. Tuck 10cm strips of thin polyethylene sheeting under perineal area of cast and tape to cast exterior. Replace when soiling occurs.

b. Clean outside of cast with dry cleanser on almost-dry cloth.

c. Pull stockinette taut, then trim and fasten to cast edges with adhesive.

d. Inspect skin for signs of irritation:
   (i) Around cast edge.
   (ii) Under cast – pull skin taut and inspect under cast, using a torch for illumination.

e. Reach up under cast and massage accessible skin.

f. Using a bedpan: roll the patient onto bedpan; place pillow in lumbosacral area.

5. Turn the patient in a body/spica cast:

a. Move the patient to the side of the bed, using a steady, even, pulling movement.

b. Place pillows along the other side of the bed; one for the chest and two (lengthwise) for the legs.

c. Instruct the patient to place his arms at his side or above his head.

d. Turn the patient as a unit. Avoid twisting the patient in the cast.

e. Turn the patient toward the leg not encased in plaster or towards the unoperated side if both legs are in plaster.
   (i) One nurse stands at other side of bed to receive the patient's shoulders.
   (ii) Second nurse supports leg in plaster while the third nurse supports the patient's back as he is turned.
   (iii) *Do not grasp cross bar of spica cast to move the patient*. The purpose of the bar is to strengthen the cast.
   (iv) Turn the patient in body cast to a prone position twice daily – provides postural drainage of bronchial tree; relieves pressure on back.

PATIENT EDUCATION

1. Check neurovascular status. Watch for symptoms of circulatory disturbance.

a. Watch for these danger signs (arm or leg cast): blueness or paleness of fingernails or toenails accompanied by pain and tightness, numbness, cold or tingling sensation.

b. Elevate the affected limb above the heart and wiggle fingers/toes.

c. Call the doctor if condition persists.

2. Prevent or reduce swelling.

a. Elevate the extremity in the cast above the level of the heart.

b. After the patient begins ambulation, encourage him to elevate the cast when he is seated.

Encourage the patient to lie down several times daily with cast elevated.

c. Prevent bedclothes from resting on cast; make use of cradles.

3. Prevent irritation at cast edge – pad edges of cast with moleskin or 'petal' the cast edges with strips of adhesive tape.

4. Teach the patient to perform isometric exercises – contracting the muscles without moving the joint, to maintain muscle strength and prevent atrophy (performed hourly when awake).

5. Exercise every joint that is not immobilized. Move the rest of the body.

6. Actively exercise joints that do not move bone fragments.

a. Leg-cast – 'Push down on the popliteal (knee) space, hold it, relax, repeat.' Move toes back and forth; bend toes down, then pull them back.

b. Arm cast – 'Make a fist, hold it, relax, repeat.' Move shoulders.

7. Avoid getting cast wet, especially padding under cast – causes skin breakdown.

8. Do not cover a leg cast with plastic or rubber boots since this causes condensation and wetting of the cast.

9. Avoid weight-bearing or stress on plaster cast for 24 hours.

10. Report to the doctor if the cast cracks or breaks; instruct the patient not to try to fix it himself.

11. Avoid walking on wet floors or pavements.

12. Do not place sharp objects under the cast.

13. To clean the cast:

a. Remove surface soil with slightly damp cloth.

b. Rub soiled areas with household scouring powder.

c. Wipe off residual moisture.

14. After cast is removed:

a. Cleanse skin with mild soap and water.

b. Apply emollient lotion to dry skin.

c. Avoid scratching the skin.

d. Gradually resume activities and exercise.

e. Elevate extremity to control swelling.

Evaluation

EXPECTED OUTCOMES

1. Patient maintains adequate tissue perfusion:

a. Minimal oedema – no swelling or pressure.

b. Intact neurovascular status – normal pulse pressure, filling time, sensation.

c. Intact skin over bony prominences.

2. Patient avoids immobility-related problems:

a. Normal body system functioning – normal bowel and urinary elimination pattern; vital signs normal; normal respiratory pattern; normal blood gases.

3. Patient participates in self-care activities to optimum ability.
4. Patient expresses feelings and fears, but maintains positive outlook and expectations.

GUIDELINES: APPLICATION OF A PLASTER CAST

EQUIPMENT

Prepare trolley with:

Plaster bandages; 5, 7.5, 10, 15, 20cm widths

Cast padding (Velband Softex)

Stockinette (tubular knitted material)

Plaster slabs (for reinforcement)

Padding for bony prominences – usually orthopaedic felt or extra layer of Velband

Knives, scissors, indelible pencil

Polyethylene sheeting or newspaper – to protect floor and patient

Disposable gloves – to protect hands of operator especially with new splinting materials

Large bucket of water at room temperature – 21 to 24°C, or as recommended by manufacturer of synthetic casting materials.

Cast finishing cream for synthetic casts as required

UNDERLYING CONSIDERATIONS

1. The application of a cast requires two or three people; one to apply the plaster (operator), one to dip and hand the plaster bandages to the operator, and a third person to hold the extremity in correct position. (Body spicas may require additional personnel.)
2. Plaster of Paris bandages and splints set in four to five minutes. This time may be altered by varying the temperature and amount of water; nonplaster splinting material usually takes longer to achieve the initial set and the technique of application varies somewhat according to the manufacturer.
3. The operator should practise cast application on a model. Plaster sets rapidly and this is a skill that requires experience.
4. There should be no movement of the extremity while the cast is being applied.
5. In general, the joints above and below the involved bone are usually immobilized.

PROCEDURE
Preparatory phase

Nursing action	Rationale
1. Spread polyethylene sheeting to protect floor and patient.	
2. Explain to the patient that there will be a feeling of warmth as the plaster is applied.	Heat is produced by crystallization as plaster sets. The reaction of water with plaster of Paris liberates heat.

3. Apply stockinette and roll padding on the limb or part to be immobilized.
   a. Apply as smoothly and snugly as possible so that each turn overlaps the preceding turn by half the width of the roll.
   b. Extra pieces of padding may be placed over bony prominences: olecranon process, malleoli, patella.

Padding is used to pad the sharp cast margins for patient comfort and to prevent pressure areas, minimize circulatory problems and enhance cast removal.

4. Having unrolled the first 10–15cm of the bandage, submerge the plaster bandage vertically in water (room temperature) for a minute or so, or until bubbles cease to rise.

Water that is too warm will accelerate setting time, may cause a burn and may result in excessive plaster loss by loosening the adhesive agents which bond the plaster to the fabric.

5. Expel excess water by squeezing (not wringing) towards the centre of the bandage; hand bandage to operator with free end hanging loose.

The cast will dry more quickly (and thus will acquire maximum strength sooner) if a well-squeezed bandage is used.

Application

Nursing action	Rationale
1. Commencing at the distal end, roll the bandage gently and evenly on the extremity, overlapping the preceding turn by half the width of the roll.	Roll inward towards the patient's body for ease of control.
2. Keep the bandage moving and in constant contact with the surface of the limb. Smooth and rub down successive layers or turns of each bandage into the layers below with the thumbs and thenar eminences (mound on the palm) in circumferential and longitudinal directions.	This keeps the cast uniformly thick. Rubbing the plaster as it is applied will form a smooth, solid and well-fused cast. Avoid indenting the cast with the fingertips since this will produce pressure sores on underlying skin.
3. Take tucks in the lower border of the bandage by lifting the bandage off the surface (without tension) and overlapping it in a V-shaped fashion.	Tucking the bandage helps to contour the cast to the changing circumference of the limb. Do not twist or reverse the bandage to change its direction since this produces sharp cutting edges.
4. Trim the cast to size with a sharp knife by pulling the plaster edge against the cutting edge of the knife.	Do not pull too vigorously on the stockinette since this may cause pressure on bony pressure points.
5. Ask the patient if there is any discomfort or pain.	If a patient complains of pain, the cast and encircling dressings should be split to avoid constriction, circulatory problems and pressure sores.
6. Write the diagnosis and date of cast application with an indelible pencil on the cast.	This is often done when a cast is applied following surgery.
7. Support the cast with the palm of the hand while moving the patient. Avoid indentations from tips of fingers.	Finger indentation on a fresh cast can produce pressure sores.

8. Expose the cast to warm, circulating dry air.

Avoid covering the cast when it is drying as this delays drying time and causes a rise in temperature. Usually the cast will reach its maximum temperature five to fifteen minutes after it is applied and will then cool rapidly. The ultimate cast strength is obtained after the cast is dry (up to 48 hours depending on outside temperature and humidity).

9. Clean plaster from equipment and store ready for use.

10. Synthetic casts may need to be 'finished' with application of cast hand cream.

Smooths rough exterior surface.

11. Synthetic casts may be dried with careful application of a hairdryer.

GUIDELINES: REMOVAL OF A CAST

EQUIPMENT

Plaster cutter – an electric saw with circular blade that oscillates through the plaster
Plaster spreader
Plaster knife
Scissors
Plaster shears

PROCEDURE
Preparatory phase

Nursing action

Rationale

1. Describe to the patient how and where the cast cutter will be used and the expected sensations. Turn on the cutter and allow the patient to hear the motor. Tell patient to shield eyes during procedure.

Reassures the patient that the cutter produces vibrations but not pain.

Plaster dust may be irritating to the eyes.

2. Determine whether or not the cast is padded.

An electric plaster cast cutter should not be used on unpadded casts.

3. Determine where the cut will be made. Mark, with a felt pen, the area to be cut.

The line should be in front of the lateral malleolus and behind the medial malleolus on a lower limb cast. An upper limb cast is usually split along the ulnar or flexor surface.

4. Dampen the cast along the portion to be cut.

Dampening diminishes the cloud of plaster dust.

Removal

Nursing action   **Rationale**

1. Grasp the electric cutter as illustrated (Figure
   13.3a).

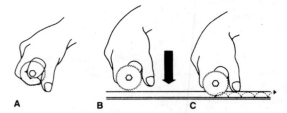

A   **B**   **C**

Figure 13.3. Operating a cast cutter (courtesy: Stryker Corporation)

2. Rest the thumb on the plaster.   The thumb serves as a depth gauge and acts as a
                                                                      guard in front of the blade.

3. Turn on the electric cutter. Push the blade firmly
   and gently through the cast while allowing the
   thumb to come in contact with the cast as the saw
   blade oscillates.

4. As the blade cuts through the plaster, a sudden
   lack of resistance is felt; plaster will 'give' (or 'dip')
   when the cut is completed.

5. Lift the cutting blade up a degree (but not out of
   the cutting groove) and advance the blade at a
   slightly higher or lower level. The cast is cut by a
   series of alternating pressure and linear
   movements along the line of the cut (Figure
   13.3b and c).

6. Avoid drawing the cutting blade along the limb in   This will cut the skin. If saw blade is in contact with
   a single motion.   padding too long, patient will feel burning sensation
                                                          on skin from rapidly oscillating blade.

7. Cut the cast on both sides. Then rock the anterior   This manoeuvre allows the operator to determine if the
   portion of the cast over the posterior portion.   cast is completely cut.

8. Insert the blades of the plaster spreader in the cut   Or spread the cast while cutting, to facilitate its
   trough. Separate the two halves with the spreader   removal.
   at several sites along the cast split. Separate the
   cast with the hands.

9. Cut through the padding and stockinette with   Use bandage scissors; place the flat blade closest to
   scissors, keeping the scissor blade that is closest   the skin.
   to the skin parallel to the skin.

10. Lift the limb carefully out of the posterior portion of the cast. Support the limb so that it is maintained in the same position as when in the cast.

When the support of the cast has been removed, stresses and strain are placed on parts that have been at rest.

After removal of cast

Nursing action

1. Cleanse the skin gently with soap and water. Blot dry. Apply a skin cream.

2. Emphasize the importance of continuing the prescribed exercises, reporting for physiotherapy, etc.

Rationale

Explain to the patient that the skin will be scaly and the limb will appear 'thin' from disuse. Reassure him that it will take a few weeks to regain normal appearance and function.

Exercises are necessary to redevelop and increase strength and function. Pain and stiffness may be expected after cast removal.

TRACTION

Traction is force applied in a specific direction. To apply the force needed to overcome the natural force or pull of muscle groups, a system of traction cords, pulleys and weights is used. Traction may be applied to the skin or to the skeletal system.

OBJECTIVES
1. Regain normal length and alignment.
2. Reduce and immobilize fracture.
3. Lessen or eliminate muscle spasm.
4. Prevent deformity.
5. Give the patient freedom for 'in bed' activities.
6. Reduce pain.

PRINCIPLES OF BALANCED (SUSPENSION) TRACTION
Balanced (suspension) traction is produced by a counterforce other than the patient's body weight. The limb balances in the traction apparatus. The line of traction on the extremity remains fairly constant despite changes in the patient's position.

PRINCIPLES OF WEIGHT AND PULLEY TRACTION
Weight and pulley traction is a form of traction in which the pull is exerted in one plane. It may utilize either skin or skeletal traction, and it may be either unilateral or bilateral. Example: Buck's extension.

METHODS OF APPLICATION
Skin traction
Acomplished by a weight that pulls on extension plaster or sponge rubber attached to the skin; traction on the skin transmits traction to the musculo-skeletal structures.
1. Skin traction is used as a temporary measure in adults; used prior to surgery in treatment of inter-trochanteric hip fracture (Buck's extension); Hamilton–Russell traction is used for applying traction to the femoral shaft with the knee flexed. Skin traction may be used definitely to treat fractures in children.
2. *Application and nursing assessment* – see pp. 816–19.

Skeletal traction
Traction applied to bone using wires, pins or tongs placed through bones; this is the most effective means of traction. It is applied by the orthopaedic surgeon under aseptic conditions.
1. Skeletal traction is used most frequently in treatment of fractures of the femur; dislocations of hips and of fractures of the cervical spine.
2. *Nursing assessment and responsibilities:*
   a. Watch for signs of infection, especially around the pin tract.
      (i) The pin should be immobile in the bone and the skin wound should be dry.
      (ii) If infection is suspected, percuss gently over the tibial tuberosity; this will elicit pain if infection is developing.
      (iii) Assess for other signs of infection: heat, redness, fever.

b. It may be necessary to clean the pin tracts using an aseptic technique to clear drainage around the skeletal pin, since plugging at this site can predispose to bacterial invasion of the tract and bone.

c. Apply a cork or pin guards over the edges of the pin.

d. Check traction apparatus at repeated intervals to see that the direction of pull is correct and the ropes are unobstructed; that weights are in proper position; and that patient is comfortable.

e. See below for nursing management.

Cervical traction
See p. 958.

Pelvic traction
Used for treatment of back disorders or injuries.

GUIDELINES: APPLICATION OF BUCK'S EXTENSION TRACTION

Buck's extension (unilateral or bilateral skin traction) is a form of skin traction used as a temporary measure to provide support and comfort to a fractured limb until definitive treatment is accomplished.

EQUIPMENT
Skin extensions
Elastic bandages, 10cm ⎫
Felt or foam padding ⎬ These are commercially available in ready-made traction kits
Spreader block or metal spreader ⎭
Pulley, traction cords and weights (2.3–3.1kg is usual – amount of weight is prescribed by doctor)
Tincture of benzoin (for adhesive traction)
Sheepskin pad
Elevator or blocks

PROCEDURE

Preparatory phase

Nursing action	Rationale
1. Place bedboard under the mattress and elevator blocks under the wheels at the foot of the bed if indicated. This depends on the size of the patient and the weight applied.	Elevating the foot of the bed (countertraction) helps prevent the patient from sliding down towards the foot of the bed.
2. Question the patient to determine previous skin conditions (contact dermatitis). Inspect skin for evidences of atrophy, abrasions and circulatory disturbances. Ensure that the patient is not allergic to elastoplast.	The skin must be in healthy condition to tolerate skin traction.
3. Make sure that the skin of the limb is clean and dry.	A clean, dry skin helps adherence of extensions.

Application

Nursing action	**Rationale**

1. For nonadhesive traction bandage:
   a. Pad both malleoli and proximal fibula.

   Pressure sores and skin necrosis may result from pressure applied directly over malleoli. Pressure over the region of the fibular head and common peroneal nerve may produce peroneal palsy and 'footdrop'.

   b. Apply Ventfoam (with the foam surface against the skin) on each side of the affected extremity, leaving a loop projecting 10–15cm beyond the sole of the foot.

2. For adhesive skin extensions.
   a. Pad both malleoli and proximal fibula. Apply tincture of benzoin to the skin.

   Tincture of benzoin may help protect the skin, although the tape adheres satisfactorily without it and some manufacturers advise against using it with these products.

   b. Gently stroke the tape onto the skin. Apply adhesive skin tape in the same manner as nonadhesive traction bandage.

   Stroking the tape onto the skin promotes skin adherence and prevents wrinkles and creases.

   c. Make 0.6–1.2cm oblique cuts along each border of the tape if necessary.

   Clipping the border of the tape allows it to conform to the contour of the leg. Uneven tension contributes to skin breakdown.

3. Have a second person elevate and support the extremity under the ankle and knee while the elastic bandage is applied (Figure 13.4). Beginning at the ankle, wrap the elastic bandage snugly over the tape up to the tibial tubercle.

   The elastic bandage improves adherence of tape to the skin and helps prevent slipping.

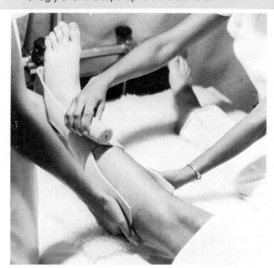

Figure 13.4. Applying an elastic bandage for Buck's extension traction

4. Attach a spreader block (or metal spreader) to the distal end of the tape. Attach a cord to the spreader block and pass it over a pulley fastened to the end of the bed (Figure 13.5).	The spreader block prevents pressure along the side of the foot. The spreader should not be too narrow (causes pressure sores on ankle) or too wide (pulls extension away from the heel).
5. Make sure knots are tied securely. Gently attach the traction weight. Release gradually.	The cord should be unobstructed; the weight should hang free of the bed and should not touch the floor.
6. Place a sheepskin pad under the leg (or use a commercial heel protector) if desired.	Sheepskin is used to reduce friction of the heel against the bed.
7. Assess the patient to ensure he is in proper alignment.	The part of the body in traction should be in line with the pull of the weight.

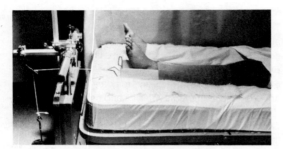

Figure 13.5. Lower limb in Buck's extension traction

NURSING ASSESSMENT OF THE PATIENT FOLLOWING APPLICATION OF BUCK'S EXTENSION

1. Palpate over area of extension daily. If area is tender to palpation, suspect skin irritation and report it immediately. The elastic bandage may have to be removed.
2. Inspect for skin irritation and pressure on:
   a. Achilles tendon.
   b. Peroneal nerve (as it passes around the neck of the fibula just below the knee).
3 Inspect dorsum of foot for loss of sensation, weakness of dorsiflexors of foot and toes, inversion of foot – may be caused by tight extensions and pressure on the common peroneal nerve.
4. Unwrap the elastic bandage and inspect leg if there is evidence of slipping of extensions.
5. Assess for complaints of persistent itching and burning.
6. Maintain the limb in a neutral position. Avoid external rotation.
7. The patient may not turn from side to side because the position of the leg on the bed will cause the bony fragments to move against each other.
8. Inspect and bathe back. To give back care instruct the patient to:
   a. Place hands on overhead trapeze (monkey pole).
   b. Bend the knee of unaffected extremity and place foot flat on bed.
   c. Push down on the uninvolved foot while at the same time pulling up on the trapeze (monkey pole) – allows the entire body and trunk to rise off the bed. The shoulders, back and buttocks must move as a single, straight unit.

NURSING PROCESS OVERVIEW (THE PATIENT IN TRACTION)

Assessment

1. Determine pathological basis for traction (e.g. muscle spasm, fracture, deformity).
2. Assess the patient's physiological and psychological status:
   a. Pain.
   b. Deformity.
   c. Swelling.
   d. Neurovascular status – paralysis, paraesthesia, pulse, colour.
   e. Emotional reactions.
   f. Understanding of treatment regimen.
   g. Skin condition – examined frequently for evidences of pressure or friction over bony prominences.
3. Examine traction equipment for safety and effectiveness.
   a. The patient is placed on a firm mattress, often with a bedboard beneath it.
   b. The cords and the pulleys should be in straight alignment.
   c. The pull should be in line with the long axis of the bone.
   d. Any factor that might reduce the pull or alter its direction must be eliminated.
      (i) Weights should hang freely.
      (ii) Cords should be unobstructed and not in contact with the bed or equipment.
      (iii) Help the patient to pull himself up in bed at frequent intervals. Traction is *not* accomplished if the knot in the rope or the footplate is touching the pulley or the foot of the bed, or if the weights are resting on the floor.
   e. The amount of weight applied in skin traction must not exceed the tolerance of the skin (approximately 3kg). The condition of the skin must be inspected frequently.
4. Evaluate the patient in skeletal traction for the possible development of infection.
   Check the patient for odour and signs of infection.
5. Review body systems for possible immobility-related problems (e.g. pneumonia, constipation, thrombophlebitis, depression).

PATIENT PROBLEMS

1. Potential for problems of immobility (musculoskeletal weakness, respiratory dysfunction, constipation) related to traction therapy.
2. Potential neurovascular compromise related to injury or traction therapy.
3. Potential skin breakdown related to pressure on soft tissue.
4. Potential infection related to bacterial invasion at skeletal traction site.

Planning and implementation

NURSING INTERVENTIONS

Maintaining effective traction therapy

1. Check traction apparatus at repeated intervals to see that the direction of pull is correct and the cords are unobstructed; that weights are in proper position; and that the patient is comfortable.
2. The cords and the pulleys should be freely movable.
3. The traction must be continuous to be effective unless prescribed as intermittent, as with pelvic traction.
4. Maintain adequate countertraction by adjustment of bed position.
5. *With fixed traction*, the patient may not be turned without disrupting the line of pull.
6. *With balanced traction*, the patient may be elevated, turned slightly and moved as desired.

NURSING ALERT

Every complaint of the patient in traction should be investigated immediately.

Maintaining normal body system functions

1. Encourage deep breathing hourly to facilitate expansion of lungs and movement of respiratory secretions.
2. Auscultate lung fields twice a day.
3. Encourage fluid intake of 2,000–2,500ml daily.
4. Provide balanced high fibre diet rich in protein; avoid excessive calcium intake.
5. Establish bowel routine through use of diet and/or stool softeners, laxatives and enemas as prescribed.
6. Encourage active exercise of uninvolved muscles and joints to maintain strength and function. Dorsiflex feet hourly to avoid development of footdrop.
7. Encourage patient participation in planning and care activities.
8. Provide diversional activities.
9. Examine the patient for development of thrombophlebitis (e.g. calf tenderness).

Retaining intact neurovascular status of immobilized extremity

1. See neurovascular compromise, p. 798.
2. Assess specific nerve functioning of peroneal nerve:

a. Have patient point big toe towards his nose.
b. Question about abnormal sensations.
c. Observe for footdrop.
3. Assess other nerves (e.g. ulnar, median, radial) that may be compressed.
4. Determine adequacy of circulation (e.g. colour, temperature, motion, capillary refill of peripheral fingers or toes).
   a. With Buck's traction the foot should be inspected for circulatory difficulties within a few minutes and then periodically after the elastic bandage has been applied.
5. Notify doctor promptly if change in neurovascular status is identified.

Maintaining intact skin without development of pressure areas
1. Examine bony prominences frequently for evidence of pressure or friction irritation.
2. Observe for skin irritation around the traction bandage.
3. Observe for pressure under the sling at the popliteal space.
4. Any complaint or burning sensation under the traction bandage should be reported immediately.
5. Special care must be given to the back at regular intervals, because the patient maintains a supine position.
6. Relieve pressure without disrupting traction effectiveness.

Avoiding infection at pin site
1. Monitor vital signs.
2. Watch for signs of infection, especially around the pin tract.
   a. The pin should be immobile in the bone and the skin wound should be dry. Small amount of serous oozing from pin site may occur.
   b. If infection is suspected, percuss gently over the tibia; this may elicit pain if infection is developing.
   c. Assess for other signs of infection: heat, redness, fever.
   If directed, clean the pin tract with sterile applicators and prescribed medication/ointment – to clear drainage at the entrance of tract and around the pin, since plugging at this site can predispose to bacterial invasion of the tract and bone.
3. Apply a cork or adhesive over the sharp edges of the pin to protect patient and care-givers from injury.

PATIENT EDUCATION
1. Teach the patient the purpose of traction therapy.
2. Delineate limitations of activity necessary to maintain effective traction.
3. Teach use of patient aids (e.g. monkey pole).
4. Instruct the patient not to adjust or modify traction apparatus.
5. Instruct the patient in activities designed to minimize effects of immobility on body systems.
6. Teach the patient necessity for reporting changes in sensations, pain, movement, etc.

Evaluation
EXPECTED OUTCOMES
1. Patient achieves effective traction therapy, immobilization and comfort:
   a. Maintains normal respiratory pattern; normal blood gases, vital signs and lung sounds.
   b. Maintains muscular strength and joint mobility; participates in exercise programme and activities of daily living.
2. Patient maintains normal neurovascular functioning – normal sensations, movement and circulatory parameters.
3. Patient shows no evidence of skin breakdown; no reddened skin from pressure.
4. Patient experiences no infection of pin site – tissue at pin site is not inflamed, red or tender beyond normal expectations; no fever.

EXTERNAL FIXATION FOR FRACTURES

External fixation is a technique of fracture immobilization in which a series of transfixing pins are inserted through bone and attached to a rigid external metal frame (Figure 13.6). The method is used mainly in the management of open fractures with severe soft tissue damage.

ADVANTAGES
1. Permits rigid support of severely comminuted open fractures, infected nonunions and infected unstable joints.
2. Facilitates wound care (frequent debridements, irrigations, dressing changes) and soft tissue reconstruction (delayed wound closure, muscle flaps, skin grafts).

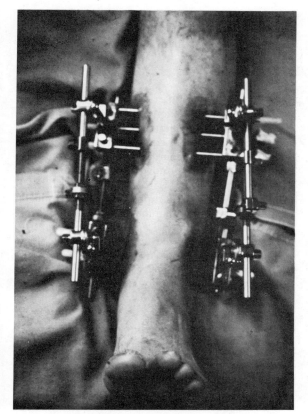

Figure 13.6. External fixation (courtesy: University of Texas Health and Science Centre, Dallas)

3. Allows early function of muscles and joints.
4. Allows early patient comfort.

PROCEDURE

Under general anaesthesia the skin is cleansed and transfixing pins are inserted through small incisions above and below the fracture and drilled through the bony cortex. Following reduction of the fracture, the appliance is tightened by adjusting and tightening the bars connecting the sets of pins.

The sharp pin heads are covered with plastic covers, cork or rubber plugs – to protect other extremity and bed linen.

Assessment

1. Determine the patient's understanding of procedure and fixation device.
2. Evaluate neurovascular status of involved body part.
3. Inspect each pin site for redness, drainage, tenderness, pain and loosening of the pin.

4. Inspect open wounds for healing, infection or devitalized tissue.
5. Assess functioning of other body systems.

PATIENT PROBLEMS

1. Anxiety and ineffective coping related to appearance of external fixation device.
2. Potential inadequate tissue perfusion and neurovascular compromise related to injury.
3. Potential infection related to open injury and skeletal pin insertion.
4. Impaired mobility and ability to perform activities of daily living related to restrictions imposed by injury and external fixator.

NURSING INTERVENTIONS
Relieving anxiety and fear related to the external fixation device

1. If possible before placement of the device, reassure the patient that although the fixator appears clumsy and cumbersome, it should not hurt once it is in place.
2. Emphasize the positive aspects of this device in treating complex musculoskeletal problems.
3. Encourage the patient to talk about reaction to the device, thereby minimizing the development of other system problems.
4. Inform the patient that he will achieve greater mobility with an external fixation device, thereby minimizing the development of other system problems.
5. Involve the patient in his care and in the management of external fixator.

Maintaining intact neurovascular status

1. See neurovascular compromise, p. 798.
2. Establish baseline of functioning for comparative monitoring. Complex musculoskeletal injuries frequently result in disruption of soft tissue functioning.

NURSING ALERT
Assess neurovascular status frequently and record findings.

3. Elevate extremity in balanced suspension traction to reduce swelling.
   a. Extremity can be suspended by hanging the fixator directly to the traction frame.
   b. Suspension is for control of oedema and not for application of traction force.
4. Notify doctor of change in neurovascular status.

Avoiding infection

1. Pin site and fixator care:
   a. Cleanse pin sites and remove crusts with sterile cotton applicator dipped in hydrogen peroxide or as directed two or three times daily – crusts formed by serous drainage can prevent fluid from draining and cause infection.
   b. Apply nonocclusive antibiotic agent around pin sites as directed.
   c. Wipe off fixator with sterile cloth dampened with sterile water.
   d. Avoid short cuts. Meticulous technique is important.
2. Wound care:
   a. The open wounds at the fracture site are usually treated by daily dressing changes.
   b. Use sterile technique.
   c. Change dressings around pins first and those underneath fixator rods last.
3. Monitor for local and systemic indicators of infection.

Promoting self-care activities

1. Encourage the patient to participate in care activities. Patient may become the 'authority' for routine care activities (e.g. pin care).
2. Assure the patient that pain associated with injury will diminish as tissue reactions to injury and manipulation resolve and healing progresses.
3. Inform the patient that the external fixator maintains the fracture in a very stable position and that the extremity can be moved. Adjustment of the fixator is done by the surgeon.
4. To move the extremity, grasp the frame and assist the patient to move. Reassure the patient that the fixator can withstand normal movement.
5. Quadriceps exercises and range-of-motion for joints are usually started on first postoperative day.
6. Patient ambulates on crutches when soft tissue swelling has diminished; weight-bearing is done only as prescribed.

PATIENT EDUCATION

1. Inspect around each pin site daily for signs of infection and loosening of pins. Watch for pain, soft tissue swelling and drainage.
2. Cleanse around each pin tract daily, using aseptic technique. *Do not touch wound with hands.*
3. Clean fixator regularly – to keep it free of dust and contamination.
4. *Do not tamper with clamps or nuts* – can alter compression and misalign fracture.

5. Review weight-bearing and other restrictions associated with injury and treatment regimen.
6. Encourage the patient to follow rehabilitation regimen.

Evaluation
EXPECTED OUTCOMES

1. Overcomes any anxiety about the external fixation device – does not appear worried about it; handles and cares for equipment with ease.
2. Maintains normal neurovascular functioning – normal sensations, movement, circulation and tissue perfusion.
3. Shows no signs of infection at pin sites or at site of open injury – no inflammation at pin site; tissue not overly tender; healing progresses as anticipated; no temperature rise or other systemic signs of infection.
4. Performs activities of daily living within limits of restrictions and uses ambulatory aids safely.

INTERNAL FIXATION DEVICE

GENERAL CONSIDERATIONS

1. Some fractures may be reduced under anaesthesia and stabilized with the surgical implantation of metal nails, nail–plate combinations, compression screw devices and intramedullary nails.
2. Surgical procedure is usually carried out as soon as possible after full medical assessment.
3. Surgical fixation of a fracture permits early mobilization of the patient thereby decreasing the adverse effects of immobilization. The metal hardware is not strong enough to permit full function of the extremity, but does facilitate maintenance of muscle strength, joint mobility and development of bony union.

Assessment

1. Carry out neurovascular check of affected extremity.
2. Monitor drainage from portable suction.

PATIENT PROBLEMS

1. Potential for injury from dislocation or loosening of fixation device related to malalignment and adverse stresses.
2. Impaired mobility related to injury and presence of fixation device.

3. Potential complications (constipation, contractures, neurovascular and respiratory problems) related to immobility.
4. Ineffective coping related to the limitations imposed by the treatment.

Planning and implementation
NURSING INTERVENTIONS
For hip fracture treated with internal fixation.

Maintaining proper alignment of extremity
1. Position affected leg as directed – usually on a pillow with mild abduction.
2. Place pillow between legs – to maintain alignment.
3. Using two persons, gently place the patient onto affected side; when lying on unoperated side, keep the affected extremity in position of abduction.

Achieving ambulation as soon as possible
1. Wrap the lower extremities with elastic compression bandages or elastic hose – increases venous velocity in legs and helps minimize dependent oedema.
2. Assist the patient into a wheelchair several times daily as prescribed – helps avoid arterial hypotension, helps maintain strength, aids pulmonary function and is beneficial psychologically.
   a. With the aid of the overhead trapeze (monkey pole) encourage the patient to move into sitting position. (Use a variable height bed.)
   b. Assist the patient to stand on the *unaffected extremity* and transfer to the chair.
   c. If weight-bearing is permitted, the patient may be encouraged to ambulate with frame, applying as much weight to extremity as is comfortable.
   d. Certain types of fractures must be supported and protected until bone union is secure and displacement of fractures unlikely. If this is the case, the patient may have to be lifted into the chair.
   e. Allow the patient to get up at his own pace; avoid hurrying.
3. Encourage the patient to participate in activities of daily living (eating, bathing, hair care) – to condition the patient for future ambulation activities and to help maintain a degree of independence.

Promoting active exercises
1. Encourage quadriceps-setting exercises hourly – the quadriceps femoris muscle extends the leg and is one of the major muscles necessary for ambulation.

2. Do heel-cord stretching of both legs and abdominal and gluteal contractions (isometric contractions). Isometric muscle contractions strengthen the muscle but do not move the joint.
3. Avoid knee contractures.
   a. Maintain the knee in a position of extension while the patient is in bed.
   b. Flex the knee in a 90° angle while the patient is in the chair. Avoid extending the knee for long periods when the patient is in a sitting position because extension produces undue strain on the fractured hip.
   c. Move the knee through assisted range-of-motion exercises.
4. Assist the patient to perform arm strengthening exercises (flexion and extension of the arms). The muscles in the shoulder girdle and upper extremities must be strong enough to bear the patient's weight while she is using the walker.
5. Assist the patient to learn to use the walker – ambulating with a non–weight-bearing (or partial weight-bearing depending on the fracture and its fixation) technique.
6. Remind the patient *not* to bear weight on the affected extremity until the surgeon gives permission and the X-rays reveal sufficient healing. Early weight-bearing before bony union occurs exerts too much stress and may cause bending or breaking of the pin, crushing of the bone, or loss of fixation due to the device cutting through the bone.

Evaluation
EXPECTED OUTCOMES
1. Maintains alignment – bony fusion occurs.
2. Transfers from bed with ease; out of bed in chair that provides good support several times a day.
3. Participates in active exercises and mobility activities; does prescribed exercises and uses ambulatory aids safely.

FRACTURES OF SPECIFIC SITES*

FRACTURE OF THE CLAVICLE (COLLAR BONE)

1. The clavicle helps to hold the shoulder upwards, outwards and backwards from the thorax.

---

* For fracture of the skull see p. 926.

2. Aim of reduction: to hold the shoulder in the position described above.
3. Most fractures of the clavicle are treated by closed reduction and immobilization accomplished by one of the following methods:
   a. Clavicular strap. (Pad axilla to prevent nerve damage from pressure.)
   b. Sling.
   c. Figure-8 bandage. Watch for tingling in hands; too tight a clavicular strap or figure-8 bandage may cause circulatory impairment.
4. Open reduction and internal fixation may be done for marked displacement and angulation of bone ends.
   a. Following surgery the patient's arm is kept in a sling.
   b. Caution patient not to elevate his arm above shoulder level until the facture has united; will impede healing of fracture.

PATIENT EDUCATION
1. Exercise elbow, wrist and fingers as soon as possible.

2. Do shoulder exercises to obtain full shoulder movement as prescribed (Figure 13.7).

FRACTURES OF THE UPPER LIMB

FRACTURES OF THE SURGICAL NECK OF THE HUMERUS (FRACTURES OF THE PROXIMAL HUMERUS)

1. Most occur from falls in which the outstretched arm strikes the ground (impacted fracture). Osteoporosis is a predisposing factor.
2. The majority of impacted fractures of the surgical neck of the humerus do not require reduction. The weight of the arm helps to correct displacement.

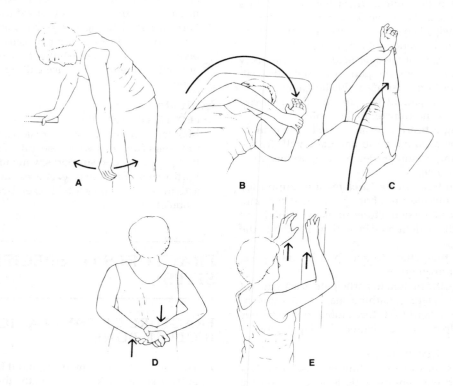

Figure 13.7. Exercises to develop range of movement of shoulder. (A) Pendulum exercise. (B) External rotation. (C) Elevation. (D) Internal rotation. In all of these, the unaffected arm is used for power. (E) Wall climbing

a. Place a soft pad under the axilla to prevent skin maceration.
b. The arm is supported by a sling bandage for comfort (Figure 13.8).
c. Advise the patient that he will sleep more comfortably when supported in an upright position.
3. Displaced fractures are treated with reduction under X-ray control, open reduction or replacement of humeral head with prosthesis.
   a. A programme of exercises is usually started four days postoperatively with emphasis on range of motion of the shoulder (see Figure 13.7).
   b. Watch for postoperative infection, a common sequela of surgery on shoulder.

PATIENT EDUCATION
Objective
Restore shoulder function and prevent adhesions.
1. Start active motion of shoulder joint early – to prevent limitation of motion and stiffness of shoulder.
2. Instruct patient to lean forward and allow affected arm to abduct and rotate (*termed pendulum exercise*) (see Figure 13.7a).

FRACTURES OF THE SHAFT OF THE HUMERUS

1. Fractures of the shaft of the humerus are most frequently caused by direct violence – falls, blows to arm, road traffic injuries.
2. Most fractures at this site can be treated nonoperatively.
3. Hanging cast is frequently applied to oblique, spiral and displaced fractures with shortening of humeral shaft.

NURSING ALERT
A hanging cast for treatment of fracture of the shaft of the humerus must be dependent (remain unsupported) to provide a traction force. Continuous traction on long axis of arm is effected by the weight of the cast. The patient must avoid supporting the elbow in the lap while seated.

4. See that the patient sleeps in a fairly upright position to maintain uninterrupted 24-hour traction.
5. Exercise fingers immediately after the application of the cast.
6. Start pendulum exercises as directed – provides active exercise of shoulder to prevent adhesions

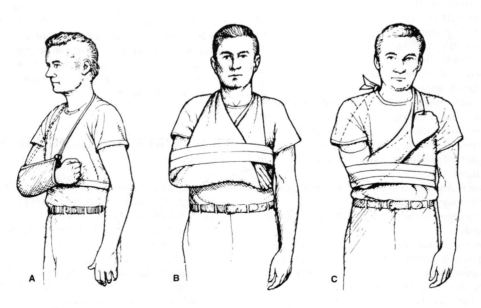

Figure 13.8. The types of immobilizing dressing used for upper humeral fractures. (A) A commercial sling which permits easy removal of the arm for exercises and is comfortable on the neck. (B) A conventional sling and bandage. (C) A stockinette Velpeau and bandage used when there is an unstable surgical neck component, because this position relaxes the pectoralis major. This is not generally available in the UK (from Rockwood, C. A. and Green, D. P. (1975) *Fractures*, J. B. Lippincott, Philadelphia)

of the shoulder joint capsule after cast removal (Figure 13.7a).

7. Open reduction and internal fixation (usually by compression plate) are performed when satisfactory alignment cannot be obtained with closed treatment, when there is associated vascular injury, and when the fracture is the result of a pathological (malignant) lesion. Internal fixation is often supplemented by methyl methacrylate (bone cement). Following a surgical procedure, the arm is placed in a sling and bandaged until bone union has taken place at the fracture site.

8. The radial nerve may be injured in this fracture because it lies immediately adjacent to the midportion of the humerus in the musculoskeletal groove.

SUPRACONDYLAR FRACTURE (ABOVE THE ELBOW)

1. This fracture is close to the median nerve and brachial artery. An injury to the brachial artery, may produce ischaemia in the flexor forearm muscles and, consequently, Volkmann's ischaemia contracture.

2. Treatment of this type of fracture varies:
   a. Alignment corrected by manipulation under general or regional anaesthesia. Fragments are usually maintained by holding elbow in an acutely flexed position after reduction. (Degree of elbow flexion is determined by amplitude of pulse.)
   b. For more severe injuries Dunlop's traction is used. The forearm is held in suspension. These methods maintain traction, keep the fracture reduced, decrease oedema and aid circulation (reduces risk of Volkmann's contracture).
   c. Open reduction and pin and screw fixation in adults may be required.

3. Watch for signs of impaired circulation in forearm and hand.
   a. Observe hand for swelling or blueness of fingernails; compare with unaffected hand.
   b. Evaluate radial pulse; if it weakens or disappears, call orthopaedic surgeon *immediately* since irreversible ischaemia may develop.

4. Assess for paraesthesia (tingling and burning sensations) in the hand – indicates nerve injury or impending ischaemia.

5. Encourage patient to move his fingers frequently.

FRACTURES AND DISLOCATIONS ABOUT THE ELBOW

1. Usually occur from direct fall on elbow or on outstretched hand with elbow in flexion. May be undisplaced or displaced (avulsion; oblique and transverse fractures; comminuted fracture; or fracture-dislocation).

2. *Undisplaced fracture* – treated by short period of immobilization in a cast with elbow in 45–90° flexion or supported with a sling and pressure dressing to the elbow.

3. *Displaced fracture* – usually treated by open reduction and internal fixation or primary excision of the proximal fragment(s).

4. Watch for signs of impaired circulation in forearm and hand. Assess for local nerve damage from injury to the median, radial or ulnar nerves.

5. Range-of-movement exercises started upon order; flexion past 90° is avoided until bone healing is demonstrated by X-ray.

NURSING ALERT
Guard against Volkmann's contracture – a severe fibrosis with resulting contracture of muscles which have become ischaemic by obstruction of the arterial flow to the forearm and hand. This complication is prevented by proper care; if allowed to develop, the results are disastrous. Following supracondylar fracture of humerus, the nurse should undertake half-hourly checks on radial pulse.

FRACTURES OF THE HEAD OF THE RADIUS

1. Usually produced by indirect trauma (fall on outstretched hand) or by direct trauma (blow).

2. *Undisplaced fracture:*
   a. Aspiration of haemarthrosis (blood in joint) at the elbow may be done to relieve pain and allow earlier range of motion.
   b. Immobilization by plaster slab or sling.

3. *Displaced fracture* – open operation with excision of radial head when indicated.
   a. Postoperatively the arm is immobilized in a posterior plaster splint and sling.
   b. Early active motion of elbow and forearm is encouraged when plaster splint is removed.

PATIENT EDUCATION

1. Encourage patient to continue *daily* programme of repetitive, progressive exercises (as prescribed). The exercise programme is designed to restore full extension and supination.
2. Instruct the patient to avoid lifting heavy objects for six weeks after sling has been discontinued.

FRACTURES OF THE SHAFTS OF RADIUS AND ULNA

1. Objective of treatment is to preserve function of forearm.
2. *Undisplaced fractures* – treated by immobilizing arm in an above elbow cast with elbow flexed 90°.
   a. Watch circulation and function of hand.
   b. Encourage active flexion and extension of fingers at frequent intervals to reduce oedema. Encourage shoulder motion.
3. *Displaced fractures* – internal fixation accomplished by compression plate or some other fixation device.
   a. Postoperatively, a closed drainage system may be used to decrease haematoma and resultant swelling.
   b. The arm is usually immobilized in plaster splints or cast until there is evidence that fracture is healing.

PATIENT EDUCATION

Encourage patient to move his fingers and the shoulder of the involved limb.

FRACTURE OF THE WRIST

1. Colles' fracture is a fracture of the radius 1.2–2.5cm above the wrist with dorsal displacement of the lower fragment.
2. Treatment usually consists of closed reduction and plaster of Paris splint or cast support.
   a. Elevate arm above level of heart for 48 hours after reduction.
   b. Watch for swelling of fingers – indicates decreased venous and lymphatic return. Check for constricting bandages or cast.
   c. Instruct patient to do finger exercises to reduce swelling and prevent stiffness.
      (i) Hold hand above level of heart.
      (ii) Move fingers from full extension to flexion (claw position). Hold to a count of two or more.
      (iii) Repeat at least ten times every half-hour

while awake – as long as hand has a tendency to swell.

FRACTURES OF THE HAND

1. Numerous injuries to the hand require extensive reconstructive surgery which is beyond the scope of this book. The reader is referred to specialized texts on the hand.
2. Objective of treatment is to regain maximum function of the hand.
3. *Undisplaced fracture of the distal phalanx:*
   a. Drainage of the haematoma under the fingernail may be necessary.
   b. Finger is splinted (to adjoining finger or by a dorsal or volar splint) – to relieve pain and to protect finger tip from further trauma.
4. *Open fractures* may be handled by Kirschner wire fixation following debridement and irrigation.

NURSING ALERT
Ensure that when splinting two fingers together, padding is inserted between each finger to prevent skin maceration.

FRACTURES OF THE LOWER LIMB

OBJECTIVES
Obtain adequate bony union with full length and normal alignment and without rotational or angular deformity.
Restore muscle power and joint motion.

FRACTURE OF THE SHAFT OF THE FEMUR

NURSING ALERT
Fracture of the shaft of the femur may be accompanied by marked, concealed blood loss.

1. Closed reduction:
   a. Fracture reduced and stabilized by means of balanced skeletal traction, using a Thomas splint with a Pearson knee flexion piece attachment (Figure 13.9).

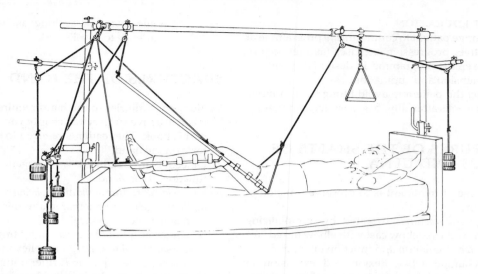

Figure 13.9. Balanced traction with Thomas leg splint with Pearson attachment

b. Thomas splint suspends the thigh; Pearson knee flexion piece attachment allows knee flexion and supports the leg below the knee.
c. Examine skin under the ring on Thomas splint.
d. Passive and active motion of knee joint may be ordered.
e. May be replaced with cast-brace (for fractures of shaft of the femur) – after two to four weeks of traction.
2. Open reduction with intramedullary (within the bone) fixation.
a. See nursing management following orthopaedic surgery (p. 834).
b. Observe for complications: postoperative infection, osteomyelitis.
c. Or a cast-brace may be used in conjunction with internal fixation of fractured femur.

4. *Treatment* (broad range of opinion on treatment of these fractures):
a. May be managed by simple manipulation and the reduction maintained by application of plaster cast (toe to groin; see Figure 13.2).
  (i) In time this long-leg cast may be replaced with a below-the-knee functional cast which permits weight-bearing and knee joint motion.
  (ii) As an alternative, a functional cast-brace (fabricated with orthoplast-like material and special hinges) may be used (Figure 13.10).
b. Or fracture may be treated by open reduction and early fixation (plate, compression plate, intramedullary nails, or other devices, or Hoffman external fixator) as indicated by aetiology, type of trauma and type of fracture.

FRACTURES OF THE TIBIA AND FIBULA

1. Treatment of tibial fractures represents a challenge; there is a high incidence of open infected fractures since the tibia lies superficially beneath the skin.
2. These fractures may require prolonged immobilization – union is slow because there is often poor blood supply to the distal part of the tibia.
3. Tibial fractures generally heal in 12 to 16 weeks; compound and comminuted fractures take longer.

FRACTURES AT THE KNEE

Fractures at the knee may involve the distal shaft of femur (supracondylar fracture), the articular surfaces (femoral condyles and/or tibial plateau fracture), or the patella. Joint and ligamentous injury occur with these fractures.

MANAGEMENT
Management may include traction, internal fixation and/or immobilization.
Knee mobility is a concern in the overall treatment of these fractures.

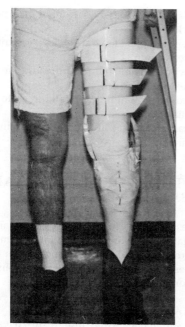

Figure 13.10. Cast-brace provides circumferential support to a segment of a fractured limb, while allowing mobility of nearby joints

NURSING MANAGEMENT

1. Elevate extremity; raise the foot of the bed.
2. Evaluate for effusion of the knee – produces marked pain.
   a. Remove pressure dressing and reapply if pain is severe. Report to doctor.
   b. Support the patient undergoing aspiration of fluid from knee joint.
3. Encourage quadriceps exercise to prevent atrophy of the thigh muscles; this also includes the unoperated leg.
4. Progressive exercises (straight leg raising, progressive resistive exercises) usually follow.
5. Weight-bearing is according to prescription. (Generally, full weight-bearing is not advised until three to four months postinjury.)

FRACTURES OF THE ANKLE

1. Fracture may occur in the distal tibia and/or fibula, medial or lateral malleoli, or superior talus, and include avulsion fracture. The fracture is generally the result of forceful twisting of the ankle and is associated with ligament disruption.
2. Treatment includes immobilization and possible open reduction and internal fixation with screws

to re-establish joint function. Weight-bearing is according to prescription.

FRACTURES OF THE FOOT

Fractures of the metatarsals and phalanges result from crush injuries of the foot. They are generally treated by immobilization with cast, splint or strapping. Partial weight-bearing is generally allowed.

REHABILITATION AFTER FRACTURE OF THE LOWER LIMB

1. Apply elastic stocking to uninvolved leg – maintains pressure on deeper leg veins, helps prevent stasis of blood, oedema and thrombophlebitis (deep vein thrombosis).
2. Elevate unaffected leg at intervals throughout day – to promote venous return.
3. Elevate affected limb to promote venous return and relieve pain.
   a. The early re-establishment of venous return helps absorb blood and tissue fluid (oedema from bleeding is a common cause of disability following fractures).
   b. Chronic oedema predisposes limb to fibrosis and ulceration.
4. Exercise as much as possible – promotes bone healing.
5. Avoid placing limb in dependent positions for prolonged periods.
6. Mobilize the patient as soon as possible. Instruct in methods of ambulation – frame, crutches and stick.
7. Physiotherapy procedures may be utilized after cast removal (heat, cold, massage, exercise) – to restore joint mobility, increase muscle strength and endurance.
8. Instruct patient to wear elastic bandage after cast is removed to support venous circulation.
9. Advise patient to move feet up and down in pedalling motion to exercise calf muscles.
10. Recommend that patient start moving affected limb under water if necessary, since water supports the limb and provides warmth, which helps promote muscle relaxation.

CAST-BRACING

A *cast-brace* (fracture-orthosis) consists of two separate weight-bearing casts (patellar weight-bearing cast on lower leg and ischial weight-bearing cast on thigh) which are joined at the knee by a pair of gliding-action hinges (see Figure 13.10). The foot and ankle joint may be included in the cast and a walking heel or boot applied; or the foot and ankle joint may be freed by a removable shoe attached to the cast by a brace joint.

The cast may be of plaster of Paris or the newer splintage materials, e.g. Bay Cast.

RATIONALE
Cast-bracing is based on the concept that weight-bearing will promote osteogenesis (bone formation).

PURPOSES AND ADVANTAGES
1. Allows motion of joints.
2. Permits progressive weight bearing.
3. Allows gradually increasing skeletal stresses and promotes fracture healing by transmission of forces through the bone.
4. Allows early return to walking (promotes patient independence).
5. Allows earlier hospital discharge.
6. Lessens detrimental effect on body physiology by shortening the period of recumbency – earlier return of bladder and bowel function, less chance of renal calculi, etc.

CLINICAL INDICATIONS
Fractures of tibia and of femoral shaft; supracondylar fractures of the femur (open or closed).
1. Tibial fracture – functional below-knee walking brace may be applied two to three weeks after fracture.
2. Femoral fracture – long leg cast-brace may be applied three to five weeks after patient has been in traction.
3. Cast-brace – applied after initial oedema has subsided and there is evidence of fracture stability.

NURSING MANAGEMENT
1. The patient may be permitted to get up 24 to 48 hours after cast is applied.
   a. As much weight is borne on affected extremity as can be tolerated.
   b. Be sure patient uses proper crutch gait (three-point gait) so that normal gait and rhythm are established.
2. Advise patient that he should be closely monitored.
   a. Angular deformity may occur during first weeks of weight-bearing.
   b. Standing weight-bearing anteroposterior and lateral X-rays are taken at intervals.
3. Watch for skin breakdown and circulatory problems.

   a. Watch for excessive swelling of exposed area of knee.
   b. Report signs of skin discoloration, numbness, breakdown.
4. Protect cast from soiling (urine and faeces) – cast may extend to groin.
5. Elevate cast when not walking – to promote venous return.
6. The cast is changed at intervals until clinical union is achieved.

FRACTURES OF THE LUMBAR AND DORSAL SPINE

Fractures of the vertebrae of the dorsal and lumbar spine may involve the vertebral body, lamina articulating processes and spinous processes or transverse processes. (Fractures of the cervical spine are discussed on p. 958.)

CLINICAL FEATURES
Severe pain in back – may radiate down legs or to the abdomen and chest.

PATHOPHYSIOLOGY
1. Fractures of the vertebral bodies may be compression fractures; they are frequently multiple and comprise the most common types of fractures of the spine.
2. A spinal cord injury may occur with fracture or dislocation of a vertebra.

AETIOLOGY
1. Indirect trauma associated with excessive loading, motion beyond physiological limits, severe muscle spasm.
2. The majority of vertebral fractures seem to be related to osteoporosis.

TREATMENT AND NURSING MANAGEMENT
Objective
Determine if there is injury to the spinal cord.
1. Assess and treat the patient for spinal cord injury.
2. Evaluate for paralytic ileus and difficulty in micturition – may occur the first few days after compression fracture of the lower dorsal or lumbar spine – may be from retroperitoneal haemorrhage.
3. Use measures to prevent risk of deep vein thrombosis complications – elevate foot of bed, apply elastic stockings, encourage active ankle motion; high risk patients may be given anticoagulant therapy.

TREATMENT
For stable injuries to vertebrae
1. Treat symptomatically for pain and encourage patient to mobilize – *or*
2. Place patient on a firm mattress and keep on bed rest until pain subsides.
   a. Encourage patient to roll from side to side; patient should not sit up during acute stage.
   b. Give analgesics and muscle relaxants as required since pain may be severe.
   c. Patient is permitted to walk with assistance (wearing shoes) when discomfort subsides.
   d. Encourage patient to do the prescribed back exercises – to increase or maintain the strength of back muscles (two to three weeks after fracture).
      (i) Exercises are prescribed that strengthen spinal extensor muscles.
      (ii) Exercises that encourage spinal flexion are contraindicated.
   e. Patient may feel better with a corset-type brace or back support when he is mobilizing; remove appliance while in bed.
   f. Patient with a more severe injury may require a more substantial back brace or cast.

For unstable fractures/displacement
1. The fracture may be reduced by postural positioning, protracted periods of immobilization, or open operation with internal fixation.
2. The patient may then be placed in a body cast for immobilization.
3. Mobilize the patient when physical examinations and X-ray evaluations determine that there is no displacement or neurological deficit.
4. Laminectomy (see p. 964) when indicated.

Assessment
1. Assess the patient for spinal cord injury (see p. 958).
2. Evaluate for paralytic ileus and difficulty in voiding – may occur the first few days after compression fracture of the lower dorsal or lumbar spine – may be from retroperitoneal haemorrhage.
   a. Assess anal sphincter tone.
   b. Observe for faecal retention.
3. Assess discomfort.

PATIENT PROBLEMS
1. Potential spinal cord injury related to fracture and/or vertebral displacement (rarely occurs with compression fractures related to osteoporosis).
2. Pain related to vertebral fracture and associated muscle spasm.
3. Potential complications related to fracture of spine and immobility.
4. Impaired mobility related to pain of fracture.
5. Constipation related to effects of pain medication, immobility and paralytic ileus.
6. Ineffective coping related to enforced immobility and inability to carry out activities of daily living.
7. Nausea, vomiting related to pain medication and possibly paralytic ileus.

Planning and implementation
NURSING INTERVENTIONS
Avoiding spinal cord injury
1. Stabilize spine during diagnostic evaluation for fracture and displacement.
2. Monitor neurological status (i.e. motion and sensations in extremities).
3. Provide nursing care according to the patient's condition and treatment regimen (e.g. laminectomy and fusion, internal fixation, casting).

Relieving pain
1. Encourage the patient to roll from side to side; the patient should not sit up during acute stage.
2. Give analgesics and muscle relaxants as required, since pain may be severe.
3. Assist the patient in application of brace or back support when he is ambulating; remove appliance while in bed.

Avoiding complications associated with spinal fracture and immobility
1. Use measures to prevent risk of thromboembolic complications – apply elastic stockings, encourage active ankle movement, given anticoagulant therapy as prescribed for patient at high risk.
2. Assist the patient to ambulate (wearing shoes) when discomfort subsides and when no neurological deficits or vertebral displacement has been determined.
3. Encourage the patient to do the prescribed back exercises.
4. Monitor bowel and bladder function.

PATIENT EDUCATION
1. Teach body mechanics for back conservation.
2. Encourage weight reduction, if applicable.
3. With fractures due to osteoporosis, teach the patient to be aware of safety factors necessary to avoid falls.

Evaluation
EXPECTED OUTCOMES
1. Patient demonstrates normal neurological func-

tion; normal sensations, motion, and strength in extremities.
2. Patient achieves pain relief.
3. Patient performs activities of daily living without complaint of pain and decreases use of analgesics.
4. Patient maintains homeostasis; no evidence of paralytic ileus, urinary stasis, constipation.

FRACTURES OF THE PELVIS

AETIOLOGY
Road traffic accidents, crush injuries and falls cause most pelvic fractures. Injury to internal organs (i.e. bladder, urethra, liver, spleen) and blood vessels (e.g. iliac arteries and veins) frequently accompany these fractures. Bleeding from bone fragments occurs also.

TREATMENT
1. Emergency management of haemorrhage and shock includes:
   a. External compression suit (G-suit) allows compression of pelvic area – provides tamponade for bleeding and immobilizes fracture. Rarely used in UK.
   b. Angiographic visualization of pelvic vascular tree – for localization of bleeding points. Bleeding artery may be occluded by an injection of autologous clotted blood deposited proximal to bleeding vessel or by balloon-tip catheter.
   c. Absence of peripheral pulses may indicate major vessel disruption (torn iliac arteries, veins, etc).
2. Existence of internal organ injury is determined and treated according to problem (e.g. ruptured bladder requires ·surgical intervention and repair).
   a. Urine is examined for blood. A cystourethrogram and intravenous urogram are performed – to detect genitourinary injuries.
3. Definitive treatment of pelvic fractures:
   a. Method of treatment depends on whether the pelvic ring has been disrupted and whether the fracture involves the weight-bearing portion of the pelvis.
   b. Pelvic fractures may be immobilized and stabilized by:
      (i) Bed rest.
      (ii) Pelvic slings.
      (iii) Skeletal traction.
      (iv) Bilateral hip spica cast.
      (v) External fixation.
      (vi) Open reduction with or without internal fixation.

Assessment
1. Determine the extent of internal injuries.
2. Palpate peripheral pulses.
3. Assess and evaluate for intra-abdominal haemorrhage – pelvic fractures may cause death from extraperitoneal and retroperitoneal haemorrhage.
4. Monitor stools and urine for blood.
5. Assess discomfort on movement and tenderness at fracture site.
6. Evaluate for other complications that are likely to develop as a result of shock, massive soft tissue injury and multiple fractures – intravascular coagulation, thromboembolic complications, fat emboli, pulmonary complications, infection from large haematomas.

PATIENT PROBLEMS
1. Potential life-threatening shock related to intra-abdominal haemorrhage and organ damage.
2. Discomfort related to fracture and soft tissue trauma.
3. Impaired mobility related to pelvic fracture and treatment regimen.
4. Coping difficulties related to limited mobility.

Planning and implementation
NURSING INTERVENTIONS
Promoting adequate tissue perfusion
1. Monitor vital signs and level of consciousness.
2. Interpret laboratory data.
3. Support vital functions as needed and prescribed.

Ensuring abdominal organ functioning
1. Monitor urine output for blood.
2. Monitor bowel function.
3. Assist the patient with therapeutic regimen prescribed for management of injury.

Relieving discomfort
See pain (alteration in comfort) related to musculoskeletal conditions, p. 797.

Promoting ambulation and activities of daily living
1. Assist the patient being treated with pelvic sling.
   a. Fold sling back over buttocks to enable the patient to use the bedpan.
   b. Reach under sling to give skin care – sheepskin

may be used to line sling to prevent pressure sores.

   c. Loosen the sling only upon doctor's request.

2. Turn the patient as a unit.
3. Encourage exercises (e.g. leg, breathing, isometric) and activities to minimize development of immobility-related problems.
4. Assist the patient with gradual resumption of activity and ambulation. Mobilization and weight-bearing are determined by X-ray and the patient's reaction to mobility.

Evaluation
EXPECTED OUTCOMES
1. Patient maintains vital functions; vital signs stable, no evidence of bleeding, and normal bowel and bladder functioning.
2. Patient achieves comfort; decreased use of analgesics and no complaint of pain.
3. Patient achieves improved mobility; ambulates with assistance and uses walking stick or frame as needed.

FRACTURES OF THE HIP

TYPES OF HIP FRACTURE
Intracapsular – femur is fractured inside the joint (femoral neck fracture)

   Extracapsular – femur fractured outside the joint (intertrochanteric fracture)

AETIOLOGY
Hip fractures frequently occur in the aged and contribute to their mortality. They occur more frequently in women, often after insignificant injuries, and are associated with osteoporosis.

TREATMENT
1. Stable fractures are usually reduced and fixed with a nail, nail-plate combination, multiple pins, screw, sliding nails, etc, by replacement of the femoral head or by a total hip arthroplasty.
2. To ensure that the patient is in as favourable a condition as possible preoperatively:
   a. Assess cardiovascular, pulmonary, renal and haematological systems.
   b. Correct fluid and electrolyte disturbances. Give intravenous infusions *slowly* – older patients with limited cardiac reserve cannot tolerate additional circulatory loading.
   c. Prevent complications (e.g. thrombophlebitis, pneumonia, fat emboli, infection, pressure sores).

Assessment
PREOPERATIVE
1. Note position of injured extremity – shortening and external rotation of affected leg.
2. Assess ability to move leg – usually unable to move leg but able to wiggle toes.
3. Assess pain – patients with fractured hip may complain of discomfort in the knee.
4. Coordinate preoperative diagnostic studies.
5. Determine if the patient is oriented to time, place and person – mental confusion may be due to underlying systemic illness, particularly to cardiopulmonary disease with inadequate cerebral oxygen transport, stroke, etc.
6. Evaluate needs for posthospital care. Notify Social Services Department – to assist planning of postoperative care to avoid unnecessary prolonged hospital care.

PATIENT PROBLEMS
1. Impaired mobility related to fracture.
2. Alteration in comfort related to fracture.
3. Knowledge deficit related to treatment regimen and expected patient participation.

Planning and implementation
NURSING INTERVENTIONS
Avoiding problems associated with immobility and fracture
1. Use anticipatory nursing techniques to avoid complications.

NURSING ALERT
Thromboembolism is the most common complication following hip fractures, and it frequently occurs without clinical signs.

   a. Prevent thromboembolism with leg exercises, elastic stockings, early ambulation.
   b. Warfarin, low-molecular-weight dextran, aspirin, or low doses of heparin given subcutaneously may be effective in reducing the incidence of venous thrombi.
   c. Elevate foot of bed 25° – to promote venous drainage.
   d. Use orienting activities to prevent confusion – clock, calendar, television, explanations and reassurance, same care-giver. (See p. 1061 for care of the confused older patient.)
   e. Prepare the bed with a monkey pole and flotation mattress.
2. Keep the skin dry and relieve pressure areas – pressure sores develop rapidly in the preopera-

tive period. (See p. 30 for prevention of pressure sores.)

  a. Check the neurovascular status of the extremity.

  b. Inspect the heel *daily* – a patient with a painful hip tends to let weight of leg press the heel against the bed; area loses sensation when blood supply diminishes and nerve endings necrose.

  c. Support leg with pillow if permitted – distributes pressure more evenly.

  d. Place a sheepskin pad under the leg.

3. Encourage the patient to move by himself as much as possible to decrease the likelihood of complications (thromboembolism, diminished cerebral perfusion, aspiration of secretions and pneumonia, gastrointestinal stasis, urinary problems, increase in bone mineral loss, pressure sores).

4. Prevent urinary tract infection.

  a. Avoid the routine use of an indwelling catheter – infection almost always follows the use of an indwelling catheter. (A urinary tract infection can cause a prolonged period of morbidity, incontinence, and confusion in the elderly.)

  b. Watch the colour, odour and volume of urinary output.

  c. Maintain a liberal fluid intake (within limits of cardiorenal function).

Promoting comfort

1. Alleviate pain.

  a. Place a pillow between the legs – to keep affected leg in a secure position.

  b. With two nurses positioned at each side of the bed, use the sheet under the patient and lift the patient off the stretcher onto the bed.

  c. Turn the patient on the affected side while supporting the shoulder and thigh, and remove the sheet.

  d. Position the patient supine. Place a pillow under the affected leg from mid-thigh to ankle and a sandbag under the pillow on the side of the patient's affected calf.

  e. Raise the head of the bed slightly, no higher than 40°.

  f. The patient may be treated with either Buck's extension or pillow positioning.

    (i) Assist with the application of Buck's extension as indicated. Buck's extension is used to afford patient mobilization and to relieve pain until the operative procedure

is performed. (Hamilton–Russell's traction may be used.)

    (ii) Check traction frequently, especially elastic bandages.

    (iii) The patient with an intracapsular fracture will assume a flexed and externally rotated position. Support extremity in this position with pillows until surgery is performed.

  g. Handle the affected extremity gently.

  h. Give analgesics as the patient's condition indicates.

2. Watch for fat embolism – characterized by fever, tachycardia, dyspnoea, and cough. (Fat embolism sometimes occurs after fractures of the long bones, particularly in elderly patients.)

PATIENT EDUCATION

1. Teach the patient to assist with turning by having her grasp the monkey pole or bedrails.

2. Encourage the patient to take deep breaths while turning.

3. Teach the use of incentive spirometer, coughing, deep-breathing and exercises, especially quadriceps setting.

4. Clarify treatment plans and discuss the patient's participation.

Evaluation

EXPECTED OUTCOMES

1. Patient shows no signs of problems related to immobility; lungs clear, skin intact, urine clear and adequate in amount.

2. Patient achieves comfort; minimal complaint of discomfort at fracture; maintains positioning.

3. Patient can explain planned treatment and participation regimen; follows directions to facilitate treatment and to prevent complications.

ORTHOPAEDIC SURGERY

SPECIAL NURSING CONSIDERATIONS

Assessment

PREOPERATIVE NURSING MANAGEMENT

1. Carry out normal assessment standards for a person undergoing surgery (see p. 45).

2. Assess nutritional status. Ensure adequate protein and calorie intake.

3. Question the patient to determine whether he has had previous therapy with corticosteroids (especially with patients with arthritis).
   a. Steroid therapy (current or past) may adversely affect the patient's response to anaesthesia.
   b. Steroids should be administered per request to cover stress of surgery.

Patient education
1. Teach patients about the following: tests and routines, coughing and deep-breathing, and immediate postoperative activities.
2. Have the patient practice voiding in bedpan or urinal in recumbent position before surgery. This helps reduce the need for postoperative catheterization.
3. Acquaint the patient with traction apparatus and the need for splints and casts – to familiarize him with postoperative environment.

POSTOPERATIVE ASSESSMENT
Immediate postoperative period
1. Evaluate the blood pressure and pulse rates frequently – rising pulse rate or slowly falling blood pressure indicates persistent bleeding or development of a state of shock.
2. Assess changes in respiratory rate or in the patient's colour – may indicate obstruction of respiratory exchange or pulmonary or cardiac complications.
3. Carry out neurovascular checks (nerve function and circulation) of affected extremity. Watch circulation distal to the part where cast, bandage or splint has been applied.
   a. Prevent constriction leading to interference with blood or nerve supply.
   b. Watch toes and fingers for healthy colour.
   c. Check pulses of affected extremity; compare with unaffected extremity.
   d. Note skin temperature – raised skin temperature may indicate bleeding or infection.

NURSING ALERT
Abnormal coolness of skin, cyanosis, rubor or pallor indicates interference with circulation.

4. Watch for excessive bleeding – orthopaedic wounds have a tendency to ooze more than other surgical wounds.
   a. Measure suction drainage if used.
   b. Anticipate up to 200–500ml of drainage in the first 24 hours, decreasing to less than 30ml per eight hours within 48 hours, depending on surgical procedure.

5. Assess for pain related to musculoskeletal surgery.
6. Watch for urinary retention – elderly men with some degree of prostatism may have difficulty in voiding.
7. Evaluate orthopaedic apparatus for safety and effectiveness.

Later postoperative period
1. Watch for development of pressure sores. See p. 30 for prevention and management.
2. Watch for complications due to prolonged disability. Venous thrombosis – see p. 341 for clinical features.
3. Assess fluid and nutritional status.
4. Watch for signs and symptoms of anaemia – especially after fracture of long bones. Haemoglobin determination usually done on third postoperative day or sooner.

PATIENT PROBLEMS
1. Pain related to musculoskeletal surgery.
2. Potential complications related to systemic responses to stresses of surgery, orthopaedic injury or immobility.
3. Potential infection related to break in skin integrity.

Planning and implementation
NURSING INTERVENTIONS
Relief of pain
1. See pain related to musculoskeletal disorder, p. 797.
2. Administer prescribed parenteral medications to control pain during the first few postoperative days.
   a. Avoid injection sites near operative site.
   b. Rotate injection sites.
   c. Muscle spasms may contribute to pain experience.

Prevention of complications
1. Monitor vital signs frequently.
2. Assess neurovascular status of involved extremity.
   a. See neurovascular compromise, p. 798.
   b. Document observations.
   c. Elevate affected extremity and apply ice packs as directed.
   d. If neurovascular problems are identified, notify surgeon and loosen cast or dressing at once.
3. Maintain sufficient pulmonary ventilation.
   a. Avoid or give respiratory depressant drugs in minimal doses.

    b. Change position every two hours – mobilizes secretions and helps prevent bronchial obstruction.
4. Encourage early resumption of activity.
5. Prevent venous complications.
    a. Encourage the patient to exercise by himself with a planned programme of exercise as soon as possible after surgery.
    b. Have the patient flex his knee, extend the knee with hip still flexed, and then lower the extremity to the bed.
    c. Encourage the patient to move fingers and toes periodically.
    d. Advise the patient to move joints that are not fixed by traction or appliance through their range of movement as fully as possible.
    e. Suggest muscle-setting exercises (quadriceps setting) if active motion is contraindicated.
    f. Wrap lower extremities with elastic bandages or apply elastic hose.
    g. Give prophylactic anticoagulants as directed.
6. Provide a normal balanced diet.
    a. Give vitamin supplements (B and C) to elderly patients or those with chronic disease as prescribed.
    b. Avoid giving large amounts of milk to orthopaedic patients on bed rest – adds to calcium pool in the body and demands more calcium excretion by the kidneys, predisposing to the formation of urinary calculi.
    c. Give iron supplements as directed.
7. Maintain urinary output by maintaining adequate fluid intake.
8. Monitor for signs and symptoms of infection.
    a. Monitor vital signs.
    b. Examine incision for redness, increased temperature and swelling.
    c. Note character of drainage.
    d. Evaluate complaints of recurrent or increasing pain.
    e. Administer antibiotic therapy as prescribed.

PATIENT EDUCATION

1. Teach the patient activities that will minimize the development of complications (e.g. turning, coughing and deep-breathing).
2. Instruct the patient in dietary considerations to facilitate healing and minimize development of constipation and renal calculi.
3. Inform the patient of techniques that facilitate moving while minimizing associated discomforts (e.g. supporting injured area and practising smooth, gentle position changes).

Evaluation
EXPECTED OUTCOMES

1. Patient achieves pain relief; utilizes pain-reduction measures and states achievement of comfort.
2. Patient demonstrates homeostasis; vital signs within normal limits and no evidence of thrombophlebitis, pressure sores, etc.
3. Patient achieves wound healing; no drainage and no signs of infection.

ARTHROPLASTY AND TOTAL JOINT REPLACEMENT

Arthroplasty is an operation to restore movement to a joint and function to the structures (muscles, ligaments, soft tissues) that control it. It may involve either replacement of the joint by a prosthesis or surgical reshaping of the bones of the joint.

Total hip replacement (total joint arthroplasty) is the replacement of a severely damaged hip with an artificial joint. Although a large number of implants are available, most consist of a metal femoral component topped by a spherical ball fitted into a plastic acetabular socket.

A total knee arthroplasty is an implant procedure in which tibial, femoral and patellar joint surfaces are replaced because of destroyed knee joint(s). Different types of implants are used, depending on degree of destruction and stability of joint (Figure 13.11).

Total joint arthroplasty is an exacting and meticulous procedure.

Bone ingrowth prosthesis designs allow for cementless fixation of the components in selected patients. Some patients require cement fixation of the components because of bone structure or condition.

CLINICAL INDICATIONS

1. For patients with unremitting pain, irreversibly damaged joints: primary degenerative arthritis (osteoarthritis); rheumatoid arthritis.
2. Selected fractures (e.g. femoral neck fracture).
3. Failure of previous reconstructive surgery (osteotomy, cup arthroplasty, femoral head replacement for complications of non-union and avascular necrosis).
4. Problems resulting from congenital hip disease.
5. Pathological fractures from metastatic cancer.
6. Joint instability.

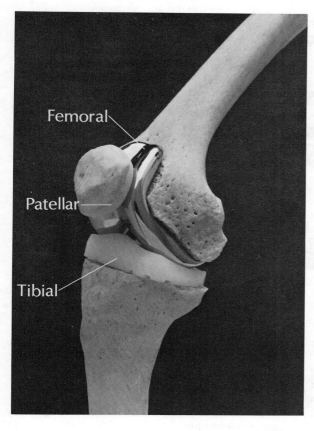

Femoral

Patellar

Tibial

Figure 13.11. Total knee replacement (courtesy: Richards Manufacturing Co. Inc.)

TREATMENT
Objectives
1. Reduce or eliminate pain.
2. Restore, improve, or maintain joint function.
3. Provide greater stability of the joint.
4. Avoid complications.

PREVENTION OF INFECTION
1. Operative area is cleaned – micro-organisms of the skin are potential cause of infection.
2. Give preoperative mediation into opposite (uninvolved) extremity.
3. Special precautions carried out in operating department to reduce particulate matter and bacterial count of air.
4. Antibiotics usually given immediately preoperatively, intraoperatively and postoperatively to reduce incidence of infection.

PREOPERATIVE NURSING INTERVENTIONS
1. Give meticulous skin preparation.
2. Administer antibiotic as prescribed.
3. Use elastic stockings to minimize development of thrombophlebitis.

4. Provide preoperative patient education.
   a. Educate the patient concerning his postoperative regimen (e.g. extended exercise programme will be carried out after surgery – atrophied muscles must be re-educated and strengthened).
   b. Teach isometric exercises (muscle setting) of quadriceps and gluteal muscles; teach active ankle motion.
   c. Fit with crutches and instruct the patient to walk without weight-bearing (if prescribed) – to develop crutch-walking ability and facilitate the patient's postoperative ambulation.
   d. Teach bed-to-wheelchair transfer without going beyond the hip flexion limits (usually 45°).
   e. Show balanced suspension apparatus, abduction splint, overhead traction frame and monkey pole – to acquaint the patient with postoperative environment.
   f. Demonstrate continuous passive motion equipment if it will be used postoperatively (see Figure 13.12).

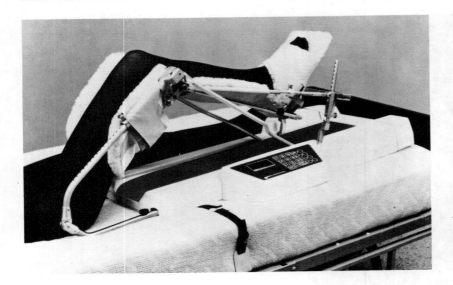

Figure 13.12. Continuous passive motion device used for postoperative total knee arthroplasty patients to facilitate range of motion (courtesy: Sutter Biomedical Inc.)

POSTOPERATIVE NURSING INTERVENTIONS
Postoperative assessment
1. Assess the patient's position for compliance with positioning prescription.
   a. Following hip arthroplasty, the patient is usually positioned flat in bed with the affected extremity held in slight abduction by either an abduction splint or pillows (may or may not be in Buck's extension) – to prevent dislocation of the prosthesis until soft tissue healing has occurred.
   b. Following knee arthroplasty, the knee may be immobilized in extension with a firm compression dressing and an adjustable soft extension splint or long-leg plaster cast.
   c. Leg may be elevated on pillows above the level of patient's heart. Alternatively, continuous passive motion may be started.

   Note: There are numerous modifications with differing requirements in the postoperative positioning of these patients.

2. Monitor the patient for signs of joint dislocation (i.e. shortened extremity, increasing discomfort, inability to move joint).
3. Assess the patient for the development of complications.
   a. Early – infection, thromboembolic complications, peroneal nerve palsy.
   b. Late – deep infection, loosening of prosthetic components, implant wear and dislocation, fracture of components.

Proper positioning and turning activities
1. Position the patient as prescribed – generally with hip arthroplasty the leg is in abduction with the use of an abduction splint or pillows.
2. Avoid acute flexion of the hip.

NURSING ALERT
The patient must not adduct or flex operated hip – may produce dislocation.

3. Turn the patient (as required by his prosthesis and condition) when indicated by surgeon.
   Following hip arthroplasty:
   a. Two nurses turn the patient on unoperated side while supporting operated hip securely in an abducted position; the entire length of leg is supported by two pillows. Use pillows to keep the leg abducted; place pillow at back for comfort.
   b. Keep bed flat except during prescribed intervals (meals) – to prevent hip flexion contraction.
      (i) The bed is usually not elevated more than 45°; placing the patient in an upright sitting position puts a strain on the hip joint and may cause dislocation.
      (ii) Support the low back with a small pillow or towel when the patient is supine – to relieve strain placed on muscles by the flat position.
   c. As the patient becomes familiar with the turning routine, assist him to change position by using overhead monkey pole.

Transfer and ambulation

1. Assist in use of the bed pan – instruct the patient to flex the unoperated hip and knee and pull up on the monkey pole to lift buttocks onto pan. Instruct the patient *NOT* to bear down on the operated hip in flexion when getting off the pan.
2. Assist in transfer from bed.
   a. *Following hip arthroplasty:*
      (i) Use an abduction splint or pillows while assisting the patient to get out of bed.
         (a) Keep the hip at maximum extension.
         (b) Instruct the patient to pivot on un-operated extremity.
         (c) Assess the patient for orthostatic hypotension.
      (ii) When the patient is ready to ambulate, teach him to advance the frame and then advance the operated extremity to the frame, bearing most of the weight on the hands.
      (iii) The patient progresses to use of crutches as directed, to prevent excessive use of hip abductors before healing occurs.
   b. *Following knee arthroplasty*, the patient may transfer out of bed into wheelchair with extension splint in place; no weight-bearing is permitted at this time.

Prevention of complications

1. Assess neurovascular status of operated extremity – check sensation, pulses, colour, and skin temperature and compare with unoperated leg.
2. Monitor blood loss – portable suction is used to decrease incidence of wound haematoma, which is a possible focus of infection.
3. Give narcotics as required the first 24 hours postoperatively and then taper to non-narcotic analgesia thereafter.
4. Encourage the patient to carry out prescribed exercise programme usually under direction of physiotherapist.
   a. Pain medication is usually given half an hour before exercise session as required.
   b. Instruct the patient to think about the motion required to contract the appropriate muscles.
   c. Encourage the patient to breathe deeply while exercising.
   d. Exercise activities depend on procedure and on condition of the patient.
      (i) Active movement of affected foot and ankle is started on the first postoperative day.
      (ii) Isometric exercise of quadriceps, gluteals, abductors is started on direction of orthopaedic surgeon.
      (iii) Flexion, extension, abduction, rotation exercises and ambulation are started upon direction of surgeon.
   e. Assist and encourage the patient during exercise.
5. Assist the patient in use of continuous passive motion equipment. Early postoperative passive exercise of joint facilitates joint healing and restoration of joint range of motion.
6. Use anticipatory nursing measures to prevent complications.
   a. Thromboembolism (major threat following reconstructive hip operations).
      (i) Continue to exercise ankles and legs – accelerates blood flow and prevents venous stasis.
      (ii) Antiembolic stockings for uninvolved extremity – to increase venous velocity; elastic stocking applied to operated extremity when elastic compression dressing is removed.
      (iii) Check for calf oedema, tenderness, local pain.
      (iv) Heparin, warfarin, aspirin – may be used for thromboembolic prophylaxis.
   b. Infection:
      (i) Give antimicrobials as directed.
      (ii) Watch for elevation of temperature and inspect wound at intervals.
      (iii) Infection may not become apparent until months or years after surgery.
      (iv) Deep infection almost always requires removal of implant.
   c. Complicating medical conditions (cardiac, gastrointestinal, genitourinary).
   d. Dislocation of prosthesis, fatigue fracture of metal component, avascular necrosis or dead bone caused by loss of blood supply, heterotrophic ossification (formation of bone in periprosthetic space).

PATIENT EDUCATION

Instruct the patient as follows:
1. Continue to wear elastic stockings after going home until full activities are resumed.
2. Avoid excessive hip adduction, flexion and rotation.
   a. Avoid sitting in low chair/toilet seat.
   b. Keep knees apart; do *not* cross legs.
   c. Limit sitting to 30 minutes at a time – to minimize hip flexion and the risk of prosthetic

dislocation and to prevent hip stiffness and flexion contracture.
3. Continue quadriceps setting and range-of-movement exercises as directed.
   a. Have a *daily* programme of stretching, exercise and rest throughout lifetime.
   b. Acquire a stationary bicycle if possible.
   c. Do not participate in any activity placing undue or sudden stress on joint (jogging, jumping, lifting heavy loads, becoming obese, excessive bending and twisting).
   d. Use a walking stick when taking fairly long walks.
4. Use self-help and energy-saving devices.
   a. Handrails by toilet.
   b. Raised toilet seat if there is some residual hip flexion problem.
   c. Bar-type stool for shower and kitchen work.
5. Lie prone twice daily for 30 minutes.
6. Report for follow-up evaluation and testing; supportive equipment (crutches, walking stick) is modified as needed.
7. Take prophylactic antibiotic if undergoing any procedure known to cause bacteraemia (tooth extraction, manipulation of genitourinary tract).

AMPUTATION

LOWER LIMB AMPUTATION

GENERAL CONSIDERATIONS
Conditions warranting amputation
1. Inadequate tissue perfusion as a result of diabetes mellitus or other vascular disease.
2. Trauma.
3. Malignant tumour.
4. Congenital deformities.
5. Uncontrolled infection (usually in bone).

Treatment
1. Level of amputation is determined by estimation of maximum viable tissue and development of a functional stump.
2. Modern trend is toward selecting most distal amputation level consistent with wound healing.

Preoperative assessment
1. Haemodynamic evaluation – arterial blood flow evaluated by Doppler pressure measurements and xenon 133 flow studies – for accurate and optimum amputation level determination.
2. Culture and sensitivity tests of draining wounds. Control of gangrene or advancing infection preoperatively is sought.
3. Evaluation of sound (contralateral) extremity.
4. Evaluation of cardiovascular, respiratory, renal, and other body systems to determine preoperative condition of the patient.
5. Evaluation of the patient's and family's emotional response to amputation.
   a. Anticipation of relief of pain related to amputation is frequent.
   b. Distress at anticipated loss of body part exhibited by patient and family.

PATIENT PROBLEMS
1. Anxiety related to proposed amputation.
2. Alteration in comfort related to primary condition requiring amputation.
3. Alteration in mobility related to general muscle weakness and projected use of ambulatory aids.
4. Health and nutritional deficits related to chronic condition and impending major surgery.
5. Knowledge deficit related to expected participation in projected rehabilitation programme.

Planning and implementation
NURSING INTERVENTIONS
Objective
To have the patient attain his highest physical and emotional level in preparation for wearing a prosthesis (artificial limb) and/or attaining mobility by other means.

Reduction of anxiety
1. Support the patient psychologically. Knowing what to expect helps reduce anxiety.
2. Amputation may be viewed as a surgical reconstructive procedure and as the first step in rehabilitation for the patient who has had prolonged periods of disability from peripheral vascular disease.
3. Avoid unrealistic and misleading reassurance – management of a prosthesis can be slow and painful.

Relief of pain
1. Instruct patient on use of pain-modifying techniques.
2. Inform the patient of the availability of postoperative pain medication.
3. Explain to the patient that he may continue to 'feel' the foot for a time; this sensation may be

helpful for the placement of the prosthetic foot while he is learning to use the prosthesis.

Incorporation of effective position changes and ambulation with use of ambulatory aids

1. Encourage the patient to reposition self every one or two hours with an awareness of body positioning to avoid contractures.
2. Have the patient strengthen the muscles of the upper extremity, trunk and abdomen as a preparation for crutch walking. (Develop arm extensors and shoulder depressors, which are the muscle groups needed for crutch walking.) Instruct the patient as follows:
   a. Flex and extend arms while holding traction weights.
   b. Do push-ups from a prone position.
   c. Do sit-ups from a seated position.
3. Teach the patient to use ambulatory aids preoperatively – prepares for postoperative mobility, maintains mobility and arm function and instils confidence.

Establishing maximal health status prior to surgery

1. Assess laboratory reports for optimal values (e.g. haematology, urinalysis and blood chemistries are within normal limits).
2. Encourage balanced diet with adequate protein to enhance wound healing.
3. Evaluate each body system for adequacy of function.

Preoperative activities to enhance recovery

1. Clarify plans for management of perioperative and postoperative periods as outlined by the surgeon.
2. Address concerns expressed about the possibilities of obtaining and using a prosthesis – not all amputees can benefit from a prosthesis.
   a. Diabetes mellitus, heart disease, infection, cerebrovascular accident, chronic obstructive pulmonary disease, peripheral vascular disease, and increasing age are factors limiting full rehabilitation.
   b. Wound breakdown, infection and delay in healing of amputation stump are significant limiting factors.
3. Introduce the patient to physiotherapist.
4. Encourage the patient to attain his highest physical and emotional level in preparation for wearing a prosthesis (artificial extremity) and/or attaining mobility by other means.
5. Explain various phases of rehabilitation involved – active participation in rehabilitation is essential for a successful outcome.
6. Teach postoperative routines (i.e. turn, cough, deep-breathe, etc).

TREATMENT

1. The surgeon creates a residual limb (stump) which is functional (with stability), nontender, pressure tolerant and not susceptible to tissue breakdown. The skin, soft tissue and scar placement are considered. The type of dressing used postoperatively will depend on the surgeon and limb-fitting centre; either a rigid plaster or firm crêpe dressing may be used.
2. A closed, rigid plaster dressing applied immediately after surgery provides for the attachment of a prosthetic extension (pylon) and a prosthetic foot immediately or within 10 to 30 days.
3. The rigid dressing controls oedema, supports circulation, minimizes pain on movement, helps shape the residual limb and promotes healing. It allows earlier fitting of the prosthesis, shortens the interval between amputation and walking, and is of tremendous psychological value to the patient.
4. Although the rigid dressing is used, early weight-bearing is not always desirable in patients with severe peripheral vascular disease.
5. A soft dressing permits wound inspection and may be used with compression dressings or external splints.
6. Prevention of complications associated with a major operation and facilitation of early rehabilitation are essential to prevent prolonged disability.

NURSING ALERT

Amputation of the lower extremity can be a life-threatening procedure, especially for patients over 60 with peripheral vascular disease. Significant mobility accompanies above-knee amputations because of associated poor health and disease as well as the complications of sepsis and malnutrition and the physiological insult of amputation.

Postoperative assessment

1. Watch for signs and symptoms of haemorrhage.
   a. Keep tourniquet (in view) attached to end of bed – to apply to residual limb (stump) if excessive bleeding occurs.
   b. Monitor suction drainage.
2. Monitor the patient's general physiological response to anaesthesia, surgery and immobility.

3. Evaluate the patient's pain (see p. 797).
    a. Anticipate complaint of pain and sensation located in the missing limb ('phantom pain').
    b. Narcotics may not relieve these sensations; physical treatments (e.g. bandaging, temperature changes) and transcutaneous nerve stimulation (TENS) may be useful.

PATIENT PROBLEMS
1. Potential haemorrhage related to inadequate/disrupted surgical haemostasis.
2. Ineffective coping related to change in body image and alteration in mobility.
3. Potential contracture deformity related to positioning and inactivity.
4. Alteration in ambulatory stability related to muscle weakness and change in body-weight distribution.
5. Residual limb conditioning related to oedema and postoperative tissue responses.
6. Lack of knowledge related to management of residual limb (stump) and prosthesis.

Planning and implementation
NURSING INTERVENTIONS
Minimal blood loss
1. Raise foot of bed slightly to elevate residual limb. Do not flex the patient's hips by elevating stump on pillow since this will produce a hip flexion contracture.
2. Monitor the patient for systemic symptoms of excessive blood loss.
3. Maintain accurate record of bloody drainage on dressings and in drainage system.
4. Reinforce dressing as required using aseptic technique.

Body image adjustment
1. Accept the frustrations and behaviour of the patient.
    a. The patient views amputation as death of part of his body; expect some depression and withdrawal.
    b. The self-image has to be adjusted after amputation. It will take time for the patient to make this modification.
2. Exhibit a positive approach combined with physiotherapy; this helps improve the patient's outlook on his potential.

Prevention of contractures
1. Prevent deformities in the immediate postoperative period. Contracture of the next joint above an amputation is a frequent complication.

Deformities include flexion and abduction.
    a. Avoid pillows under stump, hips or between legs.
    b. Encourage the patient to turn from side to side.
    c. Place the patient in prone position twice daily – to stretch the flexor muscles and prevent flexion contracture of the hip.
        (i) Keep the patient's legs close together – to prevent abduction deformity.
        (ii) Place pillow under abdomen and residual limb while the patient is prone.
2. Encourage the patient to move residual limb – to avoid contractures.
3. Start range-of-movement exercises – contracture deformities develop rapidly and cause serious problems in management of a prosthesis.

Pre-ambulation training
1. Start the patient on standing and ambulation activities.
    a. The timing depends on age, general physical status, condition of remaining foot, etc.
    b. The patient may stand by his bed within 48 hours postoperatively with rigid dressing attached and the prosthetic foot touching down (no weight-bearing) – helps minimize fear of pain and promotes confidence of the patient in his ability to handle himself.
2. Muscle-strengthening and balancing exercises – to strengthen muscles, mobilize joints and increase balance sense. Instruct the patient as follows (stand behind the patient and stabilize him at the waist, if necessary):
    a. Arise from chair and stand.
    b. Stand on toes while holding on to a chair.
    c. Bend the knee while holding on to a chair.
    d. Balance on one leg without support.
    e. Hop on one foot while holding on to a chair.

Residual limb conditioning
1. Bandage residual limb with elastic bandage to control oedema and to form a firm, conical shape for prosthesis fitting.
    a. Bandaging generally begins one to three days after surgery.
    b. Use 5 to 18cm elastic bandages for above-knee amputation and 5 to 10cm bandages for below-knee amputation.
    c. Use diagonal figure-8 bandaging technique (Figure 13.13).
    d. Wrap distal to proximal to maintain pressure gradient and to control oedema.
    e. Begin wrapping with minimal tension and in-

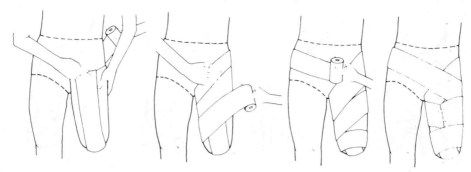

Figure 13.13. Shrinking and shaping the stump in a conical form helps ensure comfort and fit of the prosthetic device. Bandaging supports the soft tissue and minimizes the formation of oedema fluid while the stump is in a dependent position

crease as wound heals and sutures are removed.

f. Flatten skin at ends of incision to ensure conical stump shape.

g. Apply bandages snugly to adductor area to prevent formation of adductor roll.

h. Rebandage if the patient complains of more pain – dressing is probably too tight.

i. Keep residual limb bandaged at all times except when bathing.

j. Prosthesis is measured and fitted when maximum shrinkage occurs.

2. Include the patient in stump-bandaging activities.

3. Air splint may be applied to residual limb to control oedema.

4. Encourage exercises to strengthen muscles necessary for ambulation – hip flexion, abduction, adduction and extension.

5. Teach the patient to avoid long periods of sitting with limb flexed – minimizes the development of dependent oedema, flexion contractures, and pressure areas.

6. Have the patient do residual limb-conditioning exercises – to harden the residual limb.

a. The patient pushes the residual limb against a soft pillow.

b. Gradually he pushes residual limb against harder surfaces.

c. Teach the patient to message the residual limb to soften the scar, decrease tenderness, and improve vascularity.

(i) Massage is usually started when healing takes place.

(ii) Initially, massage is usually done by physiotherapist.

Note: Some limb-fitting centres now prefer that the stump is left exposed and unshaped following surgery.

Self-care of residual limb

1. Wash healed residual limb daily with soap and water, removing all soap residue.

2. Avoid soaking residual limb because it results in oedema.

3. Inspect residual limb daily for potential and actual skin breakdown.

4. Bandage residual limb at all times.

5. Rebandage residual limb a couple of times a day and as necessary demonstrating skilful ability, resulting in smooth, graded tension dressing.

Avoidance of complications

1. Make sure that the residual limb remains in the plaster cast socket during the patient's hospitalization; if the socket inadvertently comes off, excessive oedema will form very rapidly, causing a delay in rehabilitation.

a. Rebandage the residual limb immediately with elastic compression bandage (Figure 13.14).

b. Prepare for immediate reapplication of cast socket.

2. Control pain. Assess for development of complications: increasing residual limb pain, haematoma, odour emanating from cast, infection, residual limb necrosis. Keep the patient active – decreases occurrence of phantom-limb pain.

a. If the patient is not a candidate for prosthesis/ ambulation, teach him to participate in self-care activities in a special wheelchair designed for amputees.

b. Reassure the patient that phantom-limb sensation (painful sensation that amputated foot is still there) will soon pass.

3. Protect the residual limb from infection.

a. Use plastic material to protect dressing if the patient is incontinent.

b. Wash residual limb with mild soap and water.

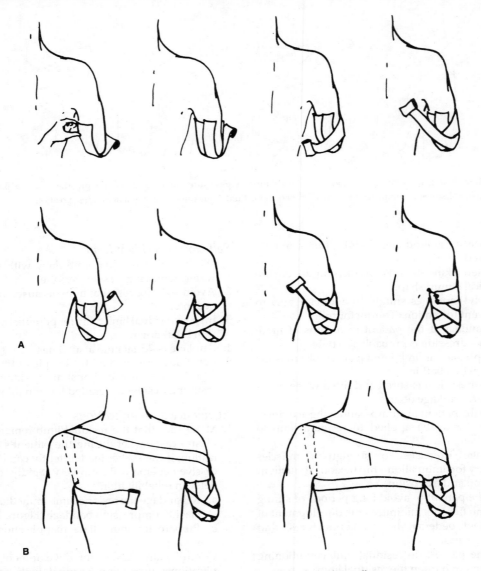

Figure 13.14. (A) Steps in the application of an elastic bandage to a standard or long above-elbow stump.
(B) An elastic bandage applied to a short above-elbow stump usually must be wrapped one or more times through the normal axilla to hold the stump wrapping in place (from: Bender, L. F. (1974) *Prostheses and Rehabilitation after Arm Amputation*. Courtesy: Charles C. Thomas, Springfield, Illinois)

4. Observe and protect the remaining foot from injury.
   a. Examine remaining foot and malleoli daily.
   b. Keep pressure (bedclothes) off foot.
5. Watch for deterioration of remaining leg – from disuse, poor vascular supply, foot trauma. (Obliterative arteriosclerotic vascular disease may necessitate *bilateral* lower extremity amputation.)

PATIENT EDUCATION
1. The patient will require rehabilitation services to learn mobility skills, transfers, wheelchair or car use, etc.
2. Progressive ambulation following first change of dressing is carried out under the supervision of physiotherapist or nurse. Gait training is continued under the direction of physiotherapist.

3. A going-home prosthesis is fitted as soon as possible following surgery. The permanent prosthesis is fitted when the residual limb is fully conditioned.

Evaluation
EXPECTED OUTCOMES
1. Avoids excessive blood loss following surgery; haematology values in normal range.
2. Exhibits behaviour indicating self-esteem and adjustment to altered mobility patterns; participates in self-care activities; learns use of mobility aids; has realistic future orientation.
3. Avoids development of contractures; exercises residual limb; avoids positions that encourage contracture development; spends increasing time prone to inhibit flexion contracture.
4. Demonstrates standing balance and ambulatory stability; increase in muscle strength, increased ambulatory ability.
5. Participates in residual limb conditioning; wraps stump with elastic dressing skilfully.
6. Demonstrates ability to care for residual limb and prosthesis; washes residual limb daily, inspects residual limb for skin pressure or breakdown, keeps residual limb wrapped at all times, works with physiotherapist and orthotist to obtain optimal fit and function.

UPPER LIMB AMPUTATION

INDICATIONS
1. Trauma (acute injury, electrical burns, frostbite).
2. Congenital malformations.
3. Malignant tumours.

TREATMENT
See Lower Limb Amputation, p. 840.

Postoperative assessment
1. Assess the patient's response to surgery and potential haemorrhage. Monitor drainage.
2. Evaluate the patient's pain (see p. 797).

PATIENT PROBLEMS
1. Potential problems related to surgery (e.g. haemorrhage, infection).
2. Ineffective coping related to change in body image and decreased independence.
3. Potential contracture deformity related to joint immobility.
4. Knowledge deficit related to management of residual limb, one-handed aids and prosthesis.

NURSING INTERVENTIONS
Avoiding postoperative complications
1. When the patient returns from the operating room he will have either a rigid plaster of Paris socket with provision for the application of a temporary prosthesis or a conventional compression bandage in place.
2. Monitor the amount and character of the suction drainage – used to eliminate haematoma and approximate the tissues.

Adaptation to altered body image
1. Give the patient psychological support to help him adapt to changes in his lifestyle. Listen to his fears and concerns. The patient will have impaired personal body image, loss of sensory input and inadequate motor output.
2. Psychological problems (denial, withdrawal) – responses influenced by support and encouragement of rehabilitation team, by early introduction of one-handed activities and by discussion of prosthetic options and capabilities.
3. Start the patient on one-handed self-care activities as soon as possible – to promote independence. Occupational therapist teaches self-feeding, bathing, grooming, etc.

Prevention of contractures
1. Encourage active movement of residual limb after mobility restrictions have been removed.
   Exercises are carried out to prevent contracture, obtain full range of movement, combat muscle atrophy, increase muscle strength, and prepare residual limb for prosthesis.
   a. Muscle setting, joint mobilizing, range-of movement exercises are performed as soon as tolerated – to strengthen muscles and joints (under direction of physiotherapist).
   b. Exercise muscles of both shoulders – an upper extremity amputee uses both shoulders to operate prosthesis.
   c. Carry out postural exercises – loss of weight of amputated extremity may produce postural abnormality.
2. Assess for residual limb contraction or residual limb contour problems.

Residual limb care (upper extremity)
1. Assist with dressing change and inspect wound.
   a. *Rigid dressing:*
   A plaster socket with temporary prosthetic device is applied – increases the patient's endurance, allows early prosthetic training and fitting of permanent prosthetic device.

b. *Compression dressing:*
  (i) Rebandage the residual limb three to four times daily – to maintain proper tension in the bandage and to reduce the fluid and shape the residual limb so that a prosthesis may be fitted.
  (ii) Keep residual limb snugly bandaged with elastic bandage for 24-hour period except for periods of bathing and exercise.
  (iii) Teach the patient and his family the correct technique of application since residual limb bandaging will be continued until the permanent prosthesis is fitted (six weeks to one year).

Self-care activities

1. Discuss the available prosthetic replacement (by orthotist, physiotherapist). The fitting of the prosthesis depends on the level of amputation, age of the patient and whether weakness or limitation of range of movement of joints proximal to amputation site is present.
  a. The patient will require instruction in putting on and removing prosthesis, control of prosthesis, etc.
  b. Ultimate patient rehabilitation ideally requires the services and supervision of rehabilitation team at a comprehensive medical rehabilitation unit.
2. Demonstrate aids to independence (one-handed knife for cutting, elastic shoelaces, one-handed methods of functioning) – usually done in co-operation with occupational therapist.
3. Teach how to assess for skin problems – from irritants in prosthetic components, lack of ventilation.

PATIENT EDUCATION

Instruct the patient to maintain careful residual limb hygiene to prevent skin irritation and infection.

1. Wash and dry residual limb thoroughly at least twice daily.
2. Wear residual limb sock. Change daily (and wash immediately) – to absorb perspiration and avoid direct contact between prosthetic socket and skin.
3. Avoid wrinkles in residual limb sock – may irritate skin.
4. Wipe the socket of prosthesis with damp cloth upon removal in evening.
5. Wear cotton T-shirt – to prevent contact between skin and shoulder harness and to absorb perspiration. Change daily.
6. Inspect the skin under harness for pressure, irritation, and abrasion.
7. Launder the washable portions of the harness as often as necessary; if practical, have two harnesses so that one can be laundered while the other is worn.
8. Have prosthesis checked periodically.

Evaluation
EXPECTED OUTCOMES

1. Patient avoids problems related to amputation; haematology values normal; residual limb heals without infection.
2. Patient exhibits adjustment to change in body image and functions independently; uses residual limb, and one-arm aids as necessary.
3. Patient avoids development of joint contracture; exercises joint routinely, obtains full range of movement, maintains muscle strength.
4. Patient demonstrates ability to care for residual limb, prosthesis and self; washes residual limb daily, bandages residual limb to shrink and shape it, uses self-help aids as needed.

SPECIFIC ORTHOPAEDIC CONDITIONS

LOW BACK PAIN

Low back pain is characterized by acute pain in the low back associated with severe spasm of the paraspinal muscles, often with radiation.

Muscle spasm is a condition in which muscles are painfully contracted.

AETIOLOGY (MULTIPLE CAUSES)

1. Mechanical (joint, muscular or ligamentous strain).
2. Congenital malformations.
3. Degenerative disc disease; acute herniation of discs.
4. Poor posture; obesity.
5. Lack of physical activity and exercise.
6. Arthritic conditions.
7. Predisposing endocrine and systemic diseases.
8. Diseases of bone (Paget's disease, metastatic carcinoma).
9. Infections of disc spaces or vertebrae.
10. Spinal cord tumours.

DIAGNOSTIC EVALUATION

1. History – to determine when, where and how the pain occurs and its relationship to activity and rest; to rule out medical causes.
2. Neurological evaluation – to spot localized weakness of extremities and reflex and sensory loss; to exclude neurogenic disease.
3. Evaluation of muscular system – for changes in strength, tone and flexibility of key posture muscles.
4. Electromyography – to record changes in electric potential of muscle and of nerve leading to it.
5. X-ray – of lumbar spine (anteroposterior, lateral and oblique).
6. Bone scan – to detect early malignant or infectious conditions.

TREATMENT AND NURSING MANAGEMENT
Objectives
Relieve muscle spasm.
Gain normal elasticity of affected muscles.
Return normal joint movement.
Correct underlying conditions.

1. Advise the patient to rest in bed in a semi-upright position (hips and knees flexed) – to relieve painful muscle and ligament sprain, heal soft tissue injury, remove stress from lumbar sacral area, relieve tension on sciatic nerves and open the posterior part of the intervertebral spaces:
   a. Acute spasm should subside in three to seven days if there is no nerve involvement or other serious underlying disease.
   b. Do prescribed isometric exercises hourly while on bed rest if possible.
2. Use heat or ice to relax muscle spasm and relieve discomfort. Follow heat by massage.
3. Medications:
   a. Give oral pain medication and muscle relaxants.
   b. Inject painful trigger points with hydrocortisone/xylocaine for pain relief (by doctor).
   c. Use parenteral pain medication in acute severe pain syndromes.
4. Pelvic traction and manipulation may be used.
5. Lumbosacral support may be used – provides abdominal compression and decreases load on lumbar intervertebral discs.
6. Transcutaneous nerve stimulation (TENS) may be helpful.
7. Psychiatric intervention may be needed for the patient with chronic depression, anxiety and low back syndrome.
   a. The patient may undergo psychological testing (Minnesota Multiphasic Personality Inventory [MMPI]).
   b. Psychotropic medication may be used for treatment of depression and anxiety, which potentiate pain.
8. Myelogram if patient shows no improvement after seven to 10 days of conservative treatment, when there is a neurological deficit, intractable pain, loss of bowel or bladder control: operative intervention may be necessary.

NURSING INTERVENTIONS
Relief of discomfort
See pain (alteration in comfort) related to musculoskeletal disorders, p. 797.

1. Advise the patient to rest in bed. (Rest in bed may eliminate the need for pain medications.)
2. Keep pillow between flexed knees while in side-lying position.
3. Apply moist warm heat (moist towels) as prescribed.
4. Administer pain medications and muscle relaxants as prescribed.

Resumption of activities
See psychological and social problems related to musculoskeletal problems, p. 798.

1. Encourage the patient to discuss problems that may be contributing to his backache.
2. Advise the patient to start activity as soon as possible – activity speeds recovery and helps prevent loss of muscle function.
3. Encourage the patient to do prescribed back exercises (Figure 13.15). Exercise keeps postural muscles strong, helps recondition the back and abdominal musculature and serves as an outlet for emotional tension.

PATIENT EDUCATION
Instruct the patient as follows:

1. Tension can contribute to spasm in the back muscles.
2. Avoid prolonged standing, walking, sitting and driving.
3. Rest at intervals throughout the day.
4. Avoid assuming tense, cramped positions. Avoid forward flexion.
5. Use a hard plywood board under a firm mattress.
6. Pick up objects or loads correctly:
   a. Maintain a straight spine.
   b. Flex knees and hips while stooping – places stress on bony components rather than on soft tissues.
7. Continue with the exercise programme, which

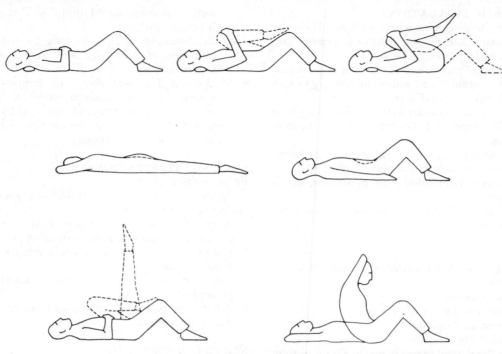

Figure 13.15. Back exercises are designed to strengthen abdominal muscles and stretch the contracted back muscles. They help keep posture muscles strong and flexible and aid in reducing nervous tension which increases low back pain

should be supervised and reviewed frequently. Continue with generalized conditioning of body (walking, swimming).

8. Reduce weight if indicated.

9. Reinforce with the patient that standing, sitting, lying and lifting properly are necessary for a healthy back, and daily exercise is important in the prevention of back problems.

RHEUMATOID ARTHRITIS

Rheumatoid arthritis is a chronic systemic disease primarily affecting connective tissue in any or all of the body systems. It is characterized most prominently by recurrent inflammation involving the synovium, or lining of the joints, that leads to destructive changes in the joints. The cause is unknown and the course is variable.

Assessment

CLINICAL FEATURES

1. Inflammation of the joints characterized by pain, swelling, heat, redness and limitation of function.

2. Subcutaneous nodules over bony prominences, bursae and tendon sheaths.

3. Enlarged lymph nodes; particularly nodes draining inflamed joints.

4. Constitutional symptoms (may accompany or precede arthropathy):
   a. Easy fatiguability and malaise.
   b. Fever.
   c. Weight loss, general weakness.
   d. Anaemia.

PATHOPHYSIOLOGY UNDERLYING JOINT DESTRUCTION

Inflammation of joint (synovitis) → synovial effusion → granulation tissue covering articular cartilage (pannus) → joint capsular and subchondral bone destruction → pain → loss of mobility of joint → muscular weakness about the joint → damage of tendons and ligaments → joint instability and deformity → joint malfunction and disuse → muscular atrophy and contracture deformity.

DIAGNOSTIC EVALUATION

1. History, physical examination.

2. Laboratory tests.
   a. Blood count (most patients are anaemic).
   b. Tests which reveal disease activity and provide guidelines for therapy include:

(i) C-reactive protein test (CRP) – positive in rheumatoid arthritis.

(ii) Erythrocyte sedimentation rate – elevated during periods of active arthritis.

c. Tests for rheumatoid factor in the serum: positive in 70–80 per cent of patients with rheumatoid arthritis:

(i) Latex fixation test.

(ii) Antinuclear antibody test.

d. Serum protein electrophoresis – increased globulins (gamma and alpha globulins); decreased albumin.

3. Roentgenograms of involved joints – to determine extent, rate of progress and structural changes within bones; reveals swelling of soft tissue, erosion of bone at articular margins, narrowing of joint space.

4. Thermography – pinpoints areas of inflammation and increased metabolic activity in the body by pictorially recording (mapping) the heat emitted from the skin over the affected areas.

5. Synovial fluid analysis – to distinguish between inflammatory, traumatic or degenerative arthritis.

6. Arthroscopy – endoscopic examination of knee joint; allows observation of synovial lining, articular cartilage and menisci; permits examination of knee during passive movements and allows biopsy under direct vision; detects pathology earlier than other methods.

TREATMENT AND NURSING MANAGEMENT
Objective
Maintain independence and prevent crippling deformities by:
1. Controlling synovitis.
2. Maintaining joint mobility and muscle power.
3. Relieving pain and promoting comfort.
4. Decreasing the activity of the disease.
5. Educating and helping the patient and family to adjust to a chronic disability.

The treatment programme includes rest, exercise, drug therapy and patient education.

PATIENT PROBLEMS
1. Pain and stiffness related to joint and muscle inflammation, degeneration and deformity.
2. Impaired physical mobility related to pain, deformity and muscle atrophy.
3. Reduction in self-care activities (feeding, bathing/ hygiene, dressing/grooming, toileting) related to fatigue, pain and deformity.
4. Weight loss, anorexia related to reduced nutritional intake.
5. Disturbance in self-concept and alteration in body image related to deformity and loss of independence.

Planning and implementation
NURSING INTERVENTIONS
Relief of pain and discomfort
1. Regular rest at specified periods is needed to relieve pain and control fatigue – arthritis affects the whole body.
   a. Complete bed rest for patients with active widespread inflammatory disease.
   b. Have the patient rest in a recumbent position (one pillow under head) on a firm mattress – to take the weight off the joints.
   c. Advise the patient to establish one or more daytime rest periods of 30 to 60 minutes.
   d. Encourage the patient to rest in bed eight or nine hours at night.
   e. Instruct the patient to lie in prone position twice daily to prevent hip flexion and knee contractures.
   f. Pillows should not be placed under painful joints – promotes flexion contractures.
2. Painful inflamed joints may be rested with splints – to decrease synovitis locally; to reduce pain, stiffness, and swelling (in wrists and fingers); and to rest inflamed joints in optimum position and to prevent/correct deformities (Figure 13.16).

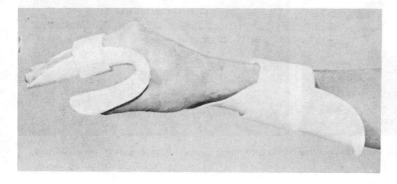

Figure 13.16. Rest splint for hand. Rest of the hand is important when soft tissues are acutely inflamed. Instruct the patient to maintain full range of motion of all joints and maintain tendon excursion while wearing a rest splint to prevent loss of important hand function (Courtesy: Western Pennsylvania Hospital, Pittsburgh, PA)

a. Use correctly designed splints: a 'working' splint (Figure 13.17) for daytime, to allow continuing function despite a painful joint, and a 'resting' splint for night-time may be indicated.
   (i) A resting splint is used at night to keep knee in extension.
   (ii) The wrist is splinted with slight dorsi-flexion – useful in patients with carpal tunnel syndrome (compression of median nerve within carpal canal).
b. Splints may need modifications as joint structures change.
c. Metatarsal bars or pads (for shoes), inserts or custom-made shoes may be used to decrease pressure on painful arthritic feet.
d. Cervical collar to prevent cervical motion may help if patient has painful neck.
e. Exercise is usually prescribed with splinting – to prevent joint deterioration and muscle weakness.

3. Use of transcutaneous electrical nerve stimulation (TENS).
4. Hot and/or cold applications reduce joint pain and swelling.
   a. Apply moist heat (15 to 30 minutes) to reduce muscle spasm and postrest stiffness; provide as much relief from pain as possible so that exercise programme can be carried out.
      (i) Take warm bath or shower upon arising – shortens period of morning stiffness.
      (ii) Use hot paraffin baths for fingers, hands.
   b. Use cold packs or ice when indicated for hot, swollen, acutely inflamed joints; heat is some-times contraindicated when a joint is acutely inflamed. Cold will relieve swelling and pain and help restore function. (Keep commercial cold packs in freezer.)
   c. Employ gentle massage to relax muscles.
   d. Take joints through range of motion after heat treatments.
5. Anti-inflammatory/analgesic medication as pre-scribed (see p. 852).

Increased physical mobility and muscle strength

1. Regular exercises to maintain function of all joints, to strengthen muscles that support the joints, to improve circulation and to promote endurance.
   a. Encourage the patient to follow a prescribed *daily* programme of exercise composed of con-ditioning exercises and specific exercises for particular joint problems (after inflammatory process is controlled).
      (i) Avoid *excessive* exercise.
      (ii) Stop exercise before tiring.
      (iii) Pain lasting more than half an hour after activity indicates that exercise is too vigor-ous; decrease, but do not stop activity.
      (iv) Exercise slowly and smoothly in short, frequent sessions.
   b. See that the patient performs isometric exer-cises – to help prevent muscle atrophy, which contributes to joint instability.
   c. Have the patient move joints through full range of movement once or twice a day to prevent loss of joint motion.
      (i) Assist the patient in performing required joint motion if necessary.

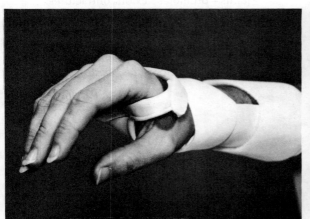
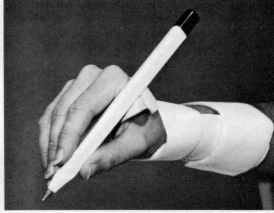

Figure 13.17. Arthritic cock-up splint is a type of working splint that allows continuing function despite a painful joint (courtesy: Western Pennsylvania Hospital, Pittsburgh, PA)

(ii) Avoid grasping painful joints; grasp belly of muscle.

d. Have the patient do progressive resistive exercises – for muscle building, after joint inflammation has been controlled.

2. Crutches or walking stick held in hand opposite affected knee/hip can be used – to reduce the load on the affected knee/hip.

3. Proper positioning to prevent flexion contractures of hips, knees, neck.

Optimal independence in activities of daily living

1. Self-help devices can be used to help with daily activities:
   a. Eating utensils with built-up handles.
   b. Raised chair seats, toilet seats.
   c. Special fastenings on clothing.
   d. Dressing sticks, extended shoe horns.
2. Allow extra time for the patient to perform activities, assisting only if necessary.

Improved nutritional intake

1. Offer well-balanced diet to include foods high in fibre, protein, iron and vitamin C.
2. Encourage weight loss, if the patient is obese, to prevent excess stress on weight-bearing joints (hips and knees).

Positive self-image

1. Maintain a supportive relationship – successful management usually requires a long period of treatment.
2. Discuss nature of disease and positive expectations of treatment; encourage the patient to set goals.
3. Adopt a positive but realistic attitude.
4. Emphasize that something can and will be done to relieve the patient's pain and mobilize his joints.
   a. Encourage him to express his feelings – the patient becomes hostile and angry because of chronic pain, stiffness and loss of mobility.
   b. Let the patient know that you are aware of his fears and that his future is important to the health team.
5. Try to modify or adapt to stress-producing situations.
6. Promote independence in activities of daily living (see above).
7. Encourage the patient to participate in social activities, hobbies, and family activities.
8. Allow the patient to participate in decision-making concerning treatment plan.

PATIENT EDUCATION
The patient should be able to:

1. Understand the disease, accept the realities of arthritis, and live within the limits imposed by it.
   a. Learn the nature of the disease and its treatment.
   b. Have confidence in his doctor and treatment programme.
   c. Avoid 'miracle cures', dietary fads, drugs not prescribed by the doctor and other forms of 'quackery'.
   d. Report to the doctor or clinic *regularly* for evaluation; have regular medical and functional re-evaluation to determine if there is any loss of joint function.
2. Maintain independence.
   a. Rely on his own capabilities.
   b. Participate in as many activities as possible without producing fatigue.
   c. Conserve energy and simplify daily activities using self-help devices, work simplification methods and energy-saving methods.
   d. Work at an even pace.
   e. Alternate periods of work, exercise and rest. Avoid overdoing on good days.
   f. Alternate sitting and standing tasks; do not remain seated too long.
3. Take the medication exactly as prescribed, on a regular schedule (Table 13.1).
   a. Aspirin is the primary drug (used for its anti-inflammatory effect). It must be taken over a long period and at high doses to achieve desired response. Long-term use does *not* lead to addiction.
   b. Report ringing in the ears or decreased hearing, since this is a guide in controlling dosage.
   c. Watch for symptoms of gastric irritation.
   d. Take with food (a buffering agent).
4. Use prescribed heat or cold treatments for muscle relaxation and relief of pain.
   a. Take a warm shower or bath upon arising to relieve morning stiffness; rest in bed 20 to 30 minutes after warm bath.
   b. If heat or cold treatment intensifies pain, discontinue and notify doctor.
   c. Try an electric blanket to ascertain its usefulness in relieving morning stiffness.
5. Do the prescribed exercises to preserve joint movement and to gain muscular strength and coordination.
   a. Exercise also in water (pool; bath) – water provides buoyancy, support and relaxation;

Table 13.1 Drugs used in rheumatoid arthritis

Drug	Action	Nursing implication and assessment for drug intolerance
Anti-inflammatory agents *Salicylates* Acetylsalicylic acid: Aspirin (may be buffered or enteric coated)	An example of a prostaglandin inhibitor – drugs of this group form the cornerstone of treatment Exerts anti-inflammatory effect Optimum dosage will produce blood salicylate levels of 20–25mg/100ml Can be used in combination with other analgesics and anti-inflammatory agents	Take salicylates with antacid or milk to protect against gastric irritation Watch for complaints of tinnitus, gastric intolerance or gastrointestinal bleeding and purpuric tendencies

Phenylbutazone (Butazolidin)	Nonsteroidal antirheumatic agents for adjunctive treatment of rheumatoid arthritis
	Exerts analgesic, anti-inflammatory action
	Sometimes remarkably effective in control of articular symptoms
	Patient should be under close medical supervision
	Can cause salt and water retention
	Usually used only for short periods
		Observe for untoward effects
		Gastrointestinal effects:
		  Nausea, vomiting, epigastric distress, precipitation and reactivation of peptic ulcer
		Haematological effects:
		  Bone marrow depression, anaemia, leucopenia, agranulocytosis, thrombocytopenia purpura
		  Irreversible blood element depression may occur rapidly despite careful supervision and frequent testing
		May precipitate gout

Indomethacin (Indocid) Ibuprofen (Brufen)	Additionally available as suppositories Anti-inflammatory action	Gastrointestinal effects, CNS effects Headache Epigastric distress. Less so than other drugs of this group

Antimalarial compounds
  Hydroxychloroquine sulphate (Plaquenil)
	Appears to be no rational basis for the comparative success of these drugs	Stress that patient should have regular ophthalmological examination every 4–6 months; *drug has potential retinal effects*
		Toxic effects:
		  Headache, dizziness, gastrointestinal complaints, ocular toxicity and retinopathy

Gold salts
  Gold sodium thiomalate
  Myocrisin
	Gold salts are useful when rheumatoid activity is uncontrolled by previous therapy
	Gold salt therapy is cumulative with slow onset of beneficial effects
	Mechanism of action unknown; exerts an inflammatory-suppressive effect
	Can produce a long-sustained remission when treatment continued indefinitely
		Toxic effects:
		  Dermatitis, stomatitis, nephritis, blood dyscrasias
		Before administering, shake the vial vigorously
		Administer deep intramuscularly into the ventrogluteal area to avoid local irritation or necrosis of nerves, a potential lethal complication of injection

Corticosteroids
  Prednisolone
  Adrenocorticotrophic hormone
    (ACTH)

Corticosteroids used in treatment of incapacitating active rheumatoid arthritis when other conservative measures fail to control the disease	Toxic effects:
	Osteoporosis and fractures
	Gastric ulcers, organic psychosis, infection
Use of corticosteroids for long periods has wide range of adverse effects	Hirsutism, acne, moon face, abnormal fat deposition, oedema, emotional disorders, menstrual disorders
Steroids should be used with caution in small doses and for limited periods	

Intra-articular corticosteroid injections

Given when rheumatoid arthritic reaction has been suppressed and one or two joints are not responding to treatment	An inflamed joint may respond to local injection when it has failed to come under control with other general systemic measures
Given when only one or two joints affected	Joints most amenable to corticosteroid injections are ankles, knees, hips, shoulders and hands
Given to patient with extremely painful joints so he can undergo physiotherapy	
Relieves pain, benefit may last from weeks to months	

Immunosuppressive drugs
  Cyclophosphamide
  Endoxane
  Azathioprine (Imuran)

Mechanism underlying action of these drugs not known; thought to affect the production of antibodies at the cellular level	*Highly toxic:*
	Bone marrow depression, gastrointestinal ulceration
Suppress autoimmune mechanism	Skin rashes, alopecia
Used only in advanced rheumatic arthritis that is unresponsive to conventional therapy	*Reduces patient's resistance to infections*
	Patient must be monitored with weekly blood evaluation and urinalysis
These drugs have teratogenic potential	Advise patient of contraceptive measures

muscles are exercised while joints are supported by water.

b. Review *Handbook for Patients* which has specific exercise instructions. Available from: Arthritic and Rheumatism Council, 8/10 Charing Cross Road, London WC2. (Other publications are also available.)

6. Conserve energy:
   a. Pace himself when doing activities.
   b. Delegate jobs to others when possible.
   c. Avoid rushing.
   d. Organize and arrange materials, utensils and tools.
   e. Simplify all activities.
   f. Perform any activity lasting more than 10 minutes in a seated position.

7. Protect joints from further damage.
   a. Consciously maintain correct posture – pain and swelling cause one to assume a position of deformity, which makes muscles work harder.
   b. Lower himself gently into a chair, using the sidearms. Collapsing into a chair produces knee and hip joint trauma.
   c. Use an elevated chair if knee and hip joints are affected.
   d. Straighten up before walking.
   e. Avoid tension and stress on fingers and thumb joints.
   f. Avoid obesity, which places greater strain on weight-bearing joints.
   g. Use a walking stick – to reduce load and impact on diseased joint.
   h. Always use large joints to perform activities.
   i. Slide objects instead of lifting them.
   j. Respect pain – do on 'good' days, don't do on 'bad' days.

Some doctors may wish patients to wear stretch nylon gloves at night to relieve numbness and tingling of fingers.

8. Seek sexual counselling (position and techniques) if arthritic involvement is a barrier to

sexual performance. See, e.g., Sexual Personal Relationships of the Disabled, 14 Peto Place, London NW1 4DT.

9. Surgical procedures are available for relief of pain and deformity (when recommended by doctor).
   a. Osteotomy.
   b. Synovectomy.
   c. Total joint replacement (see pp. 836–40 for discussion).
10. The therapeutic programme must be maintained for a lifetime; there is no cure at this time.

Evaluation
EXPECTED OUTCOMES
1. Patient achieves relief of joint pain and stiffness; no overt evidence of joint inflammation; can move joint with ease.
2. Demonstrates increased mobility and muscle strength; ambulates without manual assistance.
3. Achieves independence in self-care activities, including transporting self outside of home environment.
4. Maintains optimal nutrition, keeping body weight between ideal and 10 per cent over ideal body weight.
5. Develops and maintains a positive self-concept, expressing feelings and socializing with family and friends.
6. Describes disease and treatment plan, adhering to plan as prescribed.

GOUT

Gout is a disease manifested by an acute inflammation of a joint; it is caused by the deposit of uric acid crystals in joints and connective tissues.
1. *Uric acid* – end-product of purine metabolism derived from both dietary sources and endogenous synthesis.
2. *Hyperuricaemia* – persistent elevation of urates in the blood usually found in gout patients. It is caused by overproduction or underexcretion of uric acid.
3. *Tophi* – deposits of urates in the tissues about the joints or on the ear; development of tophi related to duration of disease, degree of hyperuricaemia and renal function status.

TYPES OF GOUT
1. *Primary gout* – due to a genetic defect of purine metabolism; occurs most often in men over 40.
2. *Secondary gout* (an acquired disease) – hyperuri-

caemia occurs in conditions in which there is an increase in cell turnover (leukaemia, multiple myeloma, psoriasis) and in cell breakdown, or because of impaired renal excretion of uric acid. May be precipitated by prolonged ingestion of diuretic agents, aspirin, trauma, treatment of myeloproliferative diseases, alcohol.

Assessment
CLINICAL FEATURES
Acute gout
1. Sudden onset of severe pain in one or more peripheral joints – may be accompanied by intense inflammation, swelling and tenderness.
   a. First joint of great toe is susceptible; later, other joints of foot are affected.
   b. Joints of feet, ankles, knees, wrist and elbow commonly affected.
2. Fever 38.3° to 39.4°C.
3. Attacks involving the same joints tend to recur; variable lengths of time between attacks.

Chronic gout
1. Development of tophi, external (skin) and/or internal – may become ulcerated and infected.
2. Renal complications – 40 per cent of gout patients develop urate renal calculi.
3. Joint deformity.

DIAGNOSTIC EVALUATION
1. Clinical history.
2. Therapeutic response to colchicine.
3. Serial elevations of serum uric acid.
4. Identification of uric acid crystals in synovial fluid – obtained by arthrocentesis (aspiration of fluid from a joint cavity).
5. Marked increase in urinary uric acid levels.

PATIENT PROBLEMS
1. Severe pain related to joint inflammation.
2. Alteration in pattern of urinary elimination related to renal calculi.
3. Alteration in skin integrity related to tophi formation.

Planning and implementation
NURSING INTERVENTIONS
Relief of joint pain
1. Immobilize and elevate affected joint(s); encourage the patient to rest, since early ambulation may precipitate a recurrence.
2. Give colchicine *early* in attack – suppresses inflammatory manifestations of acute gout; useful

in establishing diagnosis, since it gives dramatic relief if patient has gout.

  a. An initial dose of colchicine is given and is followed by doses every one or two hours until the pain disappears and gastrointestinal symptoms develop (nausea, vomiting, abdominal cramping, diarrhoea).

  b. Colchicine produces diarrhoea – stop drug temporarily until diarrhoea subsides. Drug may be given intravenously.

  c. A maintenance dose of colchicine may be given as soon as diarrhoea stops; it is given as a prophylactic agent against recurrent gouty arthritis.

  d. Colchicine may be given before and after surgery to patients with gout – reduces the incidence of acute attacks of gouty arthritis precipitated by operative procedures.

3. Alternative forms of therapy:

  a. Phenylbutazone (Butazolidin) or oxyphen-butazone or indomethacin (Indocid) are other drugs given during the acute stage of gout – these drugs reduce the fever and have an anti-inflammatory and analgesic effect (particularly Indocid).

  b. Fenoprofen, ibuprofen (nonsteroidal anti-inflammatory agents, NSAIDs) – also effective in acute gout (see p. 854).

4. Give additional analgesic for severe pain if necessary.

Adequate urinary elimination

1. Encourage large fluid intake (at least 3,000ml/day) to maintain high urinary volume and promote urinary urate excretion.
2. Monitor intake and output.
3. Avoid foods high in purine content – sardines, anchovies, shellfish, organ meats.
4. Maintain an alkaline urine to prevent uric acid precipitation in the urinary system.

  a. Eat alkaline-ash foods, such as milk, potatoes, citrus fruits.

  b. Give sodium bicarbonate or citrate solution to maintain high urinary pH.

Skin integrity

1. Provide adequate skin hygienic measures.
2. Prevent trauma to tophaceous areas.
3. Cover draining tophi and apply topical antibiotic ointment as directed.
4. Avoid restrictive clothing around tophi.
5. Tophi may be surgically removed.

PATIENT EDUCATION

1. Take medications as prescribed for acute gouty attacks.
2. Take medications for chronic gout, even if asymptomatic, to lower uric acid level.

  a. Allopurinol (Zyloric), a xanthine oxidase inhibitor – interferes with final stages of conversion of purines to uric acid, thus inhibiting production of uric acid.

    (i) Dosage based on serum uric acid levels.

    (ii) Is drug of choice for chronic gout.

    (iii) Takes several weeks before therapeutic effect is noted.

    (iv) Side-effects – rash, bone marrow depression, gastrointestinal disturbances.

  b. Give uricosuric agents for urate-lowering therapy – acts on renal tubule to inhibit urate reabsorption and thereby increases urinary excretion of urate and lowers the serum urate level; prevents formation of new tophi and reduces size of those already present. Drug selection depends on the mechanism of hyperuricaemia.

    (i) Probenecid (Benemid). Side-effects – headache, gastrointestinal disturbances, skin rash.

    (ii) Sulphinpyrazone (Anturan). Side-effects – gastrointestinal disturbances (including peptic ulcer), skin rash, haematological side-effects.

    (iii) Give after meals or with antacids if there are gastric side-effects.

3. Avoid foods rich in purine content; avoid excessive alcohol content. Eat foods high in alkaline-ash content.
4. Maintain a high fluid intake to sustain high urinary volume – minimizes urate precipitation in urinary tract.
5. Avoid fasting (to lose weight or when on alcoholic spree) – fasting has been found to increase the serum uric acid level.
6. Avoid crash diets – rapid reduction of weight may increase the serum uric acid level; slow weight reduction reduces the serum urate level without inducing an acute attack.
7. Avoid aspirin, diuretics and other drugs that interfere with uric acid excretion.
8. Avoid or cope with stress – emotional, physical (e.g. trauma, surgery).
9. Seek medical attention and begin prompt treatment early during an acute attack. Repeated attacks lead to joint deformity and immobility.

Evaluation

EXPECTED OUTCOMES
1. Achieves relief of pain by following comfort measures and adhering to drug regimen for acute gout.
2. Maintains adequate renal function by increasing fluids – no evidence of renal calculi; adequate intake and output.
3. Prevents recurrence of attacks by avoiding certain drugs, lowering food purines, and avoiding stress.
4. Complies with treatment regimen in the absence of acute attacks.
5. Maintains skin integrity; tophi, if present, are not ulcerated or infected.
6. Describes disease stages (acute and chronic) and appropriate treatment for each stage.

SYSTEMIC LUPUS ERYTHEMATOSUS

Systemic lupus erythematosus (SLE) is a chronic, inflammatory, autoimmune disease involving multiple organ systems and producing widespread damage to connective tissues, blood vessels, serosal surfaces and mucous membranes.

Discoid lupus erythematosus (DLE) is a chronic eruption of the skin, which, although often disfiguring, does not pose a threat to life. DLE may later become systemic.

CLINICAL FEATURES
1. Aetiology is not understood – evidence indicates that immune, genetic and viral factors play a role. There is also a drug-induced form of SLE (procainamide and hydralazine are most common offenders).
2. Most frequently found in young women with signs and symptoms referable to the joints and skin.
3. Is characterized by spontaneous remissions and exacerbations.
4. Often difficult to validate diagnosis.

Assessment

CLINICAL FEATURES
(Multiple organ involvement is explained by the deposit of antigen–antibody complexes throughout the body – kidneys, skin, brain, heart and joints.)
1. Vary greatly, since they can affect any or every organ system; mimic many other diseases.
2. Arthritis and arthralgia, fever, skin rash, alopecia and involvement of serosal surfaces (pleurisy and pericarditis).
3. Skin manifestations:
   a. Malar rash, alopecia, dermal vasculitis, Raynaud's phenomenon, purpura.
   b. Facial rash with butterfly distribution over bridge of nose and malar bone prominences.
   c. Similar lesions over neck, chest, upper and lower extremities – may become pruritic and scaly.
   d. Brittleness or loss of scalp hair.
   e. Photosensitivity with rashes developing after sun exposure.
4. Generalized lymphadenopathy, anaemia, leucopenia, thrombocytopenia.
5. Long-continued low-grade fever.
6. Cardiopulmonary involvement (pericarditis, myocarditis, pleural effusion).
7. Renal involvement (proteinuria, haematuria, renal insufficiency and failure) – leading cause of death.
8. Central nervous system involvement (convulsive disorders, abnormalities in mental function and cranial nerves, depression, emotional lability, neurosis, psychosis).

DIAGNOSTIC EVALUATION
(Many laboratory abnormalities may be found.)
1. Clinically documented multisystem disease.
2. Documentation of presence of antinuclear antibodies – positive fluorescent antinuclear antibody test.
3. Tests for complement (decrease) and antibodies to DNA.
4. Erythrocyte sedimentation rate – elevated during exacerbation.
5. Tests for serum rheumatoid factor (Rose and Latex) – often elevated during exacerbation.
6. Complete blood and renal function studies.

PATIENT PROBLEMS
1. Alteration in skin and mucous membrane integrity related to rash and vascular lesions.
2. Alteration in metabolism related to fever, fatigue and anorexia.
3. Disturbance in self-image related to skin rash, fatigue or joint deformity.
4. Alteration in comfort – pain and stiffness related to joint and muscle inflammation.
5. Anticipatory grieving related to unpredictability of chronic, potentially fatal disease.
6. Self-care deficit related to fatigue, weakness, pain and joint deformity.

7. Alteration in nutrition related to anorexia, weight loss and anaemia.

If multiple organ involvement is present, additional diagnoses would be identified (e.g., alteration in urinary elimination, cardiac output, etc).

Planning and implementation

NURSING INTERVENTIONS

Skin integrity

1. Keep skin clean; avoid powders and other irritants.
2. Avoid sunlight and ultraviolet lighting by wearing a hat, sunglasses and long-sleeved clothing; use sunscreens (sun can precipitate exacerbation).
3. Topical corticosteroid creams or ointments may be prescribed for use as necessary to decrease inflammation.
4. Antimalarials (hydroxychloroquine [Plaquenil]) may be used to control skin manifestations. Patient should be examined by ophthalmologist at least twice yearly because drug may cause retinal degeneration, resulting in visual impairment.
5. Provide meticulous mouth care to prevent or care for oral and mucous lesions.

Decreased fatigue and anorexia and normal body temperature

1. Provide frequent rest periods combined with 10 to 12 hours of sleep each night.
2. Utilize principles of energy conservation (see discussion under Rheumatoid Arthritis, p. 848).
3. Give antipyretics as needed to reduce fever.

Positive self-image

1. Provide emotional support – use realistic but optimistic approach.
2. Refer to beautician for skin make-up to cover lesions.
3. Patient may require psychiatric intervention if severe depression persists.

Relief of joint pain and discomfort

1. Daily exercise regimen balanced with frequent rest periods.
2. Salicylates or nonsteroidal anti-inflammatory agents – for arthritis and arthralgia:
   a. Patient should take salicylates on a regular schedule so that adequate blood levels are maintained.
   b. See treatment of arthritis, p. 849.
3. Corticosteroids (prednisone) – used for suppressing inflammation and thus relieving severe symptoms.
   a. Observe patient carefully – may be difficult to distinguish between drug effects and those of SLE.
   b. See p. 853 for discussion of side-effects of steroids.

Psychosocial adjustment

1. Allow the patient to ventilate feelings.
2. Identify and use support systems – family, friends, etc.
3. See Positive Self-image, above.

Optimal independence in activities of daily living

See Rheumatoid Arthritis, p. 848.

Improved nutritional intake

1. Eat well-balanced meals, including foods high in iron, protein and vitamin C unless otherwise contraindicated (as in renal complications).
2. Supplemental vitamin and iron therapy may be prescribed.

PATIENT EDUCATION

1. Obtain physical and emotional rest; fatigue and depression are fairly common.
2. Eat a well-balanced diet.
3. Avoid whatever you know may aggravate the condition.
   a. Avoid sun exposure – sunlight may worsen dermal lesions and precipitate a flare-up of the disease. Use a sunscreen when exposure to sun is necessary.
   b. Avoid any drugs except those prescribed by doctor; avoid using hair sprays and hair colouring agents.
   c. Avoid taking contraceptive pills – anovulatory drugs may precipitate lupus syndrome in susceptible person.
4. Use positive coping mechanisms or seek counselling to deal with stress – emotional turmoil may precipitate a flare-up.
5. Make-up may conceal facial lesions and scarring.
6. Report to the doctor immediately any worsening of symptoms – fever, cough, skin rash, increasing joint pain, etc. SLE also compromises the ability to fight infection.
7. Report onset of new signs and symptoms that may indicate additional complications of nephritis, congestive heart failure, central nervous system involvement, etc.

8. Seek medical attention for any concurrent illness (e.g., upper respiratory infection, urinary tract infection, etc). Any illness, surgery, pregnancy, trauma may precipitate an exacerbation.
9. Observe for and report side-effects of drugs – salicylates, nonsteroidal anti-inflammatory agents, corticosteroids, immunosuppressive agents (given as last resort to decrease SLE manifestation).

Evaluation
EXPECTED OUTCOMES
1. Maintains skin integrity; no skin breakdown or scarring.
2. Achieves decreased fatigue and increased appetite; maintains body temperature within normal range.
3. Develops and maintains a positive self-concept, expressing feelings and socializing with family and friends.
4. Achieves relief of joint pain and discomfort; no overt evidence of joint inflammation.
5. Accepts the course of disease, adhering to treatment plan as prescribed.
6. Avoids stress-producing situations, thus preventing exacerbations and additional complications of SLE.
7. Maintains optimal nutrition, eating well-balanced diet; haemoglobin and haematocrit within low-normal range.
8. Achieves independence in self-care activities, including transporting self outside of home environment.
9. Describes variable course of disease and treatment regimen.

SYSTEMIC SCLEROSIS

Systemic sclerosis is a disease of unknown aetiology characterized by hardening and/or thickening of the skin (scleroderma) and fibrotic, degenerative and inflammatory changes with vascular insufficiency resulting in joint changes and dysfunction of certain internal organs (gastrointestinal tract, heart, lungs, kidneys). There are several forms of localized scleroderma.

CLINICAL FEATURES
1. Thought to be an autoimmune disease.
2. Affects women more often than men, usually between the ages of 30 and 50.
3. Has a variable course, with spontaneous remissions and exacerbations.

4. Prognosis not as good as for lupus or other connective tissue diseases.

Assessment
CLINICAL FEATURES
1. The disease usually starts insidiously on hands and face:
   a. Painless pitting oedema of fingers, hands, feet, legs, face; oedema gradually replaced by thickening and tightening of skin, which acquires a tense, wrinkle-free, bound-down appearance.
   b. Wrinkles and lines are obliterated.
   c. Skin is dry – sweat secretion over involved area is suppressed.
   d. Face appears mask-like, immobile and expressionless; mouth becomes rigid ('bird mouth').
   e. Condition spreads slowly; extremities become stiff and immobile; the fingers semiflexed, immobile and useless, and the hands claw-like.
2. Detectable clinical changes may occur in the internal organs (treated symptomatically).
   a. Heart becomes fibrotic – causing congestive heart failure, arrhythmias and conduction disturbances, angina.
   b. Oesophagus is hardened, with disruption of normal oesophageal peristalsis – gastro-oesophageal reflux, with heartburn and dysphagia.
   c. Pulmonary fibrosis/pulmonary hypertension.
   d. Intestines become hardened – digestive disturbances.
   e. Progressive renal failure may occur (leading cause of death).
   f. Variety of other disturbances develop, including Raynaud's phenomenon, arthritis and polymyositis (inflammation of skeletal muscle).
3. C-R-O-S-T syndrome is common:
   Calcinosis
   Raynaud's
   Oesophagitis
   Sclerodactyly
   Telangiectasias

PATIENT PROBLEMS
See problems of patient with lupus erythematosus, p. 856.
   In addition, the following major problems may occur:
1. Alteration in nutrition (less than body requirements) related to difficulty in swallowing from oesophagitis.

2. Alteration in skin integrity related to scleroderma.
3. Alteration in tissue perfusion related to Raynaud's phenomenon.

Planning and implementation
NURSING INTERVENTIONS
Improved nutritional intake
1. Elevate head of bed while eating and for at least one hour after eating.
2. Give antacids before or after meals and at bedtime to decrease dyspepsia.
3. Provide foods that are soft, yet form a bolus (e.g., mashed potatoes, puddings).
4. Offer well-balanced diet with supplement of protein, iron and vitamin C.
5. Provide nutritional counselling if severe bowel involvement or evidence of malabsorption is present.

Skin integrity
1. Lubricate skin with topical creams and petrolatum lubricants to prevent fissuring and ulceration.
2. Avoid soap and drying agents.
3. Monitor body temperature carefully as sweat secretion is decreased.

Optimum tissue perfusion to skin and body organs
1. Avoid exposure to cold and trauma to hand (aggravates Raynaud's phenomenon).
2. Vasoactive drugs and anti-inflammatory agents may be helpful in increasing blood flow.

See also discussion under systemic lupus erythematosus, p. 856.

Evaluation
EXPECTED OUTCOMES
1. Patient maintains optimal nutrition, keeping body weight within normal range for age and body build.
2. Avoids reflux from oesophagitis by compliance with treatment regimen.
3. Maintains skin integrity; no evidence of fissures or ulcerations from dryness.
4. Complies with health instruction to prevent exacerbation of Raynaud's phenomenon, thus increasing tissue perfusion.

OSTEOARTHRITIS (DEGENERATIVE JOINT DISEASE; ARTHROSIS)

Osteoarthritis, the most common of all joint diseases, is degeneration of the articular cartilage in the joints. It is characterized by bony spur formation at the edges of the joint surfaces and by thickening of the capsule and the synovial membrane.

UNDERLYING PRINCIPLES
1. Osteoarthritis is to be regarded essentially as a senescent process – the result of prolonged wear and tear of the joint surfaces which produce changes not only in the bony structures but also in the cartilaginous and soft tissue components of the joints.
2. The tests for rheumatoid factor are usually negative, the blood count and erythrocyte sedimentation rate are normal and systemic manifestations are absent.
3. The nature of the disease should be explained to the patient and he should be reassured that the disease is usually not progressive or incapacitating unless there is severe involvement of weight-bearing joints.

PREDISPOSING FACTORS
1. Ageing – occurs mainly in middle aged and elderly.
2. Trauma – mild or continuous irritation.
3. Obesity – places unnatural strain on joints.
4. Excessive joint use – strenuous physical labour.
5. Systemic diseases.
6. Genetic influences.
7. Anatomic abnormality; malalignment.

Assessment
CLINICAL FEATURES
1. Pain and swelling in one, two or more joints, particularly after activity.
2. Stiffness (occurs less frequently than in rheumatoid arthritis).
3. Limitation of joint motion and muscle spasm; particularly in weight-bearing and finger joints.
4. Heberden's nodes – nodular bony enlargements that occur on the distal joints of some or all of the fingers.
5. Bouchard's nodes – nodular bony enlargements that occur on the proximal joints of some or all of the fingers.
6. Crepitus – audible, grating sound produced by bony irregularities within joint.
7. Primary joints involved – hips, knees, vertebrae and fingers.

DIAGNOSTIC EVALUATION
Radiographic examination demonstrates bony hypertrophy, spur formation and cartilage disruption.

PATIENT PROBLEMS

1. Pain related to joint degeneration and muscle spasm.
2. Impaired physical mobility related to pain and limited joint movement.
3. Reduction in self-care activities (feeding, bathing/hygiene, dressing/grooming, toileting) related to pain and limited joint movement.

Planning and implementation

NURSING INTERVENTIONS

Relief of pain and discomfort

1. Give anti-inflammatory agents as prescribed when synovial inflammation is present; also used for analgesic effect.
2. Give analgesics for pain control.
3. Provide rest for involved joints – excessive use aggravates the symptoms and accelerates degeneration.
   a. Use splints, braces, cervical collars, traction, lumbosacral corsets as necessary.
   b. Have prescribed rest periods in recumbent position.
4. Advise the patient to avoid activities that precipitate pain.
5. Use heat – relieves pain, muscle spasm and stiffness and allows a more effective follow-up exercise programme.
6. Support the patient undergoing intra-articular (into the joint) injections of long-acting steroids.
7. Teach the patient to use correct posture and body mechanics.
8. Advise the patient to sleep with a rolled terry towel under the neck – for relief of cervical osteoarthritis.
9. Have the patient use crutches, braces or walking stick when indicated – to reduce weight-bearing stress on hips and knees.
   Hold stick in hand on side opposite that of involved hip/knee.
10. Encourage the use of postural exercises to correct poor posture.
11. Have the patient wear corrective shoes and metatarsal supports for foot disorders – also helps in the treatment of arthritis of the knee.
12. Stress the importance of a weight reduction programme under nursing and medical supervision – to decrease stress on weight-bearing joints.
13. Teach the patient to avoid engaging in excessive activity and unusual exercise or effort.
14. Support the patient undergoing orthopaedic surgery for unremitting pain and disabling arthritis of joints.

   a. Repair of joint-supporting structures (tendon repairs).
   b. Debridement of loose bodies (cartilage, bone, large spurs).
   c. Osteotomy to redistribute joint forces; arthrodesis (fusion of joint).
   d. Joint replacement (hip, knee, ankle, shoulder, elbow).
15. Use transcutaneous electrical nerve stimulation (TENS) as prescribed.

Increased physical mobility

1. Keep active as much as possible without causing pain; avoid activities that cause pain.
2. Use range of movement exercises to maintain joint mobility and muscle tone for joint support, to prevent capsular and tendon tightening, and to prevent deformities.
3. Avoid flexion and adduction deformities – if deformities are avoided, pain is more likely to disappear.
4. Use isometric exercises and graded exercises to improve muscle strength around the involved joint.

Optimal independence in activities of daily living

See Rheumatoid Arthritis, p. 848.

Evaluation

EXPECTED OUTCOMES

1. Patient achieves relief of joint pain.
2. Patient demonstrates increased mobility; ambulates without manual assistance.
3. Patient achieves independence in self-care activities, including transporting self outside of home environment.
4. Patient describes disease and treatment plan, adhering to plan as prescribed.

BONE TUMOURS

PATHOPHYSIOLOGY

Benign bone tumours

Osteochondroma, chondroma and osteoclastoma (benign giant cell tumours) are examples of some benign bone tumours. Malignant transformation occurs with some.

Malignant bone tumours

1. Chondrosarcoma and osteosarcoma are examples of primary malignant bone tumours. Haematogenous spread to the lung occurs.

2. Multiple myeloma is a malignant neoplasm arising from the bone marrow.

Metastatic bone tumours

Metastatic bone tumours are most frequently associated with cancers of the breast, the prostate and the lung (primary malignancy site).

Assessment

1. Assess for pain in the involved bone – from effects of tumour (destruction, erosion and expansion of bone).
   a. Generally mild to constant pain which may be worse at night or with activity.
   b. Pain will be acute with fracture.
   c. Neurological symptoms may present with nerve root compression.
2. Limitation movement and joint effusion.
3. Significant weight loss (an ominous finding).
4. Physical findings:
   a. Palpable, tender, fixed bony mass.
   b. Increase in skin temperature over mass.
   c. Venous distention.
5. Sites of occurrence – lower end of femur, upper ends of tibia and humerus.
6. Sites of metastases – lung, other bone, local recurrence, brain.

DIAGNOSTIC EVALUATION

1. X-ray will usually reveal bone tumour.
2. Bone scan – helpful in detecting initial extent of malignancy, planning therapy, defining level of amputation and following course of radiation/chemotherapy.
3. Serum alkaline phosphatase – usually increased.
4. Open biopsy of bone and permanent tissue section – to confirm suspected diagnosis.
5. Intravenous urogram and creatine clearance – to evaluate renal function.
6. Chest X-ray and lung scan – to determine if metastases are present.

PATIENT PROBLEMS

1. Alteration in comfort related to bone tumour.
2. Potential for pathological fracture related to bone tumour and immobility.
3. Alteration in emotional status related to diagnosis and treatment regimen.
4. Alteration in ability to perform self-care activities related to pathology.

Planning and implementation

NURSING INTERVENTIONS

Relief of pain

See pain (alteration in comfort) related to musculoskeletal problems, p. 797.

1. Administer pain medications 30 minutes before ambulation or other uncomfortable movement.
2. Support painful extremities on pillows.

Prevention of pathological fractures

1. Assist the patient in movement with gentleness and patience.
2. Avoid jarring the patient or bed.
3. Support joints when repositioning the patient.
4. Guard the patient to avoid falls.
5. Create a hazard-free environment.

Strengthening of coping abilities

See psychological and social problems associated with musculoskeletal problems, p. 798.

1. Create a supportive environment.
2. Utilize psychological support services as needed.

Promotion of self-care activities

1. Encourage the patient to help self.
2. Allow sufficient time for the patient to complete tasks.
3. Space activities to avoid fatigue.
4. Assist the patient as needed.

TREATMENT AND NURSING MANAGEMENT

Objective

Destroy or remove malignant tissue by the most effective method possible.

Assumption

The treatment of osteogenic sarcoma requires a multidisciplinary approach, preferably in a cancer treatment centre.

1. Surgical ablation of the tumour (requires amputation of extremity) – to achieve local control of primary lesion. Usually requires a radical approach, removing the affected bone and if possible the proximal joint. (See Nursing Management Following Amputation, p. 842.)
2. Chemotherapy – to eradicate micrometastatic lesions.
   a. Chemotherapy used in combination to achieve a greater patient response at a lower toxicity rate and to minimize potential problems of drug resistance.
   b. Chemotherapy usually started three weeks after surgical treatment.
   c. Combinations of chemotherapeutic agents

may be given in varying courses separated by rest periods.

(i) Vincristine, high dose methotrexate with citrovorum factor, Adriamycin and cyclophosphamide in various combinations.

    (a) Vincristine – given intravenously before methotrexate infusion – may promote methotrexate uptake by tumour cells.

    (b) High-dose methotrexate – given by infusion to destroy malignant cells.

    (c) Citrovorum factor – 'rescue' of the patient from methotrexate by allowing larger doses of methotrexate; prevents excess toxicity.

(ii) Or Adriamycin (antitumour antibiotic) given in high doses; may be given alone or in combination with other agents.

    (a) Nausea and vomiting may occur the day after drug administration.

    (b) Appears to have cardiotoxic effect – administration followed by ECG, serum glutamic oxaloacetic transaminase (SGOT), serum creatine phosphokinase (CPK) monitoring.

(iii) Chemotherapy may be used in combination with radiation therapy.

(iv) Or immunotherapeutic approach may be selected.

(v) Hormone therapy may be used with metastatic tumours of the breast and prostate.

(vi) Prophylactic lung irradiation may be carried out – to suppress metastases.

(vii) Thoracotomy (pulmonary resection) – for treatment of pulmonary metastases.

(viii) If pathological fracture occurs, the fracture is managed with open reduction and internal fixation or other fracture treatment method.

3. See Nursing Management of Patient Undergoing Chemotherapy, p. 1036.

a. Encourage patient who has to cope with discomfort from disagreeable toxic effects, alopecia and uncertain outcome of disease.

b. Oropharyngeal mucositis of oral membranes is a frequent severe manifestation of gastrointestinal toxicity of methotrexate.

(i) Instruct patient to cleanse mouth regularly. Cleanse mouth after eating and at bedtime.

(ii) Stomatitis with superinfection of oral membranes with *Candida albicans* – may be controlled with oral nystatin.

(iii) Bone marrow depression (leucopenia and thrombocytopenia) – may require platelet transfusion.

4. Orthopaedic surgical procedures may be carried out to implant a prosthetic replacement of the area affected by the tumour. This work is still experimental but enables the patient to retain his normal body features.

Evaluation
EXPECTED OUTCOMES

1. Achieves comfort; uses medications and/or other treatments to reduce discomfort and states increased comfort.

OSTEOPOROSIS

Osteoporosis is a state in which there is a reduction in the amount of normal bony material in the skeleton. It is characterized by generalized loss of density and tensile strength throughout the skeleton.

CAUSES

1. Postmenopausal or 'senile' osteoporosis – there is a relationship between bone loss and reduction of oestrogen levels after menopause.
2. Immobilization from injury or inactivity.
3. Nutritional disorders; malabsorption syndrome (extensive diverticulitis).
4. Endocrine disorders; Cushing's syndrome, hyperparathyroidism, large doses of steroids (secondary osteoporosis).

CLINICAL FEATURES

Majority of patients have no symptoms.

1. Back pain.
   a. Sharp, severe pain aggravated by motion – usually due to vertebral fracture.
   b. Dull ache in lower thoracic/lumbar region.
2. Tendency to kyphosis; loss of stature – postmenopausal women may lose 2–15cm) in height from vertebral compression.
3. Tendency to fractures – vertebral bodies, upper femur, humerus and distal portion of forearm.
4. Renal calculi – from hypercalcaemia.

NURSING ALERT
Osteoporotic bone fragility leads to vertebral collapse and hip fractures. It is the principal cause of fractures in the aged (as a result of minimal or questionable trauma).

DIAGNOSTIC EVALUATION

1. X-rays – show increased radiolucency of bones.
2. Bone biopsy – may be necessary to rule out malignant disease.

TREATMENT AND NURSING MANAGEMENT
Objectives
Keep the patient active.
Provide optimal nutrition.
Prevent fractures.

1. Administer short-term oestrogen therapy as directed – appears to slow progression of bone loss, relieve osteoporotic pain and provide positive calcium–phosphorus balance.
   a. Oestrogen may produce breast and endometrial hyperplasia.
   b. Oral oestrogen appears to increase risk for vascular accidents and thromboembolic disease.
   c. Oestrogens may be contraindicated in high-risk patients (e.g., strong family history or previous malignancy of breast/endometrium).
2. See that the patient understands that the diet must supply adequate vitamin D, calcium (milk, milk products) and protein – to encourage bone mineralization. Vitamin D is necessary for calcium absorption. Calcium supplementation (calcium carbonate and multivitamins; for vitamin D) may be required if dietary measures are not successful.
3. Ensure daily exercise (walking) to prevent bone demineralization.
4. For vertebral compression fractures from osteoporosis.
   a. Give analgesics as required.
   b. Provide bracing and support when needed – to allow as much activity as possible as early as possible.

PATIENT EDUCATION
Instruct the patient as follows:

1. Sleep with a bedboard under the mattress.
2. Make environment safe to prevent falls.
3. Increase muscle tone of trunk flexors and extensors by isometric exercises.
4. Keep physically active to strengthen muscles and prevent disuse atrophy and further bone demineralization.
5. Weigh periodically – indicates whether or not disease is stabilized.
6. Bend and lift correctly to avoid compression fractures of vertebral bodies.
7. Have daily outdoor activity – to provide vitamin D (sunlight) and stimulate osteoblastic cells.

8. Oestrogen replacement therapy should be considered for women with premature menopause (surgical or spontaneous) – to arrest or prevent bone loss.

OSTEITIS DEFORMANS (PAGET'S DISEASE OF BONE)

Osteitis deformans is a bone disease of unknown cause marked by excessive bone resorption (bone loss) and disordered formation of bone. Increased bone turnover and loss of normal bone architecture are characteristic. In time the involved bone becomes sclerotic and brittle.

GENERAL FACTORS

1. Bony overgrowth and deformities occur and sometimes cause pressure on soft tissue structures.
2. May develop in any part of the skeleton – usually the skull, vertebral column, pelvis or long bones.
3. Eventually produces marked hypertrophy and bowing of the long bones and irregular deformities of the flat bones.
4. Increased blood flow to affected bone(s) may lead to increased cardiac output and high-output cardiac failure.

NURSING ALERT
Osteitis deformans predisposes to spontaneous fractures and malignant bone tumours.

CLINICAL FEATURES

1. Bone pain; tenderness on pressure.
2. Bone deformity:
   a. Bowing of femur and tibia.
   b. Kyphosis – producing a decrease in height.
3. Enlargement of the skull.
4. Deafness – from pronounced thickening of skull and bony overgrowth which impinges on vital structures.

DIAGNOSTIC EVALUATION

1. Skeletal X-rays – involved bones appear to be expanded and have greater than normal density.
2. Serum alkaline phosphatase (serves as index of bone resorption) – markedly elevated.
3. 24 hour urinary hydroxyproline excretion – used to assess skeletal metabolic activity; reflects increased bone resorption.
4. Bone scan – to evaluate location and activity of disease.

TREATMENT AND NURSING MANAGEMENT

1. No particular treatment is recommended in patient without symptoms.
2. Agents used to suppress clinical manifestations (particularly bone pain):
   a. Calcitonin – a polypeptide hormone comprising 32 amino acids – retards bone resorption by decreasing the number and activity of osteoclasts.
   b. Salmon calcitonin (Calsynar) and porcine (Calcitare) is available for clinical use.
      (i) Improves or relieves bone pain and produces a fall in serum alkaline phosphatase and urinary hydroxyproline secretion (showing its effect on osteoclasts); halts progression of bone lesions.
      (ii) Nausea may be a side-effect of drug.
      (iii) Patient may be taught to give his own injection.
   c. Mithramycin (Mithracin) – cytotoxic antibiotic that appears to have a hypocalcaemic effect; reduces urinary calcium and hydroxyproline levels; gives symptomatic improvement (relief of bone pain and headaches).
      (i) Hepatic, renal and haemorrhagic toxicity associated with this drug.
      (ii) Drug is given by intravenous injection and patient is monitored for signs of toxicity by measurement of platelet counts, etc.
   d. A diphosphate, sodium etidronate (EHDP) – used in inhibiting excessive bone resorption; reduces levels of both total urinary hydroxyproline and serum alkaline phosphatase; produces remission of clinical symptoms.
3. Supportive and symptomatic treatment:
   a. Give salicylates – to combat pain; may reduce hypercalcaemia.
   b. Small fractional doses of X-ray irradiation – to relieve pain.
   c. Watch for occurrence of fractures – stress fractures occur with minimal trauma.
      (i) Fractures usually treated with internal fixation.
      (ii) Avoid immobilization – increases hazard of hypercalcaemia and stone formation.
      (iii) For temporary immobilization due to fracture, limit calcium intake and provide high fluid intake – to avoid serious hypercalcaemia and the development of renal calculi.
   d. Watch for evidence of bone sarcoma (see p. 860).

FURTHER READING

BOOKS

Apley, A.G. (1982) *Systems of Orthopaedics and Fractures*, Butterworths, London.

Bedbrook, S.L.R.G. (ed.) (1985) *Lifetime Care of the Paraplegic Patient*, Churchill Livingstone, Edinburgh.

Betts-Symonds, G. (1984) *Fractures*, Macmillan, London.

Bradley, D. (1984) *Accident and Emergency Nursing*, Baillière Tindall, Eastbourne.

Brown, P. (1981) *Basic Facts in Orthopaedics*, Blackwell, Oxford.

— (1983) *Basic Facts of Fracture*, Blackwell, Oxford.

Brunner, N. (1983) *Orthopaedic Nursing*, C.V. Mosby, London.

Crawford Adams, J. (1983) *Outline of Fractures*, Churchill Livingstone, Edinburgh.

— (1986) *Outline of Orthopaedics*, Churchill Livingstone, Edinburgh.

Curry, H. (1983) *Essentials of Rheumatology*, Pitman, London.

Duckworth, T. (1984), *Lecture Notes on Orthopaedics and Fractures*, Blackwell, Oxford.

Edwards, J. and Hughes, G. (1985) *Lecture Notes on Rheumatology*, Blackwell, Oxford.

Farrell, J. (1982) *Illustrated Guide to Orthopaedic Nursing*, Lippincott, Philadelphia.

Hughes, S. (1983) *Astons Short Textbook of Orthopaedics and Traumatology*, Hodder & Stoughton, Sevenoaks.

Julien, D. (1986) *Learning to Care on the Orthopaedic Ward*, Hodder & Stoughton, Sevenoaks.

Kennedy, J.M. (1974) *Orthopaedic Splints and Appliances*, C.V. Mosby, London.

Larson, C.B. and Gould, M. (1974) *Orthopaedic Nursing*, C.V. Mosby, London.

Miller, M. and Miller, J. (1985) *Orthopaedics and Accidents Illustrated*, Hodder & Stoughton, Sevenoaks.

Mourad, A. (1980) *Nursing Care of Adults with Orthopaedic Conditions*, Wiley, Chichester.

Piggs, S. (1986) *Rheumatology Nursing*, Wiley, Chichester.

Pinney, E. (1983) *Orthopaedic Nursing*, Baillière Tindall, Eastbourne.

Porter, R.W. (1983) *Understanding Back Pain*, Churchill Livingstone, Edinburgh.

Powell, M. (1986) *Orthopaedic Nursing and Rehabilitation*, Churchill Livingstone, Edinburgh.

Roaf, R. and Hodkinson, L.J. (1980) *Textbook of Orthopaedic Nursing*, Blackwell Scientific, Oxford.

Smith & Nephew Medical (1979) *Plaster of Paris Technique*, Smith & Nephew.

Stewart, J.D.M. (1975) *Traction and Orthopaedic Appliances*, Churchill Livingstone, Edinburgh.

Swinson, D.R. and Swinburn, W.R. (1980) *Rheumatology*, Hodder & Stoughton, Sevenoaks.

Wright, V. and Haslock, I. (1977) *Rheumatism for Nurses*, Heinemann Medical, London.

ARTICLES

Amputation

Chadwick, S.J.D. (1986) Restoring dignity and mobility in the amputee, *Geriatric Medicine*, Vol. 16, No. 7, pp. 43–6.

Chung, D. (1983) Nursing care study – a move towards the end (leg amputation), *Journal of District Nursing*, Vol. 1, No. 8, pp. 20–1.

Clarke-Williams, M.J. (1978) The problems of the lower limb amputee, *The Practitioner*, Vol. 220, No. 1319, pp. 703–7.

Datta, P.K. (1982) Lower limb amputations – the last resort, *Nursing Mirror*, Vol. 154, pp. 41–3.

Grandy, E.D. and Veich, G. (1984) Help the amputee stand on his own again, *Nursing*, Vol. 14, No. 7, pp. 46–9.

Hamilton, A. (1979) Upper limb amputees, *Nursing*, Vol. 1, August, pp. 232–7.

Iveson-Iveson, J. (1981) Amputation, *Nursing Mirror*, Vol. 152, No. 26, pp. 34–5.

Kerstein, M.D. *et al.* (1975) What influence does age have on rehabilitation of amputee? *Geriatrics*, Vol. 30, No. 12, pp. 67–71.

Lockstone, C. (1983) Nursing care study – a lower limb amputee, *Nursing Times*, Vol. 79, pp. 23–5.

Smith, V. (1986) Below-knee amputation, *Nursing Mirror*, Vol. 160, pp. 54–6.

Southcombe, A. (1982) Hindquarter amputation, *Nursing Times*, Vol. 78, No. 45, pp. 1889–94.

Symposium (1980) Limb replacement and limb rehabilitation, *Annals of the Royal College of Surgeons of England*, Vol. 62, pp. 87–105.

Arthritis and rheumatology

Bradlow, A. (1983) Rheumatic disease in the elderly, *Geriatric Medicine*, Vol. 13, No. 2, pp. 137–41.

Burckhardt, C.S. (1985) The impact of arthritis on quality of life, *Nursing Research*, Vol. 34, No. 1, pp. 11–16.

Charter, R.A., *et al.* (1985) The nature of arthritis pain, *British Journal of Rheumatology*, Vol. 24, No. 1, pp. 53–60.

Chesson, S. (1984) Social and emotional aspects of rheumatoid arthritis, *Nursing*, Vol. 2, No. 31, pp. 914–5.

Clinical Forum (1981) Rheumatology, *Nursing Mirror*, Vol. 153, No. 20, Supplement.

Fox, J. (1980) Revision arthroplasty of the hip, *Nursing Times*, Vol. 76, pp. 1930–3.

Hall, M.R.P. (1980) Rheumatoid arthritis: minimising the side-effects of long-term therapy, *Geriatric Medicine*, Vol. 10, No. 2, pp. 81–9.

Hart, D. and Mann, F. (1982) Acupuncture in rheumatic disorders. *Arthritis and Rheumatism Council Magazine*, Vol. 53, pp. 6–9.

Hawkes, K.L. (1984) Rheumatoid arthritis – a personal account, *Nursing*, Vol. 2, No. 31, p. 918.

Hosking, S. (1984) Rheumatoid arthritis – fundamental nursing care, *Nursing*, Vol. 2, No. 31, pp. 900–1.

LeGallez, P. (1984) Patient education and self-management, *Nursing*, Vol. 2, No. 31, pp. 916–7.

MacFarlane, A. (1985) When givers prove unkind – arthritis sufferer's personal story, *Nursing Mirror*, Vol. 161, No. 14, pp. 36–7.

MacLennan, W.J. (1985) Rheumatoid arthritis, *Geriatric Medicine*, Vol. 15, No. 4, pp. 22–8.

Back pain/problems

Howie, C. (1987) Back breaking – work takes its toll, *Health Service Journal*, Vol. 97, No. 5032, pp. 34–5.

Markham, D.E. (1979) Low back pain – its aetiology and management, *Nursing*, Vol. 1, No. 3, pp. 129–31.

McCall, J.M. (1985) Back pain – a preventive programme for nurses, *Nurse Education Today*, Vol. 5, No. 2, pp. 78–80.

Raine, G. (1984) The scale of the problem, *Mims Magazine*, 1 June, p. 11.

Rastrick, A. (1981) Nurses with back pain, *Nursing Times*, Vol. 77, No. 20, pp. 853–6.

Rogers, S. (1985) Back pain – shouldering the load, *Nursing Times*, Vol. 81, No. 3, pp. 24–9.

Ruddick, D. (1979) Osteopathy and back pain, *Nursing*, Vol. 1, No. 3, pp. 150–2.

Stubbs, D.A., Rivers, P.M., Hudson, M.P. and Worringham, M.A. (1981) Back pain research, *Nursing Times*, Vol. 77, No. 20, pp. 857–8.

Fractures

Beherens, F. and Searle, K. (1986) External fixation of the tibia, *Journal of Bone and Joint Surgery*, Vol. 68B, pp. 246–54.

Colbert, S. (1979) Fractures, *Nursing*, Vol. 1, July, pp. 174–9.

Downes, E.M. and Watson, J. (1984) Development of the iron-cored electromagnet for the treatment of non-union and delayed union, *Journal of Bone and Joint Surgery*, Vol. 66B, pp. 754–9.

Hunt, D.M. (1980) New material for the immobilization of fractures, *British Journal of Hospital Medicine*, Vol. 24, pp. 273–5.

Lewis, M. (1979) Nursing care of fractures, *Nursing*, Vol. 1, July, pp. 185–9.

Massie, S. (1980) Cast bracing of femoral shaft fractures, *Nursing Times*, Vol. 76, No. 15, pp. 630–1.

Rogers, E.C. (1979) Paralysed patients and their nursing care, *Nursing*, Vol. 1, August, pp. 207–13.

Sarmianto, A. (1974) Fracture bracing, *Clinical Orthopaedic Journal*, Vol. 102, pp. 152–8.

Silver, J.B. (1983) Immediate management of spinal injury, *British Journal of Hospital Medicine*, Vol. 29, No. 5, pp. 412–25.

Williams, J.G.P. (1979) Sports injuries, *Nursing*, Vol. 1, July, pp. 158–62.

Wytch, R. and Mitchell, C. (1986) Getting plastered, *Nursing Times*, Vol. 82, No. 36, pp. 48–50.

Musculoskeletal tumours

Kasner, K. (1983) Bone metastases, *Nursing*, Vol. 2, No. 12, pp. 346–8.

Sweetman, R. (1980) Tumours of bone and their treatment today, *British Journal of Hospital Medicine*, Vol. 24, pp. 452–6.

Thomson, L. (1979) Cancer chemotherapy, *Nursing Times*, Vol. 75, No. 33, pp. 9–12, and Vol. 75, No. 47, pp. 17–20.

14

Care of the Patient with an Ear Disorder

EAR CARE SPECIALISTS

DEFINITIONS

1. *Otologist* – a doctor who specializes in the diagnosis and treatment (medical and surgical) of problems of the ear.
2. *Audiological physician* – a medical consultant who has overall responsibility for the rehabilitation of the hearing-impaired.
3. *Hearing therapist* – an individual who, working as part of a multidisciplinary team, specializes in assessing, implementing and evaluating the rehabilitation needs of the hearing-impaired adult. This includes help with communication skills.
4. *Physiological measurement technician (audiology)* – an individual who specializes in performing audiometric and vestibular tests, and the selection and fitting of hearing aids.

5. *Otolaryngologist* – doctor who specializes in problems related to the ear, nose and throat.

PHYSIOLOGICAL PRINCIPLES OF HEARING

1. Sound waves are transformed from airborne vibrations to mechanical stimulation of endolymphatic fluid; this is accomplished by the conductive ability of the eardrum and ossicles.
2. From the oval window, bordered by the annular ligament, impulses are received by the stapes footplate from the incus, malleus and drum membrane.
3. The ratio of the small oval window to the large tympanic membrane is 1:22; this, combined with the vibratory action of the ossicles, means a great increase in force from the air to the inner ear fluids.
4. When there is a disturbance in the above relationships, the result is a loss of hearing.
5. A lag phase is normal after sound waves stimulate the oval window and before the final effect of the stimulus reaches the round window.

TYPES OF DEAFNESS

1. *Conductive deafness* – a hearing loss due to an impairment of the outer or middle ear, that is, the conducting apparatus, or both. If causative problem cannot be corrected, a hearing aid may help.
2. *Sensorineural or perceptive deafness* – a hearing loss due to a defect of the inner ear or nerve pathways, that is, the perceiving apparatus. Sensitivity to and discrimination of sounds are impaired. Hearing aids can be helpful.
3. *Mixed deafness* – a combination of the above occurring in the same ear.

Assessment

NURSING HISTORY

Most ear diseases cause some hearing loss. The nursing history should include questions designed to assess hearing levels and identify communication problems. It is possible to make a superficial assessment of the hearing ability while conversing with the patient at this time.

HEARING TESTS

TUNING FORK TESTS

1. A unique and inexpensive instrument that can differentiate between conductive and perceptive deafness (Table 14.1).
2. A 256 or 512Hz tuning fork is preferred. When a low frequency fork is used, the patient can find it difficult to determine whether the vibration is felt or heard. Too high a frequency fork can produce a sound which fades quickly.
3. By striking the fork on your knee rather than on the heel of a shoe or on a hard object, a better patient response will be obtained. (Striking fork on a hard surface will result in overtones.)

Weber test (valuable when hearing loss is unilateral)

1. Place tuning fork on the forehead so that hearing in the two ears may be compared.
2. The vibrating tuning fork is held against the midline of the skull, usually the forehead, and the patient is asked to say in which ear he hears the fork.
3. If patient indicates he hears vibrations in the middle of his head:
   a. This may be normal.
   b. This may be deafness of equal quality in both ears.
4. Variations imply hearing inequality.
   a. In conductive hearing loss, bone-conducted sounds shift to poorer ear.
   b. In sensorineural hearing loss, sounds are louder in the better ear (because patient cannot hear any better than the nerve will allow, and the nerve in the poorer ear is damaged).

Rinne test (compares hearing by bone conduction with hearing by air conduction)

1. The base of the vibrating tuning fork is held on the mastoid process of the ear being tested until the patient indicates he can no longer hear it (bone conduction). It is then immediately removed and held close to the auditory canal (air conduction).
2. The patient is asked where he heard the sound better or longer.

AUDIOMETRY

Pure tone audiometry

See Figures 14.1 and 14.2.
1. The sound stimulus consists of a pure tone (a note of one frequency) (See p. 870).
2. Decibel (dB) – the unit of measurement of loudness or sound intensity.
3. The louder the tone required before the patient hears it, the greater the hearing loss.
4. The test is performed in a soundproof room.
5. The patient is asked to put on earphones and to signal:

Table 14.1 Comparison of tuning fork tests

Ear condition	Weber test	Rinne test
Normal, no hearing loss	No shifting of sounds laterally	Sound perceived longer by *air* conduction
Conductive loss	Shifting of sounds to poorer ear	Sound perceived as long or longer by *bone* conduction
Sensorineural loss	Shifting of sounds to better ear	Sound perceived longer by *air* conduction

a. When he hears the tone, and
b. When the tone disappears. (One ear is tested at a time.)
6. Air conduction is measured by applying tone directly to external auditory opening.
7. Bone conduction is measured when stimulus is applied directly to the mastoid process.

Evaluation

1. 20dB is considered the lower limit of normal. A young adult with normal hearing has a loss of 0dB.
2. In conductive deafness the hearing is better by bone conduction than air conduction (an air-borne gap) (see Figure 14.1).
3. In sensorineural deafness the hearing loss by air conduction closely follows the loss by bone conduction (see Figure 14.2). Acoustic trauma characteristically causes a maximum loss at 4kHz (4,000Hz).

Speech audiometry

1. The spoken word is used to test hearing.
2. The words or sentences used should contain all the vowels and consonants of normal speech.
3. The test is performed in a soundproof room.
4. A number of phonetically balanced words are played from a tape at known loudness levels.
5. The patient repeats the words as he hears them and a graph is plotted from his score.

Evaluation

1. In conductive deafness the patient can hear at least 50 per cent of the words correctly if the sound is sufficiently loud (100 per cent may be achieved at 65dB).
2. In sensorineural deafness speech discrimination is reduced as amplification increases beyond 90dB. Usually, an intensity of about 75dB is needed before 50 per cent is scored.

Impedance audiometry (tympanometry)

1. This is an objective test, the patient does not need to indicate his response!
2. A low-frequency tone is introduced into the external canal via a probe which makes a seal in the canal.
3. Attached to the probe is a pump which can alter the air pressure in the canal and so change the stiffness of the ear drum.
4. The amount of sound reflected by the ear drum and middle ear structures (their resistance to the sound) is measured automatically via equipment

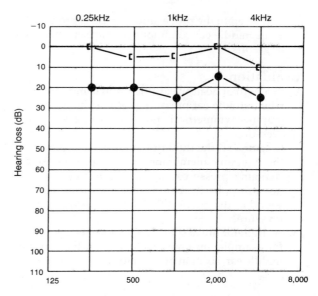

Figure 14.1. An audiogram with reduced air conduction (AC) levels (at least 15dB poorer than bone conduction (BC) levels) and essentially normal bone conduction levels is said to represent a conductive hearing loss: (AC) ●–●; (BC) [–[(from Goodhill, V. (1979) *Ear Diseases, Deafness and Dizziness*, Harper & Row, New York)

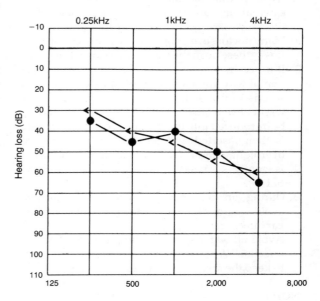

Figure 14.2. When AC = BC ± 10db, the audiogram is reported to represent a sensorineural hearing loss: (AC) ●–●; (BC) <–< (from Goodhill, V. (1979) *Ear Diseases, Deafness and Dizziness*, Harper & Row, New York)

connected to the probe, and a graph is produced. Some middle ear conditions produce characteristic graphs.

Evaluation

1. In a normal healthy ear, the drum is most mobile when middle ear pressure is atmospheric, so the graph is symmetrical and there is a peak at zero pressure.
2. In 'glue ear' the fluid in the middle ear prevents the tympanic membrane moving in response to changing pressures and middle ear pressure is not atmospheric; there is increased resistance to sound so the graph is flat and can show negative pressure.
3. A large amount of sound being reflected suggests, for example, an immobile eardrum, fluid in the middle ear, fixation of the stapes.

PATIENT EDUCATION

HYGIENE

1. Avoid putting matches, toothpicks, etc, into the external auditory canal (danger of possible infection and damage to the ear canal and drum). Many doctors even object to the use of cotton-bud tips as these push the wax further down the canal.
2. If it becomes necessary to remove an accumulation of wax, the most effective and least harmful way is to use sodium bicarbonate ear drops or warm olive oil drops. These preparations should be introduced into the meatus, a cotton wool plug is then inserted and left for several hours or overnight. After three nights of treatment the ear is gently syringed with warm water (see pp. 871–3).
3. During an upper respiratory tract infection, avoid vigorous blowing of the nose, since middle ear infection can result.
4. Avoid all water sports in the presence of an ear infection. When bathing or washing the hair, try to keep the area dry and use an ear plug.

NOISE

1. Excess noise is detrimental to health and decreases work efficiency; conversely, elimination of noise or substitution of pleasant, soft music increases work efficiency.

2. The decibel (dB) is the unit of measurement of sound intensity.
   a. Leaves rustling in a breeze – 10dB.
   b. Quiet room – 40dB.
   c. Ordinary conversation – 50dB.
   d. Heavy traffic – 80dB.
3. Frequency – number of sound waves emanating from a source per second. This is described as hertz (Hz) or cycles per second.
4. Pitch is related to frequency:
   a. For example – 100Hz is low pitch; 10,000Hz is high pitch.
   b. A healthy young adult can distinguish frequencies from 16 to 20,000Hz.
   c. Frequencies significant for speech range from 500 to 2,000Hz.
5. Health implications:
   a. Individuals react differently to noise.
   b. The noise level in the home should not exceed 35–40dB.
   c. Very loud electrical music can damage hearing.
   d. Employers are legally obliged to provide adequate suppression, protection and instruction if their workforce is exposed to noise. Noise levels should be measured, and exposed personnel must wear some form of ear defender (plugs or muffs) and be exposed for as short a time as is possible.
   e. Noise-induced hearing loss is a recognized industrial disease in certain occupations.
   f. Profound deafness can result from a single exposure to a very loud noise, e.g. bomb blast.

PROBLEMS AFFECTING THE EXTERNAL EAR

OTITIS EXTERNA (INFLAMMATION OF THE EXTERNAL EAR)

Assessment
CAUSES

1. Bacterial infection, e.g. furunculosis (boil), which may be due to scratching.
2. Fungal infection (likely in repeated use of antibiotic drops for discharge from the middle ear).
3. Non-infective (allergic) dermatitis, e.g. due to jewellery, shampoo.

CLINICAL FEATURES (DEPEND ON CAUSE)
1. Pain – moving or even touching the auricle intensifies pain.
2. Tissues may be oedematous.
3. Discharge (otorrhoea).
4. Intense itching.
5. Reduced hearing.

Planning and implementation
TREATMENT AND NURSING INTERVENTIONS
1. Administer an analgesic for pain.
2. Apply heat for comfort.
3. Instil ear drops for anti-inflammatory (steroid) and/or anti-infection (antibiotic) effect if prescribed.
4. Caution patient to avoid showering or swimming until infection is cleared.
5. Warn the patient if the preparation stains clothing or linen.
6. Whenever possible, an aural swab is taken for culture and sensitivity.
7. Advise patient on correct measures to maintain ear health and hygiene.
8. Maintain good communication.

Evaluation
EXPECTED OUTCOMES
1. Patient remains free from pain, discharge, itching and oedema. Previous level of hearing is regained.
2. The patient indicates an awareness of how to avoid recurrence, and shows knowledge of good ear health and hygiene practices.

CERUMEN IN EAR CANAL

1. Accumulated earwax does *not* have to be removed unless it becomes impacted and causes a problem.
2. To irrigate ear canal, see Guidelines, below.

FOREIGN BODIES IN EXTERNAL CANAL

1. Usually self-inserted by young child, or mentally handicapped person.
2. Insects: treat by instilling olive oil-drops to smother insect, which then will float out.
3. Vegetable foreign bodies (peas):
   a. Irrigation is contraindicated because vegetable matter absorbs water, which would further wedge foreign body in ear canal.
   b. Unskilled people should not attempt to remove foreign body because:
      (i) It may be forced into bony portion of the canal.
      (ii) The canal skin may be perforated.
      (iii) The eardrum may be perforated.
   c. Removal should be done skilfully with instruments by a medical officer; if the patient is very young, general anaesthesia is required.

GUIDELINES: IRRIGATING THE EXTERNAL AUDITORY CANAL

PURPOSES
1. Facilitate removal of cerumen or foreign bodies.
2. Remove discharge from the canal (rare).

NURSING ALERT
The procedure should be prescribed by a doctor. Ask the patient if he has a history of ear discharge, disease or surgery, or if he has ever has a perforation or other complications from a previous ear irrigation. If the reply is affirmative, check with the doctor before proceeding with the irrigation. This is usually only performed by a trained nurse.

EQUIPMENT AND SOLUTIONS

See Figure 14.3.

Type and amount of solution required, e.g. solution sodium bicarbonate (4–5g/100ml), normal saline or tapwater.

Tray containing:

Protective towels.

Cotton-wool balls and cotton applicators

Bowl containing solution

Lotion thermometer

Otoscope

Metal ear syringe or irrigating container with rubber syringe, e.g. Higginson's

Paper bag for disposable cotton

Kidney dish or container to catch the return flow of solution

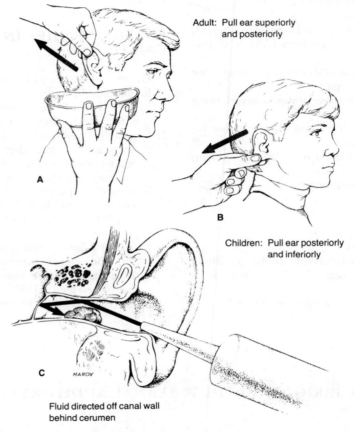

Adult: Pull ear superiorly and posteriorly

Children: Pull ear posteriorly and inferiorly

Fluid directed off canal wall behind cerumen

Figure 14.3. Ear irrigation. (A) The external auditory canal in the adult can best be exposed by pulling the earlobe upwards and backwards. (B) The same exposure can be achieved in the child by gently pulling the auricle of the ear downwards and backwards. (C) An enlarged diagram showing the direction of the irrigating fluid against the side of the canal. Note: This is more effective in dislodging cerumen than if the flow of solution were to be directed straight into the canal.

PROCEDURE

Preparatory phase

1. After explaining procedure to patient, place him in appropriate position, i.e. sitting or lying with head tilted towards affected ear.
2. Place protective towelling over shoulder.

Performance phase

Nursing action

Rationale

1. Use a cotton-wool applicator to remove any discharge on outer ear.

To prevent carrying discharge deeper into canal.

2. Place kidney dish close to the patient's head and under the ear.

To provide a receptacle to receive irrigating solution.

3. Test temperature of solution with the lotion thermometer. Should be 38°C.

More comfortable for patient; solutions that are hot or cold are most uncomfortable and may initiate a feeling of dizziness.

4. Use otoscope to ascertain whether impaction is due to a foreign hygroscopic (attracts or absorbs moisture) body before proceeding.

If water contacts such a substance, it may cause it to swell and produce intense pain.

5. Gently pull the outer ear upwards and backwards (adult); downwards and backwards (child).

To straighten ear canal.

6. Place tip of syringe or irrigating catheter at opening of ear; gently direct stream of fluid against sides of posterior/superior wall of the canal.

To permit direction for inflow and outflow; if stream is directed forcefully against eardrum, it is possible to rupture it.

7. Observe for signs of pain or dizziness.

If they occur, discontinue treatment.

8. Procedure should be complete within 10 minutes.

Failure indicates wax or foreign body so impacted that other measures are necessary.

Follow-up phase

1. Dry external ear with cotton-wool applicator.
2. Remove soiled towels, etc. and make patient comfortable.
3. Record: time of irrigation, type and amount of solution used, nature of return flow, effect of treatment.
4. Escort patient back to the doctor so that the ear can be re-examined:
   a. If the wax has been removed the eardrum can now be clearly seen.
   b. If the wax remains, ear drops, such as sodium bicarbonate, will be prescribed for several days to soften and loosen the wax before re-irrigation is attempted. If a foreign body remains, removal may be attempted by the medical officer using the microscope and suction apparatus.

PROBLEMS AFFECTING THE MIDDLE EAR

ACUTE SUPPURATIVE OTITIS MEDIA

Acute suppurative otitis media is an inflammation of the middle ear caused by the entrance of pathogenic organisms. Normally the middle ear is sterile in its environs. Commoner in children than in adults.

AETIOLOGY
Due to infection: haemolytic *Streptococcus*, *Pneumococcus*, *Staphylococcus*, influenza bacillus.

MODE OF ENTRY
1. Eustachian tube – ascending infection during an upper respiratory tract infection.
2. Auditory canal – if drum is perforated.

3. Rarely, following a fracture of the skull, or blood-borne.

Assessment

CLINICAL FEATURES

1. Variable – may be mild or severe.
2. Pain is usually the first symptom – may be in and around the ear and it may be intense. May be relieved by spontaneous perforation of the drum or by myringotomy.
3. Fever – may be caused by a virus; in some patients temperature may rise to 40.0–40.6°C.
4. Headache, difficulty hearing, tinnitus, anorexia, nausea and vomiting.
5. If the tympanic membrane has ruptured – otorrhoea (discharge).
6. Most sufferers are nursed at home. Adequate information must be given to parents or other carers.

Planning and implementation

TREATMENT AND NURSING MANAGEMENT

1. Varies with virulence of bacteria, efficiency of therapy and resistance of patient.
2. Usually the drug of choice is penicillin (by injection if necessary) or amoxycillin unless the patient is allergic to it, in which case erythromycin is used. It is essential that the full course is taken (stress this point when giving instructions).
3. Analgesia and local heat are comfort measures which may permit patient to rest more comfortably if pain is a problem. (Sedation is usually avoided, for it may interfere with the early detection of intracranial complications.)
4. If the disease is at an early stage, some doctors believe the most effective therapy is to administer decongestants via nasal drops or by mouth. The patient is also asked to yawn frequently and swallowing is encouraged by giving some boiled sweets to suck (remembering oral health). These measures all help to reopen the blocked Eustachian tube.
5. If there is otorrhoea then aural toilet, with cotton-wool-dressed applicators, is necessary three to four times daily to remove the discharge from the canal and external ear.
6. *Myringotomy* – an incision made into the posterior inferior aspect of the tympanic membrane (to relieve pressure and drain pus from the middle ear infection) is rarely done.

NURSING ALERT

1. *With wide-spectrum antibiotic therapy, acute otitis media may be become subacute with continued purulent discharge.*
2. *Recognize that symptoms such as headache, slow pulse, vomiting and vertigo are significant and should be reported.*
3. *Secondary complications may involve the mastoid process or even the brain, producing meningitis or brain abscess.*

Evaluation

EXPECTED OUTCOMES

1. Relief from all local and systemic problems – otorrhoea, pain, fever, anorexia.
2. Previous hearing level is regained.
3. No evidence of secondary complications, subacute or chronic disease.
4. Complete courses of medication taken; greater knowledge of reason for disease and treatments understood by patient.

SECRETORY OTITIS MEDIA (GLUE EAR)

Fluid filling the middle ear is the commonest cause of deafness in Caucasian children. The operation (myringotomy) to remove this glue-like fluid is the commonest operation in the UK.

CAUSES

1. The cause of glue ear is unknown. It is not certain that the 'glue' remains in the middle ear because (a) it is too thick to drain out, or (b) it cannot drain because the Eustachian tube is blocked, and this blockage is the cause of the glue accumulating. Eustachian blockage can occur if there is adenoid hypertrophy, allergy or a postnasal tumour.
2. Inadequate treatment of acute suppurative otitis media has been identified as a cause in some instances.

ALTERED PHYSIOLOGY

1. Retracted eardrum – Eustachian tube is blocked; middle ear pressure is no longer atmospheric.
2. Collection of fluid or glue in the middle ear – passage of sound waves affected.

Assessment

CLINICAL FEATURES

1. Hearing loss – usually noticed by parents or teacher. Sometimes noted at school screening audiometry.
2. Pain – seldom a feature.

DIAGNOSTIC EVALUATION

1. Eardrum – usually retracted, immobile, dull in colour.
2. Tuning fork tests – conductive hearing loss.
3. Impedance audiometry (tympanometry) – flat curve (position or shape of eardrum does not change in response to pressure changes).
4. Pure tone audiometry – a hearing loss of 30dB over the low frequencies.

Planning and implementation
MEDICAL TREATMENT

1. Aimed at re-opening the Eustachian tube by:
   a. Vasoconstricting nasal drops or sprays, e.g. ephedrine.
   b. Oral preparations, e.g. antihistamines which will shrink the nasal mucosa.
   c. Adequate information about method and frequency of taking the above.
2. Treatment of any underlying cause, e.g. allergy.

Evaluation
EXPECTED OUTCOMES

1. Eustachian tube re-opens; fluid drains out of the middle ear.
2. Hearing returns to previous level.

SURGICAL TREATMENT

1. Incision under general anaesthetic of the eardrum (myringotomy) and aspiration of fluid.
2. A small plastic grommet is inserted into the tympanic membrane. This remains patent and preserves the necessary aeration of the middle ear until the Eustachian tube re-opens.
3. The grommet is eventually extruded into the external auditory meatus after which the tympanic membrane heals, or it is removed surgically. A grommet can remain *in situ* for up to 18 months.

Nursing interventions

1. Adequate preoperative and postoperative care and preparation. This is frequently performed as a 'day case' so that time is limited. Presence of a parent is invaluable throughout stay.
2. Water should not enter the ear canal. Advise the parents that as long as the grommet remains:
   a. To protect the ear/ears with ear plugs or pieces of cotton-wool smeared with Vaseline when the child is bathing or having the hair washed.
   b. No water sports until the surgeon gives definite approval.
3. Show the parents and child a grommet (they are the people likely to find it if it is extruded).
4. Such a common condition and treatment warrants the provision of an information leaflet or booklet for the parents and child.

Evaluation
EXPECTED OUTCOMES

1. Grommet remains in place until Eustachian tube is functioning normally.
2. Hearing returns to previous level, often immediately.
3. Parents and child demonstrate knowledge of need to prevent water entering the ear canal, the need for regular attendance at outpatient clinics and are aware of good practices in relation to ear health and hygiene.

CHRONIC SUPPURATIVE OTITIS MEDIA

Chronic suppurative otitis media occurs as a result of repeated bouts of otitis media. This condition often begins in childhood and continues into adult life.

TYPES
Safe (tubo-tympanic)

1. Central perforation of the eardrum.
2. Associated with upper respiratory tract infection, e.g. sinusitis, which should be treated.
3. May be damage to the ossicles especially the incus (has a poor blood supply).
4. Not associated with serious complications.

Unsafe (attico-antral)

1. Marginal perforation.
2. Longstanding retraction of the eardrum due to Eustachian tube blockage results in the formation of cholesteatoma (keratinizing squamous epithelium). As cholesteatoma enlarges it fills the middle ear and mastoid, eroding the structures.
3. If untreated, it is likely to result in serious complications, e.g. meningitis, temporal lobe abscess.

CAUSES

1. A strain of organism which is resistant to the antibiotic used.
2. A particularly virulent strain of organism.
3. Poor management of acute suppurative otitis media.
4. Longstanding Eustachian tube dysfunction.

Assessment
CLINICAL FEATURES
Symptoms are often minimal: deafness; discharge (continuous or intermittent, usually offensive).

DIAGNOSTIC EVALUATION
1. Presence of above features, which can be seen on examination.
2. X-rays to note mastoid pathology and extent of cholesteatoma.
3. Audiometry – conductive hearing loss (sensorineural also if cochlea has been eroded).

Planning and implementation
TREATMENT AND NURSING MANAGEMENT
Medical
1. Antibiotic therapy (systemic):
   a. Often effective in simple chronic otitis media.
   b. Sometimes disappointing when certain resistant organisms are involved.
2. Aural toilet:
   a. All debris is removed using cotton-wool dressed applicators (a nursing intervention) or by a doctor using the microscope and suction.
   b. Topical applications, e.g. powder (acid boric and iodine) for excessive discharge.
   c. Teach patient self-care – how to remove debris from entrance to ear canal, apply any medication, change cotton-wool if in position at entrance to canal.

Evaluation
EXPECTED OUTCOMES
1. Patient demonstrates ability to practise self-care competently and safely.
2. Safe: discharge ceases, perforation heals, hearing levels improve in some instances.
3. Unsafe: dangerous complications avoided.
4. Incomplete resolution – surgery necessary.

Surgical
Surgery is indicated when:
1. Ear is no longer clean and dry.
2. Cholesteatoma is present (usually).
3. There is increasing deafness or discharge.
4. Complications occur or are likely to occur, e.g. facial nerve paralysis, meningitis, temporal lobe abscess.

EAR SURGERY

NURSING ALERT
1. *Performed under a general anaesthetic using the binocular operating microscope. Small operating area so a bloodless field is required – often achieved by the anaesthetist using controlled hypotension. Extra vigilance postoperatively until previous blood pressure levels reached.*
2. *Paralysis of the facial nerve (VII cranial) is a potential complication of middle and inner ear surgery. Check nerve function by asking the patient to close both eyes, wrinkle nose and smile at regular intervals. Any assymmetry to be reported at once. Paralysis of delayed onset, due to haematoma, oedema or pressure from a pack, can occur.*
3. *Advise the patient against blowing the nose, sneezing (with mouth closed), air travel, underground train travel, lifts in very high buildings after reconstructive surgery – changes in pressure can dislodge graft or prosthesis. Exact time will be given by surgeon.*

Planning and implementation
NURSING INTERVENTIONS
All of the following will not apply to every ear operation performed. An individual assessment of each patient and his response to the specific surgery performed will enable the relevant problem to be identified and care planned, implemented and evaluated accordingly.

PREOPERATIVE ASSESSMENT AND INTERVENTIONS
1. Identify problems in communication (almost all ear disease is accompanied by hearing impairment). All involved in care must be aware of any communication difficulty. Facilitate lip reading if this is used; ensure any hearing aid is in good working order. Familiarize patient with any environmental aid available in the area, for example, television aid, telephone aid, loop system. Tact and patience are essential. Ensure effective two-way communication is established and maintained.
2. Anxiety – natural response to hospitalization and surgery, made worse by communication difficulties. Sufficient detailed information and discussion about preoperative and postoperative events given. Written information can be a useful supplement to follow verbal explanations; it is not an effective substitute.

3. Local preparation to reduce infection.
   a. Hair removal depends upon position of the incision and wishes of the surgeon. Three types of incision:
      (i) Postaural – behind the pinna. Usually 2–4cm of hair needs to be removed.
      (ii) Endaural – in front of and around top of the pinna. Usually 2–4cm of hair needs to be removed.
      (iii) Endomeatal or permeatal – posterior skin of the ear canal is incised; cannot be seen externally. No hair removal required.
   b. Wash hair if necessary (and desired; will be unable to do this for at least one week after surgery).

POSTOPERATIVE INTERVENTIONS

1. Prevention of potential haemorrhage and haematoma achieved by use of a pressure dressing for 24 to 48 hours if a postaural or endaural incision has been made (a drain is seldom required). Check that dressing is neither too tight nor too loose, and check for the presence of haemorrhage.
2. 'Giddiness' due to relief of pressure when a large pressure dressing is removed is common – this dressing is best removed with the patient in bed.
3. Wound will need protecting from any spectacle arms once pressure dressing is removed – light gauze type dressing usually sufficient.
4. Ear canal and any open cavity (radical mastoidectomy) usually packed with ribbon gauze impregnated with bismuth iodoform and paraffin paste (BIPP) which may remain for several weeks – prevent contact with water and maintain cleanliness by using cotton-wool plugs, which are changed as necessary.
5. Potential vertigo, nausea and vomiting – vestibular apparatus is often temporarily disturbed by the surgery. Antiemetics and not moving the head quickly are valuable aids in reducing these side-effects. Mobilization must be gradual, and adequate supervision and support provided if a safe environment is to be maintained. Ensure adequate hydration and nutrition is maintained.
6. Pain – adequate relief of pain. Position used which will minimize pain and enhance healing (lateral position with the operated ear uppermost is usually preferred).
7. Hearing level likely to be further reduced while pack-dressing is in place – maintain good two-way communication.
8. Bilateral ear disease and hearing loss – insert any hearing aid used in unoperated ear as soon as possible.
9. Observe for possible complications:
   a. Facial nerve paralysis.
   b. Infection – operation area.
   c. Infection – spread to brain, e.g. meningitis.
10. Most people are well enough to be discharged home by the third day following surgery. Discharge advice should include the following information:
    a. Advise patient to avoid contact, for two weeks, with people (or places) where an upper respiratory tract infection may be present. If contacted, such an infection can travel to the middle ear.
    b. No water sports or return to work/school until medical approval is given.
    c. Take precautions, for example, use of cotton-wool or ear plugs to avoid water entering ear when bathing, washing hair for at least two weeks after surgery.
    d. Driving is contraindicated if there is any vertigo.
    e. Any copious, purulent, offensive or blood-stained discharge indicates the need for medical treatment.
    f. Date, place and time for suture and pack removal.
    g. Demonstrate clean technique used when changing any cotton-wool plug (supply some cotton-wool for this purpose).
    h. Complete any course of medication prescribed.

Evaluation
EXPECTED OUTCOMES
1. Safe environment maintained; mobility regained.
2. Relief from pain, vertigo and nausea achieved.
3. Hearing improved (when applicable) and good two-way communication achieved.
4. Complications, e.g. infection, haemorrhage, facial nerve paralysis, avoided or identified at the earliest opportunity and so enable effective treatment to be instigated.
5. Eradication of disease.
6. Adequate information given and absorbed by the patient to enable effective self-care to be practised following discharge.

OPERATIONS FOR CHRONIC SUPPURATIVE OTITIS MEDIA
MYRINGOPLASTY
Myringoplasty is the repair of a perforated eardrum.
1. Causes of perforation:

a. Infection (acute or chronic suppurative otitis media) is the most frequent cause of a perforated eardrum.

b. Trauma due to, for example, blast effect of high explosives, foreign objects. Most traumatic perforations heal spontaneously.

2. Conductive deafness and restrictions on taking part in water sports (increased risk of otitis media) often reasons for patient seeking surgical repair.

3. Perforation allows ease of access to middle ear by microorganisms.

4. Commonest grafting material for this operation is a piece of fascia from the temporalis muscle.

5. Postaural or endaural approach can be used. If a permeatal approach is made a separate incision (above the ear) is required to obtain the graft.

6. Advise the patient to avoid pressure change situations until the exact time given by surgeon.

OSSICULOPLASTY

Ossiculoplasty is the repair of the ossicular chain using, for example, a homograft or reshaping and repositioning the patient's own ossicles.

1. Repair is needed because:
   a. Ossicles damaged, due to:
      (i) Repeated attacks of otitis media causing erosion.
      (ii) Trauma, causing fracture or displacement.
   b. Lack of continuity in the ossicular chain – conductive deafness.

2. For this operation an endaural or permeatal incision is used.

3. Advise the patient to avoid pressure change situations until the exact time given by surgeon.

TYMPANOPLASTY

Tympanoplasty combines myringoplasty and ossiculoplasty.

1. This operation is needed when there is:
   a. Disease, trauma or surgical excision resulting in absence of all or part of eardrum and ossicular chain.
   b. Conductive deafness due to disruption of conducting apparatus.

2. The ease with which microorganisms can enter middle ear increases risk of otitis media. Water sports are not encouraged.

3. An endaural incision is likely to be used for this operation.

4. All existing disease in the ear is removed before reconstruction is carried out.

5. Advise the patient to avoid pressure change situations.

CORTICAL MASTOIDECTOMY

The air cells of the mastoid cavity are removed and a single cavity formed. The middle ear is undisturbed.

1. This operation is performed when there is:
   a. Otitis media with persistent discharge (the mastoid cells acting as a reservoir for pus).
   b. Mastoiditis with abscess formation (rare).
   c. The need to gain surgical exposure, for example, to facial nerve.
   d. Conductive deafness, perforated eardrum, depending on cause.

2. A postaural approach is usually practised. If necessary, a small drain is inserted – removed when drainage has ceased.

3. If perforation present it may heal spontaneously when the infection resolves and the wound heals.

MODIFIED RADICAL MASTOIDECTOMY

1. Performed for chronic suppurative otitis media and/or cholesteatoma.

2. Disease process is localized to the upper part of the middle ear (attic) and mastoid antrum.

3. Conductive deafness, otorrhoea (varying degrees) and perforation of eardrum are usually present.

4. Extent of tissue removed depends on extent of disease. Every effort is made to preserve as much of the eardrum and ossicles (hence hearing) as is possible.

5. An endaural or postaural approach is used.

6. The wall which divides the mastoid antrum from the posterior wall of the ear canal is removed.

7. The procedure is very similar to the attico-antrostomy operation.

RADICAL MASTOIDECTOMY

The disease is cleared from the middle ear and mastoid antrum leaving one large, smooth cavity which communicates with the external ear canal. Eardrum, malleus and incus are removed (stapes left).

1. This operation is performed for:
   a. Chronic unsafe suppurative otitis media.
   b. Diffuse cholesteatoma.
   c. Complications of chronic otitis media, for example, facial nerve paralysis, extradural abscess.
   d. Removal of malignant disease of the middle ear.

2. Effects will depend on the disease process.

3. To promote healing a graft, for example, temporalis fascia, is used to line the cavity and an antiseptic pack such as BIPP is inserted.

4. The major aim of the operation is to provide a safe ear, which is also dry. Hearing will be poor.

5. A postauricular approach is likely to be used.
6. Precautions to prevent water entering the cavity must always be practised.
7. Regular long-term follow-up for cleaning the cavity (in outpatients) is necessary.

COMBINED APPROACH TYMPANOPLASTY

1. Combines tympanoplasty with mastoidectomy.
2. An extended postauricular and permeatal incisions are likely to be used.
3. More of the ear is preserved and so the potential for reconstructing conducting mechanism and retaining function exists, and an open cavity is avoided.
4. Very careful selection and follow-up of patient is necessary – closed cavity so that recurrent infection or cholesteatoma cannot be seen.

OTOSCLEROSIS AND STAPEDECTOMY

Otosclerosis is a form of deafness caused by the formation of new spongy bone in the labyrinth, fixation of the stapes and prevention of sound transmission through the ossicles to the inner fluids.

Assessment

INCIDENCE AND CLINICAL FEATURES

1. Cause is unknown.
2. Occurs more commonly in women than men; commoner in Caucasians; both ears are usually affected.
3. Has a hereditary basis.
4. Patient presents a history of slow, progressive hearing loss with no middle ear infection. Pregnancy may cause the hearing loss to increase rapidly.
5. A frequent complaint is tinnitus.

DIAGNOSTIC EVALUATION

1. Audiometry findings substantiate hearing loss.
2. Bone conduction is much better than air condition. Reduced tuning fork transmission by air, whereas there is intensification of bone conduction sound when tuning fork handle is placed over the mastoid bone.

Planning and implementation

TREATMENT

Medical

Provision of a hearing aid and hearing therapy.

Surgical – stapedectomy

A stapedectomy involves renewing all or part of the stapes and replacing it with a prosthesis to maintain continuity of sound conduction. The defect in the oval window is closed with either a fat or vein graft.

TYPES OF PROSTHESIS

1. Stainless steel piston or wire.
2. Teflon piston.

NURSING INTERVENTIONS

1. Observe for indications of infection – fever, headache, severe pain (and vertigo if labyrinthitis is present) and for facial nerve paralysis.
2. Position patient postoperatively as desired by doctor.
   a. Some surgeons prefer that the patient be positioned with operated ear uppermost to maintain position of graft and prosthesis.
   b. Others prefer that patient be lying on operated ear to permit drainage.
   c. Still others advocate that the patient assume the most comfortable position.
3. Administer antimotion medications and sedatives if patient experiences vertigo, nystagmus or nausea.
4. Assist patient when he first tries to walk; he may feel dizzy for the first few days. He should avoid sudden head movements; mobilization is gradual to reduce vertigo.
5. Instruct patient not to blow his nose; air may be forced up the Eustachian tube and disturb the operation site.
6. No water must get into the ear until healing has taken place.
7. Administer analgesics as prescribed.
8. Advise patient that it may be weeks before full effect of surgery is determined as far as hearing is concerned. At first, hearing may be impaired because of tissue oedema, packing, etc.
9. Note that while patient may be ready for discharge in two or three days, packing is not removed until the sixth or seventh day, in the outpatient's department.
10. Instruct patient as follows:
    a. Do not play vigorous sports.
    b. Do not blow nose or go into situations where middle ear pressure is likely to change, e.g. aeroplanes, underground trains, high and rapid lifts, until the surgeon considers it safe (at least one month).
    c. Protect ears when going outdoors for the first week and avoid loud noises.

d. Avoid crowds or exposure to colds so that upper respiratory infection is prevented.

Evaluation
EXPECTED OUTCOMES
1. Relief from pain, vertigo, nausea. A safe environment maintained and total mobility achieved.
2. Hearing restored to normal.
3. Avoidance or early identification of any complications.
4. Adequate information received to enable effective self-care after discharge.

PROBLEMS AFFECTING THE INNER EAR

MÉNIÈRE'S DISEASE (ENDOLYMPHATIC HYDROPS)

Ménière's disease involves the inner ear and causes a triad of symptoms: vertigo, sensorineural hearing loss and tinnitus.

AETIOLOGY
1. Ménière's syndrome stems from labyrinthine dysfunction.
2. Suggested theories as to the cause of this syndrome:
   a. Increase in pressure of endolymph.
   b. Emotional or endocrine disturbance.
   c. Vasomotor changes causing a spasm of the internal auditory artery.

Assessment
CLINICAL FEATURES
During attack
1. Dizziness, tinnitus and reduced hearing occur on involved side.
2. Patient complains of headache, nausea, vomiting, incoordination, the room appears to spin around him.
3. Sudden movement of the head may precipitate vertigo and vomiting.
4. The most comfortable position for the patient is lying down.
5. Vertigo attacks may last several hours or all day, and leave the patient feeling miserable and exhausted.

After or between attacks
1. Patient behaves normally; may continue his work and usual daily activities.
2. Only complaint may be tinnitus or impaired hearing.

DIAGNOSTIC EVALUATION
Caloric test
1. Useful in differentiating Ménière's syndrome from intracranial lesion.
2. Fluid, which is first 7°C above body temperature, then 7°C below, is instilled into the auditory canal to stimulate the semicircular canals in the inner ear.
3. a. Normal response – nystagmus for two minutes.
   b. Ménière's disease – reduced or abnormal response.

Planning and implementation
MEDICAL TREATMENT AND NURSING INTERVENTIONS
1. Thorough explanations – patient often associates symptoms with brain damage. Adequate information and teaching to enable effective self-care by the patient. Hospitalization during an attack is rare.
2. Smoking should be avoided – nicotine is a vasoconstrictor.
3. Diuretics and low salt diet – to reduce volume of endolymph.
4. Labyrinthine sedatives, e.g. prochlorperazine – suppress vertigo attacks.
5. Vasodilating drugs, e.g. betahistine – increase cochlear blood flow.
6. Stress management, e.g. relaxation techniques taught – if related to cause.
7. During an attack:
   a. Maintain safe environment – lie patient down (bed, sofa or floor).
   b. Reduce vertigo, nausea and vomiting – sedatives, a minimum of body movements.
   c. Promote rest – minimal noise, light, interruptions.
   d. Maintain comfort – help with hygiene.
8. When attack is over, help with gradual mobilization.

SURGICAL TREATMENT
1. Surgery to the endolymphatic sac – when there is still useful hearing. Sac can be decompressed, drained or connected via a shunt to the subarachnoid space to reduce volume of endolymph.

2. Ultrasound destruction of labyrinth – some risk of cochlear damage but usually relief from vertigo is achieved.
3. Labyrinth destruction – when there is no useful hearing, and disabling vertigo. Labyrinthectomy usually gives complete relief from vertigo but the cochlea is also destroyed.

NURSING INTERVENTIONS
1. See pp. 876–7 for fuller details of actual and potential problems.
2. All of the above are performed via a postauricular incision – pressure bandage present for 24 to 48 hours postoperatively.
3. Observation for facial nerve paralysis – report any abnormality at once.
4. Mobilization assistance required – vertigo may occur.
5. Long-term vertigo – physiotherapist can teach Cooksey-Cawthorne head and neck exercises.

Evaluation
EXPECTED OUTCOMES
1. Relief from vertigo and tinnitus.
2. Preservation of existing hearing.

PRESBYCUSIS

A progressive, usually bilateral, sensorineural loss of hearing in the older individual that occurs with the ageing process.

TREATMENT
There is no effective medical or surgical treatment.

NURSING MANAGEMENT
1. Hearing aids may only serve to confuse and upset the patient. When indicated, the patient should be advised by an otologist in collaboration with a hearing therapist. A hearing therapist can be of great help in improving communication skills and quality of life.
2. Environmental aids should be considered, such as a telephone amplifier, radio and television earphone attachments, or flashing lights instead of a door or telephone bell.
3. Understanding, patience and help from family members is important.
4. 'Cupping' the hand in the back of the ear may help funnel sound toward the ear canal. See also next section.

COMMUNICATING WITH A PERSON WHO HAS A HEARING IMPAIRMENT

WHEN THE PERSON IS ABLE TO LIP-READ
1. Face the person as directly as possible when speaking.
2. Place yourself in good light so that he can see your face and mouth clearly.
3. Do not chew, smoke or have anything in your mouth when speaking.
4. Speak slowly and enunciate distinctly.
5. Provide contextual clues that will assist him in following your speech. For example, point to a tray if you are talking about the food on it.
6. To verify that he understands your message, write it for him to read. (That is, if you doubt that he is understanding you.)
7. Do not shout – distorts face and lip movements; can cause physical discomfort to patient suffering from recruitment.
8. Check that any hearing aid is working properly.

WHEN IT IS DIFFICULT UNDERSTANDING THE PERSON SPEAKING
1. Pay attention when the person speaks; his facial and physical gestures may help you understand what he is saying.
2. Exchange conversation with him where it is possible to anticipate his replies – this is particularly helpful in your initial contact with him and may help you become familiar with his speech peculiarities.
3. Anticipate context of his speech to assist in interpreting what he is saying.
4. If unable to understand him, resort to writing or include in your conversation someone who does understand him; request that he repeat that which is not understood, or write it down.
5. Practise your lip-reading skills.

INFORMATION SOURCES

Breakthrough Trust, The Link Room, Charles W. Gillett Centre, Selly Oak Colleges, Birmingham B29 6LE

British Association of the Hard of Hearing, 6 Great James Street, London WC1 3DA

British Deaf Association, 38 Victoria Place, Carlisle CA1 1HU

British Tinnitus Association, c/o Royal National Institute for the Deaf, 105 Gower Street, London WC1E 6AH *or* 9a Clairmont Gardens, Glasgow G3 7LW

DHSS, *General Guidance for Hearing Aid Users* (booklet)

Local education authorities, Many authorities make provision for sign language, lip-reading and finger-spelling instruction.

Ménière's Group, BAHOH, 7–11 Armstrong Road, London W3 7JL

National Association for Deafened People, c/o D W Calvert, 45 Broadway West, York YO1 4JN

National Deaf Children's Society, 45 Hereford Road, London W2 3DA

Royal National Institute for the Deaf, 105 Gower Street, London WC1E 6AH *or* 9a Clairmont Gardens, Glasgow G3 7LW

The Post Office, *Help for the Handicapped* (leaflet)

FURTHER READING

BOOKS

Ballantyne, J. and Martin, J.A.M. (1984) *Deafness* (4th edn), Churchill Livingstone, Edinburgh.

Bloom, F. (1978) *Our Deaf Children into the 80s*, Gresham Publications, London.

Bull, T.R. (1974). *A Colour Atlas of ENT*, Wolfe Medical Publications, London.

Innes, A.J. and Gates, N. (1985) *ENT Surgery and Disorders: With Notes on Nursing Care and Clinical Management*, Faber & Faber, London.

Lysons, K. (1984) *Hearing Impairment*, Woodhead-Faulkner, Cambridge.

Mawson, S.R. and Ludman, H. (1979) *Diseases of the Ear* (4th edn), Edward Arnold, London.

Reid, M. (1984) *Educating Hearing-Impaired Children*. Open University Press, Milton Keynes.

Royal College of Nursing (1986) *Guidelines for Nurses Working with the Hearing-Impaired in Hospital*, Royal College of Nursing, London.

Serra, A.M., Bailey, C.M. and Jackson, P. (1986) *Ear, Nose and Throat Nursing*, Blackwell Scientific Publications, Oxford.

Stokes, D. (1985) *Learning to Care on the ENT Ward*, Hodder & Stoughton, London.

Watts, W.J. (ed.) (1983) *Rehabilitation and Acquired Deafness*, Croom Helm, London.

ARTICLES

Communication

Langham-Brown, S.J. (1981) Problems of communication in patient care, *Nursing Times*, Vol. 77, No. 24, pp. 1035–7.

Cooke, J. (1986) Deafness; lip service, *Nursing Times*, Vol. 82, No. 1, p. 45.

Hanawal, A. and Troutman, K. (1984) If your patient has a hearing aid, *American Journal of Nursing*, Vol. 84, No. 7, pp. 900–1.

Jackson, J. (1986) 'Don't shout nurse!', *Geriatric Nursing*, Vol. 16, No. 3, pp. 12–13.

Meadows, E. (1981) Communication breakdown, *Nursing Mirror*, Vol. 153, No. 5, pp. 16–18.

Morgan, R.H. (1983) Breaking through the sound barrier. *Nursing 83*, Vol. 13, No. 6, pp. 24–8.

Taylor, J. (1986) What did he say, nurse? *NAT News*, Vol. 23, No. 8, pp. 14–7.

Hearing conservation and loss

Anderson, W. (1980) Sleeping giants: towards an understanding of the needs of deaf people, *Health Libraries Review*, Vol. 1, pp. 83–7.

Bull, P. (1987) Noise measurement. *Occupational Health*, Vol. 39, No. 6, pp. 192–5.

Garvey, J. (1983) The occupational health nurse and hearing conservation, *Nursing Times*, Vol. 79, No. 40, pp. 25–7.

Harris, M., Lamont, M. and Thomas, A. (1986) Hearing loss and family life, *Community Care*, 22 July, pp. 22–4.

Klein, D. (1983). Hearing impairment in children, *Nursing*, Vol. 2, No. 18, pp. 517–8.

Levene, B. (1983) Hearing loss – the invisible disability, *Nursing*, Vol. 2, No. 18, pp. 525–9.

Pedley, K. (1988) Earlier referral of adult patients with hearing loss. *Update* Vol. 36, No. 3, pp. 1837–40.

Investigations

Bellman, S. (1986) Hearing screening in infancy, *Archives of Disease in Childhood*, Vol. 61, pp. 637–8.

Hodges, M. (1983) Screening secondary school children, *Nursing Times*, Vol. 79, No. 35, pp. 53–4.

Johnson, A. (1986) Screening tests for hearing and visual impairment: how and when are they done. *Health Visitor*, Vol. 59, pp. 140–1.

Logan, S. (1988) Social services for deaf and hearing impaired clients: a review of the literature. *Health and Social Work*, Vol. 13, No. 2, pp. 106–13.

Ludman, H. (1983) Investigation of inner ear disorders, *Hospital Update*, Vol. 9, No. 1, pp. 37–8, 42, 44, 49–51.

McCormick, B. (1986) Screening for hearing impairment in the first year of life, *Midwife, Health Visitor & Community Nurse*, Vol. 22, pp. 199–202.

Moulds, A. and Maclean, D. (1987) Earache in a 6-year-old. *Update*, Vol. 34, No. 4, pp. 411–15.

Nursing care studies

Bridges, M. (1982) Extended cortical mastoidectomy and tympanoplasty for chronic otitis media (theatre nursing care study), *Nursing Times*, Vol. 78, No. 3, pp. 101–107.

Callery, P. (1981) Nursing care study – tonsillectomy, adenoidectomy and myringotomy, *Nursing Times*, Vol. 77, No. 28, pp. 1201–4.

Spence, H. (1981) The mask of deafness (nursing care study), *Nursing Times*, Vol. 77, No. 20, pp. 859–65.

Treatments and complications

Brooks, D.C. (1988) How to syringe ears. *Update*, Vol. 36, No. 1, pp. 1408–12.

Clark, W.C. *et al.* (1985) Nonsurgical management of small and intracanalicular acoustic tumors, *Neurosurgery*, Vol. 16, No. 6, pp. 801–3.

Prasad, K.S. (1984) Cardiac depression on syringing the ear. A case report, *The Journal of Laryngology and Otology*, Vol. 98, p. 1013.

Rougheen, M.J. (1983) Ear syringing, *Nursing*, Vol. 2, No. 18, pp. 530–1.

Shreeve, C. (1985) Ear wax solvents, *Nursing Mirror*, Vol. 159, No. 5, p. 33.

Windle Taylor, P.C. (1980) Superficial cerebral venous thrombosis following mastoid surgery, *The Journal of Laryngology and Otology*, Vol. 94, pp. 317–20.

Wright, A. (1985) Ménière's syndrome, *British Journal of Hospital Medicine*, Vol. 34, No. 6, pp. 366–70.

15

Care of the Patient with an Eye Disorder

EYE CARE SPECIALISTS

DEFINITIONS
Ophthalmologist or oculist
An ophthalmologist or oculist is a doctor who specializes in the investigations and treatment of eye diseases and defects, performing surgery when necessary, or prescribing other types of treatment, including spectacles.

Optician
1. A dispensing optician is a maker or seller of spectacles or optical instruments; one who makes and adjusts spectacles in accordance with the prescription of the oculist.
2. An ophthalmic optician specializes in sight testing and eye examination. He can prescribe glasses and recognize, but not treat, eye disease.

NORMAL VISION AND REFRACTIVE ERRORS

VISION
Vision is the passage of parallel rays of light from an object through the cornea, aqueous fluid, crystalline lens and vitreous body to the retina and its appreciation in the cerebral cortex.
1. Normal vision – emmetropia. Light coming from an object at a distance of 6m or more are brought to focus on the retina by the cornea and lens, without the use of accommodation (Figure 15.1).
2. Defective vision – ametropia. This is generally applied to errors of refraction.

ERRORS OF REFRACTION
Myopia – shortsightedness
Light coming from an object at a distance of 6m or more are brought to focus in front of the retina.

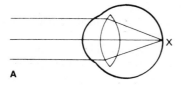
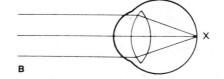

Figure 15.1. (A) Normal vision. (B) No correction necessary

Correction
Concave lenses (Figure 15.2).

Hypermetropia – longsightedness
Light coming from an object at a distance of 6m or more brought to focus on the back of the retina.

Correction
Convex lenses (Figure 15.3).

Astigmatism
Uneven curvature of the cornea, causing the patient to be unable to focus horizontal and vertical rays of light on the retina at the same time.

Correction
Cylindrical lenses.

ACCOMMODATION
In accommodation, the focusing apparatus of the eye adjusts to objects at different distances by means of increasing and decreasing the convexity of the lens – the lens has the power of accommodation; the ciliary muscle is the muscle of accommodation.

Presbyopia
Near vision is impaired. Lens loses its elasticity with advancing years. Subject cannot focus near objects on the retina (will read at arm's length).

Correction
Convex lenses for reading and close work.

EXAMINATION AND DIAGNOSTIC PROCEDURES

EXTERNAL EXAMINATION
Includes examination of eye and adnexa.

Visual acuity
Visual acuity is tested (using Snellen's test type) in all cases of eye conditions, including ophthalmic emergencies and on admission to hospital.
1. Each eye is tested separately; if patient wears glasses for distance vision, he is asked to keep them on. Note if patient is wearing contact lenses when testing vision.
2. Other eye covered by occluder.
3. Letters or objects are of a size that can be seen by normal eye at a distance of 6m from the chart.
4. Letters appear in rows and are arranged from above down, so that the normal eye can see them at distances of 60, 36, 24, 18, 12, 9, 6, 5m.

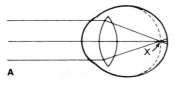
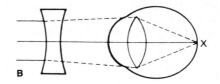

Figure 15.2. (A) Myopic eye. (B) Correction: concave lens

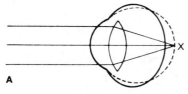
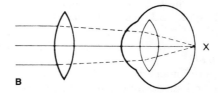

Figure 15.3. (A) Hypermetropic eye. (B) Correction: convex lens

5. When a person can identify letters of the size 6 line at 6m, his eye is said to have 6/6 vision.

6. If the letters of the size 60 cannot be read at 6m, the patient is moved towards the chart 1m at a time.

7. If the vision is less than 1/60 patient is asked to count fingers (CF) or failing this he is asked to appreciate hand movements (HM) or perceive light (PL). When this is absent, the eye is blind (NPL).

In testing the vision of a young child or adult who does not understand written English, another suitable method to use is the 'E' test. A further test is the Sheridan-Gardiner test, based on Stycar charts which are composed of nine standard Snellen's letters without serifs.

Visual fields

Performed to determine function of retina, optic nerve and optic pathways.

1. Equipment – perimeter, tangent screen, light source and test objects.

2. Fields:
   a. Peripheral – useful in detecting disorders that cause constriction of peripheral vision in one or both eyes.
      (i) Patient is seated at a perimeter with chin supported on a rest.
      (ii) Each eye is examined in turn, the other being covered by a spring occluder. The patient focuses with the unoccluded eye on a spot in the central portion of the perimeter.
      (iii) A test object (white spot) is brought in from the side at 12–15° intervals throughout 360°.
      (iv) The patient is asked to signal when he sees the test object.
      (v) The object is passed along the same meridian from the seeing to the nonseeing segment and the patient is asked to signal when it disappears.
   b. Central:
      (i) Patient is seated 1m from a black tangent screen mounted on a wall.
      (ii) Each eye is tested in turn for central vision, including the determination of blind spot and scotoma (visual field defect).

Colour vision test

Performed to determine a person's ability to perceive primary colours and shades of colour; it is particularly significant for individuals whose occupation requires normal colour perception: transportation workers, nurses, doctors, artists, interior decorators, pilots etc.

1. Equipment: Ishihara colour test plates – 32 plates in book form consisting of dots of primary colours printed on a background of similar dots in a confusion of colours.

2. Procedure:
   a. Various plates are presented to the patient at reading distance under specified illumination (usually daylight).
   b. The patterns may be numbers or a winding line which the normal eye can perceive instantly, but which are confusing to the person with a colour perception defect.

3. Outcome:
   a. Colour blindness – person unable to perceive numbers or winding lines.
   b. Red–green blindness – 8 per cent males; 0.4 per cent females.
   c. Blue–yellow blindness – rare.

Refraction

A clinical measurement of the error of focus in an eye.

In children:

1. Usually accomplished by instilling a mydriatic drop with cycloplegic effect (atropine or cyclopentolate) into the lower conjunctival sac.

2. The ciliary muscle is relaxed.

3. Accommodative power is lowered (cycloplegia).

4. The pupil is dilated (mydriasis), which facilitates the examination.

In adults:

No mydriatic/cycloplegic required.

The refractive state of the eye can be determined as follows:

1. Objectively – via retinoscopy.

2. Subjectively – trial of lenses to arrive at the best visual image.

INTERNAL EXAMINATION

Ophthalmoscopic examination

The interior of the eye is examined where a beam of light is reflected through the pupil, which is usually dilated with drops, but, if undesirable, examination can be made through the small aperture. The examiner uses either a direct or indirect ophthalmoscope.

1. Defects that may be detected:
   a. Media – cataracts, vitreous opacities.
   b. Choroid – tumours, inflammation.
   c. Retinal blood vessels – pathological changes as

in diabetes mellitus, hypertension, degeneration.
d. Retina – detachment, scars.
e. Optic disc (blindspot) – glaucous cupping.

Gonioscopy

Direct visualization of the function of the iris and cornea (angle of the anterior chamber).
1. Equipment – local anaesthetic drops, gonioscope (goniolens), slit lamp (biomicroscope). Methylcellulose (artificial tears) drops.
2. Procedure:
   a. Local anaesthetic drop instilled into the eye.
   b. The gonioscope (goniolens) is placed over the cornea, methylcellulose drops instilled between the cornea and goniolens.
   c. The patient fixes his gaze as the examiner views the anterior chamber through the slit lamp.

Tonometry

The measurement of intraocular pressure, used as one of the diagnostic criteria for glaucoma, can be determined by using the Goldmann applanation tonometer which fits on the slit lamp. This method is considered the most effective. If the patient is confined to bed, and for use in domiciliary work, then either the Perkins hand-held tonometer or the Schiøtz tonometer may be used.

Applanation tonometry

1. After instillation of local anaesthetic drops – amethocaine 1 per cent – the cornea is stained with fluorescein.
2. Record the intraocular pressure by registering the force required to flatten an area of the cornea. Average normal pressure of the eye using this method is between 11 and 18mmHg.

GUIDELINES: ASSISTING THE PATIENT UNDERGOING SCHIØTZ TONOMETRY

Schiøtz tonometry is the measuring of the intraocular pressure by means of placing a sensitive, hand-held instrument (Schiøtz tonometer; Figures 15.4 and 15.5) on the centre of the cornea. The average normal reading is 18–22mm/Hg. This procedure can be performed by a trained ophthalmic nurse or a doctor.

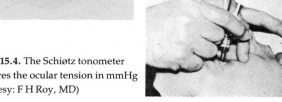

Figure 15.4. The Schiøtz tonometer measures the ocular tension in mmHg (Courtesy: F H Roy, MD)

PROCEDURE
Preparatory phase
Explain the procedure to the patient and ensure that he is comfortable and relaxed. The patient sits either in a tilt-type chair (tilted back) or lying down on examination couch, and is asked to look upward. Record results in patient's case notes.

EQUIPMENT
Patient's case notes
Schiøtz tonometer
Amethocaine drops 1 per cent
Cleansing lotion
Absorbent tissues

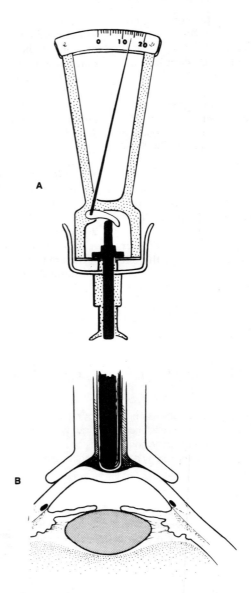

Figure 15.5. (A) Schiøtz tonometer in which the plunger (in black) measures the ease of indentation of cornea. (B) Indentation of the anaesthetized cornea by the plunger of the tonometer in order to measure ocular tension (Newell, F. W., *Ophthalmology: Principles and Concepts* (4th edn), C. V. Mosby, St Louis)

Nursing action	Rationale
1. Clean the plunger of the tonometer.	To render it clinically clean and avoid infection.
2. Amethocaine drops 1 per cent instilled in both eyes.	This will produce corneal anaesthesia within a minute.

Nursing action	Rationale
3. Place the sterile plunger of the tonometer gently on the centre of the cornea.	Pressure from the eye will be transferred to the sensitive measuring indicators.
4. Repeat for other eye.	
5. Ask patient to keep both eyes closed and with absorbent tissue wipe away any secretion.	To avoid secretions on the cheek, ensuring comfort of the patient.
6. Tell patient not to rub his eyes.	The cornea is still anaesthetized; painful abrasions can result from the natural tendency to rub the eyes due to the unusual numb sensation.
7. Record results in patient's case notes.	

GUIDELINES: INSTILLATION OF EYEDROPS

PURPOSES
1. Dilate or constrict the pupil.
2. Relieve pain and discomfort.
3. Act as an antiseptic in cleansing the eye.
4. Combat infection; to relieve inflammation.

EQUIPMENT
Patient's prescription sheet
Prescribed drops
5cm × 5cm gauze/lint squares or absorbent tissues

PROCEDURE
Preparatory phase
1. Inform the patient of the need and reason for instilling eyedrops and explain the effects to him.
2. The patient may sit in a chair with adjustable head rest, or lie down on couch or in bed with one pillow supporting his head. Whenever possible, the nurse should stand behind the patient; if this is inconvenient, then on the left or right side, as appropriate.

Nursing action	Rationale
1. Check patient's name.	For proper patient identification.
2. Check prescription sheet and drops for correct medication and strength, expiry date and clarity of drops.	To avoid medication error and prevent toxicity and irritation.
3. Check prescription sheet designating which eye requires treatment: RIGHT EYE ⎱ LEFT EYE ⎬ No abbreviations used BOTH EYES ⎰	To avoid the drops being instilled into incorrect eye.
4. Wash hands prior to instilling drops.	Good hygiene.

5. Check glass eyedropper, squeeze rubber cap to allow drops to come to the tip.	Provides an effective and safe vehicle for transmission of drops.
6. Prevent drops from flowing back into bulb end.	Loose particles of rubber may slip into medication.
7. Using a swab between forefinger and thumb, pull lower lid down gently.	To expose inner surface of lid and fornix.
8. Instruct patient to look up.	To prevent medication from going on to the sensitive cornea.
9. Instil one drop only into the centre of lower lid (lower fornix).	More than one drop at a time will overflow down patient's cheek.
10. Release eyelid and ask patient to close both eyes gently, not to squeeze them.	Closing lids allows medication to be distributed evenly over eye; squeezing would express medication.
11. Wipe excess solution with swab.	Instruct patient not to rub eye.
12. Wash hands after instilling drop.	To prevent transferring micro-organisms to self and other patients.
13. Record on patient's prescription sheet – medication, strength, which eye and time.	

Note: Eye ointments are frequently used – procedure is similar to instillation of drops. Ointment from tube is gently squeezed as a ribbon of medication along lower eyelid (from inside out) with care taken not to touch eye with end of tube. A separate applicator may be used to reduce contamination in multidose used tubes.

GUIDELINES: IRRIGATION OF THE EYE

REASONS FOR IRRIGATING
1. Irrigate chemicals or foreign bodies from the eye.
2. Remove secretions from the conjunctival sac.
3. Provide moisture on the surface of the eyes of an unconscious patient.

EQUIPMENT
1. For small amounts of solution – an eyedropper.
2. For larger amount of solution – undine or plastic beaker with prescribed solution.
3. For copious use (chemical burns) – intravenous set with sterile normal saline.
4. Receiver.

PROCEDURE
Preparatory phase
1. Verify that you have the correct patient; check chart, address patient by name.
2. The patient may sit or lie in the dorsal recumbent (supine) position.
3. Have patient tilt head towards the side of the affected eye.

Nursing action

1. Bathe eyelashes and eyelids before irrigating the conjunctiva with prescribed solution at room temperature.

2. Place a receiver on the affected side of the face to catch outflow. If possible ask the patient to hold in position.

3. Evert the lower and upper eyelids.

4. Instruct patient to look up, down and from side to side when irrigating; avoid touching any part of eye with appliance.

5. Allow irrigating fluid to flow from inner to outer canthus along conjunctival sac.

6. Use only enough force to flush secretions from conjunctiva (allow patient to hold receiver near the eye to catch fluid).

7. Occasionally have patient close his eyes.

Rationale

Any material on the lids and lashes can be removed before exposing the conjunctiva.

This involves the patient and gives him a sense of control.

The inner parts of the eyelids are less sensitive than the cornea.

To prevent injury – never touch the cornea.

This prevents the solution from flowing towards the lacrimal sac, duct and nose which would aid in transmitting infection.

Too much force may be injurious to the eye tissues. (Involve patient in his treatment).

This allows upper lid to meet lower lid with the possibility of dislodging additional particles.

Follow-up phase

Nursing action

1. Swab patient's eye (closed) and dry face with gauze or cotton wool.

2. Record type and amount of fluid used as well as its effects on the patient.

Rationale

Make patient comfortable.

EYE INJURIES (TRAUMA TO THE EYE)

PATIENT EDUCATION AND PREVENTIVE MEASURES

1. Appropriate glasses should be used for protection against very bright light, sun shining on snow, fumes of sprays or chemicals, etc.

2. Goggles should be worn if there is danger of flying gravel (power-mower lawn cutting), flying wood chips (while chopping wood), flying metal or glass particles (in machine factory); during use of laser and ultraviolet light.

3. Children should be reminded of dangers of sling shots, gun pellets, fireworks ('sparklers'), darts, arrows, etc.

4. Eyeglasses and sunglasses should have impact-resistant lenses.

5. Many schools and colleges have laws which require all students to use industrial-quality safety eye wear in workshops/laboratories.

6. Anhydrous ammonia used as agricultural fertilizer is a very destructive agent. Goggles must

be worn when handling this chemical. Sufficient water for irrigating the eye should always be present.

7. Ideally, protective lenses or goggles ought to be worn when using a hammer, mowing the lawn, etc. They are also highly recommended in various sports – hockey, tennis, hunting, etc.

8. The Health and Safety at Work Act requires people in certain occupations to wear suitable eye protection.

TREATMENT AND NURSING MANAGEMENT

1. Irrigate eye with saline solution, or universal buffer solution if chemical burns.

2. Have sterile fluorescein strips available for staining the cornea; the greenish dye facilitates detection of abrasion or ulcer.

3. Irrigate eye again with saline or prescribed solution.

4. Assist doctor in determining extent of injury; treat accordingly.

5. Encourage follow-up care.

TYPES OF EYE INJURY

Acid or alkali burns

1. Prevalence of hair sprays and other spray products have caused an increase in the incidence of chemical eye burns (chemical conjunctivitis and keratitis).

2. Acid or alkali on lids or in eye creates an emergency.

3. Action:
   a. Copiously flush the lids, conjunctivae and cornea.
      (i) Immerse patient's head in a bowl or sink filled with water.
      (ii) Flush the eye with syringe if available, or
      (iii) Hold patient's head with eye open under running water.
   b. Flush continuously for at least 15 minutes.

4. As soon as possible have a doctor see patient for further treatment.

Actinic trauma

1. Excessive sunlight (or other strong light such as a sun lamp, bright sun on snow) can cause ultra-violet-ray damage to the cornea. Welder's flash or arc eye occurs when electric arc welders or welder's mate are exposed to the ultraviolet light.

2. Damage may be superficial and resolve in 48 hours; however, punctate keratitis may develop.

3. An ophthalmologist should be consulted immediately.

4. Treatment:
   a. Reassure patient.
   b. Instil anaesthetic drops (e.g. amethocaine 1 per cent) as prescribed.
   c. Cover both eyes with eyepads.
   d. Report to ophthalmologist.

Contusions and haematoma

Injury caused by blow with blunt object:

1. Haemorrhage into orbit from trauma (black eye).

2. Bleeding into tissues of orbit produces discoloration of lids and surrounding skin, resulting in swelling.

3. The eyeball itself may have sustained injury.

4. Treatment.
   a. It is best to refer all cases to an ophthalmologist for full examination.
   b. Apply cold compresses for first 24 hours.
   c. Admission to hospital if serious injury to the eyeball.

Corneal abrasion

1. Can be detected through staining with fluorescein strips.

2. Pain can be relieved with local anaesthetic drops or by eyepad over eye for 24 to 36 hours. Local anaesthetic drops, though very useful in relieving discomfort, can mask symptoms that may otherwise be noted. In some instances they also delay the healing process of the corneal epithelium.

3. Infection prevented by application of antibiotic drops and/or ointment.

4. A firm pad and bandage are placed over the closed eye for 24 hours to promote healing. Mydriatic drops may also be used to rest the eye, i.e. Mydrilate 1 per cent.

5. Complication to be guarded against – corneal ulcer (see p. 897).

Foreign bodies

Dust particles, tiny insects, etc, frequently cause considerable discomfort to the sensitive conjunctiva and cornea.

Note: All eye emergency patients should have visual acuity checked in each eye both with and without glasses, as part of history taking and preliminary examination *prior to any* form of treatment.

GUIDELINES: REMOVING A PARTICLE FROM THE EYE (WHEN IT IS LODGED UNDERNEATH THE UPPER EYELID)

See Figure 15.6.

EQUIPMENT

Local anaesthetic drops – e.g. amethocaine 1 per cent
Saline
Corneal loupe (lens) and binocular loupe (lens)
Fluorescein strips
Cotton wool applicator sticks
Antibiotic preparation – drops/ointment

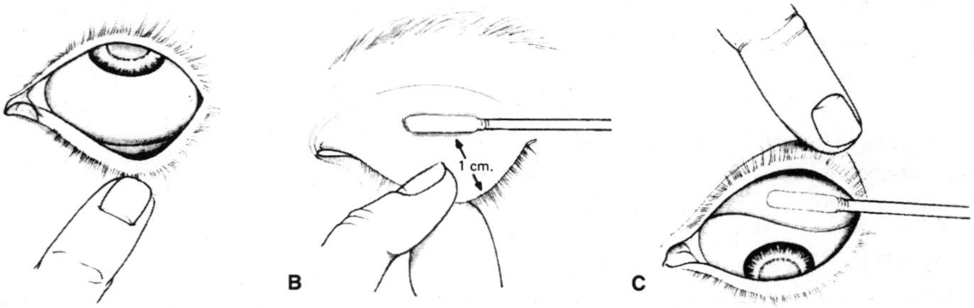

Figure 15.6. Removing a particle from the eye when it is lodged underneath the upper eyelid

PROCEDURE

Nursing action	Rationale
1. As patient looks upwards evert lower lid to expose the conjunctival sac (see Figure 15.6A).	Dust particles are often washed downwards by the upper lid.
2. With cotton applicator dipped in saline, gently attempt to remove particle.	Wipe gently across inner lid – from inside out. Use binocular loupe if necessary.
3. If offending particle cannot be seen, proceed to examine upper lid.	
4. Ask patient to look downwards while you evert the upper lid, standing behind the patient.	Serves as a safety measure since cornea is away from area of activity. Looking downwards relaxes the levator muscle which is attached to the upper border of the tarsal plate.
5. Encourage patient to relax, move slowly and reassure him that it will not hurt.	This will prevent squeezing the eyelids shut, a manoeuvre which contracts the orbicularis muscle, making eversion of lid impossible.
6. Evert by grasping upper eyelashes with fingers and place index finger of other hand on outer surface of the lid; pull lid outwards and upwards and remove finger.	Particles may be washed under the lid; visual exposure assists in detection. Eyelid will remain everted by itself.

7. With cotton applicator moistened in saline, gently remove particle (see Figure 15.6C).

NURSING ALERT

It is very important to take a history and record visual acuity. Determine what the nature of the particle is: wood? (fungus infection may result); metal? What kind – magnetic? copper? Was it a projectile? If particle cannot be seen underneath eyelids, it may have become embedded on the cornea – examine cornea using corneal loupe. If seen refer to ophthalmologist. Always stain eye with fluorescein in case the particle has caused a corneal abrasion.

GUIDELINES: REMOVING CONTACT LENSES

PURPOSE
Since contact lenses are designed to be worn while awake, if a person is injured and incapacitated due to accident, sickness or other cause, the lenses should be removed.

NURSING ALERT

1. If the injured person is unconscious or unable to remove his lenses an optician (technician) or ophthalmologist should be called.
2. If expert professional help is not available and the lenses must be removed:
   a. Determine the type of lens.
      (i) Small corneal lenses are most widely used. The diameter is less than the coloured part of the eye.
      (ii) Larger scleral lenses are worn by a few. These cover the front part of the eye.
   b. When not to remove lenses: If coloured part of the eye is not visible when opening the eyelids, await the arrival of an optician or ophthalmologist.

PROCEDURE
Preparatory phase
1. Since the patient will undoubtedly be in the recumbent position, it is acceptable to remove the lens while he is in this position.
2. Wash your hands thoroughly.

Corneal lens
Nursing action
1. For right eye, stand on right side of patient so hands will have easier access to eye.
2. Lightly place left thumb on upper eyelid; right thumb on lower eyelid close to the edge and parallel with lids (Figure 15.7A). Thumbs are placed in a leverage position on the eyelids.
3. Gently pull lids apart and observe if contact lens is visible (Figure 15.7B). If contact lens is not visible, wait for an experienced practitioner.
4. If lens is visible, it should slide with the movement of the eyelids while thumbs are still kept at the edges of the eyelids.

5. Gently open the lids wider beyond the edge of the lens and maintain this position.
6. Press gently downwards with right thumb on eyeball (Figure 15.7C). This should cause the contact lens to tip up on one edge.
7. Then slide the eyelids and thumbs together gently (Figure 15.7D). The lens should slide out between the lids, where it can be taken off.
8. FORCE SHOULD NOT BE USED! Cornea may be irreparably damaged.
9. If lens can be seen but cannot be removed, gently slide it to the white sclera.
10. For left eye, move to left side of patient and repeat.
11. Contact lens sucker may be used.

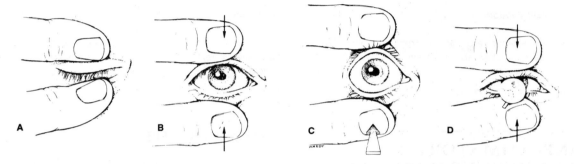

Figure 15.7. Removing corneal contact lens

Scleral lens
Nursing action
1. For right eye, stand on right side of patient.
2. Place left index finger parallel with and at the edge of the lower eyelid (Figure 15.8A).
3. Press the lid downwards and backwards until the edge of the scleral lens becomes visible (Figure 15.8B)
4. Maintain pressure but pull finger with lower lid towards the patient's right ear (Figure 15.8C). This should cause the lid to slide under the lens. Avoid force.
5. Grasp scleral lens with right finger and thumb.

Soft contact lenses
Nursing action
May be removed by gently grasping them between the fingers. This is rarely necessary, since soft contact lens may remain on the eye for many hours without harm. An ophthalmologist can be called to remove lenses if the patient is unable to do so. **Note**: If the contact lens cannot be removed with relative ease, discontinue efforts and wait for the ophthalmologist to remove them.

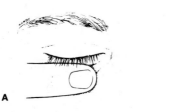 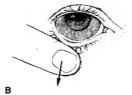 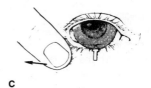

A   B   C

Figure 15.8. Removing scleral contact lens

Disposition of lenses

Nursing action

1. When lenses are found and removed, place in a case or bottle; label 'right' and 'left'.

Rationale

Since right and left lenses are often different, storing them with proper labels will be appreciated by the patient.

INFLAMMATORY CONDITIONS OF THE EYE

SUPERFICIAL LID INFECTIONS

1. *Blepharitis* – infection of eyelid margins, with crusting, redness and irritation.
2. *Hordeolum* (stye) – infection of eyelash follicle.
3. *Chalazion* – infection of a meibomian gland.

TREATMENT
Blepharitis
1. Cleanse lid margins by applying hot moist compresses three to four times daily.
2. Carefully wipe loose crusts away from lashes; apply antibiotic ointment and/or drops.

Stye
1. Remove offending eyelash.
2. Apply heat, antibiotic ointment. Continue treatment for several days until infection clears. Keep patient's hands away from eyes and wash hands after eye care.

Chalazion
Chronic chalazion may require incision and curettage.

CONJUNCTIVITIS

Conjunctivitis is an inflammation of the conjunctiva resulting from an allergy, from bacterial, viral or rickettsial infection, or from physical or chemical trauma.

CLINICAL FEATURES
1. Redness, pain/discomfort, swelling, lacrimation, photophobia.
2. Discharge, according to offending organism – abundant purulence indicates infection caused by pneumococcus or gonococcus.

TREATMENT AND NURSING MANAGEMENT
1. Conjunctival swab to determine causative organism.
2. Bathe eye with saline. If profuse discharge, irrigation may be performed.
3. Instil drops, apply ointment as prescribed – to clear infection in one to three days.
4. Prevent dissemination of infection to other eye or other persons.
   a. Wash hands before and after treatment.
   b. Restrict washcloth and towels to infected eye and change frequently.
5. Give patient dark glasses to wear (*never cover with eyepad or plastic shade*).

UVEITIS

Uveitis is inflammation of the uveal tract (iris, ciliary body, choroid).

CLASSIFICATION
1. Location:
   a. Anterior uveitis – iritis, iridocyclitis.
   b. Posterior uveitis – choroiditis, chorioretinitis.
   c. Panuveitis – entire uveal tract.
2. Granulomatous or nongranulomatous:

Details	Granulomatous	Nongranulomatous
Location:	Any part, mostly posterior	Anterior
Onset:	Insidious	Acute
Pain:	None or minimal	Marked
Circumcorneal flush:	Minimal	Present
Course:	Chronic	Acute
Prognosis:	Poor	Good

COMPLICATIONS
1. Anterior uveitis – adhesions which impede aqueous flow, leading to secondary glaucoma. May cause cataracts.
2. Posterior uveitis – adhesions impede aqueous flow from posterior to anterior uvea, causing metabolic disturbances of the lens and leading to cataracts.
3. Retinal detachment may result from traction exerted on retina by vitreous strands.

TREATMENT
1. Directed to specific type of uveitis.
2. Atropine drops – to reduce likelihood of adhesions forming between iris and lens.
3. Steroids, locally – for anti-inflammatory and antiallergic action. Steroids, systemically, occasionally.
4. Analgesic – for pain.

SYMPATHETIC OPHTHALMIA

Sympathetic ophthalmia is a severe granulomatous bilateral uveitis that may occur after any surgical or traumatic perforation involving the uveal tract. Rare, but *severe*.

CLINICAL FEATURES
Photophobia, blurring vision and injection ('bloodshot') in sympathizing eye.

TREATMENT
1. Administer corticosteroids, locally and systemically, to reduce the amount of intraocular scarring.
2. Instil atropine drops to prevent adhesions between iris and lens.
3. Possibility of preventive enucleation of originally injured eye before sympathetic ophthalmia occurs.

NURSING MANAGEMENT
1. Understand the patient's condition and the objectives desired for him by the ophthalmologist.
2. Recognize the difficult decision facing the patient if enucleation approach is suggested.
3. Assess the psychosocial implications of the individual situation, offer sustaining support and collaborate in planning immediate and long-term aims.

CORNEAL ULCER

Keratitis is an inflammation of the cornea, which when combined with a loss of substance results in corneal ulcer.

CLINICAL FEATURES
1. Pain, marked photophobia, increased lacrimation, reduced vision.
2. Injected ('bloodshot') eye.
3. When a corneal ulcer progresses deeper to involve iris, iritis develops; pus forms in the anterior chamber and collects as a white or yellow deposit (hypopyon) behind the cornea.
4. If cornea perforates, iris may prolapse through cornea.

TREATMENT AND NURSING MANAGEMENT
1. Prevention is much easier than treatment.
   a. Foreign bodies must be removed quickly.
   b. Corneal abrasions must be treated promptly.
2. Suggest the wearing of dark glasses to relieve photophobia.
3. Explain to patient that the doctor may administer mydriatics preparatory to examining the eye, may instil topical anaesthetic to relieve pain and will instil fluorescein to outline ulcer.
4. Administer antibiotic or chemotherapeutic agent as prescribed for specific type of infection.
5. Apply heat to the eye.
6. Administer systemic antibiotics when prescribed.

NURSING ALERT
Always question patient about allergies to medications, prior to treatment, whether topical or systemic drugs prescribed.

EYE DISORDERS POSSIBLY REQUIRING SURGERY

Assessment
PATIENT PROBLEMS
1. Alteration in visual sensory perception related to disease/trauma or ophthalmic postoperative condition.
2. Fear of blindness related to diminishing vision caused by trauma/disease.
3. Disturbance in self-concept related to exaggerated feeling of inadequacy because of limited vision.
4. Social isolation related to reduced contacts with people because of impaired vision.
5. Self-care deficit related to reduced vision.
6. Activity limitation related to concern because of impaired vision.
7. Lack of knowledge of physical and psychological preparation for eye surgery.
8. Potential for injury related to limited vision.

Planning and implementation
NURSING INTERVENTIONS
Reduction in anxiety
1. Recognize that dependence on sight is exaggerated when faced with possible diminution or loss of sight.
2. Observe that the concern of the patient may be manifested as fear, depression, tension, resentment, anger and even rejection.
3. Encourage the patient to express his feelings in order to determine the underlying problems.
4. Demonstrate interest, sympathy and understanding, but try not to be oversolicitous.
5. Recognize individual differences which affect the method of dealing with anxiety.
6. Reassure patient that rehabilitative programmes and personnel are available if his condition requires them.

Increase in self-care activities
1. Always orientate the new patient with diminished vision to his surroundings, his room and the people in his immediate environment.
2. Encourage the patient to care for himself so that he will be self-sufficient and not feel that he is a burden.
3. Supervise him as he attempts to feed himself so that he does not become discouraged.
4. Promote proper elimination by adequate diet, laxatives or suppositories as required.

5. Provide a rest period daily.
6. For safety reasons, discourage smoking.
7. Caution the patient against rubbing his eyes or wiping them with soiled tissue or handkerchief.
8. Maintain a safe environment that is free of obstacles such as footstools or loose rugs.
9. Doors should be completely open or closed.

Preoperative preparation
1. In preparation for general anaesthesia, evacuation of the lower bowel may be indicated with glycerine suppositories administered the night before operation.
2. Ensure patient's hair has been washed. Arrange long hair of female patient so that it may be conveniently out of the way.
3. Cut eyelashes of affected eye if ordered by doctor, using small curved blunt-ended scissors, blades covered with petroleum jelly so that lashes will adhere to them and not drop into the patient's eye.
4. Check local hospital policy regarding preoperative skin preparation; in many hospitals, this is done in the operating theatre.
5. Remove dentures, artificial eyes and any other prostheses before patient goes to the operating theatre.
6. The doctor may prescribe preoperative antibiotic eyedrops to reduce the risk of infection. An eyeswab might also be requested for culture and sensitivity.
7. Instruct the patient regarding postoperative restrictions – these will be specific for each type of surgery. Inform him he will have an eyepad, shield or both when he returns from the operating theatre.
8. Make sure the eye specified on the consent form and eye to be operated upon are the same, and marked by the doctor (skin).
9. Instil prescribed preoperative drops in the correct eye.

Postoperative recovery
1. Place the patient in the dorsal recumbent position with a pillow under his head or permit him to lie on unoperated side.
2. Position bed rails (cot sides) if policy of the hospital; this offers the patient a sense of security.
3. Place a call bell within easy reach of the patient; have him call the nurse rather than risk stress or strain in an attempt to be self-sufficient.
4. Direct anyone who enters his room to announce himself; also, let patient know when you are leaving the room. Otherwise he may be left talking to himself.

5. Avoid disturbing the patient's head with such activities as combing the hair; delay combing the hair until the patient is allowed out of bed.

NURSING ALERT
For eye patients requiring bed rest, e.g. following keratoplasty, injury, retinal detachment surgery, measures should be taken to prevent pulmonary and/or circulatory complications. This may include passive exercises, antiembolic stockings, special positioning etc.

PATIENT EDUCATION
1. Consult ophthalmologist before recommending diversional or recreational therapy that is not fatiguing to the eyes – no reading; television in moderation; radio.
2. Recognize the soothing, relaxing effect of soft pastels for the wall and ceiling colours.
3. Regulate lights so that they are not too bright and do not produce a glare.
4. Inform the patient before he leaves hospital regarding medications, eye glasses, follow-up visits, type of work he can do and when he can do it.
5. Instruct the patient or family as follows on instillation of eye medications and proper cleansing of eyes:
   a. Wash hands before and after treating eyes.
   b. To clean around the eye, use sterile, wet gauze and wipe gently across lid from inner corner to outer corner.
   c. To apply medications, pull down lower lid, have patient look up and place eye drop in middle of inside of lower lid; place ribbon of ointment along the entire length of the inside of lid (from inside to outside).
   d. Apply protective covering – eyepad or shield over the operated eye at bedtime.
6. Inform patient of large print books, talking books/tapes, records, machines and where available.
7. Initiate follow-up visits with ophthalmologist. The nurse makes the first appointment for the patient.
8. Upon discharge from hospital, check the following with patient/family:
   a. Does the patient have a return appointment date with doctor confirmed?
   b. Does he have his medications properly identified and labelled? Does he (or responsible member of family) know how to use his prescribed medication?
   c. Does the patient understand the restrictions placed on him and the reasons for them?

Evaluation
EXPECTED OUTCOMES
1. Patient demonstrates improved vision in accordance with expectations of surgery.
2. Shows no sign of infection or other postoperative complications.
3. Experiences no discomforts; does not complain of pain.
4. Manages self-care with minimum of assistance.
5. Carries walking stick/cane to prevent possible falls – with increasing age, walking unescorted may not be possible.
6. Describes precautions that must be taken as safety measures and enumerates symptoms that may occur if complications develop.
7. Appears relaxed and positive concerning outcome of surgery.

CORNEAL TRANSPLANTATION (KERATOPLASTY)

Keratoplasty is the transplantation of a donor cornea to repair corneal scarring, or deformed cornea, as in keratoconus.

TYPES OF GRAFT
1. Full thickness – most common.
2. Partial thickness – lamellar.

DONOR CORNEA
Preferably cornea of donor eyes should be used within 48 to 72 hours after donation. A procedure – cryopreservation – is sometimes used. The cornea, which is cut in the eye bank laboratory from the enucleated eye, is placed in McCarthy Kaufman medium. This preserves the cornea for up to 10 days.

PREOPERATIVE NURSING CARE
Reducing preoperative anxiety
1. Psychological preparation for surgery is simplified because the patient is usually optimistic about the immediate transplant.
2. If cultural or spiritual concerns need to be voiced by the patient, the nurse, and possibly the hospital chaplain, should be available so that the patient faces surgery in the best frame of mind possible.

POSTOPERATIVE NURSING CARE
Reducing postoperative anxiety
1. Apply eye coverings as ordered by doctor. Sometimes (rare these days) both eyes may be covered.
2. Recognize that healing is slow, due to the avascularity of the cornea.

Keeping eye pressure at safe level

This is to protect the eye from loss of aqueous fluid or from injury because of the possibility of dislocating the newly transplanted cornea.

1. Prevent sudden turning of the head.
2. Minimize those activities or sources of irritants which may cause sneezing (dusting or sweeping, heavily scented flowers, sprays) (no pepper on meal trays).
3. Avoid conversation which annoys or disturbs the patient; caution visitors not to upset the patient, since emotional disturbances may increase his intraocular pressure.
4. Instruct patient not to sleep on operated side.

Recognize the differences between care requirements of the patient having a full thickness corneal or a lamellar transplant

1. Full thickness type:
   a. May need longer bed rest.
   b. Restrict the patient's activities according to doctor's specifications: the patient may be bathed and provided with bedpan/commode.
   c. Allow patient to raise his head slightly towards unoperated side.
   d. Initiate passive range of motion activities and deep breathing exercises to prevent circulatory and pulmonary complications.
2. Lamellar type:
   a. With doctor's sanction, help the patient out of bed and into chair.
   b. Keep the patient's eye covered according to doctor's orders.

Preventing complications

1. Avoid urinary retention by providing adequate fluids.
2. Prevent constipation or straining during defaecation by avoiding constipating foods and maintaining adequate hydration.
3. Administer analgesics as necessary to relieve pain.
4. Report unrelieved pain since it may indicate that graft has slipped, that haemorrhage is occurring (hyphaema), or possible early infection, inflammation or postoperative (secondary) glaucoma.
5. Introduce additional activities gradually each day, but continue to avoid those which require straining.
6. Emphasize the importance of follow-up visits to ophthalmologist.

NURSING ALERT

For eye patients requiring bed rest, e.g. following keratoplasty, injury, retinal detachment surgery, measures should be taken to prevent pulmonary and/or circulatory complications. This may include passive range of motion activities, antiembolic stockings, special positioning.

DETACHED RETINA

Retinal detachment is the detachment of the sensory retina from the pigment epithelium of the retina.

ALTERED PHYSIOLOGY

1. The retina perceives light and transmits impulses from its nerve cells to the optic nerve.
2. Tears or holes in the retina may result rapidly from trauma, highly myopic subjects, systemic and metabolic conditions, degenerative process (e.g. macular degeneration).
3. A tear in the retina allows vitreous and transudate from choroid vessels to seep behind the retina and separate it from the pigment epithelium.

CLINICAL FEATURES

1. Patient complains of flashes of light or blurred vision due to stimulation of the retina by vitreous pull.
2. He notes sensation of particles moving in his line of vision (normally most individuals can see floating filaments when looking at a light background).
3. Delineated areas of vision may be blank (a relative scotoma); there is no perception of pain.
4. A sensation of a veil-like coating coming down, coming up, or sideways in front of the eye may be present.
   a. This veil-like coating or shadow, is often misinterpreted as a drooping eyelid or elevated cheek.
   b. Straight-ahead vision (central vision) may remain good in early stages.
5. Unless the retinal holes are sealed, the retina will progressively detach and ultimately there is a loss of central vision as well as peripheral vision.
6. Retinal detachments do not cure themselves; they must be corrected surgically.

DIAGNOSTIC EVALUATION

The diagnosis is confirmed by the patient's history and binocular ophthalmoscopy.

TREATMENT
Surgical intervention
Goal: To seal the retinal hole, thereby ensuring that the retina will adhere to the retinal pigment epithelium.

Types of surgery
1. Electrodiathermy – the passing of an electrode needle through the sclera to allow subretinal fluid to escape. An exudate forms from the pigment epithelium, adhering it to the retina.
2. Cryosurgery or retinal cryopexy – a supercooled probe is touched to the sclera, causing minimal damage; as a result of scarring, the pigment epithelium adheres to the retina.
3. Photocoagulation – a light beam (either laser or xenon arc) is passed through the dilated pupil, causing a small burn and producing an exudate between the pigment epithelium and retina.
4. Scleral buckling – a technique whereby the sclera is shortened to allow a buckling to occur which forces the pigment epithelium closer to the retina by implanting a silicone plombe or encircling band.
5. Insertion of SFG – gas sulphahexafluoride or silicone oil (internal tamponade) – both used to maintain internal retinochoroidal apposition.

Prognosis
1. Untreated, incomplete retinal detachment progresses to complete retinal detachment and legal blindness in that eye.
2. Surgical re-attachment by surgical intervention is completely successful in approximately 75 per cent of cases. Secondary operations are usually required.
3. Return of visual acuity with a re-attached retina depends on:
   a. Amount of retina detached prior to surgery.
   b. Whether the macula was detached.
   c. Length of time the retina was detached.
   d. Amount of external distortion caused by scleral buckling.
   e. Possible macular damage as a result of diathermy or cryocoagulation.
4. Retinal tears that may lead to retinal detachment may be present in the other eye. These often require surgical treatment by cryocoagulation, photocoagulation or scleral buckling.
5. Two possible complications to watch for and guard against are glaucoma and infection.

NURSING INTERVENTIONS
Preoperative care
1. Recognize the significance of emotional care during this time of stress and restriction.
2. Instruct the patient to remain quiet to prevent further detachment of the retina.
3. Explain what is to be expected before and after the operation. Tell the patient:
   a. That the eyelids and surrounding area may be swollen and bruised.
   b. That he may have an eye covering after the operation.
4. Administer sedation and tranquillizing drug for comfort and relief of anxiety.

Postoperative care
1. Positioning may be prescribed after the operation according to individual need, as prescribed by the surgeon. Usually the patient is permitted out of bed.
2. Take precautions to avoid bumping the patient's head, thus causing the retina to detach further.
3. Following general anaesthesia, the patient is encouraged to breathe deeply but not to cough since this will increase eye pressure. Vomiting must be avoided.
4. Allow additional activity according to progress following treatment.
5. Provide for diversional therapy, since this patient often becomes depressed.
6. Hospitalization is minimal unless the patient's condition requires additional attention.

PATIENT EDUCATION
1. When the patient goes home, ensure he is able to care for himself; he may care for all bodily needs in an unhurried manner, being careful to avoid falls, jerks and bumps.
2. It is advisable to take precautions and moderate activities to avoid accidental injury.
3. Watching television, looking at friends and using eyes in straight-line vision are harmless, but rapid eye movement, as in reading, should be avoided for several weeks.
4. Avoid straining and bending head below waist; driving is restricted.
5. Use meticulous cleanliness in giving eye medications.
6. The first follow-up visit to the ophthalmologist should take place in two weeks and other visits at longer intervals thereafter.
7. Within three weeks, light activities may be pursued; in six weeks, athletic and heavier activities are usually possible.

8. Acquaint the patient with the symptoms that indicate a recurrence of the detachment; floating spots, flashing light, progressive shadow. If they occur, recommend that the patient contact his doctor.

CATARACTS

A cataract is an opacity of the crystalline lens and its capsule; it is one of the leading causes of temporary blindness, particularly in the elderly.

PREDISPOSING FACTORS

1. A cataract may be present at birth (congenital cataract).
2. May be due as a result of disease such as diabetes mellitus or trauma in young subjects.
3. Can be the result of poison (toxic cataract).
4. Most commonly, cataract occurs in adults past middle age (senile cataract) as a result of the ageing process.

ALTERED PHYSIOLOGY

1. Normally the lens is a semi-solid body of clear, gelatinous protein encased in a capsule lying behind the iris, in front of the vitreous; the lens processes refractive powers (approximately one-fifth of the total).
2. Chemical changes in the lens protein may cause coagulation; as a result, the lens loses its pristine transparency and gradually become opaque.
3. Physical changes result in a swelling of the fibres, which in turn causes a distortion of the image.
4. Metabolic changes that reduce vitamins C and B_{12} in the lens may be instrumental in forming opacities.
5. Although a cataract may be readily diagnosed, the basic cause of a senile cataract is unknown.

CLINICAL FEATURES

1. Alterations in vision are noted.
   a. Objects seem distorted and blurred.
   b. Glare annoys the patient when there are bright lights.
   c. Visual loss is gradual, but eventually the opacity becomes complete.
2. The pupil, usually black, becomes grey and later milky-white.

TREATMENT

1. Surgical removal of the lens is indicated.
2. Proper time for cataract removal is determined by patient's eyesight, occupation, general health and convenience.

3. Usually a patient with one cataract can manage without surgery.
4. If cataract occurs in both eyes, he need not suffer blindness before he can be helped by surgery.
5. Following surgery and the healing process, the patient is fitted with appropriate spectacle lenses or contact lenses.
6. Intraocular lens implants may be implanted at the time of cataract extraction or as an independent procedure.

EXTRACAPSULAR EXTRACTION

1. This surgery is conservative; it is simple to perform and may be done under local or general anaesthetic.
2. The lens capsule is incised and the lens matter is withdrawn.
3. Usually performed for traumatic cataract.
4. Also performed when posterior intraocular lens is inserted.
5. The posterior capsule is left in place. This may interfere with vision, and to prevent a second operation (surgery), YAG capsulotomy, using a laser beam is performed. This is done in the outpatient clinic.
6. A standard size incision (18–20mm) is used.

INTRACAPSULAR EXTRACTION (CURRENTLY UNIVERSALLY ACCEPTED METHOD)

1. In this surgery, the lens as well as the capsule is removed through an 18mm incision.
2. Cryosurgery may be used as the technique for this operation; a pencil-like instrument with a metal probe is cooled to about −35°C; when the lens capsule is available after dissection, the cryosurgical instrument touches the lens and freezes to it so that the lens is easily pulled out.
3. Approximately one to three days of hospitalization are required, although this time is being reduced considerably and varies depending on the surgeon's preference, on the number and size of sutures used and on the patient's occupation and reliability.

NURSING INTERVENTIONS

Preoperative care

1. Make the patient comfortable in his new surroundings:
   a. Explain the plan of care.
   b. Escort the patient as he walks around the unit.
2. Allay his concerns, if he has any, regarding surgery:
   a. Determine how he feels about his operation.
   b. Assess his knowledge level regarding the

purpose of surgery and his expectations afterwards.

  c. Encourage his questions and provide the answers.

3. Reduce the conjunctival bacterial count to minimize the chance of postoperative infection:

  a. Obtain conjunctival culture if ordered.

  b. Administer local antibiotics as prescribed.

  c. Employ aseptic technique in any eye treatment or procedure.

  d. Instruct patient not to touch his eyes.

4. Introduce rehabilitative measures that the patient will practise postoperatively:

  a. Following general anaesthesia, instruct patient to take deep breaths, move extremities without jerking his head.

  b. Point out the hazard of squeezing the eyelids shut. Teach him how to close his eyes slowly.

5. Prepare the eye to be operated upon in the immediate preoperative period:

  a. Instil mydriatic if prescribed.

  b. Note whether pupil dilates after instillation of mydriatic.

6. Determine whether a properly identified and executed consent for operation and anaesthesia has been obtained. There should be no discrepancies between the patient's understanding of the surgery and the informed consent for surgery and anaesthesia.

7. Administrate preoperative medications.

  a. Sedatives.

  b. Antiemetics.

  c. Narcotics.

  d. Ocular hypotensive agents (if intraocular pressure raised).

    (i) Cholinesterase inhibitors – acetazolamide (Diamox).

    (ii) Osmotic hypotensives.

      (a) Oral – glycerine.

      (b) Intravenous – mannitol.

Postoperative care

1. Prevent pressure build-up within the eye (intraocular) which may exert stress on the sutures.

  a. Admonish patient to refrain from coughing or sneezing.

  b. Advise patient to avoid rapid movement, but allow him to turn to the unoperated side.

  c. Admonish patient not to bend from the waist.

2. Promote comfort of the patient and reorientate him to surroundings.

  a. Allow patient to turn on unoperated side to relieve back strain.

  b. Offer analgesics as prescribed to control pain; report severe pain to doctor.

  c. Instruct those who enter room to announce themselves and to inform patient when leaving room.

  d. Provide a quiet environment to promote patient's relaxation.

  e. Allow patient to be ambulatory as permitted by doctor.

3. Control symptoms that may lead to serious complications.

  a. Sudden pain in the eye may be due to a ruptured vessel or suture and may lead to haemorrhage, iris prolapse or infection – inform doctor immediately.

  b. Nausea may lead to vomiting and increase intraocular pressure – administer antiemetic drugs as prescribed.

PHACOEMULSIFICATION

See Figure 15.9.

1. Overview of this type of surgery: phacoemulsification is the mechanical breaking up (emulsifying) of the lens by a hollow needle vibrating at 40,000 cycles per second.

  a. The needle tip moves forwards and backwards.

  b. It is powered by an ultrasound generator to produce the frequency necessary to emulsify the cataract.

  c. This action is coupled with simultaneous irrigation and aspiration of the emulsified particles from the anterior chamber through the needle tip.

  d. Only a 2–3mm incision is required and the actual procedure takes 20 to 30 minutes (performed by a specially trained ophthalmic surgeon).

  e. Hospitalization of about two days is usually required.

  f. Normal activities may be resumed the day after surgery.

  g. Contact lenses can be used in about three to six weeks.

2. Criteria to be met for this operation:

  a. Pupil must be able to dilate fully.

  b. Anterior chamber must be deep enough to accommodate the manipulation of the probe-aspirator.

  c. Cornea should be healthy.

  d. The highly sophisticated phacoemulsifier utilizes expensive materials which are resupplied for each use.

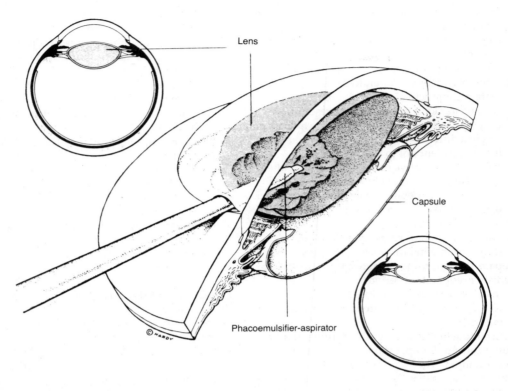

Figure 15.9. Cataract is shown in orb at upper left. Kelman ultrasonic needle (Cavitron Corps) is inserted through 2–3mm incision at corneal–scleral junction to emulsify lens cortex and nucleus and aspirate them. Righthand drawing shows cataract removed and posterior capsule intact. Cataract surgery requires a 19–20mm incision (copyright June 1975, the American Journal of Nursing Co.; reproduced with permission from *American Journal of Nursing*, Vol. 75, No. 6)

3. Preoperative nursing management:
   a. Take advantage of the opportunity to discuss fears, concerns and any questions patient may have regarding his surgery; patient is usually admitted the day before surgery.
   b. Acquaint the patient with his surroundings and his plan of care; provide him with information regarding postoperative care, since this is more flexible and liberal than for other kinds of cataract surgery.
   c. Prepare the patient to receive intravenous Diamox 500mg on the day of surgery to decrease intraocular pressure. If intraocular pressure remains elevated, the operation is postponed.
   d. Administer prescribed eyedrops to dilate the pupil and to paralyse the muscle of accommodation (ciliary muscle).
   e. Administer sedation, antiemetics and/or narcotics as in intracapsular cataract extraction (see p. 902).
4. Postoperative nursing management:
   a. Remove the eyepad; patient is allowed out of bed when fully recovered from anaesthesia.
   b. Administer eye medications as prescribed; these may be to prevent infection and to keep posterior capsule in place.
   c. Offer analgesic if he is in any discomfort.
   d. Remind the patient to use his eyedrops upon discharge from hospital, usually the first or second postoperatively.
   e. Explain the time plan for his permanent lenses and describe the need for and use of temporary lenses.
5. Considerations and possible disadvantages:
   a. The posterior lens capsule may later opacify; a

percentage of these patients (25 to 30 per cent) may require YAG capsulotomy procedure.

b. The cornea may be affected by high frequency vibrations during operation, which may later cause degeneration of the cornea.

c. Possible complications include infection, haemorrhage and fluid (aqueous) leakage from the eye.

INTRAOCULAR LENS

See Figure 15.10.

1. Basic concepts:
   a. This is the implementation of a synthetic lens – designed for distance vision, the patient wears prescribed glasses for reading and near vision.
   b. Intraocular lens implant is an alternative to sight correction with glasses or contact lenses for the aphacic patient.
   c. Sophisticated calculations are required to determine the power or prescription for lens:
      (i) Corneal curvature.
      (ii) Depth of anterior chamber.
      (iii) Axial length of eyeball (by diagnostic ultrasound).
   d. Unilateral cataract: objective is to leave patient slightly myopic (nearsighted), and to permit binocular vision, preventing an intolerable double vision.
      (i) Operated eye used for reading.
      (ii) Unoperated eye is used for distance vision.
   e. Bilateral cataract: objective is to leave the patient emmetropic (all rays of light focus perfectly on retina).

   (i) Vision is for good distance.
   (ii) Glasses required for reading.
   f. Hypermetropia (long or farsightedness) is avoided in implanting a lens because the image would be magnified and cause visual difficulty.
   g. Astigmatism is corrected with spectacles.

2. Insertion of intraocular lens.
   a. There are a number of types of intraocular lens available.
   b. Polymethyl methacrylate is a common durable compound from which such lenses are made.
   c. Various methods of fixation are being used, including (i) fastening by sutures or clips; (ii) holding in place in the way that a hub cap is fitted to the rim of a tyre; and (iii) sealing within the anterior and posterior capsule after extracapsular extraction (capsular fixation). The second method (no sutures) usually requires miotic eye drops (pilocarpine) to keep the iris from dilating too widely – thereby causing displacement of the implant.

3. Advantages of intraocular lens:
   a. Provides an alternative to individuals who cannot wear contact lenses or cataract glasses.
   b. Cannot be lost or misplaced like conventional glasses; does not need to be replaced.
   c. Provides a permanent form of near normal vision.

4. Complications (specific to implantation):
   a. Iritis or vitritis – can be controlled with steroids.
   b. Rosy vision, due to keeping pupil from full

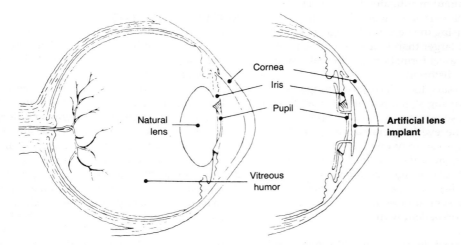

Natural lens

Cornea
Iris
Pupil

Artificial lens implant

Vitreous humor

Figure 15.10. Lefthand drawing indicates position of natural lens; drawing on right shows artificial lens implant following removal of cataract

constriction; excessive light enters pupil, causing a dazzling of macula.

c. Degeneration of cornea, chronic uveitis (see p. 897).

d. Malposition or dislocation of lens.

PATIENT EDUCATION

During rehabilitative phase of cataract extraction:

1. Encourage the patient to be independent:
   a. Assist patient in getting around his room, locating needed personal items, utilizing bathroom facilities.
   b. Gradually increase his activities each day.
2. Demonstrate to the patient and a responsible member of his family how to administer eye medications.
3. Promote patient's interest in diversional activities as he recuperates; try to prevent him becoming bored.
4. Acquaint the patient with the step-by-step requirements of a healthy convalescence.
   a. The use of dark glasses after the eye dressings are removed.
   b. Hospitalization – usually one to three days following intracapsular extraction.
   c. Fitting for temporary corrective lenses for the first six weeks if prescribed.
   d. Application of eye shield or pad over the eye at night to avoid accidental injury during sleep.
   e. Prescription for permanent lenses six to eight weeks after surgery for intracapsular extraction.
   f. Prescription for contact lenses about three to six weeks after phacoemulsification.
5. Assist the patient in adjusting to the spectacles:
   a. If spectacles are to be worn they will be quite thick, causing the perceived image to be about one-third larger than that seen by the patient before cataract formation; peripheral vision is markedly distorted.
   b. It is necessary to relearn space judgement – walking, using stairs, reaching for articles on the table, such as a cup of tea or coffee.
   c. If only one eye is operated for cataract, the patient can use only one eye at a time, with spectacles, since the operated eye has a 30 per cent increase in image size and the unoperated eye still has 'normal'-sized images, which cannot be superimposed.
6. Familiarize the patient with contact lenses, if this is his choice.
   a. With contact lenses, magnification is only about 8 to 10 per cent; peripheral vision is not distorted.
   b. Since the image size difference between an aphacic eye with a contact lens and the unoperated eye is only 8 to 10 per cent, both eyes can be used together.
   c. Space judgement presents little difficulty.
   d. There may be problems if the patient has difficulty applying lenses, has a tremor of the hands, or if there are hygienic problems which could cause swelling and infection.
7. Recognize that with an intraocular lens magnification problems are negligible. Both the operated eye and the unoperated eye can work together after cataract surgery with lens implantation.

GLAUCOMA

Glaucoma is a condition in which the pressure within the eyeball is higher than average; it is associated with progressive visual field loss. If allowed to proceed untreated will lead to atrophy of the optic nerve and eventual blindness.

INCIDENCE

1. Glaucoma is the cause of blindness in one in every seven people who become blind.
2. The incidence of glaucoma is increasing as the number of people in our population rises.
3. It is estimated that about 2 per cent of people over the age of 40 years in Britain have glaucoma.
4. People with family history of glaucoma are more susceptible than others.

ALTERED PHYSIOLOGY

1. Pressure within the eye is determined by the rate of aqueous production by the ciliary processes of the ciliary body, and the resistance to outflow of aqueous from the eye.
2. Inflow of aqueous is through the posterior chamber and pupil; outflow is at the meshwork located at the juncture of iris and cornea. Clogging at the meshwork by blood fibrin, or inflammatory cells account for the build up of pressure which produces secondary glaucoma.
3. Thickening of the meshwork appears spontaneously in those older individuals who appear to have hereditary predisposition; chronic simple glaucoma results and is the most common type.
4. When the iris is abnormally anterior and its root blocks the angle, cutting off aqueous outflow, pressure is increased – acute glaucoma results; this is the least frequent type.

CLASSIFICATIONS

1. Primary glaucoma.
    a. Angle closure (narrow angle, closed angle, acute congestive glaucoma) – acute or sub-acute.
    b. Open angle (wide angle, chronic simple glaucoma) – chronic.
2. Primary congenital or infantile (buphthalmos, hydrophthalmos).
3. Secondary – due to other ocular disease, injury, neoplasms or following surgery.

DIAGNOSTIC EVALUATION

1. Because of relative ease of developing glaucoma, unless a person past 40 years has a complete medical (physical) examination periodically, including measurement of eye pressure (tonometry), the condition may not be discovered until it is considerably advanced (chronic simple type).
2. Tonometry (see Figure 15.1): a reading of 24–32mmHg suggests glaucoma.
3. Gonioscopy – an examination of angle of eye, differentiates angle closure from open angle type glaucoma.
4. Tonography – application of electronic tonometer with a special device that records intraocular tension over a period of four minutes. Also gives indication of aqueous flow.
5. Mydriatic test – pupil is fully dilated using a mydriatic of short duration, i.e. Mydrilate 1 per cent or by confining the patient to a dark room for an hour. Full mydriasis causes a significant rise in the intraocular pressure, confirming the diagnosis.
6. Examination of optic disc and blood vessels by means of ophthalmoscopy.
7. Visual field examination – perimeter or tangent screen.

ACUTE (ANGLE-CLOSURE) GLAUCOMA

CLINICAL FEATURES

1. With intraocular pressure increasing rapidly, severe pain occurs in and around eye.
2. Artificial lights appear to have rainbow colours around them (halos).
3. Vision becomes cloudy, blurred.
4. Pupils semidilated and fixed; nausea and vomiting may occur.
5. Although onset may be insidious, severity of symptoms may develop within hours to include disturbances suggestive of gastrointestinal, sinus, neurological and dental problems as well as eye pain.
6. If untreated, irreversible blindness may result.

MEDICAL TREATMENT

Miotic drops (parasympathomimetics)

Action – pupil contracts, iris is drawn away from cornea; aqueous may drain through lymph spaces (meshworks) into canal of Schlemm. Drops usually used are shown in Table 15.1.

Carbonic anhydrase inhibitors

Action – restricts action of enzyme which is necessary to produce aqueous. Tablets that may be used are shown in Table 15.2.

Hyperosmotic agents

See Table 15.3.

SURGICAL TREATMENT

Peripheral iridectomy (sector or keyhole) – usually the operation of choice – an incision through corneal–scleral junction so that portion of iris may be drawn out and excised.

Table 15.1 Miotic drops

Drops	Action	Effect and precautions
Pilocarpine hydrochloride	Acts directly on myoneural junction	Action lasts six to eight hours
Carbachol	Acts directly on myoneural junction	Used if pilocarpine is ineffective
Physostigmine salicylate	Cholinesterase inhibitor	Action lasts six to eight hours: allergenic, unstable, short in action
Timolol	Beta-blocker suppresses formation of aqueous	Used twice daily

Table 15.2   Carbonic anhydrase inhibitors

Drug	Action	Effect and precautions
Acetazolamide (Diamox) Ethoxzolamide (Cardrase) Dichlorphenamide (Daranide)	Carbonic anhydrase inhibitor	Decreases production of aqueous CAUTION: Side-effects – gastric disorders, shortness of breath, dermatitis, tingling of extremities, acidosis, ureteral stones

Table 15.3   Hyperosmotic agents

Medication	Action	Effect and precautions
Intravenous mannitol urea	Reduces intraocular pressure by increasing blood osmolality	Useful in treatment of acute attacks and preoperatively
Oral glycerol		Safer than intravenous method

Result: iris is prevented from bulging forwards and causing the angle at cornea and iris to be crowded. Consequently, drainage is facilitated and intraocular pressure is reduced and there is relief of pupillary block.

Others that may be performed: iridencleisis and trabeculectomy.

CHRONIC (OPEN-ANGLE) GLAUCOMA

CLINICAL FEATURES
1. Insidious – mild discomfort (tired feeling in eye).
2. Slowly developing impairment of peripheral vision.
3. Possible halos around lights.
4. Progressive loss of visual field and cupping of optic disc.

TREATMENT
Medical
1. Often treated with a combination of miotic drops and carbonic anhydrase inhibitors.
2. Remission may occur; however, patient should continue to see ophthalmologist at three- to six-month intervals.
3. If medical treatment is not successful, surgery may be required, but delayed as long as possible.

Surgical
Surgery may be performed.

Objective
Provide filtering of fluid in order to decrease intraocular pressure.
1. Cyclocryosurgery.
2. Trabeculectomy.
3. YAG iridotomy.
4. YAG trabeculaplasty.

NURSING MANAGEMENT
Operative procedures are mainly performed under general anaesthesia.
1. Patient remains in recovery room until vital signs are stable and until he has orientated to time and place.
2. Administer analgesic or narcotics if required as prescribed.
3. Assist the patient in getting out of bed the first time: usually the patient is ambulatory the day after operation.
4. Provide adequate suitable diet to eliminate straining on defaecation.
5. Remind patient of periodic eye check-up since pressure changes may occur.

PATIENT EDUCATION
1. Even though glaucoma cannot be cured, it can be controlled.
2. Circumstances that may increase intraocular pressure are to be avoided, if possible.
   a. Emotional upsets – worry, fear, excitement, anger.

b. Constricting clothing such as tight collar, belt, girdle.

c. Exertion such as snow shovelling, pushing, heavy lifting.

d. Upper respiratory tract infections.

3. Recommended activities:

a. Exercise in moderation to maintain general well being.

b. Moderate use of eyes for reading and watching television.

c. Maintenance of regular bowel habits (straining on defaecation causes increased intraocular pressure.

d. Continuous daily use of eye medications as prescribed.

e. Normal intake of fluids is not restricted even for alcohol or coffee unless these are known to increase eye pressure in the particular patient.

f. Check-ups with ophthalmologist in order to keep condition under control.

g. Wearing a medical identification tag indicating patient has glaucoma or glaucoma identification and treatment card, similar to steroid cards.

NURSING CARE OF THE NONSEEING PATIENT

1. Upon entering the room of a nonseeing patient, address him by his name; use a clear, natural voice.

a. Tell him your name and that you are a nurse.

b. Indicate why you are there; do not touch him before he knows you are there.

c. Inform his family and other visitors of this procedure when entering the room of the patient (or approaching bedside) so that he is not startled.

2. Acquaint the patient with his surroundings if he is in an environment new to him.

a. If he is in bed:

(i) Take his hand and show him how to find the call bell and how to use it.

(ii) Help him in using wash basin, soap and towel; tell him you have drawn the bed curtains when he should need privacy.

b. If he is out of bed: assist him to acquaint himself with his surroundings, chairs, bed, doors, bedside table and where his personal things are kept.

3. Guide him when walking:

a. First, remember not to direct the visually handicapped person by steering him from behind – he may bump into things.

b. Walk *slightly* ahead of him and have him place his hand in the space at the bend of your elbow, walk normally, at an *unhurried* pace.

c. Describe where you are walking and inform him when you are going through a narrow passage or are approaching a curb, steps or an incline.

d. Inform him that you are leading him to the bed, chair or toilet and permit him to feel the front of the object with his knees or hands.

NURSING ALERT

Never permit a nonseeing patient to smoke in bed unattended. If he insists on smoking, have some responsible person remain with him until the cigar, cigarette or pipe is extinguished.

e. Assist him with his food; explain position of food on plate.

4. If for any reason a patient has both eyes bandaged (very rare these days) postoperatively, bed rails *may be used*. If so:

a. Hold the patient's hand as you direct him to feel the side rails.

b. Tell him the side rails are there to remind him not to attempt to get out of bed unassisted.

c. Place the bell cord within easy reach and inform the patient that someone will answer his bell when he signals. If call light is multipurpose, place a piece of tape over the nurse signal area so that the patient can feel the proper switch.

5. Assist the patient in enjoying his meals:

a. Read the proposed menu and have him make his own selection within his dietary prescription.

b. Help him to assume a comfortable position when the tray arrives.

c. Guide his hand to show him where the utensils, plate, cup, etc, are located. Describe food placement on the tray in terms of the face of a clock. If feeding patient, describe food; hot, cold, colour, flavour.

d. Plan to have the various items of food always arranged in the same pattern on the tray, so that he will know for example where the salad, beverage, bread, etc, are. On his plate the servings should be placed in a specific arrangement so that he knows the meat, vegetables, etc, are in a certain place.

e. Assist him by cutting the meat into bite-size pieces, buttering the bread, adding sugar, milk/cream to tea or coffee. Permit him to do as much for himself as he can without embarrassing himself by spilling or knocking food onto the floor.

f. Provide pleasant conversation or radio background music to make mealtime a satisfying time.
6. Gain his co-operation when he is taking medications:
   a. Tell him you have his medication ready for him; indicate how many tablets there are and that they are in a tiny medication container.
   b. Offer him half a glass of water or fruit juice to assist in swallowing the tablets.
   c. Tell him what the medication is for, if he asks.
7. Attend to the psychological and sociological needs of the person with no vision.
   a. Recognize that time does not pass as rapidly when one is inactive.
   b. When giving care, mention day of week, date, time and always involve patient in the conversation.
   c. Plan for him to have diversions that interest him – radio, talking books, braille books, visitors, television.
   d. Take time to stop and converse with him.

INFORMATION SOURCES

British Contact Lens Association, 51 Strathyre Avenue, Norbury, London SW16 4RF

British Talking Book Service for the Blind, Nuffield Library, Mount Pleasant, Alperton, Wembley, Middlesex HA0 1RR

British Wireless for the Blind Fund, 226 Great Portland Street, London W1N 6AA

Catholic Blind Institute, Christopher Grange Centre, Youens Way, East Prestcott Road, Liverpool L14 2EW

Greater London Fund for the Blind, 2 Wyndham Place, London W1H 2AQ

Guide Dogs for Blind Association, 9–11 Park Street, Windsor, Berks

Jewish Blind Society, 1 Craven Hill, Lancaster Gate, London W2 3EW

London Association for the Blind, 14–16 Verney Road, London SE16 2DZ

National Association of Deaf, Blind and Rubella Handicapped, 164 Cromwell Lane, Coventry CV4 8AP

National Library for the Blind, 35 Great Smith Street, London SW1 3BU

Royal Commonwealth Society for the Blind, Commonwealth House, Heath Road, Haywards Heath, Sussex

Royal National Institute for the Blind, 294 Great Portland Street, London W1N 6AA

The Royal London Society for the Blind, 105–109 Salisbury Road, London NW6 6RH

FURTHER READING

BOOKS

Awdry, P. and Nicholls, C.S. (1985) Cataract, Faber & Faber, London.

Bache, J.B., Armitt, C.R. and Tobiss, J.R. (1985) A Colour Atlas of Nursing Procedures in Accident and Emergencies, Wolfe Medical, London.

Bankes Kennerley, J.L. (1987) Clinical Ophthalmology: A Textbook and Colour Atlas, Churchill Livingstone, Edinburgh.

Chapman, E.K. (1978) Visually Handicapped Children and Young People, Routledge & Kegan Paul, London.

Chawla, H.B. (1981) Essential Ophthalmology, Churchill Livingstone, Edinburgh.

Coakes, R.L. and Holme Sellors, P.J. (1985) An Outline of Ophthalmology, Wright, Bristol.

Darling, V.H. and Thorpe, M.R. (1981) Ophthalmic Nursing (2nd edn), Baillière Tindall, London.

Dorrell, E. (1978) Surgery of the Eye, Blackwell, Oxford.

Englestein, J.M. (ed.) (1984) Cataract Surgery, Grune & Stratton, New York.

Gaston, H. and Elkington, A.R. (1986) Ophthalmology for Nurses, Croom Helm, London.

Hamano, H. and Ruben, M. (1985) Contact Lenses – A Guide to Successful Wear and Tear, Martin Dunitz, London.

Last, R.J. (1968) Eugene Wolff's Anatomy of the Eye and Orbit (6th edn), Lewis, London.

Leydbecker, W. and Crick, R.P. (1981) All About Glaucoma, Faber & Faber, London.

Lim, S.M. and Constable, I.J. (1979) Colour Atlas of Ophthalmology, Kimpton, London.

Luntz, M.H., Harrison, R. and Schenker, H.I. (1984) Glaucoma Surgery, Williams & Wilkins, Baltimore.

Lyall, M.G. (1985) The Illustrated Textbook of Ophthalmology, Phoenix Scientific, London.

Miller, S.J.H. (1984) Parsons Diseases of the Eye (17th edn), Churchill Livingstone, Edinburgh.

Parr, J. (1978) *Introduction to Ophthalmology*, Oxford University Press, Oxford.

Rooke, F.C.E., Rothwell, P.J. and Woodhouse, D.F. (1980) *Ophthalmic Nursing, Its Practice and Management*, Churchill Livingstone, Edinburgh.

Sachsenwerger, R. (1984) *Illustrated Handbook of Ophthalmology*, Wright, Bristol.

Thomas, P. (1978) *Pharmacology of the Eye*, Lloyd-Luke, London.

Trevor-Roper, P.D. (1986) *Lecture Notes on Ophthalmology* (6th edn), Blackwell, Oxford.

Trockel, S.L. (1983) *YAG Laser Ophthalmic Microsurgery*, Appleton-Century-Crofts, Connecticut.

Vaughan, D. and Asbury, T. (1983) *General Ophthalmology* (10th edn), Lange, Los Altos, California.

Wybar, K. and Muir, M.K. (1984) *Ophthalmology* (3rd edn), Baillière Tindall, London.

Youngson, R.M. (1984) *Everything You Need To Know About Contact Lenses*, Sheldon Press, London.

ARTICLES

Anatomy and physiology

Bissett, P. (1978) The six senses – 1. Light. *Nursing Mirror*, Supplement, vol. 146, No. 1.

Voke, J. (1983) The visual pathway, *Nursing Mirror*, Vol. 156, pp. 46–7.

Cornea

Gallagher, M.A. (1981) Corneal transplantation, *American Journal of Nursing*, Vol. 90, pp. 48–9.

Josse, E. (1984) Corneal abscess from soft contact lenses, *Nursing Times*, Supplement, Vol. 80, pp. 3–4.

General

Forman, S. (1983) Good eyesight – a natural sight, *Nursing Mirror*, Vol. 157, pp. 24–6.

Fyfe, J. and Ellebroek, D. (1984) Colour vision defects and the school nurse, *Nursing Times*, Vol. 80, pp. 48–9.

Hughes Lamb, B. (1981) Caring for the visually handicapped, *Nursing*, Vol. 28, pp. 1221–4.

Kennedy, J. and Heywood, M. (1980) I see what I feel, *New Scientist*, vol. 91, pp. 386–9.

Rawlings, T. (1984) Out of sight, *Nursing Times*, Vol. 80, pp. 38–9.

Rowell, M. (1981) Let me see the future, *Nursing*, Vol. 28, pp. 1212–6.

Treplin, M.C.W. and Arnott, E.J. (1978) Use of the microscope in ophthalmics, *Nursing Mirror*, Vol. 147, pp. 30–3.

Voke, J. (1980) Acting on impulse (colour vision), *Nursing Mirror*, Vol. 151, pp. 35–7.

— (1981) Laser therapy, *Nursing Mirror*, Vol. 152, pp. 32–4.

— (1982) Screening for visual diseases, *Nursing Mirror*, Vol. 155, pp. 30–2.

— (1983) The eyes have it, *Nursing Mirror*, Vol. 157, pp. 53–5.

Glaucoma

Murray, A. (1979) The problem of glaucoma, *Medical News*, 12 April, pp. 8–9.

Travers, J.P. (1978) Primary open glaucoma, *Nursing Times*, Vol. 74, pp. 103–4.

Infection

Boyd-Monk, H. (1982) Conjunctivitis, *Nursing*, Vol. 12, p. 67.

Marsh, R.J. (1979) Ophthalmic herpes zoster, *Nursing Times*, Vol. 75, pp. 240–3.

Lens

Brown, N. (1979) The A–Z of cataract treatment, *Geriatric Nursing*, Vol. 9, pp. 55–9.

Traynor, M.J. (1981) Day care cataract surgery, *Nursing Times*, Vol. 77, pp. 1024–5.

Retina

MacFayden, J.S. (1980) Caring for the patient with a primary retinal detachment, *American Journal Of Nursing*, Vol. 79, pp. 53–4.

Trauma

Bowman, K. (1983) Blindness following a fall at work, *Nursing Times*, Vol. 79, pp. 53–4.

— (1983) Claiming benefits, *Nursing Times*, Vol. 79, pp. 32–3.

Fletcher, D. (1981) Intraocular foreign bodies – an eye for treatment, *Nursing Mirror*, Vol. 152, pp. 34–5.

Mitchell, D.R. (1978) Treatment of eye injuries, *Nursing Mirror*, Vol. 146, pp. 17–18.

Tumulty, G. and Rester, M.M. (1984) Eye trauma, *American Journal of Nursing*, Vol. 6, pp. 740–4.

16

Care of the Patient with a Neurological Disorder

DIAGNOSIS OF NEUROLOGICAL CONDITIONS

RADIOLOGICAL PROCEDURES

Skull X-ray

Skull X-ray reveals shape, density, vascular markings, intracranial calcification, fractures and some tumours.

Computerized axial tomography (CAT scan)

Computerized axial tomography is an imaging method in which the head is scanned in successive layers by a narrow beam of X-ray. It provides a cross-sectional view of the brain and distinguishes differences in the densities of various brain tissues. A computer printout is obtained of the absorption values of the tissues in the plane that is being scanned. This same information is also shown on a cathode ray tube for additional radiological evaluation.

1. Lesions are seen as variations in tissue density

differing from the surrounding normal brain tissue.

2. Abnormalities of tissue density indicate possible tumour masses, brain infarction, ventricular displacement; useful in patients with head injury, suspected brain tumour, hydrocephalus.

3. May be done with intravenous contrast medium enhancement to give more accurately defined boundaries of certain lesions and indicate presence of otherwise undetectable lesions.

4. Patient preparation:
   a. The doctor should inquire about allergies and any previous adverse reaction to contrast agent.
   b. No special preparation is required; this is a noninvasive technique that can be done on an outpatient basis.
   c. Explain to the patient that he must lie perfectly still while the testing is being carried out; he cannot talk or move his face as this distorts the picture.

Positron emission tomography (PET)
This is a computer-based imaging technique that permits study of the brain's metabolism and function; displays pictures of metabolic and biochemical activity within the brain as thinking, speaking, hearing and other activities occur.

Magnetic resonance imaging (MRI)
This diagnostic imaging method uses a magnetic field (rather than ionizing radiation) to produce images of the body. It is extremely sensitive in detecting abnormalities in the brain, especially biochemical assessment.

Cerebral angiography
X-ray study of the vascular system of the brain (cerebral circulation) by the injection of contrast material into a selected artery. This may be done under local or general anaesthetic.

1. Contrast material may be injected into common carotid, vertebral or subclavian artery, or arch of the aorta. Selective catheterization may be done via a femoral or brachial artery.

2. After injection of selected artery, X-rays are made of arterial and venous phases of circulation through brain and head.

3. Useful in demonstrating position of arteries, intracranial aneurysms, presence or absence of abnormal vasculature, haematomas, tumours. This extra information about the positioning of vascular structures is particularly helpful to the surgeon, who has to make decisions about which operative route to take through brain tissue.

4. Nursing responsibilities/support:
   a. *Before angiogram – under general anaesthetic:*
      (i) Reinforce the doctor's explanation of the procedure and what will happen in the X-ray department.
      (ii) Ensure the doctor has obtained consent for the procedure.
      (iii) Fast the patient following the guidelines of the anaesthetist.
      (iv) Prepare the patient for anaesthetic according to local policy.
   b. *Before angiogram – using local anaesthetic* (see (i) and (ii) above):
      (i) Withhold meal preceding test.
      (ii) Patient may be prescribed sedation. This should be given by the nurse before patient goes to X-ray department. This may help minimize intensity of burning sensation felt along course of injected vessel.
      (iii) If possible, patient should be accompanied throughout the procedure by a nurse who he knows.
      (iv) Patient should be informed that he should try to lie quietly during the injection of contrast medium and that a burning sensation, lasting for a few seconds, may be felt behind the eyes, or in the mouth.
   c. *Following angiogram (performed under either method):*
      (i) Make repeated observations for neurological deficits – motor or sensory deterioration, alterations in level of responsiveness, weakness on one side, speech disturbances, dysrhythmias, blood pressure fluctuation, disturbances of pupillary function.
      (ii) Observe injection site for haematoma formation; apply an ice cap intermittently – to relieve swelling and discomfort.
      (iii) Evaluate peripheral pulses – changes may develop if there is haematoma formation at puncture site or embolization to a distant artery.
      (iv) Note colour and temperature of involved extremity.

Brain scan
Following intake (oral or intravenous) of radiopharmaceutical, the radioactivity subsequently transmitted through the skull is scanned by a rectilinear scanner which prints out a picture based on the number of counts received from the brain as it scans (or a gamma camera, which prints out image

without actually scanning, may be used; this is a more recent imaging device).

1. Patient is treated with potassium perchlorate to block the radiopharmaceutical uptake in the thyroid, salivary glands, choroid plexus and gastrointestinal mucosa.
2. Brain scanning is useful in early detection and evaluation of intracranial neoplasms, stroke, abscess, follow-up of surgical or radiotherapy of brain.
3. This test is based on the principal that a radiopharmaceutical may diffuse through a disrupted blood–brain barrier into the abnormal cerebral tissue. (Normal brain tissue is relatively impermeable.) There is an increased uptake of radioactive material at the site of pathology.
4. Nursing responsibility:
   a. Explain to patient that he will be expected to lie quietly during the procedure.
   b. This is a noninvasive procedure.

Air studies
A gaseous replacement of the fluid within the ventricles and subarachnoid systems as a contrast medium because air is less dense than fluid to roentgen rays.

Note: These investigations are now rarely used since the introduction of computerized axial tomography.

1. *Pneumoencephalogram* – withdrawal of cerebrospinal fluid and injection of air or other gas by means of a lumbar puncture.
   a. Demonstrates ventricular system and subarachnoid space overlying the hemispheres and basal cisterns.
   b. Useful in diagnosing degenerative cerebral atrophy and in detecting mass lesions at the base of the brain, e.g. pituitary tumours.
2. *Fractional pneumoencephalogram* – withdrawal of small amounts of fluid and injection of small amounts of air to visualize the ventricular system.
3. *Ventriculogram* – withdrawal of cerebrospinal fluid and injection of air, gas or contrast medium directly into the lateral ventricles through openings in the skull.
   a. Trephines (burr holes) are made through a scalp incision; ventricles are punctured by a special needle.
   b. The cerebrospinal fluid is replaced with air, the cannulae are withdrawn and the scalp wounds are closed.
   c. If a lesion is present, there is a change in the size, shape or position of the ventricular, subarachnoid or cisternal spaces.

4. *Nursing management following pneumoencephalogram or ventriculogram:*
   a. Watch the patient for increasing intracranial pressure.
      (i) Disturbances of intracranial pressure may cause serious complications.
      (ii) Prepare for ventricular tap and prompt decompression.
   b. Take vital signs as frequently as clinical condition indicates and until stabilized.
   c. Assess for complaints of headache, fever and for signs of shock.
      (i) Place ice cap on head intermittently.
      (ii) Give analgesics as directed – duration of headache depends on the speed with which the intracranial air is absorbed. Headache is reduced if patient lies flat in bed.
      (iii) Nausea and vomiting may follow air studies.
      (iv) Parenteral fluids may be necessary for first 24 hours.
5. Procedure done under general anaesthetic. Patient preparation before pneumoencephalogram.
   a. Fast following guidelines of anaesthetist responsible.
   b. Reinforce doctor's explanation.
   c. Prepare patient for anaesthetic, in accordance with hospital policy.
   d. Patient may be nursed head-down to minimize headache.

Echoencephalography
The recording of echoes from the deep structures within the skull (generated by the transmission of ultrasound (high frequency) waves) to determine the position of midline structures of the brain and the distance from the midline to the lateral ventricular wall or the third ventricular wall.

1. Useful for detecting a shift of the cerebral midline structures caused by subdural haematoma, intracerebral haemorrhage, massive cerebral infarction and neoplasms; can display dilation of ventricles; useful in evaluation of hydrocephalus.
2. Ultrasonic transducers are positioned over specified areas of the head; the echoes are imaged and stored on the oscilloscope.
3. Nursing responsibilities:
   a. There is no special patient preparation.
   b. Explain that this is a noninvasive test and that some type of gel (electrode jelly) may be used to eliminate the air gap between the transducer and the head.

Note: This test is still used in some hospitals, but needs a skilled operator to obtain an accurate echo image. It has been somewhat superseded by computerized axial tomography.

Myelography and radiculography

The injection of contrast medium into the spinal subarachnoid space, usually by lumbar puncture for radiological examination, outlines the spinal subarachnoid space and shows distortion of the spinal cord or dural sac by tumours, cysts, prolapsed intravertebral discs or other lesions.

1. After injection of the contrast medium, the head of the table is tilted down and the course of the contrast medium is observed radioscopically.
2. Contrast material may be removed after test completion by syringe and needle aspiration; patient may complain of sharp pain down leg during aspiration if a nerve root has been aspirated against a needle point – needle point is rotated or an adjustment in needle depth is made.

   Because the newer, water-soluble contrast agents are easily absorbed by the cerebrospinal fluid, it is not usual to remove them at the end of the procedure.
3. Nursing responsibilities:
   a. *Before test:*
      (i) Reinforce doctor's explanation of procedure; explain that it is not usually painful and that the X-ray table will be tilted in varying positions during the study.
      (ii) Omit the meal preceding myelography/ radiculography.
      (iii) Patient's legs may be wrapped with elastic compression bandages to eliminate hypotension during procedure.
      (iv) Patient may be given light sedative prior to test to help him cope with a rather lengthy (two-hour) procedure.
   b. *Post-test:*

NURSING ALERT

The care given post-test depends upon the type of contrast medium used during the investigation. Commonly this will be a water-based solution, e.g. Amipaque. The patient will return from the X-ray department sitting upright in bed and should remain so for at least the next six hours.

During this time the contrast will be reabsorbed by the cerebrospinal fluid. There is a danger of the patient having a fit if the patient lies flat, as this allows the contrast medium to move upwards into the brain where it acts as an irritant.

(i) Advise patient to drink liberal quantities of fluid – for rehydration and replacement of cerebrospinal fluid and to decrease incidence of postlumbar puncture headache (thought to be due to escape of spinal fluid through puncture site).
(ii) Assess neurological and vital signs; note motor and sensory deviations from normal.
(iii) Check on patient's ability to micturate.
(iv) Observe for fever, stiff neck, photophobia or other signs of chemical or bacterial meningitis.
(v) Observe for uncontrolled movements of lower limbs; if severe, the patient may need to be given diazepam.

Note: The terms *radiculography* and *myelography* are often used interchangeably. However, the term radiculography should be used when the lower nerve roots (cauda equina) have been examined, whereas myelography refers to examination of the spinal cord itself.

Discography

Injection of radio-opaque substance directly into the intervertebral disc. This study can be used in patients suspected of having herniated disc disease, but is infrequently done.

ELECTROENCEPHALOGRAPHY (EEG)

Records, by means of electrodes applied on the scalp surface (or by microelectrodes placed within brain tissue), the electrical activity which is generated in the brain.

1. Provides physiological assessment of cerebral activity; useful in diagnosis of the epilepsies.
2. Electrodes are arranged on the scalp to permit the recording of activity in various head regions; the amplified activity of the neurones is recorded on a continuously moving paper sheet.
   a. For baseline recording the patient lies quietly with his eyes closed.
   b. For activation procedures (done to elicit abnormal electrical activities) patient may be asked to hyperventilate for three to four minutes, look at a bright flashing light or receive an injection of medication (Metrazol).
   c. EEG may also be made during sleep and upon awakening.
3. Pharyngeal (electrode inserted through nose; rests on mucosa of pharyngeal roof) and sphenoidal (inserted transcutaneously with tips resting on sphenoid bone near foramen ovale)

Table 16.1   Neurological examination of cranial nerves

Nerve	Equipment	Clinical examination
1. Olfactory	Four small bottles of volatile oils, such as (1) peppermint, (2) oil of cloves, (3) coffee, (4) aniseed	Instruct the patient to sniff and to identify the odours. Each nostril is tested separately. The patient is asked if he perceives the smell and if he can identify it
2. Optic	Ophthalmoscope	In a darkened room the patient is asked to look straight ahead at a distant object while the examiner looks for papilloedema, optic atrophy and retinal and vascular lesions Special equipment is used for examination of visual fields. Eye chart is used to check visual acuity
3. Oculomotor 4. Trochlear 5. Abducens	Torch	Because of close association, these nerves are examined collectively. They innervate pupil and upper eyelid and are responsible for extraocular muscle movements
6. Trigeminal	Test tube of hot water Test tube of ice water Wisp of cotton wool Pin	*Sensory branch* – Vertex to chin tested for sensations of pain, touch and temperature. This includes reflex reaction of cornea to wisp of cotton *Motor branch* – Ability to bite is tested
7. Facial	Four small bottles with solutions which are salty, sweet, sour and bitter (Four wet cotton applicators)	Observe symmetry of face and ability to contract facial muscles. Instruct patient to taste and identify substance used. He should rinse his mouth well between each drop of solution. This is a test for the anterior two-thirds of the tongue
8. Acoustic	Tuning fork	Tests for hearing, air and bone conduction
9. Glossopharyngeal	Cotton applicator stick	Test posterior one-third of the tongue for taste and also check for gag reflex
10. Vagus	Tongue depressor	Checking voice sounds, observing symmetry of soft palate will give suggestion of function of vagus
11. Spinal accessory		Since this innervates the sternocleidomastoid and the trapezius muscles, the patient will be instructed to turn and to move his head and to elevate shoulders with and without resistance
12. Hypoglossal		Observe tongue movements

electrodes are used when epileptogenic area is inaccessible to conventional scalp preparation.

4. Patient preparation for routine recording:
   a. Antiepileptic medication and tranquillizers may be withheld before EEG – many departments prefer patients to continue with medication and allow for this when interpreting EEG patterns.
   b. Reassure patient that he will not receive an electrical shock, that the EEG takes approximately 45 to 60 minutes (more for a sleep EEG), and that the EEG is *not* a form of treatment or a test of intelligence or insanity.

ELECTROMYOGRAPHY (EMG)

The introduction of needle electrodes into the skeletal muscles to study changes in electric potential of muscles and nerves leading to them. These are shown on an oscilloscope and amplified by a loudspeaker for simultaneous visual and auditory analysis and comparison.

1. Useful in determining the presence of a neuromuscular disorder; helps distinguish weakness due to neuropathy from that due to other causes.
2. Nursing responsibilities:
   a. No special patient preparation is required.
   b. Explain to the patient that he will experience a sensation similar to that of an intramuscular injection as the needle is inserted into the muscle. Muscles examined may ache slightly for a short time.

EVOKED POTENTIAL STUDIES

These studies involve the changes and responses in brain waves recorded from scalp electrodes that are evoked (elicited) by the introduction of an external stimulus (visual, auditory, somatosensory).

1. These evoked changes are detected with the aid of computing devices, which extract, display and store the signal.
2. These studies are based on the concept that any insult/dysfunction that can alter neuronal metabolism or disturb membrane function may change evoked electrical activity.
   a. Visual evoked responses – the patient looks at visual stimulus (flashing light); the average of several hundred stimuli are recorded by EEG leads over the occiput and the transit time from the retina to the occipital area is measured (in milliseconds), using computer averaging methods.
   b. Auditory evoked responses – auditory stimulus (repetitive auditory click) is presented, and its transit time up the brain stem into the cortex is measured. Specific lesions in auditory pathway will modify or delay the response.
   c. Somatosensory evoked response – peripheral nerves stimulated percutaneously. Transit time up the spinal cord to the sensory cortex of the brain is measured and recorded from scalp electrodes. Test is used to detect deficit in spinal cord, to measure conduction in spinal cord and to monitor cord function during operative procedures.

NERVE CONDUCTION STUDIES

These studies are performed by stimulating a peripheral nerve at several points along its course and recording the muscle action potential or the sensory action potential that results. This test assesses how well the nerve transmits its electrical impulses.

CRANIAL NERVE TESTS

For neurological examinations for testing cranial nerves see Table 16.1. These tests are performed by a doctor.

LUMBAR PUNCTURE

Insertion of a needle into lumbar subarachnoid space and withdrawal of cerebrospinal fluid for diagnostic and therapeutic purposes.

GUIDELINES: ASSISTING THE PATIENT UNDERGOING A LUMBAR PUNCTURE

See Figure 16.1.

PURPOSES

1. Obtain cerebrospinal fluid for examination (microbiological, serological, cytological or chemical analysis), e.g. diagnosing meningitis.
2. Relieve cerebrospinal pressure, e.g. following neurosurgery.
3. Determine the presence or absence of blood in the spinal fluid, e.g. diagnosing subarachnoid haemorrhage.

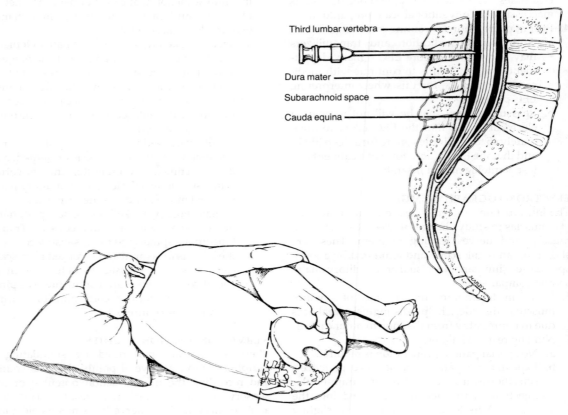

Third lumbar vertebra

Dura mater

Subarachnoid space

Cauda equina

Figure 16.1. Technique of lumbar puncture

EQUIPMENT

Sterile lumbar puncture set
Sterile gloves
Xylocaine 1–2 per cent
Skin antiseptic
Elastoplast

PROCEDURE

Note: During a lumbar puncture the nurse's prime responsibility is for the comfort and reassurance of the patient. Her secondary responsibility is to assist the doctor to perform the procedure under aseptic conditions. It is impossible for one nurse to fulfil both these responsibilities successfully.

Preparatory phase

Nursing action	**Rationale**
1. Give a step-by-step resumé of the procedure.	Reassures patient and gains his cooperation.

For lying position (see Figure 16.1):

2. Position the patient on his side with a pillow under his head. He should be lying on a firm surface.

3. Instruct the patient to arch the lumbar segment of his back and draw his knees up to his abdomen, clasping his knees with his hands.

This posture offers maximum widening of the interspinous spaces and affords easier entry into the subarachnoid space.

4. Assist the patient in maintaining his position by supporting him behind the knees and neck. Assist the patient to maintain the posture throughout the examination.

Supporting the patient helps prevent sudden movements which can produce a traumatic (bloody) tap and thus impede correct diagnosis.

For sitting position:

5. Have the patient straddle a straight-back chair (facing the back) and rest his head against his arms, which are folded on the back of the chair.

In obese patients and those who have difficulty in assuming an arched side-lying position, this posture may allow more accurate identification of the spinous processes and interspaces.

Performance phase (by the doctor)

Doctor/Nursing action

Rationale

1. The skin is prepared with antiseptic solution and the skin and subcutaneous spaces are infiltrated with local anaesthetic agent.

To reduce discomfort felt by the patient on insertion of spinal needle.

2. A spinal puncture needle is introduced between L3–L4 or L4–L5 interspace. The needle is advanced until the 'give' of the ligamentum flavum is felt and the needle enters the subarachnoid space. The manometer is attached to the spinal puncture needle.

L3–L4 or L4–L5 interspace is *below* the level of the spinal cord.

3. After the needle enters the subarachnoid space, the doctor may ask the nurse to help the patient to slowly straighten his legs.

This manoeuvre prevents a false increase in intraspinal pressure. Muscle tension and compression of the abdomen give falsely high pressures.

4. Instruct the patient to breathe quietly (not to hold his breath or strain).

Hyperventilation may lower a truly elevated pressure.

5. The initial pressure reading is obtained by measuring the level of the fluid column after it comes to rest.

With respiration there is normally some fluctuation of spinal fluid in the manometer. Normal range of spinal fluid pressure with patient in the lateral position is 70–180mmH$_2$O.

6. About 2–3ml of spinal fluid is placed in each of three sterile test tubes for observation, comparison and laboratory analysis.

Spinal fluid should be clear and colourless.

QUECKENSTEDT TEST

NURSING ALERT
This test is not done if an intracranial lesion is suspected.

Nursing action	Rationale
1. The nurse is asked by the doctor to compress the jugular vein or veins for 10 seconds.	This test is made when a spinal subarachnoid block is suspected (tumour; vertebral fracture or dislocation). In normal people there is a rapid rise in pressure of cerebrospinal fluid in response to jugular compression with rapid return to normal when the compression is released. If the pressure rises and falls slowly, there is evidence of a block due to a lesion's compressing the spinal subarachnoid pathways.
2. Pressure readings are made at 10-second intervals.	
3. After the needle is withdrawn, a sticking plaster is applied to the puncture site.	

Follow-up phase

Nursing action	Rationale
1. Record (a) procedure, (b) appearance of spinal fluid, (c) whether or not specimens were sent to laboratory, (d) spinal pressure readings, and (e) condition and reaction of patients.	
2. Allow the patient to find the most comfortable position in bed and to mobilize when he feels ready to.	
3. Administer prescribed analgesia for headache if necessary.	Some patients suffer from postpuncture headache which is thought to be caused by the leakage of spinal fluid at the puncture site. This headache can be minimized by the patient remaining flat or lying slightly head-down.

SPECIAL NEUROLOGICAL NURSING CONSIDERATIONS

NURSING MANAGEMENT OF THE PATIENT WITH RAISED INTRACRANIAL PRESSURE

INTRACRANIAL PRESSURE (ICP)
In the normal, conscious person, ICP is present and is continually fluctuating: falling when the head is raised and rising when it is lowered. Activities such as coughing or straining a stool, cause the ICP to rise sharply, but transiently.

Normal ICP measures: 80–180mm of water, 0–15mmHg.

Pathophysiology: is explained by modified Monro-Kellie hypothesis, which states: 'the skull, a rigid compartment, is filled to capacity with essentially non-compressible contents – brain tissue, intravascular blood and cerebrospinal fluid. If any of these three increases in volume, another must decrease or else intracranial pressure will rise' (Hickey, 1986).

CAUSES
1. Head injury.
2. Cerebral oedema.
3. Abscess or inflammation.
4. Haemorrhage.

5. Brain tumour.
6. Cranial surgery.
7. Hydrocephalus.

Note: The term 'space occupying lesion' (SOL) is often used when signs of raised intracranial pressure (RICP) are present, but no precise diagnosis has been made.

Nursing assessment

1. RICP can result in a wide variety of signs and symptoms in the patient, depending upon whether the increase in pressure on the brain is generalized (e.g. cerebral oedema) or localized (e.g. haematoma). The most life-threatening situation occurs when the RICP is directed towards the brain stem, as occurs during tentorial herniation.
2. There is a classic triad of events that often accompany an increase in ICP:
   a. Rising systolic blood pressure.
   b. Widening of pulse pressure.
   c. Bradycardia.
   However, this classic triad does not always occur and any marked change in observations, whatever the combination, should be reported to a senior nurse or doctor.
3. If RICP is to be detected early, then a wide range of assessment criteria need to be used by the nursing staff.

NEUROLOGICAL OBSERVATIONS

The Glasgow Coma Scale provides an objective method of assessment of the patient's conscious level, which indicates the overall brain function or dysfunction. The Coma Scale is usually included in a neurological observation chart, which also allows for the recording of pupil size and reaction, blood pressure, pulse, temperature, respiratory rate and limb movements (see Figure 16.2).

The responsibility for neurological observations, in most cases, will rest with the nurse. The interpretation of these observations will give the first indication to the medical staff that the intracranial pressure of the patient is rising, a potentially life-threatening situation, which may require rapid surgical intervention. It is important that nurses are competent at carrying out neurological observations accurately, and further reading is advised, as identified at the end of this chapter, to supplement the following information.

The Glasgow Coma Scale uses three types of behaviour to assess conscious level. Eye opening, verbal response and motor response. Each is assessed independently and recorded in the form of a graph on the chart.

1. Eye opening:
   a. Spontaneously – when approaching patient, observe whether eyes are open or closed.
   b. To speech – if eyes are closed, but open when patient is spoken to by name, record this as eye-opening to speech.
   c. To pain – if both of the above are unsuccessful, apply painful stimulus by applying pressure to fingernail bed. Record as eye-opening to pain if this results in patient opening his eyes.
   d. None – record as none if all of the above are unsuccessful.
2. Best verbal response – this section relates to the patient's level of orientation and should be modified if the patient has a known speech disorder.
   a. Orientated conversation.
   b. Confused conversation: ask patient several simple questions related to self, time, place and general facts. If orientated, patient should be able to give correct answers – allow for minor mistakes. If answers totally wrong, then record as confused.
   c. Inappropriate words – patient cannot participate in conversation and only says one or two words.
   d. Incomprehensible sounds – record this if moans and grunts are recorded in response to painful stimuli.
   e. No verbal response – record this, if patient produces no sounds in response to painful stimuli.
3. Motor response – arm, not leg responses are used. If arm responses are different then best arm response is used.
   a. Obeying commands – patient asked to perform a simple task, e.g. stick out tongue. If the patient does not respond, then painful stimuli are applied to supraorbital region, and response observed.
   b. Localize pain – patient focuses on source of irritation/pain, lifting arm in an attempt to remove it.
   c. Flexion to pain – pressure to nail bed produces flexion of the arm, i.e. bending elbow and withdrawing hand.
   d. Extension to pain – pressure to nail bed produces straightening of the elbow.
   e. None – record this if (b), (c) or (d) are not present.

PUPIL REACTION

1. Pupil reaction is tested using a pen torch.

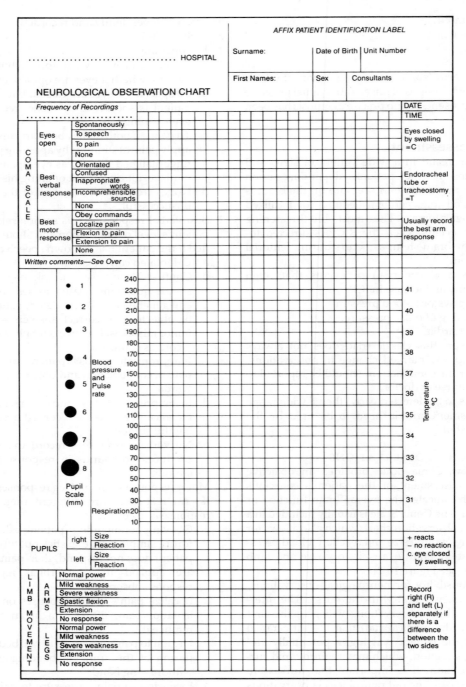

Figure 16.2. Example of neurological observation chart that includes the Glasgow Coma Scale. (Reproduced by courtesy of Butterworth and Co., London, from Campkin and Turner, *Neurological Anaesthesia and Intensive Care*)

2. Torch should be shone in each eye separately.
3. Patient should not be in a brightly lit environment, for accuracy.
4. Pupils should be equal in size and respond briskly to the light, by becoming smaller in size.
5. Record right and left pupil response and an estimate of the size of the pupil before it was tested.

LIMB MOVEMENT

1. As well as assessing the best motor response as part of the Coma Scale, it is necessary to observe limb movements to detect damage to motor pathways.
2. Both limbs should be tested, but only recorded separately if there is a difference.
3. If, on the Coma Scale, patient is able to obey commands, then ask patient to demonstrate the power of his arms by squeezing both your hands as tightly as possible. Power of the legs can be tested by asking the patient to push against your hands with his feet.
4. If, on the Coma Scale, patient is responding to pain, then this can be used to elicit response of extension or no response in limbs (see section 3 above.)

NURSING ALERT

1. *Know the patient's baseline condition; all observations should be compared to this.*
2. *Carry out repeated regular assessments – to determine improvement or deterioration.*
3. *Keep nursing staff constant to patient and at changeover of shift nurse assessment should be carried out jointly to ensure continuity of judgement.*
4. *Never omit a planned set of observations in kindness to the patient if he is asleep. ICP can rise rapidly in some cases, especially following head injury, and can produce an emergency situation within minutes.*

CLINICAL FEATURES

1. Change in Coma Scale (see Figure 16.2):
   a. If patient is fully alert he should be able to open eyes spontaneously to sounds, be orientated to name, time and place, and obey any commands, e.g. to squeeze nurse's fingers.
   b. Watch for sudden changes in condition – quietness to restlessness, orientation to no verbal response, obeying commands to no movement even with painful stimuli applied.
   c. Progressive deterioriation is a serious sign that may require immediate surgical intervention.
2. Changes in vital signs:
   a. Pulse changes – slowing rate to 60 or below; increasing rate to 100 or above.

b. Respiratory irregularities; slowing of rate with lengthening periods of apnoea; Cheyne–Stokes or Kussmaul breathing.
   c. Rising blood pressure or widening pulse pressure (the difference between systolic and diastolic blood pressure).
   d. Moderately elevated temperature.
3. Headache.
4. Vomiting.
5. Pupillary changes – increasing pressure or an expanding clot can displace the brain against the oculomotor or optic nerve.
   a. Observe size, reaction to light, deviation from midline.
   b. Look for dilating or nonreacting pupil(s), which may also be unequal.

INTRACRANIAL PRESSURE MONITORING

Intracranial pressure monitoring may be used where available.
1. Cannula (or catheter) is inserted into ventricle or subdural space and attached to a pressure transducer and recordings are then made.
   Normal level: 1–10mmHg.
   Slight increase: 11–20mmHg.
   Moderate increase: 21–40mmHg.
   Severely increased: more than 40mmHg.*
2. Effect of increased intracranial pressure on brain function varies; the cause of intracranial hypertension appears more important than the degree of pressure.
3. A change in the position of the head (e.g., flattening of bed to give care), endotracheal aspiration, hyperventilation or compression of jugular veins (head falling to one side) may markedly increase intracranial pressure.

MANAGEMENT OF INTRACRANIAL PRESSURE

1. Controlled ventilation:
   a. Hyperventilation with volume respirator – reduces blood volume in brain, causing vasoconstriction of cerebral vasculature which decreases intracranial pressure.
   b. Avoid hypoxia.
2. Osmotic diuretics (mannitol, glycerol) – given to dehydrate brain and reduce cerebral oedema (lowers intracranial pressure).
   a. Observe for electrolyte disturbances (particularly hyponatraemia) and dehydration.
   b. Make sure that indwelling catheter is in bladder since dehydrating agents produce diuresis.

---

* Horton, J.M. (1975) The immediate care of head injuries, *Anaesthesia*, 30: 212–18.

3. Steroids (dexamethasone): have dramatic effect in lowering cerebral oedema of brain tumour; appears less effective in head injury.
4. Hypothermia to reduce cerebral metabolic need for oxygen and glucose.
5. Keep the head of the bed elevated 30 to 45° (some neurosurgeons prefer the patient kept flat).
6. Removal of cerebrospinal fluid – can be removed from lateral ventricle when the patient is being monitored.
7. Prepare for surgical intervention if patient's condition deteriorates.

GUIDELINES: ADMINISTERING A TEPID SPONGE FOR FEVER

Fever is an abnormal elevation of body temperature.

A tepid sponge is the bathing of the body with tepid water (or alcohol and water) for a period of time to reduce fever. It is particularly effective in neurological conditions in which there is a disturbance of the temperature-regulating centre. Fever increases both intracranial pressure and the rate of development of cerebral oedema.

CAUSES
1. Infection.
2. Disturbance of temperature-regulating centre (trauma, central nervous system haemorrhage).
3. Tumours; diseases of blood-forming organs.
4. Heat stroke.
5. Drug toxicity; allergens.
6. Delirium tremens.

PURPOSE
To reduce body temperature when fever in itself may be deleterious.

EQUIPMENT
Basin of tepid water 21.1–29.1°C
   or
Basin of alcohol (25 per cent saturated with tepid water)
Bath blanket
Towels
Flannels/sponges/J cloths (×7)

NURSING ALERT
Make certain that the patient is adequately hydrated; unrecognized dehydration can result in decreased circulating blood volume, causing peripheral vasoconstriction which prevents heat loss.

PROCEDURE
Preparatory phase

Nursing action	Rationale
1. Place bath blanket over patient.	To prevent bedclothes becoming wet.
2. Remove top bedding.	

Performance phase

Nursing action	Rationale
1. Take temperature, pulse and respiration before starting sponge.	This serves as a baseline for determining effectiveness of treatment.

2. Give antipyretic medication as directed 15 to 20 minutes before starting sponge.
  a. Acetylsalicylic acid or
  b. Chlorpromazine.
	There is a more rapid reduction of fever when sponging is combined with administration of antipyretic medication.
	a. Has an anti-inflammatory, antipyretic or analgesic action.
	b. Controls shivering.

3. Place a wetted flannel on neck and in groin and each axilla.	The application of cold over superficial large blood vessels aids in lowering body temperature.
4. Expose the body area to be sponged. Place a towel under area. Sponge using circular movements.	Vaporization of water removes heat from the surface of the skin. Alcohol vaporizes at a lower temperature and removes heat from the skin more rapidly. Tepid water and alcohol are highly effective in producing vasodilation and evaporation of heat from skin.
5. If the patient's skin feels cold to the touch, apply skin friction to bring the blood to the surface.	
6. Bathe each extremity (5 minutes); bathe entire back and buttocks (5 to 10 minutes); bathe trunk and abdomen (5 minutes).	The fever sponge should not exceed 30 minutes.
7. Allow a fan to blow over the patient while sponging him if temperature is high.	Increased air movement augments heat loss.
8. Watch for extreme shivering. Cover the patient and wait a few minutes before proceeding with sponge.	Shivering may raise heat production.
9. Stop sponge if cyanosis, mottling, chilling do not stop when friction (rubbing) is applied to the skin.	These symptoms indicate a change in vasomotor tone.

Follow-up phase

Nursing action	Rationale
1. Remove bath blanket and change sheet. Place a dry gown on patient.	To ensure patient comfort
2. Record temperature and pulse rate 10 to 15 minutes after sponge is finished.	Post-sponge temperature indicates whether or not treatment has been effective.

CLASSIFICATION OF HEAD INJURIES

In the past, head injuries were often classified as being 'open', i.e. a skull fracture present, or 'closed', i.e. no skull fracture present. This method of classification was not very useful as it did not indicate how the injury had occurred or what the subsequent damage to the brain might be. It is now more usual to classify injuries in relation to the type of injury that has occurred.

Type 1: Blunt or acceleration/deceleration injury, e.g. head hits ground or plank hits head.

Type 2: Crush or compression injury, e.g. car falls off jack onto head or head caught between wall and vehicle.

Type 3: Sharp or penetrating injury, e.g. sharp instrument lodged in head or low velocity bullet.

Type 4: High velocity penetrating injury, e.g. rifle bullet.

EFFECTS OF INJURY ON SCALP, SKULL AND BRAIN

Types 1 and 2

1. Scalp – abrasions, contusions, haematoma, lacerations.
2. Skull:
   a. Fractures tend to be linear and are particularly dangerous if they cross vascular paths, e.g. temporal fracture.
   b. Fractures may be severe, but underlying brain damage relatively minor.
   c. Basal skull fractures can lead to cerebrospinal fluid leaks from ear, i.e. rhinorrhoea.
3. Brain – injury tends to be diffuse and can lead to concussion. Concussion is a disturbance or loss of consciousness associated with a variable period of amnesia for events before or after the incident. The most accurate assessment of severity of concussion can be made by measuring the length of time the post-traumatic amnesia (PTA) persists.
   For example:
   Minor concussion – PTA <24 hours
   Major concussion – PTA >24 hours to 1 month.
   The severity of the concussion leads to an indication of severity of underlying brain damage. May be due to contrecoup injury.

Types 3 and 4

1. Scalp:
   a. Tend to get puncture wounds and lacerations.

b. Often difficult to locate and small compared to underlying injury.
2. Skull – tendency to depressed skull fractures.
3. Brain:
   a. Type 3:
      (i) Damage tends to be more focal and surrounding penetrating instrument.
      (ii) Usually little or no concussion.
      (iii) Focal contusion or laceration.
      (iv) Effect depends on site and extent of focal injury, e.g. hemiplegia if motor area effected.
   b. Type 4:
      (i) The shock waves generated by the high velocity bullet travelling through the brain tissue leads to severe laceration which is more widespread than size of apparent injury would suggest.
      (ii) Usually fatal.

NURSING MANAGEMENT OF THE PATIENT WITH A HEAD INJURY

Assessment

CLINICAL FEATURES

1. Unconsciousness or disturbance in consciousness.
2. Headache.
3. Vertigo.
4. Confusion or delirium.
5. Changes in body temperature.
6. Respiratory irregularities.
7. Symptoms of shock – coldness, pallor, perspiring, falling blood pressure.
8. Pupillary abnormalities.

Planning and implementation

IMMEDIATE MANAGEMENT IN THE ACCIDENT AND EMERGENCY DEPARTMENT

NURSING ALERT

Regard every patient who has a head injury as having a potential spinal cord injury.

1. Maintain an open airway and ensure maximum respiratory function – oxygen deprivation and an excess of carbon dioxide may produce cerebral hypoxia and cause cerebral oedema with subsequent irreparable damage.
   a. Employ adequate suctioning procedures – patient may have aspirated blood and mucus from face and head injuries and the naso-

pharynx may be flooded with gastric contents – leads to pneumonitis which contributes to respiratory acidosis.

b. Ensure adequate oxygenation and humidification.

c. Assist with endotracheal intubation if patient is comatose.

d. Place patient in a semiprone head-level position to transport him from the accident and emergency department to the ward.

2. Determine the baseline condition of the patient; start neurological observation records.

a. Glasgow Coma Scale (see Figure 16.2). See also Nursing Management of a Patient with Raised Intracranial Pressure (p. 920).

b. Determine presence of headache, double vision, nausea or vomiting.

c. Evaluate pupil size and reaction to light.

d. Measure blood pressure, pulse, respirations.

e. Evaluate movement and strength of extremities.

f. Assess for injuries to other organ systems.

3. Obtain as accurate a history as possible from patient or observer.

a. What caused the injury? A high velocity missile? Object striking the head? A fall?

b. What were the direction and force of the blow?

c. *Was there loss of consciousness?* How long? Could the patient be aroused?

d. Is there any amnesia?

e. Was there any bleeding from eyes, ears, nose, mouth?

f. Was there paralysis or flaccidity of the extremities?

g. Are there any pupillary changes?

4. Be aware that convulsive seizures may occur.

TREATMENT AND NURSING MANAGEMENT*
Objectives
Observe for signs of raised intracranial pressure (see previous section).

Observe the patient constantly for the development of focal or generalized deficits of function that indicate need for surgical intervention.

1. Support the airway – small degrees of anoxia rapidly increase cerebral dysfunction and brain swelling.

a. Assist medical staff to carry out blood gas studies – to determine respiratory adequacy and assess effects of therapy.

b. Prepare for endotracheal intubation or

---

* See also nursing management of the unconscious patient (p. 929).

tracheostomy and ventilatory assistance if indicated.

c. Position the patient in a semiprone, three-quarters prone or prone position with his head level – improves oxygen and carbon dioxide exchange and prevents aspiration of secretions or blood.

d. Turn the patient from side to side – to prevent stasis of secretions in lungs and pressure on skin.

2. Observe, evaluate and carry out repeated neurological observations to determine minute-to-minute, hour-to-hour changes in patient's status and intracranial pressure.

NURSING ALERT
A change in the level of responsiveness/consciousness is the most sensitive indicator of improvement or deterioration. The level of responsiveness may change from minute to minute.

a. Observe and record:
   (i) Use Glasgow Coma Scale (Figure 16.2).
   (ii) Changes in vital signs.
   (iii) Motor strength.
   (iv) Pupillary changes.

b. See The Patient with Increasing Intracranial Pressure (p. 920).

3. Give fluids and electrolytes as prescribed by the medical staff. The patient may be kept slightly dehydrated to reduce extracellular fluid volume and cerebral oedema.

a. Do not give fluids by mouth to an unconscious patient.

b. Keep an accurate intake and output record.

c. Give nasogastric feeds if patient is unable to swallow after several days.

d. Be aware that patients with severe head injuries commonly develop stress ulcers which may produce severe gastrointestinal bleeding. This should be reported to medical staff at once.

e. Give prescribed intravenous infusions slowly (except mannitol which is given quickly). Overhydration may lead to cerebral oedema.

f. If the patient is unconscious it may be necessary to insert indwelling urinary catheter for assessment of urinary volume and to prevent restlessness from distended bladder.

Note: See also management of an unconscious patient (p. 929).

4. Control rising temperature with fans, tepid sponging and minimal amounts of bed clothing – to lower the metabolic requirements of the brain.

5. Give prescribed medication to treat cerebral oedema.
   a. Hyperosmolar solution (mannitol) given by intravenous infusion to dehydrate the brain and reduce cerebral oedema.
   b. Steroids (dexamethasone) may be given.
6. Observe ears and nose for leakage of cerebrospinal fluid – may indicate basilar skull fracture.

NURSING ALERT
Cerebrospinal fluid leakage may mask the usual clinical signs of an expanding intracranial haematoma by preventing brain compression.

   a. Tape sterile cotton pad under nose or loosely against ear to collect drainage.
   b. Elevate head of bed approximately 30° as directed – to reduce intracranial pressure and promote spontaneous closure of leak (some neurosurgeons prefer that the bed be kept flat).
   c. Persistence of cerebrospinal fluid otorrhoea or rhinorrhoea usually requires surgical intervention.
7. Patient may need to be treated for shock – from associated injuries of chest, abdomen, pelvis, fractures.
   a. Medical staff may require intravenous fluids, plasma or dextran, until blood transfusions can be started; these should be given as prescribed.
   b. Hourly urinary volume measurements (via indwelling catheter).
8. Support the patient during periods of restlessness.
   a. Avoid restraints; straining increases intracranial pressure.
   b. Medical staff may prescribe chloral hydrate or promazine hydrochloride (Sparine). Narcotics and sedatives should not be given as these will mask levels of responsiveness.
   c. Maintain as quiet an environment as possible.
   d. Elevate head of bed 15° unless otherwise indicated to help reduce cerebral oedema (some neurosurgeons prefer that the bed be kept flat).
   e. Be aware that restlessness may be caused by cerebral hypoxia, respiratory obstruction, pain from fractured extremities, tight cast or bandages, extradural haematoma, or distended bladder.
9. Give phenytoin (Epanutin) or phenobarbitone as prescribed – for control of seizures.
10. Protect the eyes from corneal irritation.
11. Carry out rehabilitation techniques.
    a. Put all extremities through range of motion exercises.
    b. Position the patient correctly to prevent contractures.
    c. Keep the skin dry, clean and free of pressure – to prevent pressure sores.
    d. Ensure a well-balanced diet.
    e. Gradually increase physical and mental activity (including resumption of increasingly difficult mental tasks).
12. Be aware of after-effects of head injury – usually directly related to the severity of the injury:
    a. Headache.
    b. Dizziness and vertigo.
    c. Emotional instability or irritability.
    d. Brain damage, which may lead to permanent physical disabilities.
    e. Post-traumatic epilepsy.
    f. Diabetes insipidus.
    g. Hydrocephalus.
    h. Post-traumatic neuroses and psychoses.

PATIENT EDUCATION
1. Encourage patient to continue his rehabilitation programme following discharge; improvement in status may continue up to three or more years following injury.
2. Headache may be the most reliable guide to recovery; use a second pillow/backrest at night.
3. Encourage patient to return gradually to usual activities.
4. Family may need help in setting limits for injured patient's impulses (anger, etc) and in realistically evaluating his capabilities. Family may have difficulty in understanding and accepting alterations in patient's behaviour.
5. May be useful for patient and family to contact local branch of Headway, a self-help organization which aims to help with problems of all kinds following a head injury: Headway, 17 Clumber Avenue, Sherwood Rise, Nottingham NG5 1AG.

Evaluation
EXPECTED OUTCOMES
1. Patient attains or maintains effective breathing, ventilation, and brain oxygenation – arterial blood gases within normal limits; normal breath sounds upon auscultation; spontaneous breathing without ventilatory assistance.
2. Patient becomes increasingly more responsive and oriented to environment – opens eyes spontaneously; responds to questions appropriately;

obeys simple commands; oriented to time, place and person.

3. Patient attains/maintains nutritional status – requests and takes fluids by mouth; maintains weight within expected limits.
4. Patient demonstrates continuing progress toward recovery.
5. Patient shows no evidence of physical or psychological complications – absence of seizures; less frequent outbursts of irritability or instability; beginning ability to remember names and recognize faces; reduced headache.

NURSING MANAGEMENT OF THE UNCONSCIOUS PATIENT

CLINICAL PROBLEMS

There are two major threats to the unconscious patient:
1. The disease or trauma that produced unconsciousness.
2. The threat of the unconscious state.

Assessment

CLINICAL FEATURES

Evaluate:
1. Responses to command or painful stimulus:
   a. Eye opening.
   b. Verbal responses.
   c. Motor responses.
2. Pupil reaction to light: size, equality; eye movement.
3. Swallowing reflexes; deep tendon reflexes.
4. Patterns of respiration (normal, Kussmaul, Cheyne-Stokes, apnoeic, etc).
5. Neck stiffness.
6. Head (for trauma); mouth, nose, ears for blood, cerebrospinal fluid.
7. Heart, lungs, abdomen.

PATIENT PROBLEMS

1. Ineffective airway clearance related to accumulation of secretions.
2. Potential for deepening level of unconsciousness related to change in intracranial homeostasis.
3. Alteration in fluid and electrolyte balance and reduced nutritional intake related to inability to take fluid and foods.
4. Potential for complications related to the unconscious state.

Planning and implementation
TREATMENT AND NURSING MANAGEMENT
Objectives
To assume the protective reflexes for the patient until he is aware of himself and can function in his environment.

Establish and maintain an adequate airway

1. Place the patient in a three-quarter prone or semiprone position with his face clear from obstruction – prevents the tongue from obstructing the airway, encourages drainage of respiratory secretions and promotes oxygen and carbon dioxide exchange.
2. Insert oral airway if tongue is paralysed or is obstructing airway – an obstructed airway increases intracranial pressure. This is considered a short-term measure.
3. Prepare for insertion of cuffed endotracheal tube if patient's condition requires – endotracheal intubation is more effective in permitting positive pressure ventilation. The cuffed tube seals off the digestive tract, preventing aspiration and allowing efficient removal of tracheobronchial secretions.
4. The medical staff (usually anaesthetist) may wish to use oxygen therapy, positive pressure assisted breathing techniques or mechanical ventilation with a ventilator when there is indication of impending respiratory failure.
5. Keep the airway free of secretions with efficient suctioning – in the absence of the cough and swallowing reflexes, secretions rapidly accumulate in the posterior pharynx and upper trachea and can pave the way to fatal respiratory complications.
   a. Attach sterile suction catheter to suction equipment.
   b. Do not apply suction while inserting the catheter.
   c. When catheter is at desired level turn the suction on and slowly withdraw catheter with a twisting motion of the thumb and forefinger.
   d. Gently turn the head from side to side while suctioning.
      (i) During suctioning the airway is effectively blocked, therefore limit tracheal aspiration to intervals of a few seconds.
      (ii) Allow patient to rest between aspirations.
      (iii) Oxygenate the patient between aspirations as required.
6. The medical staff will carry out periodic measurements of arterial Po_2 and Pco_2 (blood gases) to determine efficiency of treatment.

7. It may be necessary for the patient to have a tracheostomy if there is evidence of inadequate respiratory exchange or if it is likely that the patient will need artificial ventilation for more than a week.

Assess the level of responsiveness

Maintain a constant assessment of patient using Glasgow Coma Scale (see Figure 16.2). Unconscious patients may deteriorate rapidly from numerous clinical causes.

Evaluate the progression of vital signs

1. Know the patient's baseline vital signs and alert the medical staff if there are significant fluctuations of blood pressure and instability of the pulse and respiratory cycle – fluctuations of vital signs indicate a change in intracranial pressure.
2. Take blood pressure readings, pulse and respiratory rates and temperature at frequently special intervals until there is evidence of stabilization.

Maintain fluid and electrolyte balance

1. Give intravenous fluids as indicated. Serial laboratory electrolyte evaluations are made by the medical staff when the patient is maintained on intravenous fluids to ensure proper balance.
2. Initiate nasogastric feedings – feeding through a gastric tube ensures better nutrition than does intravenous feeding. Paralytic ileus is fairly frequent in the unconscious patient, and a nasogastric tube assists in gastric decompression.
   a. Insert small gastric tube through nose into stomach.
   b. Aspirate stomach before each feeding. It may be necessary to replace aspirate fluid, down the nasogastric tube, particularly if more than 50ml is being aspirated; this is to prevent both loss of fluid and electrolytes. If aspirated residual exceeds 50ml, the patient may be developing an ileus. Gastric distension and vomiting may result.
   c. Feeds (Clinifeed or a made-up preparation from the hospital diet kitchen) should be gradually increased until 400–500ml are given at each feeding.
   d. Give 2,000–2,500ml of fluid (according to patient's condition, remember head-injured patients may have their fluid intake restricted to 1,500ml).
   e. Rinse the tube with water after each feeding.
   f. Patient who has sustained a head injury will need a high-protein nasogastric feed, as head injury can cause cell metabolism to increase.

Give nursing support as the patient's changing condition indicates

1. Be aware of the varying phases of restlessness – a certain degree of restlessness may be favourable, since it may indicate the patient is regaining consciousness. However, restlessness is quite common in cerebral anoxia or when there is a partially obstructed airway, distended bladder, overlooked bleeding or fracture; it may be a manifestation of brain injury.
   a. Have adequate lighting in the room to prevent hallucinations as the patient regains consciousness.
   b. Pad side rails or use other devices to protect patient.
   c. Avoid sedating the patient.
   d. Avoid restraints if at all possible.
   e. Speak softly to the patient, calling him by name.
   f. Touch him as gently as possible.
2. Keep the skin clean, dry and free of pressure – unconscious patients are susceptible to formation of pressure sores.
3. Clip patient's nails to prevent excoriation of the skin.
4. Put all extremities through range of movement exercises four times daily – contracture deformities develop early in unconscious patients.
5. Turn the patient from side to side at regular intervals – turning relieves pressure areas and helps keep lungs clear by mobilizing secretions. Prolonged pressure on extremities produces nerve palsies.
6. Observe the patient for indication of an over-distended bladder.
   a. Utilize external sheath catheter (condom catheter) for male patient.
   b. If patient is unable to micturate, insert indwelling catheter with continuous drainage – infection invariably follows prolonged use of an indwelling catheter that is attached to straight drainage.
   c. Tape the catheter on the abdomen or horizontally to the side of the male patient and to the inner thigh of the female patient – to prevent urethral compression (male) and traction on the urethra.
7. Protect the eyes from corneal irritation – the cornea functions as a shield. If the eyes remain open for long periods, corneal drying, irritation and ulceration are apt to result.

a. Make sure patient's eye is not rubbing against bedding if blinking and corneal reflexes are absent.

b. Inspect the size of pupils and condition of eyes with a flashlight.

c. Remove contact lenses if worn.

d. Irrigate eyes with sterile prescribed solution and instil artificial tear drops in each eye – prevents glazing and corneal ulceration.

e. It may be necessary to carefully tape down the eyelids with a strip of hypoallergic tape or 'Steri-Strip'.

f. Prepare for temporary tarsorrhaphy (suturing of eyelids in closed position) if unconscious state is prolonged.

8. Protect the patient during convulsive seizures (see p. 948) – patient with head injury is a potential candidate for convulsive seizures.

   a. Protect the patient from self-injury.

   b. Observe the patient during the seizure and record observations.

   c. Regular mouth care and care of teeth. It may be necessary to remove full or partial dentures.

   d. Give prescribed anticonvulsant medications through the nasogastric tube.

9. Be alert for the development of complications.

   a. Respiratory complications (infections, aspiration, obstruction, atelectasis).

   b. Fluid and electrolyte imbalance.

   c. Infection (urinary, pressure sores, central nervous system).

   d. Bladder and gastrointestinal distension.

   e. Convulsive seizures.

10. Be aware that the patient will feel uneasy concerning his period of unconsciousness when he gains awareness of what has happened.

11. Encourage the family to become involved in small areas of the care if they want to.

Evaluation

EXPECTED OUTCOMES

1. Patient maintains clear airway – coughs up secretions; no crackles on lung auscultation; responds to appropriate stimuli.

2. Patient attains/maintains adequate fluid, electrolyte and nutritional status – swallowing reflexes normal; no clinical signs of dehydration; normal serum electrolyte values; bowel sound heard upon auscultation; minimal weight loss.

3. Patient is free of preventable complications – absence of pressure sores, contractures, overdistended bladder, corneal irritation, etc.

NURSING MANAGEMENT OF THE PATIENT UNDERGOING INTRACRANIAL SURGERY

Craniotomy is the surgical opening of the skull to remove a tumour, relieve intracranial pressure, evacuate a blood clot or stop haemorrhage.

Craniectomy is excision of a portion of the skull.

Cranioplasty is repair of a cranial defect.

Planning and implementation

TREATMENT AND NURSING MANAGEMENT

Preoperative care

Objective

Determine the precise location of the lesion (clot, tumour, aneurysm).

1. Assist the patient undergoing diagnostic tests and frequent neurological examinations.

2. Evaluate and record patient's symptoms and signs (paralysis, aphasia) preoperatively in order to make postoperative comparisons.

3. Support the patient with neurological motor and sensory defects.

   a. Position paralysed extremities to prevent contracture deformities.

   b. Familiarize the blind patient with his environment.

      (i) Personnel entering room should announce themselves – helps patient understand incoming stimuli.

      (ii) Help patient to assume an active role in his care.

   c. Assist the aphasic patient to communicate by means of picture cards, writing materials, etc.

   d. Protect the confused patient.

      (i) Remove disturbing environmental stimuli.

      (ii) Keep patient oriented to time and place; place wall calendar and clock where patient can see them.

   e. Instruct and encourage the patient and family about the impending surgery – to relieve anxiety and tension.

4. Prepare the patient physically for surgery.

   a. Reassure patient about the fact that his head will be shaved (usually in the theatre), but a wig is made available on the NHS.

   b. The hair is often washed the night before surgery.

   c. It is unusual for enemas to be given as straining upon defaecation raises intracranial pressure.

   d. Give medications and treatment as indicated:

      (i) Steroids – to decrease cerebral oedema.

      (ii) May be necessary to insert indwelling

catheter – as dehydrating agents are usually given during operation.

Postoperative care
Objectives

Watch for life-threatening complications, namely increasing intracranial pressure from oedema and bleeding.

Improve the functional status of the patient.

1. Establish proper respiratory exchange – to eliminate systemic hypercarbia and anoxia which increase cerebral oedema.
   a. Keep the patient in a lateral or a semiprone position – to facilitate respiratory exchange.
   b. Employ tracheopharyngeal suction – to remove secretions.
   c. Elevate the head of the bed 30cm after the patient is conscious – to aid venous drainage of the brain (some neurosurgeons prefer patient to be kept flat).
   d. See that the patient has nothing by mouth until an active coughing and swallowing reflex is demonstrated.
2. Assess patient's level of responsiveness.
   a. Use Glasgow Coma Scale (see Figure 16.2).
   b. Observation of patient's spontaneous activity:
      (i) Verbal or other communication.
      (ii) Changes in posture (frequency).
      (iii) Breathing pattern.
      (iv) Retching, vomiting.
      (v) Restlessness, twitching, tremors, convulsions.

NURSING INTERVENTIONS

1. Keep the patient's temperature within normal limits during postoperative period – temperature control may be lost in certain neurological states; a higher temperature increases the metabolic demands of the brain and can also lead to convulsions.
   a. Take rectal temperature at specified intervals. Extremities may be cold and dry due to paralysis of heat-losing mechanisms (vasodilation and sweating).
   b. Employ measures to reduce excessive fever when present.
      (i) Remove blankets; place loin cloth over patient.
      (ii) Aspirin suppositories may be prescribed (high fever of central origin is less responsive to salicylates).
      (iii) Apply ice bags to axilla and groin – application of cold over large superficial vessel helps lower body temperature.
      (iv) Give tepid water or alcohol sponge (see p. 924).
      (v) Use a fan blowing on patient – to increase surface cooling.
      (vi) Medical staff may prescribe chlorpromazine or promazine (Sparine) – prevents excessive shivering.
2. Evaluate for signs and symptoms of increasing intracranial pressure.
   a. Assess patient (minute by minute, hour by hour) for:
      (i) Diminished response to stimuli.
      (ii) Fluctuations of vital signs.
      (iii) Restlessness.
      (iv) Weakness and paralysis of extremities.
      (v) Increasing headache.
      (vi) Changes or disturbances of vision; dilated pupils.
   b. Control postoperative cerebral oedema.
      (i) Medical staff may prefer patient to be kept *slightly* underhydrated – to combat cerebral oedema.
      (ii) Record urinary specific gravity at intervals – especially indicated for surgery of the pituitary and hypothalamus to detect diabetes insipidus.
      (iii) Evaluate electrolyte status:
         (a) Early postoperative weight gain indicates fluid retention; a greater than estimated loss of weight indicates negative water balance.
         (b) Loss of sodium and chlorides will produce weakness, lethargy and coma.
         (c) Low potassium will cause confusion and lower level of responsiveness.
      (iv) Give steroids and osmotic dehydrating agents in selected cases, in postoperative period, according to doctor's instructions.
      (v) Institute hypothermia procedures (see above) to decrease brain metabolism.
      (vi) Elevate head of bed 20–30° to reduce intracranial pressure and to facilitate respiration (some neurosurgeons prefer patient to be kept flat).
3. Perform supportive measures until the patient is able to care for himself.
   a. Change position frequently since pain and pressure responses are variable.
   b. Give analgesics that do not mask level of responsiveness – i.e. codeine based drugs.
   c. Support the patient if convulsive seizures occur (see p. 948).
   d. Relieve signs of periorbital oedema.

(i) Bathe eyes frequently with normal saline.

(ii) Watch for signs of keratitis if cornea has no sensation.

e. Put extremities through range of motion exercises.

f. Use aseptic measures in management of indwelling urethral catheter.

g. Evaluate and support patient during episodes of restlessness.

(i) Evaluate for airway obstruction, distended bladder, meningeal irritation from bloody cerebrospinal fluid.

(ii) Pad patient's hands and bed rails – to protect from injury.

h. Watch for leakage of cerebrospinal fluid since there is ever present danger of meningitis.

(i) Differentiate between cerebrospinal fluid and mucus.

(a) Collect fluid on Dextrostix – if cerebrospinal fluid is present, indicator will have positive reaction since cerebrospinal fluid contains sugar.

(b) Assess for moderate elevation of temperature and mild neck rigidity.

(ii) It may be necessary to keep cerebrospinal pressure low by periodic lumbar puncture – to reduce cerebrospinal fluid pressure and decrease its force against the wound. Following post fossa operations, frequent lumbar punctures are performed to remove blood-stained cerebrospinal fluid and therefore decrease meningeal irritation and headache.

i. Reinforce blood-stained dressings with sterile dressing; blood-soaked dressings act as a culture medium for bacteria.

j. Evaluate patient with hypophysectomy (surgery on pituitary) for diabetes insipidus.

(i) Keep input and output record.

(ii) Evaluate specific gravity of all urine passed.

(iii) Weigh daily.

4. Assess for complications.

a. Intracranial haemorrhage. (Postoperative bleeding may be intraventricular, intracerebral, intracerebellar, subdural or extradural.)

(i) Watch for progressive impairment of state of responsiveness, signs of increasing intracranial pressure.

(ii) Prepare patient for CAT scanning.

(iii) Prepare patient for reoperation and evacuation of haematoma.

b. Brain oedema/infarction.

c. Postoperative meningitis.

d. Wound infections (scalp, bone flap) – wound may have to be reopened.

e. Pulmonary complications.

f. Epilepsy. (There is a greater risk of epilepsy with supratentorial operations.)

(i) Give prescribed anticonvulsants on a long-term basis.

(ii) Watch for status epilepticus which may occur after any intracranial operation.

g. Gastrointestinal ulceration (signs and symptoms of haemorrhage and perforation or both).

BELL'S PALSY

Bell's palsy (facial paralysis) is due to peripheral involvement of the seventh cranial nerve (facial) on one side, producing weakness or paralysis of the facial muscles.

Assessment
CLINICAL FEATURES

1. Distortion of face – from paralysis of facial muscles.

2. Feeling of numbness in face.

3. Eye problems:

a. Insensitive cornea (from denervation) – may be damaged without usual warning symptoms of pain.

b. Epiphora (overflow of tears down the cheek) – from keratitis caused by drying of cornea and lack of blink reflex; laxity of lower eyelid may alter proper drainage of tears.

c. Or decreased tear production – may lead to a dry eye which is predisposed to infection.

4. Difficulty with articulation of words, due to facial paralysis.

5. Pain – behind ear or in face.

CLINICAL MANIFESTATIONS

1. The aetiology of Bell's palsy is unknown. The three theories of possible aetiological causes (and combinations thereof) are vascular ischaemia, viral (herpes simplex; herpes zoster) and autoimmune disease.

2. It is more likely to occur in diabetic people than in non-diabetics.

3. Bell's palsy can produce grotesque disfigurement with accompanying physical and emotional stress.

4. There is no clear method of determining the prognosis at the time of onset of paralysis.

DIAGNOSTIC EVALUATION
1. History of acute onset.
2. Tests of cranial nerve function.
3. Electrodiagnostic study of facial muscles through electromyography – electrodes placed over branches of facial nerve; facial muscles observed for movement.

COMPLICATIONS
1. Corneal ulceration; blindness.
2. Facial weakness.
3. Facial spasm with contracture and synkinesis (unintentional movement).
4. Crocodile tearing.

Planning and implementation
TREATMENT AND NURSING MANAGEMENT
Objectives
Maintain muscle tone of the face.
Prevent or minimize denervation.
1. Give steroid therapy (prednisone) – may be helpful in reducing inflammation and oedema, which reduces vascular compression and permits restoration of blood circulation in the nerve; early administration appears to diminish severity of disease and mitigate pain.
2. Promote pain relief.
   a. Give salicylates or codeine as indicated.
   b. Apply heat to involved side of face – to provide comfort and to stimulate blood perfusion through facial muscles.
3. Protect the involved eye – facial paralysis may abolish the blinking reflex; eye is vulnerable to dust and foreign particles.

NURSING ALERT
Keratitis is a major threat to a patient with Bell's palsy.

   a. Protect the cornea with preparation of artificial tears.
   b. Use mild eyewash several times a day during acute stage as directed.
   c. Use eye ointment at bedtime – helps to keep eyes closed during sleep by sticking the lashes together.
   d. See that patient wears a protective patch, particularly at night.
      (i) Patch may eventually abrade cornea as paretic (incompletely paralysed) eyelids are difficult to keep closed.
      (ii) Eyelids may have to be sutured together.
   e. Instruct patient to use protective glasses (wraparound sunglasses or goggles) to decrease normal evaporation from eye.

4. Start facial massage (if no nerve tenderness present) several times daily to help maintain muscle tone.
   a. Teach patient to massage his face with gentle upward motion.
   b. Electrical stimulation to face (by physiotherapist) may or may not be prescribed.

PATIENT EDUCATION
1. Reassure patient that spontaneous recovery occurs in majority of patients; usually within three to five weeks.
2. Keep the face warm.
3. Teach facial exercises – to prevent facial muscle atrophy and to improve strength of remaining innervated muscles. Do the following while looking in a mirror.
   a. Wrinkle forehead.
   b. Close eyes.
   c. Purse lips.
   d. Move mouth from side to side.
   e. Blow out cheeks.
   f. Whistle.
4. Reinforce teaching concerning eye care (see above).

TRIGEMINAL NEURALGIA (TIC DOLOREUX)

Trigeminal neuralgia (tic doreux) is a condition of the fifth cranial nerve, characterized by sudden paroxysms of lancing or burning pain (alternating with periods of complete comfort) in the distribution of one or more branches of the trigeminal nerve.

AETIOLOGY
Unknown – may be related to compression of nerve near to brain stem.

Assessment
CLINICAL FEATURES
1. Sudden and severe pain appearing without warning – in distribution of one or more branches of trigeminal nerve (Figure 16.3).
2. Numerous individual flashes of pain, usually on one side, ending abruptly.
3. Attacks often precipitated by pressure on, or stimulation of, a trigger point, the terminals of the affected branches. (Movement of the face, talking, chewing, yawning, swallowing, shaving, cold wind, may precipitate an agonizing attack.)

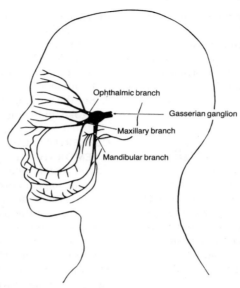

Figure 16.3. Main divisions of the trigeminal nerve are ophthalmic, maxillary and mandibular. Sensory root fibres arise in the Gasserian ganglion.

Planning and implementation
NURSING INTERVENTIONS
Objective
Give pain relief without loss of function.
1. Instruct patient to avoid exposing affected cheek to sudden cold if this is known to trigger the nerve – iced drinks, cold wind, swimming in cold water.
2. Drug therapy (antiepileptic drugs):
   a. Carbamazepine (Tegretol) or phenytoin (Epanutin) – relieves and prevents pain in some patients.
   b. Serum levels of drug monitored to avoid drug toxicity.
   c. Observe for evidence of haematological, hepatic, renal and skin reactions.
3. Surgical approach to treatment – used after medical treatment fails to give relief.
   a. Objective – to provide optimum pain relief with minimum impairment.
   b. Alcohol injection of ganglion or peripheral branches produces temporary chemical destruction of affected nerves.
      (i) Pain returns after nerve regeneration; usually six to 19 months.
      (ii) Usually produces complete anaesthesia.
   c. Radiofrequency lesions – percutaneous electrocoagulation of the Gasserian ganglion and its rootlets – introduction of needle electrode through foramen ovale to the desired portion of the trigeminal root; low voltage stimulation applied to electrode and a lesion is made. Carefully controlled electrical currents destroy enough of sensory portion of nerve to relieve pain without damaging touch sensation or motor function of face.
      (i) Root selection is made by conscious patient's response to electrical stimulation.
      (ii) Abolishes pain, but leaves touch sensation intact.
      (iii) Permanent relief expected in most patients.
   d. Open surgical procedures (not done in the first instance).
      (i) Peripheral neurectomy (excision of part of a nerve).
         (a) Usually done in patients whose pain is from first division of nerve.
         (b) Gives more prolonged relief than alcohol injection.
      (ii) Open surgical retrogasserian rhizotomy (destruction of retrogasserian rootlets).
         (a) Gasserian ganglion lies in the middle fossa and may be reached by a subtemporal, intradural or extradural route.
         (b) Following operation, patient has a complete loss of sensation in the distribution of the divided nerve fibres.

(c) See nursing management following craniotomy, p. 931.

(d) Complications: paraesthesiae (burning, stinging, numbness, discomfort in and around eye, herpetic lesions of the face, keratitis and corneal ulceration).

CEREBROVASCULAR DISEASE

Cerebrovascular disease refers to any functional abnormality of the central nervous system caused by interference with normal blood supply to the brain. The pathology may involve an artery, a vein or both, when the cerebral circulation becomes impaired as a result of partial or complete occlusion of a blood vessel or haemorrhage resulting from a tear in the vessel wall.

CEREBROVASCULAR DISEASE FROM IMPAIRMENT OF CEREBRAL CIRCULATION
Transient ischaemic attacks (TIAs)
Transient episodes of cerebral dysfunction commonly manifested by a sudden loss of motor, sensory or visual function, lasting minutes up to an hour or more, but no longer than 24 hours.
1. Causes – temporary impairment of blood flow to the brain by atherosclerosis of vessels supplying the brain, or obstruction of cerebral microcirculation by small embolus.
2. Treatment:
   a. Antiplatelet aggregation drugs (e.g. aspirin or persantin) – when problem is related to platelet aggregation.
   b. Anticoagulant therapy (heparin, warfarin).
   c. Angiography – to identify surgically treatable lesions, e.g. carotid stenosis.
   d. Surgical intervention – to increase blood flow to brain:
      (i) Carotid endarterectomy.
      (ii) Extracranial/intracranial anastomosis – provides revascularization of brain.

Cerebral thrombosis
Usually produces transient loss of speech, visual disturbance, hemiplegia or paraesthesia in one half of the body, which may precede severe paralysis. (See nursing management of the patient with a stroke.)

Cerebral embolism
Caused by heart disease (infective endocarditis, rheumatic heart disease, prosthetic heart valves, myocardial infarction) or pulmonary emboli.
1. Embolism usually lodges in middle cerebral artery or its branches where it disrupts circulation.
2. Symptoms – sudden onset of hemiparesis or hemiplegia.
3. See the nursing management of the patient with a stroke, in the discussion which follows.

CEREBROVASCULAR DISEASE FROM HAEMORRHAGE
Extradural haemorrhage
Haemorrhage occurring outside the dura mater:
1. This is considered a life-threatening emergency.
2. See care of the patient with head injury for principles of immediate care (p. 926).

Subdural haemorrhage
Haemorrhage occurring beneath the dura mater. See care of the patient with a head injury (p. 926).

Subarachnoid haemorrhage
Haemorrhage occurring in the subarachnoid space – may result from leaking aneurysm, congenital arteriovenous malformation, hypertension, tumour or trauma. See treatment of subarachnoid haemorrhage, p. 943.

Intracerebral haemorrhage
Haemorrhage occurring within the brain substance – usually from hypertension, cerebral atherosclerosis, aneurysm, etc.

STROKE OR CEREBROVASCULAR ACCIDENT (CVA)

A stroke (cerebrovascular accident) is a condition in which the blood supply to the brain is reduced as a result of transient ischaemic attacks, cerebral thrombosis, cerebral embolism, intracerebral or subarachnoid haemorrhage.

Assessment
CLINICAL FEATURES OF IMPENDING STROKE
1. Memory impairment, vertigo, headache, syncope, blurring of vision, etc.
2. Focal or neurological signs – hemiparesis or hemiplegia, aphasia, homonymous hemianopia, ataxia, cranial nerve palsies, stupor, coma.

RISK FACTORS
1. Hypertension.
2. Previous transient ischaemic attacks.

3. Cardiac disease (atherosclerotic/valvular heart disease, dysrhythmias).
4. Advanced age.
5. Diabetes.
6. Oral contraceptives.
7. Cigarette smoking.

Planning and implementation
NURSING INTERVENTIONS
The acute phase: Period of altered consciousness
Objectives
Monitor and preserve vital functions.
Ensure adequate cerebral perfusion of oxygen.
Reorientate the patient when he regains awareness.

1. See the nursing management of the unconscious patient (p. 929).
2. Carry out a nursing assessment of the following:
   a. A change in the level of responsiveness as evidenced by movement, resistance to changes of position and response to stimulation.
   b. Presence or absence of voluntary or involuntary movements of the extremities; tone of the muscles; body posture and the position of the head.
   c. Stiffness or flaccidity of the neck.
   d. Comparison of pupils as to size, reaction to light and ocular position.
   e. Colour of the face and extremities; temperature and moisture of the skin.
   f. Quality and rates of pulse and respiration; body temperature and arterial pressure.
   g. Volume of fluids ingested or administered via a nasogastric tube and volume of urine excreted each 24 hours.
3. Ensure an adequate perfusion pressure so that oxygenated blood can reach the brain.
   a. Maintain blood pressure and cardiac output – to sustain cerebral blood flow.
   b. Watch for evidence of myocardial infarction, dysrhythmias and congestive heart failure; dysrhythmia may reduce cerebral blood flow and produce cardiac arrest.
   c. Ensure hydration; dehydration may reduce blood viscosity and thereby improve cerebral blood flow.
4. Reorient the patient when he begins to regain consciousness.
   a. Expect some dysphasia if patient has right-sided hemiplegia.
   b. Reassure patient that he has not lost his mind and that he will receive help with communication (speech therapist).
   c. *Talk* to the patient while caring for him.

d. Make every effort to understand the patient.
e. Maintain a calm and accepting manner during periods of emotional lability.
5. Remove indwelling catheter as soon as patient is conscious.
   a. Offer bedpan or urinal at scheduled short intervals.
   b. Lengthen time intervals as more bladder control is gained.
6. Prepare for surgical intervention if indicated – to halt potential occlusive lesions and restore circulation.
7. The following may be amenable to surgical intervention:
   a. Intracerebral haematoma (from any cause).
   b. Cerebral aneurysm.
   c. Acute and chronic subdural haematomas.
   d. Arteriovenous malformation (angiomas).

Rehabilitation phase
Nursing staff will be part of the rehabilitation team which includes physiotherapists, occupational therapists, speech therapists and clinical psychologists. It is important that at all times the nursing staff reinforce the exercises and rehabilitation programmes designed by other members of the team.

Objectives
Prevent deformities.
Retrain the affected arm and leg.
Help the patient gain independence in activities of daily living.

1. Position the patient in bed correctly – to prevent contractures, relieve pressure and maintain good body alignment. (These principles of positioning are also carried out during the unconscious phase; see Figures 16.4 and 16.5.)
   a. It is useful to lie the patient on the affected side to prevent flexion of arm and hip. Be aware many patients find this difficult to tolerate (see Figure 16.5).
   b. Changing the patient's position in bed can be best achieved by rolling the patient from side to side. This promotes a sense of security for the patient and is less tiring (Figure 16.6).

NURSING ALERT
Do not pull on the patient's affected arm, because the shoulder is susceptible to injury.

The patient should be fully on his side

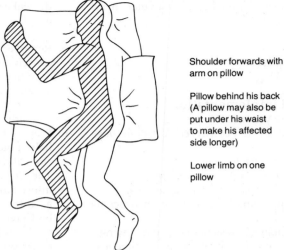

Shoulder forwards with arm on pillow

Pillow behind his back (A pillow may also be put under his waist to make his affected side longer)

Lower limb on one pillow

DO NOT put anything in the patient's affected hand or under the sole of his foot

Figure 16.4. Lying on the unaffected side. (Courtesy of Myco (1983) *Nursing Care of the Hemiplegic Stroke Patient*, Harper & Row, London)

His head is slightly forward

His trunk is straight and supported by a pillow

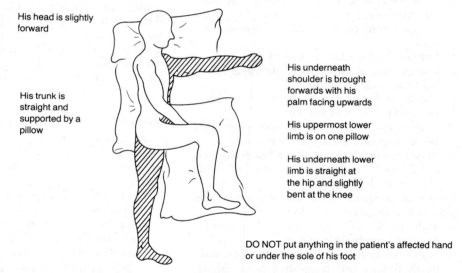

His underneath shoulder is brought forwards with his palm facing upwards

His uppermost lower limb is on one pillow

His underneath lower limb is straight at the hip and slightly bent at the knee

DO NOT put anything in the patient's affected hand or under the sole of his foot

Figure 16.5. Lying on the affected side (shaded area). (Courtesy of Myco (1983) *Nursing Care of the Hemiplegic Stroke Patient*, Harper & Row, London)

2. Exercise the affected extremities passively and carry out range of movement exercises four to five times daily – to prevent contracture development in the paralysed extremity, to prevent further deterioration of neuromuscular system, to stretch soft tissues and to enhance circulation.
   a. Involve family in exercise programme since care of a stroke patient requires time and effort.
   b. Remind the patient to exercise unaffected limbs at intervals throughout the day – to prevent contracture development in the normal limbs.
   c. Teach patient to put his unaffected leg under the affected one in order to move and turn himself.
   d. Instruct the patient to move his affected arm (and hand) with his good hand.

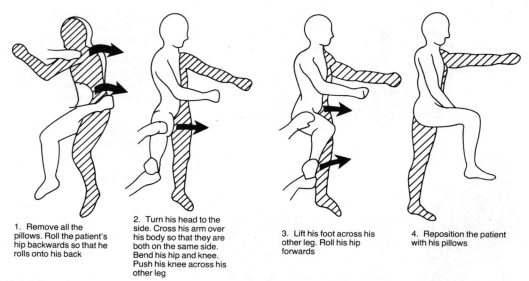

1. Remove all the pillows. Roll the patient's hip backwards so that he rolls onto his back

2. Turn his head to the side. Cross his arm over his body so that they are both on the same side. Bend his hip and knee. Push his knee across his other leg

3. Lift his foot across his other leg. Roll his hip forwards

4. Reposition the patient with his pillows

Figure 16.6. Rolling the patient over. (Courtesy of Myco (1983) *Nursing Care of the Hemiplegic Stroke Patient*, Harper & Row, London)

3. Adjust nursing approach to the patient's condition.
   a. Test for hemianopia (defective vision in half of the visual field).
      (i) Show patient an object placed to one side and ask if he can identify it.
      (ii) Hemianopia is evident if patient fails to see the object on the correct side, but responds by looking towards it on the other side. (Visual field is likely to be limited on the right if patient has right hemiplegia.)
   b. Place call light, bedside table, etc, on the side of his awareness.
   c. Approach the bed from the uninvolved side.
   d. Encourage the patient to turn his head from side to side to obtain the full view of a normal visual field.
   e. Have patient wear his spectacles.
   f. For patient with dysarthria (difficulty in articulating speech) and dysphagia (difficulty in swallowing):
      (i) Give nasogastric tube feeding if indicated.
      (ii) Give food and fluids from uninvolved side (if patient has droop of mouth). Semi-solid food may be easier to swallow.
      (iii) Remind patient to chew on unaffected side.
      (iv) Inspect patient's mouth for food collecting between cheek and gums on involved side; frequent oral hygiene is necessary.
   g. See p. 942 for nursing management of patient with aphasia.
4. Maintain bladder and bowel programme.
5. Assist the patient in getting out of bed as soon as balance returns (Figure 16.7). When planning a mobilization programme for the patient the following points should be considered: overall physical condition; current degree of mobility; physical strength; level of comprehension; and motivation.
   a. To develop sitting balance:
      (i) Slowly assist patient to a sitting position.
      (ii) Place patient's feet on floor (or on the seat of a chair).
      (iii) Place the patient's unaffected hand behind him – to assist in maintaining balance.
      (iv) Stand in front of patient – to help him maintain this posture. Watch for postural hypotension.
      (v) Assess for change in colour, shortness of breath, profuse perspiration – indications that patient should be placed back in dorsal position.
      (vi) Increase sitting time as rapidly as patient's condition permits.
   b. To develop standing balance:
      (i) Put walking shoes with strong shank on patient for all ambulation activities. (If shoes not available, it is safer for patient

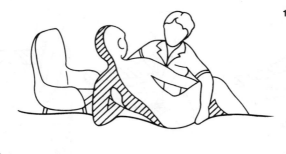

1. Place the chair on the affected side at the head end of the bed.
   Roll the patient onto his affected side

   Hold the patient with one arm under the affected shoulder and your hand over the shoulder blade and your other arm around his legs.

   Swing his legs over the side of the bed and bring him to sitting.

   Rearrange clothes, etc.

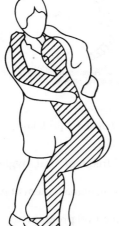

2. Rock or wriggle him to the edge of the bed. Place your hands over his shoulder blades with his arms resting on yours. He must not grip his hands together or he will pull your neck.
   Make sure both of his feet are flat on the floor, KEEP YOUR BACK STRAIGHT! And bend your knees. Wedge his feet and knees with yours.

3. Bring both of his shoulders well forwards to get his body weight over both feet.
   DO NOT LIFT HIM.
   Use your weight to counterbalance his by pressing downwards and forwards on his shoulders and leaning slightly backwards to bring him up to standing.
   With his shoulders fixed by your hands and his knees fixed by yours pivot him round, keep his shoulders forward and lower him down into the chair.

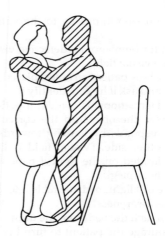

Figure 16.7. Getting out of bed. (Courtesy of Myco (1983) *Nursing Care of the Hemiplegic Stroke Patient*, Harper & Row, London)

to walk in bare feet rather than slippers.)
(ii) See Figure 16.7.
(iii) Stand behind patient and stabilize him at waist level.
(iv) Assess for dizziness, pallor and increasing pulse rate.
(v)   Assist patient to achieve standing balance at frequent intervals throughout the day.
(iv) Help the patient begin walking as soon as standing balance is achieved (using parallel bars).
(vii) Encourage patient to look at his feet occasionally – proprioceptive loss may accompany hemiplegia.

6. Encourage patient to perform his self-care activities as soon as possible. The occupational therapist should be involved in assessing and helping the patient with this.
   a. Set realistic goals and add a new task daily if possible.
   b. Have the patient immediately transfer all self-care activities to the unaffected side. Teach one-handed methods.
   c. Encourage him to brush his teeth, comb his hair and bathe and feed himself.

d. Help the patient to dress himself for ambulatory activities.
   (i) Instruct family to bring clothing that is one size larger than usually worn.
   (ii) Have patient dress himself (with assistance if necessary) while seated – to achieve better balance.
   (iii) Use clothing with front fasteners; stretch fabrics are preferable.
   (iv) Teach only one activity at a time.
7. Assist in securing supportive devices if needed – most patients develop spasticity of lower extremity and will lack motor control.
   a. The physiotherapist may secure posterior knee splint if patient has a weakened or absent quadriceps muscle – gives better balance and helps prevent loss of position sense.
   b. The physiotherapist may secure an adjustable aluminium tripod when patient is able to walk alone.
8. The physiotherapist may advise the use of a sling on the paralysed arm when patient is in upright position, if arm is flaccid or if patient complains of arm pain and heaviness.
   a. Remove sling frequently and exercise arm.
   b. Encourage patient to interlace his fingers, placing the palms together. With elbows extended, lift both arms above head repeatedly throughout day.
   c. When seated, keep the affected arm and hand elevated with a pillow.
   d. Encourage patient to flex and extend his wrist and fingers with unaffected hand at frequent intervals.
9. Secure a wheelchair of the correct size, with brakes that the patient can manage if he is unable to ambulate (physiotherapist will advise on this).
   a. Place wheelchair on patient's unaffected side; allows him to see wheelchair and lead with the stronger leg.
   b. Lock wheelchair brake and remove pedals. Instruct the patient as follows:
      (i) Lean forward, placing weight over strong leg. Push up with strong arm and foot.
      (ii) Place most of the weight on the strong leg while keeping weak knee locked.
      (iii) Pivot in the direction of the stronger leg; bring weak leg over to stronger leg. Maintain standing position a few moments.
      (iv) Lower body into chair gradually, using strong arm and leg.
      (v) Push wheelchair with uninvolved leg.

10. Prepare the patient for discharge. Home assessment is carried out by occupational therapist.
    a. Some patients will have to be transferred to rehabilitation centres for further therapy.
    b. Encourage patient to keep active, adhere to his exercise programme and remain as self-sufficient as possible.

FAMILY/PATIENT EDUCATION
Instruct the family as follows; with the help and advice of other members of the health care team.
1. Expect some emotional lability and some degree of brain damage if the patient has had a more severe stroke.
   a. Patient may cry easily; this does not necessarily imply unhappiness.
   b. Hemiplegic patients may be easily confused, forgetful, discouraged, hostile, uncooperative, withdrawn and dependent.
   c. Support him psychologically; hemiplegia has a tremendous psychological impact on the patient (and his family).
2. Avoid doing those things for the patient that he can do for himself.
3. Be supportive and sympathetic but firm and direct.
4. Install handrails by the toilet and bath or shower and put safety rails on the bed.
5. Obtain self-help devices to assist in activities of daily living; modify and adapt devices and 'gadgets' to meet individual patient's needs (occupational therapist can advise on these); e.g. nonslip mat under plate; plate guard to keep food from being pushed off plate.
6. See that patient has rest periods.
7. Set realistic goals.
8. The patient will need to attend outpatient clinics.
9. Take advantage of community services.

Evaluation
EXPECTED OUTCOMES
1. Patient obtains optimum mobility:
   a. Exercises affected/unaffected extremities; free of contractures.
   b. Attains sitting balance and transfers to wheelchair.
   c. Shows beginning ability to walk with reciprocal pattern.
2. Patient compensates for sensory deficits – feeds self; turns head to compensate for visual field deficits; remembers to look at feet occasionally; achieves increasing ability in self-care.
3. Patient communicates needs and wants to others – uses gestures when word-finding is difficult;

able to make needs known; watches facial expression/body language for nonverbal communication; attends classes with speech–language pathologist.

4. Patient attains/maintains bladder control – signals desire to urinate; transfers to bedside commode; absence of retention; absence of bacteriuria.
5. Patient attains/maintains bowel control – signals desire to defaecate; transfers to bedside commode; absence of faecal soiling/constipation.
6. Patient acquires increasing independence in self-care.
7. Patient copes with changes in lifestyle – uses cues and memory aids; has printed list of sequencing steps for activities; returns to some previous social interests/activities.
8. Patient demonstrates lessening emotional lability.

APHASIA

Aphasia is a disturbance of language resulting from cerebral dysfunction. It may involve impairment of the ability to read and write as well as to speak, listen and comprehend. The term 'aphasia' strictly indicates a complete loss of function, whereas 'dysphasia' implies partial loss; however, the prefixes a- and dys- are often used interchangeably.

The term 'dysarthria' is used when a patient has difficulty with the articulation of words (slurred speech). This is due to damage of the cranial nerves which control the movement of the soft palate and tongue. The patient has no difficulty with selecting words or understanding words.

CAUSES
1. Traumatic head injury.
2. Cerebrovascular accident.
3. Tumour.
4. Cerebral abscess.

TYPES OF APHASIA
1. Motor aphasia or expressive aphasia – loss of ability to express one's thoughts in speech and writing; person understands what is said to him but he cannot produce sequence of movements necessary to utter words.
2. Sensory aphasia or receptive aphasia – inability to comprehend spoken or written language.
3. Central or global aphasia – a combination of both motor and sensory aphasia.

NURSING MANAGEMENT
Principle
There are a variety of symptoms and disorders underlying aphasia. Therefore, the treatment is individualized.

Objective
Stimulate attempts at communication.
1. Determine the communication abilities of the patient – usually done by speech therapist.
2. Give the patient as much psychological security as possible.
3. Give the patient plenty of *time* to speak and respond; he cannot sort out incoming messages and formulate a response under pressure.
   a. Speak slowly while making eye contact with the patient.
   b. Face the patient.
   c. Avoid talking too fast, too loudly or too much.
   d. Use short sentences; pause; see if he indicates that he understands.
   e. Supplement speech with gestures when indicated.
   f. Talk to him while caring for him. Know his former interests.
   g. Be consistent – by using the same wording each time instructions are given and questions are asked.
4. Keep the environment relaxed.
5. Keep distractions at a minimum – damaged input pathways cannot sort out distracting stimuli in the environment.
6. Use as many sensory channels as possible.
   a. Supplement auditory stimulation with visual stimulation.
   b. Use visual aids (pictures); ask patient to point to and name what he sees.
   c. Use games, television, tape-recorders, cassettes, to stimulate his interest.
   d. Encourage patient to use any form of communication – gestures, writing, drawing – until his speech begins to return.
   e. Elicit responses from patient, e.g. 'Please nod your head if you understand.' Reinforce every correct response.
7. Give support by assuring the patient that there is nothing wrong with his intelligence.
   a. Treat him as an intelligent adult.
   b. Accept the patient as he is now; avoid artificial praise.
   c. Maintain a calm, accepting and deliberate manner especially during periods of emotional lability.
8. Encourage the patient to socialize with his family and friends.

a. Seek the help of other people to read aloud, play games, do puzzles.

b. Keep him in the social world, e.g. have his grandchildren visit.

9. Watch the patient for clues and gestures if his speech is unintelligible or jargon-like.

a. Continue to listen to him.

b. Nod and make neutral statements occasionally.

c. Shift the topic when appropriate to provide another point of interest and frame of reference.

10. Observe the patient during the course of his daily schedule for clues to evaluate and assess his progress.

FAMILY/PATIENT EDUCATION
1. See items 1–10 above.
2. The patient's ability to speak may vary from day to day. Fatigue has an adverse effect on speech.
3. The patient is likely to become terribly frustrated by his inability to communicate; ignore swearing and abusive language.
4. Aphasia can also involve the patient's understanding. Some people cannot express themselves but can comprehend the spoken or written word; others can speak but do not understand; while some who do neither may respond to gesture and actions.

SUBARACHNOID HAEMORRHAGE

Subarachnoid haemorrhage is bleeding into the subarachnoid space.

CAUSES
1. Ruptured aneurysm.
2. Head injury.
3. Arteriovenous malformation.
4. Primary or metastatic brain tumours.
5. Haemorrhagic disorders – leukaemia, aplastic anaemia, anticoagulant therapy, etc.
6. Hypertensive vascular disease.
7. No specific cause identified.

CLINICAL FEATURES
May occur with or without premonitory signs; related to location, site and rate of development of haemorrhage.
1. Abrupt onset of intense headache.
2. Photophobia.
3. Unconsciousness (unfavourable prognosis).
4. Convulsions.

5. Varying abnormalities in vital signs; neurological impairment – depending on severity of haemorrhage; site of bleeding usually determines neurological signs.
6. Hemiplegia.
7. Stiff neck; back pain.
8. Dizziness and vomiting.

TREATMENT AND NURSING MANAGEMENT
Objectives
Determine cause of bleeding.
Survive effects of bleeding.
Prevent immediate and long-term rebleeding.
1. Place patient on strict bed rest for approximately six weeks.
2. Support patient undergoing lumbar puncture to confirm diagnosis (see p. 917).
3. Support patient undergoing cerebral angiography (to identify source of bleeding (see p. 913)).
4. Give prescribed medications, usually dexamethasone and tranexamic acid if haemorrhage from an aneurysm or arteriovenous malformation.

CEREBRAL ANEURYSM (INTRACRANIAL ANEURYSM)

A cerebral aneurysm is a sac formed by dilation of the walls of an artery within the head.

AETIOLOGY
1. Congenital defect of vessel wall (most common).
2. Arteriosclerosis – reflects an acquired defect in vessel wall with subsequent weakness of wall.
3. Trauma.
4. Syphilis (rare).
5. Mycosis (rare).
6. Vasculitis secondary to drug addiction (heroin).

Assessment
CLINICAL FEATURES
1. Due to leakage from or rupture of aneurysm.
   a. Headache – usually severe and of sudden onset, usually frontal; disturbances of consciousness.
   b. Pain and rigidity in back of neck and spine.
   c. Visual disturbances – visual loss, diplopia (double vision), ptosis (drooping of upper eyelid).
   d. Tinnitus (ringing in the ears).
   e. Dizziness; nausea and vomiting.
   f. Hemiparesis (muscular weakness affecting one side of body) or hemiplegia (paralysis of one side of body).

2. Due to compression of cranial nerve or brain substance by large, unruptured aneurysm.

DIAGNOSTIC TESTS

1. Lumbar puncture – to confirm presence of blood in cerebrospinal fluid.
2. Cerebral angiography – to determine presence and location of aneurysm(s) and cerebrovascular spasm.
3. CAT scan – may be used to rule out any other structural lesions (see p. 912).

Planning and implementation

TREATMENT

Objective

Prevent recurrent bleeding from aneurysm – incidence of mortality and morbidity increases with each subsequent bleed. Depending on the neurological status of the patient following the initial bleed, this objective can be achieved by surgical intervention or medical treatment.

Surgical intervention

Patients with no or only minor neurological deficits, e.g. cranial nerve palsy, are usually referred for surgery.

1. Intracranial procedures:
   a. Clipping the aneurysm across its neck to isolate aneurysm from blood vessel.
   b. Clip-wrap procedure – patching and reinforcing the defect in the media of the vessel wall as well as positioning a clip across the neck of the aneurysm.
   c. Wrapping aneurysms that have no clearly defined neck with single butter muslin, gauze, muscel or plastic material.
   d. See nursing management of patient following craniotomy (p. 931).
2. Extracranial procedure: ligation of carotid artery in neck – to reduce pressure in the aneurysm and reduce the danger of rupture and haemorrhage.

Medical treatment

Patients not suitable for surgery.

1. Restriction of activities to prevent a sudden rise in blood pressure – usually achieved by bed rest for approximately six weeks.
2. Drugs – dexamethasone and tranexamic acid (an antifibrinolytic) and hypertensive agents may be given, but hypertension should be reduced gradually.

NURSING CARE – PRIOR TO SURGERY OR DURING MEDICAL TREATMENT

Underlying principles

1. To provide a quiet, nonstressful setting – activity, pain, stress, anxiety may elevate blood pressure and initiate further bleeding; highest incidence of recurrence is 10 to 14 days following first bleed.
2. Monitor patient's neurological condition using Glasgow Coma Scale (see Figure 16.2, p. 922).
3. Assess for complications of bed rest.
4. When allowed, mobilize gently – if headache returns with mobilization, patient should be helped back to bed immediately.
5. Administer prescribed codeine-based analgesia regularly to reduce headache.
6. Help patient to avoid straining at stool – give stool softeners. Some doctors allow patients out of bed to use a commode, as this is less stressful.
7. Dim lighting to reduce photophobia.
8. Give patients and relatives an opportunity to discuss anxieties.
9. Allow patient to find most comfortable position in bed. (Some doctors specify the number of pillows to be used.)

NURSING CARE FOLLOWING SURGERY

See nursing care of a patient following intracranial surgery, p. 931.

Evaluation

EXPECTED OUTCOMES

1. Patient avoids recurrent bleeding; avoids doing Valsalva manoeuvre; complies with restrictions of bed rest.
2. Patient shows absence of complications; vital signs within acceptable range.
3. Patient experiences relief of headache.

BRAIN ABSCESS

A brain abscess is a localized collection of pus within the brain tissues.

AETIOLOGY

1. By direct invasion of the brain.
   a. Cerebral trauma or surgery.
   b. Spread of infection from otitis media, mastoiditis, osteomyelitis of skull.
2. By spread of infection from other organs (remote from the brain) via the bloodstream or metastatic spread.
   a. From the lung – pneumonia, bronchiectasis, lung abscess, tuberculosis.
   b. From the heart – infective endocarditis, congenital heart disease.
   c. From other organs – septicaemia, pelvic abscess.

NURSING ALERT
Have a high degree of suspicion of brain abscess when neurological signs and symptoms develop in a person with a recent history of sinus or ear infection.

CLINICAL FEATURES
Caused by major alterations of intracranial mass dynamics (oedema, brain shift), by infection or by location of the abscess.
1. Headache – may be from increased intracranial pressure; worse in arm.
2. Focal neurological signs (depending on site of abscess) – weakness of arm or leg, visual impairment, focal epileptic seizures, papilloedema.
3. Fever and leucocytosis; temperature may be subnormal when there is a thick-walled abscess.
4. Change in patient's mental alertness.

TREATMENT AND NURSING MANAGEMENT
Objective
Eliminate the abscess.
1. Observe patient for increased intracranial pressure (p. 920) – cerebral oedema surrounds an acute brain abscess and may produce sudden increase of intracranial pressure.
   a. Secondary midbrain and brain stem compression can lead to rapid coma and death.
   b. Patient may be given dexamethasone for cerebral oedema.
   c. Keep neurological observation record, using the Glasgow Coma Scale (see Figure 16.2).
2. Give prescribed antibiotic therapy – to reduce the virulence of or to eliminate organism. Large doses of the appropriate antibiotic may be given to penetrate the abscess cavity until the lesion becomes encapsulated and ready for surgical intervention.
3. Assist in diagnostic studies for determining accurate localization of abscess; laboratory studies, computerized axial tomography and repeated neurological examinations.
4. Record seizures if they occur (see p. 948). Patient may receive anticonvulsant medication as a prophylactic measure.
5. Prepare for surgical intervention (the definitive treatment).
   a. Drainage of abscess through burr holes.
   b. Craniotomy with elevation of bone flap and removal of abscess. (See nursing management of patient undergoing intracranial surgery, p. 931.)
6. Support the patient during repeated X-ray studies following treatment to ascertain if infection has been eradicated.

   a. Relapse is common.
   b. Mortality rate is fairly high.
   c. Neurological defects following treatment of brain abscess include hemiparesis, seizures, visual defects, cranial nerve palsies and learning problems in children.
   d. Prognosis is related to the neurological status of the patient when therapy is begun.

PATIENT EDUCATION
1. It is important that the anticonvulsant medication be taken on a daily basis as prescribed.
2. *Prevention:* treat otitis media, mastoiditis, sinusitis and other systemic infections to prevent brain abscess.

BRAIN TUMOUR

A brain tumour is a localized intracranial lesion which occupies space within the skull and tends to cause a rise in intracranial pressure.

INCIDENCE
1. Tumours of the brain originate in the brain (including the roots of the cranial nerves and the meninges) in about 80 per cent of all patients with this problem. The remaining 20 per cent are metastatic tumours from outside the brain.
2. Tumours may be benign or malignant; however, any mass within closed cranial vault may be lethal.
3. The greatest incidence of brain tumours occurs between the ages of 30 and 50 years.

CLASSIFICATION
1. *Tumours arising from covering of brain:*
   Meningioma – encapsulated, well-defined, growing outside the brain tissue; compresses rather than invades brain. Benign.
2. *Tumours developing in or on the cranial nerves:*
   a. Acoustic neuroma – derived from sheath of acoustic nerve. Benign.
3. *Tumours originating in the brain connective tissue:*
   Gliomas – infiltrating tumours that may invade any portion of brain. Most common type of brain tumour. Malignant.
   a. Astrocytoma
   b. Oligodendroglioma } Subclassified according
   c. Microglioma } to predominating cells
   d. Medullablastoma } (histology)
   e. Ependymoma
4. *Metastatic lesions* – most common primary site is lung or breast.

5. *Tumours of the ductless glands:*
   a. Pituitary.
   b. Pineal.
6. *Blood vessel tumours:*
   Haemangioblastoma.
7. *Tumours in children* – thought to be congenital.

CLINICAL FEATURES
General symptoms
1. Brain tumour is usually characterized by a *progressive* course of symptoms over a period of time.
2. Brain tumours manifest themselves by:
   a. *Symptoms due to increased intracranial pressure:*
      (i) Headache – intensified by activity that increases intracranial pressure (stooping, straining).
      (ii) Vomiting, unrelated to food intake – usually due to irritation of vagal centres in medulla.
      (iii) Papilloedema – oedema of optic nerve disc.
      (iv) Mental clouding, lethargy.
   b. *Symptoms due to local effects of tumour's interference with specific regions of the brain:*
      (i) Motor abnormalities – rigidity, lack of coordination, weakness, convulsive seizures.
      (ii) Sensory abnormalities – aberrations in smell, vision, hearing.

Manifestations according to site
1. *Frontal lobe tumour:*
   a. Mental changes (memory loss, euphoria, personality changes, loss of interest, moral laxity).
   b. Headache.
   c. Focal seizures.
   d. Hemiparesis or aphasia.
   e. Failing or blurring vision.
   f. Impairment of sphincter control.
2. *Temporal lobe:*
   a. Focal epileptic seizures.
   b. Dysphasia or aphasia.
   c. Papilloedema.
   d. Headache.
   e. Behaviour disorders.
3. *Parietal lobe tumours:*
   a. Motor seizures.
   b. Sensory loss or visual impairment.
   c. Jacksonian convulsions.
4. *Occipital tumours:*
   a. Visual impairment and visual hallucinations.
   b. Focal seizures.

5. *Cerebellar tumours* (common brain tumours of childhood):
   a. Disturbances of equilibrium and coordination.
   b. Early development of increasing intracranial pressure, often due to hydrocephalus, and papilloedema.
6. *Tumours of brain stem:*
   Symptoms of cranial nerve palsies (dysphagia, dysphonia, nystagmus, ataxia in extremities).
7. *Tumours of the third ventricle:*
   Symptoms arise from increasing intracranial pressure – due to disturbance of cerebrospinal fluid flow, leading to hydrocephalus.

DIAGNOSTIC EVALUATION
Objective
Determine the precise location of the tumour.
1. X-ray of skull – to demonstrate intracranial calcification, displacement of calcified pineal gland, signs of increased intracranial pressure, bone destruction.
2. X-ray of chest – metastatic brain tumours are associated with many primary or metastatic lung tumours.
3. Brain scan – abnormal amount of radioactive material will be present in area of tumour and can be localized with scintillation counter.
4. Computed tomography – gives information concerning number, size, density of lesion(s) and extent of secondary cerebral oedema; provides information about ventricular system.
5. Angiography – to determine vascularity of lesion.
6. Neurological examination – to determine area(s) of involvement.
7. Audiometry or vestibular function studies – performed when acoustic neuroma is suspected.

TREATMENT
Objectives
Remove the tumour and cure the patient (if possible).
Achieve palliation by partial tumour removal and by decompression, radiation or chemotherapy or combinations of these.

Problems affecting treatment
1. Effectiveness of treatment depends on type and site of tumour; many tumours are in vital or inaccessible areas (brain stem tumours); even biopsies in such locations can produce unacceptable disabilities.
2. Nonencapsulated and infiltrating tumours make complete removal almost impossible; resulting

neurological defects (blindness, paralysis) would be too severe.

3. Cures may be obtained in certain tumours (meningiomas, acoustic neuromas, pituitary adenomas, dermoids, astrocytomas) if they are treated early.

Principles of treatment

1. Brain tumours require different therapeutic approaches depending on cell type and location and on age and condition of the patient. Each patient (and his lesion) is evaluated individually and the therapeutic programme designed accordingly.
2. Treatment usually involves a multidisciplinary approach including surgery, radiotherapy and chemotherapy.
3. Surgical approaches include total tumour excision, decompression, cerebrospinal fluid-vascular shunt. (See p. 931 for nursing management of patient undergoing intracranial surgery.)
4. Support the patient undergoing radiation.
   a. Give steroids (dexamethasone) as directed – to reduce cerebral oedema associated with brain tumours.
   b. Steroids may be introduced prior to therapy and withdrawn gradually as soon as definitive local treatment (surgery/radiation) has demonstrated clinical results.
   c. Local radiation to tumour is usually carried out, except in cases of medullablastoma, when total central nervous system radiation is carried out.
   d. Observe for headache, nausea and vomiting occurring during course of radiotherapy.
   e. Loss of hair may be expected; regrowth may be expected after several weeks.
   f. See Nursing Care of the Patient receiving Radiotherapy (p. 1039).
5. Encourage the patient undergoing chemotherapy.
   a. Chemotherapeutic drugs may be given singly or in combination (BCNU, vincristine, mithramycin, methotrexate, etc).
   b. Dosages of chemotherapeutic drugs may be limited by their toxicity.
   c. Assess patient for signs and symptoms of drug toxicity; bone marrow depression, liver function abnormality, etc.
   d. See Nursing Care of the Patient receiving Chemotherapy (Chapter 18, p. 1036).
   e. See Care of the Patient with Cancer (Chapter 18, p. 1023).
6. Management of patient with brain metastases from systemic cancer (lung, breast, malignant melanoma, leukaemia).
   a. Patients with systemic tumours may function well until tumour metastasizes to nervous system and rapidly produces frightening and disabling symptoms (motor loss, cranial neuropathies, intellectual impairment, convulsive seizures).
   b. Metastases to brain are commonly multiple and often unresectable.
   c. Therapeutic approach includes surgery, radiotherapy and chemotherapy; palliation more effective if treatment is started before major neurological deficits develop.
   d. See Care of the Patient with Cancer (Chapter 18, p. 1023).

THE EPILEPSIES

The epilepsies are paroxysmal transient disturbances of brain function that may be manifested as episodic impairment or loss of consciousness that may or may not be associated with convulsions, sensory phenomena, erratic behaviour or a combination of all of these.

The basic problem is thought to be due to an electrical disturbance in the nerve cells in one section of the brain that causes them to give off abnormal, recurrent, uncontrolled electrical discharges, which may remain localized or spread throughout the brain.

CAUSES

The underlying disorder of the brain may be structural, chemical or physiological or a combination of all three.

1. Head/brain injury.
2. Congenital anomalies; inherited metabolic errors.
3. Infectious disorders (meningitis, encephalitis).
4. Vascular disturbances.
5. Metabolic or nutritional disturbances.
6. Brain tumour.
7. Degenerative disorders.
8. Genetic disorders.
9. Idiopathic (cause unknown).

Assessment

CLINICAL FEATURES

1. Loss of consciousness.
2. Disturbances of the mind.
3. Excess or loss of muscle tone or movement.
4. Disorders of sensation or special senses.
5. Disturbances of the autonomic functions of the body, e.g. incontinence.

DIAGNOSTIC EVALUATION

1. History of seizures (as noted by patient and observers).
2. Electroencephalograph (EEG) – finds and measures brain electrical discharge pattern; useful in locating the site where epileptic discharge begins, its spread, intensity, duration; helps classify seizure type.

INTERNATIONAL CLASSIFICATION OF EPILEPTIC SEIZURES*

Partial seizures (seizures beginning locally)

1. Partial seizures with elementary symptomatology (generally without impairment of consciousness).
   a. With motor symptoms (includes Jacksonian seizures).
   b. With special sensory or somatosensory symptoms, e.g. hallucinations.
   c. With autonomic symptoms.
2. Partial seizures with complex symptomatology (generally with impairment of consciousness). (Temporal lobe or psychomotor seizures.)
   a. With impairment of consciousness only.
   b. With cognitive symptomatology.
   c. With affective symptomatology.

Generalized seizures (bilaterally symmetrical and without local onset)

1. Absences (petit mal).
2. Bilateral massive epileptic myoclonus.
3. Infantile spasms.
4. Clonic seizures.
5. Tonic seizures.
6. Tonic-clonic seizures (grand mal).
7. Atonic seizures.
8. Akinetic seizures.

The other two types of epileptic seizures are: unilateral seizures (or predominantly unilateral) and unclassified epileptic seizures (due to incomplete data). See below.

Note: The terms 'fit', 'seizure' and 'convulsion' are often used interchangeably; essentially they all mean the same thing.

NURSING MANAGEMENT OF THE PATIENT HAVING A CONVULSION

A convulsion is an involuntary contraction, or a

---

* Abstracted from: Gastaut, H. (1970) Clinical and electroencephalographical classification of epileptic seizures, *Epilepsia*, Vol. 11, pp. 102–13.

series of contractions, of muscles resulting from abnormal cerebral stimulation (see treatment and nursing management of the epilepsies, p. 949).

Planning and implementation

NURSING INTERVENTIONS

Objective

Prevent injury to the patient.

1. Observe and record the progression of symptoms during the seizure.
   a. State whether or not the beginning of the attack was observed.
   b. Note the following:
      (i) The first thing the patient does in an attack – where the movements or stiffness starts; position of eyeballs and head.
      (ii) The type of movements of the part involved.
      (iii) The parts involved (turn back covers and expose patient).
      (iv) Pupillary changes.
      (v) Incontinence of urine and faeces.
      (vi) Duration of each phase of the attack.
      (vii) Unconsciousness, if present, and its duration.
      (viii) Any obvious paralysis or weakness of arms or legs after the attack (Todd's paresis).
      (ix) Inability to speak after the attack.
      (x) Whether or not the patient sleeps after the attack.
2. Support the patient during the convulsive seizure.
   a. Ensure an adequate airway (if possible, turn patient onto his side).
      (i) When jaws are clenched in spasm do not attempt to pry open to insert a mouth gag.
      (ii) When respiration returns to normal following the seizure and the patient becomes flaccid, turn his head to the side to facilitate drainage of mucus and saliva.
      (iii) Try to hold the lower jaw forward when the patient is in flaccid stage.
   b. Try to protect the patient from injuring himself.
      (i) Protect his head with a folded blanket/pad to prevent head injury.
      (ii) Loosen constrictive clothing.
      (iii) Patient should not be restrained forcibly as this will increase muscular spasm and may lead to joint dislocation.
   c. Give the patient privacy and protect him from curious onlookers.

d. Stay with patient until he is fully conscious.
e. Reorient him to his environment when he awakens.
f. Handle the patient with calm persuasion and gentle restraint when seizures are characterized by disturbed behaviour.

TREATMENT AND NURSING MANAGEMENT
Objectives
Determine and treat (if possible) the primary underlying cause of the seizures, e.g. 30 per cent of all adults having seizures for the first time have a brain tumour.

Prevent a recurrence of seizures and therefore allow the patient to live a normal life.

Gain an understanding of the patient and his relationship to his environment.

1. Emphasize the importance of *regularity* in taking the prescribed antiepileptic medication to reduce number and/or severity of seizures.
   a. Objective of drug therapy: to suppress seizure activity with minimum dosage of medication and without side-effects.
   b. Drug therapy is regarded as a form of control; not a cure.
      (i) The choice of drug(s) is determined by the type of seizure.
      (ii) The dosage is adjusted according to patient's clinical response and plasma drug concentration.
      (iii) See Table 16.2 for list of drugs in current use.
   c. Treatment is usually started with one drug; the dose is increased slowly until seizures are controlled or toxic symptoms develop. A second (or rarely a third) drug is added in the same manner if one drug fails to give control.
   d. Serum plasma concentration of antiepileptic drug is measured to serve as a guide to drug therapy; helps to individualize drug regimen and to detect patient noncompliance.

NURSING ALERT
The patient should not stop taking his antiepileptic medication without medical supervision since sudden withdrawal can cause an increase in seizure frequency or precipitate the development of status epilepticus.

   e. Patient should watch for toxic effects of antiepileptic medication – drowsiness, gingival hyperplasia, nervousness, visual difficulties, motor incoordination, staggering, ataxia, bone

Table 16.2 Anticonvulsant drugs

Chemical class	Indications	Drugs		Company
		Generic name	Trade name	
Hydantoins	Generalized convulsive seizures; all forms of partial seizures	Phenytoin Mephenytoin Ethotoin	Dilantin Mesantoin Peganone	Parke-Davis Sandoz Abbott
Barbiturates	Generalized convulsive seizures; all forms of partial seizures	Phenobarbitone Primidone	Luminal Mysoline	Winthrop ICI
Oxazolidinediones	Generalized non-convulsive seizures (absences)	Troxidone Paramethadione	Tridione Paradione	Abbott Abbott
Succinamides	Generalized non-convulsive seizures (absences)	Ethosuximide	Zarontin	Parke-Davis
Dibenzoazepine	Partial seizures with complex symptomatology; generalized convulsive seizures	Carbamazepine	Tegretol	Geigy
Benzodiazepines	Generalized non-convulsive seizures	Diazepam Clonazepam	Valium Rivofril	Roche Roche
	Generalized convulsive seizures; all forms of partial seizures	Sodium valproate	Epilim	Reckitt-Labaz

marrow depression leading to blood dyscrasias.

   (i) Advise patient to avoid taking medication on an empty stomach; gastritis is apt to occur, especially with phenytoin (Epanutin).

   (ii) Instruct patient to brush teeth frequently and massage gums to prevent gingival infection.

   (iii) Patient should be advised to avoid alcohol.

2. Neurosurgical management of the epilepsies, although available, is not widely used.

   Surgical procedures performed when attacks are frontal in origin, in an area that can be excised without producing unacceptable neurological deficits (or increasing deficits already present) and when treatment with drugs is ineffective.

   (i) Cortical resection – excision of affected area of cortex (based on cortical EEG findings, preoperative studies and pattern of seizures).

     (a) Temporal lobectomy (temporal lobe most frequently involved).

     (b) Excision of epileptogenic foci in other lobe carried out less frequently.

     (c) Postoperative care is similar to that of other neurosurgical patients (see p. 932); in addition, patient is continued on antiepileptic drugs until time proves that seizure tendency has been removed.

     (d) Postoperative rehabilitation will be required to help patient attain psychosocial independence and a meaningful lifestyle.

   (ii) Stereotactic procedures – technique of placing a discrete lesion in a particular brain site to destroy epileptogenic foci.

PATIENT EDUCATION

1. Encourage the patient to study himself and his environment to determine what specific factors precipitate his seizures – illness, emotional stress, physical stress, hyperventilation, altered sleep patterns, photosensitivity or other sensory stimuli, etc.

2. The medication must be taken daily to prevent seizures; medication may have to be adjusted due to recurrent illness, weight gain, increase in stress, etc. Anticonvulsant medication is known to decrease the effectiveness of the contraceptive pill and this should be discussed with family planning doctor. Seizures may worsen premenstrually.

3. Practise *regularity* and *moderation* in daily activities; diet, exercise, rest, avoidance of certain stimulating stresses.

  a. Have regular hours for sleep.

  b. Avoid emotional overstimulation (watching late TV, etc).

  c. Avoid alcohol when seizures are known to follow alcoholic intake.

  d. Seek help (if necessary) during periods of crisis – death in family, divorce, etc.

4. Report any changes in health status – easy bruising, purpura, bleeding gums, jaundice, fever, recurrent infections or dermatosis.

5. Have follow-up urinalysis and blood studies.

6. Stress the importance of activity, both physical and mental. Activity tends to inhibit, not stimulate, epileptic seizures.

7. Reorient the attitude of patient and family to the disease.

  a. Help the family to understand that the patient has experienced rejection, anxiety (due to unpredictable seizure activity), feelings of being 'different'.

  b. Encourage patient or family to discuss feelings and attitudes about epilepsy.

  c. Epilepsy can be *controlled*; it is not insanity or a supernatural condition.

8. Have a wallet card and wear a medical-alert bracelet indicating that the wearer has epilepsy.

9. Learn of the services and publications of:

> British Epilepsy Association
> National Headquarters
> New Wokingham Road
> Wokingham
> Berkshire

Evaluation

EXPECTED OUTCOMES

1. Patient maintains control of seizures; takes medication as prescribed.

2. Patient copes with fears and achieves improved psychosocial adjustment.

3. Patient demonstrates an understanding of the disorder.

4. Patient identifies and avoid stressors that may increase susceptibility to seizures.

5. Patient carries identification card or wears medical-alert bracelet indicating nature of disorder and possibility of seizures.

STATUS EPILEPTICUS

Status epilepticus (acute prolonged repetitive seizure activity) is a series of generalized convulsions without return to consciousness between attacks.

UNDERLYING CONSIDERATIONS

1. Status epilepticus is considered a serious medical emergency. It has a high mortality and morbidity rate (subsequent mental retardation or neurological defects).
2. Common factors that precipitate status epilepticus include withdrawal of antiepileptic medication, fever and intercurrent infection.
3. Convulsive status epilepticus may be brought on by other conditions (cerebrovascular disease, head trauma, anoxic factors, metabolic abnormalities).

MEDICAL AND NURSING TREATMENT
Objectives
Stop the seizures as quickly as possible.
Ensure adequate cerebral oxygenation.
Maintain the patient in a seizure-free state.

1. Maintain an adequate airway.
2. Adequate oxygenation should be ensured – there is some respiratory arrest at height of each seizure which produces venous congestion and hypoxia of the brain.
3. Antiepileptic drugs may be given by continuous intravenous infusion.

NURSING ALERT
Epanutin (phenytoin) must never be given via intravenous infusion as it precipitates in all solutions. It must be given directly into a vein by a doctor.

4. It may be necessary to paralyse and ventilate patients in status epilepticus.
5. Monitor vital and neurological signs at regular periods.
6. Assist with electroencephalographic monitoring – this may have to be done in the patient's room with a portable machine.

PARKINSON'S DISEASE

Parkinson's disease is a progressive neurological disorder affecting the brain centres responsible for control of movement. It is characterized by bradykinesia (slowness of movement), tremor and muscle stiffness or rigidity. It is a disease most commonly found in the elderly.

PATHOPHYSIOLOGY
The major lesion appears to be loss of melanin pigment and degeneration of neurones in the substantia nigra of the brain. Levels of the neurotransmitter dopamine are reduced in this area.

AETIOLOGY
1. Unknown.
2. Viruses, encephalitis, cerebrovascular disease and certain metallic poisons have been suspected.
3. Theory advanced that there is an imbalance of two neurochemical systems, cholinergic and dopaminergic, and that the symptoms of parkinsonism are caused by overactivity or underactivity of one or the other of these systems.
4. Genetic susceptibility (positive family history).

Assessment
CLINICAL FEATURES
1. Bradykinesia (dyskinesia, hypokinesia) – usually becomes the most disabling symptom.
2. Tremor – tends to decrease or disappear on purposeful movement.
3. Rigidity, particularly of large joints.
4. Muscle weakness – affecting eating, chewing, swallowing, speaking, writing.
5. Mask-like facial expression; unblinking eyes.
6. Depression.
7. Dementia.

Planning and implementation
TREATMENT AND NURSING MANAGEMENT
Treatment is based on a combination of drug therapy, physical therapy and rehabilitation techniques, and patient and family education.

Objective
Keep the patient functionally useful and productive as long as possible.

Principles behind use of drug therapy
1. Drugs decrease symptoms, but do not halt progress of the disease; drug regimen changes as disease progresses.
2. Drug therapy is aimed at redressing balance in the brain between the neurotransmitters dopamine and acetylcholine. This usually means dopaminergic drugs are given to increase dopamine levels (see pathophysiology above) or anticholinergic drugs are given to inhibit the effects of acetylcholine.

Drug therapy
1. *Levodopa (L-dopa) therapy:*
   a. Levodopa (an amino acid which is depleted in the substance of the brain involved in nerve transmission in patients with parkinsonism) is given in increasing doses until patient's tolerance is reached; it relieves rigidity in majority of patients and usually improves tremor.

b. Levodopa must be given in large enough doses and for a long enough time to build up an effective and stable blood level.

c. Dosage is increased gradually until maximum therapeutic effect is achieved and side-effects appear – nausea, vomiting, anorexia, postural hypotension, mental changes (confusion, agitation, mood alterations), cardiac dysrhythmias, twitching.

d. Give levodopa after meals.

e. Beneficial effects most pronounced in first few years of treatment; adverse effects may increase with continued use.

(i) Abnormal involuntary movements – typically choreoathetoid in nature, affecting face and mouth initially, and then involving body and extremities.

(ii) On–off phenomena – sudden episodes of immobility.

f. Levodopa is not a cure for parkinsonism but is effective in controlling patient's symptoms, particularly bradykinesia and rigidity.

2. *Levodopa in combination with carbidopa* – carbidopa (a selective dopa decarboxylase inhibitor) reduces the peripheral metabolism of dopa; administration of carbidopa with levodopa makes more levodopa available for transport to the brain.

Sinemet (combination of carbidopa and levodopa) – potentiates therapeutic effects of levodopa; appears to achieve a therapeutic effect with much lower dose of levodopa and thus reduces incidence of side-effects.

Madopar – a combination of levodopa and beseride.

3. *Anticholinergic agents* – counteract the action of acetylcholine in the central nervous system.

a. Anticholinergics are given for patients with mild disability, who have poor response or sensitivity to levodopa; or they may be used in combination with levodopa.

b. Frequently used anticholinergics include:

(i) Benzhexol hydrochloride (Artane).

(ii) Orphenadrine hydrochloride (Disipal).

(iii) Procyclidine hydrochloride (Kemadrin).

(iv) Benztropine (Cogentin).

c. Assess for side-effects of anticholinergic agents – dryness of mouth, blurred vision, urinary retention, constipation, mental confusion.

4. *Antihistaminic compounds* – may be effective for tremor.

5. *Antidepressants* – may be given to reduce depression which frequently accompanies parkinsonism and the drug therapy.

6. *Tranquillizers* – may be given for nervousness and irritability.

Physiotherapy (supervised by physiotherapist)

1. Encourage patient to continue on an exercise and physiotherapy programme to increase muscle strength, improve coordination and dexterity, treat muscular rigidity and prevent contractures.

2. Emphasize the importance of a *daily* exercise programme (walk, ride stationary bike, swim, garden) – to maintain joint mobility.

Advise patient to:

a. Exercise each joint daily.

b. Lengthen stride when walking; swing arms while walking – loosens arms and shoulders and lessens fatigue.

c. Practise breathing exercises – to mobilize rib cage.

3. Advise patient to do stretching exercises (stretch–hold–relax) to loosen the joint structures.

4. Encourage patient to take warm baths, massage and passive and active exercises – to help relax muscles and relieve painful muscle spasms that accompany rigidity.

5. Advise patient to have frequent rest periods – patient becomes fatigued and frustrated by his symptoms.

6. Try to have patient seen by a physiotherapist on a regular basis – reinforces his programme, introduces new programme of exercises.

Psychological support

1. Help patient establish achievable goals (improvement of health and mobility, lessening of tremors).

2. Encourage patient to be an *active* participant in his therapy and in social and recreational events – parkinsonism tends to lead to depression and withdrawal.

3. Have a planned programme of activity throughout day – prevents daytime sleeping, disinterest and apathy.

4. Re-emphasize that disability can be prevented or delayed; offer realistic reassurance.

5. Try to dispel anxiety and fears of patient that may be as disabling to him as his disease.

Surgical intervention

1. Thalamotomy – stereotaxic placement of a lesion in the small area of the brain where the tremors originate; area is inactivated by heat, freezing or other methods – relieves contralateral tremor and rigidity of extremity.

2. Does not alter course of progressive Parkinson's

disease, but can help some patients with the unilateral syndrome (tremor and rigidity on one side of body).

3. Recent developments have shown that it may be beneficial to use stereotactic surgery to implant fetal brain cells into the basal ganglia. This treatment is essentially at an experimental stage and raises many ethical issues yet to be clarified.

4. See p. 931 for the nursing management of the patient undergoing intracranial surgery.

PATIENT EDUCATION

1. See drug therapy, physiotherapy and psychological support given above.

2. Patient avoids a high protein diet when taking levodopa since a high protein meal can block the effects of levodopa in some patients.

3. Suggest the patient tries the following routine when feet and legs seem to be 'glued' to the floor.
   a. Raise head.
   b. Raise toes (eliminates muscle spasm).
   c. Rock from side to side while bending knees slightly.
   d. Or raise arms in a sudden, short motion.

4. Patient attempts to get out of a chair quickly, placing feet well apart, to overcome pull of gravity.

5. Advise patient and his family to learn about services of: Parkinson's Disease Society, 36 Portland Place, London W1.

Evaluation

EXPECTED OUTCOMES

1. Patient achieves improved physical mobility; exercises and walks daily.

2. Patient maintains satisfactory nutritional status; eats slowly and without choking.

3. Patient demonstrates improved verbal communication; practises speech exercises.

4. Patient achieves self-care; allows enough time to carry out activities and uses assistive devices when necessary.

5. Patient can explain the purpose of drug therapy; adheres to the prescribed regimen.

MULTIPLE SCLEROSIS

Multiple sclerosis (MS) is a chronic, frequently progressive disease of the central nervous system characterized by the occurrence of small patches of demyelination of the central nervous system white matter, in association with inflammation and gliosis.

1. Demyelination results in disordered transmission of nerve impulses. (*Demyelination* refers to the destruction of myelin, the fatty and protein materials that ensheathes certain nerve fibres in the brain and spinal cord.)

2. Although the cause and pathogenesis of MS are unknown, it is believed that immune abnormalities are related to the disease, infection by a slow virus, or a combination of these two.

INCIDENCE

Multiple sclerosis is one of the commonest neurological diseases and primarily affects young adults (20 to 40 years of age). It occurs in temperate climates, particularly in the northern hemisphere and is rare in the tropics. However, a number of these patients have little or no disability for many years after diagnosis.

Assessment

CLINICAL FEATURES

The signs and symptoms reflect the location and areas of demyelinization within the central nervous system. Patients with MS have a wide range of clinical symptoms; there is great variability in the course of the disease, with many remissions and exacerbations.

1. Weakness and sensory disturbances.
2. Abnormal reflexes, either absent or exaggerated.
3. Visual disturbances; impaired vision, diplopia.
4. Tremor, ataxia, incoordination.
5. Paraesthesiae.
6. Sphincter impairment.
7. Impaired vibration and position sense.
8. Emotional lability; euphoria, depression.
9. Slurring of speech.

Planning and implementation

TREATMENT AND NURSING MANAGEMENT

Objectives

Keep the patient as active and functional as possible in order to lead a purposeful life.

Relieve the patient's symptoms and provide him with continuing support.

Note: Many patients are managed at home, often with the help of the district nurse. They are usually admitted to hospital when exacerbations or complications occur, or when family circumstances necessitate it.

Strengthen muscles and prevent and treat muscle spasticity

Spasticity interferes with normal function.

1. Patient should do muscle-stretching exercises

daily – to minimize joint contractures. The opinions of neurologists differ as to the extent and value of physiotherapy to prevent muscle spasticity.
2. Drugs: muscle relaxants (diazepam); antispasmodic agents (Liorésal).
3. Advise patient to avoid muscle fatigue.
4. Utilize braces, crutches, Zimmer frames to keep patient ambulant for as long as possible.

Avoid skin pressure and immobility
Since there is usually sensory loss, pressure sores accompany severe spasticity in an immobile patient.
1. Relieve pressure.
   a. Change position at least every two hours if patient is in bed.
   b. Change position every 30 minutes if in wheelchair.
   c. Use flotation pad, sheepskin, ripple mattress and other aids to distribute pressure away from bony points and over a wider area.
   d. Teach patient to inspect pressure areas (using a long-handled mirror for posterior sites) for evidences of redness and heat.
2. Avoid skin trauma, heat, cold and pressure.
3. Give careful attention to sacral and perineal hygiene.
4. See p. 30 for discussion of prevention and treatment of pressure sores.

Assist patient to overcome effects of incoordination (caused by motor dysfunction)
1. Teach patient to walk with feet wider apart – to widen his base of support and increase his walking stability.
2. Have patient use a stick or Zimmer frame.
3. Utilize wrist cuffs, eating utensils – to help overcome incoordination of upper extremities.

Support the patient with bladder disturbances
Bladder dysfunction may lead to progressive renal failure.
1. See care of the patient with a neurogenic bladder, p. 642.
2. Assess for urinary retention.
   a. Catheterize patient; insert indwelling catheter only if absolutely necessary.
   b. Give urinary antiseptics – to reduce incidence of infection.
3. Ensure adequate fluid intake (3–5 litres daily) – to reduce urinary bacterial count, minimize precipitation of urinary crystals and stone formation and encrustation of the lumen of the indwelling urethral catheter.

4. Support the patient who has urinary incontinence (or frequency and urgency).
   Female patient:
   a. Set up a micturition time schedule; every one-and-a-half to two hours initially, with lengthening time intervals if regimen is successful.
   b. Encourage the patient to drink a measured amount of fluid every two hours.
   c. Have the patient try to micturate 30 minutes after drinking.
   d. Use slipper bedpan at night; set alarm clock for patient with diminished warning sensation.
   e. For permanent urinary incontinence, urine may have to be diverted by means of ileal conduit.
   Male patient:
   a. See a, b and c, under female patient, above.
   b. Use urinal at night.
   c. For permanent incontinence, patient may wear external sheath or condom appliance for urine collection.

Place the patient on a bowel programme if he has bowel incontinence
1. Establish a programme of *regularity*.
   a. Have patient eat regularly scheduled meals.
   b. Establish bowel evacuation at *same time each day*.
2. Insert a glycerine suppository into the rectum 30 minutes before scheduled bowel evacuation time – *after* eating a meal (preferably after breakfast).
3. Advise patient to attempt to have a bowel movement within 30 minutes of eating, using as normal a position for defaecation as possible.
   a. Instruct patient to bear down and contract abdominal muscles.
   b. Teach patient to apply pressure to abdomen with hands – to assist with defaecation.
4. After this routine is established, mechanical stimulation with the suppository may not be necessary.

Treat the patient with appropriate therapy during periods of exacerbation
The residual effects of the disease may increase with each exacerbation. Neurologists differ in their approach to treatment during periods of exacerbation – some of the following may be used.
1. ACTH may be given for short periods during acute exacerbations – may reduce severity of episode.
2. Encourage bed rest for a few days during acute

exacerbation – continued activity appears to worsen attack.

3. Try to have patient avoid any known factor that causes exacerbation – allergy, infection, cold, heat, bathing in hot water.
4. Aim to prevent permanent damage; continue with range of movement exercises, specific muscle exercises, etc, as physical strength permits.
5. Take corrective action for each new problem as it rises.
6. Invent, adapt and modify equipment that can be used for self-help devices so that patient will not lose ground.

Help patient with visual disturbances and impaired movements of the eyeballs

1. Utilize eye patch, frosted lens – to block visual impulses of one eye when patient has diplopia (double vision).
2. Prism glasses may be useful for bedridden person.
3. For person who has impaired eyesight or who is unable to hold book, turn pages or read regular print, secure books and magazines recorded on discs, tape cassettes, page turning machines; usually provided by the occupational therapy department.

Help patient with speech and swallowing difficulties

Cranial nerves which control both the articulation of speech and swallowing are often affected.

1. Secure services of speech therapist to strengthen muscles and improve dysarthria (slurred speech).
2. Observe for inhalation of food particles due to impaired swallowing.
3. It is often easier for patients to swallow strong-tasting food, fizzy drinks, cold food, e.g. ice cream, and food of a semi-solid consistency.
4. May need to supplement intake with nasogastric feeds overnight if fluid and nutrition intake becomes inadequate.

PATIENT EDUCATION

1. Review objectives of treatment and nursing management given above.
2. Help the family (and patient) understand the stresses imposed by multiple sclerosis and that patients adapt to illness in many ways – denial, depression, withdrawal, inactivity, resentment, etc.
3. Patient may have feelings of alienation from family, others, work and social life; he feels that his personal worth is lessened.
   a. Try to keep him in the mainstream of life as much as possible.
   b. Contact local branch of Multiple Sclerosis Society, 286 Munster Road, London SW6 6AP, for services, publications and contact with other MS patients.
   c. Encourage patient to keep up social interests and activities.
4. Try to keep up the activities (physical, social, etc) that patient is able to do; once lost, certain abilities are almost impossible to regain.
   a. Physical abilities may vary from day to day.
   b. Devise modifications that will allow continuance of certain activities; obtain gadgets and adaptive devices for self-help (mail-order gift companies, medical supply catalogues, rehabilitation literature).
5. Try to avoid physical and emotional stresses – may worsen symptoms and impair performance.
6. Assist the patient to accept his new identity as a handicapped person and cope with the disruption in his life.
7. Keep channels of communication open.
8. Offer meaningful and realistic short-term goals – to achieve a sense of purpose.
9. Patient should try to avoid hot weather or hot baths as this often makes disabilities worse.
10. Advise patients on how to adapt to sexual dysfunction. They may find it helpful to contact local branch of SPOD (Association to Aid the Sexual and Personal Relationships of People with a Disability), 286 Camden Road, London N7 0BJ.
11. Female patients should know that pregnancy and childbirth may precipitate a relapse of the disease.

Evaluation
EXPECTED OUTCOMES

1. Patient demonstrates improved neurological functioning; has increased mobility; uses techniques to improve coordination.
2. Patient copes with bladder dysfunction; has a workable voiding schedule; able to catheterize self.
3. Patient attains bowel control.
4. Patient demonstrates intact skin; changes position to relieve pressure.
5. Patient achieves some independence in self-care.
6. Patient verbalizes ways to adapt to sexual dysfunction.
7. Patient uses coping strategies.

MYASTHENIA GRAVIS

Myasthenia gravis is a disorder of neuromuscular transmission in the voluntary muscles of the body characterized by excessive fatiguability of muscle function.

ALTERED PHYSIOLOGY

Defect in transmission of impulses from nerve to muscle cells which may be due to inadequate synthesis or release of acetylcholine at the neuromuscular junction.

Assessment

CLINICAL FEATURES

1. Diplopia (double vision), ptosis (drooping of one or both eyelids) – from involvement of ocular muscles.
2. Sleepy, mask-like expression – from involvement of facial muscles.
3. Speech weakness, choking, aspiration of food – from weakness of laryngeal and pharnygeal muscles.
4. Muscle weakness characteristically worse after effort and improved by rest; may involve any striated muscle. Respiratory muscles may become weakened leading to the need for short-term ventilation.

DIAGNOSTIC EVALUATION

1. Pharmacological test:
   a. Edrophonium (Tensilon) test – intravenous injection of edrophonium may relieve weakness markedly in 30 seconds; useful for patients with ocular, facial or oropharygeal weakness.
   b. Neostigmine methylsulphate (Prostigmin) test – given to evaluate extremity strength; positive result evidenced by increase in muscular strength about 30 minutes after injection; permits measurement of changes in strength of all muscles.
2. Electromyographic testing (EMG) to check muscle fatiguability.
3. Chest X-ray – to rule out thymoma (tumour of the thymus).

Planning and implementation

TREATMENT AND NURSING MANAGEMENT

Objective

Increase muscle strength and protect patient during times of muscle weakness.

Primary drug therapy

1. Anticholinesterase drugs – will increase response of muscles to nerve impulses and improve strength; by temporarily inhibiting acetylcholinesterase at the neuromuscular junction, they enhance the action of acetylcholine there.
   a. Neostigmine bromide (Prostigmin).
   b. Neostigmine methylsulphate (Prostigmin) (injectable).
   c. Pyridostigmine bromide (Mestinon).
2. Drug given exactly on time to control symptoms; a delay in drug administration may result in patient's losing his ability to swallow.
3. Toxicity and side-effects of anticholinesterase:
   a. Gastrointestinal – abdominal cramps, nausea, vomiting, diarrhoea.
      (i) Drug may be taken with small amount of milk, crackers or other buffering substance or after meals.
      (ii) Side-effects may be ameliorated or prevented by addition of atropine or atropine-like drugs to regimen.
      (iii) Give diphenoxylate hydrochloride (Lomotil) for diarrhoea.
   b. Skeletal – fasciculations (fine twitching), spasm, weakness.
   c. Central nervous system – irritability, anxiety, insomnia, headache, dysarthria, syncope, coma, convulsions.
   d. Other – increased salivation and lacrimation, increased bronchial secretions, moist skin.

NURSING ALERT
Watch for increase in muscle weakness within one hour after taking anticholinesterase drug; be alert for signs of respiratory embarrassment.

4. After medication adjustment has been made, patient learns to take his medication when necessary. Individual doses may vary with physical or emotional stress, intercurrent infection, etc.
5. Timespan Mestinon may be taken at bedtime for its prolonged effect.
6. Sedatives and tranquillizing drugs are given with caution; may aggravate hypoxia and hypercapnia and cause respiratory and cardiac depression.
7. Anticholinesterase drugs are not to be taken with morphine, ether, quinine (commercial cold preparations), procainamide and certain antibiotics.
8. Corticosteroid therapy may be of benefit to patient with severe, generalized myasthenia; patient may exhibit a marked further decrease in strength during course of ACTH therapy, but will generally develop a remission.

Surgical intervention (thymectomy)

May give improvement or remission of the disease, especially in patients with follicular hyperplasia of the thymus gland who are under 40 and have had myasthenia for less than five years.

1. May be carried out by transcervical or sternal-splitting procedure.
2. Preoperative evaluation includes assessment of respiratory status (tidal volume, vital capacity), muscular strength and patient's chewing, swallowing and ocular movements.
3. Postoperative nursing management (in intensive care unit) includes:
   a. Monitoring and caring for patient on mechanical ventilator, if needed.
   b. Continuing assessment of ventilatory function.
   c. Temporary cessation of anticholinesterase medications.

Crises in myasthenia gravis

Sudden exacerbation of weakness that may endanger life.

1. Sudden respiratory distress combined with varying signs of dysphagia (difficulty in swallowing), dysarthria (difficulty in speaking), eyelid ptosis and diplopia are indications of impending crisis.
2. Types of crises in myasthenia gravis:
   a. Myasthenic crisis – may result from natural deterioration of disease, emotional upset, upper respiratory infection, surgery or trauma; or may be brought about by ACTH therapy.
      Patient may be temporarily resistant to anticholinesterase drugs or may need increased dosage.
   b. Cholinergic crisis – from overmedication with anticholinergic drugs.
   c. Brittle crisis – occurs with an unpredictable response to drugs and is not controlled by increasing or decreasing anticholinesterase therapy.
3. Nursing and medical management during crisis:
   a. Place patient in intensive care unit for constant monitoring – myasthenia gravis is a disease of rapidly fluctuating intensity and patient is on verge of respiratory arrest.
   b. Provide ventilatory assistance when muscles of respiration and swallowing become involved.
      (i) Suction patient as indicated – *aspiration is a common problem*.
      (ii) Prepare patient for tracheostomy.

(iii) Appropriate antibiotic therapy will be prescribed if respiratory infection is a contributing factor.
   c. Determine the time of onset of symptoms in relation to the last dose of anticholinesterase – may show whether patient is undermedicated or having a cholinergic reaction.
      Tensilon may be given to differentiate type of crisis; Tensilon (intravenous) improves patient in myasthenic crisis, temporarily worsens patient in cholinergic crisis and is unpredictable in brittle crisis.
   d. Appropriate drugs as determined by patient's status:
      (i) For myasthenic crisis: neostigmine methylsulphate (Prostigmin) administered parenterally if patient is in true myasthenic crisis.
      (ii) For cholinergic crisis: atropine may be given to reduce excessive secretions; all anticholinesterase drugs are withdrawn.
   e. Administer fluids, medication and food via nasogastric tube if patient is unable to swallow.
   f. Avoid giving enemas – may cause sudden collapse.
   g. Develop a communication system for patient on ventilator (or if he is too weak to speak).
      (i) Try to read lips of patient.
      (ii) Use picture cards, hand signals, etc.
      (iii) Give hand bell to patient.
   h. Give continuing psychological support since patient is usually alert and anxious. Reassure him that the crisis will pass and that he will not be left alone.

PATIENT EDUCATION

Instruct the patient as follows:

1. Know the basic facts about anticholinergic drugs: action, reason for and importance of timing, dosage adjustment, symptoms of overdose and toxic effects. Know the drugs that interact with anticholinesterase drugs.
2. Try to prevent factors (emotional upset, infections) which may increase weakness and precipitate myasthenic crisis.
3. Wear an identification bracelet signifying that you have myasthenia gravis.
4. Have mealtimes coincide with peak of anticholinesterase effect (when swallowing ability is best); have standby suction available in home if swallowing difficulties occur. (Use a blender when necessary.)

5. Wear an eyepatch over one eye (alternating from side to side) if diplopia occurs.
6. Avoid vigorous physical activity and other factors leading to fatigue.
7. Avoid contracting colds and influenza – respiratory infections are extremely dangerous to the myasthenic individual.
8. Avoid excessive heat and cold (lying in sun for long period); weak spells may follow long exposure to excessive heat/cold.
9. Advise the dentist that you are myasthenic since lignocaine is usually not well tolerated.
10. Rest when fatigue sets in; do not force yourself to continue with an activity.

ACUTE INFECTIOUS POLYNEURITIS (LANDRY–GUILLAIN–BARRÉ SYNDROME)

Acute infectious polyneuritis is a clinical syndrome of unknown cause involving the nervous system and characterized by paraesthesiae of the extremities and by muscle weakness or paralysis. It may be due to an allergic or immunological reaction and is frequently preceded by an infection.

Assessment
CLINICAL FEATURES
1. Muscle weakness of legs – may progress to rapidly ascending paralysis involving the trunk, upper extremities and facial muscles (complete paralysis).
2. Paraesthesia (tingling and numbness) of lower extremities.
3. Difficulty in chewing, swallowing and talking – from cranial nerve involvement.
4. Absence of deep tendon reflexes.

Planning and implementation
TREATMENT AND NURSING MANAGEMENT
Objective
Support respiration when rapidly ascending paralysis develops.
1. Monitor vital capacity since respiratory failure is a common cause of death.
   a. Watch for breathlessness while talking, shallow and irregular breathing, increasing pulse rate and *change* in the respiratory pattern.
   b. Patient may need to be placed on a mechanical ventilator when respiratory insufficiency occurs.

   c. The heart may need to be monitored for dysrhythmias.
2. Feed patient via nasogastric tube if he is unable to swallow.
3. Watch for urinary retention – thought to be due to involvement of autonomic fibres passing through the sacral nerve roots.
4. Give corticosteroids and/or immunosuppressive therapy according to therapeutic plan; may be of value if given early in course of disease; relapse may occur after corticosteroids are withdrawn.
5. Put extremities through range of motion; use nursing support to prevent contractures, pressure sores. (See Rehabilitation Nursing, Chapter 2.)
6. Patient may complain of pain in muscles and altered skin sensations which are painful.

PATIENT EDUCATION
There may be a rather lengthy convalescence; patients usually recover in three to six months; a few have sequelae up to several years. Some patients remain severely disabled.

All patients need a planned rehabilitation programme if they are to achieve their full potential.

Evaluation
EXPECTED OUTCOMES
1. Patient achieves effective breathing pattern; no signs of respiratory failure or aspiration.
2. Patient swallows without choking.
3. Patient demonstrates improved mobility; moves feet and legs and participates in reconditioning exercises.
4. Patient is free of complications; shows normal skin integrity and is free of autonomic disturbances.

FRACTURES AND DISLOCATIONS OF THE SPINE

UNDERLYING CONSIDERATIONS
1. Fractures of the spine are serious because of danger of injury to the spinal cord.
2. Fractures appear most frequently in fifth, sixth and seventh cervical vertebrae, the twelfth thoracic and the first lumbar vertebrae – there is a greater range of mobility of the vertebral column in these areas.
3. Spinal cord injury may follow an injury without vertebral interruption (e.g., hyperflexion neck injury/whiplash injury).

CAUSES

1. Trauma – car and motorcycle accidents, falls, diving and surfing injuries, trampoline injuries – may cause compression, contusion or laceration of the cord, haemorrhage into its substance, or compression of its vascular supply.
2. Infections or inflammatory arthritis – producing spontaneous dislocations of cervical spine.
3. Prior laminectomy.
4. Pathological fractures from metastatic deposits in vertebrae.

Assessment

CLINICAL FEATURES

1. Severe pain in back, especially on movement.
2. Tenderness directly over localized area of injury.

NURSING ALERT

Injury to the spinal cord may produce paralysis of the body below the level of the lesion.

Planning and implementation

TREATMENT AND NURSING MANAGEMENT

Objectives

Reduce the fracture and obtain immobilization of the spine as soon as possible to prevent cord damage.

Observe for symptoms of progressive neurological damage.

1. Maintain the airway and ventilate the patient, if necessary.
   a. Respiratory problems are frequently seen in quadriplegic patient.
   b. Patients with cervical spinal cord injuries may have paralysis of intercostal and abdominal muscles.
   c. Assess strength of cough.
   d. Measure vital capacity.
2. Evaluate the patient constantly for motor and sensory changes – motor and sensory loss occurs from cord oedema, transection of cord.
   a. Direct the patient to move his toes or turn his feet.
   b. Pinch the skin, starting at shoulder level and progressing down the sides of both extremities.
      (i) Ascertain when patient feels pinching sensation.
      (ii) Record findings – for subsequent comparison.
      (iii) Note presence or absence of a level of sweating.
      (iv) Note that any evidence of neurological

deterioration raises suspicion of cord oedema or postoperative haematoma (in operative patients) – indicates need for immediate surgical intervention.
3. Transfer the patient to a Stryker frame or electric turning bed. (If none is available, place on a firm mattress with a bedboard under the mattress.)
   a. Keep patient in an extended position – do not allow body to be twisted or turned (log roll turn)
   b. Place patient (who is strapped to a transfer board) directly on the posterior frame of a Stryker frame.
   c. Place a blanket roll between the patient's legs.
   d. Place anterior frame in position. Secure frame straps.
   e. Turn the patient to the prone position.
   f. Remove frame straps, head bandage and posterior frame. Remove transfer board.
4. *For patient with fracture or injury of cervical vertebrae:*
   a. To manage a cervical spine injury there must be immediate immobilization, early reduction and stabilization.
   b. Immobility of vertebral column may be obtained by plaster cast, cervical collar, traction or skeletal traction with skull tongs (Crutchfield, Gardner–Wells) or halo-skeletal fixation.
   c. Use of skull tongs – achieves both reduction and immobilization of fracture or dislocation.
      Objective: To obtain a steady pull along the long axis of the cervical spine while the head is in a neutral position.
      (i) Tongs inserted in outer table of the cranium; under local anaesthesia.
      (ii) Initially 4.5–9kg (or more) of traction is applied, depending on patient's size and the degree of displacement.
      (iii) The traction is gradually increased by addition of weights – as the amount of traction is increased, the spaces between the intervertebral discs widen and the vertebrae slip back into position. Reduction will take place after correct alignment has been regained.
      (iv) X-rays are made every few hours until the fracture is reduced.
      (v) When reduction is obtained the weights are gradually removed and X-rays are taken again to verify reduction.
      (vi) Elevate head of bed (if patient is on regular bed) – patient's body serves as

a counterweight to that applied by traction weight.

    (a) Keep traction tongs several centimetres from top of bed and allow weights to hang free – to prevent interference with traction.

    (b) Give tranquillizers for apprehension and restlessness.

(vii) Watch for signs of infection, including drainage from stab wounds.

(viii) Check back of head periodically for signs of pressure.

(ix) Relieve pressure on back by pressing down on the mattress with one hand.

(x) If possible, turn patient on his side while he is being fed to minimize possibility of aspiration.

(xi) Duration of cervical traction depends on severity and mechanism of injury; usually a minimum of six weeks.

(xii) Fitted moulded collar usually applied when patient is mobilized after traction is removed.

d. Halo-skeletal traction – consists of a skeletal traction device attached to the skull by pins that penetrate the skin and external skull table and are connected to a plaster body cast by an adjustable steel frame.

    (i) Anticipate some inflammation and drainage around the pin sites; patient may experience a slight headache or minor pain around the skull pins for several days following application.

    (ii) Cleanse around the pin sites daily and shorten patient's hair periodically.

e. Patient may require open reduction (surgery); measures will still have to be taken to maintain reduction.

5. Report immediately any decrease in neurological function.

a. Keep a neurological assessment record.

b. Observe for symptoms of progressive neurological damage – symptoms of cord compression depend on level at which compression occurs. Clinical symptoms of cord compression are indistinguishable from those of cord oedema.

    (i) Loss of sensation.

    (ii) Inability to move extremities.

6. Prepare for laminectomy if progressive symptoms of cord compression occur which permits direct exploration and decompression of cord. Surgeons differ in their opinions about the value of direct exploration.

7. Evaluate for presence of spinal shock – spinal shock represents a sudden loss of continuity between spinal cord and higher nerve centres. There is a complete loss of all reflex, motor, sensory and autonomic activity below the level of the lesion.

a. Falling blood pressure.

b. Paralysis of body below level of cord injury.

c. Bladder distension – from paralysis of bladder.

d. Bowel distension – caused by depression of reflexes; retroperitoneal haemorrhage may occur with fracture of low back, producing paralytic ileus.

8. Maintain the patient's body defences until shock remits and the system has recovered from the traumatic insult. (Spinal shock is temporary, but may last several weeks.)

a. Support the airway, especially in cervical cord injury.

b. Support circulation – give blood transfusions as indicated.

c. Avoid overdistension of bladder – after spinal injury the bladder may lack functional nerve supply; overstretching of bladder may produce permanent damage. (Urinary tract infection is common cause of death after spinal injury.)

    (i) Insert indwelling catheter early in acute phase.

    (ii) Remove catheter as soon as possible.

    (iii) Initiate bladder training regimen.

d. Treat for acute gastric dilation and ileus.

    (i) Observe for abdominal distension and listen with stethoscope for presence or absence of peristaltic sounds.

    (ii) Initiate gastric suction to reduce distension and prevent vomiting and aspiration.

    (iii) Give neostigmine methylsulphate – for severe bowel distension.

    (iv) Administer rectal tube to relieve gaseous distension.

    (v) Give intravenous infusions for fluid replacement.

    (vi) Place patient on bowel training regimen as required.

9. Prevent pressure sores – inadequate peripheral circulation from spinal shock can cause pressure ulcer to develop within six hours.

a. Patients with initial vasovagal instability as well as associated injury may not be able to tolerate positional changes because of episodes of cardiopulmonary arrest.

b. Pressure on the denervated skin will sooner or later result in tissue breakdown.

c. *Objective:* to avoid ischaemia of the skin. Turn every two hours using turning frame, if patient can be turned.
   (i) Use electric turning bed (Stoke–Egerton).
   (ii) Inspect vulnerable skin areas.

10. Maintain patient in proper alignment to prevent contracture deformities.

Dorsal or supine position:

a. Position feet against padded footboard – to prevent footdrop.

b. Be sure there is a space between end of mattress and foot of bed – to allow for free suspension of the heels.

c. Apply trochanter rolls from crest of ilium to midthigh of both extremities – to prevent external rotation of the hip joints.

d. Initiate passive range of movement exercises for affected extremities within 48 to 72 hours *upon instruction* – to preserve joint motion.

e. Ambulate only upon instruction – if patient has partial cord function, activity may produce further cord injury.

11. Assess for complications:

a. Vein thrombosis or pulmonary embolism – from immobilization, muscular and vasomotor paralysis, factors affecting blood coagulation (hypoproteinaemia, infection, etc).

b. Hyperthermia – during period of spinal shock, patient does not perspire on the paralysed portions of his body since sympathetic activity is blocked.

c. Autonomic hyperreflexia or autonomic dysreflexia – from exaggerated autonomic responses to stimuli (distended bladder or bowel, stimulation of skin by pressure sore, catheter manipulation); may be accompanied by immediate and dangerous elevation of arterial blood pressure.
   (i) Syndrome characterized by severe headache, profuse sweating, flushing of skin above level of lesion, bradycardia, severe hypertension.
   (ii) Treatment.

NURSING ALERT
Hyperreflexia is considered an emergency.

Objective: to remove the triggering stimulus.
   (a) Place patient in 45° or sitting position – to help lower the blood pressure.

(b) Drain the bladder. (Do not irrigate catheter with more than 30ml of irrigating solution.)

(c) Remove any other stimuli that may be triggering episodes; cold air, object on skin, etc.

(d) Make a note of what caused the attack, patient is apt to have another episode of hyperreflexia.

d. Contractures.

e. Kidney and bladder infections.

f. Depression.

12. See paraplegia for psychological support, p. 965.

13. Employ active rehabilitation procedures when patient's spine is stable enough to assume upright position.

a. Programme is designed according to neurological deficit.

b. *Objective:* to strengthen muscles still innervated or when return of function is evident.
   (i) Muscle strengthening exercises for shoulder depressors, maintenance of sitting balance, getting up and down from wheelchair, or whatever is possible for individual patient.
   (ii) Period of immobilization determined by patient's condition (usually six weeks on a turning frame and six weeks of gradual mobilization with brace or cast, depending on level of lesion, etc).

Evaluation
EXPECTED OUTCOMES

1. Patient maintains effective respiratory functioning; respiratory rate and arterial blood gases within acceptable limits.

2. Patient shows no evidence of progressive neurological damage/deficits.

3. Patient absence of preventable complications; demonstrates intact skin; absence of respiratory, infectious complications.

4. Patient demonstrates beginning adjustment to impaired physical mobility; performs exercises within limits of disability.

5. For further information, see paraplegia, page 965.

PROLAPSED INTRAVERTEBRAL DISC (SLIPPED DISC)

Prolapse or herniation of the intravertebral disc is a protrusion of the nucleus pulposus through the annulus fibrosus, with subsequent nerve compression.

TYPES OF DISC HERNIATION

1. Cervical.
2. Thoracic (rare).
3. Lumbar.

CAUSES

1. Degeneration.
2. Trauma (accidents, strain, repeated minor stresses).
3. Congenital predisposition.

Assessment

CLINICAL FEATURES

Depend on location, size, rate of development (acute or chronic) and effect on surrounding structures.

Cervical disc

1. Pain and stiffness in neck, top of shoulders and in region of scapulae.
2. Pain in upper extremities and head.
3. Paraesthesia and numbness of upper extremities.

Lumbar disc

1. Low back pain accompanied by varying degrees of sensory and motor impairment.
2. Pain in buttock and thigh radiating to calf and ankle – aggravated by actions that increase intraspinal pressure (sneezing, straining).
3. Postural deformity of lumbar spine.
4. Pain induced by stretching sciatic nerve.
   a. Place patient on his back with his knees straight.
   b. Raise the unflexed leg (one at a time).
   c. This manoeuvre causes stretching of sciatic nerve that is transmitted to nerve roots, producing pain that radiates into the leg.
   d. Patient will experience little or no pain if leg is raised while bent at the knee since this relaxes tension on sciatic nerve.
   e. Lasègue sign – pain with straight-leg raising and absence of pain with bent-leg raising.
5. Muscle weakness.
6. Alterations in tendon reflexes.
7. Sensory loss.
8. Occasional impairment of bladder function.

DIAGNOSTIC EVALUATION

1. X-ray of spine – to rule out other lesions that cause similar signs and symptoms.
2. Myelogram/radiculogram – demonstrates area of pressure and localizes herniation of disc; disc protrusion is seen as indentation of dye.

Planning and implementation

TREATMENT AND NURSING MANAGEMENT

Cervical disc (usually occurs at C5–6 or C6–7)
Objectives
Rest and immobilize the cervical spine to allow for healing of soft tissues.
Reduce inflammation in supporting tissues and affected nerve roots in the cervical spine.

1. Immobilize and rest the cervical spine by one of the following methods:
   a. Cervical collar – allows maximal opening of intervertebral foramina.
      (i) Collar should hold the head in a neutral or slightly extended position. Important that the collar is fitted by an expert, e.g. physiotherapist.
      (ii) Inspect under the collar at intervals for skin rash or friction.
      (iii) In acute herniation the collar may have to be worn night and day until pain subsides (two to three weeks).
      (iv) Cervical isometric exercises are started when patient is pain-free – to strengthen neck musculature in preparation for 'weaning' from collar.
   b. Cervical traction – increases vertebral separation and thus relieves pressure on nerve (Figure 16.8).
      (i) Cervical traction should be comfortable.
      (ii) Patient must be relaxed.
      (iii) Keep head of bed elevated and make sure that traction is in alignment.
      (iv) Inspect for skin burns from cervical halter; pad under the halter as necessary.
      (v) Encourage male patient not to shave since beard offers a form of padding; shaving may cause irritation.
   c. Bed rest – reduces inflammation and oedema in soft tissues around disc, relieving pressure on nerve roots; relieves cervical spine of supporting weight of head.
2. Muscle relaxants may be prescribed to control muscle spasm and allow for patient comfort.
3. Give analgesics and sedatives to control discomfort and anxiety often associated with a cervical disc lesion.
4. Prepare for surgical intervention if significant neurological deficit from nerve root compression occurs, for unremitting and recurrent pain or for signs of cord compression.
5. *Discharge planning and patient education* (cervical disc). It may take six weeks to recuperate from significant disc lesions. Advise the patient as follows:

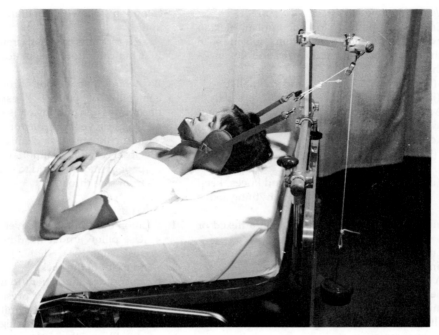

Figure 16.8. Cervical traction. The patient should be assessed for pressure sores developing under chin or occiput. The head of the bed is elevated to provide countertraction

a. Avoid extreme flexion, extension and rotation of the cervical spine while working.
b. Keep head in a neutral position while sleeping.
   (i) Pillow should be filled with feathers or down.
   (ii) Sleep on side or back; do not sleep prone.
   (iii) Avoid excessive neck flexion – do not prop up in bed with several pillows.
c. Avoid excessive car journeys during acute phase – vibration has adverse effect on spine.

Lumbar disc (majority of herniations occur at L4–L5 or L5–S1 interspace)
Objectives
Relieve the pain and slow the progress of the disease.
Increase the functional ability of the patient.
1. Encourage the patient to remain on bed rest – disc is freed from stress when the patient is horizontal.
   a. Place patient in position of comfort – usually upright with moderate hip and knee flexion.
   b. Place hinged bedboard under mattress – to limit spinal flexion.
   c. Help patient to ambulate (usually after two weeks of bed rest) when inflammatory reaction and oedema from disc herniation have subsided.
   d. Use corset or brace if necessary to mobilize patient (for obese patient with poor abdominal musculature).
2. Use of appropriate drug therapy:
   a. Analgesic agents to relieve patient's acute pain.
   b. Anti-inflammatory agents.
      Systemic steroids (dexamethasone).
3. Utilization of heat and massage by physiotherapist to relax muscle spasm.
4. Watch for development of neurological deficit.
   a. Muscle weakness and atrophy.
   b. Loss of sensory and motor function.
   c. Unrelieved acute pain.
5. Have the patient increase his activities gradually if his symptoms abate.
6. Prepare for surgical intervention when indicated (laminectomy with removal of ruptured disc). Indications for operative intervention include compression of cauda equina (motor and sensory paresis, loss of sphincter control), nerve root compression and lack of response to conservative therapy.
   a. Patients with multilevel involvement may have recurrences of pain and disability and may require reoperation(s).
   b. Spinal fusion may be required on reoperation.

7. *Discharge planning and patient education:*
   a. Encourage patient to do lumbar flexion exercises after acute symptoms subside – to strengthen abdominal muscles and flexors of the spine.
      (i) Start exercises gently and gradually.
      (ii) Discontinue exercises if pain worsens.
   b. Advise patient to sleep on side with knees and hips in position of flexion (pillow between knees).
      (i) Do not sleep in prone position – hyper-extends the spine.
      (ii) Pick up loads correctly (bend knees, keep back straight, avoid lifting anything above the elbows).
      (iii) Avoid lifting while back is in a flexed or rotated position.
   c. Encourage proper posture while standing, sitting, walking and working.
   d. A lumbar sacral support (corset) may be necessary for persons with poor abdominal musculature – serves to pull in abdomen and alter lumbar-sacral curve, which relieves strain on ligaments.

MANAGEMENT OF THE PATIENT FOLLOWING A LAMINECTOMY

Laminectomy is the removal of the lamina to expose the spinal cord in the spinal canal. It allows inspection of the spinal canal and identification and removal of pathology and compression from the cord and roots.

INDICATIONS FOR A LAMINECTOMY
1. As an emergency procedure to prevent irreversible neurological damage.
2. For progressive central nervous system involvement with muscular weakness and atrophy.
3. For recurring episodes of pain or unrelieved acute pain (intervertebral disc).

POSTOPERATIVE NURSING MANAGEMENT
Objective
Provide a stable spine to meet the functional demands of the body. (See also the preoperative principles for patient undergoing orthopaedic surgery, p. 834.

Cervical disc
1. Check neurological and vital signs at frequent intervals – there is always the possibility of respiratory difficulty, paralysis and urinary retention following operation on the cervical spine.
2. Assess for signs of urinary retention – may be the first indication of a haematoma at the operative site.
3. Be aware that a sore throat will be a major complaint of patient – especially if anterior decompression and fusion is performed.
   a. Do not give any spray or throat lozenges that numb the throat since this may cause choking.
   b. Observe for pulmonary secretions since patient may be afraid to cough because of pain from sore throat.

Lumbar disc
1. Position the patient effectively:
   a. Use pillow under head and elevate the knee rest slightly – slight knee flexion relaxes muscles of the back.
   b. Encourage the patient to move and turn from side to side to relieve pressure.
      (i) Turn patient as a unit (log rolling); place pillow between his legs while turning.
      (ii) Place pillow between legs when patient is lying on his side.
      (iii) Avoid extreme knee flexion when patient is on side.
2. Encourage early ambulation as soon as patient is able. To get patient out of bed:
   a. Raise head of bed as patient lies on his side.
   b. Encourage patient to move to the edge of the bed.
   c. Help patient to raise himself (with feet hanging over side of bed) to a full sitting position.
   d. Caution him to sit and stand with one smooth motion.
3. Give analgesics and sedatives to relieve pain and anxiety; discomfort in immediate postoperative period may vary from mild to severe pain.
4. Explain to the patient that there may be varying degrees of pain and sensory manifestations in the legs (sciatica type pain) due to temporary inflammatory changes, oedema and swelling of compressed nerve for some time following the operation.
5. Be alert for postoperative complications of infection.
6. Be alert for urinary retention. It may be necessary to allow the patient to get out of bed for toilet purposes, to avoid unnecessary catheterization.

PATIENT EDUCATION
1. It may take six weeks for ligamentous attachments of the muscles and skin to heal.

2. Instruct the patient as follows:
   a. Increase activities as tolerated – move up to the point of individual tolerance.
   b. Avoid activities that produce flexion strain on the spine – stair climbing, sitting in a car.
   c. Have scheduled rest periods.
   d. Apply heat to back when indicated – helps absorb exudates in the tissues; warm bathing is helpful.
   e. Avoid heavy work for two to three months after surgery.
   f. Resume exercises to strengthen abdominal and erector spinae muscles as directed.
   g. A brace or corset may have to be worn if back pain persists.
3. See patient education for herniation of intervertebral disc, p. 961.

PARAPLEGIA

Paraplegia is loss of movement and sensation in the lower extremities.

Quadriplegia is loss of movement and sensation involving both upper and lower extremities and the whole trunk.

CAUSES
1. Trauma – accidents, gunshot wounds, sporting injuries.
2. Spinal cord lesions (intervertebral disc, tumour, vascular lesions).
3. Multiple sclerosis.
4. Infections and abscesses of spinal cord.
5. Congenital defects.

NURSING MANAGEMENT
1. See the nursing management of patient with spinal cord injuries for immediate management principles, p. 959.
2. Understand the psychological significance of the disability.
   a. Support the patient through his stages of adjustment to injury – shock and disbelief, denial, depression, grief, etc.
   b. Allow the patient to work through his feelings about his disability at his own pace (unless his responses continue to be exaggerated or maladaptive).
      (i) Realization of the finality of paraplegia or quadriplegia may prolong the grief process.
      (ii) Patient experiences a loss of self-esteem in areas of self-identity, sexual identity and social and emotional roles.
   c. Be aware that the patient may take one of two courses:
      (i) Acceptance of disability leading to development of realistic goals for the future.
      (ii) Rejection of disability – may exhibit self-destructive neglect, noncompliance with therapeutic programme.
      Patient may require supportive psychotherapy and additional recreational therapy to prevent social and intellectual isolation.
3. Prepare for weight-bearing activities – patient with complete cord severance should start early weight bearing to decrease osteoporotic changes in long bones and to reduce incidence of urinary infections and the formation of renal calculi.
   a. Antiembolic or elastic stockings may be applied to prevent pooling of blood. A patient with a spinal cord paralysis lacks vasomotor tone in the lower extremities and will become hypotensive in the upright position.
   b. A tilt-table may be used – to help patient overcome vasomotor instability and tolerate upright posture.
      (i) Start with elevation of 45° and gradually increase angle of elevation over a period of days.
      (ii) Take blood pressure immediately before and as soon as patient is positioned on tilt-table.
      (iii) Observe for nausea and excessive perspiration.
   c. Or use high-back reclining wheelchair with extension leg rests; raise backrest slowly and lower leg rest gradually over a period of seven to ten days.
4. Initiate bladder training programme.
   a. Give meticulous attention to indwelling catheter.
   b. See Problems with micturition, p. 15.
5. Start bowel training programme.
   a. Objective is to obtain reflex bowel evacuation by conditioning.
   b. See Problems with defaecation, p. 16.
6. The physiotherapy programme will aim towards building the unaffected part of body to optimal strength – to prepare for ambulation with braces and crutches.
   Encourage patient to continue with muscle strengthening exercises for hands, arms, shoul-

ders, chest, spine, abdomen and neck – patient must bear full weight on these muscles.

7. Prevent the complications of paraplegic disorders.

a. Infection of urinary tract; urinary calculi; urethrocutaneous fistula.
   (i) Prevent overdistension of the bladder.
   (ii) Maintain continuous urinary drainage using a three-way system or, as some centres prefer, carry out intermittent catheterization as instructed.
   (iii) Frequent specimens of urine should be sent for culture and sensitivity analysis.
   (iv) Encourage fluid intake of at least 4,000ml/24 hours; urinary output should be 2,000ml/24 hours.
   (v) Prevent periurethral abscess formation and urethrocutaneous fistula – in male patient, tape the penis horizontally to the side to prevent pressure and kinking of the urethra on the catheter at the penoscrotal angle.

b. Development of pressure sores.
   (i) Some surgeons prefer patient to be nursed on a Stryker frame – prevents pressure on heels and other bony prominences and facilitates turning. If not on Stryker frame, patient is turned manually, preferably by three or four nurses, so that the patient may be turned in 'one piece', maintaining proper alignment of the vertebral column.
   (ii) Turn every two hours; give skin care immediately after turning.
   (iii) Give special attention to the perineal area.
   (iv) Prevent development of hypoproteinaemia.
       (a) Give high vitamin, high protein, high calorie diet.
       (b) Give high protein formula as in-between-meal feedings.
   (v) It is important that the patient maintains a normal haemoglobin and normal red blood cell count.

c. Abdominal distension; reflex ileus; faecal impaction.
   (i) Use rectal tube and intestinal decompression for patients with high cervical and thoracic cord lesions.
       Omit gas-forming foods and liquids.
   (ii) Ensure total evacuation of faecal material from lower bowel every day.
       (a) Give enemas or colonic irrigation.
       (b) Employ regular digital examination of

rectum – to determine presence of impacted faecal material.
   (c) Keep patient on bowel training programme.

d. Ankylosis of joints; contractures; spasticity.
   (i) Start passive exercises and range of motion early in course of treatment.
   (ii) Position patient in functional positions.
   (iii) Use splints and supports for spastic joints as indicated by patient's condition and on the advice of the physiotherapist and medical staff.

e. Autonomic dysreflexia (see p. 961).

8. Support the counselling services provided for the patient.

a. Rehabilitation engineering services – provide a greater range of self-help and mobility devices.

b. Occupational therapy – selects and utilizes devices which can aid patient in mealtime, dressing and other activities.

c. Vocational assessment and rehabilitation counselling.

d. Sexual counselling.
   (i) Most cord-injured people can have some form of meaningful sexual relationship; patient may want and require counselling on positions, techniques, etc.
   (ii) Female patient may experience little sensation during intercourse, but fertility and ability to bear children are usually not affected. Refer patient to SPOD, 286 Camden Road, London N7 0BJ.

e. Family may require counselling and social services to help them cope with burden of spinal cord injury on their lifestyle and socioeconomic status.

INTRACTABLE PAIN

Intractable pain is pain that causes incapacitation of function and that cannot be relieved satisfactorily by drugs short of drug addiction or large doses of sedation.

CAUSES
1. Malignant disease (especially of cervix, bladder, prostate, lower bowel).
2. Trigeminal neuralgia.
3. Postherpetic neuralgia following an attack of herpes zoster (shingles).
4. Uncontrollable ischaemia or other forms of tissue destruction.

NEUROSURGICAL PROCEDURES FOR MANAGEMENT OF INTRACTABLE PAIN

Objective
Interrupt the pathways by which the painful sensations are perceived.

Posterior spinal rhizotomy
Surgical interruption of selected posterior spinal nerve roots between the ganglion and the cord. This results in sensory deficit (loss of sensation).

Sensation may gradually return after one to two years, and even more distressingly severe paraesthesiae or dysaesthesiae (pain induced by touch) may appear later.

Chemical rhizotomy
Injection of alcohol (phenol) into the subarachnoid space; medication is manoeuvred over affected nerve roots by tilting the patient to achieve desired level. The patient's perception of pain is absent but motor nerve root sensations are not.

Cordotomy
Surgical interruption of the anterolateral quadrant of the spinal cord for the relief of intractable pain.
1. Obliterates pain and temperature sense but leaves motor function intact.
2. May be done by (a) open operation (via laminectomy) or by (b) percutaneous needle insertion. An electrode is introduced through the spinal needle and a lesion produced by a radio frequency current at the desired level. This is useful for patient who cannot tolerate a laminectomy.
3. Cordotomy is helpful for patients with unilateral pain of malignant origin, especially of thorax, abdomen or lower extremities.
4. Nursing management following cordotomy:
   a. See management of the patient following a laminectomy, p. 964, for principles of care also relevant to these operations.
   b. Watch for complications:
      (i) Respiratory.
         (a) Observe for loss of volume of voice and fatigue.
         (b) Medical staff should monitor arterial blood gases. Patients with reduced oxygen levels may require oxygen at night until blood gas levels return to normal. (Patient may ventilate adequately while awake but may experience progressive hypercarbia and hypoxia while asleep.)

(c) Assisted mechanical ventilation may be required.
      (ii) Urinary retention (usually transient).
      (iii) Ipsilateral (on the same side) leg weakness – usually disappears in a few days.
      (iv) Haemorrhage – may produce motor and sensory loss; immediate surgical intervention is indicated.
         Test motion, strength and sensation of each extremity every few hours during the first 48 hours.
   c. Feel patient's skin temperature at intervals to ascertain skin temperature changes.
   d. Watch for development of pressure sores.
      (i) Teach patient to inspect his skin using a hand mirror to view hard-to-see areas.
      (ii) Place patient on bladder training programme if high cervical procedure has caused loss of bladder control.
5. Family and patient education:
   a. Protect patient against external temperature changes and extremes of weather; he may not be aware of sunburn/frostbite.
   b. Test bath water before getting in tub.
   c. Avoid constricting clothing that impairs circulation.
   d. Sexual function is usually impaired in males.

Sympathectomy
Interrupts afferent pathways in the sympathetic division of the autonomic nervous system, used to control pain from causalgia and peripheral vascular disorders (eliminates vasospasm and improves peripheral blood supply).

Procedures altering patient's response to pain
1. Thalamotomy – destruction (unilaterally or bilaterally) of specific cell groups within thalamus. It is accomplished through burr holes – a lesion is produced by radiofrequency current, cryosurgery, etc. This technique is useful for pain of central origin.

Suppression of pain by electrical stimulation (pain modulation; neuromodulation)
Neuromodulation is the suppression of pain by the application of an electronic device to modify nervous system function. It is accomplished by (1) transcutaneous electrical nerve stimulation (TENS) or (2) dorsal column stimulation.
1. *Underlying principles:*
   a. This therapy is based on the gate control theory that nondestructive stimuli can interfere with the transmission of pain within the central nervous system. It is thought to relieve

pain by preventing pain messages from reaching the brain. The exact mechanics are not yet fully known.

b. It is nondestructive in nature and does not carry the potential risks of weakness, numbness, dysaesthesia, bladder/bowel incontinence, impotence or irreversibility as do destructive surgical procedures for pain relief.

c. The system consists of a pulse generator (containing the power source and electronics of the system), a pair of electric cables and two flexible electrodes which transfer the stimulating signal.

d. *Objective:* help the patient live with his pain without permitting it to affect his life adversely.

2. *Transcutaneous electrical nerve stimulation* (TENS) – passage of small electrical currents through the skin for the purpose of relieving pain.

a. Electrodes are placed over or around patient's pain area or on any peripheral nerve pathway.

b. Procedure:
   (i) The skin is washed with mild soap and water and dried thoroughly to reduce skin resistance.
   (ii) Electrode gel is applied to the electrodes, which are then placed over the nerves that serve the painful area.
   (iii) The patient operates the amplitude control until stimulation is felt (buzzing or tingling feeling). The amplitude is increased until the sensation is strong but not uncomfortable. Patient then adjusts the rate and pulse width control.
   (iv) The patient is taught to control the amplitude, frequency and duration of stimulation.

c. *Patient education:*
   (i) Give the patient the instruction booklet provided by the manufacturing company.
   (ii) Batteries must be replaced whenever levels of stimulation cannot be achieved.
   (iii) The electrodes are washed with alcohol and water after each use. The pulse generator and cables are wiped clean with a damp cloth moistened with alcohol/water solution.
   (iv) Apply talcum powder to the cables periodically to prevent tangling.
   (v) Avoid getting the pulse generator wet; avoid pulling or kinking of the cable wire.

3. *Dorsal column stimulation* – is a method for the relief of chronic intractable pain that uses an implanted device that allows the patient to apply pulsed electrical stimulation to the dorsal aspect of the spinal cord.

a. The unit consists of a radiofrequency stimulation transmitter, a transmitter antenna, a radiofrequency receiver and a stimulation lead.

b. The battery-powered transmitter and antenna are worn externally while the receiver and lead are implanted.

   A laminectomy is performed above the highest level of pain input for the placement of the electrode in the subdural space. A small subcutaneous pocket is developed over the clavicular area (site may vary) for placement of receiver. The two are connected by a subcutaneous tunnel.

c. A careful preoperative evaluation is performed to select patient who will benefit from dorsal column stimulation – history, physical examination, pain questionnaire, examination to determine areas of pain involvement, psychological and psychiatric evaluation and a trial of transcutaneous stimulation.
   (i) Trial of transcutaneous stimulation (see above) gives opportunity for patient to receive stimulation sensation – to test his tolerance of the sensation, his ability to operate the system and the efficacy of the system.
   (ii) It is essential that the patient understand that the stimulator will replace drugs and that it is installed for a lifetime.

d. Postoperative nursing management.
   (i) See p. 964 for the nursing management following a laminectomy.
   (ii) Assess for paraplegia, quadriplegia and urinary incontinence.
   (iii) Evaluate extremities for leg movement hourly. Report any decrease in movement immediately.
   (iv) Look for leakage of cerebrospinal fluid at laminectomy site – dura is opened in surgery.
   (v) Give medication as prescribed for relief of wound pain.
   (vi) Medical staff will withdraw narcotics as rapidly as possible.
   (vii) Help patient to become independently involved with his activities of daily living as rapidly as possible – inactivity serves to compound his problems.
   (viii) Look for signs of infection at implantation site – dorsal column stimulator is a foreign body within the patient.

(ix) The dorsal column stimulation system may be tested when the patient is fully alert; initial testing may not be accurate because of overlying bandage at receiver site.

e. *Patient education:*

(i) Give the patient the manufacturer's instruction booklet to acquaint him with his system.

The stimulation transmitter has four basic controls: two for the patient to use during operation of the system and two for the doctor to use when determining the voltage the patient will receive.

(ii) The patient is taught the method of attaching the antenna to the skin (and proper skin care), use of battery pack and how to make and modify dorsal column stimulation settings.

(a) Antenna is secured in place by an adhesive disc centred over the implanted receiver. (The antenna site is cleansed daily and the adhesive discs are changed daily.)

(b) Connect transmitter to antenna and adjust settings slowly to the point at which the patient first feels a definite sensation and the stimulation results in the desired effect.

(c) Encourage patient to try different stimulation frequencies to determine which frequency gives best pain relief.

(d) Have the patient keep a record of stimulation use.

(e) Instruct the patient that postural changes will cause changes in stimulation intensity.

(f) Warn patient not to adjust doctor's controls.

(g) Instruct patient to keep several batteries in reserve; battery life depends on extent of use. Patient should be instructed in battery changing procedure.

(h) Clean transmitter and antenna with gauze pad moistened with equal amounts of water and alcohol. (See instruction booklet.)

FURTHER READING

BOOKS

Bannister, R. (ed.) (1985) *Brain's Clinical Neurology*, Oxford University Press, Oxford.

BACUP (1988) *Understanding Tumours of the Brain*, BACUP, London.

Conway-Rutkowski, B.L. (1982) *Carini and Owens' Neurological and Neurosurgical Nursing* (8th edn), C.V. Mosby, London.

Evans, C.D. (1981) *Rehabilitation After Severe Head Injury*, Churchill Livingstone, Edinburgh.

Forsythe, E. (1979) *Living with Multiple Sclerosis*, Faber & Faber, London.

Hickey, J. (1986) *The Clinical Practice of Neuromedical and Neurosurgical Nursing* (2nd edn), Lippincott, Philadelphia.

Jennett, B. (1986) *An Introduction to Neurosurgery* (4th edn), Heinemann, London.

Myco, F. (1983) *Nursing Care of the Hemiplegic Stroke Patient*, Harper & Row, London.

Purchese, G. and Allan, D. (1984) *Neuromedical and Neurosurgical Nursing* (2nd edn), Baillière Tindall, Eastbourne.

ARTICLES

Epilepsy

Barry, K. and Teixeira, S. (1983) The role of the nurse in the diagnostic classification and management of epileptic seizures, *Journal of Neurosurgical Nursing*, Vol. 15, No. 4, pp. 243–9.

Lindsay, M. (1983) Never mind the label, *Nursing Mirror*, Vol. 156, pp. 18–19.

Head injury/neurosurgical nursing

Allan, D. (1984) Glasgow Coma Scale, *Nursing Mirror*, Vol. 158, pp. 32, 34.

Bannister, C.M. (1980) Extracranial–intracranial anastomoses: Keeping the lifelines open, *Nursing Mirror*, Vol. 151, pp. 44–6.

Boortz-Marx, R. (1985) Factors affecting intracranial pressure: A descriptive study, *Journal of Neurosurgical Nursing*, Vol. 17, No. 2, pp. 89–94.

Davenport-Fortune, P. and Dunnum, L.R. (1985) Professional nursing care of the patient with raised intracranial pressure: Planned or hit or miss?, *Journal of Neurosurgical Nursing*, Vol. 17, No. 6, pp. 367–70.

Ford-Krauss, M. (1980) Management of patients with brain tumours, *Nursing*, Vol. 1, No. 9, pp. 383–8.

Johnson, L.K. (1983) If your patient has increased intracranial pressure, your goal should be: no surprises, *Nursing* (US), Vol. 13, No. 6, pp. 58–63.

Wong, J. (1984) Care of the unconscious patient; a problem-orientated approach, *Journal of Neurosurgical Nursing*, Vol. 16, No. 3, pp. 145–54.

Multiple sclerosis

Anderson, E.D. (1983) The challenge of multiple sclerosis, *Nursing*, Vol. 2, No. 16, pp. 459–62.

Wise, G. (1985) Learning to live with multiple sclerosis, *Nursing Times*, Vol. 81, pp. 37–40.

Parkinson's disease

Gibberd, F.B. (1985) The treatment of parkinson's

disease – a consumer's view, *Health Trends*, Vol. 17, No. 1, pp. 19–21.

Lannon, M.C. (1986) Comprehensive care of the patient with parkinson's disease, *Journal of Neuroscience Nursing*, Vol. 18, No. 3, pp. 121–31.

Spinal surgery

Pellatt, G.C. (1983) Spinal lesions, *Nursing*, Vol. 2, No. 16, pp. 481, 482, 484.

Trigeminal neuralgia

Lindsay, M. (1983) Trigeminal neuralgia, *Nursing*, Vol. 2, No. 15, pp. 451–2.

THE INFECTION PROCESS

Communicable diseases are those which are spread (1) from person to person, either directly or indirectly, (2) from animal to person and (3) from insect to person. A sporadic outbreak of a disease is one which occurs in scattered, isolated cases. An epidemic is an outbreak of many cases of the same illness in one area. A pandemic outbreak is a series of epidemics throughout the world. An endemic illness is one which constantly occurs in one area.

CAUSATIVE AGENT
1. Bacteria.
2. Virus.
3. Rickettsia.

4. Chlamydia.
5. Protozoa.
6. Fungus.
7. Helminth.

The effect of these is modified by:
1. Pathogenicity (the ability to cause disease).
2. Virulence (disease severity) and invasiveness (the ability to enter and move through tissue).
3. Dose (number of organisms needed to initiate infection).
4. Organism specificity (host preference) antigenic variations.
5. Production of toxins.

RESERVOIR
(The environment in which the causative agent is found.)
1. Human – man is the reservoir of diseases that are more dangerous to humans than to other species.
2. Animal – responsible for infestations due to trophozoites, worms, etc.
3. Non-animal – street dust, garden soil, house dust.

MODE OF ESCAPE FROM THE RESERVOIR
1. From the respiratory tract – most common in man.
2. From the gastrointestinal tract.
3. From the genitourinary tract.
4. From open lesions.
5. From blood.
6. By mechanical escape (includes bites of insects).

MODE OF TRANSMISSION TO THE NEXT HOST
By contact transmission
1. Direct contact (person to person).
2. Indirect contact (usually an inanimate object, e.g. crockery, bed linen).
3. Droplet contact (from coughing, sneezing or close conversational contact).

By indirect transmission (contaminated items)
1. Food – salmonella.
2. Water – shigellosis, legionella.
3. Drugs – pseudomonas from infected lotions and ointments; bacteraemia from contaminated infusion products.
4. Blood – hepatitis B, or non-A non-B hepatitis.

Airborne transmission
1. Droplet nuclei (residue of evaporated droplets that remain suspended in the air).
2. Dust particles in the air containing the infective agent.
3. Organisms shed into the environment from skin, hair, perineal area, wounds.

Vector-borne transmission
By contaminated or infected arthropods such as flies, mosquitoes, ticks etc.

MODE OF ENTRY OF ORGANISMS INTO THE HUMAN BODY
1. Respiratory tract.
2. Gastrointestinal tract (oral–faecal route).
3. Genitourinary tract.
4. Direct infection of mucous membranes or skin.

SUSCEPTIBLE HOST
Illness following entry of infection into the body depends on:
1. Age, sex and genetic constitution of the host.
2. Absent or abnormal immunoglobulins.
3. Depletion or impairment of T-lymphocyte function.
4. Presence of leucopenia; efficiency of reticulo-endothelial system.
5. Presence of underlying disease.
6. Administration of steroids, radiation or antibiotics may influence the response of the host to infection.
7. Dosage and virulence of the organisms, also the length of exposure.
8. Inherent susceptibility.
9. Nutritional status, fitness, environmental factors.
10. Individual's general physical, mental and emotional status.

EMERGING PROBLEMS IN COMMUNICABLE DISEASES
1. Increase in number of different organisms that are developing resistance to increasing numbers of available antibiotics.
2. Increasing number of travellers from foreign countries, holiday-makers, business executives and also immigrants, who may have been in contact with a disease which may be incubating, but not producing any signs or symptoms until they reach their home country.
3. Increasing number of persons in a state of immunosuppression. These people, who have been treated for some forms of cancer, or who have received organ transplants, are now surviving from the illness, but are susceptible to invasion by any type of organism, including those usually considered non-pathogenic.

IMMUNITY
Immunity is the resistance that an individual has against disease.

1. Specific immunity to a particular organism implies that an individual has either generated the appropriate antibody in his own body (active immunity) or received ready-made antibodies from another source (passive immunity).
2. Immunity may be natural (not obtained through previous contact with the infectious agent) or acquired.
3. Acquired immunity may be active or passive.

Passive immunity

Passive immunity to a disease is a state of relative temporary protection produced by the actual injection of serum containing antibodies which have formed in a host other than the individual himself.

There are three types of preparations:
1. Standard human immune serum globulin.
2. Special human immune serum globulin with a known antibody content for specific infections.
3. Animal antiserum or antitoxins.

Active immunity

Active immunity is an immunity that has been produced by the stimulation of the body to produce its own antibodies.
1. It may be produced by clinical infection (the person gets the disease) or by subclinical infection (by coming in contact with the disease).
2. By the introduction of live or killed organisms or their antigens.
3. The organisms have been treated by heating or by chemical inactivation to destroy their harmful properties without destroying their ability to stimulate antibody protection.

NURSING PROCESS OVERVIEW

Assessment
HISTORY
Points which should be included:
1. Is this a local or systemic infection? Were there any prodromal symptoms and when did these first occur?
2. Has the patient or close family/friends travelled abroad recently?
3. Has there been any contact with animals or animal products? Cat scratches or exposure to birds?
4. Any illness which has lowered the body's defence mechanism?

5. What drugs have been taken?
6. Vaccination/immunization history?

CLINICAL FEATURES AND INVESTIGATIONS
1. Assess the patient for features of infection – productive cough, skin and mucous membrane lesions, fever, diarrhoea, dysuria, vomiting, purulent discharges.
2. Obtain or assist in obtaining specimens of blood, urine, faeces, sputum, nose and throat swabs, swabs from pyogenic discharges for bacteriological and microscopic examination.
3. Assist in obtaining specimens of blood, cerebrospinal fluid, bone marrow and other body fluids or tissue for cytological, serological and bacteriological tests.
4. Assist in appropriate skin tests for specific diagnostic reactions.

PATIENT PROBLEMS
1. Fluid and electrolyte balance related to fever, nausea, vomiting and excessive sweating.
2. Fever caused by the body's defence reaction to invading organism.
3. Discomfort (generalized malaise, aching, headache) related to the effects of infection.
4. Potential for spread of infection.
5. Potential respiratory insufficiency related to lung congestion (if the infection affects the respiratory system).
6. Potential alteration in elimination (diarrhoea, urinary frequency, dysuria).
7. Potential for serious systemic complications (abscess formation, perforations, septicaemia).
8. Psychological problems associated with isolation procedures, particularly if the patient is unable to understand about his condition and treatment.

Planning and implementation
IMPLEMENTATION OF NURSING PLAN TO CONTROL THE INFECTION IN THE PATIENT
1. Administer the appropriate antibiotic agents as directed.
2. Assist in administering specific immune therapy, if available, e.g. immune antiserum, gamma globulin, antitoxin, etc, and observe the patient for evidence of drug or serum sensitivity.
3. Avoid damage to body barriers:
   a. Avoid invasive procedures as much as possible.
   b. Give special care to intravenous and arterial puncture sites, etc.

ENSURING ADEQUATE HOMEOSTASIS
1. Ensure adequate hydration in the event of ex-

cessive fluid loss because of sweating, diarrhoea, vomiting.
   a. Encourage liberal fluid intake.
   b. Prepare for the administration of intravenous fluids as required.
2. Reduce the fever when indicated (it is often important to watch the temperature curve).
   a. Administer antipyretic drugs as prescribed.
   b. Tepid sponge the patient as required.
   c. Use electric fans, light bedclothes supported by a bed cradle, and cotton nightclothes.
3. Measure and record body temperature, pulse and respiration at frequent intervals.
4. Measure arterial blood pressure at regular intervals if the patient shows a tendency to vascular collapse.
5. Weigh the patient periodically, preferably at the same hour of the day.

MEASURES TO PREVENT SPREAD OF INFECTION TO OTHERS
1. *Wash hands immediately after contact with each patient and after every contact with material that may be contaminated and potentially infectious.*
   a. Wash hands even if sterile gloves are used.
   b. Wear gloves for direct exposure to blood, drainage or secretions.
2. Plan what you are going to do *before* the initial patient contact.
3. Carry out isolation precautions as required to prevent spread of micro-organisms among patients, personnel and visitors.
4. Observe asepsis as indicated.
5. Use high-efficiency disposable mask, covering nose and mouth, when indicated.
   a. Use mask only once and discard in appropriate receptacle.
   b. Refrain from handling mask while in use.
6. Use gown when required to prevent soiling of clothing.
   a. Use gown once and discard in appropriate receptacle.
   b. Use sterile gown in certain instances (extensive burns; wounds).
   c. Collect linen in water-soluble bags; double-bag and mark 'Isolation'.
7. Use gloves when indicated by the patient's condition.
   a. Disposable, single-use gloves should be worn.
   b. Use once and discard in appropriate receptacle.
8. Handle needles and syringes with *extreme* care because it is usually not known which patient's blood is contaminated with hepatitis virus or other micro-organisms.
   a. Place used needles in a labelled, puncture-resistant container; do not bend or break by hand.
   b. Blood spills should be cleaned up promptly with a solution of 5.25 per cent sodium hypochlorite solution diluted 1:10 with water.
9. Disinfect and handle wastes with all due precautions.
10. Handle bed linens and fomites with care.
11. Carry out concurrent disinfection of fomites.
12. Control dissemination of infectious droplets.
   a. Encourage the patient to cover nose and mouth when coughing or sneezing.
   b. Wrap contaminated tissues and articles in paper before disposal.
13. Control dust:
   a. Avoid creating aerosols (e.g., shaking bed linens).
   b. Require damp dusting of furniture and wet vacuum cleaning of floors.
   c. Maintain cleanliness of surroundings; wash soil from walls as soon as it appears.
   d. Reduce to a minimum the activity of personnel in the patient's room.
14. Ventilate the patient's room properly with a system that directs room air to the outside. Keep the door to the room closed.

PREVENTION OF OVERWHELMING INFECTION IN THE IMMUNOSUPPRESSED PATIENT
1. Use meticulous hand-washing techniques before each patient contact as well as between patient-care activities to different body sites.
2. Tell the patient to request all personnel/visitors to wash their hands before touching him.
3. Give *prompt* attention to fever.
4. Use a private room; people with known infections should not enter.
5. Do not use invasive devices unless absolutely necessary; use only under aseptic conditions.
6. Control water supplies (pitcher, sink) and ice machine. Dispose of open containers on a periodic basis; remember that every item in the room is potentially dangerous.
7. Teach the patient about personal hygiene and the signs and symptoms of infection.
8. Bathe the patient with antiseptic solution, paying special attention to axillary and perineal areas.
9. Give attention to proper housekeeping procedures.

10. Offer low microbial foods and beverages when indicated – fresh fruits and vegetables, cold sliced meat/rare meat can increase bacterial colonization.
11. Be aware of the patient's emotional state.

RELIEF OF SYMPTOMS OF INFECTION
1. Combat generalized aching and malaise.
   a. Utilize warm applications and massage as indicated.
   b. Apply cold compresses for headache.
   c. Administer analgesic medications as prescribed.
   d. Attend to oral hygiene.
   e. Limit physical activity.
2. Relieve cough.
   a. Humidify inspired air.
   b. Administer hot gargles and throat irrigations.
   c. Supply expectorants or cough depressants as indicated and prescribed.

ENHANCEMENT OF COPING MECHANISMS TO PROMOTE ADAPTATION
1. Develop a trusting relationship with the patient and family.
   a. Spend unhurried time with the patient.
   b. Show sensitivity to the patient's feelings; avoid showing repulsion.
   c. Employ a nonjudgemental approach to the patient with sexually transmitted disease.
   d. Lend encouragement to the patient faced with prospect of prolonged convalescence.
2. Relieve anxiety and depression of patient/family.
   a. Recognize loneliness of the isolated patient.
   b. Employ active listening without interruption; accept the patient's feelings and thoughts without judgement.
   c. Give appropriate feedback.
   d. Include the patient in decision making.
   e. Encourage family to communicate feelings, expressions of support and affection.

PATIENT EDUCATION
Provide a comprehensive patient education programme to include:
1. Availability and importance of prophylactic immunization.
2. Manner in which communicable diseases are spread, and the methods of avoiding spread.
3. Importance of seeking medical advice in the event of a febrile illness or unusual skin eruption.
4. Importance of environmental cleanliness and personal hygiene.
5. Means of preventing contamination of food and water supplies.
   a. Discipline, cleanliness and inspection of food handlers.
   b. Dangers of 'perishable' foods; the identity of food that tends to promote bacterial growth; the methods of food preservation.
   c. Significance of milk pasteurization.
   d. Necessity for adequate length of time of cooking, and reaching required temperature for certain foods, e.g., frozen chickens must be completely thawed before cooking, to ensure all parts reach the required temperature.
   e. Dangers associated with polluted waterways, and the proper toilet facilities on holiday and residential boats.
   f. Importance of meat inspection.

Evaluation
EXPECTED OUTCOMES
1. The patient co-operates in taking the prescribed medication and other aspects of the treatment programme.
2. Achievement of a normal fluid and electrolyte balance, temperature; adequate appetite and fluid intake, normal elimination, respiration.
3. Feeling of well-being returns; patient is able to undertake the activities of daily living with decreasing amount of help.
4. The patient is able to understand about the cause and outcome of the disease, and special precautions which are necessary now and in the future to protect self and others.
5. Talks through any special anxieties or concerns about the illness, or personal problems.

SCHEDULE OF VACCINATION AND IMMUNIZATION PROCEDURES

See Table 17.1.

ISOLATION OR PRECAUTIONS FOR PATIENTS WITH COMMUNICABLE DISEASES

STRICT ISOLATION
1. Private room is essential, and the door must be kept closed.

Table 17.1 Schedule of vaccination and immunization procedures (taken from DHSS Revised Schedule 1988)

Age	Vaccine	Interval	Notes
During first year of life	Diphtheria, whooping cough, tetanus Oral poliomyelitis vaccine	Three doses: commencing at 3 months; second dose after an interval of 6–8 weeks; third dose after an interval of 4–6 months	If whooping cough vaccine is contraindicated, or declined by the parent, diphtheria and tetanus vaccine should be given
During second year of life	Measles vaccine. Measles/mumps/rubella (MMR) vaccine was introduced in October 1988 for children of both sexes	There should be an interval of not less than 3 weeks after any other live vaccine	*Contraindication:* Immune deficient states
At school entry or entry to nursery school	Diphtheria, tetanus vaccination Oral poliomyelitis vaccine	Preferably an interval of at least 3 years after completing basic course	
Between 10 and 14 years of age	BCG vaccination	There should be an interval of not less than 3 weeks between BCG and rubella vaccination	For tuberculin-negative children For tuberculin-negative contacts it may be given at any age
Between 10 and 14 years of age. Girls only	Rubella vaccine		Should be offered to all girls whether or not there is a history of rubella
On leaving school, before employment or entering further education	Reinforcing dose tetanus Oral poliomyelitis vaccine		
Adult life	Poliomyelitis vaccine for previously unvaccinated adults	Oral vaccine. Three doses: 6–8 weeks between first and second dose; 4–6 months between second and third dose	For travellers to countries where poliomyelitis is endemic
	Rubella vaccine for susceptible women of child-bearing age		Adult women of childbearing age should be tested for rubella antibodies. Seronegative women should be offered rubella vaccination. Pregnancy must be excluded before vaccination. Patient must be warned not to become pregnant for 1 month after immunization
	Active immunization against tetanus for previously unvaccinated adults	Three doses: 6–8 weeks between first and second doses; third dose 6 months later	

2. Gowns must be worn by all people entering the room.
3. Masks must be worn by all people entering the room.
4. Hands must be washed on entering and leaving the room.
5. Gloves must be worn by all people entering the room.
6. 'Double-bag' technique for soiled dressings.
7. Needles and syringes must be placed in a special 'sharps' box, which must be sealed before being removed from the room for incineration.

Diseases requiring strict isolation
Pulmonary anthrax
Burns infected with staphylococcus or group A streptococcus
Diphtheria
Staphylococcal enteritis
Hepatitis A and B
Melioidosis
Plague
Staphylococcal pneumonia
Rabies
Congenital rubella
Generalized vaccinia

Note: All patients admitted with pyrexia of unknown origin (PUO) who have recently returned from tropical countries, or have been in contact with people who have returned from the tropics, should be isolated with strict precautions until a firm diagnosis is made.

Patients suffering from Lassa fever, Marburg disease or others which require strict isolation may be transferred to a designated isolation unit, where special facilities are available.

RESPIRATORY ISOLATION
1. Private room is necessary, and the door must be kept closed.
2. Gowns are not necessary.
3. Masks must be worn by all people entering the room who are susceptible to the disease.
4. Hands must be washed on entering and leaving the room.
5. Gloves are not necessary.
6. The patient should cough or spit into a disposable tissue held close to his mouth, and then discard this into an impervious bag, which must be sealed before being removed for incineration.
7. Special provision must be made for washing up cutlery and crockery, if disposable articles are not available.

Diseases requiring respiratory isolation
Measles
Meningococcal meningitis
Mumps
Whooping cough (pertussis)
Adult rubella
Herpes zoster
Open pulmonary tuberculosis
Chickenpox
Venezuelan equine encephalomyelitis

ENTERIC PRECAUTIONS
1. Private room necessary for children only.
2. Gowns must be worn by all people having direct contact with the patient.
3. Masks are not necessary.
4. Hands must be washed on entering and leaving the room.
5. Gloves must be worn by all people having direct contact with the patient or with articles contaminated with faecal material.
6. Disposable urinals, bedpans and potties should be used and should be macerated in the machine immediately after use.

Diseases requiring enteric precautions
Cholera
Staphylococcal enterocolitis
Gastroenteritis caused by enteropathogenic or enterotoxic *E. coli*
Salmonella
Shigella
Hepatitis, viral, type A, B, or type non-A, non-B
Typhoid fever (special precautions may be necessary for the disposal of faeces)

WOUND AND SKIN PRECAUTIONS
1. Private room is desirable but not essential.
2. Gowns must be worn by all people having direct contact with the patient.
3. Masks are not necessary except during wound dressing.
4. Hands must be washed on entering and leaving the room.
5. Gloves must be worn by all people having direct contact with the infected area.
6. Special precautions are necessary for instruments, dressings and linen.

Diseases requiring wound and skin precautions
1. Burns that are infected, except those infected with *Staphylococcus aureus* or group A streptococcus that are not covered or not adequately contained by dressings (see Strict Isolation, above).

2. Gas gangrene (due to *Clostridium perfringens*).
3. Herpes zoster, localized.
4. Melioidosis, extrapulmonary with draining sinuses.
5. Plague, bubonic.
6. Puerperal sepsis – group A streptococcus, vaginal discharge.
7. Wound and skin infections that are not covered by dressings or that have copious purulent drainage that is not contained by dressings, except those infected with *S. aureus* or group A streptococcus, which require strict isolation.
8. Wound and skin infections that are covered by dressings so that the discharge is adequately contained, including those infected with *S. aureus* or group A streptococcus; minor wound infection, such as stitch abscesses, need only secretion precautions.

DISCHARGE PRECAUTIONS
Secretion precautions – lesions
1. Use a 'no-touch' dressing technique (do not touch the wound or dressings with the hands) when changing dressings on these lesions.
2. Employ proper handwashing procedures.
3. Wash hands before and after patient contact; use sterile equipment when changing dressings; double-bag soiled dressing and equipment.
4. These precautions apply only with lesions from which there is a discharge.

Diseases: duration of precautions
1. Actinomycosis, draining lesions – for duration of drainage.
2. Anthrax, cutaneous – until culture-negative.
3. Brucellosis, draining lesions – for duration of drainage.
4. Burn, skin and wound infections, minor – for duration of drainage.
5. Candidiasis, mucocutaneous – for duration of illness.
6. Coccidioidomycosis, draining lesion – for duration of drainage.
7. Conjunctivitis, acute bacterial (including gonococcal) – until 24 hours after start of effective therapy.
8. Conjunctivitis, viral – for duration of illness.
9. Gonococcal ophthalmia neonatorum – until 24 hours after start of effective therapy.
10. Gonorrhoea – until 24 hours after start of effective therapy.
11. Granuloma inguinale – for duration of illness.
12. *Herpesvirus hominis* (herpes simplex), except disseminated neonatal disease – for duration of

illness. For disseminated neonatal disease, see Strict Isolation, p. 977; for oral *H. hominis* disease, see Secretion Precautions, Oral, below.
13. Keratoconjunctivitis, infectious – for duration of illness.
14. Listeriosis – for duration of illness.
15. Lymphogranuloma venereum – for duration of illness.
16. Nocardiosis, draining lesions – for duration of illness.
17. Orf – for duration of illness.
18. Syphilis, mucocutaneous – until 24 hours after start of effective therapy.
19. Trachoma, acute – for duration of illness.
20. Tuberculosis, extrapulmonary draining lesion – for duration of drainage.
21. Tularaemia, draining lesion – for duration of drainage.

Secretion precautions – oral
1. The diseases listed in this section can be spread to susceptible people by contact with oral secretions.
2. Attention should be given to the proper disposal of oral secretions to prevent spread of infection.
3. Instruct the patient to cough or spit into disposable tissues held close to the mouth; discard tissues in an impervious (impenetrable) bag at the bedside.
4. If the patient has nasotracheal suction or tracheotomy, the suction catheter and gloves should be placed in an impervious bag for disposal.
5. Seal the bag before discarding for incineration.

Diseases: duration of precautions
1. Herpangina – for duration of hospitalization.
2. Herpes oralis – for duration of illness.
3. Infectious mononucleosis – for duration of illness.
4. Melioidosis, pulmonary – for duration of illness.
5. Mycoplasma pneumonia – for duration of illness.
6. Pneumonia, bacterial, if not covered elsewhere – for duration of illness.
7. Psittacosis – for duration of illness. (It may be desirable to place patient with acute psittacosis who is coughing and raising sputum in respiratory isolation.)
8. Q fever – for duration of illness.
9. Respiratory infectious disease, acute (if not covered elsewhere) – for duration of illness.
10. Scarlet fever – until 24 hours after start of effective therapy.
11. Streptococcal pharyngitis – until 24 hours after start of effective therapy.

Excretion precautions

1. The diseases listed in this section can be spread to susceptible people through the oral route by contact with faecal excretions from a person infected with the organism.
2. Strict attention should be paid to careful handwashing following any patient contact and especially following contact with excretions.
3. Instruct the patient on the necessity of careful handwashing after defaecation.
4. Make sure there is proper sanitary disposal of excretions; a standard sewage system is adequate.

Diseases: duration of precautions

1. Amoebiasis – for duration of illness.
2. *C. perfringens (C. welchii)* food poisoning – for duration of illness.
3. Enterobiasis – for duration of illness.
4. Giardiasis – for duration of illness.
5. Hand, foot and mouth disease – for duration of hospitalization.
6. Herpangina – for duration of hospitalization.
7. Infectious lymphocytosis – for duration of hospitalization.
8. Leptospirosis (urine only) – for duration of hospitalization.
9. Meningitis, aseptic – for duration of hospitalization.
10. Pleurodynia – for duration of hospitalization.
11. Poliomyelitis – for duration of hospitalization.
12. Staphylococcal food poisoning – for duration of symptoms.
13. Tapeworm disease (only with *Hymenolepsis nana* and *Taenia solium* [pork]) – for duration of illness.
14. Viral diseases, other (ECHO or Coxsackie gastro-enteritis, pericarditis, myocarditis, meningitis) – for duration of hospitalization.

Blood precautions

1. The diseases in this category are associated with circulation of the aetiological agent in blood; be aware of the route of transmission.
2. Blood precautions should be taken for the duration of clinical disease or for as long as the aetiological agent can be demonstrated in the blood. Blood precautions should be taken with anyone who is HBs Ag-positive.
3. Disposable needles and syringe should be used for patients in isolation. They must *not* be reused.
4. Used needles need not be recapped; they should be placed in a prominently labelled, impervious, puncture-resistant container designated for this purpose. Needles should not be purposefully bent, because accidental needle puncture may occur.
5. Used syringes should be placed in an impervious bag. Both needle and syringe bags should be incinerated or autoclaved before discarding.
6. Rinse reusable needles and syringes thoroughly in cold water after use; place the needle in a puncture-resistant rigid container; wrap syringes and needles using double-bag technique and return to proper department for decontamination and sterilization.
7. These specifications pertain to needle and syringe precautions and to labelling of blood specimens. Also label blood specimens with patient's diagnosis so that necessary precautions will be taken.
8. If doctors, nurses, technicians accidently puncture their skin with a used needle, this fact must be reported immediately in accordance with the particular hospital procedure.

Diseases: duration of precautions

1. Arthropod-borne viral fever (dengue, etc) – for duration of hospitalization.
2. Hepatitis, viral, type A, B, type non-A, non-B – for duration of hospitalization.
3. Malaria – for duration of hospitalization.
4. AIDS (HIV) – probably for life.

PROTECTIVE ISOLATION

1. Private room is necessary, door must be kept closed.
2. Gowns should be sterile and must be worn by all people entering the room.
3. Masks must be worn by all people entering the room.
4. Hands must be washed on entering and leaving the room.
5. Gloves to be used routinely by all personnel having direct contact with the patient.
6. Caps and overshoes may be necessary.
7. Transportation of the patient should be strictly curtailed to avoid possible exposure to infection.

Diseases that require protective isolation

Agranulocytosis
Extensive noninfected burns
Extensive sterile dermatitis
Immune deficiency; immunosuppressive drugs
Leukaemia
Lymphoma

EPIDEMIOLOGY, THERAPY AND CONTROL OF COMMUNICABLE INFECTIONS
See Table 17.2.

Table 17.2   Epidemiology, therapy and control of communicable diseases

Disease	Infective organism	Infectious sources	Entry site	Method of spread
Amoebiasis	*Entamoeba histolytica*	Contaminated water and food	Gastrointestinal tract	Patients and carriers; faecal/oral route
Bacillary dysentery	*Shigella* group	Contaminated water and food	Gastrointestinal tract	Patients and carriers; faecal/oral route
Brucellosis	*Brucella melitensis* and related organisms	Milk, meat, tissues, blood, absorbed fetuses and placentas from infected cattle, goats, horses, pigs	Gastrointestinal tract	Ingestion of or contact with infective material
Chancroid	Ducrey bacillus	Human cases and carriers	Genitalia	Direct sexual contact
Chickenpox (varicella)	Virus	Human cases	Probably nasopharynx	Probably respiratory droplets
Diphtheria	*Corynebacterium diphtheriae*	Human cases and carriers; fomites; raw milk	Nasopharynx	Nasal and oral secretions; respiratory droplets
Encephalitis, epidemic (eastern and western equine)	Viruses	Chicken and wildbird mites; horses; hibernating garter snakes	Skin	Mosquitoes
Gonorrhoea	*Neisseria gonorrhoeae*	Urethral and vaginal secretions	Urethral or vaginal mucosa; pharynx; rectum	Sexual activity
Granuloma inguinale	Donovan body (bacillus)	Infectious exudate	External genitalia; cervix	Sexual intercourse
Type A hepatitis	Hepatitis A virus	Person-to-person contact; contaminated food or water; faeces; blood; urine	Gastrointestinal tract; skin	Faecal/oral route; ingestion of or parenteral inoculation with infected blood or blood products
Type B hepatitis	Hepatitis B virus	Infected blood donor; contaminated injection equipment	Skin	Parenteral injection of human blood, plasma, thrombin, fibrinogen, packed cells, and other blood products from an infected person; contaminated needles and syringes; venereal contact

Incubation period	Chemotherapy*	Prophylaxis
Variable	Metronidazole; emetine; chloroquine; diiodohydroxyquin; chlortetracycline	Detection of carriers and their removal from food handling; plumbing safeguards
24—48 hours	Ampicillin; chloramphenicol; tetracycline	Detection and control of carriers; inspection of food handlers; decontamination of water supplies
6—14 days	Tetracycline and streptomycin	Milk pasteurization; control of infection in animals
2—5 days	Sulphonamides; streptomycin; tetracycline	Effective case-finding and treatment of infection
14—16 days	None	Zoster immune globulin (ZIG) (an investigational drug) provided by Centre for Disease Control to high-risk susceptible children exposed to varicella zoster within 72 hours
2—5 days	Diphtheria antitoxin; penicillin; erythromycin	Active immunization with diphtheria toxoid
Variable	None	Eastern equine encephalitis vaccine, dried (available from Centre for Disease Control)
2—9 days	Penicillin G, preceded by probenecid	Chemotherapy of carriers and contacts; case-finding and treatment of patients
Unknown, presumably 8—80 days	Tetracyclines; erythromycin	Chemotherapy of carriers and contacts; case-finding and treatment of patients
2—6 weeks	None	Enteric and blood precautions for infected cases; immunization with gamma globulin
6 weeks to 6 months	None	Screening of blood donors; avoidance of unnecessary use of blood and blood derivatives

(continued)

Table 17.2   Continued

Disease	Infective organism	Infectious sources	Entry site	Method of spread
Infectious mononucleosis	E-B virus	Human cases and carriers	Mouth	Probably oral/ pharyngeal route; via blood transfusion in susceptible recipients
Influenza	Virus (types A and B)	Human cases; animal reservoir	Respiratory tract	Respiratory
Lymphogranuloma venereum	*Chlamydia trachomatis*	Human cases	External genitalia; urethral or vaginal mucosa	Sexual intercourse; indirect contact with contaminated articles/clothing
Malaria	*Plasmodium vivax, falciparum, malariae,* and *ovale*	Human cases	Skin	Mosquitoes (Anopheles)
Measles	Virus	Human cases	Respiratory mucosa	Nasopharyngeal secretions
Meningococcal meningitis	*Neisseria meningitidis*	Human cases and carriers	Nasopharynx; tonsils	Respiratory droplets
Mumps	Virus	Human cases (early)	Upper respiratory tract	Respiratory droplets
Paratyphoid fever	*Salmonella paratyphi* A and B and related organisms	Contaminated food, milk, water; rectal tubes; barium enemas	Gastrointestinal tract	Infected urine and faeces
Pneumococcal pneumonia	*Streptococcus pneumoniae*	Human carriers; patient's own pharynx	Respiratory mucosa	Respiratory droplets
Poliomyelitis	Polioviruses (types I, II, III)	Human cases and carriers	Gastrointestinal tract	Infected faeces; pharyngeal secretions
Rocky Mountain spotted fever	*Rickettsia rickettsii*	Infected wild rodents, dogs, wood ticks, dog ticks	Skin	Tick bites
Rubella (German measles)	Virus	Human case	Respiratory mucosa	Nasopharyngeal secretions

Incubation period	Chemotherapy*	Prophylaxis
2–6 weeks	None	None
24–72 hours	None	Specific virus vaccine
5–21 days	Tetracyclines	Case-finding and treatment of infection
Variable, depending on strain	Chloroquine; primaquine; amodiaquine; quinine; proguanil	Co-ordinated measures for wide-scale mosquito control; prompt detection and effective treatment of cases; suppressive drugs in malarious areas
8–13 days	None	Measles vaccine
2–10 days	Penicillin; chloramphenicol	Meningococcal polysaccharide vaccine to people at risk; rifampicin for carriers or contacts
12–26 (av. 18) days	None	Live mumps vaccine
7–24 days	Chloramphenicol; ampicillin; sulpha-trimethoprim	Control of public water sources, food vendors, food handlers, treatment of carriers
Variable	Penicillin	Control of upper respiratory infections; avoidance of alcoholic intoxication
7–12 days	None	Wide-scale application of parenteral (Salk) and oral (Sabin) poliovirus vaccines; case isolation
3–10 days	Tetracyclines; chloramphenicol	Avoidance of tick-infested areas, or wearing of protective clothing in such areas; frequent search for and prompt removal of ticks from body; specific vaccination of exposed people
14–21 days	None	Rubella virus vaccine; immune serum globulin (human) given to contacts of rubella. Rubella in early stages of pregnancy legally recognized as indication for abortion

(continued)

Table 17.2 Continued

Disease	Infective organism	Infectious sources	Entry site	Method of spread
Scarlet fever	*Streptococcus haemolyticus*	Human cases; infected food	Pharynx	Nasal and oral secretions
Syphilis	*Treponema pallidum*	Infected exudate or blood	External genitalia; cervix; mucosal surfaces; placenta	Sexual activity; contact with open lesions; blood transfusion; transplacental inoculation
Tetanus	*Clostridium tetani*	Contaminated soil	Penetrating and crush wounds	Horse and cattle faeces
Trichinosis	*Trichinella spiralis*	Infected pigs	Gastrointestinal tract	Ingestion of infected pork, undercooked
Tuberculosis	*Mycobacterium tuberculosis*	Sputum from human cases; milk from infected cows (rare in UK)	Respiratory mucosa	Sputum; respiratory droplets
Tularaemia	*Pasteurella tularensis*	Wild rodents and rabbits	Eyes; skin; gastrointestinal tract	Handling infected animals; ingestion of undercooked infected meat; drinking contaminated water; bites from infected flies, ticks
Typhoid fever	*Salmonella typhi*	Contaminated food and water	Gastrointestinal tract	Infected urine and faeces
Typhus, endemic	*Rickettsia typhi (mooseri)*	Infected rodents	Skin	Flea bites
Whooping cough (pertussis)	*Bordetella pertussis*	Human cases	Respiratory tract	Infected bronchial secretions

Incubation period	Chemotherapy*	Prophylaxis
3–5 days	Penicillin	Case isolation; prophylactic chemotherapy with penicillin; asepsis during obstetrical procedures; specific chemoprophylaxis for people with rheumatic fever
10–70 days	Penicillin; erythromycin; tetracycline	Case-finding by means of routine serological testing and other methods; adequate treatment of infected individuals
4–21 days (average 10 days)	Tetanus immune globulin (human) [TIG]	Wound debridement; toxoid booster injections for patients previously immunized; tetanus toxoid and tetanus immune globulin (separate sites and separate syringes) for non-immune people
2–28 days	None	Regulation of pig breeders; adequate meat inspection; thorough cooking of pork
Variable	Isoniazid; ethambutol; rifampicin; streptomycin	Early discovery and adequate treatment of active cases; milk pasteurization
1–10 days	Streptomycin; tetracyclines; chloramphenicol	Use of rubber gloves when skinning/handling potentially infectious wild animals; avoidance of contact with potentially infected rodents; adequate cooking of wild rabbit dishes; vaccination of hunters, butchers, laboratory workers risking heavy exposure
1–3 weeks	Chloramphenicol; ampicillin; sulpha-trimethoprim	Decontamination of water sources; milk pasteurization; individual vaccination of high-risk people; control of carriers
1–2 weeks	Tetracyclines; chloramphenicol	Delousing procedures; case quarantine
Commonly 7 days	Erythromycin, ampicillin	Active immunization with vaccine; case isolation

* Research developments produce changes in drug therapy. The reader is referred to drug brochures and digests to keep abreast of changing dosages and uses.

SEXUALLY TRANSMITTED DISEASES

The number of people infected with one (or more) of the sexually transmitted diseases throughout the world seems to be increasing. The term 'venereal diseases' was used earlier in this century, and consisted of the three 'classical' diseases, syphilis, gonorrhoea and chancroid.

It has now been established that there are many infections which can be spread by sexual contact, which may be by vaginal, anal or oral intercourse. These include: nonspecific urethritis (NSU); hepatitis B virus; human immunodeficiency virus (HIV); chlamydia trachomatis; trichomonas vaginalis; Epstein-Barr virus; scabies; pubic lice; and several others.

GONORRHOEA

Gonorrhoea is an infection involving the mucous membrane of the genitourinary tract; it is caused by the gonococcus *Neisseria gonorrhoeae*. It is an infectious disease which is transmitted sexually, the exception being gonococcal ophthalmia of the newborn. It may be acquired by sexual intercourse, orogenital, and/or anogenital contacts between members of the opposite sexes as well as members of the same sex.

EPIDEMIOLOGY
1. Changes in sexual behaviour; liberalization of attitudes.
2. Sexual contact at earlier ages.
3. Greater personal mobility.
4. Greater use of the Pill for contraception, rather than a condom.

CLINICAL PROBLEMS
1. Gonorrhoea is increasing in the UK. There were 48,393 new cases in England in 1983.
2. Gonorrhoea has a short incubation period which permits rapid spread; a high percentage of infected females are symptom-free.
3. Syphilis and gonorrhoea are frequently observed in the same patient.
4. Gonorrhoea is becoming increasingly resistant to penicillin in some countries.

COMPLICATIONS
1. Sterility in women; pelvic infection.
2. Secondary foci of infection may develop in any organ system – disseminated gonorrhoea, gonococcal arthritis, tenosynovitis, bursitis, endocarditis, pelvic infection, meningitis, lesions of the skin, severe proctitis, postgonococcal urethritis (male).

CLINICAL FEATURES
NURSING ALERT
80 per cent of women who have the disease may be asymptomatic and unaware that they are infected. There is a fairly high incidence of asymptomatic males with gonorrhoea.

Women (small percentage)
1. Vaginal discharge.
2. Urinary frequency and pain.
3. Pelvic infection, when gonococcus spreads through fallopian tubes (salpingitis):
   a. Fever
   b. Nausea and vomiting
   c. Lower abdominal pain
4. Gonococcal septicaemia.

Men (incubation period three to four days or longer)
1. Painful urination; mucopurulent urethral discharge.
2. Spread of infection to posterior urethra, prostate, seminal vesicles and epididymis.
3. Prostatitis.
4. Pelvic pain and fever.
5. Epididymitis.
   a. Severe pain, tenderness and swelling.
6. Postgonococcal urethritis and urethral stricture become major problems in male.

Anal manifestations
1. Anal itching and irritation – erythema and oedema of anal crypts.
2. Painful defaecation.
3. Sensation of rectal fullness; anal discharge.

Oral manifestations
May be affected by gonorrhoeal process directly (direct contact of oral cavity with infecting organisms) or indirectly (secondary to infection elsewhere in the body).

The majority of pharyngeal infections are asymptomatic.
1. Sore throat/pharyngeal inflammation.
2. Lips – may show intensely painful ulcerative inflammation.
3. Gingiva – erythematous, spongy and tender.
4. Tongue – red and dry with ulcerations or swollen and glazed with eroded areas.
5. Soft palate and uvula – reddened and oedematous.

6. Oropharynx – may be covered with vesicles.

DIAGNOSTIC EVALUATION
Women
Culture specimen obtained from the cervix and anal canal and inoculated on separate Modified Thayer–Martin (MTM) culture plates.

Men
1. Smear of urethral exudate for microscopic examination.
2. In homosexuals: additional culture specimens obtained from anal canal and pharynx and inoculated on Modified Thayer–Martin culture plates.
3. Culture of oral cavity with Thayer–Martin medium (sugar fermentation required) if indicated.

TREATMENT
Objective
Eradicate the organism.
1. Uncomplicated gonococcal infection:
   Penicillin is the drug of choice, given on one occasion with a total dose of 2.4 mega units; some centres use 4.8 mega units in a divided dose.
   This is preceded by probenecid given by mouth, half an hour before the injections. Probenecid prevents the rapid excretion of penicillin by the kidneys.
   As there is a possibility of an anaphylactic reaction following this penicillin injection, the patient should remain in the clinic for half an hour and appropriate emergency drugs should be available.
2. Alternative regimens:
   a. Oral therapy: ampicillin by mouth together with probenecid.
   b. Therapy for patients allergic to penicillin or probenecid or with history of previous anaphylactic reactions.
      (i) Tetracycline hydrochloride by mouth on a four-day schedule – or
      (ii) Spectinomycin hydrochloride intramuscularly in a single injection.
3. Treatment of sexual contacts: same treatment as for gonorrhoea.
4. Follow-up – imperative due to a higher resistance of *Neisseria* gonococci to antibiotics.
   Culture should be obtained from appropriate sites seven to 14 days after completion of treatment.
5. Secure serological test for syphilis at time of diagnosis.
6. Patients with gonorrhoea who also have syphilis must be given additional treatment depending on stage of syphilis.
7. Treatment of complications of gonorrhoea (endocarditis, bacteraemia, arthritis, etc) is individualized.

NURSING ISOLATION PROCEDURE
Use secretion precautions for duration of illness (until lesions stop draining).

PRINCIPLES OF CONTROL
1. Gonorrhoea is not a notifiable disease; careful records are kept by sexually transmitted disease clinics, and contacts are traced by specially trained personnel.
2. Each patient should be interviewed for names of contacts. Conduct interview and record history in nonjudgemental, empathetic manner.
3. Contacts of known gonorrhoea cases should be investigated; known contacts should be treated.
4. The patient should be instructed to avoid reinfection by sexual activity with untreated previous sexual partners until they have been tested and treated.

PATIENT EDUCATION
1. Sexually transmitted diseases are acquired by sexual contact (vaginal sexual intercourse, anal intercourse, oral intercourse) and by close and direct contact with an infected person.
2. A person who thinks that he or she may have a sexually transmitted disease or who has been exposed to someone who might have it should have a check-up. Immediate treatment should be sought if symptoms develop.
3. Anyone who is sexually active with a number of sexual partners should have regular check-ups.
4. Washing the sex organs (before and after sexual contact) and the use of a condom may give limited protection against a sexually transmitted disease.
5. Birth control pills and intrauterine devices give no protection against a sexually transmitted disease.
6. Gonorrhoea and syphilis are different diseases, caused by different germs; they attack the body in different ways but are spread in the same manner. A person may have both gonorrhoea and syphilis at the same time.
7. There appears to be no natural or acquired immunity to gonorrhoea and syphilis. A person can get gonorrhoea and syphilis again and again.
8. Pregnant women may pass infection of syphilis to unborn child. Pregnant women may pass gonorrhoea to baby during the birth process.
9. Bacteria from gonorrhoea may enter the bloodstream and affect joints, joint linings, heart valves, etc.

URETHRITIS FROM GONORRHOEA

AETIOLOGY
1. *Neisseria gonorrhoeae* – the specific organism.
2. Transmitted through sexual contact.
3. More and more asymptomatic carriers are being recognized.

CLINICAL FEATURES
Male
1. Inflammation of meatal orifice; burning on urination; *may be asymptomatic.*
2. Urethral discharge – scant and serous to thick, yellowish pus (four to 10 days or longer after sexual exposure).

Female
1. Purulent urethral discharge.
2. Frequency, urgency, nocturia.
3. Red, swollen urinary meatus.
4. Pelvic infection accompanied by abdominal pain.
5. Often is asymptomatic.

COMPLICATIONS (LOCAL)
1. Male – periurethritis, prostatitis, epididymitis, urethral stricture, sterility due to vasoepididymal duct obstruction.
2. Female – pelvic infection, abscess of greater vestibular glands (Bartholin's glands), urethral stricture.

TREATMENT AND PATIENT EDUCATION
1. See p. 987 for treatment of gonorrhoea.
2. Instruct the patient to avoid sexual activity with untreated previous sexual partners until they have been treated and examined to prevent reinfection.
3. Emphasize that the patient must return in four to seven days to assess results and determine if there is need for further treatment and tests.
4. Urge the patient to encourage any sexual contacts to come forward for treatment.

SYPHILIS

Syphilis is a chronic infectious multisystem disease caused by *Treponema pallidum* (a spirochaete). It is acquired by sexual contact or may be congenital in origin.

INCIDENCE
1. Most prevalent in teenagers and young adults.
2. More prevalent in males than females.
3. More prevalent in large urban centres.
4. Promiscuity and indiscretion are factors.

EPIDEMIOLOGY
Tracing the source and spread of infections by interviewing known patients for sex contacts.
1. Interviewing and re-interviewing every reported patient with syphilis for sex contacts.
2. Rapid investigation to identify contacts for examination within a minimal time period.
3. Identifying and conducting blood tests of other people who by definition (suspect or associate) are possibly involved sexually in an infectious chain (cluster procedure). (Promiscuous people have somewhat similar sexual behaviour patterns.)
4. Epidemiological (preventive or prophylactic) treatment of sexual contacts and infectious syphilis cases.
5. All pregnant women are screened for syphilis as a routine.

CLINICAL FEATURES
Syphilis is capable of destroying tissue in almost any organ in the body; it thus produces a wide variety of clinical manifestations.

Stages of untreated syphilis
Incubation period
1. Ten to 90 days; average 21 days.
2. No symptoms or lesions.
3. Spirochaetaemia is present; patient's blood is infective.

Primary (early) syphilis
1. Most infectious stage; lasting one to six weeks.
2. Features include:
   a. Chancre or primary sore – appears at the site where the treponema enters the body (glans penis, scrotum, cervix, labia, anus, lips, mouth, tonsils, eyelids, nipple).
      Chancre remains for short time and heals without treatment (three to six weeks), leaving a thin atrophic scar.
   b. Enlargement of regional lymph nodes.

NURSING ALERT
Syphilis should be suspected when an indolent, painless ulceration appears on the body.

Secondary syphilis
1. Lesion appears six to eight weeks after onset of primary lesion; may involve any cutaneous or mucosal surface of the body as well as any organ.
2. Skin lesions – bilaterally symmetrical in distribution, polymorphous (macular, papular, follicular, pustular).
   a. Moist papules occur most frequently in

anogenital region (condylomata) and in mouth.
- b. Lesions of mouth, throat and cervix (mucous patches) frequently occur in secondary stage.
- c. Generalized patchy hair loss on scalp.
3. Generalized lymphadenopathy.
4. Arthritic and bone pain.
5. Acute iritis.
6. Hoarseness, chronic sore throat.

Late syphilis

(Clinically destructive stage after latent period) – features may occur 10 to 30 years after exposure; recovery unpredictable.
1. Granulomatous lesions appear in skin, bones, liver, cardiovascular system and central nervous system.
2. Syphilis will mainly affect cardiovascular system (aneurysm of ascending aorta, aortic insufficiency), central nervous system and skeletal system.

DIAGNOSTIC EVALUATION
There are two types of serological tests.

Nontreponemal or reagin tests
To detect antibody-like substances, called reagin, found in serum of infected patient; these tests are not always specific and there may be false–positive reactions.
1. Flocculation tests – a reaction in which a suspension of antibody particles when added to serum, plasma or spinal fluid containing antibody will form small, usually visible clumps, or floccules.
   - a. Venereal disease research laboratory (VDRL).
   - b. Kline.
   - c. Kahn.
   - d. Hinton.
   - e. Mazzini.
2. Complement fixation tests – involves bringing together an active complement, an antigen and its antibody under proper temperature and time conditions.
   - a. Kolmer.
   - b. Wasserman.
3. Rapid reagin tests – specific-purpose tests using flocculation procedures on plasma or serum; used as a rough screening guide.

Treponemal tests
Test for detection of treponemal antibody produced in response to syphilitic infection.
1. *Treponema pallidum* immobilization test (TPI)
2. Fluorescent treponemal antibody test (FTA)
3. Fluorescent treponemal antibody absorption test

(FTA-ABS) – the standard test in most national health laboratories.

TREATMENT (FOR EARLY SYPHILIS)
1. Give benzathine penicillin G (intramuscularly) – drug of choice because it provides effective treatment in a single visit – or aqueous procaine penicillin G (intramuscularly) for eight days.
   - a. Screen for history of previous reaction to penicillin; reaction can occur in patient with negative history.
   - b. Patient should be detained 30 minutes after administration of parenteral penicillin in case of development of anaphylactoid reaction.
2. Patients who are allergic to penicillin may be given tetracycline or erythromycin.
3. Post-treatment follow-up is essential – treatment failures do occur and retreatment is required, followed by quantitative VDRL at one, three, six and 12 months.
4. Jarisch–Herxheimer reaction – a reaction appearing within hours after initiating treatment of syphilis (particularly in the secondary stage) and subsiding within 24 hours; consists of transient fever and flu-like symptoms of malaise, chills, headache and myalgia. It may involve release of endotoxin-killed treponemes or from an allergic phenomenon.
   - a. Managed by bed rest and aspirin.
   - b. Warn patient that this reaction may be expected.

NURSING ISOLATION PROCEDURES
Secretion precautions for mucocutaneous features until 24 hours after initiation of effective therapy.

PREVENTION AND PATIENT EDUCATION
1. All patients known to have been exposed to syphilitic lesion should be treated.
2. Preventive treatment should be given before or after exposure.
3. Programme of public health and sex education should be conducted.
4. Patient should be instructed to refrain from sexual intercourse with previous partners not under treatment.
5. Mass serological examinations of special groups with known high incidence of sexually transmitted disease should be conducted. (Also, see AIDS, p. 1011, and hepatitis B, p. 507.)

SUMMARY OF SEXUALLY TRANSMITTED DISEASES

See Table 17.3.

Table 17.3   Sexually transmitted diseases summary

Disease	Aetiology	Prevalence	Clinical presentation
Gonorrhoea	*Neisseria gonorrhoeae* A nonmotile, Gram-negative diplococcus; 0.6–1.0µm in diameter	In 1983, there were 48,393 new cases, the majority of which were in the 20–24 and 25–34 age groups	Men have dysuria, frequency and urethral discharge that is usually purulent and often more severe in the morning. Women experience vaginal discharge and cystitis; 5–20 per cent of men and about 60 per cent of women have no symptoms
Syphilis	*Treponema pallidum* A motile spirochaete with 6–14 spirals and ends pointed with finely spiral terminal filaments; 6–15µm in length.	In 1983, there were 1,934 new cases of primary syphilis, and 80 cases of congenital syphilis	*Primary syphilis:* classical chancre is a painless, eroded papule with a raised, indurated border. Atypical lesions are common; multiple lesions may occur. Extragenital chancres may appear on any part of body. Unilateral or bilateral lymphadenopathy may accompany. *Secondary syphilis:* Various cutaneous and mucous membrane lesions, alopecia, generalized lymphadenopathy, mild constitutional symptoms
Nongonococcal urethritis (NGU)	1. *Chlamydia trachomatis* – estimated to cause NGU in about 50 per cent of cases An obligate intracellular parasite. Diameter 250–500nm 2. *Ureaplasma urealyticum* – estimated by some workers to cause NGU in about 30 per cent of cases A mycoplasma of the T strain, less than 150nm in diameter. 3. *Other aetiological agents* – estimated to cause NGU in 10–20 per cent of cases: a. *Trichomonas vaginalis* b. *Candida albicans* c. Herpes simplex d. Coliform bacteria	Age distribution of nongonococcal urethritis parallels that of other sexually transmitted diseases, notably gonorrhoea. Recurrences are very common. In 1982, there were 134,079 cases reported	Urethral discharge varies from profusely purulent to slightly mucoid. Dysuria may or may not be present. In half of the cases, the incubation period appears to exceed 10 days. Some men may have asymptomatic infection

Diagnosis	Therapy	Complications
Presumptive identification – Microscopic identification of typical Gram-negative, intracellular diplococci on smear of urethral exudate from men or endocervical material from women, OR positive oxidase reaction of typical colonies from specimen obtained from anterior urethra, endocervix or anal canal, and inoculated on Modified Thayer–Martin medium	Aqueous procaine penicillin G, 4.8 million units intramuscularly at two sites with 1g of probenecid orally, OR tetracycline HCl, 0.5g orally 4 times a day for 5 days, 10g total, OR ampicillin, 3.5g or amoxicillin, 3g, either with 1g of probenecid orally.	Epididymitis Pharyngitis Meningitis Septicaemia Arthritis Endocarditis Conjunctivitis in newborn Pelvic inflammatory disease (PID)
Demonstration of *T. pallidum* from exudate of primary or secondary lesions by darkfield microscopy. Typical lesions, reactive reagin test for syphilis (VDRL or RPR) and FAT/ABS will confirm except in early primary cases	Benzathine penicillin G, 2.4 million units intramuscularly at one visit, OR Aqueous procaine penicillin G, 4.8 million units total: 600,000 units intramuscularly daily for 8 days, OR tetracycline HCl, 500mg orally 4 times a day for 15 days.	Late syphilis Congenital syphilis
Clinical picture of dysuria and/or urethral discharge; discharge on examination; polymorphonuclear leucocytes or urethral smear negative for *Neisseria gonorrhoeae* and negative culture for gonorrhoea on Modified Thayer–Martin medium	Tetracycline, 500mg 4 times a day for 7–21 days. Many clinicians recommend similar therapy for sexual consorts.	Epididymitis Prostatitis Proctitis Cervicitis Salpingitis Reiter's disease Ophthalmia neonatorum

(continued)

Table 17.3 Continued

Disease	Aetiology	Prevalence	Clinical presentation
Trichomoniasis	*Trichomonas vaginalis* A motile protozoan with 4 anterior flagella and a short, undulating membrane; 5–15µm in length	Colonization rates are higher among women than men. In 1983, there were 18,274 cases reported	From no signs or symptoms to erythema and oedema of external genitalia and frothy greenish-grey vaginal discharge. Granular vaginitis may include punctuate haemorrhages and may involve the cervix. Most men are asymptomatic, though some may present with urethritis
Genital herpes infection	Herpes virus – type 2 A spherical DNA virus, enveloped, with cubic symmetry; 150nm	Prevalent among adolescents, young adults, and the sexually active. In 1983, there were 16,534 cases reported	Vesicular lesions on vulva, perineum, vagina and cervix in women; lesions on penile shaft, prepuce, glans penis and (less frequently) scrotum and perineum in men. Recurrent infections. Tender adenopathy, dysuria and constitutional signs more common with primary infections than those recurring
Vulvovaginal candidiasis	*Candida albicans* A dimorphic Gram-positive fungus that appears as oval, budding yeast cells, has hyphae and pseudohyphae; 3 × 6µm	Saprophytic in the oropharyngeal and gastrointestinal tracts in 50 per cent of the population and in the vagina in 20 per cent of nonpregnant women. In 1983, there were 57,876 cases reported	Vulva is usually erythematous and oedematous. Vaginal discharge, when present, may be thick and white, resembling cottage cheese. Occasionally discharge is thin and watery. Satellite lesions may spread to the groin. Many women have no symptoms. Sexual partners may develop balanitis or cutaneous lesions on penis
Corynebacterium vaginale vaginitis or *Haemophilus vaginalis* vaginitis	*Corynebacterium vaginale* or *Haemophilus vaginalis* Gram-negative pleomorphic coccobacillus, precise taxonomy not decided: measures 1–3µm × 0.4–0.7µm	Cultured from 23–96 per cent of women with vaginitis. Recovered from 0–52 per cent of asymptomatic women.	Homogenous, relatively thin, occasionally frothy vaginal discharge, usually grey-white. Punctate haemorrhages and vulvar irritation are occasionally seen. Between 10 per cent and 40 per cent of culture-positive patients have no symptoms
Pediculosis pubis	*Phthirus pubis* Pubic louse, an oval, greyish insect which becomes reddish-brown when engorged with blood, 1–4mm in length.	Age group of patients affected by pubic lice parallels that of patients with gonorrhoea. Transmitted during sexual intercourse, very rarely by bedding or clothing. In 1983, there were 9,093 cases reported	Erythematous, itching papules. Nits or adult lice adhering to pubic hair or hair around the anus, abdomen and thighs

Diagnosis	Therapy	Complications
Microscopic examination of wet mount of vaginal discharge. Cervical smears may show the parasite Culture methods are available	Oral metronidazole 2 immediately orally, OR 250 mg 3 times a day for 7 days. Advise patient against consuming alcohol. Treat steady sex partners Oral nimorazole 2g immediately given with food, for resistant cases	Rare Epididymitis Prostatitis
Clinical appearance of herpetic lesions Cervical smears from lesions, stained to show multinucleated giant cells with intranuclear inclusion bodies Tissue culture	No specific therapy is available. Symptoms may be relieved by warm baths	Keratitis Encephalitis Neonatal herpes infection
Microscopic examination of gram-stained smears of introital or vaginal wall scrapings. Microscopic examination of wet mount of vaginal discharge. Culture on Sabouraud's modified agar	Nystatin vaginal suppositories twice a day for 7–14 days, OR miconazole vaginal cream 4 times a day, for 7 days. Discuss with patient predisposing factors and means of avoiding a recurrence Clotrimazole can be used as an alternative to nystatin	Nil
Clinical picture, microscopic examination, and culture. Gram stain of vaginal exudate may show tiny, Gram-negative coccobacilli ('clue cells') adhering to vaginal epithelial cells, although specificity of this finding is low. Wet mount far less sensitive than Gram stain	Oral ampicillin 500mg 4 times a day for 7–10 days (examine patient for syphilis or gonorrhoea before prescribing this regimen, because ampicillin may mask symptoms), OR oral metronidazole 250mg 3 times a day for 7 days.	Nil
Clinical observation of lice OR microscopically, by identification of nits at base of hair	1 per cent Y-benzene hexachloride lotion, 25 per cent benzyl benzoate lotion Combine with appropriate antibiotics if secondary infection is noted	Rare Impetigo Furunculosis Pustular eczema

(continued)

Table 17.3   Continued

Disease	Aetiology	Prevalence	Clinical presentation
Scabies	*Sarcoptes scabiei* The adult female mite is 300–400µm long and has 4 pairs of short legs. Posterior legs end in long bristles. Male is 100–200µm in length	Transmitted via close bodily contact, often incidental to coitus, infested bedding and clothing. In 1984, there were 2,192 cases reported	Linear burrows 1–10mm in length, often with a red papule which contains the mite. Scratching may produce excoriation. Most common sites are finger webs, wrists, elbows, ankles, penis. Night-time itching is characteristic
Genital warts (*Condyloma acuminata*)	Human papillomavirus. A small DNA virus, icosahedral, of the papovavirus group.	Age distribution of venereal papillomatous lesions parallels that of patients with gonorrhoea. In 1983, there were 37,899 cases reported	Flesh-coloured to pinkish papillary or sessile growths which occur around the vulva, introitus, vagina, cervix, perineum, anus, anal canal, urethra and glans penis
Chancroid	*Haemophilus ducreyi* A coccobacillus that is nonmotile, non-acid-fast, Gram-negative. Size 1–1.5µm × 0.6µm	May occur in conjunction with other genital infections, particularly genital herpes and syphilis.	A ragged, tender ulcer that is not indurated ('soft chancre'), its base covered with grey or yellow necrotic exudate. May be multiple ulcers. Tender inguinal adenopathy, usually unilateral. Women contacts are usually asymptomatic
Lymphogranuloma venereum	*Chlamydia trachomatis* An obligate intracellular parasite. Diameter 250–500nm	This is common in tropical and subtropical areas; 36 cases were reported in the UK in 1983	Primary lesion is an evanescent, painless vesicle or superficial nonindurated ulcer on the genitalia. Adenopathy of the regional lymph nodes is common. A frank purulent proctocolitis may signal rectal involvement. Rare
Granuloma inguinale	*Calymmatobacterium granulomatis* A nonmotile coccobacillus that is Gram-negative. Size 2µm × 0.8µm	Fairly common in a few underdeveloped nations. In 1983, there were 21 cases reported	Single or multiple subcutaneous nodules may erode through the skin, producing clean granulomatous, beefy-red lesions (usually painless)
Hepatitis B infection	Hepatitis virus – type B A virus of probable DNA nucleic acid content, 26µm or less	Common among homosexuals and prostitutes	Onset is usually insidious, with vague abdominal discomfort, anorexia, nausea, arthralgia, which often progresses to jaundice. Fever may be absent or mild. Asymptomatic, anicteric hepatitis may occur

Diagnosis	Therapy	Complications
Identifying the burrows and microscopic identification of the mites	25 per cent Benzyl benzoate lotion Y-benzene hexachloride crotomiton Combine with appropriate antibiotics if secondary infection is noted. Trace and treat family, domestic and sex contacts	Impetigo Pustular eczema
Clinical appearance Histology Electron microscopy	Podophyllin 10–25 per cent in tincture of benzoin, applied weekly Electrocautery Curettage Cryotherapy	Rare Malignant change
Clinical appearance Exclude possibility of syphilis through absence of indurated lesions and negative darkfield. Gram-stained exudate from lesion or aspirates from nodes may reveal short, Gram-negative rods, OR culture on blood agar or media with blood derivatives	Sulphasoxazole 1g orally 4 times a day OR tetracycline 500mg 4 times a day for 10–14 days OR Kanamycin 500mg intramuscularly twice a day for 10–14 days, OR streptomycin 500mg intramuscularly twice a day for 10–14 days. Fluctuating gland masses will call for aspiration	Chronic fistulas of gland masses in groin
Clinical picture Complement fixation test (CFT), significantly positive with a titre of 1:16 or higher in more than 80 per cent of cases Material for Frei skin test is no longer available	Tetracycline 500mg orally 4 times a day for 2–3 weeks OR sulphasoxazole 4g orally, followed by 500mg 4 times a day for 3 weeks. Fluctuating gland masses indicate a need for aspiration	Rare Elephantiasis Rectal strictures producing tenesmus, pain and constipation Men: ulcerative and fistular lesions of urethra, penis, scrotum Women: ulcerative genital lesions
Clinical picture Intracytoplasmic rods ('Donovan's bodies') in large mononuclear cell from biopsy material stained with Giemsa or Wright's stain	Tetracycline 500mg orally 4 times a day for 2–3 weeks OR gentamicin 40 mg intramuscularly twice a day for 2 weeks	Rare Elephantiasis Urethral, vaginal or rectal stricture from cicatrix following healing. Massed pelvic glands; occasional bony involvement
Detection of hepatitis B surface antigen (HBsAg) in blood by radioimmunoassay, passive haemagglutination, or other techniques	Symptomatic	Death Carriers (rare) Cirrhosis (late and rare)

BACTERIAL INFECTIONS

NOSOCOMIAL (HOSPITAL-ASSOCIATED) INFECTIONS

Nosocomial infections are those which are acquired during hospitalization, and the infection was neither present, nor incubating at the time of admission. The major cause of such infections are Gram-negative bacteria, particularly *Staphylococcus aureus*.

PREDISPOSING EVENTS

1. Most Gram-negative bacilli are not invasive in normal hosts; they are opportunistic bacteria that become invasive in people with diminishing defence mechanisms and in people with serious underlying disorders.
2. Diagnostic and treatment procedures (tubes, catheters, etc) result in disruption of usual protective barriers normally provided by the skin and mucous membranes.
3. The advent of potent immunosuppressive drugs, cytotoxic drugs, steroids, radiotherapy and previous splenectomy contribute to diminishing the defence mechanisms of the patient.

NURSING ALERT
People over 70 are at high risk of acquiring a nosocomial infection.

4. Patients in intensive care units are at risk because of underlying conditions that compromise host defences, frequent exposure to invasive procedures, close proximity to other susceptible/at-risk patients that allows opportunity for cross-infection, and resistant micro-organisms in intensive care unit environment.
5. The following contribute to the development of Gram-negative infections:
   a. Genitourinary tract – indwelling catheters, instrumentation, urinary obstruction.
   b. Gastrointestinal tract – from obstruction, perforation, neoplasia, abscesses, diverticuli.
   c. Biliary tract – cholangitis, obstruction (stones), surgical procedures.
   d. Prolonged hospitalization.
   e. Changing microbial flora.
   f. Emergence of antibiotic-resistant bacteria.
   g. Reproductive system – abortion, instrumentation, postpartum period.
   h. Vascular system – venous cutdowns, intravenous catheters, intracardiac pacemakers, prosthetic heart valves, total parenteral nutrition, indwelling arterial lines, pressure-monitoring devices, surgical procedures.
   i. Skin – wound infections, burns, pressure sores.
   j. Respiratory tract – aspiration, tracheostomy, mechanical ventilation.

PREVENTION
1. *Handwashing by personnel and patient – fundamental to the control of all infections.*
2. Isolation precautions for immunosuppressed patients.
3. Strict aseptic technique for all diagnostic/therapeutic procedures – wounds, tracheostomies, tube drainage, catheters, intravenous therapy, cardiac pacing, ventilatory equipment.
   a. Avoid invasive procedures as much as possible.
   b. Anchor intravenous catheter securely to prevent movement in vein; avoid prolonged intravenous therapy.
4. Use nursing surveillance to prevent cross-infection.
5. Monitoring sterilization procedures and cleaning practices.
6. Try to avoid putting together two patients with indwelling catheters in the same room.
   a. Use closed urinary drainage system if an indwelling catheter is required.
   b. Regard outside of catheter and drainage bag as highly contaminated.

BACTERAEMIA

Bacteraemia means bacterial invasion of the bloodstream. Septic shock is circulatory collapse occurring as a result of a severe infection (usually as a result of Gram-negative enteric bacilli).

CLINICAL FEATURES
1. Rigors and a rapid rise in temperature.

NURSING ALERT
Pyrexia may be absent in the severely shocked or elderly patient.

2. Warm, dry, flushed skin (during early stage).
3. Deteriorating mental status – due to reduction in cerebral blood flow.

4. *Hypotension and shock:*
   a. Tachycardia/tachypnoea.
   b. Cool, clammy skin/peripheral cyanosis.
   c. Decreasing pulse pressure.
   d. Oliguria.
   e. Vascular collapse – death may occur as a result of vascular collapse.
5. Intravascular coagulation.

NURSING INTERVENTIONS
Instituting appropriate treatment of bacteraemia
1. Examine the patient carefully to identify source of sepsis.
   a. Assist with collection of blood culture – to identify aetiological agent and for sensitivity testing.
   b. Obtain other smears and culture as indicated.
2. Administer appropriate antibiotic – give promptly when the patient is too ill to await result of culture.
   a. Therapy is usually started before bacteriological diagnosis is made because of seriousness of illness.
   b. The choice of antibiotic therapy also depends on the patterns of resistance in the patient's environment.
3. Remove any foreign source of possible infection (when possible) – venous or bladder catheters.
4. Assist with surgical drainage of localized infection (abscesses, infected sites).

Establishing tissue and organ perfusion and recovery from shock
1. Monitor vital signs; pulse and respiration; temperature; blood pressure; appearance of skin and mucous membranes; fluid balance (urine output should be recorded hourly if possible). Focus assessment of the patient on the trends and patterns of change.
2. Assist in setting up and maintaining the administration of adequate blood and fluids to correct fluid and electrolyte disturbances.
3. Administer oxygen to keep arterial Po_2 at desired level. Arrange for monitoring of blood gas and pH levels.
4. Monitor for signs of mental confusion or alterations in conscious level.
5. Monitor for signs of disseminated intravascular coagulation (see p. 396).
6. Administer the appropriate antibiotics and drugs ordered to maintain blood pressure or treat cardiac failure.

7. Take the appropriate nursing actions to prevent the spread of infection.

STAPHYLOCOCCAL INFECTIONS

Staphylococci are responsible for a wide variety of infections. They cause most superficial infections, but they also produce serious infections of the lungs, pleural space, bones, kidneys and surgical wounds.

EXAMPLES OF STAPHYLOCOCCAL DISEASE
1. *Skin and soft tissue infections* – furuncles (boils), impetigo, carbuncles, cellulitis, abscesses, infected lacerations.
2. *Invasion of lymphatics* – axillary, cervical, mediastinal, retroperitoneal and subdiaphragmatic abscesses.
3. *Invasion of bloodstream* – endocarditis, pneumonitis, empyema, perinephritic abscess, hepatic abscess, splenic abscess, staphylococcal enteritis, septic arthritis, meningitis, osteomyelitis, generalized septicaemia.

INFECTIOUS AGENT
Various strains of coagulase-positive staphylococci (*Staphylococcus aureus*). It has been estimated that between 20 to 40 per cent of *Staphylococcus aureus* infections in hospitals are resistant to methicillin and many other antibiotics.

MODES OF TRANSMISSION
1. Direct hand transfer.
2. Ingestion of food.
3. Nasal secretions, draining wound, asymptomatic carrier.
4. Break in skin/mucous membrane.
5. Aerosolization during dressing changes.
6. Vascular access sites (intravenous lines, drug abusers).

HOSPITAL STAPHYLOCOCCAL INFECTIONS
(Include all of the above infections.)

Susceptible hospital patients
1. Chronically ill or debilitated patients.
2. Patients receiving systemic steroids or cancer chemotherapy.
3. Patients undergoing major or prolonged surgery.
4. Infants in the nursery.
5. Patients with impairment of skin integrity (dermatoses, burns, abrasions).

Prevention and control

1. All staff working in a surgical area, and also in a ward where a patient has a pressure sore, should adhere to the guidelines of the hospital regarding handwashing, the use of plastic aprons and aseptic dressing technique.
2. It may be advisable for staff working in high-risk areas to have nasal swabs taken, as a carrier state is possible.
3. If a patient is found to be infected, ideally he should be discharged home, if he is fit enough. There is no risk to healthy relatives outside the hospital.

   If the patient is not fit for discharge, he should be transferred to an isolation unit, or a single side room. If more than one case occurs, the ward may be closed to further admissions. Gowns and effective handwashing facilities, and use of antiseptic hand rubs should be used particularly by staff who may be visiting patients in other parts of the ward or hospital, e.g. doctors, physiotherapists.
4. If an infected patient is transferred from another hospital, it is essential that the receiving hospital is notified in advance so that special preparations can be made. Also, ambulance staff and porters should wear protective gowns.
5. A receiving hospital should be notified if an apparently uninfected patient is transferred from an area where other cases have occurred.
6. Staff who have worked with infected patients should be screened before transferring to another area. Antiseptic bath and hair washing may be advised.

SPECIFIC THERAPY FOR STAPHYLOCOCCAL INFECTIONS (SYSTEMIC)

1. Penicillinase-resistant penicillins (oxacillin, methicillin, nafcillin) and the cephalosporins (cephalothin) are antistaphylococcal drugs and are selected according to sensitivity studies.
   a. Intravenous administration is usually selected because of the large doses of drug required.
   b. Serious staphylococcal infections may require four to six weeks of treatment.
2. Provide supportive care – surgical measures, pain relief, treatment of fever, etc.

PREVENTIVE MEASURES AND PATIENT EDUCATION

1. Public should be educated concerning personal hygiene.
2. People with draining lesions should be isolated from their group and treated.

STREPTOCOCCAL INFECTIONS

Most streptococcal infections in humans are caused by group A streptococci. Streptococci gain entrance to the body primarily through the upper respiratory tract or skin; transmission is by people with streptococcal infections or by asymptomatic carriers.

BETA-HAEMOLYTIC STREPTOCOCCAL INFECTIONS

1. Streptococcal pharyngitis ('strep' sore throat).
2. Wound and skin infections – impetigo, puerperal infections, cellulitis, erysipelas.
3. Scarlet fever (streptococcal throat with a rash which occurs if infectious agent produces erythrogenic toxin to which patient is not immune).
4. Sinusitis, otitis media, mastoiditis, peritonsillar abscess.
5. Pericarditis, arthritis, peritonitis, meningitis.
6. Pneumonia and empyema.

POSTSTREPTOCOCCAL DISEASES (SEQUELAE OF HAEMOLYTIC STREPTOCOCCI)

1. Rheumatic fever.
2. Acute glomerulonephritis.

DIAGNOSTIC EVALUATION

1. Throat culture and sensitivity test.
2. Culture from wounds.

TREATMENT AND NURSING INTERVENTIONS

1. Penicillin is the drug of choice in streptococcal infections (except enterococcal streptococci); several forms are available.
   a. Therapy should be continued for at least 10 days – to eliminate the organism, cases of rheumatic fever and to help prevent further spread of streptococci.
   b. Cephalosporins or erythromycin may be used for penicillin-sensitive patients.
2. Make sure the patient understands the importance of completing the course of antibiotic treatment.

NURSING ISOLATION PROCEDURES

Streptococcal disease (group A):

1. Burns – strict isolation, wound and skin precautions or secretion precautions (depending on extent of infection) until wounds or lesions stop draining.
2. Endometritis (puerperal sepsis) – wound and skin

precautions until 24 hours after initiation of effective therapy.

3. Pharyngitis – secretion precautions until 24 hours after initiation of effective therapy.

4. Pneumonia – strict isolation until 24 hours after initiation of effective therapy.

5. Scarlet fever – secretion precautions until 24 hours after initiation of effective therapy.

6. Skin infection – strict isolation, wound and skin precautions or secretion precautions (depending of extent of infection) until wounds or lesions stop draining.

7. Wound infection – strict isolation, wound and skin precautions or secretion precautions (depending on the extent of infection) until wound stops draining.

8. Streptococcal disease (not group A) unless covered elsewhere – none.

PREVENTIVE MEASURES AND PATIENT EDUCATION

1. Public should be educated concerning the relationship of streptococcal infections to heart disease and glomerulonephritis.

2. Pasteurize milk.

3. Food handlers should be instructed about hygienic procedures.

4. Obstetrical patients should be protected from personnel or visitors with respiratory or skin infections.

5. Long-term penicillin prophylaxis may be used for high-risk individuals (rheumatic heart disease).

TUBERCULOSIS

Tuberculosis is an infectious disease caused by the tubercle bacillus, *Mycobacterium tuberculosis*. It usually invades the lungs, but it also involves, and sometimes produces gross lesions in other isolated organs, or it may be widespread. The incidence of tuberculosis in the UK has decreased from 77,511 new cases in 1919, with over 46,000 deaths, to 5,877 new cases in 1984, with 698 deaths.

TRANSMISSION

1. The term *Mycobacterium* is descriptive of the organism, which is a bacterium that resembles a fungus. The organisms multiply slowly and are characterized as acid-fast aerobic organisms which can be killed by heat, sunshine, drying and ultraviolet light.

2. Tuberculosis is an airborne disease transmitted by droplet nuclei, usually within the respiratory tract of a person with active ulcerative lesions who expels them during coughing, talking, sneezing or singing.

3. When an uninfected person inhales the droplet-containing air, the organism is carried into the lung to the pulmonary alveoli.

PATHOLOGY

1. A primary complex consists of the original site of the infection, together with the reaction occurring in the regional lymph nodes. When the primary focus is in the lungs, the hilar glands are those which are affected.

2. These changes occur within about six weeks and may be asymptomatic.

3. The primary lesion in the lungs usually heals. A systemic reaction occurs and this includes the development of a degree of immunity, and of a positive reaction to a tuberculin test, e.g., Mantoux test.

4. The lung lesion may become smaller and calcify. It may be evident on chest X-ray when it is completely quiescent. It may proceed to necrosis of tissue, causing caseation and cavitation.

5. The initial lesion may progress:
   a. By invasion of adjacent tissues.
   b. By invasion of the bloodstream.
   c. Via the bronchial tree.

6. In children the hilar nodes may cause compression of the lobar bronchi, which may result in a collapsed lobe, and the subsequent development of bronchiectasis.

7. Postprimary infection refers to any development of tuberculosis after the first few weeks of the original infection. It may occur about two years after the original infection, but may be many years later.

CONDITIONS CONTRIBUTING TO THE DEVELOPMENT OF TUBERCULOSIS

1. General physical debilitation.

2. Constant exposure to active tubercle bacilli.

3. Lowered resistance because of:
   a. Presence of other disease (diabetes, silicosis, etc).
   b. Age; over 30.

4. Immune deficiency diseases.

5. Recent gastrointestinal surgery.

6. Steroid therapy.

7. Alcoholism.

8. Pregnancy.

CLINICAL FEATURES

Patient may be asymptomatic or may have insidious symptoms that are ignored.

1. Generalized systemic signs and symptoms:
   a. Fatigue, anorexia, loss of weight and strength, low grade fever, irregular menses.
   b. Some patients have acute febrile illness, chills, generalized influenza-like symptoms.
2. Pulmonary signs and symptoms.
   a. Cough (imperceptible onset) progressing in frequency and producing mucoid or muco-purulent sputum.
   b. Haemoptysis; chest pain.
3. Extrapulmonary tuberculosis: mycobacterium can infect any organ in the body (pleura, lymph nodes, genitourinary tract, bones, joints, peritoneum, meninges, etc).

DIAGNOSTIC EVALUATION

1. Sputum smear and culture – diagnosis made by finding the acid-fast bacilli in sputum obtained by coughing and expectoration. If little sputum is present, gastric aspiration should be carried out first thing in the morning, to obtain sputum which has been swallowed during the night. The culture involves incubation on a plate of Dover's medium for three weeks.
2. Tuberculin skin test – inoculation of tubercle bacillus extract (tuberculin) into the intradermal layer of the inner aspect of the forearm.
3. Multiple puncture tests – introduction of tuberculin into the skin by multiple puncture.
4. Chest X-ray.
5. Biopsy of pulmonary nodules.
6. Culture of aspirate of pleural effusion if this is present.

TREATMENT

Objective

Eliminate all viable tubercle bacilli.

1. Administer prescribed antituberculosis drugs (Table 17.4).
   a. A combination of drugs is given to reduce viable microbial organisms as rapidly as possible and to minimize the chance of persistence of drug-resistant organisms.
   b. Chemotherapy is prolonged to eliminate all organisms, since the tubercle bacillus multiplies slowly.
   c. There are 11 antituberculosis drugs currently on the market; isoniazid (INH), ethambutol (EMB), rifampicin and streptomycin (SM) are the drugs most commonly used for initial treatment (first time drugs).
   d. Intensive triple drug regimen for initial therapy: Streptomycin (intramuscularly) with oral administration of isoniazid and ethambutol (for 30 to 90 days) – followed by maintenance therapy with isoniazid and ethambutol for a minimum of 24 months after sputum cultures have been converted from positive to negative.
   e. A variety of combinations of antituberculosis drugs have been used with success.
2. Majority of patients improve rapidly after antituberculosis therapy is begun; symptoms abate and number of acid-fast bacilli on sputum smear decreases.

NURSING ISOLATION PROCEDURE

Respiratory isolation for patients with open pulmonary tuberculosis.

PREVENTION OF SPREAD OF INFECTION

Objectives

Identify, notify and effectively treat infected patients.

Trace the source of the infection of newly notified cases.

Screen the families and close contacts of newly notified cases, by means of chest X-rays and Mantoux tests.

1. Promote a vaccination programme for all schoolchildren at the age of 13 years (see Table 17.1, p. 976).
2. Vaccinate newborn babies if either parent has pulmonary tuberculosis.
3. Screen immigrants coming from countries where there is known to be a high rate of tuberculosis.
4. Teach the patient and the family about the disease.
   a. Teach the patient to cover nose and mouth when coughing or sneezing with disposable tissues, which should be burnt after use.
   b. Teach the patient and family about the principles of nutrition. Ensure that there is sufficient financial income for a good diet to be provided.
5. A number of patients suffering from tuberculosis may have associated medical or social problems. Alcoholism should be treated at the appropriate specialist clinic. Patients with psychiatric or social problems often need prolonged help.

   Patients whose housing and social conditions are satisfactory may be admitted to hospital for four to eight weeks, so that assessment of the effectiveness of drug therapy is possible, following the initial diagnostic procedures. Those with alcoholic, psychiatric or social problems may be in hospital for several months.

ACTINOMYCOSIS

Actinomycosis is a chronic, suppurating, granulomatous disease. The usual pathogen in man is an anaerobic, Gram-positive, branching, filamentous bacterium,* *Actinomyces israelii*, a normal commensal that may be found in the tonsillar crypts, dental caries and colon of apparently healthy people. Minor trauma, aspiration or surgical manipulation may initiate the infectious process.

PATHOLOGY
1. The characteristic lesions are firmly indurated granulomas which spread slowly to adjacent tissues and break down focally to form multiple sinus tracts which penetrate to the surface.
2. The exudate from the sinus tracts contains the characteristic sulphur granules which are visible masses of the organisms.

CLINICAL FEATURES
Actinomycosis involves three major forms of infection:
1. *Cervicofacial type* – swelling about the teeth, sub-maxillary region, and neck producing a flat, hard, painless tumour mass which is fixed firmly to the jawbone. Granuloma ultimately breaks down and becomes riddled with abscesses which perforate externally.
2. *Abdominal type* – soft tissue mass or draining sinus in the abdominal wall or flank; the ileocaecal area is the most common site of gastrointestinal involvement with sinus tracts and extension to bone, muscles and other intra-abdominal structures.
3. *Thoracic type* – acute and chronic inflammatory reaction may involve lungs, pleura, mediastinum, chest wall and pericardium, producing chest pain, fever, cough and haemoptysis.

DIAGNOSTIC EVALUATION
Culture and histological identification of affected tissue.

TREATMENT
1. Give penicillin (drug of choice) – therapy should be continued for weeks to months to prevent recurrence; alternative antibiotics are given if the patient is allergic to penicillin.

---

* Actinomycosis has traditionally been classified as a mycotic or fungal disease because it characteristically resembles the deep mycoses, but the actinomycetes are now classified as bacteria.

2. Surgical drainage, resection of damaged tissue and excision of sinuses and fistulous tracts may be required.

NURSING ISOLATION PROCEDURES
Secretion precautions until wounds and lesions stop draining.

PATIENT EDUCATION
1. Encourage good dental hygiene to reduce infection around teeth.
2. There appears to be a relationship between intra-uterine device use and colonization or infection of the genital tract with *Actinomyces*, especially when pelvic infection is present.

BOTULISM

Botulism is a type of poisoning which affects the central nervous system; it is caused by eating food in which *Clostridium botulinum* has grown and produced toxins. The organism is widely distributed in soil. Human intoxication usually follows ingestion of contaminated foods preserved in jars and tins. It is very rare in the UK.

CLINICAL FEATURES
Usually begin 12 to 36 hours after ingestion of contaminated food.
1. Nausea and vomiting.
2. Blurred vision; diplopia.
3. Dizziness.
4. Severe dryness of mouth and throat.
5. Difficulty in speaking and swallowing.
6. Respiratory paralysis with progressive muscle paralysis; botulinal toxins may diminish release of acetylcholine at the neuromuscular junction – extraocular, pharyngeal and extremity paralysis follow.

COURSE
1. Variable; illness may be prolonged, with a high risk of superinfection and fatal outcome.
2. Recovery in survivors may be prolonged.

CLINICAL EVALUATION
1. Electromyography – to differentiate botulism from atypical Guillain–Barré syndrome.
2. Mouse-toxin neutralization test – for detection of botulinal toxin; patient's serum sent to laboratory that has capacity for performing this test.
3. Examination of faecal samples – examined for botulinal toxin.

Table 17.4   Drug therapy of tuberculosis*

Drugs and dosage	Excretion	Relatively common reactions	Less common reactions	Mode of action
1. Isoniazid 5 mg/kg/bodyweight by mouth (usually 300mg as single dose)	Renal Hepatic	Peripheral neuritis Hepatic dysfunction	Central nervous system effects: insomnia, headache, restlessness, psychosis, increased reflexes, muscle twitching, paraesthesiae, convulsions (high dosage), drowsiness, excitement, delay in micturition Optic neuritis and optic atrophy Constipation, dryness of mouth, allergic reactions, hepatitis, agranulocytosis, exfoliative dermatitis, rheumatic symptoms	Interferes with DNA synthesis and intermediary metabolism
2. Ethambutol 15mg/kg by mouth (usually given as single dose)	Renal	Optic neuritis	Anaphylactoid reaction, dermatitis, pruritus, joint pain, anorexia, fever, headache, dizziness, mental symptoms, peripheral neuritis, elevated uric acid, liver damage	Inhibits RNA synthesis and phosphate metabolism
3. Rifampicin 600mg/day by mouth	Hepatic	Gastrointestinal upset	Headache, drowsiness, ataxia, mental symptoms, visual disturbances, weakness, fever, pain in extremities, numbness, hypersensitivity, urticaria, rash, eosinophilia, sore mouth, hepatitis, thrombocytopenia, leucopenia, anaemia, immunosuppression, renal damage, elevated uric acid	Inhibits RNA polymerase, blocking DNA-directed RNA synthesis
4. Streptomycin 1g/day or 2–3 times/week intramuscularly	Renal	Eighth nerve toxicity, vertigo, tinnitus, dizziness, deafness Paraesthesiae of hands, tongue and face	Pyrexia, headache, dermatitis, pruritus, renal insufficiency, transient dermal anaesthesia, nausea and vomiting	Inhibits protein synthesis by direct action on ribosomes
5. Aminosalicylic acid 4g three times a day by mouth (sodium salt should be 5g three times a day by mouth)	Renal	Gastrointestinal toxicity; nausea, vomiting, anorexia, diarrhoea	Fever, jaundice, pruritus, hypoprothrombinaemia, dermatitis, hypothyroidism, renal insufficiency, anaphylactoid reaction, hepatitis	Unknown

* From Mayock, R.I. and Macgregor, R.R. (1976) Diagnosis, prevention and early therapy of tuberculosis, in Dowling, H.F. (ed.) *Disease-a-Month*, May. Copyright © 1976 by Year Book Medical Publishers, Chicago. Used by permission.

6. Ethionamide 0.5g or 1g by mouth daily in one dose	Rapidly inactivat- ed site? Little free drug excreted in urine	Gastrointestinal toxicity; anorexia, nausea, vomiting, diarrhoea	Hepatotoxicity, purpura, gynaecomastia, impotence, peripheral neuropathy, psychic depression, drowsiness, asthenia, acne, allergic skin rash, difficulty in diabetic control, renal impairment	Inhibits protein synthesis
7. Pyrazinamide 0.5–1.0g three times a day by mouth	Renal	Hepatotoxicity Uric acid retention	Gout, arthralgia, anorexia, nausea and vomiting, dysuria, malaise, fever	Unknown
8. Kanamycin 1.0g intramuscularly 3–5 times weekly	Renal	Eighth nerve toxicity; dizziness, tinnitus, deafness Renal irritation; albuminuria, cells and casts Local irritation and pain	Renal damage, eosinophilia, allergic dermatitis, fever, headache, paraesthesiae	Inhibits protein synthesis
9. Cycloserine 250 mg every 12 hours	Renal	Central nervous system toxicity; headache, vertigo, lethargy, tremor, dysarthria, apraxia, coma, behavioural changes, psychotic episodes, convulsions Allergic dermatitis		May inhibit cell wall synthesis
10. Capreomycin 15mg/kg/day, usually 1g	Renal	Renal damage, vestibular damage, local pain, eosinophilia, rash, fever	Anaphylaxis	Inhibits protein synthesis
11. Viomycin 1g every 12h 2 days/week intramuscularly	Renal	Renal impairment: albuminuria, cells and casts Eighth nerve toxicity: dizziness, tinnitus, deafness Allergic reactions with eosinophilia (skin, fever, etc)	Fluid retention with oedema, renal damage, electrocardiographic abnormalities, electrolyte pattern disturbances	Inhibits protein synthesis

TREATMENT AND NURSING INTERVENTIONS
Objectives
Prevent respiratory failure.
Eliminate the toxin and C. botulinum *from the gastro-intestinal tract.*

1. Give intensive respiratory support – death is frequently due to onset of respiratory failure.
   a. Prepare for tracheotomy, mechanical ventilation.
   b. Carry out blood gas determinations as necessary.
2. Give cathartics, enemas and gastric lavage (when these can be safely administered) – to eliminate unabsorbed toxin and *C. botulinum* from the gastrointestinal tract.

3. Administer trivalent ABE antitoxin as directed (has a high reaction rate).
   a. Determine if there is a history of allergy, asthma, hay fever.
   b. Perform a skin test for sensitivity.
   c. Have ventilatory equipment and emergency drugs ready in event of life-threatening reaction.
4. Guanidine hydrochloride may be administered – enhances the release of acetylcholine from the nerve terminals; not as effective in overcoming respiratory paralysis as it is in combating paralysis of extremities and extraocular muscles.
5. Treat superimposed infections with antibiotics if necessary.

6. Provide ECG monitoring to detect signs of cardiac arrest.
7. During the convalescent period, ensure that both patient and relatives know that there is often a prevalence of persistent symptoms for a year or more, such as tiredness, weakness and dyspnoea.

PREVENTION AND PATIENT EDUCATION

1. Home canners should be taught how to prevent botulism.
2. Home-canned foods should be inspected before being eaten – foods contaminated with *C. botulinum* look soft, contain gas bubbles and give off an odour of decay. However, this is not always certain.
3. Canned foods should be boiled for 10 to 20 minutes and stirred thoroughly before serving – toxin is heat-labile and is destroyed by proper cooking of foods.
4. Be careful in preparing food for canning at high attitudes since it is difficult to provide a temperature high enough to destroy the spores of *C. botulinum*. Use pressure cooker method of canning at high altitudes.

NURSING ISOLATION PROCEDURE

No precautions are necessary. Botulism is an intoxication, not an infection.

TETANUS (LOCKJAW)

Tetanus is an acute disease caused by *Clostridium tetani* (tetanus bacillus), spores of which are introduced into the body when an injury becomes contaminated with soil, street dust or animal or human faeces. The bacillus is an anaerobe (cannot live in presence of oxygen).

CLINICAL FEATURES

Caused by potent neurotoxins elaborated by *C. tetani* which have a special affinity for nervous tissue.
1. Rigidity of muscles; muscle spasms of both flexor and extensor muscle groups.
   a. Trismus – painful spasms of masticatory muscles; difficulty in opening the mouth (lockjaw).
   b. Risus sardonicus – grinning expression produced by spasm of facial muscles.
   c. Recurrent tetanic spasms of almost every muscle group in body – involvement of respiratory muscles may lead to respiratory failure.

2. Hyperirritability; restlessness, headache, low-grade fever.
3. Hyperactive reflexes.

TREATMENT AND NURSING INTERVENTIONS
Objective
Prevent the disease from developing.
1. Consider every break in the skin as a potential portal of entry for *C. tetani*.
   a. Tetanus-prone wounds – compound fractures; gunshot injuries; burns; foreign bodies; wounds contaminated with soil or faeces; wounds neglected for more than 24 hours; puncture wounds; wounds infected with other micro-organisms; wounds from induced abortions; wounds made by dirty hypodermic needles (drug addicts).

NURSING ALERT
Tetanus-prone wounds are those in which there has been an invasion of soil or faeces or those involving a severe traumatic injury. Tetanus may develop from an insignificant wound contaminated by soil.

   b. Wash and clean the wound thoroughly.
2. Treatment depends on the immunization status of the patient. Consider nature and age of wound and conditions under which it occurred.
   a. For previously immunized patient:
      (i) Tetanus toxoid (adsorbed) according to manufacturer's directions.
      (ii) Tetanus immune globulin (human) (TIG), as directed.
         Tetanus toxoid and TIG given with separate syringes at different sites.
      (iii) Immediate debridement of the wound.
      (iv) Antibiotic therapy, usually penicillin.
   b. For patient with no previous immunization (or if immunization is in doubt):
      (i) Tetanus toxoid – course of three injections.
      (ii) TIG or antitoxin as directed.
      (iii) Immediate debridement of wound.
      (iv) Antibiotic therapy – tetanus organism sensitive to tetracycline and penicillin.
   c. Equine or bovine antitoxin is usually *not* given because of high incidence of allergic and anaphylactic reactions. *If used, its administration must be preceded by careful screening for sensitivity according to manufacturer's directions.*

TREATMENT OF TETANUS
Objective
Prevent respiratory and cardiovascular complications.
   1. Maintain an adequate airway – tetanic spasm of

larynx, pharynx and respiratory muscles usually occurs during convulsions and may lead to asphyxia and death.

a. Prepare for insertion of a cuffed endotracheal tube – laryngeal spasms cause airway obstruction, inadequate pulmonary ventilation, hypoxia, cyanosis and death.

b. Prepare patient for tracheotomy – relieves laryngeal dyspnoea, reduces risk of aspiration, and permits speedy application of controlled ventilation.

c. Maintain patient on mechanical ventilation.

d. Aspirate secretions as necessary – observe aspirate and keep a record of its appearance to assess for signs of pulmonary infection (e.g., sputum becomes coloured).

e. Curariform drugs (with mechanical ventilation) may be needed to maintain an adequate airway.

2. Provide cardiac monitoring – overactivity of sympathetic nervous system may lead to 'sympathetic crisis' and death.

a. Watch for isolated unexplained tachycardia, temporary hypertension, premature ventricular contractions, sweating.

b. Requires aggressive physiological monitoring and pharmacological treatment (propranolol to control tachycardia; phentolamine to control hypertensive episodes).

3. Keep vein open – for infusions and in the event of respiratory/cardiac arrest.

NURSING ALERT

The hearing of the patient with respiratory paralysis may be acute. Do not make unguarded comments in his presence.

4. Give TIG (human) in an effort to neutralize the toxins and to ensure that appropriate circulating levels will be present when the wound is debrided.

5. Carry out effective wound care; debride all necrotic tissue – necrotic tissue favours growth of tetanus bacillus.

6. Give antibiotics (penicillin) – to eradicate persisting *C. tetani* and other pathogens from the wound.

7. Maintain the fluid and electrolyte balance.

8. Support the patient during tetanic spasm and convulsions – due to the action of toxins in the cells of central nervous system; mortality rate of patients with frequent and severe spasms is high.

9. Provide for continuing observation of the patient.

a. Plan nursing management for minimal patient disturbance – tactile stimulation may promote spasms.

(i) Place patient in a quiet room.

(ii) Avoid sudden stimuli and light – slightest stimulation may trigger paroxysmal spasms.

(iii) Be alert for the development of fractures of the vertebral bodies, which may occur with severe spasm.

(iv) Give muscle relaxants, sedatives, anticonvulsants – to treat muscle rigidity and convulsions.

(v) Keep vein open – for infusions and in the event of cardiac/respiratory arrest.

b. See Chapter 16, Care of the Patient with a Neurological Disorder, for management of both the patient with convulsive seizures and the unconscious patient.

10. After recovery the patient should receive the primary immunization series (for tetanus) plus booster dose every 10 years.

NURSING ISOLATION PROCEDURE

No isolation or precautions are required but a side room is normally used for quietness.

GAS GANGRENE

Gas gangrene is a severe infection caused by Gram-positive clostridia which may complicate compound fractures and contused or lacerated wounds. Several species of clostridia (*C. welchii*, *C. perfringens*, *C. septicum*, *C. novyi*, *C. histolyticum*, *C. sporogenes*) and others may produce gas gangrene. These organisms are anaerobes and spore-formers and are normally found in the intestinal tract of man and in soil.

ALTERED PHYSIOLOGY

Injury → bacteria (clostridia) invade devitalized tissue, especially where blood supply is compromised → bacteria multiply and produce toxins → toxins cause haemolysis, vessel thrombosis and damage to myocardium, liver and kidneys.

CLINICAL FEATURES

1. Sudden and severe pain at site of injury – caused by gas and oedema in the tissues.

2. Rapid, feeble pulse progressing to circulatory collapse – death from toxaemia is frequent.

3. Anaemia (from haemolysis); prostration; apprehension.
4. Delirium and stupor.
5. Appearance of wound:
   a. Skin is white and tense initially; colour then progresses to a dusky hue.
   b. Crepitus (crackling) – produced by gas in the tissue.
   c. Vesicles appear; are filled with red, watery fluid.
   d. Muscle is dark red and oedematous; contains red, watery, foul-smelling fluid.
   e. Gas bubbles seen emanating from tissues – toxins ferment muscle sugar; produce acid and gas, which digest muscle protein. (Obvious gangrene is present.)

TREATMENT AND NURSING INTERVENTIONS
1. Prepare patient for surgical removal and debridement of necrotic tissue – this is preventive as well as curative.
   a. Early excision of all devitalized and infected tissue with wide incisions will render wound unsuitable for growth of clostridium.
   b. Extensive incisions (once infection has developed) in affected part allow air to inhibit growth of anaerobic organisms.
2. Place patient in hyperbaric oxygen chamber if available – increases the dissolved oxygen in the arterial system by increasing the partial pressure of the oxygen breathed by the patient; may interrupt toxin formation and microbial replication (reproduction).
3. Give antibiotic therapy (penicillin; tetracyclines; chloramphenicol) – may prevent spread of infection.
4. Support the patient with toxaemic features – gas bacillus infection produces an intense toxaemia.
   a. Monitor central venous pressure and urinary output.
   b. Give intravenous fluids to support cardiovascular system; maintain fluid and electrolyte balance.
5. Antiserum may be of value.

ISOLATION NURSING PROCEDURE
Use wound and skin precautions until the wound stops draining.

TYPHOID FEVER

Typhoid fever is a bacterial infection transmitted by contaminated water, milk, shellfish or other foods. It is caused by *Salmonella typhi*, which is harboured in human excreta. Today it is spread chiefly by carriers, patients who have recovered from the fever, but whose stools or urine may spread these bacilli for years. The ingestion of infected oysters or shellfish taken from waters contaminated by offshore sewage disposal units is another source of infection. There is increased incidence of typhoid fever acquired during foreign travel.

Its characteristic lesion consists of ulcers which form in the ileum and colon, and its distinctive clinical features consist of long-continued fever, rose-spot rash, enlarged spleen, slow pulse and leucopenia.

ALTERED PHYSIOLOGY
Organism enters body by gastrointestinal tract; it invades the walls of gastrointestinal tract, leading to bacteraemia which localizes in mesenteric lymph nodes, in the masses of lymphatic tissue in the mucous membrane of the intestinal wall (Peyer's patches), and in small, solitary lymph follicles in the ileum and colon; ulceration of the intestines may ensue.

CLINICAL FEATURES
Gradual onset
1. Severe headache, malaise, muscle pains, nonproductive cough.
2. Chills and fever; temperature rises slowly, reaching highest level in three to seven days (40–41°C).
3. Pulse is full and slow in comparison to height of fever; may have distinct dicrotic wave.
4. Skin eruption – irregularly spaced small rose spots on abdomen, chest, back. Each spot fades over a period of three to four days.
5. Epistaxis may occur.

Second week
1. Fever remains consistently high.
2. Abdominal distension and tenderness; constipation or diarrhoea.
3. Delirium in severe infections – from severe toxaemia.

Third week
Gradual decline in fever and subsidence of symptoms.

DIAGNOSTIC EVALUATION
1. White blood count – leucopenia is a distinctive haematological feature, but is not always present.

2. Blood culture – positive for organism after first week.
3. Stool culture – positive for organism after first week.
4. Urine culture – organism may or may not be present.
5. Blood serum agglutination test usually becomes positive by end of second week.

TREATMENT AND NURSING INTERVENTIONS
Objectives
Give supportive care.
Observe for haemorrhage and perforation.
1. Give specific treatment for typhoid.
   a. Chloramphenicol as directed. Monitor blood count to detect chloramphenicol toxicity.
   b. Combination of sulphamethoxazole and trimethoprim (Septrin) may be given for chloramphenicol-resistant strains of typhoid.
   c. Ampicillin or amoxicillin are also in use.
2. Give supportive care – typhoid fever is a nursing challenge.
   a. Support patient during period of toxaemia – patient may be drowsy, partially incontinent or delirious.
   b. Give steroids if prescribed for toxic or delirious patients.
   c. Prepare for blood transfusions if indicated.
   d. Take rectal temperature every two to four hours.
      (i) Give tepid sponge for temperature of 40°C or more.
      (ii) Encourage a high fluid intake.
   e. Watch for bladder distension – patient may lose urge to micturate during toxic state. Keep input and output record.
   f. Observe for retention of faeces.
      (i) Enemas are given under *low* pressure to diminish chance of intestinal perforation.
      (ii) Relieve distension with rectal tube, inserted for a short time.
   g. Give a high calorie, low residue diet during febrile stage.
3. Watch for complications which can occur after an apparent clinical cure.
   a. *Intestinal haemorrhage* – from erosion of blood vessel in ulcerated small intestine (occurs in 10 per cent of patients).
      (i) Clinical features:
         (a) Apprehension, sweating, pallor.
         (b) Weak, rapid pulse; narrowing pulse pressure.
         (c) Hypotension.
         (d) Bloody or tarry stools.

(ii) Treatment:
   (a) Withhold food.
   (b) Give blood transfusions.
b. *Perforation of intestine* – from erosion of one of the ulcers; most common during third week.
   (i) Symptoms:
      (a) Sudden, sharp abdominal pain – may stop suddenly.
      (b) Abdominal rigidity.
      (c) Shock.
   (ii) Treatment:
      Prepare for intestinal decompression procedure, intravenous fluids and surgical intervention if conservative measures do not produce clinical improvement.

ISOLATION NURSING PROCEDURE
Use enteric precautions until three successive cultures of faeces taken after cessation of antibiotics are negative for *S. typhi*. Disposable bedpans may be used. Nondisposable bedpans should be disinfected in a steam sterilizer.

PREVENTION AND PATIENT EDUCATION
1. Prevention: typhoid vaccine, one subcutaneous injection followed by second injection four or more weeks later; booster injection every three years.
2. Maintain environmental hygiene.
   a. Protect and purify water supplies.
   b. Employ sanitary waste disposal techniques.
   c. Pasteurize milk and dairy products; refrigerate while transporting.
   d. Supervise foods served, especially raw foods.
   e. Ensure that food handlers use handwashing facilities.
3. Patient must be followed with routine stool culture after recovery to detect the development of the carrier state – approximately 2 to 5 per cent of typhoid patients become permanent carriers, harbouring the organism and excreting it in their urine and stools.
   a. Carriers may be given ampicillin – to attempt to abolish carrier state (there is evidence that treating certain patients with salmonella in their stools may prolong the carrier state).
   b. Positive stool culture after six to 12 months indicates a carrier.
   c. Carriers must not become food or milk handlers.
4. Education of the patient is essential. The Medical Officer for Environmental Health (MOEH) will usually visit the home.

SALMONELLA INFECTIONS (SALMONELLOSIS)

Salmonellosis is a form of food poisoning characterized by acute gastroenteritis; it is caused by certain species of the genus *Salmonella*. The patient is infected via the oral route by contaminated food or drink.

Infectious agent – 1,500 known serotypes of salmonella – most common in the UK are *S. typhimurium, S. enteritidis, S. agona, S. heidelberg* and *S. hadar*.

NURSING ALERT

Common food offenders causing salmonella infections include commercially processed meat pies, poultry (especially turkey), sausage (lightly cooked), foods containing egg or egg products and unpasteurized milk or dairy products.

CLINICAL FEATURES

1. Diarrhoea – sudden onset of frequent, bulky stools followed by profuse, watery diarrhoea; may lead to marked dehydration.
2. Abdominal pain.
3. Nausea and vomiting.
4. Fever.
5. Other features due to infectious agent localizing in any body tissue – abscesses, cholecystitis, arthritis, endocarditis, meningitis, pericarditis, pneumonia, pyelonephritis.

DIAGNOSTIC EVALUATION

Culture of faeces, blood and urine.

TREATMENT AND NURSING INTERVENTIONS
Objective
Prevent dehydration and electrolyte imbalance.
Treatment is supportive:
1. Restrict food until nausea and vomiting subside.
2. Offer clear liquids as tolerated.
3. Correct fluid and electrolyte depletion with intravenous infusions.
4. Avoid giving antimotility drugs, since a slowed peristaltic action may extend the period of infection by interfering with the cleansing mechanism of diarrhoea.
5. Treatment is similar to that for typhoid fever if patient has focal (abscess) or systemic infection.

NURSING ISOLATION PROCEDURE

Use enteric precautions for duration of illness.

PREVENTIVE MEASURES AND PATIENT EDUCATION

1. Food service workers should have training courses and ongoing in-service training in facts about food-borne illnesses, avoidance of food contamination, food storage methods, cleaning of food preparation and service areas, and maintenance of good personal hygiene.
2. Raw eggs or egg drinks should not be eaten, nor should cracked or dirty eggs be used.
3. All foods from animal sources, especially fowl, egg products and meat dishes, should be thoroughly cooked.
4. Foods should be refrigerated during storage and should be protected against insects/rodents.
5. Any person handling food should be instructed to wash hands after toilet use, before and after food preparation.
6. Chicks, ducklings and turtles (as well as other domestic animals and pets) are sources of infection.
7. The patient must wash his hands after toilet use, particularly during illness and carrier state (two to four weeks) – to prevent infection of others.
8. Diarrhoea in infants should be investigated immediately, since salmonellae play an important role, particularly in infants less than one year old.

SHIGELLOSIS (BACILLARY DYSENTERY)

Shigellosis, an acute bacterial disease of the intestinal tract, includes a group of enteric infections caused by bacilli of the *Shigella* group of which there are four types: *S. sonnei* (most common in the UK), *S. dysenteriae, S. boydii, S. flexneri*. The source of infection is faeces from an infected person. The route of spread is faecal/oral. Shigellosis may also be of sexual origin.

CLINICAL FEATURES

1. Fever and headache.
2. Abdominal cramps.
3. Severe prostration.
4. Persistent diarrhoea – passage of varying amounts of blood, mucus and pus.

DIAGNOSTIC EVALUATION

Isolation of *Shigella* from faeces or rectal swabs.

TREATMENT AND NURSING INTERVENTIONS
Objectives
Provide aggressive treatment for the patient.
Prevent the spread of shigellosis to the patient's contacts,
i.e., to eliminate the carrier state.

1. Determine the type of shigella – organism is recovered from patient's stool.
2. Do sensitivity testing for selection of antibiotic – multi-resistance to antibiotics is common.
3. Give antibiotics which are absorbed from intestinal tract (neomycin, tetracyclines, chloramphenicol) – may shorten duration of illness. Avoid antimotility drugs as they may abolish antibiotic effectiveness.
4. Maintain fluid and electrolyte balance – to prevent profound dehydration owing to an excessively great loss of salts in the diarrhoeic stools.
   a. Assess weight loss, skin elasticity, dryness of mucous membranes, urinary volume, vital signs.
   b. Weigh daily and measure urinary volume.
5. Offer clear fluids during acute stage of illness.
6. Carry out epidemiology studies of every patient in whom the organism is found.
   a. Ask if patient has been recent traveller to Middle or Far East or has had contacts with travellers from these countries.
   b. Notify local authorities.

NURSING ISOLATION PROCEDURE
Use enteric precautions until three consecutive cultures of faeces taken 24 hours apart after cessation of antibiotic therapy are negative for infecting strain.

PREVENTIVE MEASURES AND PATIENT EDUCATION
1. See Patient Education for typhoid fever, p. 1007.
2. Programme of fly control.
3. Surveillance of water sanitation; adequate sewage disposal.
4. Detection and treatment of carriers.
5. Handwashing after defaecation.

MENINGOCOCCAL MENINGITIS (CEREBROSPINAL FEVER)

Meningitis is inflammation of the meninges, or coverings of the brain; may be caused by bacterial, mycobacterial or viral agents.

Meningococcal meningitis is an acute bacterial infectious disease caused by the meningococcus, *Neisseria meningitidis*. It starts as an infection of the nasopharynx or the tonsils and is followed by meningococcal septicaemia, which extends to the meninges of the brain and the upper region of the spinal cord. There are several distinct immunological strains of the meningococcus, but the groups A, B and C are the most important.

CLINICAL FEATURES
Symptoms result first from infection and then from increased intracranial pressure.
1. High fever.
2. Nausea and vomiting.
3. Headache, irritability, confusion, delirium, convulsions.
4. Neck, shoulder and back stiffness.
5. Appearance of petechiae (usually on legs); may progress to large ecchymotic or purpuric lesions.
6. Resistance to neck flexion.
   a. Positive Kernig's sign – when lying with the thigh flexed on the abdomen, patient cannot completely extend his leg (a sign of meningeal irritation).
   b. Positive Brudzinski's sign – when the patient's neck is flexed on the chest, flexion of the knees and hips is produced. When passive flexion of the lower extremity on one side is made, a similar movement will be seen on the contralateral (opposite) extremity.

SOURCE OF INFECTION
Human cases and carriers.

METHOD OF SPREAD
By contact or droplet infection.

DIAGNOSTIC EVALUATION
Organism usually demonstrated by smear and culture of cerebrospinal fluid, oropharynx and blood.

CLINICAL FEATURES
1. Meningococcus may localize in the brain, skin or joint synovia.
2. Predisposing factors include otitis media, mastoiditis, sickle cell anaemia (or other haemoglobinopathies), recent neurosurgical procedures, head trauma, respiratory infection, immunological defects.
3. The disease occurs in winter and spring months; epidemics are most apt to occur when people live in crowded quarters.

TREATMENT AND NURSING INTERVENTIONS
Objective
Observe and treat for vasomotor shock and collapse.
1. Support patient undergoing diagnostic lumbar puncture – cerebrospinal fluid will usually be cloudy with elevated pressure.
2. Give specific drug therapy, depending on culture and sensitivity results – initially by intravenous route; therapy continued for minimum of 10 days.

a. Penicillin G (drug of choice); chloramphenicol for patients allergic to penicillin.
b. Most antibiotics enter cerebrospinal fluid and central nervous system inefficiently.
3. Maintain a clear airway – altered consciousness may lead to airway obstruction.
   a. Carry out arterial blood gas determinations.
   b. Provide oral airway or cuffed endotracheal tube or tracheotomy as patient's condition indicates.
   c. Administer oxygen to maintain arterial Po_2 at desired levels.

VIRAL INFECTIONS

INFLUENZA

Influenza is an acute infectious disease caused by an RNA-containing myxovirus. It is characterized by respiratory and constitutional symptoms. Epidemics of influenza develop rapidly; there is a fairly high mortality rate among the elderly and those debilitated by chronic disease.

AETIOLOGY
1. The primary factor in the aetiology of influenza is a filtrable virus of which three major strains have been isolated, designated types A, B and C.
2. The numerous variants within a given type are called subtypes.
3. Group A appears to be the most virulent and is responsible for the most recent epidemics.
4. Influenza appears to become epidemic when antibody levels wane or when the antigens of prevalent influenza viruses have changed enough to render the population susceptible.
5. Transmission is by close contact or by droplets from the respiratory tract of an infected person.

CLINICAL COURSE
1. The virus is airborne and multiplies in the upper respiratory tract – selected invasion of nasal, tracheal and bronchial mucosal cells.
2. Influenza virus damages the ciliated epithelium of the tracheobronchial tree, rendering the patient vulnerable to the development of secondary invaders such as pneumococci or staphylococci, *Haemophilus influenzae*, streptococci and other organisms.

CLINICAL FEATURES
1. Fever: 39–40°C.
2. Headache and profound malaise.
3. Respiratory features – dry cough, sore throat, nasal obstruction and discharge.
4. Muscular aches – especially in back and legs.

TREATMENT AND NURSING INTERVENTIONS
Objectives
Offer the patient supportive therapy.
Prevent and treat complications (respiratory, cardiac, neurological).
1. Give aspirin or aspirin compounds every four hours for fever, headache and myalgia.
2. Offer cough syrup for dry, hacking cough.
3. Use a vaporizer – to reduce irritation to respiratory mucosa.
4. Give liberal fluid intake.
5. Watch for dyspnoea in early course of influenza – points to bronchopneumonia, which is a potentially life-threatening disease.
   a. Pneumonia may also be of viral, mixed viral or bacterial origin.
   b. Treat pneumonia.
      (i) Obtain cultures of throat, blood and sputum immediately.
      (ii) Give antibiotic therapy as required – usually penicillin G or erythromycin.
      (iii) Assess for vasomotor collapse.
      (iv) Observe for acute respiratory failure.
      (v) Initiate tracheal suctioning, tracheal intubation and assisted ventilation as required.
6. Assess for neurological complications – from direct invasion of the nervous system or by autoimmune response (hypersensitivity) in the nervous system.
7. Watch for development of myocarditis.

PREVENTION
1. Vaccination.
   a. Active immunization consists of a single dose of vaccine (influenza virus vaccine, bivalent) for either primary or annual booster vaccination.
   b. Dose volumes are specified in manufacturer's labelling.
   c. Influenza vaccine should be given by mid-November.
2. Vaccination is recommended for people who have such chronic conditions as:
   a. Heart disease of any aetiology, particularly with mitral stenosis or cardiac insufficiency.
   b. Chronic bronchopulmonary diseases, such as

asthma, chronic bronchitis, bronchiectasis, tuberculosis and emphysema.

  c. Chronic renal disease.
  d. Diabetes mellitus and other chronic metabolic disorders.
3. Vaccination recommended for older people (over 65) – excess mortality in older age groups.
4. Selective use of antiviral agents.
  a. Amantadine hydrochloride has been used for prevention and modification of influenza caused by type A influenza viruses.
  b. To be effective, amantadine should be given prior to and for the duration of exposure to type A influenza virus.
  c. Patients with high priority for antiviral therapy include:
    (i) Patients with chronic respiratory, cardiovascular, etc, disease.
    (ii) Patients hospitalized for treatment of other illnesses.
    (iii) Elderly people residing in nursing homes or other institutions.
5. Vaccination should be repeated when a new strain of virus appears.

NURSING ISOLATION PROCEDURES
Usually none. There may be some instances when respiratory isolation of patients with influenza is indicated, especially if the diagnosis can be made on or soon after admission.

PATIENT EDUCATION
1. The risk of developing influenza is related to crowding and close contacts of groups of individuals.
2. Restrict visiting privileges within health care facilities during epidemics – to minimize chance of introducing influenza.
3. It appears wise to humidify home and office air and to discourage cigarette smoking for high-risk people.

ACQUIRED IMMUNODEFICIENCY SYNDROME (AIDS)

Acquired immunodeficiency syndrome (AIDS) is a rare but severe disorder of the immune system, resulting in impairment of the normal response to infection, due to the irreversible damage of the subgroup of T-lymphocytes, known as T-helpers (Th) which normally promote the response to infection. There are also T-suppressor (Ts) cells which normally regulate the immune response to infection. As a result of this disorder there is an imbalance of Th cells to Ts cells.

AETIOLOGY
The disease has been shown to be caused by a closely related group of retroviruses. The first one, isolated in France in 1983, was called lymphadenopathy-associated virus (LAV). In America, it was called human T-cell lymphotrophic virus type III (HTLV III). Others have been named AIDS-related virus (ARV) and immunodeficiency associated virus (IDAV). In the future, the term human immunodeficiency virus (HIV) will probably be adopted. The disease is spread by sexual contact and by parenteral inoculation with infected blood and body fluids.

It is necessary for people to understand that although AIDS is comparatively rare, there are many people who are infected with HIV, and can therefore pass it on, and who may develop AIDS later on. Accurate figures are difficult to obtain, but in November 1987, the number of people with AIDS worldwide who had been reported to the World Health Organization was almost 64,000; the number of people infected with HIV was estimated to be 10 million. One organization in the UK estimates the number of HIV-positive people to be 30,000 to 50,000.

AT RISK
1. Homosexual and bisexual men who practise anal intercourse.
2. Women whose partners are bisexual.
3. Haemophiliacs who have previously been treated with infected blood or blood products.
4. Intravenous drug addicts.
5. Babies born to female drug addicts or partners of bisexual infected men.
6. Anyone who is sexually active.

Note: The majority of those infected with LAV/HTLV III have so far remained well, but the proportion of LAV/HTLV III infections which lead to clinical disease is still uncertain. In the UK it is currently estimated that one in three seropositive individuals may become ill and one in ten develop AIDS (Advisory Committee on Dangerous Pathogens, June 1986).

CLINICAL FEATURES
Prodromal phase
1. Fatigue, malaise.
2. Fever and night sweats.
3. Weight loss.

4. Lymphadenopathy which may continue for a long time.
5. Persistent diarrhoea may occur.
6. Persistent infection with *Candida* of the mouth and oesophagus.
7. Reactivation of latent herpes virus.
8. Blue or brown spots on the skin which may indicate Kaposi's sarcoma (Figure 17.1).

Appearance of AIDS
(Usually this is because of opportunist infections.)
1. Pulmonary symptoms – dyspnoea, hypoxaemia, chest pain – due to *Pneumocystis carinii*, but can also be due to legionella and cytomegalovirus infections.
2. Neurological symptoms – confusion, headaches, dementia – from infections such as toxoplasma.
3. Gastrointestinal symptoms – diarrhoea, weight loss, malnutrition, from infections such as salmonellosis, *Candida albicans*, *Toxoplasma gondii*, giardiasis, cryptosporidium.

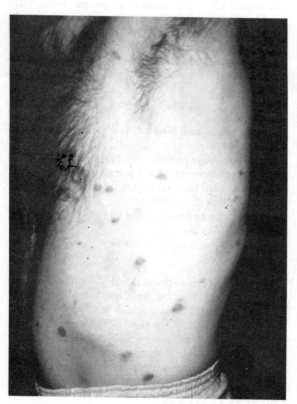

Figure 17.1. Lesions from Kaposi's sarcoma of a patient with acquired immunodeficiency syndrome (AIDS) (courtesy of Henry Masur, MD, Clinical Center, National Institutes of Health)

4. Hepatic symptoms from hepatitis B infection.
5. Malignancies – Kaposi's sarcoma. This is a rare and aggressive tumour which involves the skin, lymphatic nodes and gastrointestinal tract.
6. If a woman is HIV-positive it is inadvisable for her to become pregnant.
   a. Because pregnancy may speed up the development of AIDS, causing a greatly reduced life expectancy.
   b. The HIV virus can cross the placental barrier, and the baby may be born with HIV antibodies. After six months, about 50 per cent of such babies may be found to be negative, as the maternal antibodies disappear, but the remainder are then at risk of developing AIDS in childhood.

   It is thought that HIV can be transmitted by breast milk, so in the UK breastfeeding is contraindicated. In third world countries where artificial feeding facilities are very poor indeed, decisions will have to be made carefully.

Note: After the initial infection and incubation period, a few people may develop an illness similar to infective mononucleosis; lymphadenopathy may persist for some time; and there may be some of the symptoms mentioned above. However, a proportion of these people will return to normal health, and an altered Th/Ts ratio will disappear.

DIAGNOSTIC EVALUATION
1. No previous history of immunosuppressive disease or therapy.
2. Immunological evaluation – altered Th/Ts ratio; antibodies.
3. The virus has been detected in semen, vaginal fluid, saliva, tears, urine.
4. Stool specimens may show enteric pathogens.

TREATMENT AND NURSING INTERVENTIONS
Combating infection and providing physiological support
1. Give prescribed treatment for opportunist infections; some pathogens are not sensitive to currently available drugs.
2. Be on the alert for opportunist infections which often occur in patients who are recovering from an acute episode of a febrile illness.
3. Watch for signs of relapse after therapy is discontinued.
4. Monitor the results of blood and bone marrow tests.
5. Assist the medical staff in attempts to improve the

immunodeficient state. Various treatments which are being evaluated include:

a. Interferon – a protein existing in minute quantities in the body, known for its antiviral and antitumour activity; different types of interferon are being evaluated.
b. Thymic hormones.
c. Transfer factor.
d. Interleukin II – this stimulates gamma-interferon production, and also has a role in the proliferation and differentiation of T-lymphocytes.
e. Plasmapheresis and bone marrow transplant.
f. Zidovudine (Retrovir) is being used for some people suffering from severe effects of AIDS, and seems to be increasing their life expectancy. This drug has to be taken on a strict four-hourly routine, which includes a night time dose, which some people find difficult as their sleep is constantly disturbed.

6. Support the patient undergoing treatment for malignancies:
   a. Kaposi's sarcoma:
      (i) Radiotherapy for patients with limited disease.
      (ii) Chemotherapy; single chemotherapy for patients with slowly progressive disease and combination chemotherapy for patients with more rapid disease dissemination.
         (a) Chemotherapy may need to be prolonged.
         (b) Toxicity of chemotherapy may be more profound than expected.
   b. Other malignancies are treated symptomatically.

Providing psychosocial support

1. Be aware of the prejudices which are present in some members of society about drug addicts and homosexuals, often because of lack of knowledge and understanding.
2. Three things needed by the patient are:
   a. Acceptance.
   b. Befriending.
   c. Compassion by the carers. Many patients have lost their family contacts.
3. Know the available resources:
   a. Terence Higgins Trust, BM AIDS, London WC1N 3XX.
   b. Gay Switchboard, BM Switchboard, London WC1N 3XX (tel: 01 837 7324).
   c. London Friend, 274 Upper Street, London N1 (tel: 01 359 7371).

d. Haemophilia Society, PO Box 9, 16 Trinity Street, London SE1 1DE (tel: 01 407 1010).

4. Arrange for special counselling to help the patient through the initial reaction to the illness, as psychological consequences are often severe.
5. Be able to answer any queries simply. Have leaflets from the Health Education Council available for patients and friends.

PREVENTION/PATIENT EDUCATION

1. People with symptoms suggestive of AIDS and those at increased risk from AIDS should refrain from donating blood.
2. Provide information about the need to modify certain sexual behaviour.
   a. Avoid anonymous sex.
   b. Sexual relations should be with one person. Condoms should be used.
   c. Refrain from oral and anal sex.
3. Promotion of good health, by diet, exercise and rest.

INFECTIOUS MONONUCLEOSIS

Infectious mononucleosis ('mono'; glandular fever) is an acute infectious disease of the lymphatic system caused by the Epstein–Barr virus, a member of the herpes group. Cytomegalovirus infection can produce a clinical picture closely resembling infectious mononucleosis.

INCIDENCE AND TRANSMISSION

1. Occurs mainly between ages of 14 and 30; high frequency of occurrence in college students and military population.
2. The virus is excreted in saliva of patients with active disease or of those who are carriers, and is spread by intimate personal contact. It can also be transmitted by blood transfusion.

CLINICAL FEATURES

May be vague and masquerade as those of leukaemia, hepatitis, drug rash.
1. Fever.
2. Sore throat.
3. Skin rash – faint erythematous or maculopapular eruption on trunk and proximal extremities.
4. Lymphadenopathy.
5. Bilateral periorbital oedema.
6. Enlargement of the spleen.

DIAGNOSTIC EVALUATION
1. Blood smears – show lymphocytosis and atypical lymphocytes.
2. Heterophil antibody agglutination test – increase in titre.
3. Rising EBV antibody (Epstein–Barr virus titre).
4. Abnormal liver function tests.

TREATMENT AND NURSING INTERVENTIONS
1. The treatment is symptomatic and supportive.
   a. Encourage patient to obtain additional rest and a nutritious diet.
   b. Give aspirin for headache, muscle pains and chills.
2. Observe for complications – rupture of spleen, Guillain–Barré syndrome causing respiratory failure, glottic oedema and hepatic failure.
3. Steroids may be helpful in severe cases.

PATIENT EDUCATION
1. Patient is to avoid strenuous exercise – exertion or trauma may cause rupture of spleen. (Competitive sports should be avoided until full recovery.)
2. Observe for upper quadrant pain radiating to shoulder with signs of peritoneal irritation – evidence of splenic rupture.
3. Prepare for exploratory laparotomy.

NURSING ISOLATION PROCEDURES
Secretion precautions for duration of the illness.

ARTHROPOD-BORNE VIRAL ENCEPHALITIS

Encephalitis (inflammation of the brain) may be caused by a number of agents, including viruses, bacteria and chemicals. The viral encephalitides comprise a group of acute infections that affect predominantly the nervous system (brain, spinal cord and meninges). Each variety is caused by a specific virus. For each of these viruses there exists a particular animal reservoir, and each finds its access to man through the bite of a particular species of bloodsucking arthropod, e.g., mosquitoes, ticks.

OCCURRENCE
1. In the UK, the only form due to organism of this group is benign lymphocytic meningitis.
2. Travellers from tropical or subtropical countries may have different types, e.g., St Louis encephalitis from the USA, Murray Valley encephalitis from Australia.

MODE OF TRANSMISSION
Bite of infective arthropod.

CLINICAL FEATURES (VARIABLE)
Acute onset:
1. High fever.
2. Severe headache.
3. Signs of meningeal and spinal cord irritation.
4. Disorientation; coma – convulsions in infants.

DIAGNOSTIC EVALUATION
1. Lumbar puncture – reveals lymphocytosis in cerebrospinal fluid.
2. Rising titre of complement-fixing or neutralizing antibodies.

TREATMENT AND NURSING INTERVENTIONS
1. There is no specific therapy for arthropod-borne viral encephalitis.
2. Reduce intracranial pressure.
   a. Assist patient undergoing repeated lumbar punctures if cerebrospinal fluid pressure is elevated.
   b. Give intravenous mannitol or a urea-invert sugar preparation to reduce intracranial pressure.
3. Maintain the airway – use mechanical ventilation as required.
4. Control convulsive seizures.
5. Support patient during periods of prolonged coma.
6. Ensure adequate nutrition.
   a. Give intravenous nutrition for 48–72 hours if patient is comatose.
   b. Feed via nasogastric tube if patient remains in coma.

PATIENT EDUCATION
1. Control arthropods.
2. Give passive protection (human or animal serum) to accidentally exposed workers.

NURSING ISOLATION PROCEDURES
No isolation or precautions are necessary.

RABIES

Rabies is an acute severe viral infection affecting the central nervous system, which is transmitted to humans from the saliva of an infected animal, usually through a bite, but it can also occur through mucous membrane, but not intact skin. Animals most likely to be affected are dogs, cats, foxes and bats. No cases of rabies originating in England and Wales have been reported since 1902, but there have been 12 cases of imported rabies since 1946. In 1976, there were 11,552 cases of animal rabies in France and West Germany, and rabies has spread throughout Europe.

INCUBATION PERIOD
1. In humans, the incubation period varies from two to nine weeks, but may occasionally be shorter or very much longer.
2. The incubation period tends to be shorter if the bite is on the face or neck and also tends to be shorter in children than in adults.

CLINICAL FEATURES
Prodromal stage
1. Headache and nausea.
2. Fever.
3. Malaise, loss of appetite, mental depression.
4. Pain and paraesthesia in the bitten area, and an abnormal sensation radiating proximally from the site of the wound.

The disease may then develop in one of two forms:

Stage of excitement
1. Intermittent episodes of excitement, alternating with periods of alert calm.
2. Hydrophobia.
3. Hallucinations.
4. Severe spasms of throat and respiratory muscles.
5. Paralysis, coma and death may supervene.

Paralytic stage
1. Signs of ascending flaccid paralysis with sphincter involvement and sensory disturbances.
2. Death results from respiratory and bulbar paralysis.

DIAGNOSTIC EVALUATION
1. History of exposure and development of characteristic symptoms.
2. Demonstration of rabies antigen in corneal smears and skin biopsy material.
3. Isolation of rabies virus from specimens of saliva, cerebrospinal fluid and other secretions. These specimens should be sent to Virus Reference Laboratory, Colindale.

PREVENTION
1. Control of all animals brought into the UK. Strict quarantine regulations are in force, and heavy penalties are incurred if these regulations are ignored.
2. Prophylactic vaccination of anybody in contact with animals from abroad, or those travelling to high-risk areas who may be in contact with animals. Health workers likely to come in contact with patients suffering from rabies.

PROPHYLACTIC MANAGEMENT OF THE PATIENT
Total treatment of the wound
1. Thorough cleansing of the wound with soap and water.
2. Instillation and infiltration of human rabies immunoglobulin (HRIG) in and around the wound.
3. Tetanus prophylaxis and antibiotics given as necessary.

Systemic treatment
1. Passive immunization with HRIG which provides rapid protection.
2. Active vaccination with human diploid cell vaccine (HDCV) should be given by deep subcutaneous or intramuscular injection on day 0 (the day of the first dose), followed by further doses on days 3, 7, 14, 30 and 90. This provides longer-acting protection.

If the treatment is commenced because of a suspected rabid animal, and the animal does not develop rabies after 10 days, the treatment to the patient can be discontinued.

RICKETTSIAL INFECTIONS

Q FEVER

Q fever is an influenzal-like illness with signs of atypical pneumonia. It is spread by infected livestock, and possibly by unpasteurized milk.

AETIOLOGY
1. The organism responsible for Q fever is *Coxiella burneti*, and was originally isolated in Australia in 1937.
2. Although infected cattle are the main source, the organism has also been isolated from pigeons, domestic poultry and migrating wild birds.

OCCURRENCE
1. Mainly confined to agricultural countries with the exception of Scandinavia and New Zealand.

2. About 100 human cases are confirmed annually in the UK, mostly among farm workers, abattoir workers and veterinary surgeons.

CLINICAL FEATURES
1. Incubation period of about 19 days.
2. Sudden onset of headache, shivering, pains in the legs and anorexia.
3. Dry cough.
4. Sometimes, appearance on X-ray resembling an atypical pneumonia. Lung lesions may vary considerably.
5. Intermittent or remittent fever lasting from two days to three weeks.

DIAGNOSTIC EVALUATION
1. Patient's history.
2. Positive complement fixation test.

TREATMENT AND NURSING INTERVENTIONS
1. Chloramphenicol or tetracyclines for seven to ten days, according to the time for the pyrexia to subside.
2. Give analgesics as required for pain in legs or chest.
3. Maintain upright posture in bed, physiotherapy as required.
4. Convalescence is usually uneventful, and the mortality rate is low.

PREVENTION
1. Pasteurization of milk.
2. Wearing of gloves during calving or lambing, especially for those who handle the placenta.

PROTOZOAN DISEASES

MALARIA

Malaria is an acute infectious disease caused by protozoa which strongly resemble leukocytes. Transmission is by way of an intermediate host (the bite of an infective female *Anopheles* mosquito). Malaria has also been transmitted via blood transfusions and from the use of shared needles and syringes by drug addicts.

AETIOLOGY
Four species of malaria parasites – grouped under generic name *Plasmodium*, each causing a different type of malaria. The parasite has a complicated life cycle. Not all patients demonstrate classical cycles of fever and chills.
1. *P. vivax* – causes benign tertian malaria with a 36 to 48-hour cycle of chills and fever.
2. *P. falciparum* – causes falciparum or malignant tertian malaria (36 to 48-hour cycle)
   a. This is the most serious type of malaria because of development of high parasitic densities in the blood.
   b. Infected red cells tend to agglutinate and form microemboli.
3. *P. malariae* – causes quartan malaria with fever and chills every third day.
4. *P. ovale* – less common form of malaria.

CLINICAL FEATURES
1. Paroxysms of shaking chills; rapidly rising fever.
2. Profuse sweating; headache.
3. Splenomegaly, hepatomegaly, orthostatic hypotension, anaemia.
4. Paroxysms may last about 12 hours after which cycle may be repeated daily, every other day or every third day.

DIAGNOSTIC EVALUATION
1. Demonstration of malaria parasites in blood films by microscopic examination – microscopic examination confirms presence, species and density of parasites.
2. Residence in or travel from an endemic area is an important diagnostic clue.

CLINICAL PROBLEMS
1. Malaria causes more disability and a heavier economic burden than any other parasitic disease.
2. In much of Southeast Asia, *P. falciparum* infections are increasingly drug-resistant.
3. Mosquitoes evolve resistance against insecticides.
4. The use of antimalarial drugs depends on the stage of the life-cycle of the parasite which is affected; malarial parasites can evolve drug-resistant forms.
5. The number of imported cases into the UK is rising. In 1967, there were 111 notifications in England and Wales; in 1984, there were 1,934 cases of malaria in the UK, with six deaths.

TREATMENT AND NURSING INTERVENTIONS
Objective
Destroy the blood trophozoites and schizonts that cause the signs, symptoms and the pathological effects that characterize the disease.
1. Determine the species of parasite infecting the

patient by obtaining a blood film. The most favourable time for discovery of the parasite is during, or 12 to 18 hours after, a chill.

2. Give specific therapy.
   a. *P. vivax* (mostly from India and SE Asia) – chloroquine; primaquine; or a combination of these two drugs.
   b. *P. falciparum* (from SE Asia and the Far East). There is a problem because of drug resistance, therefore a combination of drugs is used.
      (i) (a) Quinine sulphate.
          (b) Pyrimethamine (Daraprim).
          (c) Sulphadiazine, *or*
      (ii) (a) Quinine sulphate.
           (b) Tetracycline.
      Also sulformethoxine with pyrimethamine (Sulphadoxine).

3. Give supportive nursing care.
   a. Record regular observations of the patient.
   b. Keep fluid balance charts to identify signs of:
      (i) Pulmonary oedema.
      (ii) Renal symptoms.
   c. Arrange for daily blood tests for estimating serum quinine, bilirubin, blood urea nitrogen concentrations, parasitic count and packed red cells.
   d. If there are any signs of respiratory or renal involvement, arrange for blood gases and plasma electrolytes.
   e. Consider a patient with severe falciparum malaria as a medical emergency.
      (i) Prepare for intermittent intravenous infusions of quinine.
      (ii) Watch for neurological toxicity from quinine – twitching, delirium, confusion, convulsions and coma.
      (iii) Oxygen may be necessary if tissue anoxia is present.
      (iv) Watch for jaundice – this is related to the density of the malarial parasites in the blood; also, abnormality of hepatic function is common in falciparum malaria.

4. Evaluate the degree of anaemia – this is related to the severity of the infection.

5. Watch for abnormal bleeding – nose bleeds, oozing from venepuncture sites, passage of blood in the stools. This may be due to either decreased production of clotting factors by a damaged liver or to disseminated intravascular coagulation.

NURSING ISOLATION PRECAUTIONS

1. Blood precautions for duration of hospitalization.
2. Screened rooms in tropical climates.

PREVENTIVE MEASURES AND PATIENT EDUCATION

1. In tropical areas, mosquito bites should be prevented.
   a. Effective repellents should be used.
   b. Houses should be sprayed with insecticide.
   c. Use bed netting.
   d. Install wire mesh screens across all windows.
2. Control and destroy mosquitoes.
   a. Drain and fill breeding places.
   b. Control mosquitoes in an epidemic area by aerial or ground ultra low volume applications of insecticides such as malathion or naled.
3. Give malaria prophylaxis to people residing in or travelling to endemic areas (chemoprophylaxis). It is important that the malarial parasite is not resistant to the particular drug, and that the drug is taken regularly during exposure and for four weeks afterwards. The following drugs may be used: chloroquine two tablets (300mg) once weekly; proguanil (Paludrine) 100mg daily; pyrimethamine (Daraprim) one to two tablets (25–50mg) once weekly; mepacrine one tablet (100mg) daily, commencing 14 days before exposure so as to build up a blood concentration to an effective level; quinine one tablet (250–300mg) daily.
4. Treat all new cases of malaria.

PARASITIC INFECTIONS

AMOEBIASIS (AMOEBIC DYSENTERY)

Amoebiasis is a worldwide parasitic disease which is responsible for multiple medical-surgical problems. It is caused by the protozoa *Entamoeba histolytica* and is acquired by ingestion of the cyst stage of *E. histolytica* in food or water contaminated by infected human faeces.

INCIDENCE

1. Occurs as an endemic infection of man in most regions of the world.
2. In the UK it only occurs in travellers from tropical areas.

PATHOLOGICAL INSIGHTS

1. *E. histolytica* lives in the large intestine and feeds mainly on bacteria.

2. Amoeba may be located in the bowel lumen and intestinal wall or outside the gastrointestinal tract.
   a. Trophozoites develop from viable cysts in small intestine.
   b. Trophozoites may erode intestinal mucosa, invade the bloodstream and travel to the liver via the portal circulation.
   c. Amoebas can produce abscesses and other serious complications.

CLINICAL FEATURES
1. Diarrhoea – watery, foul-smelling stools, often containing blood-streaked mucus.
2. Colicky, abdominal pain.

DIAGNOSTIC EVALUATION
1. Stool specimen for *E. histolytica*.(Trophozoites or cysts may be found in the faeces.)
   a. Several stool specimens should be collected daily.
   b. Stool specimen should be examined *immediately* for trophozoites.
2. Positive serological tests (indirect haemagglutination test and indirect fluorescent antibody test).
3. Examination of exudate from liver abscess for trophozoites.

COMPLICATIONS
1. Liver abscess.
2. Lung suppuration.
3. Meningoencephalitis.
4. Intestinal obstruction, rupture of colon; peritonitis.
5. Amoeboma (amoebic granuloma found in caecum, rectum, transverse colon, sigmoid).

TREATMENT AND NURSING INTERVENTIONS
Objectives
Give specific therapy.
Support the patient's general condition.
1. Specific therapy – metronidazole (Flagyl) produces cessation of diarrhoea and discharge of parasite from stools.
   Serial follow-up of stools is necessary.
2. Keep patient on bed rest if diarrhoea is acute.
3. Prepare for aspiration of liver abscess.
   Dehydroemetine or emetine plus chloroquine phosphate may be given for hepatic abscess.
4. Offer non-irritating, low residue bland foods – weak tea, broth, rice, toast, soft-cooked eggs.
5. Give intravenous infusions as indicated to correct fluid and electrolyte imbalance resulting from severe diarrhoea.

NURSING ISOLATION PROCEDURES
Excretion precautions (p. 979) for the duration of illness.

PATIENT EDUATION
1. Provide sanitation and safe water supplies. Water should be boiled or chlorinated.
2. Control the fly population in homes.
3. Avoid ground-grown vegetables, e.g. lettuce, when travelling in areas where amoebiasis is endemic.

FUNGAL INFECTIONS

MYCOSES AND HISTOPLASMOSIS

Fungi are primitive organisms that take their nourishment from living plants and animals and from decaying organic material. The three main types of mycoses (fungal infections), determined by the tissue level at which the fungus settles, are:
1. Systemic or deep mycoses – primarily involve the internal organs, usually centring in the lungs.
2. Subcutaneous mycoses – involve the skin, subcutaneous tissue and sometimes the bone.
3. Superficial or cutaneous mycoses – grow in outer layer of skin (epidermis), in hair and in nails.

Histoplasmosis is a chronic systemic fungus infection caused by a spore-bearing mould called *Histoplasma capsulatum*. This highly infectious mycosis is transmitted by airborne dust which contains *H. capsulatum* spores. (Partially decayed droppings of pigeons, chickens and birds offer an excellent medium for growth of this fungus.)

In the UK the most important fungal infections are:
1. *Candida albicans*, which may cause a comparatively mild problem, but which may be very troublesome in debilitated patients or those receiving chemotherapy.
2. Ringworm, which is usually passed on from infected household pets. Griseofulvin is the usual treatment for this.
3. Tinea pedis (athlete's foot), which is widespread among schoolchildren and others visiting communal swimming baths.
4. *Cryptococcus neoformans*, which causes a form of meningitis. It is an infection associated with pigeon's nests and pigeon's droppings.

HELMINTHIC INFESTATIONS

TRICHINOSIS

Trichinosis is infestation by the parasite *Trichinella spiralis*, one of the roundworms. It is acquired by consuming infected meat, usually pork.

CLINICAL COURSE
1. Tiny embryos of the parasite *T. spiralis* become encysted in the muscle fibres of an infected pig.
2. These calcified cysts appear in meat (chiefly pork); resemble tiny grains of sand.
3. If insufficiently cooked pork is eaten, the embryos are set free by the gastric juice and develop in the intestine during the following week, becoming adult worms 3–4mm long.
4. These worms make their way into the mucous membranes and there produce myriad embryos (larvae) (period of invasion).
5. The larvae, carried by the bloodstream and their own activity, migrate to all parts of the body (period of migration).
6. The larvae gradually become encysted in striated skeletal muscle.

CLINICAL FEATURES
Intestinal stage
1. Malaise.
2. Gastrointestinal complaints, diarrhoea.
3. Mild fever – progresses to high and spiking by third week.
4. Nausea and vomiting.

Muscular invasion (symptoms derive from inflammatory process developing in the muscles)
1. Oedema of the eyelids; scleral haemorrhages; pain on eye motion.
2. Generalized pain and soreness in the muscles (myalgia).
3. Cardiac irregularities (occasional) – from trichinae in the heart muscle; may be fatal.
4. Difficulty in breathing, masticating, swallowing, speaking.

DIAGNOSTIC EVALUATION
1. Biopsy specimen of muscle – reveals larvae. (Deltoid, biceps, gastrocnemius muscles are sites of biopsy.)
2. Positive serological tests (precipitin, complement-fixation, bentonite-flocculation, fluorescent-antibody) – demonstrable titres three to four weeks after infection.
3. Rising eosinophil count – appears in second week.
4. Positive skin test.

TREATMENT AND NURSING INTERVENTIONS
The treatment is symptomatic; there is no satisfactory treatment.
1. Thiabendazole (Mintezol) – may produce clinical improvement and prevent or minimize effects of illness.
   Adverse effects – nausea, vertigo, vomiting, rash.
2. Corticosteroid agents may be given to relieve symptoms in the acute stage.
3. Keep the patient on bed rest until he experiences some relief of symptoms.
4. Give analgesics to relieve muscle pain.
5. Carry out ECG evaluations to determine evidence of myocarditis.

NURSING ISOLATION PROCEDURES
None required.

PREVENTION AND PATIENT EDUCATION
1. The public should be educated regarding the importance of thoroughly cooking all pork and pork products, especially sausage. There should be no trace of pink in cooked pork.
2. Smoking, pickling, seasoning and spicing do not make pork safe unless it is cooked (especially homemade sausage).
3. Minced beef may be contaminated by a meat grinder that has been used for pork.
4. Waste intended for feed for pigs should be cooked.
5. Pork should be inspected to determine if disease is present.
6. This disease was more prevalent in the USA than in the UK, but now the numbers of cases are diminishing. This is thought to be due to the increasing use of freezers, as the cysts are readily destroyed by low temperatures.

HOOKWORM DISEASE

Hookworm disease (ancylostomiasis; 'ground itch') is the result of infestation of the small intestine by one of two quite similar roundworms about 1.2cm long. Two species are parasitic in the human intestinal tract:
1. *Necator americanus* (predominant species in the USA).

2. *Ancylostoma duodenale.*

The infection is usually contracted by penetration of the skin by infected larvae in the soil.

INCIDENCE

This is a common problem in the tropics, particularly among barefoot workers. Estimates suggest that about one-sixth of the world's population may be affected, about 500 million people. In a two-year study of immigrant schoolchildren in Birmingham in 1968–70, 37 per cent were found to be infected.

CLINICAL COURSE

1. Hookworm eggs are passed in human faeces onto the ground (indiscriminate defaecation habits). Eggs develop into infective larvae.
2. The larvae enter through the mouth if the individual eats with dirty hands, or they *bore through the skin of bare feet* ('ground itch').
3. After gaining access to the blood or lymph vessels, they are carried via the blood to the lungs, migrate from the pulmonary capillaries into the alveoli, reach the pharynx and are swallowed, maturing to adult forms in the bowel.

CLINICAL FEATURES

1. Dermatitis ('ground itch') – occurs at site where larvae penetrate skin.
2. *Gastrointestinal symptoms* – maturation of worms in the intestine is usually marked by onset of diarrhoea and other gastrointestinal symptoms.
   a. Nausea and vomiting.
   b. Flatulence, diarrhoea or constipation.
3. Low-grade fever.
4. *Severe anaemia* and hypoalbuminaemia – the worms attach to intestinal mucosa and suck blood; a single adult worm can extract 0.05ml of blood daily. The patient's iron stores become depleted. A low serum protein often develops (protein malnutrition).
   Severe anaemia may produce:
   a. Symptoms of heart failure.
   b. Tachycardia.
   c. Poor growth and development.
5. *Dry cough and dyspnoea* – from rupture of larvae through the capillary bed and their dissemination throughout the bronchial tree.

DIAGNOSTIC EVALUATION

1. History of anaemia and malnutrition.
2. Recovery and identification of the eggs in faeces.

TREATMENT AND NURSING INTERVENTIONS

1. Specific therapy – one of the following drugs:
   a. Bephenium hydroxynaphthoate (Alcopar).
   b. Pyrantel pamoate (Antiminth).
   c. Tetrachloroethylene.
2. Ensure that the patient is eating a nutritious diet – hookworm disease occurs in people suffering from malnutrition.
   a. Correct anaemia prior to therapy for worms in patients with severe anaemia.
   b. Give protein and iron supplementation – to aid in correction of anaemia.

NURSING ISOLATION PROCEDURES

None required.

PREVENTION AND PATIENT EDUCATION

1. Dispose of excreta in a sanitary manner; this is an important facet of health education.
2. Instruct the patient to wear shoes at all times.
3. Night soil (human excrement used as fertilizer) and sewage effluents should not be used for fertilizer.

ASCARIASIS (ROUNDWORM INFESTATION)

Ascariasis is an infection caused by *Ascaris lumbricoides* (intestinal roundworm). It is characterized by an early pulmonary invasion from larval migration and a later more prolonged intestinal phase.

INCIDENCE

Although this is more common in the tropics, the distribution is worldwide, and infections occur in western Europe.

CLINICAL COURSE

1. Indiscriminate defaecation in streets, fields and doorways provides a major source of infective eggs.
2. Infection may be contracted from eating raw vegetables when night soil is used for fertilizer; water pollution may cause water transmission.
3. Eggs are swallowed and pass into intestine where they hatch into larvae.
4. Larvae penetrate the intestinal mucosa and enter lymphatics and blood vessels.
5. After reaching the lungs, they pierce the capillary wall, crawl up the trachea, are swallowed and are returned to the small intestine where they grow, mature and mate.

CLINICAL FEATURES

1. *Pulmonary phase* – cough, fever and blood-tinged sputum.
2. *Intestinal phase* – masses of worms cause gastrointestinal discomfort, colicky and epigastric pain.

NURSING ALERT
Large masses of worms may migrate into various organs of the body and cause obstruction (to trachea, bronchi, bile duct, appendix, pancreatic duct).

DIAGNOSTIC EVALUATION
1. Stool specimen – for detection of ova and worms in stool.
2. Patient occasionally vomits a worm.

TREATMENT
One of the following may be given:
1. Piperazine citrate, bephenium hydroxynaphthoate, tetramisole.
2. Follow-up stool examination should be done one to two weeks after treatment.

NURSING ISOLATION PROCEDURES
None required.

PREVENTIVE MEASURES AND PATIENT EDUCATION
1. All patients with infestations should be treated.
2. Adequate toilet facilities should be provided.
3. The importance of personal hygiene should be explained.

THREADWORM

The threadworm (*Oxyuris vermicularis*) causes the most common form of intestinal roundworm infestation in the UK and is most prevalent in children.

CLINICAL PROBLEMS
1. One threadworm may produce 5,000–15,000 eggs.
2. Ingested eggs hatch in the small intestine; embryos reach adulthood in the caecum.
3. The gravid female worm migrates down the large intestine and deposits eggs on the skin of the perianal area.
4. The eggs that survive are ingested and reach maturity in two to six weeks in the gastrointestinal tract.
5. Scratching leads to contamination of the hands and nails; hand to mouth contact results in reinfection.
6. Infective eggs may contaminate food and drink, bed linen, dust, etc.

CLINICAL FEATURES
Threadworm-infected person may be asymptomatic.
1. Intense itching (nocturnal) above the anus – from nocturnal migration of gravid females from anus and deposition of eggs in perianal folds of skin.

2. Restlessness; nervousness.
3. Vaginitis – from threadworm migration into the vagina.

DIAGNOSTIC EVALUATION
1. Anal impressions on sellotape taken in the morning before going to toilet or bathing when ova deposited during the night would be removed (Figure 17.2).

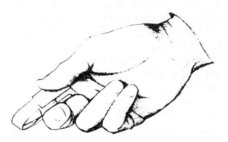

Figure 17.2. Most suitable method of finding eggs in perianal areas. Bend sellotape back over index finger with sticky side out (courtesy of *Forum on Infection*.) Prepared slides are also available

    a. A family member may be taught the method so that the test may be carried out first thing in the morning.
    b. Wash hands thoroughly.
2. Detection (inspection) of characteristic eggs about the anus.

TREATMENT
Drugs include:
1. Piperazine citrate (Antepar) – requires multiple doses.
2. Thiabendazole (Mintezol).
3. Mebendazole (Vermox).

PREVENTION OF REINFECTION; PATIENT EDUCATION
1. All members of the family should be treated, or reinfection is apt to occur. Treat on the same day to eliminate cross-infection.
2. To prevent reinfection:
    a. Cut fingernails short – eggs may be obtained from beneath the nails of infected person.
       (i) Avoid nail biting.
      (ii) Wash hands frequently during treatment period.
     (iii) Scrub nails with a brush, especially before going to bed.
    b. Wash hands with soap and water after using toilet and before meals.

c. Wash around anal area upon rising (after diagnostic test).

d. Apply salve or ointment to anal area – to prevent dispersal of eggs.

e. Infected child should wear snug-fitting cotton pants – to discourage contact of hands with perianal region and contamination of bed linen.

f. See that infected person sleeps alone.

g. Handle bedding and nightwear carefully – there are large numbers of infective eggs in a contaminated house that cause reinfection.

h. Clean sleeping quarters frequently.

i. Reassure mother and family that threadworms are not a sign of poor hygiene or housekeeping.

FURTHER READING

BOOKS

Benenson, A.S. (ed.) (1985) *Control of Communicable Diseases in Man* (14th edn), American Public Health Association, Washington DC.

Benn, R.A.V. (1986) *Aids to Microbiology and Infectious Diseases*, Churchill Livingstone, Edinburgh and London.

Brettle, R.P. and Thomson, M. (1984) *Infection and Communicable Diseases*, William Heinemann Medical Books, London.

Brewis, R.A.L. (1985) *Lecture Notes on Respiratory Disease*, Blackwell Scientific, Oxford.

Dick, G. (1978) *Immunization*, Update Publications, Guildford.

Gillies, R.R. (1978) *Lecture Notes on Medical Microbiology*, Blackwell Scientific, Oxford.

Hare, R. and Cook, M. (1984) *Bacteriology and Immunity for Nurses*, Churchill Livingstone, Edinburgh and London.

Muir Gray, J.A. (1979) *Man Against Disease*, Oxford University Press, Oxford.

Parry, W.H. (1979) *Communicable Diseases*, Unibooks, Hodder and Stoughton, London.

DHSS (1977) *Memorandum on Rabies*, HMSO, London.

— (1986) *LAV/HTLV III – The Causative Agent of AIDS. Revised Guidelines*, HMSO, London.

— (1986) *Information and Guidance on AIDS for Local Authority Staff*, HMSO, London.

— (1988) *Immunization Schedule*, HMSO, London.

ARTICLES
AIDS

Geddes, A.M. (1986) Risks of AIDS to health care workers, *British Medical Journal*, Vol. 292, 15 March, p. 711.

Miller, D. *et al.* (1986) HTLV III: Should testing ever be routine? *British Medical Journal*, Vol. 292, 5 April, pp. 941–3.

Morton, A.D. and McManus, I.C. (1986) Attitudes to, and knowledge about AIDS – a lack of correlation, *British Medical Journal*, Vol. 293, 8 November, p. 1212.

Pozniak, A.L. *et al.* (1986) Clinical and bronchoscopic diagnosis of suspected pneumonia related to AIDS, *British Medical Journal*, Vol. 293, 27 September, pp. 797–9.

General

Ayton, M. (1981) National surveillance of communicable diseases, *Nursing*, Vol. 1, No. 29, pp. 1248–51.

Collins, B.J. (1981) The spread of infection, *Nursing*, Vol. 1, No. 29, pp. 1252–4.

Gardner, S.D. (1986) In pursuit of the perfect rabies vaccine, *British Medical Journal*, Vol. 293, 30 August, pp. 490–92.

Iveson-Iveson, J. (1979) Prevention and how to stay healthy, *Nursing Mirror*, Vol. 149, No. 19, p. 18.

— (1980) Student's forum: infectious diseases, *Nursing Mirror*, Vol. 151, No. 8, pp. 26–8.

Keay, E. (1981) Coppetts Wood, an infectious diseases unit, *Nursing*, Vol. 1, No. 29, pp. 1273–7.

Sanderson, P.J. (1986) Staying one jump ahead of resistant *Staph.aureus*, *British Medical Journal*, Vol. 293, 6 September, p. 620.

Strange, J.L. (1980) Hospitals should do the sick no harm, *Nursing Times*, Vol. 76, No. 51, *Supplements* pp. 1–4.

Reports from the Public Health Laboratory Service Communicable Disease Surveillance Centre (1986) *British Medical Journal*:

a. Measles and diphtheria, Vol. 292, 24 April, pp. 1385–6.

b. Malaria and AIDS, Vol. 292, 31 May, pp. 1447–8.

c. Salmonella, Vol. 292, 21 June, pp. 1655–6.

d. Chickenpox, Vol. 293, 2 August, pp. 326–7.

e. Tetanus, Vol. 293, 13 September, pp. 680–82.

Hepatitis

Tedder, R.S. (1981) Hepatitis B, *Nursing*, Vol. 1, No. 29, pp. 1284–8.

Parasitology

Maunder, J.W. (1981) Parasitology, *Nursing*, Vol. 1, No. 29, pp. 1290–91.

18

Care of the Patient with Cancer

GENERAL CONSIDERATIONS

THE REALITIES OF CANCER

1. One-third of all cancer patients are cured.
2. Improved treatment methods enable patients with cancer to live longer, more comfortably and more productively.
3. Most cancer patients spend almost all their time away from hospitals and only come to the hospital intermittently for treatment.
4. More intense efforts at patient rehabilitation are proving effective.
5. Research continues unabated, and, as findings accumulate, prospects for specific cures are encouraging.
6. The public trend is to be aware of health and patient education. People are now more aware of the possible predisposing factors.
7. Screening to provide the early detection of cancer is becoming more widely available.
8. More patients are able to be cared for at home because of better symptom control, with more physical and psychological support for both the patient and relatives by specialist nurses and doctors.

CANCER'S WARNING SIGNALS

C hange in bowel or bladder habits
A sore that does not heal
U nusual bleeding or discharge
T hickening or lump in breast or elsewhere
I ndigestion or difficulty in swallowing
O bvious change in wart or mole
N agging cough or hoarseness

BENIGN AND MALIGNANT TUMOURS

See Table 18.1.

Table 18.1   Characteristics of benign and malignant tumours

	Benign	Malignant
Type of cell	Adult	Young
Nature	Closely resembles parent tissue	Tends to be anaplastic (reverting to primitive cells)
Growth	Slow	Rapid, usually
Encapsulated	Often	Never
Effect on surrounding tissue	Never invades	Invades widely
Localization	Remains at original site	Nonlocalized – forms secondary growths by metastasis
Recurrence after removal	Does not tend to recur	Tends to recur

METASTASIS

1. Direct invasion – tumours do not just expand, but may infiltrate between the surrounding tissue cells, causing disorganization and destruction.
2. Lymphatic spread – malignant cells may invade the lymphatic system and grow as a column or be broken off and carried as the embolus to the draining lymph node.
3. Blood spread – tumour cells may enter the bloodstream from the lymphatics or invade blood cells directly.
4. Cavity spread – a tumour may spread from one structure to another across cavities, often in a fluid medium such as pleural or peritoneal fluid, urine or cerebrospinal fluid.

INCIDENCE

1. The annual death toll from malignancy in the UK is at least 146,000 and accounts for 22 per cent of all deaths.
2. Cancer occurs at any age. Although rare in the young, it remains the second largest killer of children and young people. It strikes with increasing frequency as age advances.
3. There were about 200,000 new cases of cancer diagnosed in 1987.
4. No organ in the body is exempt for cancer death rates by site and sex (Figure 18.1).

DIAGNOSTIC EVALUATION

Many techniques may be used to diagnose tumours, depending upon their site. These include:
1. Full physical examination.
2. Haematology, e.g., full blood count, urea and electrolytes, biochemical tests.
3. Radiology, e.g., straight X-rays, lymphography, arteriography, mammography, tomography.
4. Radioisotopes, e.g., radioactive iodine scans.

5. Computerized tomography (CT scanning).
6. Ultrasound.
7. Nuclear magnetic resonance imaging (NMRI).
8. Endoscopy and biopsy.
9. Cytology, e.g., cervical smear, urine for cytology.
10. Liver scan.
11. Direct tumour biopsy, e.g. breast lump.

STAGING

Various staging systems available which indicate the extent of the tumour. TNM system is the most common:

T = primary tumour, scale 1–4 indicates size.
N = regional nodes, scale 1–4 indicates extent of local spread.
M = distant metastases: 0 = none; 1 = exist.

TREATMENT

1. Methods of treatment include surgery, radiotherapy, radioactive substances (including radioisotopes), various drugs (pharmaceuticals and hormones) and immunotherapy (see pp. 1043–44).
2. Method of treatment will depend on the type of malignancy, stage, localization or spread, condition of patient, and the doctor; a single method or combination of methods may be required.

SURGERY

1. *Biopsy* – a piece of tissue is cut out surgically from the questionable area and sent to pathology laboratory for diagnostic verification.
2. *Preventive or prophylactic surgery* – removal of lesions which, if left in the body, are apt to develop into cancer. Example: polyps in rectum may lead to cancer of colon.
3. *Palliative surgery* – a type of surgery which

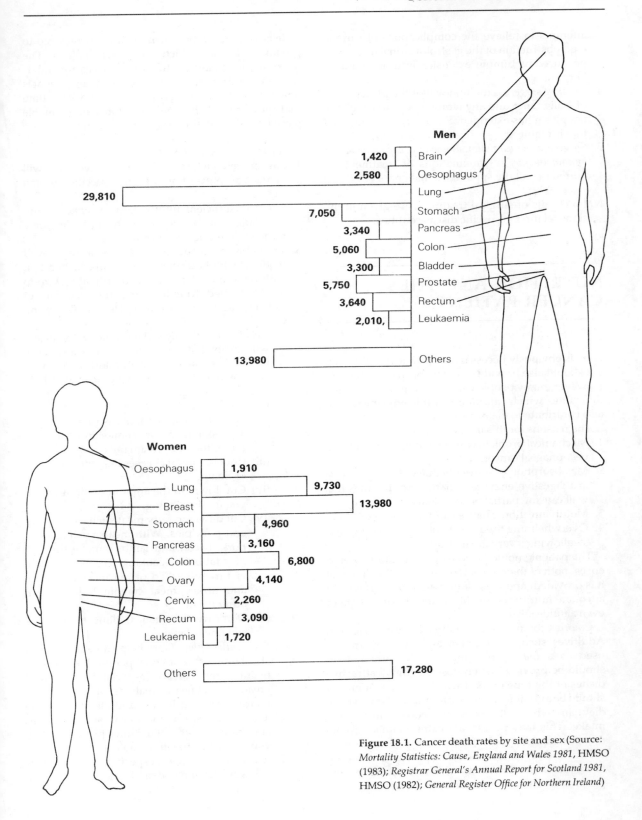

Men

1,420 Brain
2,580 Oesophagus
29,810 Lung
7,050 Stomach
3,340 Pancreas
5,060 Colon
3,300 Bladder
5,750 Prostate
3,640 Rectum
2,010, Leukaemia

13,980 Others

Women

Oesophagus 1,910
Lung 9,730
Breast 13,980
Stomach 4,960
Pancreas 3,160
Colon 6,800
Ovary 4,140
Cervix 2,260
Rectum 3,090
Leukaemia 1,720

Others 17,280

Figure 18.1. Cancer death rates by site and sex (Source: *Mortality Statistics: Cause, England and Wales 1981*, HMSO (1983); *Registrar General's Annual Report for Scotland 1981*, HMSO (1982); *General Register Office for Northern Ireland*)

attempts to relieve the complications of cancer, e.g., obstruction of the gastrointestinal tract, pain produced by tumour extension into surrounding nerves.

4. *Curative surgery* – the removal of the primary site of malignancy and any lymph nodes to which the neoplasm has extended. Such surgery may be all that is required.

5. *Surgery combined with radiotherapy, chemotherapy or immunotherapy* – combinations of treatment required to halt the spread of a malignancy.

Note: Details of surgical treatment are given in the sections relating to specific disease entities.

NUTRITION AND THE CANCER PATIENT

Food is obviously necessary for physical well-being, but should also provide an enjoyable part of the day. However, many people with cancer may have eating difficulties which can diminish this enjoyment and also contribute to malnutrition.

The reasons for this include:
1. Mechanical problems associated with mouth and oesophageal cancer.
2. Malabsorption of nutrients due to lack of necessary digestive enzymes; changes in the intestinal wall causing partial or complete obstruction.
3. Mouth infections, nausea and diarrhoea.
4. Overwhelming tiredness which makes eating and swallowing a very great effort.

The patient should be consulted about his preferences, both of the type of food and also the time that it is provided, and reassurance should be given that adequate nutrition is readily available with a light or even a fluid-only diet.

Calories for providing energy are often lacking. Additives such as Complan and Build-up can be used as a meal replacement, but 'normal' food should be provided when possible. Small attractive dishes of the type of food which the patient enjoys should be available. Planning for this will involve the dietitian, who will ensure the correct nutritional intake. This may necessitate extra vitamin supplements in liquid or tablet form.

Fruit and vegetables should be provided according to the particular problems which this patient is experiencing, e.g. constipation or diarrhoea.

Relatives should be consulted and encouraged to provide delicacies which the patient enjoys. The nurse should make sure that the relatives are understanding, and not hurt or discouraged if the patient is unable to eat their carefully prepared food at the time that they bring it. It should be stored in a suitable place until the patient feels ready to eat it.

NUTRITION AND CANCER

1. No concrete dietary advice can be given that will guarantee prevention of any specific human cancer.
2. There is sufficient information to make recommendations that are likely to provide some measure of reducing cancer risk.
3. The following nutritional guidelines are approved by the Health Education Council in collaboration with the Cancer Education Co-ordinating Group of the United Kingdom and the Republic of Ireland, and the Scottish Health Education Group.
   a. *Avoid being overweight.* The advice given below will mean that you will be eating less fatty foods. This will reduce your calorie intake and, combined with regular exercise, it will help you to lose weight.
   b. *Cut down on fats.*
      (i) Spread less butter or margarine.
      (ii) Try skimmed or semi-skimmed milk rather than full cream milk.
      (iii) Choose low fat cheeses like cottage cheese or Edam.
      (iv) Cut down on the amount of oils and lard you use in cooking.
      (v) Cut down on fatty meat such as sausages and pork pies. With meats such as beef, pork, bacon and lamb, remove the surplus fat before cooking. Try fish, chicken or turkey instead of red meats. Chicken and turkey meat contain less fat than other meat.
      (vi) Don't fry too often. Grilling, roasting or stewing is better.
   c. *Eat plenty of fibre.* Fibre helps the digestion. It also helps prevent constipation. Fibre comes mainly from bread (especially wholemeal bread), breakfast cereals (especially whole grain), peas and beans, and also from some leafy vegetables, wholewheat pasta, potatoes and fruit. If your diet includes plenty of these you will get all the fibre you need.
   d. *Avoid too much alcohol,* especially spirits such as whiskey, gin and vodka. Reduce consumption of beer.

There is, of course, no guarantee that by following this advice you'll protect yourself against any form of cancer. But you may reduce the risk of some forms, and in any case it's all good advice for your general health. It certainly won't do any harm. The occasional feast won't do you much harm either. It's what you eat regularly that counts.

CHEMOTHERAPY

Value of chemotherapy in treating a malignancy:
1. As yet no *one* drug is available to cure all malignant tumours.
2. Chemotherapeutic agents are most useful in the treatment of leukaemias, Hodgkin's disease, lymphomas, Ewing's tumour, Wilm's tumour, testicular tumours and retinoblastomas.
3. Recent work has demonstrated the value of using chemotherapeutic agents in combination with surgery and/or radiotherapy in tumours where the recurrence risk is high.
4. Chemotherapy may also be used to relieve symptoms in those patients in whom surgery or radiotherapy is no longer beneficial.
5. Combinations of chemotherapeutic agents are often more effective and no more toxic than single agents.
6. Precise timing in administering these drugs is vital to achieve the optimum effect.
7. Some chemotherapeutic agents have unpleasant systemic effects. It is imperative that the nurse knows what these are and how to minimize them.

PHARMACOLOGICAL ACTION
See Table 18.2.

1. These drugs are capable of destroying young, rapidly multiplying cells, such as malignant cells.
2. They interfere with manufacture of nucleic acids (inhibit the chain of synthesis or function of DNA and RNA) so that cellular growth and reproduction are inhibited.
3. Since many normal cells in the body also grow rapidly and have short life spans (e.g., bone marrow, gastrointestinal tract lining, hair follicles), many chemotherapeutic agents directly attack these normal cells. Herein lies the challenge.

METHOD OF ADMINISTRATION
Drugs may be given orally, subcutaneously, intravenously, intramuscularly, intra-arterially or intrathecally depending on the drug.

Intravenous administration
1. See Principles of Intravenous Therapy, p. 71. Additional specific concerns related to administration of chemotherapeutic agents include the following:
   a. In general, avoid venepuncture in an arm where:
      (i) Dissection of the axillary nodes has been performed.
      (ii) Radiotherapy has caused marked fibrosis in the axillary area.
   b. Avoid areas of sclerosis, thrombosis or scar formation.
   c. Avoid prolonged tourniquet application in order to prevent cutaneous haemorrhage.
2. If a small focal haematoma develops during insertion of needle into a vein, do not use this avenue for administration of toxic chemotherapeutic agents because of the danger of extravasation.
3. Maintain constant supervision during administration of potentially locally toxic chemotherapeutic agents.
4. If any doubt exists regarding vein patency or safety of drug administration, discontinue administration.
5. It is better to prevent *extravasation* than to treat it.
   a. Symptoms: pain (severe enough to cause patient to cry out); area may appear red, mottled and/or swollen – often leading to necrosis; may need skin grafting.
   b. Treatment
      (i) Apply ice compresses to slow down local tissue metabolism – or apply hydrocortisone to affected area. Keep area clean.
      (ii) Some individuals recommend local infiltration of the involved area with an anti-inflammatory agent, i.e., hydrocortisone.
      (iii) Later, warm compresses may be applied; local management as indicated.
   c. If only a small amount of drug is extravasated and frank necrosis does not occur, phlebitis may still result, causing pain for several days and/or induration at the site that may last for weeks or months.
6. Observe for occurrences other than extravasation:
   a. Intraluminal
      (i) Symptoms:
         (a) Patient may describe sensations of pain, stretching or pressure within the

(continued on p. 1036)

Table 18.2   Commercially available anticancer drugs

Drug	Toxicity	Nursing implications
Alkylating agents Busulphan (Myleran)	1. Bone marrow depression.	Observe for infection, bleeding, anaemia
	2. Gynacomastia Amenorrhoea Impotence	Inform patient and give psychological support, contraceptive advice
	3. Skin pigmentation	Inform patient
	4. Pulmonary fibrosis (long term)	Steroids usually given
Chlorambucil (Leukeran)	1. Bone marrow depression	Observe for infection, bleeding, anaemia
	2. Nausea and vomiting (high dose)	Dietary control. Encourage fluids. Give antiemetics
	3. Chromosomal damage (long term)	Inform patient and give psychological support
	4. Pulmonary complications (long term)	Baseline chest X-ray. Check chest X-ray prior to each treatment. Observation for onset of symptoms. Warn anaesthetist before surgery
Cyclophosphamide (Endoxana, Cytoxan)	1. Bone marrow depression	Observe for infection, bleeding, anaemia
	2. Nausea and vomiting	Dietary control. Encourage fluids. Give antiemetics
	3. Stomatitis	Oral hygiene. Bland diet
	4. Alopecia	Inform patient. Arrange wig
	5. Alteration in taste (immediate)	Use of flavourings, e.g. suck sweets
	6. Chemical cystitis	Maintain adequate fluid intake, advise twice normal intake
	7. Hot flushes, dizziness (immediate)	Warn patient, give injection slowly
Dacarbazine (DTIC, DIC)	1. Bone marrow depression	Observe for infection, bleeding, anaemia
	2. Nausea, vomiting and diarrhoea (short term)	Dietary control. Encourage fluids. Give antiemetics
	3. Alopecia (rare)	Inform patient. Arrange wig
	4. Flu-like syndrome	Observe for and treat symptoms
	5. Pain along course of vein if given in a too concentrated solution, too rapidly	Give by infusion over 30–60 minutes and may be given by very slow injection with frequent saline flushes whenever pain occurs. Always distinguish from extravasation. Dilute injection further (if pharmacologically acceptable)
	6. Facial flushing, especially in sunlight	Inform patient
	7. Hepatotoxicity	Observe for signs of jaundice, test urine for bilirubin, monitor liver function tests *Avoid extravasation*
Ifosfamide (Mitoxana, Holoxan)	1. Haematuria	Increase fluid intake before and after treatment including intravenous fluids. Test urine for blood. Mesna given concurrently will offer protection of the bladder mucosa with cyclophosphamide and ifosfamide
	2. Nausea and vomiting	Dietary control. Encourage fluids. Give antiemetics
	3. Alopecia	Inform patient. Arrange wig

	4. Mild bone marrow depression	Observe for infection, bleeding, anaemia
	5. Antidiuretic (short term)	Monitor fluid output. Intravenous diuretics
Melphalan, phenylalanine mustard, L-PAM (Alkeran)	1. Bone marrow depression	Observe for infection, bleeding, anaemia
	2. Nausea and vomiting (with high doses)	Dietary control. Encourage fluids. Give antiemetics
	3. Alopecia (with high doses)	Inform patient. Arrange wig
Nitrogen mustard (Mustine)	1. Bone marrow depression	Observe for infection, bleeding, anaemia
	2. Nausea and vomiting (rapid onset and severe)	Dietary control. Encourage fluids. Give antiemetics.
	3. Metallic taste or smell (immediate)	Inform patient, offer sweets to suck
	4. Amenorrhoea, impaired spermatogenesis	Inform patient, offer contraceptive advice
		Avoid extravasation
		Protect eyes and skin of person administering drug
Triethylene triphosphamide (Thiotepa)	1. Bone marrow depression	Observe for infection, bleeding, anaemia
	2. Very rare nausea	Dietary control. Encourage fluids. Give antiemetics
	3. Very rare allergic reaction	Regular observations
Nitrosurea-alkylating agent Carmustine (BCNU)	1. Delayed bone marrow depression (4–6 weeks)	Maintain awareness of possible infection, bleeding, anaemia
	2. Nausea and vomiting (severe)	Dietary control. Encourage fluids. Give antiemetics
	3. Gynaecomastia	Inform patient
	4. Facial flushing	Warn patient
	5. Venous pain	Administer slowly by infusion over 1–2 hours
Antimetabolites Azathioprine (Imuran)	1. Vomiting (with high dose)	Dietary control. Encourage fluids. Give antiemetics
	2. Diarrhoea (with high dose)	Dietary control. Encourage fluids. Antidiarrhoeal drugs
	3. Bone marrow depression	Observe for infection, bleeding, anaemia
	4. Susceptible to viruses	Observe for infection
	5. Hepatotoxic	Observe for signs of jaundice. Test urine for bilirubin. Monitor liver function tests
Cytosine arabinoside (Ara-C, Cytosar, Cytarbarine)	1. Bone marrow depression	Observe for infection, bleeding, anaemia
	2. Nausea and vomiting	Dietary control. Encourage fluids. Give antiemetics
	3. Flu-like syndrome	Observe for and treat symptoms
	4. Stomatitis	Oral hygiene. Bland diet
	5. Hyperuricaemia	Observe urinary output
5-Fluorouracil (5-FU)	1. Bone marrow depression	Observe for infection, bleeding, anaemia
	2. Nausea and vomiting	Dietary control. Encourage fluids. Give antiemetics
	3. Stomatitis	Oral hygiene. Bland diet

(continued)

Table 18.2   Continued

Drug	Toxicity	Nursing implications
	4. Diarrhoea	Dietary control. Encourage fluids. Antidiarrhoeal drugs
	5. Hyperpigmentation	Inform patient. Avoid bright sunlight
	6. Alopecia (rare)	Inform patient. Arrange wig
	7. Discoloration of veins with prolonged infusions	Explain reason to patient
Hydroxyurea	1. Bone marrow depression	Observe for infection, bleeding, anaemia
	2. Nausea and vomiting	Dietary control. Encourage fluids. Give antiemetics
	3. Stomatitis	Oral hygiene. Bland diet
	4. Anorexia	Small, appetizing meals
	5. Alopecia (rare)	Inform patient. Arrange wig
	6. Erythema, rash, pruritis	No perfumed soap. Encourage skin cleanliness
6-Mercaptopurine (6-MP)	1. Bone marrow depression	Observe for infection, bleeding, anaemia
	2. Nausea (mild)	Dietary control. Encourage fluids. Give antiemetics
	3. Stomatitis (high dose)	Oral hygiene. Bland diet
	4. Diarrhoea (high dose)	Dietary control. Encourage fluids. Antidiarrhoeal drugs.
	5. Liver dysfunction	Observe for jaundice. Test for bilirubin in urine. Monitor liver function tests
Methotrexate	1. Bone marrow depression	Observe for infection, bleeding, anaemia
	2. Nausea and vomiting (rare, mild)	Dietary control. Encourage fluids. Give antiemetics
	3. Stomatitis, mucosal ulceration	Oral hygiene. Bland diet. Folinic acid rescue
	4. Diarrhoea (rare, mild)	Dietary control. Encourage fluids. Antidiarrhoeal drugs
	5. Skin rash	Calamine lotion or steroid cream, avoid bright sunlight
	6. Nephrotoxicity	Encourage fluids. Observe urinary output, monitor renal function
	7. Hepatotoxicity	Observe for jaundice. Test urine for bilirubin. Monitor liver function tests
Procarbazine (Natulan) (monoamine oxidase inhibitor)	1. Bone marrow depression	Observe for infection, bleeding, anaemia
	2. Nausea and vomiting	Dietary control. Encourage fluids. Give antiemetics
	3. Mild CNS toxicity	Observe and report
	4. MAO inhibitor	No alcohol, cheese, Marmite, yoghurt, sedatives, narcotics, tricyclic antidepressants or antihistamines
	5. Flu-like syndrome	Warn patient. Usually resolves during initial treatment. Treat symptoms
6-Thioguanine (6-TG)	1. Bone marrow depression	Observe for infection, bleeding, anaemia
	2. Nausea and vomiting (rare, mild)	Dietary control. Encourage fluids. Give antiemetics
	3. Diarrhoea (rare, mild)	Antidiarrhoeal drugs

Antibiotics		
Bleomycin	1. Fever and chills	Observe for and treat symptoms. Intravenous steroids at time of administration
	2. Skin reactions	Inform patient, treat symptomatically. Report to doctor
	3. Stomatitis	Oral hygiene. Bland diet
	4. Alopecia (rare)	Inform patient. Arrange wig
	5. Nausea and vomiting (rare, mild)	Dietary control. Encourage fluids. Give antiemetics
	6. Pulmonary fibrosis	Regular chest X-ray and lung function tests. Monitor total dose of drug
	7. Tumour pain	Give analgesics. Warn patient
	8. Anaphylaxis (rare)	Emergency equipment to hand. Close observations
		Protect eyes and skin of person administering drug
Dactinomycin (actinomycin D, Cosmegen)	1. Bone marrow depression	Observe for infection, bleeding, anaemia
	2. Nausea and vomiting	Dietary control. Encourage fluids. Give antiemetics
	3. Anorexia	Small appetizing meals
	4. Stomatitis	Oral hygiene. Bland diet
	5. Diarrhoea	Dietary control. Encourage fluids. Antidiarrhoeal drugs
	6. Skin pigmentation. Reactivation of DXT site	Inform patient, avoid bright sunlight
	7. Alopecia	Inform patient. Arrange wig
	8. Mental depression (rare)	Psychological support
		Avoid extravasation
Daunorubicin, Rubidomycin (Cerubidin)	1. Bone marrow depression	Observe for infection, bleeding, anaemia
	2. Alopecia	Inform patient. Arrange wig
	3. Nausea and vomiting	Dietary control. Encourage fluids. Give antiemetics
	4. Stomatitis	Oral hygiene. Bland diet
	5. Red urine	Inform patient
	6. Fever	Inform patient. Treat symptoms
	7. Congestive cardiac failure	ECG essential predose. Observe and report symptoms of cardiac failure. Monitor total dose of drug
	8. Reactivation of DXT site	Inform patient, avoid bright sunlight
		Avoid extravasation
Doxorubicin	1. Alopecia	Inform patient. Arrange wig. Scalp cooling will substantially reduce alopecia, unless hepatic disease is present. If present, plasma filtration rate is slowed down and this drug stays in circulation for longer.
	2. Bone marrow depression	Observe for infection, bleeding, anaemia
	3. Nausea and vomiting	Dietary control. Encourage fluids. Give antiemetics

(continued)

Table 18.2 Continued

Drug	Toxicity	Nursing implications
	4. Stomatitis	Oral hygiene. Bland diet
	5. Diarrhoea	Dietary control. Encourage fluids. Antidiarrhoeal drugs
	6. Fever (rare)	Inform patient. Treat symptoms
	7. Red urine (up to 12 days)	Inform patient
	8. Cardiotoxicity	ECG essential predose. Monitor for signs and symptoms of cardiac failure. Monitor total dose of drug
		Avoid extravasation
Epirubicin (Pharmorubicin)	1. Red urine	Warn patient
	2. Stomatitis	Oral hygiene. Bland diet
	3. Nausea and vomiting	Dietary control. Encourage fluids. Give antiemetics
	4. Reactivation of DXT sites	Inform patient. Avoid bright sunlight
	5. Bone marrow depression	Observe for infection, bleeding, anaemia
	6. Alopecia	Inform patient. Arrange wig
		Avoid extravasation
Mithramycin (Mithracin)	1. Nausea and vomiting	Dietary control. Encourage fluids. Give antiemetics
	2. Metallic taste	Inform patient, offer sweets to suck
	3. Stomatitis (daily doses)	Oral hygiene. Bland diet
	4. Diarrhoea	Dietary control. Encourage fluids. Antidiarrhoeal drugs
	5. Haemorrhagic epistaxis	Stop bleeding. Apply ice packs, etc. Report to doctor
	6. Hypocalcaemia (often intentional)	Observe for increased neural and muscular excitability
	7. Hepatotoxicity	Observe for jaundice. Test urine for bilirubin. Monitor liver function tests
	8. Headache, depression, drowsiness, fever	Inform patient. Careful observation. Treat symptoms
	9. Nephrotoxicity (rare)	Monitor fluid balance and renal function
		Avoid extravasation
Mitomycin C (Mutamycin)	1. Bone marrow depression (delayed)	Observe for infection, bleeding, anaemia
	2. Nausea and vomiting	Dietary control. Encourage fluids. Give antiemetics
	3. Stomatitis	Oral hygiene. Bland diet
	4. Lethargy	Supportive care at approx. 3–4 weeks
	5. Pruritis	Apply antipruritic cream
		Avoid extravasation
Streptozotocin (Zanosar) (Nitrosurea with broad antibiotic properties)	1. Burning of the vein bolus injection	Give by infusion over 15 minutes to 6 hours
	2. Hypoglycaemia	Observe for dizziness, pallor, sweating, confusion. Monitor blood glucose levels
	3. Nausea and vomiting	Dietary control. Encourage fluids. Give antiemetics

	4. Renal tubule toxicity (long term)	Adequate hydration and lower dose in patients with pre-existing renal disease. Monitor renal function
	5. Hepatotoxicity	Observe for jaundice. Test urine for bilirubin. Monitor liver function tests
		Avoid extravasation
Vinca alkaloids Vinblastine (Velbe, Velban)	1. Bone marrow depression	Observe for infection, bleeding, anaemia
	2. Nausea and vomiting (mild)	Dietary control. Encourage fluids. Give antiemetics
	3. Alopecia (high dose only)	Inform patient. Arrange wig
	4. Peripheral neuritis	Report symptoms. Observe for paraesthesia, numbness, ataxia
	5. Constipation, abdominal pain	Give mild aperients
	6. Jaw pain (short term), tumour pain	Inform patient. Give analgesics
	7. Cold sensation along vein	Inform patient
		Avoid extravasation
Vincristine (Oncovin)	1. Alopecia (high dose)	Inform patient. Arrange wig
	2. Peripheral neuritis	Report symptoms. Observe for paraesthesia, numbness, ataxia
	3. Constipation, abdominal pain	Give mild aperients
	4. Polyuria (rare)	Observe urinary output
	5. Cold sensation along vein	Inform patient
	6. Jaw pain	Inform patient. Give analgesics
		Avoid extravasation
Vindesine (Eldisine)	1. Bone marrow depression	Observe for infection, bleeding and anaemia
	2. Alopecia (slow onset but may be total)	Inform patient. Offer wig
	3. Cumulative neurotoxicity	Observation to determine severity. Reassure patient that symptoms will usually disappear 5–6 weeks after stopping treatment
	4. Abdominal cramps, constipation	Warn patient of possibility. Prophylactic aperients. Observe for early signs
	5. Transient jaw pain	Administer analgesics. Reassure patient that effect will pass
	6. Cold sensation along vein	Inform patient
	7. Phlebitis	Warn patient. Observe for signs.
		Avoid extravasation
Other agents L-asparaginase	1. Anaphylaxis	Emergency equipment ready. Hydrocortisone and chlorphericramine (Piriton) ready. Treat symptoms, e.g. fever
	2. Malaise, anorexia	Psychological support, small appetizing meals
	3. Hepatotoxicity	Observe for jaundice. Test veins for bilirubin. Monitor liver function tests

(continued)

Table 18.2   Continued

Drug	Toxicity	Nursing implications
	4. Hyperglycaemia	Observe for symptoms, e.g. thirst. Monitor urine and blood glucose levels
	5. CNS toxicity, confusion, depression, coma	Observe for symptoms. Report to doctor
	6. High number of patients show an allergic reaction	Warn patient. Observe for signs
	7. Hypoalbuminaemia	Examine for oedema. Monitor blood levels
Carboplatin (Paraplatin)	1. Nausea and vomiting	Dietary control. Encourage fluids. Give antiemetics
	2. Very rare allergic reaction	Regular observations
	3. Bone marrow depression	Observe for infection, bleeding, anaemia
	4. Nephrotoxicity	Encourage fluids. Observe urinary output. Monitor renal function
Cisplatinum	1. Bone marrow depression	Observe for infection, bleeding, anaemia
	2. Nausea and persistent vomiting	Dietary control. Encourage fluids. Give antiemetics
	3. Diarrhoea at higher doses	Dietary control. Encourage fluids. Antidiarrhoeal drugs
	4. Metallic taste	Offer strongly flavoured sweet during injection
	5. Nephrotoxicity, particularly high doses	Monitor renal function before treatment. Record fluid intake and output during treatment. Adequate hydration, including intravenous fluid, sometimes using forced diuresis to maintain output. Test urine for pH – alkalinization may be required during treatment
	6. Otological, tinnitus, high frequency hearing loss	Baseline audiology testing. Document patient reporting tinnitus
	7. Peripheral neuropathy	Inform patient. Monitor symptoms, e.g. numbness, paraesthesia
	8. Hyperuricaemia	Observe urinary output. Encourage fluid intake
	9. Analphylaxis, increased risk as treatment proceeds	Observe patient. Emergency equipment and drugs ready
Etoposide (Vepesid)	1. Severe hypotension if infused rapidly	Slow infusion over 30 minutes
	2. Nausea and vomiting (very mild, worse with oral preparations)	Dietary control. Encourage fluids. Give antiemetics
	3. Alopecia (usually total)	Inform patient. Arrange wig
	4. Bone marrow depression (predominantly leucopenia)	Observe for infection, bleeding, anaemia
Mitozantrone (Novantrone)	1. Green discoloration of urine for 24 hours	Inform patient
	2. Mild phlebitis and blue discoloration of vein	Inform patient. Slow administration of drugs. Symptomatic relief using heparinoid creams

	3. Bone marrow depression	Observe for infection, bleeding and anaemia
C Parvum (Coparvax)	1. Fever	Observe for and treat symptoms
	2. Abdominal pain	Adequate analgesia
	3. Nausea and vomiting	Dietary control. Encourage fluids. Give antiemetics

Hormones
Oestrogens

Diethylstilboestrol (DES)	1. Nausea	Dietary control. Encourage fluids. Give antiemetics
Ethinyloestradiol		
Stilboestrol	2. Fluid retention	Avoid salt and salty foods. Encourage movement. Avoid injections
	3. Feminization	Inform patient. Give psychological support
	4. Hypercalcaemia	Rehydration with forced diuresis
	5. Uterine bleeding	Inform patient

Antioestrogens

Tamoxifen (Nolvadex)	1. Nausea and vomiting	Dietary control. Encourage fluids. Give antiemetics
	2. Fluid retention	Avoid salt and salty foods. Encourage movement. Avoid injections
	3. Hypercalcaemia	Rehydration with forced diuresis
	4. Photosensitivity of skin	Avoid exposure to sunlight

Androgens

Nandrolone	1. Coarse facial hair	Remove with depilatory cream. Avoid shaving
Phenyl propionate (Durabolin)		
Drostanolone (Masteril)	2. Thinning of scalp hair	Inform patient
	3. Hoarse, deep voice	Inform patient
	4. Oily skin, acne	Strict cleansing. Use astringent
	5. Increased libido	Inform patient

Antiandrogens

Cyproterone acetate	1. Fatigue	Avoid sedative drugs
	2. Gynaecomastia	Inform patient
	3. Weight gain	Dietary control

Progesterones

Hydroxyprogesterone	1. Nausea	Inform patient
Medroxyprogesterone (Provera)	2. Headache	Give analgesics
Norethisterone (Primolut-depot)	3. Fluid retention	Avoid salt and salty foods. Encourage movement. Avoid injections
	4. Hypercalcaemia	Rehydration with forced diuresis

Corticosteroids

Prednisone	1. Local oedema, 'moon face'	Inform patient
Prednisolone	2. Fluid retention	Avoid salt and salty foods. Encourage movement. Avoid injections
	3. Hypertension	Regular blood pressure recording

(continued)

Table 18.2 Continued

Drug	Toxicity	Nursing implications
	4. Osteoporosis	High calcium, high protein diet
	5. Impaired hearing	Inform patient. Discuss safety measures
	6. Gastrointestinal disturbance	Give antacids. Observe for haematemesis and melaena
	7. Diabetes mellitus	Observe for polyuria and polydipsia. Routine urine testing
	8. Changes in mood	Careful observation
	9. Susceptibility to infection	Strict attention to hygiene

vessel, originating near venepuncture site or 7.5–12.5cm along vein course.

(b) Discoloration – deep blue or purple 5–10cm proximal to venepuncture site.

(ii) Treatment: wait and observe; change puncture site or discontinue administration of drug.

b. Subcutaneous tissue:
   (i) Symptoms:
   Itching, muscle cramp, pressure within arm, possible urticaria.
   (ii) Treatment:
      (a) Wait and observe; change puncture site, or discontinue administration of drug.
      (b) Notify doctor if systemic effects are observed.

Isolated perfusion

A seldom-used technique whereby large doses of cytotoxic drugs are administered to an isolated extremity, organ or region of the body (excluding systemic circulation).

Intra-arterial infusion

The introduction percutaneously of a catheter into a major artery followed by the continuous administration (by means of a pump) of a chemotherapeutic agent. Treatment may be continued over several days.

NURSING CARE OF THE PATIENT RECEIVING CHEMOTHERAPY

Objectives

1. The patient will be mentally and physically relaxed prior to the administration of the drugs.

2. The side-effects of the drugs should be minimized as far as possible.

3. Nursing staff should be fully conversant with the storage, preparation, administration, therapeutic and toxic effects of these drugs, and the precautions which are necessary to safeguard the patient and themselves.

Assessment

The problems may include:

1. *Fear and apprehension.* The patient may be afraid of the actual administration of the drugs, but there may be a greater fear of the immediate side-effects and possible long-term effects in the future.

2. *Depression.* This may occur if the patient is likely to have a change of body image due to alopecia and weight loss. Also, depression can occur while the patient is coming to terms with the diagnosis of cancer.

3. *Gastrointestinal problems.* These are common and associated with particular drugs. The problems are likely to be mouth infections, nausea, vomiting, diarrhoea, constipation, anorexia.

4. *Clotting deficiency.* This is due to bone marrow depression, and may cause bruising or bleeding.

5. *Epithelial breakdown.* This means an increased tendency to pressure sores, and also oral lesions.

6. *Pain.* This is discussed in detail in Care of the Patient with Advanced Cancer, p. 1046.

Planning and implementation

1. Establish a good nurse/patient relationship. This will enable the patient to express his fears and anxieties, and allow the nurse to give full explanation of procedures. Encourage participation in planning immediate and future care. Be sensitive to patient's nonverbal communication. Try to identify the level of knowledge which the patient

has about his illness and his wish for further information.

2. Provide diversional and recreational therapy by the most suitable methods for the individual patient, and social contact with other patients.

3. Before treatment commences, the patient should be told if his drug regimen will cause alopecia, and advice given about obtaining a wig if the patient wishes. This is especially important for female patients, who, although they have been told about this previously, are deeply shocked when their hair literally falls out in handfuls. A head scarf may be preferred and the nurse should encourage an interest in the choice of colours and patterns.

4. The dietitian should see the patient to discuss food preferences, and give advice about maintaining adequate nutritional levels to prevent loss of weight. Pride in personal appearance should be encouraged.

5. The drug regimen should be carefully planned for the patient so that antiemetics are given prior to treatment. A fluid balance chart should be maintained if vomiting is severe, and four-hourly reassessment of the situation is necessary. The environment should be free from sights, smells and sounds which could cause nausea. If the particular drugs predispose to constipation, a mild aperient may be given to prevent this situation occurring.

6. Ensure that the doctor's request for a blood count has been carried out, and that the results are available before treatment is carried out, and between treatments.
   a. Check the patient's skin, mouth and throat daily for signs of bleeding.
   b. Record the patient's temperature daily.
   c. Avoid intramuscular injections. If they are unavoidable, apply firm site pressure afterwards.
   d. Warn the patient to avoid cuts and, for a man, suggest the use of an electric razor.

7. Assess pressure areas on a regular basis, using either a recognized scale, or one which has been formulated particularly for the needs of this type of patient. Encourage the patient to move and change position, and provide suitable aids to prevent pressure (see Prevention of Pressure Sores, p. 30).

8. Promote the comfort of the patient by ensuring adequate facilities and help with washing, bathing and elimination. Frequent mouthwashes and treatment for oral *Candida albicans* should be given. Clean linen should be provided regularly, and a duvet rather than blankets used if this is

more comfortable. Provide plenty of fluids which are most suitable for the patient, avoiding sour drinks.

Evaluation
EXPECTED OUTCOMES

1. Patient will feel both physically and psychologically prepared to have chemotherapy. He will have received sufficient information to allow him to participate in his own care.

2. Patient will be provided with a wig at the beginning of treatment. This will give him confidence to interact with others and feel socially acceptable.

3. Gastrointestinal problems will be minimized.

4. Signs of bone marrow depression will be detected early and appropriate action will be taken.

5. Patient's skin will remain intact. Any potential problems will be treated.

6. Patient will be comfortable and pain-free, and the oral mucosa will be intact.

RADIATION DIAGNOSIS AND THERAPY

Radiation is frequently used in diagnosing and treating cancer.

SOURCES OF RADIATION

1. Naturally occuring radioactivity, e.g. radium.
2. Artificially produced radioactivity, e.g. radioisotopes.
   a. X-ray machines.
   b. Teletherapy.
   c. Implants and applicators, e.g. caesium, iridium.
   d. Unsealed radioactive sources, e.g. iodine; intracavity, e.g. gold.

DEFINITIONS

1. Nuclide – any atomic entity capable of existing for a measurable lifetime, usually more than 10^{-9} seconds.
2. Radionuclide (radioactive nuclide) – one that disintegrates with the emission of particular or electromagnetic radiations.
3. Radioactivity – the disintegration of the atom which gives up energy in the form of rays or particles.
4. Isotope – an element whose nucleus contains a

fixed number of protons but has a differing number of neutrons, thereby changing its weight.

a. Optimal ratio between proton and neutrons is stable.

b. By using nuclear reactors, it is possible to bombard a stable isotope with additional free neutrons.

c. Most radioisotopes emit:

   (i) Particulate radiation – small fragments of the nucleus having mass and size (alpha and beta particles).

   (ii) Electromagnetic radiations – rays that have no mass (X-rays).

5. Radioactive decay or disintegration:

a. The rate of decay varies from isotope to isotope.

b. 'Half-life' or decay rate is the time required to reduce a particular radioactive substance by one-half of its atoms, thereby reducing it to half of its initial activity.

   Example: radium-225 – half-life of over 1,600 years.

c. A radioisotope administered to a patient in unsealed form has a relatively short life and is essentially inactive after therapeutic use has been completed.

   Example: iodine-131 – half-life about eight days.

d. Longer-lasting isotopes are implanted temporarily in the patient in a sealed container.

   Example: caesium-137 – half-life 32 years.

6. Alpha-rays. These are the least penetrating form of ionizing radiation. They comprise of two protons and two neutrons.

7. Beta-rays. These are comprised of electrons and are fast-moving particles. Used for skin lesions, breast wall tumours etc.

8. Gamma-rays. These rays are very penetrating, and are emitted in short wavelengths. Used to treat tumours of the bladder, bronchus, bowel etc.

9. Epilation. The hair follicles are destroyed, so causing the hair to fall out. This effect may be temporary or permanent.

10. Erythema. This is caused by vasodilation in the dermis. The skin becomes red and sore, and may blister.

11. Desquamation. Dry or moist skin, which peels off.

12. Necrosis. Death of healthy tissue caused by radiation damage.

13. Telangiectasia. Dilated capillaries giving the appearance of blood blisters on the surface of the skin.

14. Tenesmus. Painful passing of a stool.

15. Radiation enteritis. Inflammation of the small intestine due to radiotherapy.

16. Proctitis. Inflammation of the rectum due to radiotherapy.

17. Simulation. This is a diagnostic X-ray taken before the commencement of treatment, within treatment conditions. From the information received, a paper representation of the treatment is planned and charted.

18. Units of measurement (activity):

a. Bequerel (Bq) – basic unit for measuring the amount of activity in a radioactive sample.

19. Units for measuring radiation exposure or absorption:

a. Gray (Gy) – unit to measure absorbed dose (1 gray = 100 rads).

b. Sievert (Sv) – units of measurement of radiation, dose equivalent, which relates to biological effectiveness.

c. A useful unit is the mega-bequerel (MBq), which is 10^6 bequerels.

BIOLOGICAL ASPECTS AND CLINICAL APPLICATION
Nature and indications for use

1. Individualized to produce effective ionization within a tumour while avoiding unnecessary irradiation of normal structures.

2. a. Low voltage – keV (thousand electron volts).
   b. Super voltage – MeV (million electron volts).

3. Tissues most likely to respond to radiation exposure – those originating from reticuloendothelial tissues (leukaemia, lymphomas) and those from embryonal tissues (teratomas).

4. Tissues least likely to respond – bone and muscle.

Factors affecting the benefit of radiation exposure vs risk of tissue damage

1. *Dose rate* – a prescribed dose causes less tissue destruction if given in small amounts over a long period of time rather than given all at once.

2. *Area of body exposure* – the larger the area exposed, the greater the effect.

3. *Cell susceptibility:*

a. Greater susceptibility – rapidly dividing cells with no specialized function (e.g., lymphocytes and germ cells).

b. Lesser susceptibility – nondividing cells and highly differentiated cells (e.g., nerve or muscle cells).

4. *Biological variability* – individual differences play a role in human susceptibility. Examples:

a. Healthy person more responsive than malnourished individual.
b. Skin is especially vulnerable to radiation injury.
c. Bone marrow is very radiosensitive; therefore, such damage is potentially the most lethal.
d. Radiation cataracts result from excessive eye exposure.
e. Lung fibrosis occurs following injudicious radiation of chest.

Symptoms of radiation syndrome – high level
Major portion of body exposed to large doses of irradiation in a short period of time.
1. Prodromal – nausea, vomiting, malaise.
2. Latent – symptoms subside.
3. Illness – general malaise, epilation (hair loss), haemorrhage (petechiae, nose-bleed), pallor, diarrhoea, inflammation of mouth and throat, leucopenia.
4. Recovery or death.

Symptoms of radiation syndrome – low level
Low levels of radiation over a long period of time.
Examples:
1. Radiologists – may acquire leukaemia.
2. Clock dial painters – may develop sarcomas (from radium-containing luminizing paint).
3. Gonad exposure to radiation – may affect progeny.

Radiological precautions during radiography or radiotherapy
1. No one is permitted in the room where a patient is undergoing radiography or radiotherapy.
2. Fail-safe mechanisms must be provided to avoid accidental exposure to radiation.
3. Appropriate lead shielding should be used to protect the patient's most vulnerable areas, e.g. lungs, gonads.

NURSING CARE OF THE PATIENT RECEIVING RADIOTHERAPY
Objectives
The patient will:
1. Be both mentally and physically prepared before treatment is begun.
2. Have had an opportunity to express his fears and anxieties regarding treatment.
3. Be given sufficient information to enable him to participate in his own care.
The nurse will understand the implications of radiotherapy, have an understanding of the side-effects and be able to anticipate and treat these accordingly, thus enhancing the comfort of the patient.

Assessment
The patient's problems may include:
1. Anxiety about the actual treatment and the side-effects associated with it.
2. Skin disorders, e.g. erythema, desquamation.
3. Nausea and vomiting during treatment.
4. Diarrhoea and bowel problems, e.g. proctitis.
5. Mucous membrane damage.
6. Pain.
7. Bone marrow depression.
8. Tiredness and depression.
9. Dietary problems.
10. Alopecia.
11. Bladder and urinary disturbances, e.g. frequency of micturition, cystitis, dribbling, haematuria.

Planning and implementation
1. a. Assess the level of understanding of the patient about radiotherapy, and offer the appropriate information. Allow time for discussion and reassurance.
   b. Take him to the radiotherapy area and introduce him to the staff before treatment commences.
   c. Explain that although he will be alone during actual treatment, he will be able to speak to the radiographer.
   d. Explain that treatment itself is not painful, and that it is important for him to remain still during this time, to allow the exact area to receive treatment.
2. a. Explain the skin changes that may occur during treatment, and that precautions will be taken to avoid aggravation of these, e.g. the treated area should:
      (i) Not be rubbed or scratched.
      (ii) Be protected from sunlight and heat.
      (iii) Only be washed with warm water. Soap and talcum powder should not be used as these may contain heavy metal particles which increase the effect of radiation on the skin.
   b. Avoid the use of adhesive tape to the skin.
   c. Encourage the patient to wear cotton clothing.
   d. Keep the room at a cool temperature.
   e. Use light bedclothes and a bedcradle if necessary.
   f. Evaluate the skin frequently. If serious

changes occur, treatment may have to be discontinued temporarily.

3. a. Avoid sights, smells and environment which may predispose to nausea and vomiting.
    b. Give antiemetics prior to treatment and on a regular basis.
    c. Monitor the fluid and electrolyte balance.
    d. Help the patient to select the most appropriate food, e.g. avoiding oily and spicy food.

4. a. Explain that it is normal for bowel changes to occur during and sometimes following treatment. But observations should be made for signs of severe diarrhoea and dehydration, colic, blood and mucus in the stools, and pain on passing a stool.
    b. Provide a suitable choice of diet, reducing the amount of vegetables, and avoid pulses, fruit and wholemeal bread during treatment.
    c. Give antidiarrhoeal medication as prescribed.
    d. If symptoms are severe, treatment may need to be discontinued temporarily.

5. a. Observe the state of the patient's mouth daily, looking for signs of candida, ulceration etc.
    b. Explain to the patient that he may experience taste aberrations during treatment.
    c. Administer aspirin gargles/mucilage if soreness is a problem.
    d. Provide a soft diet, if dysphagia is present.
    e. Encourage the patient to stop smoking, and drinking spirits and eating spicy foods, and to rinse his mouth after every meal with a mild mouth wash.

6. a. Monitor any pain which the patient is experiencing, and determine the type and cause, e.g. due to soreness of skin, colic or actual cancer pain, and carry out the appropriate nursing intervention, or administer the drugs which have been prescribed.
    b. Liaise with the radiotherapy department, so that necessary analgesia can be given at least half an hour before treatment.
    c. Give a mild sedative if necessary.
    d. Contact doctor if pain is persistent.

7. a. Observe the patient's skin for signs of bruising, telangiectasia.
    b. Note the results of the patient's blood count.
    c. Protect the patient from sources of infection, and record temperature, pulse and respiration rates.
    d. Avoid giving intramuscular injections.
    e. Encourage the patient to use an electric razor, to avoid the risk of skin damage.
    f. Record the appropriate observations if the

patient is having a blood transfusion to correct blood problems.

8. a. Explain to the patient that a feeling of tiredness and depression commonly occurs during and following radiotherapy treatment, and that you understand his worries.
    b. Allow the patient time to rest during the day.
    c. Ask doctor to prescribe a mild night sedation to ensure a good night's sleep.
    d. Restrict visitors if the patient is becoming very tired.

9. a. Provide dietary restrictions to relieve symptoms of radiation enteritis, e.g. it may be necessary to administer a diet free from gluten, protein or lactose to avoid or overcome absorption problems.
    b. Invite the dietitian to visit the patient and help in his choices.
    c. Vitamin supplements may be prescribed.
    d. Encourage fluids and food replacements, e.g. Complan, Build-up.
    e. If dietary disturbances are severe, nasogastric or parenteral feeding may be necessary.

10. a. A full explanation should be given to the patient that he will lose his hair from the area that is being treated. This may be a permanent loss and can be particularly distressing for the patient receiving cranial radiation.
    b. A wig should be ordered immediately, and women should be encouraged to wear an attractive head scarf until the wig arrives.

11. a. Offer the patient regular bed pans, commodes or ensure that the patient can get to the lavatory easily.
    b. Treat any urinary tract infections according to the doctor's wishes. Encourage good fluid intake.
    c. Ensure that the patient is not left in soiled linen.
    d. Ask the doctor to prescribe a drug to improve bladder muscle tone, if this is appropriate.
    e. Possibly restrict fluid intake during the latter part of the day to avoid nocturia.
    f. Reassure patient that haematuria is a common occurrence at this stage of treatment.

Evaluation
EXPECTED OUTCOMES

1. Patient feels both mentally and physically relaxed prior to treatment. He is able to discuss his fears and anxieties and will have been given a full explanation about his treatment.
2. Patient is free from skin manifestations and side-

effects. Any potential skin breakdown will have been detected and treated accordingly.

3. Patient is free from nausea and vomiting; any signs will have been treated accordingly.
4. Patient is free from diarrhoea.
5. Patient is free from oral mucosal damage.
6. Patient is pain-free.
7. Blood tests for signs of bone marrow depression will have been carried out, and necessary precautions and treatment given, so that adverse effects are prevented.
8. Patient is able to rest, sleep and feel relaxed.
9. Adequate nutritional levels have been maintained in a way which is acceptable and enjoyable for the patient.
10. If necessary, the patient has accepted his alopecia, and has maintained a pride in his appearance.
11. Patient is free from bladder and urinary problems, any potential problems having been identified early, and appropriate treatment initiated.

CRANIAL RADIATION

Patients receiving cranial radiation will have specific problems related to their treatment:
1. Alopecia has been discussed previously.
2. The patient may have signs of raised intracranial pressure, e.g. a rise in blood pressure, and decrease in respiration rate.
3. Other symptoms include nausea, vomiting, headache, fits. Dexamethasone, which reduces oedema, may be prescribed by the doctor to alleviate or reduce these symptoms. An anticonvulsant may also be prescribed.
4. After a few weeks, the patient may show signs of depression or even confusion. It is important to offer explanation and reassurance to both the patient and relatives; the latter may be particularly distressed at this change in personality.

EFFECTS OF RADIOTHERAPY ON FERTILITY, PREGNANCY AND SEXUALITY

It is devastating for any person to be faced with the knowledge that they have cancer and need radiotherapy treatment. However, it can be equally devastating to think that they may be rendered sterile following treatment; nurses should be fully aware of this problem.

Radiotherapy treatment *will* have an effect on the fertility of both men and women. Spermatogonia are radiosensitive, but mature spermatozoa are fairly radioresistant. Therefore the dosage of treatment will determine the effect. A similar effect occurs with women. If an area near the gonads is being treated, lead shields should be used for protection (this applies to both men and women). Infertility may not be permanent; normal function may return some time after treatment is completed.

If a woman who has had radiotherapy wishes to conceive – and provided that her fertility has not been impaired – she should wait for a period of two years. This will enable her to regain her strength, and for the doctor to monitor her disease.

If, however, she does become pregnant during this time, careful counselling will be given to enable her to decide whether or not to continue with the pregnancy. It is therefore very important that advice about contraception is given to all women of childbearing age who are receiving radiotherapy. The oral contraceptive pill may be contraindicated with some types of cancer which are hormone-dependent. Careful counselling and sympathy is needed for any woman in this situation.

Other sexual problems may include impotence in men, and lack of libido in both men and women.

It is important that the health care team gives appropriate information to patients about the possible side-effects of radiotherapy treatment. It is vital that all questions and anxieties are discussed. If a nurse is unable to give satisfactory answers, it is her responsibility to find a suitable person to help the patient.

RADIOISOTOPE THERAPY

TELETHERAPY
This utilizes gamma-rays from a radioactive source which is kept in a shielded unit and placed at a distance from the patient.
1. Radioisotope cobalt-60 delivers radiation similar to that produced by supervoltage X-ray apparatus. Emits gamma-rays. Half-life is five years.
2. Cobalt-60 therapy unit requires extra shielding because rays are being emitted constantly. Because gamma-rays cannot be absorbed entirely, personnel are advised to spend the minimum time in the area.
3. Advantages of cobalt over conventional X-rays:
   a. Skin problems are significantly reduced.
   b. Bone or cartilage involvement is lessened.
   c. Electronic circuits are not required.
4. Disadvantages of cobalt:
   a. Because it has a half-life of five years, it is necessary to replace the cobalt machine.
   b. Radiation energy cannot be varied.
   c. Cost of room shielding is high.

PLESIOTHERAPY
External moulds
A packaged and screened container in which a radioisotope can be placed and applied to the skin surface.

1. Cobalt can be applied in this manner to small areas, as in the treatment of carcinoma of the lip, larynx, ear, etc.
2. Yttrium-90 – emits gamma-rays; half-life 2.5 days; used for shallow irradiation of eye neoplasms. Can also be used for treatment of rheumatoid arthritis in injection form.
3. Strontium-90 – emits beta-rays; half-life 28 years; also used for irradiation of eye neoplasms.

Intracavity isotope therapy
1. Liquid isotopes introduced into the pleural cavity to treat malignant effusion, e.g. gold-198 – emits, gamma- and beta-rays; half-life 2.7 days; also used to treat carcinoma of the bladder.
2. Solid sources, e.g. caesium-137 – emits gamma-rays; half-life 32 years; used to treat gynaecological tumours of uterus and cervix.
3. Phosphorus-32 – emits beta-rays; half-life 14 days; used in polycythaemia rubravera.

Interstitial isotope therapy
1. Radioactive needles, seeds, tubes or wires can be implanted directly into tumour tissue, e.g. cobalt-60, caesium-137, gold-198 and irridium-192.
2. Implants may be temporary or permanent. They may be supplementary to surgery, or to external beam radiation.
3. Radioactive solutions may be injected directly into the tumour or surrounding tissue. Colloidal solution of radioactive gold-198 is one of the most commonly used solutions.

Internal irradiation
Oral ingestion of radioiodine-131 – used in carcinoma of the thyroid; emits beta- and gamma-rays; half-life eight days. It is possible to ablate the thyroid gland with radioactive iodine; following this, thyroid replacement therapy is necessary.

NURSING MANAGEMENT OF THE PATIENT RECEIVING RADIOISOTOPES

IDENTIFICATION OF THE PATIENT AS A RADIATION SOURCE
1. Place a radioactive symbol at the end of the bed or outside his room.
2. Identify the chart cover, doctor's and nurse's order sheets and special radiation instruction sheet with the radioactive symbol.
3. For patients receiving the most minute quantities of tracer radioisotopes, such identification (see above) is not necessary.
4. Personnel who may be exposed to penetrating radiation (X-rays or gamma rays) should wear radiation badges on front of the body.

RADIATION INSTRUCTION SHEET
1. Type of radioactivity used.
2. Time of insertion.
3. Anticipated time of removal.
4. Precautions to follow.
5. Whom to notify when in doubt or in an emergency.

FACTORS AFFECTING THE AMOUNT OF RADIATION
1. *Amount* of radioactivity present, 37, 74, 111mBq, etc.
2. The *distance* of the nurse from the patient.

Note: The inverse square law applies: doubling the distance from a radiation source cuts intensity received to one-fourth.

3. Amount of *time* spent in actual contact with patient.
4. Degree of *shielding* utilized.
   Chosen according to type of radiation – alpha, beta, gamma (Figure 18.2).
5. Amount of *body area exposed* to radiation.

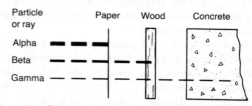

Figure 18.2. Relative penetration of alpha, beta and gamma radiation (source: US Atomic Energy Commission)

NURSING ALERT
During the period of greatest radioactivity (24 to 72 hours), limit amount of time spent with the patient to that required for essential care. Require patient to remain in his bed or room during course of treatment.

VITAL NURSING MEASURES IN CARING FOR THE PATIENT WITH INTERNAL RADIATION
Principles – speed, time, safety, distance, organization.

1. Be acquainted with the nomenclature describing dissipation of radioisotopes.
   a. *Physical half-life* – a constant rate in which one-half of radioactivity is dissipated in a given time.
   b. *Biological half-life* – the time it takes for a radio-isotope to disappear from the body via normal metabolic processes.
   c. *Effective half-life* – a combination of physical half-life and biological half-life.
2. Recognize that an isotope that is completely dispersed throughout the body (or a major portion of it) is less hazardous to an organ or tissue than an isotope concentrated by the body into a limited area.
3. Recognize that an isotope that is excreted rapidly is less hazardous than radium, which may be kept in the body for long periods.
4. Take appropriate measures associated with *sealed sources of radiation* implanted within a patient (sealed internal radiation).
   a. Do not remain within 1m of the patient any longer than required to give essential care.
   b. Know that the casing material absorbs all alpha radiation and most beta radiation, but that a hazard concerning gamma radiation may exist.
   c. Do not linger longer than necessary in giving patient care, even though all precautions are followed.
   d. Be alert for implants that may have become loosened (those inserted in cavities that have access to the exterior), e.g., check the kidney dish following mouth care for a patient with an oral implant.
   e. Notify the radiologist of any implant that has moved out of position.
   f. Utilize long-handled forceps or tongs and hold at arm's length when picking up any accidentally dislodged radium needle, seeds, tubes, etc., that may appear on dressings, bed, or floor. *Never pick up a radioactive source with your hands.*
   g. Do not discard any dressings or linens unless sure that no radioactive source is present.
   h. Wash hands with soap and water after caring for a patient who is being treated with a radioisotope. When wearing gloves, wash them with soap and water before removing them.

Note: This is not necessary for sealed sources.

   i. Encourage patients who are ambulatory to remain in their own rooms.
   j. Upon discharge of a patient, it is a good policy for the radiologist to check the room with a Geiger counter to be certain that all radioactive materials have been removed.
   k. Continue radiation precautions, when a patient has a permanent implant, until the radiologist declares precautions unnecessary. (See p. 1039 for nursing care of the patient receiving radiotherapy.)
5. Before removing a sealed source, e.g. caesium, give a full explanation to the patient about the procedure. Administer an analgesic or muscle relaxant prior to the removal of the implant. Entonox may also be appropriate.
6. Restrict visitors to two per patient. An explanation for this action should be given. Pregnant women and children under 16 should be discouraged from visiting.
7. Organization of nursing care is essential when caring for a patient with an internal source of radiation, so that the care is carried out within the time limits, and as few people as possible are involved.
8. Take appropriate measures associated with *unsealed sources*; radioactivity may be (1) widely spread in the body, (2) localized or (3) present in any body tissue or fluid.
   Examples:
   a. *Radioactive iodine.*
      (i) Circulates in bloodstream, excreted by kidneys – urine and blood contain radioactive material.
      (ii) Can be secreted by sweat glands.
      (iii) May be found in vomit of patient who recently took oral dose.
   b. *Radioactive colloidal gold.*
      (i) May be noted in wound seepage as pink, red or purple stain following intracavity injection.
      (ii) May be noted in small amounts in urine.
   c. *Radioactive phosphorus solution.*
      Be alert for contamination from excreta (urine and faeces) and vomitus.

IMMUNOTHERAPY

The immune system of the body has the ability to recognize and to defend itself against infection and invasion by foreign cells such as those of cancer. The immune system may be weakened or overwhelmed by the invasion of foreign cells so that it cannot function effectively.

Immunotherapy employs the immune mechanism of the body to combat cancer and overcome it. The immunotherapeutic approach to cancer is based on the fact that most tumours provoke an immune response (such as anti-tumour activity, production of tumour antigens) in the patient (host).

Although it is still considered investigational, significant research in immunotherapy is going on and progress is being made.

OBJECTIVES OF IMMUNOTHERAPY

1. To treat successfully the cancer patient.
2. To challenge and to induce mobilization of the patient's immune defences by utilizing a chemical or microbial agent to which the patient has previously been sensitized.
   a. This produces a delayed hypersensitivity response that can be employed against the cancer.
   b. Once developed in this way, immunocompetence (either alone or in combination with radiotherapy, chemotherapy or surgery) can fight the cancer.

VARIOUS APPROACHES TO IMMUNOTHERAPY
Active specific immunotherapy

1. Utilization of the patient's own immune mechanisms to reject or control his own malignant cells.
2. To date, active immunization, used alone, appears incapable of boosting the immune mechanism in the patient with advanced disseminated cancer.

Active nonspecific immunotherapy

1. Primarily activates macrophages and enhances delayed hypersensitivity of cellular immunity.
2. Utilization of bacteria or bacterial products as an immunological adjuvant to enhance the immune response.
   a. *BCG* is a live attenuated strain of tubercle bacillus.
   b. *C. parvum* is a killed anaerobe.
3. These agents are easy to distribute widely, and the responses achieved in patients with melanoma and several other solid tumours, as well as acute leukaemia, make them attractive for a large number of therapy protocols.

Passive-adoptive immunotherapy

1. Utilization of the immunity of a competent donor.
2. The use of hyperimmune serum for rubella (pass-

ive) or for immunodeficiency diseases (adoptive) appears possible.

Example: immune RNA and lymphocyte transfer factor (LTF).
3. Again, further study is needed.

Adjunctive immunotherapy

Because the above immunotherapeutic approaches appear inadequate, immunotherapy may be best utilized as an adjunct to other methods (and even following curative methods, to eliminate the few remaining malignant cells).

1. *Immunotherapy and surgery*.
   a. Following surgical removal of the bulk of a tumour, immunotherapy may be effective in attacking small foci of cancer cells.
   b. Whereas surgery is directed towards larger primary tumours, immunotherapy can control small foci of metastatic disease at distant sites.
2. *Immunochemotherapy*.
   a. Timing is critical in successfully combining immunotherapy with chemotherapy.
   b. Cancer chemotherapeutic drugs are often immunosuppressive, but certain chemotherapeutic agents actually stimulate the immune response to some antigens.
3. *Immunoradiotherapy*.
   a. A problem associated with chemotherapy and radiotherapy is that they attack normal cells as well as cancer cells; because of the selectivity of immunotherapy, it could logically be combined with these other methods.
   b. If the patient is given tumour-specific antibodies that are attached to isotopes, large doses of radiation could be directed to tumour cells; this would combine the destructive effects of radiation with the specificity of immunotherapy.

BIOLOGICAL RESPONSE MODIFIERS

Biological response modifiers are agents or approaches which modify the relation between tumour and host with the aim of providing therapeutic benefit. The refinement and evolution of immunotherapy to biological response modifiers has been made possible by advances in genetic engineering and hybridoma technology. The production of large amounts of relatively pure biological agents has become available for clinical trials. Interferons are prototypes of biological response modifiers.

Biological response modifiers which have been used in clinical trials include:

1. *Interferon:* this is a major determinant of natural kill cells, the main function being to inhibit viral and cellular replication. This is a normal response of lymphocytes to all viral infections.
2. *Immunomodulating agents:* nonspecific immuno-therapeutic agents.
3. *Lymphokines and cytokines:* low molecular weight lymphocytes, for example, interleukin 2.
4. *Thymosins:* belong to the group of active, non-specific immunotherapy. It plays a part as a thy-mic hormone by converting featureless null cells into T cells.
5. *Antigens:* manipulated to stimulate immunity, for example, irradiation is used to weaken the viabil-ity of tumour cells and then the patients are treated with extracts of their own tumour cells.
6. *Monoclonal antibodies:* these have a role in localiz-ing the tumour and also have the potential to act as tumour markers. There is also a possibility of chemotherapy and radiotherapy targeting. They have also been used in the purging of autologous bone marrow before it is reintroduced into the patient.

Modifiers may be administered orally, intralesion-ally, intradermally, intravenously or intravesically. Local, systemic or allergic side-effects may occur.

NURSING MANAGEMENT

1. Patient education to ensure that patient and fam-ily members understand purpose of treatment.
2. Monitoring and management of side-effects related to treatment.

BONE MARROW TRANSPLANTATION

Bone marrow transplantation is a therapeutic option in acute lymphocytic leukaemia (second remission), acute non-lymphocytic leukaemia (first and second remission) and chronic myelogenous leukaemia (primary chronic phase).

It is the only potentially curative treatment for chronic myelogenous leukaemia and acute non-lymphocytic leukaemia in second remission. Best results are achieved in the chronic phase of chronic myelogenous leukaemia. It allows for higher doses of cytotoxic drugs and radiation to be administered to eliminate the disease.

There are two types:

1. Allogeneic transplants, usually from a sibling.
2. Autologous transplants in which the patient's own marrow is reinfused.

Marrow ablative doses of chemotherapy and/or total body irradiation are administered, followed by the intravenous reinfusions of the previously harvested marrow cells.

The problems that occur in transplantation are:

1. Graft-versus-host (G-V-H) disease.
2. Infection.
3. Graft rejection.

MEDICAL AND NURSING MANAGEMENT OF TREATMENT COMPLICATIONS

Leukostasis

1. Signs and symptoms:
   a. Increased intracranial pressure and respir-atory dysfunction.
2. Medical management:
   a. Administration of fluids, allopurinol and chemotherapy.
   b. Prophylactic radiation to the central nervous system and mechanical removal of blast cells by leucopheresis may be prescribed.
3. Nursing management:
   a. Assessment of changes in clinical status.
   b. Patient education, including reasons for im-mediate intervention.
   c. Emotional support to patient and family.

Bleeding

1. Signs and symptoms:
   a. Petechiae and bruising.
   b. Disseminated intravascular coagulation with bleeding gums, epistaxis, menorrhagia, haematuria and gastrointestinal bleeding.
2. Medical management:
   a. Monitoring of signs and symptoms of in-creased bleeding.
   b. Replacement of clotting factors by the admin-istration of fresh frozen plasma or coagulation factors.
   c. Chemotherapy to control the underlying disease.
3. Nursing management:
   a. Assessing changes in patient's condition and initiating early intervention.
   b. Monitoring blood counts and coagulation studies.

c. Minimizing blood loss.
d. Assessing blood loss.
e. Educating patient and family, including reasons for treatment.
f. Offering emotional support.

Infection

1. Signs and symptoms:
   a. Classic signs and symptoms of infection may be absent in the neutropenic patient.
   b. Elevated temperature is often the first or only sign.
2. Medical management: Broad-spectrum antibiotics which may be continued until marrow recovery, even if temperature returns to normal. Amphotericin may be added if the temperature is not controlled by antibiotics after one week.
3. Nursing management:
   a. Ensuring good hygiene and allowing patient opportunities to rest.
   b. Assessment and observation to identify infection at its earliest stage.
   c. Reduction of exposure to potential infections.
   d. Reverse barrier isolation if appropriate.

HYPERTHERMIA

Hyperthermia utilizes artificially induced high temperatures in the treatment of cancer. Heat kills malignant cells by inhibiting the production of DNA, RNA and protein. Tumour cells lack the ability to repair DNA damaged by heat. Tumours are often necrotic and outgrow blood supply, which leads to heat being trapped in the tumour and the sparing of normal tissue. Cells in the relatively radioresistant S-phase are killed and radiosensitized by heat. Hypoxic tumour cells may be more sensitive to heat. Heat increases the cells' need for oxygen by increasing the metabolic rate, which the blood supply cannot meet. Heat also inhibits the repair of radiation damage and thus increases the radiation effect. The addition of hyperthermia to chemotherapy may enhance cell-killing potential. Local heat can increase the effect of chemotherapy in a tumour by increasing the blood supply. It may also increase the permeability of cell membranes and allow greater drug penetration. Heat may also stimulate the immune system.

TREATMENT METHODS

Treatment may be:
1. Local or regional.
2. Whole-body hyperthermia.

Local or regional

The heat may be produced by radiofrequency, microwaves or ultrasound. Probes may be inserted into the tumour or the patient may sit in a cylindrical machine. Regional heating has been tried using heated blood for treatment of extremities. Perfusing organs with heated solution has also been used.

Whole-body hyperthermia

Whole-body hyperthermia has been used to treat widespread disease. Temperature in excess of 42°C is not used in order to avoid heat necrosis. The patient may be immersed in heated water, hot paraffin wax or a heated suit.

Nursing management

Potential problems in whole-body hyperthermia include fatigue, hypotension, peripheral neuropathy, nausea, vomiting and diarrhoea. Sedation and fluid replacement are usually required.
1. Patient education is required to ensure that patient understands the reasons for the treatment and the specific method of heating.
2. When probes are used, a dry dressing may be applied and the site should be inspected for signs of infection.
3. Constipation should be prevented as heat may be retained in the stools.
4. Patients need to be carefully observed during treatment and fluid intake should be encouraged after treatment.

CARE OF THE PATIENT WITH ADVANCED CANCER

Objectives

1. The patient with advanced cancer is aware of and has accepted his problems. He is able to talk about these and discuss his fears and anxieties with the person that he wishes to talk to.
2. The patient's physical problems are identified and treated accordingly, enabling him to enjoy the optimum quality of life in his own manner.

Assessment

The problems may include:

1. Frustration because of loss of physical strength and independence, and inability to pursue purposeful or diversional activities.
2. The patient may be unable to maintain adequate nutritional levels (see Nutrition and the Cancer Patient p. 1026).
3. Discomfort and pain should be assessed frequently, using a pain assessment chart.
4. Inability to sleep.
5. Inability of the patient to maintain personal hygiene due to weakness, paralysis, pain, lethargy.
6. The patient may experience foul odours from wound/tumour breakdown, vaginal or rectal discharges.
7. Difficulty with breathing due to increased bronchial secretions, or an irritating cough.
8. Side-effects from radiotherapy.
9. Difficulties with elimination.
10. The patient may be at risk from skin breakdown and pressure sores.
11. The patient may be at risk from haemorrhage.

Planning and implementation

1. Arrange for relatives, friends or staff to plan outings, walks or other activities with the patient. Encourage him to express any unfulfilled ambitions, and discuss ways of achieving these.

    Be aware that antisocial tendencies and withdrawal may occur, and help to restore patient's self-esteem when these episodes pass. Plan treatments and nursing intervention to allow uninterrupted time for pursuing special interests.
2. See Nutrition and the Cancer Patient, p. 1026.
3. a. In conjunction with the medical staff plan the type and frequency of suitable analgesic, anti-inflammatory, sedative or other drugs to prevent pain and discomfort, after looking carefully at the pain assessment chart kept by the patient. 'Pain is what the patient says it is, and he experiences it when he says he does' (McCaffery, 1972).
    b. Reassess the efficacy of the drug regimen, and consult with the medical staff in increasing the dose or frequency as required. The nurse should observe the patient for signs of clock-watching. This can be an indication the pain is not fully controlled. Watch for difficulty and reluctance in moving and observe facial expression.
    c. Assess the possibility of pain due to causes other than cancer, such as constipation, retention of urine and muscular spasm, and initiate appropriate nursing measures.
    d. The use of a syringe driver to administer drugs continuously, often removes a fear from the patient that his next dose of drugs may be delayed, and so help him to relax.
    e. Most importantly, the nurse should listen to the patient, reassure him that she understands his pain, and is working with him to achieve the most effective way of preventing it.
4. It is essential that the patient achieves a full night's sleep, free from pain (see Drugs Used For Pain Control, Table 18.3, p. 1049, Helping the Patient to Rest and Sleep, p. 40).
5. a. Assist the patient with bathing or washing.
    b. Offer the patient fresh nightwear, and ensure a good supply of fresh bed linen.
    c. Keep the room at a temperature most acceptable to the patient.
6. Plan to provide an odour-free environment.
    a. Ascertain the source of the odour. Help the patient to maintain a high standard of personal hygiene.
    b. Provide good ventilation, and the use of air fresheners as necessary.
    c. Provide ample clean linen.
    d. When changing dressings:
        (i) Arrange the time carefully, to avoid meal times and visiting times.
        (ii) Consider the use of anti-odour dressings, e.g. charcoal.
        (iii) Remove soiled dressings promptly.
        (iv) Use close fitting dressings for fistulae, e.g. colostomy bags.
    e. Antiseptic douches can be used for a patient with rectal or vaginal discharge.
    f. Help the patient to come to terms with the situation. Avoid facial expressions which can make the patient feel embarrassed.
7. An irritating cough or difficulty with breathing can cause great distress to the patient.
    a. Position the patient in a position most comfortable for him and use sufficient and appropriate pillows.
    b. Encourage the physiotherapist to visit the patient and assist with breathing exercises etc.
    c. Administer humidifiers to loosen secretions.
    d. For an irritating cough, give a prescribed cough suppressant or analgesic.

e. If there is noisy breathing due to increased bronchial secretions, give prescribed drug, e.g. hyoscine, and also gentle suction if this is tolerated by the patient.

8. a. Radiation sickness – administer sedatives, antiemetics, and antihistamines as prescribed. Encourage a good fluid intake.

   b. Offer small frequent meals, and record any vomiting.

   c. Observe skin for signs of erythema or moist desquamation.

   d. Keep skin clean, use only warm water. Do not use perfumed soap or talc.

   e. Treat dry red skin with topical hydrocortisone cream.

   f. Offer medicated mouth washes as required.

   g. Protect skin from heat and sunlight, and encourage patient to wear loose-fitting clothing.

   h. Give antidiarrhoeal medication if necessary, and avoid foods which aggravate the problem, e.g. stewed fruit.

   i. Bone marrow depression means that the patient is very vulnerable to infection. Watch for an increase in temperature and for signs of bleeding. Be aware of the patient's blood count.

9. a. Assess any problems the patient has with elimination, and keep a chart if incontinence is a problem.

      See Helping a Patient with Elimination, in Rehabilitation Concepts, Chapter 2.

10. a. Encourage the patient to change position regularly, or turn him two-hourly if he is unable to move himself.

    b. Provide aids to relieve pressure, e.g. special mattresses, sheepskins, etc.

    c. Control oedema of extremities by elevating the feet, and use a bed cradle to relieve pressure.

11. a. Ensure that staff are aware of the risk of haemorrhage in certain patients.

    b. Monitor vital signs to detect increase in pulse rate and drop in blood pressure.

    c. Apply pressure if active bleeding occurs, or employ other emergency haemorrhage control methods.

    d. Note and record approximate amount of blood loss, and notify doctor.

    e. Comfort and reassure patient, and remove stained linen.

    f. Prepare patient and equipment for platelet or whole blood transfusion, or cauterization or ligation as necessary.

Evaluation
EXPECTED OUTCOMES

1. Patient's quality of life remains purposeful until his death.
2. Patient maintains adequate nutritional levels.
3. Patient is free from pain, or in control of his pain.
4. Patient is both mentally and physically relaxed and able to sleep.
5. Patient is assisted to maintain, or maintains his own, high standard of personal hygiene.
6. Patient is odour-free, and therefore not embarrassed, and feels socially acceptable.
7. Patient is able to breathe without difficulty or discomfort, and is free from noisy breathing.
8. Patient experiences minimal side-effects from radiotherapy.
9. Patient is in control of elimination functions, or appropriate measures are taken to achieve comfort.
10. Skin remains intact, and the patient is free from pressure sores.
11. Signs of haemorrhage are detected early, and staff will carry out appropriate procedures.

PAIN CONTROL

ANALGESIC DRUGS

1. Non-opioid drugs. These include aspirin, paracetamol, naproxen.
2. Weak opioid drugs. These include codeine, dihydrocodeine, dextropropoxyphene, pentazocine.
3. High-efficacy opioid drugs, including morphine, diamorphine, methadone, pethidine, omnopon.

It is a myth that all cancer patients need strong opioid drugs, but these should be freely available if needed, as they are an excellent method of controlling cancer pain.

Many people believe that patients become addicted to such drugs. However, they will be administered in adequate dosages which will be carefully increased as necessary. If a patient is repeatedly asking for more drugs, this is because the drug itself is not effective for the type of pain which the patient is experiencing, or the dose is not large enough.

NURSING ALERT
Tolerance to opioid analgesia is slow to develop; however, nurses must realize that elderly, debilitated patients have increased sensitivity. Avoid this cycle: opioid drug → drowsiness → less food and fluid → dehydration → nausea and vomiting → increased pain more opioids → resumption of cycle.

It is not only analgesic drugs which can be used to control pain. Many others can be used as adjuvant therapy (Table 18.3).

NONPHARMACOLOGICAL METHODS OF PAIN CONTROL

1. Alcohol injections to block nerve pathways.
2. Localized radiotherapy.
3. Presacral neurectomy for visceral pain.
4. Cordotomy for intractable pain.
5. Neurosurgical nerve interruptions.
6. Local anaesthetic, e.g. lignocaine, applied topically.

Table 18.3   Drugs used to control pain

Drug	Action	Nursing implications
Muscle relaxants e.g. diazepam	Mental relaxation Emotional calm Relieves agitation	1. Occasional dizziness, confusion, drowsiness 2. Dry mouth 3. Observe for postural hypotension 4. Patient may develop a tolerance for the drug
Hypnotics e.g. temazepam	Induces and promotes sleep	1. This is a short-acting drug and therefore would be contraindicated in patients who normally wake early 2. A hangover or headache is uncommon with such a drug 3. Appropriate for elderly patients
Corticosteroids e.g. dexamethasone	Anti-inflammatory Gives the patient a feeling of well-being Increases appetite	1. If the patient is unable to take the prescribed dose of drug, the doctor should be informed immediately 2. Test urine regularly for glucose and protein 3. Observe for signs of gastric irritation 4. Observe vital signs and record daily 5. If patient is going home with these drugs, ensure he has a steroid card and understands fully point 1 6. Remember that steroids mask infection
Antidepressants e.g. amitriptyline	Elevates patient's mood Sedative action	1. Sedative action may be more intense at start of drug administration 2. Do not stop drug abruptly 3. Assess for dry mouth, postural hypotension, constipation 4. Observe for difficulty with micturition 5. Observe for signs of agitation, tremulousness, visual hallucinations
Nitrous oxide and oxygen (Entonox)	Fast-acting method of inducing analgesia Gives a feeling of well-being	1. A nurse should always be present when this is being used 2. Very useful for painful procedures e.g. catheterization, dressings

7. Massage.
8. Localized heat treatment.
9. Diversional therapy, e.g. music or relaxation.
10. Any other method which the patient may find helpful, such as reflexology, acupuncture.
11. Visualization.

PSYCHOSOCIAL SUPPORT OF THE DYING PATIENT

REACTIONS OF THE PATIENT TO DYING*
1. Period of denial allows patient to mobilize his defences.
2. Patient will exhibit withdrawal and avoidance of subject of death.
3. Usually a temporary defence to be replaced in time by partial acceptance.
4. Patient may talk of death and then change topic abruptly.
5. Patient may be in a temporary state of shock.

Stage of anger
1. Denial may be replaced by anger, rage, envy and resentment.
2. Anger may be displaced and projected into environment.
   a. Anger frequently directed at hospital staff. (Avoid reacting personally to this anger.)
   b. Try to tolerate rational and irrational anger. Patient may experience considerable relief in expressing anger.

Stage of bargaining
Bargaining is an attempt to postpone the inevitable and to extend life.

Stage of depression
1. This is a stage in which the patient is preparing himself to accept the loss of everything and every-one he loves.
2. Patient may be undergoing anticipatory grief to prepare himself for the final separation; may mourn the loss of meaningful people in his life.
   a. Allow the patient to express his sorrow – helps make the final acceptance easier.
   b. Sit with the patient.

* Adapted from Kübler-Ross, E. (1970) *On Death and Dying*, New York, Macmillan.

Stage of acceptance
1. Patient is neither depressed nor angry about his impending death; he bows to the sentence.
2. May contemplate his demise with quiet accept-ance and expectation – detachment may make death easier.
3. During this stage patient may be almost devoid of feelings – his circle of interest diminishes.
4. Patient will sleep and rest more – does not desire news or visitors from outside world.
5. Patient may just wish someone to hold his hand – reassures him that he is not forgotten.
6. Patient may reach the point where death comes as a relief.
7. Family may require more support during this stage.

CARE AND SUPPORT
Nursing a patient in the terminal stage of illness means that it is necessary to have a very positive approach to care, and also to take into consideration the emotional support needed not only for the patient but also for the relatives and carers. This includes the medical and nursing staff, who have usually formed a very special relationship with the patient and family. Mutual support is necessary at this time.

CARE AND SUPPORT OF THE PATIENT
Objectives
1. The patient has accepted the fact of impending death.
2. The patient has been given time to talk about death, and to express his fears and anxieties.
3. The spiritual needs of the patient are met.
4. The patient is able to achieve death with dignity.
5. The family and carers are given support.
6. The health care team caring for the patient are supported.

Assessment
1. The patient may feel isolated and lonely.
2. The patient may feel anxious and afraid about his impending death.
3. The patient may experience behavioural and per-sonality changes when faced with the prospect of death.
4. The patient may be holding on to false hopes.
5. The patient may have business affairs, un-resolved problems, problems with human relationships to settle before he dies.

6. The patient may have spiritual needs which need to be met before his death.
7. The patient may have day-to-day complaints which need attention.

Planning and implementation

1. a. Build up a good nurse/patient relationship. Use individualized patient care to allow the patient to become close to the nurse. Personal involvement is necessary if human interaction is to be supportive.
   b. Create a suitable environment for the patient. Ask the patient if he wishes to be nursed in a ward or in a side room. Dying patients sometimes want company, and do not want to be alone. If good pain and symptom control is achieved, the patient may express a wish to die at home. Full consideration and help should be given in this case.
   c. Make time for the patient; he needs the feeling of care and support.
   d. Allow unrestricted visiting. The presence of relatives will help to take away some of the feeling of isolation. If the patient is in a side room, a comfortable camp bed may be provided for the spouse/partner to stay during the night if desired.
2. Allow the patient to talk freely about death if he wishes. Encourage him to explore his feelings or fears and be prepared to share one's thoughts if asked. Some patients may find talking about death very difficult, and may prefer to write down their thoughts. The patient may ask the nurse to talk to his family as he feels unable to start to bring up this difficult subject.
3. Ensure that staff and relatives are aware that the patient may have a period of deep depression, or anger, or even aggression, and that they support him during this time. Reassure the patient that these feelings are normal and are understood.
4. Do not give the patient false hope when he has reached the stage of acceptance. This will only confuse him and he will not have peace of mind. If the patient has not reached the stage of acceptance, his hold on hope may be helping him, and should not be taken away.
   Discourage the family from giving the patient false hopes. Explain to them the importance of peace of mind and what it means to the patient.
5. Ask the patient if he has any outstanding affairs that need attention. Do not give the impression of prying into his personal affairs, but offer to arrange any help that is required, such as the social worker or legal counsellor.

6. The patient should have been asked about his religious belief during the initial assessment, and should be asked if he wishes someone from his church/community to visit him. If the patient has not been in contact with any religious group for many years, he may find great help from the hospital chaplain who makes regular visits to everyone in the ward, and rediscover some long forgotten beliefs from childhood.
7. Be prepared to accept criticism from the patient, who may be irritable and discontented at times; in particular, show great patience when getting him into a really comfortable position. Allow the patient to make decisions about what he wishes to do.

CARE OF THE FAMILY AND CARERS

Assessment

1. The family/carers may be experiencing anticipatory grief.
2. The needs and feelings of the family need to be understood by others in the health care team.
3. The family may wish to participate in patient care.
4. The family will be faced with practical problems and decisions prior to, and following, the patient's death.

Planning and implementation

1. a. The nurse should try to build up a good relationship with the family/carers, and respect their opinions about management of care.
   b. Identify the stages that the family are going through, e.g. anger, guilt, depression, etc. Reassure them that these are normal reactions to the situation.
   c. Be nonjudgemental about the family; offer help and support, both personally and with the help of other professionals, volunteers or self-help groups.
2. a. Accept feelings and attitudes of the family, which can include ambivalent feelings towards the dying member, overt or suppressed hostility interwoven with guilt feelings or self-blame.
   b. Projection of these feelings on to medical or nursing staff.
   c. Submission or excessive courtesy may mask hostility. Recognize that all members of a family may react differently, and that apparent lack of interest may mask deep emotional feelings.

3. Ensure that the family understand that they are very welcome to participate in any part of the care of the patient that they wish to. This may be just giving drinks, for example, but it can also include helping with a bed bath or any other procedures. This will help them to feel that they are still a part of the patient's life, and that it has not been taken away from them by professionals.

Allow the family to have time and privacy with the patient. Also, encourage them to talk to the patient if he is unconscious, and to hold his hand.

4. Be aware that the family may be anticipating financial problems, and may worry about the formalities and arrangements that have to be made after death. Be able to give them any information that they request, and arrange for them to see the social worker, particularly if they are experiencing financial hardship with frequent or long-distance travelling to the hospital.

Do not let them feel embarrassed about asking very basic questions about making a will, registering a death and funeral arrangements. Assure them that help will be available, and that they are always welcome to contact or return to see the ward staff at any time.

After the patient's death, explain that bereavement counselling is available, and give names and telephone numbers of appropriate people.

Evaluation
EXPECTED OUTCOMES
1. The patient has a sense of security and trust.
2. The patient has peace of mind and a feeling of acceptance.
3. The patient is assured that his behaviour, fears and feelings are normal at this time and are understood and accepted by family and staff.
4. The patient has been able to finalize and put into order any affairs and achieved his goals.
5. Any complaints or grievances are dealt with, and the patient is satisfied that action has been taken.
6. The family are allowed to grieve and react in the manner in which they wish, and reassured that this is normal and acceptable.

CARE OF THE HEALTH CARE TEAM

Assessment
1. The health care team may find it difficult to come to terms with the death of a patient.
2. The health care team may withdraw from the presence of death.

Planning and implementation
1. a. Identify one's own feelings about death and dying. One cannot help the patient fully until this has happened, and the carer can accept her own mortality.
   b. Encourage other members of the team to discuss their own feelings, and allow a respite from the situation if they are feeling overwhelmed.
   c. Ensure that all staff have adequate rest, relaxation and recreation, and perhaps arrange for a social outing or break if there has been a particularly difficult time.
   d. Assess and correct one's own biases and fears.
   e. Watch emotional responses to the challenge of incurable disease and 'difficult families'.
2. a. Help staff to realize the inevitability of death as a completion of life. It is normal for fears and anxieties to occur to everyone, and these should be faced and openly discussed.
   b. Ensure that nobody is afraid or ashamed of asking for help, and that this is forthcoming in whatever form is necessary.

Evaluation
EXPECTED OUTCOMES
1. The family and carers have been able to participate in whatever way they wished in the care of the patient, to give them a feeling of comfort.
2. The patient, family, carers and staff have been able to explore, face up to, express and discuss their feelings to one person or in a group, and have gained emotional strength and insight from this.

FURTHER READING

BOOKS
General

Barker, G.H. (1983) *Chemotherapy of Gynaecological Malignancies*, Castle House, Tunbridge Wells, Kent.

— (1986) *Basic Gynaecological Oncology*, Castle House, Tunbridge Wells, Kent.

Becker, T.M. (1981) *Cancer Chemotherapy. A Manual for Nurses*, Little Brown, Boston.

Beyers, M., Durburg, S. and Werner, J. (1984) *Complete Guide to Cancer Nursing*, Edward Arnold, London.

Bouchard-Kurtz, R. and Speese-Owens, N. (1981) *Nursing Care of the Cancer Patient*, C.V. Mosby, London.

Burns, N. (1982) *Nursing and Cancer*, W.B. Saunders, Eastbourne.

Capra, L. (1984) *Care of the Cancer Patient*, Macmillan, London.

Chernecy, C. and Ramsey, P. (1984) *Critical Care of Nursing the Client with Cancer*, Appleton Century Crofts, New York.

Green, J.A. *et. al.* (1983) *Medical Oncology Pocket Consultant*, Blackwell Scientific, Oxford.

Johnson, B.L. and Gross, J. (1985) *Handbook of Oncology Nursing*, John Wiley, Chichester.

Leahy, I., Germain, J. and Varricchio, C. (1979) *The Nurse and Radiotherapy, A Manual for Daily Care*, C.V. Mosby, London.

Lochead, J. (1983) *Care of the Patient in Radiotherapy*, Blackwell Scientific, Oxford.

Lowry, S. (1974) *Fundamentals of Radiation Therapy*, English Universities Press, Sevenoaks, Kent.

Marks-Maran, D. and Pope, B. (1985) *Breast Cancer and Counselling*, Blackwell Scientific, Oxford.

Regnard, C. and Davies, A. (1986) *A Guide to Symptom Relief in Advanced Cancer* (2nd edn), Haigh & Hochland, Manchester.

Royal Marsden Hospital (1988) *Clinical Nursing Procedures* (2nd edn), Harper & Row, London.

Tiffany, R. (1988) *Oncology for Nurses and Health Care Professionals* (2nd edn), Vols 1 & 2, Harper & Row, London.

— (1978) *Cancer Nursing Medical*, Faber & Faber, London.

— (1979) *Cancer Nursing Radiotherapy*, Faber & Faber, London.

— (1980) *Cancer Nursing Surgical*, Faber & Faber, London.

— (1981) *Cancer Nursing Update*, Baillière Tindall, Eastbourne.

Yasko, J.M. (1980) *Care of the Client Receiving External Radiation Therapy*, Prentice-Hall, Englewood Cliffs, NJ.

— (1983) *Guidelines for Cancer Care*, Prentice-Hall, Englewood Cliffs, NJ.

Terminal care

Charles-Edwards, A. (1986) *The Nursing Care of the Dying Patient*, Beaconsfield Publications, Beaconsfield.

Doyle, D. (1983) *Coping with a Dying Relative*, Macdonald, London.

— (1984) *Palliative Care. The Management of Far Advanced Illness*, Croom Helm, Beckenham, Kent.

Hector, W. and Whitfield, S. (1982) *Nursing Care for the Dying Patient and the Family*, Heinemann, London.

Kubler-Ross, E. (1975) *Death. The Final Stage of Growth*, Simon & Schuster, New York.

McCaffery, M. (1983) *Nursing the Patient in Pain*, Harper & Row, London.

Neuberger, J. (1987) *Caring for Dying People of Different Faiths*, Austin Cornish, London.

Parkes, C.M. (1986) *Bereavement. Studies of Grief in Adult Life*, Tavistock Methuen ABP, London.

Regnard, C. and Davies, A. (1986) *A Guide to Symptom Relief in Advanced Cancer*. Haigh & Hochland, Manchester.

Robbins, J. (1989) *Care for the Dying Patient and Family* (2nd edn), Harper & Row, London.

Saunders, C. and Baines, M. (1983) *The Management of Terminal Disease*, Oxford University Press, Oxford.

Saunders, C. (1984) *Management of Terminal Malignant Disease*, Edward Arnold, London.

Spilling, R. (1986) *Terminal Care at Home*, Oxford University Press, Oxford.

Stott, N. and Finlay, L. (1984) *Care of the Dying*, Churchill Livingstone, Edinburgh.

Twycross, R. (1984) *Oral Morphine in Advanced Cancer*, Beaconsfield Publications, Beaconsfield.

Twycross, R. and Lack, S. (1983) *Symptom Control in Far Advanced Cancer. Pain Relief*, Pitman, London.

— (1984) *Therapeutics in Terminal Cancer*, Churchill Livingstone, Edinburgh.

ARTICLES

Alternative medicine

Dobbs, B.Z. (1985) Alternative health approaches, *Nursing Mirror*, Vol. 160, No. 9, pp. 41–2.

Sims, S.E.R. (1987) Relaxation (selective review of literature), *Journal of Advanced Nursing*, Vol. 12, No. 5, pp. 583–91.

Chemotherapy

Speechley, V. (1987) Recent advances in cancer chemotherapy, *Nursing*, Vol. 3, No. 20, pp. 743–7.

Warren, K. (1988) 'Will I be sick, nurse?' *Nursing Times*, Vol. 84, No. 11, pp. 30–2.

Nursing care

David, J. (1987) Quality measure for oncology nursing, *Senior Nurse*, Vol. 6, No. 4, pp. 42–5.

Douglas, S. (1985) Crisis in care – the most stressful speciality, *Nursing Times*, Vol. 161, No. 18, pp. 32–4.

Fitzgerald, V. and Sims, R. (1987) A positive approach, *Nursing Times, Community Outlook*, Vol. 83, No. 45, pp. 16–21.

Gabriel, J. (1987) Improving care in oncology out-patients, *Senior Nurse*, Vol. 7, No. 4, pp. 8–9.

Houlton, E. (1987) Coping with cancer at home, *Nursing*, Vol. 3, No. 20, pp. 752–4.

Lyall, J. (1988) Life after cancer, *Nursing Times*, Vol. 84, No. 11, pp. 26–9.

Meikle, J. (1987) Symptom control in the cancer patient, *Nursing*, Vol. 3, No. 20, pp. 739–42.

Richardson, A. (1987) A process standard for oral care, *Nursing Times*, Vol. 83, No. 31, pp. 38–40.

Webb, P. (1985) Getting to the heart of cancer, *Nursing Mirror*, Vol. 160, No. 5, pp. 40–2.

— (1987) Patient education, *Nursing*, Vol. 3, No. 20, pp. 748–50.

Webster, M. (1981) Communicating with dying patients, *Nursing Times*, Vol. 77, No. 23, pp. 999–1002.

Nutrition

Holmes, S. (1987) Nutritional problems in the cancer patient, *Nursing*, Vol. 3, No. 20, pp. 733–7.

Sutton, A. (1988) Dietetics supplement – cancer cachexia, *Nursing Times*, Vol. 84, No. 2, pp. 65–6.

Sexuality

Coughlan, V. (1987) Dear nurse, *Nursing Times*, Vol. 83, No. 42, pp. 32–4.

David, J. and Speechley, V. (1987) Scalp cooling to avoid alopecia, *Nursing Times*, Vol. 83, No. 32, pp. 37–8.

19

Care of the Ageing Person

Definitions

Ageing

A normal process of time-related changes that occur throughout life; old age is a normal part of human development and is the final phase of the life cycle.

Geriatrics

The branch of health science concerned with the study and treatment of problems and diseases associated with ageing.

Gerontology

The study of the ageing process and its effect on older people.

HEALTH MAINTENANCE AND PREVENTIVE CARE

Objective

Maintain a state of physical, mental and social well-being, and enable the individual to retain a state of independence in physical and psychological functioning.

1. Encourage forward planning for retirement in consultation with partner or family. This should include:
   a. Planning for retirement income. In addition to the state pension, contributory or noncontributory schemes are provided by many firms, or private insurance schemes are available.
   b. Planning for retirement housing. Full consideration must be given to this. A smaller house in the same area, which is easy to maintain, has adequate heating facilities and is within easy reach of a shopping area. It is unwise for aged people to move to some apparently 'ideal' location in the country or at the sea, where they have no relatives or friends, and where the demands on the social services may already be excessive.
   c. Attendance at preretirement courses (which cover the above and much more).
   d. Planning for retirement activities and hobbies.
2. Encourage a positive approach to health, by providing information about the facilities which are available for detecting signs indicating potential problems or diseases at a very early stage.

a. At special over-60s clinics for well people run by the local health authority or by general practitioners in health centres. The tests may include blood pressure reading, blood tests for anaemia, glucose level and blood urea estimation; chest radiograph, mammogram, urine testing; basic sight tests with referral for estimation of intraocular pressure if necessary.

Hearing tests and information about the provision of hearing aids, telephone accessories such as amplifiers and flashing light call indicators.

b. Health visitors who are attached to a general practice can identify all the old people registered with the doctor and provide information and help for those who have no need to visit the surgery, as well as those who attend for medical advice.

c. Because a person is old, it is not inevitable that they suffer from ill health. Any disorders should be treated.

3. Provide information about the high risk of accidents due to falls. These may be due to locomotor disabilities, environmental risks, poor lighting and poor eyesight, as well as pathological conditions. Help should be available to give advice about particular danger areas in any house and special equipment which can be provided to minimize these hazards. Working areas should be arranged so that bending down and stretching above head height are avoided. In the house ensure that there is easy access to toilet and baths.

To prevent falls:

a. Efforts must be made to ensure a steady gait.

b. Encourage the wearing of proper shoes rather than slippers.

c. Good foot care and chiropody services are essential.

d. Hands should be kept free for holding onto rails or supports rather than carrying articles.

4. Recreational activities should be encouraged. These may be run by a day centre, or by various social or welfare organizations. Occupational facilities at home should be discussed. Help with gardening can be very important for men, who often have difficulty in adjusting to retirement.

5. Statutory and voluntary services should be used. These include:

a. The primary health care team, i.e., general practitioner, who will be the key person in treating overt and latent physical and mental ill health; health visitor who gives health education advice and information about available services and benefits, and also identifies present and future problems; the community nurse who carries out care, possibly only helping with bathing or carrying out the complete care of a helpless patient. The community nurse identifies problems and initiates other services, e.g., home helps, Meals on Wheels. The community doctor acts as co-ordinator.

b. Chiropodist, optician and dental care.

c. Home helps – an hourly charge is made for this according to patient's income.

d. Meals on Wheels is a statutory service, but this may be supported financially and with voluntary support by Age Concern, WRVS, schools, etc. British Red Cross helps with transport, social clubs and visiting. Youth groups help with home decorating and gardening. Lunch clubs may be held in an old people's day centre, or in a residential home or in a village hall.

e. Day centres may be run by the social services department or by voluntary organizations. These provide meals at reduced prices, and occupational and recreational facilities. Volunteers may help with transport.

f. Day hospitals, which are usually run by the hospital, where, as well as the facilities which are available at the day centre, there is also medical assessment, bathing facilities, medical and nursing care and physiotherapy and occupational therapy. Transport facilities are provided by the ambulance service.

g. Good neighbour schemes. These are run by many different groups, e.g., churches, Women's Institutes, young wives groups; they have many different functions, the main one is to make contact with an elderly person who needs some sort of support, e.g., someone to talk to, help with shopping. An emergency call system, e.g., a card in the window, may be available. In any post office, there is a list of voluntary services available. Many areas have a branch of Age Concern, which organizes a great deal of help through various resources.

6. Financial help is available through social security. It must be explained that this is not charity but an entitlement. Rent or rate rebates, via the local authority, pay-as-you-go schemes for heating costs or additional supplementary benefit for heating costs.

7. For aged people who need continuous care in their own homes, a constant attendance allowance may be payable.

a. Outings and holidays – some social service

departments arrange subsidized or free holidays for the elderly, and various organizations have schemes (see p. 1068).

b. Travel concessions may vary in different areas, e.g., in greater London free bus travel is available. In other areas, a special card can be purchased, which entitles the holder to half-price fares. British Rail also reduce fares for this age group. It is important that older people keep in touch with their friends and relations, so full advantage should be taken of these concessions.

NUTRITIONAL CONSIDERATIONS FOR THE AGED

1. Nutritional requirements of the aged are similar to those of adults, except that energy intake should be reduced.
   a. Energy needs diminish with age, both metabolic rate and activity decrease, so that energy requirements of the aged are reduced.
   b. The energy intake is adjusted on an individual basis to maintain normal weight.
   c. Protein requirements are not reduced but protein utilization may be less efficient in old age.
   d. Calcium intake should be as great as that of a younger person – high incidence of osteoporosis in older women.
   e. Older people usually have inadequate intake of calcium, ascorbic acid and riboflavin due to insufficiency of milk, fruit and vegetables in the diet.
2. Nutritional deficiencies are frequently encountered in the aged.
   a. Vitamin C and K deficiencies – ecchymoses due to capillary fragility.
   b. Vitamin A deficiency – fissuring of skin around mouth.
   c. Vitamin B deficiency – glossitis, angular stomatitis, megaloblastic anaemia – B_{12} and folic acid deficiency.
   d. Vitamin D deficiency – osteomalacia.
   e. Mineral deficiencies – demineralization of bone.
3. Factors affecting nutritional habits of the aged.
   a. Food habits of a lifetime.
   b. Social factors (eating alone). Transport may be arranged to take the elderly patient to a day centre or lunch club.
   c. Food fads.
   d. Poor dental health; ill-fitting dentures.
   e. Shopping problems.
   f. Reduced income and financial problems; high cost of many protein foods.
   g. Lack of motivation for meal planning and food preparation.
   h. Decreased appeal of food – loss of taste buds; less acute sense of smell.
   i. Difficulty with preparation of food because of stiff hands and lack of mobility.
   j. Mental deterioration and memory loss – meals may be omitted.
4. Fluid intake should be at least 1.5 litres daily. It is essential that this is not decreased because of the fear of incontinence. This will aggravate the problem.

BODILY CHANGES ASSOCIATED WITH AGEING

GENERAL PRINCIPLES
1. Ageing occurs at all levels of bodily function – cellular, organic and systemic. Almost every organ loses functional capacity.
2. There is a reduction of reserve capacity due to actual loss of individual cells in various organ tissues of the body. The ageing body lacks reserve power (see below).
3. Ageing proceeds at different rates in different systems in the same individual.
4. In general, adjustment to physiological changes is made by reducing the level of activity.

CHANGES IN HOMEOSTASIS
Homeostasis is the ability of the body to restore equilibrium.
1. Decrease in functional capacity and efficiency of co-ordinating systems within the body.
2. Progressively limited capacity to respond to stress.
3. Diminution of functional reserve – person more vulnerable to disease, death more likely; more time required for body to return to normal after illness.
4. Temperature regulation less efficient, causing increased risk of hypothermia.

CHANGES IN THE NERVOUS SYSTEM
1. Progressive loss of brain cells and their fibres, brain compensates for this.
2. Progressive atrophy of the convolutions (gyri) of

the brain surface and consequent widening and deepening of the spaces (sulci) between the convolutions.
3. Decrease in blood flow to the brain.
4. Loss of postural reflexes causing unsteadiness of gait.
5. Slower reaction time; more time required for decision making.
6. Gradual failing of memory (particularly short-term memory).
7. Personality changes – appear to be related to blood supply to brain as well as to changes in nervous system.

CHANGES IN SKIN AND SUBCUTANEOUS TISSUES
1. Epidermis thins generally, although it may thicken in some areas.
2. Dermis becomes relatively dehydrated and loses strength and elasticity; skin is prone to excessive dryness and itching.
3. Blood flow to peripheral areas of body decreases.
4. Loss of subcutaneous fat gives characteristic appearance to skin – folds, lines, wrinkles, slackness.
5. Focal pigmentary discolorations occur.
6. Ecchymoses may appear – due to greater fragility of the dermal and subcutaneous vessels.
7. Sweating decreases.
8. Thickening and hardening of nails.

CHANGES IN MUSCULOSKELETAL SYSTEM
1. Lessening of muscular strength, endurance and agility.
2. Postural changes – from structural changes in ligaments, joints and bones. Ligaments calcify and ossify; joints stiffen from erosion of cartilaginous joint surfaces; ossification and degenerative changes occur in synovium (lining of joint cavities).
3. Increase in curvature of spine.
4. Bone changes – bones become porous and lighter and lose much of their density (see Osteoporosis, p. 862).

CHANGES IN THE SPECIAL SENSES
1. Vision – decrease in visual acuity and in ability to accommodate to light; falling off of lateral vision, receding clarity.
   Clinical problems include presbyopia (impaired vision due to ageing), senile cataract, glaucoma.
2. Hearing – loss of some hearing ability; inability to hear higher pitches; greater difficulty in hearing normal ranges of sound.

3. Voice – lower volume; slower rate of speech.
4. Smell and taste – dulling of sense of smell; decrease in number of taste buds.
5. Less acute sensations of touch; slowing of reflexes.

CHANGES IN THE CARDIOVASCULAR SYSTEM
Heart
1. Effectiveness of pumping action of heart is reduced.
2. Cardiac output and stroke volume decreases.
3. With diminishing cardiac reserve the heart reacts poorly to stress.
4. Fat deposits around heart may increase; thickening and loss of flexibility of valves due to sclerosis and fibrosis.
5. Blood flow through the coronary arteries may be lessened.

Vascular
1. Progressive chemical and anatomical changes in arteries, with an increase in cholesterol, other lipids and calcium.
2. Elastic fibres progressively straighten, fray, split and fragment.
3. As aorta becomes less elastic and there is increasing resistance to blood flow, systolic hypertension may develop.
4. Increased tendency to varicose veins.

CHANGES IN THE RESPIRATORY SYSTEM
1. Elasticity of lungs and chest wall decreases – partly due to an alteration in the structure of collagen. Calcification of cartilage of rib cage.
2. Less oxygen diffusion – due to increase in collagen and scar tissue in lung and to decrease in blood flow to the lung.
3. Reduction in amount of blood flow to lungs – contributes to dysrhythmias.
4. Decline in total lung capacity and concurrent increase in residual volume – producing decrease in function.

CHANGES IN THE GASTROINTESTINAL SYSTEM
1. Gastrointestinal function impeded by loss of teeth, impaired swallowing mechanism and diminishing gastric and enzyme secretions.
2. Tooth decay is increased because of decreased saliva.
3. Less absorption of nutrients and minerals.
4. Reduced motility of stomach.
5. Decreasing peristalsis – due to generalized weakness of muscle activity; constipation is a common complaint.

CHANGES IN THE URINARY SYSTEM

1. Decrease in kidney function and adaptability. (See p. 15 on Helping the Patient with Elimination, in Chapter 2, Rehabilitation Concepts.)
2. Reduction of blood flow to kidneys – due to decrease in cardiac output and increase in peripheral resistance.
3. Diminished filtration rate and tubular function.
4. Structural changes in kidneys. Loss of glomeruli may be 50 per cent.

METABOLIC CHANGES

1. Production of gonadal hormones is reduced; cortisol secretions decrease.
2. Decline in production of thyroid-stimulating hormone of pituitary and of thyroid hormones secreted by thyroid gland.
3. Glucose tolerance curve tends towards that of the diabetic. Reduced production of insulin.
4. Decline in ability to adapt or respond to stress.
5. Liver enzymes less efficient.

CHANGES IN THE REPRODUCTIVE SYSTEM

1. Sexual desires and capabilities, though modified, may remain in late life.
2. Cessation of sexual activity is due in part to decline of physical health in one or both partners or to death of partner.

PSYCHOSOCIAL INFLUENCE OF AGEING ON HEALTH

PSYCHOSOCIAL ASPECTS

Both physical and mental health are inter-related with psychosocial aspects of ageing.

1. Decrease in self-esteem due to loss of:
   a. Earning power. Although many people will have paid into voluntary pension schemes as well as the compulsory contribution into the national pension scheme, and so will be receiving a definite weekly amount, this often does not keep up with the rise in inflation. It is difficult for an elderly person to find a small, part-time job, and there is the possibility of the retirement pension being decreased if earnings exceed a certain amount. If Supplementary Benefit has to be provided, this may give a feeling of inadequacy, and that this is accepting charity.
   b. Status and work role. An older person may feel that the regard and respect which they received was due to their role at work and not due to themselves. This may cause them to withdraw and disengage from the mainstream of life.
   c. Social roles and resources because of loss of contact with work colleagues.
   d. Family and friends through death or moving away.
2. Lack of meaningful activity.
3. Negative stereotype or prejudices of society against the aged. There is, perhaps, too much emphasis on the concept of the retired and aged person being a burden on society and becoming increasingly dependent, physically and financially, for all their needs. The positive side of ageing, and the contribution which older people can make, needs to be stressed. This has been shown by the 'Grey Panther' movement in America.
4. Loss of cognitive functioning (thinking, perceiving, remembering) may be caused by lack of interest or concentration.
5. Decline in mental and physical capabilities – poor short-term memory, loss of speed and agility.
6. Sensory disabilities – these make individuals suspicious and distrustful of others.

PHYSICAL DISABILITIES AFFECTING ADAPTATION

1. Perceptual impairment.
2. Hearing losses – lead to depression and suspiciousness.
3. Lack of sexual desire and capacity.
4. Loss of speed and psychomotor response – inability to travel.
5. Subjective awareness of ageing.
6. Cultural devaluation.
7. Slowing down of psychological processes.
8. Personality defects exaggerated. Eccentric and hysterical trends become more obvious.

THEORIES OF ADAPTIVE TECHNIQUES EMPLOYED BY THE AGED

Some of these are contentious.

1. Disengagement – mutual withdrawal between individual and society; can produce chronic depression.
2. Activity.
3. Paranoid retreat.
4. Integration – person accepts ageing and ages gracefully.

5. Adherence to specific routine with resistance to change (helps failing memory).

DISEASE ASPECTS OF AGEING

GENERAL EFFECTS

1. Manifestations of disease are modified by old age.
2. More than one disease may be present – over 40 per cent of ageing people have more than one illness.
3. Aged persons respond to treatment more slowly and to a lesser degree. ·
4. There is less resistance to stress – one major illness lowers resistance and allows other illnesses to appear.
5. Illnesses tend to cluster during closing years of the very old person's life – chain reaction of one degenerative process leading to another and finally to death.

SPECIFIC ASPECTS

1. Most common diseases are those of circulatory system and atherosclerosis.
   Arterial disease causes cardiac, renal and neurological problems.
2. Aged people are more vulnerable to acute infections of respiratory tract – increasing numbers have chronic lung disease.
3. They are prone to gastrointestinal diseases, particularly functional diseases.
4. Incidence of cancer increases – may be of many years' duration.
5. There are changes in arterial walls (arteriosclerosis), in joint spaces (arthritis) and in functioning of certain endocrine glands (diabetes).
6. Hypothalamic temperature regulation less efficient – increased risk of hypothermia.
7. Loss of muscle tone, affecting limbs, bladder and bowels.

DRUG THERAPY AND THE AGED

FACTORS ALTERING DRUG RESPONSE IN THE AGED

1. Diminished production of liver enzymes that break down substances, including drugs; major-

ity of drugs are metabolized and detoxified by the liver.
2. Increase in circulation time (due to reduced cardiac efficiency) may have cumulative effect.
3. Diminished kidney function – lower rate of elimination leads to drug accumulation and toxicity.
4. Decrease in amount of gastric acid inhibits absorption of acid-requiring drugs.
5. Diminished ability to maintain homeostatic balance.

NURSING IMPLICATIONS

1. Be aware that drug effect is more pronounced in old people. The potential for adverse reactions, interactions and medication-induced disease is greater.
   a. Old people may not be able to handle multiple medications or may omit to take them.
   b. They appear to be more sensitive to digoxin, diuretics, aspirin, warfarin, oral hypoglycaemic drugs, sedatives, analgesics etc.
   c. The more medications that the patient takes, the greater is the risk of drug interactions and reactions.
2. Obtain a medical and drug history.
   a. Check nutritional status.
   b. Ask what over-the-counter medications the patient is taking (laxatives, antacids, aspirin); these may affect the interaction of prescribed drugs.
   c. Assess for alcohol usage.
3. Usually the doctor will hold the dosage to lowest effective amount; doses may be given further apart.
   a. Reinforce verbal instructions with written instructions to the patient, family and primary care team, using words the patient can understand.
   b. Write what the drug is used for – e.g. 'to stop indigestion after meals'.
   c. Explain possible side-effects.
   d. Be sure the drug name and instructions for taking it are typed in large letters on the label, and that containers can be opened easily.
   e. Arrange drug schedule to coincide with a regular activity (arising, eating, retiring) – helps patient to remember to take drug.
   f. Arrange some sort of check-off system.
   g. List all the medications that the patient is taking, and put this list in prominent place, e.g. stuck to kitchen cupboard door.
4. Carry out periodic drug review.
   a. Ask patient to bring medication with him on next visit to doctor or clinic.

b. Assess for patient compliance, response to therapy, possible side-effects, drug interactions.

THE 'CONFUSED' AGED PERSON

1. Changes in mental status may be the first sign of illness in the older person.
   a. Expect an underlying physical cause in any patient who has *sudden* changes in intellectual functioning.
   b. Confusion and disorientation may be first sign of infection, pneumonia, cardiac failure, coronary occlusion, electrolyte imbalance, stroke, dehydration, anaemia, malignancy.
2. Ageing is not synonymous with senility – senile dementia is a *degenerative* disease of the older person.
3. A new environment may bring on confused behaviour without physiological causes.
   a. Be optimistic over this turn of events; act on the assumption that this behaviour is temporary.
   b. Accept the person as he is now, without judgement or criticism.
   c. Pay attention to what the patient is saying – often a person who is considered confused is only transiently so and much of what he is saying makes sense.
   d. Call the person by name each time a contact is made; touch the patient when you speak to him.
      (i) Talk directly to him.
      (ii) Answer questions in simple, short sentences.
   e. Tell the person who you are, and why you are there.
   f. Keep the patient oriented with respect to time and place.
      (i) Remind him of time, dates and place each morning and whenever necessary.
      (ii) Keep a calendar and clock, both with easily readable numbers, within his range of vision.
      (iii) Keep the room well lighted to reduce confusion and fear.
   g. Have the patient's personal belongings where he can see and use them.
   h. Maintain a calm environment. Remove unduly stressful stimuli.
   i. Arrange for visits from others to counteract isolation.
      (i) Have family sit by bed so patient can see and touch them.
      (ii) Use services of a volunteer if no family is available.
   j. Attempt to alleviate the patient's anxiety.
      (i) Hold the patient's hand – many aged persons have no one to touch them.
      (ii) Use warm baths, warm milk, back massage and understanding and compassion.
   k. See that the patient wears his glasses, and that they are clean, also dentures or other prostheses. Check that hearing aid is working.
   Note: Be sure he is drinking enough fluids.
4. Avoid endorsing confused behaviour.
   a. Do not agree with confused statements.
   b. Avoid letting the patient 'ramble'. Direct him back to reality.
   c. Be consistent. Each member of the health care team should know the nursing objective and use the same approach.
5. Plan the patient's daily activities and adhere to the plan to promote security.

PSYCHIATRIC AND COGNITIVE DISORDERS

The psychiatric disorders of late life are a major cause of chronic ill health and disability. Incidence increases with age; disorders include depression, paranoid reactions and dementias.

DEPRESSION (DISORDER OF MOOD)
Most common emotional disorder of the aged, occurring in 20 to 30 per cent of elderly.
1. Characterized in late life by apathy, sense of hopelessness and exhaustion; loss of interest and somatic complaints. It may result from accumulation of many unavoidable and real losses (see above).
2. Depression may be masked as a cognitive disturbance in older people.
3. Older people (who make up 11 per cent of population) account for about 25 per cent of reported suicides.

Assessment
1. Look for physical signs and symptoms that may be the cause of depression.
2. Take a drug (including alcohol) history; many drugs can cause depression in the elderly.

Nursing interventions

1. Have an awareness that the depressed older person may be mislabelled as 'demented'.
2. Allow the patient to release anger, guilt and grief.
3. Treatment consists of psychotherapy, drugs and occasionally, electroconvulsive therapy.

PARANOIA

Characterized by suspicion and ideas of persecution (second most common psychiatric disturbance among the aged).

1. More common among older people with sensory deficits and those who are 'loners'.
2. Management – appropriate medication, supportive therapeutic relationships, hearing aid/glasses to decrease sensory isolation and development of social network.

DEMENTIAS

Progressive deterioration of intellectual functioning. (Refer to a psychiatric nursing textbook for discussion of the types of dementias.)

ALZHEIMER'S DISEASE (SENILE DEMENTIA)

Alzheimer's disease is a specific illness characterized by progressive deterioriation of memory, cognitive functioning and the ability for self-care. The cause of this disease is unknown. (There is also a presenile type of Alzheimer's disease, affecting the 40 to 60 age group, in which there seems to be a genetic link.)

Possibly one in ten people in the 65 to 70 age group may show signs of dementia, rising to one in five of those over 80 years.

PATHOPHYSIOLOGY

1. Changes occur in the proteins of the nerve cells of the cerebral cortex, which lead to abnormal, tangled fibres (neurofibrillary tangles) and characteristic senile plaques (degenerated nerve cell pieces which form around a core in the cerebral cortex).
2. Research scientists have shown that there is evidence of progressive decrease in the activity of the enzyme choline acetyltransferase (ChAT) and possibly also somatostatin in the cerebral cortex. Choline acetyltransferase is a crucial ingredient in the chemical process that produces acetylcholine, a neurotransmitter involved in learning and memory as well as in the parasympathetic nervous system.
3. There is also a marked loss of brain cells in part of the base of the brain.

Assessment

CLINICAL FEATURES

1. Significant forgetfulness.
2. Deterioration of higher cognitive function with loss of ability to read, to write, to calculate and eventually to speak intelligently.
3. Personality changes.
4. Disorders of motor function, including disorder of gait; incontinence.

DIAGNOSTIC EVALUATION

Probable Alzheimer's disease diagnosis based on clinically determined dementia confirmed by:

1. Neuropsychological tests.
2. Two or more cognitive deficits.
3. Progressive worsening of memory and other cognitive functions.
4. No disturbances of consciousness.
5. Onset between ages of 40 and 90 (most often after age 65).
6. Absence of systemic disorders or other brain disorders that could cause progressive deficits in memory and cognition.

MANAGEMENT

Maintaining the patient's current abilities in optimal state

1. No treatment presently known to prevent or arrest underlying pathological process.
2. Management of concomitant physical health problems to prevent excess disability/worsening of behaviour.
3. Behavioural interventions are used to manage memory problems and intellectual dysfunction.
4. Continuing monitoring for signs and symptoms of illness.

PATIENT PROBLEMS

1. Ineffective family coping related to burdens imposed by Alzheimer's disease.
2. Loss of cognitive function and memory related to physiological alterations in brain tissue.
3. Catastrophic behaviour related to cognitive, intellectual and memory dysfunction.
4. Alterations in sleep/rest patterns related to effects of disease.
5. Incontinence related to cognitive deterioration.
6. Impaired communication (verbal) related to loss of word recognition or meaning.
7. Diversional activity deficit related to lack of awareness.
8. Activities of living related to loss of memory function and cognitive awareness.
9. Ineffective coping related to awareness in early stages of disease that memory is fading.

Planning and implementation
NURSING INTERVENTIONS
Objective
The family receives knowledge and support and acquires skill in handling their loved one and in coping with stresses imposed by Alzheimer's disease.

Teaching and supporting the family
1. Encourage family to become part of a support group that functions to educate about latest developments in Alzheimer's disease; this helps them to know, anticipate and plan for changes.
2. Tell family what to expect:
   a. Encourage family to do legal and financial planning.
   b. Keep them informed about changes in the patient.
3. Help carer to maintain own physical and mental well-being.
   a. Encourage scheduling of *regular* respite care from the demands of a '36-hour day'.
   b. Discuss with carer the need to plan for personal fulfilment outside the relationship with the patient.
4. Assist the carer's family to identify and work through their feelings:
   a. Encourage expressions of grief, frustration, anger, loss – helps the family to know that these feelings are normal.
   b. Acknowledge problem behaviours ('shadowing' carer, combativeness, accusations, excessive demands, frequent somatic complaints) before they exist.
   c. Talk about skills needed to prevent or moderate catastrophic reactions of patient (see below).
5. Support family's decision to place the patient in an extended care facility; problems that are especially difficult for family are aggression, delusions, hallucinations, confusion and inability to provide self-care. Help the family cope with inevitable feelings of grief.

Enhancing, preserving or compensating for loss of cognitive function
1. See that the patient has sufficient sensory input that is recognized as friendly.
   a. Be sure that all sensory deficits are corrected; glasses and hearing aid on; teeth in.
   b. Approach in front of patient; avoid suddenly appearing from behind.
   c. Gain eye contact; speak slowly and in short sentences.

d. Keep the patient oriented to time, place and person *repeatedly*.
   (i) Speak the patient's name; then touch his hand or arm.
   (ii) Introduce yourself (again and again); show your name tag.
   e. Keep conversation at close range.
   (i) Do not move around while talking to the patient.
   (ii) Make short, frequent contacts.
   (iii) Pay attention to what the patient is saying – much of what he is saying makes sense.
   f. Use nonverbal (body language) communication: gestures, eye contact, smiles, friendliness, gentle touch.
2. Provide aids to help maintain or stimulate cognitive functioning.
   a. Keep frequently used articles in a definite place.
   b. Keep a calendar and clock, both with easily readable numbers, within range of vision.
   c. Give written information; use lists; mark calendar.
   d. Use pictures plus written communication.
   e. Label frequently used items.
3. Extend the person's life space.
   a. Encourage family to bring in pictures, family album, etc. since familiar objects promote a sense of continuity, aid memory, and provide security and comfort.
   b. Use pictures, music, colour, indoor gardens, etc. to enhance the environment.
   c. Read newspaper headlines. Discuss current events.
   d. Take the patient outdoors; encourage family to take him to a restaurant, shopping centre, etc.
   e. Use sensory retraining (seeing, tasting, touching, smelling, hearing).
4. Maintain activities as close to normal as possible.
   a. Keep environment ordered, predictable and failure-free.
   b. Assist the patient to continue daily routine, physical activities and social contacts.
   c. Arrange for visits from others to counteract isolation.
   (i) Use services of a volunteer who can visit regularly if no family is available.
   (ii) Work with family toward specific goals.

Maintaining consistent environment and avoiding threatening situations
1. Keep the environment consistent and failure-free.
   a. Respect the patient's territorial rights.

b. Do not move the patient's personal belongings.

c. Avoid changing rooms – difficult for marginally oriented person to cope with change.

d. Place the patient's personal belongings where he can see and use them.

e. Allow the patient to 'hoard' a few things; do not dispose of them.

2. Avoid overestimating the patient's ability; mental and physical tasks beyond his capacity produce anxiety, frustration, and anger.

3. Reassure the patient that he is safe; remind him that you are caring for him when he repeatedly calls out, asks for 'Mother', etc.

4. Study individual to recognize tolerance level to stimulation.

a. Avoid excessive stimulation that precipitates a reaction.

b. Avoid telling the patient to 'try harder', 'try to remember', etc.

c. Remove tasks that precipitate frustration.

d. Give positive directions.

5. Remain calm when the patient becomes upset.

a. Expect some anger, passivity, frustration and dependency.

b. Change focus of interaction; *use distraction.*

c. Avoid restricting movement – may lead to agitation.

6. Help the patient maintain dignity and self-respect.

a. Avoid talking about confused person in his presence.

b. Explain what is happening and when it will happen.

c. Encourage independence as much as possible.

Promoting safety and reducing anxiety

1. Attempt to deal positively with wandering behaviour.

a. Evaluate for underlying pathology (cardiac decompensation).

b. Ascertain if the patient is trying to satisfy a need (hunger, warmth).

c. Study environment and identify potential threats to safety because patient is at risk for falls, burns and accidents.

d. Restructure environment to improve well-being.

e. Allow the patient mobility without jeopardizing safety.

f. Try to engage the patient in a more stimulating activity because boredom and tension may be the basis of wandering.

g. Give directions or suggestions if the patient appears lost.

h. Have the patient wear identification bracelet (name, address, telephone number).

i. Have an alarm system/special locks to prevent wandering away from home.

2. Attempt to alleviate the patient's anxiety and restlessness.

a. Try 'laying on of hands' – touching, stroking, hugging; many aged people have no one to touch them.

b. Use warm milk, warm baths, back massage and also understanding and compassion as therapeutic methods.

c. Give the patient gentle and constant reassurance.

d. Schedule the patient's daily activities and adhere to the schedule – order and predictability reduce anxiety and promote security.

e. Be consistent. Each member of the health care team should know the patient's goals and use the same approach.

f. Give 'permission' to express grief, anger and hostility.

3. Maintain a normal day and night pattern.

a. Encourage the patient to dress in clean, attractive (colour-co-ordinated) clothes daily – the wearing of nightwear during the day confuses the concepts of day and night.

b. See that the patient wears shoes – not slippers.

c. Encourage the patient to *walk* and not use the wheelchair, which limits his environment.

d. Encourage the patient to eat at a table and not at the bedside.

e. Encourage the patient to stay awake during the day. Keep him physically active.

f. Keep the room well-lighted to reduce confusion and fear; use a night-light to reduce risk of 'sundowning' (worsening of a condition at night).

g. Reorient the patient during periods of sleeplessness.

Managing bladder and bowel incontinence

1. See p. 15 for discussion of how to prevent bladder and bowel incontinence.

2. Keep a record of the patient's voiding and defaecation patterns.

3. Maintain the patient on a *regular* voiding and defaecation schedule.

a. Colour code or mark the bathroom door.

b. Take the patient to the bathroom on schedule.

c. Keep bathroom light on at night.

d. Avoid long-acting sedatives or hypnotics – may prevent the patient from awakening at night.
4. Provide special disposable undergarments that trap wetness away from the skin if incontinence cannot be managed by above measures.

Evaluation

EXPECTED OUTCOMES

1. Family uses positive coping mechanisms while living with a patient with Alzheimer's disease; belongs to a support group; verbalizes that they may have to place the patient in an extended-care facility.
2. Patient uses some compensatory mechanisms for loss of cognitive function.
3. Family tries to avoid situations that precipitate catastrophic behaviour.
4. Family attempts to prevent alterations in sleep and rest patterns and wandering behaviour; has made the patient's environment 'safe'; demonstrates ability to calm the patient during periods of agitation.
5. Family adheres to a bladder and bowel training schedule; the patient is free of bladder and bowel incontinence.

CARE OF THE AGED PERSON IN LONG-TERM ACCOMMODATION

Long-term accommodation may be run by the local health authority or privately.

1. Private homes may be:
   a. Rest homes for the older person who needs hotel type accommodation but not nursing care. Residents must be mobile and continent. Help with bathing is usually available, but night attendance is not always possible.
   b. Nursing homes for people who need nursing care. They are supervised by a trained nurse 24 hours a day.
2. Local authority accommodation may be:
   a. Sheltered accommodation (statutory service), individual flats, bungalows or bedsitters with washing and cooking facilities, with a warden in charge. There may be communal dining room facilities for some meals and a lounge for social gatherings. A call system is often installed.

   b. Part III accommodation (old people's homes, statutory service). Residents must be continent and mobile, i.e., able to transfer and be wheelchair independent. Care attendants are employed to help with general tasks, bathing, dressing, etc. A community nurse usually visits if nursing care is required for a time.
   c. Health authority geriatric ward or unit – all types of problems will be nursed – acute (diagnostic and fast rehabilitation) and long term (slow rehabilitation and total care). Physical and psychological care is provided. Social admissions may be taken on a short-term basis to give relatives a break.

With the health and local authority accommodation, a deduction is made from the state pension. A small portion of the pension is always given to the patient for their own personal use. With private homes, the patient is responsible for the whole cost. If, through rising prices, a long-term resident is unable to meet the increased fees financial help may be available. Any aged person who remains in a National Health Service (NHS) hospital for longer than six weeks, has his state pension reduced until he is discharged.

Note: It is essential that the team approach to the care of the aged person is carried out, so the expertise of various members of the team may contribute to the physical, psychological and social side of care.

NURSING THE AGED PATIENT IN A GERIATRIC WARD

ESSENTIAL GUIDELINES

Patients may be in a long-term geriatric ward for many years, and this is their *home*. All efforts must be made to make the ward as homelike as possible. A plan of care for each patient must be formulated, and the care which is received by each patient must be evaluated frequently and regularly (case conferences). *Positive, individualized patient care is essential.*

The geriatric ward should be:

1. Purpose built, or efficiently adapted for the particular needs of the aged patient, and heated to the temperature required by them rather than the staff.
2. Within easy access for visiting, taking into account that the patients' friends and relatives may belong to the same age group.

3. Have a good outlook, be preferably on a ground floor, so that the patient feels a contact with the outside world.
4. Have clearly identifiable toilet facilities within easy reach of sleeping and day room areas. Commodes should always be used in preference to bed pans.
5. Facilities for a degree of privacy, and also maintenance of dignity during toilet and nursing procedures.
6. Television and radio should be used positively and not as background noise.
7. Be free from hazards, e.g., slippery floors.
8. Avoid restrictive equipment – cot sides, fixed chair fronts, restrainers.
   See Rehabilitation Concepts (p. 9) for more detail.

Nursing care must be:
1. Geared to the particular needs of the aged patient. Routine must be flexible and adjusted to the needs of the individual patient, e.g., there may be considerable variation in sleeping patterns. It is not necessary for all patients to be woken up or put to bed at the same time.
2. Carried out by staff who are sympathetic to the needs of the aged patients, who have skills needed for these patients, who are open minded and aware of current research and ideas, and willing to implement new procedures if they are in the interests of their patients.
3. Planned so that a full range of medical and surgical investigations and care must be available, but it is essential that the terminal stage of old age must be peaceful, dignified, free from pain or discomfort, and that overvigorous methods of treatment are very carefully considered, before causing the patient added stress. Positive planning for the latter stages of any illness are essential and the very best medical and nursing care is required at this stage. See Rehabilitation Concepts for care of bladder, bowels and help with dressing.
4. Planned to add life to years and not years to life.

NURSING CARE OF THE AGED PERSON IN HIS OWN HOME

The full resources of the health service and the social services should be used to enable aged people to remain in their own homes or with relatives if they wish. It is essential that these resources are known to them, and include financial help, home help services, Meals on Wheels, as well as all the resources available through the primary care team, such as equipment.

ESSENTIAL GUIDELINES
1. Members of the care team are entering the house at the invitation of the patient and their approach to the patient and the relatives should reflect this fact. They should therefore try to preserve an empathic and nonjudgemental approach.
2. Team management of the care of the older person is necessary, and regular case conferences by members of the primary health care team should examine all aspects of care. Many teams may designate one member to be the prime carer. This person may make an assessment visit and then act as co-ordinator for the various services. This person may be the health visitor initially, but in the course of time, if the elderly person's physical condition deteriorates, it may be more appropriate for the district nursing sister to assume this role.
3. Adaptations to the house should be carried out where necessary, to provide extra safety measures, and also increase the mobility of the patient. Facilities for the safe and easy storage and preparation of food must be available.
4. The method of heating the house should be carefully considered, because of the danger of hypothermia, the risk of fire and also from the financial point of view.
5. If relatives are living with the patient, they should be given full support and encouragement. Holiday admissions to a geriatric unit should be available and may provide a welcome break for both the patient and the relatives. It is essential that both the patient and the relatives have an area of privacy at home, where they can have visitors, and where the various members of the family can have their own hobbies without constant interference. As already mentioned, planning for retirement and old age should take place with information from various sources, and after consultation with the family.
6. If the older person is living on his own, some method of summoning help must be available, e.g., card in the window, alarm bell or light. Neighbours should be aware of the fact of this person being on his own.
7. If adequate help can be given, many older

people can safely remain in their own homes, in familiar surroundings with the maximum degree of independence.

SUMMARY OF PRINCIPLES UNDERLYING THE NURSING MANAGEMENT OF THE AGED PATIENT

1. Growth and adaptation continue to occur when the individual's strengths and potential are recognized and reinforced.
2. Nursing care must be individualized, taking into consideration the patient's past experiences, needs and individual goals.
3. Assess the data to determine the older person's health status; establish a nursing care plan.
4. Realistic and attainable goals, which are understood by the patient, are set to help him gain a sense of accomplishment and purpose.
   a. Have an optimistic view of ageing and the older person.
   b. Goals should be set with the knowledge and co-operation of the patient.
   c. The underlying goal is independence or partial independence in activities of daily living.
   d. Keep communicating to the patient and family the planned goals of his care.
   e. Support his belief in his own inner resources.
   f. Prepare the older individual to meet own needs after leaving the hospital.
5. The patient should be an active participant in his own plan of care.
   a. Learn something about the patient before the initial encounter; find out the patient's strengths.
   b. Consult the patient's preferences.
   c. Concentrate on what the patient can do.
   d. Ask the patient's opinions.
   e. Encourage the patient to keep control over his life and to make choices and decisions.
   f. Avoid making decisions for him; this promotes low self-esteem, dependency and depression.
   g. Praise even minimal achievements.
   h. Support the patient during periods of anxiety; allow expression of troubles and difficulties.
   i. Urge the patient to remain active, direct attention to gains being made and on the controls the patient still retains.
6. Nursing activities should be done *with* the patient rather than *for* him.
7. The medical and nursing management of the patient will take into account the physiological and psychological constraints imposed by the ageing process.
8. The individuality of the patient should be encouraged – to preserve his identity and sense of control.
   a. Respect the patient's personal space or territorial boundaries.
   b. Encourage the patient to have and use personal possessions that help bridge the gap between past and present.
   c. Respect the right to self-direction.
   d. Allow the person to take some risks (i.e., live alone) when benefits can outweigh risks.
   e. Give the patient *time* to express his feelings.
   f. Help him retain the social graces.
   g. Help him cope with thoughts of death.
9. Older people should be kept in the mainstream of life to prevent physical, emotional and mental deterioration.
   a. Avoid removing the element of challenge. Encourage contact with others.
   b. Give dignity and privacy for personal relationships with opposite sex and expression of sexual needs.
   c. Work out a friendship system to prevent loneliness and isolation.
   d. Stimulate mental acuity and sensory input – minimizes preoccupation with body monitoring.
   e. Encourage physical activity.
   f. Share your world with the patient.
   g. Remember the patient's preferences; accept his idiosyncrasies.
   h. Provide opportunities for him to do some activities of daily living.
   i. Encourage the patient to feed/help other residents.
   j. Provide meaningful diversional activity.
   k. Give the patient something to look forward to.
10. The particular abilities of the patient should be used.
    a. Select activities that are in keeping with life-long interests.
    b. Do not attempt to alter lifelong character and behaviour patterns.
    c. Give the patient time to listen, to learn, and to adapt.

d. Help the patient to learn new ways to maintain independence.

11. Act as an advocate of the older person, ensuring that they are helped to obtain the statutory benefits which are available to them; that advantage is not taken of their frailties by unscrupulous salesmen; that minor disabilities are not ignored or dismissed without adequate investigation, with remarks that this is only to be expected at this age and has to be put up with.

12. Evaluate the patient's progress toward attainment of goals.

ADVISORY SERVICES AND USEFUL ADDRESSES

Age Concern, Bernard Sunley House, 60 Pitcairn Road, Mitcham, Surrey CR4 3LL.

Association of Crossroads Care Attendance Schemes Ltd, 94 Coton Road, Rugby, Warwickshire CV21 4LN.

British Deaf Association, 38 Victoria Place, Carlisle, Cumbria CA1 1HU.

British Diabetic Association, 10 Queen Anne Street, London W1.

British Society for Research on Ageing, Dept. of Medicine, Leeds University LS1 3EX.

Chest, Heart and Stroke Association, Tavistock House North, Tavistock Square, London WC1H 9JE.

Disabled Living Foundation, 380–384 Harrow Road, London W9 2HU.

Distressed Gentlefolks Aid Association, Vicarage Gate House, Vicarage Gate, London W8 4AQ.

Elderly Invalids Fund (Counsel and Care for the Elderly), 131 Middlesex Street, London E1 7JF.

Extend, 3 The Boulevard, Sheringham, Norfolk NR26 8LJ.

Friends of the Elderly and Gentlefolk's Help, 42 Ebury Street, London SW1 0LZ.

Health Education Council, 78 New Oxford Street, London WC1A 1AH.

Help the Aged, St James Walk, London EC1.

National Corporation for the Care of Old People, Nuffield Lodge, Regents Park, London NW1 4RS.

Parkinson's Disease Society, 36 Portland Place, London W1N 3DG.

Royal College of Nursing Society of Geriatric Nursing, 20 Cavendish Square, London W1M 0AB.

Royal Society of Health, 38a St Georges Drive, London SW1.

Women's Royal Voluntary Service, 17 Old Park Lane, London W1Y 4AJ.

FURTHER READING

BOOKS

Butler, A. (1985) *Ageing: Recent Advances and Creative Responses*, Croom Helm, London.

Chartered Society of Physiotherapy (1980) *Handling the Handicapped*, Woodhead-Faulkner, Cambridge.

Coni, N., Davison, W. and Webster, S. (1988) *Lecture Notes on Geriatrics*. 3rd edition. Blackwell Scientific, Oxford.

Cormack, D. (1985) *Geriatric Nursing*, Blackwell Scientific, Oxford.

Darnborough, A. and Kinrade, D. (1978) *Directory of the Disabled*, Woodhead-Faulkner, Cambridge.

DHSS (1981) *Growing Older*, Her Majesty's Stationery Office, London.

Eliopoulos, C. (1979) *Geriatric Nursing*, Harper & Row, London.

Eliott, J. R. (1975) *Living in Hospital – The Social Needs of People in Long-Term Care*, King Edwards Hospital Fund, London.

Fillenbaum, G. (1984) *The Well-being of the Elderly*, WHO, Geneva.

Foott, S. (1977) *Handicapped at Home*, Design Centre Book, London.

Goldsmith, S. (1976) *Designing for the Disabled*, RIBA Publications, London.

Greengross, S. (1985) *Ageing: An Adventure in Living*, Souvenir Press, London.

Hale, G. (1979) *The Source Book for the Disabled*, Paddington Press, London.

Mace, N. L. and Rabins, P. V. (1985) *The 36-Hour Day: Caring at Home for Confused Elderly People*, Hodder & Stoughton, London.

Meredith Davis, B. (1979) *Community Health, Preventative Medicine and Social Services*, Baillière Tindall, London.

Mitchell, L. (1984) *Healthy Living over 55*, John Murray, London.

Todd, H. (1980) *Old Age – A Register of Social Research*, Centre for Policy on Ageing, High Wycombe, Bucks.

Wells, T. J. (1980) *Problems in Geriatric Nursing Care*, Churchill Livingstone, Edinburgh.

Wright, S. G. (1985) *Building and Using a Model of Nursing*, Edward Arnold, London.

— (1987) *Nursing the Older Patient*, Harper & Row, London.

ARTICLES

Aspects of ageing

Altschul, A. (1986) The elderly make the world go round, *British Journal of Geriatric Nursing*, Vol. 6, No. 2, pp. 26–7.

Bloomfield, K. (1986) Ask the family, *Nursing Times*, Vol. 82, No. 11, pp. 28–30.

Haywood, S. (1986) Private homes in perspective, *Health Services Journal*, Vol. 96, No. 5010, pp. 1020–21.

Herbert, R. (1986) The biology of ageing – the maintenance of homeostasis, *Geriatric Nursing*, Vol. 6, No. 3, 14–16.

Hernandez, M. and Miller, J. (1986) How to reduce falls, *Geriatric Nursing*, Vol. 7, No. 2, pp. 97–102.

Jackson, J. (1986) Don't shout, nurse, *Geriatric Nursing*, Vol. 6, No. 3, pp. 12–13.

Mathieson, A. (1986) Old people and drugs, *Nursing Times*, Vol. 82, No. 2, pp. 22–5.

Roberts, A. (1986) Social aspects of ageing – systems of life, *Nursing Times*, Vol. 82, No. 24, pp. 43–6.

Wade, V. and Bowling, A. (1986) Appropriate use of drugs by elderly people, *Journal of Advanced Nursing*, Vol. 11, No. 1, pp. 47–55.

Whall, A. (1986) Alcoholism in older adults, *Journal of Gerontological Nursing*, Vol. 12, No. 1, p. 36.

Community services

Buck, G. (1986) Old but not forgotten, *Health Service Journal*, Vol. 96, No. 5002, p. 758.

Lodge, B. (1986) Domestic bliss for the elderly, *Health Service Journal*, Vol. 96, No. 5017, pp. 1166–7.

Stone, M. (1986) Home is where the help is, *Nursing Times*, Vol. 82, No. 14, pp. 31–2.

— (1986) Keeping care at home, *Health Service Journal*, Vol. 96, No. 5001, p. 730.

Hospital services

Beveridge, C. (1986) Catering for health can save money, *Health Services Journal*, Vol. 96, No. 5013, p. 1110.

Reader, D. and Wright, S. (1986) Providing an information service, *Geriatric Nursing*, Vol. 6, No. 4, pp. 27–9.

Thorne, T. and Harvey, K. (1986) Short hospital breaks, *Nursing Times*, Vol. 82, No. 21, pp. 28–31.

Incontinence

Blannin, J. (1984) Nursing care of the incontinent patient, *Nursing*, Vol. 2, No. 28, Supplement, pp. 3–4.

— (1987) Men's problems, *Nursing Times Community Outlook*, February, pp. 27–9.

Copperwheat, M. (1985) Putting continence into practice, *Geriatric Nursing*, Vol. 5, No. 3, pp. 4–8.

Fader, M. (1987) Assessing continence in the elderly, *Geriatric Nursing and Home Care*, Vol. 7, No. 1, pp. 10–12.

Hamilton, B. (1984) Incontinence aids, *Nursing*, Vol. 2, No. 28, Supplement, pp. 3–4.

Kinder, R. B. (1987) Long-term urethral catheterisation in the elderly, *British Medical Journal*, Vol. 294, No. 6575, pp. 792–3.

Norton, C. (1984) Incontinence – challenging speciality, *Nursing Mirror*, Clinical Forum, Vol. 159, No. 19, pp. xiv–xvii.

— (1985) Incontinence in the elderly, Part 5, *Nursing Times*, Vol. 81, No. 5, Supplement, pp. 17–20.

— (1987) Continence and the older person, *Geriatric Nursing and Home Care*, Vol. 7, No. 3, pp. 9–13.

Mental illness

Adams, J. (1986) Reality orientation: a nursing approach, *Geriatric Nursing*, Vol. 6, No. 3, pp. 21–3.

Rowles, H. (1986) We didn't know the half, *Geriatric Nursing*, Vol. 6, No. 4, pp. 24–6.

Willcock, G. K. (1985) Current concepts in Alzheimer's disease, *Modern Medicine*, Vol. 30, No. 7, p. 13.

Preventive care

Corbett, D. (1986) Elderly screening – a cost-effective GP clinic, *Geriatric Medicine*, Vol. 16, No. 4, pp. 40–42.

Hyatt, R. (1986) How to spot the elderly alcoholic, *Geriatric Medicine*, Vol. 16, No. 1, pp. 32–6.

Social services

Garrett, G. (1986) Pensions and benefits for the elderly and their carers, *Professional Nurse*, Vol. 12, No. 1, pp. 6–10.

Graham, A. (1986) Out in the cold, *Nursing Times*, Vol. 82, No. 10, pp. 19–20.

20

Care of the Patient Admitted as an Emergency

EMERGENCY MANAGEMENT*

Emergency management refers to the care given to patients with urgent and critical needs.

PRINCIPLES OF ASSESSMENT AND EMERGENCY MANAGEMENT
Underlying consideration
Injuries or conditions interfering with vital physiological function take precedence. Treat the potentially life-threatening problems first.

Objectives
Preserve life.
Prevent deterioration before definitive treatment can be
   given.
Restore patient to useful living.

1. Maintain a patent airway, employing resuscitation measures if necessary. Use the recovery position to prevent inhalation of vomit in the unconscious patient. Assess for chest injuries with subsequent airway obstruction.
2. Assess and restore cardiac output.
3. Control haemorrhage.
4. Prevent and treat shock; maintain or restore effective circulation.
5. Carry out a rapid assessment of the patient's physical condition; the clinical course of the injured or seriously ill patient is not static.
6. Protect wounds with sterile dressings.
7. Splint suspected fractures (including fractures of cervical spine in patients with head or spinal injuries).
8. Record patient's vital signs, including blood pressure, pulse, level of consciousness and pupil reactions.
9. Check to see if patient has a Medic Alert or similar identification designating allergies or drugs.

OBTAINING DATA (HISTORY)
If possible, a brief history of the accident/illness is taken from the patient or the person accompanying him – relative, ambulance man, neighbour.

1. What were the circumstances, forces, location and time of injury?
2. What was the health status of the patient before the accident or illness?
3. Is there a past history of illness?
4. Is patient currently taking any medications – especially hormones, insulin, digitalis, anti-coagulants?
5. Does he have any allergies or bleeding tendencies?
6. Is he under a general practitioner?
7. When did he last eat or drink? (Important if an anaesthetic is to be given.)

PSYCHOLOGICAL MANAGEMENT OF PATIENTS AND FAMILIES IN EMERGENCIES
Underlying consideration
Body trauma is an insult to physiological and psychological homeostasis; it requires both physiological and psychological healing.

Objective
Prevent psychological incapacity following trauma.

1. Understand and accept the basic anxieties of the acutely traumatized patient. Be aware of the patient's fear of death, mutilation and isolation.
2. Understand and support the patient's feelings concerning his loss of control (emotional, physical and intellectual).
3. Be prepared to handle all aspects of acute trauma; know what to expect and what to do – alleviates nurse's anxieties and increases patient's confidence.
4. Maintain and convey optimism and concern for the welfare of the patient.
5. Caution the family not to be shocked or horrified by the patient's condition; encourage them to reassure the patient.
6. Accept the rights of the patient and family to have their own feelings.
7. Maintain a calm and reassuring manner – helps emotionally distressed patient or family to mobilize their psychological resources.
8. Assist the family to cope with sudden and unexpected death. Some helpful measures include the following:
   a. Take the family to a private place.
   b. Talk to all of the family together with the doctor.
   c. Assure family that everything possible was done.
   d. Allow family to talk about the deceased and what he meant to them – permits ventilation of feelings of loss.
   e. Avoid volunteering unnecessary information (patient was drinking, etc.)

---

* This section will deal mainly with emergency nursing care of patients with trauma and other conditions not found elsewhere in this book. Nursing care of the patient with an acute heart condition is found in Chapter 5, and nursing care of the patient with acute respiratory problems in Chapter 4.

f. Avoid giving sedation to family members – may mask or delay the grieving process which is necessary to achieve emotional equilibrium and prevent prolonged depression.

g. Allow family members to view the body if they wish to do so (if body is not mutilated).

AIRWAY MANAGEMENT AND ARTIFICIAL VENTILATION

Artificial ventilation is accomplished by means of mouth-to-mouth and mouth-to-nose resuscitation (described in Guidelines which follow), a bag-mask unit or tracheal intubation. Artificial ventilation is instituted on a person who is not breathing; if he is unresponsive and without a palpable carotid or femoral pulse, external cardiac massage should be started. (Airway management and artificial ventilation are discussed in detail under Care of the Patient with a Respiratory Disorder, p. 91.

GUIDELINES: GIVING MOUTH-TO-MOUTH AND MOUTH-TO-NOSE RESUSCITATION*

Performance phase

Nursing action	Rationale
OPEN THE AIRWAY	
1. Place the patient on his back, unless any solid or liquid obstruction to the airway exists. In this case, turn the patient and clear obstruction.	
2. Tilt the patient's head backwards as far as possible by placing one hand beneath the patient's neck and the other hand on his forehead.	In an unconscious, supine patient, the base of the tongue falls against the posterior wall of the pharynx, obstructing airflow into the trachea.
3. .Lift the neck with one hand and tilt the head backwards by pressure with the other hand on the patient's forehead.	This extends the neck and lifts the tongue away from the posterior pharynx; the mouth opens, and the obstruction of the airway is relieved, since the tongue no longer occludes the back of the throat. This may be all that is necessary as breathing re-establishes; otherwise absence of breathing requires further action.

Mouth-to-mouth ventilation

Nursing action	Rationale
VENTILATE THE PATIENT	
1. Pinch the patient's nostrils together with the thumb and index finger of the other hand while also continuing to exert pressure on the forehead to maintain the backward tilt.	Pinching the nose prevents air loss during ventilation.
2. Open your mouth wide. Take a deep breath. Make a tight seal with your mouth around the patient's mouth and blow into his mouth.	

* From (1974) Standards for cardiopulmonary resuscitation (CPR) and emergency cardiac care (ECC), *JAMA*, Vol. 227, pp. 837–51.

3. For the *initial* ventilatory manoeuvre, give the patient four quick full breaths without allowing time for full lung deflation between breaths.

To flush the lungs with oxygenated air. Adequacy of ventilation is ensured by seeing the patient's chest rise and fall.

4. Remove your mouth from the patient's and allow him to exhale passively.

5. Repeat this cycle once every five seconds as long as respiratory inadequacy persists (12 ventilations per minute).

Mouth-to-nose ventilation

This is performed when it is impossible to open the patient's mouth, when it is impossible to ventilate through his mouth, when his mouth is seriously injured, or when it is difficult to achieve a tight seal around the mouth.

Performance phase

Nursing action	**Rationale**
1. Tilt the patient's head with one hand on the forehead while using the other hand to lift the lower jaw and close the mouth, sealing the lips with the thumb.	
2. Take a deep breath. Seal your lips around the patient's nose and blow in until you feel his lungs expand.	
3. Remove your mouth from the patient's nose and allow him to exhale passively.	Watch his chest fall when he exhales. It may be necessary to open the patient's lips to allow air to escape during exhalation since the soft palate may cause nasopharyngeal obstruction.
4. Repeat the cycle every five seconds (12 ventilations per minute).	

HAEMORRHAGE

EMERGENCY MANAGEMENT
Objective
Maintain an adequate circulating blood volume.

1. Remove the patient's clothing as necessary quickly and carry out a rapid physical examination.
2. Apply firm pressure over the wound or the bleeding point; almost all bleeding can be stopped by direct pressure. Be aware of underlying fractures or foreign bodies in the wound; do not apply pressure over these.
3. Apply a firm pressure dressing. Elevate the injured part to stop bleeding if possible. Seek medical help urgently.
4. An intravenous cannula is inserted by the doctor to provide means of blood replacement. Blood samples are withdrawn for analysis, grouping and cross-matching. Fluid given may include isotonic electrolyte solutions, plasma and blood, depending on clinical estimates of type and volume of fluids lost.

   The rate of infusion depends on severity of blood loss and clinical evidence of hypovolaemia.

5. The following steps are taken for internal bleeding:
   a. Whole blood or plasma expanders are given at the rate of blood loss.
   b. Prepare patient immediately for the operating theatre.
6. Be alert to the possibility of cardiac arrest; patients who haemorrhage are candidates for cardiac arrest caused by hypovolaemia with secondary anoxia.

SHOCK

Shock is the condition in which there is loss of effective circulating blood volume; inadequate organ and tissue perfusion result, leading to derangements of cellular function.

CLINICAL FEATURES
1. Decreasing arterial pressure (systolic pressure usually falls more rapidly than diastolic pressure).
2. Increasing pulse rate.
3. Cold, clammy skin; prostration.
4. Pallor; circumoral pallor.
5. Alterations of mental status.
6. Suppression of kidney function.

EMERGENCY MANAGEMENT
Objectives
Restore and maintain tissue perfusion.
Correct physiological abnormalities.
1. Establish and maintain airway and breathing. Give oxygen as prescribed if available to augment oxygen-carrying capacity of arterial blood.
2. Keep patient flat and raise legs if possible.
3. Protect against heat loss without applying warmth from external source.
4. Control bleeding.
5. Handle the patient with care and immobilize injuries.
6. Reassure and comfort the patient.
7. Maintain circulatory blood volume with rapid fluid and blood replacement to correct hypotension.
   a. A central venous catheter may be inserted by the doctor in or near the right atrium to serve for fluid replacement (continuous central venous pressure reading gives direction and degree of change from baseline reading and the catheter is also a vehicle for emergency fluid volume replacement).
   b. Intravenous catheter(s) or needles are inserted by the doctor. Two catheters may be

necessary for rapid replacement in profound shock; emphasis is on volume replacement. Blood for specimens (arterial blood gases, urea and electrolytes, group, cross-match and haematocrit) are taken by the doctor. Intravenous infusion is started at a fast rate until the central venous pressure rises 5cm H_2O above baseline measurement or until there is improvement of condition.
   (i) Glucose in normal saline or lactated Ringer's solution is used to restore circulation and to serve as an adjunct to whole blood.
   (ii) Use plasma volume expanders if indicated until blood can be obtained.
   (iii) Start blood transfusion as soon as available – especially in patients with multiple or penetrating injuries.
   (iv) Control haemorrhage; haemorrhage will increase the shock state.
   (v) Maintain the systolic blood pressure at at least 80–90mmHg via fluid and blood volume replacement.
   (vi) Serial haematocrit examinations are carried out if continued bleeding is suspected.
8. A urinary catheter may be inserted. Urinary volume reveals adequacy of kidney perfusion (30–50ml/hour minimum).
9. A rapid physical examination is carried out by the doctor to determine the cause of shock.
10. Maintain nursing surveillance of blood pressure, heart and respiratory rate, skin temperature and central venous pressure, and urinary output to assess patient response to treatment – keep accurate charts of these recordings.
11. Continue to maintain a flat position for the patient, with legs elevated to promote return of venous blood to the heart. This position is contraindicated in patients with head, leg and pelvic injuries.
12. Give specific drugs as directed.
13. Support the defence mechanisms of the body.
    a. Continue to reassure and comfort the patient.
    b. Relieve the pain by giving cautious analgesics as prescribed, make the patient comfortable and stabilize injuries with support.
    c. Maintain body temperature:
       (i) Too much heat produces vasodilatation, which counteracts the body's compensatory mechanism of vasoconstriction and also increases fluid loss by perspiration.
       (ii) Too little heat slows the heart and re-

duces the cardiac output, as well as enhancing peripheral vascular collapse.

(iii) A patient who is in septic shock should be kept cool since high fever will increase cellular metabolic effects of shock.

WOUNDS

Wounds (injury to tissues) vary from minor lacerations to severe crushing injuries.

UNDERLYING CONSIDERATIONS

Life-threatening problems such as airway obstruction, haemorrhage and shock must be dealt with before the wound is treated.

EMERGENCY MANAGEMENT

Objectives

Control haemorrhage.
Avoid complications.
Promote rapid healing.
Minimize scarring and prevent deformity.

1. Control bleeding (see Haemorrhage, p. 1073).
2. Observe wound for foreign bodies or underlying fractures. Superficial contamination can be washed off; embedded particles are removed by the doctor.
3. Apply a clean emergency dressing (not cotton wool).
4. Seek medical advice on bleeding, foreign bodies, prevention of infection in dirty wounds, suitable treatment to promote healing and tetanus prevention.
5. Cleanse and shave around the wound as required using Savlon or other agent.
6. The wound may be sutured by the doctor if primary closure is indicated (depends on nature of wound, length of time since injury was sustained, degree of contamination, vascularity of tissues). The doctor may infiltrate with local anaesthesia intradermally through the wound margins or by regional block.
7. Apply dressing – to protect wound; may serve as a

splint and as a reminder to patient that he has to keep the dressing dry.

8. Give tetanus and antibiotics prophylactically, as prescribed.

TETANUS PROPHYLAXIS IN WOUND MANAGEMENT

All wounds need adequate examination and cleaning which should include the removal by the doctor of all dead and potentially dead tissue and all foreign bodies.

Specific tetanus prophylaxis

All wounds can be divided into 'clean' and 'dirty'. A 'dirty' wound is any wound sustained out of doors that draws blood, was inflicted more than six hours previously or was inflicted while dealing with soil, raw meat, skins or animals. A 'clean' wound is one which is inflicted indoors less than six hours previously. Patients can be divided into four groups according to their immune state.

1. A – Patients who are immune because their tetanus prophylaxis is up-to-date and their last injection was not more than five years previously.
2. B – Patients who have been immunized and have had a booster dose within the last 10 years.
3. C – Patients who have been immunized but have not had a booster dose for 10 years or more.
4. D – Patients who have never had a complete course of tetanus toxoid.

TETANUS PROPHYLAXIS PROCEDURE

See Table 20.1.

Course of tetanus toxoid – for complete active immunization a full course of three injections of absorbed tetanus vaccine is given. The initial dose of 0.5ml; a booster dose of 0.5ml is given six to 12 weeks later and a final booster dose of 0.5ml six to 12 months later. Immunity will not have reached a satisfactory level until after the second injection. After a course of three injections, immunity will be satisfactory for five years but depends on the severity of the injury.

Table 20.1 Tetanus prophylaxis procedure

Clean wound	Immune state	Dirty wound
Nil	A	Nil, unless booster advised by doctor
Tetanus toxoid booster	B	Tetanus toxoid booster
Tetanus toxoid booster	C	Tetanus toxoid booster and antibiotic
Course of tetanus toxoid	D	Course of tetanus toxoid and antibiotic

Antibiotic prophylaxis

Antibiotic prophylaxis will be either penicillin or erythromycin. A course giving adequate serum levels for three to five days is suggested. Triplopen is often used for patient who are not allergic to penicillin.

Immediate passive protection (Humotet)

When immediate passive protection is required human tetanus immunoglobulin can be given. If given with tetanus vaccine, it must be injected into a different site with a different syringe and needle. Indications for the use of Humotet are all highly tetanus-prone wounds, e.g., penetrating wounds, wounds with dead tissue, wounds which occur in association with farm or garden dirt or animal faeces.

Anaphylactic shock

Adrenaline injection (BP) should be available during prophylactic procedures for treatment of anaphylactic shock. In addition, a steroid (e.g. hydrocortisone) and an antihistamine (e.g. Piriton) should be available to overcome the allergic reaction. All these are given as prescribed.

INTRA-ABDOMINAL INJURIES

Intra-abdominal injuries may be either penetrating or blunt.

PENETRATING ABDOMINAL INJURIES

Penetrating abdominal injuries (gunshot wounds, stab wounds, etc) are frequently serious and usually require surgery.

EMERGENCY MANAGEMENT
Objectives
Control the bleeding.
Maintain the blood volume until surgery can be performed.
1. Obtain a history of the event as this may indicate the site of an injury.
2. Observe pulse and respiration. Be prepared to resuscitate if necessary.
3. Control external bleeding and apply a clean emergency dressing.

4. Keep the patient flat and comfortable, raise the knees, head and shoulders slightly if the patient is not in shock.
5. Reassure the patient, stay with him and seek medical help urgently.
6. Keep the patient still since movement may fragment a clot in a large vessel and produce massive haemorrhage. Remove clothing away from the wound.
7. Assess for signs and symptoms of haemorrhage. Haemorrhage frequently accompanies abdominal injury, especially if the liver and spleen have been traumatized.
   Control the shock and maintain the blood volume until surgery can be performed.
   a. Apply compression to external bleeding wounds.
   b. Intravenous catheter(s) are inserted by the doctor for rapid fluid replacement to restore circulatory dynamics.
   c. Watch for occurrence of shock after an initial positive response to transfusion therapy; this is often the first sign of internal haemorrhage.
8. Aspirate the stomach contents with nasogastric tube – also helps detect gastric wounds and prevents lung complications from aspiration.
9. Cover protruding abdominal viscera with sterile saline dressings to protect viscera from drying.
   a. Flex patient's knees since this position will prevent further protrusion.
   b. Withhold oral fluids to prevent increased peristalsis and vomiting.
10. Insert indwelling urethral catheter to ascertain the presence of haematuria and to monitor the urinary output.
11. Keep records of the patient's vital signs, urinary output, central venous pressure readings (when indicated) and neurological status.
12. Carry out tetanus prophylaxis as prescribed.
13. Give broad spectrum antibiotic as directed to prevent infection since bacterial contamination is a frequent complication (depending on history and nature of wound).
14. Prepare for surgery if patient shows evidence of shock, bleeding, wound haemorrhage, free air, burst abdomen, haematuria.

BLUNT ABDOMINAL TRAUMA

UNDERLYING CONSIDERATIONS
1. Trauma to the abdomen is frequently associated with extra-abdominal injuries – chest, head and extremities.

2. The incidence of delayed trauma-related complications is greater than that associated with penetrating injuries; this is especially true of blunt injuries involving the liver, kidneys, spleen and pancreas.

CLINICAL FEATURES

1. Pain; particularly on movement.
2. Rebound tenderness; maximal point of tenderness.
3. Guarding.
4. Diminishing or absent bowel sounds.

EMERGENCY MANAGEMENT

1. Take a detailed history (frequently unobtainable, inaccurate and misleading); obtain all possible data about the following:
   a. Method of injury.
   b. Time of onset of symptoms.
   c. Passenger location (driver frequently sustains spleen/liver rupture).
   d. Recent food intake.
   e. Bleeding tendencies.
   f. Concurrent disease. Medications.
   g. Past medical problems.
   h. Immunization history, with attention to tetanus.
   i. Allergies.
2. The medical officer will carry out examination (inspection, palpation, auscultation and percussion of the abdomen).
   a. Look for chest injuries, especially fracture of lower ribs.
   b. Avoid moving the patient until initial assessment is done – movement may fragment a clot in a large vessel and produce massive haemorrhage.
   c. Inspect front, flanks and back for bluish discoloration, asymmetry, abrasions, contusions.
   d. Assess for signs and symptoms of haemorrhage; haemorrhage frequently accompanies abdominal injury, especially if the liver has been traumatized.
   e. Note tenderness, guarding, rigidity, spasm.
   f. Look for increasing abdominal distension. Measure abdominal girth at umbilical level upon admission – serves as a baseline from which changes can be determined.
   g. Avoid giving analgesics during observation period – may mask clinical picture.
3. Monitor vital signs frequently and carefully – may be the only clue to intra-abdominal bleeding.
4. The patient may require a chest X-ray, perhaps an abdominal X-ray if the time permits. Blood samples will be taken by the doctor for grouping, cross-matching, full cell count, urea and electrolytes. Urinalysis for protein and blood is important, and monitor urine output.
5. Prepare for insertion of nasogastric tube – to prevent vomiting and subsequent aspiration; helpful in decompressing (removing air) from the gastrointestinal tract.
6. Patient may be admitted for observation or exploratory laparotomy.

CRUSH INJURIES

Crush injuries occur when a person is crushed beneath debris, run over or compressed by machinery.

CLINICAL FEATURES

1. Oligaemic shock – due to extravasation of blood and plasma into injured tissues after compression has been released.
2. Paralysis of part, erythema and blistering of skin – damaged part (usually an extremity) becomes swollen, tense, hard.
3. Renal dysfunction – prolonged hypotension causes kidney damage and acute renal insufficiency.

EMERGENCY MANAGEMENT

1. Control shock.
2. Observe carefully for acute renal insufficiency – injury to back may cause severe kidney damage.
3. Support major soft tissue injuries to control pain.
4. Elevate the extremity, if possible.
5. Administer medication for pain and anxiety, as prescribed.

CHEST INJURIES

Injuries to the chest can be dire emergencies and are potentially life-threatening because of disturbances to cardiorespiratory physiology. See Chapters 4 and 5 for a more complete discussion of chest injuries.

EMERGENCY MANAGEMENT
Objective
Restore normal cardiorespiratory function as rapidly as possible.

1. Maintain a clear airway and be prepared to commence resuscitation if necessary.
2. Keep the patient semi-upright, well supported to aid breathing unless he is in shock. Inclining the chest over towards the injured side will reduce involvement of the uninjured lung.
3. Any open wound of the chest must be sealed urgently by hand – or some available dressing – to prevent air from being sucked in. A polythene bag makes an excellent temporary seal for this type of wound.
4. Examine the chest wall movements. Any flail segment should be immobilized by splinting the segment with the forearm of the same side, held firmly across the loose segment by broad bandages.
5. Observe the pulse, respiratory rate, skin colour and levels of consciousness, and treat for shock.
6. Obtain a history and seek medical help.
7. Undress patient completely in order to evaluate respiratory pattern and to look for other injuries; multiple injuries frequently occur with chest injuries.
   a. Is the chest wall intact?
   b. Are there active respiratory movements and lung expansion?
   c. What is the respiratory rate?
   d. Is there shortness of breath, inspiratory or expiratory stridor, cyanosis or pain?
   e. Determine if the patient is ventilating properly. Auscultate both sides of the chest.
8. *Priorities:*
   a. Ensure the airway is open.
   b. Perform a rapid physical examination to detect associated injuries.
   c. Assist with insertion of a tube into the chest cavity if indicated.
   d. Elevate the head and chest unless the patient is in shock.
   e. Prepare for blood transfusion; patients with severe thoracic injuries need blood to replace that which has been lost in the pleural cavity.

SUCKING WOUNDS

Air passes through hole in the chest wall (from stab or bullet wound, etc), causing the lungs to collapse and the mediastinum to shift. There is an audible passage of air from the wound during inspiration and expiration.

1. Instruct the patient to exhale.
2. Cover the wound with pad and a pressure bandage maintained by circumferential strapping – prevents further shifting of mediastinum and allows for airtight closure of wound.
3. The medical officer will insert chest tube connected to an underwater-seal drainage system – pneumothorax almost invariably accompanies these wounds.
   a. The skin is cleansed and infiltrated with a local anaesthetic by the doctor.
   b. A small incision is made between the fifth and sixth intercostal space in the midaxillary line.
   c. The chest tube is inserted and sutured in place.
   d. Chest tube is attached to a closed underwater-seal drainage system to evacuate blood and air and to measure blood loss.
4. Continue to assess respiratory status. Treat the patient symptomatically until surgical closure of the chest wall wound can be carried out.

FLAIL CHEST

Usually results from multiple rib fractures, which cause instability of the chest wall and subsequent respiratory impairment.

1. Immobilize the flail portion of the chest by stabilizing it with the hands and then applying a pressure dressing with adhesive strapping.
2. Prepare for endotracheal intubation plus mechanical ventilation with volume-controlled ventilator to expand the lungs and give adequate oxygenation and to promote stability of the chest wall once the patient is anaesthetized.
3. Assist with insertion of tube into the chest cavity.
4. A central venous catheter is inserted.
   a. Blood is taken for haemoglobin, haematocrit determinations, grouping and cross-matching.
   b. Monitor central venous pressure.
   c. Administer intravenous fluids as indicated.
5. Arterial blood for blood gas analysis is taken to determine the physiological effects of the flail chest.

TENSION PNEUMOTHORAX

Occurs when air enters the pleural cavity and produces displacement of the heart and mediastinum to the uninvolved side (with resultant severe cardiorespiratory embarrassment).

1. Assess the patient for dyspnoea, chest pain,

tachycardia and diminished or absent breath sounds on the involved side.

2. Assist with insertion of a chest drain to which an underwater-seal bottle is attached to prevent back flow of fluid and air into the pleural space.

HAEMOTHORAX

An accumulation of blood in the pleural cavity which can cause collapse of the lung and hypovolaemia or shock.

1. Assess the patient. Note any increase in pulse rate, decrease in blood pressure or signs of bleeding and shock.
2. Assist with the insertion of a chest tube. Attach the tube to an underwater-seal drainage system.
3. Blood volume is restored by giving blood and fluids, as prescribed.
4. Prepare for emergency thoracotomy for operative control of bleeding, particularly if large haemothorax is present.

CARDIAC TAMPONADE

Compression of the heart resulting from excessive fluid within the pericardial sac. It is the result of intrapericardial injury secondary to blunt or penetrating trauma.

1. Assess for falling blood pressure, pulsus paradoxus and reluctance on the part of the patient to lie down.
2. Assist with pericardiocentesis.
3. Monitor the electrocardiogram (ECG) and central venous pressure.
4. Prepare for thoracotomy if there is continuing evidence of bleeding into the pericardium.
5. Blood is taken for cross-match for possible blood transfusion.
6. Hypovolaemia is corrected with intravenous fluids, as prescribed.

HEAD INJURIES

Head injuries are classified as open or closed injuries. About 15 to 20 per cent of all patients who come to emergency departments for treatment have some form of head trauma. (See Chapter 16 for a more complete discussion of treatment of head injuries.)

EMERGENCY MANAGEMENT

NURSING ALERT
Exercise care when moving the patient's head and neck. Fracture of the cervical spine frequently accompanies a head injury.

1. Maintain the airway and breathing – hypoxia and hypercapnia can increase brain swelling and cell damage. Be prepared to commence resuscitation if necessary.
2. Check for a head wound with bleeding and control this with pressure over an emergency dressing. Be aware of any underlying fractures or foreign bodies, and avoid these.
3. Check the level of consciousness by response to speech, commands or pain. Maintain this observation every few minutes.
4. Apply a cervical collar. Always suspect a neck injury unless proven otherwise.
5. Observe for shock, bleeding or serous fluid discharged from the ears or nose, or swelling of the face or eye sockets. These may indicate serious skull injury.
6. Observe pupil size and reaction to light. Unequal pupils or no reaction to light may indicate raised intercranial pressure.
7. Turn the unconscious patient as quickly as possible to the recovery position unless resuscitation is required. This position will help to prevent the inhalation of any vomit.
8. Obtain a history and get medical help urgently.
9. In hospital, clear the respiratory passages via suctioning.
10. Ensure adequate oxygenation and humidification. (Hypoxia of the brain, which leads to increased intracranial pressure, is the most frequent cause of death following head injury.)
11. Assist with endotracheal intubation if patient is comatose (after determining that a cervical neck injury is not present).
12. Utilize assisted ventilation if necessary. (The brain is very sensitive to lack of oxygen.)
13. Control haemorrhage and shock.
    a. Shock is rarely the result of head injury – it usually has some other cause.
    b. Marked intracranial bleeding in an adult usually produces hypertension.
14. Determine the baseline condition of the patient – serves as a basis for comparison as patient's condition changes.

a. Assess level of responsiveness. Record exactly what patient does and can do on command.
b. Determine the presence of headache, double vision, nausea, vomiting.
c. Assess pupil size and reaction to light.
d. Measure blood pressure, pulse, respirations.
e. Assess for signs of rising intracranial pressure – deterioration in level of responsiveness, slowing of pulse, rising systolic pressure, increasing pulse pressure, changes in pattern of respiration, dilating, nonreacting pupils.
f. Assess motion and strength of extremities.
g. Assess for injuries to other organ systems.

15. Look for changes in patient's condition. (*Change in level of responsiveness is the most sensitive sign of improvement or deterioration.*)
16. Utilize intracranial monitoring (if available) – for recognition of increased intracranial hypertension and to help guide the use of hyperosmotic agents (mannitol, glycerol) to lower elevated intracranial pressure.
17. Prepare for computed tomography or angiography – gives information useful for achieving a precise diagnosis.
18. Prepare for surgical intervention – for depressed fracture or bleeding.

SPINAL CORD INJURY

Spinal cord injury may vary from a mild cord concussion with transient numbness to full trans-section of the cord with immediate and permanent quadriplegia. The most common sites are the cervical areas C5, C6 and C7 and the junction of the thoracic and lumbar vertebrae (T12, L1).

Any person with a head, neck or back injury should be suspected of having a potential spinal cord injury until the suspicion is proved groundless.

CLINICAL FEATURES

1. Total sensory loss and motor paralysis below level of injury.
2. Loss of bowel and bladder control; usually urinary retention and bladder distension.
3. Loss of sweating and vasomotor tone below level of cord lesion.

4. Marked reduction of blood pressure – from loss of peripheral and vascular resistance.
5. Neck pain.

EMERGENCY MANAGEMENT

1. *Keep the patient still and do not move him*, unless any danger cannot be removed.
2. Seek medical help urgently; the patient will require the transportation, equipment and assistance available with an ambulance.
3. Check the following to obtain an accurate diagnosis:
   a. The patient can move his own limbs.
   b. Sensation to the hands and feet.
   c. The level at which pain occurs in the spine.
   d. The history;
4. Apply a cervical collar to maintain head and neck stability.
5. If possible, secure the legs together at the ankles and knees. A spinal board may be applied by the ambulance crew prior to moving the patient. Alternatively, the patient should be lifted onto a firm stretcher by the blanket method by *at least six people. The patient must be moved as little as possible and kept in a straight line.*
6. Reassure the patient to allay fears as the patient will be frightened and shocked. It is very important to talk to the patient throughout, to provide information on what is happening and to gain information on his condition.
7. Treat for shock.
8. In hospital, immobilize the patient. Keep him on a hard, flat stretcher or trolley.

NURSING ALERT
A spinal cord injury can be made worse during the acute phase of injury. Proper handling is an immediate priority.

   a. Do not move the spine; keep the back straight – flexion or extension can aggravate the cord injury.
   b. Keep the head and neck in line with the body, supported each side by sandbags or rolled blankets. A cervical collar may help to support the head and neck.
9. Assist the doctor to assess and examine patient for level of spinal cord injury and associated injuries; the presence of spinal shock may make assessment difficult.
   a. Test for sensory impairment.
   b. Record vital signs of pulse, blood pressure and level of consciousness.
10. Assess the patient's respiratory exchange. Pre-

pare for tracheostomy if there is a high cervical lesion.

11. The doctor may introduce nasogastric tube – to prevent and treat paralytic ileus, gastric and intestinal distension.

12. Catheterize the patient – patient with spinal cord injury cannot empty his bladder.

13. Prepare patient for skeletal traction (Crutchfield tongs) if he has a cervical spinal cord injury – to obtain anatomical alignment and reposition dislocated facets.

14. Prepare for surgery, if required.

MULTIPLE INJURIES

UNDERLYING CONSIDERATIONS

1. *Evidence* of gross trauma may be slight or may be completely absent. The injury regarded as the *least significant* may be the *most lethal*.

2. Any injury interfering with a vital physiological function is an immediate threat to life and has highest priority for immediate treatment (obstructed airway, haemorrhage).

3. The patient should be completely undressed and a rapid physical examination should be carried out as quickly as possible after the airway has been established.

4. Mortality in patients with multiple injuries is related to the severity of the injuries and the number of systems and organs involved.

EMERGENCY MANAGEMENT
Objectives
Determine the extent of injuries.
Establish priorities of treatment.

Carry out a *rapid* physical examination to determine if patient is breathing, bleeding or in shock; determine the status of his responsiveness and if he has severe wounds or fracture deformities.

1. Establish an open airway.*
   a. Ask conscious patient if he is having difficulty in breathing. Ask if he has chest pain.
   b. Apply suction to clear the trachea and bronchial tree.
   c. Insert oropharyngeal airway – to prevent occlusion by tongue.
   d. Ventilate the patient (bag-mask system).
   e. Prepare for endotracheal intubation if adequate airway cannot be maintained.
   f. Suspect serious intrathoracic injuries if respiratory distress continues after adequate airway has been established. See pp. 1077–9 for management of chest injuries.
   g. Administer oxygen if required.

2. Assess cardiac function and treat cardiac arrest – hypoxia, metabolic acidosis and chest trauma may precipitate cardiac arrest.*
   a. For cardiac arrest, start closed chest compression and ventilation.
   b. Sodium bicarbonate is given (intravenously) by the doctor to compensate for acidosis if indicated – severely traumatized patients with respiratory and circulatory embarrassment will have some degree of metabolic acidosis.

3. Control haemorrhage.*
   a. Apply pressure over bleeding points if haemorrhage is overt.
   b. Expect significant blood loss in patient with fracture of shaft of femur, with multiple fractures or with major pelvic trauma.
   c. Prepare for immediate surgical intervention if patient is bleeding internally.

4. Prevent and treat hypovolaemic shock.
   a. Intravenous catheters (or needles) are inserted by the doctor; blood for laboratory studies is taken as directed (typing and cross-matching, baseline complete blood count, electrolytes, urea, glucose, prothrombin time). Infusions are commenced as required.
   b. A central venous catheter is introduced by the doctor to monitor patient's response to fluid infusion and to prevent fluid overload.
   c. Monitor urinary output (via catheter) – gives indication of adequacy of fluid replacement.
   d. Monitor ECG.
   e. Continue clinical evaluation to observe for improvement or deterioration in level of responsiveness, skin warmth, speed of capillary filling.
   f. Be prepared for immediate surgical intervention if patient does not respond to fluids or blood. Inability to restore blood pressure and circulatory volume in patient usually indicates major internal bleeding.

5. Assess for head and neck injuries (p. 1079).
   Make definite statements concerning baseline neurological status of patient (level of responsiveness, size and reactivity of pupils, motor power, reflexes).

---

* Imperative life-saving procedures are performed simultaneously by the emergency team.

6. Splint fractures to prevent further trauma to soft tissues and blood vessels and to relieve pain; note presence or absence of pulses in fractured extremities.
7. Assist with insertion of nasogastric tube if upper gastrointestinal bleeding is suspected or if gaseous distension of stomach develops – will decrease incidence of vomiting and aspiration.
8. Prepare for laparotomy if patient shows continuing signs of haemorrhage and deterioration.
9. Continue to monitor urinary output hourly – reflects cardiac output and state of perfusion of visceral organs.
   a. Assess for haematuria and oliguria.
   b. Record measurements on a chart.
10. Evaluate patient for other injuries and institute appropriate treatment, as prescribed, including tetanus immunization. (See wound treatment, p. 1075.)

FRACTURES

A fracture is a break in the continuity of the bone. Fractures are classified as either open or closed. In open fractures, the broken ends are in direct contact with the exterior and can therefore become infected.

EMERGENCY MANAGEMENT
1. Keep the patient still to prevent aggravation of the injury.
2. Look for bleeding, wounds, deformity, foreign bodies and the site of pain. Comparison with the uninjured side is useful.
3. Control bleeding from compound fractures by direct pressure around the wound. Apply a clean dressing when possible.
4. Assess circulation to the injured limb by checking the colour, warmth, pulse and sensation.
5. Immobilize the injury using splintage material and bandages as available. Inflatable splints may be available on the ambulance. The uninjured limb is often used as a splint.
6. Careful lifting and handling is essential to reduce pain and shock. All fractures should be transported well supported on a firm surface.
7. Give immediate attention to the patient's general condition, especially if the patient is admitted with multiple injuries.

8. Control haemorrhage.
9. Treat for shock. This may result from blood loss or prolonged severe pain.
10. Give analgesics as prescribed to control pain.
11. Inspect the fractured part(s).
    a. Remove clothing as necessary, with minimal movement.
    b. Look for angulation, shortening and rotation.
    c. Check the state of the limb:
       (i) That the circulation to the limb is intact.
       (ii) That the sensations of the limb are normal.
       (iii) Which movements of the limb are affected.
       (iv) The amount of swelling and bruising.
       (v) The amount of skin damage if an open fracture.
    d. Handle the fractured limb gently and as little as possible. Retain the limb supported on a firm surface.
12. Apply a sterile saline dressing if the fracture is an open one.
13. X-rays will be ordered to estimate the extent of the injury and to help plan the treatment.
14. For detailed account of treatment of individual fractures, see Chapter 13 on care of the patient with a musculoskeletal disorder.

BURNS

FIRST AID MANAGEMENT
Stop burning process to prevent further tissue destruction by immersion in cold water.
1. Remove patient from source of burn or smoke.
2. Flush with cold water any clothing saturated with boiling water, then remove carefully. Clothing charred by flames should not be removed, but flushed with cold water.
3. Immerse the burn in cold water for as long as necessary to ease pain. Cold water inhibits capillary permeability and thereby suppresses or prevents oedema, blister formation and tissue destruction.
4. Cover the burn with a clean dressing.
5. Keep patient warm, and get medical help.

Chemical burns
1. Irrigate copiously with large quantities of running water (except for burns caused by phosphorus).
2. Cover with loosely applied clean cloth.

Electrical burns

Electrical energy affects all tissues that it traverses – may cause sepsis and gangrene of extremity due to thrombosis of the blood vessels.

1. Remove electrical source by switching off or disconnecting the supply.
2. Treat for coma, circulatory and respiratory collapse.
3. Treat the injuries as for a heat burn.

TREATMENT OF BURNS IN THE EMERGENCY DEPARTMENT

Objectives

Maintain ventilation and circulation.
Prevent or treat shock and acute renal failure.
Relieve pain and prevent infection.

General

1. Assist with assessment of thermal injuries to determine the extent of burns and their probable depth. The area of burn can be assessed using the 'rule of nines' technique as a percentage of total body area. Depth can be assessed into three categories: superficial, partial thickness and full-thickness (see Chapter 11).
2. Determine the history.
   a. Circumstances of accident.
   b. Age and previous health condition (e.g., diabetes, renal disease, etc.).
   c. Time, place and mechanism of injury.
   d. Mental status.
   e. Care given patient before coming to casualty department.
3. Carry out rapid physical examination.
   a. Assess for hoarseness of voice and respiratory stridor (in patients with head and neck burns). Anticipate oedema formation.
   b. Look for other injuries especially in patients burned from automobile accidents or explosions.
4. Use rigid asepsis (cap, mask, gown, sterile gloves) when indicated.
5. Treat for shock. Keep patient warm to prevent hypothermia.
   a. Blood is taken for grouping, cross-matching and blood gas samples.
   b. Intravenous fluids are commenced and a cutdown is sometimes necessary through unburned skin.
      (i) Patient loses significant intravascular protein, salt and water during the first few hours after burn, plasma volume is greatly reduced.
      (ii) See Fluid Therapy Following a Burn (p. 769).
      (iii) Record fluids given on the appropriate chart.
6. Insert indwelling urinary catheter to assess urine volume, pH, specific gravity, sugar, acetone. Measure volume hourly. Observe for haemoglobinuria.
7. Assist in care of the burn wound.
   a. Avoid further damage and contamination. Take swabs for bacteriological examination.
   b. Treat the burn either by the open method (if admission is to a specialist burns unit) or with dressings. The use of sterile drapes or towels to protect the burn throughout will reduce the risk of infection.
8. Give analgesic as prescribed.
   a. Patients with extensive superficial burns will complain of pain because of irritated hypersensitive nerve endings.
   b. Occasionally patients with deep burns may require no medication during shock period because of destruction of nerve endings in burned tissue.
9. Start a record of vital observations.
10. Systemic antibiotics may be given – for burn wound sepsis.
11. Administer tetanus immune globulin (Humotet) for immediate protection or toxoid if previously immunized.
12. Nasogastric tube may be passed to help reduce gastrointestinal content because risk of reduced gastric motility may accompany extensive burns.
13. Children with burns covering more than 10 per cent of the body surface and adults with more than 15 per cent will require hospital admission and intravenous fluids.
14. Patients with critical burns should be treated at a burn centre or in a burn unit.

Inhalation burns

1. Establish adequate airway, maintain adequate oxygenation, especially for patients with major burns and for the elderly.
2. Prepare for endotracheal intubation or early tracheostomy in the following circumstances:
   a. Patients with deep burns of face, neck and respiratory tract; injuries from inhalation of gases.
   b. Stridor and inadequate respiratory exchange.
   c. Patient unable to handle tracheobronchial secretions.
3. Give oxygen as required since carbon monoxide poisoning may accompany inhalation burns.

EYE INJURIES

BASIC ASSUMPTIONS
1. All ocular injuries are potentially serious.
2. Suspect a penetrating ocular injury with every eye wound until suspicion is proved incorrect.

EMERGENCY MANAGEMENT
1. Try to keep the patient calm, seated and prevent him from rubbing the affected eye.
2. A provisional examination will reveal the depth of injury.
3. A saline wash can help some injuries, usually of value for loose foreign bodies with no penetration of cornea.
4. Cover the eye with a pad and retain this with a bandage or strapping.
5. Seek medical aid as soon as possible.

CORNEAL ABRASION

Injury to the cornea which goes no deeper than the epithelium.
1. Instil amethocaine 0.25 per cent solution as requested – to relieve pain and facilitate eye examination.
2. Stain the cornea with fluorescein – to detect existence of an abrasion and its extent.
   a. Gently touch conjictiva of lower lid with edge of fluorescein paper strip.
   b. The exposed (damaged) layers of epithelium will take the stain and turn green; undamaged areas remain unstained.
3. Chloramphenicol drops will prevent infection and can be used by the patient at home.
4. The eyelids are sealed closed to prevent abrasion of the cornea on the eyepad. This seal can be achieved by smoothing tulle-gras over both lids while closed. Apply a pad and bandage over this.
5. Give oral analgesic as prescribed – abrasions of the cornea are painful.
6. Advise patient to rest his eyes for 24 hours for greater comfort; the corneal epithelium usually heals in 24 to 48 hours.
7. Instruct the patient to return to ophthalmologist the following day for dressing change and inspection of eye for evidence of infection or ulcer formation.

CONTUSION

Black eye; haemorrhage into the orbit from trauma; hyphema (haemorrhage into anterior chamber of eye).
1. Contusions usually clear slowly and without treatment.
   a. Apply cold compresses intermittently for first 24 hours to control pain and swelling.
   b. Apply warm compresses (after 24 hours) intermittently.
2. Place patient on bed rest with both eyes bandaged for hyphema.
3. Chloramphenicol eye drops to prevent infection may be recommended for the time needed for healing.

FOREIGN BODIES LODGED IN CORNEA

Treatment by ophthalmologist or emergency department doctor.
1. Instil sterile anaesthetic as prescribed into the conjunctival sac – to facilitate examination.
2. Ophthalmologist will remove superficial particles with a moist cotton-tipped applicator; foreign body removed with a spud or similar instrument.
3. Apply eye pad and reinforce instruction to return to ophthalmologist the following day to determine if healing is occurring.

PENETRATING INJURIES TO THE EYE

1. Cover eye with sterile dressing and call ophthalmologist.
   a. Intraocular foreign bodies should be removed as soon as possible; they cause damage by disintegration or become encapsulated by fibrous tissue.
   b. Apply eye patch lightly – pressure of pad may cause further penetration.
2. Give sedative – analgesic combination as directed; have patient lie quietly until ophthalmologist arrives.
3. Give tetanus prophylaxis for any penetrating eye injury.
4. Give oral antibiotics as prescribed.

BURNS OF THE EYE

Cause drying of the cornea with resulting chronic conjunctivitis and corneal ulceration.

1. *Thermal burns* (associated with face or body burns).
   a. Call ophthalmologist urgently.
   b. Normal saline washes and local anaesthetic drops as prescribed will ease pain when required.
2. *Chemical burns* – may be either acid or alkali in nature. Both cause intense pain and inflammation.
   a. *Irrigate eye with copious amounts of water* – holding the patient's eye directly under running water with lids retracted by gauze flats is the best way to irrigate the eye when immediate irrigation is required.
   b. Irrigate for 20 to 30 minutes.
   c. Repeat irrigation every 15 to 20 minutes (using regular eye irrigation equipment) until patient is seen by ophthalmologist.
   d. Control severe pain thereafter with systemic analgesics as prescribed.
   e. Patient may be hospitalized for treatment to enhance healing.

HEAT STROKE

Heat stroke is a medical emergency caused by failure of the heat-regulating mechanisms of the body when the temperature–humidity index is high. People who are not acclimatized to heat exposure, the elderly and those with cardiovascular problems are particularly vulnerable.

CLINICAL FEATURES
1. Headache and visual disturbances.
2. Dizziness and nausea.
3. Hot, flushed, dry skin.
4. Weak, rapid and irregular pulse.
5. Sudden loss of consciousness.
6. High fever.
7. Cessation of sweating.
8. Muscle cramping.

EMERGENCY MANAGEMENT
Objective
Reduce high temperature as rapidly as possible.
1. Reduce the body temperature (rectal) to 39°C as rapidly as possible, using one or more of the following methods.
   a. Place the patient in a cool environment.
   b. Remove top clothing. Sponge patient liberally with water at room temperature.
   c. Place electric fan so that it blows on patient since air movement increases evaporation.
2. Administer oxygen by face mask if cyanosis is present.
3. An intravenous infusion may be started by the doctor; the prescribed rate is usually slow because of the danger of pulmonary oedema.
4. Give antipyretics as prescribed.
5. Measure urinary output – acute tubular necrosis is a complication of heat stroke.
6. Advise patient to avoid immediate re-exposure to high temperatures (after his condition has stabilized). Patient may remain hypersensitive to high temperatures for considerable length of time.

HEAT EXHAUSTION

Heat exhaustion occurs when water and salt are lost from the body in excessive amounts during sweating, and not adequately replaced. Hot environments combined with work or exercise are the usual cause, although the body temperature may remain normal because the temperature-regulating centre maintains control of heat loss.

CLINICAL FEATURES
1. Physical tiredness with restlessness.
2. Pallor, cold clammy skin.
3. Dizziness and fainting.
4. Muscular cramps.
5. Weak, rapid pulse.
6. Rapid, shallow breathing.

EMERGENCY MANAGEMENT
Objective
Restore the fluid and electrolyte balance.
1. Place the patient in a cool environment to reduce sweating.
2. Oral fluids can be administered to the conscious

patient provided he can tolerate anything by mouth.

3. Safeguard the airway in unconscious patients and observe breathing. Artificial ventilation will be necessary if breathing fails.
4. Obtain medical help urgently.
5. In hospital, intravenous fluids and electrolytes would be ordered for all unconscious patients and those who cannot take enough by mouth to correct the depletion.

COLD INJURIES AND HYPOTHERMIA

UNDERLYING CONSIDERATIONS
1. The extent of injury from exposure to cold is not always known when the patient is seen initially. A frozen extremity appears white, yellow-white or mottled blue-white and is hard, cold and insensitive to touch.
2. Colour changes (purple: cyanosis) after rewarming may be transient *or* they may indicate pressure within the fascial compartment.

EMERGENCY MANAGEMENT
Objective
Restore normal body temperature.
1. Do not allow the patient to walk if lower extremities are involved.
2. Remove all constrictive clothing.
3. Rewarm extremity slowly in warm-water bath of 32–41°C or by skin-to-skin contact – early thawing appears to give better chance for maximum tissue preservation.
   a. Handle parts gently to avoid further mechanical injury.
   b. Protect thawed part; do not rupture blebs.
   c. Administer analgesic for pain as prescribed – thawing process may be quite painful.
4. Give tetanus prophylaxis if indicated by associated trauma.

HYPOTHERMIA IN THE ELDERLY
Hypothermia in the elderly is a common occurrence in the winter months. The patient, often a woman living alone, sustains a fall or has an acute illness, which immobilizes her in a cold flat or house, unable to get help. It may be a varying length of time before help arrives. By this time, the patient is often dehydrated, undernourished and confused.

Objective
Restore normal body temperature by gradual warming.
1. Place the trolley in a warm part of the department and remove the patient's clothing. Show care and consideration as the patient is often upset by the state in which she finds herself, but has been unable to prevent.
2. Cover with a 'space blanket' which will retain most of the body heat.
3. Place an ordinary blanket on top.
4. Clean mouth if required, check swallowing reflex and administer warm drinks.
5. Monitor rectal temperature and aim to raise this by no more than ½–1°C per hour. Do not apply an external heat source as this may cause shock. Do not wash the patient unless badly soiled as this will remove heat from the skin.

In severe cases:
1. Oxygen with artificial respiration may be required.
2. Ventricular fibrillation may be treated by a defibrillator and cardiac massage.
3. If the patient is dehydrated, intravenous fluids will be administered, e.g., 5 per cent dextrose.
4. If necessary a central venous pressure line is established.
5. Hydrocortisone sodium succinate 100–200mg immediately; may be given intravenously followed by 100mg four-hourly.
6. Antibiotics are given if respiratory infection is present.
7. Catheterization may be necessary to check kidney function.

ANAPHYLACTIC REACTION

Anaphylactic reaction is a sudden, generalized systemic (and frequently fatal) reaction occurring within seconds to minutes after exposure to causative agent, namely, foreign sera, drugs or insect venoms.

ALTERED PHYSIOLOGY
1. An anaphylactic reaction is the result of an antigen–antibody interaction in a sensitized individual who, as a consequence of previous exposure, has developed a special type of antibody (immunoglobin) that is specific for this particular allergen.

2. The antibody immunoglobulin IgE is responsible for the great majority of immediate type human allergic responses – the individual becomes sensitive to a particular antigen after production of IgE to this antigen.

CAUSES
Penicillin, sera, other drugs, bee and wasp stings, or almost any repeatedly administered parenteral or oral therapeutic agent.

CLINICAL FEATURES
1. Diffuse erythema and feeling of warmth (with or without itching).
2. Respiratory difficulty – choking sensation, difficulty in swallowing, tightness or pain in chest, wheezing and shortness of breath, hoarseness, respiratory stridor.
3. Hives on face and upper chest – appear within first few seconds after injection. (With massive facial angio-oedema, expect that upper respiratory oedema may occur.)
4. Severe abdominal cramps, nausea, vomiting, urinary and bowel incontinence.
5. Vascular collapse; cyanosis, pallor, imperceptible pulse – circulatory failure leading to coma and death.

EMERGENCY MANAGEMENT
1. Establish and maintain an airway.
   a. Turn face to one side; support angles of mandible.
   b. The patient may need endotracheal intubation by the doctor. Suction should be available to remove secretions.
   c. Employ resuscitative measures as necessary (especially for patients with stridor and progressive pulmonary oedema).
2. Give adrenaline as directed – to provide rapid relief of hypersensitivity reaction. This should be done while another person is establishing the airway.
3. Give antihistamine drugs, e.g. chlorpheniramine maleate (Piriton) as prescribed if the patient requires adjunctive treatment – useful when asthma is present.
4. The doctor may administer hydrocortisone intravenously if the patient is having a prolonged reaction – helpful in preventing later relapses.
5. The doctor may give vasopressor agent intravenously under close observation for extreme hypotension. Titrate according to blood pressure.
6. The doctor may give aminophylline intravenously *slowly* over a 10-minute period; useful for patients with severe bronchospasm and asthmatic symptoms.
7. If patient is convulsing, the doctor may give intravenous injection of short-acting barbiturate or diazepam (Valium) over several minutes.

PREVENTIVE MEASURES AND PATIENT EDUCATION
1. Be aware of the danger of anaphylactic reactions.
2. Ask about patient's previous allergies to medications; if positive, do not give the medication or injection.
3. Question patient before giving a foreign serum or other type of antigenic agent to determine if he has had it at some earlier time.
4. Question patient concerning previous allergic reactions to food or pollen.
5. Avoid giving drugs to patients with hay fever, asthma and other allergic disorders unless absolutely necessary.
6. Avoid giving parenteral medications unless absolutely necessary; anaphylactic reactions are more likely to occur when therapeutic agent is given parenterally.
7. Do skin testing before administering foreign serum.
   a. Skin testing can precipitate anaphylaxis in highly susceptible individuals.
   b. A negative skin test does not always indicate safety.
   c. Have adrenaline on hand to control acute untoward reactions.
8. If patient is being treated as an outpatient, keep him in office, hospital or clinic at least 30 minutes after injection of any agent.
9. Caution patients who are sensitive to insect bites to carry first aid kits or kits equipped to treat insect stings. Instruct patient to report any untoward reaction that develops after he leaves the clinic, etc.
10. Encourage allergic individual to wear identification tag.

POISONING

Poison is any substance which when ingested, inhaled, absorbed, applied to the skin or developed within the body, in relatively small amounts, produces injury to the body by its chemical action.

SWALLOWED POISONS

EMERGENCY MANAGEMENT

1. Do not make the patient sick, or give him anything by mouth.
2. Obtain a history, including details of what was taken.
3. The unconscious patient should be placed in the recovery position with airway, breathing and circulation closely monitored. Resuscitation must be commenced if these vital signs fail.
4. Remove to hospital urgently, taking evidence of the poison and vomit with you.
5. Maintain the airway.
   a. Administer oxygen for respiratory depression, unconsciousness, cyanosis, shock.
   b. Administer artificial respiration if respiration fails; positive expiratory pressure applied to airway may help keep alveoli inflated.
6. Try to discover the nature of the poison. Call the Regional Poisons Information Service if an unknown toxic agent has been taken or if it is necessary to identify an antidote for a known toxic agent.
7. Consider gastric lavage or induce vomiting as the doctor directs. This can be doubtful value if attempted more than four hours after ingestion except for the recovery of salicylates which can be achieved up to 24 hours, and tricyclics up to eight hours.
8. Treat shock appropriately (see p. 1074).
9. Support the patient having convulsions; many poisons excite the central nervous system; the patient may convulse because of oxygen deprivation.
10. Monitor central venous pressure as indicated.
11. Monitor fluid and electrolyte balance.
12. Reduce elevated temperature.
13. Give specific therapy. Administer special chemical antidote (if indicated) or specific pharmacologic antagonists as prescribed.
14. Provide constant nursing surveillance and attention to the patient in a coma; coma from poisoning results from interference with brain cell function or metabolism.
    a. Maintain recovery position and a clear airway.
    b. Monitor the pulse, blood pressure and breathing, and record results. Observe skin colour for cyanosis.
    c. Monitor urinary output, via catheter if necessary, and maintain a fluid balance record. Continue intravenous fluid regimen as ordered.
    d. Aspiration of a nasogastric tube may be necessary to prevent vomiting.
15. Assist with forced alkaline diuresis, haemodialysis or peritoneal dialysis to shorten period of unconsciousness in the event of barbiturate and other hypnotic or tranquillizer poisoning.
16. Assist in securing specimens of blood, urine, stomach contents.

CORROSIVE POISONS

Types of corrosive poison

1. Acid and acid-like corrosives; sodium acid sulphate (toilet bowl cleaners), acetic acid (glacial), sulphuric acid, nitric acid, oxalic acid, hydrofluoric acid (rust removers), iodine, silver nitrate.
2. Alkali corrosives – most common are sodium hydroxide (lysol; drain cleaners), dishwasher detergents, sodium carbonate (washing soda), ammonia water, sodium hypochlorite (household bleach).

Clinical features

1. Severe pain; burning sensation in mouth and throat.
2. Painful swallowing or inability to swallow.
3. Vomiting.
4. Destruction of oral mucosa.

NURSING ALERT

Do not induce vomiting if victim has consumed a strong acid, alkali or other corrosive or hydrocarbon solvent. Do not induce vomiting if patient is unconscious or is having convulsions.

Emergency management

The first aid and hospital management, see previous column, applies to corrosive poisons, except that if the patient can swallow after ingestion of a *corrosive* poison, he may be offered milk as an emollient agent.

NONCORROSIVE POISONS

1. In hospital, remove poison from patient's stomach as soon as possible. Either:
   a. Induce vomiting by giving ipecacuanha as prescribed, or
   b. Carry out gastric lavage if less than four hours since ingestion, but not if a corrosive substance is involved.
2. A patient who has ingested hydrocarbons should have a chest X-ray done to assess for damage, e.g., chemical pneumonia.
3. Instruct family to bring unused poison to hospital for identification.

OTHER COMMON POISONS

Iron

Iron is very dangerous in small children. Desferrioxamine mesylate solution (2g to 1 litre) (a chelating agent rendering the iron harmless) is used for gastric lavage. A solution of desferrioxamine mesylate 10g to 50ml water should be left in the stomach and 2g given intramuscularly.

Paracetamol

Paracetamol can cause liver damage, often fatal, occurring several days after taking as little as 20 to 30 tablets (10–15g). It can occur without jaundice. Plasma paracetamol concentrations dictate the amount of antidote to be given, e.g., methionine, acetylcysteine or cysteamine, which all afford protection against liver damage if given within 10 to 12 hours of ingestion.

Paraquat

Paraquat is a weedkiller and is extremely toxic if taken in the concentrated form. That available for domestic use is usually much weaker. The systemic effects of swallowed concentrated paraquat are painful ulceration of the tongue, lips and fauces within a few hours, accompanied by nausea and vomiting. Later, convulsions, dyspnoea with pulmonary oedema and acute renal failure may also occur. Obtain a specimen of urine, which should confirm the diagnosis, but a more accurate level of concentration will be shown in the plasma paraquat levels. Gastric lavage is carried out and a solution of Fullers earth and magnesium sulphate is left in the stomach. Oral administration of Fullers earth over a period of 24 hours is continued. In severe cases a forced diuresis combined with charcoal haemoperfusion may also be used.

Aspirin (salicylate)

This is an analgesic with anti-inflammatory properties. Overdose interferes with prothrombin levels and causes bleeding for which vitamin K is often needed. Aspirin compounds remain in the stomach for longer periods than the other drugs, and can be removed by gastric lavage up to 12 hours or more after ingestion. Gastric irritation occurs with bleeding from any peptic ulceration. Excess salicylates will upset the blood pH and cause acidosis with electrolyte imbalance and tinnitus.

GUIDELINES: ASSISTING WITH GASTRIC LAVAGE

Gastric lavage is the aspiration of the stomach contents and washing out of the stomach by means of a gastric tube.

PURPOSES

1. Remove unabsorbed poison after poison ingestion.
2. Diagnose gastric haemorrhage.
3. Cleanse the stomach before endoscopic procedures.
4. Remove liquid or small particles of material from the stomach.

NURSING ALERT

Gastric lavage is always dangerous, especially after acid or alkali ingestion, in the presence of convulsions or after ingestion of hydrocarbons or petroleum distillates. It is dangerous after ingestion of strong corrosive agents and if the patient is distressed and dislodges the tube during the procedure. Gastric lavage must be carried out under the control of an anaesthetist if the patient is unconscious.

EQUIPMENT

Stomach tubes (large lumen)
Large irrigating syringe with adapter
Large plastic funnel with adapter to fit stomach tube
Water-soluble lubricant

Bucket for aspirate
Mouth gag; nasotracheal or endotracheal tubes with inflatable cuffs
Containers for specimens

Tap water or appropriate antidote (milk, saline solution, sodium bicarbonate solution, fruit juice, activated charcoal*)

Litmus paper to test for gastric acidity.

PROCEDURE

Nursing action

Rationale

1. Remove dental appliances and inspect oral cavity for loose teeth.

2. Measure the distance between the bridge of the nose and the xiphoid process. Note this distance along the tube.

3. Lubricate the tube with water-soluble lubricant.

4. If the patient is comatose he is intubated with a cuffed nasotracheal or endotracheal tube by a doctor.

   A cuffed endotracheal tube prevents aspiration of gastric contents.

5. Place the patient in a left lateral position with the head, neck and trunk forming a straight line. After the lavage tube is passed, the head of the table is lowered. Have standby suction available.

   This position prevents fluid from running into the trachea and keeps reflux vomitus from being aspirated.

6. Pass the tube via the oral route while keeping the head in a neutral position. Pass the tube to the distance noted, or about 50cm.

   The depth of insertion of the tube will vary with the height of the patient. If the tube enters the larynx instead of the oesophagus the patient will experience coughing and dyspnoea.

7. Aspirate the stomach contents with syringe attached to the tube before instilling water or antidote. Save the initial specimen for analysis. Test this with litmus paper for acidity before progressing.

   Aspiration is carried out to remove the stomach contents. Blue litmus will turn red if gastric acid is present.

8. Remove syringe. Attach funnel to the stomach tube or use 50ml syringe to put lavage solution in gastric tube. Volume of fluid placed in the stomach should be small.

   Overfilling of the stomach may cause regurgitation and aspiration or force the stomach contents through the pylorus.

9. Slowly elevate funnel above the patient's head and pour approximately 120–300ml of solution into funnel.

   If the syringe method is used, the turbulence from the pressure of the syringe will cause the fluid to mix with the stomach contents and assist in washing all of the mucosal surface. It is possible for poison/drugs to be trapped in the rugae of stomach.

* Activated charcoal will absorb significant quantities of many drugs and chemicals and thus retards absorption from the gastrointestinal tract.

10. Lower the funnel and siphon the gastric contents into the bucket.

11. Save samples of first two washings.

Keep first washings isolated from other washings for possible analysis.

12. Repeat lavage procedure until the returns are relatively clear.

13. At the completion of lavage:
    a. Stomach may be left empty.
    b. Antidote may be instilled in tube and allowed to remain in stomach.
    c. Aperient may be put down tube.

14. Pinch off tube during removal or maintain suction while tube is being withdrawn.

Pinching off the tube prevents aspiration and the initiation of the vomiting reflex. Keeping the patient's head lower than the body also gives this protection.

15. Give the patient an aperient if ordered.

An aperient may be given if the poison has no corrosive action on the bowel. The aperient will help remove unabsorbed material from the intestine.

INHALED POISONS

CARBON MONOXIDE POISONING
May occur as an industrial or household accident or as an attempted suicide.

Underlying principles
1. The effect of carbon monoxide is to render the haemoglobin useless as an oxygen-carrying chemical, because it unites so firmly with the pigment in place of oxygen. As a result, tissue anoxia occurs.
2. Carbon monoxide causes damage by hypoxia:
    a. Patient may appear intoxicated (result of cerebral hypoxia).
    b. Skin may be cherry red or cyanotic and pale – skin colour is *not* a reliable sign.
3. History of exposure to carbon monoxide should justify immediate treatment.

Emergency management
Objectives
Reverse cerebral and myocardial hypoxia.
Hasten carbon monoxide elimination.
1. Give 100 per cent oxygen at atmospheric or hyperbaric pressures to reverse hypoxia and accelerate elimination of carbon monoxide.
2. Observe the patient constantly – psychoses, spastic paralysis, visual disturbances and deterioration of personality may persist following resuscitation and may be symptoms of permanent central nervous system damage.

INJECTED POISONS

STINGING INSECTS
Bee, hornet, wasp.

NURSING ALERT
A patient may have an extreme sensitivity to Hymenoptera stings (bees, hornets, wasps). This constitutes an acute emergency. Stings of the head and neck are especially serious although stings in any area of the body can result in anaphylaxis.

Clinical features
1. Anaphylactic shock (p. 1086).
2. Oedema of face, lips.
3. Urticaria.
4. Itching.
5. Respiratory stridor, bronchial constriction.
6. Diarrhoea, abdominal cramps.
7. Local pain and swelling at the site of the sting.

Emergency management and patient education

1. See p. 1086 for treatment of anaphylactic shock.
2. Do not squeeze the venom sac as this may cause additional venom to be injected. Remove it carefully with tweezers. Wash the site with soapy water and apply cold (e.g. ice) to reduce pain and swelling. In the mouth, such stings are best treated by sucking an ice lolly.
3. Instruct the patient to avoid the following:
   a. Localities with stinging insects (camp and picnic sites).
   b. Going barefoot outdoors – some insects may nest on ground.
   c. Perfumes and bright colours – attract bees.

SNAKE BITE

Snake bites are fairly uncommon in the UK. The adder is the only poisonous snake native to the British Isles. Snake venoms are complex poisons. The toxic effects of snake venoms include agitation, restlessness, abdominal colic, diarrhoea and vomiting. In the UK each region has a special hospital designated to store snake antivenom. Advice should be sought from these hospitals regarding treatment and care.

The most common snake to be found is the grass snake, the bite of which is harmless, except for the local effects which include a mild inflammatory reaction with pain and swelling.

1. The patient should be laid on a trolley. Reassure – victims of snake bites may be extremely frightened.
2. Ask the patient to describe the snake in detail if possible.
3. Examine the site of the bite – usually the ankle or hand and it usually consists of two puncture marks.
4. Record temperature, pulse, respiration and blood pressure.
5. Clean the site of the bite.
6. Give antitetanus toxoid as prescribed.
7. If the snake is known to be a grass snake, the patient may be discharged. If the snake was unidentified, the patient is usually admitted overnight for observation.

FOOD POISONING

Food poisoning is a sudden illness which may occur after ingestion of contaminated food or drink.*

---

* Botulism, a serious form of food poisoning, is discussed on p. 1001 since the treatment differs and the patient requires continuing surveillance.

EMERGENCY MANAGEMENT

1. Determine the source and type of food poisoning.
   a. Have family bring suspected food to the hospital.
   b. Take the history:
      (i) How soon after eating did the symptoms occur? Immediate onset suggests chemical, plant or animal poisoning.
      (ii) What was eaten in the previous meal? Did the food have any unusual odour or taste? – Most foods causing bacterial poisoning do not have unusual odour or taste.
      (iii) Did vomiting occur? What was the appearance of the vomit?
      (iv) Did diarrhoea occur? – Usually absent with botulism, shellfish or other fish poisoning.
      (v) Are any neurological symptoms present? – Occur in botulism, chemical, plant and animal poisoning.
      (vi) Does the patient have fever? – Seen in salmonella, favism (ingestion of fava beans) and some fish poisoning.
      (vii) What is the patient's appearance?
2. Monitor vital signs on a continuing basis.
   a. Assess respiration, blood pressure, pulse and muscular activity.
   b. Weigh the patient for future comparisons.
3. Support the respiratory system. Death from respiratory paralysis can occur with botulism, fish poisoning.
4. Maintain fluid and electrolyte balance by prescribed intravenous infusion – electrolytes and water are lost as a result of vomiting and diarrhoea.
   a. Observe for oligaemic shock – from severe fluid and electrolyte losses.
   b. Assess for apathy, rapid pulse, fever, oliguria, anuria, hypotension, delirium.
   c. Get stool specimen for culture and sensitivity and for ova and parasite tests if indicated.
5. Monitor blood glucose levels by BM-stix or dextrostix.
6. Control the nausea.
   a. Give sips of weak tea, carbonated drinks, tap water for mild nausea.
   b. Give clear liquids 12 to 24 hours after nausea and vomiting subside.
   c. Graduate to a low residue bland diet.
7. Control the diarrhoea – diarrhoea may be desirable to rid body of ingested toxins.
   a. Apply warm compresses and moist, mild heat to abdomen – for comfort.

b. Give antidiarrhoeal agents as ordered – to absorb and bind toxins.

DRUG ABUSE

Drug abuse is the use of drugs for other than legitimate medical purposes. The clinical features may vary with the drug used but the underlying principles of management are essentially the same. Adopt a supportive, empathetic and realistic relationship with the patient.

ACUTE DRUG REACTION

PRIORITIES
1. Maintain adequate airway.
2. Support respiration.
3. Correct hypotension.

EMERGENCY MANAGEMENT
1. Maintain the patient's respirations.
2. Remove the drug from the stomach as soon as possible (if drug has been ingested).
   a. Induce vomiting if patient is seen *early* after ingestion, and only if the patient is conscious.
   b. Use gastric lavage if the patient is unconscious or if there is no way to determine when the drug was ingested.
      (i) In an unconscious patient, carry out this procedure only after intubation with cuffed endotracheal tube to prevent aspiration of stomach contents.
      (ii) Activated charcoal may be a useful adjunct to therapy and is used after vomiting or lavage.
3. The doctor may consider haemodialysis or peritoneal dialysis for potentially lethal poisoning.
4. Monitor the flow of urine since the drug or metabolites are excreted by the kidneys. Record the output on a fluid balance chart.
5. The doctor will do a thorough physical examination to rule out insulin shock, meningitis, subdural haematoma, stroke, trauma.
   a. Look for needle marks, constricted pupils.
   b. Examine breath for characteristic odour of alcohol, acetone, etc.
   c. Start ECG monitoring if indicated.
   d. Temperature, pulse, blood pressure are charted. Check the colour of the skin.
   e. Observe for level of consciousness and pupil reaction to light.
   f. Check the blood sugar levels using BM-stix or dextrostix for risk of hypoglycaemia.
6. Assist in the fluid replacement therapy and monitor all input of fluids by oral or parenteral route.
7. Try to obtain a history of the drug of experiences (from the person accompanying the patient or from the patient himself).
   a. Do not leave the patient alone.

Specific types of drug abuse
1. Narcotics (e.g. heroin, morphine, codeine and methadone).
2. Hallucinogens (e.g. lysergic acid diethylamide, or LSD).
3. Amphetamines (e.g. benzedrine, dexadrine).
4. Barbiturates (e.g. Nembutal, Seconal, sodium amytal).
5. Non-barbiturates (e.g. Librium, Valium)

In each of these, the priorities of emergency management apply, with additional antidote and drug therapy as indicated:
1. Narcotics are treated with naloxone hydrochloride (Narcan), a narcotic antagonist.
2. Methadone may be prescribed to ease the symptoms of heroin withdrawal if the doctor is registered to treat these patients.
3. Valium may be used to sedate patients in acute hyperactivity or convulsions.
4. Phenobarbitone could be used in barbiturate withdrawal syndrome to reduce symptoms, as abrupt withdrawal may be life-threatening.

ALCOHOLISM

ACUTE ALCOHOLISM

CLINICAL FEATURES
Caused by depressant action of alcohol on nervous system.
1. Drowsiness, inco-ordination, slurring of speech – or
2. Belligerence, grandiosity, uninhibited behaviour.
3. Odour of alcohol on breath.
4. Blood alcohol concentration.

EMERGENCY MANAGEMENT
1. Approach the patient in a nonjudgemental manner.

a. Expect patient to use mechanisms of denial and defensiveness.
b. Adapt a firm, consistent, accepting and reasonable attitude.
c. Speak calmly.
d. If patient appears drunk, he probably is drunk even though he denies any alcohol intake.

2. Allow the drowsy patient to 'sleep off' the state of alcoholic intoxication.
   a. Observe for symptoms of respiratory depression.
   b. Protect the airway.
   c. Undress the patient and cover with a blanket.

3. Examine the patient for injuries and organic disease which can easily be masked by alcoholic intoxication; alcoholics suffer more injuries than the general population.
   a. Look for symptoms of head injury. Assess the neurological status of the patient.
   b. Assess for alcoholic coma – a medical emergency.
   c. Assess for hypoglycaemia by testing with BM-stix or dextrostix if possible.

4. Admit to hospital if necessary.

DELIRIUM TREMENS (ALCOHOLIC HALLUCINOSIS)

Delirium tremens is an acute psychotic state that follows a prolonged bout of steady drinking or diminution or cessation of alcoholic intake.

CLINICAL FEATURES

1. Anxiety; uncontrollable fear.
2. Tremulousness, restlessness and agitation, irritability, insomnia.
3. Talkativeness; preoccupation.
4. Visual, tactile and auditory hallucinations (usually of a frightening nature).
5. Autonomic overactivity – tachycardia, profuse perspiration, fever.

NURSING ALERT

Delirium tremens is a serious complication and poses a threat to the life of the alcoholic patient.

EMERGENCY MANAGEMENT

Objective

Give proper sedation to enable the patient to rest and recover without the danger of injury or exhaustion.

1. Take the blood pressure since the patient's subsequent medication may depend on his blood pressure readings.

2. The doctor will carry out physical examination to identify pre-existing or contributing illnesses or injuries (cerebral injury, pneumonia).

3. A sufficient dosage of medication to produce adequate sedation may be prescribed by the doctor if it is considered safe to do so – to reduce his agitation, prevent exhaustion and promote sleep.
   a. A variety of drugs and combinations of drugs are used – chloral hydrate, diazepam (Valium).
   b. The dosage may be adjusted according to the patient's blood pressure response.

NURSING ALERT

Maintain regular assessment of the patient's airway and breathing as sedatives may, in conjunction with alcohol, cause respiratory depression.

4. Place the patient in a private room where he can be observed closely.
   a. Keep room lighted – to reduce incidence of visual hallucinations.
   b. Observe patient closely – he may become homicidal or suicidal in response to his hallucinations if he is having alcoholic hallucinations.
   c. Have someone stay with the patient as much as possible – presence of another person has a reassuring and quieting effect.
   d. Explain in detail every procedure done to the patient.
   e. Explain visual misinterpretations (illusions) – strengthens link with reality.
   f. Use restraints only as a last resort if patient is not under direct and constant observation.

5. Maintain electrolyte balance and hydration via oral or intravenous route – fluid losses may be extreme because of profuse perspiration and agitation.

6. Record temperature, pulse, respiration and blood pressure frequently (every 30 minutes in severe forms of delirium) – in anticipation of peripheral circulatory collapse and/or hyperthermia (the two most common lethal complications).

7. Phenytoin sodium (Epanutin) or other anticonvulsant drugs may be prescribed to prevent or control alcoholic or epileptic convulsions.

8. Assess respiratory, hepatic and cardiovascular status of patient – pneumonia, liver disease and cardiac failure are complications.

9. Give supplemental vitamin therapy and a high

protein diet; these patients are usually vitamin deficient.

10. Refer to alcoholic treatment centre for subsequent follow-up and rehabilitation.

PSYCHIATRIC EMERGENCY

Psychiatric emergency is a sudden serious disturbance of behaviour, affect or thought which makes the patient unable to cope with his life situation and interpersonal relationships.

BEHAVIOURAL FEATURES
The patient may be overactive, underactive or suicidal.

Overactive
1. Disturbed, unco-operative, unpredictable paranoid behaviour.
2. Anxiety and panic-like state.
3. Assaultive and destructive impulses and behaviour (patient may be noisy or disturbed).
4. Crying, depression, intense nervousness.

Underactive
1. Depression.
2. Fearfulness, detached attitude.
3. Slowing of responses.
4. Sad facial expression.

EMERGENCY MANAGEMENT
Overactive
1. Determine (from family, etc) if patient has had past mental illness, hospitalizations, injuries or serious illnesses, uses alcohol or drugs, or has experienced crises in interpersonal relationships or intrapsychic conflicts.
2. Try to gain control of the situation.
   a. Introduce yourself by name to the patient.
   b. Tell him 'I am here to help you'.
   c. Repeat patient's name from time to time.
   d. Speak in one-thought sentences. Be consistent.
   e. Give the individual space. Let him slow down by himself and allow him to become compliant.
   f. Approach the patient with a calm, confident and firm manner – this attitude is therapeutic and will help calm the patient.
   g. Be interested in and listen to the patient – encourage him to talk of his thoughts and *feelings*.
   h. Offer appropriate explanations. Tell the truth.
3. Give tranquillizer or psychotropic drug as prescribed for emergency management of functional psychosis. Chlorpromazine (Largactil) or haloperidol (Haldol) acts specifically against psychotic symptoms of thought fragmentation and perceptual and behavioural aberrations.
   a. Observe patient for one hour after initial dose to determine degree of change in psychotic behaviour.
   b. Subsequent dosages depend on patient's reaction.
   c. If behaviour is caused by hallucinogens (LSD) psychotropic drugs are not used.
4. Admit to psychiatric unit or arrange for psychiatric outpatient treatment.

Underactive
1. Listen to the patient in a calm, unhurried manner – offer follow-up services.
2. Find out if the patient is on any drugs. Give antidepressants with anti-anxiety drugs as prescribed.
3. Attempt to find out if patient has thought about or attempted suicide.
4. Anticipate that the patient may be suicidal.
5. Notify relatives about a seriously depressed patient.
6. The doctor may refer patient to hospital psychiatric unit.

Suicidal
Suicide is an act that stems from depression (from illness, loss of a loved one, loss of body integrity or status).
1. Treat the emergency condition brought about by the suicide attempt (gunshot wound, lacerations, overdose, etc.).
2. Prevent further self-injury – a patient who has made a suicidal gesture may do so again.
3. Admit to the ward for observation or to psychiatric unit.

SEXUAL ASSAULT

Rape or sexual assault is a serious attack on an individual. The patient should be seen immediately upon entrance into the emergency department.

EMERGENCY MANAGEMENT
Objectives
Give sympathetic support.
Reduce the emotional trauma of the patient.
1. Respect the privacy and sensitivity of the patient; be kind and supportive.
   a. The manner in which the patient is received and treated in the emergency department is important to the future psychological well-being of the patient. Crisis intervention should begin when the patient enters the department.
      (i) Emotional trauma may be present for weeks, months, years. Patient may go through phases of psychological reactions:
         (a) Phase of disorganization – fear, guilt, humility, anger, self-blame.
         (b) Phase of resolution (putting incident into perspective) – may have sleep disturbances, phobias, sexual fears.
      (ii) Reassure patient that anxiety is natural and that appropriate support is available from professional and community resources.
   b. Accept the emotional reactions of patient (hysteria, stoicism, overwhelmed feeling).
2. Leave clothing undisturbed. The police should be informed if the patient consents. A police surgeon is sent, accompanied by a policewoman.
3. Assist with the physical examination.
   a. Secure informed consent from patient (or parent/guardian if patient is a minor) for examination and for the taking of photographs if necessary – may be used as legal evidence.
   b. Take history *only* if patient has not already talked to police officer, social worker. Do not ask the patient to repeat the history.
   c. Record general appearance of patient – evidence of bruises, lacerations, secretions, torn and bloody clothing.
   d. Record emotional state.
   e. Assist patient to undress. Conserve dignity. Save clothing; place in plastic bag, label appropriately. Do not wash the patient until she has been seen by the police surgeon.
   f. Assist with vaginal examination.
      (i) Prepare water-moistened vaginal speculum for examination; do not use lubricant.
      (ii) Assist with securing laboratory specimens.
4. The doctor will treat associated injuries as indicated, and give patient the option of prophylaxis against venereal disease.
5. Offer antipregnancy measures if patient is of childbearing age, is using no contraceptives, and is at high risk in menstrual cycle.
6. Offer cleansing douche if patient desires.
7. Provide for follow-up services:
   a. Make appointment for follow-up surveillance for pregnancy and venereal disease.
   b. Encourage patient to return to previous level of functioning as soon as possible.
   c. Inform patient of counselling services to prevent long-term psychological effects.
   d. Patient should be accompanied by family/friend when leaving department.

NURSING IN DISASTER CONDITIONS

A disaster is a catastrophe which may be either natural or man-made in origin – produced either accidentally or by design.

NURSING FUNCTIONS IN DISASTERS
Since the nurse is delegated greater responsibilities in emergency and disaster situations, when mass casualties occur, nursing functions at such times may include:
1. Administering first aid such as artificial ventilation, cardiopulmonary resuscitation.
2. Controlling haemorrhage.
3. Treating shock.
4. Recognizing trauma to any organ or system.
5. Showing a proficiency in intravenous monitoring – in the use of equipment, fluids, medications, and central venous pressure measurements.
6. Properly and adequately cleansing and treating wounds.
7. Recognizing common fractures; bandaging and splinting.
8. Observing neurological functions.
9. Inserting nasogastric tubes for purposes of aspiration.
10. Catheterizing males and females.
11. Administering immunizing agents as prescribed.
12. Recognizing life-threatening conditions in their early stages – acute pulmonary oedema, respiratory complications, gastrointestinal bleeding.
13. Managing psychiatric emergencies. Managing psychologically disturbed persons.

SORTING (TRIAGE)

The sorting of casualties (also called *triage*) involves placing patients in categories for treatment on the basis of diagnosis and prognosis.

1. Sorting is a continuous process.
2. The most responsible and able people of the medical team are assigned sorting responsibilities.

CLASSIFICATION FOR PRIORITY IN TREATMENT

1. *Minimal treatment* – patients who can be returned to active duty immediately.
2. *Immediate treatment* – patients for whom the available expedient procedures will save life or limb.
3. *Delayed treatment* – patients who, after emergency treatment, will incur little increased risk by having surgery withheld temporarily.
4. *Expectant treatment* – critically injured patients who will be given treatment if time and facilities are available.

PRIORITIES OF TREATMENT

The following is a priority schedule which serves as a guide for establishing the flow of casualties from the disaster area through the first aid station to forward treatment centre and hospital.

First priority (individuals needing immediate attention to save life)

1. Any wound interfering with airway or causing airway obstruction. (This includes sucking chest wounds, tension pneumothorax and maxillofacial wounds in which asphyxia is present or an impending threat.)
2. Any wound requiring immediate pressure.
3. Shock due to major haemorrhage from wounds of any organ system, fractures (some of these conditions may be so urgent that immediate life-saving measures will have to be taken by the person doing the sorting).

Second priority (individuals needing early surgery)

1. Visceral injuries, including perforations of the gastrointestinal tract; wounds of the biliary and pancreatic system; wounds of the genitourinary tract; and thoracic wounds without asphyxia.
2. Vascular injuries requiring repair.
3. Closed cerebral injuries with increasing loss of consciousness.

Third priority (patients who require surgery but can tolerate a delay)

1. Spinal injuries in which decompression is required.
2. Soft-tissue wounds in which debridement is necessary, but in which muscle damage is less than major.
3. Lesser fractures and dislocations.
4. Injuries of the eyes.
5. Maxillofacial injuries without asphyxia.

IDENTIFICATION OF CASUALTIES

1. Identification is done by an emergency medical tag.
2. Place the tag directly on the body, preferably the wrist; do not attach to clothing since it may be lost.
3. Tags are written out by a clerk who accompanies the sorting officer; clerk completes admission records, clinical records and emergency tags.
4. Drugs administered are written on the tag, along with time given, and routes.
5. The nurse should be familiar with the local major accident policy.

FURTHER READING

BOOKS

Anon (1984) *Shock* (*Nursing Now* Series), Springhouse Corporation, Philadelphia.

Bache, J.B., Armitt, C.R. and Tobiss, J.R. (1985) *A Colour Atlas of Nursing Procedures in Accidents and Emergencies*, Wolfe Medical Publications, London.

Barrett, J. (1985) *Accident and Emergency Nursing*, Blackwell Scientific, Oxford.

Evans, T.R. (ed.) (1986) *ABC of Resuscitation*, British Medical Journal, Tavistock, London.

Fought, S.G. and Throwe, A.N. (1984) *Psychosocial Nursing Care of the Emergency Patient*, John Wiley, Chichester.

Joint Voluntary Aid Societies (1987) *First Aid Manual* (5th edn), St John Ambulance Association, St Andrew's Ambulance Association and British Red Cross Society, Dorling Kindersley, London.

Miller, M. and Miller, J. (1985) *Orthopaedics and Accidents Illustrated*, Hodder & Stoughton, Sevenoaks.

Templeton, J. and Wilson, R.I. (1983) *Lecture Notes on Trauma*, Blackwell Scientific, Oxford.

Walsh, M. (1986) *Accident and Emergency Nursing: A New Approach*, William Heinemann, London.

Westaby, S. (1985) *Wound Care*, William Heinemann, London.

ARTICLES

Assault

Walsh, M. (1986) Counting the bruises (violence in A & E), *Nursing Times*, Vol. 82, pp. 62–4.

— (1986) On the front line (violence in A & E), *Nursing Times*, Vol. 82, pp. 55–6.

Cold injuries and hypothermia

Shennan, V. (1985) How to recognise and prevent hypothermia, *New Age*, Vol. X, No. 32, pp. 16–17.

Drug and alcohol abuse

Gardner, R. (1983) Psychiatric aspects of self-poisoning, *Hospital Update*, Vol. X, April, pp. 485–91.

Strickland, S. (1986) Critical health issues in the workplace (alcohol and substance abuse), *American Association of Occupational Health and Nursing Journal*, Vol. 34, No. 9, pp. 443–4.

Emergency management

Anon (1984) Emergency care for myocardial infarction, choking, seizures, poisoning and near-drowning, *Nursing Life*, July/August, pp. 36–9.

— (1986) New CPR guidelines: bicarb now a last resort. *American Journal of Nursing*, Vol. 86, No. 8, p. 889.

Baskett, P. (1986) ABC of resuscitation. The ethics of resuscitation, *British Medical Journal*, Vol. 293, pp. 189–90.

Busfield, J. (1980) Be prepared for anything! *Nursing Mirror* (Supplement), November, pp. ii–v.

Harris, M. (1986) ABC of resuscitation. Drowning and near-drowning, *British Medical Journal*, Vol. 293, pp. 122–4.

Pearce, C. (1986) The challenge of change: application in a specific care setting, *Senior Nurse*, Vol. 5, No. 3, p. 33.

Simons, R. (1986) ABC of Resuscitation. Training manikins. *British Medical Journal*, Vol. 292 p. 1509–1513.

Simons, R. and Howell, T. (1986) ABC of resuscitation. The airway at risk, *British Medical Journal*, Vol. 292, pp. 1722–6.

Thompson, J. (1986) Nursing diagnosis: an overview and application to emergency nursing, *Journal of Emergency Nursing*, Vol. 12, No. 4, pp. 218–24.

Wilson, D. (1980) Extending a helping hand, *Nursing Mirror* (Supplement), November, pp. viii–xii.

— (1980) Teamwork – an essential part of A and E, *Nursing Mirror* (Supplement), November, pp. xv–xxi.

Wynne, G. (1986) ABC of resuscitation. Training and retention of skills, *British Medical Journal*, Vol. 293, pp. 30–32.

Zideman, D. (1986) ABC of resuscitation. Resuscitation of infants and children, *British Medical Journal*, Vol. 292, pp. 1584–8.

Fractures

Dunn, J. (1985) Fracture of the tibia and fibula, *New Zealand Nursing Journal*, Vol. 78, No. 12, pp. 25–8.

Genge, M. (1986) Orthopaedic trauma: pelvic fractures, *Orthopaedic Nursing*, Vol. 5, No. 1, pp. 11–19.

Worlock, P. *et al.* (1986) Patterns of fractures in accidental and non-accidental injury in children: a comparative study, *British Medical Journal*, Vol. 293, pp. 100–2.

Head injuries

Allan, D. (1986) Management of the head-injured patient (by accident and emergency nurses), *Nursing Times*, Vol. 82, pp. 36–9.

Pentland, B. *et al.* (1986) Head injury in the elderly, *Age and Ageing*, Vol. 15, No. 4, pp. 193–202.

Multiple injuries

Barber, J.S. (1986) Immunological responses to trauma, *Critical Care Quarterly*, Vol. 9, No. 1, pp. 57–67.

Smith, S. (1986) Care of the multi-injured patient. A nursing perspective, *Care of the Critically Ill*, Vol. 2, No. 1, pp. 28–9.

Nursing in disasters

Shea, K.G. (1986) Natural disaster: personal preparedness, *Association of Operating Room Nurses Journal*, Vol. 43, No. 6, pp.1226–38.

Shea, K. and Hesterly, S. (1986) Disaster nursing: paredness in the OR, *Association of Operating Room Nurses Journal*, Vol. 43, No. 6, pp.1240–1, 1243–7.

Shock

Beckwith, N. and Carriere, S. (1985) Fluid resuscitation in trauma: an update, *Journal of Emergency Nursing*, Vol. 11, No. 6, pp. 293–9.

Wounds

Johnson, A. (1986) Modern concepts of wound management (review of wound dressings), *Practical Diabetes*, Vol. 3, No. 1, pp. 20–23.

McMahon, B. (1986) Self-inflicted wounds, *Nursing: The Add-on Journal of Clinical Nursing*, Vol. 3, No. 6, pp. 222–4.

Stewert, A. (1985) Factors affecting wound healing, *Professional Nurse*, Vol. 5, No. 1, pp. 11–19.

Index

Note on page references: Italic type indicates illustrations.

KT-489

LIBREX-

Imprint

The Deutsche Nationalbibliothek lists this publication in the Deutsche Nationalbibliografie; detailed bibliographical data are available on the internet at http://dnb.d-nb.de.

ISBN 978-3-03768-098-8
© 2012 by Braun Publishing AG
www.braun-publishing.ch

1st edition 2012

Editorial staff: Julia Chromow, Sara Dame, Lisa Rogers, Chris van Uffelen
Translation: Lisa Rogers
Graphic concept and layout: Michaela Prinz, Berlin

500 x Art in Public

Chris van Uffelen

BRAUN

Content

Antiquity

Medieval Art

Renaissance

Baroque / Rococo

Classicism / Historicism

Classical Modernity

Modernity

Contemporary

Art

Antiquity
Renaissance
Baroque
Rococo
Historicism/
Classicism
Modernity
Contemporary
Medieval

Preface
Chris van Uffelen

Works of art on display in the public realm have always featured amongst the greatest achievements of mankind. In earlier cultures, these works indicated a social consensus or belief or were of importance for cult practices. Even today, art in public functions as an important, identifying feature, providing an opportunity for the open expression of ideas. This book traces the history of public art, by considering works of art on permanent display within the public realm. Temporary works have been omitted from this book, along with art in private space and interior art. However, these rules have been fairly generously interpreted. Examples of "transient" work, made only to disappear over time are viewed as "permanently in the past". Works of art that are today housed in museums but that were originally (presumably) conceived for public space have been included, along with those in museum gardens and unfenced, open spaces as these are so similar to works exhibited in open park space, it was felt that exclusion was not justified. It is also likely that a few of the (Antique period) works included were not originally in the public realm, but these have been included in an effort to portray important styles. A further criterion considered was the "freedom of panorama", this allows the public to freely publish or discuss public works of art; this includes the freedom to interact with the art work, which is, of course, an important attribute of "Art in Public". However, not every land has freedom of panorama, this means that the "public" work in these countries is, to all intents and purposes, not in public. Artists who come from countries without the freedom of panorama laws are featured in this book but the works published are usually those situated in countries where freedom of panorama is a given. Around 150 works explain the history of public art over 4,500 years of historical eras and styles. 350 examples are from the 1960s to present day, allowing an in-depth look at contemporary works. The historical examples figuratively portray parts of history, depicting governors or rulers of the time or fulfill ancient decorative criteria. However, even the modern, space-defining function of art in public can be found in historical examples. This all comes seamlessly together to provide a non-stop history of art, aligned more with contemporary works.

Great Sphinx of Giza
unknown

Completion: 26th c. BC. **Technique:** stone. **Location:** Giza, Egypt

This monolithic sculpture of a reclining or couchant "Sphinx" in Giza is the largest monolith statue in the world. It is estimated that it was sculpted during the reign of the Pharaoh Chefren, between 2558–2532 BC. It is located beside the valley temple and the causeway leading to the mortuary temple beside the pyramid. The nose of the "Sphinx" was already gone in the 15th century and after the Giza Necropolis was abandoned, the Sphinx became buried up to its shoulders in sand.

Chefren was the fourth Pharaoh of the fourth dynasty. He was the son of Cheops and took over the throne from his brother, who reigned for about one decade after their father's death. It was under orders from Chefren that the second largest pyramid was built (Cheops' is three meters larger) in the Giza Necropolis complex and, most likely, the "Great Sphinx" as well. The "Great Sphinx" is cut out of the same stone quarrel, which was used for the pyramid.

Photo: Mavila2 / Wikimedia Commons

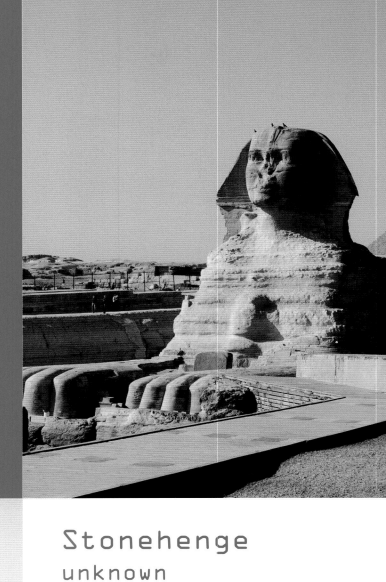

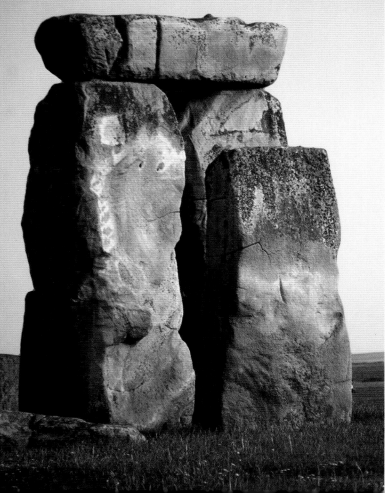

Stonehenge
unknown

Completion: 2800 BC–1800 BC. **Technique:** stone. **Location:** Salisbury, United Kingdom.

The stones used to make "Stonehenge" are believed to be from the Prescelly Mountains, roughly 240 miles away. The stones weigh up to four tons each and about 80 were used, in total. It is speculated that the stones were dragged by roller or sledge from the inland, before being floated around the coast of Wales and then down the river Avon, after which they were then dragged over land before being floated down the river Wylye to Salisbury.

No one can say for certain why "Stonehenge" was built, but it is most commonly attributed to the druids. However, this was later disproved, because the site was created some 2,000 years before the druids. Other theories suggest that it was more likely to have been built by the people of the late Neolithic period, named Beaker Folk, after their use of pottery drinking vessels. It was most likely a place for religious ceremonies though it has also been suggested it was used as an astronomical observatory and calendar.

Photo: Chris van Uffelen

Mortuary Temple of Hatshepsut
Senenmut

Completion: 1460 BC. **Technique:** stone. **Location:** Deir el-Bahari, Egypt.

The "Mortuary Temple of Hatshepsut" is the best-preserved temple in the Deir el-Bahari, the "Northern Monastery", near the city of Luxor. It consists of three layers of terraces with colonnaded fronts, is 30 meters high and is reached by long ramps that were once graced with gardens. Most of the original statue ornaments are missing – Osiris statues in front of the pillars of the upper colonnade, the sphinx avenues in front of the court, as well as the figures of Pharaoh Hatshepsut.

Senenmut was an architect and government official of the 18th dynasty who probably died in the 16th year of Hatshepsut's reign (1463 BC). The joint tomb of his parents, discovered in the mid-1930s, reveals much more about him, than those of most non-royals. It is likely that he began working as a priest-scholar but by the end of his life he had been awarded 88 titles, like "High steward of the King" and "Custodian of Amun". Senenmut had constructed a tomb for himself near Hatshepsut's mortuary temple.

Photos: Olaf Tausch / Wikimedia Commons (a.); Daniel Fafard (Dreamdan) / Wikimedia Commons (b.)

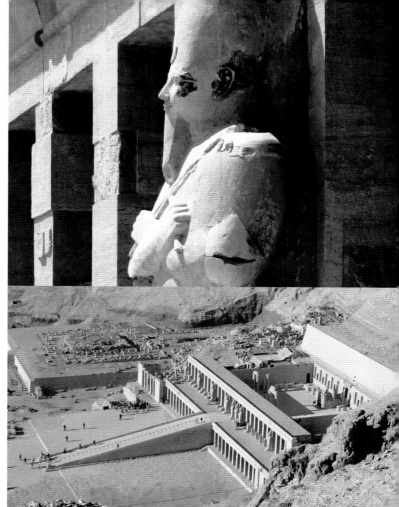

Lion Gate
unknown

Completion: 1250 BC. **Technique:** stone, bronze. **Location:** Mycenae, Greece.

This main gate provides access to the ancient town of Mycenae. It is made of just four stones, two posts, 3.10 meters high, the lintel stone, which weighs 12 tons, and a triangle-stone. Two lions are carved above the gate – the first monumental figurative sculpture of Europe. The lions are the central piece of the composition and stand with their forefeet on altars that support a column, symbolic of the Mycenae-kings. The missing heads of the lions are believed to have been made of bronze.

In the late Bronze Age, Mycenae, 90 kilometers south-west of Athens, became one of the centers of Greek culture. The Cretan culture at this time (up to 1450 BC) was centrally organized, consisting of several independent city-kingdoms, Thebes was also of great importance at this time. These cultural centers faded in around 1200 BC, possibly due to Doric invasions. Excavations began in 1802.

Photos: Ken Russell Salvador / Wikimedia Commons (a.); Chris van Uffelen (b.)

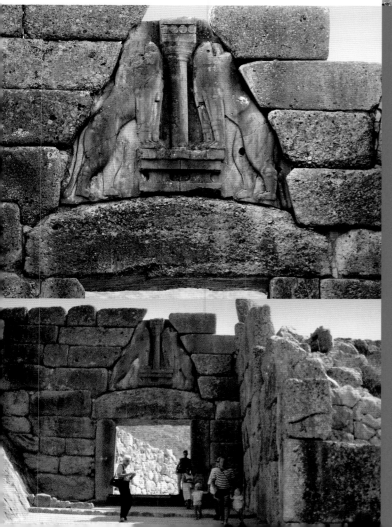

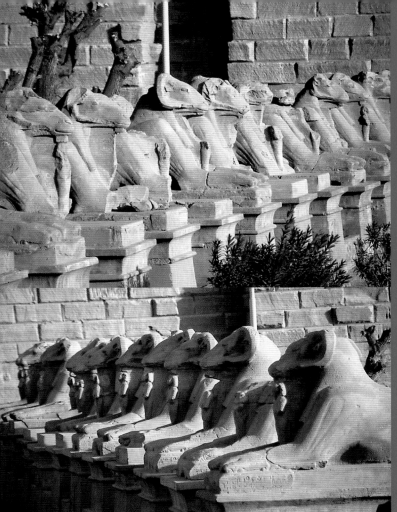

Ram-Sphinxes
unknown

Completion: early 13th c. BC. **Technique:** sandstone. **Location:** Karnak, Egypt.

The "Ram-Sphinxes" have the body of a lion, the head of a Ram and they are symbols of Amun. Amun became the god of Thebes in the 11th dynasty and when Thebes was chosen as new capital of Egypt in the 12th dynasty. As Amun-Re he took the functions of Re, Min und Amun. He was the leader of Thebes Triad, together with his consort Mut and their son Konsuth. The temple of Amun-Re in Karnak was the largest and richest in the country.

The temple complex of Karnak was begun under the rule of Pharaoh Sestores I (1975–1965 BC) close to the Nile. It once had its own harbor, from where the holy barks were carried through the valley, guarded on both sides by the Ram-headed sphinxes. The procession route ended at the 43-meter-high, unfinished, pylon-gate. The sphinxes led to the second pylon-gate, but they had originally been placed when the first was built (fourth century BC). The second gate was built at the end of Horemhebs reign (1292 BC).

Photos: Chris van Uffelen

Luxor Obelisk
unknown

Completion: mid 13th c. BC. **Technique:** granite. **Location:** Paris, France.

The 23-meter-high obelisk, weighing 250 tons, once flanked one side of the entrance to the Luxor Temple, in Egypt, together with its twin. They were erected under Ramses II (1279–1213 BC). Luxor, called Thebes in ancient times, was founded in 1400 BC. The temple was dedicated to the Theban triad of Amun, Mut and Chons. At the annual Opet Festival, the cult statue of Amun was paraded down the Nile from the nearby Karnak Temple where it stayed for a short while in a celebration of fertility.

In 1829 both obelisks were offered to the French King Louis-Philippe by Muhammad Ali Pasha and, after travelling for two years, the first one arrived in 1833. 1836 it became the center of Place de la Concorde when Jacob Ignatz Hittoft rearranged the ensemble of Jacques-Ange Gabriel (1755). The other obelisk remained on location and was officially given back to the Egyptians in the 1990s by President François Mitterrand. The Paris twin was given a three and a half-meter-high "Pyramidion", of gilded bronze, by Pierre Bergé, compagnon of Yves Saint-Laurent, in 1998.

Photo: Chris van Uffelen

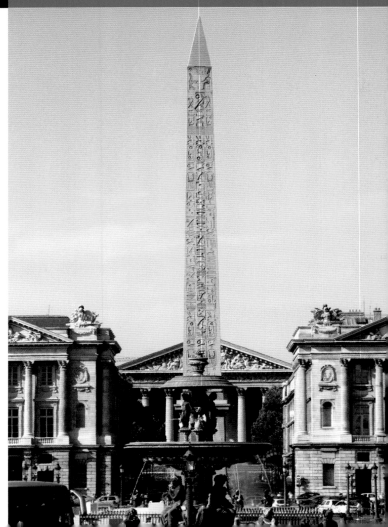

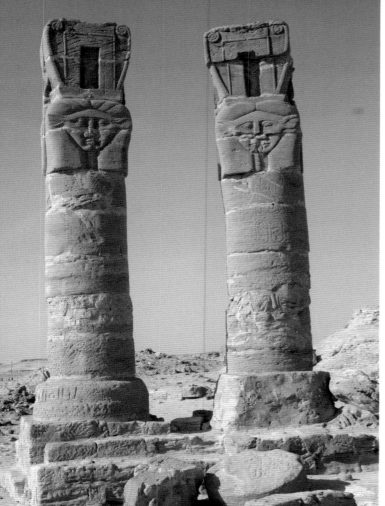

Hathor Columns
unknown

Completion: 680 BC. **Technique:** sandstone. **Location:** Barkal, Sudan.

Barkal was the most important religious center for Egyptians in Nubia. The temple "B.300" was built on the site of the older temple of Mut under the reign of Taharqa, a Pharaoh of Egypt and the Kingdom of Kush located in Northern Sudan. Mut, Hathor, Bes are all represented in this unique temple, and all can be identified in some regard with the myth of the "Eye of Re".

Hathor was a goddess, who was first depicted as a cow, she later became the goddess of the western sky and finally came to personify the principles of love, beauty, music, motherhood and joy. She was depicted with two horns on her head; these flanked a sun disc for a while and then later became volutes. Hathor is also often depicted playing the sistrum, a percussion instrument whose name comes from the Greek word "seiein" meaning "to shake".

Photos: Bertramz / Wikimedia Commons

Warrior of Hirschlanden
unknown

Completion: 6th c. BC. **Technique:** sandstone. **Location:** Hirschlanden, Germany.

The "Warrior of Hirschlanden" is a sculpture of a warrior and is made of sandstone. The statue is extremely worn and the feet have been broken off, suggesting that it stood for a long time in the elements. This is the oldest known example of a life size sculpture of the human form, north of the Alps. It is estimated to date back to the sixth century BC and comes from the Hallstatt culture. The original statue stands in the Württembergisches Landesmuseum in Stuttgart.

The Hallstatt culture spanned Central Europe and has been divided into four categories, HaA, HaB, HaC, HaD. HaA existed from 1200–1000 BC, B from 1000–800 BC, C from 800–650 BC and D from 650–475 BC. The 'real' Hallstatt period is accepted as HaC and D and corresponds to the early European Iron Age. Two culturally different areas have been identified, one to the east and the other to the west, with the dividing line running across the Czech Republic and Austria.

Photos: Harke / Wikimedia Commons

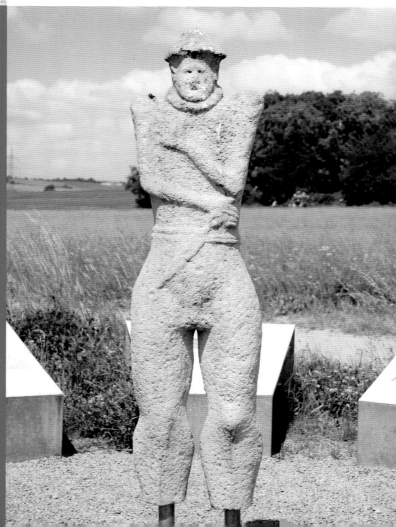

Wounded Amazon
Phidias (copy after)

Completion: 450–425 BC (copy 1st–2nd c.). **Technique:** marble, original bronze. **Location:** New York City, NY, USA.

This sculpture, a gift of John D. Rockefeller Jr., to the Metropolitan Museum of Art 1932, is a Roman copy of the Imperial period and is modeled on the Greek, bronze original. Other copies of the work of Phidias (for example in Berlin and Copenhagen) gave clues for the reconstruction of missing parts. Not a single work of Phidias survived in original and there remain only Roman copies of the most famous sculpture of ancient Greece.

Phidias was born around 500 BC in Athens and died in around 432 BC. He was a Greek sculptor, who learned his trade in the workshops of Hegias and Ageladas von Argos. His most famous works were the standing Athena Parthenos in Athens and the sitting Zeus statue in Olympia – both 12 meters high. The Zeus statue was one of the seven wonders of the ancient world. It was made of iron, wood and gypsum with a surface of gold and ivory. The workshop of Phidias in Olympia was discovered 1954.

Photo: Marie-Lan Nguyen / Wikimedia Commons

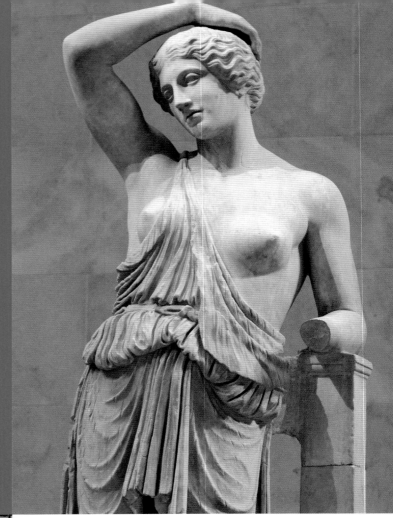

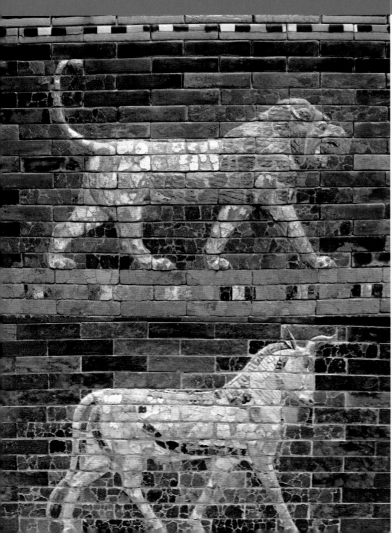

Ishtar Gate
unknown

Completion: 575 BC. **Technique:** glazed tiles. **Location:** Berlin, Germany.

This gate was dedicated to the Babylonian goddess Ishtar. It is one of the eight gates to the inner city of Babylon and was constructed by order of King Nebuchadnezzar II, on the north side of the city. It was one of the seven wonders of the ancient world until the sixth century AD. The Berlin reconstruction – only the forefront – measures 14 x 30 meters. The gate was decorated with lions, dragons and aurochs, symbolizing the gods Ishtar, Marduk and Adad.

Babylonia in central-southern Mesopotamia, today's Iraq, was an early culture that arose in the 17th century BC. The city of Babylon was first mentioned in the 23rd century BC. Its art and architecture derives from the Mesopotamian cultures of the Bronze Age. After the death of the last Assyrian ruler Assurbanipal in 675 BC, Babylonia rebelled under Nabopolassar the Chaldean and the Neo-Babylonian Empire was founded.

Photos: Gryffindor / Wikimedia Commons

Caryatids of the Erechtheion
Alkamenes (attributed)

Completion: 406 BC. **Technique:** stone. **Location:** Athens, Greece.

The roof of the south porch of the "Erechtheion" is supported by six caryatid figures. It is thought that they are the work of Alcamenes, a student of the great sculptor Phidias. The figures that can be seen today are replicas of the originals, which have been preserved in museums. One is at the British Museum and was removed from the "Erechtheion" by Lord Elgin in around 1803. This example is in a much better condition than the ones still in Greece as it was removed much earlier.

A caryatid is an architectural support that takes the form of a column, sculpted into the form of a female figure. Some of the earliest known examples were found in the treasuries of Delphi. The best known examples are those of the caryatid porch of the "Erechtheion" on the Acropolis in Athens. The practice of using caryatids was reintroduced in the Renaissance, when their use on façades became fashionable and they were also integrated into interior architecture as fireplace supports.

Photo: Chris van Uffelen

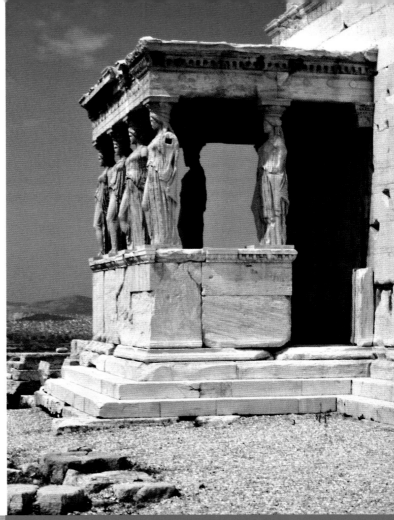

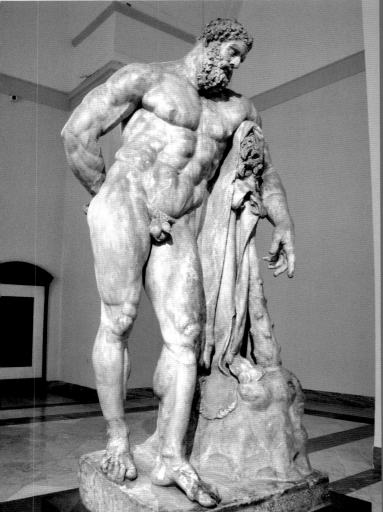

Farnese Hercules
Lysippos (copy after)

Completion: approx. 320 BC (copy 1st century BC). **Technique:** marble, original bronze. **Location:** Naples, Italy.

This statue shows Hercules leaning on his club, with the fur of a lion draped over it. His right hand holds three apples behind his back. These are both references to the tasks he was given: to kill the Nemean lion and to steel the apples of the Hesperides, guarded by a hundred-headed dragon, named Ladon. The extremely muscled figure, typical of the Late-Classic Style was first seen in around 1546 and has been copied by hundreds of artists since then.

Lysippos was born in Sicyon in approximately 370 BC and died in around 300 BC. He was the most famous scholar of Polykleitos and became court-sculpture for Alexander the Great. The National Museum in Naples houses a copy of the Hercules statue, made by Glykon, it is the most famous of over 200 known Roman copies of Greek bronzes. A copy of the head of this statue is on display in the Metropolitan Museum in New York.

Photo: Gryffindor / Wikimedia Commons

Apollo of the Belvedere
Leochares (copy after)

Completion: 350~325 BC. (copy 120~140). **Technique:** marble, original bronze. **Location:** Vatican Museums, Vatican City.

This statue of Apollo which is over two meters high is the Roman copy of a Greek sculpture. It depicts Apollo having just shot an arrow. The figure stands in a typical posture called contapposto, with most of the weight on one foot, so that the shoulders and arms twist off-axis from the hips and legs, this has the effect of making him appear relaxed and at ease.

Leochares was a Greek sculptor who lived in the fourth century BC. He worked on the construction of the Mausoleum of Maussollos at Halicarnassus and his sculptures survived only in the form of Roman copies. Besides the Apollo statue, the Diana of Versailles is also one of his most famous works. Several examples of his sculptures were placed in the Philippeion in the Altis at Olympia and Plato mentions him as a young and hard-working artist.

Photo: Marie-Lan Nguyen / Wikimedia Commons

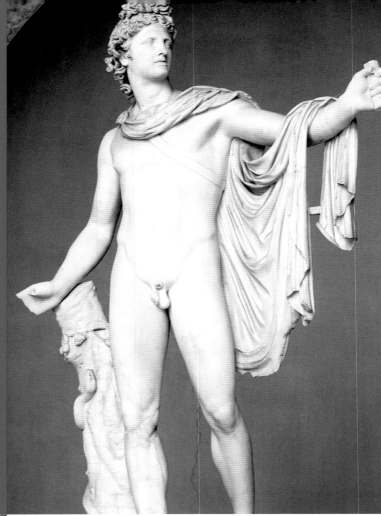

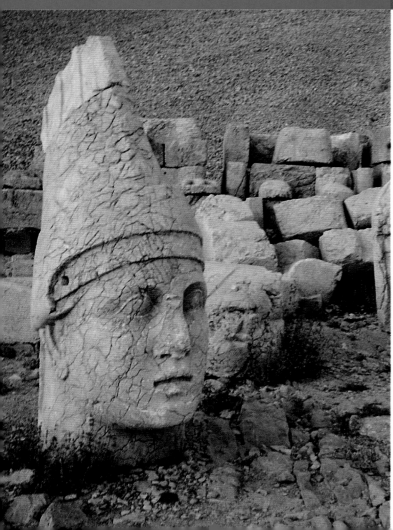

Nemrut Dağı
unknown

Completion: 1st c. BC. **Technique:** stone. **Location:** Nemrut Daği, Turkey.

Nemrut Daği is a mountain in south-east Turkey. At the summit, around what is assumed to be a tomb from the first century BC, are a large number of statues. High statues of King Antiochus I Theos of Commagene, as well as statues of eagles, lions and other gods originally flanked the tomb. The heads of the statues were removed from the bodies at some point and now lie scattered around the site. The damage to the heads is believed to have been done deliberately, probably out of religious reasons.

The site is believed to be the tomb of Antiochus I Theos of Commagene. He ordered the statues and tomb to be built before his death, an impressive religious sanctuary. During his reign as king, Antiochus created a royal cult, his birthday was celebrated on the 16th and his coronation on the tenth of each month. On these days he hosted a large feast and party. Antiochus appointed priests to continue the rituals after his death and wanted his body to be preserved and celebrated for eternity.

Photos: Tony f / Wikimedia Commons

Trajan's Column
Apollodorus of Damascus

Completion: 113 AD. **Technique:** marble. **Location:** Rome, Italy.

"Trajan's Column" is a 30-meter-high Doric column, with a five-meter-high pedestal and a frieze that winds 23 times around the shaft. The decoration on this 200-meter-long bas-relief tells the story of the Dacian wars. The senate commissioned propagandist monuments of this kind. Often there are different perspectives used in the same scene, to show more details, even though not the entire 2,500-figure story was to be seen from the ground or even from the two library wings that formerly flanked it.

Apollodorus of Damascus was a Greek engineer, architect, designer and sculptor and a favorite of Trajan. He designed the Trajan's Forum, Trajan's Thermae and the Emperor's Villa. Apollodorus made fun of Hadrian's works as architect and artist and after Hadrian became Emperor Apollodorus was banished. Shortly afterwards, he was charged with imaginary crimes and put to death. A self-portrait is kept in the Munich Glyptothek.

Photos: Chris van Uffelen

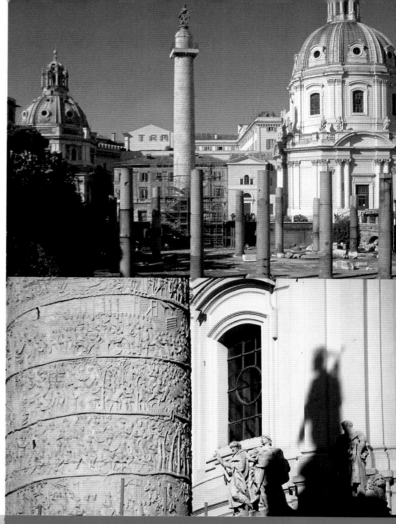

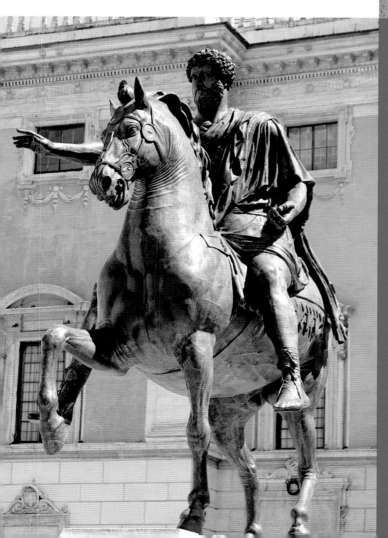

Equestrian Statue of Marcus Aurelius
unknown

Completion: 165~176 AD. **Technique:** bronze. **Location:** Rome, Italy.

Michelangelo placed this statue – its original is today exhibited in the Palazzo Nuovo – on the Capitoline Hill. It shows the Emperor Marcus Aurelius as a victorious conqueror, without any weapons but with military-robe. The work was designed according to the Platonic ideal of a philosopher-king after his victory over the Parthians. The statue is believed to have been gilded and has served as a model for hundreds of equestrian statues since the Renaissance.

This is the only equestrian statue of Roman Antiquity that survived. In the 8th century it stood in the Lateran Palace. In medieval times it was thought to be a statue of Constantine the Great and because of this, it was not melted down. In 1447 a librarian of the Vatican discovered that it was Marc Aurel and between 1536 and 1546 Michelangelo remanaged the Piazza del Campidoglio as first concept of axis for the city. He designed the paving as well but this wasn't realized until 1940 under Benito Mussolini.

Photo: Jastrow / Wikimedia Commons

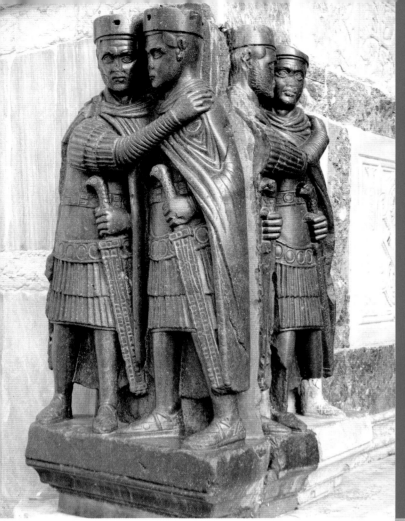

The Tetrarchs
unknown

Completion: approx. 300 AD. **Technique:** porphyry. **Location:** Venice, Italy.

The very schematic look of this work is typical of late Roman sculpture, which replaced the classical, Greek-Roman Style under Diocletian and even became characteristic for early Christian Art in the following centuries. The idea of equally ranked persons looking the same became what is now known as "Isocephaly", which is based on the idea that the sizes of the people and objects were attributed according to their importance.

"The Tetrarchs" were the four co-rulers that governed the Roman Empire for the short term of the Diocletian's reform. There were two senior and two junior emperors (taking the titles of Augusti or Caesares). A statue of them is located on the corner of St. Mark's Basilica in Venice, in this portrayal, hardly any difference can be seen between the four figures. This means that the four were of equal importance. Today the paired figures are thought to be: the Caesares Galerius and Constantius and the Augusti Diocletian and Maximian.

Photo: Nino Barbieri / Wikimedia Commons

Nok Terracotta Sculpture
unknown

Completion: 6th century AD. **Technique:** terracotta. **Location:** Nok, Nigeria.

This is an example of a Nok terracotta sculpture. The first of these was discovered in 1943, when tin mining operations began near the village of Nok in Nigeria. Since then, numerous figures of this type have been found over a large part of Nigeria. The Nok terracotta figures are typically hollow, built from coils of clay that were then fired in a kiln. The sculptural detail and the way the figures are carved suggest that the technique was developed from woodcarving techniques.

The Nok culture appeared in Nigeria around 1000 BC and died out in around 500 AD. The culture's social system is believed to have been very advanced and it is unknown why the tribe suddenly vanished. They were one of the earliest groups to begin producing life-sized terracotta sculpture. Similarities between these figures and the Yoruba Art forms have been noted, suggesting early connections between the ancient Nok tribe and the contemporary Yoruba people.

Photo: Jastrow / Wikimedia Commons

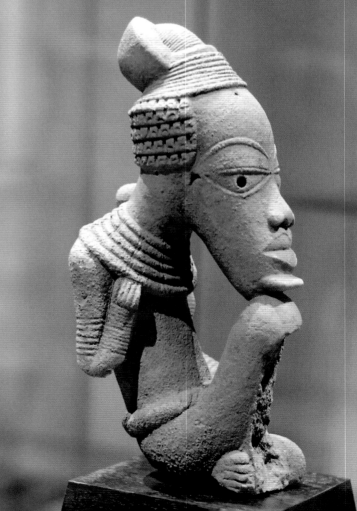

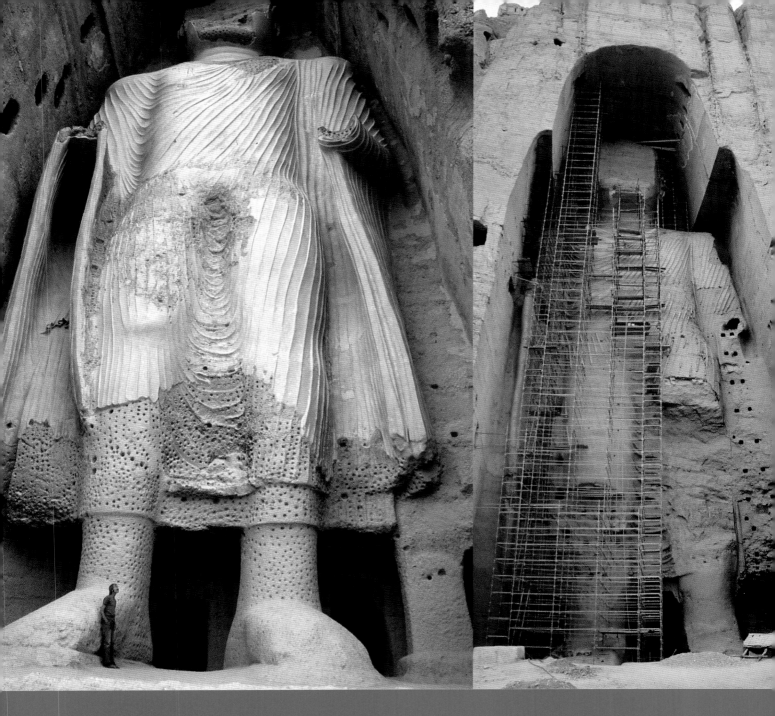

Buddhas of Bamiyan
unknown

Completion: 507 and 554 AD. **Technique:** red sandstone. **Location:** Bamiyan, Afghanistan.

The "Buddhas of Bamiyan" have been two enormous, carved statues of standing Buddhas. They were carved into the side of a hill in the Hazarajat region of central Afghanistan. The main bodies are cut directly from the sandstone cliffs but the detail was added after the carving, molded out of a mud and straw mixture and coated over with stucco to hold it in place. The lower arms were also made in this way.
The Taliban blew up the statues in 2001, after they declared them to be 'idols'.

Bamiyan lies on the Silk Road, in the Hindu Kush mountain region. The Silk Road linked the markets of China with those of Asia. Bamiyan was formerly a part of the Kingdom of Gandhara and was the site of several Buddhist monasteries. It remained a Buddhist site and a thriving center for religion, philosophy and Indian Art until the Islamic invasion in the ninth century.

Photos: Phecda109 / Wikimedia Commons

15

Jogeshwari Caves
unknown

Completion: 550. **Technique:** stone. **Location:** Mumbai, India.

The "Jogeshwari Caves" are located in the Mumbai suburbs of Jogeshwari and are amongst the earliest examples of Buddhist cave temples. These caves are not as well preserved and protected as other ancient Buddhist temples and are infested with bats. The caves are accessed by a long flight of stairs and carvings of Dattatreya, Hanuman and Ganesh line the walls. A line of carved pillars supports the caves.

The Mauryan Emperor Ashoka adopted Buddhism in around 300 BC and set out to spread the Buddhist teachings as far as possible. He had some 85,000 monuments constructed and engraved with Buddhist teachings. It was during the fourth, fifth and sixth centuries AD that India witnessed a huge resurgence of Hinduism, at the time when Hinduism became the official religion of the Gupta Empire. This resulted in a decline of the influence of the Buddhist religion.

Photo: Himanshu Sarpotdar / Wikimedia Commons

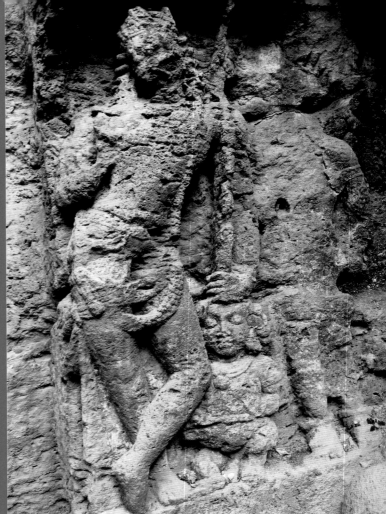

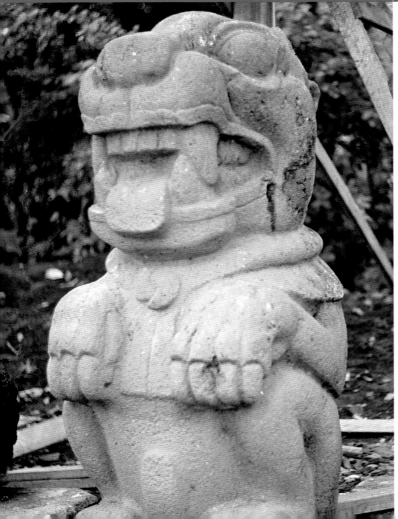

El Baúl
unknown

Completion: from 600–1000. **Technique:** stone. **Location:** Cotzumalguapa, Guatemala.

In the town of Santa Lucía in Guatemala stand huge, carved, stone heads with grotesque faces and reliefs with carved scenes. The sculptures were found at the Cotzumalguapa archaeological site, which also includes the sites of Bilbao and El Castillo. More than 200 sculptural works and carvings have been found at this site, varying in form from sculptures to decorated reliefs.

Santa Lucía Cotzumalguapa is one of the most important archaeological zones of Guatemala, located in the department of Escuintla, at the foot of the Pacific volcanic range. It is thought that this area experienced an early development going back at least to the end of the Early Pre-Classic Period (approx. 800 BC). The Cotzumalguapa archaeological project includes field archaeological research, artifact analyses and documentary research. Extensive excavations have revealed systems of bridges and causeways.

Photo: HJPD / Wikimedia Commons

Platform of Venus
unknown

Completion: 8th c. AD. **Technique:** stone. **Location:** Chichén Itzà, Mexico.

There are two structures called the "Platform of Venus" at Chichén Itzà. The first and better known one is located in the Great Plaza, a second one is located near the grave of the high priest. The platform was probably used for public addresses or rituals such as dance or sacrifice. Its base panels are inscribed with images of Kukulkan and representations of the planet Venus, which is believed to have been of great symbolic importance. The platform was originally painted in ochre, blue, red, green, and black.

Chichén Itzà is the second most visited archeological site in Mexico and is one of the most important sites linked to the Mayan culture, hundreds of buildings once stood here but today around 30 remain. The best known construction on the site is Kukulkan's Pyramid which is one of the seven wonders of the world.

Photos: HJPD / Wikimedia Commons (a.); Altairisfar / Wikimedia Commons (b.)

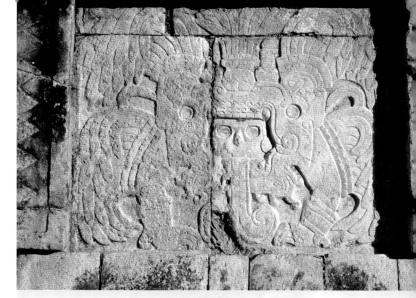

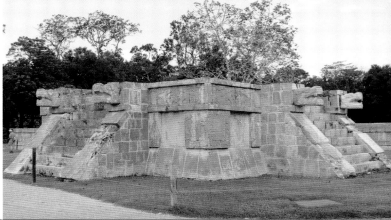

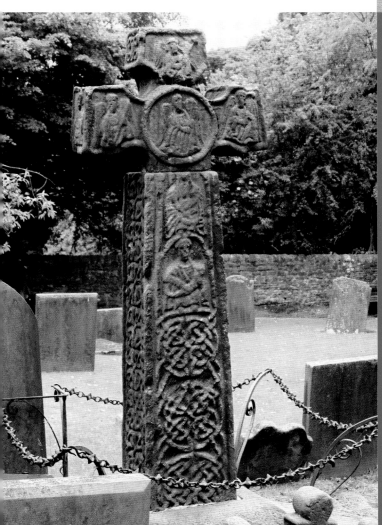

Celtic Cross
unknown

Completion: 8th c. AD. **Technique:** stone. **Location:** Eyam, United Kingdom.

Large, standing Celtic crosses made of stone can be found in graveyards and other places of religious importance throughout Ireland and Scotland, as well as other parts of Europe. There are many styles of Celtic crosses but they often have certain characteristics in common. Many feature a circular design around the cross shape or are engraved with circular patterns. Celtic crosses also often portray religious stories and were once used as a way of communicating a chosen story to a largely illiterate population.

The name "Celt" originated from the ancient Greeks, who called the barbarians of central Europe "keltoi". The Celts were a race of nomadic warriors who first emerged in Central Europe. Their descendants have roots in Italy, Greece, France, Britain and Ireland. When the Romans marched north, they conquered much of Europe before invading Britain. Much of England submitted to Roman rule; however, the Celts in Wales and Scotland resisted defeat and, along with Ireland, preserved their original Celtic culture.

Photo: Dave Pape / Wikimedia Commons

17

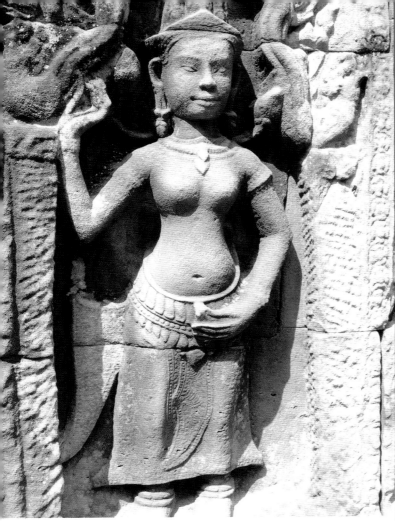

Angkor Wat
unknown

Completion: starting 802 AD. **Technique:** stone. **Location:** Angkor, Cambodia.

The ruins of Angkor are located amongst forests and farmland near modern-day Siem Reap. There are over 1,000 temples in the Angkor area, ranging from piles of brick to the magnificent "Angkor Wat", which is said to be one of the largest single religious monuments in the world. Many of the temples at Angkor have been restored, and together, they comprise the most significant site of Khmer architecture. It is thought that Angkor was the largest pre-industrial city in the world.

Angkor, between the ninth and the 12th century, served as the seat of the Khmer Empire. Between 900 and 1200 the Khmer Empire made some of the world's most impressive architecture. Around 72 important temples can still be found on this site, with the remains of several hundred smaller ones scattered across the area. Angkor lacked an official boundary but the main area is defined by a complex infrastructural system, including canals and roads.

Photo: David Wilmot / Wikimedia Commons

Goa Gajah - Elephant Cave
unknown

Completion: 9th c. AD. **Technique:** stone. **Location:** near Ubud, Indonesia.

The "Goa Gajah" or "Elephant Cave" is located on the island of Bali. The cave served as a sanctuary and the façade is made of various creatures and demons, carved directly into the rock face. The main motif was once thought to have been an elephant, giving the cave its nickname. The entrance to the cave is directly through the demon's mouth. In front of the caves are two water pools and legend has it that bathing in their waters kept the bather eternally young.

Inside the caves are several Hindu statues, one of which is of Ganesha. Ganesha is one of the best known and most widely worshipped Hindu deities. Ganesha's elephant head makes him easy to identify. He is widely revered as the lord of beginnings, the patron of the arts and sciences and the deva of intellect and wisdom. Ganesha is a popular figure in Indian Art and depictions of him vary widely.

Photo: Jack Merridew / Wikimedia Commons

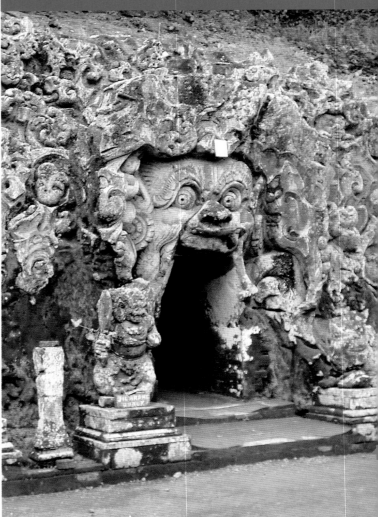

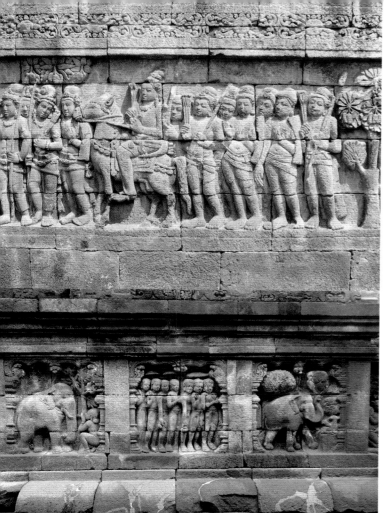

Borobudur
unknown

Completion: 842 until end of 9th c. AD. **Technique:** stone.
Location: Borobudur, Indonesia.

"Borobudur" is a Mahayana Buddhist monument in Indonesia. The monument is decorated with 2,672 panels and over 500 statues of Buddha. The site is both a place of pilgrimage and a shrine to Buddha. A pathway leads from the base of the monument and gradually ascends towards the top, through the three levels of Buddhist Cosmology, namely the world of desire, the world of forms and the world of formlessness. Evidence suggests that the site was abandoned after the Javanese conversion to Islam during the 14th century.

Mahayana is one of two main branches of Buddhism and originated in India. In the course of its history, Mahayana Buddhism spread from India to China, Japan, Vietnam, Korea, Singapore and Tibet and beliefs were anchored in seeking complete enlightenment for the benefit of all, also called Bodhisattva. This is different from attaining nirvana, which is seen as too narrow a goal as it does not seek to liberate others from their suffering.

Giant Buddha of Leshan
Haithong

Completion: 803. **Technique:** stone. **Location:** Leshan, China.

"The Giant Buddha of Leshan" is the largest, carved stone Buddha in the world. It is carved out of a cliff face, situated at the confluence of the Minjiang, Dadu and Qingyi rivers in China. Construction began in 713 and was led by a monk named Haithong, in the hope that the Buddha would calm the tormented waters of the river. Haithong is said to have gouged out his own eyes as a sign of piety when funding for the Buddha was threatened. After his death, construction was halted and the Buddha wasn't completed until 803.

This Buddha was constructed during the Tang dynasty, an imperial dynasty started by the Li family who gained power during the decline and later collapse of the Sui Empire. The estimated population during the Tang dynasty is at around 80 million people and it was largely a period of stability and progress. A wealth of poetry, paintings and literary works were created in this period as the culture developed and matured.

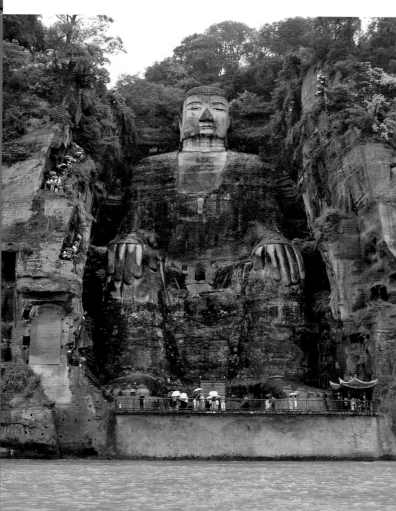

Bernward Doors
unknown

Completion: 1015. **Technique:** bronze. **Location:** Hildesheim, Germany.

The western doors of the Hildesheim Cathedral are considered major works of Ottonic Art. The doors depict scenes from the first book of Moses and the life of Christ. There is hardly any background depicted but the stereotypical figures vividly interact in scenes. They rise out of the flat relief at their feet gradually becoming fully three-dimensional form from shoulders upwards. The 'missing' background works to make the scenes more dynamic.

The artist of these doors is unknown – although the name of a Master Berenger who made the doors in Mainz at the same time is known. The Hildesheim doors are named after the bishop who commissioned them: Bernward (950/60–1022), who was in close contact with the court of the Saxon emperors. As patron of arts he commissioned important works: the doors, cross and psalter are named after him as well as the Hildesheim Christ column and the new cathedral.

Photo: Bischöfliche Pressestelle Hildesheim (bph) / Wikimedia Commons

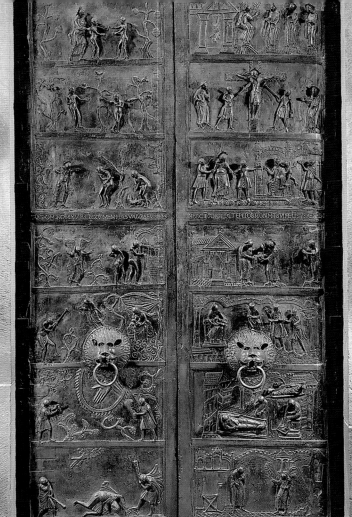

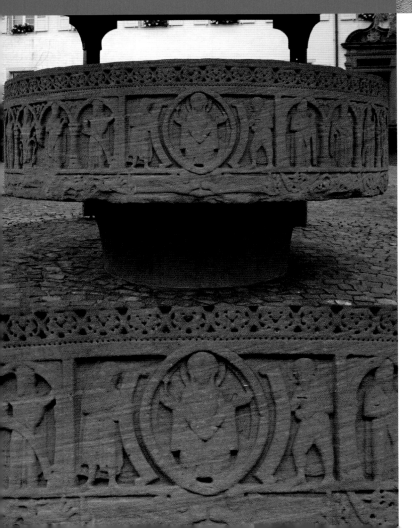

St Ulrich Basin
unknown

Completion: 11th c. **Technique:** sandstone. **Location:** Bollschweil, Germany.

This eight-ton basin, sometimes called the baptismal font, probably stood in the cloister of a medieval priory. There are three registries: palmettes above and mythical creatures below the figured zone. The main scenes show Christ in a Mandorla, a Vesics Piscis shaped aureola which surrounds the figures of Christ and the Virgin Mary in traditional Christian art and Maria pictured together with two saints and the twelve apostles.

It is not known where the basin was made, probably not in Cluny as popular legend has it. It is more likely that it was a present from the prior of Hirsau. Both Hirsau and Cluny were examples of the young monastic movements that rose all over Europe and that revitalized the knowledge and skills of the Antique world leading to early Romanesque Art.

Photos: Chris van Uffelen

Ruins of Sukhothai
unknown

Completion: 12th c. **Technique:** stone. **Location:** Sukhothai, Thailand.

There are hundreds of Buddha statues in the ancient ruins of Sukhothai, some small, some large but each of them with that famous enigmatic smile. People still come to the site and pray at the Buddha's feet, giving the site life and making it more than just a museum. The elephant carving is a motif that is repeated often around Sukhothai and Si Satchanalai temples, showing the influence of Sri Lankan religious architecture.

Sukhothai was the capital of the first Kingdom of Siam between the 13th and 14th centuries AD. It was one of the major ancient kingdoms of South-East Asia, along with the Khmer and the Mon. These three kingdoms were often at war and each one was ascendant at different times, each bringing a wealth of cultural variety to Thailand. Today, the protected site of Sukhothai includes 193 ruins, spread over 70 square kilometers of land.

Photo: Chris van Uffelen

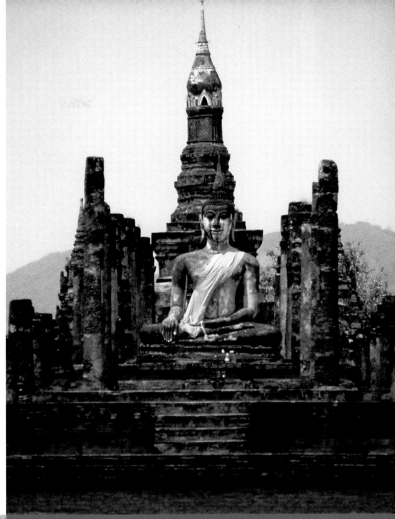

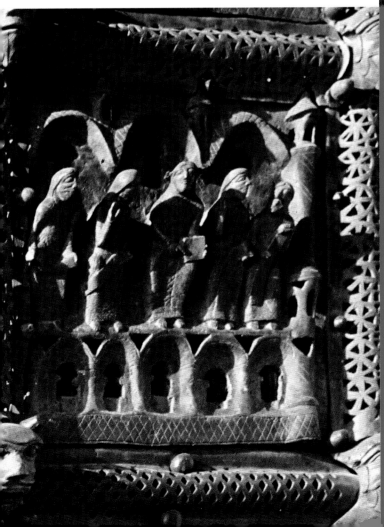

Doors of San Zeno
unknown

Completion: approx. 1100 and approx. 1200. **Technique:** bronze. **Location:** Verona, Italy.

The magnificent bronze doors of the church of San Zeno in Italy date from the 12th century and are one of the artistic highlights of Verona. The doors are decorated with 48 bronze panels depicting bible stories and the lives of the saints Michael and Zeno. The panels on the left door depict stories from the New Testament and are believed to have been created by a German artist from Hildesheim. Those on the right portray the Old Testament and were made around 100 years later by an Italian artist.

The church of San Zeno was founded in the fifth century to shelter the relics of Verona's patron saint, bishop St. Zeno. Zeno is attributed with converting Verona to Christianity and many of his sermons still survive. The church was rebuilt several centuries later and then again between 963 and 983, after Hungarian invaders destroyed it. In the 12th century the sculptors Nicolaus and Wiligelmus added reliefs to the façade. For the right door there might have been a sculptor from Verona, maybe Benedetto Antelami.

Photo: Chris van Uffelen

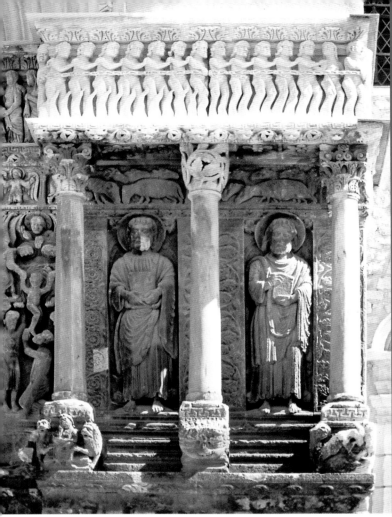

Saint Trophime Portal
unknown

Completion: approx. 1140. **Technique:** sandstone. **Location:** Arles, France.

The church that stands on this site today was first founded as an abbey and built between 1100 and 1150. The main portal is one of the most famous sculptures of Romanesque Art and led the way to the later Gothic style. The tympanum shows the last judgment. Christ is shown with the book of seven seals within the tetramorphic arrangement of the Evangelist-symbols. Angels are blowing trumpets for the last judgment. A frieze shows the twelve apostles; on their left is a procession.

Below this relief there are carved figures of saints and apostles. These are the forerunners of the embrasure figures of the Gothic Style of northern France, which began, around this time, in Saint-Denis close to Paris. From this moment onwards artists became specialists that travelled to different workplaces, taking their knowledge and sharing it over large distances.

Photo: Chris van Uffelen

Notre Dame Portal
unknown

Completion: approx. 1150. **Technique:** sandstone. **Location:** Chartres, France.

The portal of the Chartres Cathedral is the first Gothic, stepped portal where the original figures survived, as the Saint-Denis figures were lost. In contradiction to the Arles portal the large saints were more naturalist in style, new nobility replaces the earlier depictions of Romanesque joy. The figures get more independence from the building's surface but seem to be bound at the columns.

Since the 12th century the cathedral has been an important destination for pilgrims. This created a huge income, allowing the building to be constructed of the highest possible quality. The portal is one of the few parts that survived the fire of 1194 that led to the church being rebuilt as one of the earliest examples of classic Gothic Style.

Photos: Vassil / Wikimedia Commons (a.); Chris van Uffelen (b.)

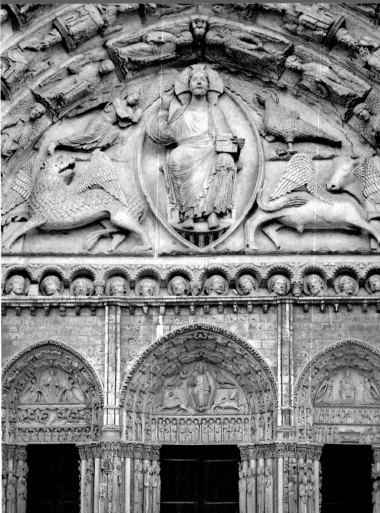

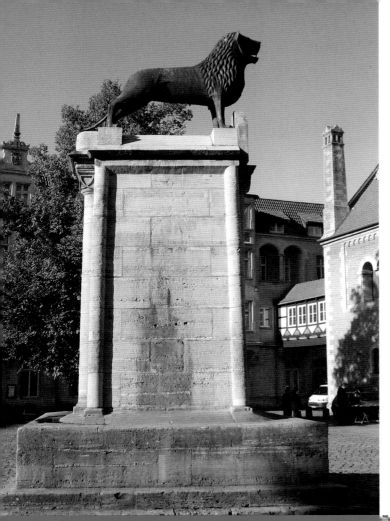

Brunswick Lion
unknown

Completion: 1166. **Technique:** bronze. **Location:** Brunswick, Germany.

This Romanesque lion stands on the Burgplatz in front of Dankwarderode Castle and Brunswick Castle and dates back to the 12th century. Henry the Lion, duke of Bavaria and Saxony was born in 1129/30 and died 1195, commissioned it as a symbol of his authority and jurisdiction. It is the first large hollow casting of a figure since antiquity. On the place there stands a replica today, while the original is on display inside the castle.

The artist is unknown but it is thought that the duke was inspired to order this work after having seen the famous Capitoline Wolf in Rome on a journey with Frederick I Barbarossa. The lion shows the same fine chasing and interest in a naturalistic look, with ribs and muscles and bones on his hind legs. It is speculated that the artist may have been a goldsmith, possibly working together with a bell founder.

Photos: C.Löser / Wikimedia Commons

Gallus Portal
unknown

Completion: approx. 1170. **Technique:** sandstone. **Location:** Basel, Switzerland.

While Gothic art was taking hold in France, the most important Romanesque sculpture of Switzerland, and probably first Romanesque portal in the German-region of Switzerland, was made. At the north side of the Basel Münster it is inscribed with an antique triumphal arche showing archaic figurative scenes. The reliefs show the four evangelists, wise and foolish virgins, angels with trumpets and rising death in the last judgment.

The intense gestures of this Romanesque work, compared with the Chartres portal, demonstrate the similarity of styles in the middle ages. The German regions are not ready yet to embrace the French style, this would come over 100 years later. This suggests that the interaction between regions is still only on a small scale and that local styles dominate. Gothic Art can be seen as the Île-de-France version of late Romanesque Art of that time.

Photo: Chris van Uffelen

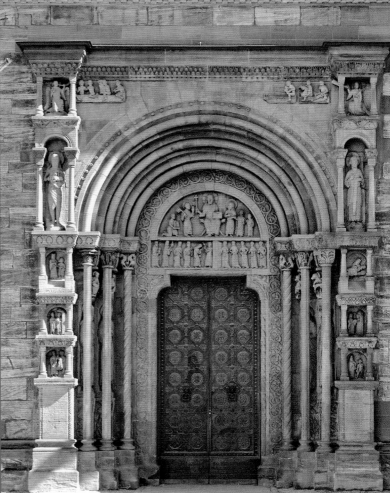

Annunciation of Reims
unknown

Completion: 1220. **Technique:** stone. **Location:** Reims, France.

The "Annunciation" on the right side of the middle west portal of the cathedral is the best known work of the workshop of Reims. The wavy hair and the large body under fine folded drapery are obviously inspired by the antique Classical Style, which must have survived from when it was introduced to Reims in the Roman times.

Up to around the year 1225 there was an artist working in one of the workshops in Reims, who can be traced in Noyon and Amiens as well. Later the "Smile of the Reims angel" can be found in Metz and from 1230 onwards in Mainz on the west chancel-screen. It travelled further to Merseburg and finally to Naumburg, where it became typical for the "Master of Naumburg".

Photo: Vassil / Wikimedia Commons

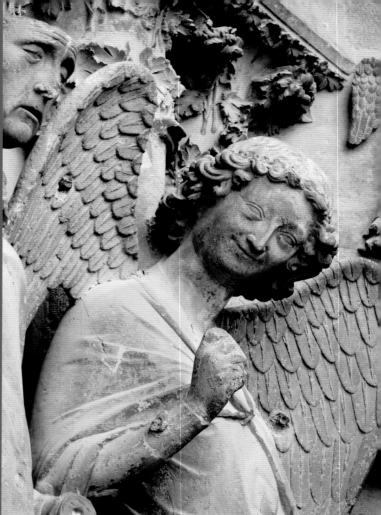

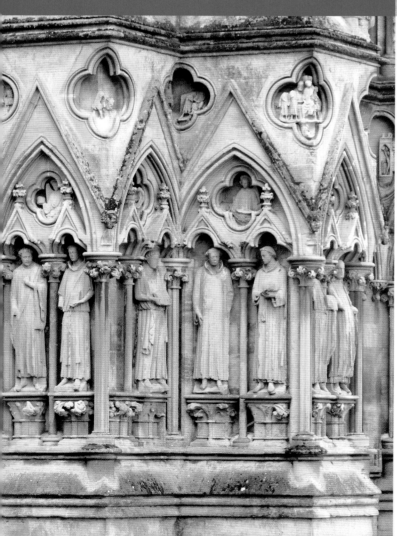

Façade Sculpture
unknown

Completion: 1230. **Technique:** stone. **Location:** Wells, United Kingdom.

Screen-façades are a specialty of English Gothic architecture, with a spread display of figures. While French sculptures are limited to the portals and a king's gallery above, this whole façade has 176 figures and 134 reliefs. The attributes of the saints were made out of metal or wood and have not survived. Besides saints and apostles there are people of both the Old and New Testament, patriarchs, priests and monks.

The figures in the lower zones did not survive the numerous iconoclasms of English history. Revolutions turning against public art are quiet common still today and always have been. For example, in France the king's galleries of Gothic cathedrals disappeared during the French revolution. Most often the iconoclasts started by destroying the eyes of the figures, as if they could really see.

Photo: Ad Meskens / Wikimeadia Commons

Synagogue
unknown

Completion: 1230. **Technique:** stone. **Location:** Strasbourg, France.

This blindfolded figure symbolizes a "Synagogue", an "Ecclesia" pendant is situated on the other side of the south-transept portal of the cathedral. The "Synagogue" is always the more interesting one of the two. The Christian church wanted to be seen as dignified, so the "Ecclesia" shows the common style elements of beauty, while the "Synagogue" representation is an example of pagan personification and portrays a more experimental style and a more sensual look, with the figure's body clearly visible under her dress.

The Strasbourg Cathedral was the hinge between French and German Gothic Style. The stone masons and sculptors all belong to various organizations who had workshops on or near to the site which they were working on. The main German workshops at this time were located in Cologne and Strasbourg as well as in Vienna, Berne and later Zurich. According to the rules of these working areas, the main workshops had the deciding voice in disputes. These workshop areas existed until 1731 when Charles VI eliminated them.

Photo: Chris van Uffelen

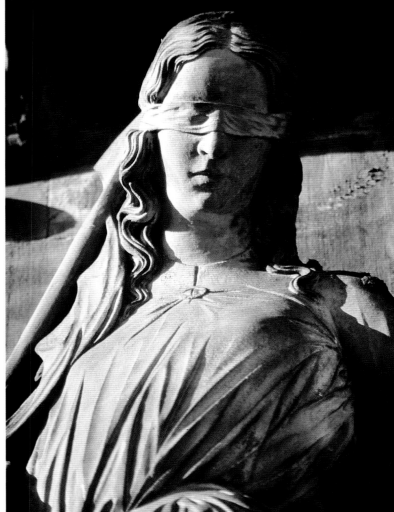

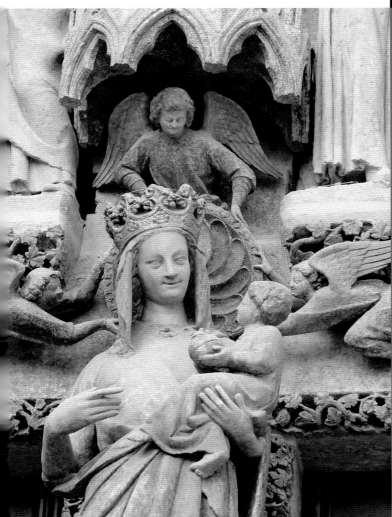

Gilded Virgin
unknown

Completion: approx. 1250. **Technique:** stone. **Location:** Amiens, France.

The "Vierge Dorée" (Gilded Virgin) on the trumeau of the south portal of the Amiens Cathedral probably replaced a sculpture of Saint Honoratus in around 1250. The former gilded Madonna is much more animated and vivid than the Reims figures. In the second half of the 13th century the drapery became more natural, responding to the bodies they covered. The folds are softer and more individualized than before. The bodies become recognizable below the textiles.

The Parisian court, where a more elegant technique arose in the mid 13th century, influences this new, softer style. Examples of work from the artist that made the "Gilded Virgin" can also be found at St. Mauritius in Tholey, where he made the figure of an angel. His "Gilded Virgin" is the first example of a figure that turns to the baby Jesus and smiles. This new idea started a new tradition of sculptures which paid more attention to portraying the strength of this mother-child relationship.

Photo: Vassil / Wikimedia Commons

Baptistry South Doors
Andrea Pisano

Completion: 1336. **Technique:** gilded bronze. **Location:** Florence, Italy.

The "South Doors" of the Florence Baptistry are made of gilded bronze. The Calimala, the guild who was responsible for the Baptistry's maintenance and decoration, commissioned the doors and they are signed and dated at the top by Andrea Pisano. Each door has 14 panels, 20 depict the life of John the Baptist and eight at the bottom are personifications of the virtues. The scenes should be read chronologically, from top to bottom and from left to right, like a book.

Andrea Pisano was an Italian sculptor and architect, born in 1290. He first worked as a goldsmith and later went on to work with Mino di Giovanni, collaborating with him on several sculptures. Pisano's best known works are in Florence. He produced a series of reliefs for the Florence Cathedral, where he was employed as master of the works. He had two sons, both of whom succeeded him as master of the works at Orvieto Cathedral.

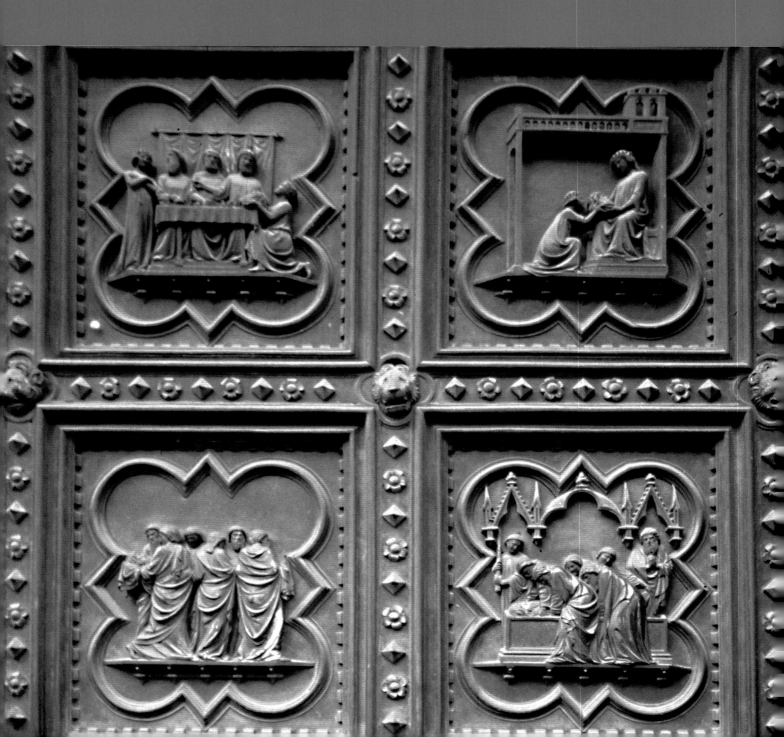

Cangrande I. della Scala
unknown

Completion: 1340. **Technique:** marble. **Location:** Verona, Italy.

The first public equestrian monuments since antiquity – though there have been some saints on horses inside churches and on façades – are the five funeral monuments of the Scaliger family, who ruled Verona in the 13th and 14th century. The Arche Scaligere next to the Santa Maria church houses copies of the sculptures, the originals are in the Castello Vecchio-museum. One of them, nowadays on the wall of the church, used to be in San Fermo Maggiore and was bought here in 1400.

Two of the artists of the five monuments are known, but the artist responsible for the pictured sculpture remains unknown. The sculpture, brought from San Fermo Maggiore, was made by Andriolo de' Santi in 1359 and the most decorated one in this group by Bonino da Campione in 1375. The latter – his name indicates he was born in an Italian enclave in Switzerland – made at least one more equestrian monument: The tomb monument of Bernabò Visconti (1363) in the Castello Sforzesco-museum in Milan. This amounts to specialization by the standards of the 14th century.

Photo: Frode Inge Helland / Wikipedia Commons

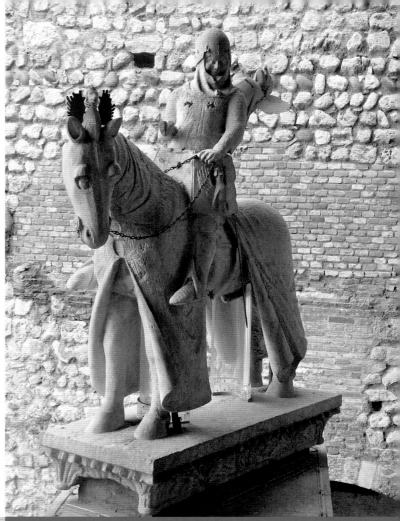

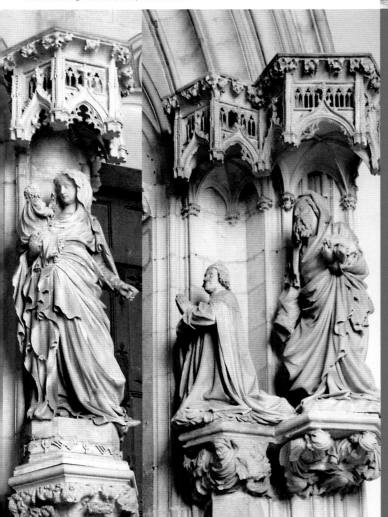

Portal Carthusian Monastry Champmol
Claus Sluter

Completion: 1391. **Technique:** stone. **Location:** Champmol, France.

This group comprises five figures of Sluter: a Madonna at the trumeau, two saints and two benefactors, one on either side of the doors. Philip the Bold and Margaret of Flanders are kneeling next to the Madonna, their patron saint leaning slightly over them. The five figures become united in one scene are typical of a new style of portal-sculpture. The smoother look, elegant movements and curved forms are typical elements of the International Gothic in the late 14th century and early 15th century.

Claus Sluter, was born in Haarlem ca. 1350 and died in Dijon in 1405/6. He was one of the founders and most important sculptor of the Burgundian School from the 14th to the 15th century. It is estimated that he would have arrived at the court of Philipp the Bold in Dijon before 1385, later becoming a public member of the workshop of Jean de Marville. In 1389 he succeeded Marville as chief of the workshop and court-artist.

Photos: Markus Golser

Moai
unknown

Completion: approx. 15th c. **Technique:** basalt, tuff. **Location:** Easter Island, Chile

At one time, there were more than 1.000 of the famous Easter Island statues, called "Moais", making it the largest ceremonial area of the South Pacific. Though their exact use is unknown, it is possible that the statues symbolized chiefs or ancestors and functioned as a link from this to the next world. Originally, they wore hats of different colors and their eyes were colored white with pupils of either black obsidian or red scoria.

The figures have been cut out of local stone and their heads are large, making up a third of the statue's height. It is believed that the statues were transported lying on their backs to their allocated place, most of them are positioned along the coast. The largest of the statues are up to ten meters high and weigh 75 tons. The age of the statues varies but most are estimated as having been made between 1250 and 1500.

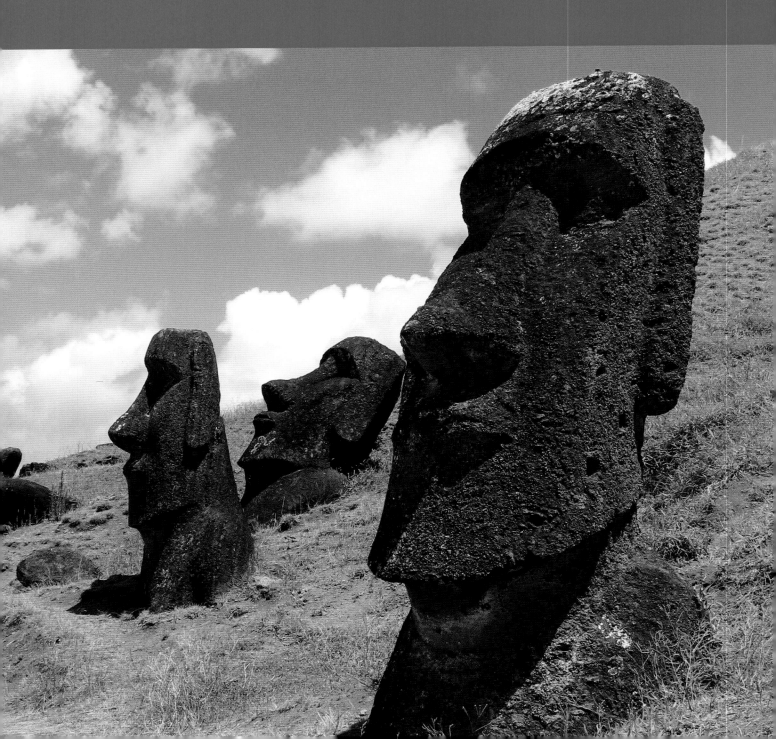

Roland
unknown

Completion: 1404. **Technique:** chalkstone. **Location:** Bremen, Germany.

This statue of "Roland" stands in front of Bremen town hall, in the market place. The five and a half-meter high sculpture is positioned against a pillar with baldachin, which measures slightly more than ten meters in total. Roland, commander and nephew of Charlemagne, was a symbol of the king's governorship. His shield, decorated with a double-headed eagle stands for the imperial immediacy of the town while the sword symbolizes the towns jurisdiction.

This stone sculpture was made to replace a wooden one that originally stood here was burned in 1366 by the soldiers of Archbishop Albert II from Brunswick-Wolfenbüttel. Like a lot of medieval (and antique) sculptures the Roland was originally painted in different colors. These were painted over with gray in the 18th century and later removed entirely. Some remnants of the paint can still be seen, giving a clue to the colors that were originally used.

Photo: Arne Hückelheim / Wikimedia Commons

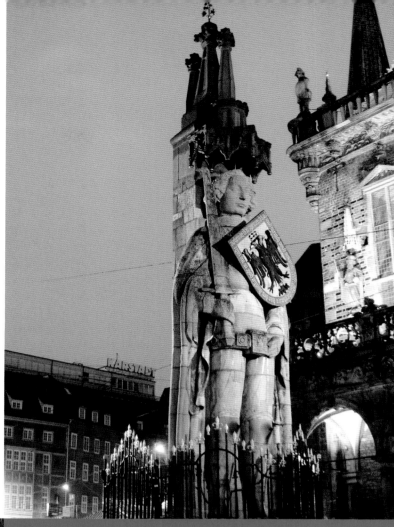

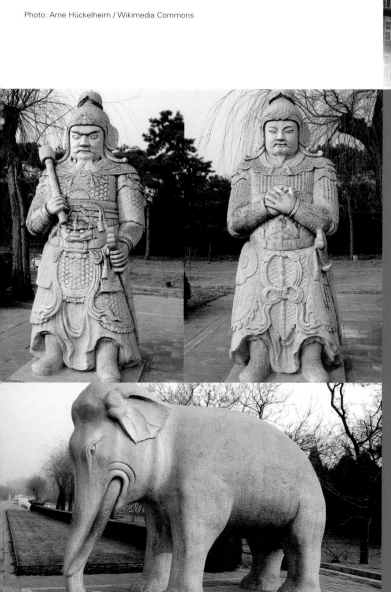

The Spirit Way,
Ming Dynasty Tombs
unknown

Completion: 1409. **Technique:** stone. **Location:** Jundu Mountains, China.

The third Ming dynasty emperor, Yongle, selected the site of the "Ming dynasty Tombs". The site was chosen according to the principles of Feng Shui. "The Spirit Way" leads into the complex and is lined with statues of guardian animals and official figures. The front gate consists of three arches and is called the "Great Red Gate". "The Spirit Way", or "Sacred Way", starts with a huge stone memorial archway positioned at the front of the area.

Emperor Yongle was responsible for moving the capital of China from Nanjing to Beijing. He then repaired the Grand Canal of China, after it had fallen into disrepair during the Yuan dynasty, allowing supplies to reach the new capital more easily. He also ordered the construction of the Forbidden City, which was the Chinese imperial palace from the Ming dynasty to the end of the Qing dynasty.

Photos: Ofol / Wikimedia Commons

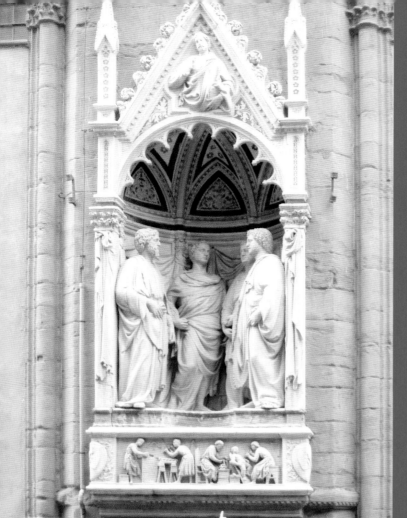

Four crowned Saints
Nanni di Banco

Completion: 1410/15. **Technique:** marble. **Location:** Florence, Italy.

In a niche of the Or San Michele are the "Four crowned Saints" (Santi Quattro Coronati), patrons of the stonemason's guild. The work was commissioned by the Maestri di Pietra e Legname, the guild of stone and woodworkers. It shows four Early Christian sculptors, who suffered a martyr's death under the Emperor Diocletian, after they refused to carve a statue of Aesculapius for him. The figures are arranged as single sculptures but are connected to each other by their gaze and gestures.

Nanni di Banco (1375–1421) trained as a stonemason in the cathedral-workshops in Florence. He was a classicist amongst the Early-Renaissance sculptors whose work was influenced more by the Antiquity than by Gothic Styles. Or San Michele was in both form and meaning a truly astonishing work and served the double function of both town granary and oratory. There are 14 niches and slots in the outer walls and each is filled by a patron saint or other figures of importance to the guild of the stonemasons.

Gaia Fountain
Jacopo della Quercia

Completion: 1419. **Technique:** stone. **Location:** Siena, Italy.

The "Gaia Fountain" originally on this site was built in around 1343 to celebrate that, after eight years of work, the site finally had water. This fountain was replaced in 1419 by Jacopo della Quercia. A copy from Tito Sarrocchi then, in turn, replaced this and the original tiles are now preserved in the Santa Maria della Scala. The "Gaia Fountain" is one of the most important works of the 1400s and displays both Gothic and Renaissance style.

Jacopo della Quercia was born around 1374. He was an Italian sculptor of the Italian Renaissance period, widely considered to be a precursor of Michelangelo. He received training from his father, who worked as a woodcarver and goldsmith. His early work is more Gothic in style, later shifting to the emerging style of the Italian Renaissance. He received numerous commissions, including for the design of the Trenta Chapel in the Basilica of San Frediano and the upper part of the baptismal font for the Siena Baptistery.

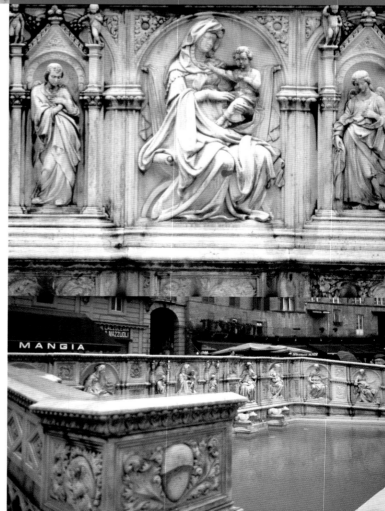

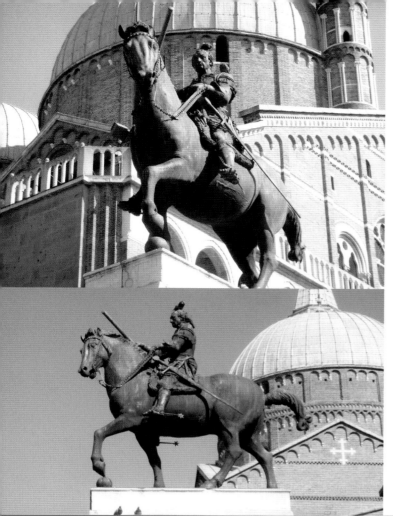

Gattamelata
Donatello

Completion: 1447. **Technique:** bronze. **Location:** Padua, Italy.

Erasmo da Narni, also known as Gattamelata, was the commander of the Venetian troops. He died in 1443 and his will decreed that a stone monument should be built in his honor. His heirs wanted to create something original and this became the first monumental, cast statue to be created since the Antiquity. The statue itself is over three meters high and nearly four meters in length. The sculptor created the design in the appearance of a Roman commander, using old portraits to achieve an accurate representation.

Donatello, born Donato di Niccolò di Betto Bardi (1386–1466), was an Italian sculptor. He studied the sculpture of the Antiquity, developing his own style around what he learned. This personal style led to Renaissance-sculpture. In his early career, Donatello created many marble sculptures, but later in his career he preferred bronze. He produced several bronze sculptures for Cosimo de Medici, one of which is a bronze of a young David, with one foot playfully positioned on the head of Goliath.

Photos: sailko / Wikimedia Commons

Gates of Paradise
Lorenzo Ghiberti

Completion: 1452. **Technique:** bronze, partly gilded. **Location:** Florence, Italy.

Ghiberti worked on the third baptistry doors for 27 years before he finally completed them. Their name was given to them by the young Michelangelo, who was so impressed by the doors that he said they were worthy of adorning the entrance to Paradise. Each of the ten reliefs depicts episodes from the Old Testament, beginning with the story of creation, the Fall and the exclusion of Adam and Eve from the Garden of Eden. The many figures show Ghiberti's talent for creating realistic figures in a wide variety of poses.

Lorenzo Ghiberti (ca. 1378–1455) was an Italian sculptor, goldsmith brass-caster and art critic. He was commissioned to decorate the north doors of the baptistry after winning a legendary art competition at the age of 23. After completing this door he was given the task of working on another door, the "Gates of Paradise". Ghiberti also worked as second master-architect in Florence with Filippo Brunelleschi. Ghiberti's artwork shows a connection between the Gothic Style and the idealism of the Renaissance.

Photo: Chris van Uffelen

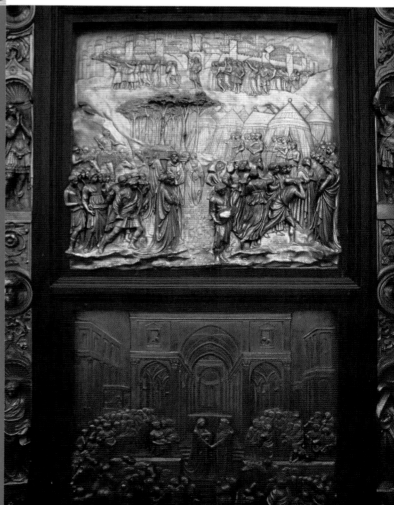

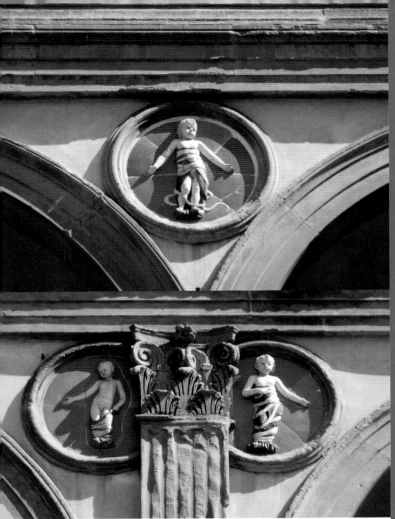

Medallions of Infants
Andrea della Robbia

Completion: 1466. **Technique:** glazed ceramic. **Location:** Florence, Italy.

The Hospital of the Innocents, a children's orphanage, designed by Filippo Brunelleschi in 1419 is one of the first examples of Renaissance architecture in Florence. The medallions on the façade were meant to be empty, but Andrea della Robbia was later commissioned to fill them with ceramics of swaddled babies. The high reliefs are made out of separate pieces. The standing infants with quiet large bodies are reminiscent of paintings of Jesus as a baby because of the way in which their arms are spread, wide open and welcoming.

Andrea della Robbia was born in Florence in 1435 and died there in 1525. He was born to a family of specialist ceramic sculptors and his uncle Luca della Robbia taught him this technique. From 1455 on he carried out his own work. Around 1470 he took over the workshop, enriching his teacher's technique with more colors. Several of his sons also later became ceramic-specialists.

Adam and Eve
Tilmann Riemenschneider

Completion: 1494. **Technique:** stone. **Location:** Würzburg, Germany.

"Adam and Eve" at the portal of the Maria-Chapel were commissioned by the city of Würzburg for the new church. The artist earned 120 pieces of gold, with the promise of 20 more if the statues were good. This was a large sum of money at the time and demonstrates the importance of these sculptures to the city. The figures of Adam and Eve are extremely correct for the late middle ages, with the muscle exactly shown beneath the skin. The original sculptures are now housed in the Mainfränkisches Museum.

Tilman Riemenschneider was born around 1460 in Heiligenstadt and died in 1531 in Würzburg. He was one of the most important wood carvers and sculptors of this time north of the Alps, became extremely successful and earned a lot of money from his trade. He was also one of the first artists who refused to paint his wood statues. Typical for his work are expressive figures and the rich fall of the folds of the clothing. In 1504 he became councilman of Würzburg, even serving as mayor between 1520 and 1524.

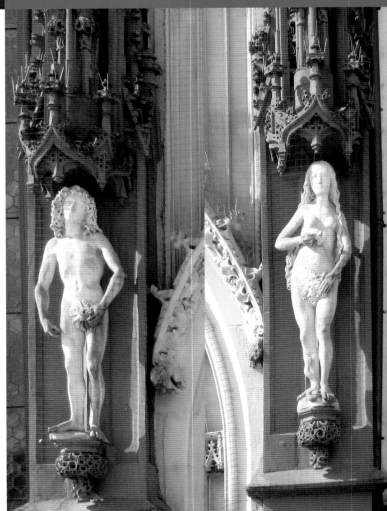

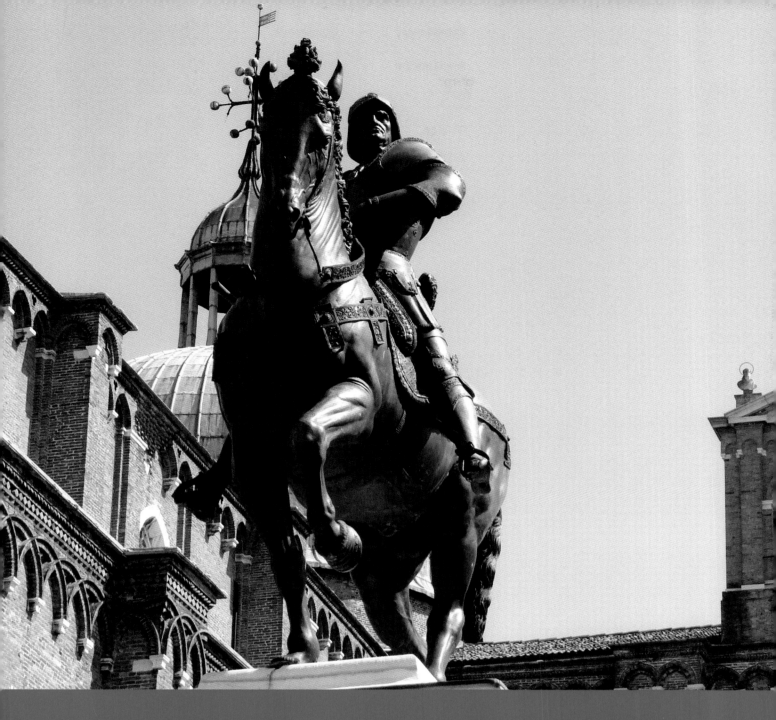

Equestrian Statue of Bartolomeo Colleoni
Andrea del Verrocchio

Completion: 1488. **Technique:** bronze. **Location:** Venice, Italy.

Colleoni, the most famous field-commander of his time, died in 1475. He bequeathed a large amount of money to the city of Venice, on the condition that an equestrian statue must be built in his honor. Verrocchio depicts the commander in a more modern, rather than classical way, riding a smaller, lighter horse than his predecessors. The tense position of the rider reflects the bravery and intrepidness that he was famous for.

Andrea del Verrocchio, also known as Andrea di Michele Cioni (ca. 1436–1488) was one of the most influential artists of the transition period between Early and High-Renaissance. For more than two decades, Verrocchio led a productive, multi-disciplinary workshop in which he created not only sculptures and paintings, but also craftwork. His most famous works were sculptural, characterized by a sense of reality, achieved through carefully applied light and shadow effects.

David
Michelangelo Buonarroti

Completion: 1504. **Technique:** marble. **Location:** Florence, Italy.

This large statue of "David" was made from one, single block that Agostino di Duccio began to work on 40 years previously, without much success. Michelangelo shows "David" neither throwing the stone nor as winner above Goliath on the ground but with the slingshot on his shoulder and the stone in his hand, looking at his antagonist, still standing relaxed in contrapposto but with muscles already flexed. Michelangelo's "David" knows and understands the task that lies before him.

Michelangelo Buonarroti was born in 1475 in Caprese and died in 1564 in Rome. He was a renowned Italian Renaissance painter, sculptor, architect, poet, and engineer. Domenico Ghirlandaio taught him painting, Bertoldo di Giovanni sculpture and Lorenzo de' Medici sent him to the Humanist academy. He led an eventful life and was much in demand, working between Rome and Florence. His idea of sculptures being already in the stone and set free by the artist and the (unintended) "non-finito" became important characteristics of his work.

Photo: Gina Sanders / Fotolia.com

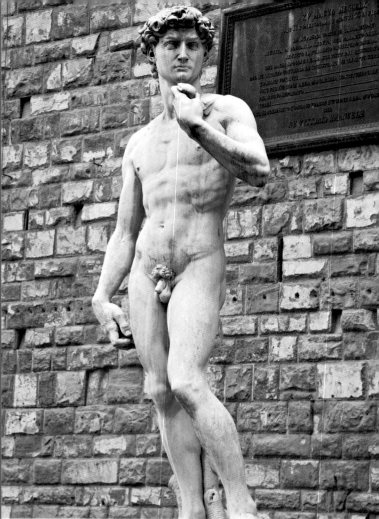

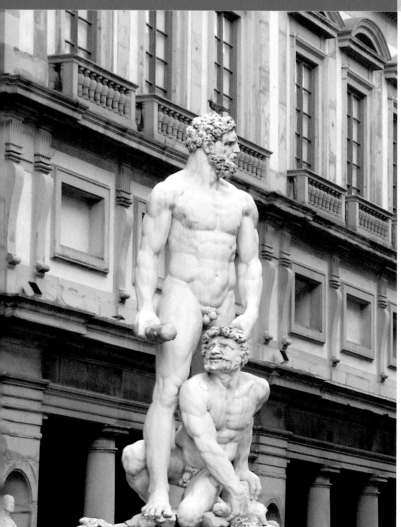

Hercules and Cacus
Baccio Bandinelli

Completion: 1534. **Technique:** marble. **Location:** Florence, Italy.

This sculpture was finished in 1534 and is situated at the entrance to the Palazzo Vecchio in Florence. The sculpture depicts Hercules, who killed the monster Cacus for stealing cattle. Hercules, who holds a club, menacingly in his hand, is pulling Cacus' head back. The sculpture was commissioned by Pope Clement VII, to mark the return of the Medici family who were forced into exile by a Republican government. The strength shown by Hercules is a symbol of the Medici family's return to power.

Baccio Bandinelli was the son of a wealthy Florentine goldsmith, he was born in 1488 and died in 1560. He was in awe of the work of Michelangelo, though his own sculptures never inspired the same fascination as those by Michelangelo. Bandinelli's "Hercules and Cacus" sculpture was ridiculed by his peers and overshadowed by Michelangelo's sculpture of David. Bandinelli was said to have been a talented teacher and opened one of the first academies at the Vatican, later creating a second, in Florence.

Photo: Jean-Christophe Benoist / Wikimedia Commons

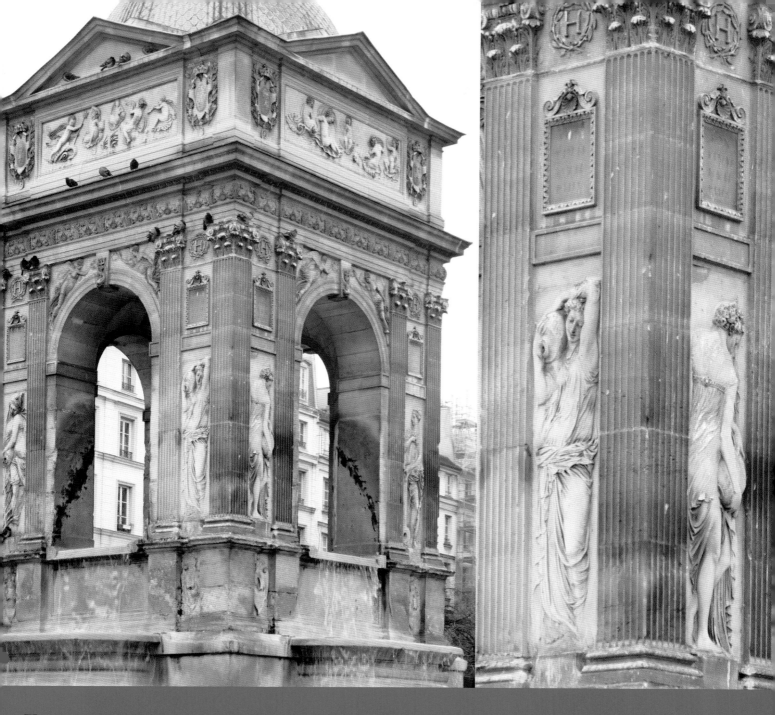

Fountain of Innocence
Jean Goujon

Completion: 1549. **Technique:** stone. **Location:** Paris, France.

This early public fountain in Paris was originally called "of the Nymphs". It was constructed between 1547 and 1550 by architect Pierre Lescot. Originally it stood along a wall but was later relocated in the late 18th century, when the church by which it stood was torn down. The architecture and sculpture are typical of the new style of the French Renaissance.

Jean Goujon, is believed to have been born before 1510 and died in approximately 1572. He was termed the "French Phidias" and was especially famous for his reliefs. It is assumed that he spent time in Italy to study the antiques and contemporary sculpture. In 1547 he became "sculptor to the king" (Henry II of France) and worked at the Castle of Anet with Philibert Delorme. From 1555 to 1562 he was architect at the Louvre.

Photos: Chris van Uffelen

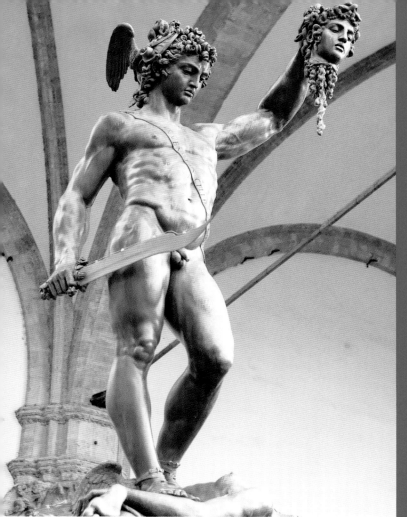

Perseus
Benvenuto Cellini

Completion: 1554. **Technique:** bronze. **Location:** Florence, Italy.

This statue of "Perseus" is situated in the Florentine Loggia dei Lanzi and is Cellini's most important work. Cosimo I de Medici commissioned it in 1545. The technically impressive casting of the main figures is considered a masterpiece of the Italian Renaissance. Depicted is the figure of Perseus, holding aloft the severed head of Medusa, while her lifeless body lies at his feet.

Benvenuto Cellini (1500–1571) is considered one of the most important sculptors since the Antiquity and the typical "uomo universale" of the Italian Renaissance. His sculptural work, writings, music and gold work showed both the style of the Renaissance and some characteristics of the Mannerists.

Rape of the Sabine Women
Giovanni da Bologna

Completion: 1583. **Technique:** marble. **Location:** Florence, Italy.

This 4.10-meter sculpture is one of the first sculptural groups that was designed to be viewed from several angles, with no 'main' view. This concept represents the Mannerist ideal of the "figura serpentinata", a spiraling sculptural design that can be viewed from every side. It is supposed that the sculptor simply wished to express the youthful power of his male figures and the tender femininity of the female figures. It stands in the Loggia dei Lanzi in Piazza della Signoria in Florence.

Giovanni da Bologna (1529–1608), was a Flemish-Italian sculptor whose work was influenced by the Florentine style of Mannerism and Early-Baroque. Bologna made numerous sculptures and fountains at the bequest of the Italian elite, in particular for the Medici family. He also made many small bronzes, which spread his style throughout Europe. Apart from Michelangelo, Bologna was one of the most important Italian sculptors of the 17th century.

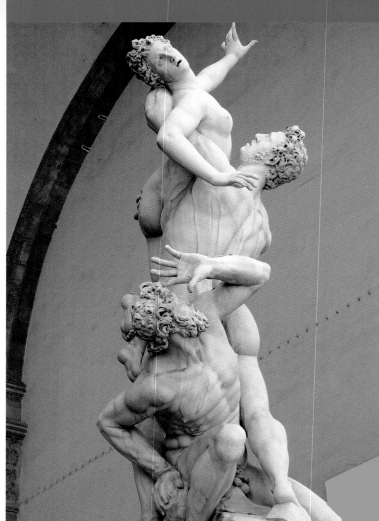

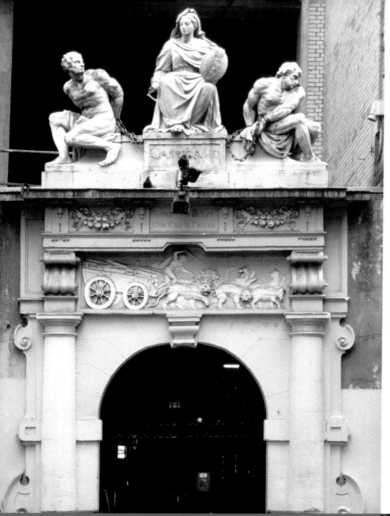

Prisongate
Hendrick de Keyser

Completion: 1603. **Technique:** stone. **Location:** Amsterdam, The Netherlands.

This gate once functioned as the outer entrance to one of the world's first prisons. The Dutch Republic replaced corporal punishment by prison labor – though the inscription "Castigatio" means corporal punishment. The prisoners had to rasp Brazilian wood to pigment, in order to make color out of it. A carriage bringing this wood is shown in the relief on the frieze. The figures above are more recent but were made in the style of the original artist's design. It is a personification of the city with its coat of arms, guarding two men in irons.

Hendrick de Keyser "the elder" was born in Utrecht in 1565 and died in Amsterdam in 1621, he was an important architect and sculptor of the Dutch Renaissance. Born into a family of sculptors, he learned his trade under the tutorage of Cornelis Bloemaert, even going with him to Amsterdam when Bloemaert became the city's architect. Later traveling to London, Inigo Jones had a great influence on de Keysers' Classicist style that turned to Mannerism in the so-called "Amsterdam Renaissance". In 1595, de Keyser was appointed the new city architect.

Photo: Chris van Uffelen

Nikko Toshogu Shrine
unknown

Completion: 1616. **Technique:** wood. **Location:** Nikko, Japan.

These carvings are on the outside of the "Nikko Toshogu Shrine" in Japan. They are carved on the Shinyosha or "Sacred Stable" and are part of a number of carved panels that express ways of life. Among the different carvings are these ones of the "Three Wise Monkeys", who "hear no evil, see no evil and speak no evil". An 11-meter-high gate is the masterpiece of the shrine. 12 pillars are colored by white pigment, and scrolling patterns are carved on the pillars.

The "Nikko Toshogu Shrine" is a UNESCO World Heritage Site. It was built for Tokugawa Ieyasu, after his death in 1616. He was an extremely powerful man and one of the most important figures in Japanese history. He requested that a shrine be created for him, so that he could continue to be the guardian of Japan even after his death. Tokugawa was the founder and first shogun of the Tokugawa shogun dynasty, which ruled from 1600 until 1868.

Photos: Chris van Uffelen (a.); Fg2 / Wikimedia Commons (b.)

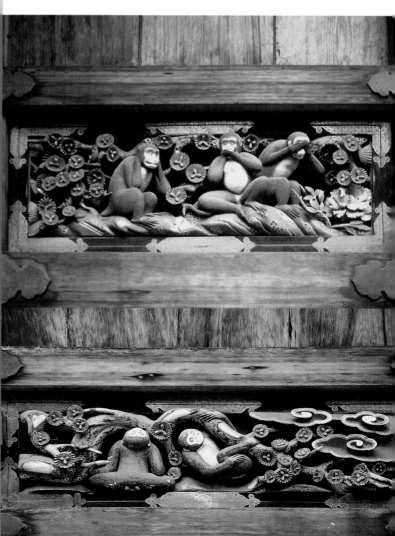

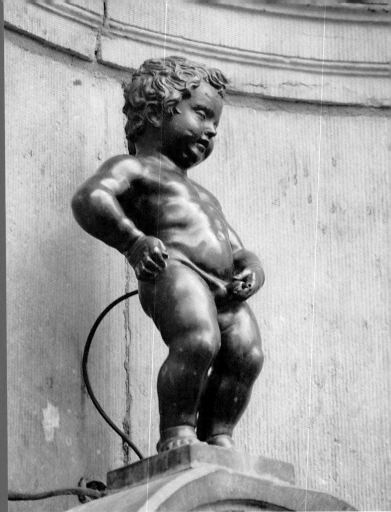

Little Man who Pees
Jerome Duquesnoy

Completion: 1619. **Technique:** bronze. **Location:** Brussels, Belgium.

The "Little Man who Pees" is a famous monument in Brussels. There are various legends about this statue. The most famous concerns Duke Godfrey III of Leuven. This two-year-old lord was taken by his troops to the battlefield, where they were fighting against the troops of Berthouts. They hung the little lord safely from a tree in his basket, as a reminder to the troops of whom they were fighting for. The little lord urinated on the heads of the Berthouts, who eventually lost the battle.

Jerome Duquesnoy was born in 1602. He trained with his brother in Rome and is believed to have then gone to Madrid, Lisbon and Paris. He later moved back to Rome and worked in a studio with his brother. He then returned to Brussels where he developed a reputation for his sculpture. In 1651 he was appointed architect and sculptor of the royal court and the same year, he carved a statue of Saint Ursula for the Notre Dame du Sablon in Brussels.

Photos CHG / Wikimedia Commons

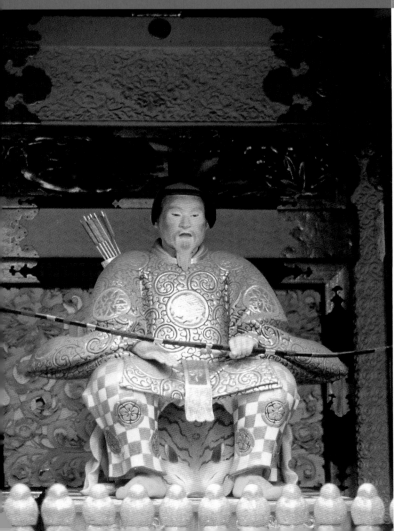

Yomeimon Gate
unknown

Completion: 1636. **Technique:** range of techniques. **Location:** Kyoto, Japan.

The Yomeimon Gate (Gate of Sunlight) is decorated with more than 500 sculptures, bringing together a range of techniques, including metal work, sculpture, metal fitting and decoration skills. The gate is a shrine, dedicated to Tokugawa Ieyasu, the founder of the Tokugawa shogunate. During the Edo period, the Tokugawa shogunate carried out stately processions passing this gate. The shrine's annual spring and autumn festivals re-enact these occasions, and are known as "The processions of a thousand warriors."

This shrine is an example of a Shinto shrine, built to house one or more Shinto kami (spirits). The building is primarily for safeguarding sacred objects and not designed as a pace of worship. The number of Shinto shrines in Japan is estimated at around 100,000 and miniature shrines called Hokura can occasionally be found along the sides of streets.

Photo: Chris van Uffelen

Fountain of the Four Rivers
Gian Lorenzo Bernini

Completion: 1651. **Technique:** marble. **Location:** Rome, Italy.

The "Fountain of the Four Rivers" (Fontana dei Quattro Fiumi) stands on the Piazza Navona and is a masterpiece of Baroque sculpture. It was built on the orders of Pope Innocent X. The fountain represents not only the known world of that time but also the Pope's claim to power over the earth. In the middle stands an obelisk surrounded by the four river gods who represent the major continents known at that time; the Nile (Africa), Danube (Europe), Ganges (Asia), and La Plata River (America).

Gian Lorenzo Bernini (1598–1680) was one of the most influential Italian sculptors and architects of the Baroque period. In the course of his life, Bernini worked for eight popes. His works stand out because of its unusually dynamic form, dramatic light-shadow effect and the figure's lively gestures and suggested movements. His architectural work often sought to combine sculpture and architecture.

Photo: Lalupa / Wikimedia Commons

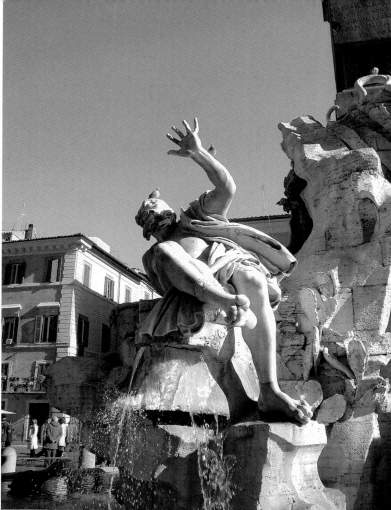

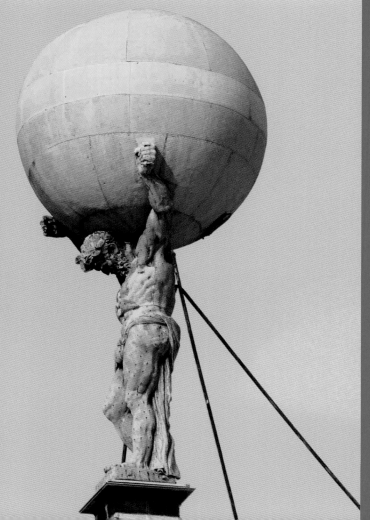

Atlas
Artus Quellinus the elder

Completion: 1665. **Technique:** bronze. **Location:** Amsterdam, The Netherlands.

Most of the sculptural decoration of the former town hall, todays Royal Palace of Amsterdam is by Quellinus. In particular, the room where judgments were announced is highly decorated. There are six large, bronze figures: Peace, Prudence, Justice, Atlas, Cautiousness and Temperance, these are located on the two outside gables. Atlas carrying the world on his shoulders is the central personification and symbolizes the burden of responsibility.

Artus Quellinus the elder was born in Antwerp in 1609 and died there in 1668. François Duquesnoy trained him in Rome and on his return in 1639 he introduced the "gran maniera greca" of his teacher, a classicizing of the Baroque style, to Northern Europe. He took over his father's workshop in 1640 and between 1648 and 1665 he worked in Amsterdam, especially on the Royal Palace, with the architect Jacob van Campen. His works, spread by etchings made by his brother, were of great influence.

Photo: Gunnar Bach Pedersen / Wikimedia Commons

Latona Fountain
André Le Nôtre (design)
Gaspard and Balthazar Marsy (sculptors)

Completion: 1670. **Technique:** red and white marble. **Location:** Versailles, Paris.

The "Latona Fountain" is constructed in the style of a huge wedding cake. It is located between the Palace of Versailles and the Grand Canal. The fountain features the Titaness Latona with her children Apollo and Diana. Legend has it that Latona turned the Lycian peasants into frogs and the frog sculptures on the second and third tier of the fountain are a reference to this. The lower tier features turtles and alligators.

The "Latona Fountain" was designed by André Le Nôtre and sculpted by Gaspard und Balthazar Marsy. The project was overseen by the architect Jules Hardouin-Mansart. André Le Nôtre (1613–1700) was a French landscape architect and the principle gardener of King Louis XIV. He was responsible for the design and construction of the park at the Palace of Versailles. Garpard (1629–1681) and Balthazar (1628–1674) Marsy were French sculptors, employed by King Louis XIV.

Photo: Chris van Uffelen

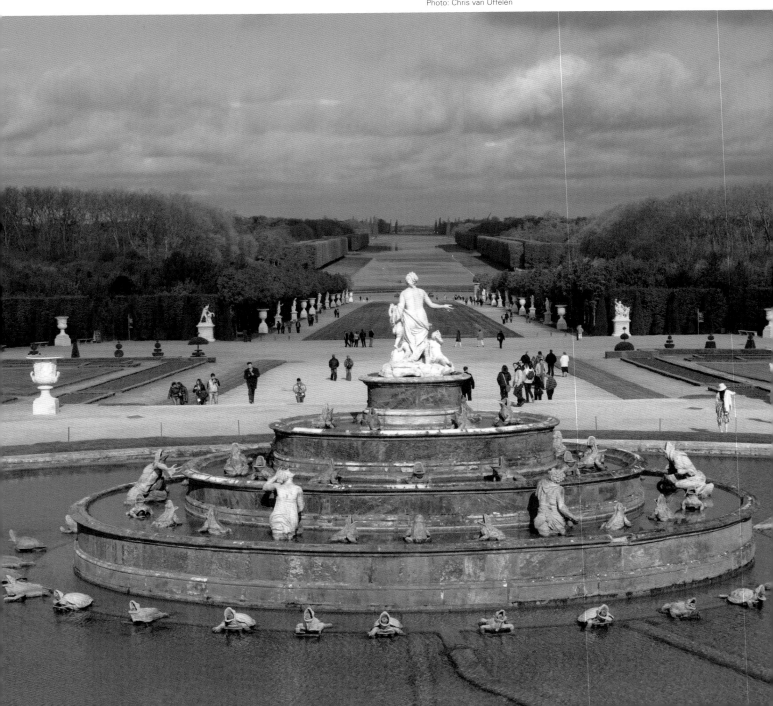

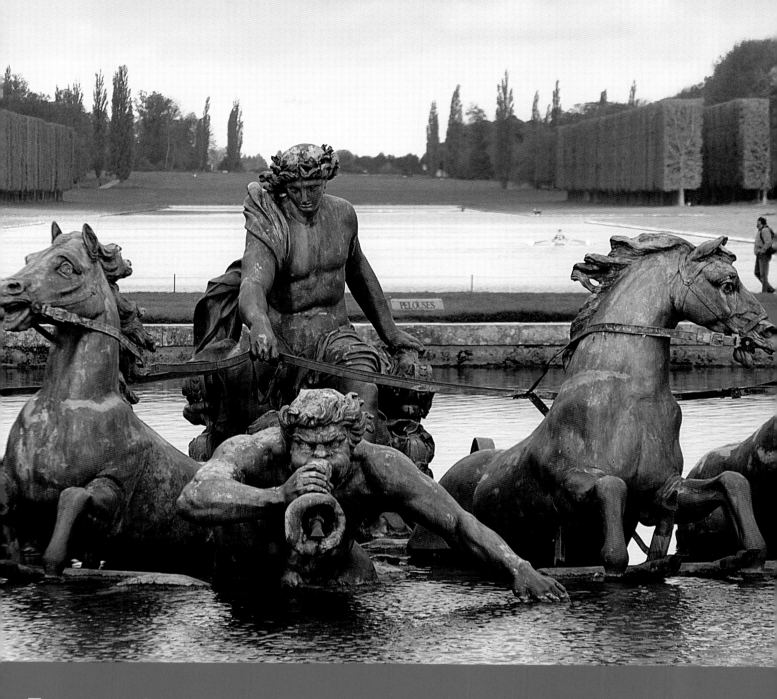

Fountain of Apollo
Jean-Baptiste Tuby

Completion: 1671. **Technique:** gilded bronze. **Location:** Versailles, France.

The "Fountain of Apollo" in the palace gardens in Versailles is situated in a prominent place, between the estate gardens and the head of the Grand Canal. Both the canal and a large number of fountains were fed with water diverted from the river Eure. The sculpture depicts Apollo emerging from the water amongst the thrashing bodies of horrible monsters. In Versailles, all of the depictions of Apollo, the sun god, also represent Louis XIV, who was also known as the "Sun King".

Jean-Baptiste Tuby was a French sculptor born in Rome in 1635. He became a French national in 1666. His most renowned work is the "Fountain of Apollo". He had a successful career in the service of Louis XIV, and became one of the most eminent sculptors of later 17th century. He concentrated his artistic activities to the decoration on the Palace of Versailles.

Photo: Chris van Uffelen

Fountain of Ceres
Thomas Regnaudin

Completion: 1679. **Technique:** gilded bronze. **Location:** Versailles, France.

The "Fountain of Ceres" was designed between 1672 and 1679 by Thomas Regnaudin and based on a drawing by Charles le Brun. Ceres, the goddess of harvests is sitting on a bed made of wheat sheaves and decorated with blueberries and roses. Ceres is the symbol of summer, complimenting the other fountains in the Versailles gardens. The Baccchus fountain represents autumn, the Saturn fountain represents winter and the Flora fountain represents spring.

Thomas Regnaudin was a French sculptor born in 1622, the son of a master mason. He trained in Moulins before entering the Paris workshop of François Anguier, where he worked on carving the tomb of Henri II de Montmorency. He was received as a member of the Royal Academy, where he became a professor in 1658 and assistant rector in 1694. His long career was largely founded on commissions from the Bâtiments du Roi, though he also received work from religious houses.

Photo: Chris van Uffelen

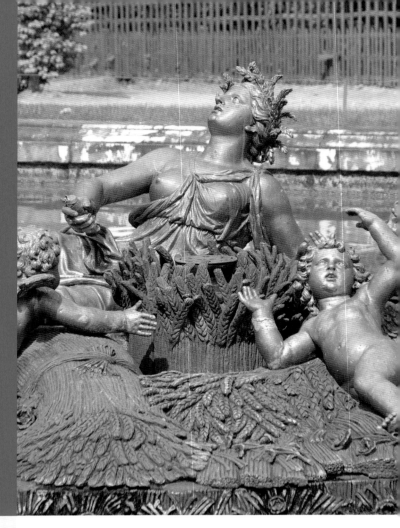

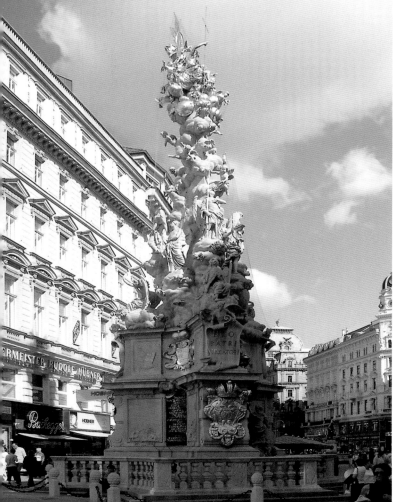

Plague Column
Matthias Rauchmüller

Completion: 1693. **Technique:** marble. **Location:** Vienna, Austria.

The "Plague Column" is located on the Grabenstraße and it is one of the city's most prominent pieces. The column was erected under the direction of Emperor Leopold I, who swore, during the plague epidemic of 1679, that if the plague should end, he would erect a mercy column. Johann Frühwirth made a provisional wooden column and Matthias Rauchmüller was then commissioned for the marble work, but he died before it was completed. Paul Strudel was eventually assigned the task of completing the work.

Matthias Rauchmüller was born in Germany in 1645, he worked in Vienna and became a very well reputed sculptor and artist. In addition to producing numerous large sculptures, ivory carvings and paintings, Rauchmüller also produced numerous drawings. Jacob von Sandrart engraved his drawings of the "Death of Sophonisbe" and the "Death of Cleopatra". Paul Strudel was born in 1648 and worked as a sculptor, engineer, architect and painter. The most important works from Strudel are large statues of white marble made for the ancestor gallery of the Habsburgs.

Photos: Chris van Uffelen

Equestrian Statue of the Great Elector Palatine
Andreas Schlüter

Completion: 1700. **Technique:** bronze. **Location:** Berlin, Germany.

This equestrian statue was originally placed on the "Long Bridge" close to the Berlin Castle. Friedrich III commissioned it, as a memorial to his father, the so-called "Great Elector Palatine", as he was one of the few people given the privilege of voting for new ruler. Schlüter formed his impression of the „Great Elector" from pictures and literature, resulting in the depiction of this a powerful, heroic figure. An influence for this work was probably the equestrian statue of Louis XIV.

Andreas Schlüter (1659/1664–1714) was a Prussian architect and sculptor. In 1694 he was summoned to Berlin by Friedrich III and appointed as court sculptor. He made several trips to France, the Netherlands and even Italy, where he acquired plaster casts of the ancient sculptures for the Berlin Academy. On these journeys he was exposed to the works of Michelangelo and Gian Lorenzo Bernini, these must have had a lasting effect on him, influencing his own work.

Photo: Chris van Uffelen

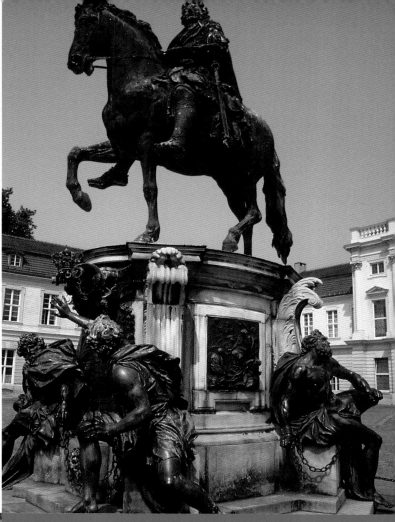

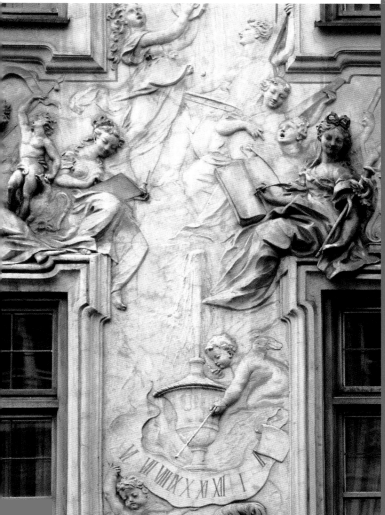

Asam House
Brothers Asam

Completion: 1733. **Technique:** stone. **Location:** Munich, Germany.

The so-called "Asam Church" (1746) was built to serve as the private chapel of these two sculptor-brothers, who then opened it to public on demand of the citizens. It is surrounded by both the "Asam House" (1733) and the "Priest's House" (1771). The façades are typical of the southern German Late-Baroque and Rococo Styles, in its rich ornamental design: the house shows allegories of the arts and joy of life as reliefs of different depth, the church tells the story of the life and deeds of Saint John of Nepomuk.

Egid Quirin Asam (1692–1750) was a plaster sculptor. Cosmas Damian Asam (1686–1739) was a painter and architect. They were sons of the painter Hans Georg Asam, and together they built this chapel, designing it as a Gesamtkunstwerk. After their father's death they realized that they would be much more successful if they offered architecture and plastering as well. Their early works strived to achieve perfect illusions, their later compositions were much freer in their arrangement.

Photo: Chris van Uffelen

Trevi Fountain
Nicola Salvi

Completion: 1762. **Technique:** travertine, marble. **Location:** Rome, Italy.

The 26-meter-high and 50-meter-wide "Trevi Fountain" (Fontana die Trevi) in Rome was built in the Late-Baroque style at a time when it was changing to the Classical style. The "Trevi Fountain" consists of a palace façade with a triumphal arch set above it. In the middle niche is the sea god Oceanus. In front of him various sea creatures are playing on a small stone island while water pours into a shallow stone basin. The theme of this work is the destructive forces of nature that threaten the work of man.

Nicola Salvi (1697–1751) was an Italian architect. The "Trevi Fountain" is his most famous work and he was occupied in completing this until his death. The fountain was finally completed in 1762, by Giuseppe Panini. He worked very strictly to the plans left by Salvi and it was only the sculpture of Oceanus that was re-designed, because Pope Benedict found the original too brutal and rough.

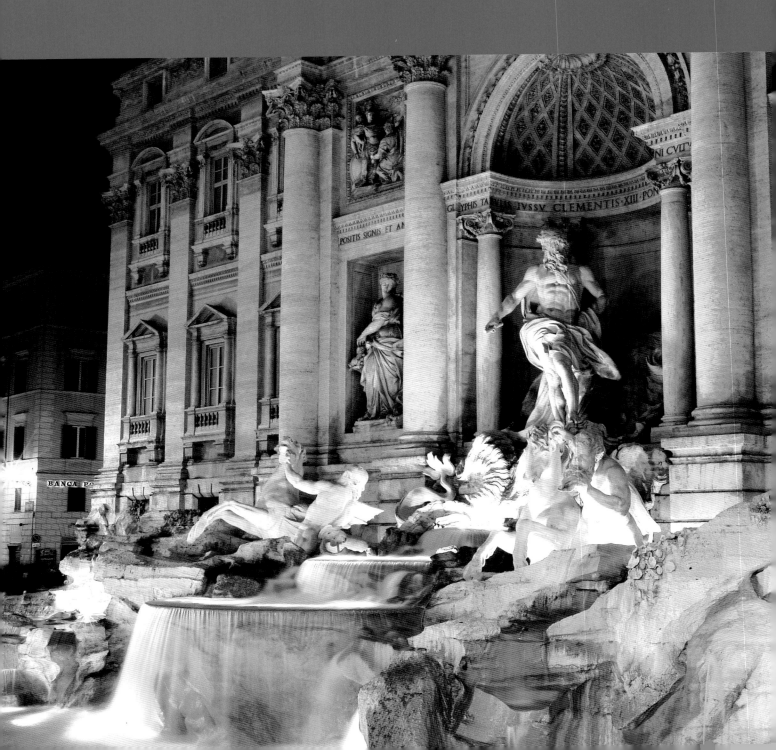

Cupid fashioning a Bow from the Club of Hercules
Edmé Bouchardon

Completion: 1739/1778. **Technique:** marble. **Location:** Versailles, France

The architect Richard Mique built this small Temple of Love in the park of the Petit Trianon. It was modeled on the temple of the Sibyl in Tivoli, for Madame de Pompadour, who was King Louis XV's concubine. The original sculpture was made in 1739 and is on display in the Louvre. Louis-Philippe Mouchy made a copy in 1778. It depicts a young man and is made in an un-idealized, naturalistic style and was inspired by an antique "Amore leaning on his Bow" in the Capitoline Museum in Rome.

Edmé Bouchardon (1698–1762) is considered to have been a leading influence in introducing Neo-Classicism to Rococo Art, sculpture and architecture. He was awarded the Rome Prize in 1722 and spent ten years in Rome, before becoming a French court-sculptor in 1732. His un-idealized Naturalism often shocked viewers but despite this he was highly admired, in particular for his equestrian monument of Louis XV on the Place de la Concorde.

Photo: Chris van Uffelen

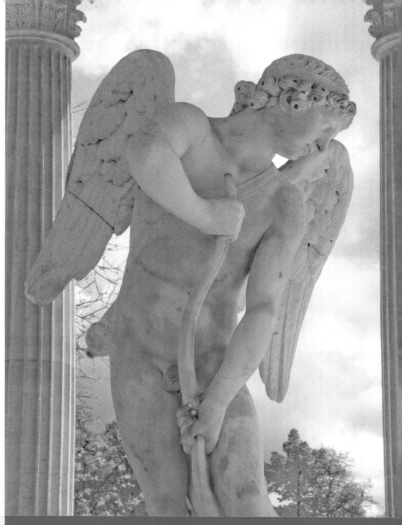

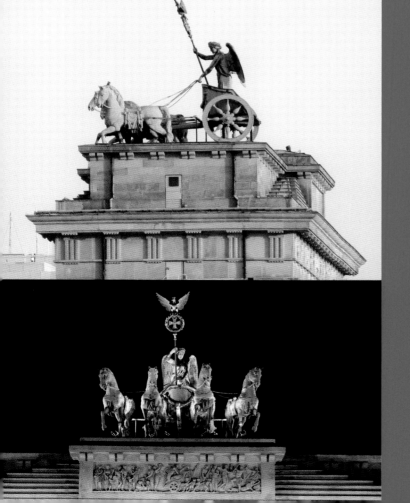

Quadriga
Johann Gottfried Schadow

Completion: 1793. **Technique:** copper. **Location:** Berlin, Germany.

The Brandenburg Gate is crowned with a five-meter-high sculpture. The sculpture portrays Victoria, the winged Goddess of Victory, standing on a war chariot being pulled towards the city by four horses. This sculpture proved to be unpopular with the people and Schadow attempted to improve it. Victoria now wears a crown of laurel leaves and carries a staff, topped with a Roman eagle. The original was destroyed in 1945 and the one that now stands in its place was created from a plaster cast of the original.

Johann Gottfried Schadow (1764–1850) was a Prussian artist and one of the most important figures of German Classicism. Schadow made memorials, tombs, statues, busts and sculptures consisting of both single figures and groups. He published theoretical and historical writing and was one of the founders of the Berlin tradition of Classicism.

Photos: Schlaier / Wikimedia Commons (a.); Chris van Uffelen (b.)

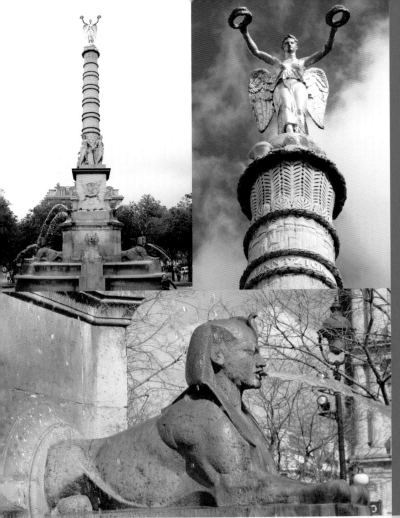

Fountain of Palms
François-Jean Bralle, Louis-Simon Boizot

Completion: 1808. **Technique:** sandstone, granite, gilded bronze.
Location: Paris, France.

The "Fountain of Palms" was one of a series of 15 fountains commissioned by Napoleon in 1806. It was designed by the engineer François-Jean Bralle. The column of the fountain is decorated with palm leaves, giving it its name. It is encircled with rings, bearing the names of military campaigns in Egypt and Italy. At the top of the column is a statue of Victory made of gilded bronze, carrying the laurels of victory. The statue is the work of the sculptor Louis-Simon Boizot.

François-Jean Bralle was born in 1750 and died in 1832. He was a French architect and engineer, best known for constructing various fountains in Paris, during the time of Napoleon Bonaparte. Bralle was commissioned to build 15 fountains in Paris; several of which are still functioning today. Louis-Simon Boizot was a French sculptor, born in 1743. He was a member of the Commission of Monuments in 1792 and from 1805 he held a chair at the Academy of Fine Arts in Paris.

Vendôme Column
Pierre-Nolasque Bergeret, Antoine-Denis Chaudet, and others

Completion: 1810. **Technique:** bronze, porphyry. **Location:** Paris, France.

The Royal Place was built by Jules Hardouin-Mansart and featured an equestrian monument of Louis XIV by François Girardon 1699. This was removed in 1792, during the French Revolution. In 1810 a 44-meter column was set on this site, made from melted-down cannons. Inspired by the Trajan column, it is crowned by a statue of Napoleon, portrayed as a Roman Caesar. The reliefs were designed by Pierre-Nolasque Bergeret and the statue by Antoine-Denis Chaudet.

Besides the Neo-Classicists Pierre-Nolasque Bergeret (1782–1863) and Antoine-Denis Chaudet (1763–1810), sculptors Jean Joseph Foucou, Louis Boizot, Bosio, Bartolini, Claude Ramey, François Rude, Edme Gaulle and others worked on this column. In 1833 the first Napoleon was replaced by one from sculptor Charles Émile Seurre and Napoleon III ordered Auguste Dumont to repeat the first. In 1871 the Paris Commune destroyed the column but in 1874 the painter Gustave Courbet was charged for compensation to fund its reconstruction.

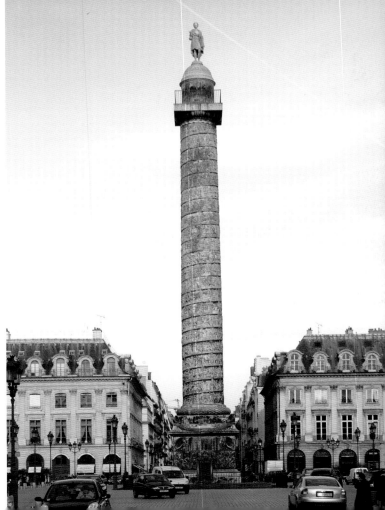

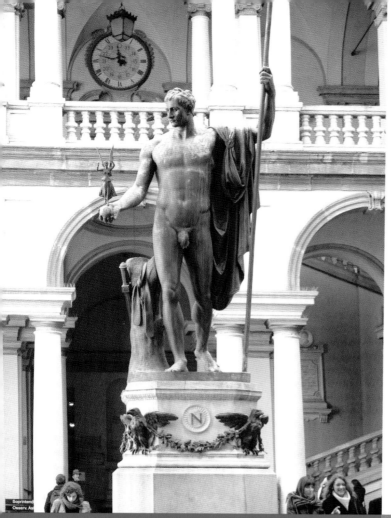

Napoleon as Mars the Peacemaker
Antonio Canova

Completion: 1811. **Technique:** bronze. **Location:** Milan, Italy.

This monumental bronze depicts the French King as the god Mars, holding a small Victoria. It was originally made in 1806 as a marble-sculpture (Apsley House, London). Canova visited Napoleon to model a bust of him 1802, which became the head of the statue. This sculptor faced the same problem every sculptor of the time faced; a man in antique clothing or even naked might look ridiculous so the figures were often idealized. However, Napoleon refused to accept this sculpture because it was too athletic.

Antonio Canova, born in 1757 in Possagno, was the most renowned sculptor of the Neo-Classic style in around 1800. His figures are of stringent composition, always to be viewed from the front and clearly lined but with smooth details and forms. Most of his works have antique references either in their form or theme. He saw studies of the naked body as the only way to return to a more natural look. He died 1822 in Venice and was buried in Possagno in the Tempio Canoviano.

Photo: Giovanni Dall'Orto / Wikimedia Commons

Waterpalace Fountain
Pierre-Simon Girard

Completion: 1811. **Technique:** cast-iron. **Location:** Paris, France.

The "Waterpalace Fountain" was made by Pierre-Simon Girard. The fountain is made of cast-iron, which was quite an accomplishment in 1811 and is one of the earliest examples of the use of cast-iron in fountains. In addition to its decorative function, the fountain served to provide water to the surrounding area. In 1867, it was moved from what is today known as the Place de la République, to La Villette, where it stands today.

Pierre-Simon Girard was born in Paris in 1765 and died in 1836. He was a French mathematician and engineer and was considered a child prodigy after he designed a water turbine at the age of just ten. Girard worked as an engineer and was in charge of the planning and construction of the Amiens Canal and the Ourcq Canal. He wrote many papers and books on fluids and the strength of materials and also produced the Dictionary of Bridges and Highways, in collaboration with Gaspard de Prony.

Photos: Romary / Wikimedia Commons (a.); Chris van Uffelen (b.)

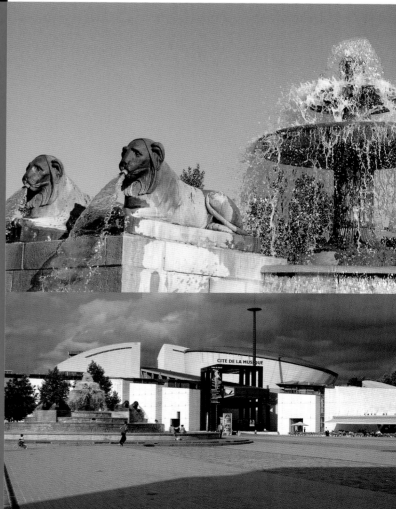

Arc de Triomphe du Carousel
François Joseph Bosio

Completion: 1828. **Technique:** bronze, gilded. **Location:** Paris, France.

The "Arc de Triomphe du Carousel" is a triumphal arch in Paris and is situated on the former site of the Tuileries Palace. It was built in commemoration of Napoleon's military victories. The monument is 19 meters high and the main arch is flanked by two smaller ones. Eight Corinthian columns are positioned around the outside, each supporting a soldier of the empire. A quadriga takes pride of place on top of the arch, depicting Peace riding in a chariot and led by gilded Victories on both sides.

François Joseph Bosio was a French sculptor, born in 1769. He was considered the best portrait sculptor in Paris and was awarded various titles and prizes, including being made a Knight of the Order of Saint Michael in 1821 and being appointed 'the Kings first sculptor'. Charles Percier, a French Neo-Classical architect and designer who was born in 1764, and Pierre François Léonard, born in 1762, designed the arch itself. The two worked in close partnership together on many projects.

Photos: Jastrow / Wikimedia Commons (b.); Chris van Uffelen (a.)

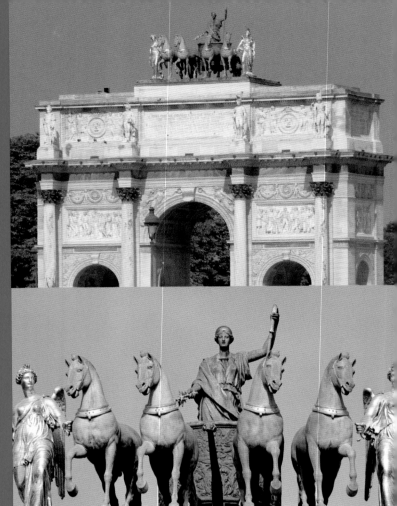

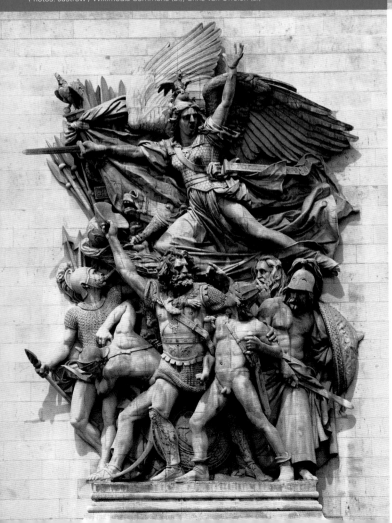

Depature of the Volunteers of 1792
François Rude

Completion: 1836. **Technique:** stone. **Location:** Paris, France.

The "Departure of the Volunteers of 1792" known as "La Marseillaise" or "Farewell song" is a relief on the right eastern post of the large Arc de Triomphe in Paris. Just a few years after the famous painting of "Freedom Leading the People" by Eugène Delacroix, Rude also turned to Romanticism in his sculpture. The frontal stage and balanced composition of Neo-Classicism is gone, most protagonists are not naked Romans but vital Gauls, with Rude's own wife – the painter Sophie Fremiet – as Marianne leading them.

François Rude was born in Dijon in 1784 and died in 1855 in Paris. He first worked as a stove-maker, before attending the Academy of Fine Arts in Paris in 1807 and later working in the workshop of Pierre Cartellier. He was awarded the Rome Prize in 1812 and formed a close contact to the painter Jacques-Louis David. From 1815 to 1827 he worked at the Royal Palace of Tervuren near Brussels.

Photos: Chris van Uffelen

Gutenberg
Bertel Thorvaldsen

Completion: 1837. **Technique:** bronze. **Location:** Mainz, Germany.

This monument is one of the first truly 'civil' monuments: of a citizen and financed by citizens, not ordered by a political leader or for a religious purpose. The first suggestion for a Gutenberg monument came in 1792 from Georg Christian Wedekind, a doctor and revolutionary. Napoleon kept the idea, but nothing was realized. A second effort led to a provisory work in 1827. Finally Ludwig Lindenschmit the elder, a painter and museum-founder, made a concept and the citizens succeeded in convincing the famous sculptor Thorvaldsen to make the statue.

Bertel Thorvaldsen was born around 1770 in Copenhagen and died there in 1844, after spending most of his life in Italy. At the age of eleven he started studying at the Copenhagen Academy. His work – a lot of portraits and mythological subjects – is famous for strictly adhering to classical norms. Upon his return to Denmark in 1838 he was received as a national hero and two years after he died the Thorvaldsen Museum, housing his work, opened next to Christiansborg.

Photo: Tobbecker / Wikimedia Commons

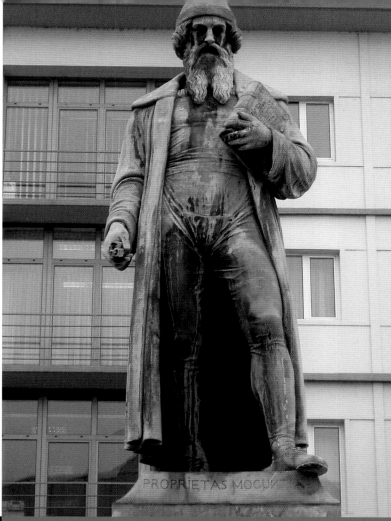

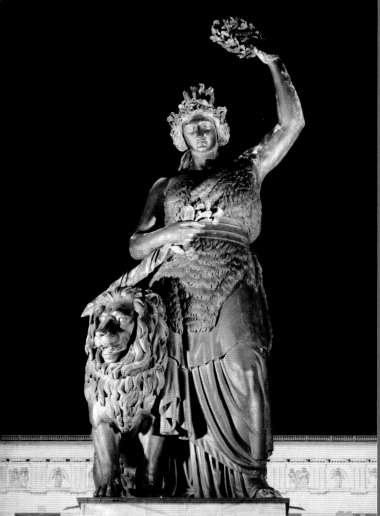

Bavaria
Ludwig Michael von Schwanthaler

Completion: 1848. **Technique:** bronze. **Location:** Munich, Germany.

This huge sculpture is 18.5 meters tall and stands on a nine-meter pedestal. It weighs almost 90 tons and was cast in bronze, in four different sections (chest, hips, lower half and lion). "Bavaria" is the female symbol and secular patron. She also personifies the area's political structure of Bavaria. A spiral staircase winds up the inside of the sculpture, ending in a viewing platform at the figure's head.

Ludwig Michael von Schwanthaler (1802–1848) is one of the most influential Neo-Classical sculptors in south Germany. The "Bavaria" in Munich is one of his most important works. He was born into a family of sculptors and received his first lessons from his father. When Schwanthaler died, he bequeathed all of his models and studies to the Munich Academy and these are now housed in the Schwanthaler Museum.

Photo: Schlaier / Wikimedia Commons

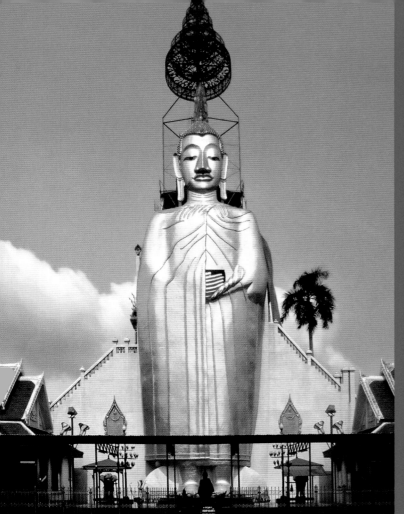

Buddha of
Wat Indrawiharn
unknown

Completion: mid 19th c. **Technique:** gold mosaic tiles. **Location:** Bangkok, Thailand.

The standing "Buddha of Wat Indrawiharn" is 32 meters tall, and could be seen from almost anywhere in the Old town, before the city was developed and modernized around it. It is now hidden behind the new buildings, built during Thailand's boom years. The Buddha was built to house relics from Sri Lanka and stands in front of a temple, founded by King Rama IV in the mid 19th century.

It is tradition in Thailand that only the king introduces new forms of Buddha sculptures, whether it be standing, sitting or any other of a variety of positions. King Rama IV, also known as King Mongkut, ruled from 1851–1868. During his reign, the pressure of Western Expansionism was felt for the first time in Siam. Mongkut embraced western innovations, earning him the name "The Father of Science and Technology".

Photo: Chris van Uffelen

The Dance
Jean-Baptiste Carpeaux

Completion: 1863. **Technique:** stone. **Location:** Paris, France.

The Paris Opera House, by architect Charles Garnier, is the architectural epitome of bourgeois representation in the Neo-Baroque style. One of the façade reliefs, "The Dance", was considered both scandalous and a celebrated masterpiece. The brief demanded a life-like depiction of three female dancers. Carpeaux's naked dancers were obviously too realistic for his time. Due to the 'wild' moving of arms and bodies and the non-idealized look of real body-parts were reminiscent of popular dance and of the indecent Can-Can.

Jean-Baptiste Carpeaux was born in 1827 in Valenciennes and died in Courbevoie in 1875. He first began his career by making models for the art industry before going on to study at the Paris Academy of Fine Arts. In 1854 he achieved the Rome Prize, before returning to Paris in 1862 when he founded his own workshop and became famous for his portraits and his life-scenes with antique topics, like the "Flora" for the Louvre-extension.

Photo: Chris van Uffelen

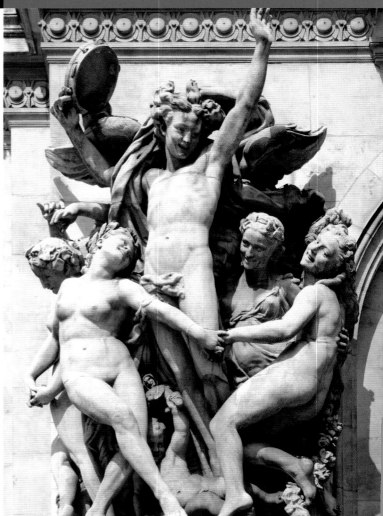

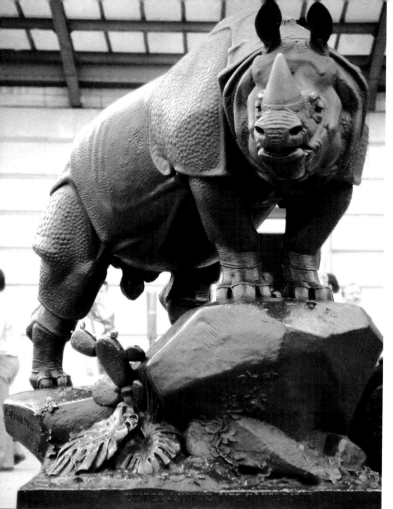

Rhinoceros
Alfred Jacquemart

Completion: 1878. **Technique:** cast-iron. **Location:** Paris, France.

For the Paris International Exposition in 1878 Jacquemart made a group of four, cast-iron animals. Intended for a fountain at the old Palais du Trocadéro, these were originally gilded and depict a horse, an elephant, a bull and a 2.86-meter-high rhinoceros. After the demolition of the palace, the sculpture was moved to the Porte de Saint-Cloud. Since 1985, the horse and elephant stand in front of the Musée d'Orsay, while the bull is in Nîmes.

Alfred Jacquemart was born in Paris in 1824 and died there in 1896. He studied at the Paris Academy and later travelled in Egypt and Turkey, where he was commissioned to create a colossal statue of Muhammad Ali of Egypt in Alexandria. He became most famous as sculptor of animals, a highly admired theme of 19th century sculpture.

Photo: Chris van Uffelen

The Binnenhof Fountain
Pierre Cuypers

Completion: 1883. **Technique:** iron, gilt, painted. **Location:** The Hague, The Netherlands.

"The Inner Court Fountain" is a work from the Dutch sculptor Pierre Cuypers and was made in 1883. It was originally intended for the Amsterdam National Museum before finally being erected on the Binnenhof. The Binnenhof is a complex of buildings in the Hague. It has been the location of meetings of the Dutch parliament, since 1446, and has been the center of Dutch politics for many centuries. The Inner Court is studded with monumental old buildings and this gilt, Neo-Gothic fountain adorns the main square.

Pierre Cuypers was a Dutch architect, born in Roermond in 1827. He studied architecture at the Royal Academy of Fine Arts and was taught by Frans Andried Durlet, Frans Stoop and Ferdinand Berckmans, who were all leaders of the Neo-Gothic architecture movement in Belgium. Cuypers' most famous architectural projects include the National Museum and the Amsterdam Central Train Station. He also designed a large number of churches and restored many important monuments.

Photos: Subarrator / Wikimedia Commons

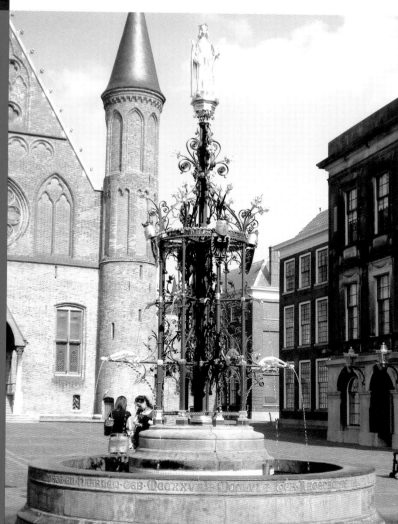

Duke of Wellington
Francis Chantrey

Completion: 1884. **Technique:** bronze. **Location:** London, United Kingdom.

This statue was created by the sculptor Francis Chantrey. It is made from melted down French cannons, seized by Wellington during his battles in the Napoleonic wars. Wellington was also known as the Iron Duke and is a national hero. At his funeral, a carriage, also made from French cannons, was used to transport him. This can still be seen in the crypt of St Paul's Cathedral.

Sir Francis Chantrey was an English sculptor. He lived during the Georgian era and donated the Chantrey Fund after his death, which allowed the purchase of works of art for the nation. He was born in Sheffield, and was placed with a woodcarver in Sheffield as an apprentice at the age of 15. Raphael Smith gave him painting lessons before he left England, moving first to Dublin, then Edinburgh and later to London. He became a successful sculptor and has numerous works displayed across the United Kingdom, Europe and America.

Photo: Rob Sandiford

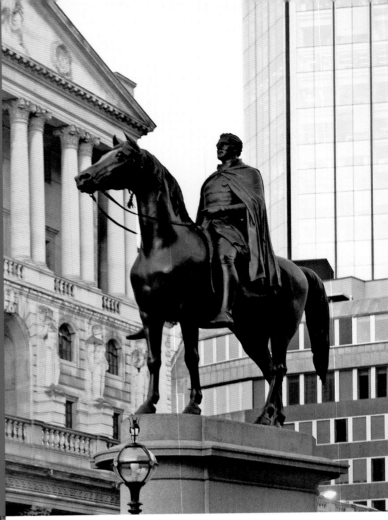

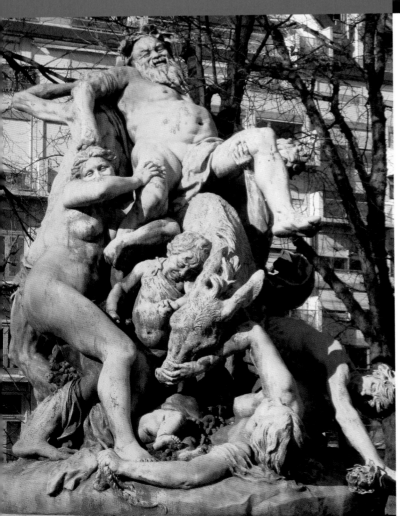

The Triumph of Silenus
Aimé-Jules Dalou

Completion: 1885. **Technique:** bronze. **Location:** Paris, France.

This sculpture, in the Jardin du Luxembourg, has a pyramidal form. Silenus, chief of the satyrs, teacher to the wine god Dionysus, rides a donkey that seems to have collapsed and Silenus himself is obviously so drunk he is about to fall off. In an extraordinary naturalistic portrayal he neither cares about this, nor about his sliding loincloth. A naked nymph is trying to hold him, laughing as well. The fingers of the nymph press deep in his flesh, showing how heavy the old god is.

Aimé-Jules Dalou was born in Paris in 1838 and died there 1902. He studied drawing as a student of Jean-Baptiste Carpeaux and was accused of taking part in the Paris Commune of 1871. As Louvre curator under Gustav Courbet he fled to England and taught at the South Kensington School of Art. He later returned to Paris after the 1879 amnesty.

Photo: Daderot / Wikimedia Commons

Statue of Liberty
Frédéric Auguste Bartholdi

Completion: 1886. **Technique:** copper-coated steel frame (original: copper-coated iron frame). **Location:** New York City, NY, USA.

The "Statue of Liberty" was a belated anniversary gift, given to America by France to mark the 100th anniversary of the Declaration of Independence in New York. It came ten years after the anniversary and was built in New York in 1886. The statue is 45 meters high and Liberty holds a stone tablet in her left hand, on which is engraved the date of the American Declaration of Independence, fourth of July 1776. In her right hand she holds a torch with a golden flame.

The best known works of the French sculptor, Frédéric Auguste Bartholdi (1834–1904) are "The Statue of Liberty", and the "Lion of Belfort", an 11-meter-high and 22-meter-long stone sculpture and landmark of the town of Belfort. Bartholdi drew inspiration for his monumental sculpture from the Colossus of Rhodes, one of the Seven Wonders of the World. Gustav Eiffel (1832–1923) was responsible constructing the iron framework for the "Statue of Liberty".

Photo: Derek Jensen / Wikimedia Commons

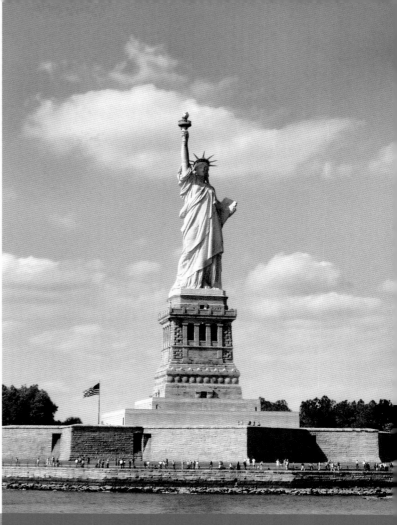

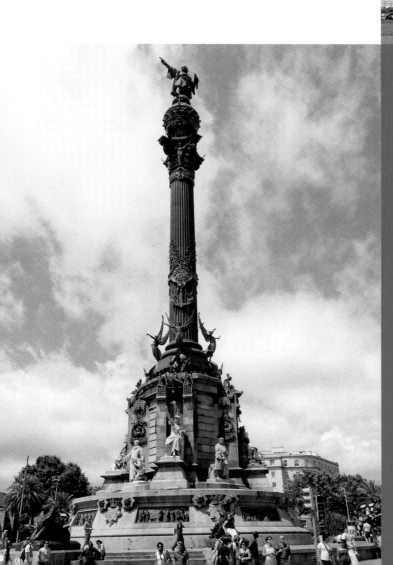

Columbus Monument
Rafael Atché i Ferré

Completion: 1888. **Technique:** bronze. **Location:** Barcelona, Spain.

The "Columbus Monument" in Barcelona is a 60-meter-high monument to Christopher Columbus. It is located on the site where Columbus returned to Spain after his first voyage to the Americas. The statue at the top of the monument is just over seven meters tall and is said to depict Columbus pointing with his right hand, towards the New World. However, when the statue was positioned, it was fixed with the hand pointing east, towards the city of Geneva.

Rafael Atché i Ferré was born in Barcelona, Spain in 1854 and died in 1923. He set up a studio with another sculptor, Carcass in 1872. He participated in the National Exhibition in Madrid in 1882 with the sculpture "The wounded Genius" and in 1884, with "The bad Thief". He is best known for his sculpture of Christopher Columbus that crowns the monument in the center of Barcelona.

Photos: Chris van Uffelen

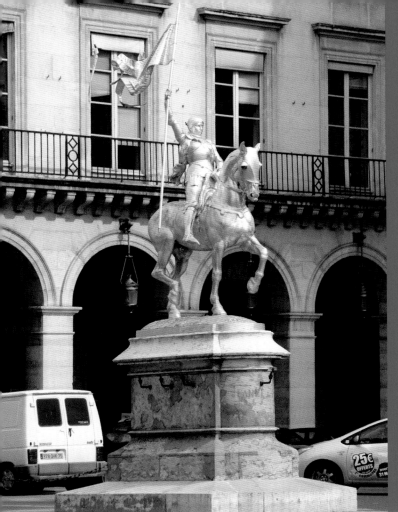

Joan of Arc
Emmanual Frémiet

Completion: 1889. **Technique:** gilded bronze. **Location:** Paris, France.

In 1872, the French government commissioned Emmanuel Frémiet to design a monument to Joan of Arc for the Place des Pyramides in Paris. Frémiet studied the design of 15th century French armor and dress in order to convey the figure within her historical context. In 1899 Frémiet was informed that his statue was under threat by ongoing underground repairs to the street. He took this opportunity to make some improvements to the statue, making Joan 20 centimeters taller and the horse's neck thinner.

Emmanual Frémiet was a French sculptor, born in Paris in 1824. His most famous work is the Joan of Arc statue in Paris. He was considered to be the leading animal sculptor of his day and exhibited his first sculpture in the Paris Salon in 1843. Frémiet received his first commission for a public monument in 1849, he went on to receive the most public monument commissions of any artist of his time. A large number of his works adorned the streets of Paris.

Photo: Chris van Uffelen

The Burghers of Calais
Auguste Rodin

Completion: 1895. **Technique:** bronze. **Location:** Calais, France (first copy).

This group of six figures shows an episode from 1347, during the Hundred Years' War. The city of Calais was under the siege from the English for over a year and Edward III offered to spare the people of the city if the six most prominent leaders would surrender themselves to execution. Rodin shows them at the moment they leave their hometown. It was one of the first monuments to be designed without a pedestal and is most famous for its different mimics and gestures.

François Auguste René Rodin was born in 1840 in Paris and died in 1917 in Meudon. His sculptural works are said to be the first examples of modern sculpture. He studied drawing and applied arts but was not admitted into the Academy, Paris' foremost school of art. In 1864 he entered the studio of Albert-Ernest Carrier-Belleuse but later left after a dispute. He studied Michelangelo's works in Italy and the Non-Finito of the Renaissance-artist became extremely important for Rodin. Putting together fragments of different projects was typical for his later work ("Hells gate").

Photos: Gryffindor / Wikimedia Commons (a.); Chris van Uffelen (b.)

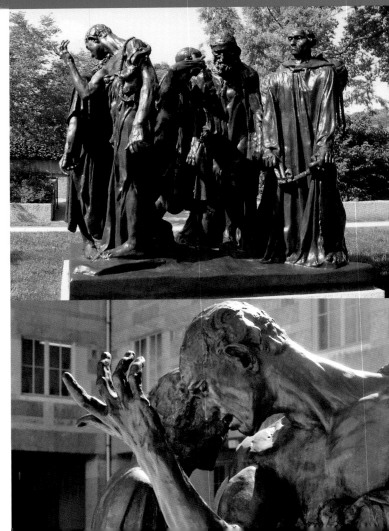

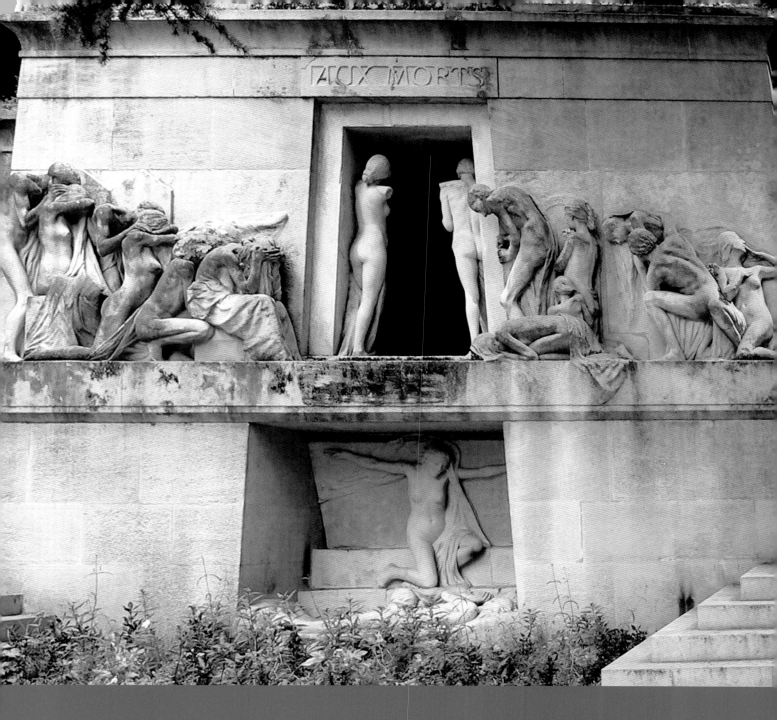

Photo: Wikimedia Commons

Cenotaph
Paul-Albert Bartholomé

Completion: 1899. **Technique:** stone. **Location:** Paris, France.

This is the main monument to all the dead souls in the Père Lachaise cemetery. The cemetery is the largest in Paris and is named after the Louis XIV's confessor. This work is a monument to all the dead and is built like a stage with an Egyptian pylon. There are carved figures, positioned around the outside, walking into the realm of the dead. Each of the individual figures is portrayed in a pose of grief, clinging to the wall of the building and to each other.

Paul-Albert Bartholomé was a French artist and sculptor, born in 1848. He was a student of Barthélémy Menno in Geneva and later worked under the direction of Jean-Léon Gérôme in Paris. Bartholomé turned to sculpture after the death of his wife Marie Louise in 1887 after carving the headstone for her grave. Another famous work by the artist is the monument to Jean-Jacques Rousseau in the Panthéon in Paris. Bartholomé is buried in the Père Lachaise cemetery as well.

Metro-Entrance
Hector Guimard

Completion: 1899. **Technique:** cast iron. **Location:** Paris, France.

These entrances were built for the first lines of the new subway in Paris; the first line opened in 1900. They are very fragile-looking constructions and it is obvious that they were inspired by nature. This is typical of the rising French Art Nouveau movement, where lamps are like glass buds, breaking out of the metal stem. The German Jugendstil, later introduced a much more geometric style to art and architecture.

Hector Guimard was born in Lyon in 1867 and died in New York in 1942. Though actually an architect, Guimard is best known for his sculptural "Metro-Entrances". He studied at the Academy in Paris and was influenced by the rationalist theories of Eugène Emmanuel Viollet-le-Duc. The Neo-Gothic influence of his tutor became as important to him as the floral decoration he found in Brussels, on the buildings of Victor Horta.

Photo: Chris van Uffelen

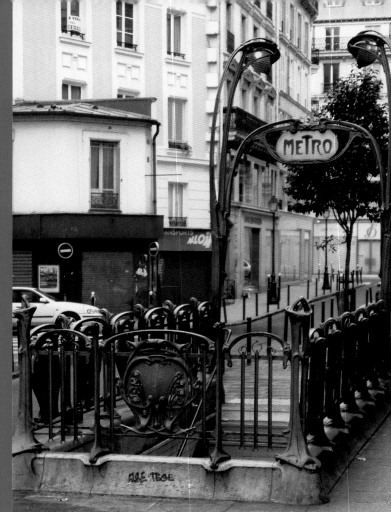

The Athena Fountain
Carl Kundmann

Completion: 1902. **Technique:** marble. **Location:** Vienna, Austria.

"The Athena Fountain" stands in front of the Parliament building in Vienna. The fountain was made by Carl Kundmann, Josef Tautenhayn and Hugo Haerdt and took nine years to complete. The four figures lying at Athena's feet are allegorical representations of the four most important rivers of the Austro-Hungarian Empire; the Danube, the Inn, the Elbe and the Vitava. The female statues represent the legislative and executive powers of the state; Athena, who is raised above them, dominates these.

Carl Kundmann was an Austrian sculptor. He is considered one of the main sculptors of the Ringstraße, a circular road around the inner city of Vienna that has a large number of sculptures and decorative works; a number of which were made by Kundmann. He was a student of Franz Lukas Bauer and Ernst Julius Hähnel in Germany before he moved to Rome to study. His most highly regarded work is the "Athena Fountain".

Photo: Chris van Uffelen

Kneeling Woman
Wilhelm Lehmbruck

Completion: 1911. **Technique:** bronze. **Location:** Duisburg, Germany.

The "Kneeling Woman" in the sculpture park of the Lehmbruck Museum is a typical work of Lehmbruck, who always positioned the naked figure – standing, kneeling, sleeping or fallen – as the central piece of his work. The figures in his sculptures express feelings or situations, his use of Expressionism appears Naturalistic but with no portrait features. His work was labeled "Degenerate Art" by the Nazi regime and so his "Kneeling Woman" (version of the MoMA, New York) was a perfect opener for the first Documenta exhibition in 1955.

Wilhelm Lehmbruck was born in Meiderich in 1881 and died in Berlin in 1919. He studied at the Dusseldorf School of Applied Arts from 1899 until 1901, at which time he changed to the Academy. In 1910 he moved to Paris and was involved with the Salon d'Automne, where most modern artists exhibited their work. From 1916 onwards he lived and taught in Zurich. In 1919 he moved to Berlin where he committed suicide.

Photo: Gerardus / Wikimedia Commons

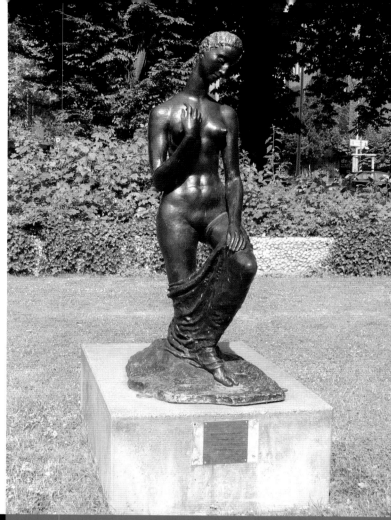

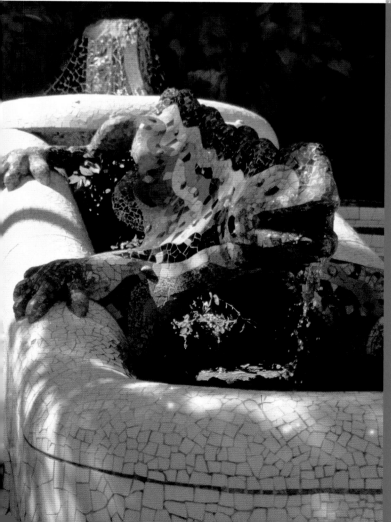

Dragon Fountain
Antoni Gaudí

Completion: 1914. **Technique:** cement, ceramic fragments. **Location:** Barcelona, Spain.

The "Dragon Fountain" is covered with a mosaic, made from blue, turquoise and orange-red tile pieces. It stands in front of a small water basin and serves as water reservoir. The dragon sits on the open stairway of the Gu_ell park, a large park of 17 hectares that was planned by Gaudí for the industrialist Eusebi Güell between 1900 and 1914. However, from the 60 that were planned, only three houses, the entrance gates with gatehouses, the stairway and the terrace were realized.

Antoni Gaudí, one of the most important representatives of modern architectural styles and the instigator of the Catalonian interpretation of the Art Nouveau Style, was born in 1852. Curving lines, uneven floors and sloping columns were all typical hallmarks of the Modern Style. Gaudí's most important works include the Sagrada Familia; he took over this project in 1883, working tirelessly on it until his death in 1926. He also built the Palau Güell, the Güell Park and took on the renovation of the Casa Batlló and the Casa Milà, all in Barcelona.

Photos: Chris van Uffelen

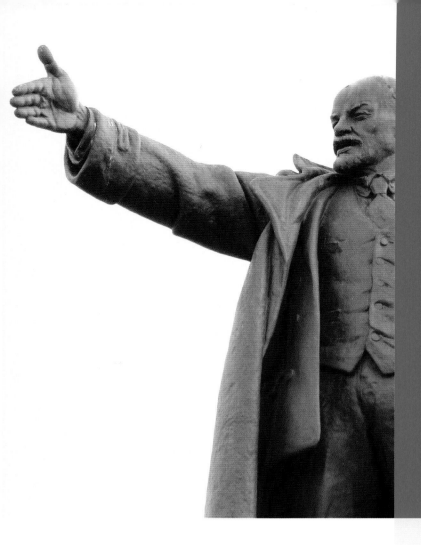

Lenin
Vladimir A. Shuchuko
Sergei A. Evseev

Completion: 1926. **Technique:** bronze. **Location:** Saint Petersburg, Russia.

This statue is one of the earliest, monumental Lenin statues and stands in front of the Finland Station in Saint Petersburg. It established a style that was followed a lot in the following decade. A similar 100-meter-high statue was planned to crown Boris Iofans giant building, the Palace of the Soviets, but was never finished. While this first Lenin statue was built two years after he died, the Stalin monuments were built during his lifetime.

Very little is known about the sculptor of this piece, Sergei A. Evseev, though the architect and designer Vladimir A. Shuchuko (1878–1939) was a well known representative of Monumental-Classicism. From 1918–1929 he was professor at the Saint Petersburg Academy of the Arts. In the early years of the Soviet Union the new state was the hope of all Modernists and also promoted Constructivist and Modernist work. In 1932 Socialist Realism became the official style.

Europa and the Bull
Carl Milles

Completion: 1926. **Technique:** bronze. **Location:** Halmstad, Sweden.

This famous depiction of "Europa and the Bull" is positioned in the center of a fountain in Halmstad's main square. Sculptor Carl Milles won a competition to design the piece and it was finished in 1926. The figure comes from Greek mythology and is taken from the story of Zeus, when he disguised himself as a bull in order to kidnap the Princess Europa, whom he had fallen in love with.

Carl Milles was a Swedish sculptor, born in 1875. He moved to Paris in around 1897, where he married and began studying art, working at the studio of Auguste Rodin. During this time, he built up a favorable reputation as a sculptor. He and his wife moved to Germany in 1904 and then later to Sweden. Milles continued to gain recognition as a sculptor and moved to America to work as sculptor in residence for George Gough Booth. Today, Milles is best known for his fountains.

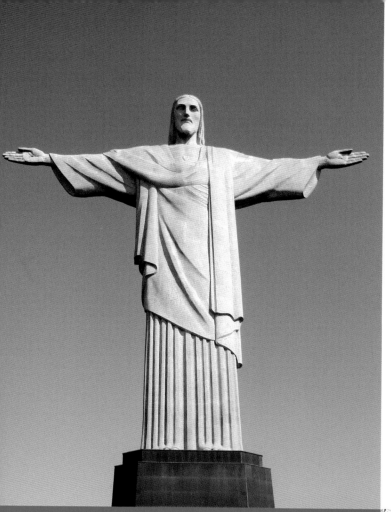

Christ the Redeemer
Heitor da Silva Costa, Paul Landowski

Completion: 1931. **Technique:** reinforced concrete, soapstone.
Location: Rio de Janeiro, Brazil.

"Christ the Redeemer" is a statue of Jesus Christ in Rio de Janeiro. It is thought to be one of the largest Art Deco statues in the world and is located at the top of the 700-meter-high Corcovado Mountain, overlooking the city. It is made of reinforced concrete and soapstone and took nine years to build. The head, fingers and eyebrows were damaged when it was struck by lightening in 2008. It was designed by Heitor da Silva Costa and sculpted by Paul Landowski.

Heitor da Silva Costa was a Brazilian engineer, born in 1873. He was an atheist who later converted to Christianity and won the competition to design a monument to Christ, commissioned by the Catholic Church. The commission of the statue was to celebrate the 100th anniversary of Brazilian independence. Paul Landowski was a French monument sculptor. He won the Rome Prize with his statue of David and went on to produce 35 monuments in the city of Paris.

Photo: Pedrohiroshi / Wikimedia Commons

Standing Woman
Gaston Lachaise

Completion: 1932. **Technique:** bronze. **Location:** Paris, France.

The "Standing Woman" is made of bronze and is one of Gaston Lachaise's most famous works. It stands in the Jardin des Tuileries in Paris. Lachaise produced many different drawings and depictions of the female figure and is said to have drawn inspiration from his wife's figure. Despite his French origins, Lachaise's work is much better known in America, where his works are in the collections of several prominent museums.

Gaston Lachaise was a French sculptor. He was born in 1882 and died in 1935. He lived in Paris and was most famous with his female nudes. His father was a cabinetmaker and Lachaise trained in decorative arts, later studying sculpture at the School of Fine Arts. Lachaise immigrated to America in 1906 and worked for H. H. Kitson, a company that made historic monuments. He moved to New York in 1912 and worked as an assistant to sculptor Paul Manship.

Photo: Janericloebe / Wikimedia Commons

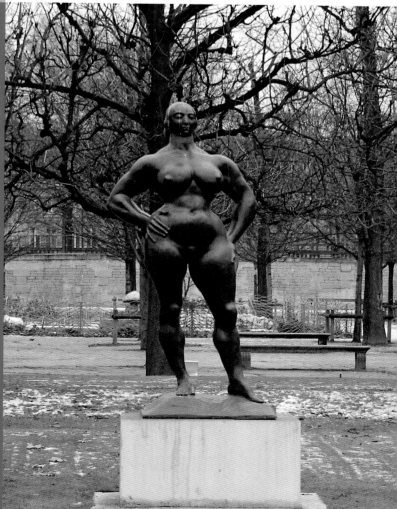

The Four Points of the Compass
Hildo Krop

Completion: 1933. **Technique:** stone. **Location:** Amsterdam, The Netherlands.

Four sculptures symbolizing Western, Eastern, Northern and Southern culture mark the ends of the two walls of a bridge in Amsterdam. A lot of bridges where built in the early 20th century extension of the city at that time by the city architect Piet Kramer. Hildo Krop, the official city sculptor, made hundreds of sculptures to decorate them. He was an early multi-style artist shifting between styles for the different bridges, so no two ever look the same.

Hildebrand Lucien Krop, known as Hildo Krop, was born in Steenwijk in 1884 and died in Amsterdam in 1970. He was working as a cook for a couple in England, when his talent was recognized. He went to study at the private Julian Academy in Paris, where a lot of artists of the upcoming Avant-garde also studied. He worked at the John Rädecker-workshop and followed Georg Kolbe to the Berlin Academy of Applied Arts. After working at the Scheepvaarthuis – the building that established the Amsterdam School of architecture 1916 – he was announced city-sculptor.

Photo: Chris van Uffelen

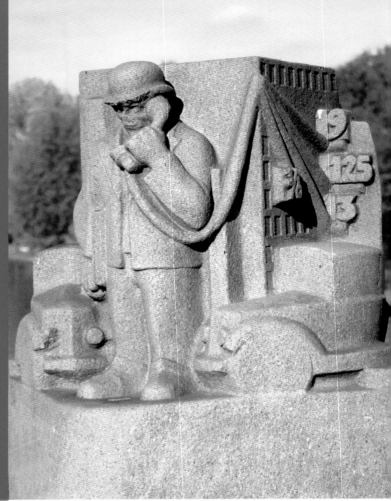

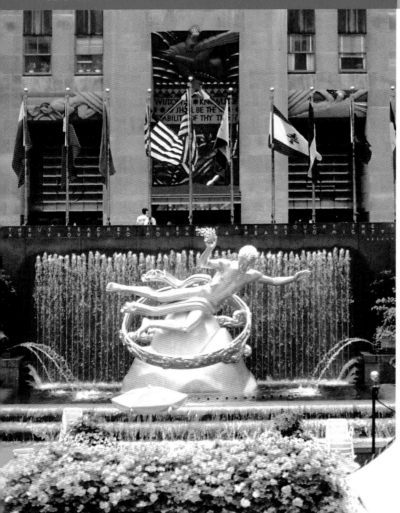

Prometheus
Paul Manship

Completion: 1934. **Technique:** gilded bronze. **Location:** New York City, NY, USA.

In the sunken plaza of the Rockefeller Center, the titan "Prometheus" flies between earth (mountain) and heavens (zodiac). He brought fire to mankind and was punished for the deed. He is a god that helped mankind – a symbolic figure for John D. Rockefeller, who saw himself as a philanthropist. The "Prometheus" corresponds with a sculpture of "Atlas" from 1937, by sculptors Lee Lawrie and Rene Paul Chambellan. A chic work of beauty that explores the Art Deco Style.

Paul Howard Manship was born in 1885 and died in 1966. He studied in Minnesota, Pennsylvania and New York City before winning the Rome Prize, after which he attended the American Academy. He became interested in Indian, Egyptian, Assyrian and Pre-classical Greek sculpture. The simplification of line and detail made his work interesting for modernists as well as for conservatives. Manship is a major precursor to Art Deco and he was also a member of the board of the Smithsonian American Art Museum.

Photos: Chris van Uffelen

The Bringer of Light
Bernhard Hoetger

Completion: 1936. **Technique:** gilt. **Location:** Bremen, Germany.

This bas-relief, is entitled the "Bringer of Light" and marks the entrance to Böttcherstraße in Bremen. It depicts the Archangel Michael fighting with the dragon. The relief was originally called "Victory to our Leader Over the Fools of Darkness" and was dedicated to Adolf Hitler. Although the artist was named one of the 'degenerate artists' by the Nazi regime, it is said that he dedicated this work to Hitler to save the famous Böttcherstraße from being destroyed by the Nazi regime.

Bernhard Hoetger (1874–1949) was a Expressionist German sculptor, painter and craftsman. After being involved in the art colonies in Darmstadt and Worpswede, Bernhard Hoetger met coffee merchant Ludwig Roselius. The biggest project of his life, the artistic design of the Böttcherstraße in Bremen, stemmed from this association. He also worked as a self-taught architect, building the connecting street between Market and Weser.

Photo: Chris van Uffelen

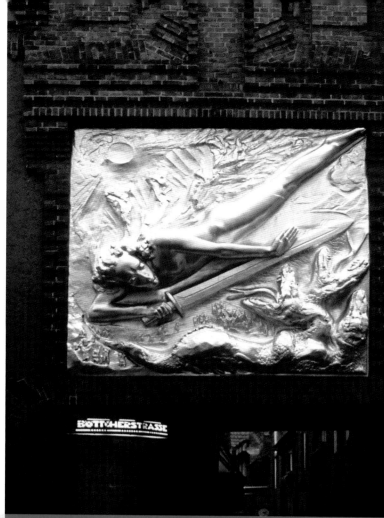

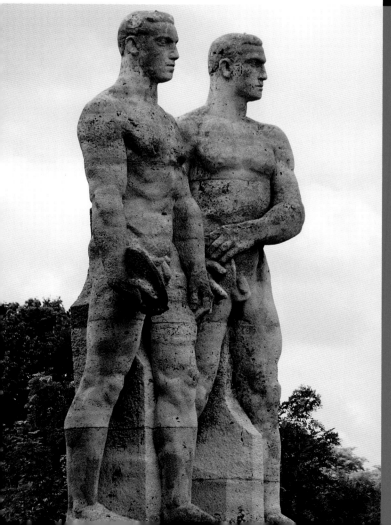

Discus Thrower
Karl Albiker

Completion: 1937. **Technique:** shell limestone. **Location:** Berlin, Germany.

The "Discus Thrower" is an example of sculpture commissioned by the Nazi regime. It is one of several sculptures of this type, located at the Olympic Stadium in Berlin. The sculpture is clearly an idealization of the human body and propagandist in nature, promoting the Nazi ideal of a superior race. There has been much discussion as to whether the sculptures should be removed but many people believe that they should not be hidden and forgotten, but rather left as a permanent reminder of the atrocities of the past.

The German sculptor Karl Albiker was born in 1878 and died in 1961. He worked as a sculptor, lithographer and taught as professor of art in Dresden. He studied at the Karlsruhe Academy of Fine Art, where he was recognized as a gifted student. He moved to Paris in the early 20th century, where he met Auguste Rodin, later training at his workshop. He returned to Germany, opening a studio in 1905. The Nazi regime approved of Albiker's ideology and he was commissioned to produce sculptures to adorn the new Olympic Stadium.

Photo: Chris van Uffelen

Endless Column
Constantin Brâncuşi

Completion: 1938. **Technique:** cast iron, steel, gilded brass, travertin. **Location:** Târgu-Jiu, Romania.

Constantin Brâncuşi's ensemble commemorates the soldiers who lost their lives defending Târgu-Jiu in World War I. The ensemble consists of the "Table of Silence", the "Gate of the Kiss" and the "Endless Column", arranged along an axis stretching from the floodplain of the Jiu River. During five decades of communist rule, the sculptures were left to languish as the landscape drastically changed around them. OLIN architects were given the task of restoring the monument, enhancing the majestic and contemplative nature of the art.

Constantin Brâncuşi was an internationally renowned Romanian sculptor, whose works have had a strong influence on numerous modernist sculptures. He was born in Romania to peasant farmers, his talent for woodcarving was eventually recognized and his then-employer financed his education at the School of Crafts in Craiova where he graduated with honors. He then enrolled in the Bucharest School of Fine Arts. In 1903 Brâncuşi traveled to Munich and later to Paris where he was invited to work in the workshop of Auguste Rodin.

Photos: Victor Bortas for OLIN

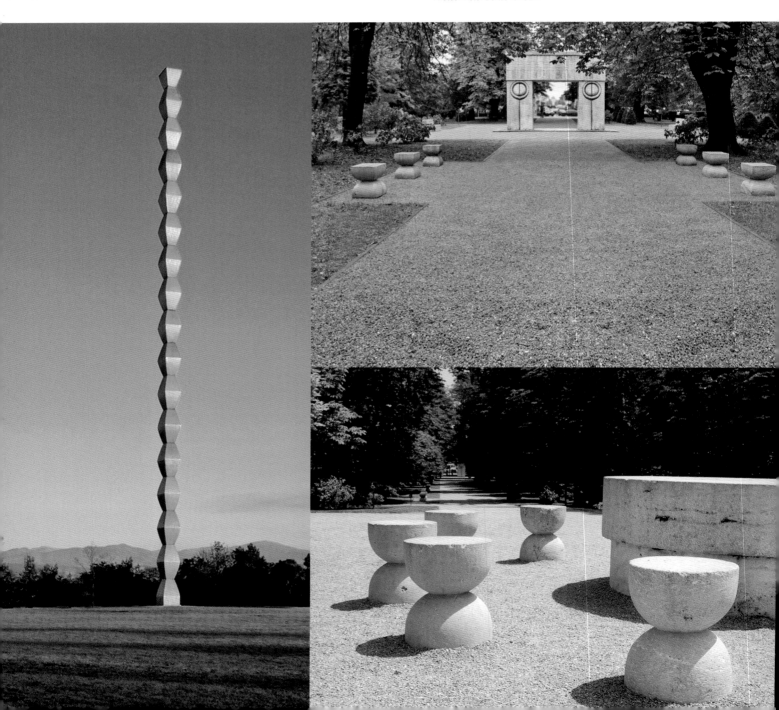

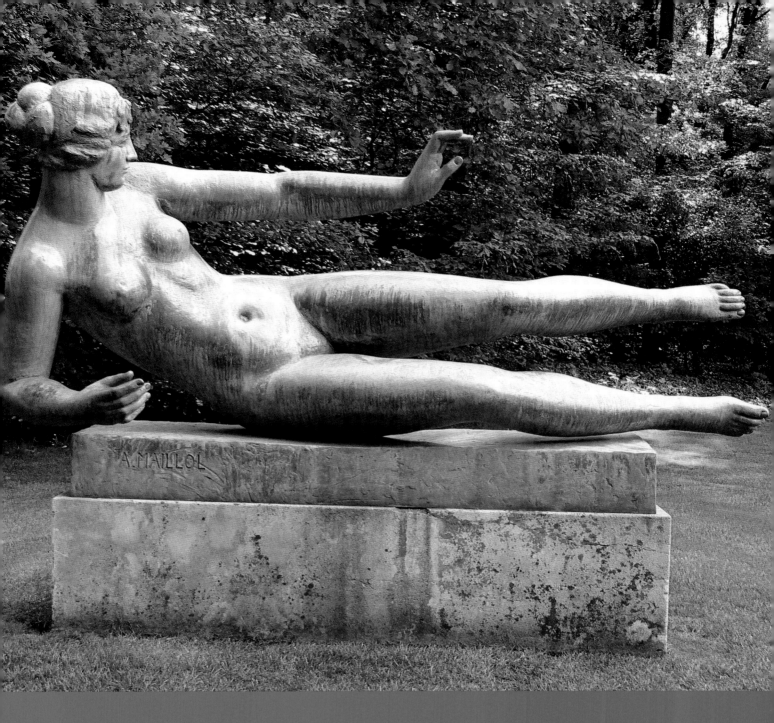

The Air
Aristides Maillol

Completion: 1939. **Technique:** stone. **Location:** Otterlo, The Netherlands.

"The Air" by Aristides Maillol is displayed in the sculpture garden at the Kröller-Müller Museum in the Netherlands. Dina Vierny was a young Jewish girl who often modeled for Maillol, Henri Matisse and Pierre Bonnard. She became an important source of inspiration for Maillol in his later work and was the model for this sculpture, which is now in the museum's permanent collection.

Aristides Maillol was an influential sculptor, born in Catalonia in 1861. He moved to Paris in 1881 to study art. After being turned down several times, he was finally accepted into the School of Fine Arts in 1885 where he studied under Jean Léon Gérôme and Alexandre Cabanel. In 1912 he was commissioned to produce a monument to Cézanne. Maillol died in a car accident in 1944, a large collection of his work is kept by the Maillol Museum in Paris which was established by his close friend and artistic model, Dina Vierny.

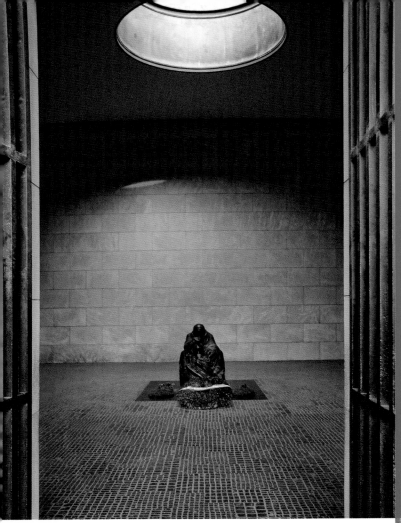

Mother with her Dead Son
Käthe Kollwitz

Completion: 1939/1993. **Technique:** bronze. **Location:** Berlin, Germany.

This sculpture stands in the New Guard House in Berlin. The building has been used as a war memorial since 1931. After the reunification of Germany, the New Guard House was re-dedicated in 1993. The memorial in the center was replaced at this time with an enlarged version of Käthe Kollwitz's "Mother with her Dead Son". It was resized by artist Harald Haacke in 1993 and now sits directly under the oculus, exposed to the rain, snow and cold. This symbolizes the suffering experience during World War.

Käthe Kollwitz was one of the most important German female sculptors of the 20th century. She was born in 1896 and began creating sculpture in 1910. Her son Peter was killed in Flanders in 1914. By 1914, Kollowitz was one of the foremost artists of her day and began to create a memorial for her dead son, she was however, unsatisfied with her design and it wasn't until twelve years later that she revisited the project. It was completed in 1931 and placed next to his grave.

Photo: Chris van Uffelen

Town Musicians of Bremen
Gerhard Marcks

Completion: 1951. **Technique:** bronze. **Location:** Bremen, Germany.

The "Town Musicians of Bremen" sculpture is inspired by a fairytale of the same name, recorded by the Brothers Grimm. Despite the title of the fairy tale the animals never actually arrive in Bremen, but a bronze statue by Gerhard Marcks depicting the "Town Musicians of Bremen" was built in 1953. The statue is made from bronze and the front hooves have become shiny over the years, as touching them is said to make wishes come true.

The German sculptor Gerhard Marcks was born in Berlin in 1889 and died in 1981. As well as sculpture, Marcks is also renowned for his drawings, lithographs and ceramic works. He was appointed as director of the University of Arts in Burg Giebichenstein where he worked until his dismissal in 1933, after his work was deemed unsuitable by the Nazi regime. After World War II, Marcks taught at the Regional Art School in Hamburg, where he taught for four years before retiring to Cologne.

Photo: Gerhard-Marcks-Stiftung, Bremen 2010

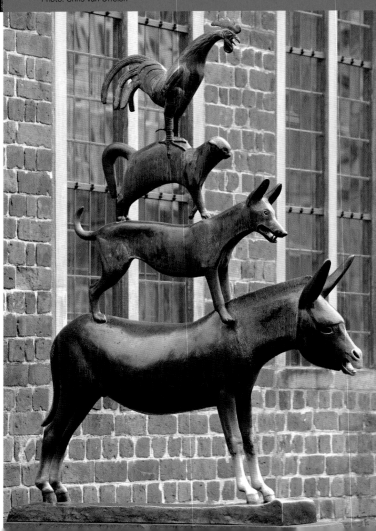

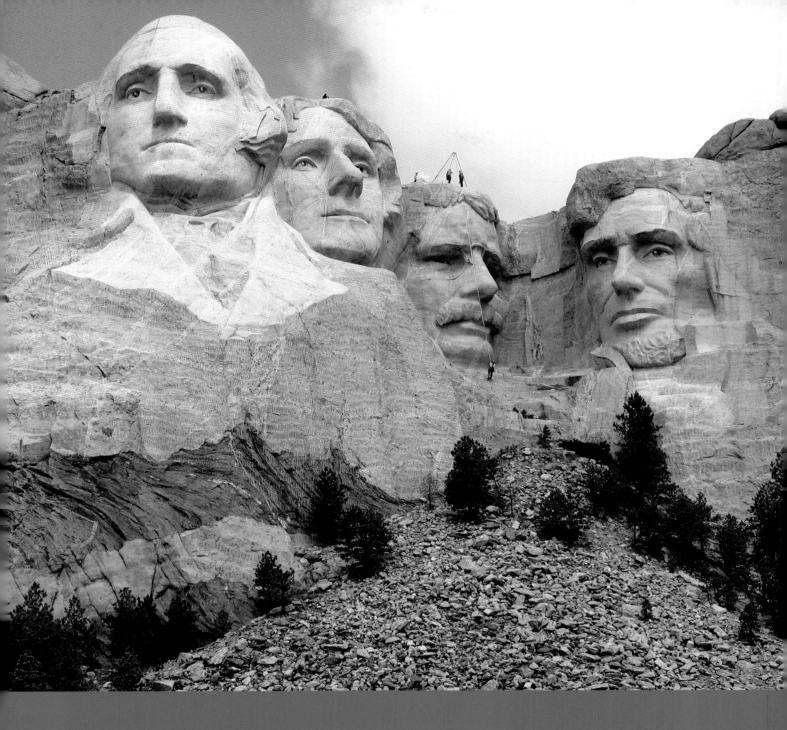

Mount Rushmore National Memorial
John Gutzon de la Mothe Borglum

Completion: 1941. **Technique:** stone. **Location:** Keystone, SD, USA.

This monument portrays the four presidents: (left to right) George Washington (1930), Thomas Jefferson (1936), Theodore Roosevelt (1939) and Abraham Lincoln (1937), each 18 meters tall and worked directly into the bedrock by dynamite, air hammer and chisel. The work was finished by Gutzon's son Lincoln Borglum. Doane Robinson first conceived the idea for a national monument at this location, carved into the mountains of South Dakota.

John Gutzon de la Mothe Borglum was born in St. Charles in 1867 and died in Chicago, 1941. He was the son of a Danish woodcarver and attended the Academy of Arts in San Francisco. He later studied at the Julian Academy in Paris and it was here that he became familiar with the work of Auguste Rodin. In 1893 he moved back to the USA, where he worked on the largest bas-relief sculpture in the world, the "Confederate Memorial Carving". This measures a staggering 12,000 square meters and was completed in 1923.

Air Bridge Memorial
Eduard Ludwig

Completion: 1951. **Technique:** concrete. **Location:** Berlin, Germany.

During the Berlin Blockade, from June 1948 to May 1949, all street and rail connections from the Western occupied zones to West Berlin, through the Soviet occupied zone were closed. At this time the Western Allies delivered supplies to the town by plane, over the so-called "Air Bridge". As a reminder of this time a memorial was built. Three ribs rise out from the memorial, pointing West towards the "Air Bridge". Two other monuments of the same design were also made; one in Frankfurt/Main, and one in Celle, where the planes took off.

Eduard Ludwig (1906–1960) was a German architect. He studied at the Bauhaus and under the tutorage of Ludwig Mies van der Rohe. After the war he worked as professor of architecture at the University of Fine Arts in Berlin as well as running his own architectural office, until his unexpected death after an accident. Ludwig's passion was building houses in the bungalow style, the impetus for this came from Mies van der Rohe and the Barcelona Pavilion.

Photo: Chris van Uffelen

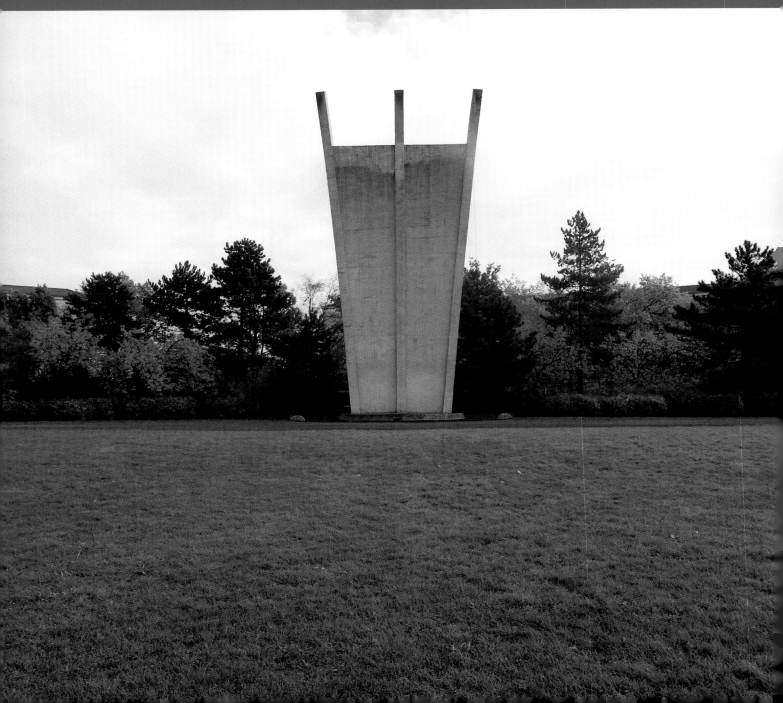

The Large Marching Flower
Fernand Léger

Completion: 1952. **Technique:** fiber-cement. **Location:** The Hague, The Netherlands.

"The Large Marching Flower" is one of the later works of French artist Fernand Léger. The artists produced both painting and sculpture throughout his career and experimented with various different styles. His early works were Cubist in style, though he also investigated Figurative and Populist style. His bold, colorful and simplified treatment of modern subject matter is often referred to as Pop Art.

Fernand Léger was a French painter, sculptor and filmmaker. He was born in Normandy in 1881 and died in 1955. Léger initially trained as an architect but later went on to study at the School of Decorative Arts in Paris. He began working seriously as an artist at the age of 25. In the 1920s, in collaboration with Amédée Ozenfant, he established a school where he taught from 1924. His early work was heavily influenced by the Cubist Style, though in his later work he developed a more figurative approach.

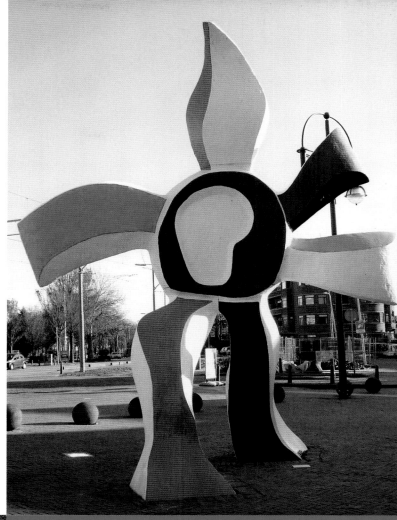

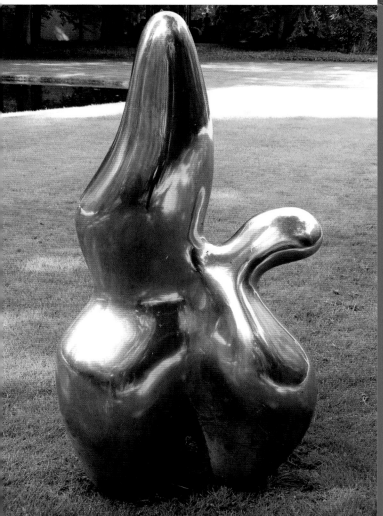

Cloud Shepherd
Hans Arp

Completion: 1953. **Technique:** bronze. **Location:** Otterlo, The Netherlands.

"Cloud Shepherd" is an abstract sculpture on display in the sculpture garden at the Kröller-Müller Museum in the Netherlands. This sculpture is arguable Arp's most famous work. It is made of pure bronze and has a very clear, carefully defined shape. The soft curves of the sculpture symbolize the wonders of nature, such as clouds, hills and lakes. It is a protest against the brutality of machinery and the greedy acquisition of wealth.

Hans Arp was a talented artist, born in 1886. He worked as a painter, poet, sculptor and abstract artist as well as experimenting with unusual materials in his art, such as torn or pasted paper. The son of a French mother and German father, Arp studied in Strasbourg before moving to Paris in 1904. He stayed only a year before going back to Germany to study at the Weimar Academy of Fine Arts. He was a founding member of the Dada movement in Zurich, his early work was more Surrealist in style, but his work later became much more abstract.

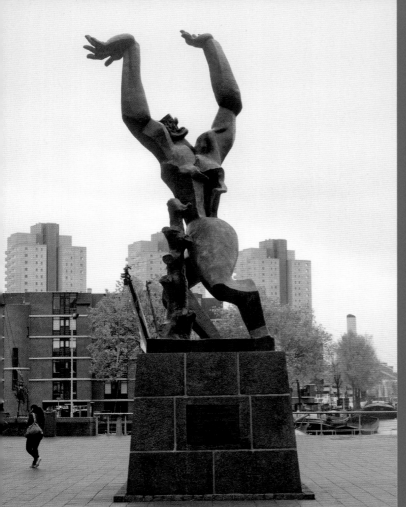

The Destroyed City
Ossip Zadkine

Completion: 1953. **Technique:** bronze. **Location:** Rotterdam, The Netherlands.

"The Destroyed City" represents a man without a heart. The piece is one of the artist's best known works and is a memorial to the destruction that occurred in the Dutch city of Rotterdam in 1940, by the German Air Force. The object of the attack was to force the Dutch to surrender, however, negotiations were already underway at the time and the German commander radioed to delay the forces. A breakdown in communications meant that this message was never delivered and the city was bombed, probably unnecessarily.

Ossip Zadkine was a Russian-born artist who lived in France. He is best known for his sculpture but also produced paintings and lithographs. Zadkine studied in London and settled in Paris in around 1910. In Paris, he became part of the Cubist Movement, but later developed his own style that was heavily influenced by African art. Zadkine taught at his own school of sculpture. His former home and studio is now the Zadkine Museum.

Photo: Chris van Uffelen

Kwakwaka'wakw Heraldic Pole
Mungo Martin

Completion: 1953. **Technique:** wood. **Location:** Vancouver, Canada.

The "Kwakwaka'wakw Heraldic Pole" is located in front of the Mungo Martin House. It is dedicated to the Kwakwaka'wakw Nations. Five figures are carved onto the totem pole – Dzunuk´wa, a wild woman holding a child in her arms, a beaver, a grizzly bear and a thunderbird who is positioned on the top of the pole. The Mungo Martin House in the background is used for ceremonial gatherings and is not open to the public.

Mungo Martin was born in British Columbia, Canada, in 1879 and died in 1962. Both he and his family belonged to the so-called "Kwakwaka'wakw Tribe". Because of his enthusiastic interest in this tribe, he attempted to preserve his knowledge of their culture in the form of woodcarvings, rituals, songs and art. Mungo was responsible for the restoration of numerous carvings, sculptures and totem poles.

Photo: Ryan Bushby (HighInBC) / Wikimedia Commons

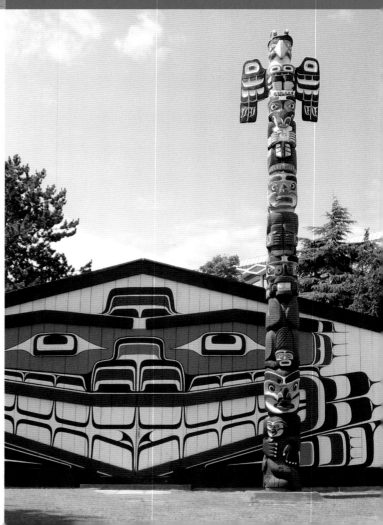

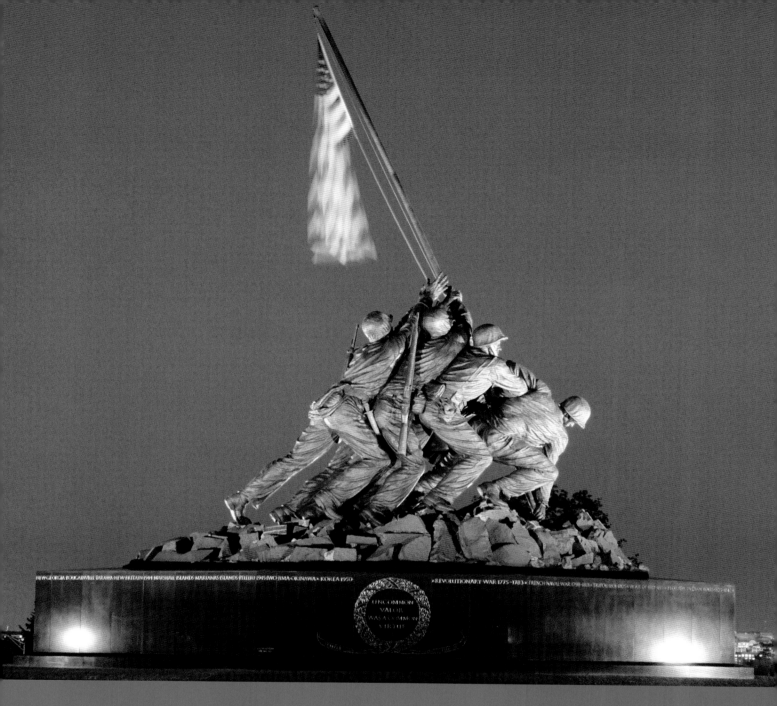

United States Marine Corps War Memorial
Felix de Weldon

Completion: 1954. **Technique:** bronze. **Location:** Arlington, VA, USA.

The "United States Marine Corps War Memorial" is situated outside the Arlington National Cemetery. The memorial is dedicated to all the members of the United States Marine Corps who have died in defense of their country since 1775. The design was based on the famous photograph "Raising the Flag on Iwo Jima", taken by Joe Rosenthal. The location and date of every Marine Corps engagement are inscribed around the base. The sculpture was officially dedicated by President Eisenhower in 1954.

Felix de Weldon was an American sculptor, whose most famous work is the "United States Marine Corps War Memorial". He was born in Vienna in 1907 and studied at the University of Vienna. He first received notice for his sculptural works at the age of 17 with his statue of Ludo Hartman, an Austrian educator and diplomat. In 1951 he moved to the historic Beacon Rock estate on Rhode Island where he lived until 1996 when he lost the property due to financial hardship. Weldon died in 2003.

Photo: US Navy / Wikimedia Commons

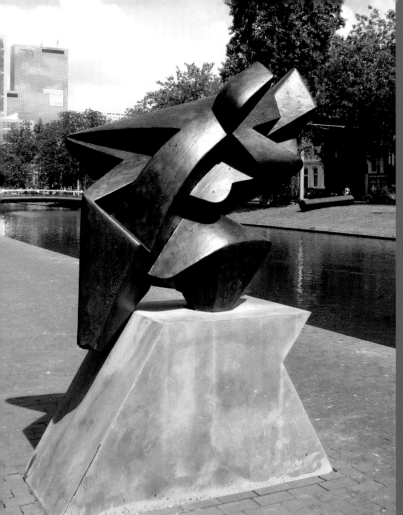

The Farewell
Umberto Mastroianni

Completion: 1955. **Technique:** bronze. **Location:** Rotterdam, The Netherlands.

"The Farewell" is an abstract sculpture, which was clearly influenced by the Cubist Style. The sculpture is dynamic, evoking ideas of movement and sharp emotion. Made out of bronze, the angles are sharp, with few carving lines, two figures are joined to form a compact shape. The figures appear to be moving away from each other, two lovers pulled apart in an embrace, one reaching outside the plinth, pulled into unknown territory.

Umberto Mastroianni was born in 1910. He was one of Italy's leading sculptors, creating towering, bronze and steel creations that are exhibited in museums and in the public realm throughout the world. As a teenager, Mastroianni traveled to Rome to study at the San Marcello Art School. Two years later he left Rome for Turin and completed his apprenticeship with the sculptor Michele Guerrisi. Mastroianni's work was figurative in style until he embraced abstraction in 1942.

Photo: K. Siereveld / Wikimedia Commons

National Monument on the Dam Square
John Rädecker, Jacobus Johannes Pieter Oud

Completion: 1956. **Technique:** travertine. **Location:** Amsterdam, The Netherlands.

This World War II monument consists of a obelisk-like, conical column, a wall and two lions. A sculpture called "Peace" features a relief which depicts four chained figures, representing suffering (one of them in the pose of Christ on the cross) and two male statues representing the resistance. The wall contains twelve urns, filled with soil from execution grounds and cemeteries. The lion is the heraldic animal of the Netherlands.

John Rädecker was born in Amsterdam in 1885 and died in 1956. He studied in Amsterdam and Rotterdam and later lived in Paris. He participated in the building-boom in Amsterdam, making various sculptural works, at the time when the Amsterdam School Style suddenly became extremely popular. His sons Han and Jan Willem finished his work on the monument while Paul Grégoire was responsible for the reliefs. The architect Jacobus Johannes Pieter Oud, (1890–1963) studied in Amsterdam and Delft and was taught by Pierre Cuypers and Theodor Fischer. He was also part of the "De Stil" group.

Photo: Phyzome / Wikimedia Commons

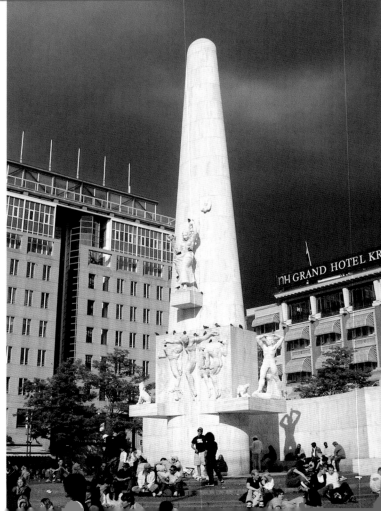

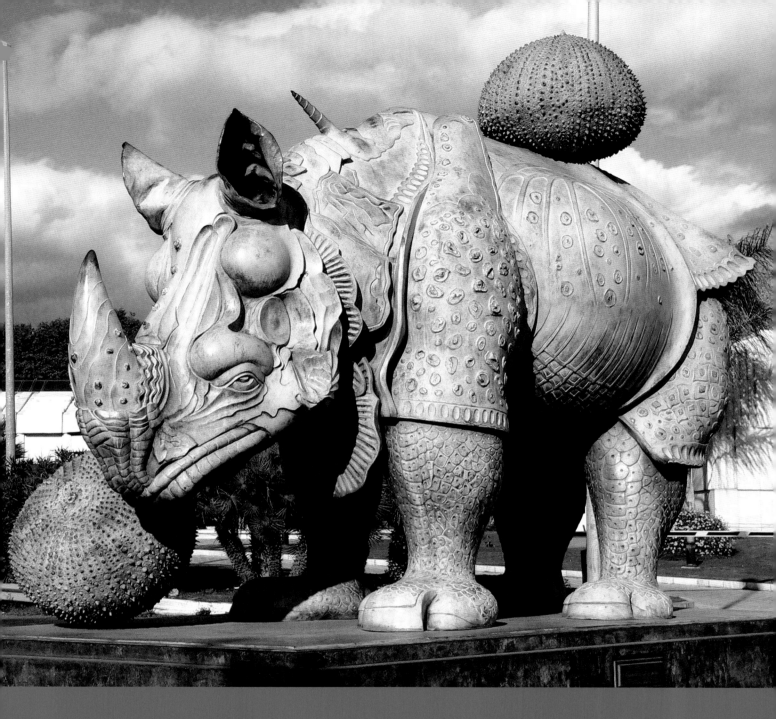

Rhinoceros Dressed in Lace
Salvador Dalí

Completion: 1956. **Technique:** bronze. **Location:** Marbella, Spain.

Salvador Dalí's "Rhinoceros Dressed in Lace" is located in Marbella, Spain and is based upon a woodcut of a rhinoceros made by German painter and printmaker Albrecht Dürer. The depiction by Dürer was not a strictly accurate one, as he had never seen an actual rhinoceros. He depicted the animal with armor-type plates covering its body; Dalí then later used this image. Dalí created the rhinoceros after filming his Surrealist film "Prodigious Adventure of the Lace Maker and the Rhinoceros".

Salvador Dalí was born in Figueres in Spain in 1904. He is most famous for his surrealist paintings and is considered one of the key figures of the Surrealist Movement. In 1931, Dalí painted one of his most famous paintings, "The Persistence of Memory". In this picture several pocket watches are depicted melting away and being eaten by ants and flies in a vast landscape of a mountain and a sea. Dalí was also involved, less famously, in other artistic media, including photography, sculpture and film.

Let us beat Swords into Ploughshares
Evgeny Viktorovich Vuchetich

Completion: 1957. **Technique:** bronze. **Location:** New York City, NY, USA.

"Let us beat Swords into Ploughshares" is named after "Swords to Ploughshares" idealism, where military weapons or technologies are converted into peaceful tools for civilian applications. The ploughshare often serves as an example of a creative tool that has benefited mankind. The sculpture was a gift from the then Soviet Union and was presented in 1959. It symbolizes man's desire to put an end to war and convert the means of destruction into creative tools that benefit society.

Evgeny Viktorovich Vuchetich was born in 1908 and was a prominent sculptor and artist in the Soviet Union. He was a promoter of Soviet Realism and was awarded many government prizes, including the Lenin Prize, Stalin Prize for Art, Order of Lenin and the Order of the Patriotic War. He was the sculptor of a number of statues "Mother Motherland", such as those in Volgograd and Kiev. He died while working on the monument in Kiev, which was completed seven years after his death.

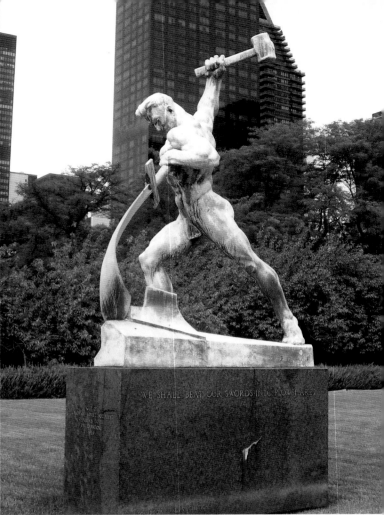

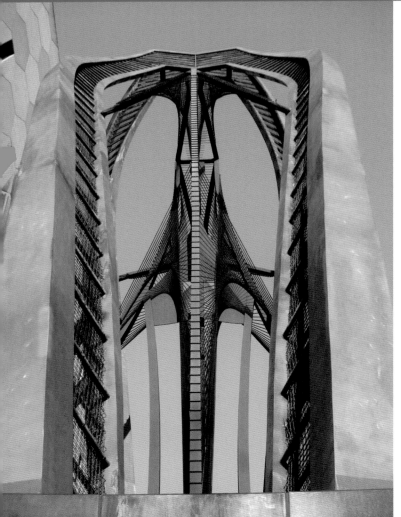

Untitled, 1957
Nuam Gabo

Completion: 1957. **Technique:** concrete, marble steel, bronze.
Location: Rotterdam, The Netherlands.

This sculpture was built outside the Bijenkorf department store in Rotterdam in 1957. The sculptor's aim was to communicate the impression of weightlessness, an unusual feature in a sculpture of this size. The gradual, directional changes in the sculpture are suggestive of movement, adding to its light, dynamic appearance. The black marble base takes an organic form, reminiscent of a trunk and anchoring the structure firmly to the ground.

Nuam Gabo was born in 1890 and is considered one of the pioneers of modern sculpture. He began to use new material, such as, acrylic, glass and plastics as opposed to the more tradition stone and bronze. He lived in Russia before moving to Germany to study medicine and then engineering. He returned to Russia in 1917 and became involved with the Russian Constructivists. He lived in various European countries and traveled extensively before settling in American in 1946, where he lived until his death in 1977.

Monument to the Discoveries
Leopoldo de Almeida, Cottinelli Telmo

Completion: 1960. **Technique:** concrete. **Location:** Lisbon, Portugal.

The "Monument to the Discoveries" is 52 meters tall and was built on the north bank of the Tagus River to commemorate the 500th anniversary of the death of Prince Henry the Navigator. It represents a three-sailed ship, ready to depart and depicts sculptures of important historical figures such as King Manuel I who is carrying a sphere. Inside is an exhibition space with temporary exhibits. The side that faces away from the river features a carved sword stretching the full height of the monument.

Architect José Ângelo Cottinelli Telmo and sculptor Leopoldo de Almeida designed this monument. De Almeida was born in 1898 and died in 1975. He was regarded as a talented artist from a very young age, accepted to study at the College of Fine Arts in London at the age of just 15. He is considered one of the most important sculptors in modern Portuguese history. José Ângelo Cottinelli Telmo was architect, photographer, musician and dance. He was born 1897 and died 1948.

Photo: Chris van Uffelen

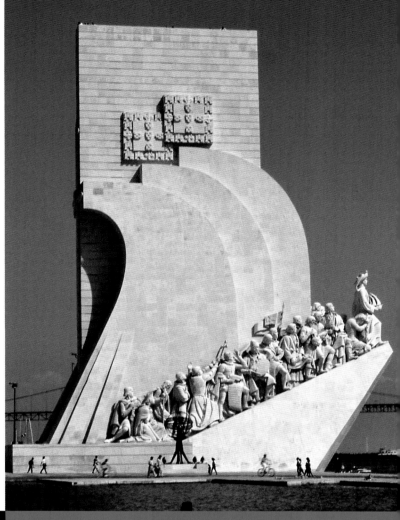

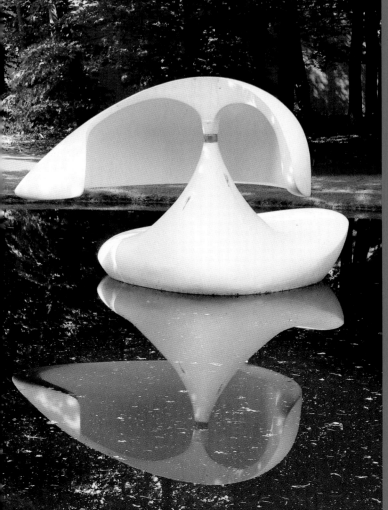

Floating Sculpture
Marta Pan

Completion: 1960. **Technique:** glass fiber reinforced polyester resin. **Location:** Otterlo, The Netherlands.

Marta Pan's "Floating Sculpture" was commissioned by the Kröller-Müller Museum in the Netherlands for a pond at the entrance of the sculpture garden that opened in June 1961. The structure is made from glass fiber reinforced, polyester resin. The top part is able to turn independently, activated by the wind. Pan has also created various other floating sculptural works that are situated in ponds in public space, including at the Lynden-Bradley Sculpture Park in Wisconsin.

Marta Pan was born in Budapest, Hungary in 1923. She studied fine arts in Budapest before moving to Paris in 1947. She became a French citizen in 1952. She met Brâncusi and Le Corbusier, who were both influential figures in France at the time and later married Andre Wogenscky, a close associate of Le Corbusier. Pan has produced numerous public sculptures, integrating them into the surrounding architecture and urban space. Her sculptures can be found in Europe, the USA, Japan and Lebanon.

Photo: Gerardus / Wikimedia Commons

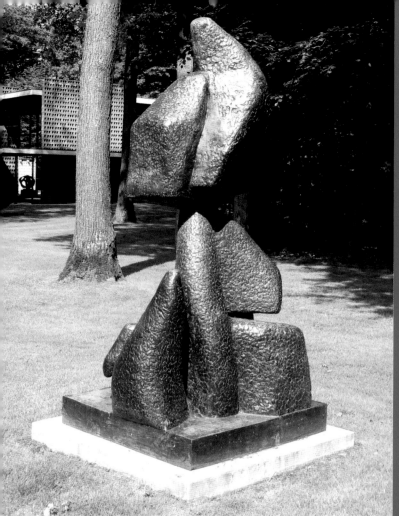

Composition
Otto Freundlich

Completion: 1961. **Technique:** bronze. **Location:** Otterlo, The Netherlands.

"Composition" by Otto Freundlich stands in the Kröller-Müller Museum sculpture park in the Netherlands. It is made from bronze and was cast in 1961, after the artist's death, although the plaster model from which it was cast was actually made in 1933. Much of Freundlich's work drew inspiration from the Cubist Style and his sculptural works were often abstract in form.

Otto Freundlich first studied dentistry but began painting and sculpting at the age of 27. He moved to Paris in 1908, returning to Germany in 1914. In 1919 he organized the first Dada exhibition in Cologne with Max Ernst and Johannes Theodor Baargeld. The Nazi regime later condemned his works and some were taken and displayed at the Nazi exhibition of Degenerate Art. In 1943 he was arrested and deported to the Majdanek Concentration Camp, where he was murdered.

Photo: Gerardus / Wikimedia Commons

The Great Musician
Henri Laurens

Completion: 1963. **Technique:** bronze. **Location:** Rotterdam, The Netherlands.

"The Great Musician" is the figure of a woman, kneeling on one knee, playing the lyre. The sculpture is an important representation of Cubist sculpture. The form allows the parts of the work to mold together, limiting the tension created by the heavy piece; the shapes of the work are sensual. The forms of the large curve of the hip, the crescent shaped arm, the strings of lyre to the point of the elbow, blend together.

Henri Laurens was born in Paris in 1885 and worked as a stonemason before becoming a sculptor. In 1899 he attended drawing classes and his early artwork was heavily influenced by the work of Auguste Rodin, in his later work he began to embrace the Cubist Style. Laurens worked with a variety of media, including collage and engraving as well as theater design and decoration. Many of his sculptures are massive in size such as the piece "L'Amphion" in Venezuela.

Photos: K. Siereveld / Wikimedia Commons

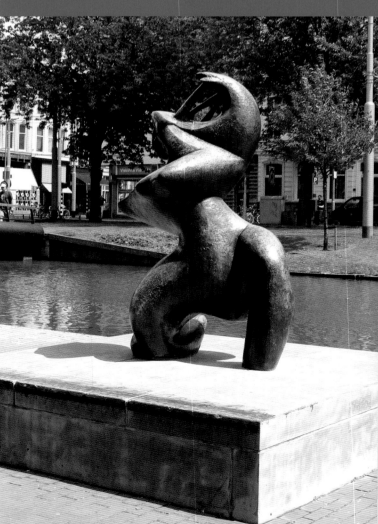

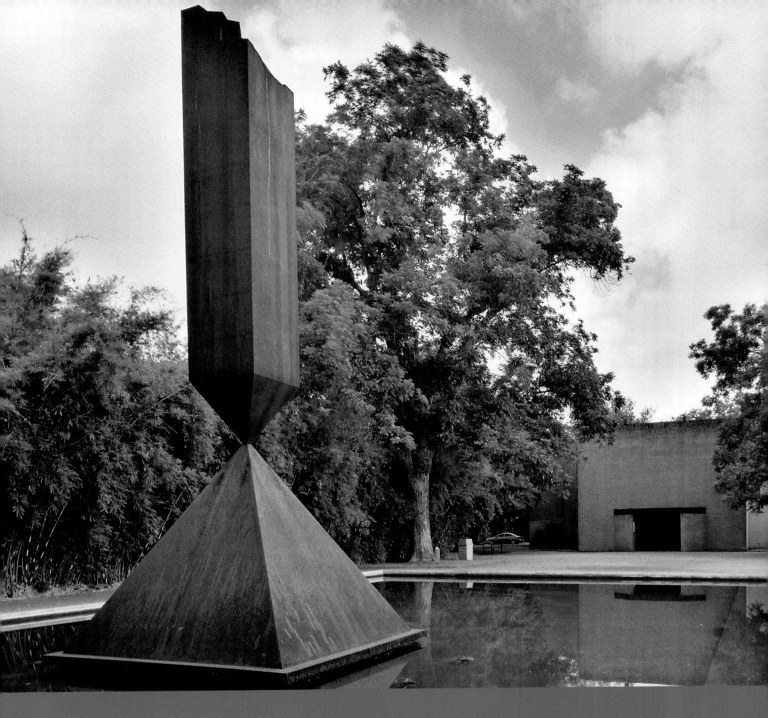

Broken Obelisk
Barnett Newman

Completion: 1963. **Technique:** Corten steel. **Location:** Houston, TX, USA.

"Broken Obelisk" is the largest of Newman's sculptures and is made of three tons of Corten steel. Newman casted several copies of this sculpture, this one is permanently installed in front of the Rothko Chapel in Houston, Texas. The Houston sculpture is dedicated to Martin Luther King Jr. and was acquired from the Corcoran Gallery of Art in Washinton D.C. When Corcoran's director, James Harithas left the gallery in 1969, Newman arranged to have his sculpture removed. John de Menil funded its relocation to Houston.

Barnett Newman was an American artist (1905–1970). He is considered to be one of the most influential figures in Abstract Expressionism and one of the foremost Color Field painters, a style of abstract painting that emerged in New York City and was inspired by European Modernism. He studied philosophy, later working in his father's business, manufacturing clothing. His work developed into a more Surrealist Style during the 1940s before later maturing into his better known, Abstract Expressionist Style.

Medea
Eduardo Paolozzi

Completion: 1964. **Technique:** steel. **Location:** Otterlo, The Netherlands.

"Medea" stands in the sculpture garden at the Kröller-Müller Museum in the Netherlands. It is one of Eduardo Paolozzi's later works and is almost robotic in form. Paolozzi first gained praise for his early bronze sculptures of the human figure. As his work developed, he embraced Surrealism and Modern Art and is often referred to as the father of Pop Art in Britain.

Artist, sculptor and printmaker Eduardo Paolozzi was born in Edinburgh in 1924. He studied at Edinburgh College of Art and later went on to study at the Slade School of Fine Art, London. His early work was influenced by the Dadaists and Surrealists in Paris, but his later work, using in bronze and steel, often resembled stylized robotic figures. His best known work is a series of mosaics on the walls of Tottenham Court Road Tube Station in London.

Photo: Gerardus / Wikimedia Commons

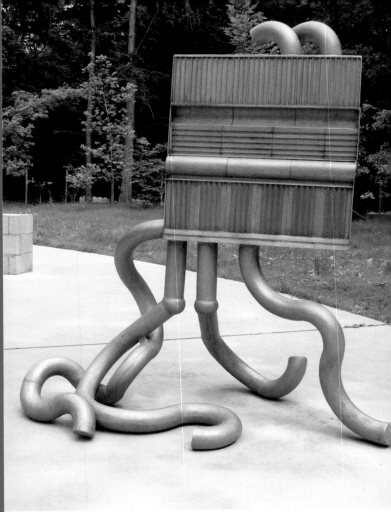

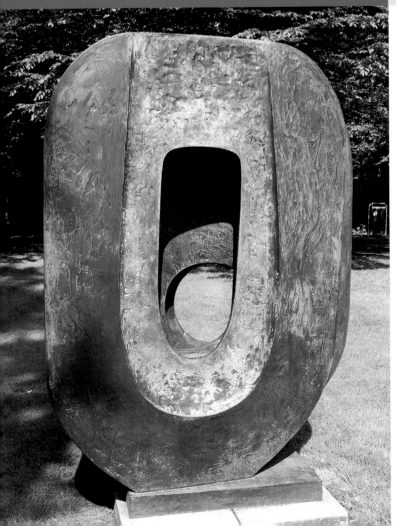

Dual Form
Barbara Hepworth

Completion: 1965. **Technique:** bronze. **Location:** Otterlo, The Netherlands.

This sculpture is part of the collection of the Kröller-Müller Museum sculpture park in the Netherlands. Hepworth's early work was naturalistic in form and it wasn't until the 1930s that her work became more abstract. As her talent developed during the 1930s and 1940s much of her work concentrated on the counter play between mass and space, this development is illustrated by the "Dual Form" sculpture. Together with Henry Moore, Hepworth was one of the leading figures of the Modern Movement in England.

Barbara Hepworth was born in Yorkshire in 1903 and was one of Britain's most famous female sculptors. She studied at the Leeds School of Art and went on to study sculpture at the Royal College of Art in London. In 1924 she received a scholarship to travel abroad and traveled to Italy to study Renaissance Art and Architecture. Hepworth's works are held in numerous museums and private collections, there are also several museums dedicated to her, including the Barbara Hepworth Museum and Sculpture Garden in St Ives.

Photo: Gerardus / Wikimedia Commons

The Gateway Arch
Eero Saarinen

Completion: 1965. **Technique:** steel, concrete. **Location:** St. Louis, MO, USA.

"The Gateway Arch" is the centerpiece of the Jefferson National Expansion Memorial in St. Louis. It symbolizes the westward expansion of the United States. It has both a height and width of just over 192 meters, making it the tallest man-made monument in the USA. The arch is located on the west bank of the Mississippi and the design is the result of a competition, held in 1947. The arch is earthquake resistant and can withstand winds of up to 240 kilometers per hour.

Eero Saarinen was a Finnish architect. He was born in 1910 and died in 1961. He immigrated to the USA at the age of 13 and grew up in Michigan, where his father was a teacher at the Cranbrook Academy of Arts. He studied in Paris and later went on to study at the Yale school of Architecture, graduating in 1934. Saarinen died of a brain tumor and his partners went on to finish his ten remaining projects, including the St. Louis arch.

Photos: Bev Sykes from Davis, CA, USA

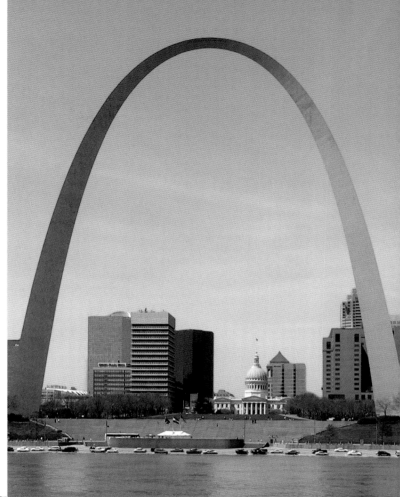

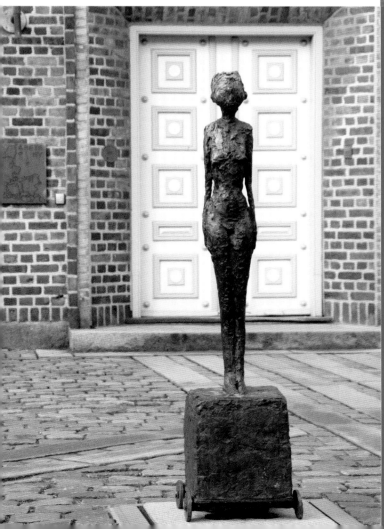

Woman on a Cart
Alberto Giacometti

Completion: 1966. **Technique:** Bronze. **Location:** Holstebro, Denmark.

This was the first sculpture purchased by the Holstebro municipality and was part of efforts to develop the town culturally. The figure is typical of Giacometti's style, his figures were often extremely slim and elongated and his work often resembles the shadows created by an object rather than the object itself. His sculpture suggests emotion with just a small amount of detail; nothing is overdone. He leaves hints for the observer rather than simply dictating an idea.

Alberto Giacometti was born in 1901 and died in 1966. He was a Swiss sculptor, painter, draughtsman and printmaker, the son of Giovanni Giacometti; a well known artist. He studied at the School of Fine Arts in Geneva before moving to Paris to study sculpture under Antoine Bourdelle. Giacometti's earlier work focused on the human head, he later progressed to full-body representations, which gradually increased in size. His later work became much more Surrealist in nature and he was awarded the Grand Prize for Sculpture at the Venice Biennial in 1962.

Photo: Tobias Scheffe - tosch / fotocommunity.com

The Fantastic Paradise
Niki de Saint Phalle with Jean Tinguely

Completion: 1966. **Technique:** fiberglass, plastic, painted iron. **Location:** Stockholm, Sweden.

This fountain was a collaboration with Jean Tinguely, who made the sculpture positioned in the middle of the fountain, amongst others. The work exists of 16 separate parts, of which the fountain is just one section. The female figures are typical of de Saint Phalle's style. Her work often explored the roles of women and she made various life-sized dolls of women as brides or giving birth. Her artistic expression of the 'everywoman' came to be known as "Nanas".

Niki de Saint Phalle was born in France in 1930 and died in 2002. Her family were thrown into financial difficulty during the Great Depression and moved to America in 1933. She enrolled at the Brearley School in New York but was expelled for drawing red fig leaves on campus statues. She graduated from Oldfields School in Maryland in 1947. She spent some time in Spain and was strongly influenced and impressed by the works of Gaudí. Her most well known pieces are her collaborations with Jean Tinguely.

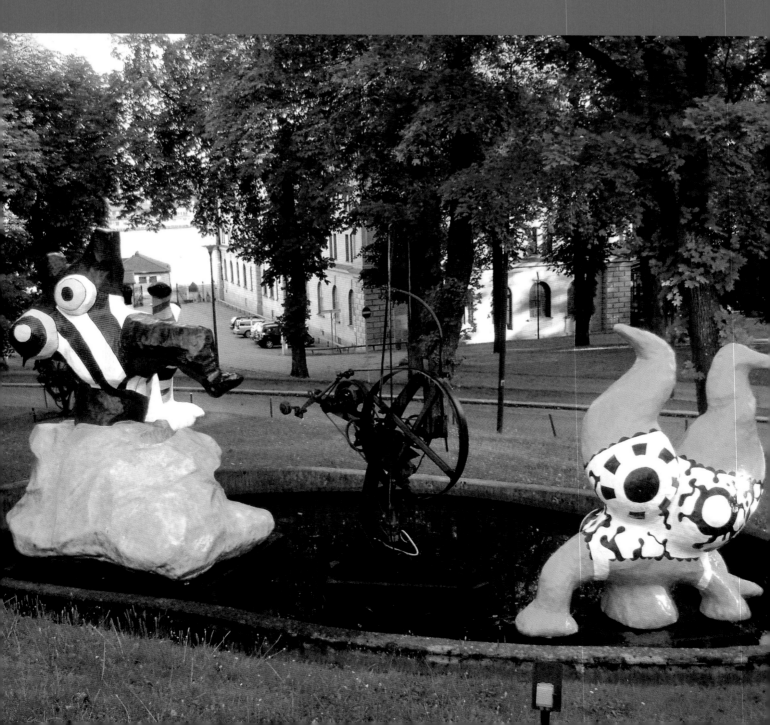

Monument to the Founding of the State
Heinrich Deutsch

Completion: 1966. **Technique:** steel. **Location:** Vienna, Austria.

This tall, steel structure is in the third district of Vienna, in the Swiss Garden. The square, metal body combines the curved pillars to form a column. The surfaces have been embellished by a design engraved on the surface. It was originally planned that a stone column should stand in this place until Deutsch came up with this steel design.

Heinrich Deutsch was born in Vienna in 1925. He is an Austrian sculptor and works with stone, bronze, metals and polyester. He has also designed ceramic sculptures and mosaics. He studied in Paris from 1948–1950 and later graduated with a degree in sculpture from the Academy of Fine Arts in Vienna in 1951.

Photo: Karsten11 / Wikimedia Commons

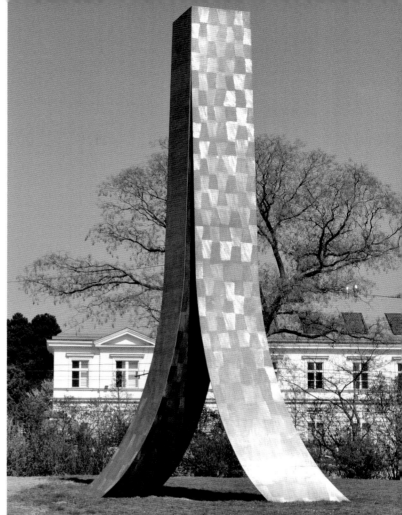

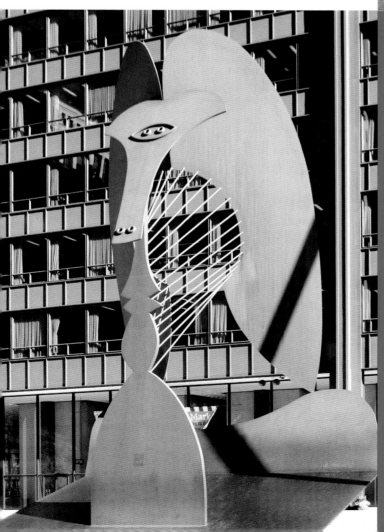

Untitled
Pablo Picasso

Completion: 1967. **Technique:** Corten steel. **Location:** Chicago, IL, USA.

The Chicago Picasso is an untitled sculpture in Cubist Style. It is made of Corten steel and is 15 meters tall. Picasso was offered 100,000 Dollars for the piece but refused it, instead giving the work as a gift to the city of Chicago. Before the arrival of the Picasso, public sculpture in Chicago was largely confined to depictions of historical figures and the Picasso sculpture was originally met with controversy, but has since become a treasured landmark in the city.

Pablo Picasso (1881–1973) was a Spanish painter and sculptor. He is undoubtedly the preeminent figure in 20th century art, best known as the co-founder, along with Georges Braque, of Cubism. Picasso was admitted to the advanced classes at the Royal Academy of Art in Barcelona at the age of just 15. His 1907 painting "Les Demoiselles d'Avignon" marked the first phases of Cubism. His later style became much more representational, with bright decorative patterns replacing the more austere compositions.

Photo: J. Crocker / Wikimedia Commons

Negev Monument
Dani Karavan

Completion: 1968. **Technique:** wind, sunlight, water, fire, desert acacias, grey concrete, text. **Location:** Beer Sheba, Israel.

This monument, dominating the desert plain, was Karavan's first environmental, site-specific sculpture and an initial work of this movement. It uses elements of nature and memory and covers an area of 10,000 square meters. The monument takes on the organic forms of the landscape and manifests them as abstract and geometric forms. The tower is pierced by holes and creates musical tones when the wind blows. Visitors become part of a comprehensive totality and are invited to engage physically with the work, using all of their senses.

Dani Karavan was born 1930 in Tel Aviv. Since the 1960s, he created large scale site specific artworks, like the "Axe Majeur" in Cergy-Pontoise, a three-kilometer-long urban sculpture north-west of Paris, which he has been working on since 1980. His work often has high political and / or historical themes, while the forms stay abstract and universal. Typical examples of his work are "The Way of Human Rights" in Nuremberg, "Passages – Homage to Walter Benjamin" in Portbou and "Murou Art Forest" in Japan.

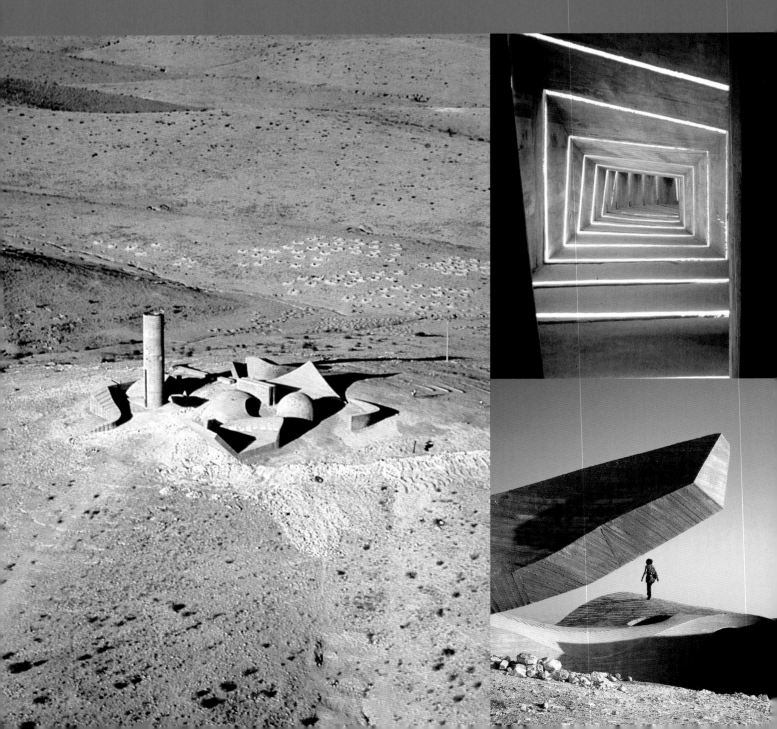

Red Cube
Isamu Noguchi

Completion: 1968. **Technique:** steel, red paint. **Location:** New York City, NY, USA.

"Red Cube" is located in front of the Harriman building in New York. It stands, surrounded on three sides by tall skyscrapers and, despite its name, is not actually a cube. It is extended along its vertical access. This draws the viewer's gaze upwards as the cube looks as if it is being stretched upwards by some visible force. The building behind the sculpture can be seen through the large hole in the middle, connecting the sculpture to the architecture.

Isamu Noguchi was an Experimental Artist; born in 1904, he died in 1988. Throughout his long career he created sculpture, garden furniture, ceramics, architectural works and set designs. He traveled throughout his life, maintaining studios in both New York and Japan. Noguchi was first recognized in America when he made a large sculpture, commissioned for the Associated Press building at the Rockefeller Center.

Photo: Chris van Uffelen

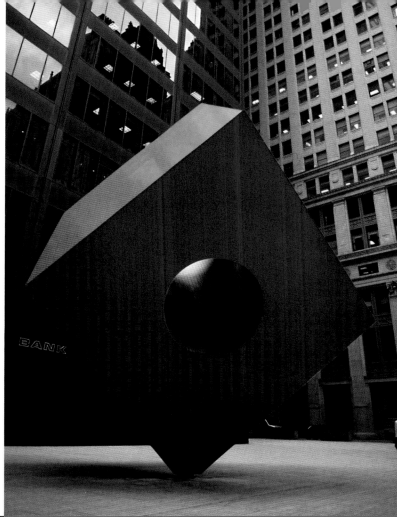

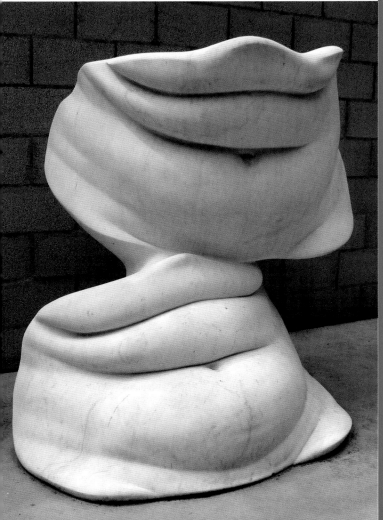

Bellies
Alina Szapocznikow

Completion: 1968. **Technique:** marble. **Location:** Otterlo, The Netherlands.

"Bellies" is a marble sculpture, one of a series by this artist depicted fragmented body parts. Szapocznikow was an innovative sculptor, using techniques and styles very advanced for her time. In 1963 she began to combine molds of body parts with sculpting materials including polyester and polyurethane, this technique was extremely innovative at the time.

Alina Szapocznikow was a Polish sculptor, born in 1926. She was a Jew and grew up in occupied Poland during the war. She was endured incarceration in concentration camps, including Auschwitz and Bergen-Belsen. After the end of the war she began training as a sculptor. In 1962 she was offered a solo show in the Polish Pavilion at the Venice Biennial. She also worked as a photographer, producing a series of 'photosculptures', each showing a wad of used chewing gum set on a tiny shelf. The gum was twisted to form a series of mini-sculptures, earning her a reputation for post-modern photography.

Photo: Gerardus / Wikimedia Commons

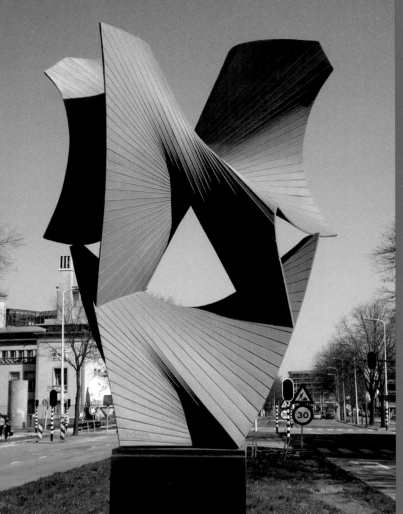

Third and Fourth Dimension
Antoine Pevsner

Completion: 1969. **Technique:** bronze. **Location:** The Hague, The Netherlands.

Antoine Pevsner's undulated sculptures attempt to explore the dimensions of space. In contradiction to the De Stijl movement, the Constructivists did not see space as a linear, endless flat grid but as a flexible, subjective abstract. According to Albert Einstein's theory of relativity, time and space get curved and bent, which is shown in the forms of this sculpture. It can be seen as an objective form carrying universal meaning.

Antoine Pevsner was born in 1884 in Klimavichy and died in Paris in 1962. He is the older brother of the artist Naum Gabo. He attended both the Kiev Art School and the Saint Petersburg Academy. In Paris he met Archipenko and Modigliani and started abstract painting. Together with his brother, he published the "Realist Manifesto" in 1920, a key text of the Constructivist that segregated geometric forms. In 1931 he, Naum, Theo van Doesburgh and Georges Vantongerloo co-founded the group Abstraction-Creation. He was also involved in the rise of Kinetic and Concrete Art.

Photo: Wikifrits / Wikimedia Commons

Flame
Oscar Niemeyer

Completion: 1969. **Technique:** steel. **Location:** Paris, France.

This sculpture stands in front of the Niemeyers Communist Party Headquarters in France and represents a flame, the symbol of the Communist Party. "Flame" consists of two, curved segments connected to a base. The form is very reduced but easy to read, due to the convex and concave shapes that functions as an universal symbol for the flicker of fire.

Oscar Niemeyer, born 1907 in Rio de Janeiro, studied architecture from 1928 until 1934 in his hometown and went on to work for the urban designer Lúcio Costa. He later met Le Corbusier when working on Brazils first modernist building, the Ministry for Health and Education. In 1945 he became a member of the Communist Party. From 1947 to 1953 he worked for Le Corbusier at the UN headquarters in New York and from 1957 to 1964 he designed Basilia, the new capital of Brazil.

Photo: Chris van Uffelen

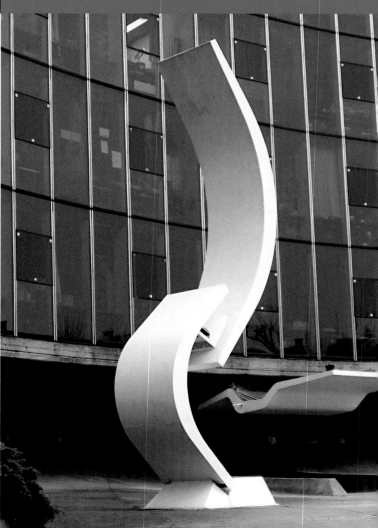

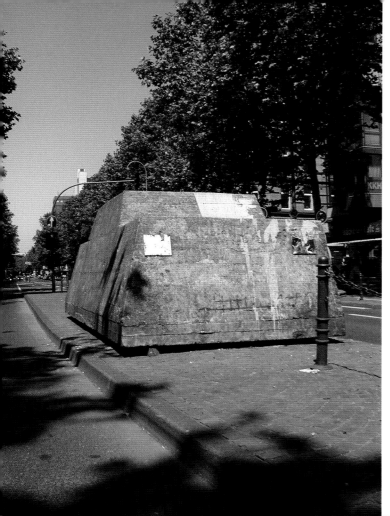

Stationary Traffic
Wolf Vostell

Completion: 1969. **Technique:** concrete, car. **Location:** Cologne, Germany.

Under this concrete skin hides an Opel Kapitän L, located on Domstraße. Originally the 15-ton object used a real parking space. After publically announcing this Happening, Vostell parked his own car on a concrete plate, he boxed it out to create an abstract silhouette and covered it in cast-concrete in two sessions. Other "Stationary Traffic"-sculptures can be found in Chicago, Malpartida de Cáceres and Berlin.

Wolf Vostell was a pioneering German artist. He was born in 1932 and worked with sculpture, video art, environmental art and painting. He was a master in techniques such as blurring and the dé-coll/age, many of his works involved objects embedded in concrete. He was also involved in Happening, with performance or street productions that are artistic in style. Vostell took part in his first Happening in Paris called "Theater is in the Streets", in 1958.

Photo: Horsch, Willy - HOWI / Wikimedia Commons

Victims Warn Us
Jozef Jankovič

Completion: 1969. **Technique:** bronze. **Location:** Banská Bystrica, Slovakia.

On a knoll near the historic center of Banská Bystrica one can see a monumental building, divided into two parts. In the middle is a passage, in which stands a large bronze sculptural group of human bodies. The figures are lying in a bunch as if they have been just exhumed. Above them stand those who survived – the same legs, arms and bodies looking ahead. This sculptural group, is entitled "Victims Warn Us". It is this sculpture in particular that makes the Monument both impressive and thought provoking.

Jozef Jankovič was born in 1937 in Bratislava, Slovakia. He studied between 1952 and 1956 at the School of Applied Arts, Bratislava. He then went on to enhance his studies at the Academy of Fine Arts, Bratislava. In 1984 he was appointed as visiting professor at the Academy of Applied Arts in Vienna. In 1990 he was appointed as chancellor at the Academy of Fine Arts, Bratislava, later becoming a professor. He has exhibited his work at various museums and institutions.

Photos: Kocal Ivan (a.), Lomnicky Jozef (b.)

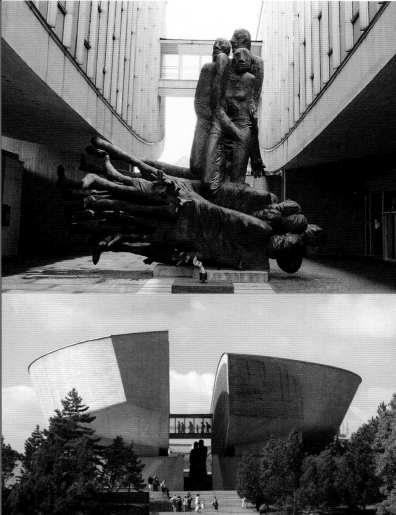

Wandering Rocks
Tony Smith

Completion: 1970. **Technique:** painted steel. **Location:** Otterlo, The Netherlands.

"Wandering Rocks" by Tony Smith is on display at the Kröller-Müller Museum sculpture park, in the Netherlands. At a glance, the painted steel forms look like they are a natural part of the landscape but close-up, their forms are too regular, too smooth. The sculpture serves as an example of how Smith combines abstract, geometric forms with a human, scale. His inspiration for this piece came from formal Japanese gardens, with their arranged stones.

Tony Smith was a minimalist sculptor. He was born in America in 1912 and died in 1980. Smith worked as a sculptor, visual artist and architectural designer. He was also a respected art theorist. His sculptures were minimalistic in style and many view him as a pioneer in the development of American Minimalist sculpture. In 1938, he began working as an office clerk for noted architect, Frank Lloyd Wright. He later worked for a short while as an architect before turning to sculpture.

Photo: Gerardus / Wikimedia Commons

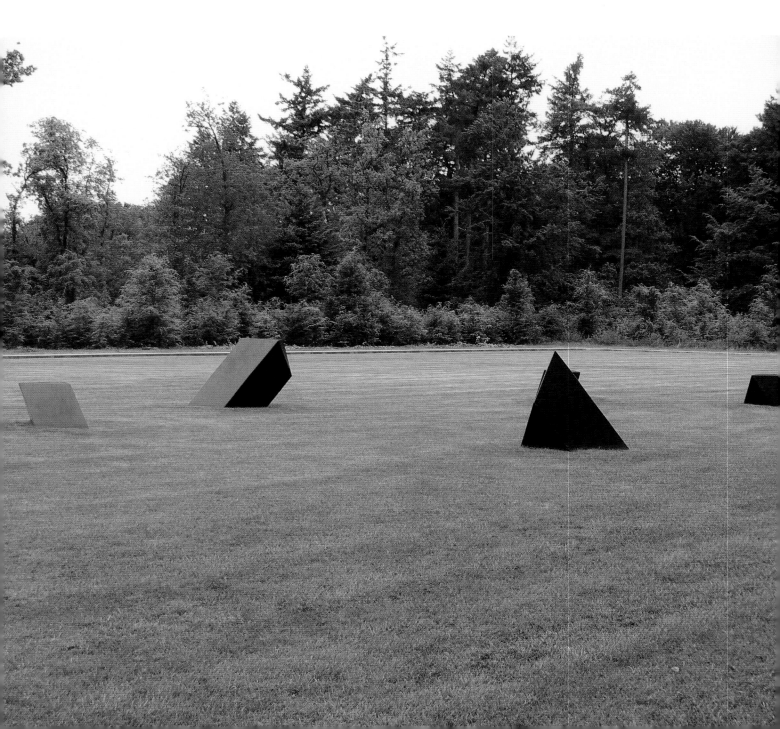

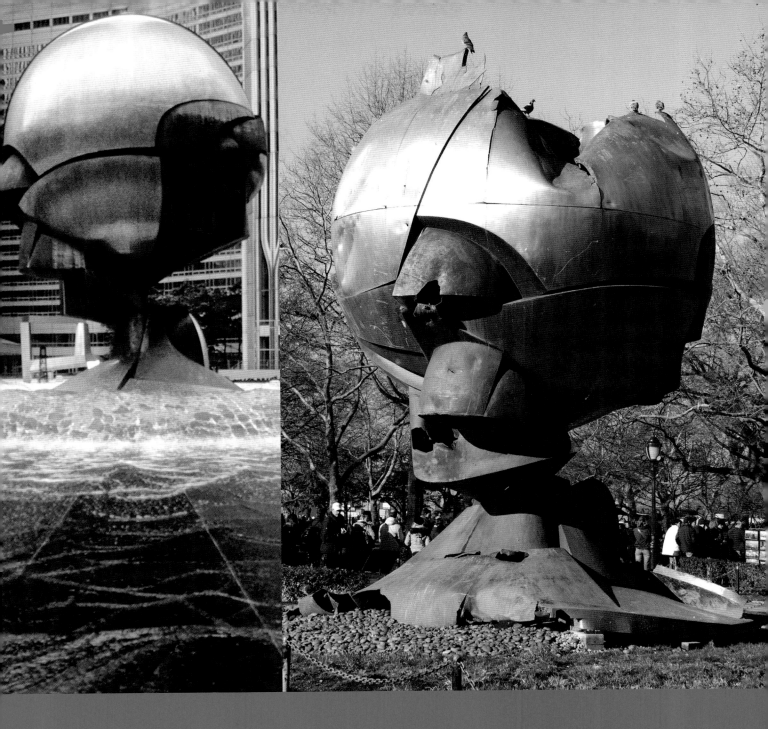

The Sphere
Fritz Koenig

Completion: 1971. **Technique:** metal. **Location:** New York City, NY, USA.

"The Sphere" is a large, metallic sculpture by German sculptor Fritz Koenig. It is currently displayed in Battery Park but once stood in the middle of Austin Tobin Plaza, the area between the World Trade Center towers. After being recovered from the rubble of the Twin Towers after the 2001 terrorist attacks, it was dismantled. Six months after the attacks it was relocated to Battery Park on a temporary basis and was later formally rededicated with an eternal flame as a memorial to the victims of 9/11.

Fritz Koenig was born in 1924, in Würzburg, Germany. In the years after World War II, he studied at the Academy of Fine Arts, graduating in 1952. Since 1964 he worked as a professor of art at the Technical University in Munich. Koenig's work has largely consisted of figures or shapes assembled from simple geometric forms, cast in metal. When he has represented human forms, these have been heavily stylized, with heads made of spheres and bodies and limbs of cylinders.

Photos: Chris van Uffelen (l.); Michele Gerarduzzi / http://twitter.com/michelegera (r.)

Blue Spiral
Louis Constantin

Completion: 1972. **Technique:** fiberglass-reinforced polyester, blue lacquer. **Location:** Munich, Germany.

This blue spiral, made of fiberglass-reinforced polyester, resembles the path of a screw as it is screwed into a surface. It was made in 1972, at the end of the artist's university studies and won the Pschorrbräu Foundation Junior Prize in 1982. The Straßenkunst Foundation bought the sculpture in 2001 and later donated it to the city of Munich. The sculpture is the largest freestanding sculpture in the city.

Louis Constantin was born in Hagen / Westfalen, Germany, in 1944. In 1966 he enrolled at the Art Academy in Paris, graduating in 1972. He went on to study at the School of Fine Arts, also in Paris, later continuing his education at the Art Academy in Munich. His work was widely exhibited, both in solo and group exhibitions, throughout the late 1970s and '80s. Since 1975, Constantin has lived and worked as artist and art teacher in Munich.

Photo: Chris van Uffelen

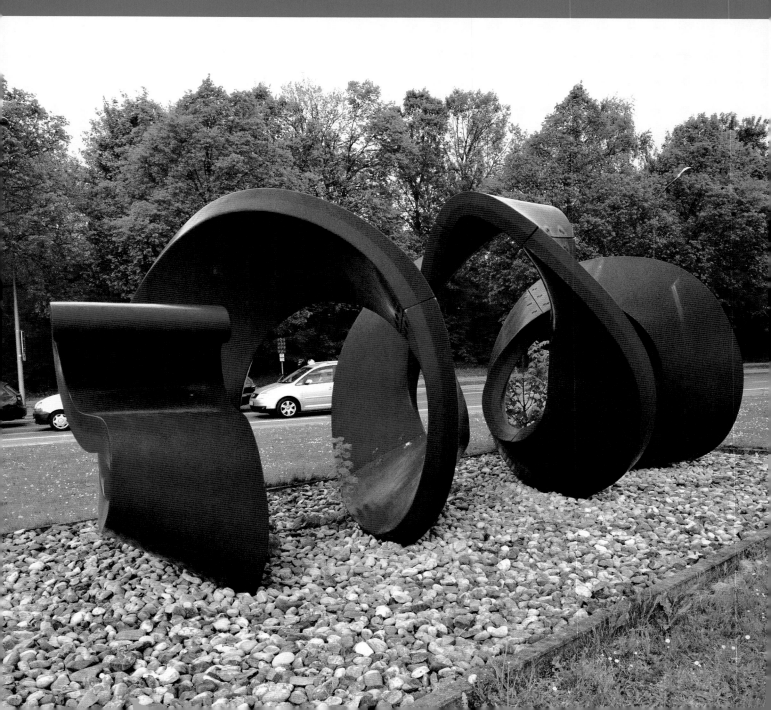

Group of Four Trees
Jean Dubuffet

Completion: 1972. **Technique:** synthetic plastic, aluminum, steel.
Location: New York City, NY, USA.

"Group of Four Trees" is a black and white sculpture that stands in front of the Chase Manhattan Bank. The irregular surfaces of the work contrast the regularity of the building behind it. The tree's canopies lean in different directions and the height of each one is different. The sculpture is made with plastic, draped over an aluminum frame; a steel armature holds the whole piece together.

Jean Dubuffet was a French painter and sculptor. He was born in 1902 and died in 1985. He disregarded traditional aesthetics and standards of beauty in his quest to produce more authentic and humanistic images. Dubuffet moved to Paris in 1918 to study painting at the Julian Academy but left after just six months. He later took over his father's wine-selling business, not returning to art properly until 1942. He painted ordinary people in ordinary situations, with a primitive style and strong use of color.

Photo: Chris van Uffelen

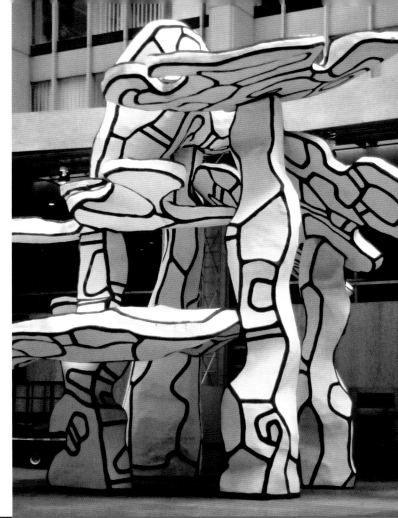

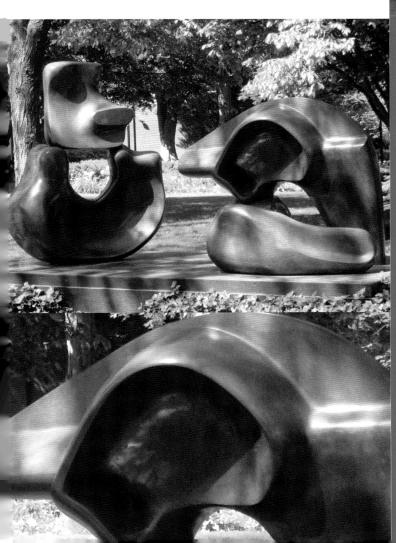

Four Piece Reclining Figure
Henry Moore

Completion: 1973. **Technique:** bronze. **Location:** Cambridge, MA, USA.

The "Four Piece Reclining Figure" is on display in the grounds of Harvard University. Moore produced many seating and reclining figures, exploring this form and interpreting it in different ways. Moore's earlier reclining figures deal with mass, while his later ones contrast the solid elements of the sculpture with the space, and he began to pierce them with opening. His later, more abstract, figures are often penetrated by holes directly through the body as Moore explored concave and convex shapes.

Henry Moore was one of Britain's most influential abstract sculptors. He was born in West Yorkshire in 1898 and showed a very early interest in sculpture and art. He worked briefly as a teacher before being called to the army when he turned 18. After the war he received a grant to study at the Leeds School of Art where he met another hugely important British sculptor, Barbara Hepworth. His early sculptures were Victorian in style but his later work became gradually much more abstract.

87

Photo: Daderot / Wikimedia Commons

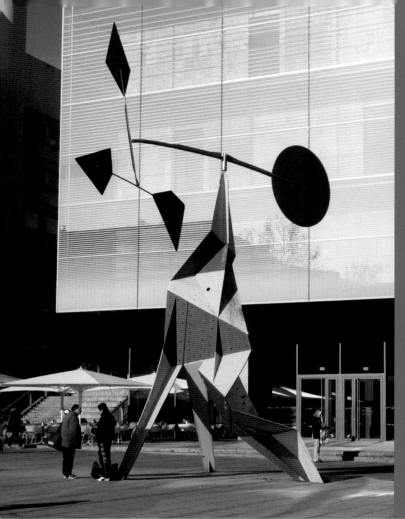

Crinkly with Red Discs
Alexander Calder

Completion: 1973. **Technique:** steel, aluminum. **Location:** Stuttgart, Germany.

"Crinkly with Red Discs" was made in 1973 and stands on the Schlossplatz in Stuttgart, Germany. This so-called "Mobile-stable" consists of many steel plates, screwed and fixed together, giving the sculpture a folded appearance. The three-legged body of the piece is colored black and white on one side while the other side is painted red and yellow. The round discs and the three, moveable aluminum sections are colored a bright red.

Alexander Calder was born in 1898 in Lawton, Pennsylvania and died in New York in 1996. He was an American sculptor who was best-known for his mobile sculptures. He first studied engineering at Stevens Institute of Technology in Hoboken, before going on to take several art courses at the Art Students League in New York. He moved to Paris in 1930, where he attended the Academy de la Grande Chaumière. He was also a member of the art group Abstraction-Creation.

Five in One
Bernard Rosenthal

Completion: 1974. **Technique:** Corten steel. **Location:** New York City, NY, USA.

This sculpture, "Five in One", by Bernard Rosenthal is made of Corten steel. It was the second of five public art sculptures created by Rosenthal and now on permanent display in New York. The sculpture consists of five interlocking discs, which represent the interconnectedness of the city's five boroughs: Bronx, Brooklyn, Manhattan, Queens and Staten Island. The sculpture was initially installed with its raw Corten steel exposed but funds were later raised to paint the "Five in One" sculpture red.

Bernard Rosenthal was born in 1914, in Illinois and is best known for a body of monumental public art sculptures, which were created over seven decades. He received his first commission for a figurative sculpture in 1939 for the International Exposition. Rosenthal constantly explored sculpture, whether it be of monumental size or just a few centimeters, in a variety of mediums including, steel, bronze, aluminum, brass, wood and concrete. He handcrafted both macquettes and many of the larger versions, himself.

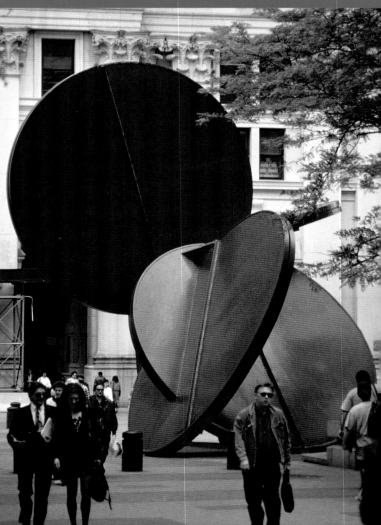

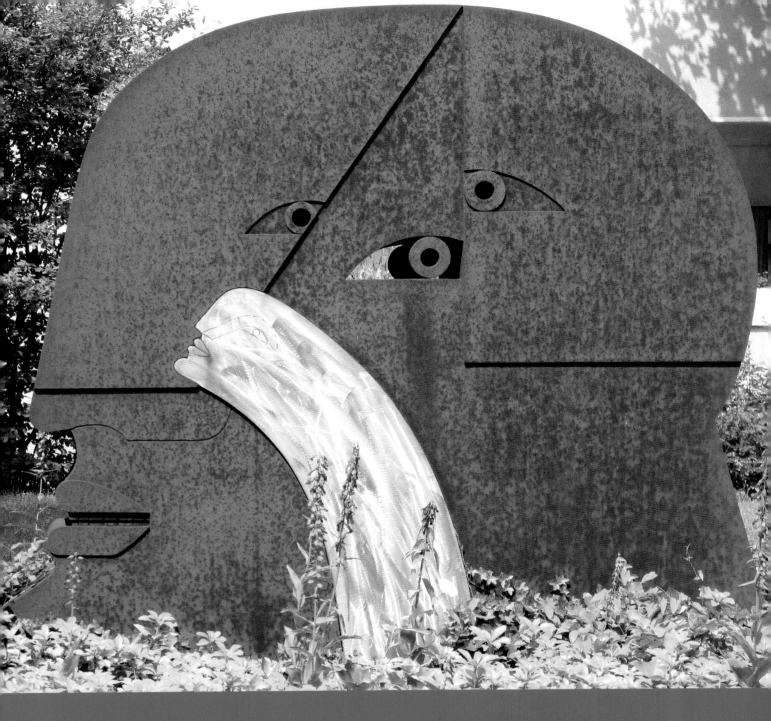

Head 73
Horst Antes

Completion: 1973. **Technique:** steel. **Location:** Essen, Germany.

The most common form by this artist is that of the "Kopffüßler" (Head-Footer) a mystical figure, that was believed to exist in the Middle Ages. Though this sculpture is not a typical example of this, it is a typical work of Antes in that it explores the head shape, the head is cut into a silhouette form with little detail, except for three eyes on the side of the head, and a smaller head inserted into the steel in as a silver stripe.

Horst Antes is a German sculptor and artist, born in 1936. He studied at the Academy of Fine Arts in Karlsruhe between 1957 and 1959 under the tutorage of influential woodcutter, HAP Grieshaber, winning both the Hanover Art Prize and the Pankofer prize in 1959. In the 1960s Antes discovered the "Kopffüßler" (Head-Footer) form, and he produced many works of this style, where a head is directly joined to legs. He won various prizes for his work and was offered a teaching post at the Academy in Karlsruhe at the age of 29.

Crystal, vertical Accent in Glass and Steel
Edvin Öhrström

Completion: 1974. **Technique:** crystal glass, steel. **Location:** Stockholm, Sweden.

This fountain-sculpture in glass and steel is 37.5 meters high, with over 80,000 glass pieces. It was the result of a competition for a sculptural focus in the city's center. Öhrström's suggestion has a richly faceted and varied sculptural form and represents a clear, constructive concept. The proportions in relation to the square are cogent and together, the sculpture and the play of water form a powerful composition. The glass and steel, make a good impression both close up and at a distance.

The Swedish sculptor Edvin Öhrström (1906–1994) is best known for his tall glass pillar at Sergels Torg and Swedish glassworks Orrefors. With a technique that Öhrström himself developed, he quickly switched to casting massive sculptures in glass but retained his characteristic expressions. Glass as a material, and its refraction of light and significance for perception, grew into a virtual obsession. Öhrström would spend the rest of his life exploring the possibilities of glass.

Photo: Sten Öhrström

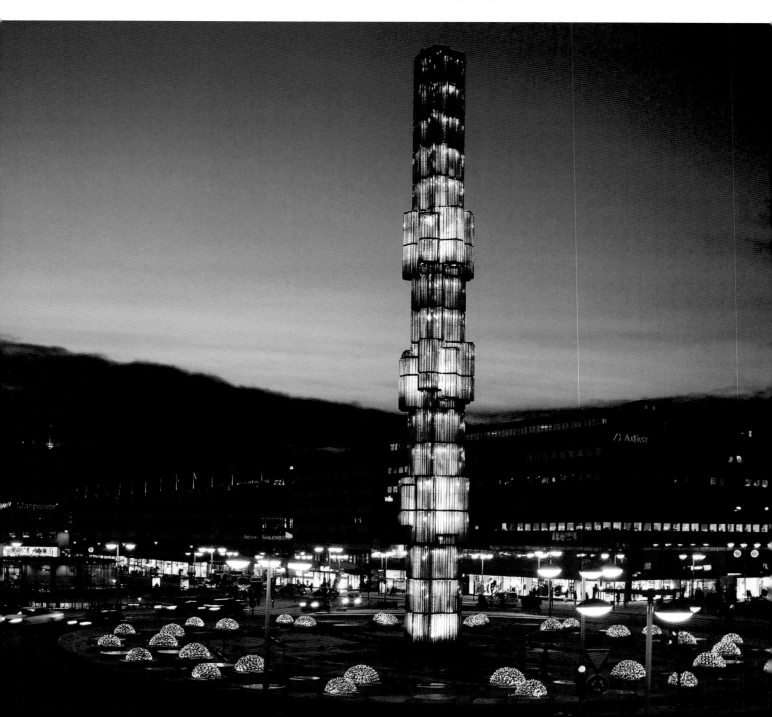

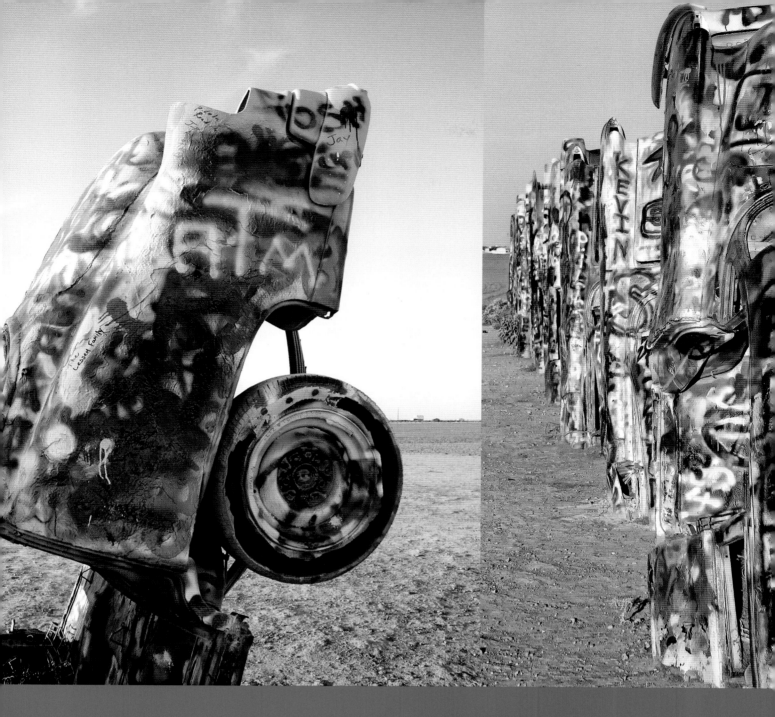

Cadillac Ranch
Ant Farm

Completion: 1974. **Technique:** Cadillac cars. **Location:** Amarillo, TX, USA.

The cars of the "Cadillac Ranch" are half buried, nose in the ground at an angle corresponding to that of the Great Pyramid of Giza. The work was created as a monument to the golden age of American automobiles and the famous Route 66. Writing on the vehicles and graffiti of any form is strongly encouraged. The cars have also periodically been painted a uniform color for various reasons; white for a TV ad campaign and black at a time of mourning and sometimes just to provide a blank canvas for new graffiti.

Chip Lord, Hudson Marquez and Doug Michels, who were a part of the art group Ant Farm, created "Cadillac Ranch". Ant Farm was an architectural, graphic arts and environmental design practice. As well as architectural works, the group was well known for its performances and media events. A fire destroyed the Ant Farm studio in 1978 and after that the group disbanded.

Photos: Roger Andres / www.rogerandres.ch

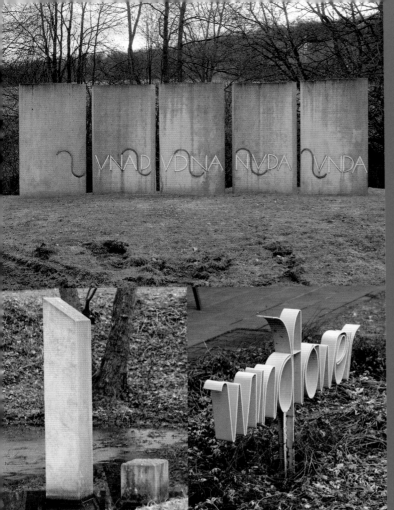

Concrete Verse
Ian Hamilton Finlay

Completion: 1975. **Technique:** marble, concrete, steel.
Location: Stuttgart, Germany.

This sculpture was made by Ian Hamilton Finlay and is located in the garden of the Max Planck Institute in Stuttgart. The work consists of seven art stations; "Ship", "VNDA", "Here Lies a Small Section of a Larger Quantity of Water", "Clouds", "Wind flower", "Waves" and "Weathercock", although the latter no longer exists. Through combining language and material, Finlay has created a philosophical place, which harmonizes well with the architectural form of the institute.

Ian Hamilton Finlay was born in the Bahamas in 1925 and died in Edinburgh in 2006. He was called up to serve in the army during the World War II and after the War's end he studied philosophy. In the 1950s he produced numerous plays for Radio and TV. From 1962 he began to develop his poetry into concrete verse. He was best known for his work "Little Sparta" a work inscribed on stone.

Photos: Chris van Uffelen

Horizontal Column
Wolfgang Kubach, Anna-Maria Wilmsen-Kubach

Completion: 1975. **Technique:** marble. **Location:** Vancouver, Canada.

This work is on display at the VanDusen Botanical Garden. It is one of 11 stone sculptures located here. The piece is made of carved marble and is intended to look more than a little inconspicuous, lying on a law of neatly mown grass. The piece has the appearance of a piece of classical architecture but the name and form play with the viewer's expectations; the strong form of the architecture has been twisted in the middle, questioning the strength of classical sculptural traditions.

Wolfgang Kubach, born 1936, died 2007 and Anna-Maria Wilmsen-Kubach, born 1937, were both German sculptors. They both studied at the Academy of Arts in Munich from 1959 to 1965. In 1965 they opened a studio in an old church in Hakenheim. They have both worked as stone sculptors since 1968. Their combined body of work pays homage to stone in all its forms and types. In 1998, they founded the Kubach-Wilmsen Foundation, this also features its own sculpture park.

Photos: Athen Ananda / Wikimedia Commons (a.); Mike Linksvayer / Wikimedia Commons (b.)

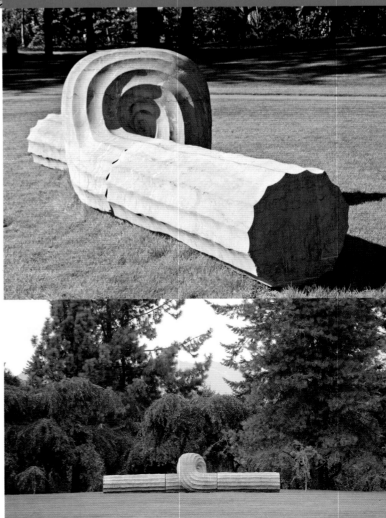

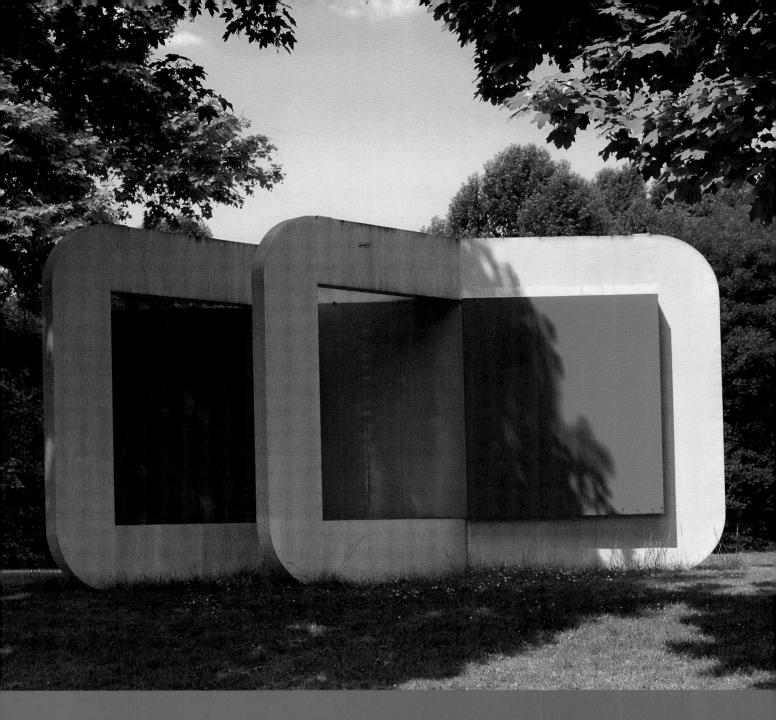

Color-Space Object
Georg Karl Pfahler

Completion: 1977. **Materials:** steel, acrylic paint. **Location:** Stuttgart, Germany.

"Color-Space Object" is situated on a small hill surrounded by green space. The sculpture seeks to engage passersby, attracting the gaze of drivers on Stuttgart's main traffic artery. The sculpture consists of two frame-like rectangles, three meters tall, four meters long and 15 centimeters thick. The rectangles offer a splash of color in the uniformly ordered park area; the framed colors become paintings within the landscape.

Georg Karl Pfahler was a German painter, artist and art lecturer. He was born in Emetzheim in Bavaria in 1926 and died in 2002. He studied at the Academy of Art in Nuremberg, where he was introduced to a new world of art, full of new styles and possibilities. He first began experimenting with painting techniques, focusing on the presence of surface texture and color. He was inspired mainly by artwork from America and Britain and longed to travel, to escape the detrimental effect of the stifling Nazi regime.

Photo: Chris van Uffelen

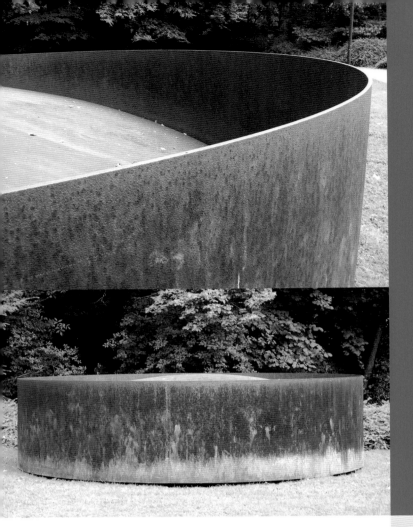

Untitled
Donald Judd

Completion: 1977. **Technique:** Corten steel. **Location:** Bottrop, Germany.

Judd's untitled works are simple, geometric, reparative forms that explore space in relation to themselves. One can view them as monochrome paintings in space. He admired Josef Albers whose paintings involved geometric, simple forms in clear colors, Judd's work achieved a three-dimensional effect through its use of shadows, whereas Albers' works remained two-dimensional and investigated color more than form.

Donald Judd was born in 1928 and died in 1994. He studied art history in Williamsburg and New York, under Rudolf Wittkower and Meyer Shapiro and later studied philosophy. He started working as a painter but quickly found the two-dimensional form uninspiring. He developed an interest in three-dimensional works, cutting the canvas or integrating objects. As a sculptor he started placing minimalized objects in rooms in an effort to make the rooms volume more noticeable. He began working on large-scale pieces in the 1970s.

Photos: Gerardus / Wikimedia Commons

Observatory
Robert Morris

Completion: 1977. **Technique:** earth, wood. **Location:** Flevoland, The Netherlands.

In 1971 Robert Morris designed an observatory for an exhibition in Velsen. In 1977 it was rebuilt on a larger scale in Flevoland. It consists of two rings of earth, the inner ring with a wooden wall. Large stones mark the sunrise, equinoxes and solstices. So the observatory is a kind of calendar, like the ones the Maya and other early cultures had. Since 1990 the Flevolandschap Foundation has been responsible for the care of the monument.

Robert Morris, born 1931 in Kansas City, is one of the two leaders of American minimalist art. Like Donald Judd, he is also an art critic. He studied in Kansas City and Portland and first began working as a painter. His interest in choreography began when he made a film about Jackson Pollok, this work led him to minimal installations. His works follows his statement "Simplicity of form is not necessarily simplicity of experience".

Photos: Lvellinga / Wikimedia Commons

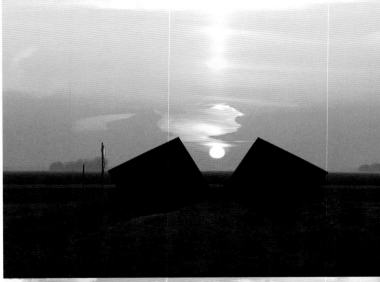

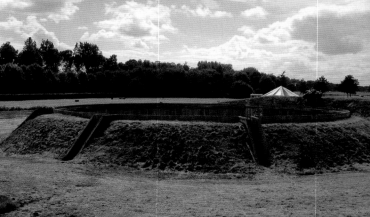

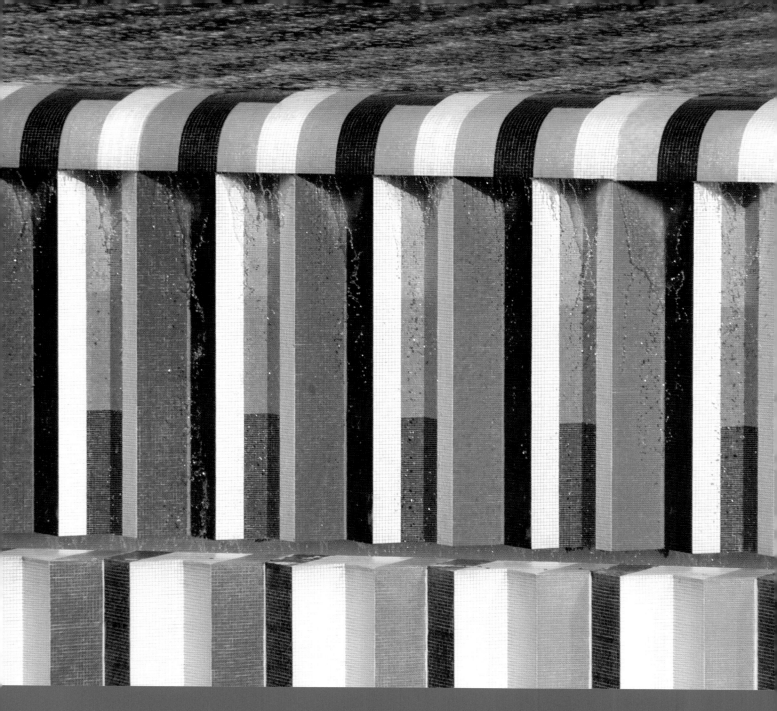

La Défense Fountain
Yaacov Agam

Completion: 1977. **Technique:** acrylic. **Location:** La Défense, France.

This musical fountain was created in 1977. The fountain's pool is made of polymorphic, mosaic surface and is comprised of 66 vertical water jets that shoot water up to 14 meters into the air. The fountain is illuminated at night and was improved with the addition of five new jets in 1991. Another famous project by Agam is the "Fire and Water Fountain" in Tel Aviv, which is located on a raised roundabout and painted in bright, rainbow colors.

Yaacov Agam was born in 1928 and is an Israeli sculptor and Experimental Artist. Agam studied at the Bezalel Academy of Art and Design in Jerusalem, before moving to France in 1951 where he still lives today. He had his first solo exhibition in 1953 and soon began establishing himself as one of the leading figures in Kinetic Art. His work is usually abstract and frequently involves the use of light and sound. His work has been exhibited at both the Guggenehim in New York and at the Museum of Modern Art in Paris.

Photo: Chris van Uffelen

The Four Seasons
Leonard French

Completion: 1978. **Technique:** stained glass panel. **Location:** Melbourne, Australia.

"The Four Seasons" is a work in stained glass by the Australian artist, Leonard French. The four colored glass panels represent the changing of the seasons and are on permanent display in the La Trobe University Sculpture Park, Bundoora Campus, Melbourne.

Leonard French is an Australian artist, born in 1928. He is best known for his major stained glass works, including a series of panels in the café and foyer of the National Library of Australia and a stained glass ceiling for the great hall at the National Gallery of Victoria. He also created a work entitled "The Legend of Sinbad the Sailor", made from seven panels and displayed in the Legend Café, Melbourne. French was awarded the Sulman Prize and has held more than 40 solo exhibitions in Australia alone.

Photos: resascup / Wikimedia Commons

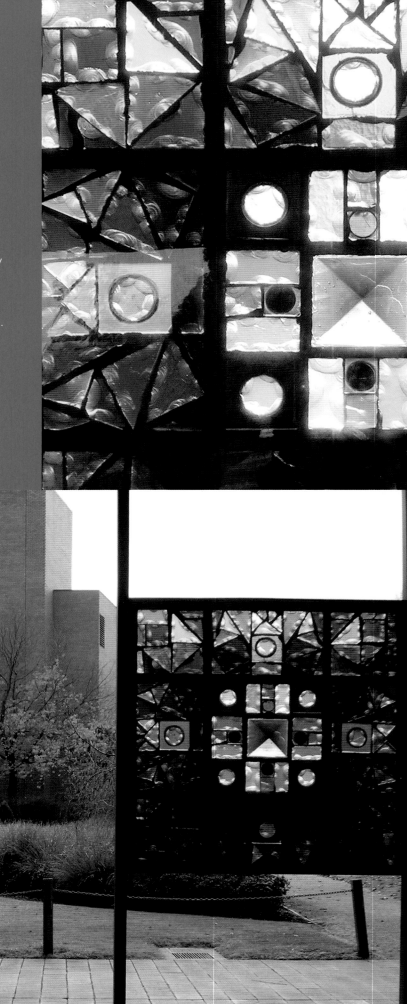

Rock Rings
Nancy Holt

Completion: 1978. **Technique:** stone masonry using Brown Mountain stone. **Location:** Bellingham, WA, USA.

"Rock Rings" is situated in the Western Washington University. Brown Mountain stone is locally sourced and the various minerals in the rock cause hues of orange, yellow, purple, brown, gray and blue. The four arches in the work are aligned on the north-south axis as calculated from the north star, Polaris. The work relates to a point in the universe, a true north. The 12 holes are aligned northeast-southwest, east-west, northwest-southeast, spatially orienting the landscape.

Nancy Holt was born in 1938 in Worcester, Massachusetts and studied at Tufts University. She is famous for her public sculptures and is associated with Earthwork, a tradition which emerged in the 1960s and coincided with the growing ecological movement in the USA, encouraging people to become more aware of the negative impact they have on the environment. Holt has exhibited work in solo exhibitions spatially and perceptually across the USA, she also produces works in other mediums, including film and photography.

Photos: Courtesy of the artist

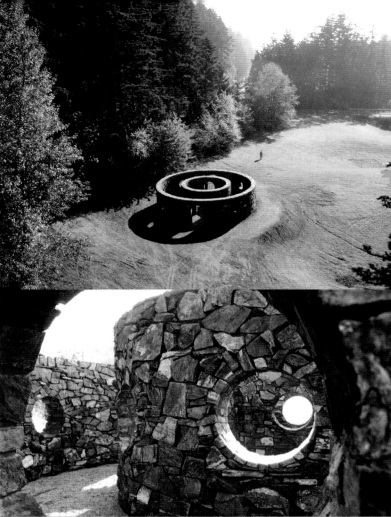

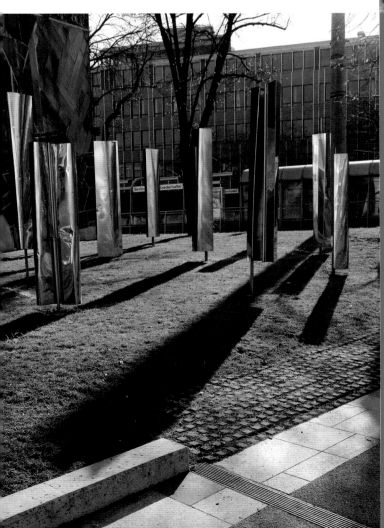

Stainless Steel Column-Forest
Karl-Heinz Franke

Completion: 1979. **Technique:** stainless steel. **Location:** Stuttgart, Germany.

The "Stainless Steel Column-Forest" by Karl-Heinz Franke was a commission from the International Art Congress in Stuttgart in 1979. The sculpture consists of 11 stainless steel objects, built in a vertical orientation. The objects are anchored directly to the ground with metal rods and are made of metal plates, approximately one millimeter thick and two meters tall. Each object was handcrafted and reflects the immediate surroundings in different ways.

Karl-Heinz Franke was born in Berlin in 1916 and died in 2006. He was a metal sculptor and painter who studied in Dessau from 1932–1937. It was during the 1960s that he first turned to sculpture. In 1984 he founded the group "Constructive Tendencies", which united artists from all over south Germany. He is best known for his stainless steel sculptures.

Photo: Chris van Uffelen

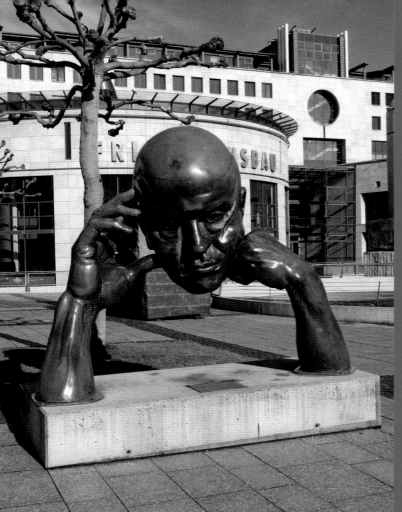

Thinking Partner
Hans-Jörg Limbach

Completion: 1980. **Technique:** bronze. **Location:** Stuttgart, Germany.

The bronze sculpture "Thinking Partner" is on loan from E. Hildebrandt and is located, after being removed from the Rotebühlplatz, on the Börsenplatz in Stuttgart. The sculpture weighs 800 kilograms and, as the name suggests, intends to give the viewer food for thought. It is comprised of a human head, supported by two hands. Its expression and gesture forge an intended connection between it and the surrounding architecture.

Hans-Jörg Limbach was a Swiss painter, drawer and sculptor. He was born in Zurich in 1928 and died in 1990. He lived in Japan from 1952 to 1955 in order to be able to devote himself to the study of Japanese sculpture and painting.

Photo: Chris van Uffelen

Bodenstück
Wilfried Hagebölling

Completion: 1980. **Technique:** Corten steel. **Location:** Mannheim, Germany.

The sculpture "Bodenstück" ("Ground Piece") was created by German sculptor Wilfried Hagebölling. This large sculpture is composed of steel plates, set at different angels but of equal sizes, positioned to appear as if they grow out of the ground itself. The sculpture aims to change a viewer's orientation and is designed with structural clarity and transparency; whether it is viewed as a three dimensional sculpture or simply as a walk through passage, is left up to the viewer.

Wilfried Hagebölling was born in 1941 in Berlin. Between 1963 and 1967 he studied at the Academy of Arts in Munich. In the 1970s and 1980s he exhibited in Paris, Germany and Asia, making him one of Germany's best known steel sculptors. Much of his early work involved competition projects, which often related to both architecture and sculpture. Hagebölling is especially well known for his large, walk-on sculptures, often located in public spaces.

Photos: Courtesy of the artist

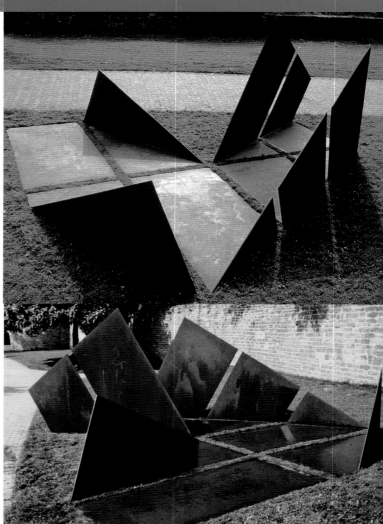

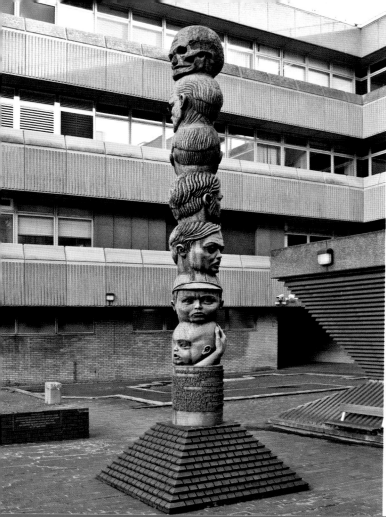

The Seven Ages of Man
Richard Kindersley

Completion: 1980. **Technique:** cast aluminum. **Location:** London, United Kingdom.

"The Seven Ages of Man" is just over seven meters tall and cast in aluminum. The sculptor drew his inspiration for the description of the seven ages of man in Shakespeare's "As You Like It". The reference to Shakespeare here is particularly poignant as the work is situated along the route that Shakespeare may have taken to reach the Globe Theater from his lodgings. Various models were used in the creation of the forms, including the artist's son.

Richard Kindersley studied lettering and sculpture at Cambridge School of Art and in his father's workshop. He set up his own studio in 1970 and has received many commissions for his sculptural works, including from Exeter University, British Telecom, Sainsbury's and Christies' Fine Art. He has also designed lettering schemes for several prominent locations, such as London Bridge, Tower Bridge and the New Crown Court Buildings in Liverpool. Kindersley has also lectured on architectural lettering and its development.

Photo: Rob Sandiford

Between
Clement Meadmore

Completion: 1980. **Technique:** Corten steel. **Location:** Perth, Australia.

"Between" is a Corten steel structure; three shapes balanced together to form a whole. Meadmore's monumental sculptures can be found in public space around the world. Their majestically twisting, strong forms bent and shaped into a huge variety of expressive shapes. Meadmore's sculptures reflect his interest in Minimalism as well as his fascination with geometry.

Clement Meadmore was born in 1929 in Melbourne Australia and died in 2005. His early work received a lot of attention and was displayed at several solo exhibitions in Melbourne and Sydney. In 1963 Meadmore moved to New York, later becoming an American citizen. As his artistic talent developed, Meadmore began to produce monumental sculptures, his early work was more minimalist in style. He later became interested in geometrical forms, employing and exploring their shapes in his sculptures.

Photo: Spinn / Wikimedia Commons

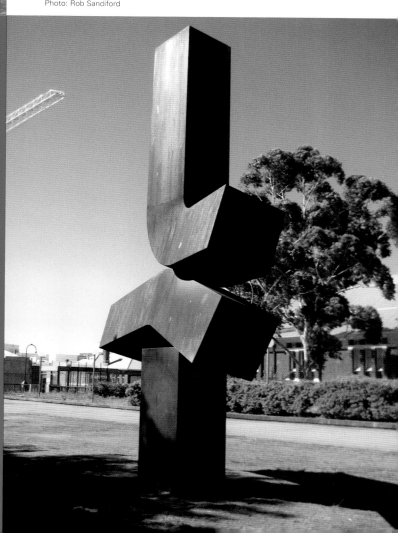

Cubi Series
David Smith

Completion: 1980. **Technique:** stainless steel. **Location:** Jerusalem, Israel.

This sculpture is one of a series of 28 "Cubi" works by the artist. Each of the works is made with stainless steel and created from a series of cubes and cylinders with spherical or flat end-caps. This series is the last artistic work made by David Smith, who died shortly after making the 28th. The first eleven "Cubi" sculptures were not completed in the order in which they are numbered, as shown by the following inscriptions Smith welded onto the base of each "Cubi".

David Smith was born in Indiana, USA in 1906. He attended Ohio University from 1924 to 1925 and then the University of Notre Dame, which he left after two weeks because there were no art courses. Smith began sculpting with wire, soldered metal and other found materials but soon began using an oxyacetylene torch to weld metal heads. The last sculpture in Smith's "Cubi Series", Cubi XXVIII, was sold at auction in 2005 for 23.8 million dollars, making it the most expensive contemporary art work ever to be sold at auction.

Photo: deror_avi / Wikimedia Commons

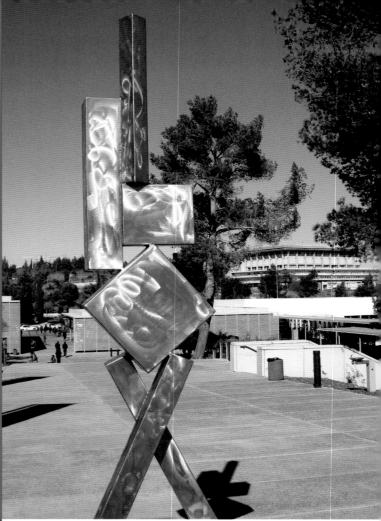

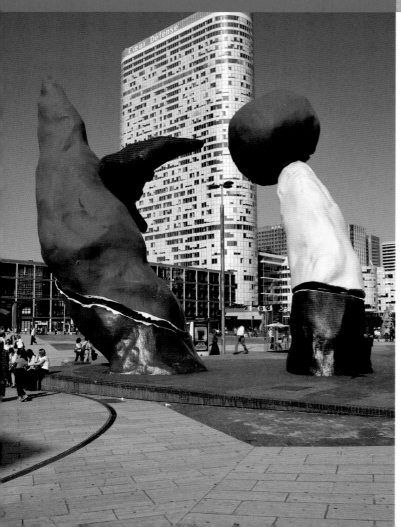

Two Fantastic Figures
Joan Miró

Completion: 1980. **Technique:** concrete. **Location:** La Défense, France.

These two large sculptures, named "Fantastic Figures", measure 11 and 12 meters and are recognizable as humans by just a few hints. An eye – just by its form and position, not by its color and proportion –, a mouth and the proportion of the head in relation to the body. Most other details remain abstract and look as if they have been formed from plasticine with troughs and hilltops, as if a giant child made them. This playful, irregular surface contrasts with the modernist architecture of La Défense.

Joan Miró was born in Barcelona in 1893, the son of a goldsmith and watchmaker, and died in Palma de Mallorca, 1983. He studied in Barcelona first, moving to Paris in 1920, where he came into contact with the Pablo Picasso-circle. His style changed from Naïve Art to Cubism and to Surrealism when working with Max Ernst. His later style drew out of all of these influences.

Photo: Chris van Uffelen

Tower
Nils Udo

Completion: 1982. **Technique:** stones. **Location:** Frenswegen, Germany.

"Tower" by Nils Udo is an example of his desire to create work that compliments and molds to its surroundings. Udo's work struggles with the fundamental contradiction of Land Art. Even Land Art, in its efforts to compliment nature and embrace it, disturbs the environment, bringing something artificial and manipulated by man into a natural space. "Tower" is a large, strong piece that almost appears as if it grew out of the land itself, the stones roughly cut and fitted together.

Nils Udo is a German painter and Land Artist who has specialized in Land Art since the 1960s. He was born in Bavaria in 1937 and one of his best known pieces of art was actually not Land Art, but was the cover to Peter Gabriels album Ovo. In 1972 he turned away from painting, concentrating on his environmental work. He began working with trees, plants and shrubs, renting land from farmers on which to create his Environmental Art.

Photo: Gerardus / Wikimedia Commons

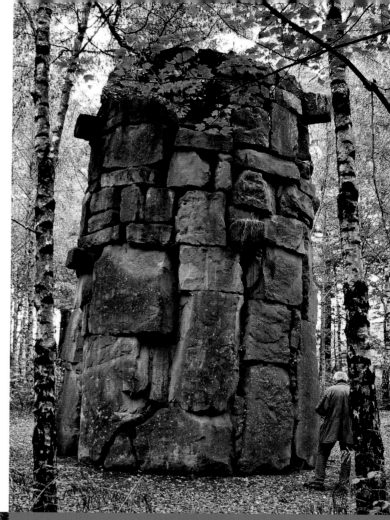

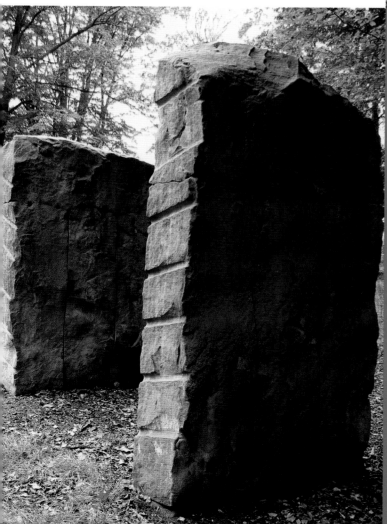

Untitled
Ulrich Rückriem

Completion: 1982. **Technique:** Bentheim sandstone. **Location:** Frenswegen, Germany.

The minimalistic form of his sculptures helped to made Rückriem famous. Because of their rough outlines, his work looks archaic at first glance, until one recognizes that there are traces of modern quarry work. The large stones are taken from a quarry, split and then put together again. He does not search for a figure within the stone like Michelangelo did, but searches for the aesthetic of the stone itself. He looks for the stones specific beauty and attempts to compliment it, like with this sculptural pair.

Ulrich Rückriem was born in 1938 in Dusseldorf. Between 1957 and 1959 he worked as a stonemason's apprentice in Düren before being employed in the workshop of the cathedral in Cologne, studying under professor Ludwig Gies. In 1967 he began to receive recognition for his detailed, wood sculptures and the following year he began to work on stone sculpture, sharing a workshop with Blinky Palermo. He currently lives in Ireland.

Photo: Gerardus / Wikimedia Commons

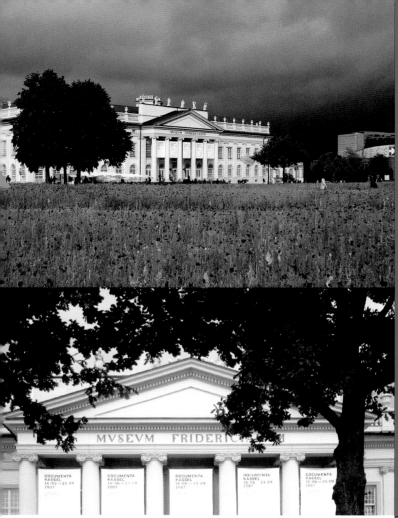

7,000 Oaks
Joseph Beuys

Completion: 1982. **Technique:** 7.000 Oaks. **Location:** Kassel, Germany.

"7,000 Oaks" was first publicly presented in 1982 at the seventh Documenta. It is a work of Land Art by Joseph Beuys. With the help of volunteers, Beuys planted 7,000 oak trees in the city of Kassel; a basalt stone accompanies each of these trees. This project has long term goals – aiming to permanently alter the living space in the city. Because of the urban environment, planting the trees was an extensive artistic and ecological project, planting ended in 1987 at the eighth Documenta exhibition.

Joseph Beuys was born in 1921 in Dusseldorf and died in 1986. He was a German sculptor, Installation Artist, art theorist, educator and performer. His work is grounded in the concepts of humanism and social philosophy. He extended the traditional definitions of art, and introduced the idea of Social Sculpture. The meaning, purpose and definition of his work have always been fiercely debated, but he is now considered one of the most influential artists of the 20th century.

Photos: Michael Wolf / fotolia.com (a.); Wasily / Wikimedia Commons (b.)

Igloo of Stone
Mario Merz

Completion: 1982. **Technique:** sandstone, metal. **Location:** Otterlo, The Netherlands.

"Igloo of Stone" is displayed in the sculpture garden at the Kröller-Müller Museum in the Netherlands. The sculpture is made from sandstone and metal and takes the traditional igloo shape. Merz began working on his series of Igloo sculptures in 1968. The sculptures show his interest in the fundamentals of human survival, shelter and man's relationship to nature. Many of his works refer to the principles of the Fibonacci series, a mathematical sequence that underlies the growth patterns of natural life.

Mario Merz was born in 1925 in Italy and died in 2003. Merz started drawing during the World War II, and was later imprisoned for his involvement in the anti fascist group, Guistizia e Libertà. His artwork was experimental and he often drew with a continuous stroke, not removing the pencil from the paper. His sculptural work often explores the relationship between nature and subject. Merz was also fascinated by architecture and the relationship between the human and occupied space.

Photos: Gerardus / Wikimedia Commons

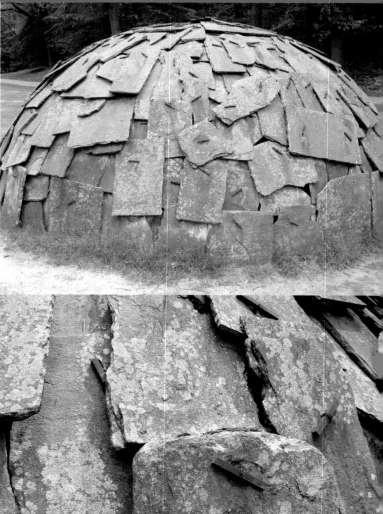

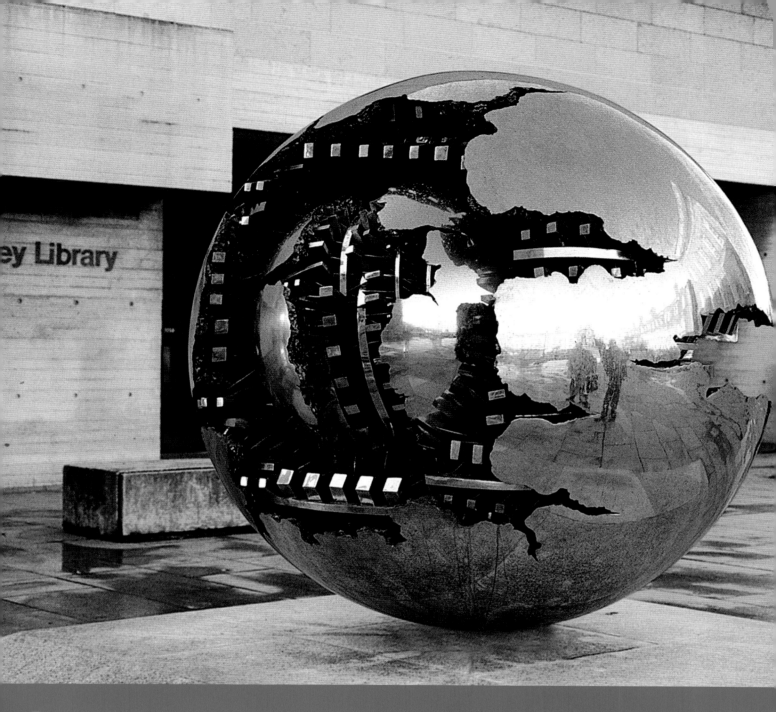

Sphere within a Sphere
Arnaldo Pomodoro

Completion: 1983. **Technique:** bronze. **Location:** Dublin, Ireland.

Arnaldo Pomodoro's work is driven by his desire to break open the perfect shape of a sphere to see what is inside. He works to destroy the form but also to simultaneously recreate it as something new. The sphere, broken open and revealed, can be vied by observers, in its new state it fulfills a need for discovery a childlike need to know what is inside a form or shape. This sculpture is located at the Trinity College, University of Dublin in Ireland.

Arnaldo Pomodoro was born in 1926. He went to live in Milan in 1954. His works have been well received by critics such as Gillo Dorfles, Guido Ballo and Franco Russoli. His statuary work is installed in squares and open spaces around the world. Pomodoro has taught in the Art Department of Stanford University, University of California at Berkeley, and Mills College. He has also applied his art to theater, and has been involved in many Italian theatrical events.

Photo: Arnaldo Pomodoro

Stravinsky Fountain
Jean Tinguely with Niki de Saint Phalle

Completion: 1983. **Technique:** metal, hoses, polyester. **Location:** Paris, France.

The "Stravinsky Fountain" is a playful public fountain next to the Centre de Pompidou in Paris. It is decorated with 16 sculptural works that move about and spray water. The fountain is 580 square meters and the sculptures were inspired by Igor Stravinsky's musical piece, "Rite of Spring". The work was built as part of a larger sculptural program, which demanded seven contemporary, sculptural fountains be built in different parts of Paris.

Jean Tinguely was a Swiss painter and sculptor who often worked in collaboration with Niki de Saint Phalle. He was born in 1925 and died in 1991. Tinguely grew up in Basel but moved to France to pursue his art career. His most famous works are kinetic sculptures, sometimes involving water. He has made several self destructing sculptures, one of which was detonated in front of an audience, in the desert near Las Vegas. His work often satirizes the overproduction of material goods in modern industrial society.

Photos: Chris van Uffelen

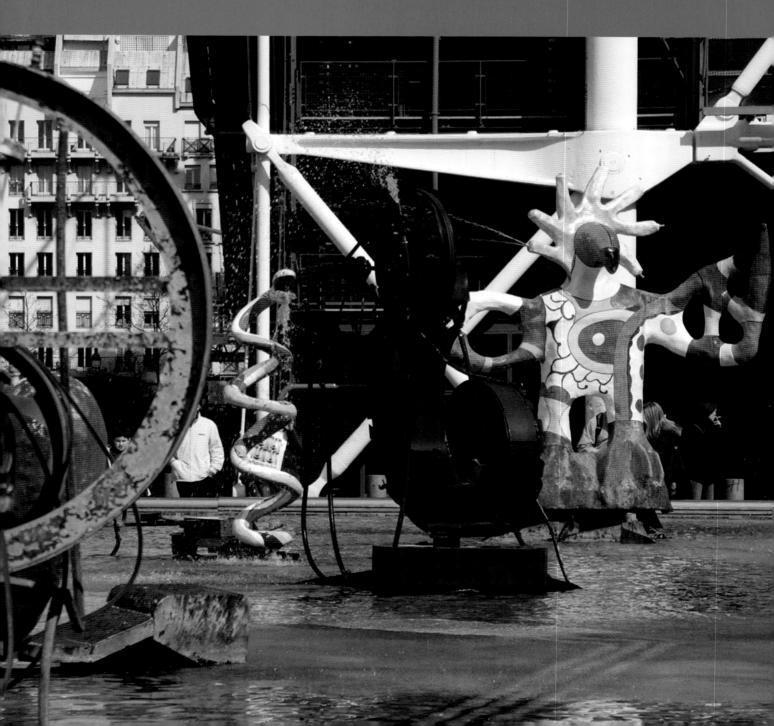

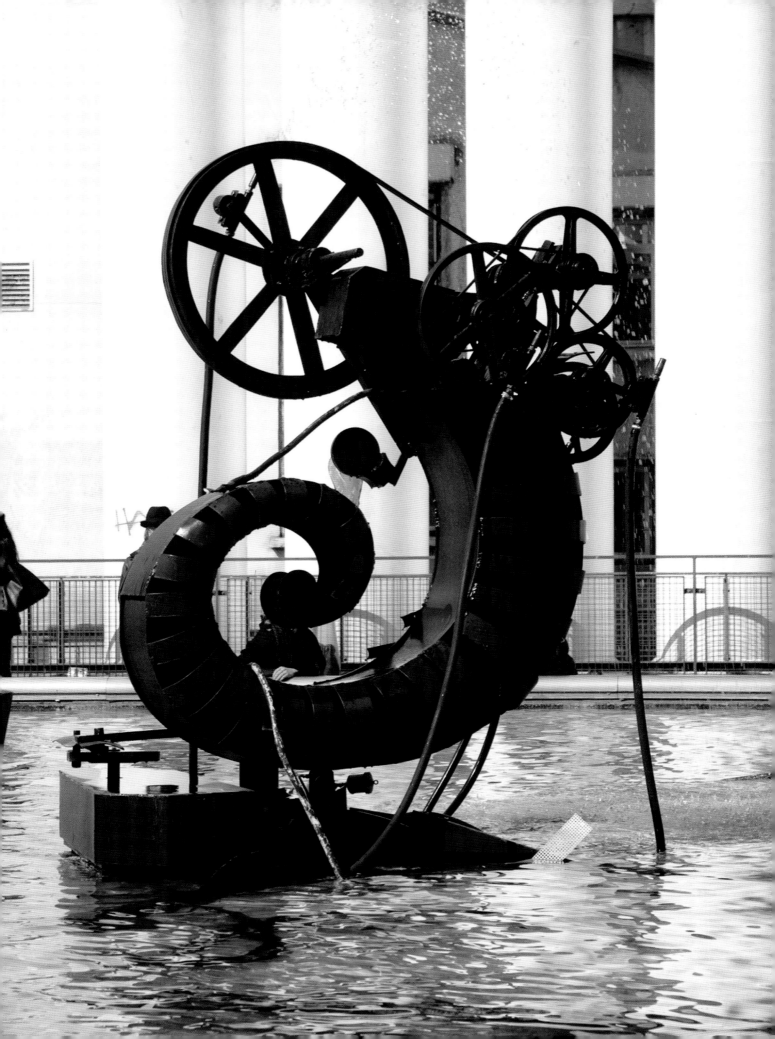

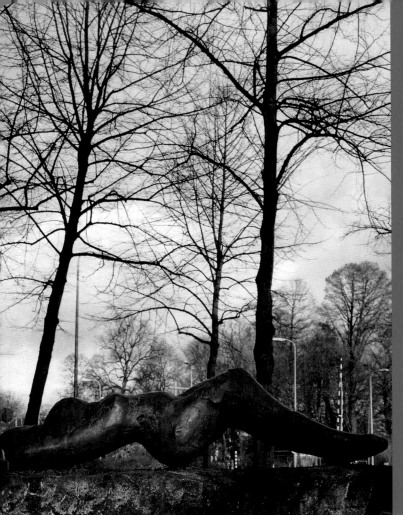

Reclining Woman
Maja van Hall

Completion: 1983. **Technique:** stone, bronze. **Location:** Utrecht, The Netherlands.

In the 1980s, when this sculpture was created, artist Maja van Hall opted for a more informal, abstract expression in material and gesture. She never entirely foreswore figuration, though, preferring the form to emerge from her subjects. The figure is made from bronze and reclines on a stone base; the figure of a woman apparently relaxing in the sun, the true nature left open to interpretation.

Maja van Hall's work is often abstract in form. She is a feminist, whose past works include a series of bound, lying and standing female figures, referring to the social restriction of women within a male dominated society. Using her personal experience as a source of creativity, Maja van Hall has built up a consistent oeuvre that pays scant heed to trends. She has allowed space for personal emotion in her sculptures, giving them a unique look.

Photo: Jannes Linders, Rotterdam

Buried Bicycle
Claes Oldenburg and Coosje van Bruggen

Completion: 1983. **Technique:** steel, aluminum, fiber-reinforced plastic, painted with polyurethane enamel. **Location:** Paris, France.

Coosje van Bruggen's thoughts on Samuel Beckett's anti-hero Molloy – who falls off his bicycle and finds himself lying in a ditch unable to recognize the object – prompted her selection of a bicycle as the subject for this piece. Her husband Claes Oldenburg decided on an invisible bicycle, with the front wheel turned slightly so that a portion would protrude above the ground, and plotted the locations of a pedal, one half of the seat, and one handlebar with a bell, using a sawed-up standard bicycle as a model.

Claes Oldenburg was born in Sweden in 1929 and is renowned for creating works of art that seek to blend fantasy and reality. Oldenburg takes objects from the everyday – a bicycle, typewriter or a flashlight and lifts them out of their usual context, forcing viewers to reassess their preconceptions of the object. Oldenburg has worked in a variety of modes, including drawing, painting, film, soft sculpture, and large scale sculpture in steel. After 1959 he was influenced by the theater.

Photos: Chris van Uffelen

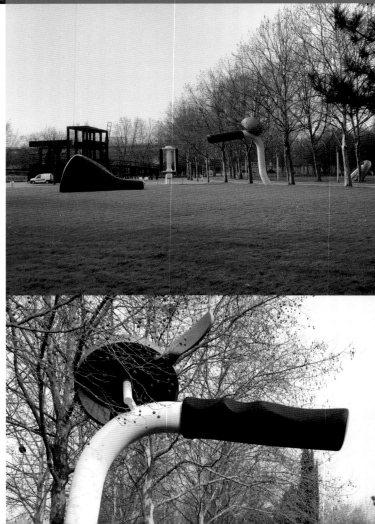

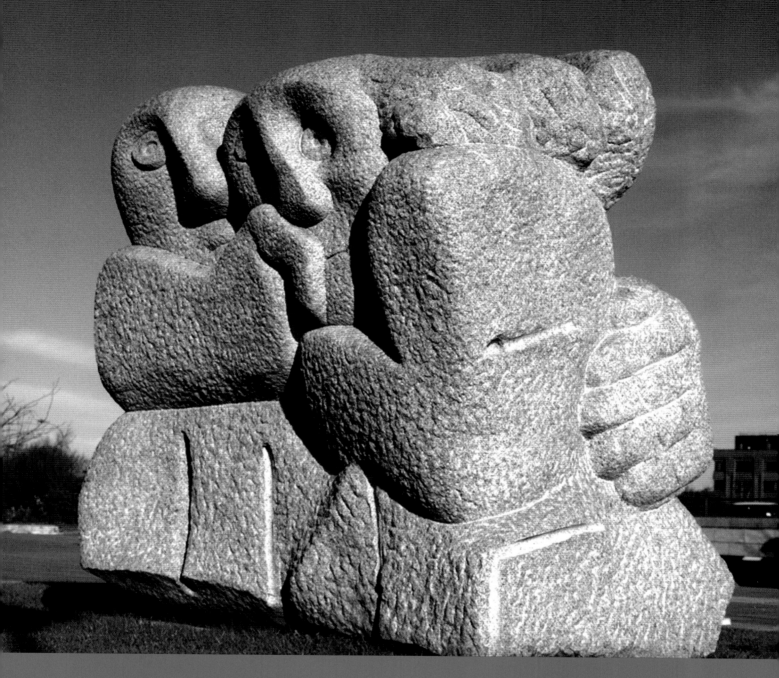

O Wert Thou in the Cauld Blast
Ronald Rae

Completion: 1984. **Technique:** granite. **Location:** Milton Keynes, United Kingdom.

This was a commission for the New Towns project and was purchased in 1999, following a major exhibition of Ronald Rae's work in the city. The sculpture is hand-carved in Creetown Scottish granite that is 391 million years old. This emotive sculpture celebrates one of Scottish poet Robert Burns' last poems, written for Jessy Lewars who nursed him during his final illness. The sculpture shows a couple comforting each other in times of trouble. In Milton Keynes the local people call it "the cuddling couple."

Ronald Rae was born in Ayr, Scotland in 1946. At the age of 15 he discovered granite. This discovery changed his life forever. Largely self-taught, he is now one of Britain's foremost sculptors, known for his powerful hand carved works in granite. Rae makes no preliminary drawings for his sculptures – instead he works intuitively to reveal what is within each stone. His sole aim is to express his care for humanity and the natural world through his sculpture. Since 1980 Rae has exhibited widely, his sculptures now in major public and private collections throughout the United Kingdom and abroad.

Pot of Gold
Jean-Pierre Raynaud

Completion: 1985. **Technique:** polyester laminate, treated steel, gilded. **Location:** Paris, France.

The "Pot of Gold" sculpture by Jean-Pierre Raynaud was made in 1985. It is one of Raynaud's most famous works and measures approximately three and a half meters in height. The sculpture is covered with gold leaf, produced by the Cartier Foundation in Paris. After being exhibited in both Japan and Berlin, the pot found a home on a pedestal in front of the Centre Pompidou in 1988.

Jean-Pierre Raynaud is a French artist, born in 1939. He actually studied horticulture but later began creating sculpture. He often uses plant pots in his sculptures and this soon became his trademark. In 1964 he exhibited his work at the Salon de la Jeune in Paris and had his first solo exhibition in 1965. In 1986 he was awarded the Grand Prize for Sculpture from the city of Paris.

Photo: Chris van Uffelen

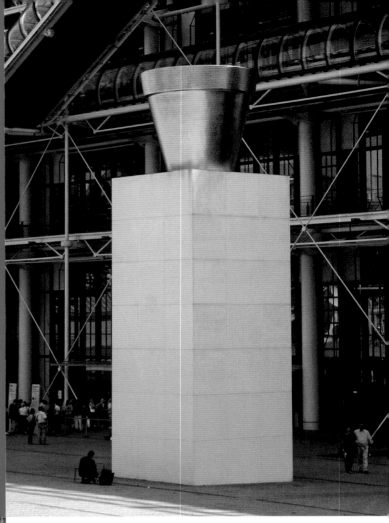

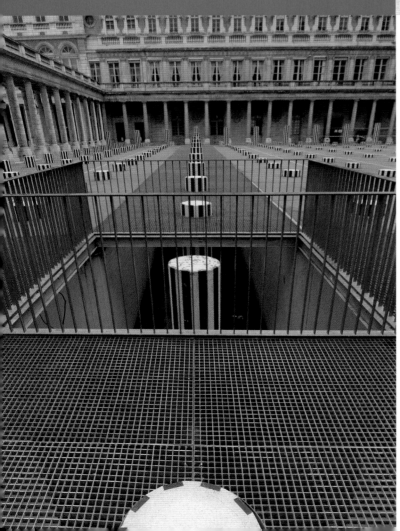

The Two Platforms
Daniel Buren

Completion: 1985. **Technique:** white and black marble. **Location:** Paris, France.

"The Two Platforms", commonly referred to as the "Buren columns", is located in the heart of the cour d'honneur of the Royal Palace, is made up of 260 black and white striped columns made of white marble from Carrera and black marble from the Pyrenees, together with a hydraulic system and a complex lighting system. Commissioned from Daniel Buren in 1985, the work has recently been restored to revive its colors and its shine. The cour d'honneur is now once again open to tourists and walkers.

Daniel Buren is a French Conceptual Artist, born in 1938. He is best known for using regular, contrasting stripes to integrate the visual surface and architectural space, visually relating art to its situation. He started by putting up hundreds of striped posters around Paris, and later in more than 100 metro stations, drawing public attention to himself through these unauthorized acts. By the 1980s Buren was exhibiting artwork in Europe, America and Japan.

Photo: Chris van Uffelen

Willow Rings
Harriet Feigenbaum

Completion: 1985. **Technique:** willow trees, landscaping.
Location: Scranton, PA, USA.

"Willow Rings" is a reclamation project. The 15 acre site is now a wetland ideal for supporting many different species of wildlife. This project was created with an artist's fellowship from National Endowment for the Arts with in-kind services from the Greater Scranton Chamber of Commerce, Scranto, Pennsylvania. The project involved willow trees, in a protective circle, enclosing a small lake in the wetland area. The young trees symbolize a new era for the area, one where the site can be reclaimed and given back to nature.

Harriet Feigenbaum attended Columbia University and the National Academy School of Fine Arts in New York. Throughout her career she has focused on sculptures and installations out-of-doors, both in rural and urban settings. Feigenbaum has developed many environmentally conscious works, spending a great deal of time in the coal mining regions of Pennsylvania. As seen in her famous Holocaust Memorial, Harriet Feigenbaum is concerned with sociopolitical issues and has exhibited extensively throughout the United States.

Photos: Courtesy of the artist

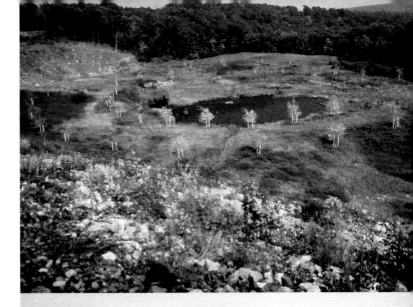

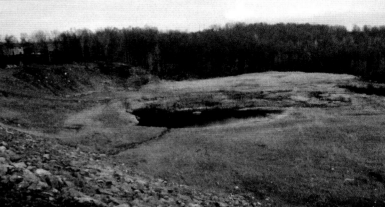

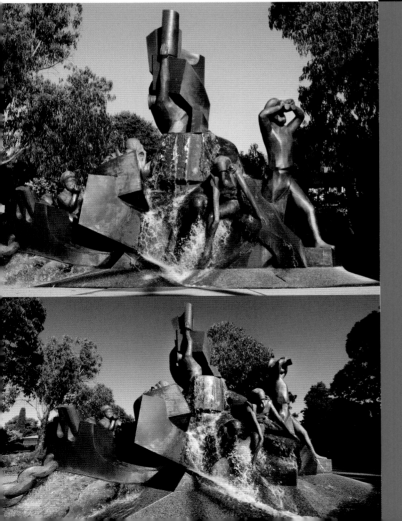

R.A.N. Memorial
Ante Dabro

Completion: 1986. **Technique:** bronze, water, concrete.
Location: Canberra, Australia.

The "Royal Australian Navy Memorial" is located on ANZAC parade, Canberra, Australia and was commissioned to celebrate the 75th Anniversary of the Royal Australian Navy. The sculpture was unveiled by Her Majesty Queen Elizabeth II on the third of March, 1986. The bronze figures show all the daily activities of navy life and are thematically complemented by the streams of water running down the sides.

Ante Dabro was born in Croatia in 1938 and migrated to Australia in 1967. He has found inspiration throughout his life in the artistic portrayal of the human figure within the European tradition, yet believes that every new work is an unending struggle with the inexpressible. A lifetime of sculpture brings fresh explorations and new challenges, but the resolution is as far away as ever. He has won numerous awards and commissions throughout the world during his long and successful career.

Photos: Lui Seselja Canberra Australia

The Double Face of the Sky
Luciano Fabro

Completion: 1986. **Technique:** marble, steel cable. **Location:** Otterlo, The Netherlands

"The Double Face of the Sky" is a large, beautifully colored piece of marble, suspended in a network of steel wires. The heavily veined stone is polished on one side and left rough on the other. "The Double Face of the Sky" refers simultaneously to the Italian sky, symbolized by the polished part, and the cloudy Dutch sky, the rougher side of the stone. Nature is of extreme importance in Fabro's work and he tackles big themes from art and culture in the wider sense, both from the past and the present.

Luciano Fabro was an Italian sculptor, Conceptualist and writer, born in Turin, 1936. He decided at the age of 12 that he wanted to become an artist and was largely self-taught Throughout his career, his artworks were accompanied by detailed writing and lecturing about its meaning. The San Francisco Museum of Modern Art held a 25-year retrospective of his work in 1992 and the Barbara Gladstone Gallery in New York has also exhibited his work in 1992.

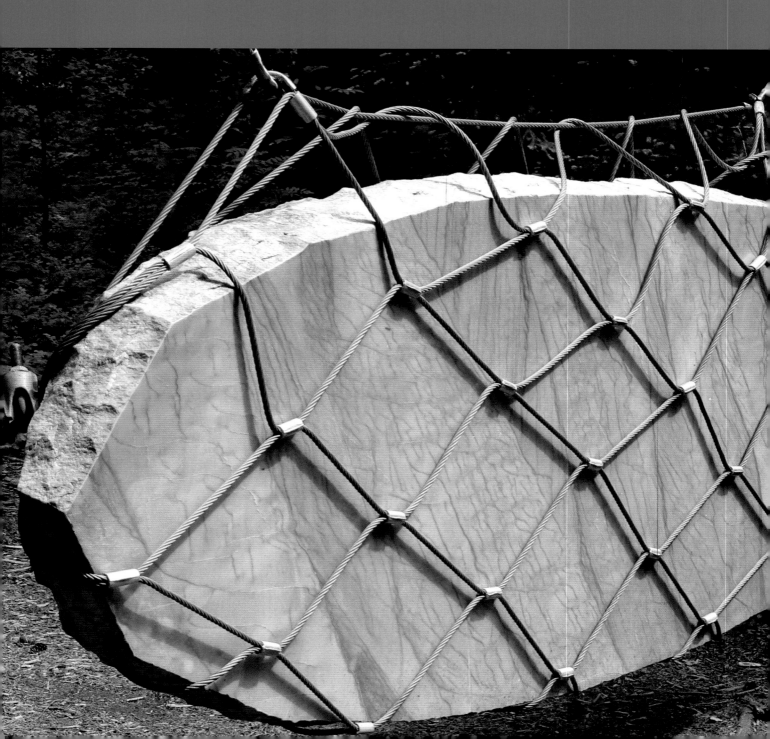

La Villette-Park Folies
Bernard Tschumi

Completion: 1986. **Technique:** painted steel. **Location:** Paris, France.

This area used to be the city's abattoir but has since been converted into a 35-hectare park. The concept has three layers: the "lines" of the path, "areas" of the gardens, and the "points" of the red folies on a grid. Most of the folies have functions, for example as kiosk or viewpoint. Besides these, they are sculptures positioned in individual spaces who refer to one another, these are inspired by the orthogonal forms of the Bauhaus Style on the one hand and of Russian Constructivism on the other.

Bernard Tschumi, born in 1944 in Lausanne, is the son of the architect Jean Tschumi. He studied in Zurich until 1969 and then began making small, modular buildings, which he also called folies. He went on to win the Parc de la Villette-competition. With his writings, teaching and buildings he is one of the leading theorists on Deconstructive Art. His La Villette work is one of the first examples of this style, using fragmentation to reinterpret or show context.

Photo: Chris van Uffelen

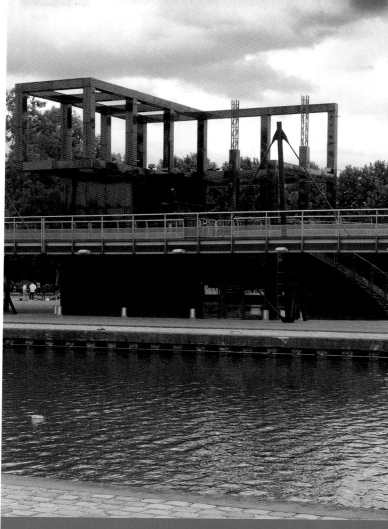

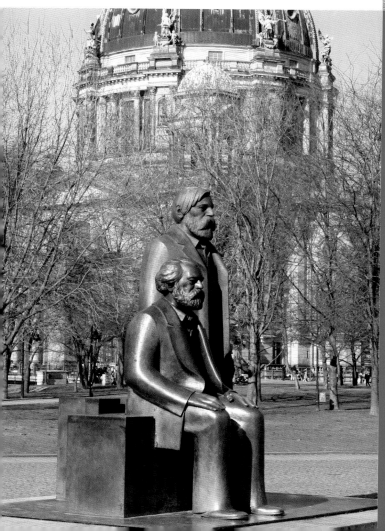

Marx-Engels-Monument and Forum
Ludwig Engelhardt

Completion: 1986. **Technique:** painted steel. **Location:** Berlin, Germany.

The whole Marx-Engels Forum was built in the former German Democratic Republic next to the Palace of the Republic. It was constructed under the supervision of the sculptor and includes various artworks, the main one being the sculpture of Karl Marx (sitting) and Friedrich Engels (standing). Since the German reunification in 1989 the appropriateness of the monument has been questioned.

Ludwig Engelhardt was born in 1924 in Saalfeld / Saale, and died in 2001 in Berlin. He first learned carpentry, from 1949–1950 before going on to study at the Berlin-Weißensee University of Art, under the tutorage of Heinrich Drake, graduating in 1956. In 1969 he taught at the Academy of Arts member, becoming head of the fine arts department in 1974, a position he held until 1978.

Photo: Bernt Rostad / Wikimedia Commons

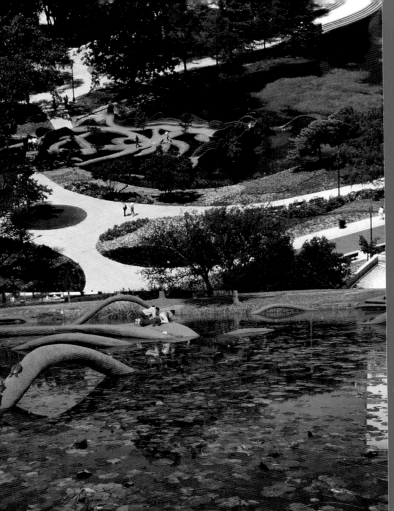

Fair Park Lagoon
Patricia Johanson

Completion: 1986. **Technique:** gunite. **Location:** Dallas, TX, USA.

"Fair Park Lagoon", one of the earliest examples of ecological artwork displayed in public, is located in Dallas, Texas. Two monumental sculptures, whose forms are inspired by plants, provide access, prevent shoreline erosion, and delineate protected wildlife habitats. Plantings filter and purify storm water while providing wildlife food and habitat. Sculptural paths, bridges islands, overlooks and seating are all incorporated into a work of art that brings visitors into intimate contact with living ecological communities.

Patricia Johanson was born in 1940. She graduated from Bennington College, Hunter College, and the City College of New York, School of Architecture. Her major projects combine art, ecology, landscaping, and infrastructure. Her most well known works include: "Endangered Garden", San Francisco; "The Draw at Sugar House" in Salt Lake City, a project that combines a safe highway crossing with flood control; and "Mary's Garden" in Scranton, Pennsylvania, which involves remediating mine-scarred land.

Photo: Courtesy of the artist

Fulcrum
Richard Serra

Completion: 1987. **Technique:** Corten steel. **Location:** London, United Kingdom.

"Fulcrum" by Richard Serra is a 17-meter-high, freestanding sculpture made of Corten steel. The sculpture is near Liverpool Street Station in London and towers over the rush-hour crowds. The design is typical of Richard Serra's Minimalist Style. The overlapping metal sheets create a small space inside, a tiny oasis of calm in the crowded street. Though not aesthetically beautiful, the size and strength of the piece gives it character, making it a landmark in the urban, corporate space.

Richard Serra is an American, Minimalist Sculptor, born in San Francisco in 1939. He first studied English Literature before going on to study art at the University of California, Santa Barbara. It wasn't until 1966 the Serra began making his first sculptures, using mainly fiberglass and rubber. Many of his later works are freestanding, large Corten steel constructions. His work is held in the collections of many museums including the Guggenheim in Bilbao and the Museum of Modern Art in New York.

Photo: Rob Sandiford

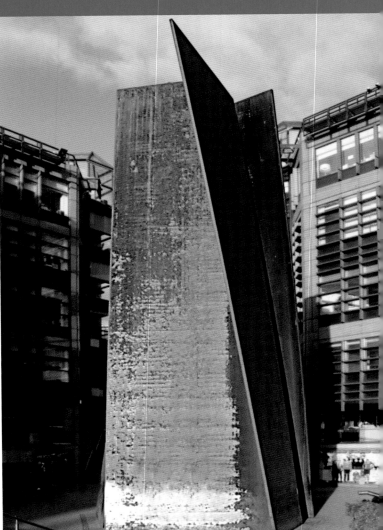

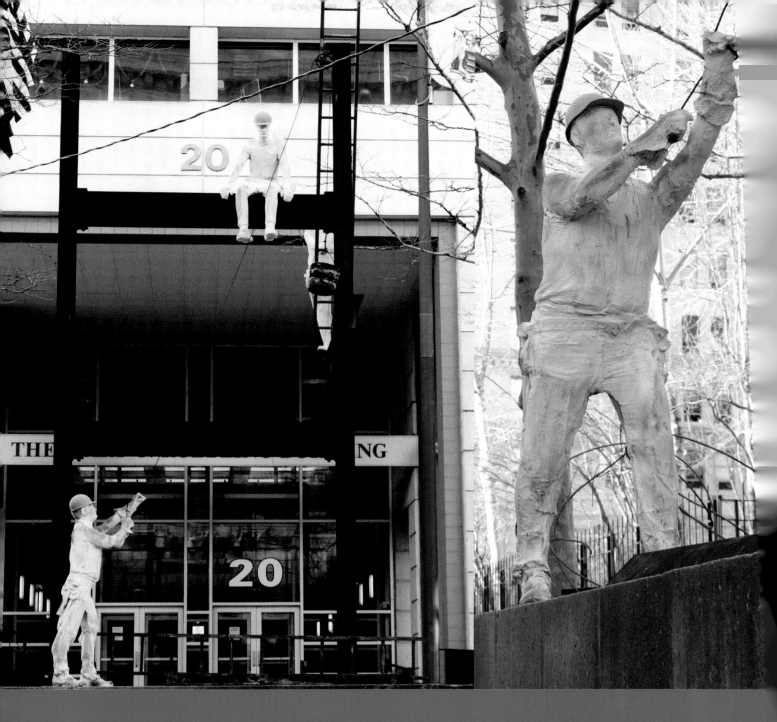

The Constructors
George Segal

Completion: 1987. **Technique:** bronze, steel. **Location:** Trenton, NJ, USA.

"The Constructors" was commissioned as part of New Jersey's Public Arts Inclusion Act, brought in 1978. This was the 36th piece to be constructed under this Act, which demands that one and a half per cent of the cost of new buildings erected by the state will be spent on public art. The sculpture centers on three bronze construction workers, working on a construction of interlocking steel beams. The sculpture is typical of George Segal's work, as his sculptures often attempted to applaud the dignity of everyday acts; like building a building.

George Segal was born in 1924 and was raised in the Bronx, before his family relocated to New Jersey. He studied at the Pratt Institute in New York and began working as an artist in 1950s, also working as a teacher at the Highland Park Community Center. He is best known for his life size sculptures of humans. Segal has been involved in creating public sculpture since 1973. His works tackle a range of subjects, including gay liberation, the Great Depression and biblical themes.

Photos: Susan Kane

Lobotchevsky
Mark di Suvero

Completion: 1987. **Technique:** steel. **Location:** Stuttgart, Germany.

This steel sculpture stands outside the adult education center in Stuttgart. It has no base, raising directly out of the concrete paving, and is reminiscent of an extended X shape. The legs are slightly tilted backwards, shifting the whole shape out of balance. Rings in the center and an arm, bent across the middle and stretching down to the floor, provides stability. The result is a balanced construction. The abstract work contrasts the surrounding architecture and adds character to the busy road intersection.

Mark di Suvero is an American Abstract Expressionist Sculptor. He was born in China in 1933 to Italian parents. The family moved to California in 1942 and he later studied philosophy at the University of California, Berkley. He moved to New York and worked in construction but was then injured in an elevator accident, in rehabilitation he began to focus his attention on sculpture. Di Suvero's work is featured in exhibitions across the world, and many of his sculptures are on display in public space.

Photo: Chris van Uffelen

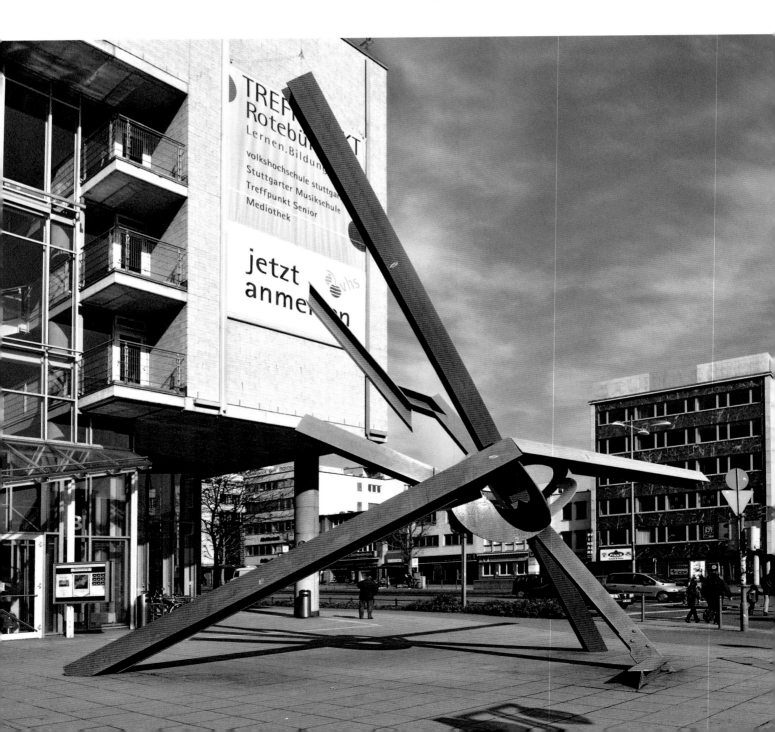

Homage to Oud and Van Doesburg
Lucien den Arend

Completion: 1987. **Technique:** concrete. **Location:** Rotterdam, The Netherlands.

In 1983 the city of Rotterdam commissioned Lucien den Arend to make a proposal for a sculpture for the subway stations on the Marconi Square on the west side of the city. Den Arend's construction is called "Homage to Oud and van Doesburg" and involves three concrete squares, each oVe is a square of seven and a half meters, 20 centimeters thick. The Spangen Housing project where Oud and van Doesburg worked is situated just around the corner from the sculpture that was named after them.

Lucien den Arend was born in Dordrecht, the Netherlands in 1943. When he was ten his family immigrated to California. He returned to Dordrecht three years later, staying for six months before returning back to America once more. He studied art and language at the California State University. He received his first sculptural commission in 1968. After graduating from university in 1969, den Arend was soon offered his first solo exhibition. He produces large sculptural works as well as landscapes sculptures.

Photos: Gerardus / Wikimedia Commons

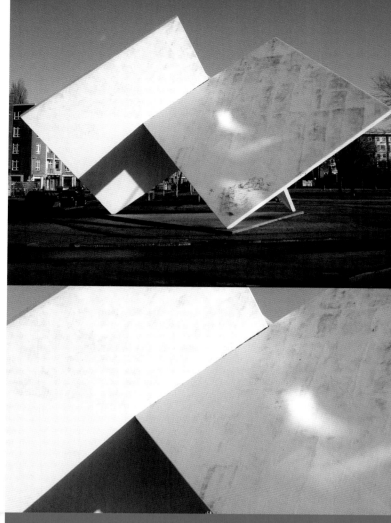

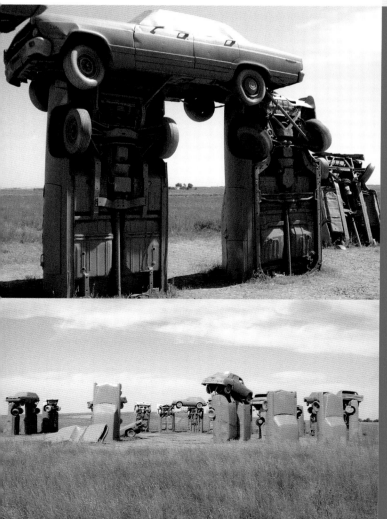

Carhenge
Jim Reinders

Completion: 1987. **Technique:** painted cars. **Location:** Alliance, NE, USA.

"Carhenge", as the name suggests, is based around the form of Stonehenge. Some of the cars are half-buried in holes of around two meters deep, while those used to form the arches are welded on; all are covered with gray spray paint. The sculpture is meant as a memorial to the artist's father and is built on the farm where he lived. The site is run and maintained by a local group called Friends of Carhenge. Additional sculptures have since been added to the site.

Jim Reinders, an artist who experimented with unusual and interesting artistic creations throughout his life, created "Carhenge". He spent some time living in England, where he had the chance to study Stonehenge. His desire to copy Stonehenge in physical size and placement was realized in the summer of 1987 with the help of many family members. Local officials threatened to tear the structure down but it was saved by local people, who have since formed the group Friends of Carhenge.

Photos: Plumbago / Wikimedia Commons

115

Rounded Blue
Rupprecht Geiger

Completion: 1987. **Technique:** lacquered aluminum. **Location:** Munich, Germany.

Rupprecht Geiger's "Rounded Blue" is a strong, single-color sculpture, typical of the artist. Geiger deliberately avoids mixed colors, using only red, blue or yellow for his sculptures. Here, it is the color that is the theme more than the shape or technique. The color works to make the material lighter in appearance. It contrasts the orange brickwork of the architecture and looks almost as if a piece of the sky has fallen, and landed, capable of rolling away at any moment.

Rupprecht Geiger was born in Munich 1908 and died in 2009. Between 1926 and 1935 he studied and taught architecture and art at academic institutions in Munich; he later worked as an architect. He served in World War II and then worked as a war illustrator in the Ukraine and Greece. He was appointed as a professor at the State Academy of Art in Dusseldorf from 1965 until 1976. His paintings and sculptures are often focused on color and characterized by geometric forms, single colors and strong contrasts.

Photo: Chris van Uffelen

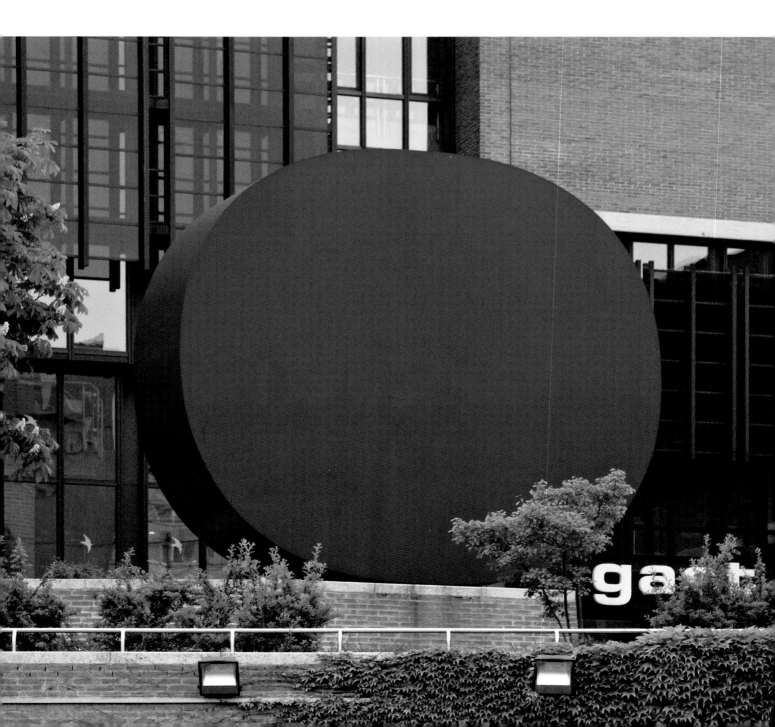

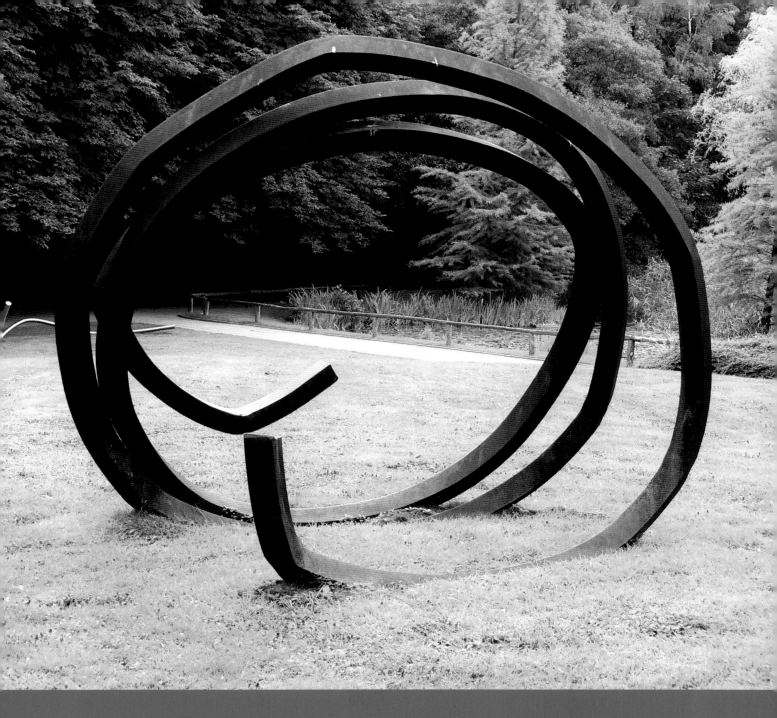

Undetermined Line
Bernar Venet

Completion: 1987. **Technique:** steel. **Location:** Bottrop, Germany.

The "Lines" series are the most spontaneous work in Venet's sculptural oeuvre. He has explored several different themes within his works and these all give very different impressions. His "Angles", "Bows" and "Diagonals" all work with exact mathematical forms whereas the "Lines" series takes the appearance more of hand-drawn gestures – begun somewhere and ending by chance somewhere else. They are undefined shapes, with the potential to evolve into something else before the eyes of the viewer.

Bernar Venet was born in France in 1941. He studied in Nizza at the School of Formative Arts and was later employed as a stage builder at the Opera House. In 1964 he participated in the "Salon Comparaison" at the Museum of Modern Art in Paris. Venet's sculptures are held in private and museum collections but many examples of his work can also be found on display in public space.

Photo: Gerardus / Wikimedia Commons

Red Dog for Landois
Keith Haring

Completion: 1987. **Technique:** steel. **Location:** Ulm, Germany.

"Red Dog for Landois" was originally located at Münster Zoo but currently stands in front of the Weishaupt Art Gallery in Ulm. The sculpture depicts a two-dimensional, fiery-red dog and is made out of steel. It was dedicated to Landois, a famous professor from Münster. The "Red Dog" shows a simplified silhouette, typical of Haring's style, with the animal's two ears positioned at a 90 degree angel to its mouth.

Keith Haring is an American artist whose artistic work was greatly influenced by graffiti. He was born in Reading, Pennsylvania in 1958 and died in 1990. He studied at the School of Visual Arts in New York and was friends with Andy Warhol. He painted walls in Amsterdam, Paris und Phoenix, amongst others and he also painted Checkpoint Charlie in Berlin in 1986. As Pop Artist he opened Pop Shops in New York and Tokyo.

Photo: Chris van Uffelen

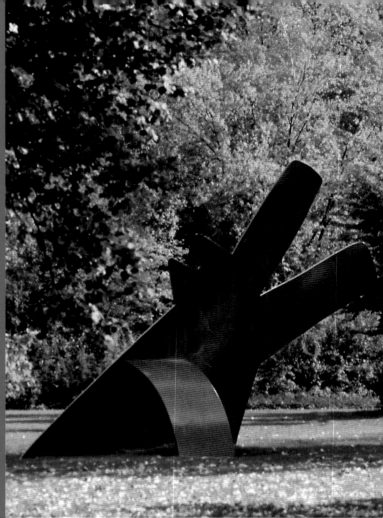

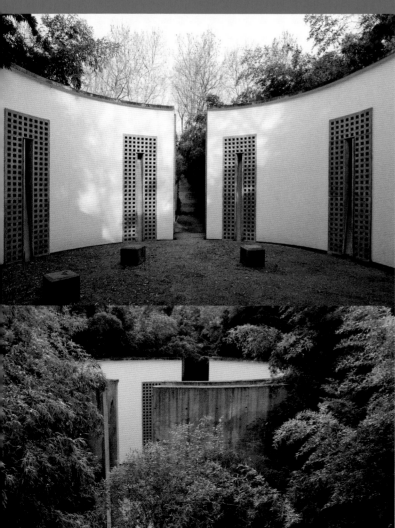

The Sound Cylinder
Bernhard Leitner

Completion: 1987. **Technique:** concrete. **Location:** Paris, France.

This work, commissioned as a piece of public art, is situated in front of the bamboo garden in the Parc de la Villette in Paris. Sounds can be heard from the outside of this room, attracting passersby. The cylindrical space serves foremost as a sound chamber, consolidating sound by means of weight and tension between the curved walls. Water runs down in narrow rivulets, trickling into a basin lower down. The sound spaces in this work are concealed behind eight, perforated concrete elements.

Bernhard Leitner was born in Austria in 1938 and studied at the University of Technology in Vienna from 1956 to 1963. He moved to New York in 1968 and worked as an urban designer before becoming associate professor at New York University. He taught at the University of Applied Arts in Vienna and was awarded the City of Vienna Prize for the Visual Arts in 1999.

Photos: Chris van Uffelen

Cherry Column
Thomas Schütte

Completion: 1987. **Technique:** sandstone, painted aluminum cherry. **Location:** Münster, Germany.

This sculpture is over six meters high and was purchased by the city of Münster where it is now on permanent display. The column is made of sandstone and the two cherries on the top are of painted aluminum. The sandstone column blends in with the architecture of Münster and appears old but is not really, like much of the surroundings. The cherries contrast the column, mixing styles and perhaps mocking classic styles and idolization.

Thomas Schütte is a German sculptor and artist, born in 1954 in Oldenburg. He studied at the Art Academy in Dusseldorf, graduating in 1981. He began sculpting in the 1980s and his first work was a series, depicting men stuck in mud. His work ranges widely, encompassing everything from small-scale models and figures to large installations. He has exhibited his work across Germany and Europe and was awarded the Golden Lion for Best Artist at the Venice Biennial in 2005.

Photo: Chris van Uffelen

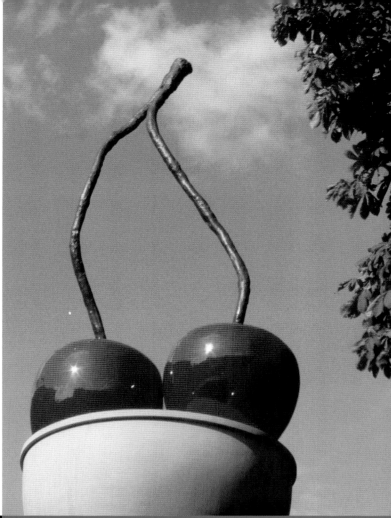

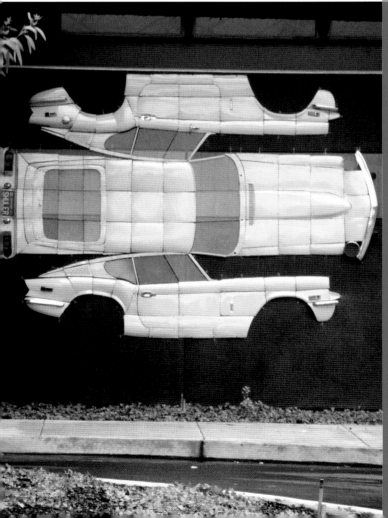

Triumph Pelt
Dustin Shuler

Completion: 1988. **Technique:** painted steel, plexiglas, chrome. **Location:** San Jose, CA, USA.

The "Triumph Pelt" is an artwork created by Dustin Shuler and is a contemporary analog to an animal hide rug, it is a trophy specimen of the modern day herd, seen migrating on the freeways. The "Triumph Pelt" is currently in the collection of the San Jose Department of Motor Vehicles and is displayed on the side of their building. It was commissioned by the California Arts Council and is one of several such works displayed across California.

Dustin Shuler was born in 1948 in Wilkinsburg, Pennsylvania. From 1968–1971 Shuler attended evening art classes at the Carnegie Institute of Technology, while also working full time for Westinghouse Electric Corporation. In 1971 he left Westinghouse and began working as a sculptor. Immigrating to California in 1973, Shuler gained recognition as a sculptor and held numerous solo exhibitions, as well as participating in various national and international group exhibitions.

Photo: Courtesy of the artist

Bird Totem
Adrian Mauriks

Completion: 1988. **Technique:** bronze. **Location:** Sydney, Australia.

"Bird Totem" consists of two tall upright shapes, which form the lower part of the sculpture. This is capped by sweeping, outstretched outlines that could be seen as wings or arms. The entire piece creates an impression of massive weight, but the height and the sharp angular forms enliven the visual effect. A surprising lightness provided by the vertical movement upwards through the center of the work provides a sense of dynamism to the large forms.

Adrian Mauriks studied as an undergraduate and later as postgraduate, at the Victoria College of the Arts in Australia, majoring in fine art. In 1997 he was invited to work in one of the guest studios at Foundation Art & Complex in Rotterdam. He has since participated in many group exhibitions such as the McClelland Sculpture Survey and Award Exhibition 2003 and 2010. Mauriks was also a finalist for the Helen Lempriere National Sculpture Award in 2006.

Photos: Adrian J Mauriks

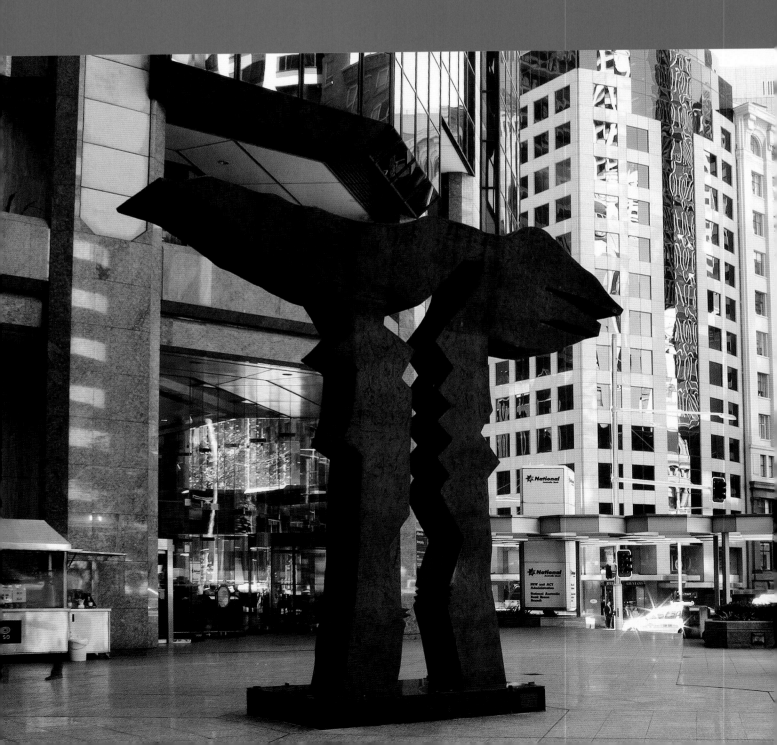

St George and the Dragon
Michael Sandle

Completion: 1988. **Technique:** bronze. **Location:** London, United Kingdom.

"St George and the Dragon" was made by Michael Sandle assisted by Uwe Buechler, Herman Berger and Simon Stringer. St George is placed on a sloping grille, on top of a tower with his spear pointed down through the grille, towards the dragon. The dragon has three brass tongues, curling threateningly around the sculpture. The piece arose from Sandle's wish to create something new that was also instantly recognizable. It also fulfilled his desire to revisit and re-evaluate the sculpture of the 19th century.

Michael Sandle was born in Dorset in 1936. He studied at the Douglas School of Art and Technology on the Isle of Man and attended evening classes at Chester College of Art during his two years National Service in the Royal Artillery. Sandle taught at leading art schools throughout the 1960s, in Alberta and British Columbia, Canada and later in Germany. He has exhibited his work widely and undertaken many commissions. In 1986 he was awarded the Rodin Grand Prize, Japan's most prestigious contemporary art award.

Photo: Rob Sandiford

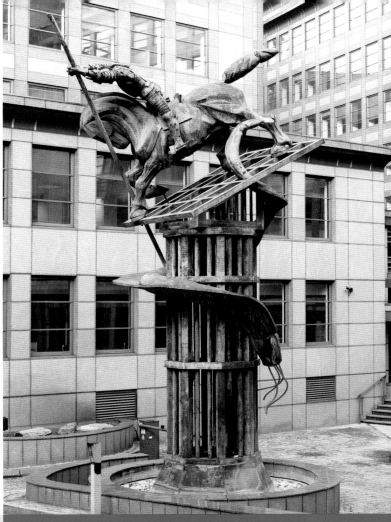

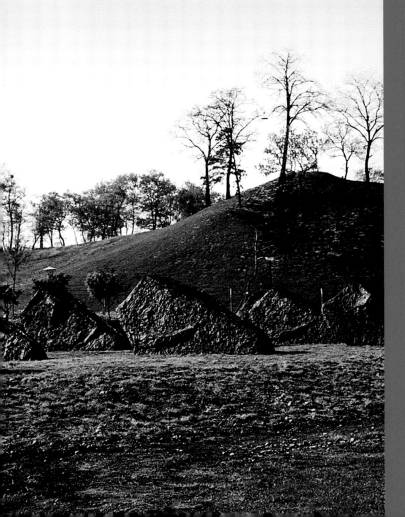

Space of Dragon
Magdalena Abakanowicz

Completion: 1988. **Technique:** bronze. **Location:** Seoul, South Korea.

This work by Magdalena Abakanowicz is part of the Olympic Park in Seoul and took part in the Olympic Arts contest. It consists of ten forms of about 220 x 450 x 220 centimeters, made of bronze and gathered together in a small group. At first glance they seem abstract, but on the second glance one recognizes them as somehow familiar; by identifying hollows as eye sockets and sharp edges as cheekbones suddenly they become identifiable as fossilized dinosaur or dragonheads.

Magdalena Abakanowicz was born in Falenty, Poland, in 1930 and studied at the Academy of Fine Arts in Warsaw, from 1950 to 1954. In the 1960s she create monumental three-dimensional, woven forms called "Abakans" and in the following decade her "Alterations" consisted of huge sculptures made out of burlap and resins. Since the 1980s Abakanowicz forms series of monumental sculptures using bronze, stone, wood and iron. The figures are metaphorical, often without heads.

Photo: Courtesy of the artist

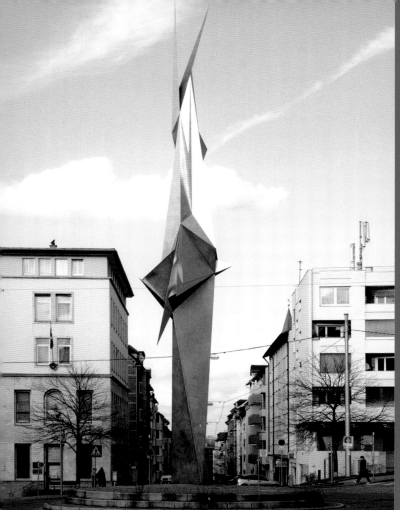

6-87/88
Erich Hauser

Completion: 1988. **Technique:** polished stainless steel.
Location: Stuttgart, Germany.

The over 18-meter-tall stainless steel sculpture, "6-87/88" is made from lots of single, triangular forms. These forms are not all the same but work together to create an elegant work that reaches up towards the sky. The whole composition of the piece offers the observer a new view from every angle. The point of the triangle is created from two large, elongated tetrahedrons, positioned against each other. The effect of the light works to soften the sharp-edged sculpture.

The German sculptor Erich Hauser, was born in 1930 and died in 2004. Hauser completed an apprenticeship as a steel engraver before he began working as a freelance artist. He received international recognition after he was awarded the Art Prize at the São Paulo Art Biennial. He was a member of the Academy of Art in Berlin from 1970–1986.

Photo: Chris van Uffelen

Untitled 1988
Richard Artschwager

Completion: 1988. **Technique:** concrete. **Location:** Rotterdam, The Netherlands.

This work is comprised of two concrete objects, 15 centimeters thick and sculpted into peaked forms. The organic forms of this sculpture contrast the urban setting and the abstract form leaves it open to wide interpretation. The piece was made specifically for this site, as part of Rotterdam's Sculptures in the City program.

Richard Artschwager was born in Washington D.C. in 1923. He studied at Cornell University and was taught painting by the Cubist painter Amédée Ozenfant. His style has been described as Hyper-realist and is often also extremely abstract. His paintings and drawings were exhibited at the Terrain gallery in 1957. He had his first solo exhibition in 1965 and participated in the annual sculptural exhibition at the Whitney Museum of Modern Art in 1968.

Photo: K. Siereveld / Wikimedia Commons

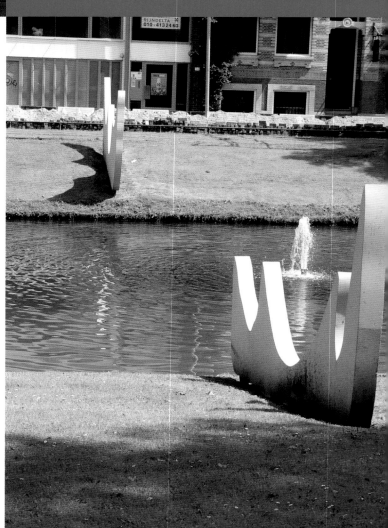

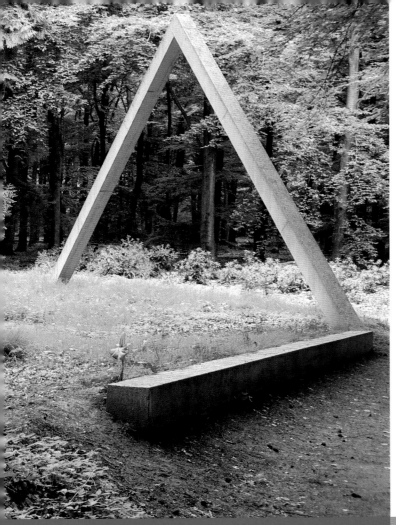

The Flat Bland
François Morellet

Completion: 1988. **Technique:** concrete. **Location:** Otterlo, The Netherlands.

"The Flat Bland" is a concrete sculpture by François Morellet. It stands in the sculpture garden of the Kröller-Müller Museum in the Netherlands. The sculpture is positioned on the conjunction of a corner, mimicking the curve of the path and turning it upside down, creating a new path in the air. The sculpture draws attention to the corner and presents another possibility, taking what is mundane and making it thought provoking. Morellet also often worked with neon tubing, creating abstract light sculptures.

François Morellet is a contemporary French sculptor, born in Maine-et-Loire in 1926. Morellet's earlier work was more figurative in style and it wasn't until the 1950s that he turned to abstraction. His work often involves simple forms; straight lines, squares and triangles, assembled as two dimensional compositions. His later work has been influential in the field of geometrical abstraction over the past 50 years.

Photo: Gerardus / Wikimedia Commons

Tibesti
Jean Verame

Completion: 1989. **Technique:** painted rocks. **Location:** Tibesti desert, Chad.

During a period of three months, Jean Verame utilized 30 tons of blue, violet, red and white paint to complete this work of Land Art. The bright colors are not meant to denaturalize the eroded rocks in any way, but to emphasize the individual vivacity of the sometimes bizarre formations, highlighting tiny individualities which may otherwise have gone unnoticed. The painted rocks stand out from the surroundings, drawing attention to themselves in the dry landscape.

Artist Jean Verame is also known as the painter of deserts, his monumental artwork is now part of the collective culture. With Land Art projects in Morocco and Chad, Verame enters into an intense dialogue with the desert. Verame's artwork is a meditative interaction with nature, interpreting what is already there into a language of color. Often compared to Christo, Jean Verame offers a different approach to contemporary painting: his mountains will last for at least 100 years.

Photo: Courtesy of the artist

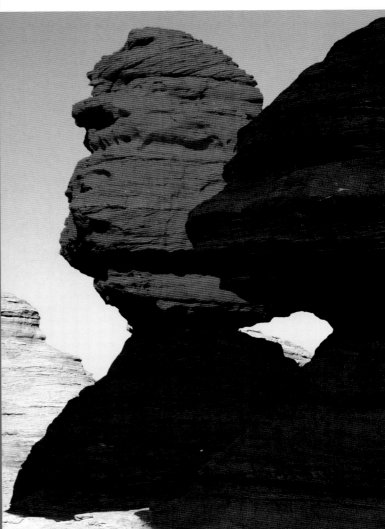

Cloud on the Great Arch
Johann Otto von Spreckelsen

Completion: 1989. **Technique:** textile. **Location:** Paris, France.

"Cloud on the Great Arch" is a work of textile art that is suspended from the "Great Arch" in Paris. The design was decided by a competition in 1982. The winners, Johann Otto von Spreckelsen and Danish engineer, Erik Reitzel wanted to create a modern "Arc de Triomphe", but as a monument to humanity and humanitarian ideals, rather than to military victories. The arch is an almost perfect cube, and is rotated slightly on its axis.

Johann Otto von Spreckelsen was a Danish architect, born in 1929. He studied at the Royal Academy of Arts in Copenhagen and was later appointed as director, a position that he held until his death in 1987. He built several churches in Denmark but is best known for "The Great Arch" in Paris. After his retirement the responsibility for finishing this project was given to his associate, Paul Andreu. Andreu is a French architect, best known for having planned numerous airports worldwide.

Photos: Chris van Uffelen

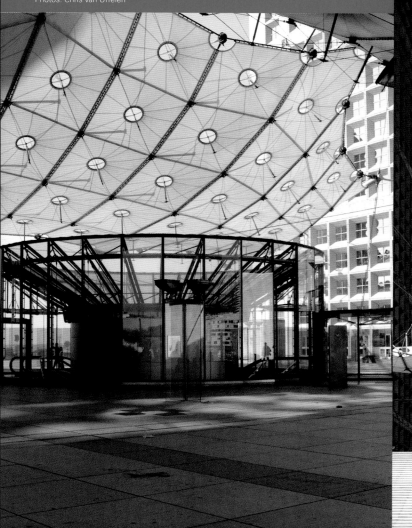

Two kinked Stele
Stefan Wewerka

Completion: 1989. **Technique:** steel. **Location:** Munich, Germany.

Standing both right and left of the tunnel entrance on the side of the motorway in Munich are these two, painted metal sculptures by Stefan Wewerka. The sculptures point specifically to areas of interest in the city, for example the Nuenhofener Berg, with its round-temple, dedicated to the memory of Air Force victims of World War II. The sculptures draw the attention of passersby to things that may otherwise have gone unnoticed.

Stefan Wewerka is the second son of the sculptor Rudolph Wewerka and was born in Wilhelmstadt in 1928. After the end of the World War II, he went to work in his father's studio for six months between 1945 and 1946. He then studied architecture at the University of Art in Berlin and built the International Student House at Eichkamp in 1949, together with Werner Rausch. Wewerka began to work building steel sculptures in 1983 and has constructed various sculptural works in public space.

Photo: Courtesy of the artist

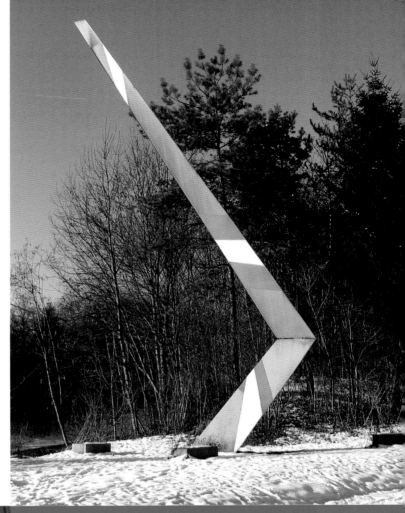

Looking Towards the Avenue
Jim Dine

Completion: 1989. **Technique:** bronze. **Location:** New York City, NY, USA.

These three bronze sculptures are a reference to the famous "Venus de Milo", one of the most famous examples of ancient Greek sculpture. They are incorporated into the fountain. The sculpting of the lower half suggests movement, as if they are wading through the water's cool depths. The sculptures are different sizes, the two smaller ones stand facing towards the 53rd Street side of the block, while the larger figure stands towards the 52nd Street side.

Jim Dine is an American Pop Artist. He first gained respect in the art world with his Happenings, which he pioneered in collaboration with Claes Oldenburg, Alan Kaprow and John Cage. The first of these events was "The Smiling Worker" in 1959. Dine is largely considered to be one of the fathers of the Pop Art movement and his work was included in the New Painting of Common Objects exhibition at the Norton Simon Museum, considered to be one of America's first Pop Art exhibitions.

Photo: Chris van Uffelen

Large Stele
Heinz Mack

Completion: 1989. **Technique:** steel. **Location:** Stuttgart, Germany.

The "Large Stele" sculpture is approximately 42 meters high and has adorned the entrance to the Mercedes Benz plant in Stuttgart since 1989. It was important for the artist that the sculpture portrayed meaning in a simple way. The vertical lines of the sculpture appear to divide the landscape. It is made from polished, stainless steel and reflects the daylight. When the light is strong enough, rays of light bounce from the structure, creating interesting patterns of light and shadow.

Heinz Mack was born in Hessen in 1931 and, from 1945 onwards, was one of Germanys most important sculptors. In 1950 he began studying at the Art Academy in Dusseldorf, later going on to study philosophy in Cologne. In 1956 he completed his education with a degree in art education. His work shows an interest in optical illusion in minimal form. He was a member of the internationally renowned Zero group and has also designed countless sculptures for public space.

Photos: Chris van Uffelen

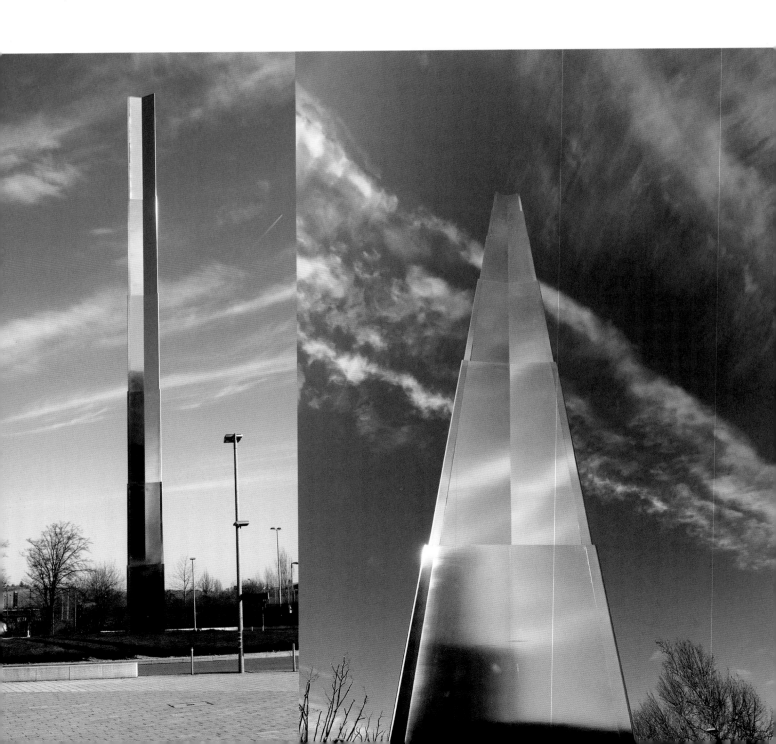

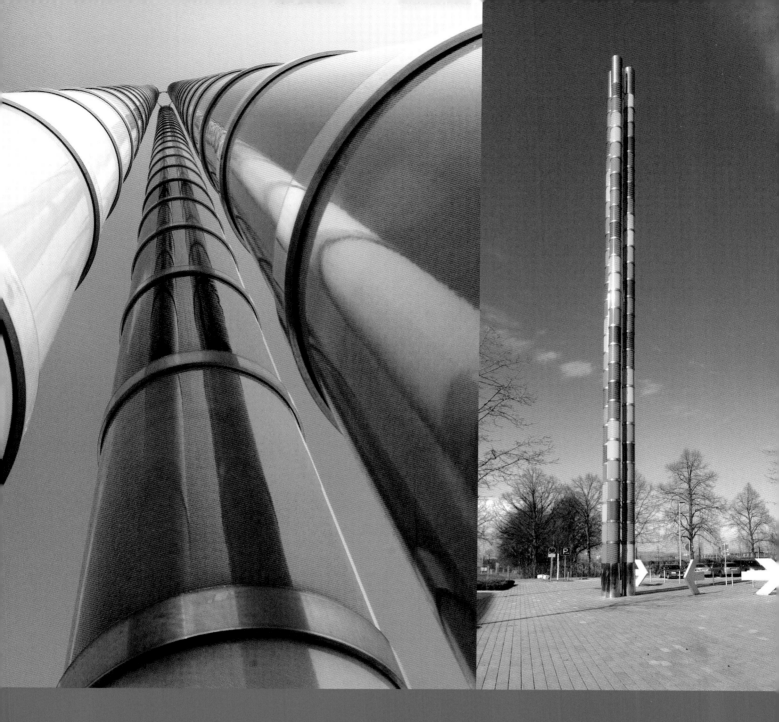

Ornamental Column - Triad
Max Bill

Completion: 1989. **Technique:** enamel on steel. **Location:** Stuttgart, Germany.

This Sculpture "Ornamental Column – Triad" was built in 1989 and references the Mercedes star in its design. The artist's goal was to combine painting, architecture and sculpture together into one art form. The colors of the sculpture are an expansion of the traditional color wheel and every column is painted with a different shade. As each column begins with a different color the spectra run against each other. To prevent the colors merging together, each of the sections is separated by a steel band.

Max Bill was a Swiss architect, artist and designer. He was born in 1908 in Switzerland and died in 1994 in Berlin. He studied at the Bauhaus Institute in Dessau, where he was taught by Wassily Kandinsky and Paul Klee. Between 1932 and 1937 he was a member of the Abstraction-Creation movement in Paris and in 1938 became a member of the International Congress of Modern Architecture. He went on to teach at the School of Applied Arts in Zurich and later co-founded the School of Design in Ulm.

Photos: Chris van Uffelen

Gateway III
Klaus Duschat

Completion: 1990. **Technique:** rusted steel. **Location:** Wilhelmshaven, Germany.

"Gateway III" stands in the northern part of Adalbert square in Wilhelmshaven, Germany. The sculpture is nearly five meters in height and made from steel. It stands in close proximity to the Art Gallery of Wilhelmshaven and is on loan from the artist. It is tilted slightly and takes the form of Roman architecture. The sculpture evokes the idea of classical architecture while at the same time revisiting and modernizing it, using industrial material to give it a new meaning.

Klaus Duschat was born in South Africa in 1955. He studied sculpture in Hanover, later going on to study at the University of Art in Berlin under sculptor, Bernhard Heiliger. Duschat founded the group Odious, together with Klaus Hartman, Gisela von Bruchhausen, Hartmut Stielow, Gustav Reinhardt and David Lee Thompson. The six artists worked together in Berlin, regularly exhibiting works as a group. Duschat often uses waste materials to create his sculptures.

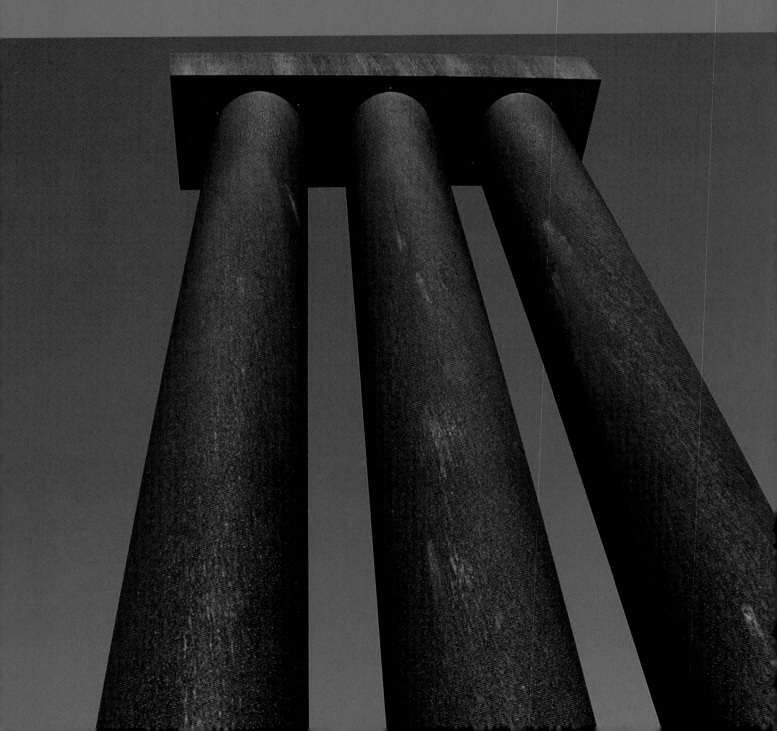

Untitled
Anne und Patrick Poirier

Completion: 1990. **Technique:** stainless steel. **Location:** Munich, Germany.

This piece is part of a four piece sculptural ensemble. The column is untitled, though the three other sections are named: the "Eye of History", the "Eye of Memory" and the "Eye of Forgetting". The ensemble stands in front of the city archives building in Munich. "Untitled" is an eight and a half meter, stainless steel column, positioned on a stone base. It is divided into seven sections, balanced unevenly one on top of each other.

Anne and Patrick Poirier are a French art duo. Anne was born in 1942 in Marseille and Patrick in 1942 in Nantes. They both studied at the School of Fine Arts in Paris, graduating in 1966. They won the Rome Prize and subsequently lived in the Villa Medici in Rome, as fellows of the French Academy in Rome. They work with a variety of artistic media, including photography, drawing, installation and monumental public sculpture. There work is often connected with memory, archeology, ruins, loss and remembering.

Photo: Chris van Uffelen

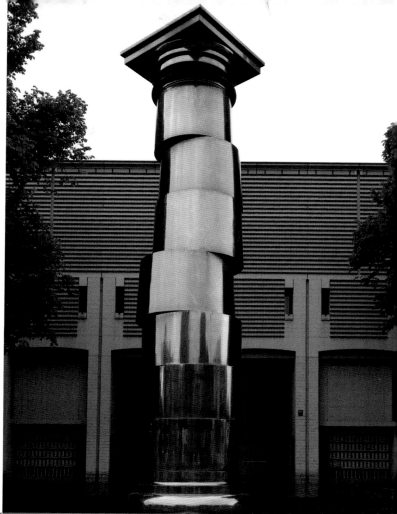

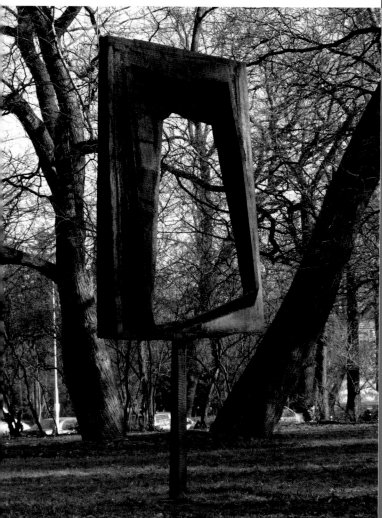

Iron Window
Ventsislav Zankov

Completion: 1990. **Technique:** iron . **Location:** Sofia, Bulgaria.

"Iron Window" was finished soon after the socialist utopia failed. The tension between iron on the one hand, and window on the other, is intensified by the act of placing it in an open, green area. The artist invites art out into public spaces, encouraging freedom of expression in the aftermath of social change. "Iron Window" is among the first works that broke free from the gravity of ideological art promoted by totalitarian power and stepped out into public space.

Ventsislav Zankov was born in 1962 in Sofia. He studied sculpture, graduating from the National Academy of Arts in Sofia, Bulgaria in 1988. He works with different media, including painting, sculpture, video, installation, performance and new media. Zankov is part of the pioneering generation of contemporary artists who promoted and worked to protect freedom of expression, after the social changes in 1989.

Photo: Courtesy of the artist

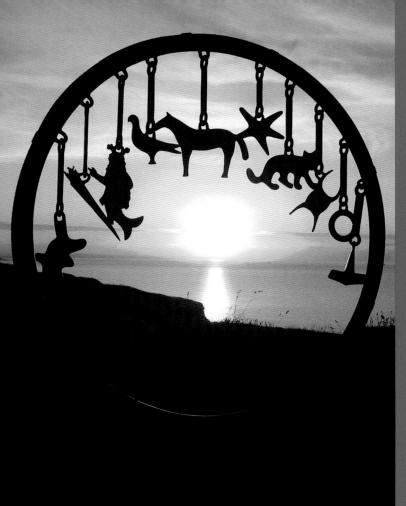

Circle on Huntcliff
Richard Farrington

Completion: 1990. **Technique:** steel. **Location:** Saltburn by the Sea, United Kingdom.

This sculpture was commissioned as a Milestone Commission from Common Ground. The project was inspired by ideas about locally distinctive features in the landscape and was the first time the artist had got involved in public art. The artist used steel rolled from the local steel rolling mill in nearby Skinningrove where he worked. He forged the sculpture himself; forging flame cut pairs of steel plates that he welded together. A local film crew documented the work in a program called Elements.

Richard Farrington was born in London in 1956. He studied at the Bath Academy of Art, graduating with a degree in sculpture in 1978. Farrington has worked as a freelance sculptor since 1984, receiving numerous commissions for both public and private works. He has exhibited his work widely, including at the Chichester Cathedral Festival exhibitions, with the Hampshire Museum Service and at the Craft Council gallery. His current work in steel explores the 'organic' potential of the material and the freedom to work spontaneously, creating exciting small scale sculptures.

Photo: Courtesy of the artist

Pre-Bell-Man
Nam June Paik

Completion: 1990. **Technique:** old TVs, radios, transistors, metal. **Location:** Frankfurt / Main, Germany.

"Pre-Bell-Man" stands outside the Communications Museum in Frankfurt / Main, Germany. The sculpture is of a mounted rider, robotic in form, atop a more classical horse form. The robot is made from scrap metal, old transistors, radios and TVs. The name is a reference to Alexander Bell, who invented the telephone and the rider is a reference to the pre-telecommunications era when riders delivered messages. At night the body of the robot is lit by brightly-colored neon lights.

Nam June Paik was an American artist, born in Korea in 1932. He died in 2006. He is thought to be the first Video Artist and worked with a variety of media throughout his career. He was trained as a classical pianist and lived in Korea until 1950 when his family had to flee from their home during the Korean War. He then lived in Japan before moving to Germany and later to America. In New York, he began working with cellist Charlotte Moorman, combining music, video and performance.

Photo: Chris van Uffelen

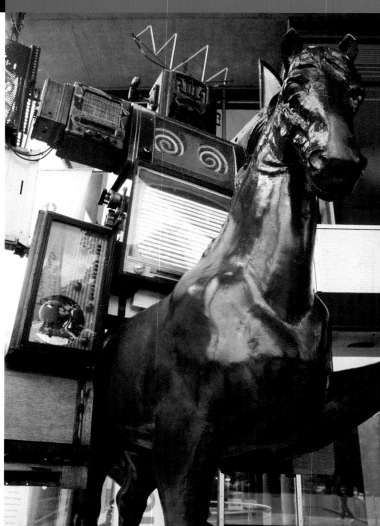

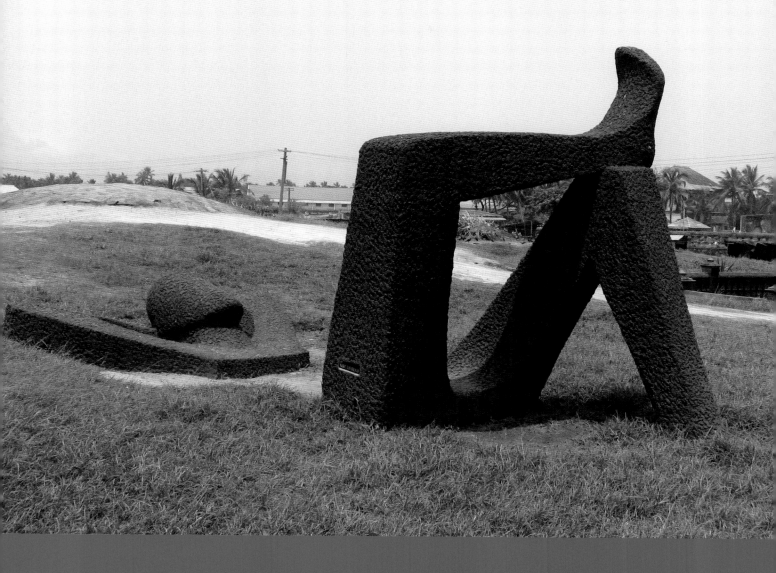

Relaxation
Kanai Kunhiraman

Completion: 1990. **Technique:** concrete. **Location:** Thiruvnanthapuram, India.

"Relaxation" is a large sculpture of a figure reclining in the sun, located on Sanghumukham Beach, Trivandrum. The sculpture is made of concrete and, as with most of Kunhiraman's sculptures, it is very large. Another of the artist's famous works, "Mermaid" is also situated along this beach and was the subject of some controversy because of her nude appearance.

Kanai Kunhiraman is one of Indian's most renowned sculptors. He was born in 1937 in the Kasargod district of Kerala, India and has been employed as Raja Shilpi's royal sculptor for over 50 years. He left home at the age of 17 and went on to study at the Government College of Arts and Crafts in Chennai. He received the Commonwealth scholarship in 1965 and traveled to England to study at the Slade School of Fine Art. On his return to India, he quickly gained a favorable reputation for his sculpture "Malampuzha Yakshi".

Video Clip Folly
Coop Himmelb(l)au

Completion: 1990. **Technique:** steel. **Location:** Delfzijl, The Netherlands..

The Folly offers space for 40 spectators. It was made as both a piece of art and platform to show videos for the "What a Wonderful World" video festival in Groningen. It was relocated to Delfzijl in 2003. The ramp, offering access to the open room functions is clamped between earth and the screen wall, like a drawn catapult.

Wolf D. Prix, born in 1942 in Vienna, Helmut Swiczinsky, born in 1944 in Pozna, and Michael Holzer, who left in 1971, established Coop Himmelb(l)au in 1968 working in the fields of architecture, art and design. The company's name is a mixture of the business abbreviation for cooperative, and the word "sky" (Himmel) and "blue" (blau) or construction (bau)". In 1988 their work was displayed at the exhibition of deconstructivist architecture, held at the MoMA.

Photos: Gerardus / Wikimedia Commons

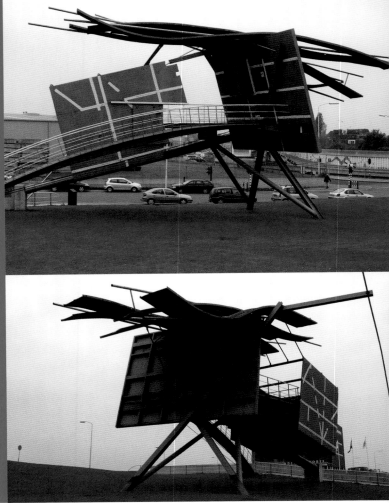

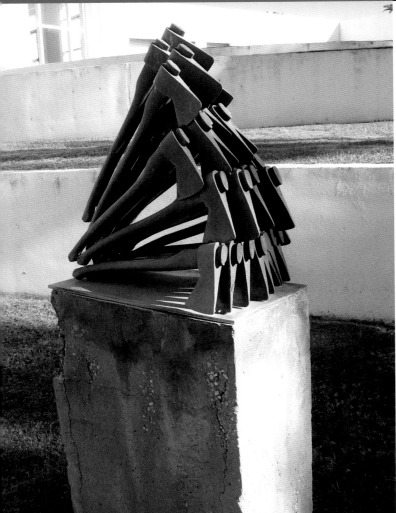

Avalanche
Arman

Completion: 1990. **Technique:** axes, stone. **Location:** Tel Aviv, Israel.

This work is on display at the Tel Aviv University Campus in Israel. It is a typical "accumulation" work of Arman in that it uses multiple copies of an identical object, putting them together to form a sculptural piece. The pieces are no longer viewed as individuals but rather as something new, they are given a new composition and a new shape, fused together as one.

Arman, Armand Pierre Fernandez, was born in France in 1928 but moved to America in the 1960s. His best known works are his "accumulations" and his "destruction / recomposition" pieces. Arman learned oil painting techniques from his father but studied philosophy and mathematics before enrolling in an arts course at the National School of Decorative Arts in Nice. He developed his "accumulations" between 1959 and 1962, putting identical objects together to create a sculptural work.

Photo: Talmoryair / Wikimedia Commons

Light of the Moon
Igor Mitoraj

Completion: 1991. **Technique:** bronze. **Location:** The Hague, The Netherlands.

Igor Mitoraj's sculptures are often classical in style. Many of his figures are masked or blindfolded, referring to loneliness and suffering. He often creates fragments, the side of a face, legs, a torso. The classically well-proportioned features reflect timeless issues of love and femininity, referring back to a lost, classical beauty.

Igor Mitoraj is a Polish artist, born in 1944. He was born in Germany but went on to study at the Academy of Fine Arts in Cracow. In 1968 he moved to Paris, where he studied at the National School of Art. Mitoraj took up sculpture after a year spent traveling around Mexico. He returned to Paris in 1974 and had his first solo exhibition in 1976, at the La Hune Gallery. He returned to Poland in 2003.

Photo: Gerardus / Wikimedia Commons

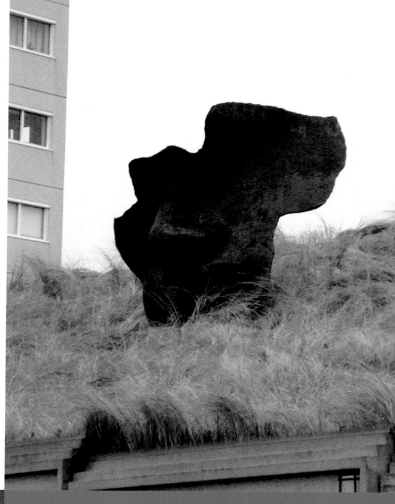

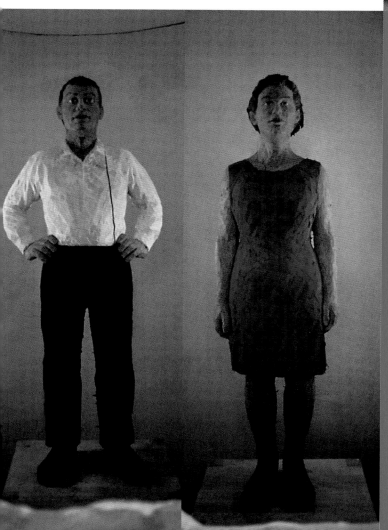

Untitled
Stephan Balkenhol

Completion: 1991. **Technique:** painted wood figures, the building from sandstone. **Location:** Frankfurt / Main, Germany.

This work stands in the garden of the Städel Museum. The piece consists of three sculptures, referencing each other in an architectural and spatial context. Two of the figures, a woman and a man, stand in a specially built house of sandstone. The third figure is made of poplar wood and stands in an niche inside the actual museum building. The sandstone house in the garden has slits in all of the walls, allowing people to see inside.

Stephan Balkenhol is a contemporary German sculptor. He was born in 1957 and studied at the University of Fine Arts in Hamburg. He was awarded the Karl Schmidt-Rottluff scholarship, allowing him to begin to realize his ambition of becoming a sculptor. He taught at the Städel Art Institute in Frankfurt / Main and was later appointed as professor at the Karlsruhe Academy of Fine Arts. Balkenhol has his own studio in Berlin and large, roughly hewn and colorfully painted wooden sculptures have become his trademark.

Photos: Chris van Uffelen

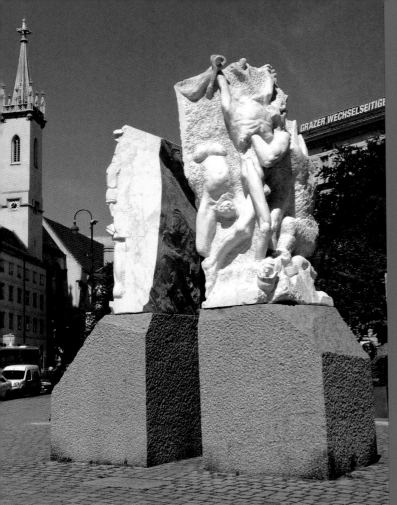

Memorial against War and Fascism
Alfred Hrdlicka

Completion: 1991. **Technique:** bronze, stone. **Location:** Vienna, Austria.

The "Memorial Against War and Fascism" is located on Helmut Zilk Platz in Vienna. At the end of the square stand the "Gates of Violence". This is made of granite, as a reminder of the thousands of prisoners in the Mauthausen concentration camp, who were forced to drag granite up the "stairs of death". The sculpture to the left commemorates the victims of the mass murders that took place in Mauthausen and in other camps. The group of figures on the right gatepost is devoted to all the victims of war.

Alfred Hrdlicka was born in Vienna in 1928 and died in 2009. He was a famous sculptor, painter and graphic artist. After the end of the World War II, he studied painting at the Academy of Fine Arts in Vienna. He gained international recognition after being invited to exhibit his work at the 32nd Venice Biennial. Hrdlicka has taught in Stuttgart, Hamburg, Berlin and Vienna and completed numerous works, significantly influencing the European "monument culture".

The Writing Place
Joseph Kosuth

Completion: 1991. **Technique:** stone. **Location:** Figeac, France.

"The Writing Place" is a huge copy of the Rosetta Stone, an Ancient Egyptian stele on which a decree is inscribed. The decree is written in three scripts: Ancient Egyptian hieroglyphs, Egyptian demotic and Ancient Greek and, because of this, was the key to the modern understanding of Egyptian Hieroglyphics. This copy is engraved on stone and can be found near to the Champollion Museum in France.

Joseph Kosuth is an American Conceptual Artist, born in Ohio in 1945. He studied fine arts at the School of Visual Arts in New York, graduating in 1967. His art tries to explore the nature of art itself, focusing on the ideas behind the production of a work of art, rather than on the work itself. He has also written several books on the nature of art and artists and has expressed the view that art is an extension of philosophy. He also refused to define art, seeing definition as destruction.

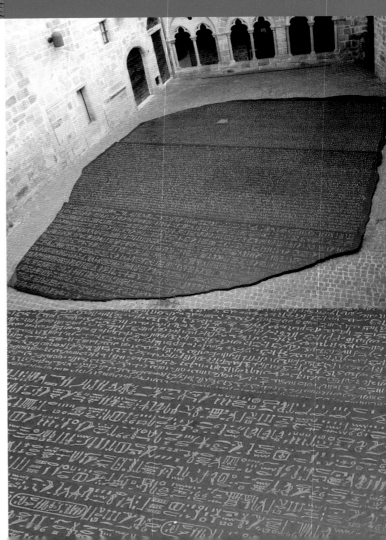

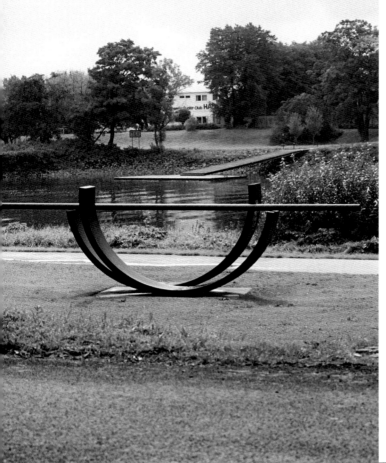

Between Tides
Jan Meyer-Rogge

Completion: 1991. **Technique:** steel. **Location:** Bremen, Germany.

Two large steel arcs combine to create a semi-circle arc. They are balanced differently so that the piece is not symmetrical and the focus shifts when viewed from different perspectives. Together, the two arcs support a round, iron rod, which balances horizontally across the piece, complimenting the horizontal line of the river's course. The work is exhibited on a permanent basis in Bremen, Germany.

Jan Meyer-Rogge was born in Hamburg in 1935. He has exhibited work in solo exhibitions throughout Germany and many of his sculptures are displayed in public areas. Meyer-Rogge studied painting at the Academy of Fine Arts in Hamburg and became a student of Karl Kluth. It wasn't until 1965 that he began sculpting. In 1981 he was offered support from the Heitland Foundation and in 1982 he was awarded the Olevano Romano scholarship. He then was granted the Edwin Scharff Prize in 1987.

Photo: Ursula Meyer-Rogge

Architectural Fragment
Petrus Spronk

Completion: 1992. **Technique:** blue stone. **Location:** Melbourne, Australia.

This work, commissioned by the city of Melbourne, is based on the Pythagoras triangle. It is manufactured in blue stone and was inspired by the artist's walks around the Greek island of Samos, where he found numerous architectural fragments lying in the landscape, like a spontaneous sculpture garden. The work hopes to inspire the viewer to look at and appreciate the architectural forms of the past and to realize that those expressions form the basis of the present architectural styles.

Petrus Spronk began working as an artist in the 1960s, concentrating mainly on working with ceramics. He gained a reputation for his high-quality, burnished broken and re-stored bowls. When the recession in the 1980s resulted in slow art sales Spronk began working as a street artist, using sand to create architectural fragments, inspired by the surrounding buildings. This led to commissions for public art works. Spronk now works in both the public sculpture and ceramic mediums.

Photos: Petrus Spronk (a.); Andy Powell, UK / Wikimedia Commons (b.)

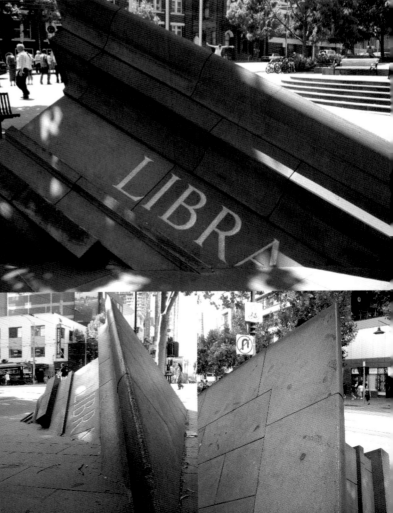

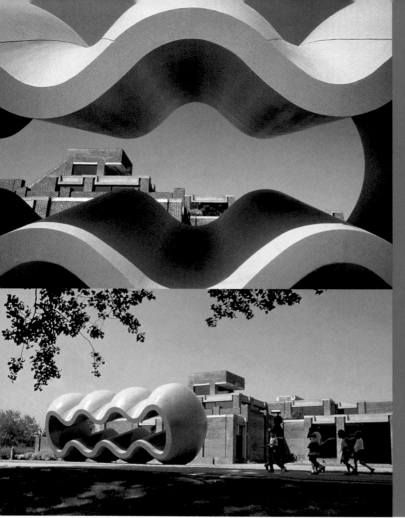

Between Fiction and Fact
Richard Deacon

Completion: 1992. **Technique:** painted steel. **Location:** Villeneuve-d'Ascq, France.

"Between Fiction and Fact" was a public commission for the LaM art park. The sculpture interacts with the museum's architecture by interpreting some of its features: its horizontality and the viewer's fragmentary and gradual discovery of the building on approach towards it. The work's snake-like form, is made from painted sheet-metal and is lying on its side. The mobility and instability of its forms engage the viewer but also aim to leave freedom of interpretation.

Richard Deacon studied at Somerset College of Art, Saint Martins College of Art and Design, London and the Royal College of Art, London. He has worked as a visiting lecturer at various art schools, including the Central School of Art and Design in London and the Chelsea School of Art. He currently works as a professor at the Art Academy in Dusseldorf. Deacon's first one-man show was held in 1978 at The Gallery, London. This led to a string of solo exhibitions, both nationally and internationally. Deacon won the Turner Prize in 1987.

Photos: Max Lerouge

Larry LaTrobe
Pamela Irving

Completion: 1992. **Technique:** bronze. **Location:** Melbourne, Australia.

This bronze life-size dog is called "Larry LaTrobe" as LaTrobe was the surname of the first Governor of Victoria, Australia. The dog stands in the City Square in Melbourne and is popular with tourists and locals, especially children, who like to be photographed sitting on its back or patting its nose. It is a mongrel dog, which means it is a combination of dog breeds. "Larry LaTrobe" is a playful work typical of Pamela Irving's whimsical style.

Pamela Irving was born in Melbourne in 1960. She graduated, with a degree in education, from Melbourne State College in 1982 and completed her master of arts by research at the University of Melbourne in 1989. Irving's work is represented in municipal, university, public and private collections in Australia and Internationally. These include Museum Victoria, Shepparton Art Gallery Collection, Artbank, Bars Studio, Russia.

Photo: Benjamin Lindner

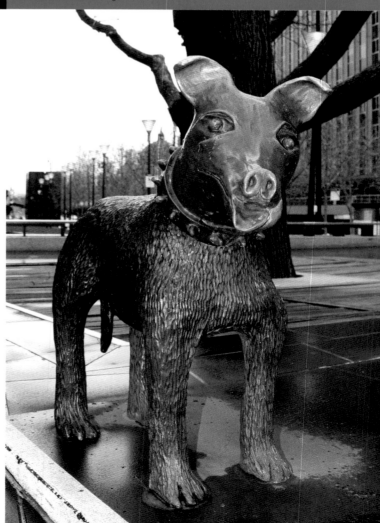

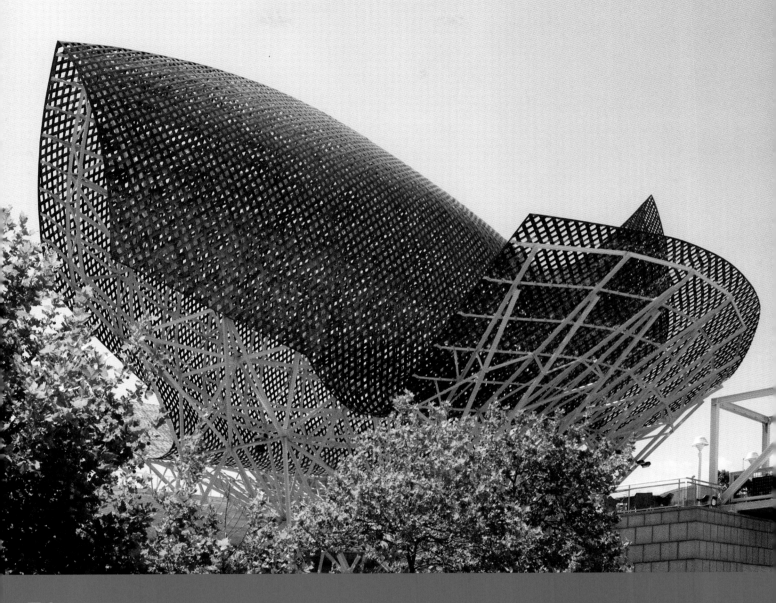

Fish
Frank Gehry

Completion: 1992. **Technique:** copper. **Location:** Barcelona, Spain.

Barcelona's golden fish sculpture sits in the Port Olympic, at the base of the Hotel Arts, one of the tallest buildings in the city. Frank O. Gehry was commissioned to produce the piece for the 1992 Summer Olympics like many of his sculptures, this has been influenced by the basic form of the fish. The sculpture faces the sea and its copper colored, shiny metal plates catch the sunlight, making it shine. The sculpture can be seen from several of Barcelona's beaches.

Frank O. Gehry is a Canadian architect, based in California. He studied at Los Angeles City College and later at the University of South California's School of Architecture, where he graduated in 1954. He is considered one of the world's most important and influential contemporary architects. His works include the Guggenheim Museum in Bilbao, the Art Gallery of Ontario and his own private residence in Santa Monica. His buildings are fundamental to Deconstructivism.

Photo: Chris van Uffelen

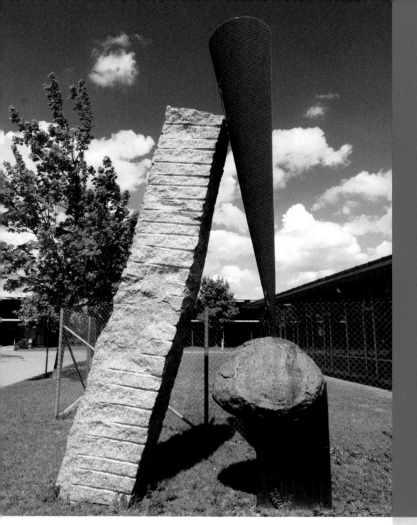

Floating Form / Inclination
Keiji Uematsu

Completion: 1992. **Technique:** steel, granite, iron. **Location:** Munich, Germany.

This piece is one of a series of similar sculptural works by Keiji Uematsu. The sculpture is made of heavy technique: iron, granite and steel, but seeks to achieve a weightless appearance. The slender form of the cone, contrasted against the solidity of the other two shapes helps to create the illusion that the cone is a weightless, balanced form. The cone is the only colored part of the ensemble, drawing attention to this finely balanced shape.

Keiji Uematsu was born in Kobe, Japan, in 1947. He studied art at Kobe University, graduating in 1969. He has been awarded various prizes for his work, including the Excellence Prize at the eighth Japan Art Festival in 1973, the 22nd Blue Culture Prize in 1998 and the Grand Prize at the sixth Asago Outdoor Sculpture exhibition in Tataragi. He has been involved in numerous solo and group exhibitions in both Asia and Europe. His recent exhibitions include "Art as Photography, Photography as Art" at Osaka Municipal museum of Modern Art in 2008.

Star Wound
Rebecca Horn

Completion: 1992. **Technique:** glass, steel. **Location:** Barcelona, Spain.

"Star Wound" sits at the junction of the Paseo Marítimo de la Barceloneta and Paseo Joan de Bourbon. It was constructed in the year Spain hosted the Olympics and is one of several works commissioned at this time. The sculpture shoots vertically upwards, just behind the sandy beach, a steel tower of four, stacked cubes. The design of this piece is supposed to honor the simple architecture of this part of the coast.

Rebecca Horn is a German Installation Artist. Her most well known works include "Unicorn", a body suit with a large horn protruding from it and "Pencil Mask", a mesh helmet with pencils attached to it, projecting outwards. She started drawing as a young child, finding it a far less confining way of expressing her emotions than the use of language. Horn mostly produces performance and installation pieces but also works with poetry and drawing.

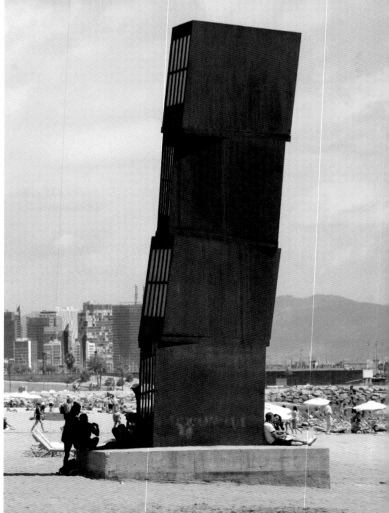

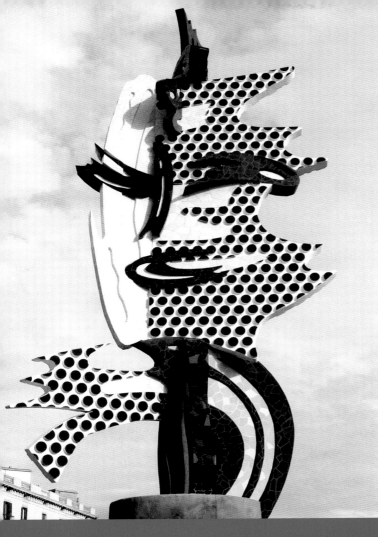

The Head of Barcelona
Roy Lichtenstein

Completion: 1992. **Technique:** concrete, ceramics. **Location:** Barcelona, Spain.

This is a sculpture designed by the famous Pop Artist, Roy Lichtenstein. It stands in the north-eastern part of the harbor in Barcelona. It is almost 20 meters tall, made of concrete and ceramics and was commissioned as part of the transformation of the wharf area in the run-up to the 1992 Olympic games.

Roy Lichtenstein was an American Pop Artist. He was born in 1923 and died in 1997. Lichtenstein was a leading figure in the new art movement, along with Jasper Johns, Andy Warhol and James Rosenquist. His most famous work was heavily influenced by advertising and comic book style. Lichtenstein began studying art during summer classes at the Art Students League of New York, before later enrolling at Ohio State University. He rose to international fame and his most famous image, "Whaam!" is in the Tate Modern in London.

Photo: Mutari / Wikimedia Commons

Structure
Sol LeWitt

Completion: 1992. **Technique:** sand-lime brick. **Location:** Ostfildern, Germany.

This large sculpture is fittingly named "Structure" and consists of four parts. It stands on the street between separate areas of the suburbs of Ostfildern and represents the four villages, which were originally separate but merged together in around 1975. This work has been developed from the basic form of a wall into a cube shape. The walls do not touch each other as the artist sought to make a logical structure from individual parts.

The American artist Sol LeWitt was born in Connecticut in 1928 and died in 2007. He studied at the Syracuse University in New York. After graduating with a Bachelor degree in Fine Arts, he was called up for service in the Korean War. In 1976 he founded the publishing house, Printed Matter, which organized the distribution and marketing of books from various artists. He also taught at the School of Visual Arts at New York University.

Photos: Chris van Uffelen

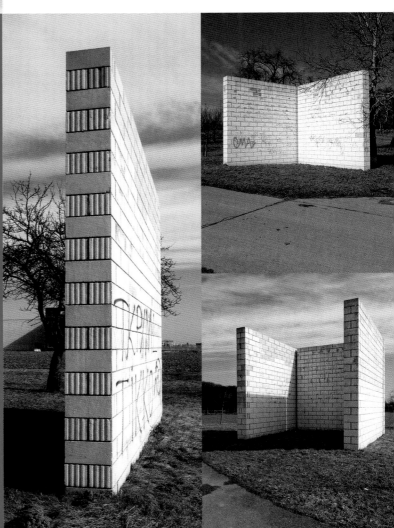

Man on Horse
Fernando Botero

Completion: 1992. **Technique:** bronze. **Location:** Jerusalem, Israel.

The sculpture "Man on Horse" is a typical 'rounded' work of Fernando Botero. It is made of bronze and stands at a height of just 24 centimeters. The figures of horse and man are disproportionately sized. The head of the horse, in comparison to its body, is too small, the legs are too wide and the rider appears to have legs of the same width as those of the horse.

Fernando Botero was born in 1932 and is one of Latin America's most famous artists. In 1951 he moved to Europe, developing his unique style around the end of the 1950s. His works mostly deal with the human form and all the facets of human life. His sculptural forms are often disproportionate, requiring the viewer to look closely and not assume that what they expect to see is what is actually there.

Photo: Wmpearl / Wikimedia Commons

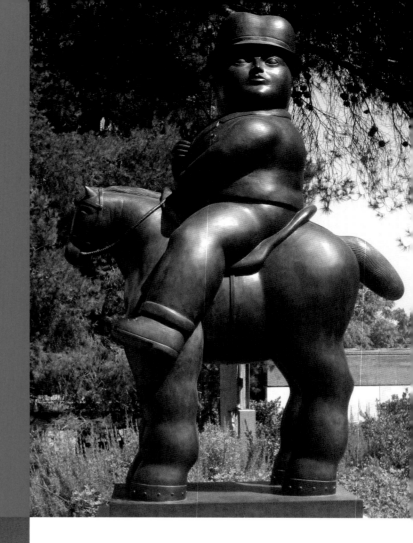

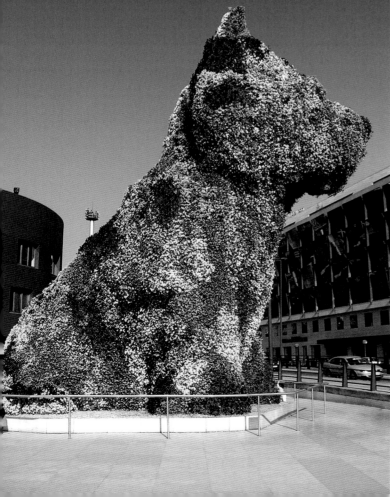

Puppy
Jeff Koons

Completion: 1992. **Technique:** planted flowers on a stainless steel armature. **Location:** Bilbao, Spain.

This floral sculpture of a west highland terrier is 13,1 meters tall, from its paws to its ears. The sculpture was formed of a stainless steel armature and holds over 25 tons of soil. It was first created in 1992 for a temporary exhibition in Germany and was later exhibited at New York City's Rockefeller Center. In 1997 the piece was purchased by the Guggenheim foundation and installed on the terrace outside the Guggenheim Museum Bilbao, it is now part of the permanent collection.

Jeff Koons is an American artist, born in 1955. He studied painting at the School of the Art Institute of Chicago and the Maryland Institute College of Art. After college, he worked as a Wall Street commodities broker while establishing himself as an artist. He is famous for his reproductions of banal objects, such as his stainless steel replicas of balloon animals. Koon holds the world record auction price work by a living artist but he divides critical opinion, with some critics labeling him as kitsch and crass.

Photo: Noebse / Wikimedia Commons

Imperia
Peter Lenk

Completion: 1993. **Technique:** cast concrete. **Location:** Constance, Germany.

The "Imperia" is a statue at the entrance of the harbor of Constance, in Germany. The work commemorates the Council of Constance that took place there between 1414 and 1418. The statue is made of concrete and is ten meters high. It weighs 18 tons, and stands on a pedestal that rotates around its axis once every three minutes. The statue depicts a woman, holding two men, one in each hand. The two men represent Pope Martin V and Emperor Sigismund.

Peter Lenk was born in 1947 in Nuremberg, Germany. He is most famous for the "Imperia" in Constance but has also attracted attention for producing other controversial sculptures, that challenge taboos. His "group-sex relief" features prominent politicians and corporate players in various states of undress and completely nude. One panel depicts German Chancellor Angela Merkel and former Chancellor Gerhard Schröder laughing and grabbing each others private parts.

Photo: Achim Mende

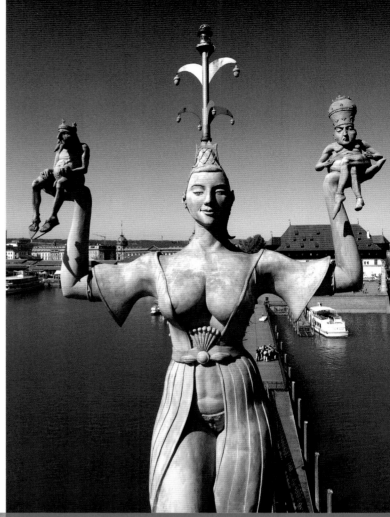

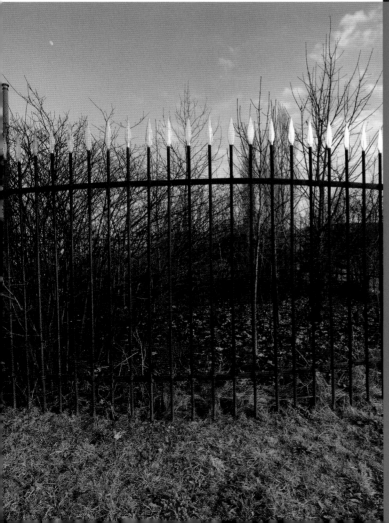

Sanctuarium
Hermann de Vries

Completion: 1993. **Technique:** partial gilded steel. **Location:** Stuttgart, Germany.

This piece is a circular, fenced off area with a diameter of 11 meters. Inside the fence undergrowth, plants and weeds can be seen, sprawling across the space. The plants and trees have no structure, young birch trees mix with bushes and other greenery. The steel rods of the enclosing fence are spaced at regular intervals and end in arrow shaped tips covered in gold leaf. The project allows the greenery in the space to grow wildly and not be domesticated like the rest of the city's green spaces.

Herman de Vries is a Dutch artist, born in 1931 and better known for his painting than sculptural works. He worked for some years as a gardener and farm laborer. In the mid 1950s he began painting formal images and his work was displayed at several solo and group exhibitions. In 1961 de Vries began to display his work in the public realm. Important exhibitions of his work were held in Würzburg and Vienna in 2005.

Photos: Chris van Uffelen

The Involved Student
Brian Hanlon

Completion: 1993. **Technique:** painted bronze. **Location:** Clifton, NJ, USA.

"The Involved Student" is a life size sculpture by Brian Hanlon. The sculpture is painted and the artist manages to communicate a sense of peace in the simple lines of the sculpture. It lies in front of the Clifton police station in New Jersey and is one of a number of public sculptures situated in this area.

Brian Hanlon studied art education and has produced over 200 works of public art, a number of which are situated in New Jersey. He started his own company, Hanlon Sculpture, in 1991. Much of his work concentrates on depicting people who have achieved greatness; he is the official sculptor for the Naismith Memorial Basketball Hall of Fame in Massachusetts. His sculptural subjects also include firemen and members of the police force.

Photo: Susan Kane

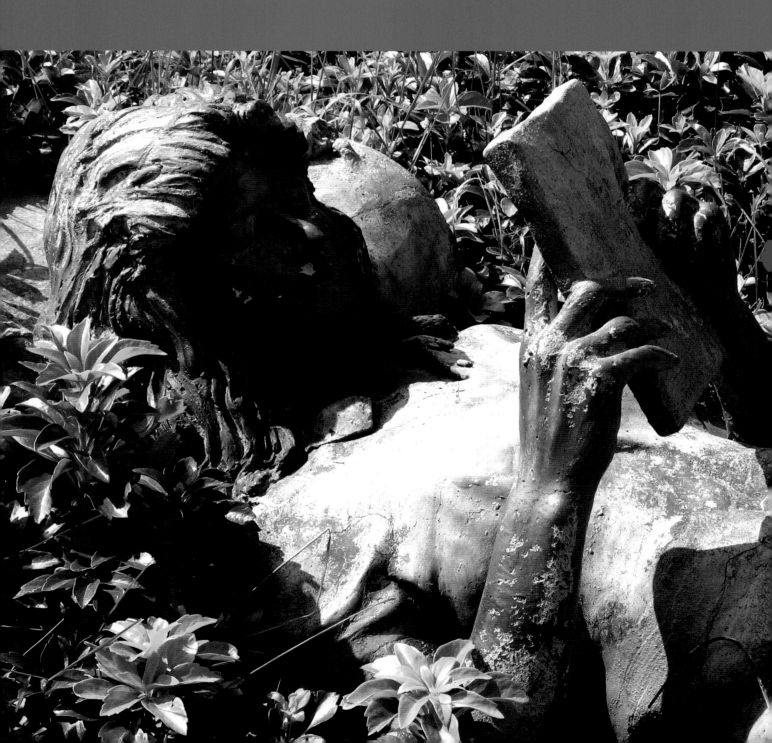

Der Grenzstein
Hans-Oiseau Kalkmann

Completion: 1993. **Technique:** Carrara marble, painted steel.
Location: Bodenburg, Germany

The "Border Stone" was made as part of the 33rd Contact Art Campaign in 1993 and was funded by the German Foreign Ministry and the IFA in Berlin. Students from Poland, Germany and former Czechoslovakia took part in the project. The bird-like stele is located on the western border of Bodenburg. The purpose of the sculpture is to serve as a visible symbol that everyone is welcome. The bird stands near the border with out-spread wings, welcoming all.

Hans-Oiseau Kalkmann, is a German sculptor, born in 1940. He has 45 sculptures on display in public and frequently works together with his son Jens Kalkmann. Kalkmann's sculptures arose in the context of Contact Art actions, bringing people together and connecting the meaning of the area to the sculpture. In this way, he creates site-specific sculptures from granite, marble, sandstone and steel. His works often relate to water, light or sound in their design.

Photo: Courtesy of the artist

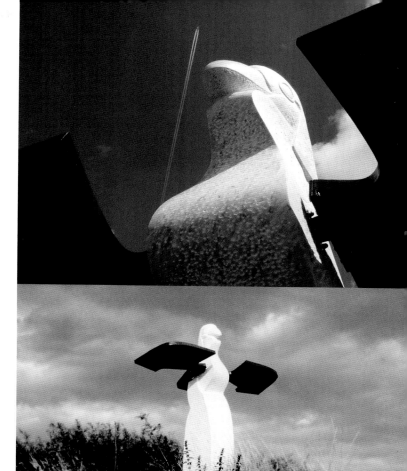

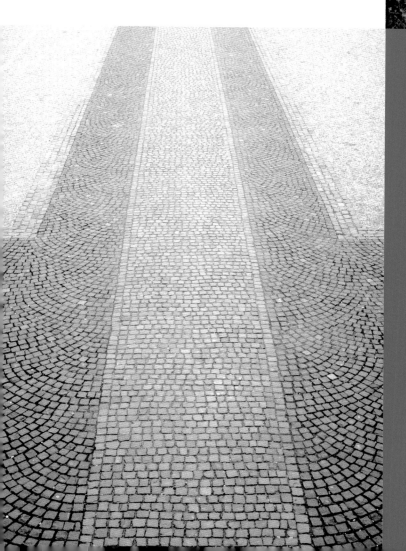

2146 stones - Monument against racism
Jochen Gerz

Completion: 1993. **Technique:** 2146 cobblestones. **Location:** Saarbrucken, Germany.

This subtle intervention, subtitled "The Invisible Monument" is a testament to hidden trauma and buried histories. Gerz, with the help of 61 Jewish communities, compiled a list of all the Jewish cemeteries in use before World War II. He removed the cobblestones from in front of Saarbrucken Castle, today a Provincial Parliament. He did this illegally, under the cover of darkness. He then carved the names on the underside of the stones before replacing them. He was discovered about half way through the process and the work was retrospectively commissioned.

Jochen Gerz is an internationally renowned German artist. He was born in Berlin in 1940. Gerz's work in public space has radically altered the relationship between art and viewer. The individual is no longer just part of the public but is made part of the work. Gerz's work details the aesthetics of a democracy in search of its cultural dimension. He has been creating his 'anti-monuments' since 1983.

Photos: Martin Blanke

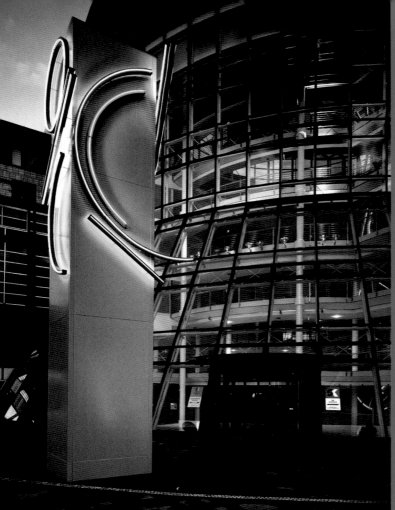

Neon for Stadtsparkasse
Stephen Antonakos

Completion: 1993. **Technique:** painted aluminum, neon.
Location: Cologne, Germany.

This work is located on the sidewalk at the entrance to the Stadtsparkasse bank. The column, with different compositions of neon forms on each side, must be walked around to be seen as a whole. It corresponds formally in its essentially multiple angles and sequences of viewpoints with neon forms that are situated in the interior of the bank.

For over 50 years Stephen Antonakos has redefined neon in his abstract installations and public works. Known also for his drawings, chapels, collages and books, he makes "real things in real spaces". He has exhibited internationally in museums and galleries including a major retrospective at the Benaki Museum in Athens, 2007. His works are included in important private and museum collections worldwide and over 50 public works are installed in the USA, Europe and Japan.

Photo: Carl Victor Dahmen, Cologne; courtesy of the artist and Kalfayan Galleries, Athens – Thessaloniki

Gate of Hope
Dan Graham

Completion: 1993. **Technique:** stainless steel, metal mesh, one-way mirror glass. **Location:** Stuttgart, Germany.

The "Gate of Hope" is a pavilion-sculpture, built for the International Garden Exhibition in 1993. The sculpture takes the geometric form of a tetrahedron. Through a missing triangular on one side and a cut-off triangle point at the back, the shape functions as a kind of corridor. The triangular sides are glazed and a grid-covered pool of water lies inside the sculpture.

Dan Graham is an American sculptor, born in Illinois in 1942. He is considered one of America's most successful Concept Artists. At the age of 22 he opened his own gallery, the John Daniels Gallery, in New York. In 1969 he taught at the University of San Diego and in 1971 at the Nova Scotia College of Arts in Halifax. Graham is best known for his pavilions, constructed out of steel and mirrored glass.

Photo: Chris van Uffelen

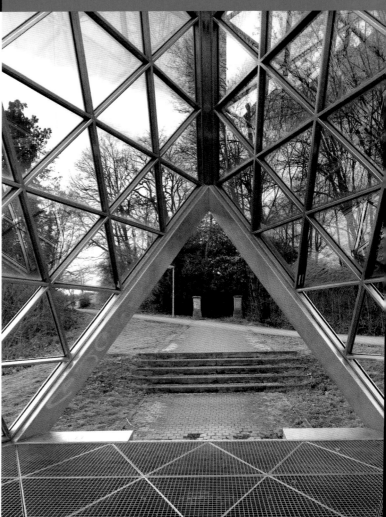

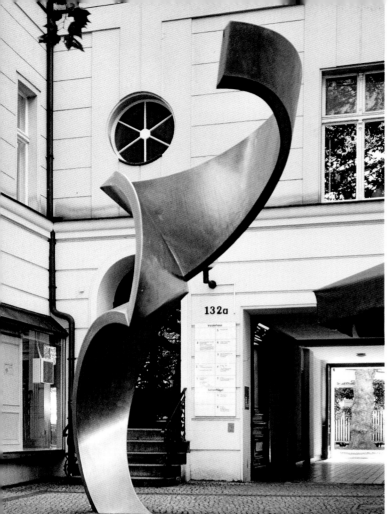

Versus
Karl Menzen

Completion: 1993. **Technique:** stainless steel. **Location:** Berlin, Germany.

"Versus" is one part of a group of artworks developed since the 1990s. Beginning with cylindrical material, the forms change playfully from concave to convex showing changing rhythms and dynamics. The sculptures represent movement within a space, appearing to overcome the heaviness of their own material, while at the same time expressing the quality of the steel from which they are made.

Karl Menzen is a German sculptor. Many of his works are of architectural scale, made from stainless and rusted steel and often situated in public space. Menzen studied material science at the Technical University in Berlin. Since 1987, he has exhibited his artwork in Germany and Sweden, as well as in Milan and Budapest. Examples of his work are displayed in Berlin, Salzgitter, Radebeul and castle Gottorf in Schleswig-Holstein.

Photo: Lars Hennings, Berlin

Bridge/Ramp
Siah Armajani

Completion: 1994. **Technique:** steel. **Location:** Stuttgart, Germany.

"Bridge/Ramp" is 58 meters long and is made of lacquered gray steel. It rests on eight supporting columns, connecting the inner courtyard of the Landesbank Baden-Württemberg with the administrative center of the bank. Above the lower gate to the second pair of pillars is a type of truss bridge construction in yellow-painted steel. The piece does not function as a bridge but rather as an indicator of architectural history.

Siah Armajani is an Iranian-born American sculptor, best known for designing the Olympic Torch for the Summer Olympics in 1996. He has also worked on other well known projects, such as the Staten Island tower and bridge and the Irene Hixon Whitney Bridge in Minnesota in the USA. His 2005 work, Fallujah, has been censored in the USA because of its critical view of the Iraq war. In 2010 he won a Fellow award, granted by United States Artists.

Photos: Chris van Uffelen

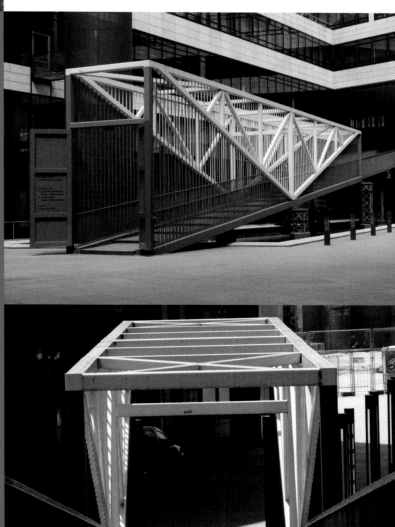

Field of Corn (with Osage Orange Trees)
Malcolm Cochran

Completion: 1994. **Technique:** Pre-cast concrete, Osage orange trees, bronze text panels. **Location:** Dublin, OH, USA.

Dublin, Ohio is changing rapidly from a relatively small, agricultural community to a busy corporate city. In the process, land that has been farmed for approximately 1,800 years is experiencing development. The site of this work is an acre and a half plot cut off from its corporate headquarter neighbors by two roads. Cochran thinks of this work as a formal memorial for corn production and a surprising roadside attraction. Five text panels mounted at ground level provide historical accounts of land use in this area.

Malcolm Cochran has created large-scale objects, installations and site specific works, which often develop in response to a particular location, since the late-1970s. He has exhibited widely in the US and Europe. Cochran's permanent public projects are in Brattleboro, Vermont; Cleveland and Columbus, Ohio; and the Hudson River Park, New York City. Since 1987 he has taught sculpture at The Ohio State University, Columbus.

Photos: Malcolm Cochran

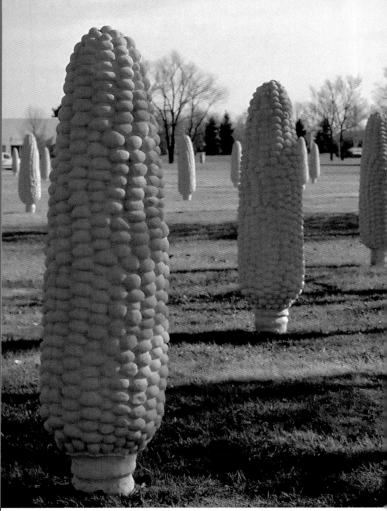

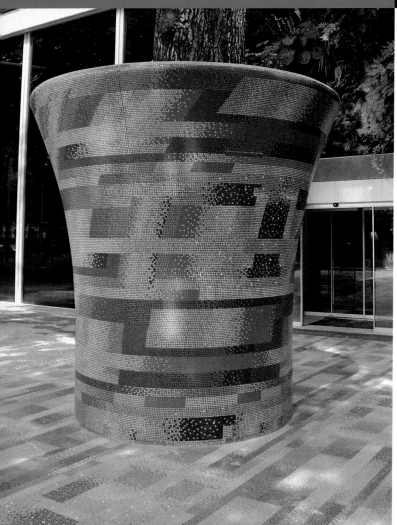

Mosaic
Alessandro Mendini

Completion: 1994. **Technique:** ceramic. **Location:** Paris, France.

This work is typical of Alessandro Mendini in that it shows a fusion of styles. The work is made of ceramic but adapts a mundane object to create something different. The fusion of colors makes the piece more an example of sculptural work than one of furniture. The fine pattern of the surroundings camouflages the plant pot, blurring the boundaries between work and surroundings.

Alessandro Mendini was born in Milan in 1931. He is an Italian designer and architect who played an important role in the development of Italian design. His work explores different cultures and forms of expression. He has created furniture, interiors, paintings and architectural works as well as writing several books and working for the magazines Domus, Casabell and Modo. He was a main figure in the Radical design movement and in 1982 he founded the Domus Academy, the first postgraduate design school.

Photo: Chris van Uffelen

Drink a Cup of Tea
Kazuo Katase

Completion: 1994. **Technique:** stones from Naoshima, aluminum, blue anodized. **Location:** Island Naoshima, Kagawa, Japan.

This permanent work is part of a series, situated in the landscape of the Benesse House Naoshima Contemporary Art Museum. The archetype was made in Switzerland in 1987, against the back drop of the Alps. The selection of the stone material always relates to the location. The bowl is either waterless or filled with rainwater. The title is taken from the words from the Zen priest Sengai. The image of the bowl becomes a sign of the presence of humanity, a metaphor for the dialectic relationship between fullness and emptiness.

Kazuo Katase was born in 1947 in Shizuoka, Japan and currently lives in Kassel, Germany. He brought with him to the West a Zen tradition enlightened by modern Japanese philosophy. Since 1973 he has been participating in national and international, solo and group exhibitions. Since 1987 his work has focused on projects that consider the connection between architecture and landscape in Germany, Europe and Japan.

Photos: Kazuo Katase, Kassel, Germany (a.); Koji Murakami, Japan (b.)

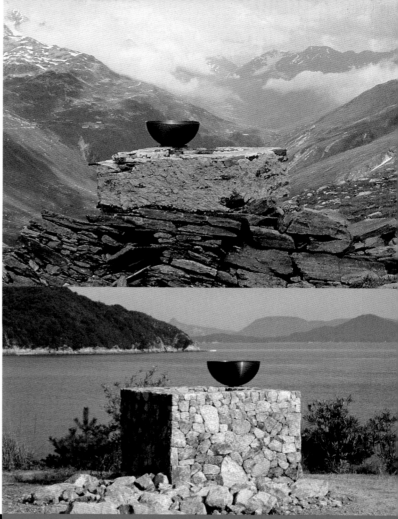

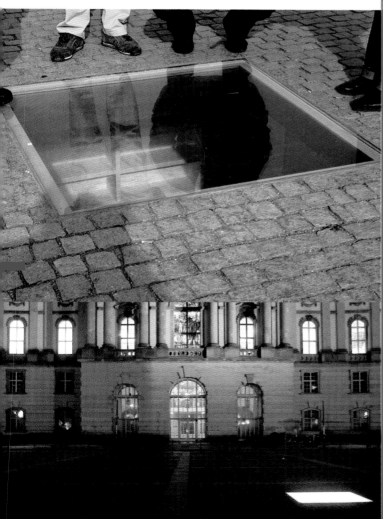

The Sunken Library
Micha Ullman

Completion: 1995. **Technique:** glass plate, bronze plate. **Location:** Berlin, Germany.

"The Sunken Library" is situated below the Bebelplatz in Berlin. This square was the site of the 1933 book burning, shortly after Hitler had assumed the role of dictator in Germany. It was created by Micha Ullman and is an underground room covered by a glass window, which is set into the cobbles of the square for people to look through. The empty bookshelves within are a reminder of the tens of thousands of books that were burnt, written by Jews, liberals and others who were not approved of by the Nazi regime.

Micha Ullman was born in Tel Aviv, to German-Jewish parents who emigrated in 1933. Between 1960 and 1964, he studied at Bezalel Academy of Art and Design, in Jerusalem. In 1965, he attended the Central School of Arts and Crafts in London, where he learned how to etch. He was awarded the Israel Prize for Sculpture in 2009 and currently lives in Ramat Hasharon, Israel. He taught at Bezalel Academy in 1970–1978 and became a visiting professor at the Academy of Arts Dusseldorf in 1976.

Photos: Chris van Uffelen

Saiki Peace Memorial Park
Eiki Danzuka, Earthscape

Completion: 1995. **Technique:** Corten steel, concrete. **Location:** Saiki-city, Japan.

This area is the site of an old naval port. The old naval facilities were dismantled and the area transformed into a public park. The large open area is covered by grass and the main spaces are defined by the white paths cutting through them. These simple pathways are dressed with river boulders as well as abstract interpretations of natural flow patterns in Saiki. In addition to these, mounds, pools and monuments were also constructed to form a harmonious whole.

Eiki Danzuka is a landscape designer. After graduating from Kuwasawa Design School in Japan he attended the Environment Art Studio, headed by artist Nobuo Sekine and founded Earthscape in 1999. Earthscape is a landscape design studio that considers the devices that create connections between humans and nature as design. They enact design works that become a platform for experience.

Photos: Koji Okumura / Forward stroke, Tokyo

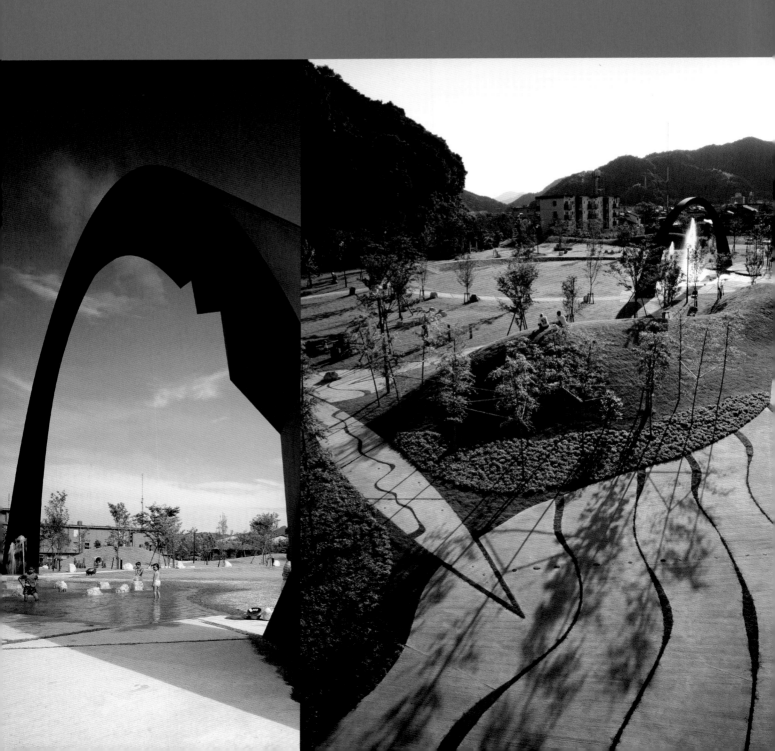

Temple of Several Cultures
Lia Versteege

Completion: 1995. **Technique:** marble. **Location:** Tijnje, The Netherlands.

This work has to do with the source of existence: life. The sculpture communicates the human strive for survival. As human beings, we have always sought for the meaning of our existence. Searching for meaning in life, people seek to be part of a bigger entity. For centuries, myths, gods and religions have offered relief. At the same time, religions have brought conflicts and wars. The "Temple of Several Cultures" is meant for people from all religious backgrounds, offering peace without discrimination.

Lia Versteege was born in Amsterdam and studied in the Hague and in Haarlem. She has produced several works in stone and steel and has been exhibiting her work since 1978 in the Netherlands, Germany, Belgium, Switzerland and Bulgaria. Versteege has also been commissioned to produce several sculptural works. She owns her own sculpture garden and is a member of the Dutch Society of Sculptors and Sculpture network.

Photo: Courtesy of the artist

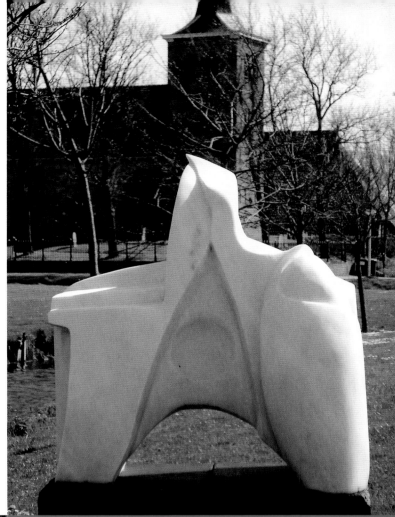

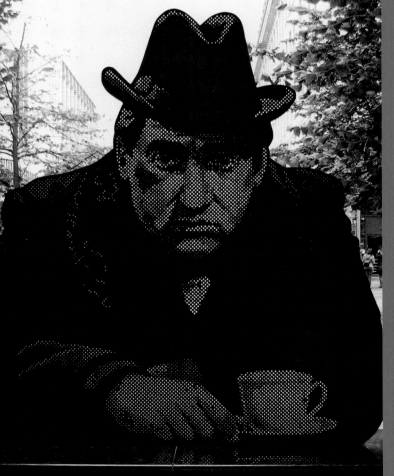

Tony Hancock Memorial
Bruce Williams

Completion: 1995. **Technique:** bronze, glass, granite. **Location:** Birmingham, United Kingdom.

This work memorializes the iconic outline of Birmingham born comedian Tony Hancock, in a single plane of bronze, pierced by hundreds of glass rods. Light sparkles in the glass to recreate the celebrity's laconic expression. The unique combination of traditional bronze, with the fleeting illusion of a photographic image, provides a fitting, permanent memorial to a star of film and television.

Bruce Williams works primarily in the public realm, creating works of art in response to commissions tendered by regional governments, public art agencies, trusts and private developers. His career has been marked by high-profile projects, often on an architectural scale. The "Tony Hancock Memorial" and "Kiss Wall" in Brighton pioneered the use of photographic imagery outdoors, a technique he has developed with laser cutting and computer driven fabrication techniques.

Photo: Courtesy of the artist

Never had a man less reason to be humb!s

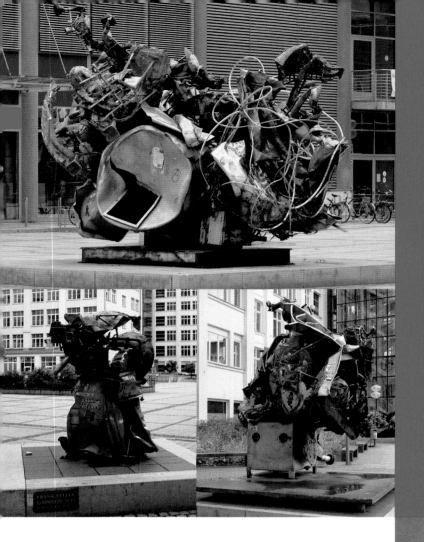

Sculptures on Ernst Abbe Platz
Frank Stella

Completion: 1995. **Technique:** steel. **Location:** Jena, Germany.

This group of five works stands on Ernst Abbe Platz in Jena, Germany. The work is abstract in style, combining a number of different forms. Each piece was made in 1995 and each has a different name; Newburgh, Bear Mountain, Fishkill, Peekskill and Garrison. Each is made of steel, apart from Bear Mountain, which also incorporates bronze.

Frank Stella is an American painter, printmaker and significant figure in the Minimalist and Abstract Movements. His work is influenced by Abstract Artists, such as Jackson Pollock. Stella studied at Princeton University, moving to New York after he graduated. His later work concentrates on the different uses of color and his print works had a strong impact on developing printmaking as an art form. In the 1980s and '90s Stella focused on producing a body of work that responded to Herman Melville's Moby Dick.

Photos: Andreas Praefcke / Wikimedia Commons

Chain to the Heavens
Peter Weidl

Completion: 1996. **Technique:** square steel tube. **Location:** Viechtach, Germany.

"Chain to the Heavens" sculpture symbolically links the building of the central Fines Administration Offices in Bavaria with the city traffic. The sculpture appears as if it has been cut out of a longer sequence; the form jutting out towards the open sky. It can be seen from all levels of the building behind it as well as from the connecting passages between the office buildings. The chain works as a visible connector between the people and traffic.

Peter Weidl was born in 1948 in Tegernsee. He studied painting at the Malschule Atelier Geitlinger and at the Academy of Fine Arts in Munich. After graduating he turned to sculpture and built up experience working in his father's workshop. Weidl's work has been widely exhibited and he has created several works that stand in public space in various locations throughout Germany.

Photos: Courtesy of the artist

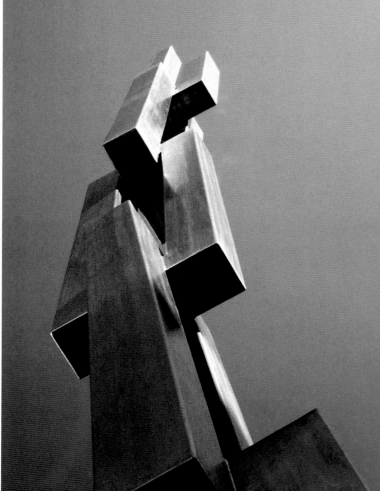

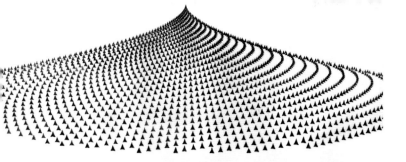

Tree Mountain — A Living Time Capsule
Agnes Denes

Completion: 1996. **Technique:** trees on manmade mountain.
Location: Ylöjärvi, Finland.

"Tree Mountain", subtitled "11,000 Trees, 11,000 people, 400 Years", measures 420 x 270 x 38 meters. The elliptical shape was planted with eleven thousand trees by eleven thousand people from all over the world at the Pinziö gravel pits near Ylöjärvi, Finland. "Tree Mountain" is protected land, to be maintained for four centuries, eventually creating a virgin forest. People who planted the trees received certificates acknowledging them as custodians of the trees for the next 24 generations.

Agnes Denes is an American artist / scholar and one of the originators of Conceptual Art. Denes has investigated the physical and social sciences and transformed her explorations into unique works of visual art. Denes was a pioneer of Ecological Art and one of the first artists to initiate the Environmental Art movement. Her work involves ecological, cultural and social issues, and are often monumental in scale. Denes has written five books and holds two honorary doctorates in fine arts.

Photos: Courtesy of the artist

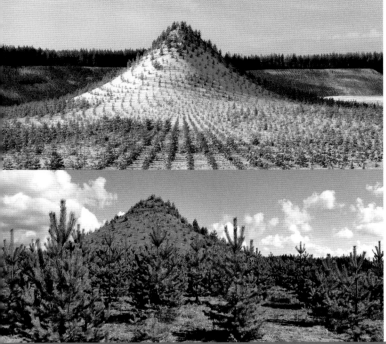

Schouwburgplein
West 8

Completion: 1996. **Technique:** steel, LED displays, glass.
Location: Rotterdam, The Netherlands.

The "Schouwburgplein" is a large, public square, located in the heart of Rotterdam. The design emphasizes the importance of empty space, opening up a panoramic view of the city's skyline. The square is designed as an interactive public place and the main features are four hydraulic lighting elements. Each of these lightweight steel structures is activated with LED displays. At night the towers are lit from the inside spreading a soft filtered light.

West 8 was founded by Adriaan Geuze in 1987 and is an award-winning international office for urban design and landscape architecture. West 8's main office is in Rotterdam but there are also branches in New York, Belgium and Toronto. The firm employs an international team of 70 architects, urban designers, landscape architects and industrial engineers. West 8 has extensive experience in large-scale urban master planning and design, landscape interventions, waterfront projects, parks, squares and gardens.

Photo: K. Siereveld / Wikimedia Commons

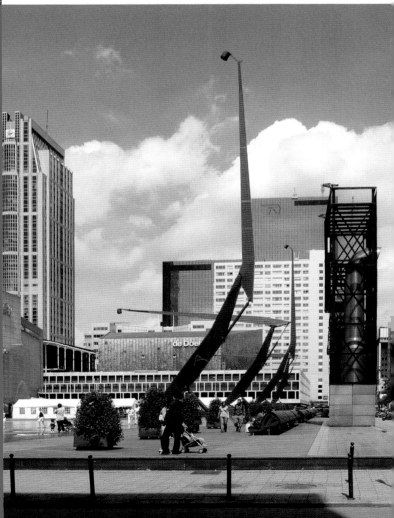

Untitled
Per Kirkeby

Completion: 1996. **Technique:** brickwork. **Location:** Copenhagen, Denmark.

Per Kirkeby's large brick sculptures can be found throughout Europe and are often on display in public space. He was commissioned to produce two small brick sculptures, one for each end of the Meldahlsgade in Copenhagen, to celebrate the city's appointment as Capital of Culture in 1996. Both pieces are more durable than the artist's other works and are made with copper copings and drip molds. The sculptures are not adapted to the surrounding architecture but deliberately stand out.

Per Kirkeby is a Danish painter, sculptor and architect born in Copenhagen in 1938. He taught at the Karlsruhe University of Fine Arts from 1978 to 1988 and was also a member of the Avant-Garde art group "Eksperimenterende Kunstskole", which dealt mainly with graphics. In 1989, he was appointed as professor at the Städel School in Frankfurt / Main, where he taught until 2000. Kirkeby is best known for his large brick sculptures.

Photo: Paul Henderson / Wikimedia Commons

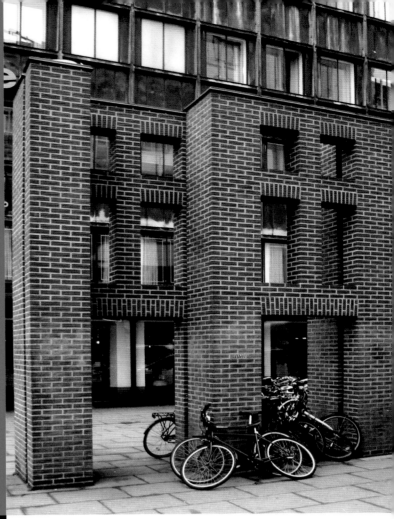

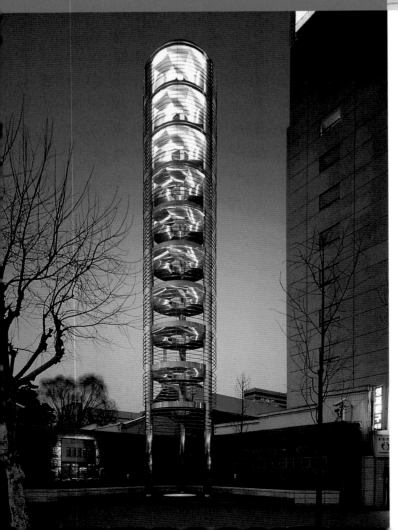

Doosan 100 Year Park
Sasaki Associates

Completion: 1996. **Technique:** stainless steel, integrated lighting, granite, stone, bronze. **Location:** Seoul, South Korea.

"Doosan 100 Year Park" celebrates the accomplishments of the Doosan Corporation, Korea's oldest company. The names of 27 subsidiary companies are inscribed on the granite wall, symbolizing both the unity and uniqueness of each company. The tower is encircled with 100, small-diameter, metal rods forming a ring around the tower as it ascends skyward. Centered directly below the tower is a time capsule. The interior of the tower is illuminated by lights positioned to create a 'cone of light' illuminating the capsule.

Sasaki Associates was founded in 1953 by Hideo Sasaki. He was also former head of landscape architecture at Harvard University and a major figure in 20th century design. Today, Sasaki Associates is an international design firm, actively engaged in virtually every aspect of the built environment. The firm's interdisciplinary structure and focus on innovation motivates professionals to connect ideas and synthesize economic reality, environmental sustainability, cultural awareness and keen aesthetic judgment.

Photo: Seung Hoon Yum

The Lost Form
Thomas Virnich

Completion: 1998. **Technique:** ceramic, paint. **Location:** Freiburg, Germany.

"The Lost form" is comprised of five sculptures, all made of ceramic and each one 110 x 100 x 200 centimeters in size. Each colored segment shows animal forms. The further away from the sculpture the observer stands, the clearer the form becomes. The artist's intention was to portray the path of evolution, to clarify biological origins. The sculpture is reminiscent of a fossil; but also brings to mind Noah and his systematical attempt to save the animals.

Thomas Virnich is a German sculptor and painter, born in Eschweiler in 1957. He studied at the Technical University in Aachen before changing to the Art Academy in Dusseldorf, where he graduated in 1985. He was awarded the Lower Saxony Art Prize in 2001. Virnich's sculptures are often large and colorful, sometimes created from waste material or rubbish. His work has been exhibited in various locations throughout Europe including at the Art Association in Arau in 2005 and Wiesbaden Museum in 2007.

Photo: Chris van Uffelen

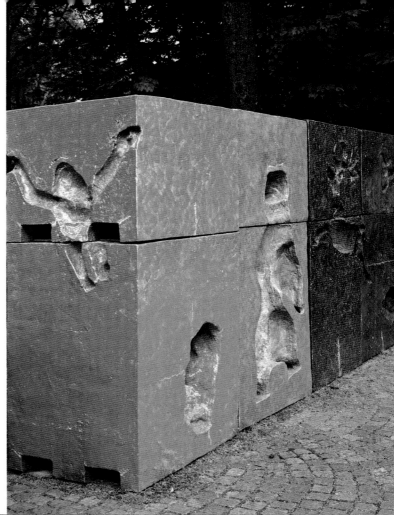

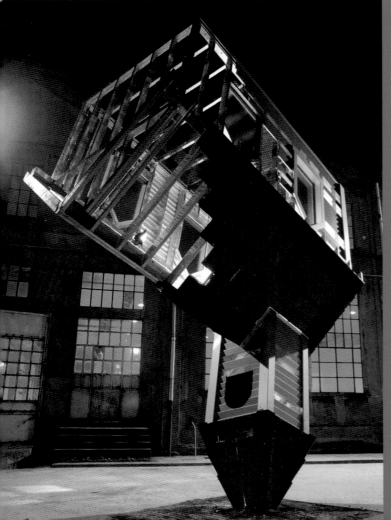

Device to Root out Evil
Dennis Oppenheim

Completion: 1997. **Technique:** galvanized steel,red Venetian glass, punch plate. **Location:** Denver, CO, USA.

This controversial work was first shown at the Venice Biennial. It was criticized by the President of Stanford University but has since become a widely respected and exhibited artwork. The artist claims that depicting a church upside down may be considered to be aggressive but not blasphemous. In the work, a country church is seen balancing on it's steeple, as if it had been lifted by a terrific force and brought to the site as a device or method of rooting out evil.

Dennis Oppenheim was born in 1938 in Washington and died in 2011. He graduated in 1965 from the School of Arts and Crafts, Oakland and from Stanford University. He has received fellowships from the Guggenheim Foundation and the National Endowment for the Arts. Oppenheim has received international attention for a body of conceptual work, which spans over four decades. He has exhibited his works internationally in galleries and museums including solo shows in Europe, North and South America and Asia.

Photo: Edward Smith

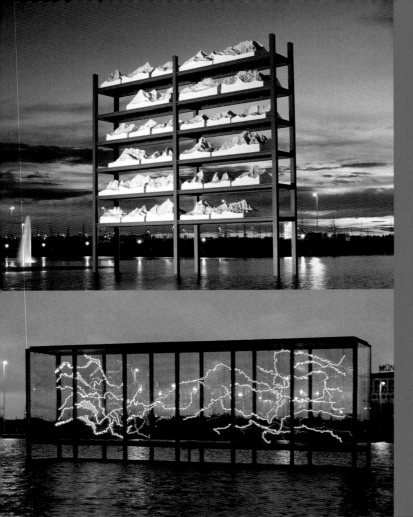

Gran Paradiso
Stephan Huber

Completion: 1997. **Technique:** steel, glass, neon, polyester.
Location: Munich, Germany.

The intermingling, so typical of Huber's biographical region-alism, evocative and aestehetic stage-like construction and ironical distancing, condenses with striking impact in his work "Gran Paradiso". The major peaks of the Alps them-selves are visible as radiantly white models. At the same time, the most important Alpine rivers can be viewed simul-taneously as a neon map in a glass cabinet.

Stephan Huber is an influential German sculptor. He was born in 1952 in Lindenberg / Allgäu. He began studying at the university in Munich in 1971 and graduated in 1976. His work combines visual force and theatrical aesthetics, psy-choanalysis and ironic detachment. Huber has participated in the eighth Documenta and the Venice Biennial 1999 and has been making sculptures for public display since 1986. He lives and works in Munich and Bidingen / Ostallgäu.

Photos: Dieter Hinrichs, Munich

Veteran's Memorial
Maryann Thompson, Charles Rose

Completion: 1997. **Technique:** Indiana limestone. **Location:** Columbus, IN, USA.

The "Veteran's Memorial" features the names of 156 veter-ans from Bartholomew County, who gave their lives during the wars of the 20th century. Their names are carved onto the pillars along with their letters and diaries. Viewers expe-rience a layered passage into the heart of the pillars, within which the recorded experience of the veterans becomes more and more intimate as one delves deeper into the space. The memorial places past occurrences and deeds within the contemporary culture of the county.

Maryann Thompson Architects was founded in 2000 by Mary-ann Thompson. Prior to that Thompson was a founding partner in the firm Thompson and Rose Architects. Maryann Thomp-son and Charles Rose emphasize the importance of viewing architecture and the site on which it is built as a unified whole. Each site is carefully studied, allowing the work to compliment the physical, ecological, cultural and historical features of the specific area, striving to create an innovative environment.

Photo: Chuck Choi, NY

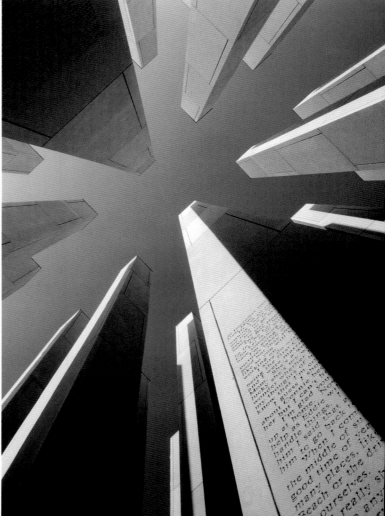

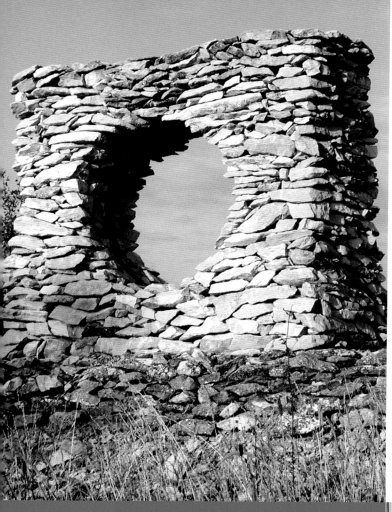

The Mistral's Hole
Harry Schaffer, Wolf Warnke

Completion: 1997. **Technique:** limestone in ancient technique of dry masonry. **Location:** Reillanne, France.

"The Mistral's Hole" is created from Provence limestone, using the dry masonry technique. It is a minimalist work of art, conceived as a pure example of Land Art. All of the material used was found and taken from directly around the site. The circle in the center of the piece frames the background around it, focusing the attention of the observer on one particular area of the view, creating a small, framed space and highlighting the beauty of the area.

Harry Schaffer was born in Switzerland in 1963. He works as a Land Artist and has held several exhibitions in Switzerland, France and Italy. He also works as an interior architect and has a studio in Basel. Wolf Warnke was born in Hamburg in 1945. He studied fine art and has lived and taught in both Germany and France. He works as a Land Artist, sculptor, painter and photographer. He was a founding member of "Gruppe Junge Kunst" in Germany and "Association Lézard" in France. Schaffer and Warnke have been creating artworks together for the past 25 years.

Thinker on a Rock
Barry Flanagan

Completion: 1997. **Technique:** bronze. **Location:** Utrecht, The Netherlands.

Barry Flanagan has explored painting, dance, and installation pieces; reacting against the formal, constructed metal sculpture that predominated when he was in art school. "Thinker on a Rock" is a reference to Rodin's famous sculpture "The Thinker". The artist combines his signature hare motif with Rodin's "Thinker", making a clever and irreverent reference to one of the world most famous sculptures. The figure of a hare appears in an endless variety of poses in Flanagan's work.

Barry Flanagan was born in 1941 in Wales. He studied at Birmingham College of Arts before attending Saint Martin's College of Art and Design in London. He graduated in 1966, going on to teach at several colleges and universities. He is famous for producing sculptures featuring a hare motif, which have been in many exhibitions, including on Park Avenue in New York. He also represented Britain at the Venice Biennial. A major exhibition of his work was shown at the Public Art Gallery Recklinghausen in Germany in 2002.

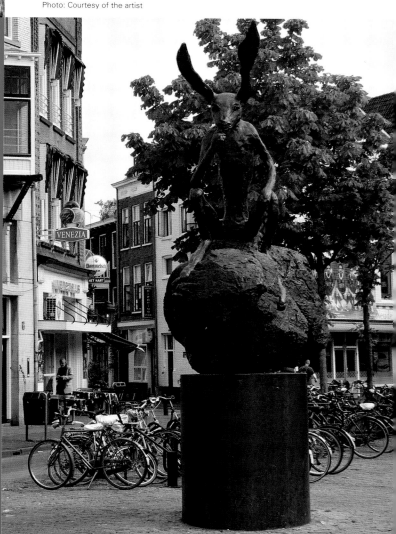

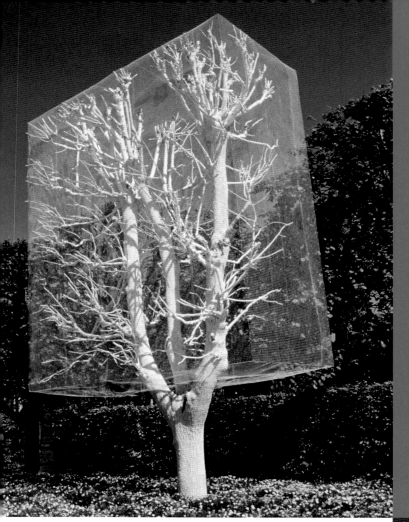

St Cloud
Edouard François

Completion: 1997. **Technique:** textile web, tree, white pigeons. **Location:** St Cloud, France.

This artwork is fittingly called "St Cloud" and was made for the magazine Marie-Claire-Maison. Edouard François' works often combine nature with design, concentrating on the textures and colors of a surface. The textile wrapping forms a frame around the tree; the silver colored branches are framed within the textile "tree house", emphasizing the beauty of something that we see every day while at the same time not altering its essential form. The tree can be absorbed into the landscape.

Edouard François was born in 1957. He is an architect, whose work focuses on the ecological, combining art, nature and architecture to create unique, "green" projects. He studied town planning at the National School of Bridges and Roads and architecture and engineering at the Paris Academy of Fine Arts. He designs buildings specifically to suit their context; chameleon-like they respond to their environment. François' best known projects include the "Building that Grows" in Montpellier and the "Flower Tower" in Paris.

Photo: Courtesy of the artist

Tulach a' tSolais
Michael Warren, Scott Tallon Walker Architects

Completion: 1998. **Technique:** concrete. **Location:** Co. Wexford, Ireland.

In the pastoral landscape of Wexford, a shaft of concrete cleaves through a green hill like a futuristic burial mound. It is a historical commemoration, marking the bicentenary of the 1798 Irish rebellion at Oulart Hill. The elementally simple monument, designed by architect Ronald Tallon and sculptor Michael Warren, rises in the middle of fields of rolling pastureland. Its walls capture the rays of the rising and setting sun, framing the view to Vinegar Hill where the uprising was subsequently quashed.

Born in Wexford in 1950, Michael Warren studied at Bath Academy of Art, Trinity College, Dublin and at the Brera Academy in Milan. He won the Alice Berger Hammerschlag scholarship and a Macaulay fellowship in 1978. Ronald Tallon is one of the leading architects in Ireland and his firm, Scott Tallon Walker Architects has won many awards for its work including the prestigious Royal Gold Medal. Ronald Tallon has won the Triennial Gold Medal of the Royal Institute of the Architects of Ireland, twice.

Photos: Scott Tallon Walker Architects

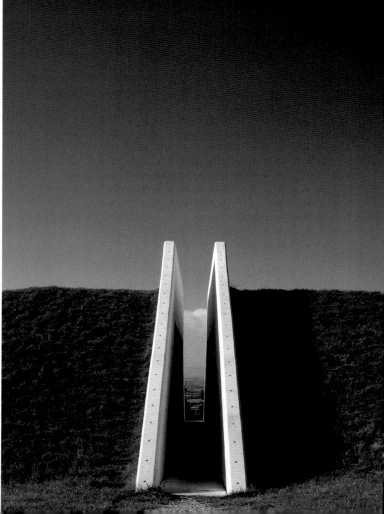

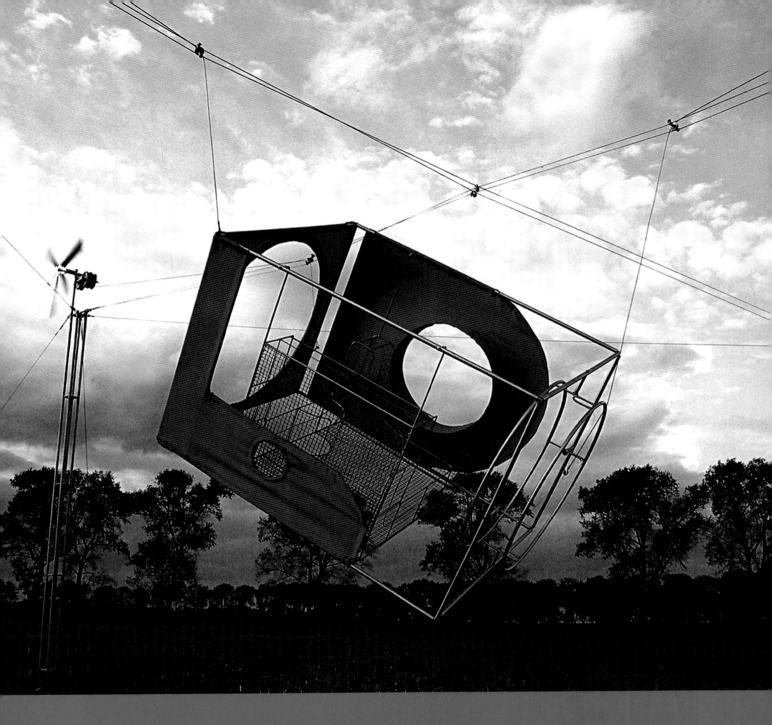

The Cloud Room
Adam Kalinowski

Completion: 1998. **Technique:** aluminum, cloth, wind turbines with reduction gears. **Location:** Bydgoszcz, Poland.

This project is a kinetic outdoor sculpture. The structure is steel and aluminum, with heavy fabric, aircraft cable and propellers. The direction of the slow movement of the form is unpredictable as it depends entirely on the wind direction and strength. The slow motion of the form is more like a dynamic levitation.

Adam Kalinowski is a contemporary Polish sculptor and artist. He has exhibited work both nationally and internationally, including at the Municipal Gallery in Poznañ, Poland and the Zacheta Gallery of Contemporary Art, Warsaw. In 2001 he also achieved third place at the tenth International design competition in Osaka, Japan for his work "The Sky Reaching Hammock". In 2008 "The Sky Reaching Railway Track" was a finalist at the International Creative Competition in London.

Forest
Snejana Simeonova

Completion: 1998. **Technique:** sandstone. **Location:** Beratzhausen, Germany.

Human intervention in the landscape is always a reflection of man's ideas. In the sculpture "Forest" the natural form of a tree is stylized and constructed in sandstone. This transformation represents diversity, where man can transform natural material. When the viewer approaches the stylized, sandstone trees, the outlines open out, resembling the shapes of branches formed by a real tree. Trees can be seen through these chiseled gaps in the stone; true nature contrasted with man-made structure.

Snejana Simeonova graduated from the Academy of Fine Arts in Sofia, Bulgaria. She has been involved in more than 25 solo exhibitions in Bulgaria, Germany, Austria and Switzerland as well as many group exhibitions in Bulgaria, Germany, China, India, Hungary and New Zealand. She works with stone, bronze, resin, paper and other media. Her sculptures are in the collections of the National Gallery in Sofia and the Sofia City Art Gallery, as well as many private collections, including in Belgium and Australia.

Photo: Courtesy of the artist

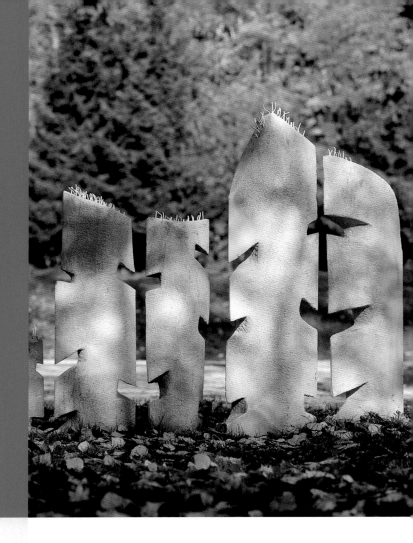

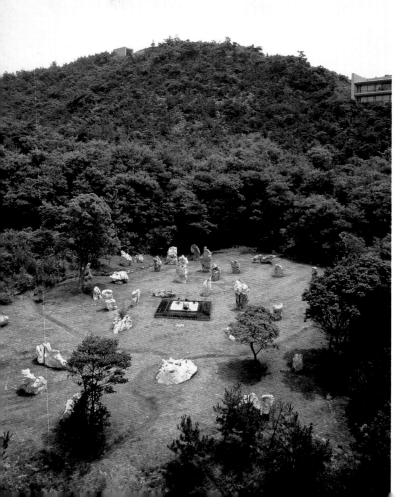

Cultural Melting Bath
Cai Guo-Qiang

Completion: 1998. **Technique:** 36 Taihu rocks, hot tub with hydrotherapy jets, bathwater infused with herbs. **Location:** Benesse House, Japan.

This piece was one of the works in Cai Guo-Qiang's first solo exhibition. The work, pictured here in Japan, gathers Taihu rocks in animal or ghostly shapes and arranges them around a small courtyard garden, in accordance with the principles of Feng Shui. Audience members are in the optimal position in terms of the natural flow of energy. By combining the separate worlds of contemporary art and Feng Shui, the artist attempts to explore an alternative methodology from that of western contemporary art.

Cai Guo-Qiang was born in 1957 in Quanzhou, China. Between 1981 and 1985 he studied at the Shanghai Theater Academy in the Department of Stage Design. He has been awarded many prizes in Europe, Asia and the USA and has been involved in various solo and group exhibitions.

Photo: Fujisuka Mitsuo

Marking pilgrims' route
Henk Rusman

Completion: 1998. **Technique:** steel. **Location:** St. Jacobiparochie, The Netherlands.

This sculpture is the marking point at the start of the pilgrimage route from St. Jabobiparochie in the Netherlands to Santiago de Compostela in Spain. The triangle, which forms the basis of this work, is two meters wide at it's base and twelve meters long. The steel triangle is molded to an arch, which represents a gateway to the pilgrims route. The gateway is embedded on a diamond shaped, granite base, in which the stylized form of a scallop shell is engraved; the European logo for the St James Way.

Henk Rusman is a Dutch sculptor, born in the Netherlands in 1950. He was educated at the City Academy in Maastricht and later at the Jan van Eyck Academy. He began working as an artist in 1978. His sculptures are often large and made using metals or stone.

Photos: Courtesy of the artist

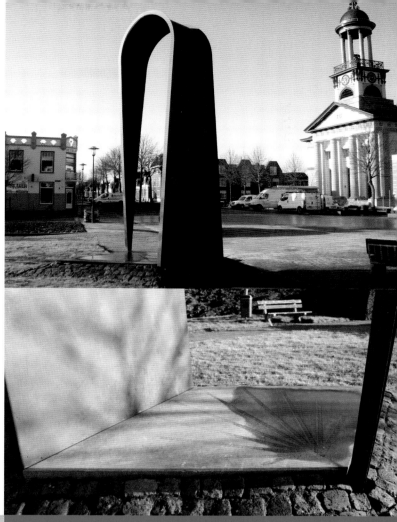

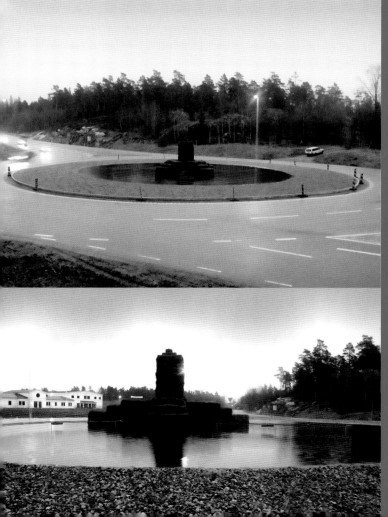

Gazebo Stairs
Karin Lind

Completion: 1998. **Technique:** ready lawnturf, pond, neon. **Location:** Mölnvik, Sweden.

This sculpture stands in the center of a roundabout at the end of a highway. It is made of living plants and greenery, giving its appearance variety throughout the year. The centerpiece is of stacked turf, rising to a height of over four meters, standing in a pond where red neon lights float above the surface. The "Gazebo Stairs" and neon light reflects in the surface of the water like a mirage, during both day and night.

Karin Lind was born in Stockholm in 1959. She studied at the University College of Arts, Crafts and Design, Stockholm and later went on to study at the Royal University College of Fine Arts, Stockholm. She also completed several minor courses at the School of Architecture. Lind works with Simon Häggblom in artist duo Simka.

Photos: Peter de Ru, Stockholm

Reflektionswand
Olaf Metzel

Completion: 1998. **Technique:** galvanized steel, prism reflectors. **Location:** Münster, Germany.

"Reflection Wall" is a large sculpture, five meters high and nine meters wide; it is clearly visible from a distance. The sculpture is sun-like in color and made of steel, similar in shape to an advertising billboard. Instead of advertisements, the gently curved wall is covered with prisms, taking the familiar and making it unfamiliar. The sculpture promotes freedom of thought and expression to passersby, inviting them to consider new perspectives.

Olaf Metzel was born in Berlin in 1952. He studied at both the Free University and the University of Art in Berlin. Since 1990 he has worked as a professor at the Academy of Arts in Munich, working as principle between 1995 and 1999. He has exhibited his work both nationally and internationally, including in Munich, Australia, Istanbul and São Paulo. Metzel also has many sculptural works on display in the public realm, in Bonn, Lisbon, Munich, Essen and Berlin. He has been awarded many prizes, including the Wilhelm Loth Prize in Darmstadt.

Stone Cycle
Julie Edwards,
Ron Thompson

Completion: 1998. **Technique:** stone carving. **Location:** Bury, United Kingdom.

Stone Cycle took a year to create. The artists worked on site for twelve months, gaining an understanding of the place, the passing of time, people and industry. This understanding is represented in the interrupted circular layout of the sculpture. Like the site, the stones had a previous life, originally quarried and cut for use as a bridge. Under the 100 years of industrial grime the artist discovered marks made by the original masons. Carved symbols were added to these marks, clues to long forgotten stories.

Julie Edwards was awarded a first class honors degree in fine art and sculpture from Nottingham University. Ron Thompson graduated with a first class honors degree in fine art from Staffordshire Polytechnic. Edwards and Thompson started the art partnership Planet Art in 1997 and have produced several collaborative works for the public realm including commissions from Birmingham City Council, British Waterways, Countryside services and Hospital Le Puy en Velay in France, amongst others.

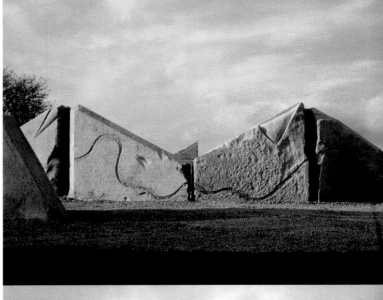

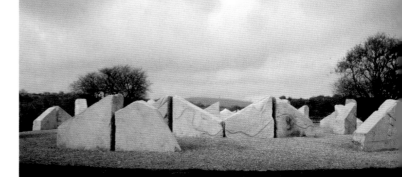

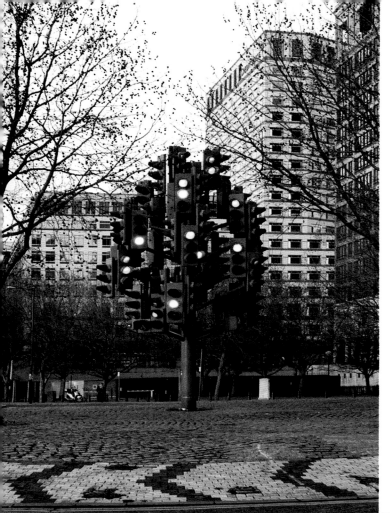

Traffic Light Tree
Pierre Vivant

Completion: 1998. **Technique:** plastic, steel, metal, lamps.
Location: London, United Kingdom.

French sculptor Pierre Vivant made the "Traffic Light Tree", following a competition run by the Public Arts Commissions Agency. The tree is situated in the middle of a roundabout in London's financial district, near Canary Wharf. The tree is eight meters tall and has 75 sets of traffic lights attached to it, controlled by a computer. The tree combines natural and artificial landscapes and the changing pattern of the lights reflect the hustle and bustle of London's financial district.

Born in Paris in 1952, Pierre Vivant has studios in Oxford and Paris and regularly exhibits his work in both England and France. Since 1984, Vivant has been undertaking commissioned work, usually of a temporary nature and conceived for specific events and locations. In 1990 he was appointed as sculptor in residence at Warwick University.

Photos: Rob Sandiford

The Angel of the North
Antony Gormley

Completion: 1998. **Technique:** steel. **Location:** Gateshead, United Kingdom.

"The Angel of the North" stands in a prominent position, on raised ground in Gateshead, near Newcastle upon Tyne. The piece was built to withstand winds of 160 kilometers per hour and 600 tons of concrete were required to anchor the sculpture to its rock foundations. The huge construction was made in three parts, costing over one million Euro; it was largely funded by the National Lottery. Though it received some criticism when it was first built, it is now considered an important landmark.

Antony Gormley was born in London in 1950. He has worked as a sculptor for over 40 years, producing some of England's most iconic public sculptures. His work often investigates the relation of the human body to space. Gormley's work has been widely exhibited in the United Kingdom, America and Europe, with solo shows in the United Kingdom including at the Serpentine, Tate and the British Museum. In 2010 he and 100 other artists signed an open letter to the United Kingdom Culture Minister, Jeremy Hunt, protesting against cutbacks in the arts.

Photos: The Halo / Wikimedia Commons (a); Tony Grist / Wikimedia Commons (b.)

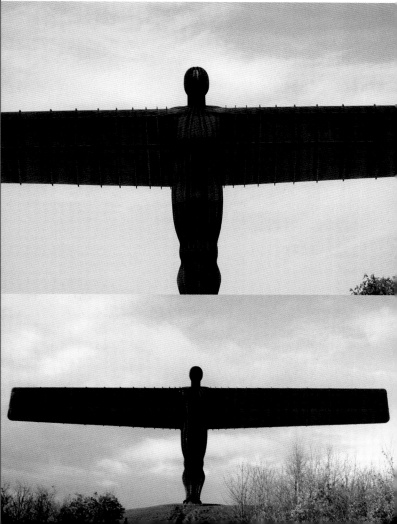

Tromsø Labyrinth
Bjarne Aasen,
Guttorm Guttomsgaard

Completion: 1998. **Technique:** stones in various sizes, fashioned and polished. **Location:** Tromsø, Norway.

The University of Tromsø is the worlds most northerly, at 70° north, and is characterized by snowy winters and polar nights from 21st November until 21st January and summers of midnight sun. The space features a labyrinthine snake that surrounds and guards a symbolic warm, luminous source in the center. The idea of the labyrinth pattern stems from arctic folklore, which is one of the youngest labyrinth cultures in the world, probably formed as a magical symbol.

Guttorm Guttormsgaard is a Norwegian artist, born in 1938. He works primarily with graphics and drawing. He has produced several works of public art and taught drawing and graphics at the National Art Academy until 1984. He currently has a gallery and workshop in an old dairy, from where he organizes exhibitions. Bjarne Aasen is a Norwegian landscape architect who is involved in many projects both within Norway and internationally.

Photos: Ola Röe

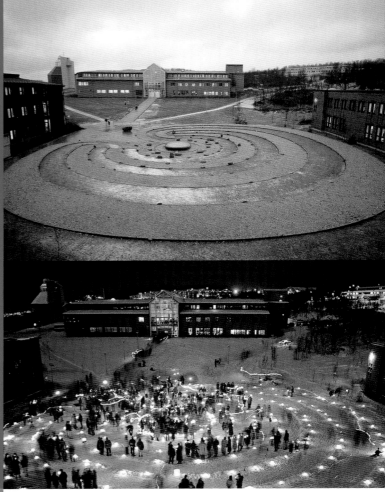

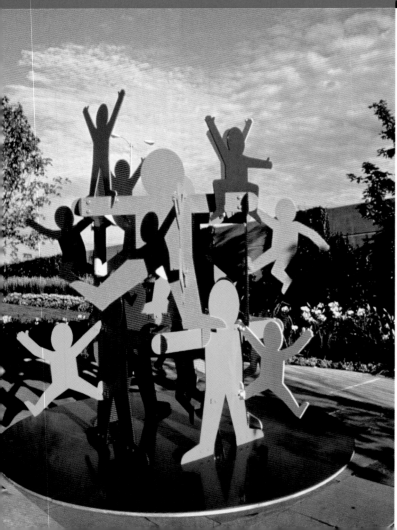

Fathers and Sons
Peter W. Michel

Completion: 1999. **Technique:** powder coated aluminum.
Location: Urbana, IL, USA.

"Fathers and Sons" is a three-meter tall painted aluminum sculpture. It represents community - a celebration of relationships and the spirit of playfulness. The colorful, interlinked figures symbolize the support structure provided by fathers, upon which their sons can play, grow and become men. It was first shown during Pier Walk '99 on Chicago's Navy Pier and is now part of the permanent collection of the Wandell Sculpture Garden in Urbana, Illinois.

Peter W. Michel was born in Schenectady, NY. He studied fine arts at Oberlin College in Ohio and architecture at MIT in Cambridge, MA. His training and work as an architect has influenced his constructivist approach to sculpture. Public sculpture highlights include showings at the Chesterwood Museum in Stockbridge MA, the Navy Pier in Chicago, Downtown Stamford CT and the Federal Reserve Board in Washington. He has recently completed commissioned work in Houston, TX, Utica and Syracuse, NY.

Photo: Courtesy of the artist

Ecce Homo
Mark Wallinger

Completion: 1999. **Technique:** resin-bonded marble dust, gold leaf, barbed wire. **Location:** London, United Kingdom.

"Ecce Homo" was the first project commissioned for the vacant fourth plinth in Trafalgar Square, in 1999. This life-size sculpture of Christ is an actual body cast of a male figure, his hands tied behind his back, naked except for a loin cloth and a crown of barbed wire. He appears vulnerable amongst the oversized imperial symbols surrounding him. The sculpture was later shown as part of Wallinger's British Pavilion installation at the 2001 Venice Biennal.

Mark Wallinger is a British artist, born in Essex in 1959. His work focuses on themes of politics, cultural identity, social class and religion and has been exhibited internationally. Wallinger's installation "State Britain", was on display at Tate Britain in 2007. Wallinger also represented Great Britain at the 2001 Venice Biennial. He has been nominated twice for the Turner Prize and was the winner in 2007. His video work "Via Dolorosa", is permanently installed in a crypt in the Duomo in Milan.

Photo: © the artist, courtesy Anthony Reynolds Gallery, photograph by Peter White

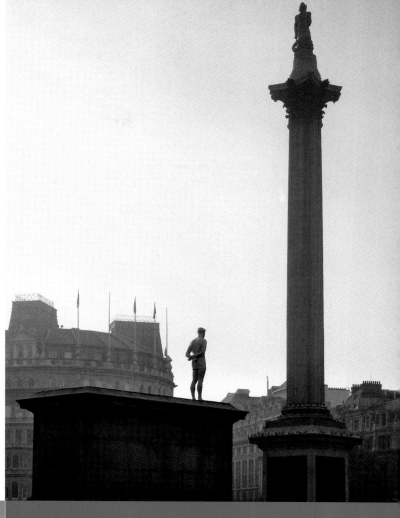

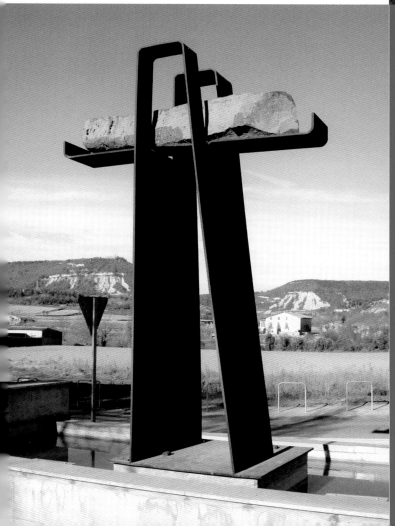

Cross of Guixa
Ernest Altes

Completion: 1999. **Technique:** steel, basalt. **Location:** Vic, Spain.

This artwork is made from metal and stone. The size and weight of the materials in the rural landscape suggest endurance and strength. The sculpture is five meters tall, two meters wide and three meters deep. The shape frames a part of the natural landscape so that the observer looks between the two iron sides a piece of the surroundings hills is framed, drawing attention to a fragment of the landscape and allowing the viewer to focus on the beauty of the view.

Ernest Altes was born in 1956 in Vic near Barcelona, Spain. As a child he was always fascinated by the nature around him. He became interested in art at the age of ten, creating sculptures from sea smoothed glass, branches and leaves. Altes had his first exhibition in 1977 and the same year began working in a foundry, learning how to work metal. He later traveled widely, visiting the Sahara dessert and experimenting with different artistic techniques. He made many sculptures in public space and collaborates with architects.

Photo: Courtesy of the artist

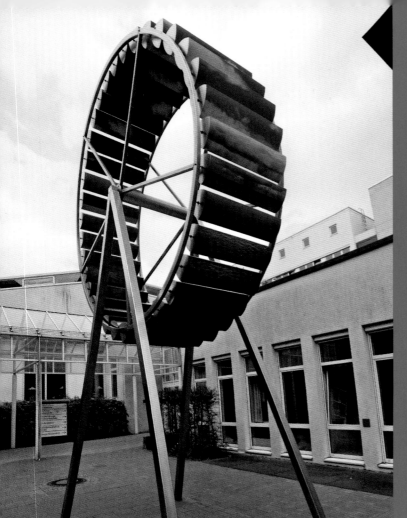

Shifting Horizons
Stefanie Zoche

Completion: 1999. **Technique:** solar propulsion, stainless steel, photo transfer prints. **Location:** Munich, Germany.

This sculpture is simultaneously reminiscent of a water wheel, sun wheel and the sky. The puzzle works to attract observers, encouraging them to stop on their way past. The wheel is propelled by solar power and the blue and cloud pattern of the paddles are made from photo print transfer. The circle symbolizes the circle of life, the continuation of nature and the journey of water as it falls from the sky and returns to the sea, only to evaporate and become, once more, part of the sky and clouds.

Stefanie Zoche is a German artist, born in Munich in 1965. She studied painting and sculpture at the School of Fine Arts in Perpignan and later studied art at the Middlesex Polytechnic in London. She has been working together with art photographer Sabine Haubitz, under the name Haubitz + Zoche, since 1998. She has exhibited her work at various solo exhibitions, including at the Fotomania Gallery in Rotterdam and the Twin Peaks Project in Sweden.

Photo: Chris van Uffelen

The Frog Prince or Waiting for the Princess
Ottmar Hörl

Completion: 1999. **Technique:** plastics. **Location:** Darmstadt, Germany.

"The Frog Prince or Waiting for the Princess" fountain is located in Darmstadt and is typical of the artist's Multiple or "Same-Art" displays, where he uses the same form again and again. The frogs are positioned in rows over a decorated, tiled floor. The idea came from the "Frog King" fairy tale, where an enchanted prince is turned into a frog and waits in a fountain for a princess to come and free him from the enchantment with a kiss.

Ottmar Hörl is a German artist and sculptor. He was born in Nauheim, Germany in 1950. He studied at the Academy of Fine Arts in Frankfurt / Main, later going on to study at the Art Academy in Dusseldorf. In 1985, he established the group " Formalhaut", with architects Gabriela Seifert and Götz Stöckman. He was appointed as a professor at the Academy of Fine Arts, Nuremberg in 1999 and promoted to president in 2005.

Photos: Chris van Uffelen

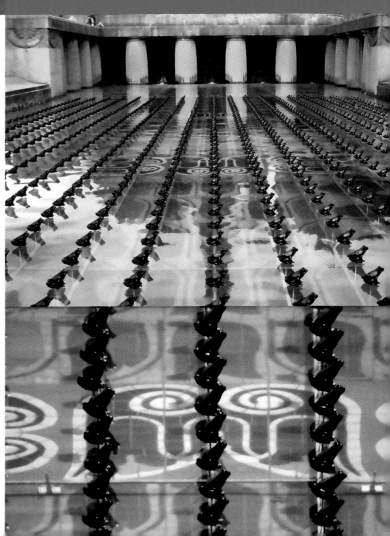

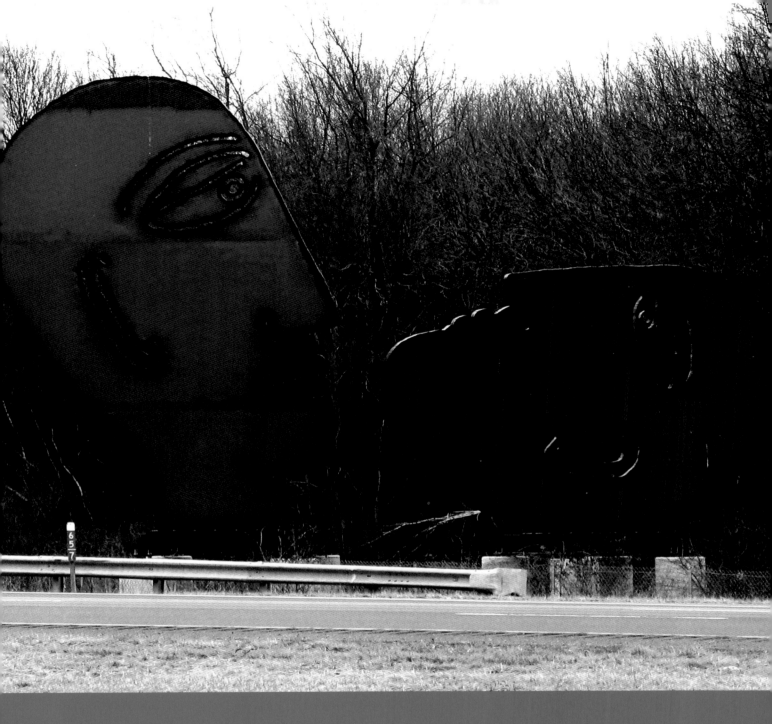

Head 2 Head
John Martini

Completion: 1999. **Technique:** steel, enamel. **Location:** Hamilton, NJ, USA.

"Head 2 Head" is located along Interstate-295 just before exit 65B. This is the largest sculptural work by artist John Martini and is over ten meters tall and eight meters long. The sculpture is made of plasma-cut and welded steel; painted black around the rim to create the effect of exposed steel and then finished with colorful enamel. The piece is a site specific work, commissioned in 1999 by the Sculpture Foundation Inc.

John Martini lives and works in both Florida and Veuxhaulles-Sur-Aube, France. His sculptures are on display in various galleries and museums both in America and internationally. His works are extensively represented in private and public collections, including the large installation, "Head 2 Head," at the Grounds for Sculpture in Hamilton, New Jersey. Martini is best known for creating large metal sculptures that are often finished with brightly colored enamel.

Photo: Susan Kane

Stain on the Vision, Summer 2048
Benni Efrat

Completion: 1999. **Technique:** zinc coated barbed wire.
Location: Tel Aviv, Israel.

This sculpture is on display in the sculpture garden of the Tel Aviv Museum of Art. It is made of barbed wire, coated in zinc and from a distance it takes on the almost cozy look of a carpet and sofa. It is only when one comes closer that the true nature of the piece can be known. The piece plays with expectations, taking the known and making it threatening and unknown. It encourages the viewer to question what is seen, not just to assume that it is really what it seems to be.

Benni Efrat is an Israeli sculptor, painter, printmaker and filmmaker. He was born in Beirut in 1936 but immigrated to Israel in 1947. He studied at the Avni Institute of Art and Design in Tel Aviv, graduating in 1961. He lived in London for ten years, between 1966 and 1976 and studied at St Martin's School of Art in London. He later settled in New York and became interested in Conceptual Art, exploring energy, space and perception in his works.

Photos: Benni Efrat / Wikimedia Commons

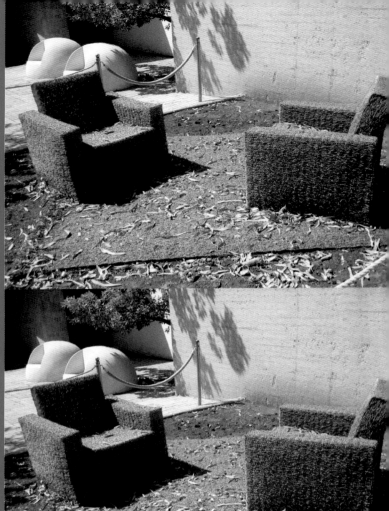

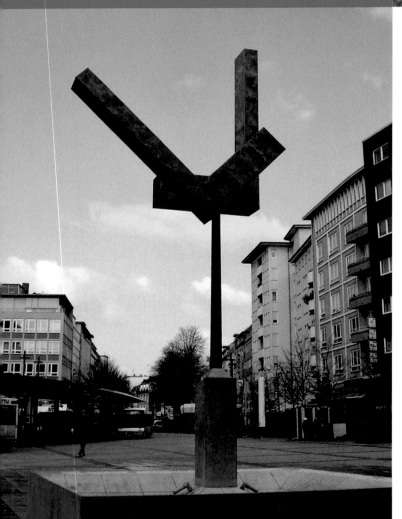

Conversation II
George Rickey

Completion: 1999. **Technique:** stainless steel. **Location:** Ludwigshafen, Germany.

This kinetic sculpture, "Conversation II" can be found in Berliner Platz in Ludwigshafen and is positioned over a granite base, filled with water. It was presented as a gift to the people of the city at the turn of the millennium by the BASF company. The two L-shapes rotate in the wind, producing either the letter L or the letter U, which together comprise the first two letters of the number plates of cars from Ludwigshafen: LU.

George Rickey is an American sculptor; he was born in Indiana in 1907 and died in 2002. He studied art at New York University, the New York Institute of Arts and the Chicago Institute of Design. Inspired by the works of Alexander Calder, he created his first kinetic works in 1945. He has since made many works of kinetic sculptures, some of which are on display in public space.

Photo: Immanuel Giel / Wikimedia Commons

Way Marker 7
Otto Herbert Hajek

Completion: 1999. **Technique:** steel, blue paint. **Location:** Stuttgart, Germany.

"Way Marker 7" is one of several works by Otto Herbert Hajek located in Stuttgart. His public sculptures often serve as way markers in the city. This one stands near the Stuttgart television tower and points towards it, drawing the attention of the viewer upwards, towards the world's first television tower.

Otto Herbert Hajek was born in 1927 in Nové Hute, Czech Republic. He studied sculpture at the Stuttgart State Academy of Art and Design in Stuttgart. Hajek participated in the second and third Documenta exhibitions in Kassel and was appointed as chairman of the German Association of Artists in 1972; a position he held until 1979. In his capacity as chairman he dedicated himself to the projection and promotion of public art. He lived in Stuttgart until his death in 2005.

Photo: Andreas Praefcke / Wikimedia Commons

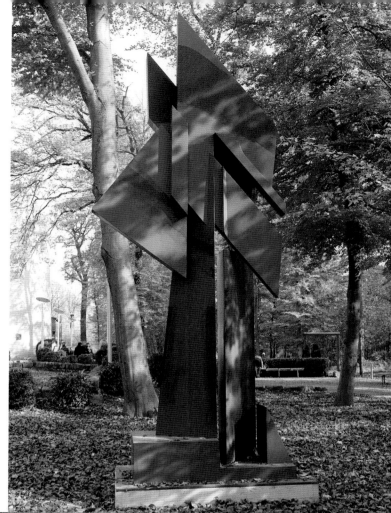

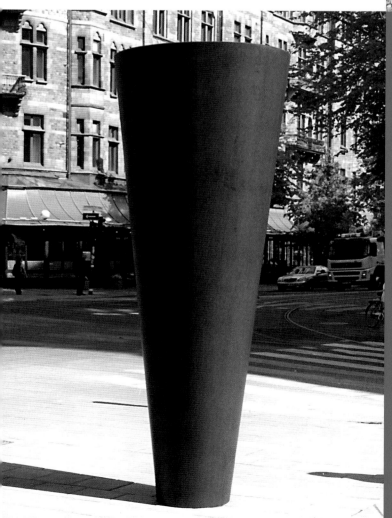

Conical Ellipse
Jene Highstein

Completion: 1999. **Technique:** Swedish black granite. **Location:** Stockholm, Sweden.

Carved from a single block of intensely black Swedish diabase, this sculpture is installed at the intersection of a busy street in the center of Stockholm. The sculpture "Conical Ellipse" rises from a small circle at its base to a larger elliptical form at the top. It is at the same time a column and a figure, its form relates to the human dimension. It is three and a half meters tall and it stands out in relation to the human form. It does not tower over the viewer, rather it acts to scale the viewer to the surrounding architecture.

Jene Highstein was born in Baltimore, USA in 1942. He studied philosophy at the University of Maryland and University of Chicago before dedicating himself to a career as an artist in 1966. His works are held in the collections of many museums in America, including the Contemporary Art Museum of Chicago and the National Gallery in Washington D.C. Highstein also works in theater and produced a theater production of Flatland for the Brooklyn Academy.

Photo: Courtesy of the artist

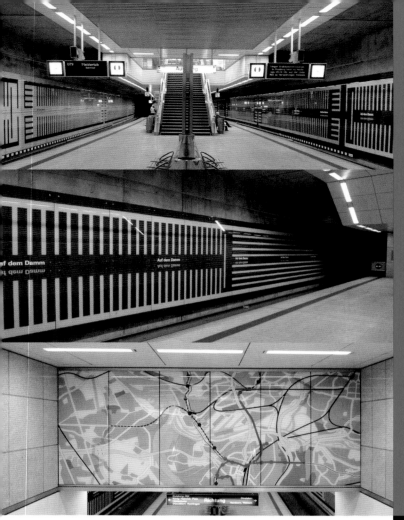

Subwaystation Duisburg
Eberhard Bosslet

Completion: 2000. **Technique:** silkscreen behind glass.
Location: Duisburg, Germany.

These two geometrically formed, colored-glass surfaces are each 85 meters long and are the main characterizing features of this underground station. The geometrical structure of the picture-screens accompany the coming, going and waiting passengers; supporting the conduct and orientation of the users on the platform. On the approaching-face of the stairs in the station is a printed image of the tunnel during the construction phase and a structural plan in the form of a city map.

Eberhard Bosslet is a German artist, born in Speyer in 1953. He studied painting in Berlin and in the 1970s changed to sculpture and three-dimensional installations. He works with different media, including paint, sculpture, and photography. Bosslet has worked with the terms of construction and housing in many different ways, within interior and exterior, public and private space. Since 1997 he has worked as professor of sculpture and spatial concept at the Academy of Fine Arts in Dresden.

Photos: Courtesy of the artist

Lichtburg
Yann Kersalé

Completion: 2000. **Technique:** neo lights. **Location:** Berlin, Germany.

French artist Yann Kersalé was commissioned to accentuate this building, built by architect Helmut Jahn, with one of his elaborate light displays. The light installation slowly changes color as it tapers up the 60-meter building. The changing pattern of the lights is designed to give the impression that the building 'breathes'. At night, red, blue, green and yellow alternate. The installation complements other areas of Kranzler Eck, such as the distinctive red and white awning of Café Kranzler.

Born in 1955, Yann Kersalé studied at the School of Fine Arts in Quimper, graduating with a higher national diploma in 1978. Kersalé began working with light soon after graduating and has since developed more than 100 projects. His installations can be seen on many buildings, including the Sony Center in Berlin and Bangkok Airport. He often works with architect Helmut Jahn and has worked on projects in Qatar, Germany and Washington.

Photo: Chris van Uffelen

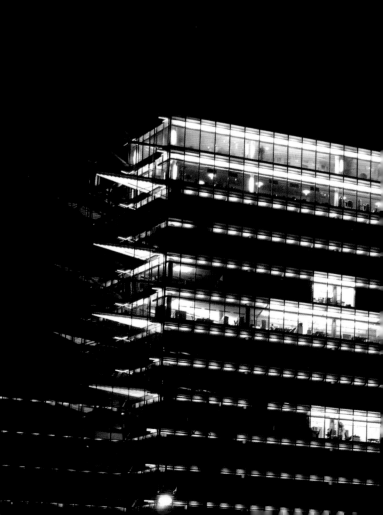

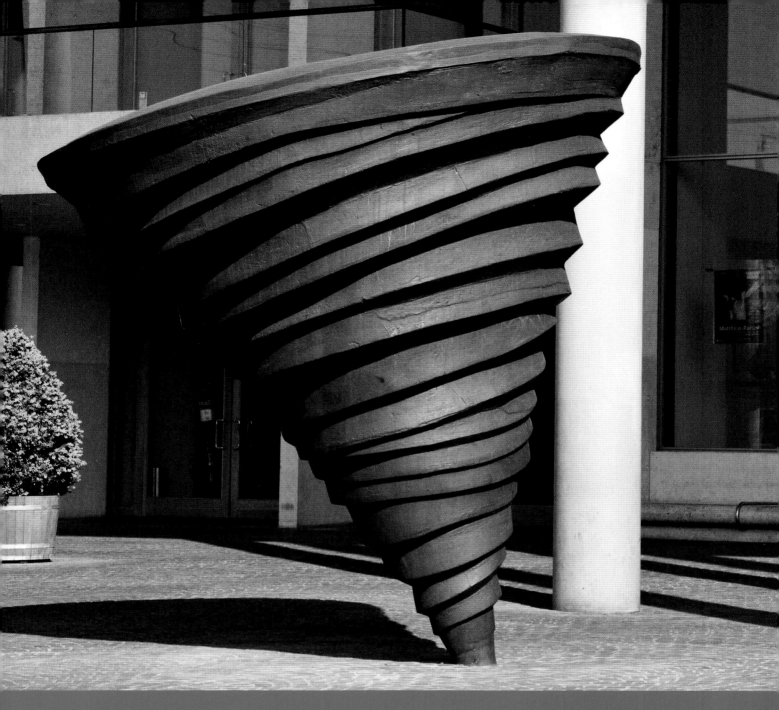

Dance with Me
Andrea Zaumseil

Completion: 2000. **Technique:** steel. **Location:** Freiburg, Germany.

This sculptural ensemble "Dance With Me" consists of four, monumental steel sculptures. The individual pieces are shaped like spinning tops and vary in height from three to four meters. They have a surprisingly light, dynamic appearance and give the impression that they could spin away from their allocated space at any moment. The artwork stands in front of the concert hall in Freiburg and is related to music, to rhythm and the expression of movement and music.

Andrea Zaumseil is a German sculptor, born in Überlingen in 1957. She studied German literature and history at the university in Constance, graduating in 1979. She then went on to study sculpture at the State Academy of Art in Stuttgart, where she graduated in 1985. She began teaching in Stuttgart in 1985 and later worked a professor of metal sculpture at the University of Art in Burg Giebichenstein. She has exhibited her work widely and produced many sculptures for public space, situated in various locations throughout Germany.

Photo: Chris van Uffelen

Sanctuary
Roddy Mathieson

Completion: 2000. **Technique:** bronze, stone. **Location:** Locheport, United Kingdom.

"Sanctuary" is a site specific work inspired by the elements of its location. Growing out of the rock like a windblown Hebridean tree, the sculpture embraces its surroundings, pointing out towards the mouth of the sea-loch, referencing local boat design and the marine environment. It evolves in form along the way, concluding with a wing – celebrating the vast Atlantic skies of Uist. Patinating in the spindrift, "Sanctuary" is maturing with the elements, capturing a sense of belonging within its environs.

Roddy Mathieson graduated with a bachelor of arts in fine art from Duncan of Jordanstone College of Art and Design. His sculpture explores our relationship with the natural world, working site specifically in bronze. He is employed at Duncan of Jordanstone, works as a freelance artist, and is director of The Mobile Foundry. This travelling sculpture foundry grew out of the Sanctuary commission, undertaking public commissions and educational projects for a variety of clients around Scotland.

Photos: Courtesy of the artist

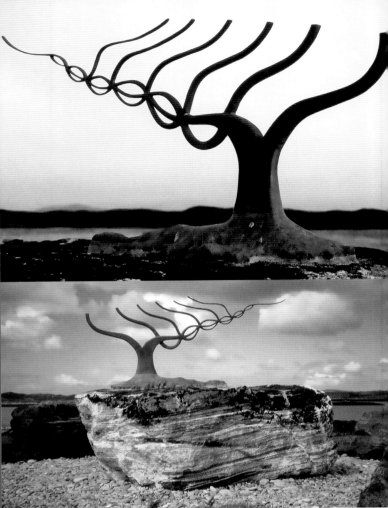

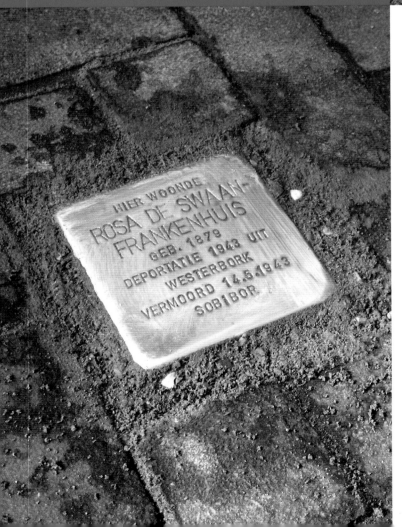

Stumbling Blocks
Gunter Demnig

Completion: 2000. **Technique:** brass. **Location:** Glanerbrug, The Netherlands.

The "Stumbling Blocks" project first began in the year 2000. Each brass block is a memorial to one of the victims of the Nazi regime in Germany. The blocks are set in the ground in front of the last known place where the victim lived. There are around 500 brass plaques across Germany, each commemorating a life that was taken. With this thought provoking project, Gunter Demnig keeps the memory of the victims alive, not allowing the atrocities of the past to be forgotten.

Gunter Demnig was born in Berlin in 1947. He studied art education at the University of Arts in Berlin until 1969 and then went on to study industrial design at the same institution. Between 1977 and 1979 he worked restoring and designing monuments and later as artistic and scientific assistant in the arts department at the University of Kassel. He opened a studio in Cologne in 1985 and in 1993 he began to plan and design the project "Stumbling Blocks". The project is coordinated by Uta Franke.

Photo: Gerardus / Wikimedia Commons

The Kiosk for Nighthawks
Jean-Michel Othoniel

Completion: 2000. **Technique:** colored glass, aluminum.
Location: Paris, France.

"The Kiosk for Nighthawks" is actually an entrance to the subway. The work is comprised of two parts; the outer part, visible from the street and an interior section. The outer section takes the form of rings, linked to each other and made from colored glass. Six pillars, made from aluminum spheres, three on each side of the subway mouth, support two domes. The domes are made of glass beads and each one is topped by a small, glass sculpture.

Jean-Michel Othoniel is a contemporary French artist. Born in Saint-Etienne he now lives and works in Paris. He first gained a reputation with a series of sculptures made from sulphur, exhibited at the ninth Documenta in Kassel, 1992. In 1993 Othoniel began to introduce glass into his work. His work is concerned with the state of materials, how they can be transformed and the stags they go through in this transformation. He uses a variety of media, including photography, film, choreography and video.

Photos: Chris van Uffelen

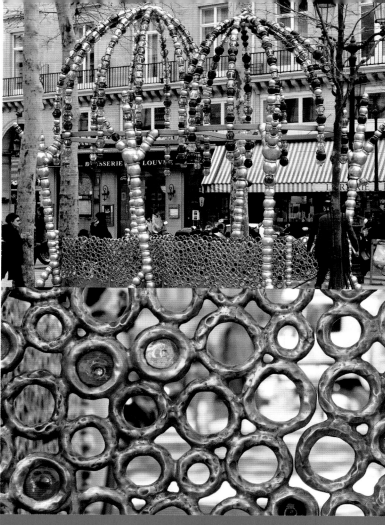

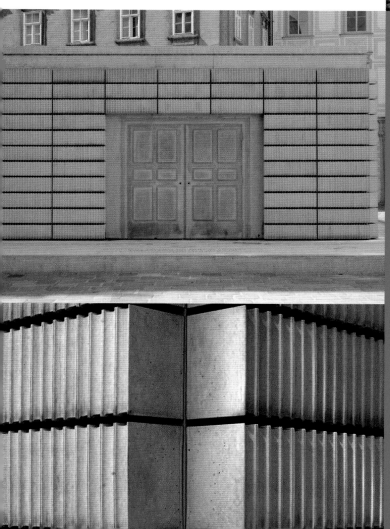

Nameless Library
Rachel Whiteread

Completion: 2000. **Technique:** steel, concrete. **Location:** Vienna, Austria.

The "Judenplatz Holocaust Memorial" is also known as the "Nameless Library" and is located in Vienna. This is the city's central monument for the Austrian Holocaust victims. The memorial is made of steel and concrete, the outside façades are library shelves, turned inside out, with the spines of the books facing inwards. The books represent the vast number of victims and the reputation of Jewish people for being "people of the book". The work was not intended to be beautiful, but to evoke tragedy and brutality.

Rachel Whiteread is a British sculptor, born in 1963. She studied painting at the Faculty of Arts and Architecture at Brighton Polytechnic, later attending the Slade School of Art. She had her first exhibition in 1987 and exhibited work at the Royal Academy's Sensation exhibition in 1997. Whiteread was also the first woman to win the Turner Prize in 1993. "House" in London is one of her best known works and is a concrete cast of the inside of an entire Victorian terraced house.

Photos: Chris van Uffelen

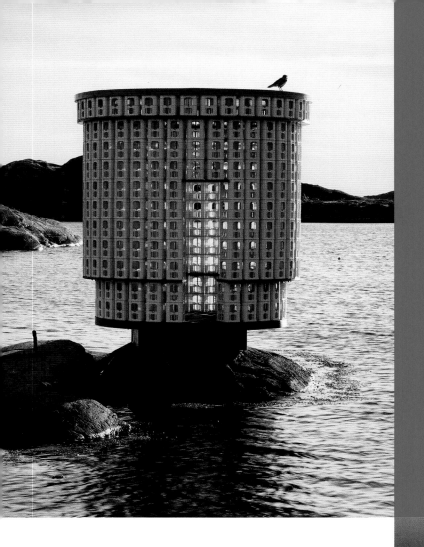

Lighthouse
Wolfgang Winter, Berthold Hoerbelt

Completion: 2000. **Technique:** green plastic bottle crates, various materials, illumination. **Location:** Skärhamn, Sweden.

"Lighthouse" is mint green in color and is made of German mineral water boxes. It can be seen easily from passing ships and from the beach. In summer it is possible to swim out and climb into it. On stormy days and at high water levels, the lighthouse and the small island are completely surrounded by the sea. The artificial material makes a striking, but surprisingly pleasant contrast to the surrounding area.

Artists, Wolfgang Winter and Berthold Hoerbelt have collaborated since 1992, under the name Winter/Hoerbelt. They aim to develop the potentials and possibilities of Installation Art and sculpture. The exploration of other artistic realms, such as music and architecture often leads to building-like sculptures or objects accompanied by sound. The use of objects that are traditionally perceived as not artistic, such as plastic crates, car tail lights or industrial materials, are often a focus for their work.

Photo: Christer Hallgren

Anzac Commemorative Site
Taylor Brammer Landscape Architects Pty Ltd.

Completion: 2000. **Technique:** sandstone, concrete, granite coble.
Location: Gallipoli, Turkey.

A site of national significance, Gallipoli has been a focus for many in their search for identity and meaning in a modern world. The design of the "Anzac Commemorative Site" reflects this by deliberately including the natural character and landscape setting that forms an integral part of the design. In doing so, the site is not perceived as one of the many memorials located at Gallipoli but as a singular and special place to gain a further understanding of the history of the site and the nations involved.

Taylor Brammer Landscape Architects is a leading proponent in the field of landscape architecture in the Sydney and metropolitan areas. Matthew Taylor is an experienced landscape and conservation landscape architect. His work, both in Australia and internationally has been recognized with a number of design awards. Iain Brammer is an experienced landscape architect. His involvement in the creation of new communities provides a strong presence in the evolution of landscape design.

Photos: Taylor Brammer Landscape Architects Pty Ltd., Australia

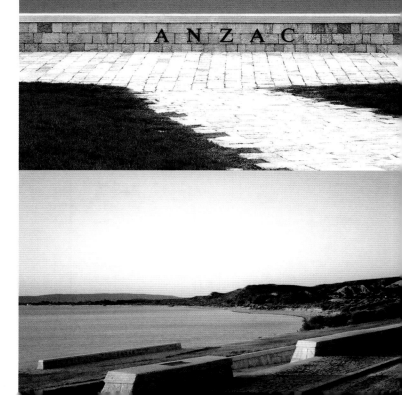

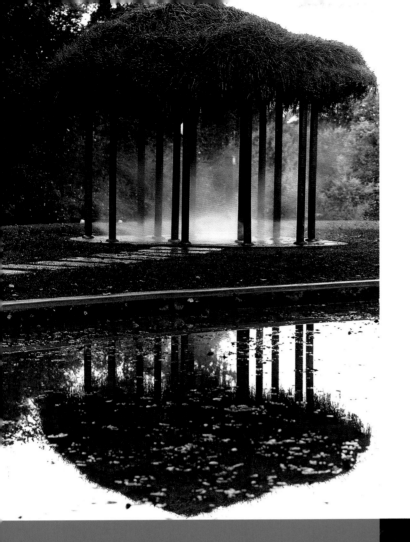

Umbrella
Monika Gora /
Gora art&landscape

Completion: 2001. **Technique:** bronze, water mist, grass. **Location:** Helsingborg, Sweden .

"Umbrella" is an abstraction of a house. Once inside the sculpture your head stays dry while your feet all the time run the risk of getting wet. The grass is irrigated by a telescopic water nozzle, which regularly pops up from the ground, the sprinkling water is spread in a wide circle around the sculpture. Now and then steam seeps out from the pillars. You experience water rising as vapor and falling down as liquid at the same time.

Monika Gora was born in 1959 and has been working as a landscape architect since 1989. Before starting her own business, Gora made several prolonged journeys around the world. She was a member of the Swedish National Council for Architecture, Form and Design until its dissolution in 2009. In her practice she has systematically chosen her own paths – both experimenting with and challenging accepted ideas and practices – at the same time searching for practical solutions. Gora often works to combine landscape architecture and public art.

Photo: Gora art&landscape, photo by Urzula Striner

Shell
Paweł Chlebek Odebek

Completion: 2001. **Technique:** marble. **Location:** Marmara, Turkey.

Marmara is an island full, not only of buildings, but also of beautiful, natural stone formations and quarries. The contrast between civilization and nature is clearly visible. "Shell" pays homage to its setting with both its topic and form. The sculpture is surrounded by buildings, but by looking through the hollowed out space in the center, the observer can see only seaside port. Because of this, observers can almost travel in time, blotting out the modern developments to just see the sea.

Paweł Chlebek Odebek comes from Poland, he graduated from the Academy of Fine Art in Cracow and was later awarded a PhD at the same institution. Odebek is mainly engaged in creating sculptures in a small village in South Poland, attempting to translate the happiness and passion he feels about life into his sculptures. He is a member of the International Sculpture Center and Sculpture Network and a chair of the regional art community. He also works as a teacher at an art school in Rzeszów.

Photos: Courtesy of the artist

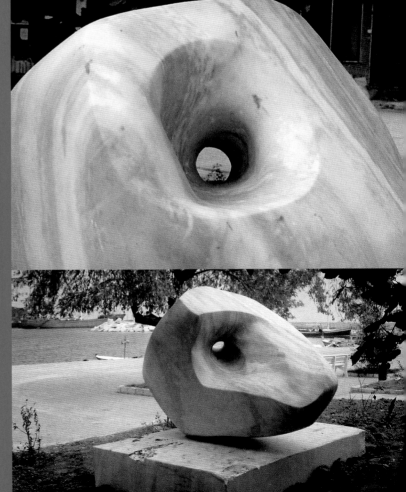

Jazzing Down the Lines
Valerie Maynard

Completion: 2001. **Technique:** steel. **Location:** Jersey City, NJ, USA.

"Jazzing Down the Lines" by Valerie Maynard is a five piece sculptural ensemble, situated at Grove Street Station in New Jersey. The work was commissioned by New Jersey Transit and is typical of Maynard's bold, expressive artwork. Each figure is playing a saxophone and the simple lines succeed in communicating feelings of passion and emotion.

Valerie Maynard was born in Harlem in 1937 and studied art at the Museum of Modern Art, the New School and at Goddard College. Her work mainly focuses on public murals, landscape photography, set designs and animated billboards. Examples of her art are featured in various private collections, including in the personal collections of Stevie Wonder and Toni Morrison. Maynard's work continuously pushes the boundaries of contemporary art.

Photos: Susan Kane

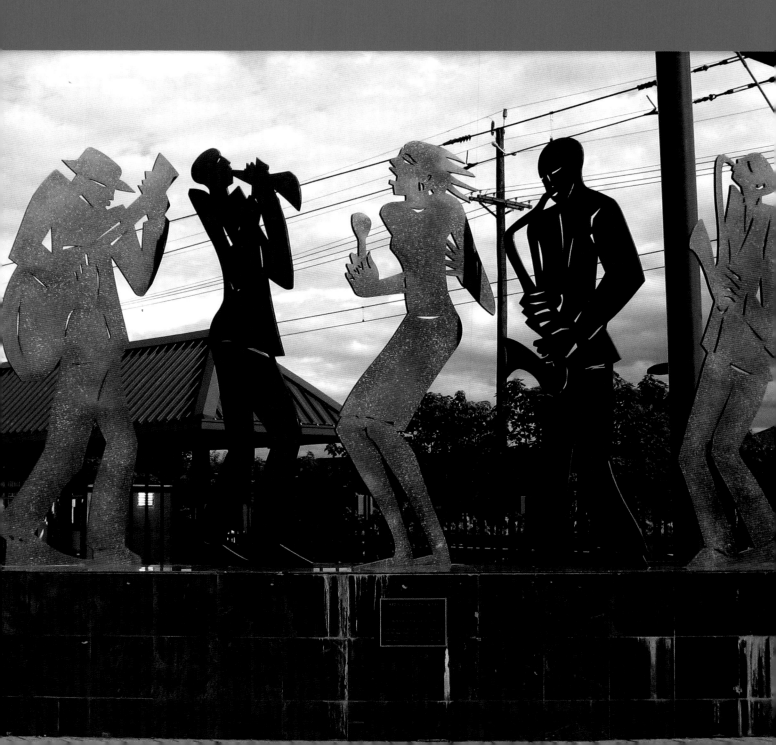

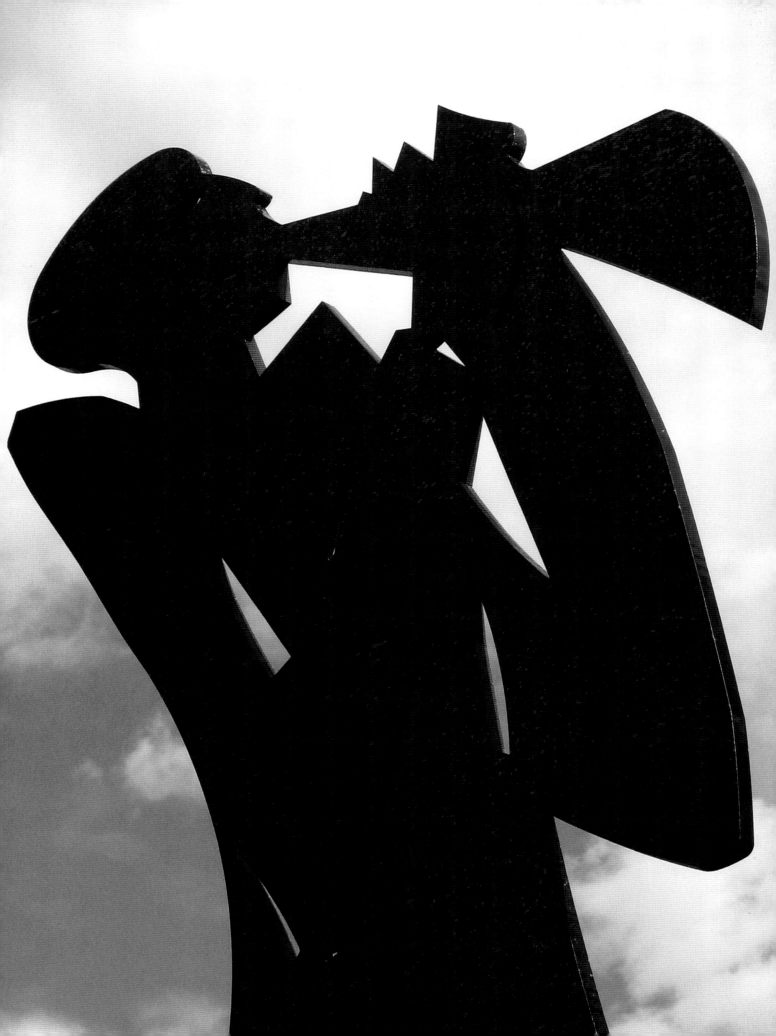

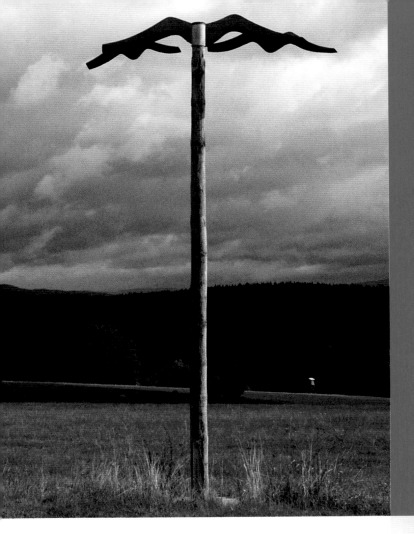

Birds
František Svátek

Completion: 2001. **Technique:** wood, metal. **Location:** Klášter Hradište nad Jizerou, Czech Republic.

This sculpture is a kinetic wind object entitled "Birds". Svátek works with different materials, including stone, glass, marble and metal. The sculpture is six meters high and was constructed using metal and wood, it stands in an open field. The wooden work is reminiscent of birds in flight, with the two sides echoing the shape of wings.

František Svátek was born 1945 in Tábor. He first attended the Technical College of Nuclear Technology in Prague, graduating in 1963. He later studied stone sculpture, graduating in 1968. Since completing his studies, Svátek has been designing kinetic sculptures, usually involving water. He has lived in Switzerland, Germany and Italy but currently lives in the Czech Republic. He has been exhibiting his work since 1988 in Italy, America, Japan and Germany.

Photos: Courtesy of the artist

Piercing
Inges Idee

Completion: 2001. **Technique:** stainless steel. **Location:** Heidenheim an der Brenz, Germany.

A large, high-grade steel ring is mounted at the level of the seventh story, on a corner of the Heidenheim an der Brenz city hall. It pierces the wall of the building to appear again on the other side of the corner, resembling an earring. The intrusion into the structure of the building contrasts with the proud adornment of a flawlessly crafted, polished-steel ring. The sculpture reflects the fact that the decoration of our bodies is an everyday phenomenon, visible on every street.

The artist collective Inges Idee was founded in Berlin in 1992 with the aim of focusing on site specific public art projects. The four members of Inges Idee are Hans Hemmert, Axel Lieber, Thomas Schmidt and Georg Zey. Since 1992, they have worked on over 200 projects, competitions and commissions. More than 50 projects have been realized as permanent artworks in international locations, including Germany, France, Sweden, Denmark, the Netherlands, Canada, Singapore, Taiwan and Japan.

Photos: Courtesy of the artist

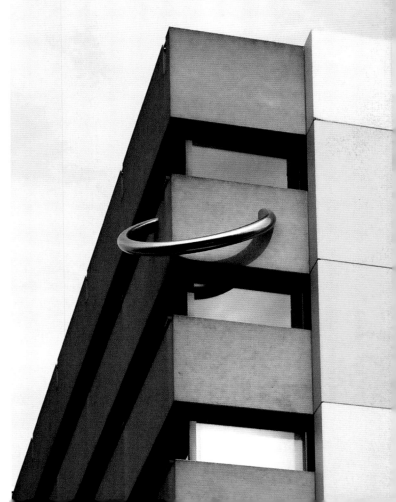

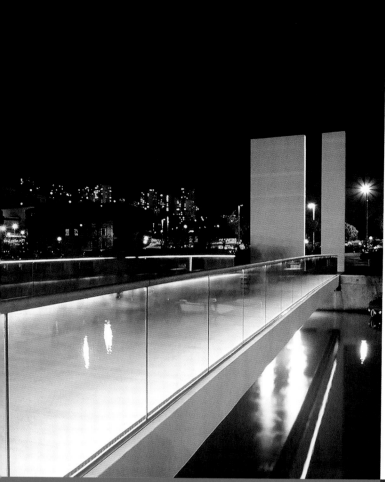

Memorial Bridge Rijeka
ƎLHD architects

Completion: 2001. **Technique:** steel, aluminum, glass, lighting.
Location: Rijeka, Croatia.

The site of the "Memorial Bridge" is in the very center of the town of Rijeka in Croatia on the canal separating the historical center from the former port area. The bridge is a monument to Croatian defenders, a place of memory as well as a place of social encounter. It is softly illuminated at night, making it a striking monument. This urban space changed the city in a physical and symbolic way, the bridge being both a new and modern structure as well as a memorial.

ƎLHD is an architecture studio that often collaborates with other firms, professionals and experts to allow the realization of a broad range of projects. ƎLHD are particularly involved in architecture, art and urban landscape projects. They have completed widely diverse projects both in Croatia and abroad.

Photo: Aljosa Brajdic

Light Score
Brigitte Kowanz

Completion: 2001. **Technique:** neon light. **Location:** Munich, Germany.

Light is not just the material or medium of this piece but is the central subject of her deliberations. The four cases each have two neon-lit sides and appear to grow out of the wall as the observer moves towards them. In each case are 15 red and 15 yellow neon tubes. These are controlled by a computer to display a specially developed pattern of light. This forms the basis for a vivid and moving play of colors in the display cases.

Brigitte Kowanz is an Austrian artist, born in Vienna in 1957. She studied at the University of Applied Arts in Vienna, graduating in 1980 and was appointed as professor of media and cross-media art at the same institution in 1997. She is best known for her work with light installations and was awarded the Otto Mauer prize in 1989. She was presented with the Austrian state Prize for Art in 2009 and currently lives and works in Vienna.

Photos: Chris van Uffelen

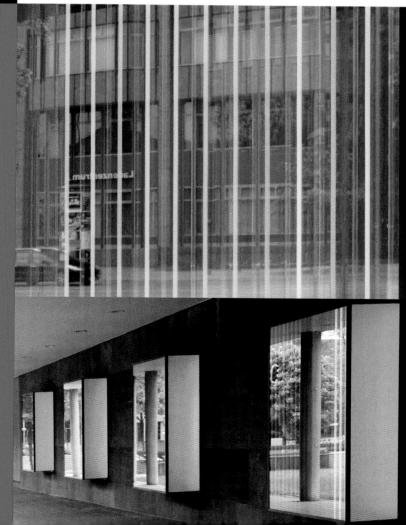

Enduring Navajo
Martha Pettigrew

Completion: 2001. **Technique:** bronze. **Location:** Loveland, CO, USA.

The "Enduring Navajo" bronze sculpture is located in Benson Park Sculpture Garden, Loveland, Colorado. It depicts the determination of the Navajo people and their continuing challenge to maintain their culture and way of life, including preservation of their unique language. The solid simplicity of the design underscores this portrayal. The half closed eyes reflect the quiet introspective nature of the Navajo people.

Martha Pettigrew is a former illustrator, she studied fine arts at the University of Nebraska. Pettigrew often works with bronze, depicting indigenous women of the South-West and Mexico, though her work also includes wildlife and equine subjects. Recent commissions include at three-meter high rearing horse, for the City of Irving, Texas, and a life-size depiction of Senator Ben Nelson and his family for the city of McCook in Nebraska. Her work is also held in various museum collections.

Photo: Courtesy of the artist

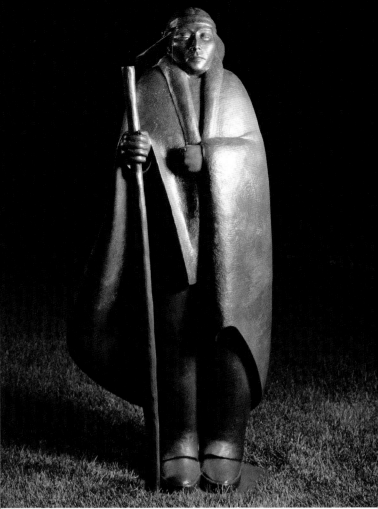

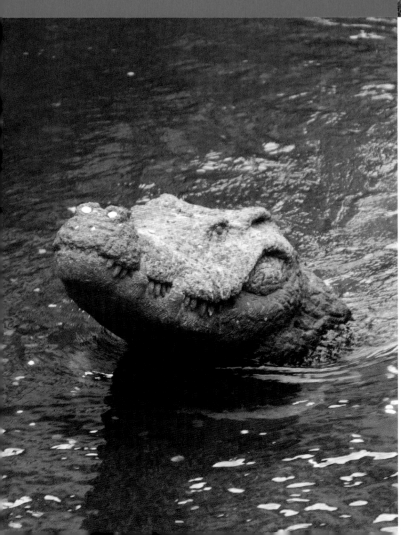

Crocodile
Ole Meinecke

Completion: 2001. **Technique:** granite, water. **Location:** Freiburg, Germany.

This stone crocodile is in one of the many small rivers that flow in and round the center of Freiburg. Made of granite, the head peers threateningly over the waterline, sharp teeth clearly visible on either side of the mouth. Artist Ole Meinecke created the crocodile as part of a semester-long study on animal head sculpture. A plaque is fixed to the stone side of the waterway; it reads "Here is a crocodile made of stone, with wide smile, but not from the Nile."

Ole Meinecke was born in Hamburg in 1967. He completed an apprenticeship in stonemasonry and sculpture in Hamburg. He worked various different jobs in Hamburg and Berlin before deciding to enroll at the Friedrich Weinbrenner Vocational School in Freiburg with the aim of becoming a fully qualified stonemason and sculptor. Meinecke has worked in Berlin since 2002.

Photo: Chris van Uffelen

The Planted Cathedral
Giuliano Mauri

Completion: 2001. **Technique:** plants. **Location:** Trento, Italy.

"The Planted Cathedral" was one of the main projects on display at the Arte Sella exhibition in 2001. The piece is the size of a Gothic cathedral and comprised of three aisles, formed by 80 columns of twisted branches. The plants grow about 50 centimeters each year and over time they will become a veritable green cathedral, covering an area of 1,230 square meters. The piece will be slowly taken over by nature, first leaving the traces of the recent dialogue with man, but later disappearing completely.

Giuliano Mauri was born in 1938 in Lodi Vecchio, Italy. He is most famous for his poetic and striking environmental interventions, called Natural Architecture. He participated in the Venice Biennial in 1976, the Milan Tiennial in 1992 and the Biennial of Penne in 1994. He works with branches and trunks of wood to build architectural works. Nature fills the gaps in the work, creating a dialogue between man and nature. The work eventually fades away and is completely reclaimed by nature.

Photo: Pava / Wikimedia Commons

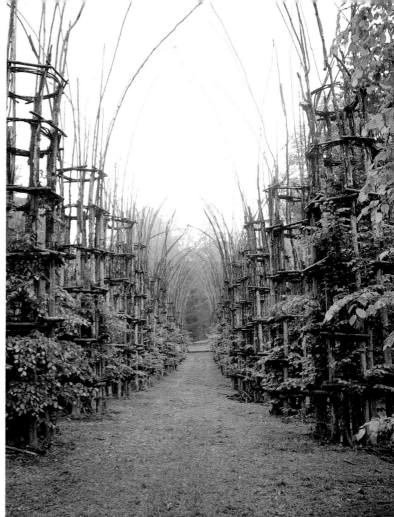

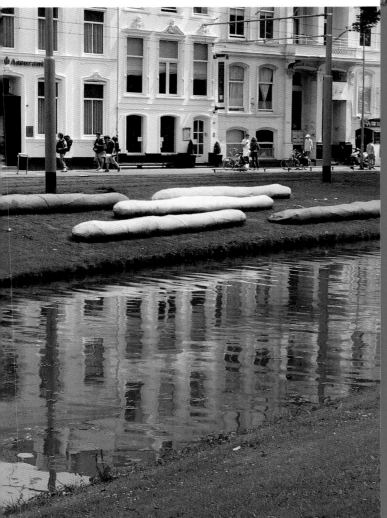

Qwertz
Franz West

Completion: 2001. **Technique:** painted aluminum. **Location:** Rotterdam, The Netherlands.

These five pastel-colored cocoons are part of Sculpture International, Rotterdam and offer a meeting and resting place along the river. The name "Qwertz" is simply the top six letters on a German keyboard, it has no obvious meaning, and makes no suggestions about the work's purpose. Each piece is made from aluminum and sprayed with colorful paint. They are known locally simply as the "Sausages".

Franz West was born in Vienna in 1947. He experimented with photography, printmaking and papier mâché even before beginning his studies at the Academy of Arts, Vienna. West has made many sculptures from papier mâché and plaster that act as human protheses, these can be attached to the human body in various ways. At his exhibitions, West left instruction to visitors on how to fit them. He has had various exhibitions in Europe and his work is often interactive, encouraging people to try it out, touch it or sit on it.

Photos: K. Siereveld / Wikimedia Commons

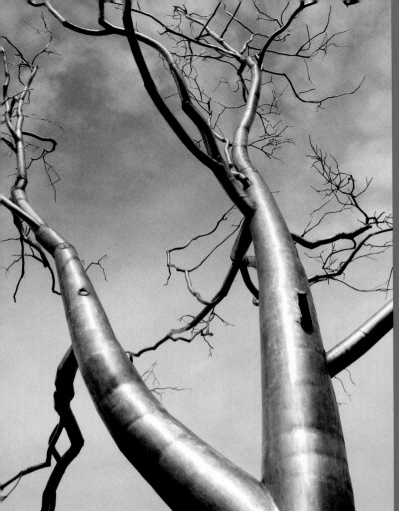

Transplant
Roxy Paine

Completion: 2001. **Technique:** stainless steel. **Location:** Cádiz, Spain.

This is one of a series of stainless steel trees, displayed in various locations, including in New York, Canada, Israel and Washington. The trees translate organic forms into steel evoking connections with industry. They are always leafless, possibly pointing towards a barren future, where pollution has finally destroyed the earth.

Roxy Paine is an American artist, born in 1966. He studied at the College of Santa Fe in New Mexico and later in New York. Paine's work concentrates on the tension between what is organic and what is man-made, between the human wish for control and nature's wish to reproduce. He has created a series of stainless steel trees and several works showing mushrooms and plant life in various states of decay. His first exhibition was at the Heron Test-Site in October 1992.

Santa Claus
Paul McCarthy

Completion: 2001. **Technique:** bronze. **Location:** Rotterdam, The Netherlands.

Though created for public display in Rotterdam, the Rotterdam Municipal Council originally deemed this bronze statue unsuitable for installation. Instead of the more traditional depictions of Santa Claus holding a Christmas tree, this sculpture is holding a giant sex toy. A butt plug to be specific. After being moved around Rotterdam, in an attempt to find a "suitable" place, the sculpture was eventually installed in the grounds of the Boijmans Van Beuningen Museum.

Paul McCarthy is a contemporary American artist. He was born in Salt Lake City in 1945 and lives and works in Los Angeles. McCarthy studied art at the San Francisco Art Institute, graduating with a Bachelor of Fine Arts in painting. He went on to study film, video and art at the University of Southern California. McCarthy is interested in everyday situations and the mess created by them, this theme is often conveyed in his work. In his early paintings, he often used food or bodily fluids as a substitute for paint.

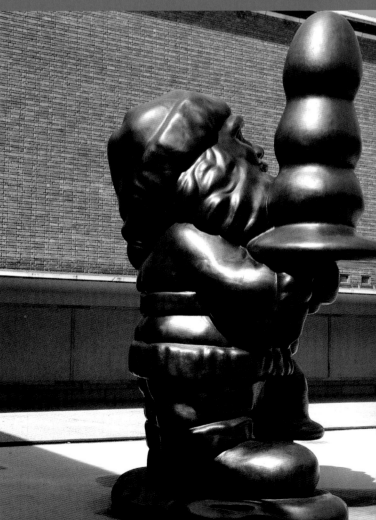

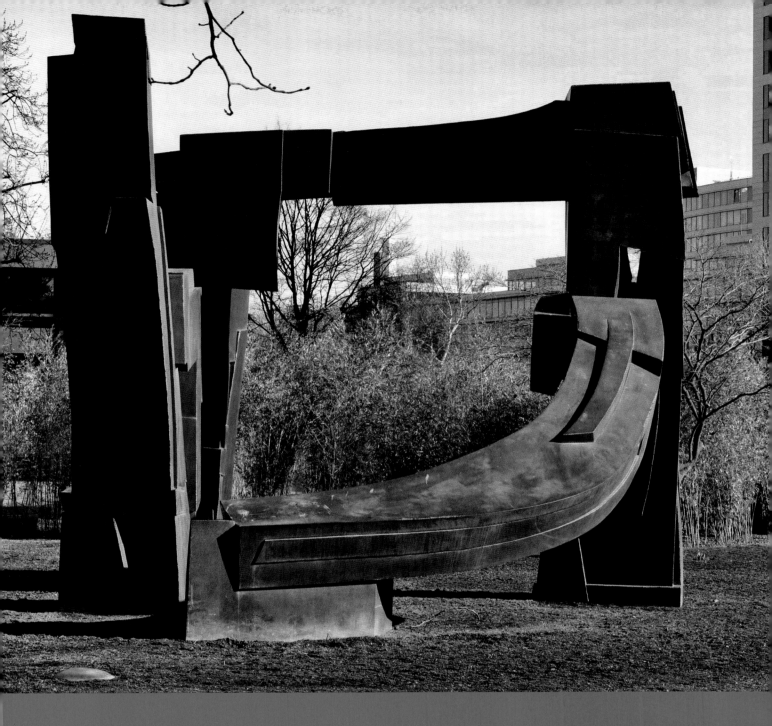

Bridge
Volker Bartsch

Completion: 2001. **Technique:** bronze. **Location:** Frankfurt / Main, Germany.

This almost ten-ton bronze sculpture has stood in front the BHF-Bank in Frankfurt since 2001. Welded bronze wire was used to create the distinctive ridges on its surface and its irregular form offers various spaces and passages to be explored. The viewer is invited to observe and touch it, walk under it, over it and round it.

Volker Bartsch is a German painter and sculptor, born in Goslar in 1953. He studied sculpture at the University of Art in Berlin, under the tutorage of Hans Nagel and Joe Lonas, graduating in 1979. He was awarded the Goslar Kaiserring scholarship in 1988 and in 1990 he won the Darmstadt Secession art prize. He has lived in Berlin since 1981, working as a freelance artist.

Wall for Peace
Clara Halter,
Jean-Michel Wilmotte

Completion: 2001. **Technique:** concrete, glass, metal. **Location:** Paris, France.

Loosely inspired by the Wailing Wall of Jerusalem, visitors are encouraged to write their messages of peace in the chinks of this wall. On the internet one can send peace-messages to the wall's thirty monitors, as well as reading the messages that others send. It depicts the word "peace" in 32 languages on columns and glass screens. The architecture aligns itself with both the Eiffel tower on one side and the Military Academy on the other.

Clara Halter was born around 1955 in Paris. She ran the publication Elements, which was the first publication for peace in the Middle East, before becoming an artist. She focuses primarily on drawing and sketching but also works with letters and signs. In 1992 she agreed for the first time to show her work to the public. Jean-Michel Wilmotte, born in Soissons in 1948, is an architect and designer. Together with Cara Halter he realized the "Peace Tower" in Saint Petersburg (2003) and the "Gates of Peace" in Hiroshima (2005).

Photo: Chris van Uffelen

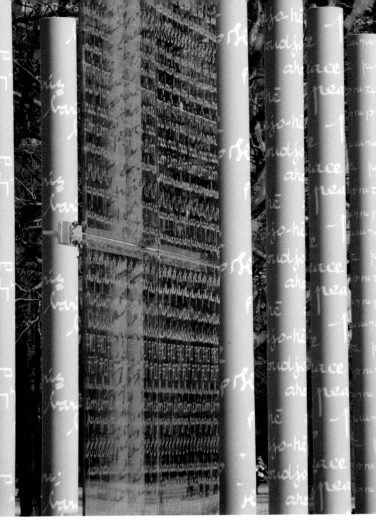

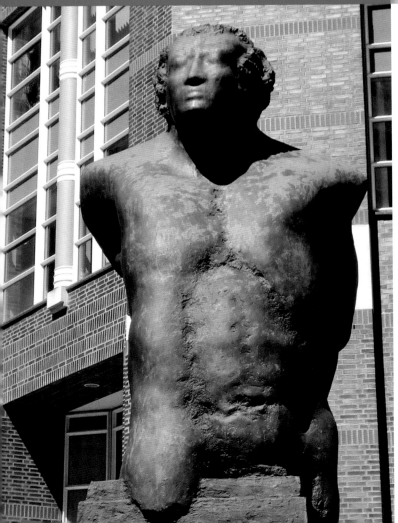

Light and Darkness
Rob Krier

Completion: 2001. **Technique:** bronze. **Location:** The Hague, The Netherlands.

The bronze sculpture, "Light and Darkness" is five and a half meters tall and weighs around three tons. The sculpture depicts two men, whose backs are fused together. This Postmodern sculpture is situated in front of the "Muzentoren" and was designed by Rob Krier in 2000.

Rob Krier is a sculptor, architect and town planner, born in Luxembourg in 1938. He studied architecture at the Technical University in Munich, graduating in 1964. He worked as an assistant at the Stuttgart School of Architecture from 1973 and 1975 and later taught architecture at the University of Technology in Vienna. He also worked as guest professor at Yale University. He is now mainly engaged in producing sculpture for display in public space. The writings of Rob and his brother Leon Krier are fundamental to Post-modernism.

Photo: Wikifrits / Wikimedia Commons

Marathon
Henk Visch

Completion: 2001. **Technique:** lacquered metal. **Location:** Rotterdam, The Netherlands.

This colorful sculpture against the monotone of the asphalt adds color to this gray, urban area. The glossy surface reflects the sunlight, making the structure extremely noticeable. Each of its many, flat surfaces are of a different color, creating a contrast. No two shades are the same, each color compliments its neighbor simply by its difference.

Henk Visch was born in the Netherlands in 1950 and is a Dutch artist and professor. He studied from 1968 to 1972 at the Academy of Art in 's-Hertogenbosch. He spent some time in New York from 1982–1983, before returning to the Netherlands and working as a lecturer at the Academy of Art in Amsterdam. He exhibited his work in the Dutch pavilion at the Venice Biennial in 1988 and participated in the tenth Documenta in Kassel in 1992. In 2005 he was appointed professor of sculpture at the Academy of Fine Arts in Münster.

Photo: K. Siereveld / Wikimedia Commons

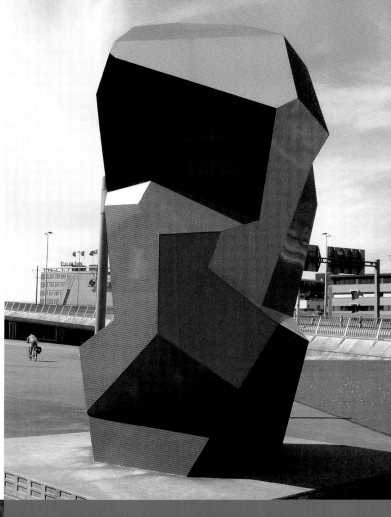

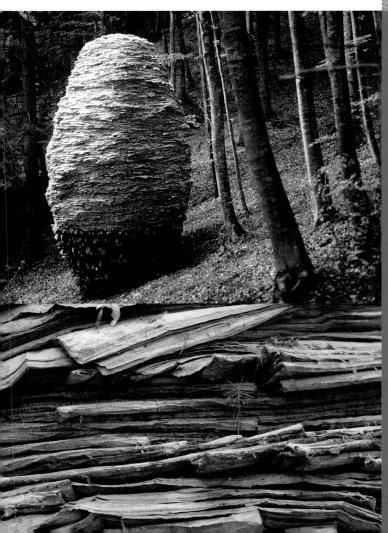

Like a hive, like an egg?
Steven Siegel

Completion: 2002. **Technique:** newspaper, wood. **Location:** Borgo Valsugana, Italy.

This piece was built in 2002 at Arte Sella, in Northern Italy. It is made of newspaper and wood and is over five meters tall. It is situated on a steep mountainside next to an eco and sculpture trail. Because the interior is framed with larch wood it is durable, even with the heavy snows it bears in the winter. It has become sort of an icon at Arte Sella, in spite of being in an out of the way location. The sculpture is covered with small larch seedlings, growing and adapting naturally to its situation.

Steven Siegel studied at different universities in the USA in the 1970s. He has been involved in many solo and group exhibitions. He builds on the rich tradition of using recycled materials and found objects to create art. Large boulders of compressed cans and plastic bottles and multilayered newspaper ridges call attention to the abundant source material, yet stand on their own as sculptural forms in the landscape, there to remind us of our impact on the landscape we inhabit.

Photos: Courtesy of the artist

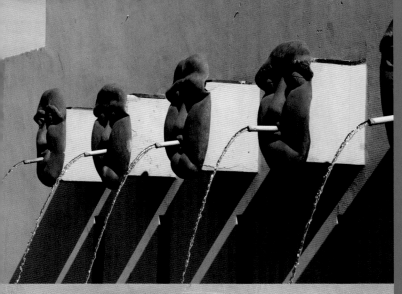

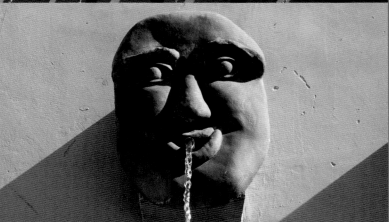

Masks Fountain
Lea Dolinsky

Completion: 2002. **Technique:** bronze . **Location:** Ganei Tikva, Israel.

The "Masks Fountain" was designed in 2002 by Lea Dolinsky, for the public Garden of Peace and Love in Ganei Tikva. It was commissioned by the Town Council and Moria-Sekely Landscape Architecture were responsible for building it. The fountain symbolizes images and expressions of people living in peace. The nine masks, cast in bronze, are fixed to a venetian-red wall at height of two and a half meters. Water is spilled through the masks in a close circle, to a pool at the garden level.

Lea Dolinsky was born in Argentina in 1942 and has lived in Israel since 1963. She studied architecture and worked as an architect from 1968–1984. Dolinsky learned art and ceramic sculpture under the tutorage of Hedwig Grossman, Immre Shrammel and Enrique Mestre. Her sculptures and environmental projects are focused on people, behavior, duality and conflicts. She has held 14 solo exhibitions both in Israel and abroad as well as contributed to 60 group exhibitions.

Photos: Courtesy of the artist

Points of View
Tony Cragg

Completion: 2002. **Material:** bronze. **Location:** Stuttgart, Germany.

Tony Cragg's work experiments with shapes and material, pushing boundaries and testing the perception of the viewers. A committee selected "Points of View", as part of the Art and Buildings initiative and it stands outside the House of History in Stuttgart. The sculpture offers a contrast to the architectural surroundings, giving the area a modern character. The subject of the sculpture is the tension between what we know and what we don't know, what we see and don't see and what we feel and don't feel.

Tony Cragg was born in Liverpool in 1949. He worked as a lab technician at the National Rubber Producers Research Association between 1966 and 1968 before studying art at Gloucestershire College of Art, Cheltenham. He received his bachelors degree from the Wimbledon College of Art and a masters from The Royal College of Arts. He began exhibiting his own work in 1977 and had his first solo exhibition at the Lisson Gallery. He later took up a teaching post at the Art Academy in Dusseldorf.

Photo: Chris van Uffelen

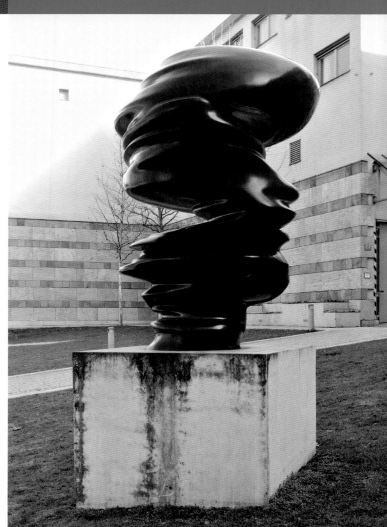

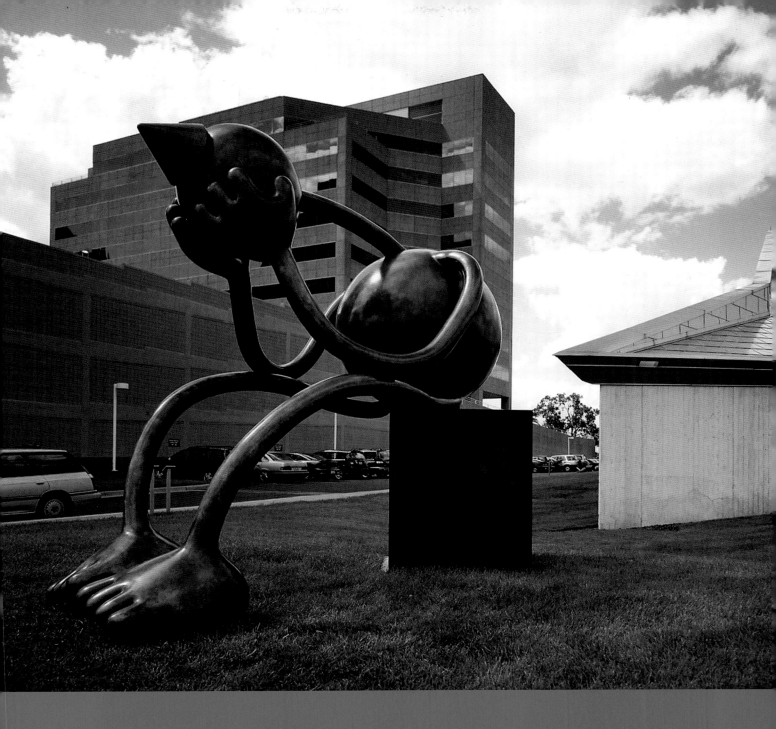

Crying Giant
Tom Otterness

Completion: 2002. **Technique:** bronze. **Location:** Kansas City, MO, USA.

The "Crying Giant" by Tom Otterness is situated in front of the Kemper Museum of Contemporary Art in Kansas. The sculpture is over three meters tall and made from cast bronze. The giant is perched on the edge of a bronze base; the powerful figure of fairytale reduced in power and alone, an unexpected figure on a Kansas embankment.

Tom Otterness is one of the country's pre-eminent public artists, with 17 public projects completed. He has been commissioned by a variety of public entities in the USA and abroad. He is included in many museum collections, among them the Solomon R. Guggenheim Museum, New York, Museum of Modern Art, New York; and the Carnegie Museum of Art, Pittsburgh, Pennsylvania.

Photo: Tom Otterness, photo by: Dan Wayne

Gottenheim Water Sculpture
Gerhard Birkhofer

Completion: 2002. **Technique:** acrylic glass. **Location:** Gottenheim, Germany.

The "Gottenheim Water Sculpture" (Wasserskulptur Gottenheim) relates in concept to the Fibonacci number sequence, thus establishing a relationship to harmony in nature. The proximity between the mathematical concepts of the Golden Ratio and Fibonacci's number sequence are used in this sculpture, the flowing water symbolizes dynamic development and continuing reality. Transparency and light whisper of the closeness of earthly elements, turning the sculpture into a symbol of harmony.

Gerhard Birkhofer was born in Ravensburg Germany, in 1947. He studied art history at the University of Freiburg and teaches at the University of Education, Freiburg since 1982. Examples of his work can be found in museums as well as private and public collections.

Photo: Courtesy of the artist

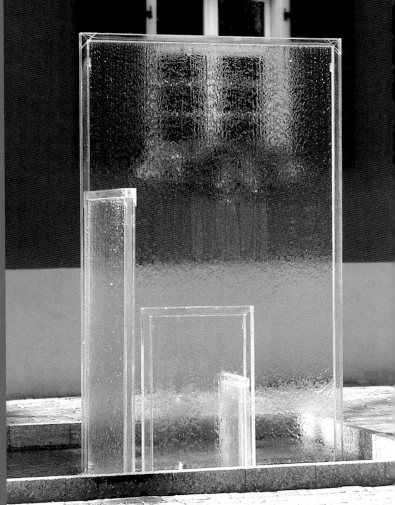

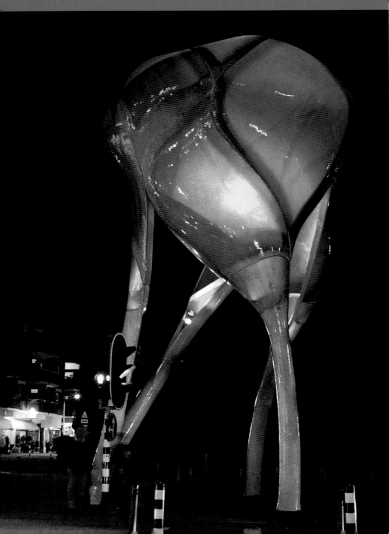

D Tower
NOX / Lars Spuybroek, Q.S. Serafijn

Completion: 2002. **Technique:** LEDs, polyepoxide. **Location:** Doetinchem, The Netherlands.

This sculpture is one part of a three-part project. Part one consists of the "lift of emotions" survey, conducted daily via the Internet for registered local residents. Part two is the "Landscape of emotion", exhibited on www.d-toren.nl. The sculpture resembles the form of an upside-down heart and shows the dominant emotion of the day, gained from the information gathered. Information is displayed using integrated LEDs: red for love, blue for happiness, yellow for fear and green for hate.

Lars Spuybroek, born in Rotterdam in 1959, is an architect and artist. He started the NOX-magazine with Maurice Nio 1991. In 1995 he founded the office NOX, which has since become renowned for non-standard architecture, deals with interactive and living forms. Q.S. Serafijn, born in 1960 in Roosendaal, is an artist and author who thinks that art should reflect society and public debates, raising new questions and ideas.

Photos: Courtesy of the artist

TT Monument
ONL / Ilona Lénárd

Completion: 2002. **Technique:** chrome metal. **Location:** Assen, The Netherlands.

The "TT Monument" is an interactive monument standing next to the TT circuit in Assen. It shows the highly abstracted form of a racer and his motorbike in movement, as an approximation of its form on the move; played about with by the frozen airstream. The chrome body is lit from below by a real-timecontrolled program that shows, by color code, what events are taking place on the circuit. Red for example, means the WCC Superbike is taking place.

Ilona Lénárd, born in Budapest in 1948, first trained as a professional actress in Budapest and then as a sculptor in Rotterdam. Kas Oosterhuis, born in Amersfoort in 1951, studied architecture at the Delft University of Technology. In 1988/1989 they came together professionally at the former studio of Theo van Doesburg in Paris. Their design studio was renamed ONL [Oosterhuis_Lénárd] in 2004. ONL is known for its innovative research on technique, architecture and life, incorporating interactivity and real time behavior.

Photos: Courtesy of the artists

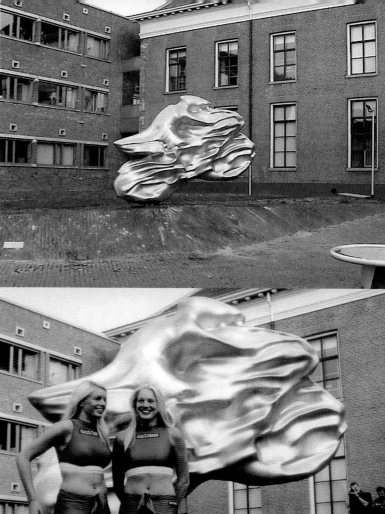

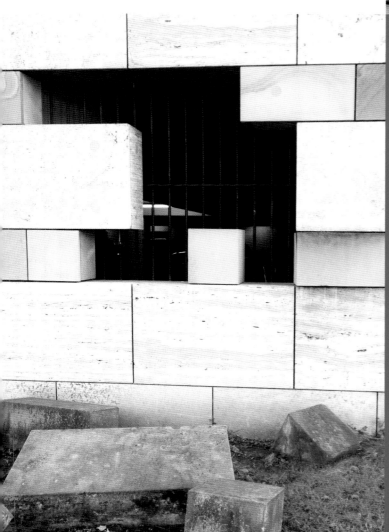

Staatsgalerie
James Stirling

Completion: 2002. **Technique:** concrete, stone. **Location:** Stuttgart, Germany.

In the same way that medieval cathedrals have their own sculpture, this work is integrated into the building as part of the Post-modern architecture. A few stones seem to have fallen out of the retaining wall in front of a parkade, under the museum. They look like they have been placed at random on the lawn. All of a sudden, the spectator recognizes the trick. The ashlar blocks on the ground are the only real stone, while the rising masonry is obviously just clad with a front of concrete.

James Stirling was an important Postmodern architect, born in 1926 he died in 1992. He studied architecture in Liverpool from 1945 to 1950 and then worked with James Gowan. During this period his work retained a technical Realism. It was after Michael Wilford became partner in 1971 that Stirling became an influential Post-modern architect. His buildings are never just influenced by the Antiquity or Neo-Classicism but respond to different styles and are always slightly tongue in cheek.

Photo: Chris van Uffelen

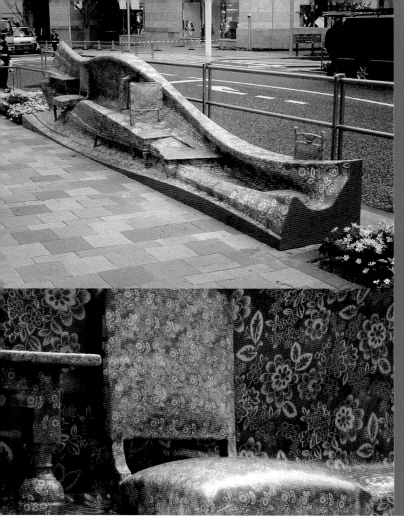

Tokyo Day-tripper
Studio Makkink & Bey

Completion: 2002. **Technique:** skin of fiberglass, printed with white flower decoration over pink colored polyester. **Location:** Tokyo, Japan.

"Day-tripper" is a seven-meter long city bench in Tokyo. The bench is based on a study of the different postures people assume on the street during the course of a day, while leaning, sitting, lounging, or squatting. Seven of these postures have been fixed and have shaped the wave-like form of this work. More formal pieces of "furniture" have been integrated into this wave – like a dining table, a coffee table or chairs. The designers have chosen to fabricate the works using a skin of fiberglass, printed with a white flower decoration over pink colored polyester.

Studio Makkink & Bey, is led by architect Rianne Makkink and designer Jurgen Bey. Supported by a design team, the practice has been in operation since 2002. Studio Makkink & Bey investigates the various domains of applied art while studying the tension between the private and public domain. The design team includes experts from various disciplines ranging from fashion and design to architecture. This mix prompts new insights and perspectives, which are used in each stage of the design process.

Photos: Courtesy of the artist

Sit and Flit
Rabbits
Rosalie

Completion: 2002. **Technique:** steel, glass reinforced plastic. **Location:** Ostfildern, Germany.

12 sitting and 12 running rabbits and a carrot make up this 25-piece ensemble, in Scharnhauser Park, a new part of Ostfildern near Stuttgart. Together with the "Wind Chime" and a fountain "Frog – Water", it formed the installation "Pleasure Garden" for a horticultural show. The shadow of the large carrot turns like a sundial with the rabbits as the numbers. Colors and simplified, iconic forms make them a part of modern pop-culture.

Born as Bugrun Müller in 1953, Rosalie is a German stage builder and painter. She studied painting, graphics and sculpture at the State Academy of Arts in Stuttgart, graduating in 1982. She has worked as a freelance artist since 1979, working in set and figure design. She was awarded the European Culture prize in 2008 by the European foundation Pro Europa.

Photo: Chris van Uffelen

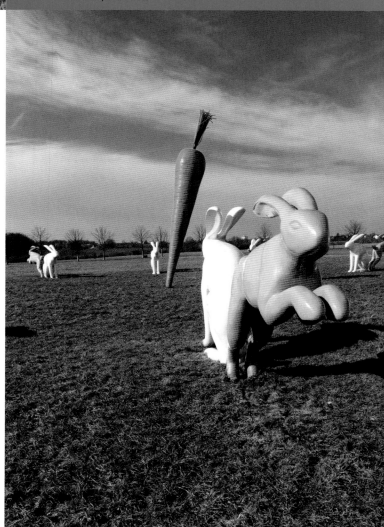

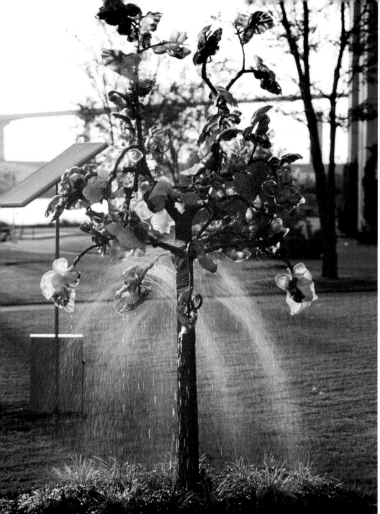

Etherea
Mara Adamitz Scrupe

Completion: 2003. **Technique:** cast-resin, illumination, solar power generating station, commercial landscape plantings. **Location:** Savannah, GA, USA.

"Etherea's" large, cast-resin tree trunks and limbs are fitted with huge hand-cast and dyed resin leaves wired for solar-powered electrical illumination. The project refers to a preference for faux foliage and landscapes in American shopping malls, theme parks and other public sites. This tree, covered with grotesquely oversized colored leaves explores ideas about contemporary public landscape design and environmental preservation.

Mara Adamitz Scrupe graduated from the Milton Avery Graduate School of the Arts at Bard College in New York and from Macalester College, Saint Paul, Minnesota. She is an environmentally and socially attuned artist and writer, creating projects about place for museums, arboretums and public landscapes and spaces. Her works have been exhibited in various solo exhibitions in the USA, Estonia, Ireland, and Lithuania. Scrupe has been awarded many fellowships and grants in the United States, Europe and Asia.

Photo: Daniel Jon Holm

Rotate
Trudi Entwistle

Completion: 2003. **Technique:** mild steel. **Location:** West Yorkshire, United Kingdom.

"Rotate" sits on a former railway line, which is now incorporated into the British National Cycle Network. The artwork was commissioned by Sustrans as part of a program to give local character to cycle paths. Twenty-eight steel hoops form an open tunnel on the circular route. The aim of the artwork was not to decorate the space but to create a mood. Cycling through, experiencing the hoops overhead and the shadows below, is designed to give the passerby an exaggerated sense of motion.

Trudi Entwistle's work is site specific, investigating how sculptural form integrates with the surrounding environment, human movement and the changing elements of light, weather, growth and decay. Her artwork is often used as a stage, hosting events ranging from theatrical production, through play and conversation, to the quiet of solitary contemplation. For more than 15 years, commissions have taken her nationally to varied locations and internationally from coast, mountain, woodland and city.

Photos: Courtesy of the artist

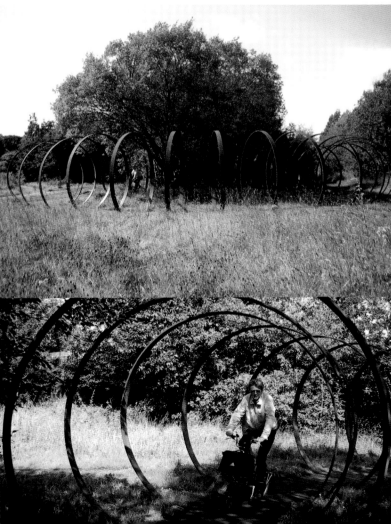

Glass Ark
Roland Fischer, Hubert Stern, Tomáš Indra and Libor Kuzd'as

Completion: 2003. **Technique:** glass, oak wood. **Location:** Bavaria, Germany.

This project is located in the national park, on Lusen Mountain in Bavaria. The shimmering green boat is made of 480 joined-together glass pieces, held in an oak wood hand. The sculpture travelled for five years, through the Bavarian Forest and the Bohemian Forest, which together make up the so-called "Woodsea of Europe". Every place where the sculpture was displayed was connected to an action; either artists' workshops, school project days, guided hikes through the national park or lectures.

Ronald Fischer and Hubert Stern created the glass arch. Fischer was born in Zwiesel in 1966 and is a co-founder of the Männerhaut studio, which opened in 1991. Stern is a glass artist who currently works in Spiegelau, Germany. The wooden hand was created by two Czech wood sculptures, Tomáš Indra und Libor Kuzd'as

Photo: WaldZeit e.V.

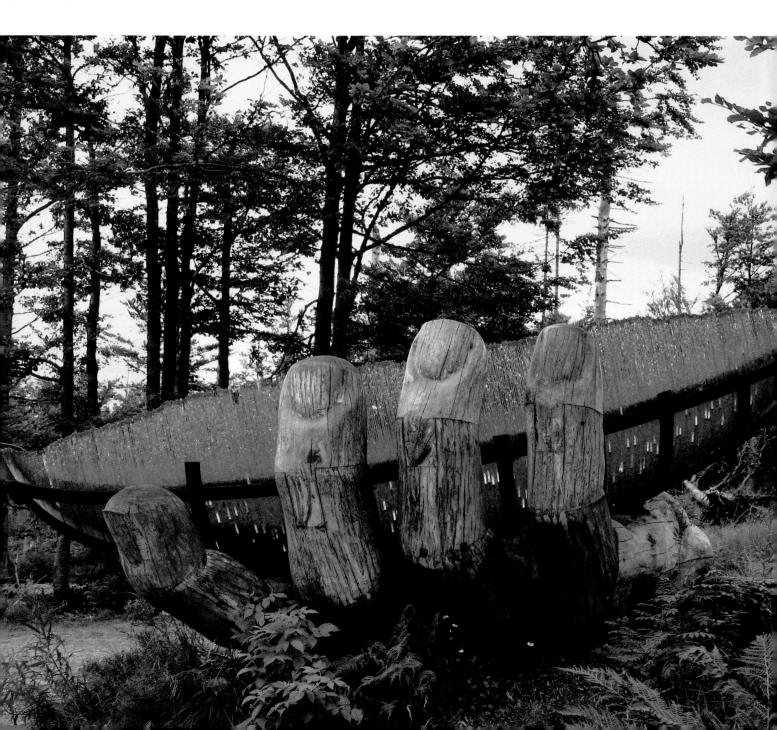

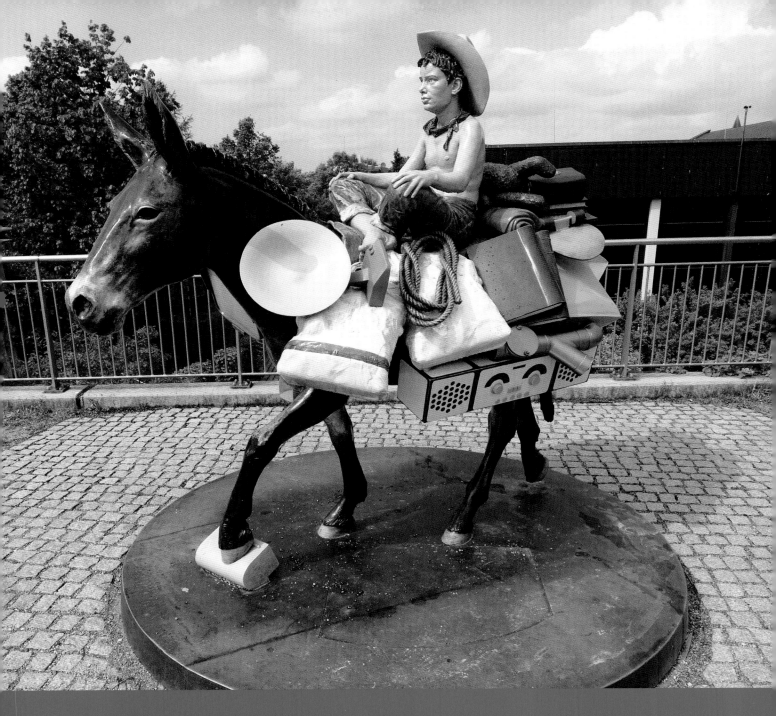

Go!
Pia Stadtbäumer

Completion: 2003. **Technique:** painted bronze. **Location:** Munich, Germany.

This painted bronze sculpture is situated in Petuel Park, Munich. It is of a heavily laden mule, packed with all manner of items and being ridden by a young boy. The sculpture humorously combines the outdated idea of traveling by means of donkey with modernity. The packages include a plastic carrier, a lamp and modern shopping bags. The sculpture is extremely tactile, making it a favorite with children visiting the park.

Pia Stadtbäumer is a German sculptor and installation artist. She studied at the Art Academy in Dusseldorf, graduating in 1988. She was appointed as a professor at the University of Art in Hamburg in 2000. She is married to sculptor Harald Klingelhöller and currently lives and works in Dusseldorf. Her work has been exhibited in both group and solo exhibitions in Germany and internationally.

Photo: Chris van Uffelen

Pavilion - Slanted Walls
Kay Winkler

Completion: 2003. **Technique:** concrete. **Location:** Munich, Germany.

This artwork is a walk-in installation by Kay Winkler. It was constructed in 2003 and was designed to allow the observer to be actively involved in the artwork. The piece cannot be fully experienced from the outside alone; the observer must enter the sculpture to gain a full perspective. The sculpture has been given a simple title "Pavilion – Slanted Walls", and the viewer is invited to consider questions raised by the piece, which is deliberately ambiguous and open to interpretation.

Kay Winkler is a German sculptor and installation artist, born in Kirchheim Teck, Germany in 1956. Between 1976 and 1979, he trained as a painter and graphic artist in Innsbruck, under the tutorage of Heinrich C. Berann, before going on to study woodcarving at a vocational college in Bischofsheim. He later continued his education in Stuttgart, studying painting at the State Academy of Art in Stuttgart; he graduated in 1988. He currently lives and works in both Munich and Berlin.

Photo: Chris van Uffelen

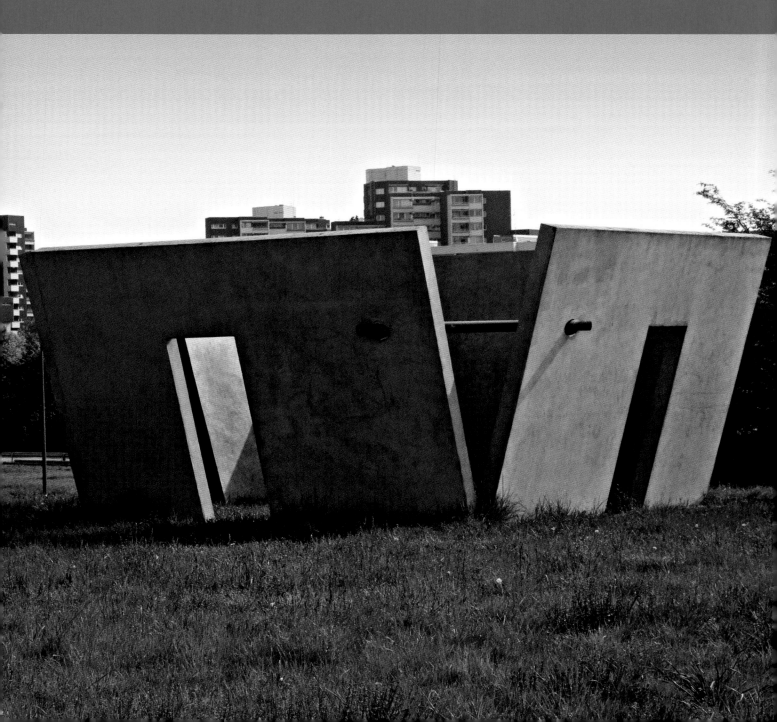

Soundchambers
Nikolaus Hirsch, Michel Müller

Completion: 2003. **Technique:** foam and audio. **Location:** Porto, Portugal.

"Soundchambers" provides a site-specific intervention in the park of Museo Serralves in Porto. By referring to a geometrical configuration of hedges, Nikolaus Hirsch and Michel Müller develop an acoustic and spatial structure that expands, diverts and bifurcates existing conditions of the park. The complex interior and exterior volumes create a hybrid space between landscape and pavilion and provide a variety of sound chambers that perform segments of a specifically developed music.

Nikolaus Hirsch is an architect and director of the Städel School Academy of Arts and Portikus in Frankfurt / Main. His projects include the award-winning Dresden Synagogue, Hinzert Document Center and Experimental Art institutions such the European Kunsthalle, United Nations Plaza in Berlin (with Anton Vidokle), Cybermohalla Hub in Delhi, and a studio structure at Rirkrit Tiravanija's The Land. His work was shown in numerous exhibitions such as Indian Highway at the Serpentine Gallery and Manifesta 7 in Bolzano.

Photos: Courtesy of the artist

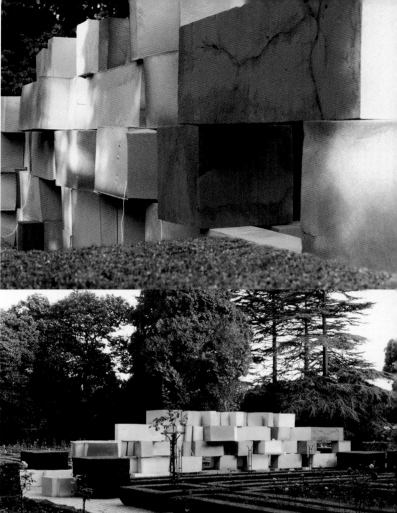

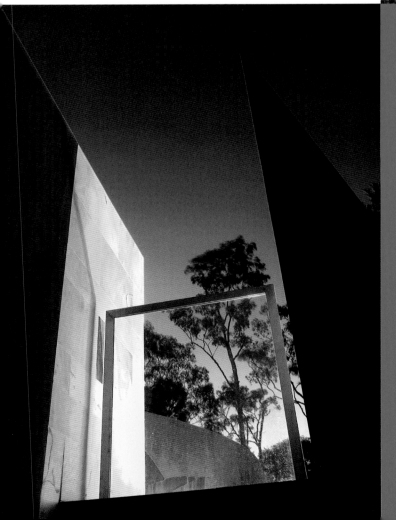

Bali Memorial
Donaldson + Warn, Architects

Completion: 2003. **Technique:** weather resistant steel, Kimberley sandstone. **Location:** Perth, Australia.

The "Bali Memorial" was commissioned in memory of the victims of the terrorist bombing in Bali and to honor individuals and institutions that provided help during the aftermath of the tragedy. The memorial is comprised of several elements arranged around two symbolic axes. The Swan river axis frames a view across the water to the ranges beyond, while the sunrise axis captures within the memorial the first rays of light on 12th October each year, illuminating the victims' names cast into a bronze plaque.

Founded in 1985, Donaldson + Warn rank among Australia's most well-known architects. Working mainly in Australia, their architecture frequently touches on the artistic. They have accomplished a wide variety of projects including residential and educational buildings, offices, interior designing, and urban planning. Their portfolio includes notable projects such as Perth Institute of Contemporary Arts, and the Tree Top Walk footbridge in Valley of the Giants Nature Park.

193

Photo: Martin Farquharson

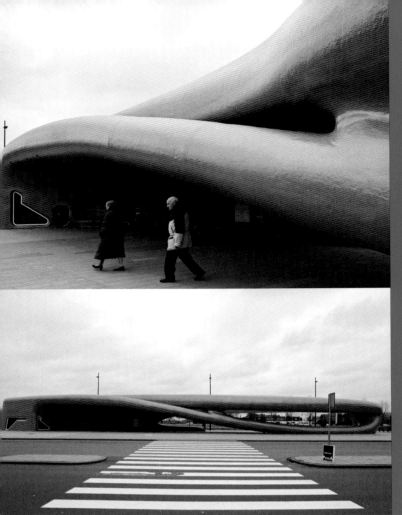

The Amazing Whale Jaw
NIO architecten

Completion: 2003. **Technique:** polystyrene foam, polyester.
Location: Hoofddorp, The Netherlands.

This work is a facilities block in a public area by Hoofddorp's Spaarne Hospital. The design is called "The Amazing Whale Jaw" and the aim was to create a strong, individual image that was less generic than what is usually offered by this type of building. It was designed in the tradition of Oscar Niemeyer as a cross between Modernism and Baroque. The building is completely made of polystyrene foam and polyester and is the world's largest structure in synthetic materials.

Maurice Nio is a well-know Dutch architect. He founded his own company, Nio architecten, in 2000 with Joan Almekinders. Nio is famous for giving life to static, mundane structures such as tunnels, industrial areas and parking lots. His work was exhibited in the solo exhibition Snake Space at the Associazione Culturale Grafio in Italy. The exhibition focused on technical spaces and included a showcase of a number of projects and also featured a special installation of robotics interacting with architectural models.

Photos: Hans Pattist

Temporal
Mike Baur

Completion: 2003. **Technique:** concrete, Corten steel. **Location:** Elgin, IL, USA.

"Temporal" molds the visual history of Elgin into the medium of concrete and steel. Water snakes down the artwork's concrete face, cutting through its pattern of jagged ridges and plains. Constructed of curving I-beams, the diagonal braces buttressing the tower become curved arms reminiscent of machinery. The massive structure responds to the hilly site, reaching the ground on three different planes, prompting the consideration of the interplay between natural geography and manmade industry.

Mike Baur is best known for his concrete and steel public sculptures, but is also prolific in smaller scale works. In 1974, while attending the University of Illinois in Urbana, he won an international competition to build a concrete sculpture in Tarragona, Spain. Baur's sculpture can be found in numerous locations in the USA including pieces in the Illinois Department of Natural Resources. Baur has exhibited in numerous museums and outdoor large-scale sculpture venues in the United States and Europe.

Photo: Courtesy of the artist

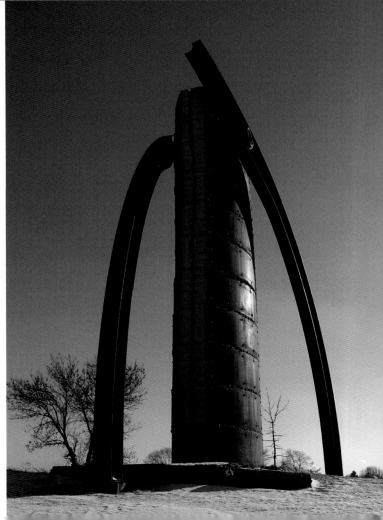

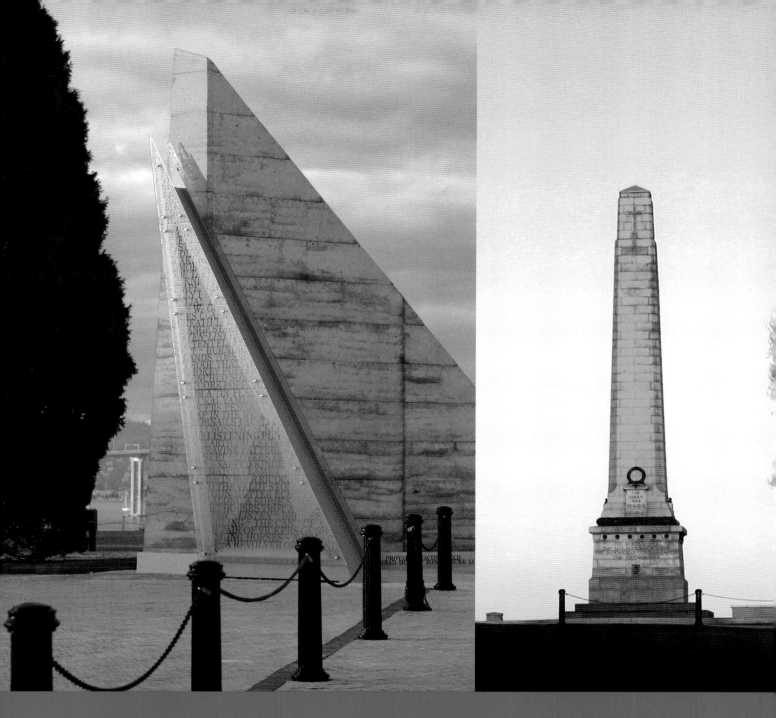

The Listening Posts -
Victoria Cross Memorial
Julie Stoneman

Completion: 2003. **Technique:** rammed earth, glass, metal, text, sound. **Location:** Hobart, Australia

To create "The Listening Posts", soil from the battle fields was mixed with soil from the soldiers' birthplaces in Tasmania, forming darker bands within the rammed earth walls. Layered glass is sandblasted with extracts from the soldier's poetry, expressing sounds of war and triggering contemplation about tragedy whilst resonating and reflecting the spiritual. The music was composed by Joe Bugdon, soundscape by Jane Stapleton and the poem "Listen" was written by Bernard Lloyd.

Stoneman's initial training was in the field of visual art, running her own ceramics design and production practice for 18 years. She became involved with Hobart City Council in 1996, being responsible for several streetscape public art projects. Julie graduated in 1999 in Queensland and has since worked for Hobart City Council on a diverse range of projects, including the redevelopment and upgrade of some significant and established urban parks in Hobart.

Photos: Julie Stoneman, Hobart

Give and Take
Peter Randall-Page

Completion: 2003. **Technique:** granite. **Location:** Newcastle upon Tyne, United Kingdom.

"Give and Take" is a sculpture by Peter Randall-Page and was commissioned by Silverlink Properties with funding from the Arts Lottery, as part of Newcastle City Council's Hidden Rivers public art program. It was installed in 2005, within an amphitheater of hard landscaping. Initially enabled by Sculpture at Goodwood and designed by the artist, in collaboration with landscape architect Ros Southern. It won the Marsh Award for Public Sculpture, selected by the Public Monuments and Sculpture Association.

Peter Randall-Page was born in 1954 and studied sculpture at Bath Academy of Art, 1973–1977. He has gained an international reputation through his sculpture, drawings and prints as well as his numerous commissions and exhibitions. Randall-Page's work is held in public and private collections throughout the world and he is represented in the permanent collections of the Tate Gallery and the British Museum. Recent projects include a major solo exhibition at the Yorkshire Sculpture Park.

Photos: Courtesy of the artist

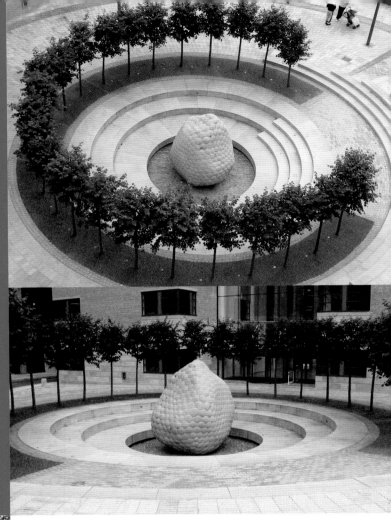

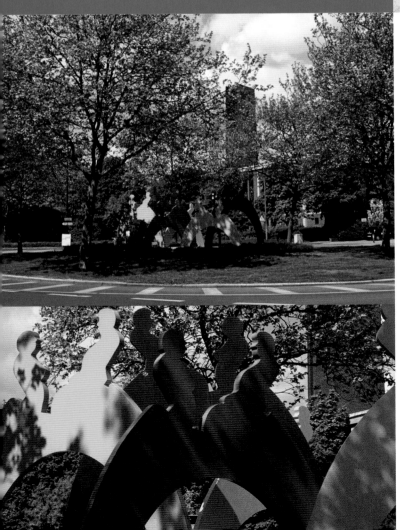

Pairs
Hans-Joachim Müller

Completion: 2003. **Technique:** steel. **Location:** Bremen, Germany.

"Pairs" is a sculpture of seven parts. The figures are brightly colored with red and yellow paint and symbolize the energy and dynamic nature of city life. The arched shape of the figures suggests connections being forged, people being brought together in some colorful celebration of life and community.

Hans-Joachim Müller was born in Donaueschingen, Germany in 1952. From 1978–1985, he studied sculpture in Bremen. In 1992, he was appointed as guest lecturer at the Academy of Art and Music, also in Bremen. His work has been exhibited at various solo exhibitions throughout Germany, and 21 examples of his sculptural work are displayed in public space.

Photos: Fliegner, Bremen

Searching for Utopia
Jan Fabre

Completion: 2003. **Technique:** bronze, silicone. **Location:** Nieuwpoort, Belgium.

This sculpture illustrates the artist's romantic feelings about journey. Like a warrior on a horse he sits on large female turtle, ready to go to sea. The oldest living animal – an oracle and a symbol for the nomad – will take him somewhere. The drawing on the tortoise shell represents a forgotten language from mythology; its form is the form of a zither, an instrument once used in ritualistic acts. Artist and animal are reaching out for Utopia, the artist delivers himself to the water, knowing he might drown.

Jan Fabre is a multi-disciplinary artist, born in Antwerp in 1958. He works as a theater and visual artist and writer. He studied at the Municipal Institute of Decorative Arts and the Royal Academy of Fine Art in Antwerp. He has his own theater company "Troubleyn", established in 1986 and his company for visual arts is called "Angelos". He became famous for his "Bic" artwork after he covered an entire building – the Tivoli castle – with drawings done with a "Bic" ballpoint pen in 1990.

Photos: Malou Swinnen; © Angelos

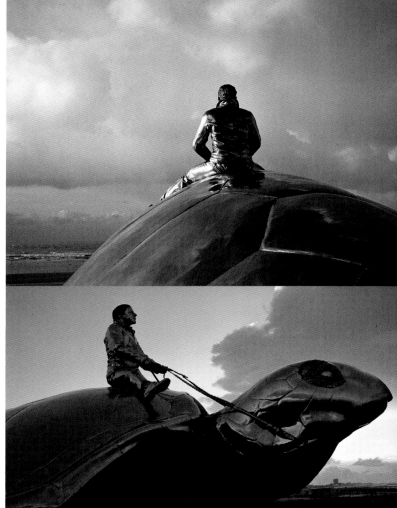

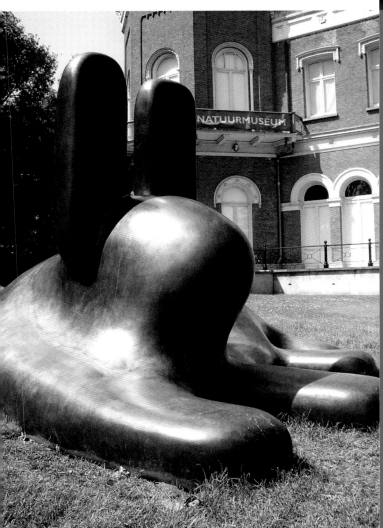

Rabbits
Tom Claassen

Completion: 2003. **Technique:** bronze. **Location:** Rotterdam, The Netherlands.

"Rabbits" is situated outside of the Kunsthal in Rotterdam. Due to the extreme enlargement, the three rabbits can almost be seen as small interruptions in a landscape, their identity as animals fading to the background; yet, at the same time Claassen's rabbits are obviously rabbits. It is this combination that gives the work its power. The rabbits seem both very satisfied and fairly disillusioned by their own state of affairs. It is this balanced state of being which seduces and catches the viewer unaware.

Tom Claassen was born in Heerlen, the Netherlands in 1964. He is most famous for his large animal sculptures that are held in both public and private collections. He was awarded the Charlotte Köhler award in 1994 as well as being nominated in 1992 for the Rome Prize award. Claassen's work has been exhibited in solo and group exhibitions throughout the Netherlands, Germany and Belgium as well as other European locations.

Photo: Tom Haartsen; courtesy Kunsthal Rotterdam

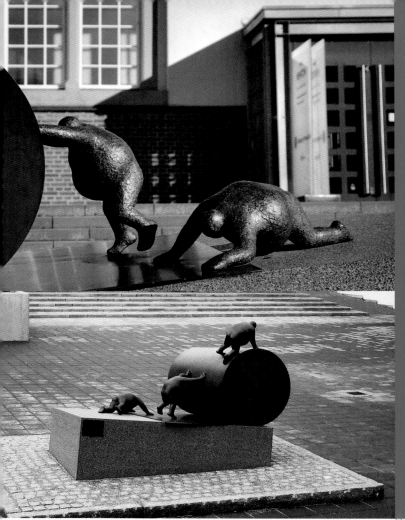

Paperworkers' Sculpture
Keld Moseholm

Completion: 2003. **Technique:** bronze, copper, granite.
Location: Silkeborg, Denmark.

The paper mill on this site closed down and this sculpture was created in memory of the mill and all the people who once worked there. The artist focused on the final product of papermaking, the paper, which in this case is a large paper roll pushed by three figures. The size of the roll suggests, in a humorous way, their efforts in finishing the process. The sculptural effect is caused by the grouping of the cylinder, the flat paper, the round figures and the movement in play with the surrounding architecture.

Keld Moseholm was born in Denmark in 1936. He was educated at The Royal Danish Academy of Fine Arts, Copenhagen and has taught at the Art Academy, Odense and a masterclass at Tom Bass Sculpture Studio School in Sydney. He has exhibited his work widely, including at the 21st International Biennial, São Paulo, Brazil in 1991 and the Danish-Indonesian exhibition, Jakarta in 1992. He has also participated in Sculpture by the Sea in Sydney and Perth, Australia since 1999. He was awarded the Balnaves Foundation Sculpture Prize in 2010.

Photos: janeby.dk (a.); courtesy of the artist (b.)

Meringue
Stefan Kern

Completion: 2003. **Technique:** stainless steel, aluminum, painted white. **Location:** Stuttgart, Germany.

The sculpture "Meringue" is just over four meters in height and was made from 32-centimeter thick steel that has been painted white. The work is made from one single tube, wound around to create a sculpture. The tube first runs perpendicular to the ground in four loops, these work together to form the base for the spiraling shape. The pipe changes direction to horizontal and the tube is organized into winding layers, drawing together at the top, the circles gradually diminishing in size.

Stefan Kern was born in Hamburg in 1966. He studied at the Städel School under Per Kirkeby, Ulrich Rückriem and Franz West. His work deals with ordinary things in extraordinary context. He either sets artificial looking objects, familiar in everyday life, into nature or streetscape or hides the artwork away by disguising it as everyday things. Despite their complex production his works always appear simple. A moment of surprise lets the spectator recognize that it is a work of art worth looking at for its autonomous form.

Photo: Chris van Uffelen

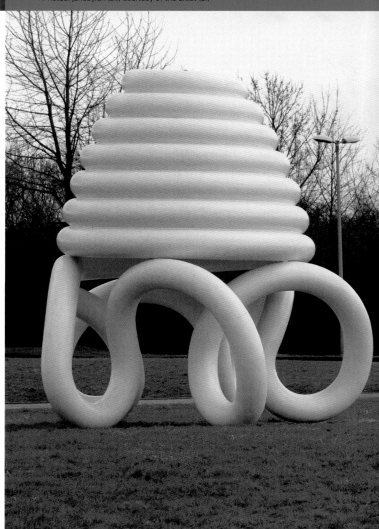

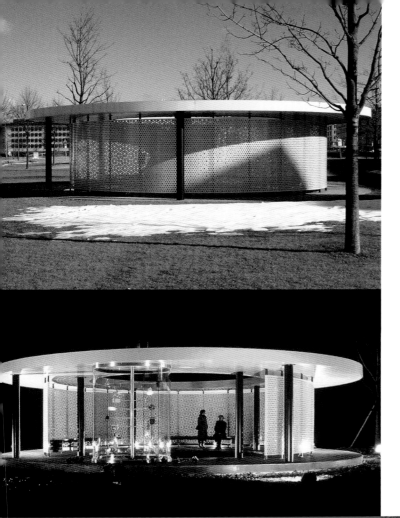

Wishing Well
Stephen Craig

Completion: 2003. **Technique:** steel, glass, plants, metal, painted wood. **Location:** Riem, Germany.

"Wishing Well" was made by artist Stephen Craig and is situated in Munich, Germany. The piece investigates the relationship between art and architecture as it can be viewed as a work of architecture or as a sculpture. "Wishing Well" is one of a series of works, and is a usable, permanent structure. The open top and permeable walls blur the definition of what is interior and what is exterior.

Stephen Craig was born in Ireland in 1960 but currently lives in Germany. He studied at Sydney College of the Arts and was awarded an bachelor of arts in visual arts, majoring in sculpture. In 1992 he received his masters in visual arts / sculpture from the Amsterdam Academy of Art. Much of Craig's work explores the interface between art and architecture. His works investigate permeability, the transition from outside to inside.

Photos: Stephen Craig (a.); Edward Beierle (b.)

Fountain
Fernando Sánchez Castillo

Completion: 2003. **Technique:** riot van. **Location:** Cádiz, Spain.

This work by Fernando Sánchez Castillo is on display in the grounds of the NMAC Foundation in Cádiz, Spain. The majority of the artist's projects take the form of toys, or games and involve a degree of audience complicity. This project is a riot van that takes on the unlikely role of fountain. The artist has transformed an object of violence and oppression into an aesthetic, decorative object. His work reflects on the different forms of monitoring and control within society, and the power associated with these.

Fernando Sánchez Castillo is a Spanish artist, born in Madrid in 1970. He works with both video and sculpture and produces sculptures that ask the viewer to consider an object in a new light. His work sometimes takes symbols of violence or oppression and subvert them, making them powerless.

Photo: Iain and Sarah / Wikimedia Commons

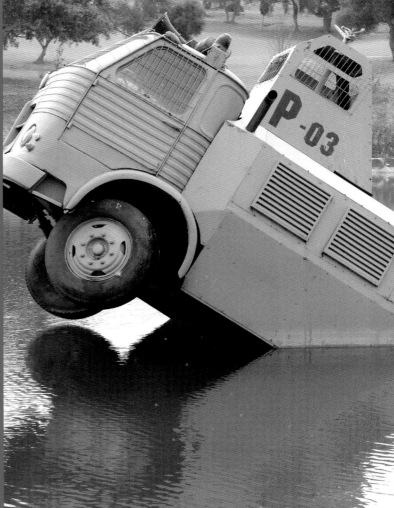

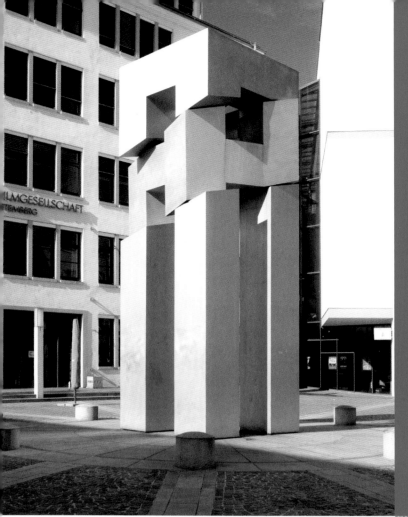

The Kinetic Project
Bernd Wilhelm Blank

Completion: 2003. **Technique:** steel, aluminum alloy. **Location:** Stuttgart, Germany.

"The Kinetic Project" uses technology developed by Bosch and is located in the middle of the Robert-Bosch-Platz in Stuttgart. The sculpture stands on a circle of gray stones, and four, seven -meter-high metal pillars rise into the air, forming a cube shape. The work is interspersed with square openings. The unusual feature of this sculpture is that the middle section turns round, driven by a wind-powered motor.

Bernd Wilhelm Blank was born in Berlin in 1935. He studied at the School of Applied Arts in Berlin-Charlottenburg, which later became the Department of Applied Arts at the University of the Arts. Blank was taught by professor Martin Dittberner, amongst others. He made his first sculpture for display in public space, in the 1950s. It is of the utmost importance to the artist that his works blend with their surroundings.

Photo: Chris van Uffelen

The Endless Staircase
Olafur Eliasson

Completion: 2004. **Technique:** steel, wood. **Location:** Munich, Germany.

"The Endless Staircase" is made of steel and wood and stands in the courtyard of the KPMG Building in Munich. Visitors can climb the steps from the bottom upwards, just like a normal staircase, except that this one has no destination, the stairs simple loop down again, bringing the visitor back to the start position. The sculpture gives character to the large courtyard and the shape of the staircase gently compliments the architecture of the surrounding building.

Olafur Eliasson was born in Copenhagen in 1967. He studied at the Royal Danish Academy of Fine Arts, graduating in 1995. He was shortlisted for the Hugo Boss-Prize in 2002 and awarded the Austrian Friedrich-Kiesler-Prize for excellence in the fields of art and architecture. He lives and works in both Berlin and Copenhagen and his work focuses primarily on physical phenomena in nature, such as light and water, movement, repetition and reflection.

Photo: Chris van Uffelen

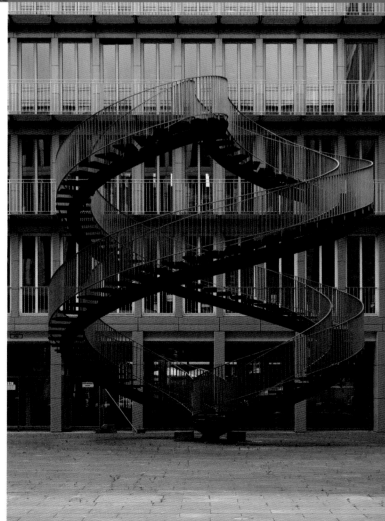

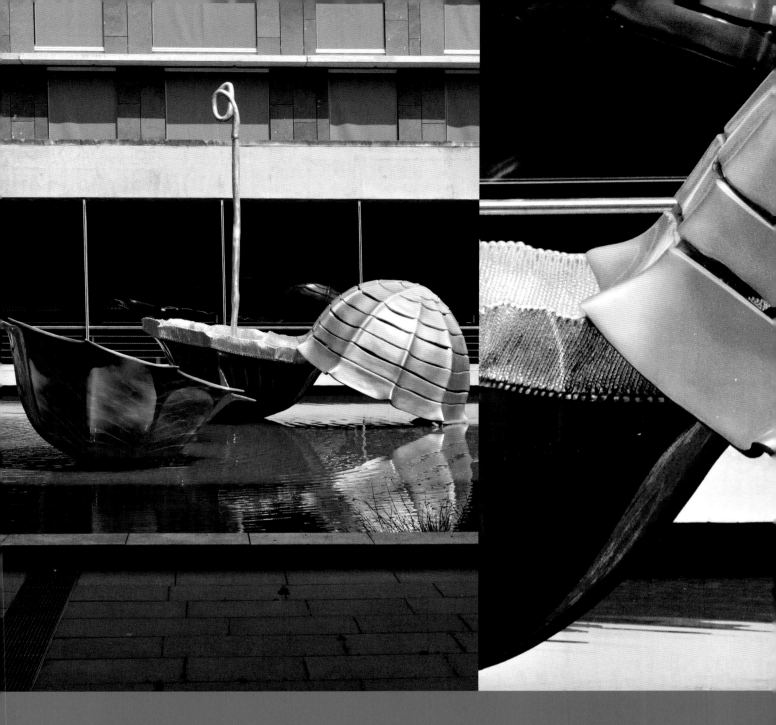

Three Umbrellas
Stephan Hasslinger

Completion: 2004. **Technique:** aluminum, ceramics. **Location:** Freiburg, Germany.

"Three Umbrellas" is comprised of an upturned blue umbrella positioned next to a gold one, with a third upturned some meters away. The sculpture has a lightweight appearance, as if the umbrellas could be blown away by the wind at any moment. The work's intrigue comes from the appealing contrast between the apparent lightness of the technique and the actual heaviness of the shapes. The colored surfaces of the sculptural ensemble are created from weatherproof, glazed ceramic.

Stephan Hasslinger was born in 1960 in Marburg, Germany. He studied sculpture at the University of Art in Bremen and was later awarded a DAAD scholarship, allowing him to study for one year at the Royal College of Art in London. He often works with steel to produce his sculptures and his work is often influenced by textile structures, giving them a modern appearance. Hasslinger currently lives and works in Freiburg.

Photos: Chris van Uffelen

The Weight of a Shadow
Wilhelm Holderied

Completion: 2004. **Technique:** steel, red paint. **Location:** Munich, Germany.

"The Weight of a Shadow" symbolizes two "Moosgeist (March ghosts)" figures that represent the local carnival festival, held in February each year. The sides of the figures have been folded outwards, opening the sculpture out and making it more abstract in form. As with many of Wilhelm Holderied's sculptures, this work plays with weight and shadow, the sides of the works lie like solid shadows on the ground, while the opened out form of the work gives it a lightweight appearance.

Wilhelm Holderied is a German painter and sculptor, born in 1940. His work focuses on various themes, including weight, weightlessness, shadows and masks. Holderied's work often considers signs and their illustrative power. He has exhibited his work widely, including at exhibitions in Munich, Berlin, New York, Chicago, San Francisco and Seoul. He has traveled widely and currently lives and works in Munich.

Photo: Chris van Uffelen

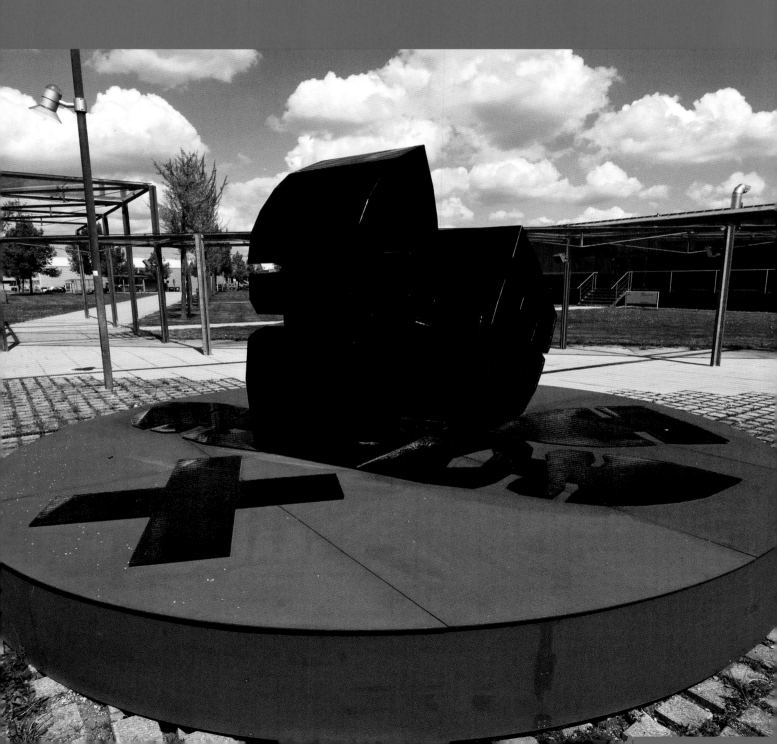

Maria, Source of Life
Hans van Houwelingen

Completion: 2004. **Technique:** marble, water. **Location:** Munich, Germany.

The Petuel Park, where this sculpture is located, is in an open area between two sections of the city. The park has been built on top of the now underground highway, dissolving the physical barrier between two neighborhoods. The artist created the work as a consideration of the idea of Mary as life-giving and life-receiving source. Mary sits in a bath made of carrara marble, receiving water from the Nymphenburger canal, which flows back into the canal from the child's hand, this cycle symbolizes a new era.

Hans van Houwelingen was born in Harlingen, the Netherlands, in 1957. He studied at Academy Minerva in Groningen between 1978 and 1984 and the Academy of Art in Amsterdam from 1985 to 1988. He has exhibited his work widely throughout the Netherlands, including at the Van Abbe Museum, and has been commissioned to produce various public works, including "The Olympic Ideal" in 2005 for the winter Olympics.

Photo: Chris van Uffelen

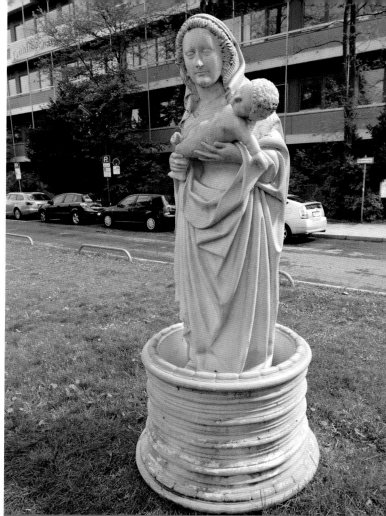

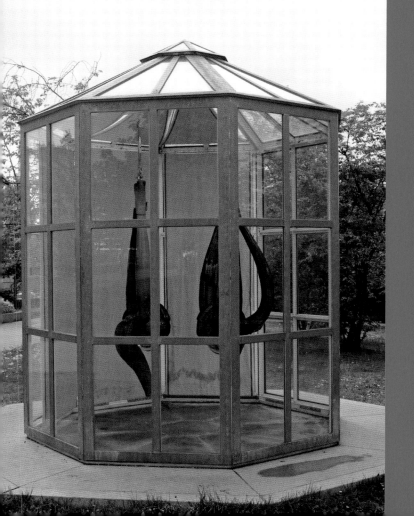

The Aviary
Raimund Kummer

Completion: 2004. **Technique:** glass. **Location:** Freiburg, Germany.

"The Aviary" stands in Petuel Park in Munich. The glass house is shaped like a green house but instead of housing plants it is home to two green-glass sculptures. The green shapes are abstract in form and resemble neither flowers nor birds, as one might expect. The green of the glass compliments the park area and the transparent windows of the house frame the sculptures, drawing the attention of passersby and encouraging them to stop and take a closer look.

Raimund Kummer was born in 1954. He initially studied painting but turned away from this art form not long after finishing his studies. He belongs to a generation of artists whose works focus on the production and presentation of art and a more expansive use of technique. With the increase of site specific public works of art, Kummer became well-established as a sculptor. He began to make excursions in Berlin and New York, seeking out interesting places. He then began developing sculpture to emphasize a given situation, highlighting what was already there with his installations.

Photos: Chris van Uffelen

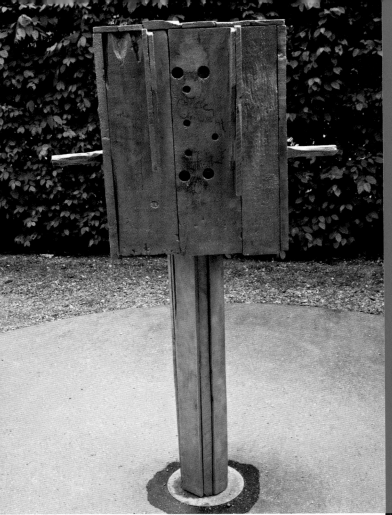

Periscope
Bogomir Ecker

Completion: 2004. **Technique:** wood, lenses, sound and video installation. **Location:** Munich, Germany.

"Periscope" stands in a corner of Petuel Park in Munich. The piece is fairly unobtrusive, no signs inform the visitor what it is and it can be easily overlooked. However, hiding within the unremarkable exterior, is a high tech periscope, giving the observer a view into the motorway that runs below. The user can see the cars whizzing past below them, the drivers completely oblivious to the fact that they are being observed. Sound accompanies the piece so that the noise of passing cars can also be heard.

Bogomir Ecker is a German sculptor, photographer and installation artist. He studied at the State Art Academy in Karlsruhe, later continuing his education at the Art Academy in Dusseldorf. He worked as professor of sculpture at the University of Art in Hamburg and then later as a professor at the University of Art in Brunswick. He was awarded the Edwin Scharff Prize of the city of Hamburg in 2001 and the Lower Saxony Art prize in 2006.

Photo: Chris van Uffelen

DNA
Mirosław Struzik

Completion: 2004. **Technique:** acid resistant stainless steel. **Location:** Wroclaw, Poland.

This sculpture, entitled "DNA", was designed for the Municipal Botanic Garden of Wroclaw University. It is made of acid-resistant stainless steel; the form twists and turns, causing the light to reflect off it at different angles, giving it a shiny, almost sparkling appearance. The sculpture represents the continuation of a cycle. The form symbolizes a spiral line of DNA code, combining masculine and feminine elements with upward dynamics, striving for further evolution.

Mirosław Struzik graduated from the Fine Arts Academy in Warsaw, Poland. In 2005 he received the Sugarman Foundation Award, an award supporting up-and-coming artists. Struzik's work mainly involves creating sculptures for public areas, for example his "Adam and Eve" sculpture, for the Skokie North shore Sculpture Park in Chicago and his "Memorial of Gratitude to World War II Victims", in Opoczno, Poland. Struzik uses various materials, including bronze, wood, stone and stainless steel.

Photo: Courtesy of the artist

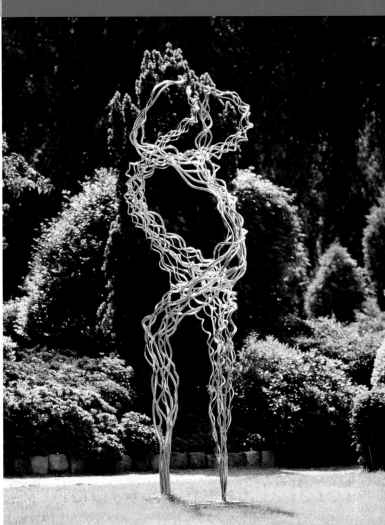

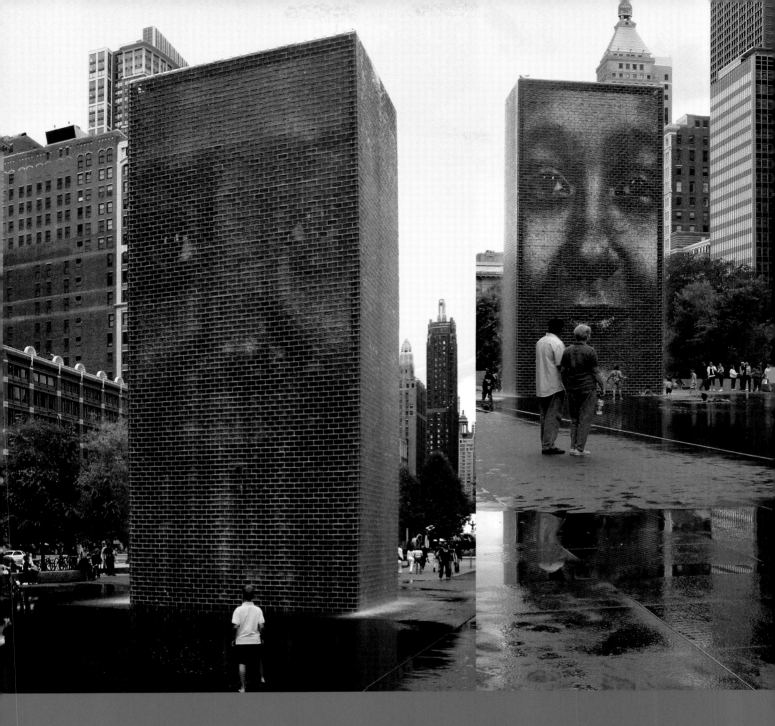

Crown Fountain
Jaume Plensa

Completion: 2004. **Technique:** black granite, glass bricks, video installation. **Location:** Chicago, IL, USA.

"Crown Fountain" is an interactive work of public art. It stands in the Loop community area and is composed of a reflecting pool made of black granite situated between two glass brick towers. Water cascades down the towers and out of a nozzle on the front face of each tower. Some of the videos displayed are of scenery, but most attention has been given to the videos featuring local residents. Hundreds of people visit the fountain in the hope of seeing themselves on one of the fountain's screens.

Jaume Plensa is a Spanish contemporary artist and sculptor, born in Barcelona in 1955. "Crown Fountain" is one of his best known projects. Another acclaimed work is "Blake" in Gateshead, a laser beam that lights up the sky over Gateshead in England on special occasions. He also created a site specific work for St Helens in Merseyside; "The Dream" was created with the help of ex-miners. He has been awarded various prizes, including the National Award of Arts by the Government of Catalonia.

Photos: Jens Rogotzki

Ancient Language
Andrew Rogers

Completion: 2004. **Technique:** volcanic rock bound with clay and bird droppings. **Location:** Atacama Desert, Chile.

"Ancient Language" was created as part of the "Rhythms of Life" (ROL) project. Two other geoglyphs, "The Ancients" and "Rhythms of Life", are also located on this site. ROL is the largest contemporary Land Art undertaking in the world – 48 structures in 13 countries across seven continents involving over 6,700 people. "Ancient Language" is 80 meters long and almost three meters high. It is constructed of volcanic rock, bound with clay and bird droppings and is located at the end of the Valle de la Luna, Atacama Desert, Chile.

Andrew Rogers is one of Australia's most distinguished and internationally renowned artists. He exhibits internationally and his critically acclaimed sculptures are in numerous private and prominent public collections across the world. Rogers has received many international bronze commissions and has created "Rhythms of Life", one of the largest Land Art undertakings in the world. His new forms are a continuing contribution to contemporary visual arts, forging new paths in the use of materials and forms.

Photo: Courtesy of the artist

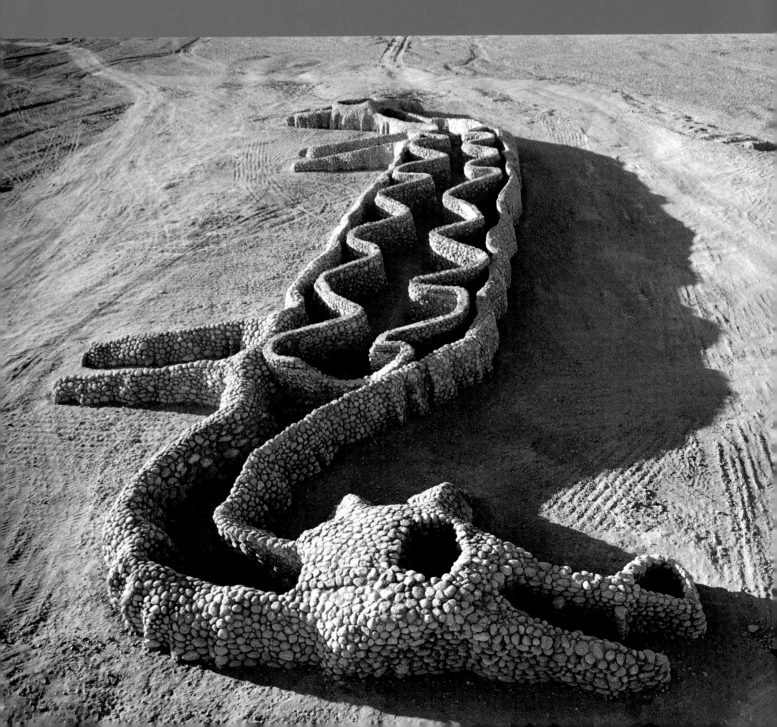

Peep-Wheel
Tom Carr

Completion: 2004. **Technique:** painted stainless steel. **Location:** Madrid, Spain.

"Peep-Wheel" is a lens pointing to infinity. The piece was conceived in 1995, to be placed in an open landscape near a road. The three brightly colored rings and radials suggest movement and an ambiguous depth, directing the viewer to a framed fragment of nature. It was built in 2004 and installed on Madrid's R II outskirt ring highway. The piece is first seen as a tiny shape in the landscape, growing in size as the observer approaches and finally framing all that lies behind it.

Tom Carr was born in Tarragona in 1956, to a Spanish mother and North-American father. He grew up in the USA, returning to Spain at 17. He studied at the University of Barcelona, receiving a bachelor of arts degree and a PhD in fine arts. Carr works primarily as a sculptor, using many different media. A lot of his works are displayed in public space and frequently explore the concepts of time and space. Carr is also included in the international program of the School of Visual Arts in New York.

Photo: Courtesy of the artist

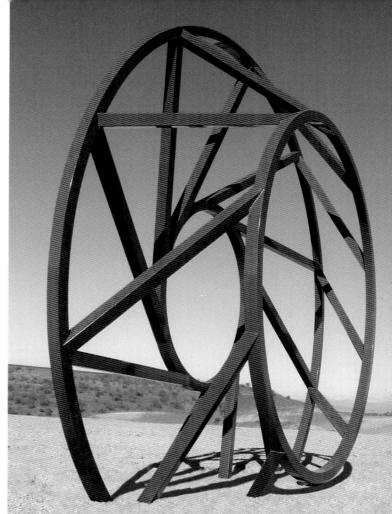

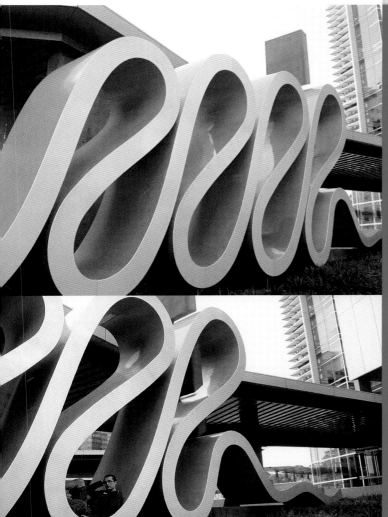

Confluence
Daniel Templeman

Completion: 2004. **Technique:** aluminum, concrete. **Location:** Brisbane, Australia.

"Confluence" was Daniel Templeman's first public art commission. The sculpture is a highly visible artwork, measuring 65 meters in length. It was completed in September 2004 and sits in the George Street forecourt of the Brisbane Magistrates Court. The sculpture was created as a part of the Art Built-In program and is made of aluminum and concrete. The artwork begins in gentle waves before building in intensity, finally cutting through a seemingly impenetrable object and then returning to its calmer state.

Daniel Templeman is a contemporary Australian sculptor. He graduated from Queensland University of Technology with honors in 1999. Since then he has been exhibiting his work around Brisbane, Australia. He has already completed two major commissions, the most recent being for Griffith University, Queensland. His work is about the gaps between which everything falls and is minimalist in form. Templeman's works are delicately balanced, testing the form and strength of the materials that he chooses.

Photos: Paleontour / Wikipedia Commons (a.); Paleontour / Wikipedia Commons (b.)

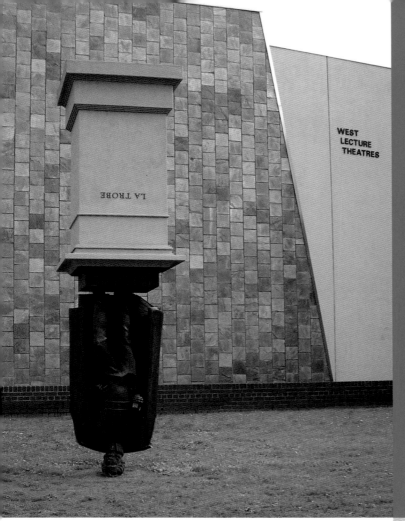

Landmark
Charles Robb

Completion: 2004. **Technique:** bronze. **Location:** Melbourne, Australia.

This sculpture is now a permanent installation at Latrobe University in Australia. The sculpture is an inverted statue of Charles Joseph Latrobe, the first Lieutenant Governor of Victoria, Australia. The artist claims that he positioned the work upside down to encourage dialogue and to correspond to the notion that universities should turn ideas on their heads. The sculpture has been the focus of much debate as some viewers have interpreted the meaning of the piece as disrespectful to Latrobe.

Currently based in Brisbane, Charles Robb has been shortlisted three times for the Helen Lempriere National Sculpture Awards and has received project grants from both Arts Queensland and the Australia Council. Robb has also widely exhibited his work, both in solo and group exhibitions, including at the Institute of Modern Art in Brisbane. Robb currently holds the position of associate lecturer in sculpture at the University of Southern Queensland, Toowoomba.

Photo: resacup / Wikimedia Commons

Cosmos
Dimitris Fortsas

Completion: 2004. **Technique:** painted steel. **Location:** Volos, Greece.

"Cosmos" was created in the context of the Olympic Games, held in Greece in 2004. The sculpture consists of five circles. Four of them are formed of human bodies and the hands of human figures, while the fifth serves as a pedestal. The composition symbolizes the idea of the cosmos and its dynamic movement, the co-existence of people, the mutual understanding and the competition as a means of encouraging new ideas and young people. In the sculpture, there is an inside space accessible to the visitor.

Dimitris Fortsas was born in 1957 in Greece. He studied painting from 1979–1983. Since 1990 he has been occupied with sculpture and design. He has participated in many group exhibitions and has realized eight personal exhibitions. His works in public space include: sculpture at Municipal Hall, Thessaloniki 2010, sculpture in Attiki Metro Station, Athens 2004 and a decorative painting of Apollo Theater, Siros 1997.

Photos: Courtesy of the artist

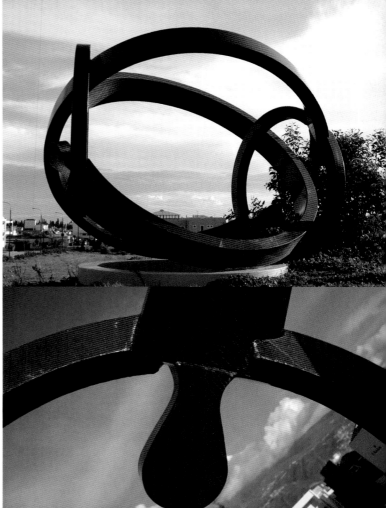

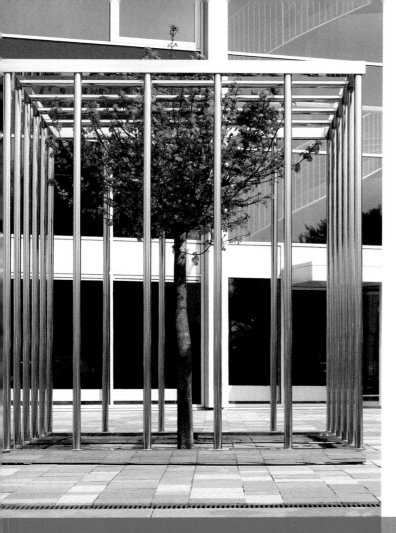

Amnestree
Ram Katzir

Completion: 2004. **Technique:** polished stainless steel, maple tree. **Location:** Utrecht, The Netherlands.

"Amnestree" is an organic sculpture that changes form with the passing seasons. Viewed from outside, one sees his / her face reflected in the polished bars; viewed from inside, one is imprisoned with the tree. The sculpture was commissioned by Amnesty International and CBK Utrecht as a monument for the Declaration of Human Rights. "Amnestree" reflects the effects of suppression on freedom and individual growth.

Ram Katzir was born in Israel in 1969. He studied sculpture and photography at The Cooper Union School of Art in New York and received a bachelors degree from the Gerrit Rietveld Academy in Amsterdam. Katzir has exhibited internationally and held many solo exhibitions, including at the Stedelijk Museum, Amsterdam, the Israel Museum, Jerusalem and Kyoto Art Center in Japan. Katzir's public sculptures have been placed in landmark locations across Europe and he is currently working on new projects for Berlin, Tokyo and Shanghai.

Photo: Allard Bovenberg; © Studio Ram Katzir

Swastika
Dhruva Mistry

Completion: 2004. **Technique:** lazer cutting of sheet metal, two sheet metal figues crossed over one another. **Location:** Dahej, Gujarat, India.

The word "Swastika" in classical Sanskrit symbolizes the energy of the sun and has auspicious connotations. The human figure in space with a convincing silhouette of front and side views extend into four directions of space. The image symbolizes energy and the movement of the sun, referring to the cosmic symbolism of the Indian Swastika. The piece is made of twelve millimeter, galvanized and painted steel. The shapes are cut using laser cutting.

Dhruva Mistry was born in 1957 in Kanjari (Central Gujarat). He studied sculpture at the Faculty of Fine Art, The Maharaja Sayajirao University of Baroda from 1974 to 1981. Mistry has shown regularly in solo exhibitions apart from being included in significant national and international group shows and exhibitions since 1979. Mistry's work has been included in numerous group shows in India and abroad. His works are held in important public and private collections in the United Kingdom, Japan and India, including the Tate and the Royal College of Art.

Photo: Courtesy of the artist

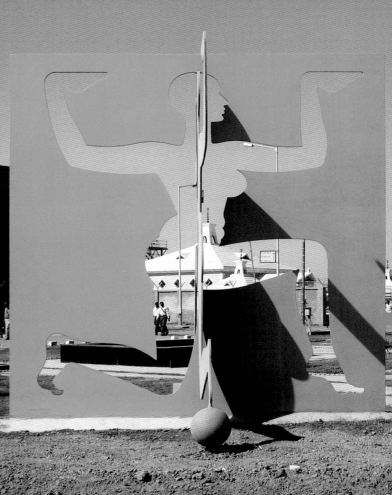

Memorial to the Murdered Jews of Europe
Peter Eisenman

Completion: 2004. **Technique:** concrete slabs. **Location:** Berlin, Germany.

This is a memorial to the victims of the Holocaust. The 19,000-square meter site is covered with concrete slabs, these are arranged in a grid pattern on the gently sloping site. Attached to the site is an underground information area, where the names of all known victims of the Holocaust are recorded. The memorial has been criticized for only representing Jewish victims. A monument to the people persecuted on the grounds of sexual orientation is situated across the street.

Peter Eisenman is a world-renowned American architect, born in New Jersey in 1932. He first became famous as a member of the New York Five, a group of five architects whose work appeared in an exhibition at the Museum of Art in 1967. Eisenman's focus on "liberating" architecture was well regarded for its theoretical standpoint but is criticized for leading to the production of buildings that have no consideration of the building's functional purpose.

Photos: Chris van Uffelen

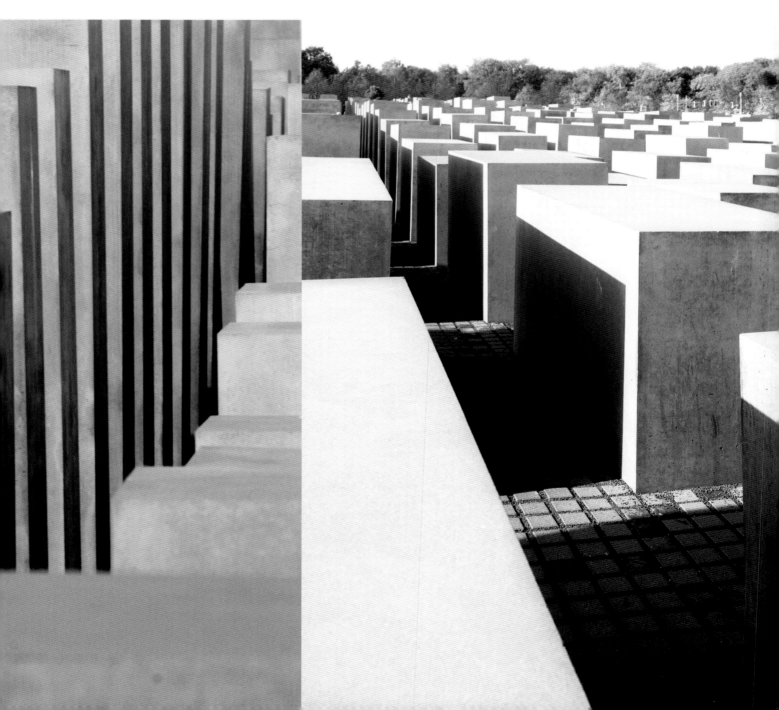

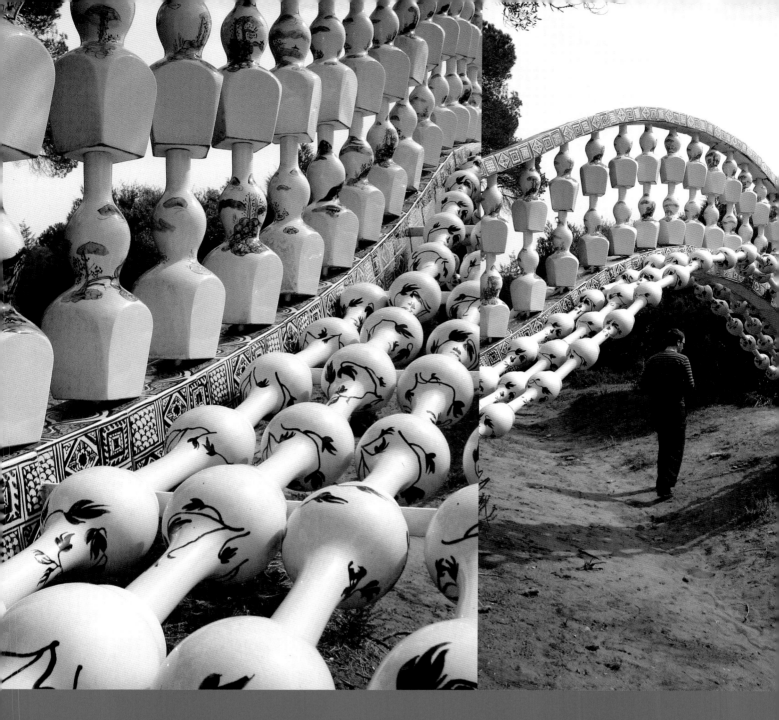

Bridge
Shen Yuan

Completion: 2004. **Technique:** ceramic. **Location:** Cádiz, Spain.

This ceramic work is on display at the NMAC Foundation in Spain. It aims to bridge the gap between two different cultures, namely Chinese and Spanish. The balustrade is comprised of two identical rows of vases, these are decorated with Chinese and Islamic motifs. At each end of the bridge is a slender, ceramic structure, patterned with the same motifs. "Bridge" is symbolic of the difficulties between cultures that must be somehow overcome.

Shen Yuan is a Chinese artist and sculptor. She was born in Fuzhou and became involved in the Avant-garde art movement in Xiamen in the late 1980s. She moved to Paris in 1990 and has lived there ever since. Yuan's work has been exhibited at both solo and group exhibitions in France, Germany, England, Switzerland, Belgium, Japan and China. She has participated in many major international exhibitions including the Guangzhou Art Triennial, Guangzhou, China, 2005.

Photos: Iain and Sarah / Wikimedia Commons

Giant Foot
Alixe Fu

Completion: 2005. **Technique:** acrylic, paint. **Location:** Pingtung, Taiwan.

Alixe Fu produces uncanny, ambiguous works that encourage viewers to take a fresh look at the ordinary body. Fu composes his work by contrasting fields of color and texture with bold colors and shapes, juxtaposed with subtle variations. Through this project Fu intends to make himself and the viewer look more closely at the constructed geographic of humankind. Poetic reinterpretations of these spaces force us to see absurdity and beauty often overlooked in ordinary sights.

Alixe Fu, born in 1961, is originally from Taiwan. He is a multi-disciplinary artist, producing work in a variety of media, such as oil, ink, acrylic, ceramic, mosaic, bronze, resin and metal. His first solo exhibition was in Taipei in 1983. His work can be found in the collections of the Museum of Daubigny, France; Fine Arts Museum, Taipei; Hong-Gah Museum, Taipei and the Museum Nakasendo in Japan. Fu has received numerous awards, including two grants from the National Foundation of the Arts in Taiwan.

Photo: LYNA Art

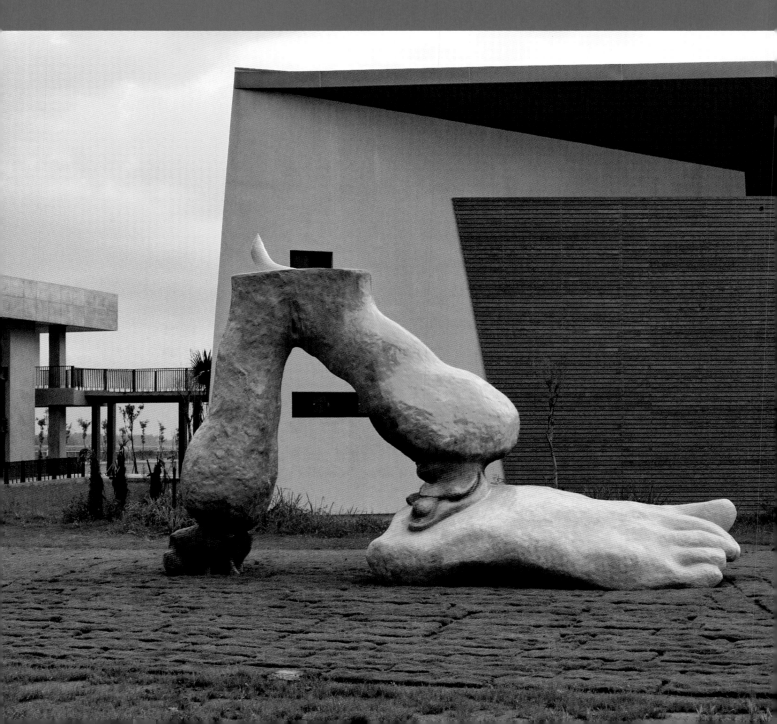

The Way to Independence
J Seward Johnson Jr.

Completion: 2005. **Technique:** painted bronze. **Location:** Morristown, NJ, USA.

This sculpture, depicting a blind man and his guide dog, was dedicated to Morris Frank in 2005. Frank was an American who lost the site in both of his eyes in an accident. In 1927 he heard of a guide dog training scheme in Switzerland and requested that a dog be trained for him, to help him regain his independence. The guide dog, Buddy, became the first "seeing eye" dog in the USA. The Seeing Eye dog center was subsequently established in America in 1929.

John Seward Johnson Jr. is an American artist. He was born in 1930 and is best known for his life-size bronze sculptures. Johnson first focused his artistic efforts on painting, but turned to sculpture in 1968. His work often depicts people in everyday situations and has been labeled as kitsch by some critics. In 1974 he founded The Sculptural Foundation, which aims to instruct talented young sculptors and also includes a foundry where both his own sculptures and sculptures from many renowned artists are cast.

Photos: Susan Kane

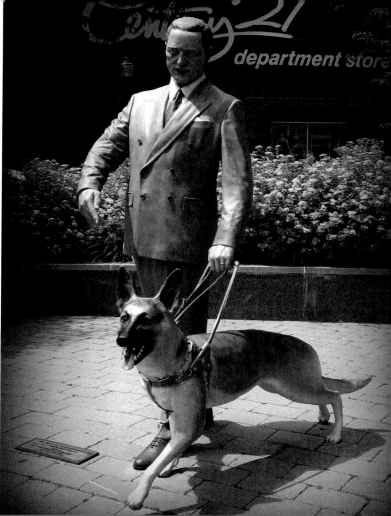

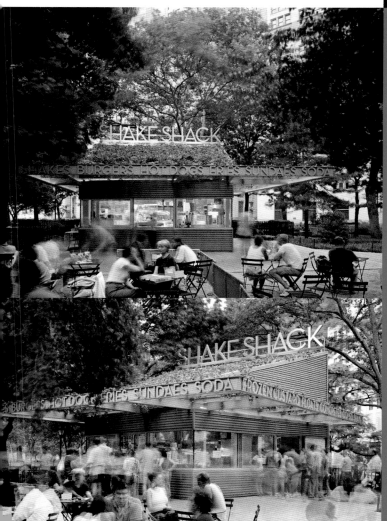

Shake Shack
SITE

Completion: 2004. **Technique:** glass, corrugated zinc, plants. **Location:** New York City, NY, USA.

The "Shake Shack" is a social architecture phenomenon in the wake of the 1990s relational aesthetics movement. The small torqued building emerged from site analysis in line with the nearby Flatiron Building and a continuous client dialogue engaging Madison Square Park and restaurateur, Danny Meyer. An oversized, cantilevered trellis, an inclined roof plane and the back wall of the structure are covered in vines.

Sculpture In The Environment is an architecture and environmental arts studio, internationally known for innovative buildings and public spaces. SITE works developing artistically distinguished and highly communicative design projects and is a collaborative team of architects, artists and designers. In the last 30 years the studio has completed works in the USA, Canada, Spain, France, Italy, England, Austria, China, Korea and Japan. Core members include Denise M.C. Lee, Sara Stracey and James Wines.

Photos: Peter Mauss / ESTO, New York

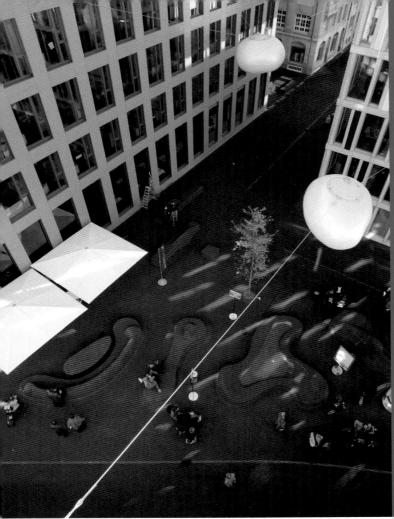

Citylounge
Carlos Martinez Archi-
tekten, Pipilotti Rist

Completion: 2005. **Technique:** traffic signs, trees, hydrocarbon polymer granulated rubber. **Location:** St. Gallen, Switzerland.

The "Citylounge" (Stadtlounge) is exhibited in the Raiffeisenquarter in St. Gallen, Switzerland. It is a blazing red, surprisingly soft floor, changing the atmosphere of the area and giving a sense of a whole rather than a sense of division. The soft silhouettes of the furniture deliver a deliberate contrast to the hard precision of the surroundings. The plants offer a contrast to the red carpet. This work has breathed new life into the quarter, the public comes to the fore and the traffic takes a back seat.

Carlos Martinez was born in 1967. He is an architect who owns and runs his own firm in Switzerland. The firm's vision is to provide affordable but individual housing projects. He has worked on other art projects, combining architecture and art. Pipilotti Rist was born in 1962 in Switzerland. She studied at the School of Applied Arts in Vienna. She has also studied audio visual communications and was been making freestyle video / audio and installations since 1986. Rist has participated in several solo and group exhibitions around the world.

Photo: Carlos Martinez, photographer: Hannes Thalmann

New Zgody Square
Piotr Lewicki and
Kazimierz Łatak

Completion: 2005. **Technique:** bronze, iron cast, galvanized steel, syenite cobblestones, concrete. **Location:** Cracow, Poland.

Zgody Square is famous as the play where the Nazi regime gathered together Jews from a nearby ghetto, to deport them to concentration camps. After the deportations, the square and the surrounding area contained many traces of the atrocities committed. Abandoned items becoming a meaningful trace of the absence of their owners. This artwork is a memorial to all those sent to the concentration camps, paying homage to the owners of those lost possessions which gained a sad significance as they lay abandoned.

Biuro Projektów Lewickiłatak, was established in 1995 by Kazimierz Latak (born 1962) and Piotr Lewicki (born 1966). Graduated from the Faculty of Architecture at Cracow University of Technology in 1990, they have been working together since 1988. Biuro Projektów Lewickiłatak is an architectural firm spezializing in planning, architecture and interior design. Between 2003 and 2009 they also ran a design workshop at Cracow Frycz-Modrzewski Academy.

Photos: Paweł Kubisztal, Cracow

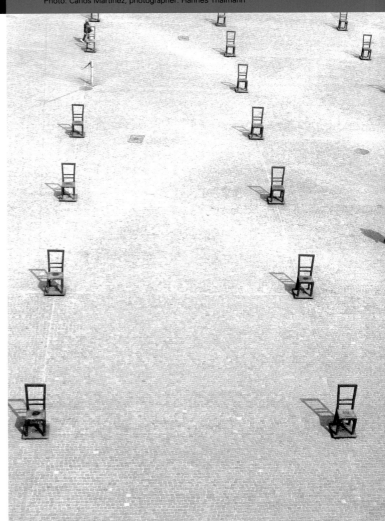

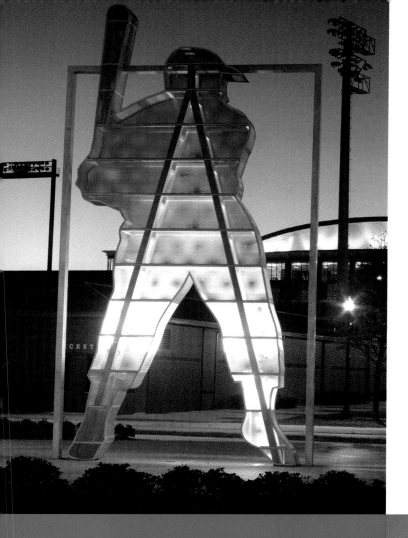

Rookie Card
Barbara Grygutis

Completion: 2005. **Technique:** aluminum and lighting. **Location:** Jacksonville, FL, USA.

"Rookie Card" is an aluminum sculpture, commissioned by the city of Jacksonville, Florida. It stands at over eight meters in height and portrays the semi-transparent silhouette of a baseball figure. It was made for the new Jacksonville Ballpark and pays tribute to the time-old immortalization of baseball players through trading cards. The sculpture is lit at night and several oversize granite baseballs provide small seating units.

Barbara Grygutis has been commissioned to create large-scale works of public art across the United States and beyond. Her numerous awards include two U.S. National Endowment for the Arts awards and second place in the International Quadrennial Competition in Faenza, Italy. She has created over seventy permanent public art installations and her work has been exhibited at The Smithsonian Institute in Washington D.C. and The Parker Collection for the Vice-President's House and the White House, Washington D.C.

Photo: Courtesy of the artist

Frame
Richard Rezac

Completion: 2005. **Technique:** glazed terracotta, commercial glazed brick, limestone, concrete. **Location:** Governors State University, IL, USA.

This sculpture acknowledges the resonant character of the rural landscape that defines the university campus. It functions in two specific ways: as a framing device that takes in the prairie from two directions, and as a two-dimensional composition, like a picture. The six ovals that penetrate the solid wall are arranged along two intersecting axes with the three medium-sized ovals positioned at eye-level. The use of green and white glazed brick promotes a merging or camouflage effect.

Richard Rezac was born in 1952. He studied between 1974 and 1982 at the Pacific Northwest College of Art in Portland, and at the Maryland Institute, College of Art in Baltimore. He has received the Guggenheim Foundation fellowship and Rome Prize fellowship at the American Academy in Rome and Louis Comfort Tiffany Award. Examples of his sculptures are held in the collections of The Art Institute of Chicago and the Museum of Contemporary Art, Chicago. He currently lives and works in Chicago.

Photos: Tom Van Eynde

The Community Chalkboard
Pete O'Shea, Robert Winstead

Completion: 2005. **Technique:** slate panels with stainless steel chalk tray. **Location:** Charlottesville, VA, USA.

Believed to be the first of its kind in the public realm of the USA, this interactive, democratic and uncensored monument to the first amendment of the US Constitution provides a venue for the practice of the right to free expression. The slate wall and podium provide a free and accessible venue for expression, allowing people from all walks of life to engage the chalkboard on a daily basis. The wall has become the symbolic destination for all public discourses in the city.

Pete O'Shea is the founder of Siteworks Studio and Robert Winstead is the principal of VMDO Architects, they often work in collaboration. O'Shea is a former faculty member of the University of Virginia School of Architecture. His work integrates architecture, engineering and landscape into holistic projects that prioritize concerns for ecological intelligence, human experience and public art. O'Shea is the recipient of numerous awards for design excellence including the prestigious Rome Prize.

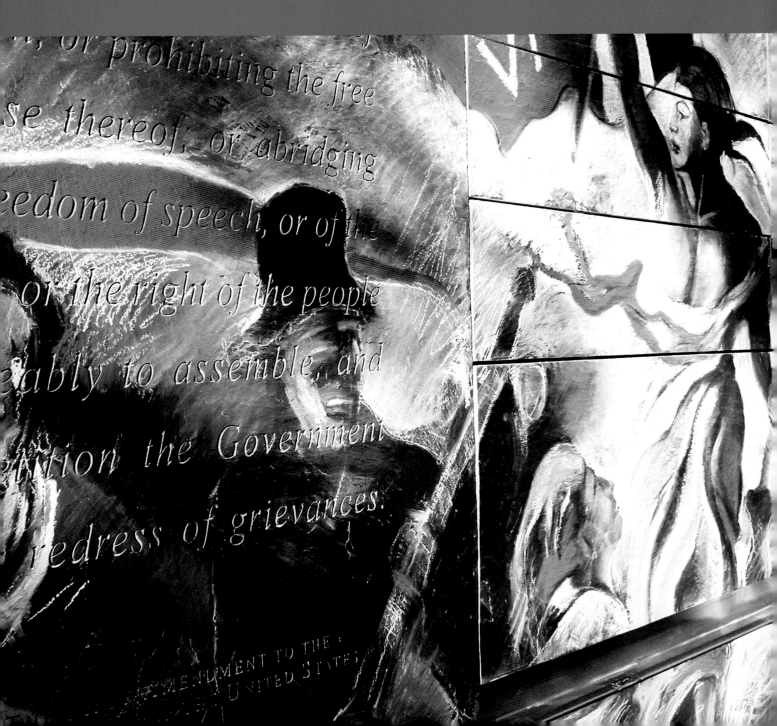

Attiki Odos
Nella Golanda,
Aspassia Kouzoupi

Completion: 2005. **Technique:** re-use of concrete pre-cast blocks, silver, white paint, reflective surfaces, collage of cut traffic signs fragments. **Location:** Athens, Greece.

"Attiki Odos" is a high-speed motorway crossing Athens. This project aimed to distort the unvaried character of the highway by recycling and using highway construction materials. The structure brings together the natural and the man-made, serving to disperse the monotony of the highway by producing micro-landscapes, which change their appearance depending on the time of day and the driver's speed. The micro-landscapes are inconspicuous poles, dragging the passenger's gaze to the wider landscape, along four kilometers.

Nella Golanda is a landscape sculptor and honorary member of the Hellenic Association of Landscape Architects. Since 1972 she has applied "Total Art" in public spaces, re-establishing the relationship between the natural and historical landscape. Aspassia Kouzoupi, is an urban landscape architect. They have worked as associates since 1994, establishing the studio Sculpted Architectural Landscapes in 2000.

Photos: Dimitris Kalapodas (a.); Johanna Weber (b.)

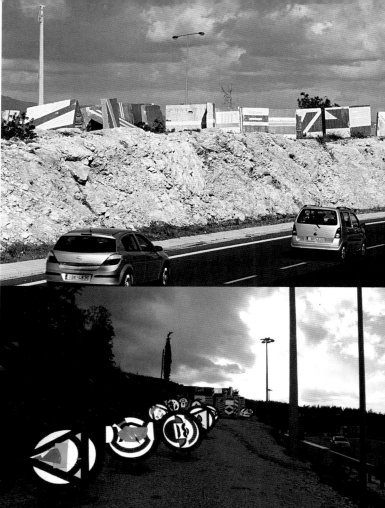

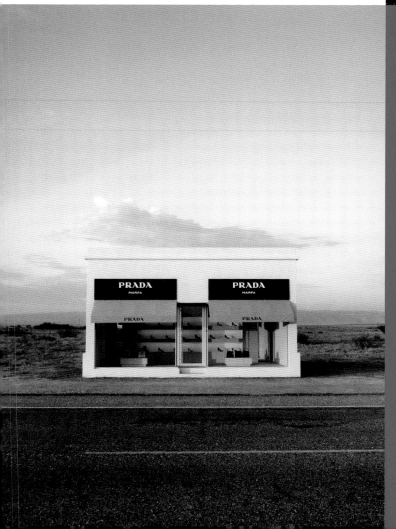

Prada Marfa
Michael Elmgreen,
Ingar Dragset

Completion: 2005. **Technique:** adobe bricks, plaster, aluminum frames, glass panes, MDF, paint, carpet, Prada shoes and bags. **Location:** Marfa, TX, USA.

"Prada Marfa" is a sculpture in Texas, designed to resemble a Prada store. On the front of the structure there are two large windows displaying Prada wares, shoes and handbags, picked out and provided by Miuccia Prada herself. The sculpture was intended never to be repaired so that it might slowly degrade back into the landscape. This was deviated from when, three days after it was completed, vandals sprayed graffiti on the exterior and broke into the building stealing bags and shoes.

Michael Elmgreen and Ingar Dragset are a collaborative duo of visual artists who currently live and work in Berlin. They are famous for producing work that has wit and subversive humor but also considers serious cultural concerns and problems. Elmgreen and Dragset met in 1995 and moved to Berlin in 1997. They won the German Government's competition in 2003 for a memorial in Tiergarten Park, Berlin, in memory of gay victims of the Nazi regime. This was unveiled in May 2008.

Photo: James Evans

River Eyelash
Stacy Levy

Completion: 2005. **Technique:** painted buoys, steel washers, pink rope. **Location:** Pittsburgh, PA, USA.

42 strands of buoys radiate out from the bulkhead of the Point State Park, like an eyelash for the city. The eyelash floats where the concrete of the city meets the edge of the water, engaging the great open surface of the Three Rivers in Pittsburgh. The eyelash changes formation in response to wind direction, speed of the currents and types of waves. The lines of buoys mimic the arched forms of the steel bridges which cross nearby, creating a bright shadow of the bridge's forms.

Stacy Levy is an artist who investigates water, clarifying the movement of rain and storm water in the landscape and making the patterns of watersheds and flowing water visible. She has both public and private commissions across America. Levy graduated from Yale University in 1984 with a bachelor of arts in sculpture and forestry and she received her masters of fine arts in 1991 from the Tyler School of Art. She attended the Architectural Association in London in 1981 and the Skowhegan School of Painting and Sculpture in 1988.

Photos: Larry Rippel

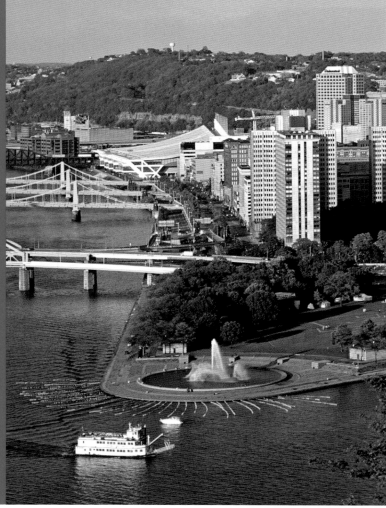

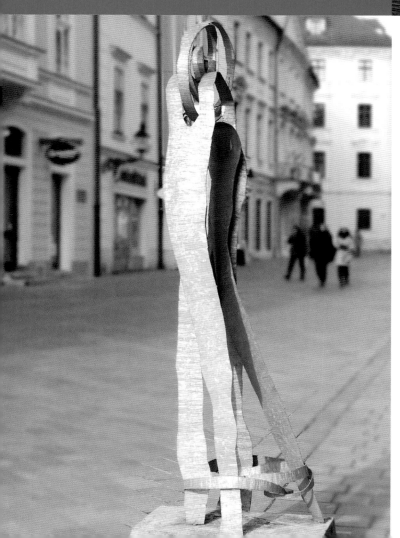

Don´t Disturb my Circles
Martin Lettrich

Completion: 2005. **Technique:** galvanized steel. **Location:** Bratislava, Slovakia.

The object "Don't Disturb my Circles" is located in the pedestrian area, in Bratislava, close to the Visual Arts Gallery. The size, material and location of the artwork ensue from the characteristics of the environment. The silhouette of the object, drawn by the different projections of the material is more compact from the lateral perspective. The composition gradually changes into circles and spiraling towards the background.

Martin Lettrich is a Slovakian sculptor, born in Bratislava in 1951. He studied at the University of Applied Arts in Prague, graduating in 1976. Selected solo exhibitions include at the Slovak Institute, CEU Budapest, Hungary, Gallery NOVA, Gallery SPP, K-Gallery Bratislava. He has also received several awards including from the Small Sculpture Biennial in Poznan, Poland.

Photos: Courtesy of the artist

Art at the Dreescher Markt
WES & Partner Schatz, Betz, Kaschke, Wehberg-Krafft

Completion: 2005. **Technique:** glass fiber reinforced plastic. **Location:** Schwerin, Germany.

Pillows provide a sense of wellbeing, comfort and warmth, as well as healthy sleep. It is the form and the dimensions of the artwork that is unusual and unexpected. Pillows as over-sized, physical space, green, orange and striped give the area a new identity and produce a positive, cheerful atmosphere in simple surroundings. Embedded in a loose grove of small trees that indicate towards the light, air and sky. Wooden chairs invite the observer to sit, to read or to discuss. A positive place, newly defined.

The work of this company encompasses the architectural design of interior and exterior spaces. Along with projects in Germany and Europe, such as the Jungfernstieg in Hamburg. WES & Partner are also planning new projects in China and Arab regions. The jury of the international book "Made in Germany – Best of Contemporary Architecture" voted WES & Partner as the best landscape architecture firm in Germany, 2008.

Photos: Courtesy of the artist

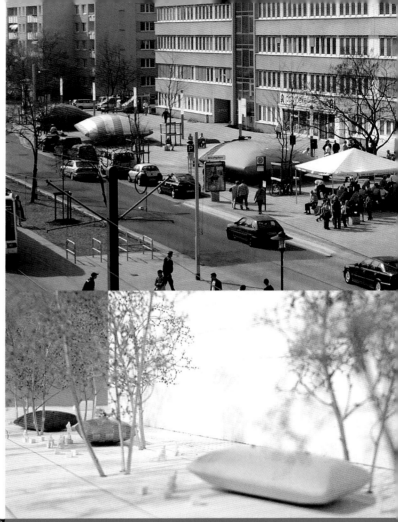

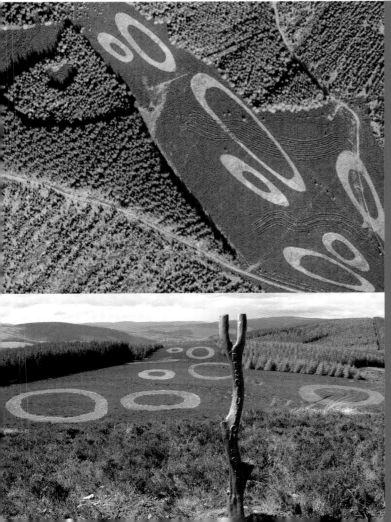

Point of Resolution
Charles Poulsen

Completion: 2005. **Technique:** heather. **Location:** Innerleithen, United Kingdom.

The lead covered branch in the foreground with the brass ring establishes a fixed viewing point – the "Point of Resolution". From this point, a series of what appear to be circles were cut in the heather. Once the viewer moves away from the resolution point it becomes apparent that what can be seen are not circles at all but huge, irregular, elongated ovals. Gradually the heather is growing back and the work will disappear. In 2011 the circles are still very visible.

Charles Poulsen has worked as a sculptor for 25 years. He has exhibited his work widely and been commissioned to produce both public and private pieces. In sculpture he works with lead and tree parts; casting, drilling, wrapping, excavating to reveal, deconstruct and rearrange. Several of his works of growing sculpture are displayed in public spaces. Poulsen uses trees, heather, bulbs, grass and found objects. Most of his installations are worked over years, while others are finished in one go.

Photos: Courtesy of the artist (a.); © The GeoInformation Group (b.)

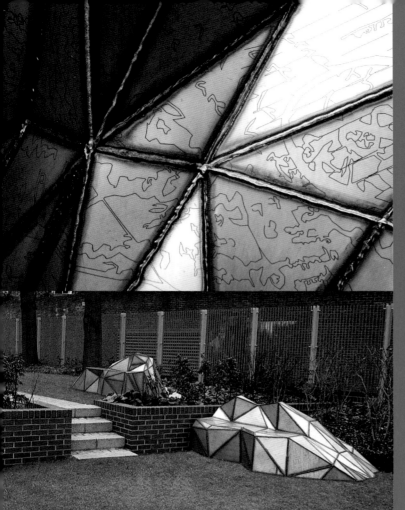

Regency Benches
Julian Mayor

Completion: 2005. **Technique:** stainless steel. **Location:** London, United Kingdom.

The form of this artwork was developed as a reaction to the site. A fluid series of volumes, which were inspired by their position near the water. The surfaces are made up of a complex series of planes that act as angled mirrors to ambient light, allowing the shapes to react to light conditions and the color and brightness of the sky. The artwork on the benches was created by students at the nearby Millbank Primary School as part of a series of workshops exploring the history of the area.

Julian Mayor is an artist and designer, based in East London. After graduating from the Royal College of Art in 2000 he worked in California as a designer for IDEO design. On returning to London in 2002 he worked for Pentagram and other design studios while starting to exhibit his own work. In 2005 he completed a series of sculptural benches for a park behind the Tate Britain Gallery in London and in 2007 a commission called "burnout" for a collector in East London.

Photos: Courtesy of the artist

Loop V
Sonja Edle von Hoeßle

Completion: 2005. **Technique:** oxidized and welded steel. **Location:** Würzburg, Germany.

This sculpture "Loop V" (Endlosschleife V) by Sonja Edle von Hoeßle is made out of steel, the surface of which has oxidized over time. The forms of the piece are exactly formulated and knowingly reminiscent of the form of geometric elements. The structure is shaped from both straight and curved sections, welded as infinite loops. Their appearance changes depending on the position of the viewer, sometimes a figure swings in an unstable position or rests on two steep peaks.

Sonja Edle von Hoeßle was born in Wiesbaden in 1960, she studied visual communication in Mainz and Würzburg. In 1996 she was awarded the Debutante Prize of the Bavarian State Ministry for Science, Research and Art. She was awarded the Cultural Award of the city of Würzburg in 2003.

Photo: Courtesy of the artist

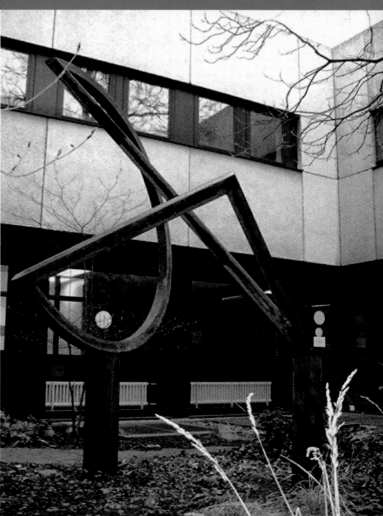

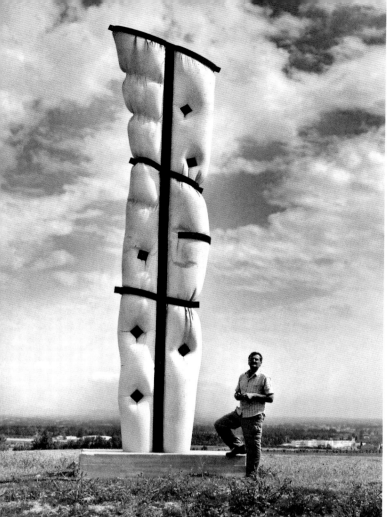

Libération
Felix Haspel

Completion: 2005. **Technique:** cast concrete, white cement, sandstone. **Location:** Tunis / Bou Argoup, Tunisia.

This sculpture was built in 2005 and dominates a hill on a Tunisian vineyard. "Libération" is widely visible and made of 38 tons of sandstone, concrete and steel, sculptured in a textile mold. Wrought iron bands encircle the sculpture. The constrained form represents a repressed people and the struggle for reform and new identity. The sculpture is in particular a monument to women, to the hope that the women of Africa may find a new identity and freedom.

Felix Haspel is a Viennese painter and sculptor, born in 1951. He graduated from the School of Applied Arts in Vienna and has been working as an artist since 1978. In 1993 he was appointed as professor at the Academy of Arts in Vienna. Haspel draws inspiration from the landscape, the effect of light on personal experience and recollection. He has been fascinated with the Maghreb and Sahara deserts since the 1980s and has spent a lot of time exploring the land and the myriad of cultures there.

Photo: Courtesy of the artist

The Echo of the Veluwe
Chris Booth

Completion: 2005. **Technique:** granite, secured with steel cable. **Location:** Otterlo, The Netherlands.

"The Echo of the Veluwe" is on display at the Kröller-Müller Museum sculpture garden in the Netherlands. The sculpture is formed from boulders of different kinds of granite, secured with steel cable. Veluwe is the Netherlands largest woodland and the sculpture draws inspiration from this place. The piece is site specific, resulting in the work truly reflecting and harmonizing with the surroundings. The artist set up a studio workshop on the site for two seasons while he completed the work.

Chris Booth is an acclaimed New Zealand sculptor, born in 1948. He studied at the School of Fine Arts in Canterbury before specializing in sculpture for two years. Booth's works are mostly made on commission and are usually monumental in form. Examples of his work can be found throughout New Zealand, Australia, Europe and North America. Booth is inspired by his religious relationship with the environment and fascinated by the prehistoric stones and other materials that can be found in nature.

Photo: Gerardus / Wikimedia Commons

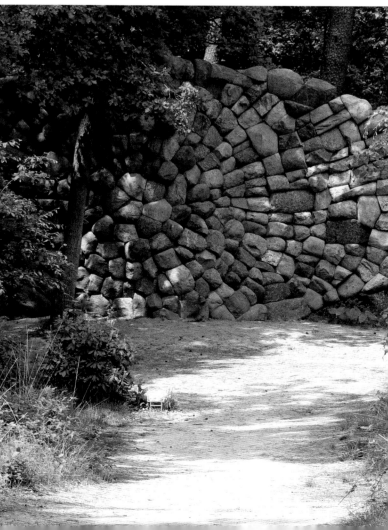

Stranger
Christopher Pöggeler

Completion: 2005. **Technique:** painted polyester. **Location:** Dusseldorf, Germany.

The "Stylit" project began in 2001 and involves sculptures of ordinary figures: a mother and child, two young lovers and a businessman, amongst others, are placed on the top of advertising pillars. The sculptures are known collectively as the "Sacred Pillars". The figures have been lifted from their everyday situation and placed on a 'pedestal' becoming visible as individuals. This sculpture of a woman carrying a small child is poignantly entitled, "Stranger".

Christopher Pöggeler was born in Münster in Germany in 1958. He studied at the Academy of Arts in Dusseldorf, graduating in 1985. In 1993 Pöggeler was awarded the city of Dusseldorf Art Award. He was appointed as a lecturer at the University of Wuppertal, in the architecture department, in 2001.

Photo: Andreas Praefcke / Wikimedia Commons

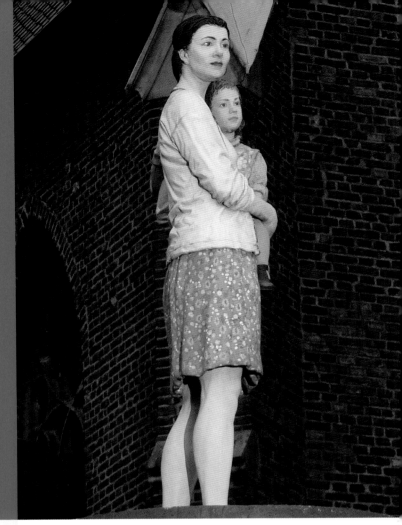

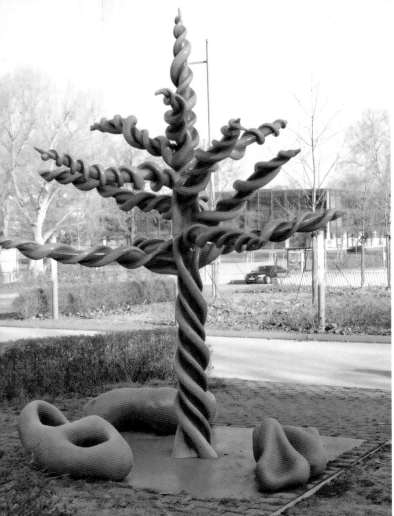

Red Tree
Mariella Mosler

Completion: 2005. **Technique:** painted steel. **Location:** Stuttgart, Germany.

This sculpture was constructed in 2005, near the footpath that reaches across the B14 road in Stuttgart. Through its soft and fluid form, it calls into memory the form of living trees, a nice touch in a place where growing a living tree is impractical. The red, glossy surface creates a contrast to the grey of the roads and the nearby greenery. The artist wanted to impel the hurrying pedestrians to stay for a moment, taking the time to really look at the work.

Mariella Mosler was born in Oldenburg in 1963. She studied art from 1985–1992 at the Art Academy in Hamburg, later going on to study philosophy. She is best known for her ornamental sand-reliefs, which always have a relationship to the space they inhabit. She participated in the tenth Documenta exhibition in 1997, which helped her achieve international recognition. She now works as a professor at the Academy of Art in Stuttgart.

Photo: Chris van Uffelen

Town Hall Square
Janet Rosenberg + Associates with Jean Pierre Morin

Completion: 2005. **Technique:** Ginko trees, concrete, boxwood, aluminum, Corten steel. **Location:** Toronto, Canada.

"Town Hall Square" is an elegant outdoor space in Yorkville, Toronto. The design of the park is a contemporary take on a French parterre, featuring bold geometrical shapes and patterns. Rows of Gingko trees in concrete disks and custom-finished pots are accented by a sculptural piece that anchors the site. The piece, by Canadian artist Jean Pierre Morin, is called "Piercing a Cloud". It is a majestic Corten and aluminum work that bears resemblance to the trees that surround it.

Janet Rosenberg + Associates / JRA is an award winning landscape architecture and urban design practice, based in Toronto. JRA is one of Canada's most distinguished design firms, recognized globally for innovative and precedent-setting landscapes. Jean Pierre Morin, born in 1951, is a Canadian sculptor and has a Bachelors degree in visual arts from the Quebec University and a masters in sculptor from the University of Montreal.

Photos: Janet Rosenberg + Associates, Toronto

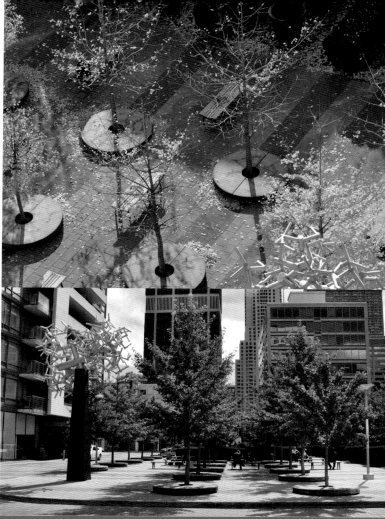

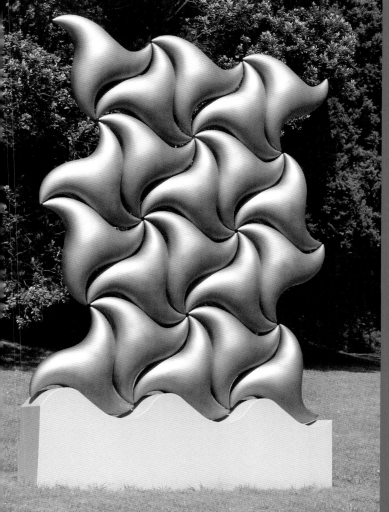

Numbers are the Language of Nature
Chiara Corbelletto

Completion: 2005. **Technique:** bronze. **Location:** Auckland, New Zealand.

This sculpture is situated in the Auckland Domain, New Zealand. It was created as part of a project initiated by Sculpture Outdoor, with support from the New Zealand Lottery Grant board. The work is an interconnected composition of repeated elements. The fluidity of these shapes works to remind the viewer of the underlying geometry of all living organisms and the symmetry of cellular forms. The fluidity of the interlocking lines stops the observer from finding one focal point where the eye can rest.

Chiara Corbelletto was born in Italy. She graduated from Modigliani Art School in Novara and subsequently graduated from the University of Milan. Corbelletto is an established artist who has extensively exhibited her work. She has various sculptural installations in public space and private collections. The central theme in Corbelletto's work is perception of space, demarcation and enclosure, space as interior and space as infinity. She currently lives and works in New Zealand.

Photo: Gadfium / Wikimedia Commons

I see what you mean
Lawrence Argent

Completion: 2005. **Technique:** composite materials, steel. **Location:** Denver, CO, USA.

This faceted bear appears as if it is pushing its nose and paws against the glass of the building attempting to peer inside the convention center to see what is happening. Both from afar and close-up, curiosity and fascination are instilled in the viewer. In light of this humorous, lighthearted play there lies perhaps an essence that reflects nature, upsetting the balance of the viewer and the viewed. The facets, plain to see on the sculpture's surface, were created from the reduction of digital data.

Lawrence Argent was born in England and trained in sculpture at the Royal Melbourne Institute of Technology. He also has an master of fine arts from the Rinehart School of Sculpture at the College of Art in Baltimore. Currently, he is professor and head of the sculpture program at the University of Denver. He is the recipient of numerous fellowships. Argent is known for his multi-media sculptures and indoor and outdoor installations. His often abstract, conceptual works strive to encourage contemplation, creating a presence that can illuminate and stimulate.

Photo: Courtesy of the artist

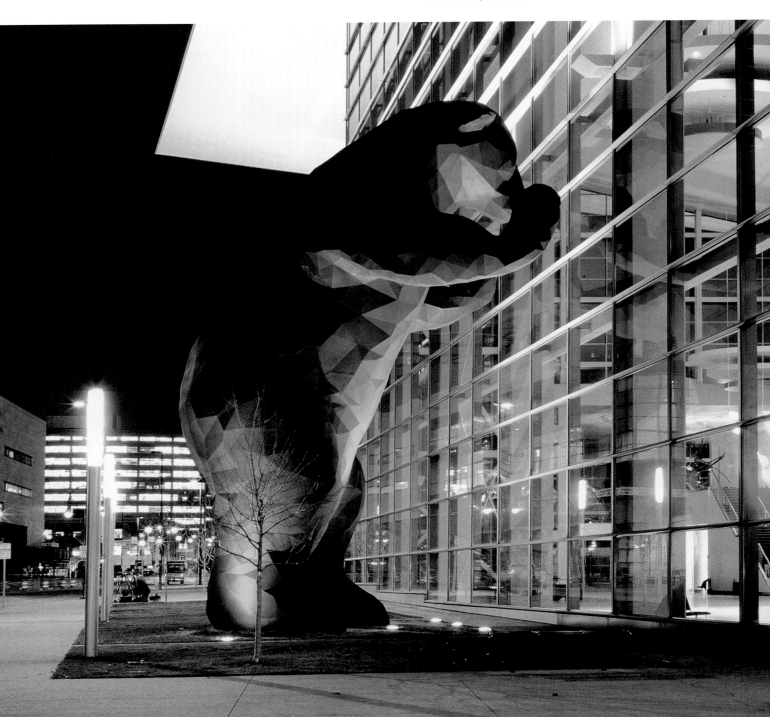

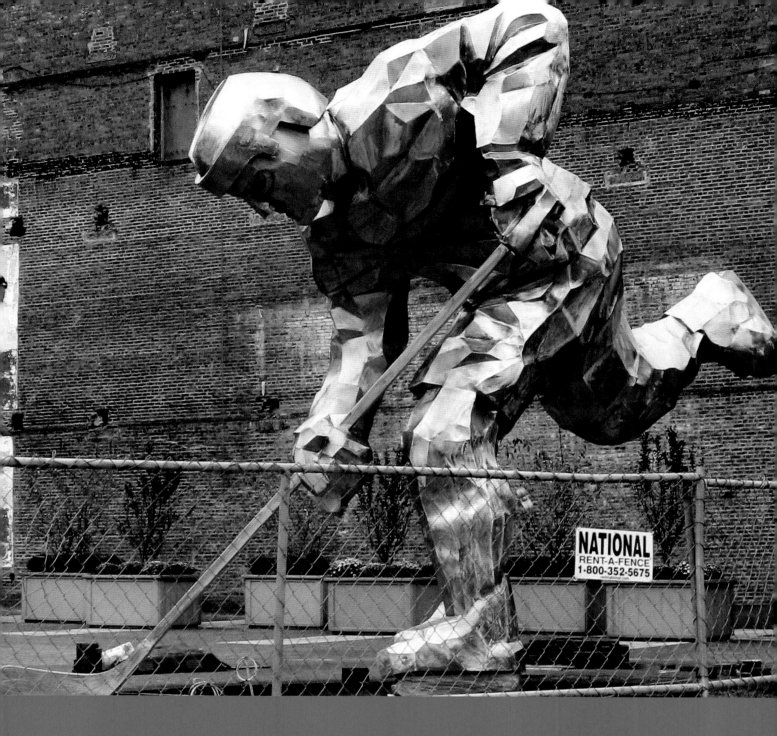

Photos: Susan Kane

Devils Sculpture
Jon Krawczyk

Completion: 2006. **Technique:** steel. **Location:** Newark, NJ, USA.

This sculpture of a hockey player is nearly seven meters tall. It is located near a new hockey arena in New Jersey and is a tribute to the Devils hockey team. The statue's faceted exterior is designed to resemble blocks of ice as they break into pieces. The many surfaces of the sculpture reflect and disperse the sunlight, giving it a moving appearance. A hockey puck, a cap and a Scott Steven's jersey have been sealed inside the sculpture to bring luck.

Jon Krawczyk is a modernist sculptor, whose sculptures investigate the human condition. He graduated from Connecticut College in 1992 and has studied fine art in various locations throughout Europe. He works mainly with bronze and steel, transforming the heavy material into dynamic sculptural works. He has been commissioned to produce over 20 works of art for various institutions and has exhibited his work across America.

Narcissus Field
Anette Merkenthaler

Completion: 2006. **Technique:** printed photographs, trees. **Location:** Freiburg, Germany.

"Narcissus Field" keeps the Narcissus flower alive all year round, so that that first feelings of spring can be experienced whatever the weather. The piece is comprised of printed photographs, pinned high in the trees of the Urachstraße in Freiburg. The work plays with expectations, bringing a feeling of spring to every season. The work also strives to demonstrate how technology and human processes can compliment nature.

Annette Merkenthaler was born in Bayrischzell in Germany in 1944. She first completed training as a ceramicist and then studied for one year at the School of Decorative Arts in Geneva. She later opened her own studio, still working with ceramics from time to time. Her first large commissioned work was "Blue Mountains"; various other commissions have followed this. Her work often involves nature and natural processes.

Photo: Chris van Uffelen

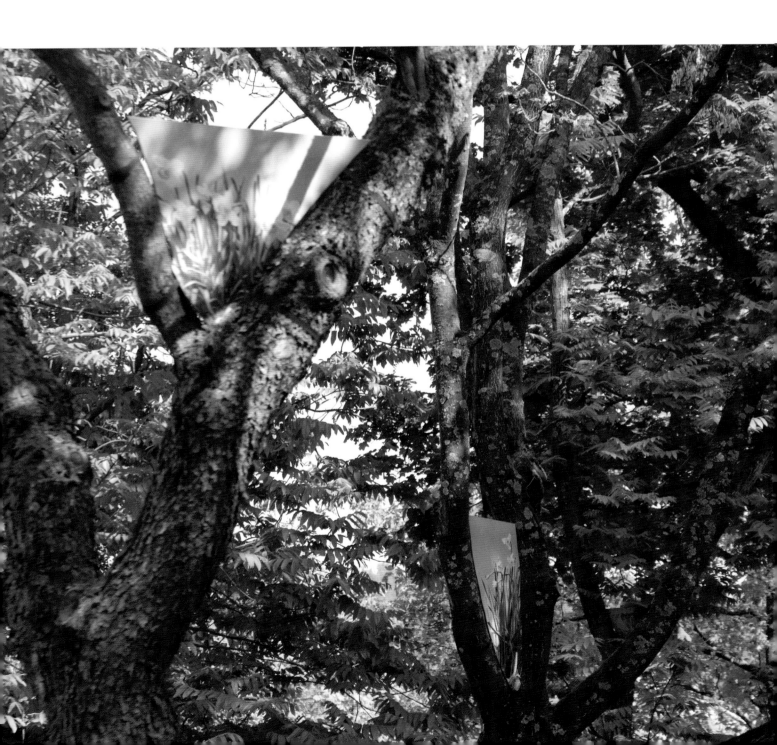

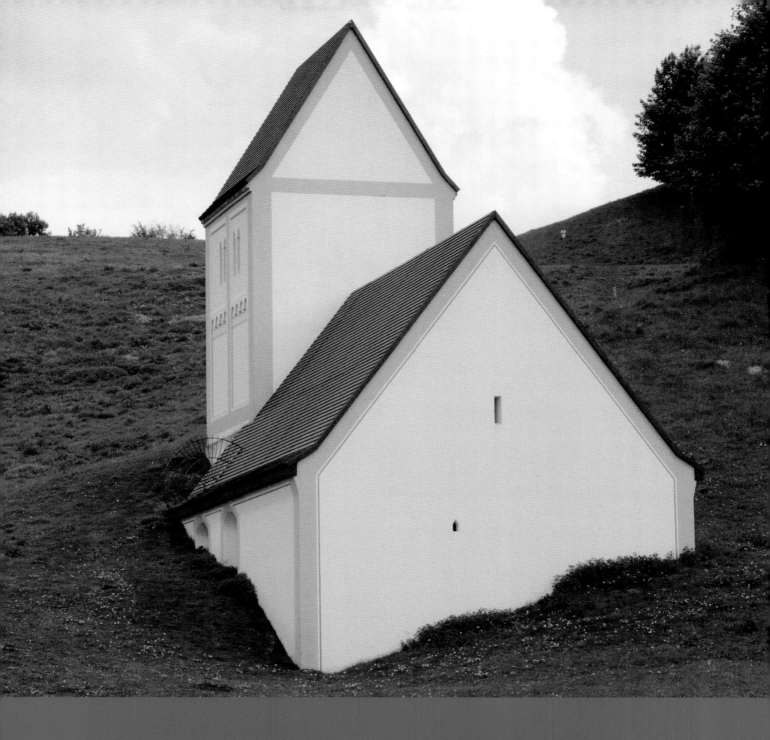

Sunken Village
Timm Ulrichs

Completion: 2006. **Technique:** concrete, silicate and emulsion paint. **Location:** Munich, Germany.

This sculpture is identical on the outside to the nearby Holy Cross Church, a small village church from the middle ages. This duplicate highlights what could have happened if the original had been left where it first stood. The sculpture is half-buried in a rubbish tip, laid over with greenery. The village of Fröttmaning, which once stood here, was sacrificed to make room for a huge rubbish tip. Only the church was moved to a new location. This sculpture highlights the dangers of modern culture and the cost of progress.

Timm Ulrichs is a German artist, born in Berlin in 1940. He first began training as an architect but quit his studies before graduating. He has been working as an artist since 1959. He was appointed as guest professor at the State University of Art in Brunswick, a position he held for one year, before being appointed as professor of sculpture and total art at the State Art Academy in Münster. He has exhibited his work widely both in Germany and internationally.

Photo: Chris van Uffelen

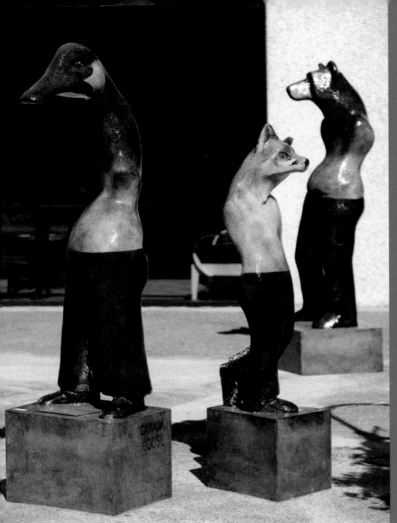

Photo: Kevin Smith

Wilderness, Wildlands and People: A Partnership for the Public
Rachelle Dowdy

Completion: 2006. **Technique:** ferro-concrete, oil based paints, sealers. **Location:** Anchorage, AK, USA.

Rachelle Dowdy's work focuses primarily on sculptures of birds and animal-human hybrids. She combines organic and industrial technique to address issues of modern life in America, often putting a spin on popular Alaskan wildlife and motifs. The Wild Foundation commissioned these four sculptures, to commemorate the eighth World Wilderness Congress, held Alaska in 2006.

Rachelle Dowdy has exhibited her work throughout the state of Alaska and taken part in a solo exhibition at the Anchorage museum. Her work is held in many public collections, including the Anchorage museum, University of Alaska's Museum of the North, and Alaska's Percent-for-Art program. Dowdy was a recipient of a Rasmuson Foundation Fellowship and was a Marie Walsh Sharpe Art foundation Summer Seminar scholar.

Allerton Mandalas
Michele Brody

Completion: 2006. **Technique:** faceted glass. **Location:** New York City, NY, USA.

The faceted glass installation, "Allerton Mandalas", is based on the MTA subway map. The word mandala is taken from Sanskrit, loosely translated it means circle. From up close, or afar, each mandala is meant to at first dazzle the viewer with color and light, then upon closer inspection, reveal a central structure inspired by the mark of subway lines themselves. Fabricated into 20 panels that are installed on the subway platform, they can be viewed from inside as well as outside the station.

Born in Brooklyn in 1967, Michele Brody received her bachelor of arts degree from Sarah Lawrence College in 1989 and a master of fine arts from the School of the Art Institute of Chicago in 1994. Utilizing her strong background in the liberal arts, she creates site-specific, mixed media installations and works of public art that are generated by the history, culture, environment, and architecture of a wide range of exhibition spaces. Brody has exhibited artwork in America, South America and Europe.

Photos: Courtesy of the artist

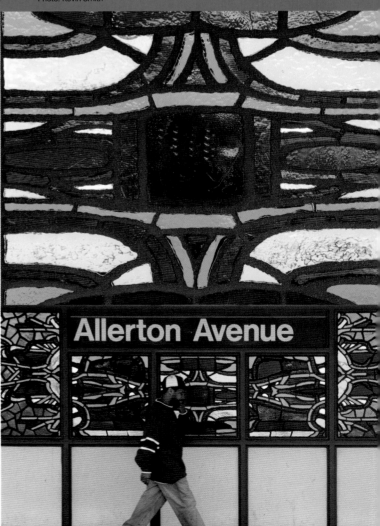

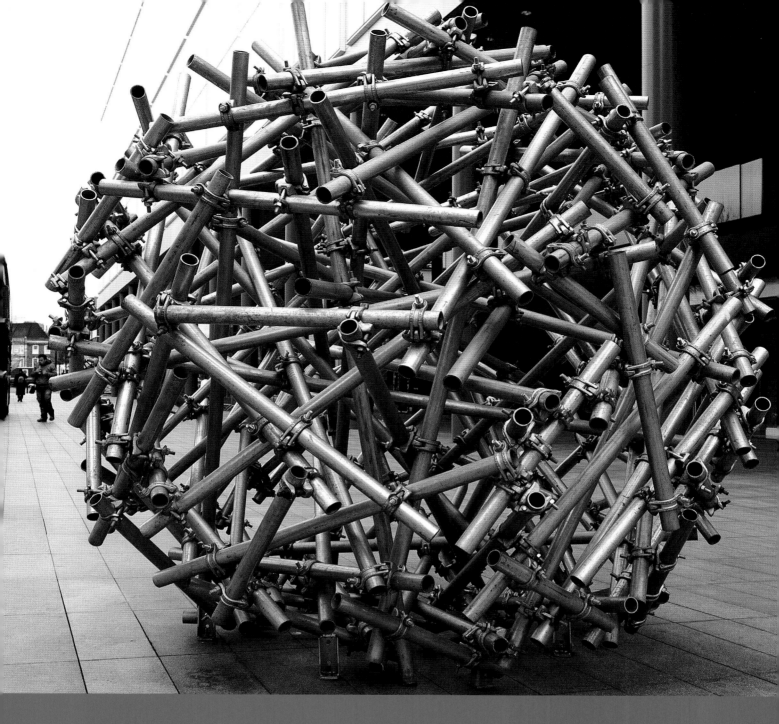

System no. 18
Julian Wild

Completion: 2006. **Technique:** galvanised steel scaffolding. **Location:** London, United Kingdom.

"System no. 18" is part of a sequential series of works. The word "System" implies a method and a sense of prevailing order. The sculpture is constructed from a configuration of random lines that have accumulated into the form of a sphere. Within the context of the re-development of Spitalfields, "System no. 18" acts as a remnant of the areas' intense building activity. The artist was interested in creating something permanent with a construction material that is normally temporary.

Julian Wild graduated from Kingston University in 1995 and is the current recipient of the Royal Borough of Kensington and Chelsea Trust Studio Bursary. Wild's work explores the use of functional materials and how just a single line or series of units can hold countless expressive possibilities. Wild has recently been commissioned to create public works for the Cass Sculpture Foundation and Radley College Oxford, amongst others. In 2005 he was shortlisted for the Jerwood Sculpture prize.

Photo: Noah Da Costa

House, House – Open Work
Werner Pokorny

Completion: 2006. **Technique:** Corten steel. **Location:** Busan, South Korea.

The Busan Biennial in 2006 in South Korea resulted in the creation of this steel sculpture: "House, House – open work". This work belongs to a group of steel sculptures, which deal with houses as an ambivalent metaphor. The work can be read as a standing, dynamic form but also noticeable is the other perspective, that of a form plunging towards the ground. Nothing is clear or simple, the meaning open to interpretation. .

Werner Pokorny was born in Mosbach, Germany. He studied at the State Academy of Art in Karlsruhe from 1971–1974, and later studied art history at Karlsruhe University. In 1988 he was awarded the Villa Romana scholarship in Florence, Italy. He worked as visiting professor at the State Academy of Art in Karlsruhe and was then later employed as professor of art at the State Academy of Art and Design, in Stuttgart. Since 1977, Pokorny had displayed his work in both solo and group exhibitions across Europe.

Photo: Kestas Svirnelis, Stuttgart

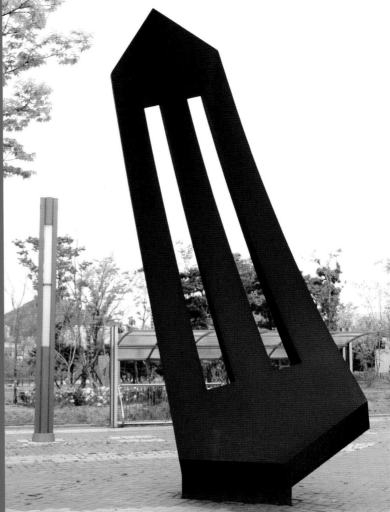

DeutzTwins
Rainer Gross

Completion: 2006. **Technique:** finely polished concrete. **Location:** Cologne, Germany.

This work is a slim construction, approximately ten meters high, made of finely sanded concrete. The side facing the Cologne Triangle shows a classical motif of the artist, a picture of the twins. In contrast to his paintings, the artist has not, however, placed the "DeutzTwins" images mirrored next to each other, but set at an angle of 90 degrees. The horizontal half of the picture serves as the base of the water basin. The vertical twin appears in contrast as a "fixed-image" over which a water spray runs.

Rainer Gross is a German artist and sculptor, born in Cologne in 1951. He moved to the USA in 1973, at which time he worked with Howard Kanovitz and later with Larry Rivers. Gross produces both painted artwork and sculpture. Much of his artwork interprets American society with allegorical and classical allusions. He is also a keen art historian, he believes in re-working old traditions and learning from past masters.

Photo: Jens Willebrand

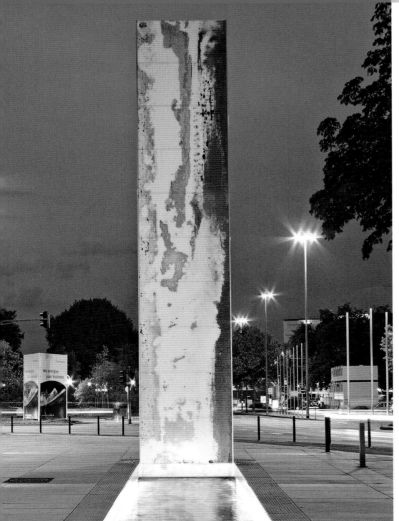

Lines of Communication
Paula Craft, John Pegg

Completion: 2006. **Technique:** concrete, steel. **Location:** London, United Kingdom.

The "Lines of Communication" for the Spitalfields Public Art project has opened up to the community an almost forgotten episode of London's 17th century history. The proposal envisaged reinterpreting and making an 18th century paper plan as a three dimensional piece, ghosted with the present day road network of the city. The process of drawing and analyzing the historic development of London has led to a rediscovery of relationships between the lost fortification "trace" and the current city.

Paula Craft and John Pegg formed craft:pegg to pursue their desire to create unique, site specific designs, revealing the culture and history of place. John Pegg trained in geology and geography at Nottingham University and holds a masters in landscape architecture from Harvard University. Paula Craft studied architecture at the University of Florida and Harvard University. Her work explores the creative interpretation of cultural heritage. Aitor Albo and Julia Putsep were also a key part of the design team.

Photo: Courtesy of the artist

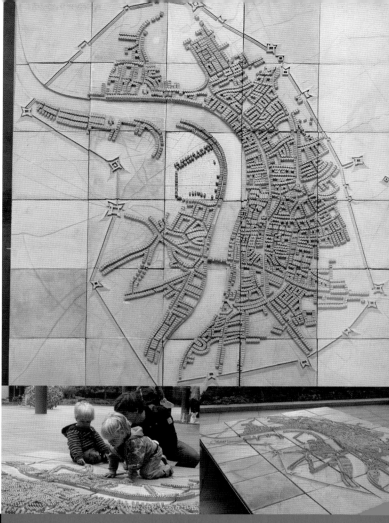

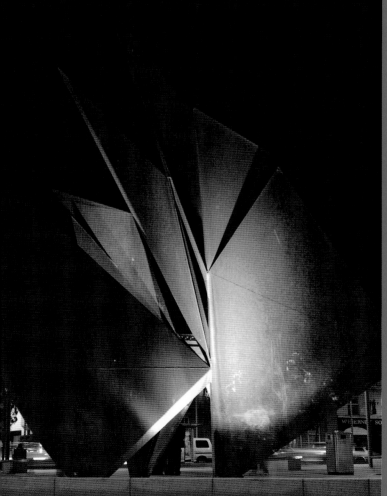

Galway Hooker
Eamonn O'Doherty

Completion: 2006. **Technique:** steel plates. **Location:** Galway, Ireland.

The "Galway Hooker", stands in the center of a large water feature in the center of Eyre Square, Galway. The square was renovated by architects, Mitchell and Associates and is a main feature of the city. Despite its suggestive name, this sculpture pays homage to a traditional type of sailing boat, the "Galway Hooker". These have long been used as a symbol for the county of Galway, this sculpture immortalizes their distinctive sail shape and seeks to honor Irish tradition.

Irish sculptor Eamonn O'Doherty was born in Derry and is one of Ireland's best known living artists. He graduated from University College Dublin with a degree in architecture and was awarded a visiting scholarship to Harvard University. O'Doherty has created many of Ireland's late 20th century public sculptures. His best known sculptural works include "Fauscailt", County Wexford, "Crann an Oir", Dublin, and the "Galway Hookers", Eyre Square. He has worked in bronze, stone and various other media.

Photo: Mitchell + Associates. Dublin

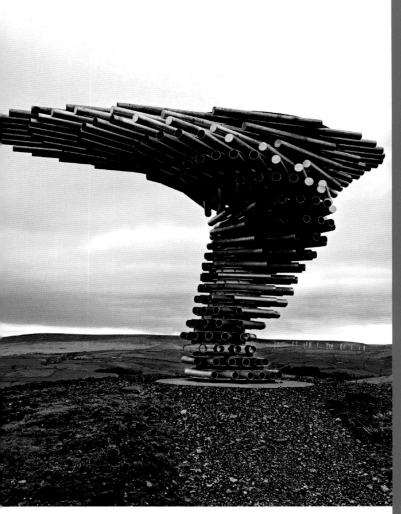

Singing Ringing Tree
Tonkin Liu

Completion: 2006. **Technique:** stacked mild steel. **Location:** Burnley, United Kingdom.

The "Singing Ringing Tree" is a musical sculpture in the landscape, constructed of stacked mild steel pipes of varying lengths, which sits on the top of a hill above Burnley. It is part of the Panopticons project, an initiative set up to explore the value of art's role in regeneration. Encouraging both locals and visitors to explore the beautiful Lancashire countryside, "Singing Ringing Tree" takes the form of a tree, bending to the winds and harnesses the energy of those winds to produce a low, tuneful song.

Tonkin Liu was founded in 2001 by Mike Tonkin and Anna Liu, who developed their practice whilst co-teaching at the Architectural Association. Their book, "Asking Looking Playing Making", published in 1999, sets out their design approach which is based on story telling, space, time and change. Projects – which range from private houses to public spaces – sit at the interface of art and architecture and are characterized by an approach which is both beautifully puritanical and seductively fanciful.

Photo: John Lyons

Circulation – Neagarimatsu
Kenji Kobayashi

Completion: 2006. **Technique:** granite stone. **Location:** Kobe, Japan.

This artwork was installed as a symbol of the reclamation project, which aimed to re-grow the landscape of the past, reinstalling the old pine trees of the area. The project also aims to provide a community space, where people can meet and spend time together. The artwork symbolizes eternity and natural circulation, the pieces of the sculpture harmonizing with the surrounding natural landscape and the wind and waves of the nearby ocean.

Kenji Kobayashi is a Japanese sculptor and architect. Born in Nagano, Japan in 1964, he studied architecture and graduated from Meiji University in 1986. In 1989, he graduated in space design from Kuwasawa Design School, later joining Kenmochi Design Associates & En Environmental Planning and Design Institute. He established Kobayashi Kenji Atelier in 1993. Kobayashi works to create garden space and art pieces with natural materials like soil, stone, water and plants.

Photos: Forward Stroke Inc./ Tokyo, Japan

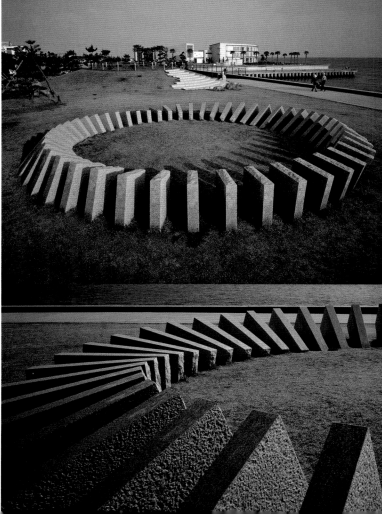

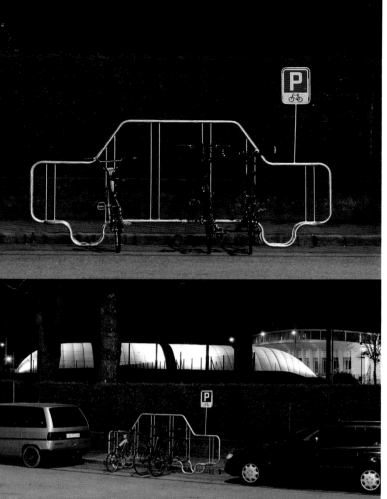

VD 003
Adrien Rovero

Completion: 2006. **Technique:** galvanised steel. **Location:** Lausanne, Switzerland.

This bike rack highlights the environmental advantages of bike riding versus car driving. It is made of metal, shaped into the simple outline of a car. The rack is the same size as one car, and in the space six bikes can be parked. The space-saving advantages of riding a bike are made obvious by this work.

Adrien Rovero was born in Switzerland in 1981. He received his masters in industrial design in 2006 from the Art Academy of Lausanne, where he now teaches. Rovero has exhibited his work widely in galleries across Europe. His work is based on an precise observation of elementary needs, where everything is an excuse for speculation. He brings together the commonplace and the extraordinary, creating unexpected solutions that are both simple and relevant.

Photos: Yann Gross & Emilie Müller

The Sum of Us
Marco Cianfanelli

Completion: 2006. **Technique:** metal. **Location:** Mogale City, South Africa

This sculpture is part of the landscape design by GreenInc. It is located at the Forum Homini boutique hotel, near the Sterkfontein Caves, outside Johannesburg. Palaeo-anthropological sites situated in the area have produced the remains of hominids dating as far back as 3.3 million years. The sculpture shows the evolution from the early ancestral skull shape into that of modern man. It states that our history, and our pre-history, is still part of us and highlights our unconscious developmental achievement.

The artist Marco Cianfanelli was born in 1970 in Johannesburg. In 1992 he graduated, with a distinction in fine art, from the University of the Witwatersrand and has special interest in computer aided design, this is portrayed in his work. He deals with new techniques and their specific looks (like pixalization) but the results never appear machine made: the result is a specific and unique piece.

Photo: GREENinc

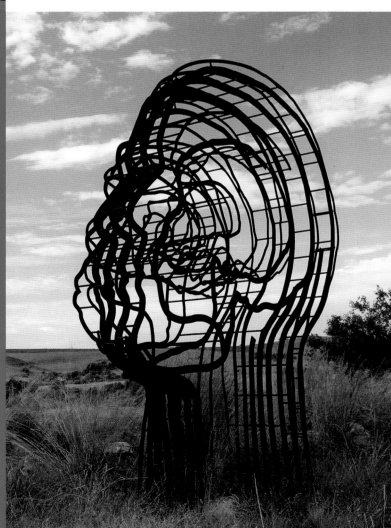

Sheepfolds
Andy Goldsworthy

Completion: 2006. **Technique:** stone. **Location:** Cumbria, United Kingdom.

"Sheep Fold" is a typical example of Andy Goldsworthy's Land Art installations. The piece aims to work with rather than against the environment. Goldsworthy has created various sheepfolds around the Lake District in the United Kingdom, he uses old sheepfolds, in varying states of disrepair, sometimes reviving old folds that have disappeared altogether but were still marked on old maps. In this way he invigorated them with new energy, incorporating his sculptural works into the designs.

Andy Goldsworthy is a British Environmental Artist. He produces site specific installations in both natural and urban settings. He was born in 1956 and worked as a farm laborer from the age of 13 until he moved to Bradford to study fine art at the Bradford College of Art, graduating in 1975. Goldsworthy's work often involves brightly colored flowers as well as mud, twigs, pinecones, snow and stone. He often works with just his bare hands, teeth and found materials as tools.

Photos: SideLong / Wikimedia Commons

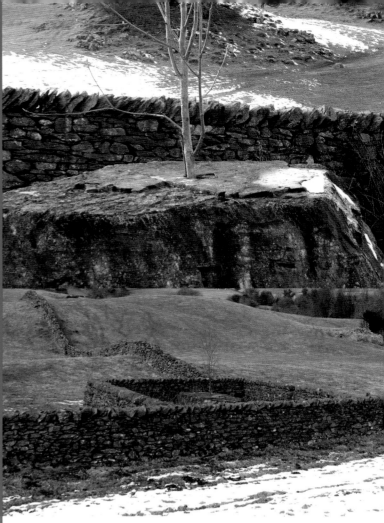

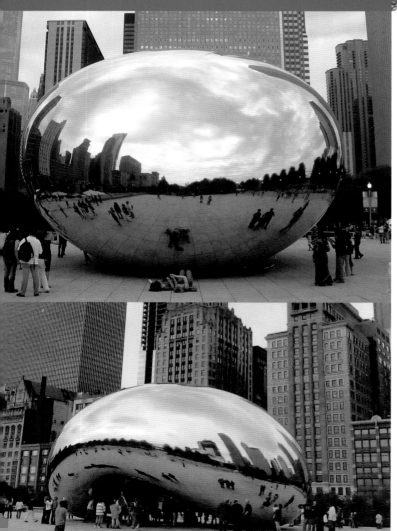

Cloud Gate
Anish Kapoor

Completion: 2006. **Technique:** stainless steel. **Location:** Chicago, IL, USA.

"Cloud Gate" is a public sculpture at the center of the AT&T Plaza in Millennium Park, Chicago. It is comprised of 168 stainless steel plates, welded together and then highly polished so that no seams are visible. The design was inspired by liquid mercury and the shape of the sculpture results in a distorted reflection of the city's skyline. Visitors can walk around and underneath the sculpture; every surface reflects the surroundings.

Anish Kapoor is an Indian sculptor, born in Mumbai in 1954. Kapoor moved to London in the early 1970s to study art and has lived there ever since. He exhibits his work internationally and his pieces are often simple, curved forms that vary in size. His work "Taratantara" is 35 meters high and installed in the Baltic Flour Mills in Gateshead. Many of his works involve reflecting surfaces and explore distortion and how a curved surface can warp a reflection so that it is almost unrecognizable.

Photos: Jens Rogotzki

Untitled
Jenny Holzer

Completion: 2006. **Technique:** neon, glass, white plastic.
Location: New York City, NY, USA.

Jenny Holzer's light installation is inside the lobby of the 7 World Trade Center in New York, though the tall, brightly lit letters can be clearly seen and read from the street. The unusually tall letters march across a wall of glass behind the security desk, the writings come from a range of different sources including E. B. White's classic book 'Here Is New York' in its entirety, a poem by Allen Ginsberg, and David Lehman's reconsideration of the World Trade Center after the first attack in 1993.

Jenny Holzer was born in Ohio in 1950 and is an American Conceptual Artist. She studied at Ohio University and the Rhode Island School of Design as well as attending the Independent Study Program at the Whitney Museum of American Art. Her work focuses mainly on the use of words and ideas, displaying them in different ways in public space. She incorporates a range of media in her work, using bronze plaques, stone benches, painted signs, sound, video and light.

Photos: Dogears / Wikimedia Commons

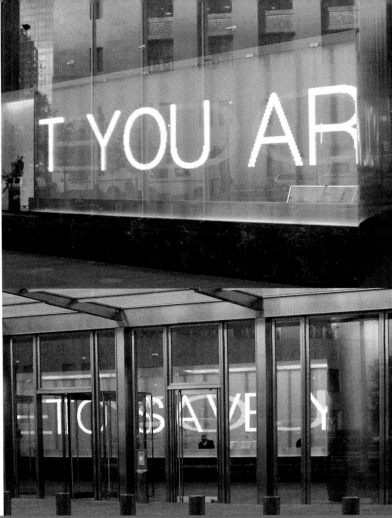

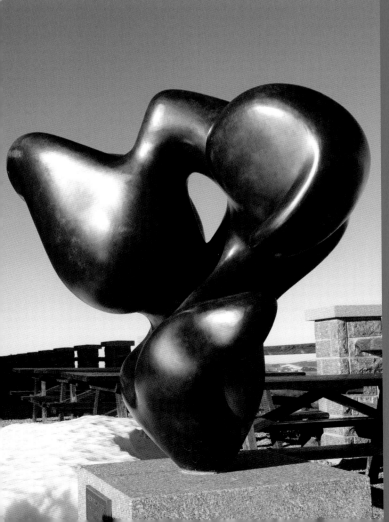

Rendez-vous
Maritta Winter

Completion: 2006. **Technique:** bronze. **Location:** Grand Ballon, Alsace, France.

This abstract, sensual form manages to be simultaneously earthy and floating at the same time. Tight lines express the power and stability of the land. The rotundity of the sculpture is reminiscent of the hilly forms of the Vosges Mountains, the nursing mother and female silkiness. Implanted on the top of the highest mountain of the Alsace, this sculpture radiates beyond the frontiers of Germany, France and Switzerland.

Born in the south-west corner of Germany in 1961, now residing in Switzerland and France, artist Maritta Winter has created a moving, powerful and timeless body of work. After attending art school in Strasbourg, she completed various figure drawing and portrait classes, as well as training in sculpting and photography. One of her biggest influences is dance, for her like an ever-present companion and a vital experience in reference to her perception of space and sensuality.

Photo: Courtesy of the artist

235

Guards of Time
Manfred Kielnhofer

Completion: 2007. **Technique:** polyester, resin. **Location:** Linz, Austria.

"Guards of Time" relates to the idea that since the beginning of time mankind has had protectors, both for historic and mystical reasons. It seems that only man himself is a potential source of danger for his own existence. In his works of art Manfred Kielnhofer deals with the natural human desire for security. Thus his oeuvre reflects genuine exploration, consideration and discussion of current as well as historic moods and sensibilities of his social environment. His works of art captivate with elaborate combinations of light and different technique.

Manfred Kielnhofer was born in Haslach an der Mühl, Austria. He is self-taught and works with many different mediums; including, painting, film, photography, installation, performance and sculpture. His work usually concerns the human figure and its different forms and movements, focusing mainly on the peculiarities of human nature. He uses the human form as a tool, either on a canvas or in a sculpture.

Photos: Courtesy of the artist

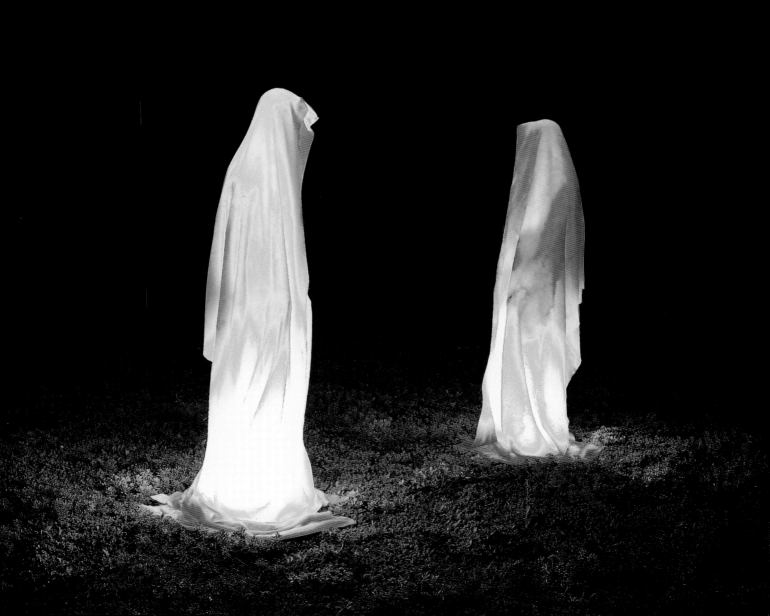

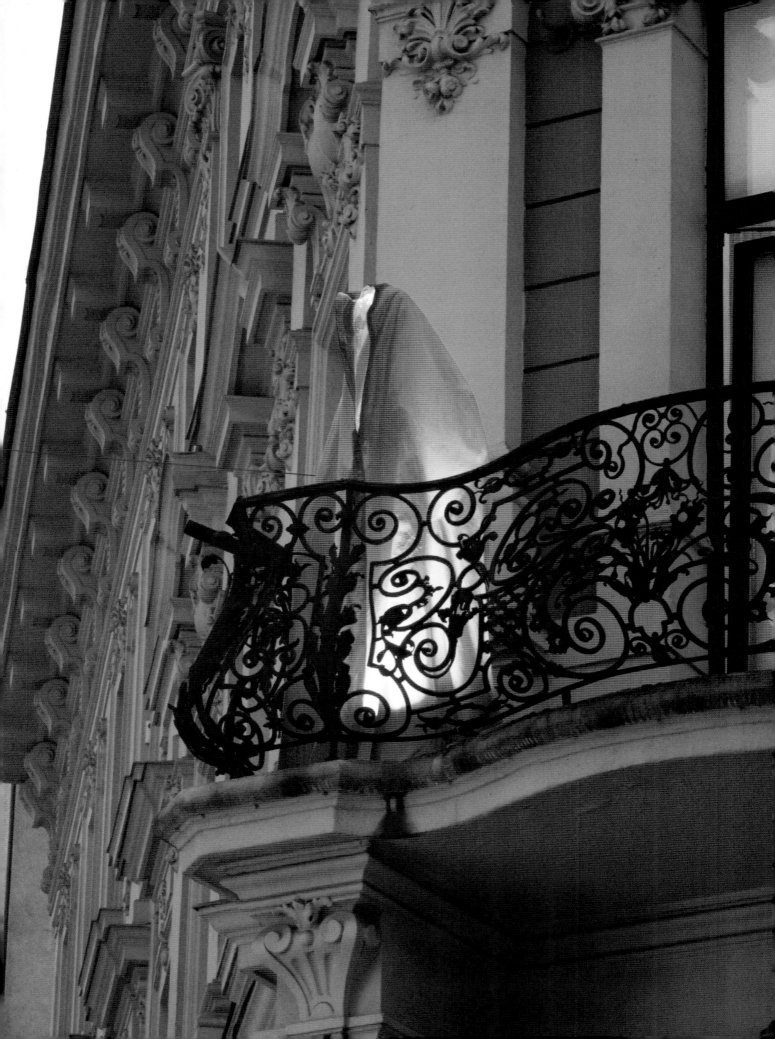

Arresting Prostitute
Gao Brothers

Completion: 2007. **Technique:** painted bronze. **Location:** Beijing, China.

"Arresting Prostitute" is a life-size piece, based on a photograph widely circulated on the Internet of police physically removing a streetwalker during an official clampdown on prostitution. For many Chinese, among them the Gao Brothers, this image represented an affront against personal freedom as well as a poignant symbol of the brutal insensitivity of an authoritarian regime. The physical rendering of the original news image challenges both the society's indifference and the authorities' casual disregard for human dignity.

The Gao Brothers are Gao Zhen, born in Jinan in 1956 and Gao Qiang, born in Jinan in 1962. They are based in Beijing and have been collaborating on installation, performance, sculpture, photography works and writing since the mid 1980s. Their artistic output has gained international recognition and they are represented in major public and private collections including those of the Pompidou Center, the China National Art Museum, the San Francisco Museum of Modern Art and the Saatchi, Steven Cohen and Sigg collections.

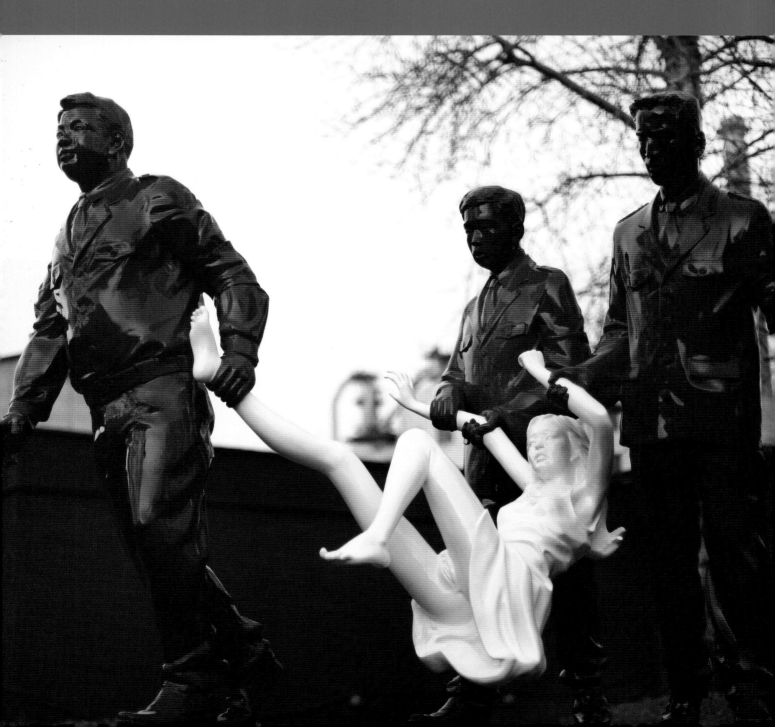

Gum
Stefan Sous and Heinke Haberland

Completion: 2007. **Technique:** marble. **Location:** Freiburg, Germany.

"Gum" is a sculptural work comprising of two marble sculptures. These are formed to represent two lumps of spat out chewing gum, their smooth indentations showing the indentations of teeth and tongue. They lie on a patch of grass outside the teeth and mouth clinic in Freiburg and function as a reminder that chewing gum is good for the teeth and mouth. A "chew meeting" was held and various people, including the artist, were invited to chew gum so that two pieces might be found, on which the sculptures could be modeled.

Stefan Sous is a German sculptor, born in Aachen in 1964. His sculptures often focus on everyday objects like chewing gum or a hand mixer. Sous takes objects apart and analyses them, remodeling them in an unexpected way. He attempts to make the hidden, visible in his work, re-introducing mechanics to the age of technology. Heinke Haberland was born in 1966 in Kiel. He studied art and graphics at the Muthesius School in Kiel and has worked in collaboration with Stefan Sous on various public art projects.

Photo: Chris van Uffelen

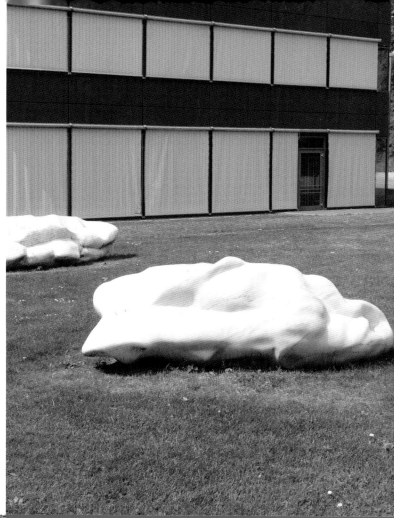

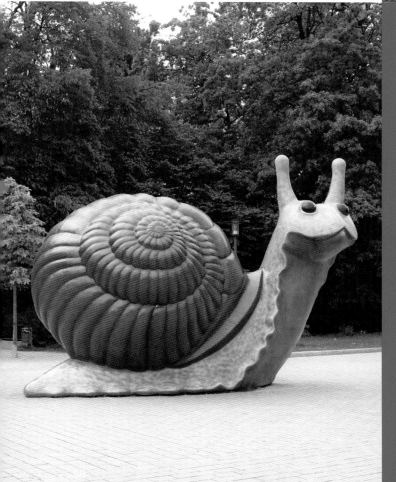

Sweet Brown Snail
Jason Rhoades with Paul McCarthy

Completion: 2007. **Technique:** painted fiberglass. **Location:** Munich, Germany.

This snail sculpture is made of painted fiberglass and stands in front of the Transport Center at the German Museum in Munich. The artist was asked to design a sculpture based on the theme of global speed. Rhoades' humorous response to this demand was to create a sculpture of the creature most often associated with the word "slow". The snail clearly has an ironic association with the transportation section of the museum and is typical of the artist's whimsical, humorous style.

Jason Rhoades was a critically acclaimed Installation Artist, considered by some to be one of the most important artists of his generation. Rhoades received his masters in fine arts from University of California, Los Angeles in 1993. His work has been exhibited internationally, including at the Whitney Biennial exhibition in 1997 and multiple galleries and museums across Europe. Paul McCarthy is a contemporary American artist, he is famous for producing Experimental Art, using his body as a paintbrush or canvas.

Photo: Chris van Uffelen

Childhood Dreams
Patrick Dougherty

Completion: 2007. **Technique:** bending tree branches and saplings. **Location:** Phoenix, AZ, USA.

While planning this work, the artist became fascinated by the shape of the barrel cactus, growing near his site at the Desert Botanical Garden in Phoenix. This work is based around the shape of that plant and the finished sculpture, entitled "Childhood Dreams", provides the visitor with a shaded interior space and a variety of desert views through its portals. The artist strives to achieve a natural look, allowing his works to slide effortlessly into the surrounding landscape.

Patrick Dougherty grew up in North Carolina. As an adult, he combined his carpentry skills with his love of nature and began to learn about primitive techniques of building and to experiment with tree saplings as construction material. In 1980 he began with small works, quickly progressing from single pieces on conventional pedestals, to monumental, site specific installations that require sticks by the truckload. To date he has built over 200 of these massive sculptures all over the world.

Photos: Adam Rodriguez

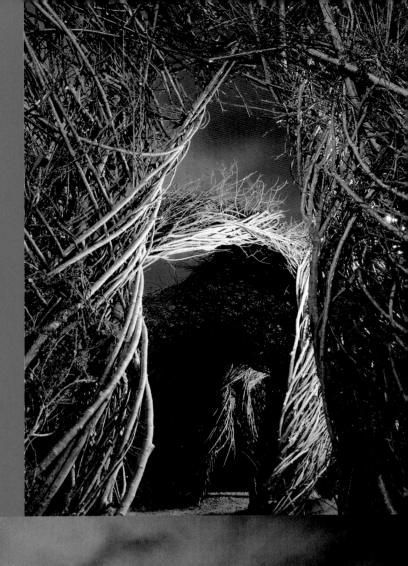

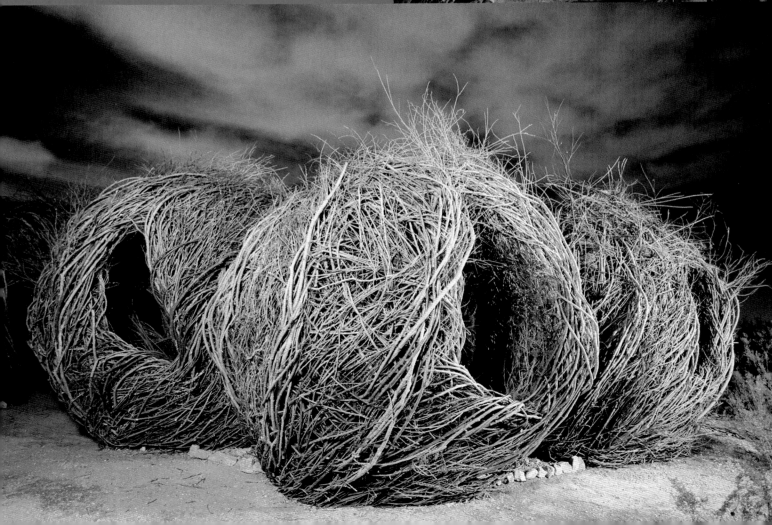

SEART Park, Sylvia Park
Isthmus Group Ltd.

Completion: 2007. **Technique:** fiberglass, steel. **Location:** Auckland, New Zealand.

This artwork is located on the underside of a motorway overpass that bisects the Sylvia Park retail center. The work was designed to enliven the space by day and night. The main design elements are simple vertical steel poles, painted with vibrant colors to bring life and excitement into the gray space. The poles are situated randomly, with rhythmic changes in height and color, and are combined with organic seats that contrast with the vertical structures.

Isthmus is a New Zealand-based design practice that works in collaboration with other professionals including architects, engineers, planners and artists to design and implement innovative public space projects. At the heart of Isthmus' practice is the desire to create meaningful landscapes from the large scale through to the detail, and to design landscapes that are enduring, vibrant, and sustainable. Many of their projects can be found in public space, and are designed as a talking point and a way of bringing life to public space.

Photo: Simon Devitt

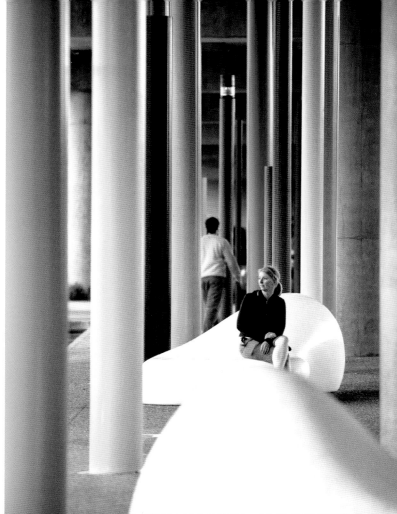

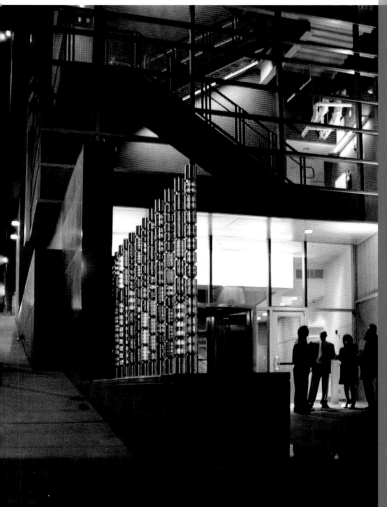

Waterwall at the University of Pittsburgh
Landworks Studio Inc.

Completion: 2007. **Technique:** stainless steel, internally lit with LED lights, water. **Location:** Pittsburgh, PA, USA.

As a landscape element in the streetscape and entry courtyard for the Biomedical Science Tower, a 'waterwall' adds to the activity along Fifth Avenue. Stainless steel sticks, located adjacent to the main entrance, are internally and colorfully lit and enlivened with water. These sticks represent the chromosome sequence of the mouse genome and celebrate the ways that research, using mice, has uncovered many of the complexities of human biology.

Michael Blier is a landscape architect and founding principal of the critically recognized design group, Landworks Studio Inc. Blier's recent work is largely urban and site specific in nature. It seeks to exploit the inherent complexities that exist at ecologically challenged sites, ecological and cultural sustainability, material tectonics, and program. Blier taught and lectured at universities throughout the USA, including Harvard University's Graduate School of Design and Rhode Island School of Design.

Photo: Payette Associates

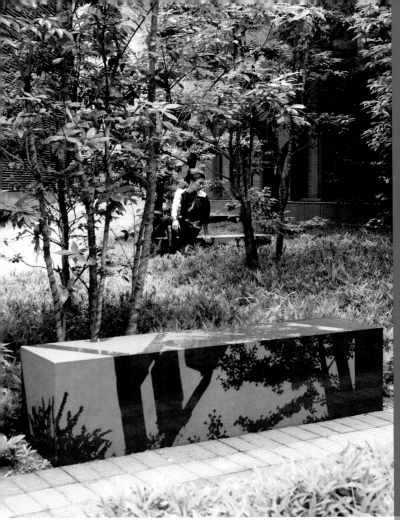

Memory Chair
Earthscape

Completion: 2007. **Technique:** carving on polished black granite.
Location: Tokyo, Japan.

"Memory Chair" stands in front of the new Central Government Building in Tokyo. Before the government building was built, the Ministry of Education building stood in its place. Earthscape engraved onto the stone chair the shadow of this building, as it was on July 11th, 2003, just before it was demolished to make way for the government building. The engraved shadow of the former building overlaps with the shadow of the current building, bringing to mind memories of the area, and the flow of time.

Earthscape is a landscape design studio. By thinking about the devices that create connections between humans and nature as design, they enact design works that become a platform for experience. With landscape design as their primary axis, Earthscape is involved in a wide array of activities, including the MHCP / Medical Herbman Cafe Project, which seeks to contribute to society through design, promoting discourse and unity within a varied society.

Photos: Shigeki Asanuma, Tokyo

Woodhenge
Tanya Preminger

Completion: 2007. **Technique:** wood. **Location:** Furstenfeld, Austria.

"Woodhenge" is a wooden replica of the famous English archeological monument Stonehenge. It was built during the Land Art festival in Austria, as part of a promenade around the town of Furstenfeld. The meaning of Stonehenge is unknown to us but it considered by many to have been a tribute to the gods. This project is made of wood, a material that contains warmth and is associated with life and growth. The wood circle expresses comradeship of people, togetherness, globalization and unity.

Tanya Preminger is a stone sculptor born in the Soviet Union in 1944. Since 1972 she has lived, worked and taught in Israel. She works using various art media: stone sculpture, landscape art, installation and photography. In the past few years Preminger has been very active in the fields of Environmental Art and Land Art, striving to connect people to nature, and improve the modern culture's relationship with the natural world. Over 50 of her sculptures are installed in Israel and overseas.

Photos: Courtesy of the artist

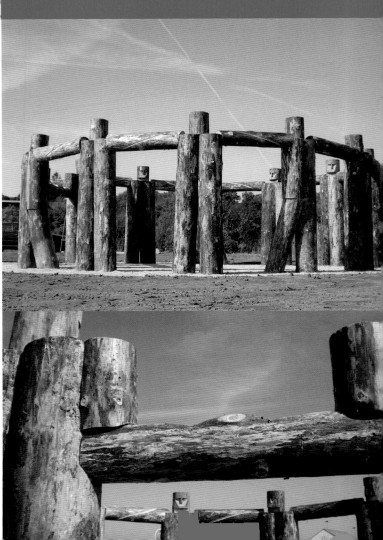

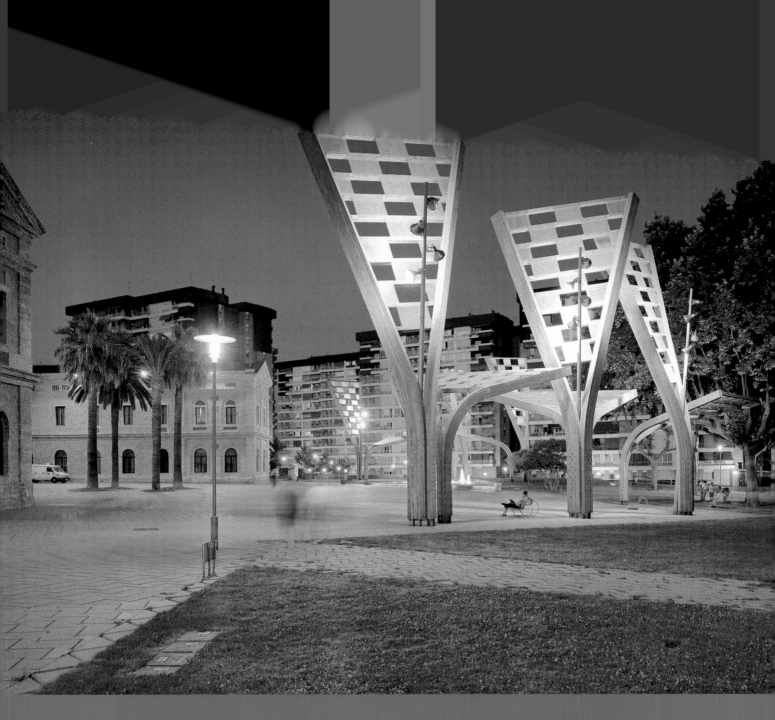

Parc Central de Nou Barris
Arriola & Fiol arquitectes / Andreu Arriola, Carmen Fiol

Completion: 2007. **Technique:** enamel on steel. **Location:** Barcelona, Spain.

The qualities of Cubism have a great potential for transposition in the field of architecture and urban planning. The design for the "Parc Central" sets out to transfer a Cubist landscape onto the cityscape. The tense volume of the Cubist plane explodes, breaks free and transforms the real three-dimensional landscape. Though fragmented, this new landscape is composed of all the parts and is open to change and extension of its form, uses and collective meanings.

Andreu Arriola and Carmen Fiol were awarded their masters degree in architecture from Columbia University in New York. From 1981–1988, they created some of the most memorable contemporary public spaces, which were awarded the Harvard University Prince of Wales Prize in 1990. The design excellence represented by this work has continued in their private practice, which has won awards in international and national competitions.

General Maister Memorial Park
Bruto, Primož Pugelj

Completion: 2007. **Technique:** iron. **Location:** Ljubno ob Savinji, Slovenia.

This memorial park is designed as an abstract three dimensional space-illustration of the northern border mountain ridges in Slovenia, which general Maister's soldiers fought for in 1918, against the Austro-Hungarian Empire. Made out of welded metal rods, the sculpture represents a stylized image of general Maister followed by his horse and soldiers. The whole embankment is protected by solid stone blocks, safeguarding the park like a stone shield.

Primož Pugelj graduated from the Academy of Fine Arts in Ljubljana in 1998, later completing his postgraduate study at the Indiana University of Pennsylvania and a masters at the Academy of Fine Arts Ljubljana. Bruto is a landscape architecture and design firm, which focuses on emphasizing the importance of functionality in modern design. Bruto works on the principle that the context of space, which can be manifested as an influence or as a guiding principle in project design is of the utmost importance.

Photos: Miran Kambič, Radovljica

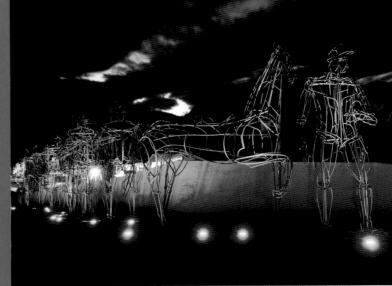

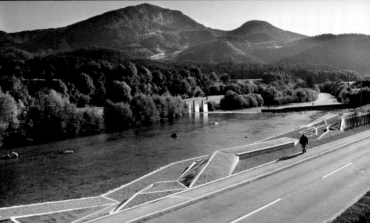

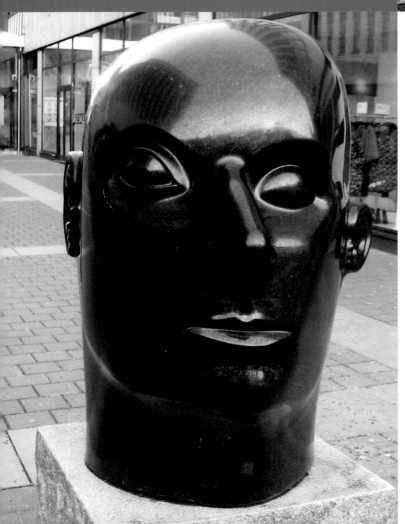

The Happy Man of Borås
Olle Brandqvist

Completion: 2007. **Technique:** stone diabase. **Location:** Borås, Sweden.

This sculpture, "The Happy Man of Borås" (Den nöjde Boråsaren), took a little over a year to create and was completed in 2007. It was then purchased by the city of Borås City in Sweden in 2008. The sculpture is carved from a diabase, a black stone, which was cut, ground and polished to create the head shape. The head itself has a height of nearly one meter and it is placed on a pedestal of light granite. This sculpture has an intimate touch and appeals to the public as it can be experienced with both hands and eyes.

Olle Brandqvist from Sweden works as both sculptor and artist. He studied at the Industrial Art School in Gothenburg and finished his studies at the University of Stockholm. He is a member of the Swedish Sculptor's Association. Some of his public works can be seen in the Church at Brommaplan, Stockholm, Mark's town hall, Kinna, as well as in Borås' city's Main Square.

Photo: Courtesy of the artist

Spitalfields Journey
David Rhys Jones

Completion: 2007. **Technique:** steel, aluminum. **Location:** London, United Kingdom.

This installation was inspired by a journey through Spitalfields, an area of London that has always been on the 'edge' geographically and socially. The sculpture is constructed of steel and aluminum and arranged in two parts. One face has a mirrored surface, reflecting the viewer and allowing them to become part of the street scene. The images within the work have been photographed locally but in selecting unusual angles and scale, the viewer is dawn into an enigmatic world. The installation was curated by Dickson Russell Art Management.

David Rhys Jones trained at Central Saint Martins College of Art and Design in London and has exhibited widely, including at the V&A Museum and the Royal Academy of Arts. He was joint winner of the Jerwood Prize in 2010 and his work is held in many private and public collections, including the Tate. Rhys Jones' artworks are based on journeys or site specific locations, and recorded using photographs and drawings. They contribute a form of social documentary, recording the mix of cultures and architecture found in the modern city.

Photo: Courtesy of the artist

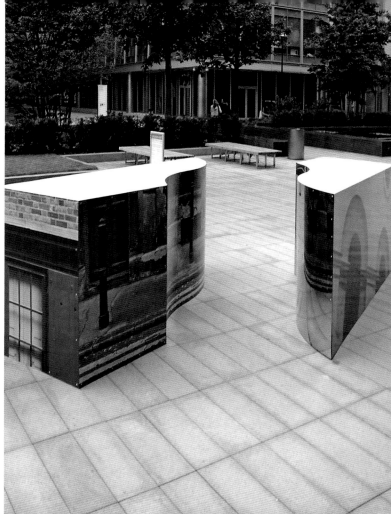

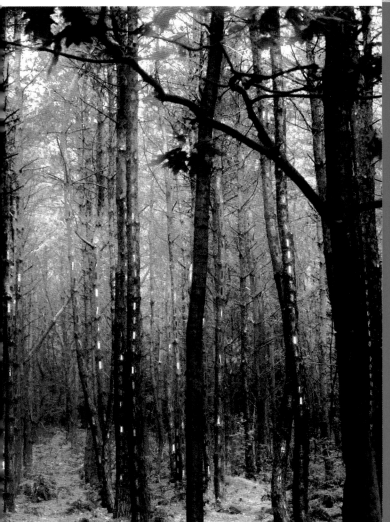

Mirrored Wood
Femke van Dam

Completion: 2007. **Technique:** 600 mirrors ciselised in 27 living trees. **Location:** Schoonoord, The Netherlands.

These strips of mirror reflect the surrounding trees, enlarging the forest space and referring to the past, a time when forests spanned most of Europe. The mirrors reflect place, modifying what the viewer sees, blurring the boundaries between what is real and what is reflection. The mirrors can also appear as drops of congealed sap, permanently stilled in their downwards journey. The trees are decorated with drops of beauty, maybe tears, paying homage to the past grandeur of the forests.

Femke van Dam was born in 1949 and worked in urban and rural planning for more than 25 years. She later returned to studying and received a bachelor of arts degree from the Academy of Fine Arts Minerva, the Netherlands. As a professional artist, she creates spatial art, inspired by the geography and the history of each particular site. She uses the landscape, natural materials and found objects to tell the story of that place. Her work is exhibited in public and private collections across Europe.

Photo: Courtesy of the artist

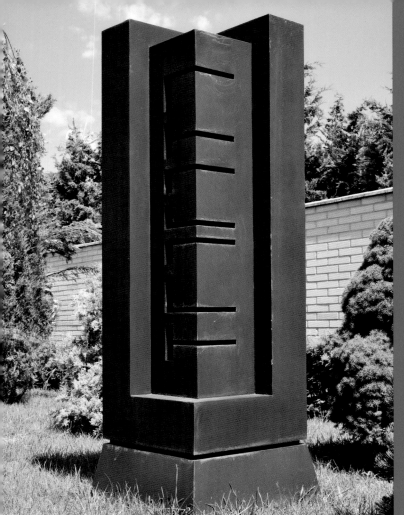

Message
Peter Roller

Completion: 2007. **Technique:** metal. **Location:** Boldog, Slovakia.

This metal sculpture, entitled "Message", is part of a series of large, metal compositions created for display in both public and private space. In these art compositions, the sculptor aimed to search for and express thought and shape connections to ancient cultures and consider how these connections are transformed in the present. Signs of writing formulate desire of humans to find their own place in the great space of the universe. The sculpture is located at the Open Gallery Jan Kukal, Boldog in Slovakia.

Peter Roller is a Slovakian artist, born in 1948. He studied at the Academy of Fine Arts in Bratislava, Slovakia, graduating in 1975. He worked as a lecturer at the Academy of Fine Arts, becoming senior lecturer in 1996. Roller works in sculpture, graphic art, object art, drawing and painting and has participated in around 40 international sculpture and object symposia throughout the world, as well as exhibiting his work at a number of solo and group exhibitions. In 2009 Roller was appointed as professor at the Academy of Fine Arts in Bratislava.

Photo: Matrin Marenčin, Bratislava

Flora
Astrid Krogh

Completion: 2007. **Technique:** neon, aluminum. **Location:** Kolding, Denmark.

"Flora", is a decoration for the Nicolai Quarter in Kolding, Denmark. In contrast to the artist's previous neon tapestries "Flora" is less patterned but still a free composition of floral ornaments. With her colorful "neon wallpapers" and her delicate luminous weavings the Danish textile designer Astrid Krogh has not only lightened up some rather dry environments, such as the Danish Parliament, many of her works are associated with the architecture of well known, international firms.

Astrid Krogh was born in 1968 in Denmark and studied at the Institute for Product Design in Denmark. She has many representations and commissions in Scandinavia, the Netherlands and Germany. Astrid Krogh works mainly with textile and light, with an emphasis on patterns, ornamentation and textile craftsmanship. Typically working on a large scale that gives the patterns and the light a physical presence. She strives to challenge and apply new materials and technologies in her field as a textile designer.

Photo: Ole Hein Pedersen

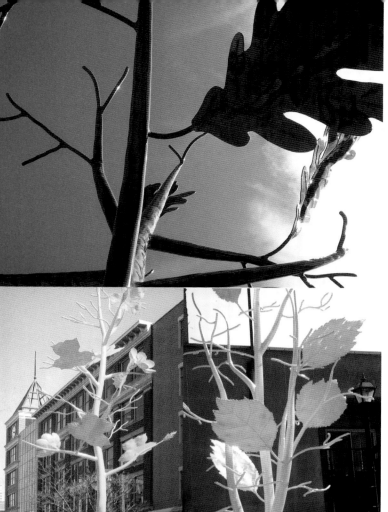

Metal Trees
Bill Hodgson

Completion: 2007. **Technique:** metal. **Location:** London, Canada.

These metal trees were commissioned for the town of London in Canada. This began with just a few trees and led to the commission of seven more, creating a veritable metal forest in downtown London. The trees are five meters tall and were first introduced in 2007. The artists aimed to add his own touch to nature, creating elaborate designs and exaggerating the branches. The project is ongoing, with new trees added every year.

Bill Hodgson learned to work metal by taking welding courses for two years at a local college. He later began making and selling his artwork from the basement of his house before increasing local demand allowed him to open a small chain of shops selling his wares. The inspiration for this project comes from the area's natural tree population. Hodgson's trees are deliberately colorful, bringing life to concrete areas of the city, reanimating the downtown area.

Photos: WayneRay Wayne Ray / Wikimedia Commons

Spidernethewood
R&Sie(n)

Completion: 2007. **Technique:** netting and wrapping trees with plastic mesh to encourage plant growth. **Location:** Nîmes, France.

This design is based on the idea of a spider's web. The architects have used netting to wrap the trees with a plastic mesh, creating a labyrinth within the branches. The web-like structure includes a 450 square meter building, attached to the web by a sliding glass door. Because of the use of glass to connect web and building, the boundaries between inside and outside become a blur. In time, the web will become lost within the wood, as the trees grow up around and become entwined with the netting.

R&Sie(n) is an architectural practice based in Paris. It was founded in 1989 by François Roche and Stéphanie Lavaux. Toshikatsi Kiuchi joined the company in 2007. The firm's architectural work seeks to articulate the real and / or fictional and the geographic situations and narrative structures that can transform these concepts. R&Sie(n) unfold their protocols through the re-staging of different kinds of contemporary relationships: aesthetical, computational, biological and even artificial.

Photo: Courtesy of the artist

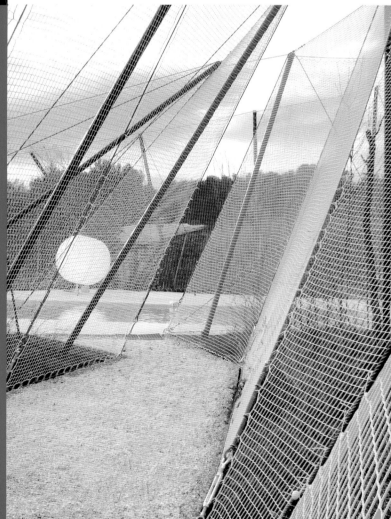

Fields of Mist
Rudi van de Wint

Completion: 2007. **Technique:** steel. **Location:** Hoogeveen, The Netherlands.

"Fields of Mist" is a posthumous work of Rudi van de Wint. It was designed by him but realized by his sons. The work is a series of four sculptures, situated along the highway near to Hoogeveen. The title refers to an old folk belief, that mythical "white women" used to roam the fields of Hoogeveen, which was why the area often appeared to be covered in a thick, white mist. These sculptures are 10 meters high and 15 meters wide, made between 2007 and 2010.

Rudi van de Wint was born in the Netherlands in 1942, he died in 2007. He studied at the Academy of Art in Amsterdam and originally focused on painting rather than sculpture. He was invited to exhibit his work at the tenth Documenta exhibition in Kassel in 1977 and it wasn't until later than he began to concentrate on sculptural and architectural work. He often created huge sculptures, using Corten steel and other metals. He died in Tenerife and a memorial was built there in his honor.

Photo: Gouwenaar / Wikimedia Commons

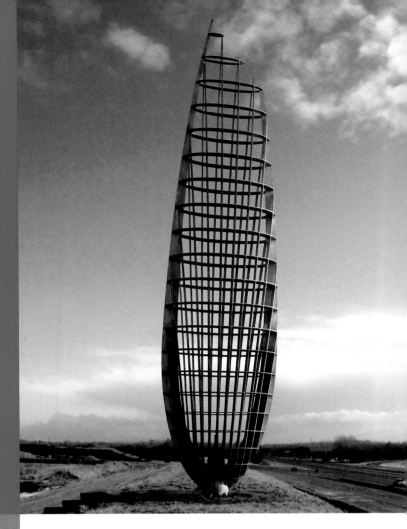

Bou
Santiago Calatrava

Completion: 2007. **Technique:** bronze. **Location:** Palma de Mallorca, Spain.

This work is made up of five blocks, reaching a height of 15 meters and with a combined weight of 40 tons. The sculpture is made from bronze and abstractly depicts the transition between sitting and standing. The supporting structure connecting the cubes represents the human spine and the two conical supports are the legs. The sculpture is clearly visible from a distance due to its height and its elevated location.

Santiago Calatrava was born in 1951 and is a famous Spanish sculptor and architect. He has offices in Zurich, Valencia, Paris and New York. His early career was focused on bridges and train stations. He went on to build the Montjuic Communications Tower in Barcelona, situated in the middle of the Olympic Site, this led to a number of new commissions and helped to gain him international recognition. He is currently building the new train station at the rebuilt World Trade Center in New York.

Photo: ILA-boy / Wikimedia Commons

One and Many
Sara Stracey

Completion: 2007. **Technique:** billion-color light-emitting diodes LED, pentagon polycarbonate channeled panels. **Location:** Tampa, FL, USA.

These colorful geometrical shapes of light can be spotted from interstate I-75. Commissioned by developer Novare-intown on behalf of Skypoint Tower, "One and Many", is a contextual landscape consisting of revealing tinted pentagon-channeled greenhouse panels and colored-light emitting diodes. The work is installed facing the Tampa Museum of Art on two recessed areas, providing a transition between the towers modern steel and concrete façade and the emerging downtown Cultural Arts District.

Sara Stracey was born in Canada in 1976 and is currently based in New York. She graduated with a masters in fine arts from Columbia University in 2008 and has a bachelors degree from the Rhode Island School of Design. Stracey has been in motion making intuitive works with and in parallel to SITE Architecture. Her works have been exhibited in National Building Museum, Venice Architecture Biennial, Musée des Beaux-Arts d'Orléans.

Photo: Courtesy of the artist

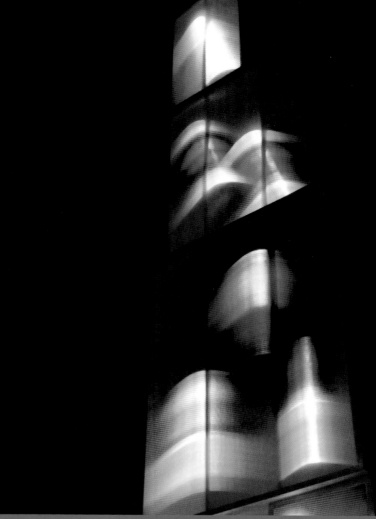

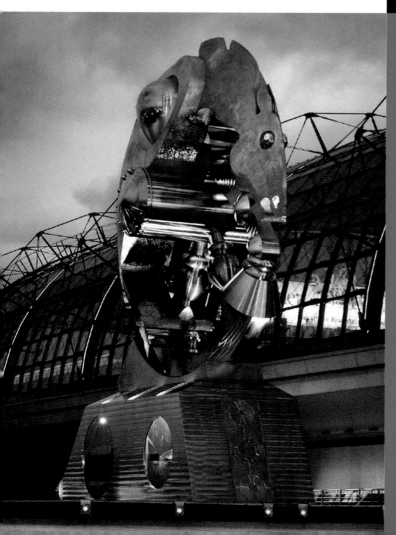

Rolling Horse
Jürgen Goertz

Completion: 2007. **Technique:** aluminum, stainless steel, iron, plastic, fiberglass installation. **Location:** Berlin, Germany.

This large sculpture, entitled "Rolling Horse", was created in 2007 and serves as an evocative monument and urban character. It stands in a public area outside Berlin's main station. The high-tech horse is made from modern material and finished with technical, engineering elements. It is geometrically constructed and rotates around its vertical axis. The movement creates the impression of something living, with a will and drive of its own.

Jürgen Goertz was born in Albrechtshagen, Posen in 1939. He studied sculpture at the Art Academy in Karlsruhe from 1963–1966, he later spent two years in London at the Camberwell College of Arts as part of a DAAD program. In 1972 he got the Rome Prize Villa Massimo. In 2005 Goertz was awarded the honorary title of guest lecturer at the New York Studio School. Between 1980 and 2001 he participated in various competitions and has been awarded several commissions for producing art in the public realm.

Photo: Wolfgang Selbach

Alittlemorelove
das änderungsatelier

Completion: 2008. **Technique:** various. **Location:** Munich, Germany.

This sculptural ensemble is made up of various different parts, including a gondola, leaning posts, an historical lantern, lions and a wall with a passage from a Thomas Mann novel "Death in Venice". The work has obvious associations with Venice, linking the title "Alittlemorelove" with romantic notions of Venice. The ensemble gives character to the flat green space, giving the area a romantic and whimsical flair.

Das änderungsatelier consists of Georg Schweitzer and Nadja Stemmer, who have been working together since 1993. Schweitzer was born in Trier in 1963. He studied at the State Academy of Art in Karlsruhe, graduating in 1990. Stemmer was born in Munich in 1966 and studied communication design and graphic design at the vocational college in Heidenheim. Schweitzer and Stemmer's work has been exhibited widely throughout Germany.

Photos: Chris van Uffelen

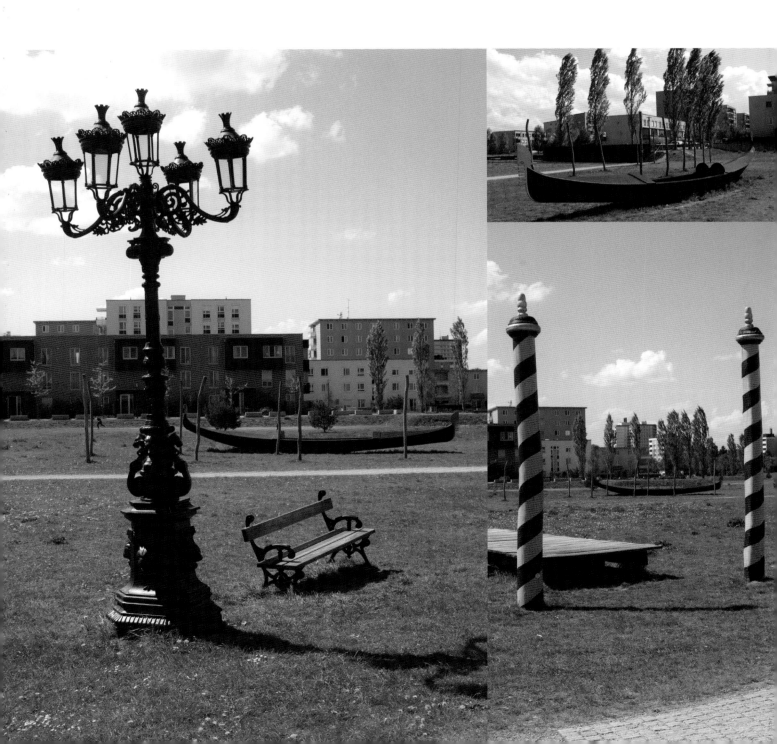

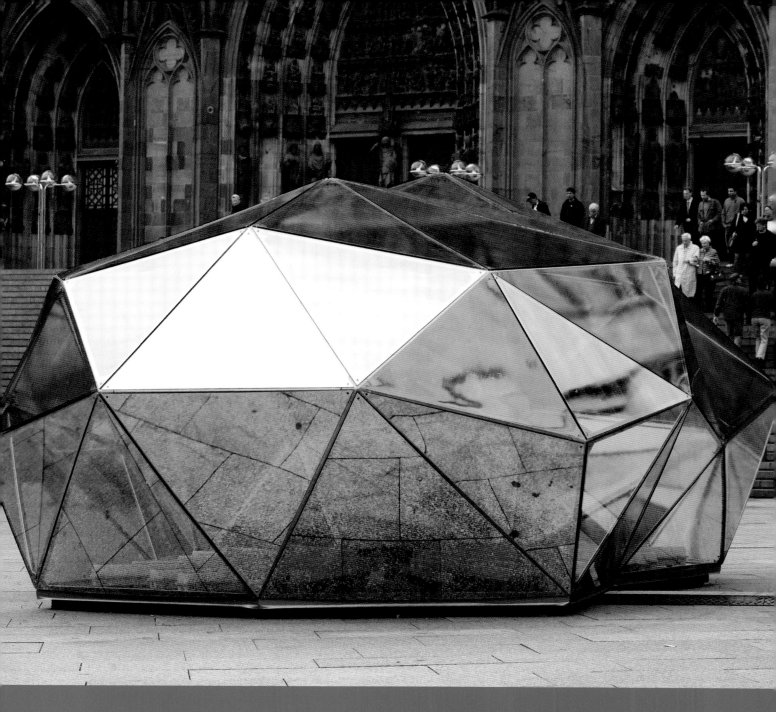

Photo: Christian Doppelgatz, Cologne

Cityscope
Marco Hemmerling

Completion: 2008. **Technique:** aluminum frame, acrylic panels, dichroic foil. **Location:** Cologne, Germany.

"Cityscope" deals with the fragmented perception of urban spaces. The bevelling structure can be seen as an urban kaleidoscope, reflecting fragmented views of the city and composing at the same time a three dimensional image of the surrounding façades. While moving around the sculpture, the images continuously change. The dichroic foil is dependent on the daylight situation and the position of the beholder. The appearance changes into complementary colors by night, when the installation is lit from inside.

Marco Hemmerling studied architecture, interior design and media management at various universities. Before setting up his studio for spatial design in Cologne, he worked for six years at Dutch firm UNStudio where he was co-head for the design and realization of the Mercedes-Benz Museum in Stuttgart. Hemmerling teaches and conducts research as professor for computer aided design in architecture and interior design at the University of Applied Sciences in Detmold.

Favela Painting
Haas&Hahn

Completion: 2008. **Technique:** paint, in-situ concrete. **Location:** Vila Cruzeiro, Brazil.

This work was the second large work to be created in Rio Cruzeiro, one of Brazil's most notorious slums. The project began in 2006, when a large mural of a boy flying a kite was realized on the side of a building, with the help of local youths. This work is situated on a massive concrete structure, built to prevent mudslides on the hill. It was painted by local youths, not only teaching them a skill, but also giving them the chance to earn some money. Tattooist Rob Admiral designed the piece.

Haas & Hahn is artistic duo Jeroen Koolhaas and Dre Urhahn. They have been working together since 2005. It was during the filming of a documentary about hip-hop in Brazil that they were inspired to take on a larger, artistic project. Painting dynamic works in the slums of Brazil, with the help of local youths. Koolhaas was born in 1977 and studied graphic design at the Design Academy in Eindhoven. Urhahn was born in 1973 and has worked as a journalist, copywriter and artist.

Photos: Courtesy of the artist

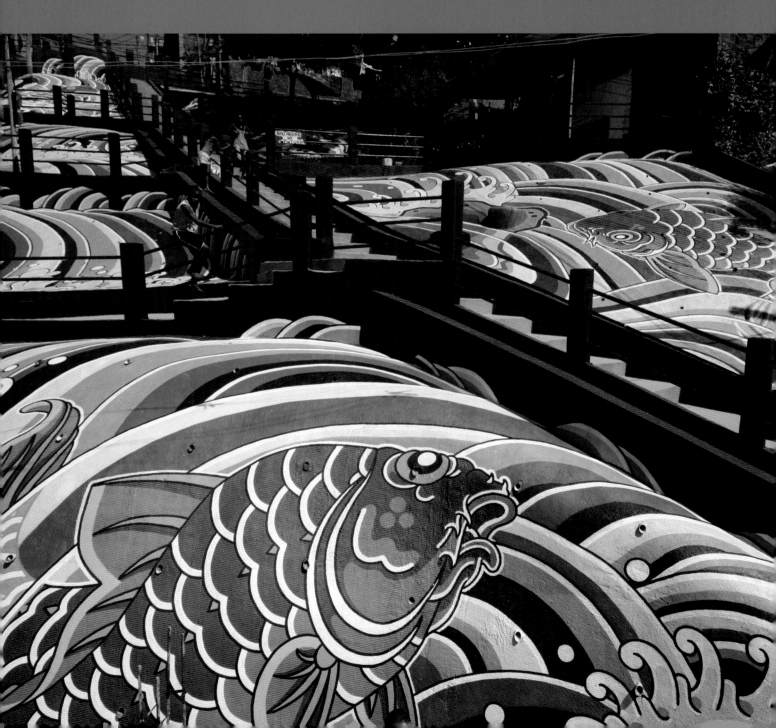

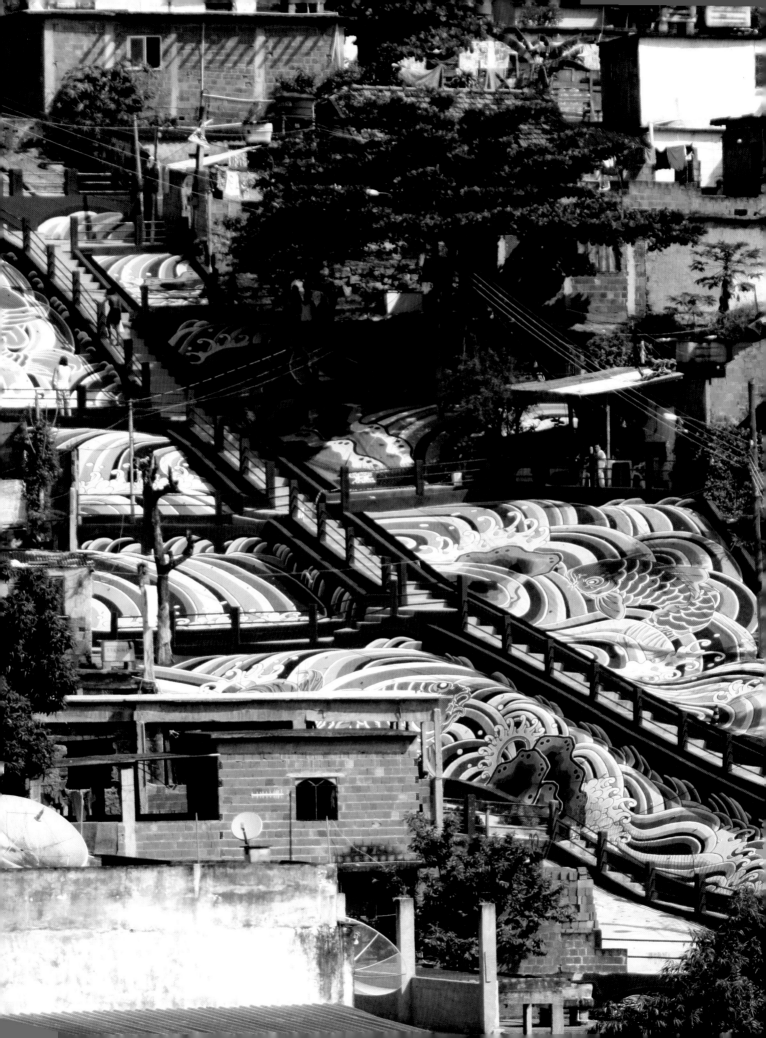

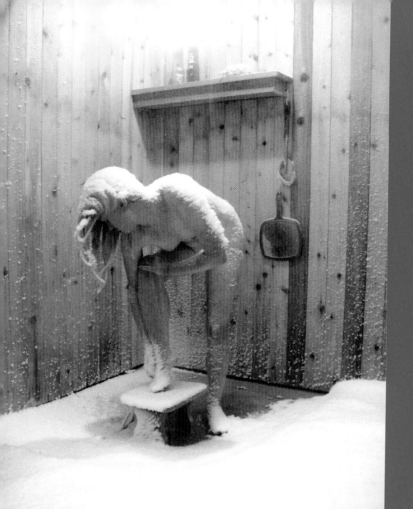

Employee Shower
Carole A. Feuerman

Completion: 2008. **Technique:** cedar wood, painted bronze, mirror, stereo system. **Location:** Hamilton, NJ, USA.

The sculptural installation "Employee Shower" is on permanent display at the Grounds for Sculpture in Hamilton. The piece is set back into a wooden area behind the restaurant in the sculpture park. Passersby hear softly playing Carly Simon music in the clearing. Curiosity brings the observer down a small path to stumble upon a sign that reads "Employee Shower", announcing an open, wooden cabana with a young woman showering in it. The viewer becomes complicit in the experience, realizing that a trick has been played.

Carole A. Feuerman was born in Connecticut in 1945. She works with bronze, resin and marble, painting her sculptures many times to achieve human-like skin tones; her work often focuses around recreating the human condition. Carole Feuerman has had six museum retrospectives to date - the most recent being her 52-piece retrospective at the El Paso Museum of Art in 2010 entitled "Earth, Water, Air, Fire". She has been awarded various awards, including the Amelia Peabody award and the Lorenzo de Medici Prize.

Photos: Courtesy of the artist

Walking to the Sky
Jonathan Borofsky

Completion: 2008. **Technique:** stainless steel, painted hybrid epoxy fiberglass composite. **Location:** Seoul, South Korea.

In 2008, Borofsky's "Walking to the Sky" was permanently installed in Seoul, South Korea. The sculpture shows a number of people scaling a soaring, stainless steel pole, tilted at an angle of 75 degrees. The figures include a young girl, a businessman and a young man, amongst others. The work is a celebration of human potential and diversity; no challenge is insurmountable. The artwork demonstrates that humanity is striving towards an unknown future with strength and determination.

Jonathan Borofsky was born in 1942, in Boston, Massachusetts. He received his masters degree at Yale School of Art and Architecture in 1966. Borofsky's artworks are installed at the Philadelphia Museum of Art and the Whitney Museum of American Art, amongst others. He has created more than 30 permanent and temporary public sculptures for cities around the world, including the 30.5-meter-tall "Molecule Man", which stands in the Spree river in Berlin; and the 21-meter-tall "Hammering Man" in Frankfurt / Main, Germany.

Photo: Courtesy of the artist

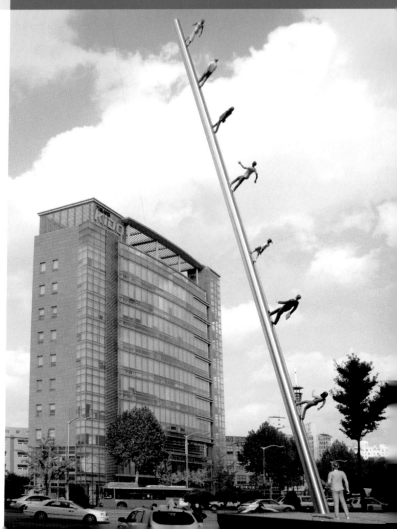

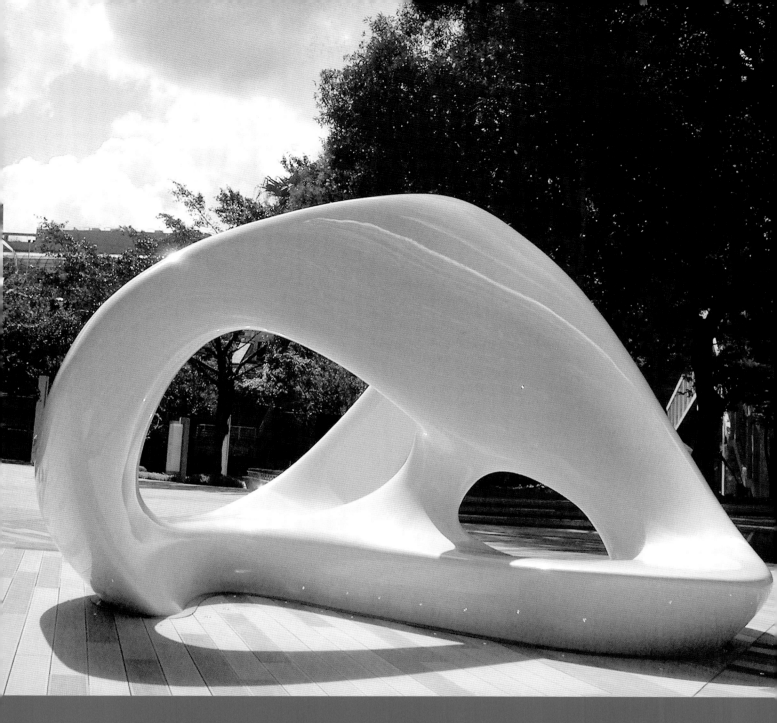

Wirl
Zaha Hadid Architects

Completion: 2008. **Technique:** EPS foam reinforced with fiberglass shell. **Location:** Hong Kong, China.

"Wirl" was conceived to reflect the intensity of a hyper-acceleratory force within an elastic tactile form. As the curvature of the surface dynamically twists and turns, dynamic form and functional furnishings are seamlessly integrated. Swells provide areas for seating while stretches in the form furnish opportunities to recline. A generous upward sweep provides shade as well as integrating a series of evolving, framed views of the surrounding environment and buildings.

Zaha Hadid was born in Baghdad in 1950. She studied at the Architectural Association School of Architecture in London. After her degree she became a partner of Rem Koolhaas and Elia Zanghalis in the Office Metropolitan Architecture. In 1980 she opened her own office. She was awarded the Pritzker Prize in 2004 and is internationally known for her professional and academic work. Each of her projects build on thirty years of research as she constantly tests the boundaries of architecture, urbanism, art and product design.

The Verdant Walk
North Design Office, Peter and Alissa North

Completion: 2008. **Technique:** aluminum, fabric, flexible solar panels, LED lights. **Location:** Cleveland, OH, USA.

"The Verdant Walk" is a response to our industrial past and new direction toward a sustainable agenda. The forms represent the promise of new technologies. In summer the forms are wrapped in translucent covers, while winter reveals their skeletal shapes. As their location changes, the forms respond to local textures and seasons. Gathered in a herd, like futurist beasts and glowing with excitement, the forms of "The Verdant Walk" invite visitors to join them as they lead the way to a green future.

North Design Office is based in Toronto, the office was established by partners Pete and Alissa North in 2005. At North Design Office, research and theory inform a process-based approach to complex urban environmental issues. Projects range in scale from site specific installations to landscape architecture to ecology, technology and urbanism strategies. A unique design strategy is created for each project, founded on an intensive exploration of site, context, and program as the mechanism for transformation.

Photos: North Design Office / Pete North, Toronto

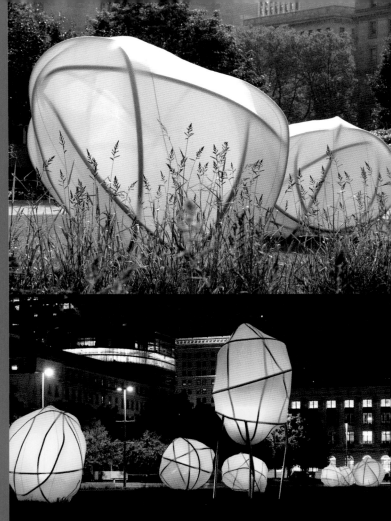

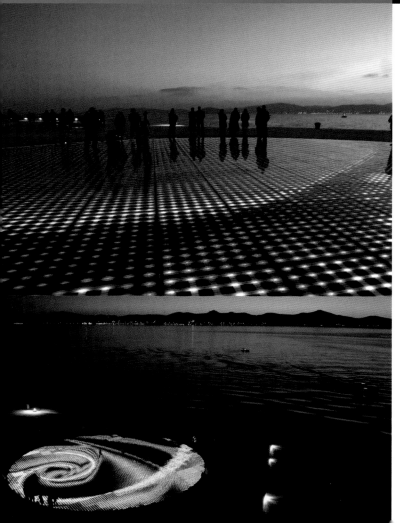

Sea Organ & Greeting to the Sun
Nikola Bašić, Ivan Stamać

Completion: 2008. **Technique:** marble, 35 calibrated steel tubes, 300 multi-layer glass panels, photovoltaic solar modules. **Location:** Zadar, Croatia.

"Sea Organ" and "Greeting to the Sun" are parts of a project involved in reshaping the promontory of the Zadar peninsula. "Sea organ" takes the form of stairs and is situated on the seafront. The stone staircase is divided into seven sections containing tubes of different diameters. The air is pushed by the waves into the tubes, which then produce sound. "Greeting to the Sun" is a circular surface, lying in the plane of the seafront pavement. Solar cells change solar energy into a spectacle of light.

Nikola Bašić is a Croatian architect. He was born in 1946, on the Croatian island of Murter and attended school in Zadar. Bašić later graduated from the Faculty of Architecture and Urbanism in Sarajevo and started his own architectural firm, Marina Projekt, in 1991. In 1995 he became the head of the architectural workshop at the University of Split. He is best known for the creation of the "Croatian Sea Organ" in Zadar, which won the European Prize for Urban Public Space.

Photos: Stipe Surać

I Wish
John R. Henry

Completion: 2008. **Technique:** steel. **Location:** Miami, FL, USA.

Commissioned by the Arison Arts Foundation for the Miami Art Museum, "I Wish" was constructed in 2008 to represent Miami in John Henry's Drawing in Space: The Peninsula Project exhibition. "I Wish", is located in Bicentennial Park at the end of the deep-water slip of the Miami seaport. To date "I Wish" competes as one of John Henry's most massive and complex pieces, weighing almost 750 kilos and standing 25 meters in height.

John R. Henry is known worldwide for his largescale public works of art, many of which are exhibited in America as well as throughout Europe and Asia. Henry has exhibited his work extensively since the early 1960s and demonstrates a definitive trademark style that is recognized internationally. He attended the University of Kentucky, University of Chicago and the Art Institute of Chicago, where he received a Ford Foundation grant. He is currently professor of art at Chattanooga State College.

Photo: Katelyn Littlejohn, Miami

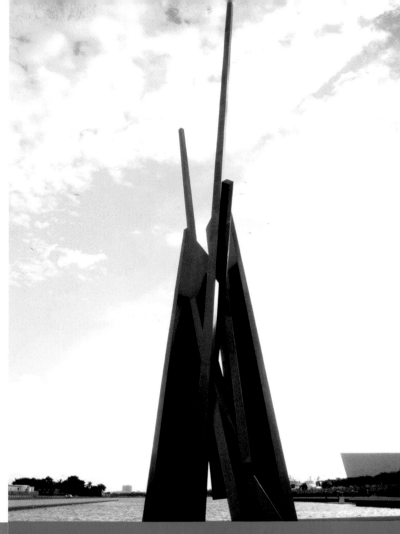

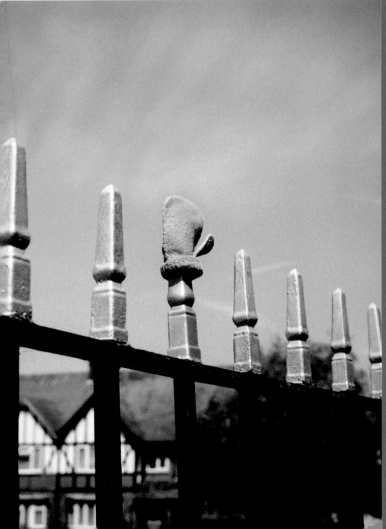

Baby Things
Tracey Emin

Completion: 2008. **Technique:** painted bronze. **Location:** Folkestone, United Kingdom.

"Baby Things" is a trail of baby clothes scattered through Folkestone. The work is made in bronze but painted to match the real thing. Emin is famous for producing autobiographical and often controversial work that speaks of teenage sex and unwanted pregnancies, often focusing on Margate, the town where she grew up. This artwork was commissioned for the Folkestone Triennial, a three-yearly art exhibition. Emin claims she created "Baby Things" because the town has the highest rate of teenage pregnancy in the United Kingdom.

Tracey Emin is a British artist. She was nominated for the Turner Prize in 1999 and exhibited "My Bed", an installation consisting of her own unmade bed, complete with used condoms and blood-stained underwear. One of her earlier works "Everyone I have ever slept with 1963–1995" gained her considerable media attention. Emin is also a panelist and speaker and has lectured at institutions all over the world about the link between creativity and autobiography.

Photo: Thierry Bal and Folkestone Triennial 2008

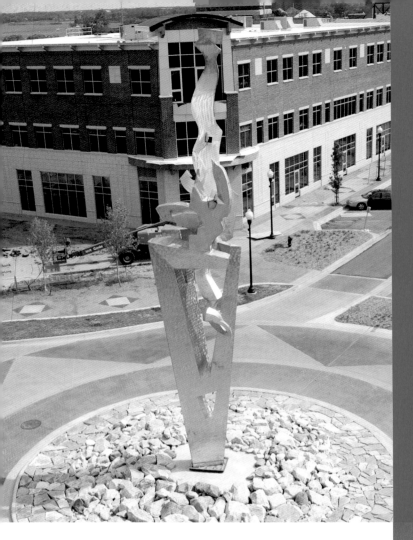

Muskegon Rising
Richard Hunt

Completion: 2008. **Technique:** welded stainless steel. **Location:** Muskegon, MI, USA.

"Muskegon Rising" was commissioned by the Community Foundation of Muskegon County as part of the city of Muskegon's downtown renewal effort. The 17-meters-tall welded stainless steel sculpture is situated on a new round-about, where it creates a point of focus and welcomes visitors into the renewed city center. The sculpture is intended as a symbol of hope and renewal for the town, bringing art to the community.

In 1971, Richard Hunt became the first African American sculptor given the honor of a retrospective at the Museum of Modern Art, New York. Hunt holds 14 honorary degrees and his work is represented internationally in major museums and collections. He has completed more public sculpture than any other artist in the country and was appointed by President Lyndon Johnson as one of the first artists to serve on the governing board of the National Endowment of the Arts. Hunt is famous for his abstract work, suggesting recognizable human, natural and architectonic forms.

Photo: Richard Hunt, Chicago, IL

GreenPix - Zero Energy Media Wall
Simone Giostra & Partners Architects

Completion: 2008. **Technique:** LEDs and photovoltaics laminated in glass panels. **Location:** Beijing, China.

The "GreenPix - Zero Energy Media Wall" was designed by Simone Giostra & Partners Architects. The wall features one of the largest color LED displays in the world and transforms the building envelop into a self-sufficient organic system, harvesting solar energy by day and using it to illuminate the screen after dark. The polycrystalline photovoltaic cells are laminated within the glass of the curtain wall and placed with changing density on the entire building's skin.

Simone Giostra graduated from the Polytechnic School of Architecture in Milan, where he earned a masters degree in architecture in 1994. He acted as project architect for the construction of several prestigious buildings in the USA and Europe. His company, Simone Giostra & Partners Architects, is based in New York and is dedicated to the investigation and performance of architecture energy technology and new media. He is associate professor at the Pratt Institute in New York.

Photo: Simone Giostra, ARUP, Ruogu

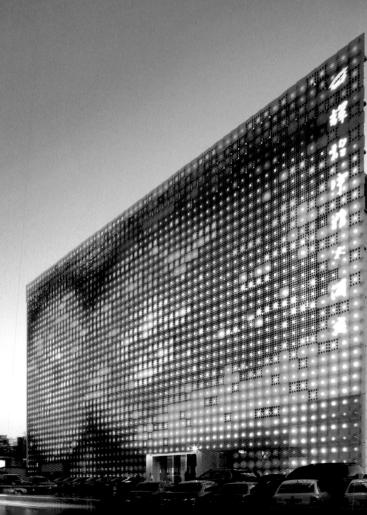

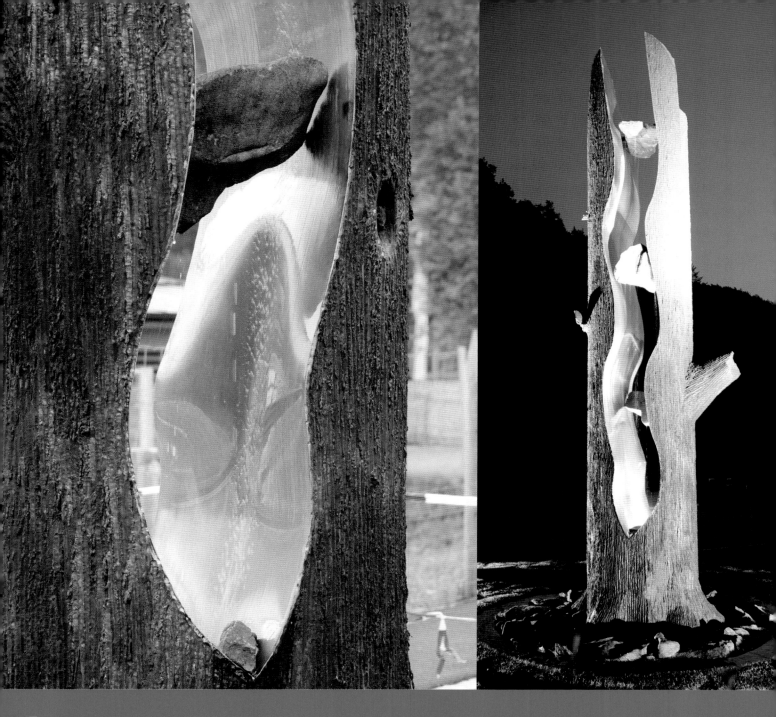

Stroke of lightning
Gerhard Fallmann

Completion: 2008. **Technique:** Corten steel, polished metal. **Location:** Türnitz, Austria.

This sculpture was built in 2008 and stands at the entrance of a new swimming pool. The sculptor was given the theme "water and wood" but other than that was left to his own devices. The sculpture he produced is six meters high and made from Corten steel. It takes the appearance of a tree trunk, with a waving line cut down through the center representing the flow of water. The inside is of polished metal and reflects the sunlight, while the inserted stones cast shadows down the inside of the trunk.

Gerhard Fallmann is an Austrian sculptor, born in 1959. He works primarily with metal. After completing an apprentice-ship as a locksmith and blacksmith in the Austrian town of Türnitz, Fallmann's creative talents were recognized, at which point he was moved to the creative department of the company. After this he began to sculpt in his spare time. After restoring an old forge belonging to a friend, Fallmann was offered space to begin creating his own sculptures on a larger scale.

Photos: Courtesy of the artist

Bellinge Gate
Søren West

Completion: 2008. **Technique:** granite, bronze. **Location:** Odense, Denmark.

The sculpture "Bellinge Gate" (Bellingeporten) with its stone benches, lamps, pavement and plantation constitutes a gateway in the center of Bellinge town. The gate connects the old marketplace with a new park that includes playground and playing fields. Back in 1880, a beautiful bronze key from the Viking period was found in a creek passing through Bellinge. This story sparked the idea of a "town gate" where visitors are presented with a large version of the ancient key – as an invitation to the town and to the park.

Søren West was born in Copenhagen in 1963. He graduated in sculpture from the Academy of Fine Arts in Odense, Denmark in 1988. West currently lives in a windmill next to Egeskov Castle, Denmark but often stays at Studio Corsanini in Carrara, Italy. His works involves fractures, cracks, acts of balance, rough matter challenging smoothness. West has produced many sculptures, which are displayed in public locations. He is also a member of many Danish artist's organizations.

Photos: Courtesy of the artist

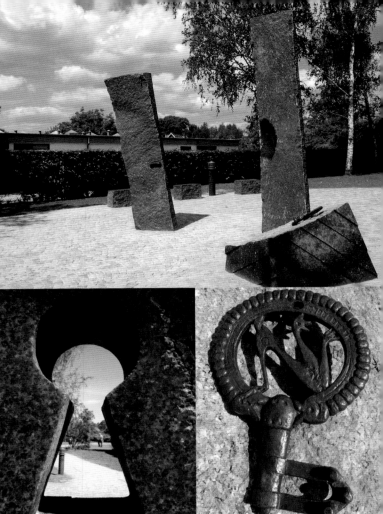

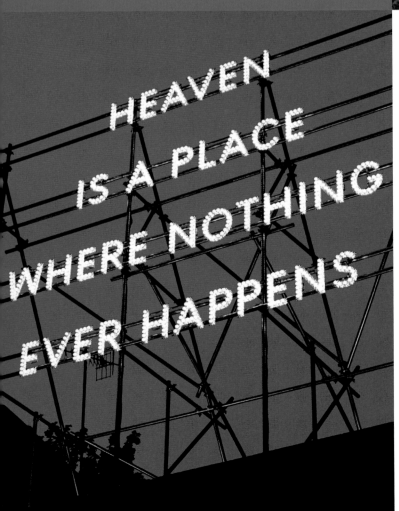

Heaven is a place where nothing ever happens
Nathan Coley

Completion: 2008. **Technique:** 480 light bulbs on scaffolding. **Location:** Folkestone, United Kingdom.

This artwork was commissioned for the Folkestone Triennial, a three-yearly art exhibition in the public realm. The sign evokes religious roadside architecture conjoined with fairground aesthetics. The artist's intention was not to produce a clear message, but that the work would be interpreted differently. For some it's a comforting message and for others it poses the question of whether heaven is the place we are promised it will be.

Nathan Coley was born in Glasgow in 1967 and studied at the Glasgow School of Art. His practice is based on an interest in public space, exploring how architecture comes to be invested with meaning. Coley works in a diverse range of media including public sculpture and photography. His previous works include a scale model of the Manchester Marks and Spencer building which was damaged by an IRA bomb and demolished, and another work focused on Pan Am Flight 103 which was blown up over Lockerbie.

Photo: Thierry Bal and Folkestone Triennail 2008

Bugscreen
Pae White

Completion: 2008. **Technique:** powder coated aluminum.
Location: Cleveland, OH, USA.

Pae White's "Bugscreen" references the tradition of red sculpture in green landscapes. It's location, Celebreeze Plaza in Cleveland, Ohio, experiences winds of up to 145 kilometers-per-hour so openness was a structural necessity. Bugscreen sits directly across the street from Claes Oldenburg's large red "Free" stamp. The artist wanted to have a conversation with these conditions; freedom, wind, bug wings and redness and also have the feeling that a folding screen just suddenly fell from the sky.

Pae White was born in 1963 in Pasadena, CA. She lives and works in Los Angeles. She received her master of fine arts from Art Center College of Design in Pasadena and her bachelor of arts from Scripps College in Claremont, CA. Recent solo exhibitions include in Cologne, Milan, New Zealand, Vancouver, London and in Los Angeles. White has also participated in several important projects involving art in the public realm, such as the Folkestone Triennial in 2008, Skulptur Projekte Münster in 2007, Whitney Biennial in 2010 and the Venice Biennial in 2009.

Photo: Mike Finn

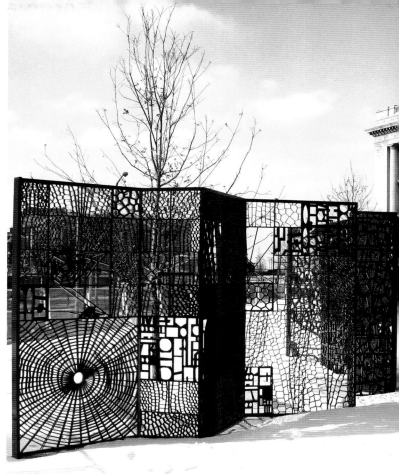

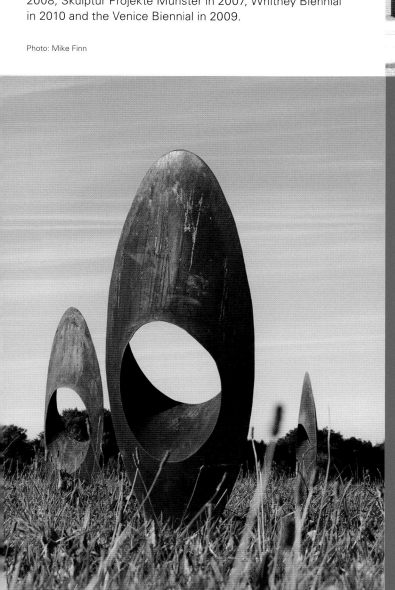

Obeles
Pieter Obels

Completion: 2008. **Technique:** Corten steel. **Location:** Devantave, Belgium.

This work is made from steel. The artist attempts to frame individual details within the landscape, giving the area new form and identity. The steel used to create this work has the advantage of providing it with an ever-changing skin. Rain and moisture in the air create rust, causing discolorations and changing the appearance over time. The intervals between the separate elements of this work and their relation to the space that surrounds them are important for retaining tension within the sculpture.

Pieter Obels works mainly with steel to create his trademark, large sculptures. He has exhibited his work widely in the Netherlands and abroad. He has also produced several commissioned pieces, for both private and public collections.

Photo: Courtesy of the artist

Wolves
Sally Matthews

Completion: 2008. **Technique:** bronze. **Location:** Stokke, Norway.

These bronze wolf sculptures are located in woodland in Fossnes, Norway. They pay homage to the declining wolf population in the country, where the number of remaining wolves is estimated at around just 30, with a proposed cull of eight in 2011. Many controversial wolf hunts have taken place in Norway in recent years and the sharp decline is due to both legal culling and illegal poaching.

Sally Matthews was born in Tamworth in 1964. She was awarded a bachelor of arts degree in fine art sculpture from Loughborough University. Matthews' gets the inspiration for her sculptures from animals. With her work she aims to capture the nature of both domesticated and wild animals, so that the spirit is clear to see as well as the form.

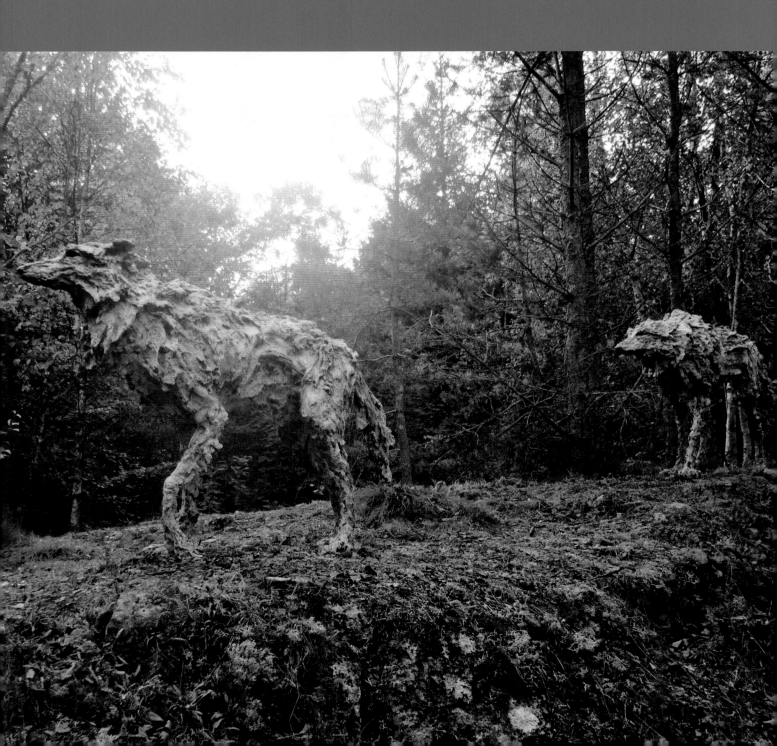

18 Holes
Richard Wilson

Completion: 2008. **Technique:** excavated concrete slabs, artificial lawn, steel, paint. **Location:** Folkestone, United Kingdom.

The X3 Beach Huts were not made of the usual wooden planking but cut from concrete slabs that previously made up the abandoned 18-hole crazy golf course located at the back of the esplanade. Each hut was made by excavating six, measured panels that came together as a series of planes or slabs. Because they are made of concrete slab, the huts are brutal in appearance, mimicking the old World War II concrete defense bunkers but their exterior surfaces still hold the color and form of the golfing game.

Richard Wilson was born in London in 1953 and studied at the London College of Printing, Hornsey College of Art and Reading University. Since his first solo exhibition in 1976, Wilson has had over 50 solo exhibitions devoted to his work around the world. Richard Wilson's fascination with architectural and perceived space has resulted in a 30-year body of work, where the observer's accepted comprehension of space is questioned and subverted. His interventions are characterized by concerns with size and structural daring.

Photo: Courtesy of the artist

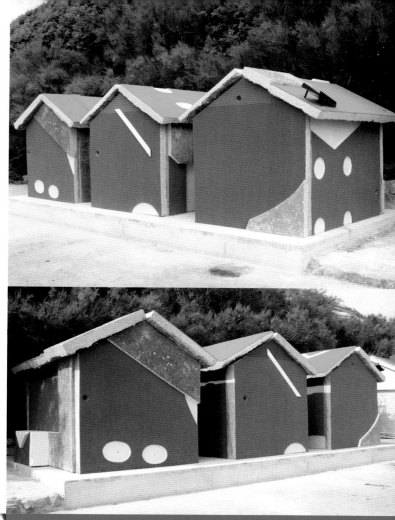

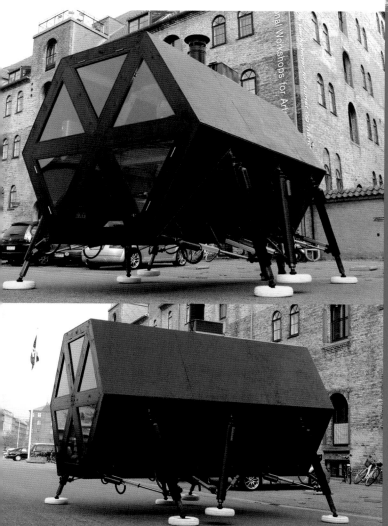

Walking House
N55

Completion: 2008. **Technique:** steel, aluminum, wood, polycarbonate. **Location:** Cambridge, United Kingdom.

"Walking House" is a modular dwelling system that enables persons to live a peaceful, nomadic life, moving slowly through the landscape or cityscape with minimal impact on the environment. It collects energy from its surroundings using solar cells and small windmills. There is a system for collecting rain water and a system for solar heated hot water. A small greenhouse unit can be added to the basic living module, to provide a substantial part of the food needed by the inhabitants.

Ion Sørvin4 is a Danish artist, activist and self-proclaimed 'closet architect', who lives out the summer months on a small houseboat moored at Copenhagen harbor. With N55, the art collective he co-founded with his wife in 1994, Sørvin has carved out a career challenging conventional notions of living, architecture and ownership. His current collaborators are architect Anne Romme and artist Sam Kronick. They have participated in several exhibitions and projects all over the world.

Photos: Courtesy of the artist

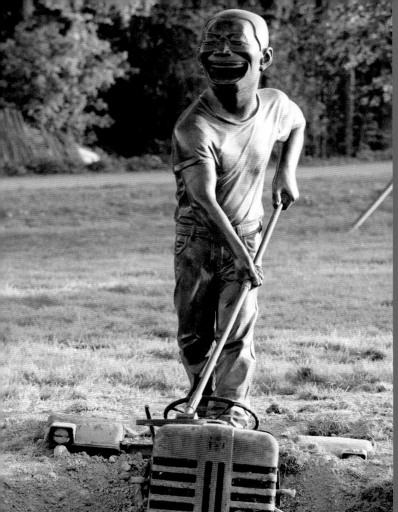

AD 3009
Yue Minjun

Completion: 2008. **Technique:** bronze, tractor. **Location:** Bramsche, Germany.

This sculpture "AD 3009" by Yue Minjun is one of many works of smiling sculpture by the artist. He depicts laughing or grinning figures going about everyday tasks, celebrating laughter. The sculpture is made of bronze and stands at over two meters in height. Minjun claims that the artwork is a monument to peace. Symbolic of the hope that in the year 3009 archeological discoveries will reveal everyday items, such as tractors and machinery and not the relics of war.

Yue Minjun is a Chinese sculptor, born in 1962 in the province of Hei Long Jiang, China. He studied oil painting at Hebei Normal University and has exhibited his work internationally. His exhibitions include at the National Museum of Fine Arts of Cuba and Venice International University. His works are held in the collections of museums across China, Korea and Europe. Minjun is most famous for his sculptures of laughing figures, grinning as they go about seemingly mundane tasks.

Photo: Courtesy Alexander Ochs Galleries Berlin I Beijing

Meeting
Wang Shugang

Completion: 2008. **Technique:** painted bronze. **Location:** Vancouver, Canada.

This sculptural work is entitled "Meeting", every crouching figure is 92 centimeters in height and each is identical in form; all cast in bronze from the same model. Each individual figure is painted in a bright red. The color red has several different cultural associations in Chinese culture. Once a color representing happiness, red is more readily associated with the terror of the Chinese Cultural Revolution and the color of the Communist Party.

Wang Shugang is a Beijing-based artist, born in Beijing in 1960. Shugang lived in the Ruhr region in Germany for ten years, returning to China at the age of 40. He currently has his own studio in Caochangdi, Beijing, an area that is home to several contemporary artists as well as many galleries and studios. Shugang's figurative sculptures express Buddhist iconography mixed with Chinese contemporary culture though his work has been influenced by the Western art tradition and contemporary Realism.

Photos: Dan Fairchild, Courtesy Alexander Ochs Galleries Berlin I Beijing

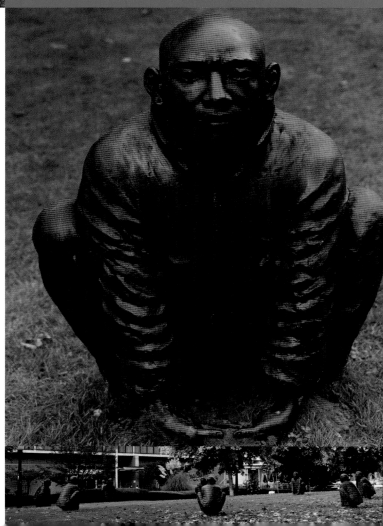

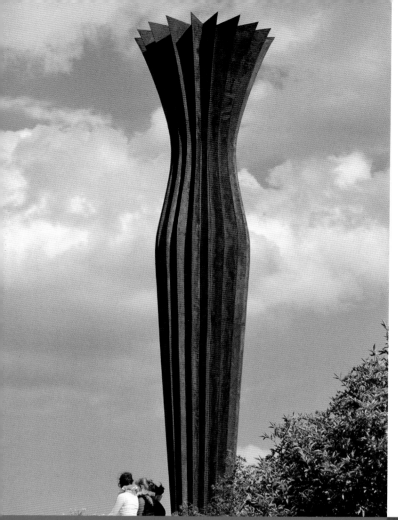

Belladonna
Herbert Mehler

Completion: 2008. **Technique:** Corten steel. **Location:** Würzburg, Germany.

"Belladonna" is a seven-meter-tall sculpture made of Corten steel. The sculpture was made in 2008 by German sculptor, Herbert Mehler. The "Belladonna" work is considered on of Mehler's major works and stands in front of the Würzburg Art Museum. As the title suggests, the form of the sculpture has obvious associations with the female form, though the lines and shape can also be interpreted as floral and are often seen as resembling the sepals of a flower.

Herbert Mehler is a German sculptor, born in Fulda in 1949. He was trained as a sculptor by his father, wood carver Franz Mehler, from 1964–1968. In 1972 he went on to study at the Academy of Fine Arts in Nuremberg, graduating in 1978. Mehler was awarded the Würzburg Culture Prize in 2007 and his work has been exhibited internationally.

Photo: Wolfgang Stenger

Oushi Zokei 2008
Keizo Ushio

Completion: 2008. **Technique:** carved granite. **Location:** Sydney, Australia.

Keizo refers to many of his sculptures by the name "Oushi Zokei". This was assigned as an overall name for Keizo's work by his main teacher, who was also a pioneer in geometrical sculpture in Japan. The name has several interpretations. Oushi can mean "deep truth", or alternatively "bull" or "steer". Ushi-o also refers to the shape of a bull's back or tail; the latter relates to the twisted forms often found in Keizo's work. Zo means "creating" or "forming", while Kei refers to "shape".

Keizo Ushio was born in Fukusaki Town, Hyogo Perfecture, Japan, in 1951. He completed his studies at Kyoto City University of Arts in 1976. Since then he has received numerous prizes and has participated in stone sculpture symposia and outdoor sculpture exhibitions throughout the world. Keizo's works are in public and private collections in many countries, including Australia, Denmark, Germany, Iceland, India, Israel, New Zealand, Spain and the United States.

Photos: Courtesy of the artist

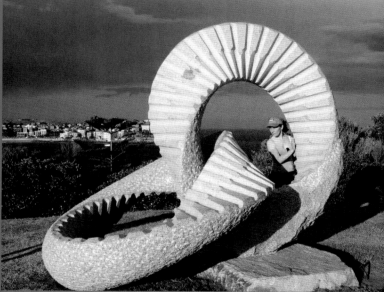

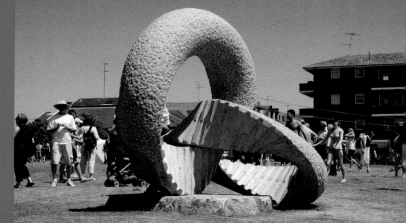

Dancing Steps Amphitheater and Star Fountain
Athena Tacha

Completion: 2008. **Technique:** glass, concrete. **Location:** Louisville, KY, USA.

The "Dancing Steps Amphitheater and Star Fountain" was designed by Environmental Artist Athena Tacha and fabricated by Architectural Glass Art. It is actually a series of fountains, running through multiple levels. A waterfall is positioned at the highest level, the water cascading down through the amphitheater before pouring into the main fountain at the base. Each element of the plaza responds to an overall spiral formation, reflected in the paving, which culminates at the star fountain.

Athena Tacha, born in Greece in 1936, received a masters in sculpture from the Athens School of Fine Arts in Greece as well as a masters in history from Oberlin College, Ohio and a doctorate in aesthetics from the Sorbonne. Tacha is best known for her environmental public sculpture, being one of the first artists to develop environmental, site specific sculpture in the early 1970s. In 1989, a retrospective of her sculptures, drawings and photography was held at the High Museum of Art in Atlanta.

Photos: Atspear / Wikimedia Commons

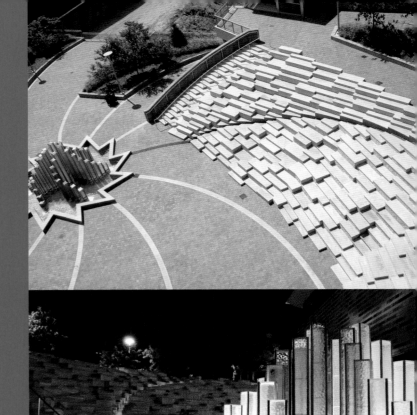

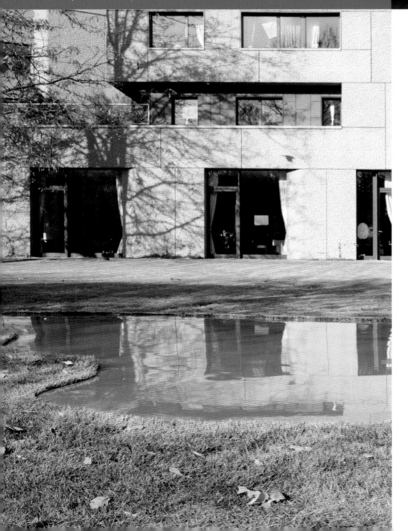

Reflecting Pool
Rainer Splitt

Completion: 2008. **Technique:** pigment, polyurethane. **Location:** Warsaw, Poland.

In the garden of the German Embassy, a giant sea of paint is sprawled across the ground. By pouring 1,600 kilograms of colored polyurethane compound, gravity and movement have created a soft-edged organic pool. The high-gloss surface appears to be of still liquid and the material seems to dissolve into its mirrored surroundings. The 'painting' evokes the movement of the viewer, helping in the simultaneous discovery of absence and presence, of fiction and reality.

Rainer Splitt was born in Celle in 1963 and studied in Brunswick, Nîmes and New York City. He has been awarded various prestigious grants and prizes including the Kunstfonds (Bonn) and the Rome Prize Villa Massimo. From 2007–2009 he was appointed as guest professor at the Karlsruhe Academy of Fine Arts. Splitt´s projects have been exhibited internationally in galleries and museums, and collected by numerous public institutions and private collections throughout Europe and the United States.

Photo: Courtesy Gallery Max Weber / Six Friedrich, Munich

Standortmitte
Lutz Fritsch

Completion: 2008. **Technique:** steel, lacquer. **Location:** Cologne and Bonn, Germany.

These sculptures stand on the two traffic islands at the beginning and end of the motorway between Cologne and Bonn. The two parts are identical in form, each 50 meters high, 90 centimeters in diameter and 22.5 kilometers away from each other. The artist intended that the observer could experience space and time, near and far, beginning and end. Both poles, which stand also as individual sculptures, can never both be seen at the same time. They are only brought together as a whole in the mind and feelings of the observer.

Lutz Fritsch was born in Cologne in 1955. He is most famous for his large sculpture "Rheinorange", located at the mouth of Rhine and Ruhr in Duisburg and the "Library in Ice", in Antarctica. His investigations of space in sculpture, drawings and photography have been exhibited at various museums and institutions both nationally and internationally. His works are represented in both public and private collections.

Photos: Lutz Fritsch, photographer: Eileen Maes

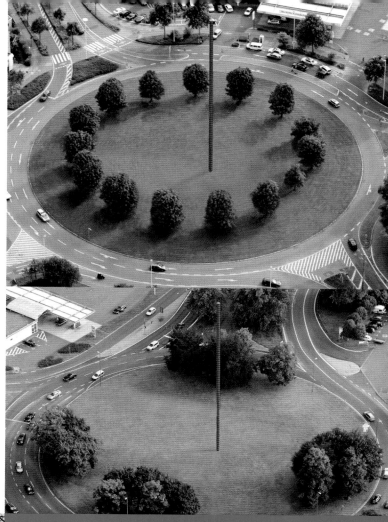

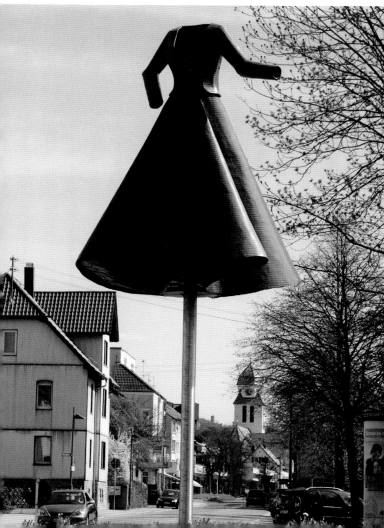

Way Marker
Anja Luithle

Completion: 2009. **Technique:** stainless steel, wire mesh, PU foam, laminated fiberglass. **Location:** Eislingen, Germany.

Anja Luithle's sculptures aim to subtly communicate the small and large occurrences of everyday life. The "Way Marker" can be seen from afar by the oncoming traffic. The sculpture stands in the middle of a roundabout, turning gently in the breeze. When it is still it indicates ambiguously in a random direction. The sculpture describes the endless circle of life, with it ambiguous choices, unexpected directions and reoccurring renewal, with all of its various opportunities.

Anja Luithle was born in Germany in 1968. She studied at the State Academy of Art in Stuttgart, graduating in 1995. She was awarded a prize for her artwork from the Stuttgart Art Academy in 1993 and a scholarship from the Art Foundation of Baden Württemburg in 1995. She has successfully exhibited work throughout Europe, including at the "Textile Structures" exhibition at the House of Modern Art in Austria and the "Four Walls" exhibition in Karlsruhe.

Photo: Chris van Uffelen

Suckling Calf
Astrid Hohorst

Completion: 2009. **Technique:** bronze. **Location:** Freiburg, Germany.

"Suckling Calf" is situated opposite the old Wiehre train station in Freiburg, Germany. It is entirely black, except for an oversized yellow tag in its ear. The tag reminds the observer of human control over animals, how we use them for food, for medical trials, or to work. The red of the base is a bright red, linking it deliberately to blood and the inevitable end faced by a calf. The calf stands with its head facing south-west and its rear facing the town.

Astrid Hohorst was born in Germany in 1961. She grew up around animals and many of her sculptures focus on her observations of animals in their natural environment. She first studied as a printer's apprentice before going on to attend the State Academy of Art in Karlsruhe, where she studied sculpture under professor Balkenhol. She has exhibited her work widely in both group and solo exhibitions, including at the Fluchtstab Gallery in Staufen im Breisgau.

Photos: Chris van Uffelen

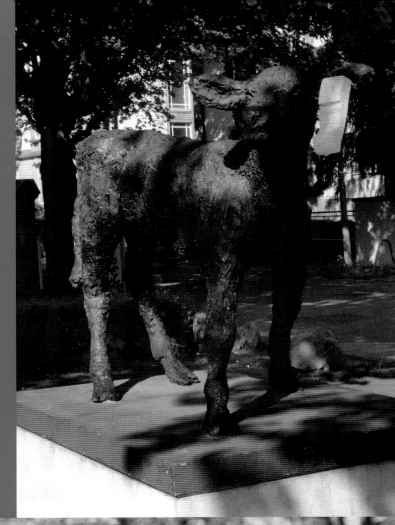

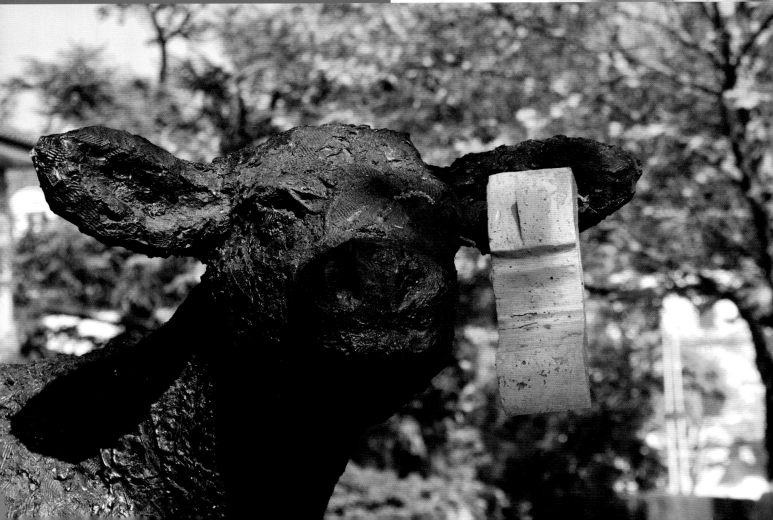

Inhale/Exhale
Phillip K Smith III

Completion: 2009. **Materials:** fiberglass, steel, concrete.
Location: La Verne, CA, USA.

This vertical fiberglass sculpture, designed as an inspiration for the student body, is a formal transformation between three identical equilateral triangles, alternately rotated 180 degrees. The form warps from its triangular faces to the tips of a triangle and back again, over ten integrated modules. The high-gloss surface reflects the surrounding environment and colors, creating an ever-changing skin as sun and the viewer move around the sculpture. Inhale/Exhale marks the University of La Verne's new Campus Center.

Phillip K Smith III explores and merges the boundaries of fine art, architecture and design. Born in Los Angeles, Smith earned a bachelor of architecture and bachelors of fine arts from Rhode Island School of Design. He confronts ideas of modern design and exploits new technologies to refine his art. An award-winning building designer, in recent years Smith has created various commissioned monumental public artworks across the USA. In 2012, Smith will install "Where the Earth and the Sky Meet," in Oklahoma City.

Photo: Courtesy of the artist

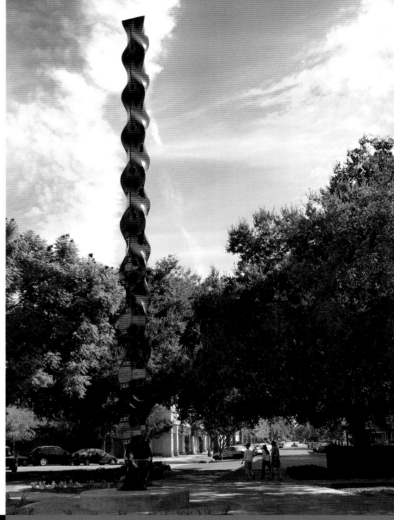

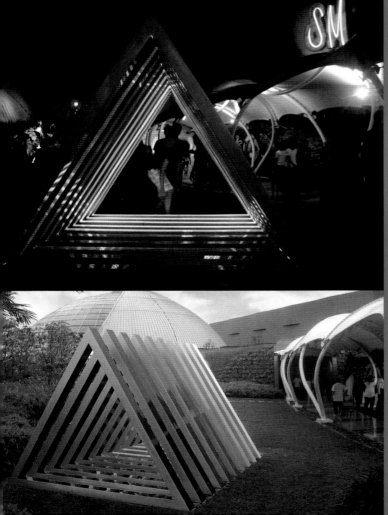

Prism 24
Joel Eugenio Epistola Ferraris

Completion: 2009. **Technique:** metal, polyester resin, paint, LED lights. **Location:** Quezon City, Philippines.

Prism 24 is located in the SM Sky Garden, SM North Edsa in Quezon City. It consists of an array of thin, prism-shaped sculpture pieces arranged to comprise a bigger prism, allowing viewers to see and play inside the inner portion of the whole tunnel-like structure. The interplay of the many contrasting colors from all surfaces show the colors of the rainbow and earth colors as well as the gradation from black to white. The work symbolizes 24 hours and reveals an interesting visual stimulus as people move around this piece of public art.

Joel Eugenio Epistola Ferraris is a self-taught artist. He studied studied architecture at the University of the Philippines. He has shown his work at five solo exhibitions and numerous group exhibitions and is director of the Ferraris Art Studio and vice chairman of the Hong Kong Mural Society. His recent projects include six interactive sculptures for the Sky Gardens in the Philippines.

Photos: joel e. ferraris

Almodóvar-Monument
Sergio García-Gasco Lominchar

Completion: 2009. **Technique:** dry, self-compacting concrete. **Location:** Castilla La Mancha, Spain.

This monument is situated in the hometown of Pedro Almodóvar, Calzada de Calatrava, in the heart of La Mancha. The competition for its design demanded that a link be forged between the birthplace of Almodóvar and his cinematographic work. The stepped form of the structure is inspired by a camera focus, as well as its shape, resolving at the same time the accessibility of the monument to be used as a meeting point or a place for concerts. The monument was constructed with dry self-compacting concrete, developed by Cemex.

Sergio arcía-Gasco Lominchar is a Spanish architect. He studied at the School of architecture of Valencia, Spain, where he graduated with honors in 2006. He currently holds a teaching and research position at this school. He has won various competitions, divided between the worlds of architecture and art. In 2005 he founded the studio Enproyecto Arquitectura, a multidisciplinary firm whose projects have received numerous awards, including the FAD national prize of architecture and the national award Valencia Crea.

Photos: Ricardo Santonja, Emilio Valverde

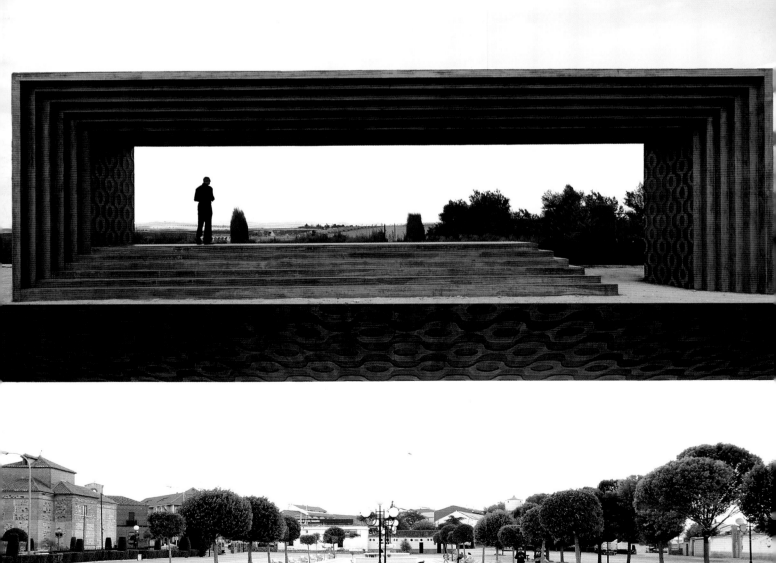

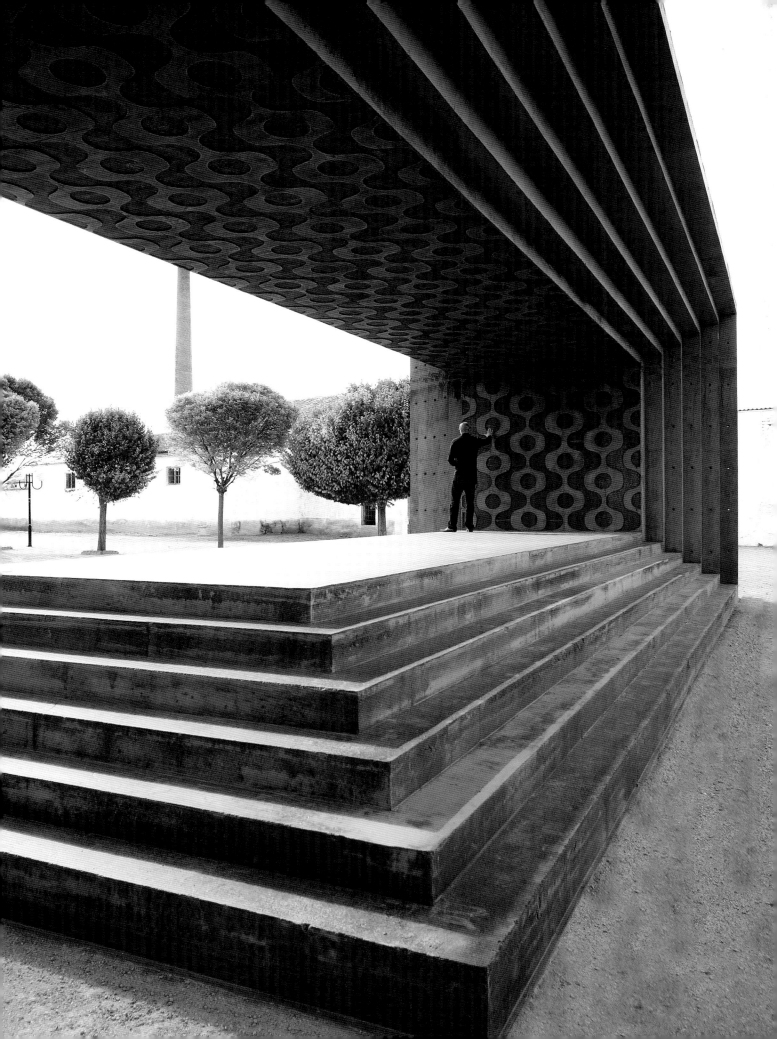

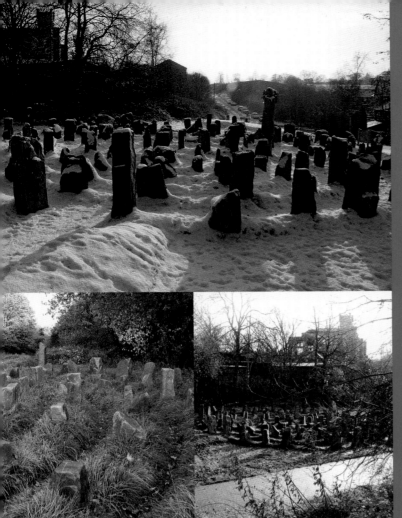

The Festival Labyrinth
Lorna Green, Jeff Teasdale

Completion: 2009. **Technique:** 150 Gritstone boulders and crushed stone, nine grasses. **Location:** Macclesfield, United Kingdom.

Lorna Green and Jeff Teasdale designed "The Festival Labyrinth", which was commissioned by and for the Bollington Festival 2009 in Cheshire, England. It also serves as a memorial to Dr. John Coope and the previous festivals he inspired. The labyrinth is constructed with local Kerridge boulders and crushed stone and has been planted with nine grasses, forming a wall between the boulders. This project was funded by the National Lottery Arts For All Awards and The Bollington Festival.

Lorna Green is a fellow of the Royal British Society of Sculptors and works mainly with public art and environmental projects. Her sculptures are site specific, considering the history, landscape and mythology of the area and mainly outdoors. Jeff Teasdale, artists-in-education, works with a variety of sculptural media, from installation pieces with stone and live willow, to smaller works using ceramics and found objects connected to the landscape around his home in the north-west of England.

Photos: Donald Judge (a.); Lorna Green (b. r., b. l.)

Optic Garden
26'10 south
Architects, Maja Marx

Completion: 2009. **Technique:** gum poles, road traffic signs, reflective tape. **Location:** Johannesburg, South Africa.

This project was commissioned by the Johannesburg Development Agency in the run up to the 2010 World Cup. The standard chevron sign is used as 'drawing material' with 195 signs planted to form an optic mass. As one rounds a bend in the approach road, the field of signs converges and aligns to reveal the outlines of a soccer playing field. Upon passing, the image fragments back into the individual signs – alluding to the temporary nature of sports events and their potential to bring people together.

26'10 south Architects is based in Johannesburg. Formed by Anne Graupner and Thorsten Deckler in 2004, the company works within diverse geographical, as well as social and economical scenarios – engaging equally in the inner-city, the suburb, informal settlements and the open landscape. Maja Marx is a Johannesburg based artist. She is known for her large scale works in South Africa and abroad, and is engaged in the optical study of landscape as experienced by the moving viewer. Her works can be seen in various South African Art Galleries.

Photo: John Hodgkiss, Johannesburg

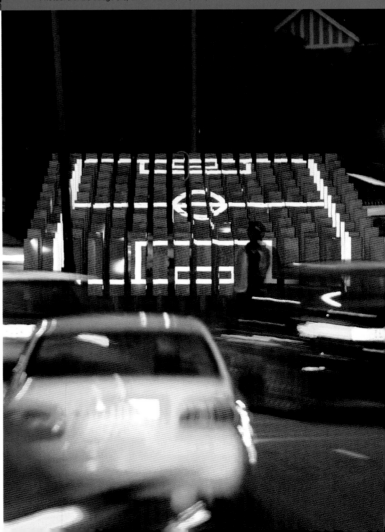

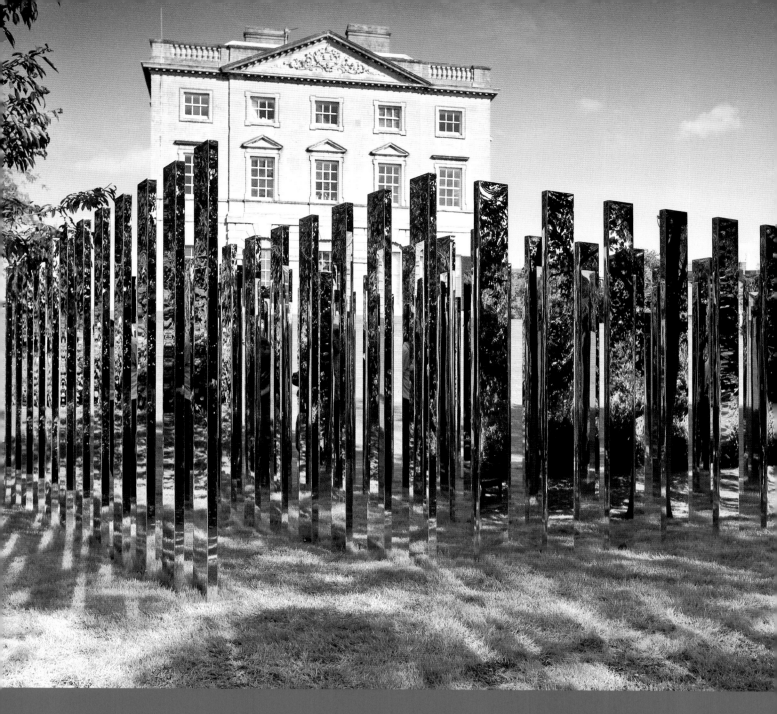

Follow Me
Jeppe Hein

Completion: 2009. **Technique:** steel frame, Alucobond, high-polished steel (super-mirror). **Location:** Bristol, United Kingdom.

Visitors enter this mirrored labyrinth at Bristol University and follow the corridor into the center of the square only to be lead out again. The mirrored surfaces reflect viewer, surrounding area and the other mirror lamellae. Actual space appears through the slots between individual lamellae, and is inserted between the mirror images. This multi-faceted reflection produces a fragmented view of the space, surrounding the viewer with an unfamiliar and disorientating situation similar to the experience of a labyrinth.

Jeppe Hein was born in 1974. He is an artist, based in Berlin and Copenhagen. He studied at the Royal Danish Academy of Fine Arts between 1997 and 2003 and at the Städel School in Frankfurt between 1999 and 2000. Hein is widely known for producing experiential and interactive artworks and has participated in many solo and group exhibitions including at the Tate Modern, London; Centre Pompidou, Paris and the Sculpture Center, New York. Hein is also cofounder of the Karriere Bar in Copenhagen, which features artworks by international artists.

Photo: Jamie Woodley, courtesy Johann König, Berlin, 303 Gallery, New York and Bristol University

Reflections > Expressions
BJ Krivanek

Completion: 2009. **Technique:** mirror-polished aluminum panels, powder-coated color, applied reflective icon graphics. **Location:** Chicago, IL, USA.

These iconographic works were created by artist BJ Krivanek and designed by Joel Breaux. They are situated above two train station platforms and comprise pivoting, mirror-polished sections. Reflections of the city are agitated and shattered by the wind and approaching trains. The fragments of symbols, icons and language shift, de-forming and re-forming. The forms show a perseverance of the creative process and the iconography is drawn from a spectrum of creative realms; visual, musical, scientific and literary.

BJ Krivanek is professor at the School of Art Institute of Chicago and principal of Krivanek+Breaux / Art+Design. His urban constructions and activations infiltrate the cityscape with metaphoric forms, integrating the languages of urban structures and spaces with the languages of communities. Krivanek has completed public commissions at the Union Rescue Mission and the 9/11 Memorial at LAX in Los Angeles. His work has been funded by the NEA and included in the National Design Triennial at the Cooper-Hewitt Museum.

Photos: Eric Craig Studios/ Chicago (a.); BJ Krivanek/ Chicago (b.)

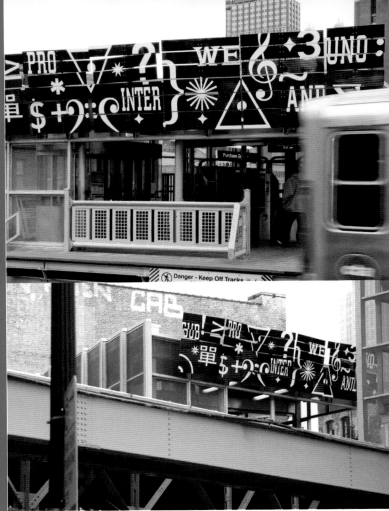

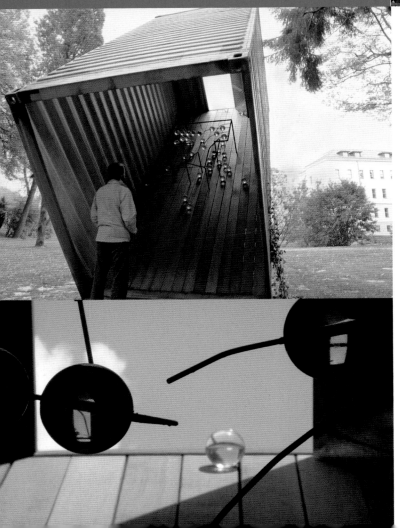

Memorial to the Victims of the Nazi Medical Trials
Dorothee Golz

Completion: 2009. **Technique:** steel, wood, acrylic glass. **Location:** Klosterneuburg, Austria.

This memorial is dedicated to the victims of Nazi medical trials. The central element is an old freight container, balanced at a 45-degree angle. When the viewer looks through the container the outline of a table and stool can be seen, as well as a broken chain of transparent spheres. The spheres symbolize a life cut short and more are strewn across the floor, to be considered together with the word "life". An open, steel door is set into the raised, short side of the container and gives an unobstructed view of the sky.

Dorothee Golz was born in Mülheim but has lived and worked in Vienna since 1988. She graduated from the School of Decorative Arts in Strasbourg in 1986, while at the same time studying art history and ethnology in Freiburg. Photography and drawing as well as sculptural works are important methods of artistic expression for Golz. She gained international fame after participating in the tenth Documenta, where she exhibited her sculpture, entitled "Hollow World", and a selection of drawings.

Photos: Courtesy of the artist

Animal Wall
Gitta Gschwendtner

Completion: 2009. **Technique:** woodcrete. **Location:** Cardiff Bay, United Kingdom.

Gschwendtner's design for this "Animal Wall" includes around 1,000 nest boxes for different bird and bat species, integrated into the fabric of the wall, separating this gated development from a public footpath. Through consultation with an ecologist, four different sized animal homes have been developed, which have been integrated in the custom made woodcrete cladding for the wall to provide an architecturally stunning and environmentally sensitive wall for Century Wharf.

Born in Germany in 1972, Gitta Gschwendtner moved to London in the early 1990s to study design at the Royal College of Art. Following graduation from the RCA in 1998, she set up her independent design studio for furniture, interior design and public art. Gschwendtner takes everyday objects and adds a touch of the unusual to provoke particular associations and memories in people. She has worked on shows for the Victoria and Albert Museum and the British Council.

Photo: Kiran Ridley

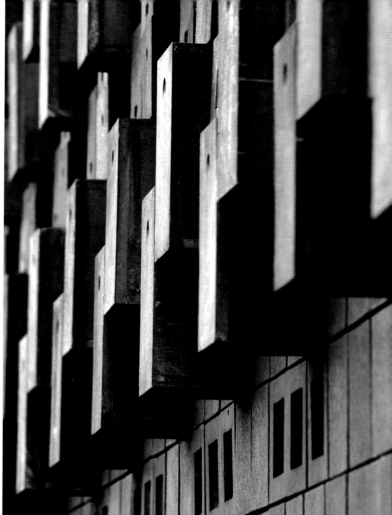

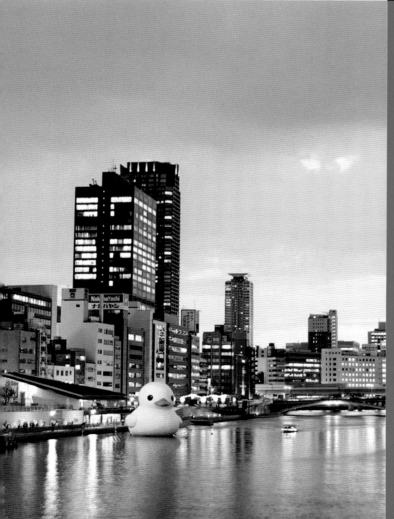

Rubber Duck
Florentijn Hofman

Completion: 2009. **Technique:** inflatable, pontoon, generator. **Location:** anywhere.

This international project by Dutch artist Florentijn Hofman aspires to be the most positive and even healing artistic statement in recent memory. Appearing in ten cities around the world, including Amsterdam, Nuremberg, São Paulo and Osaka. The "Rubber Duck", dubbed Bathzilla by some onlookers, knows no frontiers, it doesn't discriminate people and doesn't have a political connotation. It is, quite simply, what it is.

Florentijn Hofman attended the Christian Academy of Art in Kampen, where he graduated in 2000. Examples of his work include a 31-meter long straw muskrat, which was partly a satirical response to the muskrat being labeled a "big problem" in the Netherlands. Hofman sees the world as a huge playground and he can choose just about any spot or material in which to display his installations. The Loire river in France was the starting point of a project that ultimately became the giant rubber duck.

Photo: courtesy Florentijn Hofman, Osaka 2009

Garden of Hope
Jason deCaires Taylor

Completion: 2009. **Technique:** cement casting. **Location:** Cancun, Mexico.

The "Garden of Hope", depicts a young girl lying on a square of patio steps, cultivating a variety of plant pots. The sculpture lies four meters below water, in the National Marine Park, Cancun. The empty pots are planted with live coral cuttings, taken from areas of the reef damaged by storm or human activity. With this piece, the sculptor aims to promote a message of hope, portraying human intervention as positive. The young girl symbolizes a new, revitalized symbiosis with the environment.

Jason deCaires Taylor was born in 1974. He graduated from the London Institute of Art in 1998. Before working as a sculptor Taylor worked as a scuba diving instructor, this led to a strong interest in conserving underwater habitats. Experience working in Canterbury Cathedral taught him traditional stone carving techniques, which he later put to use in producing sculpture. Taylor is also the creator of the world's first, underwater sculpture park, bringing together science and art to preserve habitats.

Photo: Courtesy of the artist

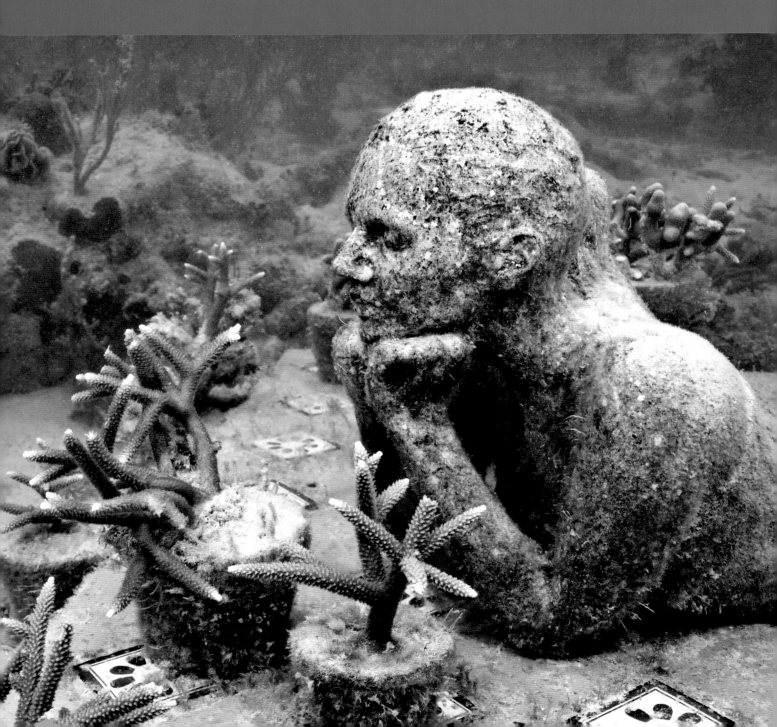

Haboob
Toma Gabor

Completion: 2009. **Technique:** fabricated steel. **Location:** Dubai, United Arab Emirates.

This work by Toma Gabor is designed not to take a concrete form and shape, but to change depending on the perspective of the viewer. Rather than a concrete shape, which can be seen and recorded in just a side glance, "Haboob" is reminiscent of a whirlwind, a swirling cloud that moves with the wind, light and fleet. The thin form of the metal work doesn't impose itself on the viewer or on the space, but announces possibility to passersby, changing in shape and form as they walk past.

Toma Gabor was born in 1966 in Trâgu-Mures, a town in the north of Romania, famous for its medieval architecture and significant traces of the Austro-Hungarian Empire. Gabor moved to the south of the country, to Bucharest, to study visual art and sculpture. Since then he has also visited Italy to study the Renaissance and Ancient Heritage. Gabor has exhibited work in Dubai and Romania and currently lives and works in Dubai.

Photo: Courtesy of the artist

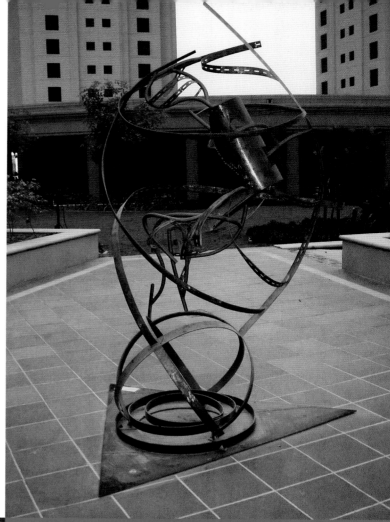

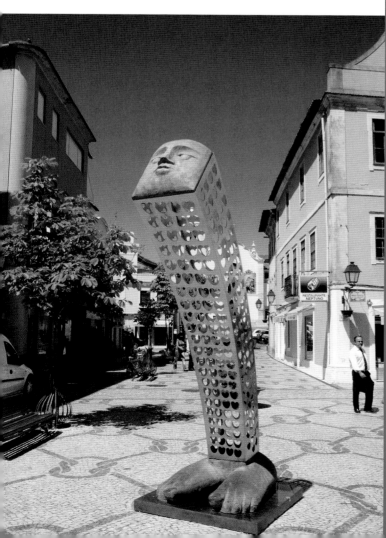

Man of the Future
Luis Queimadela

Completion: 2009. **Technique:** stainless steel, bronze, black granite. **Location:** Aveiro, Portugal.

This sculpture is called "Man of the Future", by Portuguese artist Louis Queimadela and depicts a figure with a face and feet. The body shape in between has no arms and legs. The face and feet are defined but the body is suggestive of something unfinished, a work in progress that can evolve into anything. The transparent nature of the body also aids the idea of possibility. The figure is not concrete but changeable. It is made of stainless steel, bronze and black granite and belongs to the city of Alveiro.

Louis Queimadela is a Portuguese artist who lives and works in Sao Pedro Do Sul. Queimadela has been working in the field of visual arts for over 30 years, particularly in the fields of painting and sculpture. He has over 20 public sculptures installed in various cities, museums and universities as well as works in private collections throughout Portugal.

Photo: Verarte Gallery

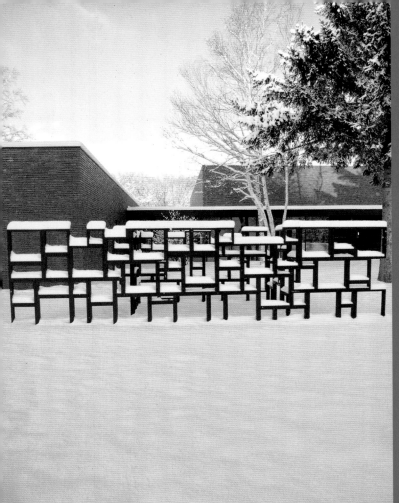

Emerging Landscape
Ryo Yamada

Completion: 2009. **Technique:** wood. **Location:** Sapporo, Japan.

This artwork is located on the northernmost island of Japan and made entirely of a set of frames. The concept is to capture the surrounding landscape. This is a space that functions not only as exterior but also interior space. There is no clear process or direction, from which to look or to enter. The changing perspective as the viewer moves changes the framed image. This allows the observer to focus on different parts of the surrounding, contemplating parts instead of the whole.

Ryo Yamada is a Japanese artist and architect. He was born in Tokyo in 1968 and educated at the Shibaura Institute of Technology, where he graduated in architectural design. He later studied art at the Tokyo University of the Arts. Yamada was awarded the Good Design Award, Japan in 2010 and the American Society Landscape Design Award in 2004.

Photo: Courtesy of the artist

Silvas Capitalis
Simparch

Completion: 2009. **Technique:** European larch. **Location:** Kielder Forest, United Kingdom.

This monumental wooden head is situated in Kielder Forest, located near the Scottish border in England. Large enough to enter into, with stairs to a second level, "Silvas Capitalis" is a pavilion for those passing through this working forest. Inspired by the history of this once fiercely contested border, and by the often anonymous, body-less Celtic Gods of Britain, this large icon induces an amplification of anthropology and myth.

Simparch is an artist collaborative begun in 1996. Uniting all of Simparch's projects is an overarching interest in the work's social potential. They specialize in creating large-scale works that take into account the specificities and histories of a given site. Simparch works to highlight how popular artistic and architectural languages, iconographies and concerns intersect.

Photos: Steve Rowell

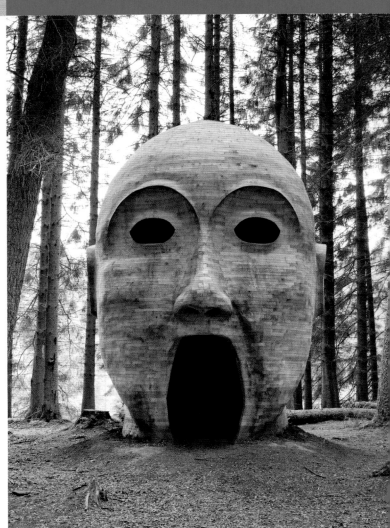

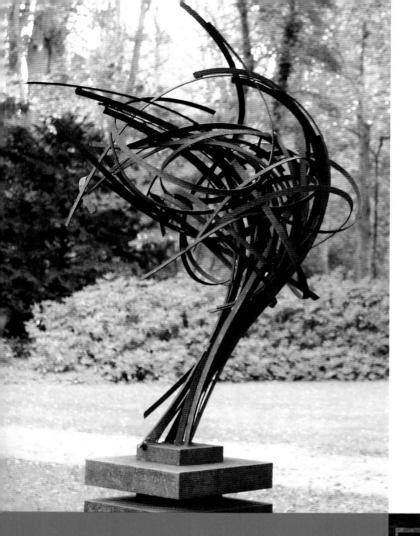

La Girouette
Kees Machielsen

Completion: 2009. **Technique:** Corten steel. **Location:** Aalsmeer, The Netherlands.

This artwork is inspired by the shape of a cockerel's plumage and intends to produce something delicate from steel. In contrast to large sculptures, solid masses of fixed shape, this work is changeable, providing the viewer with a different view when looked at from different angels and perspectives. The delicate-looking stands of the work protrude at different angles. By working and bending the steel, the artist attempts to master it, to control it with human power.

Kees Machielsen is a Dutch sculptor. He first began work as a blacksmith in 1982, setting up his own business in 1983. It wasn't until 2000 that he began working part time as a sculptor, from his own studio in Oirschot, while simultaneously working in a print shop. In 2008 he began working full time as a sculptor and blacksmith. Machielsen's work is often inspired by nature and natural forms, he creates abstract, dynamic sculpture based on what he sees.

Photo: Courtesy of the artist

The Interchange
Larry Kirkland

Completion: 2009. **Technique:** carved and engraved granite.
Location: El Paso, TX, USA.

"The Interchange" connects two buildings of a new Medical School for Texas Tech University. The pathway is engraved with the double helix of DNA. Sculptural elements of carved granite have been placed along the path, two are thresholds, defined by the image of a human head. Images of human anatomy are engraved on the granite keyholes and images of the tools of life are hidden within the floral pattern of the head. The work serves as a reminder: know the science but also know your patient as an individual.

Larry Kirkland has created over 150 large-scale, site specific installations, commissioned all over the world. Ranging from Hong Kong Central Station, to Iwate University in Japan, the American Red Cross Headquarters in Washington D.C. and the California Science Center in Los Angeles, California. Kirkland's projects are all conceived for the public realm. With his work he aims to bring an element of the unexpected to public space, making it interesting and challenging to the observer and user.

Photo: Shayne Hensley, Woodstock Georgia

In-Flux
James Brenner

Completion: 2009. **Technique:** Corten steel, glass, fiberoptic light. **Location:** Minneapolis, MN, USA .

"In-Flux" is created with steel, glass and light and explores the relationship between the internal and external form. Up close the external mass dominates. The ordered slicing of the form expresses the protective armor of the exterior. The internally illuminated glass form is revealed at a distance: a flowing jewel conveying inspiration, creativity and openness. What is revealed or concealed is in flux and depends on the viewer's vantage point. This is a site specific sculpture that relates to the community.

James Brenner is the director of Chicago Sculpture Works and a core artist for the Chicago Public Art Group. He received his masters of fine arts in Sculpture from the School of the Art Institute of Chicago. He has exhibited internationally and has sculptures in the collections of the Nathan Manilow Sculpture Park, Alfred University, New York Mills Sculpture Park, City of Chicago, Village of Wilmette, City of Minneapolis, City of Evanston, Smurfit Stone Corp, Ceridian Corp.

Photos: Sean Smuda

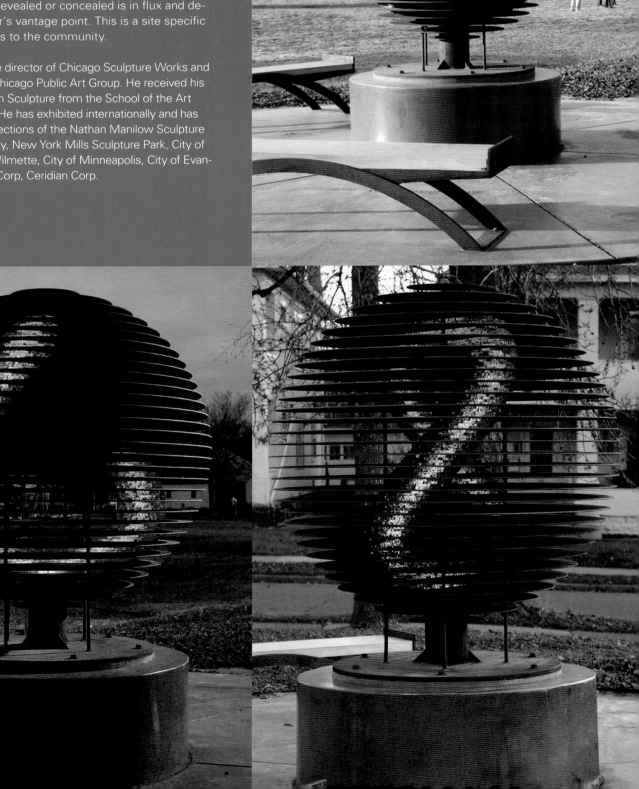

Quincy Court
Rios Clementi Hale Studios

Completion: 2009. **Technique:** steel, translucent acrylic panels, white granite. **Location:** Chicago, IL, USA.

The aim of Rios Clementi Hale Studios was to transform a street into a sculptural gathering place. The plaza features seven, tree-like canopy elements made of steel and three tones of translucent acrylic panels that are lit from above. Influenced by local honey locusts, the trees are rooted by sandblasted concrete in an abstracted leaf pattern. Concrete benches and translucent resin tables, glowing with inner lighting, rest on granite pavers. Four large leaves are seemingly scattered on the pavement.

Rios Clementi Hale Studios was established in 1985 and has since developed an international reputation for its collaborative and multi-disciplinary approach, establishing an award-winning tradition across a range of design disciplines. The designers at Rios Clementi Hale Studios create buildings, places, and products that are thoughtful, effective, and striking.

Photo: Scott Shigley, Chicago, IL

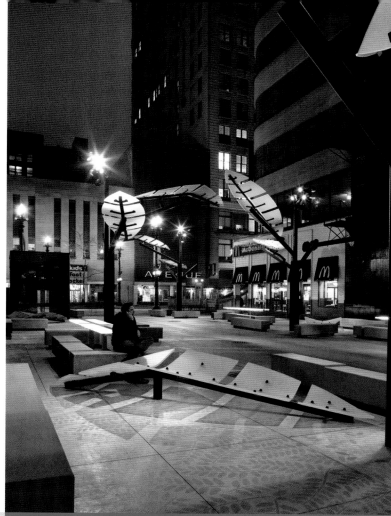

Sugar Beach
Claude Cormier, architectes paysagistes inc.

Completion: 2009. **Technique:** fiberglass umbrellas, granite bedrock with thermoplastic stripes. **Location:** Toronto, Canada.

"Sugar Beach" is made up of three distinct spaces, united by a singular conceptual reference taken from the sugar factory across the slip. The granite-paved maple-lined promenade offers a shaded route to the water's edge, with many opportunities along the way to enjoy the view. Diverse topography, offered by the candy-striped bedrock and grassy berms, provides points of elevation to view the space and surrounding lake and city context.

Claude Cormier is a second-generation Conceptualist landscape architect based in Montreal, Canada. He is a graduate of Harvard's Graduate School of Design, and studied landscape architecture at the University of Toronto and agronomy at the University of Guelph. Cormier was recently selected as an emerging voice for North America by the Architectural League of New York, as well as one of 14 international designers advancing the design field by Fast Company magazine.

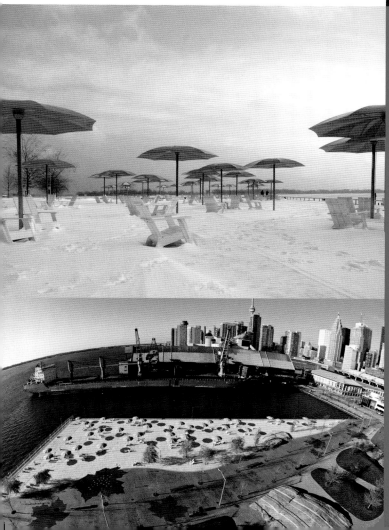

Photos: Toronto Waterfront (a.); Jessie Jackson (b.)

Poly Stella
Carsten Nicolai

Completion: 2009. **Technique:** stainless steel on alucubond, steel structure, concrete pedestal. **Location:** Tokyo, Japan.

Carsten Nicolai's work "Poly Stella" was commissioned for the public space at new square in front of Kasumigaseki Building in Chiyoda-ku, Tokyo, Japan. Its shape is a complex polyhedron. Although it seems rather manifold, the shape consists of a composition put together with a large amount of just one single element. It is thus a striking example of how a rather simple structure can lead to an extremely complex system. The sculpture operates as a prominent landmark to signify the space surrounding it.

Carsten Nicolai was born in 1965 in Karl Marx Stadt, Germany, now called Chemnitz, and is interested in various media, such as sound, image, sculpture and installation. Nicolai's work focuses on human perception, works with error and coincidence and questions artistic creative power. His fascination with natural phenomena, mathematics and physics has become an integral part of his artistic output as he considers nature as a creative power, an erratic entity that man still does not fully understand.

Photo: Daniel Klemm, Berlin; courtesy of Galerie EIGEN + ART Leipzig / Berlin and The Pace Gallery

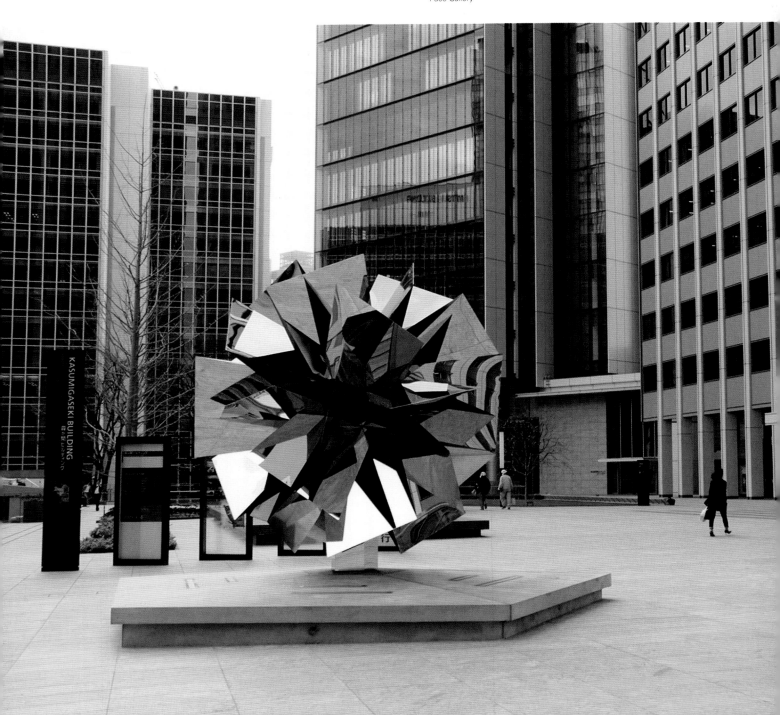

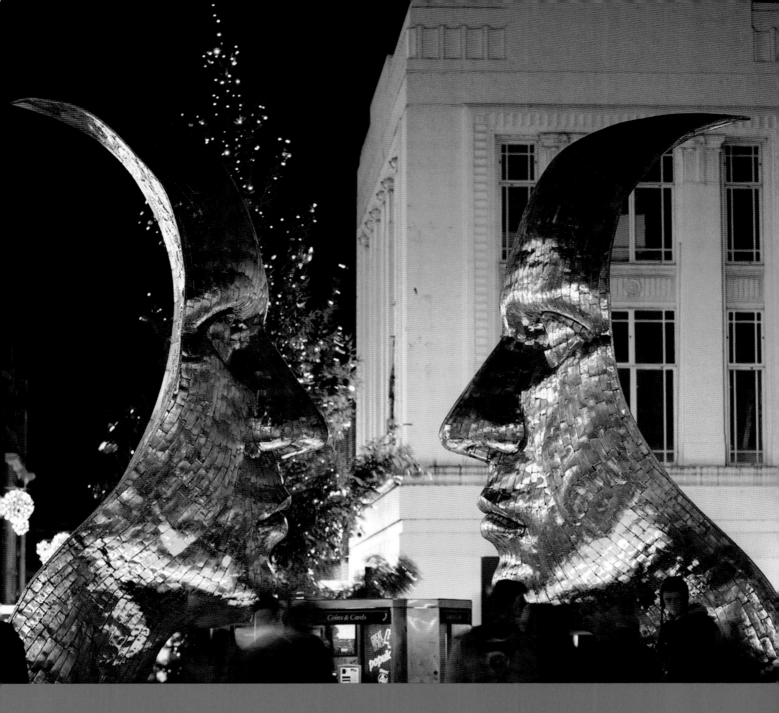

Reflections of Bedford
Rick Kirby

Completion: 2009. **Technique:** stainless steel. **Location:** Bedford, United Kingdom.

These two stainless steel sculptures "Reflections of Bedford", some six meters tall, act as a 'gateway' to the pedestrianized area in Silver Street. The faces refer to Bedford's rich multi-cultural population and its reputation for cross-cultural peace and harmony. These faces look at each other in friendship, respect and understanding.

Rick Kirby is a British sculptor, based in Hertfordshire. He studied at the Somerset College of Arts and Technology, Newport College of Art and Birmingham University. He has received several awards for his sculptural works, including first prize at the Essex Open and the Rouse Kent Public Art Award. Kirby has around 30 sculptures displayed in public place in locations all over the United Kingdom.

Photo: Clever Captures

283

Spitalfields Spirit
Paul Cox

Completion: 2009. **Technique:** plastic. **Location:** London, United Kingdom.

Paul Cox created this sculpture for the Spitalfields Public Art project. The rabbits are located in Bishop's Square and were created to pay homage to the areas history, going right back to the days when the space where the rabbits are now located was a grazing ground for cattle. The tight-knit group of grazing rabbits suggests a sense of community, creating a place for children to play and acting as a discussion point.

Paul Cox is an award-winning sculptor specializing in metal and ceramics. His work is represented internationally in private and public commissions. A nine-ton boat sculpture of Cox's was recently sold to the Cafesijian Museum in Armenia. Cox was awarded the Henry Moore scholarship, allowing him to study postgraduate sculpture at the Royal Academy Schools, London. He now lives and works in Newhaven where he works on one-off commissions and limited edition production pieces.

Photo: Rob Sandiford

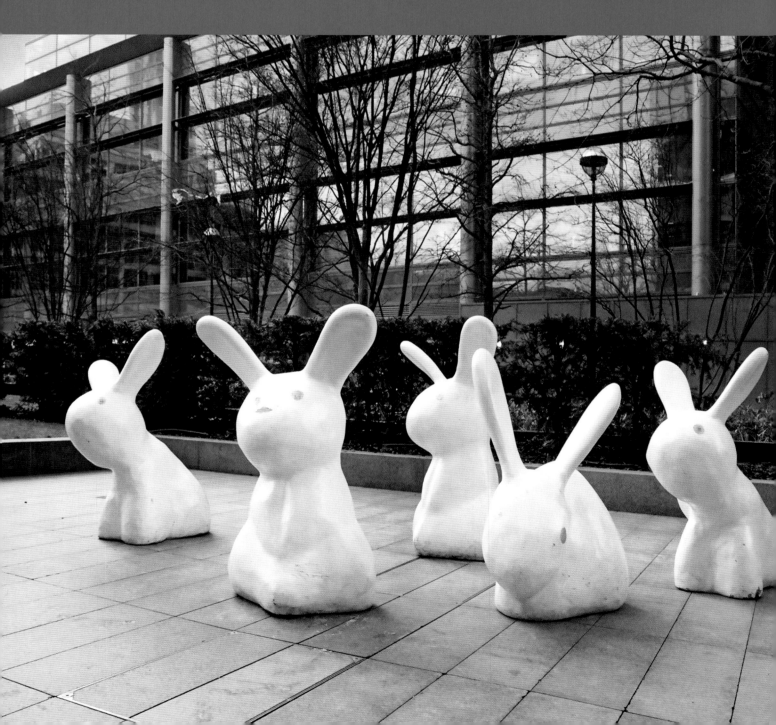

The Lost Bark of Urschanabi
Suter & Bult

Completion: 2009. **Technique:** iron, gauze, cement, lime, wood.
Location: Rantum, Germany.

Urschanabi is the ferryman of the immortal flood hero Utnapischtim in the Epic of Gilgamesh. Urschanabi must row Gilgamesh, who is on a quest to gain eternal life, across The Waters of Death to the immortal Utnapischtim. The Waters of Death can only be crossed using special ores made of stone. However, Gilgamesh destroyed these in a battle, forcing him to make 120 new ores out of wood. Each of these will only last for one paddle stroke, as they become unusable as soon as they touch the water.

Pascal Suter, born 1962 in Basel, is a self-taught sculptor who assisted at the workshop of his father Paul Suter in the 1980s. In 1997 he had his first exhibition, together with Christiane Bult. Christiane Bult, born in Basel in 1957, studied photography 1976–77 and she received her masters from University of Basel in 1990. She is largely a self-taught sculptor and had her first exhibition in 1995. Since 1997 Suter and Bult have had several interior and exterior exhibitions, both as individuals and together.

Photos: Courtesy of the artist

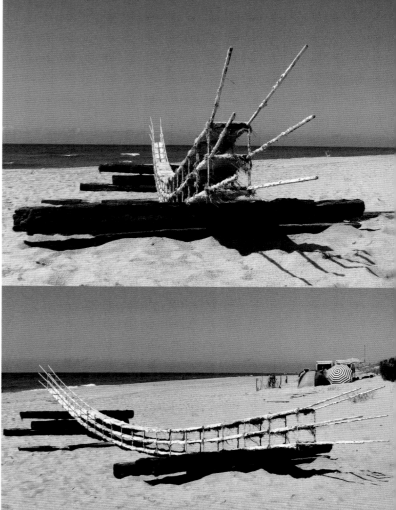

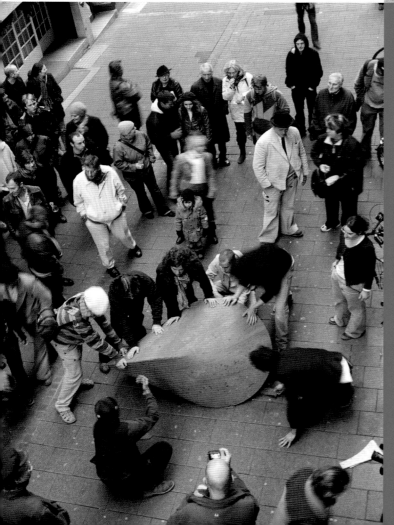

Oloid-Week
Hildegard von Homeyer, Claudia Winkler

Completion: 2009. **Technique:** Lahr sandstone. **Location:** Liestal, Switzerland.

These two stonemasons, together with colleagues from France, Germany and Switzerland, worked on a collaborative project at the Rüdenplatz in Basel, where they in turns made an "Oloid" form from a block. The "Oloid" is the only form that develops its entire surface when rolling. After being finished, the "rolling stone" was presented during a weekend in a nearby café, despite its weight of about one ton, the object still moves easily. The work was conceived in conjunction with the Paul Schatz Foundation.

Hildegard von Homeyer was born in 1983 and learned stonemasonry in the workshop of the Berner Münster. As a freelance sculptor, her work deals with questions about inverting the cube and exploring the form of the oloid. Since 2009 she has been traveling the world, working as a travelling apprentice. Claudia Winkler was born in 1983 and earned her qualification as stonemason at the Compagnons du devoir in Bordeaux. Since 2004 she has worked on the restoration of historic monuments as well as several pedagogic working projects.

285

Photos: Courtesy of the artist

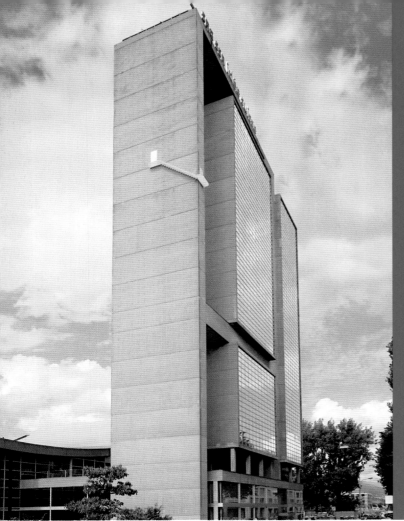

Beautiful Steps #2
Lang/Baumann

Completion: 2009. **Technique:** steel, anodized aluminum.
Location: Biel-Bienne, Switzerland.

The intervention on the façade of the Palais des Congrès was created for the Sculpture Exhibition "Utopics" and remained as a permanent piece of the city's art collection. Between two joins in the concrete wall, 36 meters above the ground, two fake doors are connected by steps. What might appear as a real architectural solution becomes doubtful when the viewer recognizes that the handrails are missing: doors and steps loose their function, becoming a form shifting between art and reality.

Lang/Baumann is Sabina Lang, born in Berne, Switzerland in 1972 and Daniel Baumann, born in 1967 in San Francisco, USA. Based in Switzerland, the two artists have been working jointly under the name Lang/Baumann or L/B since 1990. Their installations, inflatables and "real work" sculptures often have a functional aspect, such as the "Hotel Everland", a mobile structure that was placed on the roof of the Palais de Tokyo in 2007.

Photo: Courtesy of the artist

Milk Heat
Tue Greenfort

Completion: 2009. **Technique:** radiator, water pipe. **Location:** Knislinge, Sweden.

"Milk Heat" invites visitors to experience the heat of fresh milk through a conventional radiator, placed on an organic farm. The milk's heat is transferred to the building's central heating system. Livestock are responsible for 18 per cent of the greenhouse gases that cause global warming, more than cars, planes and all other forms of transport put together. The artist attempts to visualize the impact animal farming has on the environment – whether organic or not. The artist questions the sustainability of today's intensified dairy production.

Tue Greenfort was born in Holbaeck, Denmark in 1973 and currently lives and works in Berlin. He has participated in numerous international individual and group exhibitions, at the Royal Academy of Arts, London, Bonniers Konsthall, Stockholm, Secession Vienna, Witte de With, Rotterdam, Skulptur Projekte Münster and Made in Germany, Hanover 2007, amongst others.

Photos: Anders Norrsell; Courtesy Wanås Foundation, Knislinge

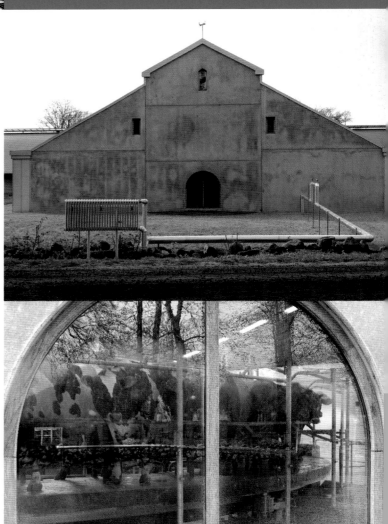

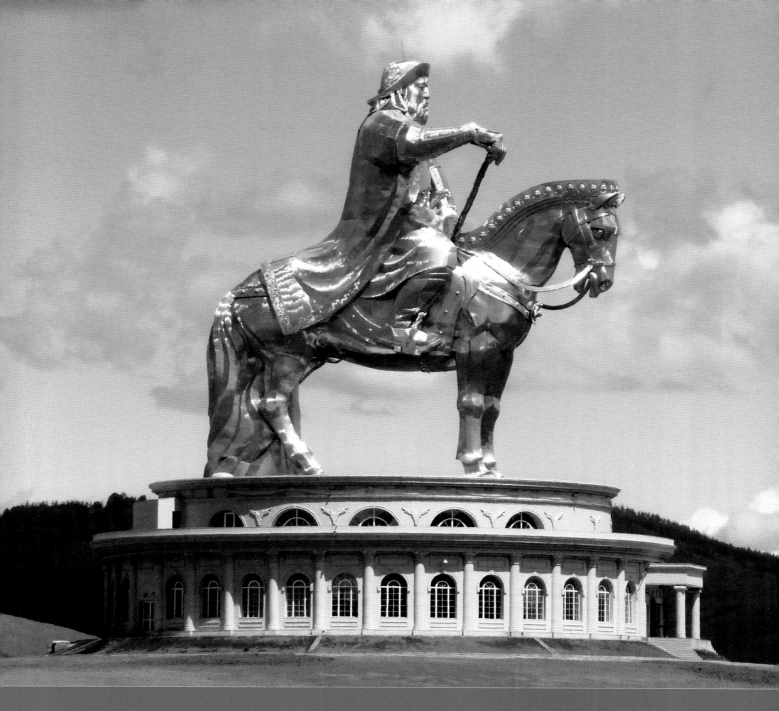

Genghis Kahn Equestrian Statue
D. Erdembileg, J. Enkhjargal

Completion: 2009. **Technique:** stainless steel, concrete. **Location:** Tsonjin Boldog, Mongolia.

This huge statue of Genghis Khan is 40 meters in height, standing on a ten-meter-high base, making it the tallest equestrian statue in the world. It is located in the place where, as legend has it, Genghis Kahn found a golden whip. The base consists of 36 columns, which serve as a memorial to the 36 kings that ruled the country between Genghis Kahn and Ligdan Kahn.

Sculptor D. Erdembileg and architect J. Enkhjargal made this statue. It is a sign of Mongolia's pride of the achievements of Ghengis Kahn. Though he is viewed unfavorably by large parts of the world, looked upon as a genocidal warlord whose military campaigns involved the massacre of civilian populations, Kahn also advanced the Mongolia Empire. He is said to have promoted religious tolerance and united many of the tribes of north-east Asia. He is revered among the Mongols because of his association with Mongol statehood and victory.

Arria
Andy Scott

Completion: 2010. **Technique:** galvanized steel. **Location:** Glasgow, United Kingdom.

This sculpture in Cumbernauld overlooks the M80 motorway in central Scotland. The design is based on the original meaning of Cumbernauld, the Gaelic "cumer nan allt", which means the coming together of waters. The female figure, with swooping arcs representing the waters, is ten meters in height and was constructed in 15 sections. She was fabricated in a welded mosaic of thousands of small sections of steel plates. The poem "Watershed", written by Jim Carruth, appears in steel letters on the base of the sculpture.

Andy Scott is a graduate of Glasgow School of Art and an Associate of the Royal British Society of Sculptors. To date he has created over 70 public sculptures and architectural detailing commissions, in a variety of media for a broad range of international clients. The practice is based on the creation of recognizable objects. Scott strives to create works that operate on varying levels of interpretation. His distinctive aesthetic combines traditional sculptural dexterity with contemporary fabrication techniques.

Photo: Steve Lindridge

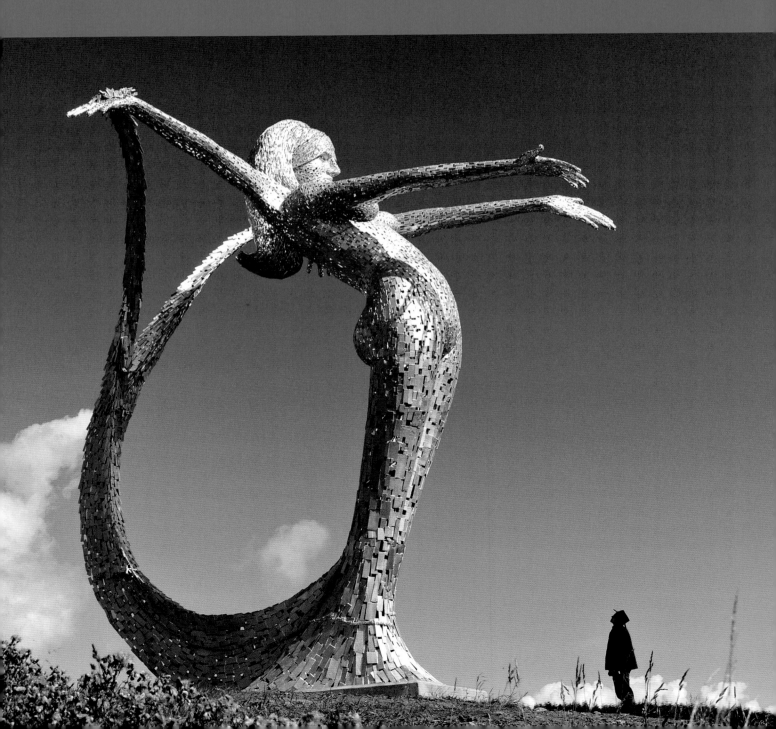

Industry-Culture
Rüdiger Stanko

Completion: 2010. **Technique:** aluminum panel with wooden frame, paint. **Location:** Heidenheim, Germany.

This colorful project was created with the help of residents and visitors in the Heidenheim area. Artist Rüdiger Stanko collected color and quantitative data and then interpreted this into the specific colors used in the sculpture. The colors reference the history and identity of the city's residents, who were asked to select colors associated with the words "culture" and "industry". The sculpture becomes symbolic of the democratic process, with decisions being made by the town, not by the artist.

Rüdiger Stanko was born in Groß-Gerau in 1958. He studied at the University of Art in Brunswick, graduating in 1985. Various examples of his work are on display in public space. His works are like colorful group portraits, expressing the particular preferences of a group of people. The colors of his sculptures are always democratically selected by gathering information through interviews and the titles of his works correspond to the specific theme: "Colors of the Future", "Colors of Home", "Colors of Luck". Stanko currently lives and works in Hanover.

Photo: Chris van Uffelen

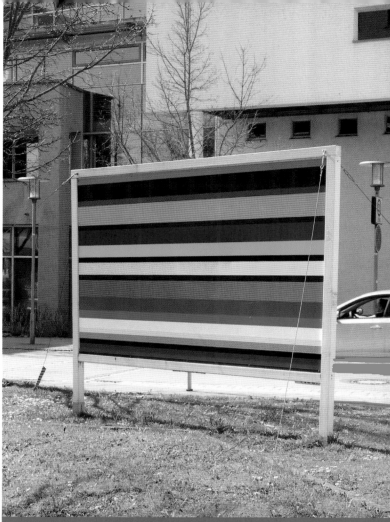

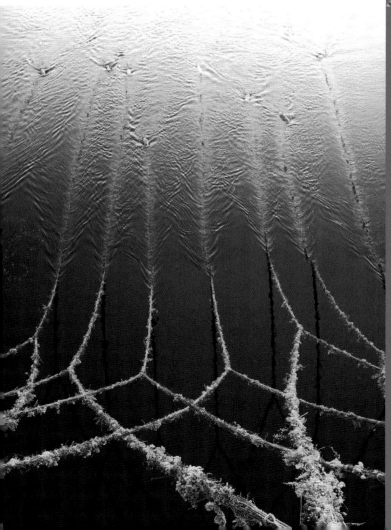

Eau Claire Currents
Roy Frank Staab

Completion: 2010. **Technique:** wild plantes, five ply jute cord, wood logs. **Location:** Eau Claire, WI, USA.

This site specific sculpture is suspended from the middle of the footbridge. The artist and students gathered wild plants and bundled them into lines, before pulling them up and into place from the river's edge. The repeated Y- shaped lines, five meters apart, layered patterns in the air before they junction into a single line and touch the water. Torpedo shaped logs on the ends are pulled and moved in a subtle way by the strong Chippewa River current.

Roy Frank Staab, born in 1941, attended Layton School of Art and received a bachelor of fine arts from UWM in 1969. He had his first professional exhibition in 1977 that permitted his work to be acquired by Museum of Modern Art, Paris and the National Foundation of Contemporary Art, Paris. He began installation art in 1979 in the south of France. In 1980 Staab moved to New York City exhibiting works-on-paper, collected by the Metropolitan Museum of Art, New York. He began to create site specific installations in nature only using all natural materials.

Photo: Courtesy of the artist

Broken Light
Daglicht & Vorm

Completion: 2010. **Technique:** halide lamps, projection light units, light and shadow. **Location:** Rotterdam, The Netherlands.

The starting point of this lighting project was a study of the duality of light - the meaning of light versus the experience of light in public places. The designers created a new optical system where the lighting creates vertical and horizontal light patterns. Together they form a total light effect, which changes constantly as the spectator follows the path. The intention of "Broken light" is to focus on the mutual influence of more types of perception, making the spectator conscious of his position as observer.

Daglicht & Vorm is a Dutch lighting design company, which investigates the possibilities of artificial and natural light. The firm takes on all aspects of the design process, from idea to concept. Dutch designer and visual artist Rudolf Teunissen founded the company. He works on lighting projects for retail and healthcare organizations as well as designing and realizing art projects in public space. The Luminare was made partnership with Thomas Linders and Marinus van der Voorden

Photo: Hans Wilschut

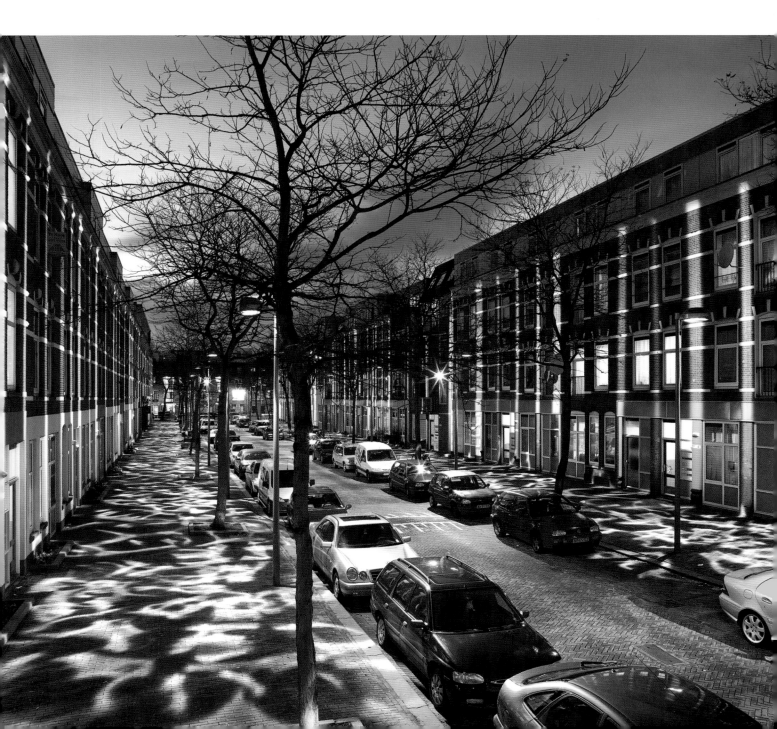

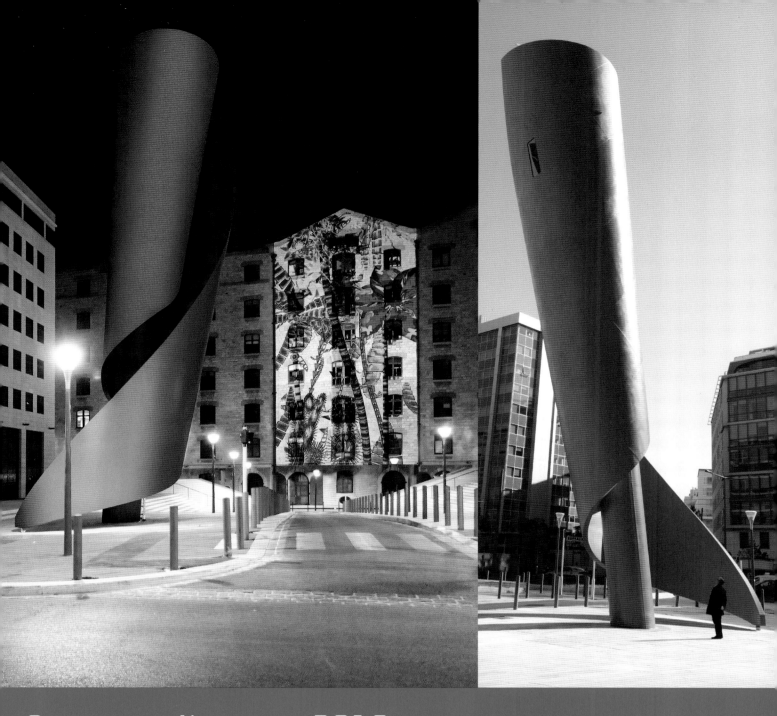

Seconde Nature 2010
Miguel Chevalier with Charles Bové

Completion: 2010. **Technique:** steel, 3 videoprojectors, PC, infrared sensor. **Location:** Marseille, France.

"Seconde Nature 2010" was commissioned by the Public Commission for Marseille-Provence 2013, European Capital of Culture commissioned by Euroméditerranée and is an 18-meters orange sculpture, whose shape is reminiscent of a shell or the large sail of a boat. As such, this sculpture is a strong sign in this urban space. Every evening a new interactive, virtual garden is projected from the sculpture onto surrounding warehouses, using Music2eye software. This virtual garden grows in an infinite variety of ways and changes following the cycle of the seasons.

Miguel Chevalier was born in Mexico City in 1959, but has been based in Paris since 1985. He graduated from the School of Fine Arts in Paris in 1981 and went on to study at the School of Decorative Arts. After graduating, he was awarded the Lavoisier scholarship and studied at the Pratt Institute, New York. Since 1978, he has focused exclusively on computers as a means of artistic expression. Chevalier continues to be a trailblazer and has proven himself one of the most significant artists on the contemporary scene.

Photos: Courtesy of the artist

The Blue Guardians
The Cracking Art Group

Completion: 2010. **Technique:** polyethylene. **Location:** Erbusco, Italy.

In 2009, the Cà del Bosco winery asked the Cracking Art Group to come up with an image of an animal, which could be presented as a group within the estate. The installation developed spontaneously, because the guardian of the vineyard requires the company of its pack to allow it to exalt its cautious role. "The Blue Guardians" observe the hillside where the visitors appear, keeping their watchful position. They resemble a diligent army, contrasting the green of the natural composition of the landscape.

The Cracking Art Group consists of Renzo Nucara, Marco Veronese, Alex Angi, Carlo Rizzetti, Kicco and William Sweetlove. Six international artists who, since the birth of Cracking Art Movement in 1993, underline the group's intention to change art history through both a strong social and environmental commitment and the revolutionary and innovative use of different plastic technique that evoke a strict relationship between natural life and artificial reality.

Photos: Tommaso Trojani

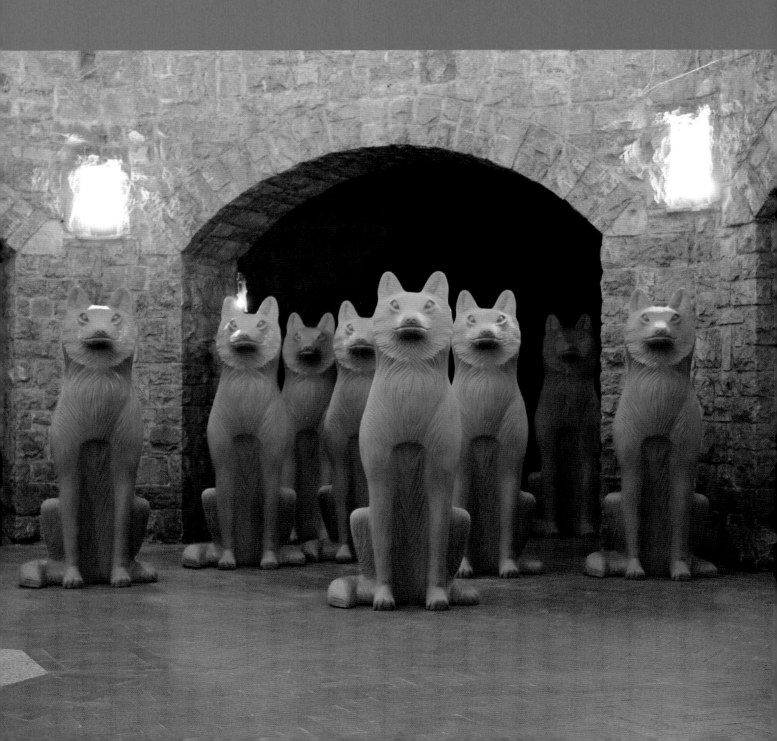

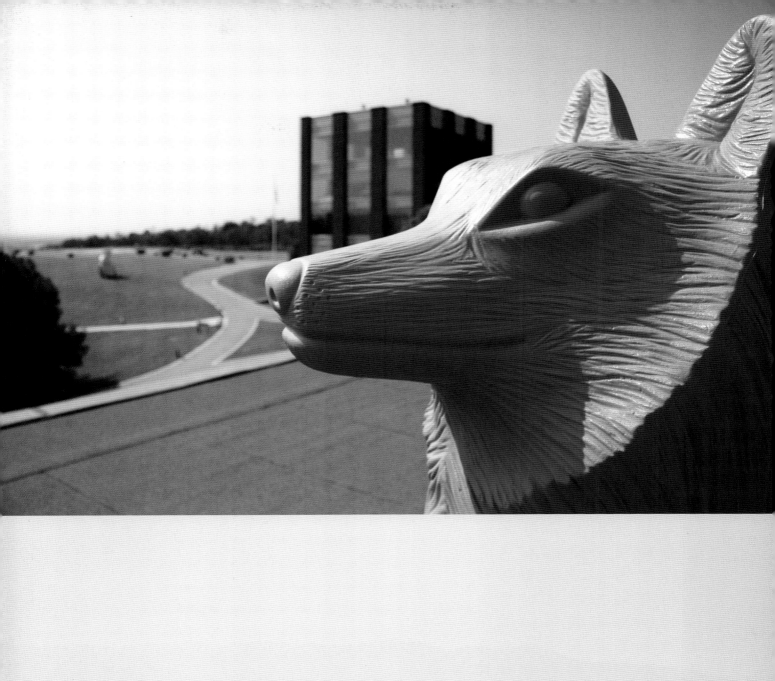
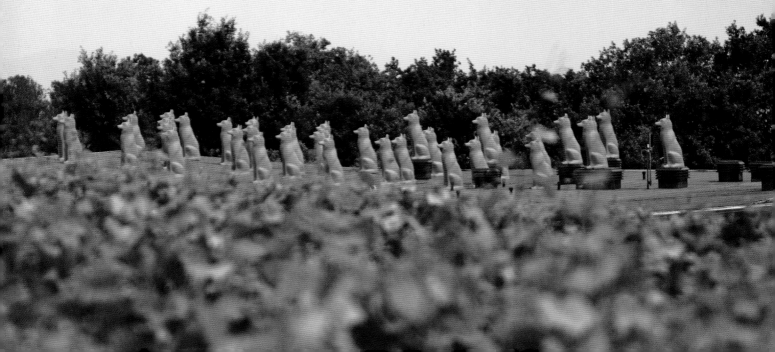

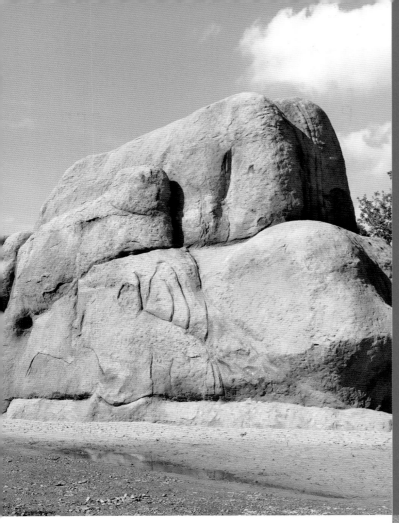

Monument for a
Forgotten Future
Olaf Nicolai, Douglas Gordon, Mogwai

Completion: 2010. **Technique:** reinforced concrete, steel.
Location: Gelsenkirchen, Germany.

This monument is a replica of a rock formation from the Joshua Tree National Park in South California. Conceptual artist Olaf Nicolai, in collaboration with Scottish artist Douglas Gordon, has established the work on the so-called "Wild Island" in Germany. A song, composed especially by Scottish band Mogwai, can be heard playing through the rock; but only when one is close enough to put one's ear to the rock wall. The work is symbolic of how the artificial can complement the natural.

This work was a collaboration between Olaf Nicolai, born 1962, Douglas Gordon, born 1966 and the Scottish music group Mogwai. Nicolai creates artificial landscapes and sculptures, many of which are centered around consumer goods and people's relationship to and use of the earth and its resources. Gordon has exhibited work internationally, including New York, London and Berlin. He works with films, texts and photography. The abiding themes of his work are memory and repetition.

Photo: EMSCHERKUNST.2010, photographer Roman Mensing

Desert Star
Carlotta Brunetti

Completion: 2010. **Technique:** granite, colored sand. **Location:** Palmer, Australia.

The work "Desert Star" was created in 2010 in Palmer, South Australia. In this work, a whole mountaintop was processed as an entire sculpture. The mountaintop is of pink granite and the artist has molded points out of red and yellow sand into the eroded earth. The piece connects the wide space and colors of the half-dried landscape. The concept of this work is one of developing space and color.

Italian-born and based in Germany, Carlotta Brunetti studied art history at the University of Florence and later studied in Munich. She has created works internationally, including in Taipei, Germany and the USA. Brunetti brings outdoor installations and indoor projects to public spaces throughout the world. Her work encourages the viewer to experience nature with fresh eyes and to reflect on the connections between urban and rural perceptions of the world.

Photo: Trevor Rodwell, Adelaide

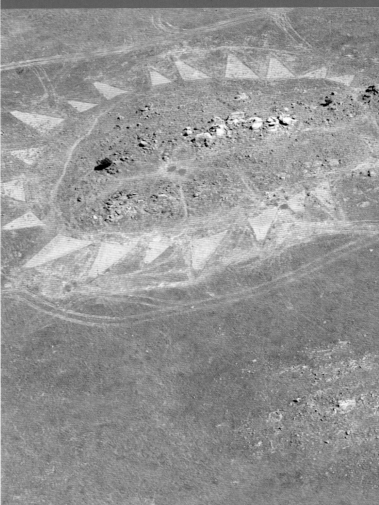

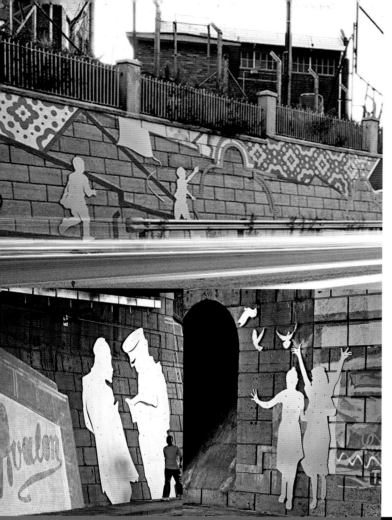

Subway Mural
Bronwyn Lace, Reg Pakari, Rookeya Gardee

Completion: 2010. **Technique:** sandblasted surfaces, plaster, paint and laser-cut steel elements. **Location:** Johannesburg, South Africa.

This mural celebrates the heritage and memory of Fordsburg and Fietas, two historic areas near Johannesburg's inner city. The making of the artwork engaged artists with roots in the area as well as past and present residents. The process started with a series of conversations, which were recorded as part of an archive of testimonies. From these stories and from artifacts, the mural was conceived as a series of historical and contemporary elements depicting ordinary characters and characterizing life.

Bronwyn Lace is an installation and performance artist based in Johannesburg. She participates in national and international projects, focusing on the role of art in the development of communities. Reg Pakari is a freelance graphic designer who grew up in Lenasia. Rookeya Gardee often works with recycled materials and memorabilia. She sees the mural project as a stepping stone for documenting and remembering.

Photos: Sean Tangney, Johannesburg

Dube TradePort entrance
Tanya de Villiers

Completion: 2010. **Technique:** concrete, slate. **Location:** Durban, South Africa.

CNdV Africa designed two unique matching entrance features or portals into King Shaka International Airport and Dube TradePort north of Durban, South Africa. The features allude to Dube TradePort as a global 'port' and 'gateway to Africa' without reverting to obvious or typical African symbolism. The slightly curved aerodynamic vertical features bow towards visitors in a universal gesture of greeting and welcome, symbolizing the many diverse cultures of Africa.

CNdV Africa specializes in landscape architectural design, urban design and planning. Tanya de Villiers has been involved in the design and coordination of a large variety of projects such as the V&A Waterfront development in Cape Town and Dube City, Durban. She was chairperson of the Institute of Landscape Architects of South Africa – Cape and served on the South African Council of the Landscape Architectural Profession.

Photos: Sean Laurenz, Durban, South Africa

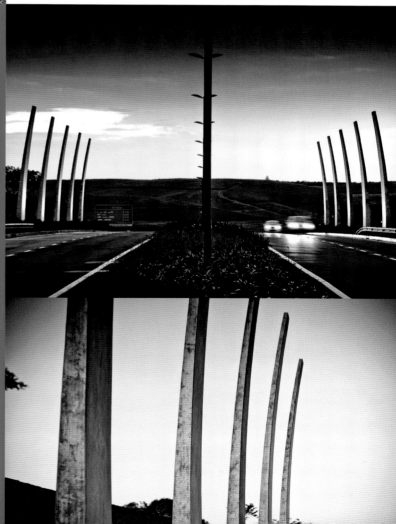

Hehe Xiexie
Zhang Huan

Completion: 2010. **Technique:** mirror finished stainless steel.
Location: Shanghai, China.

"Hehe Xiexie" is an image of two sitting pandas that symbolize dreaming, righteousness with courage, perseverance, optimism, tolerance, and generosity. One is called "Hehe", the other "Xiexie", they are made of mirror-finished stainless steel. In honor of the Shanghai International Exposition, this sculpture will be situated on the north Expo axis to serve as a permanent public sculpture near the China and Taiwan Pavilion.

Zhang Huan was born in 1965 in Anyang, China. In the 1990s he was a central figure in Avant-garde Chinese art, engaged in Conceptual Art. In 1998 he moved to New York and became a full time artist, engaging in various artistic mediums and artistic performances in major cities all over the world. Since 1998, Zhang Huan has had nearly thirty solo exhibitions in art museums, public institutions and art galleries all over the world. He currently lives in both Shanghai and New York.

Photos: Courtesy of the artist

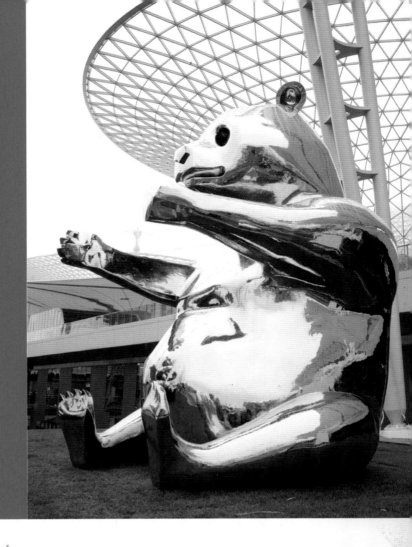

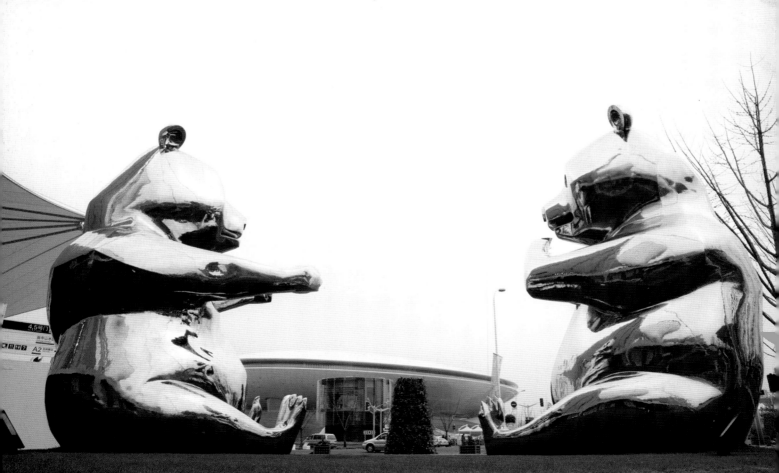

The Meadow Garden
Brodie McAllister

Completion: 2010. **Technique:** earth and turf, wildflower mix, cherry trees, steel igloo shaped arbor, hoggin paths, willow.
Location: Gloucester, United Kingdom.

Within the context of Highnam Court historical estate and landscaped gardens, this "Meadow Garden" used an area where silt from the adjacent dredged lake had been dumped and spread. The artist, with assistance from Chris Trollope, created the spiral mound at the center, allowing an overview of the property. Rings of cherry trees reinforce the circular pathways around the meadows. A path runs up to a giant igloo shaped steel arbor where willows are being trained to enclose the outer form.

Brodie McAllister is a chartered landscape architect and artist, fellow and vice president of the Landscape Institute. Formerly, he was a director of studies at the University of Gloucestershire. His experience includes major projects in the United Kingdom, Japan, the USA, Singapore, Malaysia and Brunei and he has been a juror on several national and international design competitions. He has received several national awards including in housing design, three Civic Trust, and four Royal Institute of British Architects.

Photos: Rob Keene, Gloucestershire (a.) ; Bob Train, Glucestershire (b.)

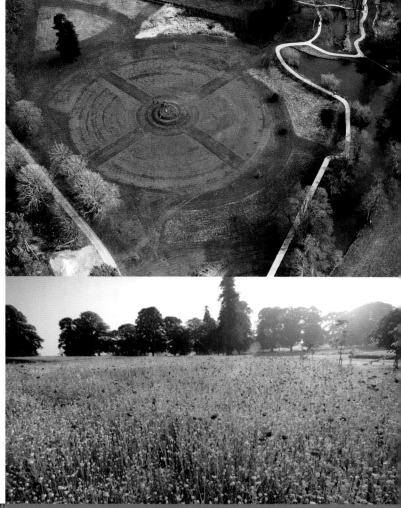

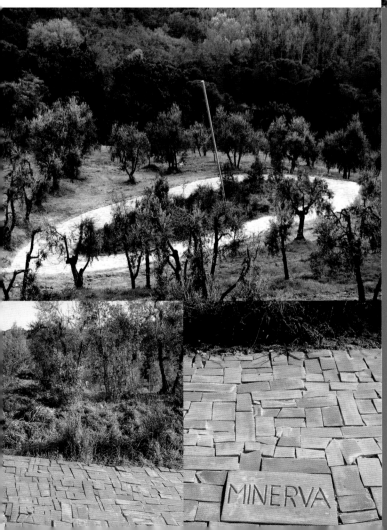

Birth by Spear
Alan Sonfist

Completion: 2010. **Technique:** concrete, oliv trees, bricks.
Location: Tuscany, Italy.

"Birth by Spear" is a visual marker of time as well as an educational forum for the community. Alan Sonfist has created a fingerprint of the original olive leaf of the original olive tree that existed 5,000 years ago. The site is five acres in size and in the center is the shape of the original olive leaf. The spear that protrudes from the ground is representative of Minerva giving birth to the olive tree. The surrounding Renaissance tiles have descriptions of the olive tree from ancient to contemporary history.

Alan Sonfist's art projects are often recreations of the environment, as it existed before man's interference. For example, in his "Time Landscape" in New York City, Sonfist replanted the kind of forest that once blanketed the whole of the city, returning an area of land to its primal state. Sonfist had a research fellowship in MIT and has had diverse solo exhibitions from the Ludwig Museum in Aachen to the Boston Museum of Fine Arts. His artwork is featured in notable collections, including the Museum of Modern Art in New York and the Philadelphia Museum of Art.

Photos: Courtesy of the artist

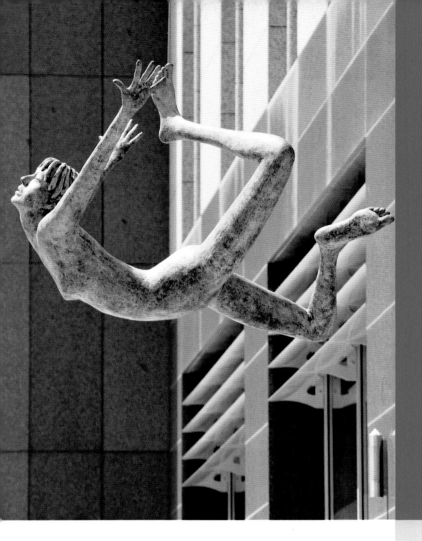

Jersey Girl
Rowan Gillespie

Completion: 2010. **Technique:** bronze. **Location:** St Helier, Jersey.

The roots of "Jersey Girl" lie in the legend of Cathleen Ní Houlihan, William Butler Yeats's personification of Ireland. The story begins in 1995 with "Aspiration" and continues with "Birdy" (1997) where we see a crouched figure about to leap from a window ledge above Crescent Hall. "Jersey Girl" (2010) shows the figure now in full flight, the dream finally realized, as she sways gently above the Esplanade, suspended from a single toe. She symbolizes the emancipation and consequent liberation of the modern woman.

Rowan Gillespie was born in the city of Dublin in 1953. He is an international renowned sculptor, whose work has been exhibited at various solo exhibitions throughout Europe and the USA. In 1997 and 2005 he participated in international exhibitions, festivals and arts fairs. Gillespie's early inspiration came from the sculptor Henry Moore and artist, Edward Munch. In 2007 Gillespie was awarded an honorary doctorate of Fine Arts from Regis University, Denver.

Photo: Roger Kohn

am/pm Shadow Lines
Strijdom van der Merwe

Completion: 2010. **Technique:** gravel and stones from the mine dumps. **Location:** Koingnaas, West Coast, South Africa.

This project was created for the De Beers Namaqualand Mining Company. 7,000 tons of earth where moved in an circle of 100 meter diameter. Each of the 14 lines are two meters high and they are grouped in five lines running from north to south and nine lines running from east to west. Because of the movement of the sun, various shadows are cast through out the day. It is a very important work in South African art history as it is the first time that a big diamond company have invested in a project like this.

Artist Strijdom van der Merwe is a recipient of the Jackson Pollock-Krasner Foundation Grant and was nominated for the Daimler Chrysler Award for Art in Public Spaces. Merwe has been invited to exhibit his work in various countries all over the world, including South Korea, Turkey, Belgium and France. He has hosted many personal exhibitions in various art galleries and public spaces in recent years and his work has been bought by numerous private and public collectors locally and abroad.

Photos: Courtesy of the artist

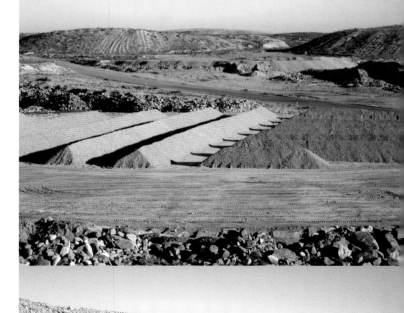

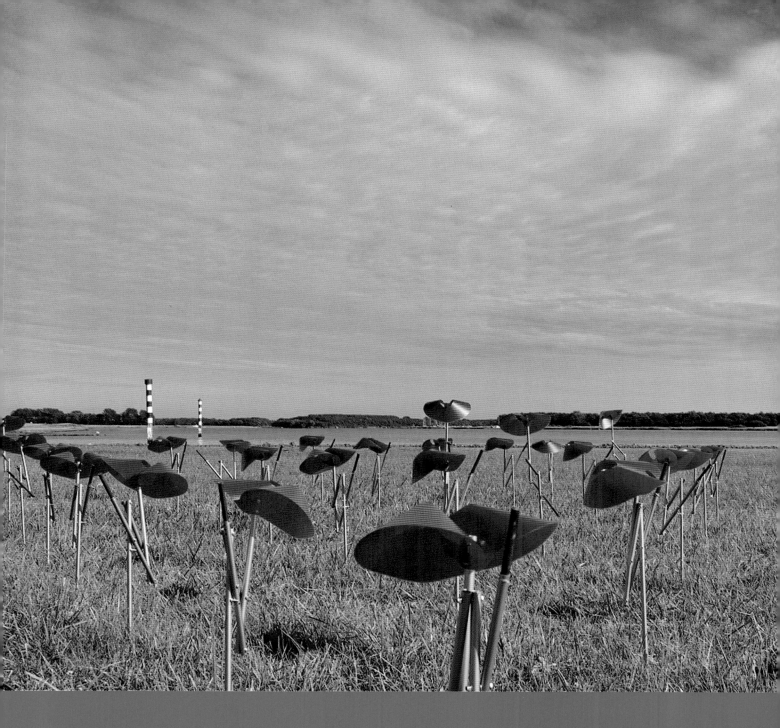

Strawberry Fields Forever
Bert Schoeren

Completion: 2010. **Technique:** aluminum, synthetics. **Location:** Kamperland, The Netherlands.

"Strawberry Fields Forever" is composed of many, individual 'berries', which move with the wind in an unpredictable manner. The red berry figures are light and transparent and can flow and wave across the field. Once the berries begin to move, the unique nature of each is revealed. Each is individual, some of them put their heads above the crowd, others refuse to move at all, some move only in groups. The view, in its entirety, brings a surprising and amusing scene.

Bert Schoeren studied industrial design engineering at the Delft University of Technology and after graduation, began working as exhibit designer at the NEMO Science and Technology Center in Amsterdam. Schoeren has designed many objects for the public realm, including street furniture; cardboard and wooden furniture for design stores, museums and galleries. He also creates sculptures in stone and bronze. Schoeren is particularly interested in Kinetic Art, sculptures that move by wind, water or solar energy.

Photo: Jürgen Kolbach

Temple of Light
Jens J. Meyer

Completion: 2010. **Technique:** cotton, elasthan, polypropylen.
Location: Lushan, China.

"Temple of Light" was created for the Forest Art China, the second World Famous Mountains Conference. The artist's vision was to highlight a place in nature with his artwork, in order to slow people down for a moment of contemplation of nature and art. People finding themselves between the gates are invited to come inside and discover the dialogue between art and nature. The sunlight opens a new level of interaction, creating constantly changing shadows and movement.

Jens J. Meyer was born in Hamburg, Germany, in 1958. Parallel to studying economic engineering, he also studied painting and sculpture. Since 1989 he has worked as a freelance artist and his work has been displayed in many exhibitions including in Indonesia, Norway, Austria, Argentina, USA and China. In 2003 he was part of the eighth Biennial in Havana, Cuba. His work is held in permanent collections across Europe and he has received various awards, including the first prize for landmark-art, Hamm in 2001.

Photo: Courtesy of the artist

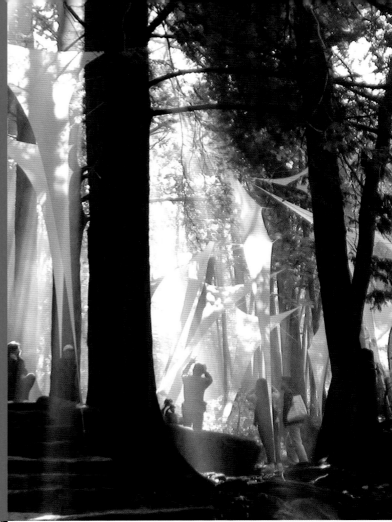

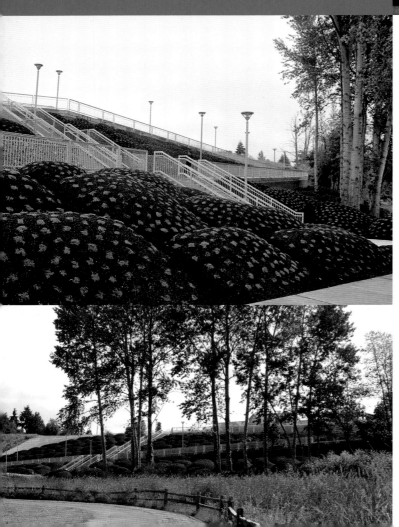

Pillow Field
Andy Cao, Xavier Perrot

Completion: 2010. **Technique:** compacted soil, plants. **Location:** White Center, WA, USA.

This permanent earthwork, "Pillow Field" is comprised of 227 mounded earth 'pillows', varying in size and shape to represent the multi-cultural diversity of White Center. The surface is unified by a soft blanket of creeping thyme, a perennial, evergreen ground cover that will maintain the mound shapes and bring a burst of vibrant pink, blossoming carpet in late spring until summer. The pillows can be viewed from many different vantage points, from the top of stairway and ramp to the ponds below.

Drawing on diverse cultural backgrounds, Cao I Perrot studio creates hybrid environments, blending art and landscape to make a place for dreaming. The projects, both temporary and permanent, cross commercial, artistic and residential boundaries, varying in size from intimate courtyards to large scale public parks, often using overlooked materials to create environments that defy specific meaning and invite the viewer into a contemplative world of color and sensuality.

Photos: Courtesy of the artist

Rhine Mosel Slate Whirlpool
Chris Drury

Completion: 2010. **Technique:** slate. **Location:** Koblenz, Germany.

This work was commissioned through the Heike Strelow Gallery in Frankfurt and created for Koblenz Garden Festival 2011. It is an earth sculpture, made from 20 tons of slate and is situated on a site above where the river Mosel flows into the Rhine, close to a fortress. The slate pieces are placed so that they appear to flow downwards, disappearing into the center. The slate under the ground here is said to give the wine of the region its distinctive taste.

Born in 1948, Chris Drury currently lives in England. He has been working as a land artist for over 30 years and has exhibited in museums and galleries worldwide as well as making permanent works in Europe, America and Japan and ephemeral works in many of the wild places of the world including Antarctica. His monograph book Silent Spaces is published by Thames and Hudson.

Photos: Courtesy of the artist

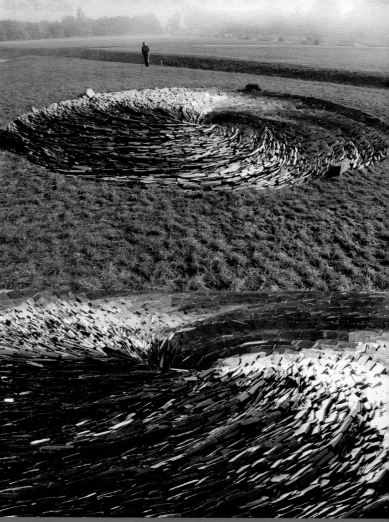

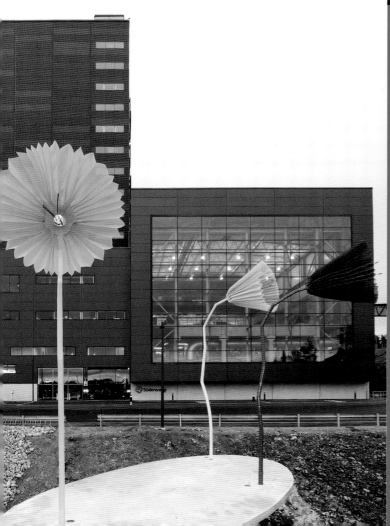

Song of the Forest
Simka

Completion: 2010. **Technique:** concrete, fiberglass, steel, polystyrene, lighting. **Location:** Södertälje, Sweden.

In front of the entrance to Söderenergi thermal power plant stand three tall flowers. Framed in an elliptical surface. The flowers rotate slowly in the wind. These can be seen both from boats in the canal and cars driving into the area. Visitors and those who work inside the plant can see them through the generous outlook at both low and high altitude. The actual flower is about one and a half meters deep and has a circumference of approximately three meters, in a folded, pleated mesh of stainless steel.

Simka is the project name for Simon Häggblom's and Karin Lind's shared artistic activities. They are involved in designing sculpture, set design and landscape architecture. The core of their work is the investigation and formation of different spaces and sites. They have several public artworks across Sweden and have exhibited work at Konstnärshuset, Öja-Landsort and Nynäshamn in Stockholm.

Photo: Antonius van Arkel, Stockholm

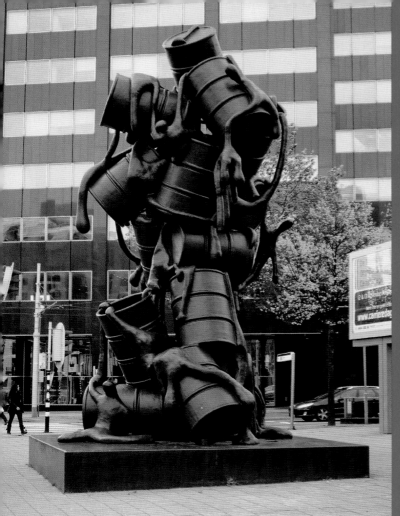

Cascade
Atelier Van Lieshout

Completion: 2010. **Technique:** polyester. **Location:** Rotterdam, The Netherlands.

This sculpture was commissioned by Sculpture International in Rotterdam. The 18 oil drums are carefully arranged to give the impression that they are cascading from the sky like a waterfall. The drums appear to be coated in a black, oily substance, dripping and oozing down the sides of the piece. At a second glance, the ooze takes the form of people, attempting to climb up or slither down. The sculpture highlights the impending exhaustion of raw materials, questioning our consumer-driven society.

Atelier Van Lieshout is a studio well known for its multi-disciplinary approach. The studio operates internationally and is involved in the fields of contemporary art, architecture and design. The workshop of the company is situated in an old warehouse in Rotterdam. The building itself is something of a monument as it one of the first concrete warehouses ever to be built, originally used to store cotton. The company has around 20 employees, working across the disciplines of sculpture, wood and metal.

Photo: Chris van Uffelen

World Travellers
Daniel Wagenblast

Completion: 2010. **Technique:** aluminum. **Location:** Stuttgart, Germany.

The "World Travellers" are three figures on a globe in the middle of a roundabout in Stuttgart-Möhringen. On the globe they look in different directions – this fits the directional function of a roundabout. They appear as giants of different sizes, traveling the global village, but there is nothing threatening about them. They do not even interact and it is doubtful if they see each other even though they are looking around.

Daniel Wagenblast, born in 1963 in Schwäbisch Gmünd, studied at the State Academy of Art and Design in Stuttgart from 1984 to 1990. Most of his work is made of ceramics and wood. Besides the "World travellers", the "Yellow Cab, N.Y." series is his most renowned work. In both series the people shown often appear to be contemplating something – looking waiting, sitting, thinking. Hints about what might have happened or is going to happen are given but no clear action is taken.

Photo: Chris van Uffelen

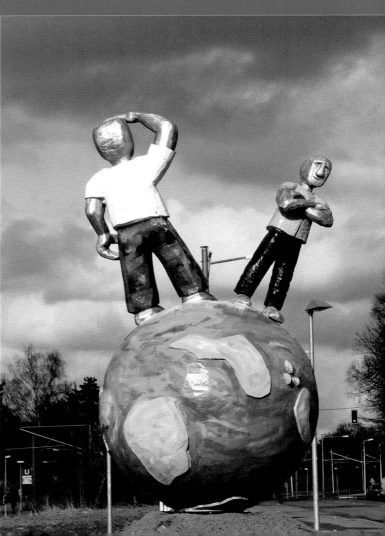

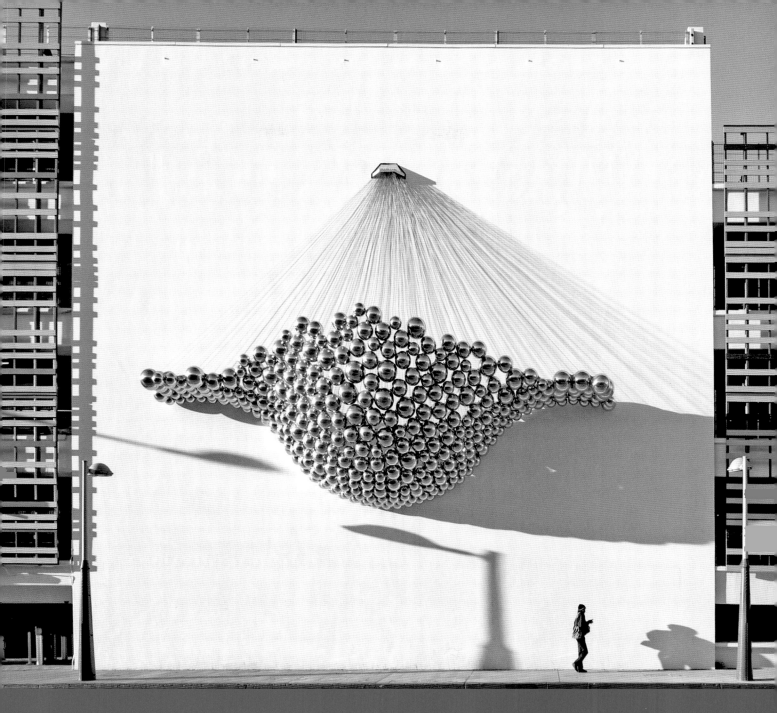

Cradle
Ball Nogues Studio

Completion: 2010. **Technique:** stainless steel. **Location:** Santa Monica, CA, USA.

An agglomeration of mirror-polished, stainless steel spheres, the sculpture operates structurally like an enormous Newton's Cradle – the ubiquitous toy found on the desktops of corporate executives. The project is an exploration in sphere packing. Each ball is suspended by a cable from a bracket on the wall and locked in position by a combination of gravity and neighboring balls while reflecting a distorted image of passersby both in cars and on foot.

Benjamin Ball and Gaston Nogues explore the nexus of art, architecture, and industrial design. Their work has been exhibited at major institutions throughout the world, including the Museum of Contemporary Art, Los Angeles; the Museum of Modern Art, New York; the Guggenheim Museum; PS1; the Los Angeles County Museum of Art; Arc en Rêve Centre d'Architecture + Musée d'Art Contemporain de Bordeaux; the Venice Biennial, the Hong Kong / Shenzhen Biennial; and the Beijing Biennial.

Photo: Lawrence Scarpa, Los Angeles

Cathedral Square
OKRA

Completion: 2010. **Technique:** light, smoke, metal. **Location:** Utrecht, The Netherlands.

The heart of the city is built on top of a castellum and the project revitalizes the significance of the origins of the city. The castellum wall, four meters underground, has a clearly recognizable and yet mysterious dividing line. Fragments of smoke come out of the gutter in the metal plates and reveal the presence of the ray of light. The line is even more visible during rain or mist and after darkness has set in.

Hans Oerlemans, Martin Knuijt, Christ-Jan van Rooij and Boudewijn Almekinders founded OKRA in 1993. The office works on national and international projects in the fields of landscape architecture, urban design, architecture, art, industrial design and graphic design, employing specialists from all these disciplines. They are specialize in shaping the urban landscape.

Photo: Ben ter Mull

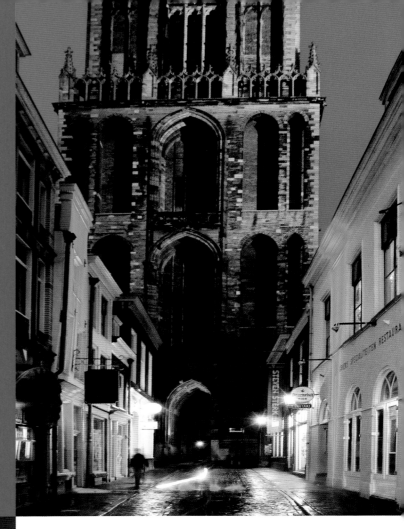

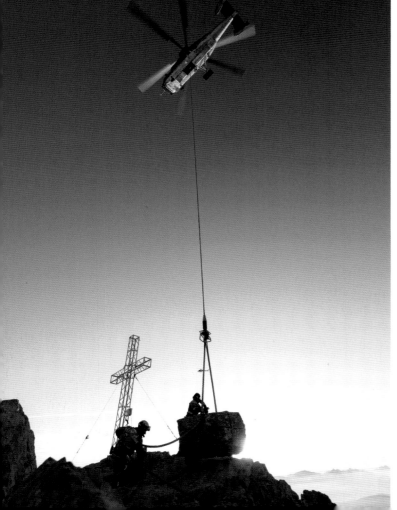

High Dachstein
Ai Weiwei

Completion: 2010. **Technique:** stone. **Location:** Dachstein Mountains, Austria.

As part of the regional culture festival, this four-ton boulder was placed on top of the High Dachstein Mountains in Austria. The rock fell from its original position in China, during the 2008 earthquake, which killed thousands of children when their schools collapsed. The stone functions as a memorial, while also posing questions about human capabilities and the forces of nature. It reminds of the work of Sisyphus, an antique hero who was made to roll a rock up a hill for the whole of eternity.

Ai Weiwei (born 1957) is a Chinese artist, curator, architect, social and cultural critic and filmmaker. He entered the Beijing Film Academy in 1978, the year that he co-founded the avant-garde art group "Stars," and in 1981 moved to New York to study at the Parsons School of Design. He returned to China in 1993 and founded the CAAW in 1997 and the architecture studio FAKE Design in 2003. Ai collaborated with Swiss architects Herzog and de Meuron as the artistic consultant on the Beijing National Stadium for the 2008 Olympics. In 2011 he was imprisoned for three months.

Photo: Herbert Raffalt

Bear One Anothers Burdens
Gennadij Jerszow

Completion: 2010. **Technique:** bronze, granite. **Location:** Gdansk - Zaspa, Poland.

This work commemorates Pope John Paul II's visit to Poland in 1987. During the Holy Mass that took place in Zaspa on the 12th June 1987, the Pope addressed thousands of attending Poles with the words "Bear one another's burdens" (Galatians 6,2), helpful words in a city governed by the iron hand of Communism. Slawoj Leszek Glodz, Archbishop of the Gdansk diocese in 2010, commissioned this sculpture. The form of the work symbolizes the beginning of the end of the communist regime.

Gennadij Jerszow was born in Chernihiv, in Ukraine, to a Ukraine-Polish family. He attended the Academy of Arts in Lviv and The National Academy of Fine Arts and Architecture in Kiev (1991–1995). During this time he also worked as an assistant, attending postgraduate doctoral studies. In 2001 he returned to Gdansk, Poland. He specializes in monumental figurative sculpture for display in public space, as well as in small bronze bass-reliefs, statues and portraits.

Photos: Dariusz Kula / Gdansk, Poland www.fotokula.pl

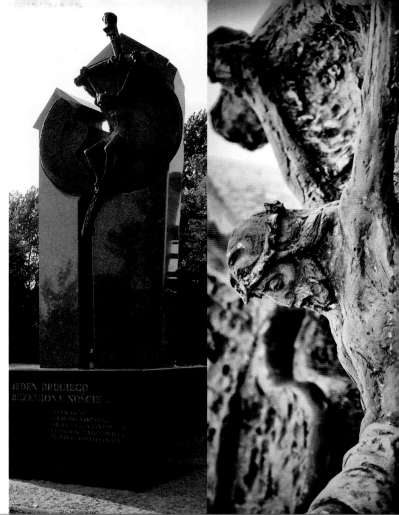

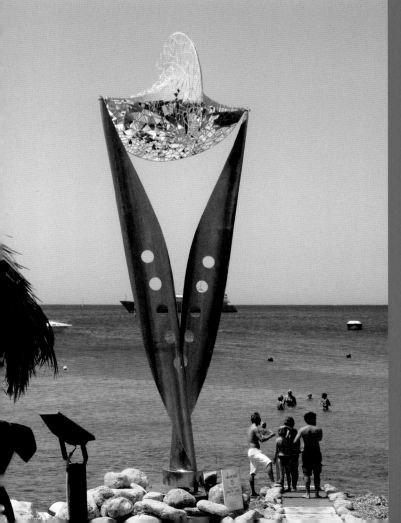

Angel del Viento
Gerhard Höhn

Completion: 2010. **Technique:** stainless steel, mirror. **Location:** Playa Cala Jondal, Ibiza, Spain.

"Angel del Viento" is a kinetic wind sculpture. It is made from stainless steel and glass and stands at over four meters high on the Playa Cala Jondal. The mirrored surfaces of the sculpture reflect the surrounding sea, sky and beach, intrinsically connecting it to the nature that surrounds it. Two different movements happen at the same time the two leaves with the five holes turn vertically, pushed by the wind. At the same time the mirror shape rotates horizontally.

Gerhard Höhn was born in Germany in 1966. He is a self-taught sculptor and has spent many years researching art of different media and styles. Höhn collaborated in several diverse artistic groups and projects and exhibited his work at various exhibitions throughout Germany as well as periodically working in stage and tradefair design. In 2003 he moved to Ibiza, Spain and has been creating kinetic wind sculptures there since 2008.

Photo: Courtesy of the artist

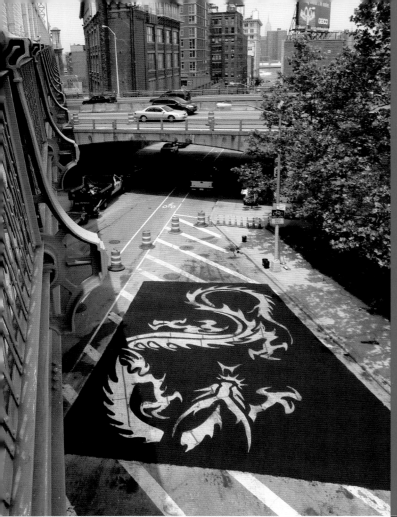

Asphalt Tattoo
Paula Meijerink, Kris Lucius

Completion: 2010. **Technique:** asphalt, crushed recycled New York glass. **Location:** New York City, NY, USA.

"Asphalt Tattoo" celebrates New York City's most ubiquitous surface and skin of the city – asphalt – as an urban carpet, it honors the surface as the carrier of all urban movement. The designers were intrigued with the ambiguity of the site, as it is wholly public but divorced from any circulation, pedestrian, bicycle, car or otherwise. Early cartographers dealt frequently with such unexplored and potentially dangerous lands and would label them as "hic sunt dracones", "there are dragons here".

The project "On Asphalt" was initiated by Paula Meijerink and is an ongoing effort to make asphalt spaces more engaging public landscapes. Meijerink is a landscape architect and founder of Wanted Landscape llc, she was on the faculty of the Harvard Design School and is currently the Gerald Sheff professor at McGill University, Montreal. Kris Lucius graduated from Harvard Design School in landscape architecture. He is a designer at Landworks Studio Inc. and teaches at the Boston Architectural College.

I Goat
Kenny Hunter

Completion: 2011. **Technique:** aluminum, paint, concrete. **Location:** London, United Kingdom.

"I Goat" in Spitalfields stands on top of a collection of packing crates, tenacious and independent. The animal featured is only a part of the composition and must be read in context with the architectonic elements. In this case the rule of base, pedestal and plinth has been deconstructed and reformed into a freestyle asymmetric composition, informed by its surroundings. The packing crate is synonymous with the movement of people and goods, associating it with the history of migrant populations in Spitalfields.

Kenny Hunter was born in Edinburgh in 1962. He studied at the Glasgow School of Art, graduating with a bachelor of arts in fine art sculpture. He was also awarded an honorary doctorate from Aberdeen University in 2008. Hunter's recent solo exhibitions include "Natural Selection" at the Yorkshire Sculpture Park, 2006; "More Light More Shadows" at the New Art Centre, 2009, and "New Prints and Editions" at The Multiple Store, 2010. His work has also been exhibited in the USA and in Germany.

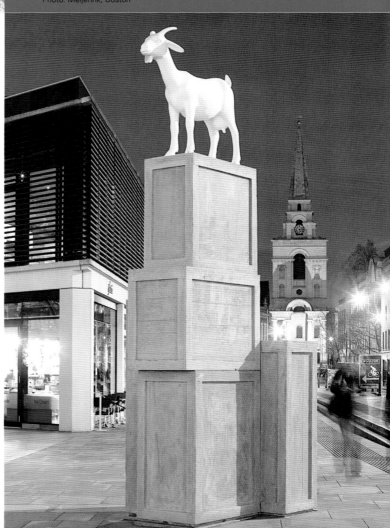

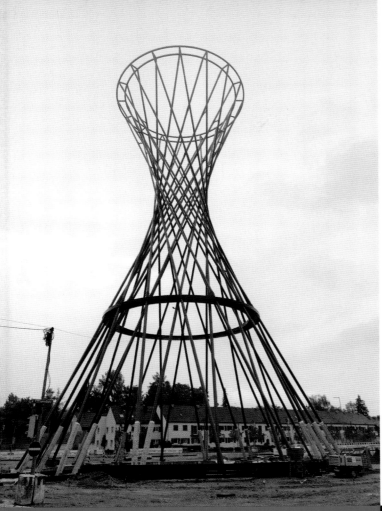

Mae West
Rita McBride

Completion: 2011. **Technique:** carbon fiber. **Location:** Munich, Germany.

"Mae West" is a sculpture by the artist Rita McBride, located on Effnerplatz in Munich. The sculpture is named after the actress Mae West and is a 52-meter-tall construction made from carbon fiber. The aim of the project was to give some character to Effnerplatz, an area of the city surrounded by heavy traffic and busy roads. The design continues the circular shape of the nearby traffic system and the shape of the neighboring high-rise buildings.

Rita McBride is an American sculptor and installation artist. She graduated from Bard College, New York, with a bachelor of arts degree before going on to study at the California Institute of the Arts in 1982, graduating with a masters of fine arts in 1987. Her large sculptural installations deal with architecture, function and communication and her work has been exhibited internationally since the end of the 1980s. Since 2003, McBride has worked as professor of sculpture at the Art Academy in Dusseldorf.

Photo: Chris van Uffelen

Tindaya Project
Eduardo Chillida

Completion: 2012. **Technique:** stone. **Location:** Fuerteventura, Spain.

In 1994 the sculptor Eduardo Chillida had the opportunity to initiate the Tindaya Project in Fuerteventura, Canary Islands. He had first envisioned the project in 1984, a sculptural work which opens a large interior space in the heart of the mountain. The sculpture was intended by the artist as a monument to tolerance, welcoming people of every color and race.

Eduardo Chillida was a Spanish Basque sculptor, born in 1924. He was famous for his large, abstract sculptures. His work is based on the idea that a sculpture is not just situated in a place, but is also a place in itself. Because of this tension, Chillida believed that a sculpture had to be an embodiment of the place it was in. He died 2002.

Photos: Daniel Díaz Font León, Spain

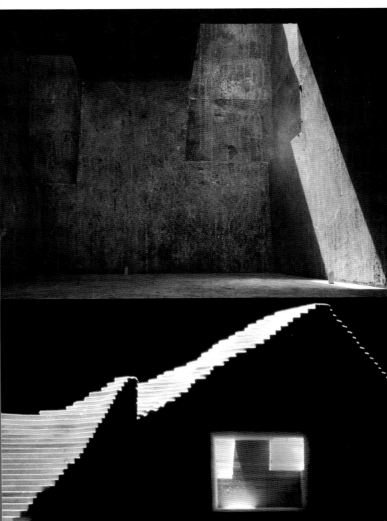

Star Axis
Charles Ross

Completion: 2012. **Technique:** granite, sandstone, earth, concrete, bronze. **Location:** New Mexico, USA.

"Star Axis" is created from star geometry. Every shape, every measure, every angle was first discovered by observation and then brought down into stone structures embedded in the land. Its chambers and tunnels provide places to spatially experience various time frames – one hour of earth's rotation and the shape of a season. By climbing the stairs in the "Star Tunnel", exactly aligned with the earth's axis, you walk through the history of the earth's shifting alignment with the stars.

Charles Ross' work is primarily involved with developing new works involving light, time and planetary motion. His work has been exhibited in numerous museums and he has created major permanent artworks in Japan, France, Costa Rica, and throughout the USA. Ross recently completed three major solar spectrum works: one for the Kauffman Foundation in Kansas City, another at the new Federal Courthouse in Tampa, Florida, and the third in collaboration with architect Riken Yamamoto for Saitama University, Japan.

Photos: Courtesy of the artist

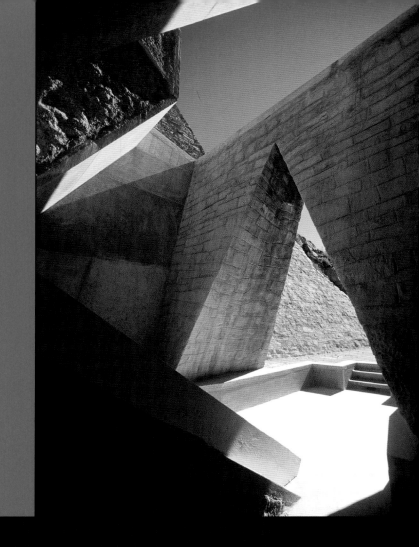

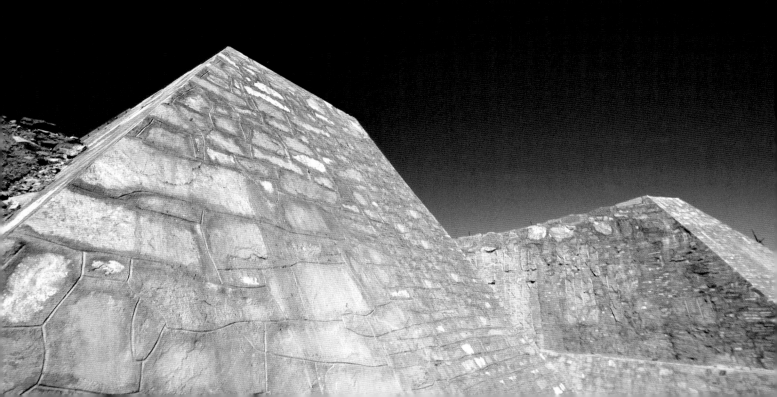

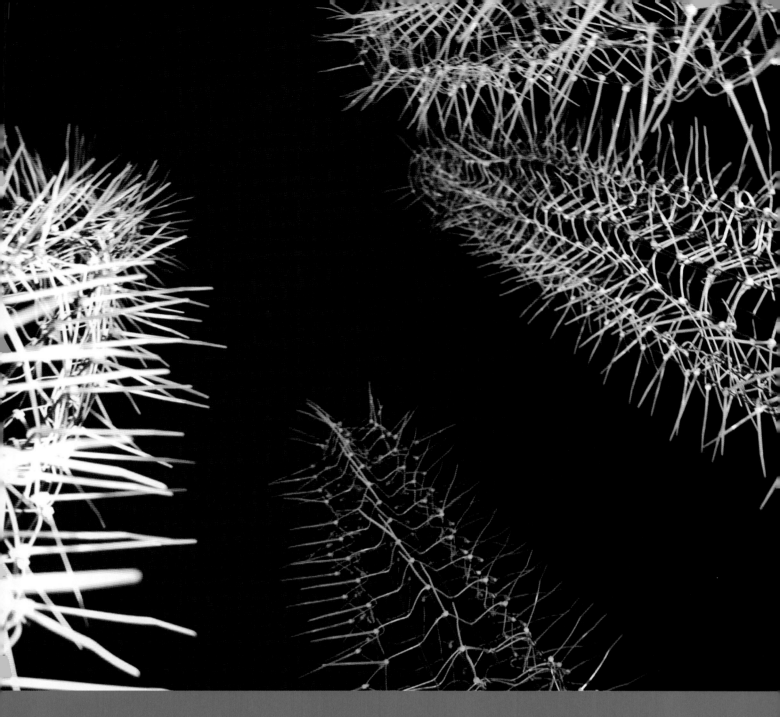

Light-Cactuses
Christoph Luckeneder

Completion: 2011. **Technique:** galvanized mesh wire, cable-ties, light-sources, color filter. **Location:** Berlin, Germany.

The inspiration for this work comes from a journey to the Saguaro National Park in America, where the artist found the "Carnegiea gigantea" cactus; which defies the hostile environment and simultaneously acts as a living water donor. This work is a collection of four "Light-Cactuses". It was made for the Festival of Light in Berlin. Each element is lit by one light source with a color filter. The artist began making cacti out of left over mesh wire, these then developed into the "Light Cactuses", which have become more realistic over time.

Christoph Luckender is a light artist. He was born in 1950 in Gramastetten, Austria. He began working as an artist in 1979, before studying at the University of Design in Linz, graduating in 1988. He has exhibited his work widely, both in solo and group exhibitions, including a 30 light objects installation at the "Islands of Light" at the Hagenberg castle close to Linz 2010/2011 and Gallery Stauber in Passau. He has been selected by a panel of judges to exhibit his work at the Triennial of Sculpture 2012 in Switzerland.

Photo: Courtesy of the artist

The Blue Trees
Konstantin Dimopoulos

Completion: 2011. **Technique:** trees, natural colourant. **Location:** Vancouver Biennale: West Vancouver, City of Richmond, City of Port Moody, Canada.

"The Blue Trees" is a social art action. Using color to transform trees, the artist makes a personal statement about their spirituality and importance to our survival. Color is used here to define space and time as well as altering the perception of the observer, combining the familiar with the unexpected. In the animal world color is used to protect and attract. "The Blue Trees" elicits a similar response from viewers.

Konstantin Dimopoulos is an artist who creates both public art installations and sculpture. His sculptures focus on color, line, form and repetition where line is used as a tool to define space. His sculptures are bold and dynamic, moved by the wind. In 2001 he was invited by the Wellington Sculpture Trust, to create a wind-driven sculpture for the City of Wellington, New Zealand. He created Pacific Grass in response to this, a work that is now an iconic sculpture. His sculptures are now in public and private collections around the world.

Photos: www.kondimopoulos.com

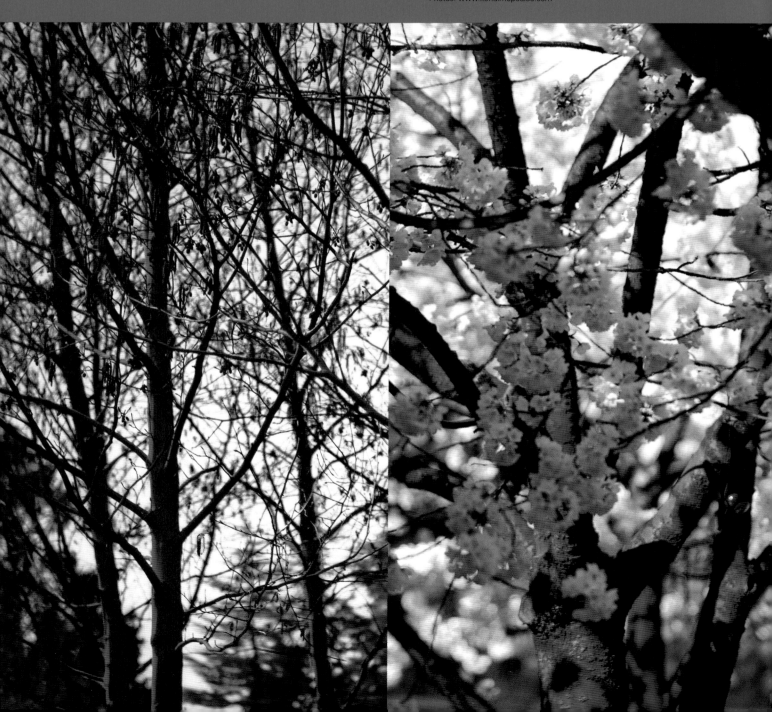

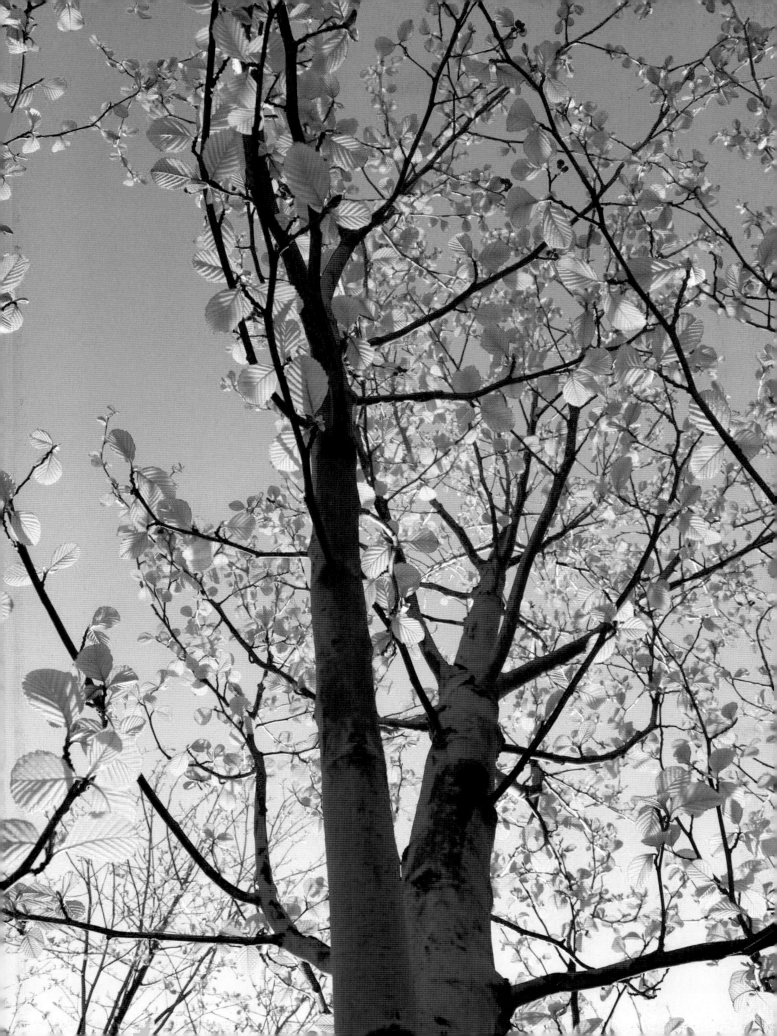

Index